Burger's Medicinal Chemistry

Fourth Edition

Part III

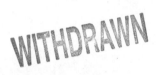

BURGER'S MEDICINAL CHEMISTRY

Fourth Edition

Part III

Edited by

MANFRED E. WOLFF

Department of Pharmaceutical Chemistry
School of Pharmacy
University of California
San Francisco, California

A WILEY-INTERSCIENCE PUBLICATION

JOHN WILEY & SONS, New York · Chichester · Brisbane · Toronto

Notice Concerning Trademark or Patent Rights.
The listing or discussion in this book of any drug in
respect to which patent or trademark rights may exist
shall not be deemed, and is not intended as
a grant of, or authority to exercise, or an
infringement of, any right or privilege protected by
such patent or trademark.

Library of Congress Cataloging in Publication Data (Revised):

Burger, Alfred, 1905– ed.
  Burger's Medicinal chemistry.

  "A Wiley-Interscience publication"
  Bibliography: p.
  Includes index.
  CONTENTS: pt. 1. The basis of medicinal chemistry.
  1. Chemistry, Pharmaceutical. 2. Chemotherapy.
I. Wolff, Manfred E. II. Title. III. Title: Medicinal
chemistry. [DNLM: 1. Chemistry, Pharmaceutical.
QV744.3 B954]

RS403.B8 1979   615'.7   78-10791
ISBN 0-471-01572-5

Printed in the United States of America

10 9 8 7 6 5 4 3 2 1

Preface

The chapters in this concluding part of *Burger's Medicinal Chemistry* highlight many aspects of our science—new areas as well as old ones, defeats as well as triumphs.

The book begins with two futuristic classes of compounds, the anti-aging drugs and the radioprotective agents. These fields are still in their infancy but will undoubtedly grow to greater importance in the coming decade. By contrast, in Chapters 50, 51, and 52 dealing with general anesthetics, local anesthetics, and analgetics, we see what has happened to fields once considered static. Here the impact of new knowledge in biochemistry, medicinal chemistry, organic chemistry, and molecular biology has resulted in tantalizing new theories and new approaches to old problems. Thus not only the newest fields but even the oldest fields in our discipline must be examined from new viewpoints made possible by advances in other sciences. It is an exciting time in which to be working.

A crucial unsolved problem in medicinal chemistry is seen in Chapter 38 on cardiac drugs. Like the antineoplastic agents, cardiac drugs have an exceptionally low therapeutic index, and frequently give rise to serious toxic effects. Our powerlessness in solving this dilemma reflects the fact that, although some success has been achieved in predicting active structures, none of our techniques, including QSAR, is of major value in forecasting the toxic effects of drugs. A better understanding of the chemical basis for drug toxicity, as already discussed in Part I, is of clear importance.

An elegant example of the effective modern practice of medicinal chemistry is presented in Chapter 48 dealing with the histamine H_2 receptor agonists and antagonists. The development of the drug cimetidine involved the application of structure-function analysis, receptor analysis, physiological studies, bioisosterism, and organic synthesis in an outstanding way. The result was not only a useful active drug, but a reduction of toxicity as well. It is the hope of the editor, contributors, and publisher that medicinal chemists all over the world will be aided in achieving similar success in their own work by the information presented in these volumes.

MANFRED E. WOLFF

San Francisco, California
June 1980

Contents

B. V. Rama Sastry
Department of Pharmacology
School of Medicine
Vanderbilt University
Nashville, Tennessee 37232, USA

Vernon G. Vernier
Pharmaceuticals Division
E. I. du Pont de Nemours & Co., Inc.
Newark, Delaware 19711, USA

John B. Stenlake
Department of Pharmaceutical
Chemistry
University of Strathclyde
Glasgow G1 1XW, Scotland

R. J. Mohrbacher
McNeil Laboratories, Inc.
Camp Hill Road
Fort Washington, Pennsylvania
19034, USA

C. Robin Ganellin and Graham J.
Durant
The Research Institute
Smith Kline & French Laboratories
Limited
Welwyn Garden City, Hertfordshire,
England

Donald T. Witiak and Richard C.
Cavestri
Division of Medicinal Chemistry
College of Pharmacy
Ohio State University
Columbus, Ohio 43210, USA

Keith W. Miller
Departments of Anesthesia and Pharmacology
Harvard Medical School and Massachusetts General Hospital
Boston, Massachusetts, USA

Bertil H. Takman and H. Jack Adams
Chemistry and Pharmacology Sections
Astra Pharmaceutical Products, Inc.
Framingham, Massachusetts 01701,
USA

M. Ross Johnson and George M.
Milne
Central Research
Pfizer Inc.
Groton, Connecticut 06340, USA

David Miller
Research Division
Beecham Pharmaceuticals
The Pinnacles, Harlow
Essex CM19 5AD, England

Julius A. Vida
Bristol-Myers Co.
International Division
345 Park Avenue
New York, New York 10022, USA

Eugene I. Isaacson
College of Pharmacy
Idaho State University
Pocatello, Idaho 83201, USA

Jaime N. Delgado
College of Pharmacy

Contents

Part I Contents

Part II Contents

Burger's Medicinal Chemistry

Fourth Edition

Part III

CHAPTER THIRTY-SIX

Anti-Aging Drugs

JASJIT S. BINDRA

Central Research
Pfizer Inc.
Groton, Connecticut 06340, USA

CONTENTS

1 INTRODUCTION

Research on aging has long been regarded as an impractical pseudoscience, and proved prolongation of life by pharmacological means apparently still remains in the realm of science fiction. It is only in recent years, with the application of scientific method and control, that experimental gerontology has begun to achieve respectability and capable scientists from many disciplines have begun to focus on aging as a disease process (1).

1

A major stimulus to this increasing interest has come from social and economic (2, 3) considerations. Welcome consequences of this interest are an improvement in the quality of research on senescence phenomena and a discernible shift from purely descriptive studies to studies on mechanism. This chapter discusses briefly some of the recent studies and theories in gerontology that have yielded significant results, and the one aspect of gerontological research that perhaps most immediately concerns the medicinal chemist, viz., the current status of agents believed to affect the aging process.

2 THEORIES OF AGING

Theories of aging are legion. In fact, one of the problems of gerontology has been that there are too many hypotheses but very few data to test them. Several books highlighting various aspects and individual theories have appeared in recent years, and many of the theories proposed to explain why aging occurs have been dealt with in comprehensive reviews (4–11). Several of the theories simply attempt to explain obvious deleterious changes associated with senescence and many are based on extremely limited evidence or even pure speculation, and must therefore be approached with caution.

Aging processes are increasingly being thought of as originating at the cellular or subcellular level, even though there is no general agreement as to the nature of these processes. However, there is no reason to believe that there is only one fundamental type of cellular or subcellular aging process. An attractive general hypothesis of aging is that senescence is primarily a cellular information loss phenomenon originating at the molecular level. Taken in the broadest sense this hypothesis may be related to any theory of aging. Interference with the flow of cellular information could occur anywhere in the sequence from DNA to RNA to protein synthesis, building up to Orgel's

cytoplasmic "error catastrophe" due to impaired protein synthesis (12–14). Alternatively, impaired cellular function due to breakdown of essential cellular components, rampant lysosomal enzyme activity, autoimmune reactions, increased crosslinking, or accumulation of lipofuscin pigments and waste products could also result in cellular information loss, ultimately manifesting itself as biologic aging.

The fundamental changes that may occur in cellular information-containing molecules can be classified into two categories: (1) an age-dependent deterioration as the result of an active "self-destruct" program or a systematic unfolding of the genetic program, and (2) a passive "wearing out" process as the result of a random accumulation of errors and injuries from environmental insults.

Strehler et al. (15) have dealt with programmed senescence rather extensively in their "codon-restriction theory" of aging, in which they propose that vital genetic code words in messages controlling protein synthesis are systematically repressed with cell aging.

In all tissues examined thus far, the rate of production of new cells is controlled by a tissue-specific antimitotic messenger molecule called a chalone (negative feedback system). Bullough (16) suggests that the onset of aging and the rate at which it proceeds are probably controlled through a chalone mechanism by a nonmitotic tissue which acts as a pacemaker. There is reason to believe that deterioration of postmitotic cells may well be a major cause of aging in mammals (17). Evidence has been presented that changes in neurons and in cells in the microvascular system are the main cause of aging in mammals (18). Since the antimitotic power of chalones is known to be strengthened by stress hormones, such as adrenaline and glucocorticoid hormones, one test of the chalone theory would be to discover whether it is possible to affect the life-span by strengthening or weakening the chalone action. The marked increase in life-span of rats on restricted caloric intake (7) has been explained on the basis of continued high level of stress hormones secretion owing to strengthened chalone action (16).

Gelfant and Smith (19) have presented a model in which cellular and tissue aging is regarded as the result of progressive transition of cycling to noncycling cells in tissues capable of proliferation. Cycling cells are regarded as cells that are actively moving through the cell cycle of periods of nuclear DNA synthesis and mitosis. A cell may be blocked at any of the intervening gaps, and remain in these noncycling states until death or until they are recalled to proliferate in response to a stimuli (20). These authors suggest that immune mechanisms may be involved in cellular aging by keeping noncycling cells in restraint. Reversal of cellular aging by hydrocortisone, an immunosuppressive agent, has been rationalized as a release of noncycling cells (19, 21). Gelfant and Grove have also shown that the ability of noncycling cells to be released to the cycling state is reduced with chronological age (22).

3   AGING OF TISSUE CULTURE CELLS

Cultured normal cells cannot be maintained indefinitely, but rather have a finite ability to replicate in vitro. This property has led to the use of diploid fibroblasts of human and chick embyro origin as in vitro models of cellular aging (6, 23, 24).

Hayflick (25) attributed the limited life-span (50 ± 10 doublings for embryonic human fibroblasts) to an intrinsic programmed expression of aging at the cellular level (clonal aging theory), and has suggested that viral transformations may be a prerequisite for conversion of such cells into permanent lines. Evidence in support of clonal aging is based on the inverse correlation existing between age of donor in vivo and life-span obtained in vitro (26, 27). Moreover, physiological rather than

chronological age appears to be important since fibroblasts from patients suffering from the premature-aging syndrome of progeria (28) and Werner's syndrome (26) have decreased growth potential in comparison with age-matched controls. Support for the view that genetic material of a given tissue is programmed to undergo a given number of cell divisions has been obtained by Daniel et al. (29–31), who studied the growth rate of mouse mammary epithelium and found it declines during serial transplantation in vivo. These authors compared transplant lines in which cells proliferated continuously with lines in which growth was restricted and showed that the decline in growth rate was related primarily to the number of cell divisions undergone rather than to the passage of metabolic time. There have been reports confirming the fact that in vitro finite life-span of human diploid cells is related to the number of cumulative population doublings and occurs independently of metabolic time (32).

Maynard-Smith (17) has summarized some results from serial transplantation technique which seem to argue against the view that clonal aging of mitotic cells is an important cause of aging. Nevertheless, limited life-span of fibroblasts has now been observed sufficiently often in different laboratories for it to be regarded as a phenomenon that calls for an explanation, whether or not aging of individuals can be attributed directly to the limited life-span of stem lines.

4   ANTI-AGING DRUGS

4.1   Impaired Protein Synthesis

The error theories are based on the assumption that aging is a consequence of progressive accumulation of errors in the protein synthesizing machinery. Errors in protein synthesis may occur at either the DNA level by mutation, single-strand breaks, or other structural changes, or at subsequent stages during transcription and translation (33, 34). Questions of age-associated alterations in DNA have been particularly difficult to pursue because of the problem of detecting subtle molecular changes at that level. Animals receiving sublethal doses of X-rays have been shown to become prematurely senile and suscepti-ble to fatal diseases. X-rays have been used to induce single-strand breaks and to ap-parently duplicate age-associated changes that occur naturally in DNA of senescent brain cells (35). However, in view of the rather remarkable ability of cells to rejoin broken strands and to replenish altered base units in DNA (36, 37) the relevancy of radiation to aging is debatable. This does not exclude the possibility , of course, that damage could build up if DNA-repair en-zymes are progressively lost (34) or if an age-associated rampant increase in the re-lease of hydrolytic enzymes occurs. Cellular aging has also been attributed to an irrever-sible nuclear protein–DNA interaction (38, 39).

Introduction of errors during translation of the DNA message into RNA and protein sequences has been suggested as a more likely basis for aging than changes in the DNA molecule itself. Orgel has recently reviewed how errors in the synthesis of RNA and information-handling enzymes can accumulate progressively, decrease the fidelity of protein synthesis, and eventually jeopardize the entire protein-synthesizing machinery ("error catastrophe") (13, 14). Frolkis has discussed the interrelationship between cell function and protein biosyn-thesis in the process of aging (40).

4.1.1 AGENTS AFFECTING PROTEIN SYN-THESIS. Agents that enhance learning and memory have been examined in geriat-rics supposedly because they act on brain RNA and protein synthesis. However, no evidence for their anti-aging effects has been obtained. 5,5-Diphenylhydantoin (36.1) reportedly prevents polyribosimal

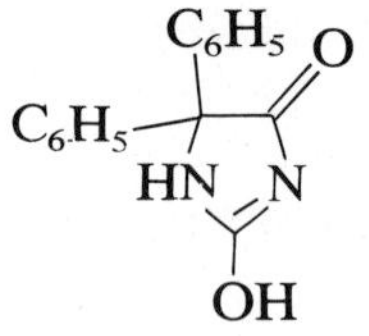

36.1

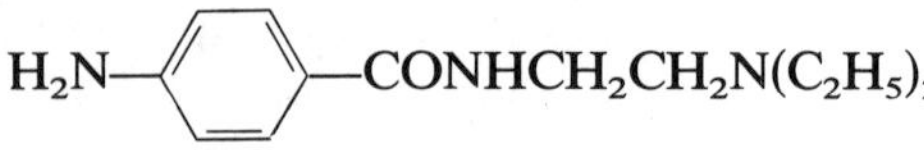

$$H_2N-C_6H_4-CONHCH_2CH_2N(C_2H_5)_2$$

36.2

disaggregation in the aging brain tissue and renders RNA more resistant to hydrolysis by RNAse. The drug has been claimed to improve the avoidance response and learn-ing retention in aged rats (41–43).

Procainamide (36.2) has been tested for learning enhancement activity in experi-mental animals of different ages and claimed to improve behavior and learning deficits in aging rats (41). Procainamide was reported to increase brain RNA content and to redistribute intracellular amino acids from the free pool to an RNA-bound form (42).

4.2 Free-Radical Damage

Free radicals are normally present in all biological systems, and can arise from a number of sources in the living system (44). Harman has suggested that free-radical mediated damage of unsaturated fatty acids and other cellular components can result in cumulative degeneration of cellular func-tion which expresses itself as aging (45–47). One consequence of free-radical attack on cell components is lipofuscin production. Lipofuscin granules are fluorescent lipopro-tein masses, appropriately called age pig-ments, which tend to accumulate with ad-vancing age, especially in postmitotic cells such as those of the brain, myocardium, skeletal muscle, and adrenals. Lipofuscin pigments may be debris left over from peroxidation of polyunsaturated lipids and their cross-linking with proteins in subcellular membranes (48), and are believed to be an important indicator of the degree of cellular insufficiency in aging (49, 50). However, there is as yet no direct evidence that they interfere with normal cell processes. The role of free radicals and lipid peroxidation in the aging process has been reviewed in detail by Gordon (51).

4.2.1 ANTIOXIDANTS AND FREE-RADICAL SCAVENGERS. Vitamin E and several chemically unrelated antioxidants and free-radical scavengers such as cysteine, 2-mercaptoethylamine (2-MEA), 2,2-diaminoethyl disulfide, vitamin C, gluthathione, butylated hydroxytoluene (BHT) (36.**3**), ethoxyquin (36.**4**) and seleno amino acids suppress lipid peroxidation of biological membranes *in vitro*, and have been tested for anti-aging effects. BHT and 2-MEA are among the most effective agents in increasing the mean life-span in animal colonies, but have no significant effect on maximum life-span (47, 52). Ethoxyquin reportedly produces a 20% increase in life-span of C3H mice (53). Several antioxidants that are ineffective in increasing survival may have achieved inadequate tissue distribution or concentration. Various combinations of vitamins C and E, cysteine, glutathione, and selenium compounds are being investigated for antioxidant therapy in humans (54).

4.2.2 MECLOFENOXATE. Meclofenoxate (centrophenoxine) (36.**5**), the *p*-chlorophenoxyacetyl ester of dimethylaminoethanol, is a geriatric therapeutic agent useful for treatment of patients suffering from confusional states, parkinsonism,

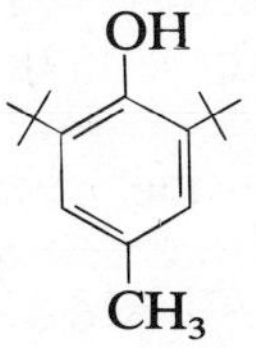

$$Cl\!-\!\bigcirc\!-\!OCH_2\overset{\overset{\text{O}}{\|}}{C}CH_2CH_2N(CH_3)_2$$

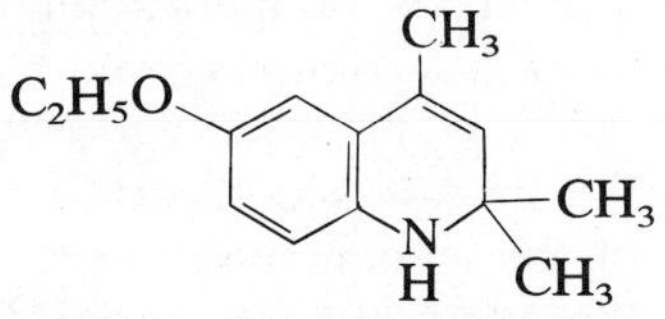

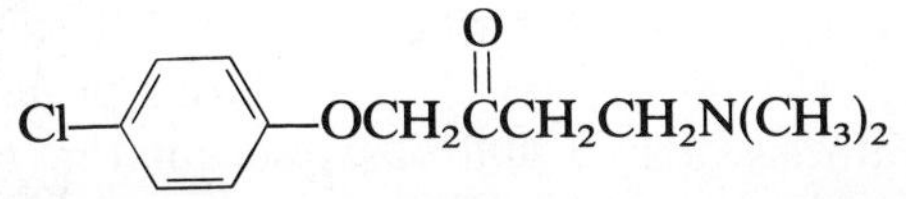

36.**5**

and other senile mental disorders. Nandy and Bourne (55, 56) have shown that meclofenoxate treatment can reverse the accumulation of lipofuscin pigments in neurons of senile guinea pigs, and suggest that reduction of lipofuscin may be one of the ways by which the drug exerts its beneficial effects on the CNS. There is also a marked reduction in the activity of a number of oxidative enzymes, as determined histochemically (56). The drug is said to promote an increase in glucose-6-phosphate dehydrogenase activity by diversion of glucose metabolism to the pentose cycle, the common pathway of glucose metabolism in cells undergoing rapid growth or multiplication, which results in an unexplained elimination of the accumulated pigments.

4.3 Lysosomes and Membrane Damage

Labilization of the lysosomal membrane and rampant lysosomal action have been suggested as a cause of cellular death during aging (57). A detailed discussion of the possible involvement of membrane breakdown in aging has been presented (58). Hochschild (58) notes that leakage of lysosomal enzymes into the cytoplasm could, in principle be responsible for several processes suggested as primary aging mechanisms, such as reduced fidelity of protein synthesis. In this context membrane damage in inositol-starved mutants of neurospora has been shown to result in synthesis of altered proteins (59). Several agents are known to stabilize lysosomal membranes (e.g., corticosteroids) (60). Cortisone (61) and hydrocortisone (62) have been shown to prolong the mitotic capacity of human embryonic fibroblasts. However,

36.**3**

36.**4**

it is as yet unclear whether corticosteroids act on aging systems by stimulating protein synthesis or by stabilizing lysosomal membranes.

4.3.1 DIMETHYLAMINOETHANOL. Hochschild proposes that alkylamino alcohols such as dimethylaminoethanol (DMAE) stabilize lysosomal membranes. Administration of DMAE to senile mice in drinking water resulted in a significant increase in their life-span (63, 64). FDA-approved clinical studies with DMAE are underway (65).

4.4 Cross-linking of Connective Tissue

4.4.1 LATHYROGENS. Agents that interfere with cross-linking of peptide chains in fibrous connective tissue macromolecules and collagen are expected to retard biological aging (66–70). Lathyrogens inhibit the oxidative deamination of free ϵ-amino groups of lysyl residues to aldehydes, which is the first step in the cross-linking of lysine residues on different peptide chains. Therefore, lathyrogenic compounds, such as β-aminopropionitrile, penicillamine (68), and semicarbazide, which prevent maturation of collagen, have been suggested as anti-aging drugs. La Bella (66) has obtained some evidence that these drugs extend the average life-span (but not the maximum life-span) of rats if given in doses sufficient to slow down cross-linking but not enough to cause undesirable side-effects. The use of penicillamine was accompanied by an inhibition of wound healing and by increased skin fragility (71, 72).

4.5 Autoimmunity

Walford (73, 74) and Burnet (75, 76) have elaborated on the idea that aging is an autoimmune phenomenon. They propose that aging is a consequence of increasing immunogenetic diversification of dividing cell populations of the body. The age-dependent decline of immunocompetence is manifested in a progressive failure of the organism's own cells to distinguish self from foreign cells with damaging immunological reaction against them ("unleashing of self-destroying process"), or the development of damaging autoimmune cell clones (forbidden clones) owing to somatic mutation of immunocytes and a decreased responsiveness to extrinsic antigens. Burnet (76) has emphasized that decreased immunologic surveillance may originate in the thymus-dependent segment of the immune system, and the latter, in turn, may depend on exhaustion of the Hayflick limit (inbuilt metabolic clock) in thymus cells and dependent tissues. Based on experiments with "nude" mice (a C3H derived strain of mice born without a thymus which suffer from immunodeficiencies similar to, but more acute than, those produced experimentally by thymectomy), Pantelouris (77) suggests that senescent normal animals have an excess of IgM antibodies over IgG antibodies. The IgM antibodies mainly produced in response to bacterial polysaccharides often cross-react with the mammal's own tissue (cross-reaction autoimmunity). This gradually increasing dependence on IgM antibodies has been correlated with involution of the thymus (78) and may be an important process in "immunologic aging," independent, though not exclusive, of forbidden clones and somatic mutations. In general, immune function does show a decline in intensity with advancing age. There is a progressive incidence of autoantibodies such as antinuclear, rheumatoid, antithyroid, and antiparietal factors in the aged (73, 79–81). This occurs despite a decrease in the numbers of antibody-forming cell precursors in both the spleen and bone marrow with increasing age (82). The current status of the immunologic theory of aging has been reviewed by Walford (83).

4.5.1 IMMUNOSUPPRESSANTS. On the basis of the autoimmune theory, Walford tested the effect of azathioprine (Imuran) (36.**6**), an immunosuppressant, on the life-span of aging mice (84). Animals receiving a daily

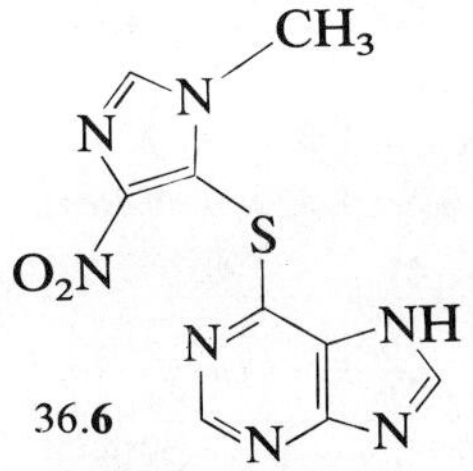

36.6 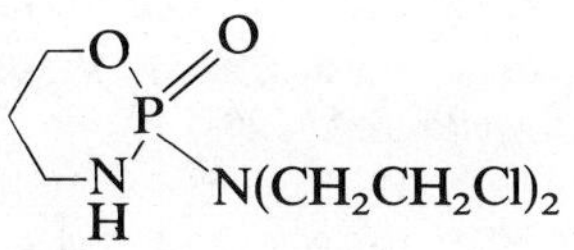   36.7

dose of 100 mg/kg of azathioprine showed
a mean survival time 10 weeks longer than
controls, but the maximum life-span (135–
140 weeks) was not affected. Similar results
were obtained with another immunosuppressant, cyclophosphamide (36.**7**) (84). It
seems probable that anti-aging therapy at
this level may be too late in the chain of
events. Moreover, suppression of the immune system may accelerate death from
other causes.

4.6   Hormonal Control of Aging

The diversity of regulatory functions performed by the hypothalamus has led to the
suggestion that age-dependent changes in
the hypothalamus are responsible for the
functional and metabolic changes associated with aging. Frolkis (85, 86) has
presented evidence that the hypothalamus
undergoes structural changes and exhibits a
decrease in functional activity with age.
There is a reduction in the activity
of neurosecretory processes and the
hypothalamic structures show an increased
sensitivity to such physiologically, active
agents as catecholamines, acetylcholine,
and insulin (85). Dilman (87) suggests that
the key process in the genetic program of
development and aging is a gradual reduction in sensitivity of the hypothalamus to
feedback control. This leads to increased
secretion of "aging hormones" and disruption of the two basic homeostatic systems
regulating reproduction and energy
metabolism. Everitt (88) has further examined the relationship between hormones
and aging, stressing the role of
hypothalamic–pituitary regulation of the

rate of aging and onset of age-related
pathology.

Chronic administration of dihydro-
tachysterol produces premature aging in
rats (89). This effect is prevented by
anabolic steroids and estrogens. Pituitary
growth hormone (90), thyroxine (91), and
plant growth hormones (92) have been administered to rats but do not influence life-
span.

4.7   Miscellaneous Agents

4.7.1   PROCAINE AND GEROVITAL H_3. The
highly controversial use of procaine hydrochloride for retarding the aging process
was first disclosed by Aslan and colleagues
in Romania during 1950 (93). Repeated
injections of procaine hydrochloride were
claimed to improve skin texture, recall,
psychomotor activity, and muscle strength
in senescent individuals. Aslan's work,
however, suffers from lack of scientific control and evaluation, and several controlled
human trials by others have been unable to
substantiate the rejuvenation claims by the
Romanian workers (94–96). The subsequent popular use of Gerovital H_3, a formulation of procaine hydrochloride containing benzoic acid and potassium
metabisulfate (93), as a "youth" drug and
rejuvenating agent appears to be equally
dubious. Gerovital H_3 has weak
monoamine oxidase inhibitor properties
(97, 98), and this probably accounts for its
reported benefits in treating depressive disorders in the elderly.

4.8   CONCLUSION

The enigma of human aging continues to
persist, although it is becoming increasingly
evident that aging may be caused by a
number of different mechanisms operating
simultaneously in the individual. There is
growing research emphasis on some
theories of aging that are especially promising. Most impressive has been the accumulation of evidence that aging is

caused, at least in part, by a progressive breakdown of the body's immunological defenses—whether programmed or random. Although on the basis of present experimental evidence it is difficult to mount a chemical attack on aging, and the available rejuvenating drugs are all of dubious utility, a clear understanding of the fundamental aging process will surely lead to a rational chemical approach to retarding human aging during the next two decades.

REFERENCES

1. A. Comfort, *Aging: The Biology of Senescence*, Holt, Rinehart & Winston, New York, 1964; *Nature*, **217**, 320 (1968).

2. B. L. Strehler, *Fed. Proc.*, **34**, 5 (1975).

3. I. S. Wright, *J. Am. Geriatr. Soc.*, **19**, 737 (1971).

4. C. G. Kormendy and A. D. Bender, *J. Pharm. Sci.*, **60** 167 (1971).

5. See also "Reports on aging", *Chem. Eng. News*, July 24, 13 (1971); March 28, 15 (1974).

6. L. Hayflick, *Fed. Proc.*, **34**, 9 (1975); *New Engl. J. Med.*, **295**, 1302 (1976).

7. S. Goldstein, *New Engl. J. Med.*, **285**, 1121 (1971).

8. F. S. La Bella, in *Search for New Drugs*, A. A. Rubin, Ed., Dekker, New York, 1972, p. 347.

9. M. Rockstein, Ed., *Theoretical Aspects of Aging*, Academic, New York, 1974.

10. C. E. Finch and L. Hayflick, Eds., *Handbook of the Biology of Aging*, Van Nostrand Reinhold, New York, 1977.

11. A. Rosenfeld, *Prolongevity*, Knopf, New York, 1976.

12. L. E. Orgel, *Proc. U.S. Natl. Acad. Sci.*, **49**, 427 (1963).

13. *Ibid.*, **67**, 1476 (1970).

14. L. E. Orgel, *Nature*, **243**, 441 (1973).

15. B. Strehler, G. Hirsch, D. Gusseck, R. Johnson, and M. Bick, *J. Theor. Biol.*, **33**, 429 (1971).

16. W. S. Bullogh, *Nature*, **229**, 608 (1971).

17. J. Maynard-Smith, in *Cell Biology in Medicine*, E. E. Bittar, Ed., Wiley, New York, 1973, p. 681.

18. L. M. Franks, *Exp. Gerontol.*, **5**, 281 (1970).

19. S. Gelfant and J. G. Smith, *Science*, **178**, 357 (1972).

20. J. J. DeCosse and S. Gelfant, *Science*, **162**, 698 (1968).

21. V. J. Cristofalo, *Advan. Gerontol. Res.*, **4**, 45 (1972).

22. S. Gelfant and G. L. Grove, in Ref. 8, p. 105.

23. L. Hayflick and P. S. Moorehead, *Exp. Cell Res.*, **25**, 585 (1961).

24. L. Hayflick, in Ref. 10, p. 159.

25. L. Hayflick, *Exp. Cell Res.*, **37**, 614 (1965).

26. G. M. Martin, C. A. Sprague, and C. J. Epstein, *Lab. Invest.*, **23**, 86 (1970).

27. S. Goldstein, J. W. Littlefield, and J. S. Soeldner, *Proc. Natl. Acad. Sci. U.S.*, **64**, 155 (1969).

28. S. Goldstein, *Lancet*, **1**, 424 (1969).

29. C. W. Daniel, K. B. DeOme, L. J. T. Young, P. B. Blair, and L. J. Franklin, *Proc. Natl. Acad. Sci. U.S.*, **61**, 52 (1968).

30. C. W. Daniel, L. J. T. Young, and D. Medina, *Exp. Gerontol.* **6**, 95 (1971).

31. C. W. Daniel and L. J. T. Young, *Exp. Cell Res.*, **65**, 27 (1971).

32. R. T. Dell'Orco, J. G. Mertens, and P. F. Kruse, *Exp. Cell Res.*, **77**, 356 (1973).

33. H. J. Curtis, *Biological Mechanisms of Aging*, Charles C. Thomas, Springfield, Ill. 1966.

34. K. L. Yielding, *Perspect. Biol. Med.*, 201 (1974).

35. S. P. Modak and G. B. Price, *Expo. Cell Res.*, **65**, 289 (1971).

36. E. Fahr, *Angew. Chem. Int. Ed.*, **8**, 578 (1969).

37. C. J. Dean, M. G. Ormerod, R. W. Serianni, and P. Alexander, *Nature*, **222**, 1042 (1969).

38. J. S. Salser and M. E. Balis, *J. Gerontol.*, **27**, 1 (1972).

39. H. P. von Hahn, *J. Gerontol.*, **21**, 291 (1966).

40. V. V. Frolkis, *Gerontologia*, **19**, 189 (1973).

41. P. Gordon, S. S. Tobin, B. Doty, and M. Nash, *J. Gerontol.*, **23**, 434 (1968).

42. P. Gordon, *Recent Advan. Biol., Psychiatr.*, **10**, 121 (1968).

43. B. Doty and R. Dalman, *Psychon. Sci.*, **14**, 109 (1969).

44. W. A. Pryor, *Sci. Am.*, **223**, 70 (1970).

45. D. Harman, *J. Gerontol.*, **23**, 476 (1968).

46. D. Harman, *J. Gerontol.*, **26**, 451 (1971).

47. D. Harman, *Agents Action*, **1**, 3 (1969).

48. A. L. Tappel, *Geriatrics*, **23**, 97 (1968).

49. B. L. Strehler, *Advan. Gerontol. Res.*, **1**, 343 (1964).

50. W. Reichel, J. Hollander, J. H. Clark, and B. L. Strehler, *J. Gerontol.*, **23**, 71 (1968).

51. P. Gordon, In Ref. 8, 61.

52. D. Harman, *Am. J. Clin. Nutr.*, **25**, 839 (1972).

53. A. Comfort, I. Youhotsky-Gore, and K. Pathmanathan, *Nature*, **229**, 254 (1971).

54. R. A. Passwater and P. A. Welker, *Am. Lab.*, **3,** 21 (1971).

55. K. Nandy and G. H. Bourne, *Nature*, **210,** 313 (1966).

56. K. Nandy, *J. Gerontol.*, **23,** 82 (1968).

57. A. Comfort, *Lancet*, **1966-II,** 1325.

58. R. Hochschild, *Exp. Gerontol.*, **6,** 153 (1971).

59. J. L. Sullivan and A. G. Debusk, *Nature New Biol.*, **243,** 72 (1973).

60. G. Weissman, in '*Lysosomes in Biology and Pathology*', Part 1, J. T. Dingle and H. B. Fell, Eds. Wiley, New York, 1969.

61. G. C. Yuan and R. S. Chang, *Proc. Soc. Exp. Biol. Med.*, **130,** 934 (1969).

62. V. Gristofalo, in '*Aging in Cell and Tissue Culture*', E. Holeckova and V. J. Gristofalo, Eds., Plenum, New York, 1970, p. 83.

63. R. Hochschild, *Exp. Gerontol.*, **8,** 185 (1973).

64. R. Hochschild, *Exp. Gerontol.*, **8,** 177 (1973).

65. Anon., *Med. World News*, Jan. 11, 13 (1974).

66. F. S. LaBella, *Gerontologist*, **8,** 13 (1968).

67. R. R. Kohn and A. M. Leash, *Exp. Mol. Pathol.*, **7,** 354 (1967).

68. A. J. Bailey, *Gerontologia*, **15,** 65 (1969).

69. F. Verzar, *Gerontologia*, **15,** 233 (1969).

70. J. Boorksten, *J. Am. Geriatr. Soc.*, **16,** 408 (1968).

71. A. Ruiz-Torres, *Arzneim.-Forsch.*, **5,** 594 (1968).

72. M. E. Nimmi and L. A. Baretta, *Science*, **150,** 905 (1965).

73. R. L. Walford, *Lancet*, **1970-II,** 1226.

74. R. L. Walford, '*Immunologic Theory of Aging*', Munksgaard, Copenhagen (1969).

75. F. M. Burnet, '*Immunological Surveillance*', Pergamon, New York (1970).

76. F. M. Burnet, *Lancet*, **1970-II,** 358.

77. E. M. Pantelouris, *Exp. Gerontol.*, **7,** 73 (1972).

78. E. M. Pantelouris, *Exp. Gerontol.*, **8,** 169 (1973).

79. M. M. Sigel and R. A. Good, Eds., *Tolerance, Autoimmunity and Aging*, Charles C Thomas, Springfield, Illinois, 1972.

80. S. Whittingham, J. D. Mathews, I. R. Mackay, A. E. Stocks, B. Ungar, and F. I. R. Martin, *Lancet*, **1971-I,** 763.

81. J. Preito Valtuena, M. I. Gonzalez Guilabert, M. A. del Pozo Perez, F. del Pozo Crespo, and R. Velasco Alonso, *Biomedicine*, **19,** 301 (1973) and references therein.

82. S. Kishimoto and T. Yanamura, *Clin. Exp. Immunol.*, **8,** 957 (1971).

83. R. L. Walford, *Fed. Proc.*, **33,** 2020 (1974).

84. R. L. Walford, *Symp. Soc. Exp. Biol.*, **21,** 351 (1967).

85. V. V. Frolkis, V. V. Berzrukov, Y. K. Duplenko, and E. D. Genis, *Exp. Gerontol.*, **7,** 169 (1972).

86. V. V. Frolkis, N. Verzhikovskaya, and G. V. Valueva, *Exp. Gerontol.*, **8,** 285 (1973).

87. V. M. Dilman, *Lancet* **1971-II,** 1211.

88. A. V. Everitt, *Exp. Gerontol.*, **8,** 265 (1973).

89. H. Selye and R. Strebel, *Proc. Soc. Exp. Biol. Med.*, **110,** 673 (1962).

90. A. V. Everitt, *J. Gerontol.*, **14,** 415 (1959).

91. A. V. Everitt, *Gerontologia*, **3,** 37 (1959).

92. A. V. Everitt, *Gerontologia*, **3,** 65 (1959).

93. For a review, see A. Aslan, in Ref. 8, p. 145.

94. P. Lüth, *J. Gerontol.*, **15,** 395 (1960).

95. G. C. Chiu, *J. Am. Med. Assoc.*, **175,** 502 (1961).

96. A. D. Bender, C. G. Kormendy, and R. Powell, *Exp. Gerontol.*, **5,** 97 (1970).

97. M. D. McFarlane, *J. Am. Geriatr. Soc.*, **21,** 414 (1973).

98. T. M. Yau, in Ref. 8., p. 157.

CHAPTER THIRTY-SEVEN

Radioprotective Drugs

WILLIAM O. FOYE

Massachusetts College of Pharmacy
Boston, Massachusetts 02115, USA

CONTENTS

1   INTRODUCTION

The protective action of certain substances against the damaging effects of ionizing radiation was first noted in 1942 by W. M. Dale. A decrease was observed in the inactivation of two enzymes by X-rays on the

11

addition of several substances, including colloidal sulfur and thiourea, to aqueous solutions of the enzymes (1). Since then, a variety of animal and plant cells have been shown to receive radiation protection from a surprising number of chemicals, although of only a few chemical or pharmacological classifications. Chemical radiation protectors, it should be pointed out, are effective only when administered prior to exposure to radiation, and should therefore be considered distinct from substances, such as bone marrow cells, that are used for restorative therapy after irradiation.

Radioprotective effects for a bacteriophage were noted in 1948 by Latarjet using thioglycolic acid, glutathione, tryptophan, cysteine, and cystine (2). Radioprotection of mice using cyanide (3), cysteine (4), and thiourea (5) was achieved shortly after, these protective effects all being attributed at the time to inhibition of or reaction with cellular enzymes. The importance of an amino group for the radioprotective action of a mercaptan was first demonstrated by Bacq et al. (6), who removed the carboxyl group of cysteine in order to liberate the amino function; the important discovery of cysteamine (β-mercaptoethylamine), still regarded as one of the most potent of the radioprotective agents, was the result.

Since 1952, other types of structures have been found with radioprotective effects, including a number of commonly used pharmacological agents, but the most effective have generally been derivatives or analogs of the aminoalkyl mercaptans. Among the pharmacological agents, serotonin and its derivatives have shown particularly potent effects. Several rather clearly defined classes of protective agents have emerged, along with a wealth of facts relating to biochemical and physiological events which the presence of the protective agents modify following irradiation. A number of hypotheses concerning the mode of action of those agents have been advanced, and it is becoming clear what cellular structures

or functions are protected by a given class of protectant. No universal explanation for the mode of protection by all classes of protectants has been made that has withstood criticism, but some cellular events appear quite reasonably related to the protection afforded by several of the more extensively investigated compounds.

Research attempts to explain the action of chemical radiation protection have involved the use of not only mammals, but plants, bacteria, distinct types of cells, and cellular components as well. This chapter attempts to list the various types of chemical structures that afford some protection against the deleterious effects of high energy ionizing radiation in mammals and to describe the more widely considered mechanisms of protection by which they may act.

2 RADIATION DAMAGE

Biologic effects of radiation have been reviewed in detail by a number of authors, including Bond et al. (7), Pizzarello and Witcofski (8), Casarett (9), Okada (10), and Dertinger and Jung (11). In general, ionizing radiation results in damage to the blood-forming organs, gastrointestinal system, or central nervous system, depending on radiation dose. Hematopoietic death from bleeding, infection, or anemia is the type usually observed from antiradiation screening of potential protectants, and follows 7–30 days after exposure to a lethal dose (~1000 rads) in mice.

Absorption of radiation energy by biological molecules has been considered to be either direct or indirect, although the distinction between them is not clear. Direct action involves absorption of radiation energy by target molecules, such as DNA or RNA, resulting in molecular damage. Indirect action involves the release of radiation energy in the environment of a target molecule with transfer of the energy to the target molecules by free radicals. These are generally considered to be the radiolytic

ducts of water, which deposit their
ergy in biological systems and create ex-
ted molecules and ions, or ultimately
emistable bioradicals, which lead to
molecular alterations and resulting loss of
normal biological activity. The following
model reactions have been suggested (12):

$$RH \rightleftarrows R\cdot + H\cdot \qquad (37.1)$$

$$RH + H\cdot \rightarrow R\cdot + H_2 \qquad (37.2)$$

In the presence of oxygen:

$$R\cdot + O_2 \rightarrow RO_2\cdot \qquad (37.3)$$

And in the presence of a sulfhydryl compound:

$$R\cdot + RSH \rightarrow RH + RS\cdot \qquad (37.4)$$

These model reactions show how molecular
oxygen sensitizes cellular molecules to radiation damage by preventing the reversal of
reaction (37.1) and producing a damaging
peroxy radical. A rapid hydrogen atom
donor, such as a thiol, is considered responsible for instantaneous repair (13).

The radiolytic products of water are hydrogen atoms, hydroxyl radicals, hydrated
electrons, and several nonradical species,
hydrogen molecules, hydrogen peroxide,
and hydronium ions:

$$H_2O \rightarrow H\cdot + OH\cdot + e_{aq}^- + H_2O_2 + H_3O^+ + H_2$$
$$(37.5)$$

Regardless of the direct or indirect transfer
of energy to a molecule, radiation inactivation can be transferred to other molecules
through coupled reactions (14). Thus a
marked amplification of radiation damage
can result. It can be seen, however, that the
presence of a sulfhydryl group, or molecule
capable of scavenging the radiolytic radicals
from irradiation of water molecules, can
bring about radiation protection.

3 ANTIRADIATION TESTING

Most testing of antiradiation agents has
employed X- or γ-rays from an external
source. These high energy radiations cause
the ejection of electrons from the atoms
through which they pass with resulting ionization. Neutrons have been used infre-
quently. Test animals most often have been
mice or rats, with guinea pigs used less
frequently. Antiradiation testing with dogs
or monkeys has been limited to the more
effective compounds as determined from
screening with mice or rats. Further information on this subject may be found in a
number of texts devoted to radiobiology
(15–17).

Various physiological effects may be observed, depending on the dose and type of
radiation, as well as on the type of animal
used. In theory, the appearance of any observable symptom of radiation damage may
be used as the basis of a testing procedure,
but in practice lethality has generally been
the criterion for protection. Sufficient numbers of animals must be employed for
statistical significance, and in the case of
mice irradiated with a lethal dose of X- or
γ-rays, a 30 day survival period is generally
observed. Testing results are expressed
most commonly as the percentage survival
for the observation period in comparison to
the survival of control animals. Another
method of expression of test data is in
terms of the dose reduction factor (DRF)
(the ratio of the radiation dose causing an
LD_{50} in the treated animals compared to
the LD_{50} from irradiation in the unprotected animals).

The dose of protective agent employed is
usually the maximum tolerated dose,
(MTD), i.e., the dose causing no deleterious effects. In a drug-screening program,
candidate compounds are usually tested at
their MTD level using a radiation dose that
is lethal to all control animals in 30 days.
The time interval between administration
of the drug and irradiation of the animals is
usually 15–30 min for intraperitoneal dosing and 30–60 min for oral dosing. Drugs
believed to act by hypoxia or other
metabolic changes must be administered
several hours prior to irradiation. Rate of

irradiation in screening programs has been done commonly at 50–250 rads/min. At lower rates, the time for maximum effectiveness of drug can be exceeded before the total dose is administered. In addition, repair processes could become significant before the irradiation is complete. Chronic radiation studies have been carried out with repeated administration of protectant, but results have been less decisive (18).

Other testing procedures used to a lesser extent include the inhibition of bacterial or plant growth and the prevention of depolymerization of polymethacrylate or polystyrene (19) or of DNA (20). Plaque-forming ability of coliphage T (21), effect on Eh potential (22), inhibition of peroxide formation of unsaturated lipids or β-carotene (22), and inhibition of chemiluminescence of γ-irradiated mouse tissue homogenates (23) have also been employed as test procedures. Protection of cells in tissue culture has also been used (24), as well as spleen colony counts (25). A review of the nonlethal test methods has been made (26).

4 PROTECTIVE COMPOUNDS

The more extensively investigated compounds have been well discussed in books by Thomson (17) and Bacq (27) and in a number of reviews. A catalog of compounds tested for radiation protection up to 1963 was compiled by Huber and Spode (28), and a handbook of radioprotective agents appeared in Russia in 1964 (29). Extensive reviews on protective agents since 1963 have been written by Balabukha (30), Foye (31), Overman and Jackson (32), Romantsev (33), Melching and Streffer (34), and more recently Klayman and Copeland (35). Reports of two international symposia on radioprotective and radiosensitizing agents have been published by Paoletti and Vertua (36) and by Moroson and Quintiliani (37). Chapters on radio-

protective agents have appeared in *Annual Reports in Medicinal Chemistry* in 1966 and 1967 (38) and in 1968 and 1970 (39). A variety of reviews on more specialized topics related to radiation biochemistry with more or less emphasis on radiation protection are available; those by Alexander and Lett (40), Silini (41), and Fahr (42) are particularly useful.

In the following discussion of structure–activity relationships, results on radioprotection of mice are compared unless otherwise stated. Relevant details concerning radiation dose, compound dose, route of administration, or strain of test animal, variations of which can alter results significantly, may be found in the original references.

4.1 THIOLS AND THIOL DERIVATIVES

2-Mercaptoethylamine (MEA, cysteamine) (37.**1**) and 2-mercaptoethylguanidine (MEG) (37.**2**) and derivatives of these structures have constituted the most effective class of radioprotective compounds. Since the initial discoveries of the protective action in mice of cysteine by Patt et al. (4) and its decarboxylated derivative MEA by Bacq et al. (6), hundreds of derivatives and analogs of the mercaptoethylamine structure have been synthesized and tested for radioprotective activity. Several structural requirements for activity in this class of compounds have become established.

$$\text{NH}_2\text{CH}_2\text{CH}_2\text{SH} \qquad \overset{\overset{\displaystyle \text{NH}_2^{+}}{\|}}{\text{NH}_2\text{CNHCH}_2\text{CH}_2\text{SH}} \cdot \text{Br}^-$$

$$\quad\; 37.\mathbf{1} \qquad\qquad\qquad 37.\mathbf{2}$$

The presence of a basic function (amino, amidino, or guanidino) located two or three carbon atoms distant from the thiol group appears to be essential. Activity drops off completely with more than a three-carbon distance (43, 44).

The presence of a free thiol group, or a thiol derivative that can be converted to a free thiol *in vivo*, is essential for high activity. Several acyl thiol derivatives (37.**3**) such as the thiosulfuric acid (45), phosphorothioic acid (46), and trithiocarbonic acid (47), most likely liberate free thiol in the animal; an increase in tissue nonprotein thiol levels results after administration of the thiosulfate and phosphorothioate of MEA (48).

$$^+NH_3CH_2CH_2SX \quad X = SO_3^-, PO_3H^-, CS_2^-$$
37.**3**

Alkylation of the nitrogen usually causes some loss of activity. The *N*-β-phenethyl and *N*-β-thienylethyl derivatives, however, have good activity (49). The *N,N*-diethyl derivative also retains much of the activity of MEA; the *N,N*-dimethyl derivative is more toxic (44). The *N,N*-dipropyl and *N,N*-diisobutyl derivatives retain a little activity, whereas the di-*n*-butyl derivative is inactive (44). Other *N*-alkyl derivatives are listed in Ref. 34. *N,N'*-Polymethylene bridging of the MEA structure provides compounds,

$$XS(CH_2)_2NH(CH_2)_nNH(CH_2)_2SX,$$

that are active where X is PO_3H_2 and *n* is 3 or 4, but inactive where X is SO_3H (50).

Alkylation of the carbon atoms has given varied results. Active compounds have been found among *C*-monoalkyl derivatives of MEA, 2-aminopropane-1-thiol (37.**4**) having moderate activity and 1-aminopropane-2-thiol (37.**5**) having good activity (51, 52). Whereas α,α-dialkyl-β-aminoethanethiols are inactive (53, 54), some β,β-dialkyl-β-aminoethane thiosulfates and phosphorothioates (37.**6**) have protective activity (55). 2-Amino-1-pentanethiol and 2-amino-3-methyl-1-butanethiol also have good activity (55). Trialkylmercaptoethylamines (54) (37.**7**), *sec*-mercaptoalkylamines (56) (37.**8**), and

2-mercapto-2-phenethylamine (57) are all inactive. Generally, the presence of phenyl groups blocks activity (58). α,α-Dimethyl-2-aminoethanethiol (37.**9**), derived from penicillamine, is not protective but is a radiosensitizer (59).

$$CH_3{-}\underset{\underset{NH_2}{|}}{CH}{-}CH_2SH \quad CH_3{-}\underset{\underset{SH}{|}}{CH}{-}CH_2NH_2$$
37.**4**   37.**5**

$$NH_2{-}\underset{\underset{R}{|}}{\overset{\overset{R}{|}}{C}}{-}CH_2SX$$
37.**6** $X = SO_3^-, SPO_3H^-$

Alkylation of the mercapto group generally results in loss of activity. The *S*-benzyl derivative of MEA has some activity, however (60).

Attempts to determine whether the stereochemical structure of the amino alkyl thiols is important have revealed that a given stereoisomer may provide greater radioprotection than the others. A small difference in activity was found for the cis and trans isomers of 2-aminocyclohexane-1-thiol (61). The cis forms of 2-mercaptocyclobutylamine and (2-mercaptocyclobutyl) methylamine have distinctly higher radioprotective ability in mice than the trans forms, but no correlation could be found between protective ability and ability to protect against either induction of DNA single-strand breaks or inacti-

$$NH_2{-}\underset{\underset{R'}{|}}{\overset{\overset{CH_3}{|}}{CH}}{-}\underset{\underset{R'}{|}}{\overset{\overset{R}{|}}{C}}{-}SH \quad NH_2{-}\underset{\underset{R}{|}}{CH}{-}\underset{\underset{SH}{|}}{CH}{-}R'$$
37.**7**   37.**8**

$$NH_2{-}CH_2{-}\underset{\underset{CH_3}{|}}{\overset{\overset{CH_3}{|}}{C}}{-}SH$$
37.**9**

vation of proliferative capacity of hamster cells *in vitro* (62). On the other hand, the trans forms are less toxic and more effective in competing for free radicals in DNA. The D and L isomers of 2-aminobutylisothiouronium bromide, a particularly effective derivative of AET, have been separated, and the D isomer is twice as active in mice as the L isomer (63). The optical isomers of dithiothreitol show a greater difference in protective ability, the D_g isomer protecting 50% of mice exposed to 650 R, whereas the L_g isomer affords no protection (64). The D_g isomer is also less toxic. The oxidized forms are also nonprotective.

Other functional groups in the MEA structure have generally caused diminution or loss of protective ability. The presence of a carboxyl group frequently causes lower activity; cysteine, for instance, has the same dose reduction factor (1.7) in mice as MEA or MEG, but a much larger dose is required (65). α-Homocysteinethiolactone has only low protective ability (66), and cystine, the disulfide, is nonprotective (4).

N-Monosubstituted derivatives of MEA containing thioureide or sulfone substituents are inactive, although sulfonic acid zwitterions, $HS(CH_2)_2NH_2^+(CH_2)_3SO_3^-$, are strongly protective (67). The presence of hydroxyl appears to favor activity; e.g., L(+)-3-amino-4-mercapto-1-butanol gives good protection to mice (68). An additional thiol group diminishes activity in a series of 2-alkyl-2-amino-1,3-propanedithiols, which show little protection in mice (67). Dithiothreitol (Cleland's reagent) (37.**10**) has low protective ability (64, 69); although Falconi et al. (69) found that an oxidized form protects 56% of mice treated, Carmack et al. (64) found no protection from the oxidized (dithiane) form. Sodium 2,3-dimercaptopropane sulfonate (Unithiol) (37.**11**), which has been studied mainly in Russia, has been claimed to be more protective and less toxic than MEA (70), however.

$$\begin{array}{cccc} CH_2 & CH & CH & CH_2 \\ | & | & | & | \\ SH & OH & OH & SH \end{array}$$

37.10

$$\begin{array}{ccc} CH_2 & CH & CH_2-SO_3Na \\ | & | & \\ SH & SH & \end{array}$$

37.11

S-Acylation of the MEA structure has provided some very active compounds, particularly where zwitterions have resulted. The thiosulfate, or Bunte salt (45), phosphorothioate (46), and trithiocarbonate (47) of MEA, all of which form zwitterions, have protective activities comparable to that of MEA. Corresponding zwitterions of MEG also give protection corresponding to that of MEG (47, 71). Of these S-acyl derivatives, the phosphorothioates have been particularly effective; S-(3-amino-2-hydroxypropyl)phosphorothioate (37.**12**) and S-(2-aminopropyl)phosphorothioate have DRF values in mice of 2.16 and 1.86, respectively, in comparison to a DRF value of 1.84 for MEA (72). S-[2-(3-Aminopropylamino)ethyl]phosphorothioate (37.**13**) (known as WR2721, from the screening program of the Walter Reed Army Institute of Research) (73) has high antiradiation activity and has been used in numerous investigations. 3-Aminopropylphosphorothioate (71), however, and N-substituted derivatives of 2-aminoethylphosphorothioate are essentially inactive (71).

A comparison of the relative activities and toxicities of thiols with the corresponding thiosulfates showed the thiosulfates to be less toxic and comparable in activity (52, 74). In a series of 2-N-alkyl-aminoethanethiols, comprising 66 compounds, the thiosulfates were generally superior to either the corresponding thiols, disulfides, or thiazolidines (74), given intraperitoneally to mice. Another comparison of the relative effectiveness of thiols with the common sulfur-covering groups, the

$$\overset{\displaystyle OH}{\underset{|}{}}$$

$$NH_2{-}CH_2{-}\overset{|}{CH}{-}CH_2{-}SPO_3H^{-} \qquad NH_2{-}CH_2{-}CH_2{-}CH_2{-}NH{-}CH_2{-}CH_2{-}SPO_3H^{-}$$

37.**12**   37.**13**

disulfide, thiosulfate, and phosphoro-thioate, was made with a series of 84 2-mercaptoacetamidine derivatives (75). Although generalities were not evident, by the intraperitoneal route the (3,5-dimethyl-1-adamantyl)methyl phosphorothioate (37.**14**) was the most effective compound. Perorally, the disulfides appeared to be superior, the most effective compound being the 1-adamantylmethyl disulfide (37.**15**). In a series of N-heterocyclic aminoethyl disulfides and aminoethanethiosulfuric acids, the thiosulfates were generally more active and less toxic than the disulfides, administered either intraperitoneally or perorally (76). The most effective compound was the 2-(2-quinoxalinylamino)ethanethiosulfate (37.**16**). It is believed that the phosphorothioate group aids in cellular transport (77).

Two inorganic phosphorothioates, diammonium amidophosphorothioate (37.**17**) and diammonium thioamidodiphosphate (37.**18**), surprisingly gave DRF values, respectively, of 2.30 and 2.16 at relatively low doses (72). Alkylation of the amidophosphorothioate lowered or eliminated activity, however (78).

In a series of straight chain aliphatic thioesters of MEA, the best protection was found with the acetyl and octanoyl derivatives (79); the benzoyl ester was essentially inactive. N-Acetyl and N,S-diacetyl MEA showed minimal activity (80). In a series of hemimercaptals of MEA derived from glycolic acid, the most active protected mice at one-half the LD_{50} dose with activity comparable to that of MEA (81).

Other basic functional groups can replace the amino group in the MEA structure to provide protective thiols. The inclusion of the guanidino group has provided very active compounds, notably 2-mercaptoethylguanidine (MEG) (37.**2**) and 2-mercaptopropylguanidine (MPG) (80). Solutions of these compounds were obtained by alkaline rearrangement of the aminoethylisothiouronium (AET) salts. When these compounds are employed for radiation protection, the hydrobromides of the 2-aminoalkylisothiouronium bromides are generally rearranged in neutral or alkaline media. This rearrangement has been termed "intratransguanylation." Thus 2-aminoethylisothiouronium bromide (AET) or 3-aminopropylisothiouronium bromide

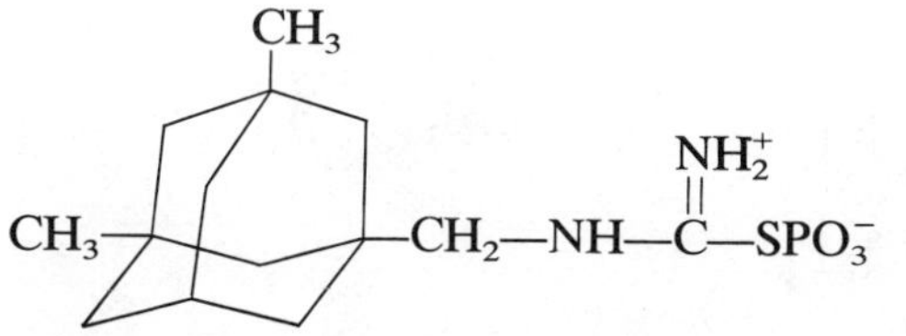

37.**14**

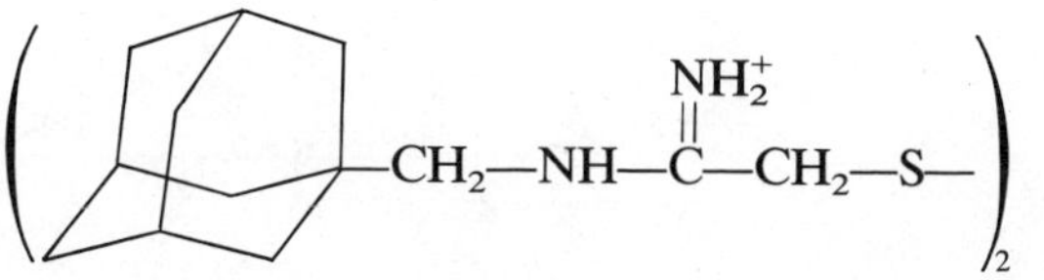

37.**15**

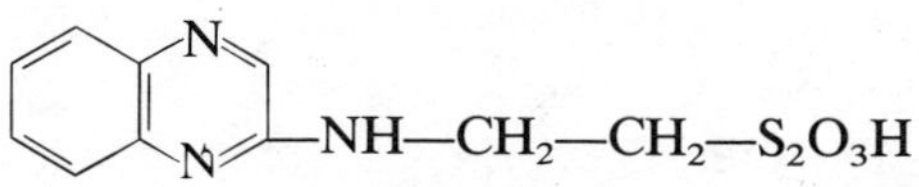

37.**16**

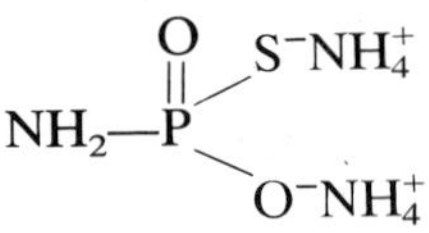

37.**17**

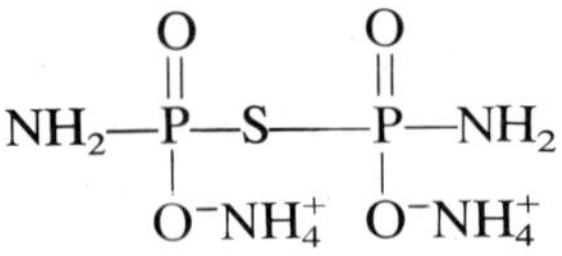

37.**18**

(APT) give solutions of MEG or MPG (equation 37.6). These compounds are generally not isolated, but may be isolated as the sulfates (82) or the trithiocarbonate esters (47).

Although AET is not subject to air oxidation, as most thiols are, it is affected by moisture, resulting in conversion to 2-amino-2-thiazoline. The disulfide, bis(2-guanidinoethyl) disulfide (GED), is readily prepared, however, and is relatively stable. With more than three carbon atoms between the amino and isothiouronium functions, rearrangement does not readily occur, and the isothiuronium salts give little protection. 2-Aminobutylthiopseudourea dihydrobromide, however, requires about one-fourth the molar quantity of AET for comparable protection in mice (63).

Replacement of the amino group by amidino has also resulted in compounds with good protective activity, particularly with Bunte salts of α-mercaptoacetamidines (83) (37.**19**). Among the most effective of the amidinoalkylthiosulfuric

acids are several terpene derivatives, including the bornyl (84) (37.**20**).

Other amidines related to MEA and MEG have been effective; 3,3'-dithiobis-(propionamidine) (85) and propionamidines containing isothiouronium groups (86), for instance, have good activity.

Use of strongly basic nitrogen heterocycles having pKa values of 10–12.5 has also provided protective compounds having the dithiocarbamate group as the sulfur-containing function. Reaction of imino-N-alkyl pyridines, pyrimidines (87), quinaldines, and acridines (88) with carbon disulfide gave imino-N-carbodithioates (37.**21**) having moderate protective effects:

Substitution of the hydrazino group for amino has not provided many active compounds. Protection of mice has been reported for N,N'-bis(mercaptoacetyl)-hydrazine (89), as well as for N-acetyl-thioglycolic hydrazide, $HSCH_2CONHNH-COCH_3$, and its disulfide (90).

Oxidation of the thiol group of the MEA structure has provided products with radioprotective properties, particularly with the disulfides. The disulfides of MEA (cystamine) and MEG (GED) are as active as the parent thiols, although GED is more toxic than MEG (91). The argument has been advanced that the thiol is the active

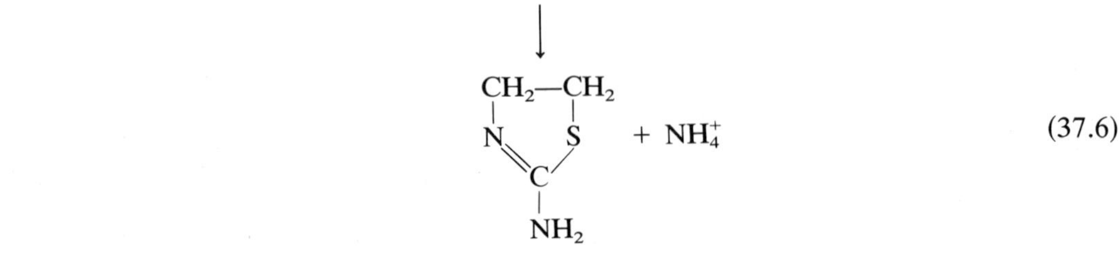

(37.6)

$R_2N—\overset{\overset{NH_2^+}{\|}}{C}—\underset{\underset{R'}{|}}{C}H—SSO_3^-$

37.**19**

$\underset{\underset{CH_3}{}}{\overset{\overset{CH_3\quad CH_3}{}}{}}$

$NH—\overset{\overset{NH_2^+}{\|}}{C}—CH_2SSO_3^-$

37.**20**

$\overset{\overset{S}{\|}}{N}=NCS^-$ with R on N

37.**21**

form of these compounds, since some *in vitro* systems protected by MEA are not protected by cystamine (92), and the reduction of cystamine to MEA during irradiation of mice has been observed (93, 94). In the case of GED, appreciable amounts of this disulfide were found *in vivo* after administration of either MEG or GED (95), however.

Cystine is nonprotective in mammals, probably because of its inability to penetrate some cellular membranes (93). Mixed disulfides of MEA have provided good protection, particularly those derived from *o*-substituted mercaptobenzenes where zwitterions are formed with carboxyl, sulfonyl, or sulfinyl anions (96) (37.**22**). It is possible, however, that *in vivo* the unsymmetrical disulfides are disproportionating to the two symmetrical disulfides, thus giving rise to cystamine. Mixed disulfides containing *N*-decyl MEA are also effective (97), as is the mixed disulfide of thiolacetic acid and *N*-acetyl MEA (98). Disulfides lacking basic groups have generally been found inactive, although a bis(butanesulfinate) disulfide (37.**23**), derived from (37.**24**) by disproportionation, was highly active (99). The bis(butanesulfinate) trisulfide was also very active, protecting 100% of mice against a lethal dose of radiation (99). Two thiocarbamoyl disulfides (37.**25**, R = H, CH$_3$) also gave good protection (100).

Higher oxidation states of the sulfur in the MEA and MEG molecules have been obtained, and some protective activity has been found with these derivatives. The thiolsulfinates of both MEA (101) and MEG (102) have been prepared, as well as

the corresponding thiolsulfonates (103) (37.**26**).

Protective activity has been reported for both the thiolsulfonate (103) and the thiolsulfinate of MEG (104), as well as for the thiolsulfonates of *N*-acetyl and *N*-decyl MEA. Taurine and hypotaurine (the SO$_3$H and SO$_2$H derivatives, respectively, of MEA), both metabolites of MEA in mice (105), provide essentially no protection (27).

Thiazolidines have been prepared from MEA or its *N*-substituted derivatives by reaction with aldehydes or ketones. A number of these thiazolidines have shown good protective activity in mice, which has been attributed to ring opening *in vivo* to give the amino thiols (106). *N*-Substituted thiazolidines having oxy or thio cycloalkyl, aryl, or heterocyclic alkyl groups (**27**) have high activity (107). Thiazolidine-4-carboxylic acid, derived from cysteine, affords 40% protection to rats (108). Thiazolidines with particularly good activity are 2-propylthiazolidine (106), the 2-(3-phenylpropionate ester) derivative (37.**28**) (109), and the *N*-pentylthiopentyl derivative (37.**29**) (110). The latter compound is active orally. 2-Aminothiazoline, which is derived from AET at pH 2.5, has protective activity (111); it is probably converted to *N*-carbamylcysteamine at pH 9.5 (112). 2-Mercaptothiazoline has been found active in two laboratories (16, 60); others have found it inactive (111, 113).

4.2 Other Sulfur-Containing Compounds

A number of dithiocarbamates have significant radioprotective effects, although

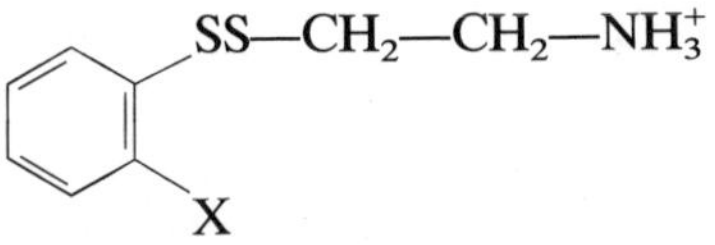

$$SS—CH_2—CH_2—NH_3^+$$

37.22   X = CO_2^-, SO_3^-, SO_2^-

$$NaO_2S—(CH_2)_4—SS—(CH_2)_4—SO_2Na$$
37.23

$$CH_3CONH—(CH_2)_2—SS—(CH_2)_4—SO_2Na$$
37.24

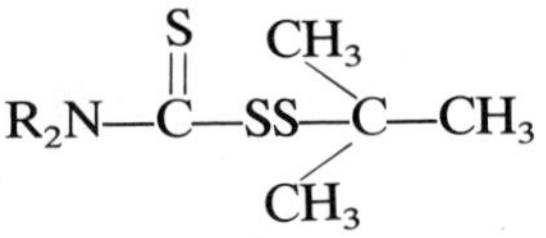

$$R_2N—\overset{S}{\overset{\|}{C}}—SS—\overset{CH_3}{\underset{CH_3}{\overset{|}{\underset{|}{C}}}}—CH_3$$
37.25

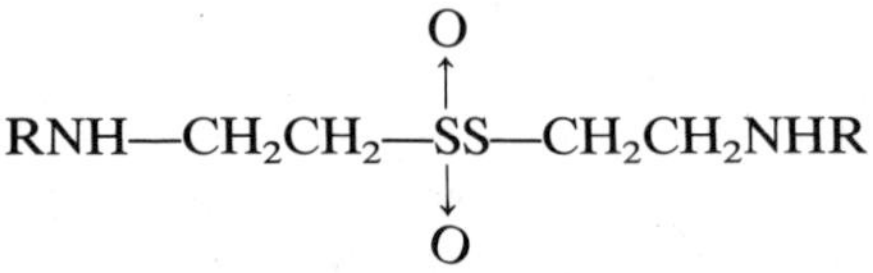

$$RNH—CH_2CH_2—\overset{O}{\underset{O}{\overset{\uparrow}{\underset{\downarrow}{SS}}}}—CH_2CH_2NHR$$

37.26   R = H, $\overset{NH_2^+}{\overset{\|}{C}}—NH_2$

$$R—O—(CH_2)_n—N\underset{S}{\diagdown}$$
37.27   R = cycloalkyl, aryl, heterocyclic

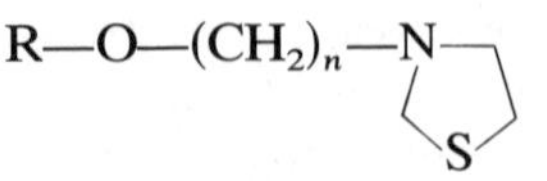

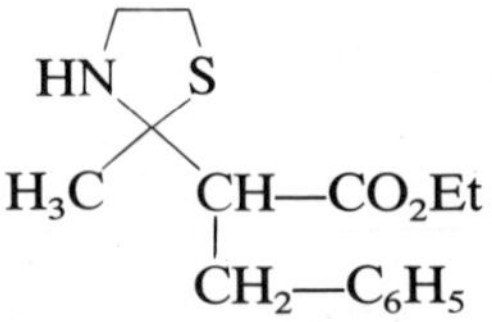

$$\underset{H_3C}{HN}\underset{CH—CO_2Et}{\diagup S}$$
$$CH_2—C_6H_5$$
37.28

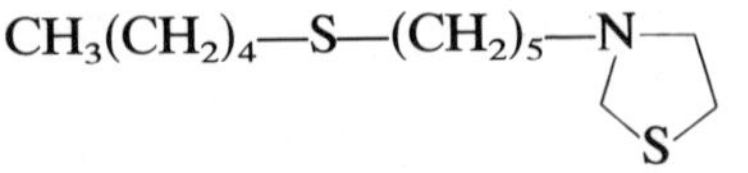

$$CH_3(CH_2)_4—S—(CH_2)_5—N\underset{S}{\diagdown}$$
37.29

the order of activity is less than that of MEA and its derivatives. The simplest compounds of this type, either with the nitrogen unsubstituted or bearing small alkyl groups, up to *n*-butyl, have shown the most activity (114, 115). 2-Methylpiperazinedithioformate (37.**30**), however, provides protection more nearly comparable to that of MEA (116). The mechanism by which the dithiocarbamates protect is believed to differ from that of the aminothiols. Xanthates have not been found protective (117). The related thiocarbamyl derivatives (37.**31**) and (37.**32**) have been reported to provide good protection (118).

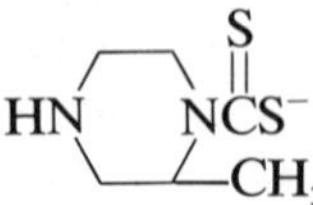

Reaction of cysteine with carbon disulfide gives the trithiocarbonate dithiocarbamate (119) (37.**33**), which is equivalent in protective activity in mice to that of MEG but is only one-third as toxic. A metabolism study in mice showed the dithiocarbamate group to be stable *in vivo* but the trithiocarbonate to be unstable (120); the dithiocarbamate is most likely the active form. Trithiocarbonates of MEG and MPG and several derivatives of MEG (37.**34**) also provided good protection to mice against a lethal dose of X-irradiation (47).

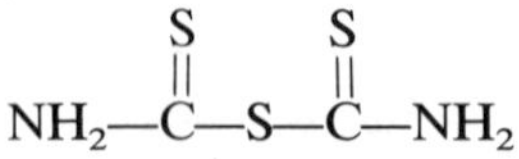

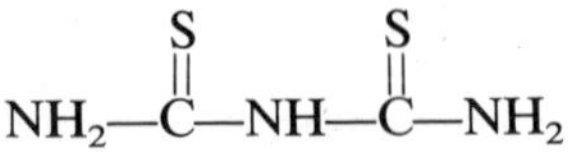

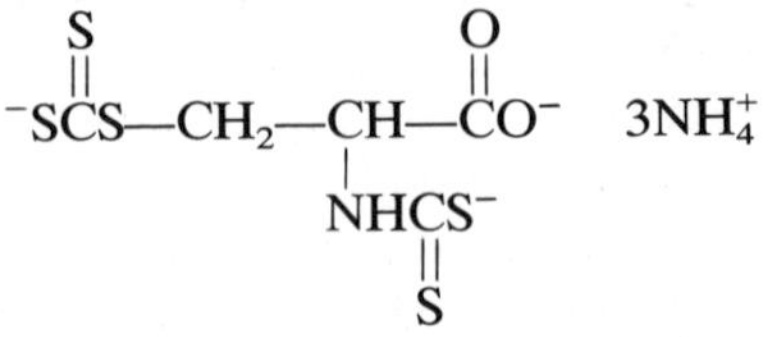

$$HN\diagup\diagdown N\overset{S}{\overset{\|}{C}}S^-$$
$$\diagdown\diagup—CH_3$$
37.30

$$NH_2—\overset{S}{\overset{\|}{C}}—S—\overset{S}{\overset{\|}{C}}—NH_2$$
37.31

$$NH_2—\overset{S}{\overset{\|}{C}}—NH—\overset{S}{\overset{\|}{C}}—NH_2$$
37.32

$$^-S\overset{S}{\overset{\|}{C}}S—CH_2—\underset{NHC S^-}{\underset{\underset{S}{\overset{\|}{}}}{\overset{|}{CH}}}—\overset{O}{\overset{\|}{C}}O^-   3NH_4^+$$
37.33

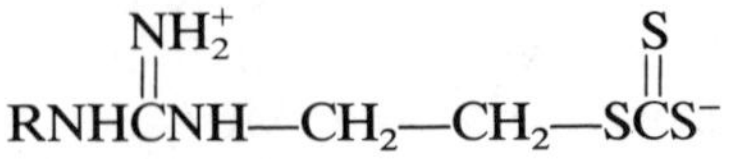

$$RNH\overset{NH_2^+}{\overset{\|}{C}}NH—CH_2—CH_2—S\overset{S}{\overset{\|}{C}}S^-$$
37.34

Thioureas and cyclic thioureas have shown only marginal or no protection. Thiourea itself protects mice only in massive doses (1800–2500 mg/kg) (5). *S*-Alkylisothioureas, with alkyls up to *n*-butyl, have shown moderate protective effects (121). Dithiooxamide is nonprotective, but symmetrical *N,N*′-dialkyldithiooxamides provide some protection (113). 1,5-Diphenylthiocarbohydrazide and several derivatives have fair activity (122).

Simple, nonbasic thiols have no value as radiation protectors. Conflicting results have been reported for the dithiol BAL as well as for thioctic acid (27). 2,3-Dithiosuccinic acid is protective in mice versus 700 R (123), but most other dithiols are inactive. 2-Mercaptoethanol protects bacteria (124) but not mice (125); it has also been found to be radiosensitizing (126).

Other sulfur-containing compounds with significant radioprotective ability include dimethyl sulfoxide (127) when given in large doses (other sulfoxides afford little or no protection). Organic thiosulfates, other than those that liberate MEA or an active derivative of MEA, have generally failed to protect. Inorganic thiosulfate is a good protector of macromolecules *in vitro* or of the mucopolysaccharides of connective tissue *in vivo* (128); it does not protect animals cells, however, because of its inability to penetrate. Sodium cysteinethiosulfate (37.**35**), derived from the cleavage of cysteine with thiosulfate ion, has good activity, being protective of the intestines and kidneys of mice (129). The related *S*-sulfocysteine, having one less sulfur atom, is almost devoid of activity (130).

$$Na^{+-}O_3SSS—CH_2—\underset{\underset{NH_2}{|}}{CH}—CO_2H$$

37.35

Mercapto acids have shown little protection, with the exception of thioglycolic acid, which is slightly protective, inactive, or sensitizing, depending on the system tested (27). The *β*-aminoethylamide of thioglycolic acid, $HSCH_2CONHCH_2CH_2NH_2$, has good activity (81), however.

Monothio acids and their derivatives are generally inactive, although several dithio acid dianions, obtained by condensation of carbon disulfide with cyanomethylene compounds (37.**36**), show some protection of mice (131). The most active of this series is the dithio acid derived from 2-cyanoacryloylpyrrolidide (37.**37**), which gives 80% protection to mice (76). Dithio esters derived from pyridinium dithioacetic acid betaine (37.**38**) also show some protection in both mice and bacteria (132).

$$\underset{R}{\overset{NC}{>}}C=C\underset{S^-K^+}{\overset{S^-K^+}{<}}$$

37.36   R = CN, CO₂Et, C₆H₅CO

37.**37**

$$\underset{\overset{||}{O}}{N—C}\ C=C\underset{S^-K^+}{\overset{S^-K^+}{}}$$

37.37

$$N^+—CH_2—\overset{\overset{S}{||}}{C}—SR \quad X^-$$

37.38

Thiols that occur naturally are not appreciably protective in animals with the exception of glutathione (133), which is moderately active. Pantoyltaurine apparently has some activity (134). Bacq (27) has presented arguments which make it appear unlikely that coenzyme A is involved in radioprotection. Both *S*-(135) and *N*-acylation (136) of MEA with *α*-amino acids, however, provide compounds with some activity.

Selenium compounds have been generally ineffective in animal tests. 2-Aminoethaneselenol, 2-aminoethaneselenosulfuric acid (52), and 2-aminoethylselenopseudourea (137) are much more toxic than the sulfur analogs and are nonprotective. Sodium selenate (138) and some selenium-containing heterocycles (139) have been claimed to be protective in rats, however. The investigation of organic selenium compounds as potential radioprotective compounds has been reviewed by Klayman (140).

4.3 Metabolic Inhibitors

Cyanide ion has been found radioprotective in a number of laboratories (3, 141), but it must be administered immediately before irradiation because of its rapid detoxication (17). It has a number of biological properties in common with thiols, such as reduction of disulfide linkages and inhibition of copper-containing enzymes, but unlike the thiols, it also inactivates cytochrome C oxidase, which controls oxygen consumption in mammals. Among other enzyme inhibitors, azide (142), hydroxylamine (143), and 3-amino-1,2,4-triazole (144) are weak protectors. The latter two compounds are inhibitors of catalase, but no relation between this effect and radioprotection was apparent (a later study with different compounds did show a correlation with catalare inhibition).

Several organic nitriles show radioprotective effects; the most effective, probably, is hydroxyacetonitrile (113). Fluoroacetate is protective (145) when sufficient time is allowed before irradiation for its conversion to fluorocitrate, an inhibitor of citrate metabolism. Other thiol group or enzyme-inhibiting agents, such as iodoacetic acid, malonic acid, mercurials, and arsenicals have no protective ability, but many of these agents have radiosensitizing effects.

4.4 Metal-Binding Agents

A number of metal-binding agents are radioprotective and are also known to inhibit enzymes. Some metal complexes imitate the action of enzymes, such as copper complexes which catalyze the decomposition of peroxides (146). These effects may play some role in radiation protection. Metal-binding agents already discussed include the dithiocarbamates as well as the aminothiols (147). EDTA protects mice only in very large doses (148), probably because very little EDTA enters the cells. 8-Hydroxyquinoline (oxine) is too toxic for animal studies, but was found highly protective in a polymer system (125). Other common metal-binding agents, such as N-nitroso-N-phenylhydroxylamine and nitrilotriacetate, show appreciable protection (149). Derivatives of 1,5-diphenylthiocarbohydrazide, avid metal binders, protect mice, rats, and dogs (122).

Some metal complexes have been tested and found to afford some protection. Iron complexes of polyamines (150) are active, as well as zinc complexes of MEA and MEG, the copper and iron complexes showing little or no activity (147). Copper complexes of diethyldithiocarbamate, dithiooxamide, and oxine, however, give less protection than the uncomplexed ligands (125). Complexes of chlorophyllin (with Co, Mg, Mn, V) are radioprotective in mice (151).

4.5 Hydroxyl-Containing Compounds

The degree of radioprotection afforded by hydroxylated compounds is of a lower order than that from thiols and thiol derivatives, but a number of alcohols and phenols have been reported with significant protective effects. Ethanol in large doses protects mice (152), and glycerol is protective in mice as well as other systems (5, 148). In tests with *E. coli*, glycerol, ethylene glycol, and methanol have significant DRF values (153).

Phenols are protective in polymethacrylate tests (125), but many of them are too toxic for animal tests. The catecholamines provide protection, possibly by lowering oxygen tension in the cells (27). The protective effects of gallic acid esters are attributed to inhibition of chain oxidation processes induced by radiation (154). Arachidoyl derivatives of pyrogallol and the naphthols have shown some activity (155). Ionol (2,6-di-*t*-butyl-4-methylphenol), injected after irradiation, prolongs life of mice and alleviates intestinal damage (156).

Organic acids provide little or no protection, but the polycarboxylic acids pyromellitic and benzenepentacarboxylic, though not mellitic acid, give good protection to mice (157). These polyionic substances are believed to protect by causing hypoxia from osmotic effects, rather than by chelating calcium ion, which also has an effect on radiation damage.

In a series of *S*-2-(3-aminopropylamino)-alkylphosphorothioates (37.**39**), which are effective protectors in mice when given orally, the presence of hydroxyl groups in the alkyl chains generally lowers effectiveness for oral administration (158), but still gives good protection by intraperitoneal injection.

$$NH_2-(CH_2)_n-NH-(CH_2)_m-SPO_3H_2$$
37.**39**

4.6   Heterocyclic Compounds

Several relatively simple heterocyclic compounds provide significant protective activity. In a series of imidazoles tested, imidazole itself, benzimidazole, and 1-naphthylmethylimidazole are the most effective compounds (159). Related imidazolidine-5-thiones are also protective (160). The cyclic analogs of AET, 2-

aminoethyl- (37.**40**) and 2-aminopropyl-thioimidazoline, are moderately protective (161).

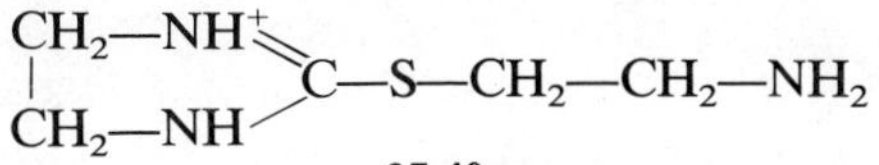

37.**40**

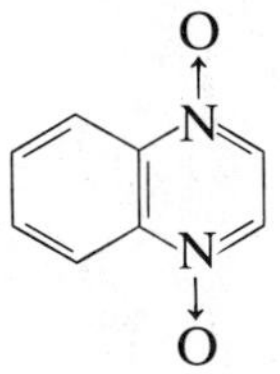

37.**41**

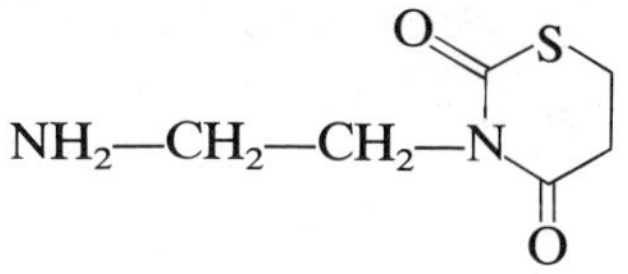

37.**42**

Of a large number of amine oxides tested for radiation protection, quinoxaline 1,4-di-*N*-oxide (**41**) (believed to act in part by radical trapping) was the most effective (162). It is protective in mice but radiosensitizing in the dog (163). 2*H*-1,3-Benzoxazine-2,4-dione (164), 3,5-diamino-1,2,4-thiadiazole (165), and 3-(β-aminoethyl)-1,3-thiazane-2,4-dione (166) (37.**42**) have some protective activity. Aminoethyl and aminomethyl purines and pyrimidines give one-third as much protection in mice as MEA (167). 8-Mercaptocaffeine and the β-aminoethyl and β-hydroxyethyl derivatives (**43**) have similar activity in mice to that of cystamine (168). These compounds also enhance hemopoiesis and decrease blood loss in irradiated animals.

Good protection is provided by 6-acyl-2, 3-dimethyl-4, 7-dimethoxybenzofurans (169) (37.**44**), and fair protection is observed for several 2-dialkyl-1,3-oxathiolanes (170). In a large series of 1,3-dithiolanes tested, moderate protection was

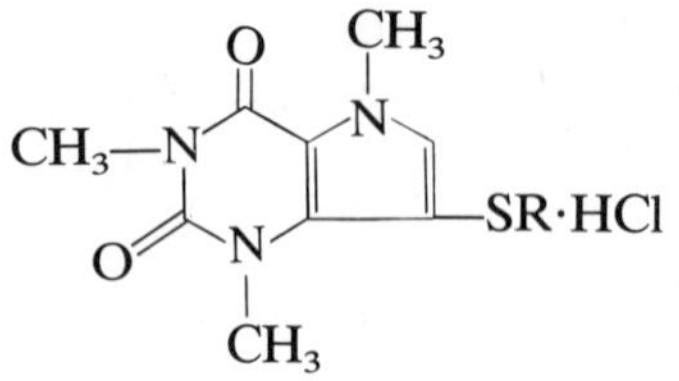

37.**43**   R = H, CH$_2$CH$_2$NH$_2$,
CH$_2$CH$_2$OH

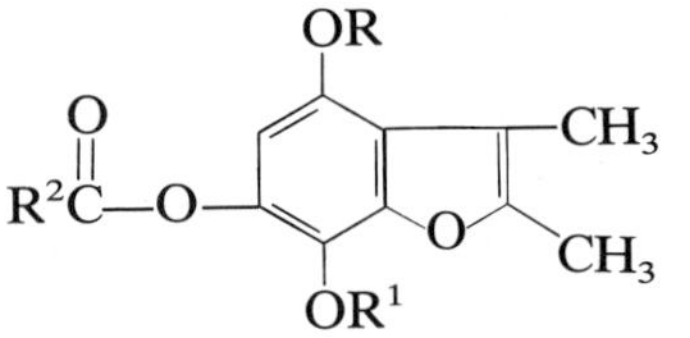

37.**44**

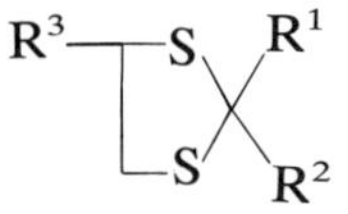

37.**45**

shown by 1,3-dithiolane itself and its 2-
and 4-methyl derivatives (171) (37.**45**).

In a series of 2,1,3-benzothiadiazoles,
the 4-hydroxy derivative (37.**46**) had the
best protective effect in mice (172), either
intraperitoneally   or   orally.   Several
aminothiazines, including 2-amino-4,6,6-
trimethyl-1,3-thiazine (37.**47**), increased
survival time in mice (173) without liberation of thiol groups. Several analgesic
pyrazolones also showed moderate protective effects, but in conjunction with MEA
gave good protection from intestinal death
(174).

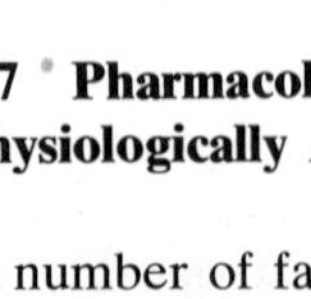

37.**46**

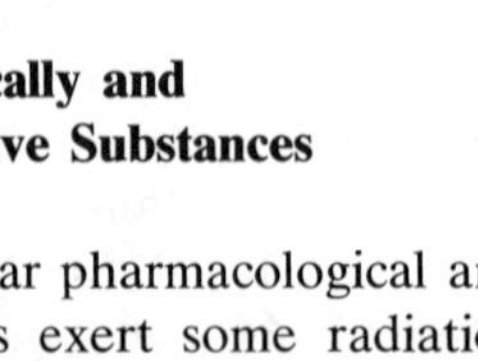

37.**47**

4.7 Pharmacologically and Physiologically Active Substances

A number of familiar pharmacological and
physiological agents exert some radiation
protection, which is generally of a lower
order of activity than that provided by the
amino thiols. A notable exception is 5-

hydroxytryptamine, which has been reported equal in activity to MEA (134, 175).
Many of these agents are believed to be
radioprotective by virtue of their ability to
lower oxygen tension in the cells or by
depression of the whole-body metabolism.

Central nervous system depressants have
only small or moderate effects as radiation
protectors. Chlorpromazine has been extensively studied, but exerts only a slight
effect. The effect is most pronounced when
the drug is given 4.5 hr prior to irradiation,
when a state of hypothermia exists (176).
Chlorprothixene is also most effective when
body temperature and metabolism are depressed (177). Reserpine is effective when
given 12–24 hr before irradiation (178),
possibly by release of serotonin and
catecholamines (179).

Central nervous system stimulants generally are nonprotective. An exception is
found with the magnesium complex of
pemoline   (2-imino-5-phenyl-4-oxazo-
lidinone), which gives moderate protection
to mice versus 750 R (180). Complamine, a
derivative of caffeine and nicotinic acid, also
has some protective ability (181).

The different classes of autonomic drugs
provide some radiation protection; the
causative factor is believed to be production of hypoxia by various mechanisms,
such as through vasodilation or reduction
of blood flow in the viscera. Epinephrine
provides   some   protection   (182),   but
norepinephrine, which decreases oxygen
tension in the spleen much less than
epinephrine, gives very little protection to
mice (183). The cholinomimetic compounds arecoline, tremorine, and oxyt-
remorine are also protective in mice (184).

p-Aminopropiophenone (PAPP) apparently protects by induction of tissue
hypoxia as well (185). It is used in relatively small quantities in combination with
other protective agents, such as MEA (186)
and AET (186–188). The radioprotection
afforded by PAPP is removed by increased
oxygen pressure during irradiation (189).

Serotonin (5-hydroxytryptamine, 5-HT), is approximately equal in protective effects to the amino thiols; it is effective, however, at a dose well below the toxic level (113), unlike the thiols. A DRF value of 1.85 has been reported (190). It is most often used as the creatinine sulfate salt. Its activity has been attributed to its vasoconstrictor effect causing hypoxia of radiosensitive tissues (191); some support for this is found in the removal of its protective action by pharmacological antagonists (192). 5-Hydroxytryptophan is comparable in activity (193), and the 5-methoxy ether (mexamine) is also a good protector, but higher alkyl ethers do not affect survival (194). Numerous indole derivatives have been prepared as radiation protectors, including 5-acetylindole (195), but none exceeds 5-HT or mexamine in potency. Serotonin and mexamine are frequently used in combinations with the amino thiols. A synergistic radioprotective effect results from a combination of AET, ATP, and serotonin in mice and rats (196).

Physiological changes can probably account for the radioprotective action of some substances. Urethane (197), estrogens (198), and colchicine (199) can stimulate blood cell production by damaging bone marrow. If irradiation is carried out while there is an increased leucocyte/lymphocyte ratio in the blood, so that a greater percentage of more radioresistant cells are present, enhanced survival may result. The effect of colchicine may also be due to inhibition of mitosis, by which more radioresistant cells might be present, but there is evidence against this supposition. Colchicine is protective only when administered 2 or 3 days prior to irradiation, by which time mitotic inhibition has ceased. Urethane and the estrogens are similar in that they must be given a day or more before irradiation. The pro-estrogen tri-*p*-anisylchloroethylene is effective when given 5–30 days prior to irradiation (200). Other inhibitors of mitosis, however, can enhance

survival; these include demecolcine (Colcemide), sodium arsenite, epinephrine, cortisone, and typhoid–paratyphoid vaccine (201).

Procaine (202) and several derivatives of procainamide, particularly the *p*-nitro derivatives (203), have shown appreciable protective activity. 4-Hydroxybutyric acid and 6-phosphonogluconolactone, substances that stimulate turnover of $NADP \cdot H_2$, a physiological reducing agent, provide protection to mice (204). An antihistamine, thenalidine, affords moderate protection (202). Alloxan protects both mice (205) and the pancreatic ultrastructure in dogs (206).

4.8   Metabolites and Naturally Occurring Compounds

A variety of compounds of these categories has been examined for radiation protection, but few really effective protectants have been found. Some polysaccharides, such as dextran (207), those extracted from typhoid and proteus organisms (208), and a lipopolysaccharide from *S. abortus* (209), provide some protection for mice, possibly by inducing phagocytosis. Bacterial endotoxins, which are lipopolysaccharides of molecular weight around 1,000,000, show relatively good protective properties in both normal (199) and germ-free mice (210), probably by decreasing blood flow in capillaries and causing tissue hypoxia (210). Typhoid–paratyphoid vaccine shows similar protective properties (211).

Vitamins and coenzymes are not appreciably protective. Pyridoxal phosphate, however, has a moderate effect (212) which may be connected with a repair rather than a protective process (213). Several thiol-containing derivatives of vitamin B_6, including 5-mercaptopyridoxine (214), are also protective. Some of the naturally occurring pyrimidine bases and nucleotides (215), including ATP (216), have an effect in mitigating radiation damage, but their value may be due to postirradiation repair. Protection from RNA, DNA, and derivatives has been claimed, but their effects are more likely due to postradiation repair (216–218). A protamine–ATP combination provides good protection to rats (219).

Among the commonly used antibiotics, the tetracyclines have shown the most favorable effects on survival rates of mice (220); this is believed due to an increase in metabolic activity. A gallate–tannin complex (221) was active probably because of its antioxidant effect. 5,7-Dihydroxyisoflavones are effective when administered to mice percutaneously but not intraperitoneally (222), presumably due to protection of the capillaries. O-β-Hydroxyethyl rutoside is also protective in mice, presumably by strengthening vascular walls and reducing bacterial invasion of the blood stream (223). The radioprotective effect of rutin and other flavonoids has been controversial.

Fluoroacetate exerts a moderate protective effect, possibly by causing an accumulation of citrate; radioprotection is coincident with a high concentration of citrate (145). It may also induce hypothermia (224–226) but this subject is controversial.

4.9   Polymeric Substances

A synthetic polymer prepared from N-vinylpyrrolidone and S-vinyl-(2,2-dimethylthiazolidyl)-N-monothiol carbamate (37.**48**) was found protective, possibly by liberation of thiol groups *in vivo* (227). Other copolymers containing isothiouronium salts, thiosulfates, and dithiocarbamate groups give appreciable protection when administered 24–48 hr prior to irradiation (228). Polyinosinic–poylcytidylic acid increases survival of mice, probably by increasing the stem cell fraction in blood-forming tissues (229). Both poly(vinyl sulfate) (230) and heparin (231), a sulfated

mucopolysaccharide, increase survival rates, possibly by affecting deoxyribonuclease activity.

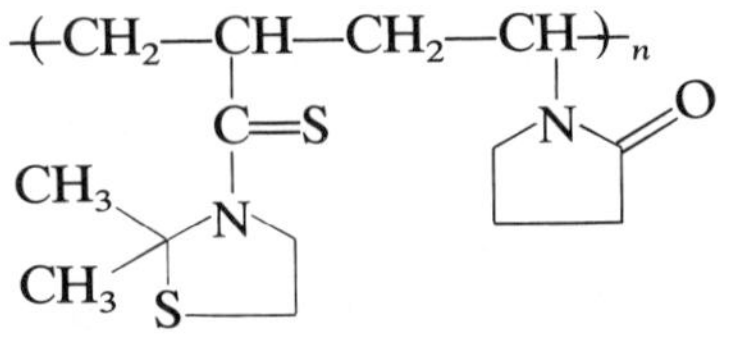

37.**48**

5   RADIOSENSITIZERS

The damaging effects of radiation may be increased in the case of high doses of a compound by the addition of the toxicity of the compound to that of the radiation. Some compounds, however, appear to have a true sensitization effect, which is often difficult to distinguish from additive toxicity (17). Some sensitizations reported may represent additive toxicities.

Several thiols related to cysteine have been recognized as sensitizers (126). These include isocysteine, β-homocysteine, and D-penicillamine; thioglycol and thioglycolic acid (232) also cause sensitization (Table 37.1). Thiamine diphosphate (233), riboflavin (234), and menadiol sodium phosphate (Synkavit) (235) act as sensitizers in animals. Demecolcine sensitizes mice when administered 12 hr prior to irradiation, probably due to intestinal damage, but is radioprotective when given 48 hr prior (236).

Many of the common thiol-binding reagents cause sensitization in animals. Increase in toxic effects after irradiation has been observed for p-chloromercuribenzoate (237), iodoacetate (238), iodoacetamide (239), and N-ethylmaleimide (239) in mice. Sensitization of mice or rats has also occurred with pentobarbital (240), nalorphrine (241), butanone peroxide (242), hematoporphyrin (243), methylhydrazine

(244), and cupric salts (245). Sensitization by cupric salts is prevented by administering thiols. Halogenated pyrimidines, particularly 5-bromo- and 5-fluorouracil (246), are consistent sensitizers. The halogenated thymidine analogs, 5-bromo- and 5-iodo-2-deoxyuridine, are apparently incorporated into DNA and produce sensitization (247). Other halogen compounds, such as chloro- and fluoroacetic acids, chloroform, and trichloroacetic acid, as well as methanesulfonate, sensitize rabbit erythrocytes to radiation (248). The role of halogenated thymidine analogs in inducing cellular radiosensitization has been reviewed (249).

A variety of compounds has sensitized bacterial cells and enzymes to radiation. Thiol-binding reagents, stable free radicals, and halogen compounds, including the halogenated pyrimidines, cause sensitization (244). Other bacterial sensitizers include hadacidin (250), chloral hydrate and other halides (251), quaternary heterocyclic salts, including phthalanilides, phenaziniums, and isoindoliniums (252), methylhydrazine (244), methylglyoxal (253), 1-(β-D-arabinofuranosyl)cytosine (254), tetracyclines (225), triacetoneamine N-oxide (256), and irradiated cupric salts (257). Many of these compounds, including cupric salts, N-oxides, and nitroxide free radicals (258), are more effective sensitizers under anoxic conditions. Compounds such as benzoquinone, nitrofurans, diamide, and oxygen, which are belived to react with free radicals of DNA or mononucleotides, are termed electron-affinic sensitizers (259). They react by radical oxidation or radical–adduct formation; the threshold for sensitization occurs at a sensitizer redox potential of ~0.3 V for oxidation of DNA radicals. Hydrogen donating species, such as MEA and other thiols, compete with sensitizers for the target free radicals. Nitro-substituted imidazoles and pyrazoles, including 37.**49**, also sensitize hypoxic bacteria and cultured mammalian cells to radiation (260).

37.**49**

6   RADIOPROTECTIVE AGENTS AND RADIOSENSITIZERS IN RADIOTHERAPY OF TUMORS

The use of radioprotective or radiosensitizing drugs to augment the effects of radiation of tumors has shown only partial benefit in animal experiments. For this type of therapy to succeed, a selective concentration of a protective drug in noncancerous tissue or of a sensitizer in cancerous tissue should be realized. Relatively few studies of such selective distribution between healthy and tumor tissue have been reported.

No distinct advantages have been observed in the use of most radioprotectors in connection with radiotherapy of tumors, usually because of protection of the tumor tissue. This has frequently been the result with MEA, cysteine, and serotonin (261) in tumor-bearing animals. Concentrations of AET in several types of tumors are lower than in normal tissues (262, 263), however. Crocker sarcoma is protected by MEA, menadiol, and nicotinamide, but not by serotonin or thiourea (264). Ehrlich ascites tumor is protected by 6-aminonicotinamide and menadiol diphosphate (264). Cysteine thiosulfate also protects Crocker sarcoma in mice (265). Heterologous RNA gives some protection to mice with Ehrlich ascites tumor but does not protect the tumor cells (266). S-2-(3-Aminopropylamino)-ethylphosphorothioate (WR 2721) (37.**13**) protects oxygenated EMT-6 mouse mammary tumors more than hypoxic cells (267), and also modifies the radiation dose required for treatment of both EMT-6 carcinoma and P-388 leukemia in mice (268), but its potential for human radiotherapy is considered questionable.

Some favorable effects have been observed in the use of radioprotectors with radiotherapy. MEA has given favorable results when used in conjunction with cyclophosphamide and X-rays in rats with Geren's carcinoma (269). Cystamine also decreased chromosomal aberrations in peripheral blood lymphocytes in uterine cancer patients (270). Although AET penetrates normal and cancerous tissue of mice to the same extent, it greatly prolongs the life of mice bearing ascites tumor cells (271). Favorable effects on irradiation of mice with Ehrlich carcinoma were reported for AET and DL-*trans*-2-aminocyclohexanethiol, but were less favorable for menadione bisulfite and an oxindole derivative (272). A combination of AET, serotonin, cysteine, and glutathione is definitely favorable to the survival of mice with Landschutz ascites tumors treated with 6000 R (273). Distributions of MEA released from the phosphorothioate and thiosulfate of MEA in various tissues have been found (274); the phosphorothioate of MEA shows a lower concentration in sarcoma M-1 than in the organs (275). The phosphorothioate of MEA also diminishes symptoms of radiation sickness in human patients undergoing radiation therapy for breast cancer (276). Also, in cancer patients, 2-mercaptopropionylglycine (37.**50**) decreases the severity of lymphopenia and decreases the number of chromosome aberrations following irradiation (277). MEA, AET, 1-cysteine, and 1-cysteine-D-glucose restore the mitotic index in X-irradiated rats bearing Yoshida sarcoma (278); 5-fluorouracil is a sensitizer. The radioprotectors do not appear to protect the tumor cells versus the effects of irradiation and 5-fluorouracil combined, however.

$$CH_3-\underset{\underset{\displaystyle SH}{|}}{CH}-\overset{\overset{\displaystyle O}{||}}{C}-NH-CH_2-CO_2H$$

37.50

Results of a more promising nature have been obtained with radiosensitizers, and some clinical use has been reported. Thymidine analogs that modify the structure of DNA, such as 5-iodo-2'-deoxyuridine, improve the effects of irradiation of tumors in both animals (279) and human patients (280). 5-Fluorouracil and 5-fluoro-2'-deoxyuridine have also been of value in advanced cancer cases (281). Actinomycin D also potentiates the therapeutic action of radiation, and has been used in radiation treatment of Wilms's tumor (282). This compound is known to complex with DNA, as does acriflavine, which is also radiosensitizing in tumor-bearing animals (283). The effect of cyclohexanol succinate is controversial, although it is apparently effective in radiotherapy of squamous carcinoma of the skin (284). Menadiol sodium phosphate concentrates selectively in some animal and human tumors, and gives favorable results in carcinoma of the bronchus (285).

Other sensitizers that show favorable effects in radiation of animal tumors include 2-butanone peroxide (286). hematoporphyrin and its copper complex (287), 6-azauracil riboside (288), the pyrimidines pentoxyl and metacil (289), 6-methylthiouracil and thyroidin (290), menadione (291), and several dihydroxy and dicarboxy thiophenes and sulfides (292). Radiosensitization of HeLaS$_3$ tumor cells *in vitro* by *N*-ethylmaleimide has been observed (293). 6-Chlorothymine also aids in reducing Ehrlich carcinoma growth in mice versus 2500 R (294), and sodium persulfate has sensitized mice with Coker sarcoma 180 (295). 1-(2-Dimethylaminoethyl)cycloheptimidazol-2(1*H*)-one (Ametahepazon) (37.**51**) is effective in increasing radiosensitivity of ascites hepatoma AH-109A in rats (296). The X-ray requirement for a murine anaplastic carcinoma is reduced by oral administration of metronidazole 36 hr prior to irradiation; the effect is attributed to direct killing of hypoxic tumor cells (297). The require-ments for a successful radiosensitizer in cancer radiotherapy have been discussed (258).

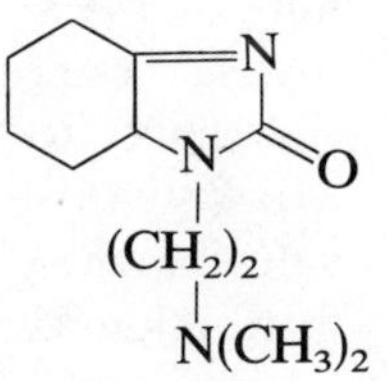

37.**51**

There has recently been an increasing use of fast neutrons for cancer therapy (298). Cysteine provides some protection against neutron damage and also aids in restoring lipid metabolism, in rats, altered by neutron irradiation (299).

7 MECHANISMS OF PROTECTIVE ACTION

The manner in which mammalian cells are protected from the damaging effects of ionizing radiation is not known in complete detail, although evidence is accumulating for several postulated pathways of radio-protection. Protection by means of radical trapping or antioxidant action, which can be demonstrated for simpler systems, such as polymers, may be operative in animal cells as well. It is also probable that other mechanisms are more important in protec-tion of cells, and that more than one mode of protection may be possible for a given type of agent. A number of the phar-macological and physiological agents de-scribed are believed to protect by anoxia; the evidence for this has been discussed (27).

Table 37.1 Sensitizing versus Protective Thiols[a]

Protective	Sensitizing	Inactive

HS—CH₂—CH—CO₂H
    |
    NH₂
Cysteine
	NH₂—CH₂—CH—CO₂H
	    |
	    SH
	Isocysteine
		CH_3
		HS—CH₂—C—CO₂H
		   |
		   NH₂
		α-Methylcysteine

HS—CH₂—CH₂—CH—CO₂H
      |
      NH₂
α-Homocysteine
	HS—CH₂—CH—CH₂—CO₂H
	    |
	    NH₂
	β-Homocysteine
		CH_3
		HS—C—CH—NH₂
		 | |
		CH₃ CH₃
		2-Methyl-3-amino-2-butanethiol

HS—CH₂—CH₂—NH₂ Cysteamine	CH_3 HS—C—CH—CO₂H | | CH₃ NH₂ Penicillamine	

HS—CH₂—CH—NH₂
   |
   CH₃
2-Amino-1-propanethiol
	HS—CH₂—CH₂—OH
	Thioglycol
		HS—CH₂—CO₂H
		Thioglycolic acid

[a] Taken mainly from Koch (126).

7.1 Protection by Anoxia or Hypoxia

Protection by producing a state of cellular anoxia or hypoxia is based on the phenomenon of the "oxygen effect," the increase by two- to threefold of the damaging effects of radiation owing to the presence of oxygen. A number of radioprotective drugs possess the physiological function of producing anoxia or severe hypoxia in various tissues; these include the catecholamines, histamine, choline esters, p-aminopropiophenone, morphine, ethyl alcohol, and nitrite. Other physiological effects, however, may contribute to their ability to protect, particularly with serotonin. Although the powerful protection afforded by this compound is not completely explained, a correlation between vasoconstrictive effects and radioprotection was found for a series of indolamines (300).

The amino thiols, notably cysteine, MEA, and AET, can decrease oxygen consumption in the cells (301), but no appreciable hypoxia exists during the protective period (302). In regard to the effect of regenerating tissues on oxygen tension, they apparently produce large amounts of catalase, which can inactivate OH· and HO$_2$· radicals as well as remove peroxide (303).

7.2 Inhibition of Free-Radical Processes

Mechanisms of protection involving "free-radical scavenging" are based on the assumption that the free radicals resulting from radiolysis of water are the main cause of radiation damage to the cells. Radioprotectors then would react with these radicals, of which H·, OH·, and HO$_2$· are known radiolysis products, and prevent chain reactions from proliferating and ultimately damaging biologically important molecules. This concept received support when a correlation was found between the protective action of about 100 substances in two systems: an aerated aqueous solution of polymethacrylate, and the mouse

(125). It is probable that radical scavenging is the primary event in the prevention of the polymer from depolymerizing (304), but it is probably not of equal importance in the cell. However, it has been calculated that concentrations of MEA necessary to protect cells by a radical scavenger mechanism would have to be at least $10^{-2}\,M$ (305); MEA gives significant protection at doses less than $3 \times 10^{-3}\,M$, assuming even distribution throughout the aqueous phase of the organism protected. Also, in yeast cells, amino thiol protectors decrease the total number of radicals but do not appear to protect the cells from the radicals arising from radiolysis of water (306).

Reaction of the sulfhydryl compounds with free radicals formed on protein molecules is a more likely possibility. Reaction rates with such radicals were measured for several radiation protectors; the fastest rates were observed for diethyldithiocarbamate, MEA, and cysteine (307) (Table 37.2). Cysteine and glutathione were found

Table 37.2 Reaction Rates of Radioprotective Substances with Serum Albumin and Glycyltryptophan Free Radicals[a]

Radioprotective Substance	Reaction Rate, l/mol sec	
	Serum Albumin	Glycyl-tryptophan
2-Mercapto-ethylamine	4.6	10.6
Thiourea	2.9	4.4
Cysteine	2.6	10.4
2-Aminoethyliso-thiouronium bromide HBr	1.7	3.3
3-Aminopropyliso-thiouronium bromide HBr	1.6	1.8
Gluthathione (reduced)	1.3	3.5
Propylgallate	1.2	0.4
Diethyldithio-carbamate	3.4×10^3	10^3

[a] From Sapezhinskii and Dontsova (307).

to accept electrons from irradiated proteins, whereas cystine and some nonsulfur compounds did not (308).

A number of antioxidant phenols, pyridines, and gallic acid esters are believed to be effective by virtue of their antioxidant action. A direct relation between radical inhibitory action and radiation protection has been observed (309).

7.3 Mixed Disulfide Hypothesis

This hypothesis of Eldjarn and Pihl (310) proposes that radioprotective thiols form mixed disulfides with thiol groups of proteins. The mixed disulfides provide protection to the thiol groups either by interfering with indirect radiation damage from radiolysis products of water (Scheme 37.1) or by facilitating energy transfer from the directly damaged protein to the administered thiol. Some arguments with this hypothesis have arisen; many thiols do not protect, and most thiols are capable of forming mixed disulfides (311). Equilibrium constants for mixed disulfide formation are high for radioprotective thiols but low for poor protectors, however (312).

In their original hypothesis, Eldjarn and Pihl proposed that the mixed disulfide bond would be cleaved by radical scavenging, but subsequent studies with protein solutions indicated that this may not be the case (313). Disulfide formation may also protect

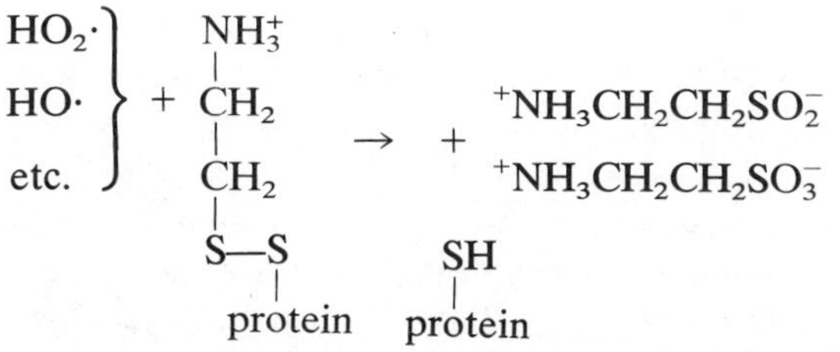

by moderating radiation-induced rearrangements (314). Radical scavenging may be an important function of the mixed disulfides (315), but mixed disulfide formation may also be a precursor for the liberation of cellular thiols, to be discussed later.

Another argument against this hypothesis is that many proteins are not damaged seriously by a dose of radiation lethal to mammals (316). Also, the nucleic acids, important target molecules of the cell nucleus, do not contain thiol or disulfide groups. The nuclear proteins involved in cell division have been proposed, however, as likely sites for mixed disulfide formation (317). RNA polymerase is particularly implicated for this process (318).

7.4 Biochemical Shock Hypothesis

A number of biochemical and physiological disturbances take place in the cells after administration of thiols, and realization of the full extent of the cellular changes produced led to the postulation of the "biochemical shock" hypothesis of Bacq (319) and others. This states that protective thiols undergo mixed disulfide formation in the cells leading to a series of disturbances including decreased oxygen consumption, decreased carbohydrate utilization, and mitotic delay by temporary inhibition of DNA and RNA synthesis, along with cardiovascular, endocrine, and permeability changes. The mitotic delay allows time for repair processes to restore normal nucleic acid synthesis.

Other metabolic effects observed after thiol administration include hypotension, hypothermia, and hypoxia (320). An increase in serotonin level has also been noted in rats following injection of aminothiols (321). Release of endogenous thiols is another metabolic effect of the radioprotective thiols. This has been caused not only by aminothiols but by serotonin and hypoxia-causing compounds, as well as by the anoxic state (322). This increase in

$$\left.\begin{array}{l} HO_2\cdot \\ HO\cdot \\ etc. \end{array}\right\} + \begin{array}{c} NH_3^+ \\ | \\ CH_2 \\ | \\ CH_2 \\ | \\ S\!-\!S \\ | \\ protein \end{array} \rightarrow + \begin{array}{c} \\ \\ ^+NH_3CH_2CH_2SO_2^- \\ ^+NH_3CH_2CH_2SO_3^- \\ \\ SH \\ | \\ protein \end{array}$$

Scheme 37.1 Postulated mechanism of protection by mixed disulfide formation of protein SH or S–S groups against the indirect action of ionizing radiation. Either of the two sulfur atoms may be attacked; in this case the interaction results in reconstitution of the target SH group [from Eldjarn and Pihl (310)].

cellular thiol content is often thirty- to forty-fold greater than the amount of thiol supplied by the protective agent. Protective effects of the amino thiols in Ehrlich ascites (323) and other tumor cells (324), as well as in mice (325), show direct correlations with the levels of nonprotein thiols. The natural radiosensitivity of mice is related to the concentration of thiol groups in the blood-forming tissues of the spleen (326), and development of radioresistance in cells is attributed to increased concentration of nonprotein-bound thiols (327), whereas radioresistance in some tumor cells is believed due to protein thiol content (328). Protection of the chromosomal apparatus in Ehrlich ascites cells by MEA is associated with the increase in nonprotein thiol levels (329). Both MEA and cystamine increase plasma, liver, and spleen concentrations of free thiols and disulfide groups (330). Radioresistance of bacterial cells is believed due to a repair system dependent on the thiol content of the cells (331). The role of endogenous thiols in repair of DNA has been reviewed (332).

7.5 Control of DNA Breakdown

The ability of the disulfides of the radioprotective aminothiols to bind reversibly to DNA, RNA, and nucleoproteins has been postulated as a result of *in vitro* studies (333). This, according to Brown (334), can result in two restorative effects: first, the loose ends of the helix resulting from single-strand rupture are held in place, so that shortening or alteration of the chain is prevented; and second, the replication rate of DNA is decreased or halted so that repair can take place before radiation-induced alterations are replicated. This binding, together with either radical scavenging (335) or repair by proton donation, can account for the protection of the nucleic acids by the aminothiols. It requires that the disulfide of the aminothiol be pres-

ent for binding, and it also explains why more than a three-carbon distance between amino and thiol functions leads to a sharp drop in protective ability. Portions of the DNA helix unprotected by histone have been found to accommodate an aliphatic chain of approximately 10 atoms; consequently, a disulfide with two or three carbons between the amino and disulfide functions would fit this exposed portion of the helix. Other strongly protective derivatives of MEA and MEG, such as the thiosulfate, phosphorothioate, trithiocarbonate, or acyl-thioesters, readily undergo disulfide formation. A recent study of the quantitative binding ability to DNA of a series of protective thiosulfates and disulfides of MEA with N-heterocyclic substituents shows that the thiosulfates do not bind at all, but there is no correlation between binding ability and protective activity of the disulfides (336).

DNA has also been protected by thiourea and propyl gallate, as well as by cysteine and cystamine, apparently by antioxidant effects (337). Another explanation for the protection of DNA by the amino thiols is that MEA renders cell membranes more resistant to radiation damage. Localization of repair enzymes and nucleases on the membrane makes it possible that radiation damage to the membrane could result in irreversible damage to DNA by nucleases, and interference with repair of DNA (338).

Other observations regarding the temporary inhibition of nucleoprotein synthesis by thiol protectors have been reported. Temporary inhibition of nuclear RNA synthesis in the radiosensitive tissue of rat thymus was found along with inhibition of thymidine phosphorylation for a short period (339). Radiosensitizers, such as penicillamine and β-mercaptoethanol, inhibited thymidine phosphorylation for a longer period. Some evidence for mixed disulfide formation with proteins, e.g., thymidine kinase, was found. Inhibition of

DNA synthesis in rat thymus, spleen, and regenerating liver by MEA and AET is believed to arise from a delay in the synthesis of relevant enzymes: nuclear RNA polymerase and thymidine-phosphorylating kinases (340). Although MEA decreases the frequency of radiation-induced single-strand breaks in DNA of mammalian cells (341), this is not considered to be the lesion responsible for the killing of E. coli cells by γ-radiation (342).

7.6   Modes of Repair

The mechanisms proposed by which radiation-produced radicals of cellular macromolecules are repaired may be stated briefly as follows: (1) hydrogen atom transfer from thiols to radicals; (2) transfer of radicals or radiation energy from macromolecules to protective agents that have undergone complex or mixed disulfide formation with the macromolecules; and (3) general radical scavenging. Repair of simple free radicals by hydrogen transfer from thiols has been observed by pulse radiolysis studies using γ-irradiated polyethylene oxide (343). The radical RS· presumably produced in irradiated neutral solutions of thiol compounds was observed as the radical complex RSSR⁻. The following scheme was proposed.

$$XH + OH \cdot \rightarrow X \cdot + H_2O$$

$$X \cdot + RSH \rightarrow XH + RS \cdot$$

$$RS \cdot + RSH \rightarrow RSSR \cdot + H^+$$

Oxygen inhibits repair by a competing process:

$$X \cdot + O_2 \rightarrow XO_2$$

Some question has arisen whether the thiol or disulfide form of the aminothiols is necessary for protection in the cells; the conclusion generally is in favor of the thiol

(344, 345). According to Cohen, however, both mercaptans and disulfides may enter rapid, repetitive hydrogen atom transfer reactions affecting radiation-induced free radicals (346). These hydrogen-transfer reactions proceed rapidly (with rate constants of 10^3–$10^6 \, M^{-1} \sec^{-1}$) and show very little free energy change, so they compete effectively with other reactions possible for free radicals. The following scheme proposed by Cohen shows how mercaptan, disulfide, and thiyl radical are all involved in the process of hydrogen transfer. It begins with hydrogen transfer from thiol to a radical:

$$X \cdot + RSH \rightarrow XH + RS \cdot$$

or from a radical to a thiyl radical or disulfide:

$$R_2\dot{C} - XH + RS \cdot \rightarrow R_2C = X + RSH$$

$$R_2\dot{C} - XH + RSSR \rightarrow R_2C = X + RSH + RS \cdot$$

In these free-radical reactions, transfer of a hydrogen atom is a chain-propagating step, and radical combination is terminating, so each molecule of sulfur compound, being used repeatedly, may negate the consequences of many radicals.

Evidence that hydrogen atom transfer from thiol to radicals produced by OH· attack is the major mode of repair has been found for the protection of thymine by cysteine (347). ESR studies have also shown direct hydrogen atom transfer from thiols to both abstraction and addition free radicals (348), and that the characteristic spectrum of irradiated cystamine, glutathione, and cystine-containing proteins is that of disulfide anions (349). ESR studies on irradiated mixtures of penicillamine disulfide and macromolecules have shown extensive transfer of radiation energy from macromolecule to disulfide (350), so it is apparent that either thiol or disulfide can provide radiation protection. Most likely, a thiol in cellular surroundings exists in equilibrium with its disulfide; this has been observed following radiation (344).

That free radicals are actually formed in irradiated animal or bacterial cells was not demonstrated until 1969 (351, 352); ESR studies showed transitory free-radical formation. These radicals probably undergo conversion to hydroperoxides or similar species quite rapidly, unless destroyed by hydrogen atom transfer from a thiol. That thiols are capable of decreasing hydroperoxide formation was shown with irradiated aqueous thymine (353).

The sites of radical formation in radiosensitive macromolecules have been postulated; the postulations generally point to sulfur functions. Although they have not yet been identified, possibilities for target SH or S–S groups exist in histones, spindle proteins, repair enzymes, or cell membranes (305). A radiochemical study of lipoic acid led to the conclusion that a single radiolytic radical generated in or near a disulfide-containing protein can denature and deactivate the molecule (354). Such radiosensitive proteins are found in the nonhistones of the chromosomal sheath, and their disruption, rather than that of nucleic acid, was believed to cause the genetic and biosynthetic malfunction of cells.

That radical scavenging does take place in the cells following irradiation appears to be mainly a function of cellular components rather than of introduced aminothiols. A study of the scavenging of diphenylpicrylhydrazyl radicals in both animal spleen and leguminous plant tissues revealed that those tissues with the higher concentration of radical scavengers were the more radioresistant (355). A correlation between ability to complex catalase, and presumably protect its iron content from radiation-induced valence change, and the radioprotective ability of a series of thiols also points to the role of cellular protectors in removing radiation-induced radicals (356).

The activity of catalase and peroxidase enzymes has also been associated with radiosensitivity in plants (357).

7.7 Role of Metal Ions

Heavy metal ions are involved in both radiation damage and protection, but their exact role is not clear. It is known that irradiation induces metal ion release in cells, which causes structural changes in nucleic acids and influences enzyme systems (358). It is also known that cupric and other heavy metal ions complex with DNA; a metal-binding agent could thus be expected to provide some shielding for damage to DNA (359). Stabilization of the oxidation state of copper in copper-containing enzymes is also regarded as important in preventing radiation damage (360). Correlations between metal-binding ability and extent of radiation protection have been found for aminothiols (361) and other metal-binding agents (362) with copper ions.

In regard to complexation of DNA by metal ions, EDTA and other chelating agents affect the extent of chromosome aberrations in irradiated dry seeds (363). In addition, presence of Cu^{2+} increases the damage to irradiated seeds, but Fe^{2+}, Zn^{2+}, Mn^{2+}, and Mg^{2+} decrease the damage. The stabilization of radiation-damaged nucleic acids is related to the electrode potentials of the ions (364).

Radioprotective properties of heavy metal ions are also known; ferrous and ferric ions protect plants (365) as well as trypsin (366). A number of metal ions (Cu^{2+}, Fe^{2+}, Fe^{3+}, Co^{2+}, Hg^+) lower radical concentrations of trypsin and reduce cysteine sulfur radicals (367). All these ions, except Hg^+, protect trypsin. Cupric ions have a protective effect for ribonuclease (368), but are sensitizing for α-amylase and catalase (369).

Catalase is a natural alleviator of radiation damage, since it removes peroxides from cells, and is damaged by a radiation dose (500 R, X-rays) just below the lethal level for rats and mice (370). A correlation has been found between the extent of radiation protection in mice by thiols and thiol derivatives and the degree of inhibition of catalase, presumably by complexation of the iron (356). It is also revealing that radiation-induced oxidation of cytosine and uracil produces radicals, but in the presence of Cu^{2+} or Fe^{3+} ions, the organic radicals do not result (371).

Mechanisms of radiation protection which involve the binding of metal ions have been proposed; these include the scavenging of ions of copper or iron to interrupt cellular oxidation initiated by radiation (372), the stabilization of the valence state of copper in copper-containing enzymes (373), and protection of metals bound to enzymes from radical attack by transient complexation by the protector (147, 374). A correlation appears to exist between the copper contents of different mammalian species and their radiosensitivity (375); and cellular copper-containing molecules undergo radiolytic damage preferentially to other molecules (376).

Evidence for possible metal-binding by protective agents was found for a series of metal-binding para-substituted phenylthioacetic acids and N-phenyldithiocarbamates containing both electron-donating and electron-withdrawing substituents. The substituents change the nature of the compounds from radioprotectant to radiosensitizer in bacterial tests (359). The effect follows the order of Hammett σ constants, with the strongest electron donors giving the greatest protection, and the strongest electron-withdrawing groups giving the greatest sensitization.

Another effect of metal ions that may be radioprotective is stimulation of mitosis by calcium and magnesium ions (377). Raising calcium levels in rats, either by injection or by parathyroid hormone, increases survival (378).

7.8 Other Mechanisms

Although a state of hypoxia sufficient to provide radiation protection is not brought about by most radioprotectors, some effect on oxygen availability and the oxidation–reduction potential of the cells does result following their administration. A correlation was observed between the duration of respiration inhibition and the radioprotective effect of cystaphos (37.**3**) (379). Several phosphorothioates were also found to induce vasodilation in the spleen, resulting in altered blood supply to the body, and decreasing tissue oxygen tensions (380). Aminoethyl and aminopropyl thiosulfates also decreased the oxidation–reduction potential in body tissues of rats and mice (381). They also increased serotonin and histamine levels, and decreased peroxide levels. Several heterocyclic compounds, including aryl derivatives of triazoline-2,5-dithione, decreased the oxygen tension in rat spleen, liver, and muscles (382); a correlation was observed between the decrease in oxygen tension and radioprotective effects of the compounds.

Radioprotective and radiosensitizing effects of various compounds have been related to an oxygen effect. A theory has been developed consisting of an "oxygen fixation hypothesis" (383), in which target free radicals react either with radical-reducing species, resulting in "chemical repair," or with radical-oxidizing species, resulting in "fixation" of radical damage to a potentially lethal form. MEA and other thiols protect by adding to the pool of radical-reducing species, resulting in enhanced repair of free-radical damage. Electron-affinic compounds radiosensitize by adding to the pool of radical-oxidizing species, enhancing free-radical damage; *N*-ethylmaleimide has a similar effect. Metal ions, however, do not alter sensitivity to radiation inactivation of bovine carbonic anhydrase by oxidizing radicals, but do exert a protective effect against inactivation by reducing radicals (384).

An explanation of the protective effects of ethanol, and other hydroxy compounds, arose from the observation that ethanol adds to thymine under γ-irradiation (385). This prevents formation of thymine dimers, deleterious to DNA. It also explains the radiation resistance of bacterial spores, and protection of bacteria in glucose medium, where hydroxy compounds are in adequate supply to add to thymine.

Other cellular effects produced by the amino thiols may be involved in the complex process of radiation protection. Release of enzymes is one such effect, and various enzymes have been released in rat plasma following introduction of either MEA or 5-mercaptopyridoxine, or by a state of hypoxia (386). Treatment with two nonprotective thiols, 2-mercaptoethanol and 4-mercaptopyridoxine, did not affect the plasma enzyme levels. The liberation of cellular thiols, discussed earlier, may be due to enzyme liberation, at least in part. Mixed disulfide formation may be a factor in this release, as suggested by the "biochemical shock hypothesis."

The radioprotective thiols protect the erythropoietic system of animals, ^{59}Fe uptake being used as the test for protection (387). MEA, AET, penicillamine, and 2-mercaptoethanol all inhibit phosphorylation of thymidine in rat thymus and spleen (388). The effect of the protective agents AET and MEA is reversible, whereas that of the two sensitizing compounds is irreversible.

Addition of MEA to mitochondria first accelerates, then slows respiration. A decrease in ATP synthesis was also noted, both in mitochondria and rat thymus nuclei, thus diminishing both respiration and

phosphorylation coupling (389). Mixed disulfide formation is believed to be involved.

Bacq and Alexander have proposed that a significant contribution to the radiobiological effects of ionizing radiation is due to cell membrane damage (16). The effect of X-rays on the permeability of Ehrlich ascites tumor cell membranes has since been studied by measuring loss of potassium from the cells (390). The radiosensitizing effects of Synkavit and excess oxygen were demonstrated by a marked loss of potassium from the irradiated cells, whereas the protective effects of MEA and 2-amino-3-methyl-butanethiol prevented this loss. Also, blocking of cell surface amino and probably thiol groups with citraconic anhydride, dimethylmaleic anhydride, and diacetyl also modified radiation damage to the cell membrane. It was suggested that radioprotection may depend on combination with cell surface protein groups which determine the surface charge and maintain the integrity of the cell membrane.

The general pharmacology of sulfur-containing radioprotective agents, and the importance of pharmacological effects in radioprotective action, has been reviewed recently (391).

REFERENCES

1. W. M. Dale, L. H. Gray, and W. J. Meredith, *Phil Trans. Roy. Soc.*, **242A,** 33 (1949).
2. R. Latarjet and E. Ephrati, *C. R. Soc. Biol.*, **142,** 497 (1948).
3. A. Herve and Z. M. Bacq, *C. R. Soc. Biol.*, **143,** 881 (1949).
4. H. M. Patt, E. B. Tyree, R. L. Straube, and D. E. Smith, *Science*, **110,** 213 (1949).
5. R. H. Mole, J. St. L. Philpot, and C. R. V. Hodges, *Nature*, **166,** 515 (1950).
6. Z. M. Bacq, A. Herve, J. Lecomte, P. Fischer, J. Blavier, G. Dechamps, H. LeBihan, and P. Rayet, *Arch. Int. Physiol.*, **59,** 442 (1951).
7. V. P. Bond, T. M. Fleidner, and J. O. Archambeau, *Mammalian Radiation Lethality*, Academic, New York, 1965.

8. D. J. Pizzarello and R. L. Witcofski, *Basic Radiation Biology*, Lea and Febiger, Philadelphia, 1967.

9. A. P. Casarett, *Radiation Biology*, Prentice-Hall, Englewood Cliffs, New Jersey, 1968.

10. S. Okada, Ed., *Radiation Biochemistry*, Vol. 1, Academic, New York, 1969.

11. H. Dertinger and H. Jung, *Molecular Radiation Biology*, Springer-Verlag, Berlin–New York, 1970.

12. P. Alexander and A. Charlesby, in *Radiation Symposium*, Z. M. Bacq and P. Alexander, Eds., Butterworths, London, 1955, p. 49.

13. T. Henriksen, *Radiat. Res.*, **27,** 694 (1966).

14. S. Okada, Ed., *Radiation Biochemistry*, Vol. 1, Academic, New York, 1969, p. 70.

15. H. A. Blair, Ed., *Biological Effects of External Radiation*, McGraw-Hill, New York, 1954.

16. Z. M. Bacq and P. Alexander, Eds., *Fundamentals of Radiobiology*, 2nd ed., Pergamon Press, Oxford, 1961.

17. J. F. Thomson, *Radiation Protection in Mammals*, Reinhold, New York, 1962.

18. H. L. Andrews, D. C. Peterson, and D. P. Jacobus, *Radiat. Res.*, **23,** 13 (1964).

19. Z. M. Bacq and P. Alexander, Eds., *Radiobiology Symposium*, Academic Press, New York, 1955.

20. W. D. Fischer, N. G. Anderson, and K. M. Wilbur, *Exp. Cell Res.*, **18,** 48 (1959).

21. G. Hotz, *Z. Naturforsch.*, **21b,** 148 (1966).

22. G. I. Gasanov, *Izv. Akad. Nauk Azerb. SSR, Ser. Biol. Med. Nauk*, **1966,** 110; through *Chem. Abstr.*, **66,** 5278 (1967).

23. K. S. Burdin, I. M. Parkomenko, Y. M. Petrusevich, and S. V. Shestakova, *Tr. Mosk. Obshch. Ispyt. Prir. Otd. Biol.*, **16** 19 (1966); through *Chem. Abstr.*, **66,** 62465 (1967).

24. B. U. Leonov and A. A. Mikhailova, *Vopr. Obshch. Radiobiol.*, **1966,** 135; through *Chem. Abstr.*, **66,** 16680 (1967).

25. J. F. Duplan and J. Fuhrer, *C. R. Soc. Biol.*, **160,** 1142 (1966).

26. D. E. Smith and J. F. Thomson, in *Methods Drug Eval.*, *Proc. Int. Symp.*, *Milan*, 1965, 1966, p. 32.

27. Z. M. Bacq, *Chemical Protection Against Ionizing Radiation*, Charles C. Thomas, Springfield, Ill., 1965.

28. R. Huber and E. Spode, *Biologisch-Chemischer Strahlenschutz*, Akademie-Verlag, Berlin, 1963.

29. L. A. Tiunov, G. A. Vasil'ev, and E. A. Val'dshtein, *Agents for Protection Against Radiation, Handbook*, Nauka, Moscow, 1964.

30. V. S. Balubukha, Ed., *Chemical Protection of the Body Against Ionizing Radiation*, Macmillan, New York, 1964.

31. W. O. Foye, "Radiation-Protective Agents in Mammals," *J. Pharm. Sci.*, **58,** 283 (1969).

32. R. R. Overman and S. J. Jackson, *Ann. Rev. Med.*, **18,** 71 (1967).

33. E. F. Romantsev, *Radiation and Chemical Protection*, Atomizdat, Moscow, 1968.

34. H. J. Melching and C. Streffer, *Progr. Drug Res.*, **9,** 11 (1966).

35. D. L. Klayman and E. S. Copeland, in *Drug Design*, Vol. VI, E. J. Ariens, Ed., Academic, New York, 1975.

36. R. Paoletti and R. Vertua, Eds., *Progress in Biochemical Pharmacology*, Vol. 1, Butterworths, Washington, D.C., 1965.

37. H. L. Moroson and M. Quintiliani, Eds., *Radiation Protection and Sensitization*, Barnes and Noble, New York, 1970.

38. W. O. Foye, *Ann. Rep. Med. Chem.*, **1966,** 324; **1967,** 330.

39. E. R. Atkinson, *Ann. Rep. Med. Chem.*, **1968,** 327; **1970,** 346.

40. P. Alexander and J. T. Lett, in *Comprehensive Biochemistry*, Vol. 27, M. Florkin and E. H. Stotz, Eds., Elsevier, New York, 1967, p. 267.

41. G. Silini, Ed., *Radiation Research*, North-Holland, Amsterdam, 1967.

42. E. Fahr, *Angew. Chem. Int. Ed. Engl.*, **8,** 578 (1969).

43. D. G. Doherty, W. T. Burnett, Jr., and R. Shapira, *Radiat. Res.*, **7,** 13 (1957).

44. H. Langendorff and R. Koch, *Strahlentherapie*, **99,** 567 (1956).

45. B. Holmberg and B. Sorbo, *Nature*, **183,** 832 (1959).

46. S. Åkerfeldt, *Acta Chem. Scand.*, **13,** 1479 (1959).

47. W. O. Foye, J. Mickles, R. N. Duvall, and J. R. Marshall, *J. Med. Chem.*, **6,** 509 (1963).

48. B. Sorbo, *Arch. Biochem. Biophys.*, **98,** 342 (1962).

49. A. F. Ferris, O. L. Salerni, and B. A. Schutz, *J. Med. Chem.*, **9,** 391 (1966).

50. J. R. Piper, C. R. Stringfellow, Jr., and T. P. Johnston, *J. Med. Chem.*, **9,** 563 (1966).

51. D. W. vanBekkum and H. T. M. Nieuwerkerk, *Int. J. Radiat. Biol.*, **7,** 473 (1963).

52. D. L. Klayman, M. M. Grenan, and D. P. Jacobus, *J. Med. Chem.*, **12,** 510 (1969).

53. F. I. Carroll, J. D. White, and M. E. Wall, *J. Org. Chem.*, **28,** 1240 (1963).

54. G. W. Stacy, B. F. Barnett, and P. L. Strong, *J. Org. Chem.*, **30**, 592 (1965).

55. J. R. Piper, C. R. Stringfellow, Jr., and T. P. Johnston, *J. Med. Chem.*, **9**, 911 (1966).

56. F. I. Carroll, J. D. White, and M. E. Wall, *J. Org. Chem.*, **28**, 1236 (1963).

57. K. Tonchev, *Nauch. Tr. Vissh. Med. Inst., Sofia*, **39**, 143 (1960); through *Chem. Abstr.*, **55**, 19007 (1961).

58. L. I. Tank, *Med. Radiol.*, **5**, 34 (1960).

59. H. Langendorff, M. Langendorff, and R. Koch, *Strahlentherapie*, **107**, 121 (1958).

60. D. P. Jacobus and T. R. Sweeney, private communication.

61. H. Irie, *Strahlentherapie*, **110**, 456 (1959).

62. R. W. Hart, R. E. Gibson, J. D. Chapman, A. P. Reuvers, B. K. Sinha, R. K. Griffith, and D. T. Witiak, *J. Med. Chem.*, **18**, 323 (1975).

63. D. G. Doherty and R. Shapira, *J. Org. Chem.*, **28**, 1339 (1963).

64. M. Carmack, C. L. Kelley, S. D. Harrison, Jr., and K. P. DuBois, *J. Med. Chem.*, **15**, 600 (1972).

65. R. L. Straube and H. M. Patt, *Proc. Soc. Exp. Biol. Med.*, **84**, 702 (1953).

66. W. Braun, E.-J. Kirnberger, G. Stille, and V. Wolf, *Strahlentherapie*, **108**, 262 (1959).

67. T. P. Johnston and C. R. Stringfellow, Jr., *J. Med. Chem.*, **9**, 921 (1966).

68. G. R. Handrick and E. R. Atkinson, *J. Med. Chem.*, **9**, 558 (1966).

69. C. Falconi, P. Scotto, and P. deFranciscis, *Experientia*, **26**, 172 (1970).

70. S. J. Arbusov, *Pharmazie*, **14**, 132 (1959).

71. S. Åkerfeldt, *Acta Radiol. Ther. Phys. Biol.*, **1**, 465 (1963).

72. S. Åkerfeldt, C. Ronnback, and A. Nelson, *Radiat. Res.*, **31**, 850 (1967).

73. J. R. Piper, C. R. Stringfellow, Jr., R. D. Elliott, and T. P. Johnston, *J. Med. Chem.*, **12**, 236 (1969).

74. R. D. Westland, M. L. Mouk, J. L. Holmes, R. A. Cooley, Jr., J. S. Hong, and M. M. Grenan, *J. Med. Chem.*, **15**, 968 (1972).

75. R. D. Westland, M. M. Merz, S. M. Alexander, L. S. Newton, L. Bauer, T. T. Conway, J. M. Barton, K. K. Khullar, and P. B. Devdhar, *J. Med. Chem.*, **15**, 1313 (1972).

76. W. O. Foye, Y. H. Lowe, and J. J. Lanzillo, *J. Pharm. Sci.*, **65**, 1247 (1976).

77. B. Shapiro, G. Kollmann, and D. Martin, *Radiat. Res.*, **44**, 421 (1970).

78. Åkerfeldt, C. Ronnback, M. Hellström, and A. Nelson, *Radiat. Res.*, **35**, 61 (1968).

79. W. O. Foye, R. N. Duvall, and J. Mickles, *J. Pharm. Sci.*, **51**, 168 (1962).

80. D. G. Doherty and W. T. Burnett, Jr., *Proc. Soc. Exp. Biol. Med.*, **89**, 312 (1955).

81. E. J. Jezequel, H. Frossard, M. Fatome, R. Perles, and P. Poutrain, *C. R. Acad. Sci., Ser. D*, **272**, 2826 (1971).

82. T. Taguchi, O. Komori, and M. Kojima, *Yakugaku Zasshi*, **81**, 1233 (1961).

83. L. Bauer and K. Sandberg, *J. Med. Chem.*, **7**, 766 (1964).

84. J. M. Barton and L. Bauer, *Can. J. Chem.*, **47**, 1233 (1969).

85. S. Robev, I. Baev, and N. Panov, *C. R. Acad. Bulg. Sci.*, **19**, 1035 (1966).

86. S. Robev, I. Baev, and N. Panov, *C. R. Acad. Bulg. Sci.*, **19**, 1143 (1966).

87. W. O. Foye and D. H. Kay, *J. Pharm. Sci.*, **57**, 345 (1968).

88. W. O. Foye, D. H. Kay, and P. R. Amin, *J. Pharm. Sci.*, **57**, 1793 (1968).

89. E. R. Atkinson, G. R. Handrick, R. J. Bruni, and F. E. Granchelli, *J. Med. Chem.*, **8**, 29 (1965).

90. F. L. Rose and A. L. Walpole, *Progr. Biochem. Pharmacol.*, **1**, 432 (1965).

91. E. E. Schwartz and B. Shapiro, *Radiat. Res.*, **13**, 780 (1960).

92. O. Vos, L. Budke, and A. J. Vergroesen, *Int. J. Radiat. Biol.*, **5**, 543 (1962).

93. P. Fischer and M. Goutier-Pirotte, *Arch. Int. Physiol.*, **62**, 76 (1954).

94. A. V. Titov, D. A. Golubentsov, and V. V. Mordukhovich, *Radiobiologiya*, **10**, 606 (1970); through *Chem. Abstr.*, **73**, 127508 (1970).

95. B. Shapiro, E. E. Schwartz, and G. Kollman, *Radiat. Res.*, **18**, 17 (1963).

96. L. Field and H. K. Kim, *J. Med. Chem.*, **9**, 397 (1966); P. K. Srivastava, L. Field, and M. M. Grenan, *J. Med. Chem.*, **18**, 798 (1975).

97. L. Field, H. K. Kim, and M. Bellas, *J. Med. Chem.*, **10**, 1166 (1967).

98. L. Field and J. D. Buckman, *J. Org. Chem.*, **32**, 3467 (1967).

99. L. Field and Y. H. Khim, *J. Med. Chem.*, **15**, 312 (1972).

100. L. Field and J. D. Buckman, *J. Org. Chem.*, **33**, 3865 (1968).

101. D. L. Klayman and G. W. A. Milne, *J. Org. Chem.*, **31**, 2349 (1966).

102. W. O. Foye, A. M. Hebb, and J. Mickles, *J. Pharm. Sci.*, **56**, 292 (1967).

103. L. Field, A. Ferretti, R. R. Crenshaw, and T. C. Owen, *J. Med. Chem.*, **7**, 39 (1964).

104. R. I. H. Wang and A. T. Hasegawa, private communication.

105. R. A. Salvador, C. Davison, and P. K. Smith, *J. Pharmacol. Exp. Ther.*, **121,** 258 (1957).

106. A. Kaluszyner, P. Czerniak, and E. D. Bergmann, *Radiat. Res.*, **14,** 23 (1961).

107. R. D. Westland, R. A. Cooley, Jr., J. L. Holmes, J. S. Hong, M. L. Lin, M. L. Zwiesler, and M. M. Grenan, *J. Med. Chem.*, **16,** 319 (1973).

108. R. Riemschneider, *Z. Naturforsch.*, **B16,** 75 (1961).

109. P. S. Farmer, C.-C. Leung, and E. M. K. Lui, *J. Med. Chem.*, **16,** 411 (1973).

110. R. D. Westland, M. H. Lin, R. A. Cooley, Jr., M. L. Zwiesler, and M. M. Grenan, *J. Med. Chem.*, **16,** 328 (1973).

111. R. Shapira, D. G. Doherty, and W. T. Burnett, Jr., *Radiat. Res.*, **7,** 22 (1957).

112. J. X. Khym, R. Shapira, and D. G. Doherty, *J. Am. Chem. Soc.*, **79,** 5663 (1957).

113. J. Doull, V. Plzak, and S. Brois, in *University of Chicago USAF Radiation Lab, Status Report*, No. 2, Aug. 1, 1961.

114. D. W. van Bekkum, *Acta Physiol. Pharmacol. Neerl.* **4,** 508 (1956).

115. W. O. Foye and J. Mickles, *J. Med. Pharm. Chem.*, **5,** 846 (1962).

116. V. Palma, G. Galli, S. Garrattini, R. Paoletti, and R. Vertua, *Arzn.-Forsch.*, **11,** 1034 (1961).

117. T. Stoichev, *Izv. Inst. Fiziol. Bulg. Akad. Nauk.*, **10,** 149 (1966); through *Chem. Abstr.*, **67,** 29697 (1967).

118. V. G. Yakovlev and V. S. Mashtakov, *Khim. Zashch. Org. Ioniz. Izluch.*, **1960,** 72; through *Chem. Abstr.*, **55,** 27649 (1961).

119. R. I. H. Wang, W. Dooley, Jr., W. O. Foye, and J. Mickles, *J. Med. Chem.*, **9,** 394 (1966).

120. W. O. Foye, R. S. F. Chu, K. A. Shah, and W. H. Parsons, *J. Pharm. Sci.*, **60,** 1839 (1971).

121. M. J. Ashwood-Smith and A. D. Smith, *Int. J. Radiat.*

122. A. A. Gorodetskii, R. G. Dubenko, P. S. Pel'kis, and E. Z. Ryabova, *Patog., Eksp. Profil. Ter. Luchevykh Porazhenii (Moscow), Sb.,* p. 179 (1964); through *Chem. Abstr.*, **64,** 989 (1966).

123. F. Cugurra and E. Balestra, *Progr. Biochem. Pharmacol.*, **1,** 507 (1965).

124. A. Hollaender and C. O. Doudney, in *Radiobiology Symposium, Liege*, 1954, Butterworths, London, 1955, p. 112.

125. P. Alexander, Z. M. Bacq, S. F. Cousens, M. Fox, A. Herve, and J. Lazar, *Radiat. Res.*, **2,** 392 (1955).

126. R. Koch, in *Advances in Radiobiology*, G. C.

DeHevesy, Ed., Oliver and Boyd, Edinburgh, 1957, p. 170.

127. M. J. Ashwood-Smith, *Int. J. Radiat. Biol.*, **3,** 41 (1961).

128. R. Brinkman, H. B. Lamberts, J. Wadel, and J. Zuideveld, *Int. J. Radiat. Biol.*, **3,** 205 (1961).

129. T. Zebro, *Acta Med. Pol.*, **7,** 83 (1966).

130. B. Hansen and B. Sorbo, *Acta Radiol.*, **56,** 141 (1961).

131. W. O. Foye and J. M. Kauffman, *J. Pharm. Sci.*, **57,** 1611 (1968).

132. W. O. Foye, Y. J. Cho, and K. H. Oh, *J. Pharm. Sci.*, **59,** 114 (1970).

133. W. H. Chapman and E. P. Cronkite, *Proc. Soc. Exp. Biol. Med.*, **75,** 318 (1950).

134. Z. M. Bacq, *Acta Radiol.*, **41,** 47 (1954).

135. W. O. Foye and R. H. Zaim, *J. Pharm. Sci.*, **53,** 906 (1964).

136. F. Bonati and U. Nuvolone, *Radiobiol. Latina*, **1,** 162 (1958).

137. S.-H. Chu and H. G. Mautner, *J. Org. Chem.*, **27,** 2899 (1962).

138. Z. M. Hollo and S. Zlatarov, *Naturwissenschaften*, **47,** 328 (1960).

139. A. Breccia, R. Badiello, A. Trenta, and M. Mattii, *Radiat. Res.*, **38,** 483 (1969).

140. D. L. Klayman, in *Organic Selenium Compounds; Their Chemistry and Biology*, D. L. Klayman and W. H. H. Gunther, Eds., Wiley, New York, 1973, p. 727.

141. J. Schubert and J. F. Markley, *Nature*, **197,** 399 (1963).

142. Z. M. Bacq and A. Herve, *Brit. J. Radiol.*, **24,** 618 (1951).

143. E. Boyland and E. Gallico, *Brit. J. Cancer*, **6,** 160 (1952).

144. R. N. Feinstein and S. Berliner, *Science*, **125,** 936 (1957).

145. Z. M. Bacq, P. Fischer, and A. Herve, *Arch. Int. Physiol.*, **66,** 75 (1958).

146. H. Sigel and H. Erlenmeyer, *Helv. Chim. Acta*, **49,** 1266 (1966).

147. W. O. Foye and J. Mickles, *Progr. Biochem. Pharmacol.*, **1,** 152 (1965).

148. Z. M. Bacq, A. Herve, and P. Fischer, *Bull. Acad. Roy. Med. Belg.* **18,** 226 (1953).

149. C. Corradi, R. Pagletti, and E. Pozza, *Atti Soc. Lomb. Sci. Med. Biol.*, **13,** 80 (1958); through *Chem. Abstr.*, **52,** 17525, (1958).

150. O. I. Smirnova, *Radiobiologiya*, **2,** 378 (1962).

151. N. Kasugai, *J. Pharm. Soc. Jap.*, **84,** 1152 (1964).

152. E. Paterson and J. J. Mathews, *Nature*, **168,** 1126 (1951).

153. J. D. Earle, *Radiat. Res.*, **19,** 234 (1963).

154. A. A. Gorodetskii, V. A. Baraboi, and V. P. Chernetskii, *Vopr. Biofiz. Mekh. Deistoya Ioniz. Radiats.*, **1964,** 159; through *Chem. Abstr.*, **63,** 18617 (1965).

155. N. P. Buu-Hoi and N. D. Xuong, *J. Org. Chem.*, **26,** 2401 (1961).

156. V. S. Nesterenko, S. I. Suminov, Y. A. Gurvich, E. L. Styskin, and S. T. Kumok, *Farmakol. Toksikol.* (Moscow), **37,** 443 (1974); through *Chem. Abstr.*, **81,** 145897 (1974).

157. J. H. Barnes, *Nature*, **205,** 816 (1965).

158. J. R. Piper, L. M. Rose, T. P. Johnston, and M. M. Grenan, *J. Med. Chem.*, **18,** 803 (1975).

159. R. Rinaldi, Y. Bernard, and M. Guilhermet, *Compt. Rend.*, **261,** 570 (1965).

160. R. Rinaldi and Y. Bernard, *Commiss. Energ. At. (Fr.), Rapp.* **1841** (1961); through *Chem. Abstr.*, **55,** 16787 (1961).

161. L. Sztanyik, V. Várterész, A. Döklen, and K. Nador, *Progr. Biochem. Pharmacol.*, **1,** 515 (1965).

162. T. J. Haley, A. M. Flesher, and L. Mavis, *Arch. Int. Pharmacodyn.*, **138,** 133 (1962).

163. T. J. Haley, W. E. Trumbull, and J. A. Cannon, *Progr. Biochem. Pharmacol.*, **1,** 359 (1965).

164. V. Wolf and W. Braun, *Arzneim.-Forsch.*, **9,** 442 (1959).

165. K. Stratton and E. M. Davis, *Int. J. Radiat. Biol.*, **5,** 105 (1962).

166. E. Campaigne and P. K. Nargund, *J. Med. Chem.*, **7,** 132 (1964).

167. I. G. Krasnykh, V. S. Shaskkov, O. Y. Magidson, E. S. Golovchinskaya, and K. A. Chkhikvadze, *Farmakol. Toksikol.* (Moscow), **24,** 572 (1961).

168. G. N. Krutovshikh, M. B. Kolesova, A. M. Rusanov, L. P. Vartanyan, and M. G. Shagoyon, *Khim.-Farm. Zh.*, **9,** 21 (1975); through *Chem. Abstr.*, **83,** 108312 (1975).

169. H. Frossard, M. Fatome, R. Royer, J. P. Lechartier, J. Guillaumel, and P. Demerseman, *Chim. Ther.*, **8,** 32 (1973).

170. J. Bitoun, H. Blancou, M. Fatome, M. Flander, H. Frossard, R. Granger, P. Joyeux, R. Perles, and Y. Robbe, *Trav. Soc. Pharm. Mont. Fr.* **33,** 147 (1973); through *Chem. Abstr.*, **80,** 127 (1974).

171. G. Grassy, A. Terol, A. Belly, Y. Robbe, J. P. Chapat, R. Granger, M. Fatome, and L. Andrieu, *Eur. J. Med. Chem.–Chim. Ther.*, **10,** 14 (1975).

172. V. G. Vladimirov, Y. E. Strelnikov, I. A. Belenkaya, Y. L. Kostyukovskii, and N. S. Tsepova, *Radiobiologiya*, **14,** 766 (1974).

173. Y. Takagi, M. Shikata, and S. Akaboshi, *Radiat. Res.*, **15,** 116 (1974).

174. A. V. Piskarev and V. S. Nesterenko, *Byull. Eksp. Biol. Med.*, **80,** 58 (1975); through *Chem. Abstr.*, **83,** 126391 (1975).

175. H. Langendorff and R. Koch, *Strahlentherapie*, **98,** 245 (1957).

176. M. Langendorff, H.-J. Melching, H. Langendorff, R. Koch, and R. Jacques, *Strahlentherapie*, **104,** 338 (1957).

177. A. Locker and H. Ellegast, *Strahlentherapie*, **129,** 273 (1966).

178. H. J. Melching and M. Langendorff, *Naturwissenschaften*, **44,** 377 (1957).

179. Z. M. Bacq and S. Liebecq-Hutter, *J. Physiol.*, **145,** 52p (1959).

180. H. Levan and D. L. Hebron, *J. Pharm. Sci.*, **57,** 1033 (1968).

181. G. Barth, H. Graebner, H. Kampmann, W. Kern, and K. Noeske, *Arzneim.-Forsch.*, **16,** 841 (1966).

182. J. L. Gray, E. J. Moulden, J. T. Tew, and H. Jensen, *Proc. Soc. Exp. Biol. Med.*, **79,** 384 (1952).

183. C. van der Meer, D. W. van Bekkum, and J. A. Cohen, *Proc. U.N. Int. Conf. Peaceful Uses At. Energy 2nd*, **23,** 42 (1958).

184. A. H. Staib and K. Effler, *Naturwissenschaften*, **53,** 583 (1966).

185. J. B. Storer and J. M. Coon, *Proc. Soc. Exp. Biol. Med.*, **74,** 202 (1950); E. F. Romantsev and N. I. Bicheikina, *Radiobiologiya*, **4,** 743 (1964).

186. J. B. Storer, *Radiat. Res.*, **47,** 537 (1971).

187. R. I. H. Wang and D. E. Davison, *U.S. Army Med. Res. Lab. Rep.*, **484** (1961); through *Chem. Abstr.*, **56,** 5082 (1962).

188. L. T. Blouin and R. R. Overman, *Radiat. Res.*, **16,** 699 (1962).

189. P. R. Salerno and H. L. Friedell, *Radiat. Res.*, **1,** 559 (1954).

190. R. A. Goepp, F. W. Fitch, and J. Doull, *Radiat. Res.*, **31,** 149 (1967).

191. C. van der Meer and D. W. van Bekkum, *Int. J. Radiat. Biol.*, **4,** 105 (1961).

192. H. A. S. van den Brenk and K. Elliott, *Nature*, **182,** 1506 (1959).

193. S. Kobayashi, W. Nakamura, and H. Eto, *Int. J. Radiat. Biol.*, **11,** 505 (1966).

194. I. G. Krasnykh, P. G. Zherebchenko, V. S. Murashova, N. N. Suvorov, N. R. Sorokina, and V. S. Shashkov, *Radiobiologiya*, **2,** 156 (1962).

195. L. Andrieu, M. Fatome, R. Granger, Y. Robbe, and A. Terol, *Eur. J. Med. Chem.–Chim. Ther.*, **9,** 453 (1974).

196. I. Baev and D. Benova, *Roentgenol. Radiol.*, **14**, 50 (1975).

197. L. J. Cole and S. R. Gospe, *Radiat. Res.*, **11**, 438 (1959).

198. H. M. Patt, R. L. Straub, E. B. Tyree, M. N. Swift, and D. E. Smith, *Am. J. Physiol.*, **159**, 269 (1949).

199. W. W. Smith and I. M. Alderman, *Radiat. Res.*, **17**, 594 (1962).

200. K. Flemming and M. Langendorff, *Strahlentherapie*, **128**, 109 (1965).

201. W. E. Rothe and M. M. Grenan, *Science*, **133**, 888 (1961).

202. J. Cheymol, J. Louw, P. Chabrier, M. Adolphe, J. Seyden, and M. Selim, *Bull. Acad. Natl. Med.* (Paris), **144**, 681 (1960).

203. G. Arnaud, H. Frossard, J.-P. Gabriel, O. Bichon, J.-M. Saucier, J. Bourdais, and M. Guillerm, *Progr. Biochem. Pharmacol.*, **1**, 467 (1965).

204. H. Laborit, M. Dana, and P. Carlo, *Progr. Biochem. Pharmacol.*, **1**, 574 (1965).

205. D. P. Doolittle and J. Watson, *Int. J. Radiat. Biol.*, **11**, 389 (1966).

206. B. W. Volk, K. F. Wellmann, and S. S. Lazarus, *Am. J. Pathol.*, **51**, 207 (1967).

207. H. Blondal, *Brit. J. Radiol.*, **30**, 219 (1957).

208. A. P. Duplischeva, K. K. Ivanov, and N. G. Silinova, *Radiobiologiya*, **6**, 318 (1966).

209. K. Flemming, Biophys, *Probl. Strahlenwirkung Jahrestag Tagungsber.*, **1965**, 138 (1966); through *Chem. Abstr.*, **67**, 50865 (1967).

210. R. Wilson, G. D. Ledney, and T. Matsuzawa, *Progr. Biochem. Pharmacol.*, **1**, 622 (1965).

211. E. J. Ainsworth and F. A. Mitchell, *Nature*, **210**, 321 (1966).

212. H. Langendorff, H.-J. Melching, and H. Rosler, *Strahlentherapie*, **113**, 603 (1960).

213. H.-J. Melching, *Strahlentherapie*, **120**, 34 (1963).

214. R. Koch, *Acta Chem. Scand.*, **12**, 1873 (1958).

215. H. Langendorff, H.-J. Melching, and C. Streffer, *Strahlentherapie*, **118**, 341 (1962).

216. R. Wagner and E. C. Silverman, *Int. J. Radiat. Biol.*, **12**, 101 (1967).

217. M. A. Tumanyan, N. G. Sinilova, A. P. Duplischeva, and K. K. Ivanov, *Radiobiologiya*, **6**, 712 (1966).

218. M. E. Roberts, C. Jones, and M. A. Gerving, *Life Sci.*, **4**, 1913 (1965).

219. T. P. Pantev, N. V. Bokova, and I. T. Nikolov, *Eksp. Med. Morfol.*, **12**, 186 (1973).

220. T. Aleksandrov, I. Nikolov, D. Krustanov, and T. Tinev, *Roentgenol. Radiol.*, **5**, 45 (1966).

221. V. A. Baraboi, *Biokhim. Progr. Tekhnol. Chai. Poizood. Akad. Nauk SSSR, Inst. Biokhim.*, **1966**, 357; through *Chem. Abstr.*, **66**, 2490 (1967).

222. J. M. Gazave, D. C. Modigliani, and G. Ligny, *Progr. Biochem. Pharmacol.*, **1**, 554 (1965).

223. V. Brueckner, *Strahlentherapie*, **145**, 732 (1973).

224. Z. M. Bacq and S. Liebecq-Hutter, *J. Physiol.* (London), **145**, 52 (1958).

225. Z. M. Bacq, M. L. Beaumariage, and S. Liebecq-Hutter, *Int. J. Radiat. Biol.*, **9**, 175 (1965).

226. J. Sikulová and L. Novák, *Int. J. Radiat. Biol.*, **17**, 587 (1970).

227. C. G. Overberger, H. Ringsdorf, and B. Avchen, *J. Med. Chem.*, **8**, 862 (1965).

228. J. Barnes, G. Esslemont, and P. Holt, *Makromol. Chem.*, **176**, 275 (1975).

229. O. V. Semina, A. G. Konnoplyannikov, and A. M. Pomerennyi, *Radiobiologiya*, **14**, 689 (1974).

230. N. P. Kharitanovich, G. A. Dokshina, V. A. Pegel, E. I. Yartsev, and V. G. Yashunskii, *Radiobiologiya*, **15**, 104 (1975).

231. V. Brueckner, *Umschau*, **73**, 607 (1973).

232. R. Lange and A. Pihl, *Int. J. Radiat. Biol.*, **3**, 249 (1961).

233. H. Langendorff, R. Koch, and U. Hagen, *Strahlentherapie*, **99**, 375 (1956).

234. S. Grigorescu, C. Nedelcu, and M. Netase, *Radiobiologiya*, **6**, 819 (1965).

235. D. H. Marrian, B. Marshall, and J. S. Mitchell, *Chemotherapia*, **3**, 225 (1961).

236. W. E. Rothe, M. M. Grenan, and S. M. Wilson, *Progr. Biochem. Pharmacol.*, **1**, 372 (1965).

237. H. M. Patt, S. H. Mayer, and D. E. Smith, *Fed. Proc.*, **11**, 118 (1952).

238. H. Langendorff and R. Koch, *Strahlentherapie*, **95**, 535 (1954).

239. H. Moroson and H. A. Spielman, *Int. J. Radiat. Biol.*, **11**, 87 (1966).

240. C. Stuart and G. Cittadini, *Minerva Fisioter. Radiobiol.*, **10**, 337 (1965).

241. G. Caprino and L. Caprino, *Minerva Fisioter. Radiobiol.*, **10**, 311 (1965).

242. L. A. Tiunov, N. A. Kachurina, and O. I. Smirnova, *Radiobiologiya*, **6**, 343 (1966).

243. G. Cittadini, *Boll. Soc. Ital. Biol. Sper.*, **41**, 360 (1965).

244. H. Moroson and D. Martin, *Nature*, **214**, 304 (1967).

245. V. G. Yakovlev, *Radiobiologiya*, **4**, 656 (1964).

246. J. S. Mitchell, *Progr. Biochem. Pharmacol.*, **1**, 335 (1965).

247. B. Djordjevic and W. Szybalski, *J. Exp. Med.*, **112**, 509 (1960).

248. M. R. Bianchi and E. Strom, *Ann. Ist. Super. Sanita*, **2,** 342 (1966).

249. J. P. Kriss, in *U.S. At. Energy Comm. Symp. Ser. No. 6*, 305 (1966).

250. R. F. Pitillo, E. R. Bannister, and E. P. Johnson, *Can. J. Microbiol.*, **12,** 17 (1966).

251. J. Burns, J. P. Garcia, M. B. Lucas, C. Moncrief, and R. F. Pitillo, *Radiat. Res.*, **25,** 460 (1965).

252. R. F. Pitillo, M. B. Lucas, and E. R. Bannister, *Radiat. Res.*, **29,** 549 (1966).

253. M. J. Ashwood-Smith, D. M. Robinson, J. H. Barnes, and B. A. Bridges, *Nature*, **216,** 137 (1967).

254. R. F. Pitillo and M. B. Lucas, *Cancer Chemother. Rep.*, **51,** 229 (1967).

255. R. F. Pitillo and M. B. Lucas, *Radiat. Res.*, **31,** 36 (1967).

256. P. T. Emmerson, *Radiat. Res.*, **30,** 841 (1967).

257. W. A. Cramp, *Radiat. Res.*, **30,** 221 (1967).

258. P. T. Emmerson and P. Howard-Flanders, *Radiat. Res.*, **26,** 54 (1965).

259. C. L. Greenstock, J. D. Chapman, J. A. Raleigh, E. Shierman, and A. P. Reuvers, *Radiat. Res.*, **59,** 556 (1974).

260. J. C. Asquith, M. E. Watts, K. Patel, C. E. Smithen, and G. E. Adam, *Radiat. Res.*, **60,** 108 (1974).

261. S. Greco, G. Gasso, and A. Billitteri, *Progr. Biochem. Pharmacol.*, **1,** 277 (1965).

262. N. I. Shapiro, E. N. Tolkacheva, I. G. Sparskaya, and V. M. Fedoseeva, *Vopr. Onkol.*, **6,** 71 (1960).

263. B. Shapiro, E. E. Schwarz, and G. Kollman, *Cancer Res.*, **23,** 223 (1963).

264. R. Koch and I. Seiter, *Arzneim.-Forsch.*, **14,** 1018 (1964).

265. T. Zebro, *Acta Med. Pol.*, **7,** 83 (1966).

266. M. Pini, L. D'Acunzo, and G. Giudici, *Strahlentherapie*, **128,** 558 (1965).

267. J. F. Utley, T. L. Phillips, L. J. Kane, M. D. Wharam, and W. M. Wara, *Radiology*, **110,** 213 (1974).

268. T. L. Phillips, L. J. Kane, and J. F. Utley, *Cancer* (Philadelphia), **32,** 528 (1973).

269. S. P. Sizenko and L. Y. Nesterovskaya, *Vopr. Eksp. Onkol. Sb.*, **263** (1965); through *Chem. Abstr.*, **65,** 7868 (1966).

270. L. B. Berlin, *Dokl. Adkad. Nauk SSSR* **195,** 998 (1970); through *Chem. Abstr.*, **74,** 72530 (1971).

271. J. R. Maisin, J. Hugon, and A. Léonard, *J. Belg. Radiol.*, **47,** 871 (1964).

272. H. Yoshihara, *Nippon Igaku Hoshasen Gakkai Zasshi*, **23,** 1 (1963); through *Chem. Abstr.*, **62,** 802 (1965).

273. J. R. Maisin, and G. Mattelin, *Bull. Cancer*, **54,** 149 (1967).

274. J. J. Kelly, K. A. Herrington, S. P. Ward, A. Meister, and O. M. Friedman, *Cancer Res.*, **27A,** 137 (1967).

275. G. M. Airapetyan, G. A. Anorova, L. N. Kublik, G. K. Otarova, M. I. Pekaskii, V. N. Stanko, L. K. Eidus, and S. P. Yarmonenko, *Med. Radiol.*, **12,** 58 (1967).

276. E. Karosiene, *Sin. Izuch. Fiziol. Akt. Veshchestv.*, *Mater. Konf.* **1971,** 47 (1971); through *Chem. Abstr.*, **79,** 7385 (1973).

277. T. Sugahara, *Advan. Antimicrob. Antineoplastic Chemother.*, *Proc. Int. Congr. Chemother., 7th*, 1971, 825 (1972); through *Chem. Abstr.*, **79,** 38697 (1973).

278. T. Ohshima and I. Tsykiyama, *Nippon Igaku Hoshasen Gakkai Zasshi*, **33,** 351 (1973); through *Chem. Abstr.*, **81,** 45486 (1974).

279. J. R. Berry and J. R. Andrews, *Radiat. Res.*, **16,** 82 (1962).

280. P. Calabresi, *Cancer Res.*, **23,** 1260 (1963).

281. C. Heidelberger and F. J. Ansfield, *Cancer Res.*, **23,** 1226 (1963).

282. S. Farber, *Cancer Chemother. Rep.*, **13,** 159 (1961).

283. H. Kurosaka, *Nippon Igaku Hoshasen Gakkai Zasshi*, **19,** 1217 (1959); through *Chem. Abstr.*, **60,** 4427 (1964).

284. E. Scolari, D. Boiti, M. Nannelli, and C. Vallechi, *Rass. Derm. Sif.*, **12,** 207 (1959).

285. T. J. Deeley, *Brit. J. Cancer*, **16,** 387 (1962).

286. L. A. Tiunov, O. I. Smirnova, N. A. Kachurina, and Z. I. Menshikova, *Med. Radiol.*, **12,** 91 (1967).

287. L. Cohen and S. Schwartz, *Cancer Res.*, **26,** 1769 (1966).

288. E. Magdon and R. Konopatzky, *Arch. Geschwultsforsch.*, **29,** 259 (1967).

289. R. I. Pol'kina, *Nespetsifich. Lek. Profil. Ter. Raka.*, **1966,** 134; through *Chem. Abstr.*, **67,** 97500 (1967).

290. V. S. Begina, *Tr. Kirgizsk. Nauchn.-Issled. Inst. Onkol. Radiol.*, **2,** 242 (1965); through *Chem. Abstr.*, **67,** 97472 (1967).

291. S. A. Baisheva, *Tr. Kayakhsk. Nauchn.-Issled. Inst. Onkol. Radiol.*, **1,** 308 (1965); through *Chem. Abstr.*, **64,** 8612 (1966).

292. M. B. Sahasrabudhe, *J. Sci. Ind. Res.*, **26,** 243 (1967).

293. M. Klimek, *Neoplasia*, **13,** 31 (1966).

294. E. Magdon, *Naturwissenschaften*, **53**, 44 (1966).

295. A. M. Lokshina, and V. N. Tugarinova, *Med. Radiol.*, **12**, 81 (1967).

296. H. Hayashi, T. Imai, N. Inoue, Y. Tabeta, and H. Okayama, *Nippon Kokuka Gakkai Zasshi*, **19**, 196 (1970); through *Chem. Abstr.*, **79**, 234 (1973).

297. J. L. Foster, P. J. Conroy, A. J. Searle, and R. L. Willson, *Brit. J. Cancer*, **33**, 485 (1976).

298. H. Tuschl, W. Klein, F. Kocsis, R. Kovac, and H. Altmann, *Stud. Biophys.* (Berlin), **50**, 55 (1975).

299. U. Georghe and A. Strungascu, *Rev. Roum. Morphol. Physiol.*, **20**, 49 (1974).

300. P. G. Zherebchenko, G. M. Airapetyan, I. G. Krasnykh, N. N. Suvorov, and A. N. Shevchenko, *Patog. Eksp. Profil. Ter. Luchev. Porazenii* (Moscow), **1964**, 193; through *Chem. Abstr.*, **64**, 2394 (1966).

301. L. Novak, *Bull. Cl. Sci. Acad. Roy. Belg.*, **52**, 633 (1966).

302. E. Y. Graevsky, I. M. Shapiro, M. M. Konstantinova, and N. F. Barakina, in *The Initial Effects of Ionizing Radiations on Cells, A Symposium*, R. J. C. Harris, Ed., Academic, New York, 1961, p. 237.

303. M. F. Popova, *Mater. Vses. Soveshch. Radiobiol. Vopr. Prir. Roli. Radiotoksinov Biol. Deistvii Ioniz. Radiats., Ist.*, **1965**, 254 (1966); through *Chem. Abstr.*, **68**, 19339 (1968).

304. P. Alexander and A. Charlesby, *Nature*, **173**, 578 (1954).

305. A. Pihl and T. Sanner, in *Radioprotection and Sensitization*, H. L. Moroson and M. Quintiliani, Eds., Barnes and Noble, New York, 1970, p. 43.

306. B. Smaller and C. E. Avery, *Nature*, **183**, 539 (1959).

307. I. I. Sapezhinskii and E. G. Dontsova, *Biofizika*, **12**, 794 (1967).

308. W.-C. Hsin, C.-L. Chang, M.-J. Yao, C.-H. Hua, and H.-C. Chin, *Sci. Sinica* (Peking), **15**, 211 (1966).

309. E. B. Burlakova, V. D. Gaintseva, L. V. Slepukhina, N. G. Khrapova, and N. M. Emanuel, *Dokl. Akad. Nauk SSSr*, **164**, 394 (1965); through *Chem. Abstr.*, **64**, 2394 (1966).

310. L. Eldjarn and A. Pihl, *J. Biol. Chem.*, **225**, 499 (1957).

311. G. Gorin, *Prog. Biochem. Pharmacol.*, **1**, 142 (1965).

312. L. Eldjarn and A. Pihl, *Radiat. Res.*, **9**, 110 (1958).

313. E. A. Dickens and B. Shapiro, *U.S. Dep. Comm. Off. Tech. Serv., P.B. Rep.* **146**, 190 (1960); through *Chem. Abstr.*, **56**, 13205 (1962).

314. G. Kollmann and B. Shapiro, *Radiat. Res.*, **27**, 474 (1966).

315. R. H. Bradford, R. Shapira, and D. G. Doherty, *Int. J. Radiat. Biol.*, **3**, 595 (1961).

316. D. Jamieson, *Nature*, **209**, 361 (1966).

317. T. Sanner and A. Pihl, *Scand. J. Clin. Lab. Invest.*, **22**, Suppl. 106, 53 (1968).

318. J. Sumegi, T. Sanner, and A. Pihl, *Int. J. Radiat. Biol.*, **20**, 397 (1971).

319. Z. M. Bacq, *Bull. Acad. Roy. Med. Belg.*, **6**, 115 (1966).

320. C. Duyckaerts and C. Liebecq, in *Radiation Protection and Sensitization*, H. Moroson and M. Quintiliani, Eds., Barnes and Noble, New York, 1970, p. 429.

321. E. N. Goncharenko, Y. B. Kudryashov, and L. I. Alieva, *Dokl. Akad. Nauk SSSR*, **184**, 1437 (1969); through *Chem. Abstr.*, **70**, 112161 (1969).

322. E. Y. Graevsky, M. M. Konstantinova, I. V. Nekrasova, O. M. Sokolova, and A. G. Tarasenko, *Radiobiologiya*, **7**, 130 (1967).

323. E. V. Gusareva, A. G. Tarasenko, and E. Y. Graevsky, *Radiobiologiya*, **8**, 721 (1968).

324. L. Revesz, H. Modig, and P. Lindfors, *Tr. Kayakhsk Nauchn.-Issled. Inst. Onkol. Radiol.*, **6**, 36 (1969); through *Chem. Abstr.*, **73**, 21940 (1970).

325. L. X. Thu, *Radiobiologiya*, **9**, 630 (1969).

326. L. X. Thu and E. Y. Graevsky, *Dokl. Akad. Nauk SSSR*, **182**, 965 (1968); through *Chem. Abstr.*, **70**, 17403 (1969).

327. H. G. Modig and L. Revesz, *Atomkernenergie*, **14**, 214 (1969).

328. M. L. Efimov and N. I. Mironemko, *Radiobiologiya*, **9**, 359 (1969).

329. A. G. Tarasenko, E. V. Gusareva, and E. Y. Graevsky, *Radiobiologiya*, **10**, 373 (1970).

330. P. Van Caneghem, *Strahlentherapie*, **137**, 231 (1969).

331. A. K. Bruce, P. A. Sansone, and T. J. MacVittie, *Radiat. Res.*, **38**, 95 (1969).

332. D. Chobanova, *Suvrem. Med.*, **25**, 33 (1974).

333. E. Jellum, *Int. J. Radiat. Biol.*, **9**, 185 (1965).

334. P. E. Brown, *Nature*, **213**, 363 (1967).

335. G. Kollman, B. Shapiro, and D. Martin, *Radiat. Res.*, **31**, 721 (1967).

336. M. Karkaria, M. S. thesis, Mass. College of Pharmacy, Boston, 1977.

337. B. P. Ivannik and N. I. Ryabchenko, *Radiobiologiya*, **6**, 913 (1966).

338. P. Alexander, C. J. Dean, A. R. Lehmann, M.

G. Ormerod, P. Felschreiber, and R. W. Serianni, in Ref. 37, p. 15.

339. E. F. Romantsev, N. N. Koshcheenko, and I. V. Fillippovich, in Ref. 37, p. 421.

340. R. Goutier and L. Baugnet-Mahieu, in Ref. 37, p. 445.

341. S. Sawada and S. Okada, *Radiat. Res.*, **39,** 553 (1969).

342. D. M. Ginsberg and H. K. Webster, *Radiat. Res.*, **39,** 421 (1969).

343. G. E. Adams, in Ref. 37, p. 3.

344. D. L. Dewey, in Ref. 37, p. 139.

345. O. Vos, G. A. Grant, and L. Budke, in Ref. 37, p. 211.

346. S. G. Cohen, in *Organosulfur Chemistry*, M. J. Janssen, Ed., Interscience, New York, 1967, p. 33.

347. H. Loman, S. Voogd, and J. Blok, *Radiat. Res.*, **42,** 437 (1970).

348. C. Nicolau and H. Dertinger, *Radiat. Res.*, **42,** 62 (1970).

349. A. D. Lenkers and M. G. Ormerod, *Nature*, **225,** 546 (1970).

350. T. Sanner, *Radiat. Res.*, **44,** 13 (1970).

351. N. J. F. Dodd and M. Ebert, *Nature*, **221,** 1245 (1969).

352. P. Kenney and B. Commoner, *Nature*, **223,** 1229 (1969).

353. V. Drasil, L. Ryznar, and P. Van Duyet, *Radiation Damage Sulphydryl Compounds*, *Proc. Panel*, 1968, 55 (1969); through *Chem. Abstr.*, **72,** 86940 (1970).

354. T. C. Owen and A. C. Wilbraham, *J. Am. Chem. Soc.*, **91,** 3365 (1969).

355. A. M. Kuzin and A. S. Gaziev, *Dokl. Akad. Nauk SSSR*, **184,** 221 (1969); through *Chem. Abstr.*, **70,** 64934 (1969).

356. W. O. Foye and M. C. M. Solis, *J. Pharm. Sci.*, **58,** 352 (1969).

357. A. T. Seisebaev and M. K. Babaeva, *Radiobiologiya*, **9,** 257 (1969).

358. H. Altmann, *Biophysik*, **1,** 329 (1964).

359. S. S. Block, D. D. Mulligan, J. P. Weidner, and D. G. Doherty, in Ref. 37, p. 163.

360. J. Schubert, *Copper and Peroxidases in Radiobiology and Medicine*, Charles C Thomas, Springfield, Ill., 1964.

361. E. C. Knoblock and W. C. Purdy, *J. Electroanal. Chem.*, **2,** 493 (1961).

362. M. M. Jones, *Nature*, **185,** 96 (1959).

363. J. Moutschen-Dahmen, M. Moutschen-Dahmen, and J. Gilot-Delhalle, *Experientia*, **25,** 998 (1969).

364. J. Kalam, *Eesti NSV Tead. Akad. Toim. Biol.*, **19,** 2533 (1970); through *Chem. Abstr.*, **72,** 97142 (1970).

365. P. A. Vlasyuk, D. M. Grodzinskii, and I. N. Gudkov, *Radiobiologiya*, **6,** 591 (1966).

366. J. A. V. Butler and A. B. Robins, *Nature*, **193,** 673 (1962).

367. B. B. Singh and M. G. Ormerod, *Int. J. Radiat. Biol.*, **10,** 369 (1966).

368. P. Riesz, *Biochem. Biophys. Res. Commun.*, **23,** 273 (1966).

369. M. Anbar and A. Levitzki, *Radiat. Res.*, **27,** 32 (1966).

370. S. Capilna, E. Ghizari, M. Stefan, and G. Petec, *Studii Cercet. Fiziol.*, **9,** 369 (1964).

371. J. Holian and W. M. Garrison, *Nature*, **212,** 394 (1966).

372. A. Albert, *Selective Toxicity*, 3rd ed., Wiley, New York, 1965, p. 248.

373. J. Schubert, *Abstr. 139th Nat. Meet. Am. Chem. Soc* **1961,** p. 9N.

374. W. Lohmann, *Progr. Biochem. Pharmacol.*, **1,** 118 (1965).

375. J. Schubert, *Nature*, **200,** 375 (1963).

376. M. Anbar, *Nature*, **200,** 376 (1963).

377. A. D. Perris, J. F. Whitfield, and R. H. Dixon, *Radiat. Res.*, **32,** 550 (1967).

378. A. D. Perris and J. F. Whitfield, *Nature* **214,** 302 (1967).

379. J. Misustova, L. Novak, and J. Kautsha, *Radiobiologiya*, **13,** 388 (1973).

380. J. M. Yuhas, J. O. Proctor, and L. H. Smith, *Radiat. Res.*, **54,** 222 (1973).

381. G. P. Bogatyrev, E. N. Goncharenko, Y. Y. Chirkov, and Y. B. Kudryashov, *Biol. Nauki,* **16,** 50 (1973); through *Chem. Abstr.*, **79,** 111626 (1973).

382. P. N. Kulyabko, N. G. Dubenko, and V. D. Konysheva, *Fiziol. Akt. Veshchestv.*, No. 4, 87 (1972); through *Chem. Abstr.*, **79,** 38542 (1973).

383. J. D. Chapman, A. P. Reuvers, J. Borsa, and C. L. Greenstock, *Radiat. Res.*, **56,** 291 (1973).

384. J. L. Redpath, R. Santus, J. Ovadia, and L. I. Grossweiner, *Int. J. Radiat. Biol.*, **28,** 243 (1975).

385. P. E. Brown, M. Calvin, and J. F. Newmark, *Science*, **151,** 68 (1966).

386. G. Plomteux, M. L. Beaumariage, Z. M. Bacq, and C. Heusghem, in Ref. 37, p. 433.

387. P. V. Vittorio, E. A. Watkins, and S. Dziubalo-Blehm, *Can. J. Physiol. Pharmacol.*, **47,** 65 (1969).

388. I. V. Fillipovich and E. F. Romantsev, *Radiobiologiya*, **8,** 800 (1968).

389. Z. I. Zhulanova, E. F. Romantsev, E. E. Kalesnikow, and E. V. Kozyreva, in Ref. 37, p. 453.

390. J. N. Mehrishi, in Ref. 37, p. 265.

391. Z. M. Bacq, Ed., "Sulfur-Containing Radioprotective Agents," Sect. 79, *International Encyclopedia of Pharmacology and Therapeutics*, Pergamon, Oxford, 1975.

CHAPTER THIRTY-EIGHT

Cardiac Drugs

RICHARD E. THOMAS

Department of Pharmacy
University of Sydney
Sydney, N.S.W. 2006 AUSTRALIA

CONTENTS

1 INTRODUCTION

The heart is affected directly or indirectly by a wide variety of drugs. Many of these agents are discussed elsewhere in this book and this chapter is therefore limited to four groups of drugs: the cardiac glycosides and related inotropic agents, the antiarrhythmic agents, the antianginal agents, and the cardiac unloading agents.

Of the drugs discussed in this chapter, the properties of the cardiac glycosides (in the form of squill) were recognized by the ancient Egyptians, the antianginal nitrate of choice was introduced in the nineteenth century, and the nonspecific antiarrhythmic drugs were discovered by accident, having been introduced for the treatment of malaria, epilepsy, or for local anesthesia. In recent years there have been major advances in our understanding of how these drugs act and in our knowledge of how best to use these drugs. Behind these advances is an expanding knowledge of the interaction of drug molecules with biological systems at the molecular level. In my opinion, it is this knowledge that is the dominant theme of medicinal chemistry. This chapter attempts to develop this theme with respect to both the pharmacodynamic and pharmacokinetic properties of drug action and to compare these properties with respect to drugs that act specifically (digitalis) and those that act nonspecifically (the quinidine-like antiarrhythmics). Finally, an attempt is made here to identify the biomolecular systems that seem likely targets in the future development of drugs affecting the heart.

The references cited in this chapter are mainly to key reviews that, in turn, provide references to the major prime sources.

2 MOLECULAR BASIS OF MYOCARDIAL CONTRACTILITY

It is appropriate to begin with a discussion of the molecular basis of excitation and contraction in the heart. Particular emphasis is given to the movement of ions across cell membranes since this forms the foundation of the medicinal chemistry of digitalis and the antiarrhythmic agents.

2.1 Transmembrane Ion Fluxes

The biophysical property that connects excitation and contraction is the electrical potential difference that exists across cell membranes: the intracellular face of the membrane is electrically negative with respect to the extracellular face.

This situation is the result of several factors, principally the following:

1. the intracellular fluid is rich in K^+ and poor in Na^+ and the reverse applies to the extracellular fluid;
2. the membrane is more permeable to K^+ than it is to Na^+;
3. the anions of the intracellular fluid are largely organic and do not diffuse through the membrane;
4. a process of active transport exists which maintains the steady-state levels of Na^+ and K^+.

As a result of the first three factors, there occurs, at least initially, a net loss of intracellular K^+ that is not balanced electrically by either an efflux of anions or an influx of other cations. As predicted by the Nernst equation, the loss of intracellular K^+ is limited by the development of an inward directed electrical gradient that balances the outward directed chemical gradient. However, there also exists a slow passive influx of Na^+ along its electrochemical gradient, and this in time would balance the efflux of K^+. This trend toward electrical neutrality is prevented by the existence of a Na^+, K^+ pump that actively transports Na^+ out of the cell in exchange for a smaller ratio of K^+ ions. A steady-state situation is therefore reached in which the extracellular fluid has a slight excess of cations and the intracellular fluid a slight excess of anions. These charges are attracted to each other and become aligned on either side of the membrane so that a charge separation or potential difference exists across the membrane. These potential differences can be measured by means of microelectrodes inserted on either side of the membrane. Where this has been done, it has been found that the potential difference varies from -20 to -100 mV. In most cardiac cells the diastolic transmembrane potential difference is about -90 mV. A more rigorous discussion of the electrophysiology of heart cells is given in Ref. 1.

An appropriate stimulus, electrical or chemical, can depolarize the membrane, presumably by causing conformational changes that open "channels" in the membrane and allow various ions, particularly Na^+, to flow into the cell and reduce the negative charge on the inner surface. In the cells of most tissues this effect is localized but may be of great importance in providing a stimulus to trigger events within the cell. In the cells of excitable tissue, depolarization can give rise to more than just a localized effect. If the stimulus reduces the transmembrane potential to a threshold value, it produces an action potential which is then transmitted in an all-or-none fashion along the entire membrane. By an all-or-none effect is meant that the action potential, once triggered, is transmitted in such a way that its size and rate of travel are independent of the initial stimulus (although they may be modified by other factors). As the action potential travels along the membrane it induces a rise in the levels of free or "activator" Ca^{2+} within the cell. The calcium ions react di-

rectly with the contractile elements to initiate the contractile process.

The relationship between ion fluxes and action potentials in the myocardium is complex and varies for different types of myocardial cell. At least eight separate ion fluxes have been reported to cross the membrane of heart cells (2). The study of these fluxes is a very recent but active field of investigation, and references to key reviews and books on this subject are given in Ref. 3. A concise but informative account is given in Ref. 4. A representation of the major ion fluxes associated with the action potential of a normal nonpacemaker cell of ventricular tissue is shown in Fig. 38.1

The action potentials of myocardial cells are of much longer duration (300–500 msec) than those of other excitable tissues and are characterized by a plateau period (phase 2). There is general agreement that depolarization in most heart cells is due to the opening of fast sodium channels, allowing for the rapid influx of Na^+ that produces the upstroke (phase 0) of the action potential. The fast Na^+ channels are blocked by tetrodotoxin (38.**1**) and kept

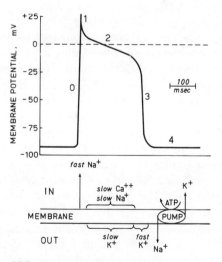

Fig. 38.1 Diagrammatic representation of an action potential of a nonautomatic ventricular cell together with the principal time-related ion fluxes.

38.1 Tetrodotoxin

open by aconitine and the veratridine alkaloids, and this is the basis for the repetitive activity induced by the latter. There is evidence that fast sodium channels are absent in cells of the sinus node.

Following depolarization (which takes about 1 msec), a partial repolarization event (phase 1) occurs as a result of closure of the fast sodium channels and an influx of chloride ions. Depolarization should also lead to a rapid efflux of K^+ as a consequence of the reduction in the electrical barrier to K^+ efflux. This occurs in nerve cells and results in rapid repolarization. However, in the heart, K^+ efflux is much slower than expected, and this leads to a reduction in the rate of repolarization. In addition, there occurs a slow inward current of cations (Na^+ and Ca^{2+}), which further delays repolarization. These two properties (reduced K^+ efflux and slow influx of Na^+ and Ca^{2+}) are the main factors that give rise to the plateau region (phase 2) which characterizes the action potentials of cardiac cells. The slow influx of Na^+ and Ca^{2+} seems to involve a common channel that is not blocked by tetrodotoxin. The final phase of repolarization (phase 3) occurs as a result of the closure of the slow inward channels for Na^+ and Ca^{2+} and the activation of one or possibly two fast outward channels for K^+. At the end of phase 3, the transmembrane potential is restored to its resting (phase 4) value but the intracellular fluid has lost K^+ and gained Na^+. If this situation is not reversed, the prerequisites for excitability (an inward electrochemical gradient for Na^+ and a transmembrane potential difference) are lost. Steady-state levels of Na^+ and K^+ are restored by the expenditure of metabolic energy which drives the Na^+,K^+ pump (Fig. 38.1). This pump utilizes ATP to actively transport Na^+ out of the cell and K^+ into the cell. The pump requires the presence of Mg^{2+} and is activated by rising concentrations of Na^+ on the inner face of the membrane and rising concentrations of K^+ on the outer face of the membrane. The pump is therefore called Na^+,K^+-ATPase. It is specifically inhibited by the cardiac glycosides and it is generally believed that the binding of cardiac glycosides to the outer face of Na^+,K^+-ATPase is the primary event that mediates their inotropic activity.

Little is known of the macromolecular mechanisms involved in the active and passive transport of ions across cell membranes but the subject is of great interest to medicinal chemists since the carrier mechanisms are all actual or potential sites for drug action. The fast sodium channel has been the subject of much speculation. It is known that conformational changes in membrane components are associated with the movement of Na^+ through the membrane and that the rate of travel of Na^+ is decreased with reduction in the transmembrane potential. All this suggests that the "channel" involves the movement of charged macromolecules and that this movement is controlled by the charge on the membrane surface. A number of models have been proposed including the opening and shutting of molecular "gates" and the movement of charged carrier molecules. Of particular interest is the concept of ionophores (literally ion carriers). These are macromolecules that possess a specific affinity for particular ions and are able to carry the ion through a lipid matrix. A number of molecules that act as ionophores have been identified. These substances appear to be able to enclose the ion in a polar cavity while presenting an outer surface that is lipophilic. Exogenous ionophores have been studied and shown to have marked physiological activity (5). Such substances are being investigated as potential therapeutic agents.

The distinction between "channels" and pumps can be misleading since all of the mechanisms described above could be applied to either system of ion movement. The word "pump" is simply an expression to describe an uphill or energy-consuming movement of an ion or other molecule.

The contraction of the heart is normally initiated by spontaneous depolarization in the pacemaker cells of the sinus node. This occurs because of a decrease in a slow outward current of K^+ during phase 4 which, in turn, results in a steady decrease in the net negative charge on the inner face of the membrane. When this reaches a threshold value (T.P., Fig. 38.22, A) it stimulates a moderately fast inward movement of Na^+ and Ca^{2+} which depolarizes the membrane. Unlike other cardiac cells, those of the sinus node do not possess a fast Na^+ channel. The action potential, once initiated, is carried by cell membranes to all cells of the myocardium, and is passed from cell to cell via the intercalated disk formed by the tight abutment of the ends of adjacent cells.

2.2 Chemistry of Contraction

Heart muscle is striated muscle and like skeletal muscle owes its property of contractility to the presence of myofibrils. Each cell (or fiber) contains many myofibrils. The basic unit of the myofibril is the sarcomere whose boundary is a disk of fibrous material known as the Z line (Fig. 38.2). Attached to the Z line is an array of thin filaments which extend from each end of the sarcomere and interdigitate with the thick filaments that lie in the central region. Since the sarcomere is roughly cylindrical, a

three-dimensional system exists in which the spacing of the filaments is hexagonal: each thick filament is surrounded by six thin filaments and vice-versa. Contraction occurs when the array of thin filaments is drawn into the matrix of thick filaments by means of cross bridges that form between the two sets of filaments.

The principal component of thick filaments is myosin. This protein has a double-strand, helically-coiled tail region and a globular head (Fig. 38.3). Enzymatically, myosin is an ATPase with the active site at the tip of the head. Molecules of myosin can be isolated, and if these are placed in a medium of low ionic strength they spontaneously recombine to form thick filaments identical to those in the sarcomere (Fig. 38.4). The arrangement of myosin in thick filaments is such that the heads project in a helical fashion with one complete turn occurring every 430 Å. It is the myosin heads that form the cross bridges during muscle contraction.

The major protein components of thin filaments are fibrous actin (F-actin), troponin, and tropomyosin. F-actin resembles a string of beads, with each bead derived from globular actin (G-actin). When molecules of G-actin are treated *in vitro* with ATP and Mg^{2+}, they combine to form a helically arrayed double strand of F-actin identical to that found in the sarcomere. If troponin and tropomyosin are then added, they become attached to the helical groove of the F-actin strand to complete the formation of the thin filament as it exists *in vivo* (Fig. 38.5).

The following type of experiment provides the model for how the contractile machinery works. If isolated molecules of myosin, or even cleaved myosin heads, are placed in a medium containing ATP and Mg^{2+}, ATP binds to the myosin heads but little or no hydrolysis to ADP occurs. If actin is then added, hydrolysis proceeds in an uncontrolled fashion until all the ATP is consumed. If troponin and tropomyosin are

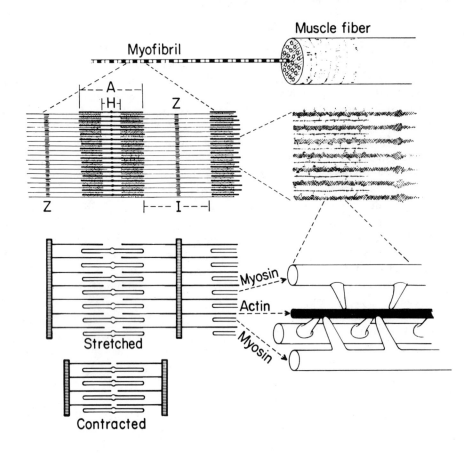

Fig. 38.2 The contractile elements of the heart. The cell (or muscle fiber) contains many myofibrils, each of which is made up of a large number of repeating units called sarcomeres. The sarcomere is delineated at each end by a Z line and is composed of overlapping thick (myosin) and thin (actin) filaments. Contraction occurs when the array of thin filaments is drawn into the matrix of thick filaments by means of cross bridge formation. (From R. F. Rushmer, *Structure and Function of the Cardiovascular System*, Saunders, Philadelphia, 1972. Used with permission.)

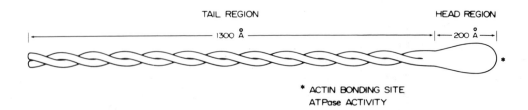

Fig. 38.3 The myosin molecule. (From N. R. Alpert and B. B. Hamrell in *Cardiac Physiology for the Clinician*, M. Vassalle, Ed., Academic, New York, 1976, Chap. 7. Used with permission.)

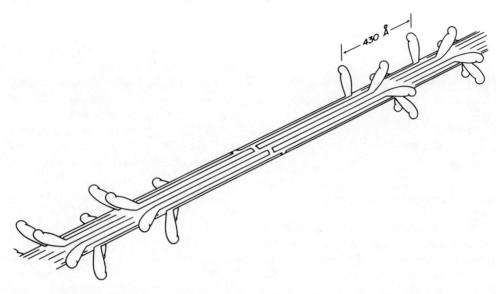

Fig. 38.4 Organization of thick filaments by tail-to-tail aggregation of myosin molecules. (From N. R. Alpert and B. B. Hamrell in *Cardiac Physiology for the Clinician*, M. Vassalle, Ed., Academic, New York, 1976, Chap. 7. Used with permission.)

also added, hydrolysis of ATP is inhibited. If Ca^{2+} is then added, in increasing concentrations, the effects of troponin–tropomyosin are progressively overcome. This effect is negligible at $10^{-7}\,M\,Ca^{2+}$ and complete at $10^{-5}\,M\,Ca^{2+}$ (Fig. 38.6), these being the respective concentrations of free Ca^{2+} that are believed to exist in the sarcomere during diastole and systole.

From experiments such as those de-scribed above and from X-ray crystallography studies, there has emerged the following concept of muscle contraction.

Following depolarization of the cell membrane, the levels of free Ca^{2+} in the cytoplasm rise from about $10^{-7}\,M$ to about $10^{-5}\,M$. Free Ca^{2+} enters the sarcomere where it combines with a subunit of troponin known as troponin C (TnC). This initiates a change in the conformation of

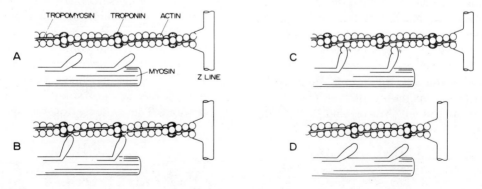

Fig. 38.5   Cyclic interaction of the globular myosin head with actin in the presence of high Ca^{2+} ($>10^{-5}\,M$), ATP, and Mg^{2+}. (From N. R. Alpert and B. B. Hamrell in *Cardiac Physiology for the Clinician*, M. Vassalle, Ed., Academic, New York, 1976. Used with permission.)

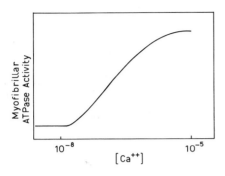

Fig. 38.6 Relationship between myofibrillar ATPase activity and Ca^{2+} concentration.

troponin that, in turn, promotes a change in the conformation of tropomyosin, thereby uncovering active sites in the helical groove of F-actin. Myosin heads containing bound ATP react with the uncovered sites to form cross bridges (Fig. 38.5B). This activates the ATPase at the tip of the myosin head. ATP is split and the energy liberated is converted to work in the form of changes in the angle of attachment of the myosin heads to actin (Fig. 38.5C) with a resultant sliding of the thin filaments into the thick filament matrix. The myosin heads then bind more ATP; this breaks the cross bridges and allows the heads to resume their former orientation (Fig. 38.5D), whereupon they recombine with a new active site on actin. The cycle continues for as long as the levels of Ca^{2+} remain elevated, and as many as 30 cycles may be performed during the course of one contraction. The process is terminated by a fall in the levels of free Ca^{2+} which results in the return of tropomyosin to its resting state in which it blocks the active sites on F-actin. A very lucid account of the events involved in muscle contraction together with key references, are given by Murray and Weber (6).

2.3   Uptake and Release of Calcium

There is no doubt that alteration in the levels of free intracellular Ca^{2+} is one of the key biological control mechanisms and seems to be related principally to the ability of Ca^{2+} to form bridges between anionic groups. This "structure forming" ability of Ca^{2+} can lead to conformational changes and molecular associations among macromolecules. Neurotransmitter–receptor interactions as well as various secretory processes appear to depend on the ability of Ca^{2+} to form ionic bridges between secretory vesicles and the plasma membrane. It is well established that the action of many hormones is mediated by stimulation of Ca^{2+} influx into cells. The control of the uptake and release of Ca^{2+} must therefore be recognized as an actual or potential instrument of drug action of great importance (7). Calcium ionophores, for example, promote insulin secretion by pancreatic cells, histamine release from basophils, and blast transformation by lymphocytes (8). For the heart, there is compelling evidence that the inotropic effects of the cardiac glycosides, the catecholamines, and agents such as dibutyryl 3,5-AMP are mediated by increased uptake of Ca^{2+}, whereas the cardiac depressant effects of verapamil (38. **2**) and lanthanum are due to inhibition of Ca^{2+} uptake (9). Under *in vitro* conditions, release of Ca^{2+} by the sarcoplasmic reticulum is facilitated by caffeine and blocked by procaine (10).

The mechanisms that control the movement of Ca^{2+} in the heart are not understood, and there is much conflicting evidence based on *in vitro* studies that may not be valid. The evidence for and against

38.2 Verapamil

the various theories is discussed in Refs. 8–13. Figure 38.7 shows the principal subcellular elements believed to be involved in Ca^{2+} storage and movement. A highly speculative representation of possible Ca^{2+} compartments and fluxes is shown in Fig. 38.8.

There is general agreement based on solid evidence that contraction is terminated by the transfer of Ca^{2+} from the sarcomere to the longitudinal tubules of the sarcoplasmic reticulum (SR). An ATP-dependent pump is required to transfer Ca^{2+} across the SR membrane. Some of the Ca^{2+} taken up by the SR is stored in the lateral and subsarcolemmal cisternae (Fig. 38.7) but some must be returned to the extracellular space to balance the uptake of Ca^{2+} that occurs during repolarization (Fig. 38.1). Movement of Ca^{2+} out of the cell is against the chemical gradient (see Fig. 38.8) and a pump is therefore required. It is not clear whether this applies to the outward movement of Ca^{2+} from the cisternae.

Unlike skeletal muscle, cardiac muscle

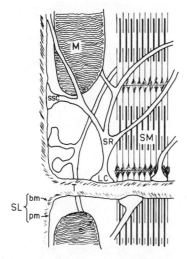

Fig. 38.7 Diagrammatic representation of a myocardial cell. M = Mitochondrion; SM = sarcomere; SR = sarcoplasmic reticulum; LC = longitudinal cisterna; SSC = subsarcolemmal cisterna; T = T-tubule; SL = sarcolemma, comprising a plasma membrane (pm) and a basement membrane (bm).

rapidly loses contractility when placed in a Ca^{2+}-free medium. It is clear from this and other evidence that extracellular Ca^{2+} plays a key role in the contraction–relaxation cycle. Some investigators believe that the increase in *free* intracellular Ca^{2+} that is needed to activate contraction is provided by Ca^{2+} drawn entirely from extracellular sources. Others believe that the influx of a small amount of extracellular Ca^{2+} stimulates the release of Ca^{2+} from intracellular stores such as those in the cisternae. The small amount of Ca^{2+} that enters the cell during phase 2 of the action potential is not sufficient to fully antagonize troponin so that some other process of Ca^{2+} uptake must be involved if extracellular Ca^{2+} is the sole source of activator Ca^{2+}. Specialized Ca^{2+} carriers (ionophores?) have been suggested as well as pinocytosis and electroneutral pumps involving exchange with either Na^+ or K^+. Various sites have been suggested as the sole or principal store of activator Ca^{2+}. Langer (12) believes that the principal store is the basement membrane of the sarcolemma. Hajdu and Leonard (8) have proposed the existence of a microdomain with a high Ca^{2+} concentration immediately external to the plasma membrane and maintained by an external pumping system or "calcium transport system." They believe that this system is operative in cardiac and skeletal muscle and possibly is general for all cells where Ca^{2+} fluxes are involved in the control of cell response. Schwartz (11) has suggested that activator Ca^{2+} may be stored by the plasma membrane and replenished, at least in part, by extracellular Ca^{2+}. This suggestion has the advantage of placing the store in a position that is under obvious control of the action potential as well as providing a unified theory to explain the action of digitalis (discussed below). Probably the most commonly held view is that activator Ca^{2+} is heterogeneous in origin, with the major portion being released from the cisternae of the SR in response to membrane

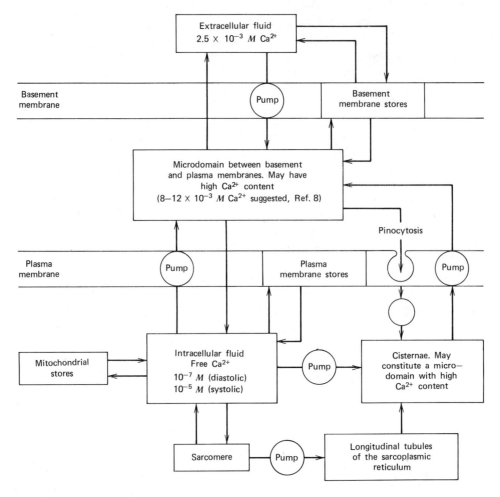

Fig. 38.8 Diagrammatic representation of the various stores and fluxes of Ca^{2+} that have been proposed for cells of the myocardium.

changes linked to depolarization of the plasma membrane (9, 10). It should be pointed out that the T system is part of the sarcolemma.

3 CARDIAC GLYCOSIDES AND RELATED INOTROPIC AGENTS

Inotropic agents are drugs that increase the force of muscle contraction. Drugs that exert an inotropic (or positive inotropic) effect on the heart are called cardiotonic agents and are divided into two classes on the basis of their mode of action. There are those that act by stimulating adenyl cyclase by either a direct effect on the enzyme system (tolbutamide, glucagon) or indirectly by stimulating the beta-adrenergic receptor (catecholamines), and there are those agents that act as cardiac glycosides do. The cardiotonic activity of the cardiac glycosides is qualitatively different from that of the catecholamines, and the two groups of drugs are used for different indications in treating heart disorders. It is interesting that both groups of drugs appear to affect the heart by altering the amount of Ca^{2+} available in the cytoplasm consequent to a primary effect at the cell membrane (9). In this chapter, only the cardiac gylcosides and related substances are discussed.

The cardiac glycosides are one of the oldest groups of drugs used in medicine. They occur naturally in a wide variety of plants and, in a nonglycoside form, in the poison of the toad. The glycosides from squill were used by the Egyptians and Romans who recognized the diuretic, emetic, and cardiotonic properties of this drug. Today the best known cardiac glycosides are those from digitalis, a genus of Scrophulariaceae found in Europe and Asia and known mainly by the species *Digitalis purpurea* or the purple foxglove. The first recorded reference to the medicinal properties of digitalis is believed to have been made in 1250, although the drug was used long before that in folk medicine, particularly by the Welsh. Because of its high toxicity and the variable content of its active principles, digitalis was rarely popular with physicians. The most notable exception was Dr. William Withering, who in 1785 published a remarkable book entitled *An Account of the Foxglove and Some of Its Medicinal Uses.* This work culminated 10 years of careful study and in it Withering described the indications for the use of the drug, the methods for establishing an appropriate dosage schedule by careful titration of the patient, and methods for collecting, preparing, and standardizing the drug. Unfortunately, his advice on how to use the drug was largely ignored and the drug fell again into disrepute until it was revived in the twentieth century. Withering believed that digitalis acted primarily as a diuretic but that it also had a profound effect on the heart and wrote, and is often quoted, "That it has a power over the motion of the heart, to a degree yet unobserved in any other medicine and that this power may be converted to salutary ends." It was not until the classic work of Cattell and Gold (14) in 1938 that it was firmly established that digitalis affected the heart primarily as a result of a direct effect on myocardial contractility.

3.1   Chemistry

3.1.1 CHEMICAL CLASSIFICATION.   Representative examples of digitalis-like cardiotonic agents are shown in Fig. 38.9; these substances may be classified into four groups.

The butenolides (also called cardenolides) contain an α,β-unsaturated lactone derived from 4-hydroxybutenoic acid (a butenolide) attached to the 17β position of a 14β-OH steroid. These agents are found in a wide variety of plants and occur usually as a glycoside. Glycosides are conjugation products of a sugar and a nonsugar portion called a genin or aglycone.

The pentadienolides (also called bufadienolides) contain a diunsaturated lactone derived from 5-hydroxypentadienoic acid (a pentadienolide) attached to the 17β position of a 14β-OH steroid. These agents are found in certain plants and in toad venom. Hellebrin (38.**5**) has been isolated from the roots of the Christmas rose and bufotalin (38.**6**) occurs both as the free genin and as the suberylarginine conjugate in the venom of the common toad *Bufo vulgaris*. Pentadienolides such as 38.**26**, 38.**27**, and 38.**28** (Fig. 38.11) occur in the bulb of the squill (*Urginea maritima* and *U. indica*, members of the Liliaceae family).

The alkaloids from Erythrophleum species are nitrogenous terpenes and, although they have a superficial resemblance to the butenolides and pentadienolides, they lack many of the structural features previously thought essential for digitalis-like activity.

The synthetic and semisynthetic digitalis analogs include a diverse group of structures, of which representative examples are shown in Fig. 38.9

Reviews of the chemistry of the cardiac glycosides and related substances are given in Refs. 15–20.

In spite of the diverse groups of structures shown in Fig. 38.9 and the promise that these hold for future therapeutic agents, only the butenolide gylcosides are used in medicine. More than 300 such cardiac glycosides have been isolated from natural products. They occur in plants usually in small amounts and as complex mixtures. The isolation, purification, and structure determination of these compounds constitute one of the great chapters in

BUTENOLIDES

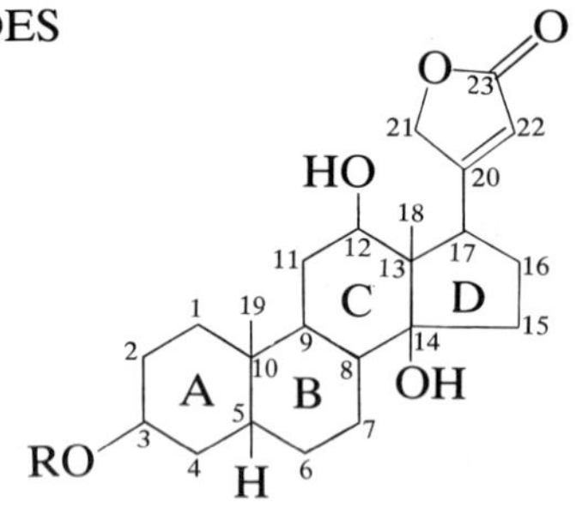

38.3 R = H: digoxigenin
38.4: R = (digitoxose)$_3$: digoxin

PENTADIENOLIDES

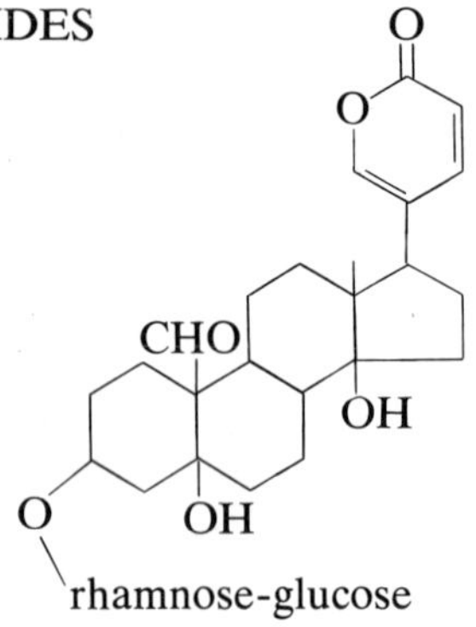

rhamnose-glucose

38.5 Hellebrin

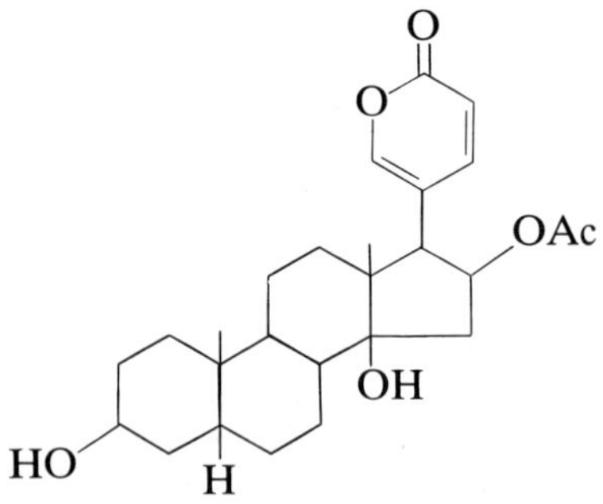

38.6 Bufotalin

ERYTHROPHLEUM ALKALOIDS

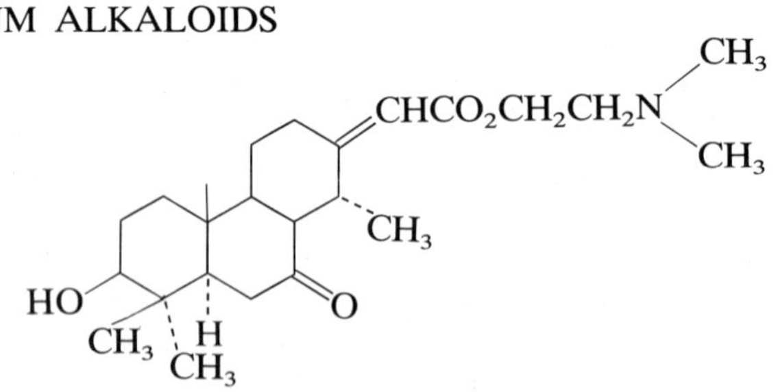

38.7 Cassaine

Fig. 38.9 A selection of substances with digitalis-like inotropic activity. Substituents shown connected to the ring system by a solid line have β orientation; those connected with a dotted line have α orientation.

SYNTHETIC AND SEMISYNTHETIC ANALOGS

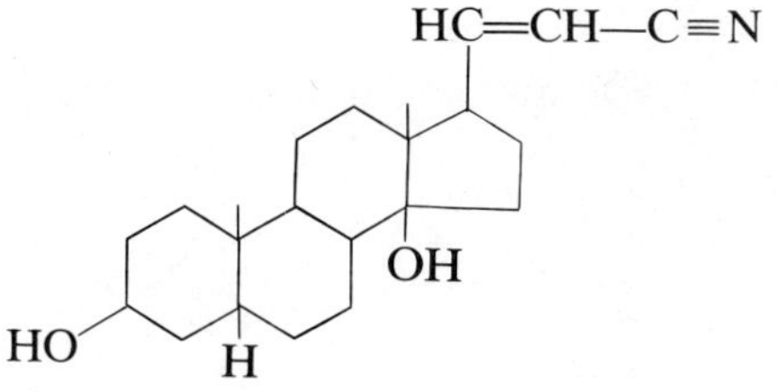

38.8

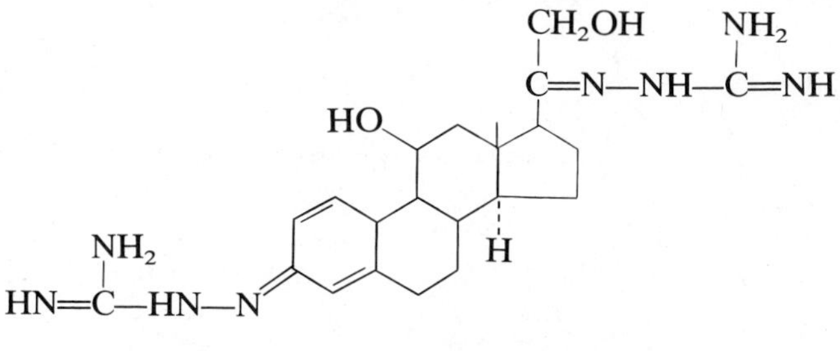

38.9   Prednisolone 3,20-bisguanylhydrazone

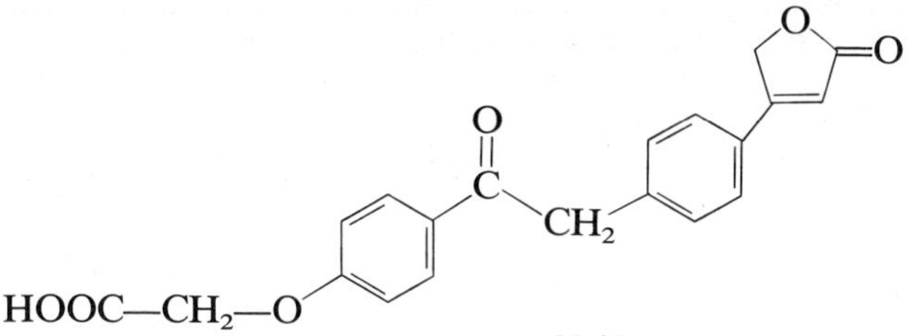

38.10

Fig. 38.9 (*Contd.*)

natural product chemistry (15–20). Of all these compounds, one glycoside, digoxin (38.4), is used almost exclusively. Lanatoside C (38.13) and ouabain (38.24) are still used but the use of digitoxin (38.17), once very popular in some countries, has virtually ceased.

3.1.2 DIGITALIS GLYCOSIDES. The digitalis glycosides belong to the butenolide class. They are obtained from a variety of digitalis species, principally from *Digitalis purpurea* (the purple foxglove) and *D. lanata* (the woolly foxglove), the latter being the source of digoxin.

The digitalis glycosides occur as complex mixtures which are divided into five series designated A, B, C, D, and E. All five series are present in *D. lanata*, where the parent or primary glycosides are referred to as lanatosides. Removal of one acetyl group and one glucose moiety yields the respective secondary glycosides, namely, digitoxin, gitoxin, digoxin, diginatin, and gitaloxin. *D. purpurea* contains only the A, B, and E series and the primary glycosides, referred to as purpurea glycosides, lack the acetyl group present in the lanatosides. The amorphous material gitalin refers to a mixture of purified glycosides obtained after cold water extraction of the leaves of *D. purpurea*. The reader's attention is drawn to the absence of digoxin in *D. purpurea*. The three principal series of digitalis glycosides (A, B, and C) are shown in Fig. 38.10).

The sources and structures of other well-known cardiac glycosides are shown in Fig. 38.11.

3.1.3 GENINS. The genins of the cardiac glycosides are distinguished from other steroids by three unusual features: a cis C/D ring junction, a 14β OH, and an α,β-unsaturated lactone attached to the 17β

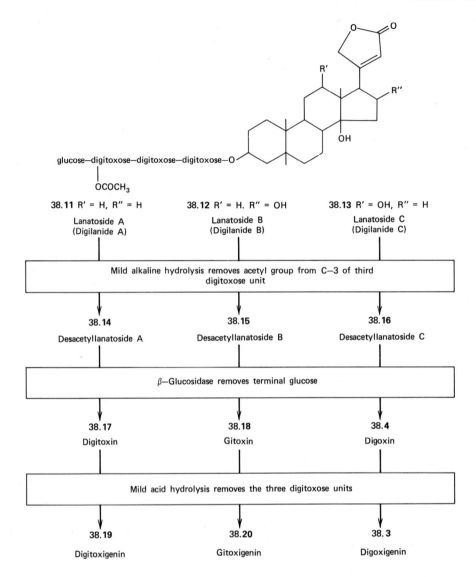

glucose–digitoxose–digitoxose–digitoxose–O

OCOCH₃

38.11 R′ = H, R″ = H	38.12 R′ = H. R″ = OH	38.13 R′ = OH, R″ = H
Lanatoside A (Digilanide A)	Lanatoside B (Digilanide B)	Lanatoside C (Digilanide C)

Mild alkaline hydrolysis removes acetyl group from C–3 of third digitoxose unit

38.14	38.15	38.16
Desacetyllanatoside A	Desacetyllanatoside B	Desacetyllanatoside C

β–Glucosidase removes terminal glucose

38.17	38.18	38.4
Digitoxin	Gitoxin	Digoxin

Mild acid hydrolysis removes the three digitoxose units

38.19	38.20	38.3
Digitoxigenin	Gitoxigenin	Digoxigenin

Fig. 38.10   Glycosides of the A, B, and C series present in *D. lanata*. This plant also contains glycosides of the D and E series. Glycosides of the A and B series are also found in *D. purpurea* where the primary glycosides (known as purpurea glycosides) are identical with desacetyllanatosides A and B.

position. If any of these features is changed, most or all of the biological activity is lost. In addition, almost all genins contain a cis A/B ring junction. A trans A/B ring junction is found in a few genins such as uzarigenin and in some cases this causes loss in biological activity. The simplest genin is digitoxigenin, and this molecule serves to illustrate the effect of the above structural features on the shape of the molecule. Figure 38.12 compares the shape of digitoxigenin with that of cholestanol, a steroid in which all ring junctions are trans. All naturally occurring cardiotonic genins possess a 3-OH group which must be β-oriented in the A/B cis series for biological activity. The sugars are attached to the genin through the 3-oxygen

Glycosides from the Seeds of *Strophanthus kombé*

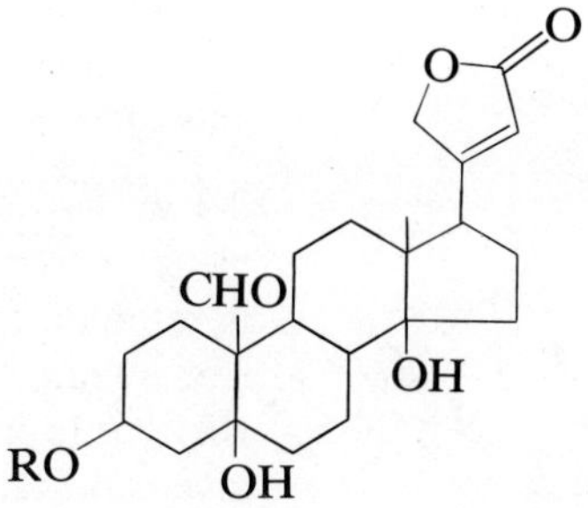

38.**21** R = glucose-cymarose: *k*-strophanthoside
38.**22** R = cymarose: k-β-strophanthin
38.**23** R = H: strophanthidin (the genin)

Glycosides from the Seeds of *Strophanthus gratus*

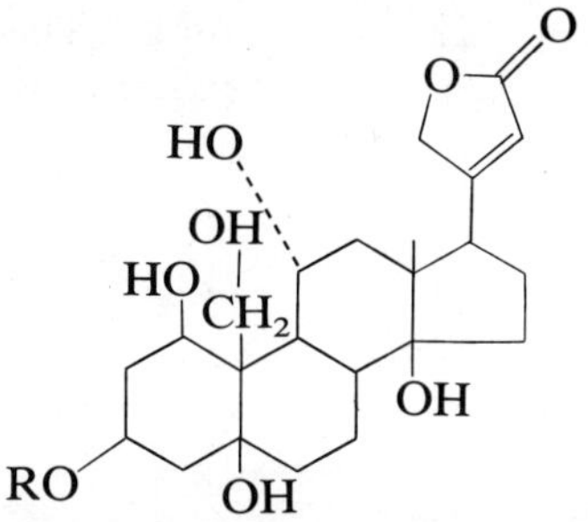

38.**24** R = rhamnose: g-strophanthin (ouabain)
38.**25** R = H: g-strophanthidin (ouabagenin)

Glycosides from the Bulbs of *Urginea maritima* (White Squill) and *U. indica* (Indian squill)

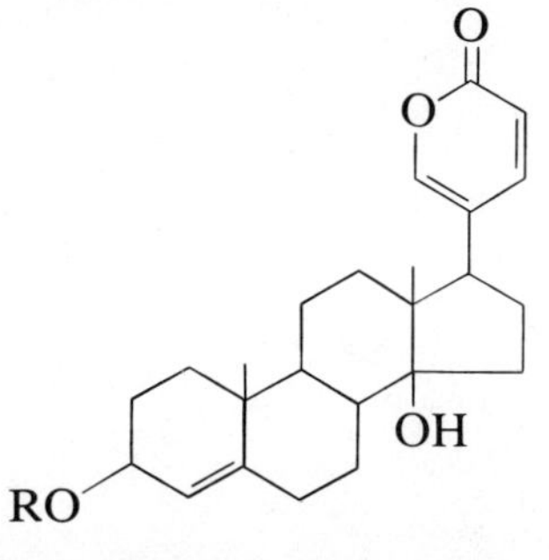

38.**26** R = glucose-rhamnose: scillaren A
38.**27** R = rhamnose: proscillaridin A
38.**28** R = H: scillaridin A (the genin)

Fig. 38.11 Structures and sources of some cardiac glycosides used in medicine. Refer to Fig. 38.14 for structural formulas of sugar components.

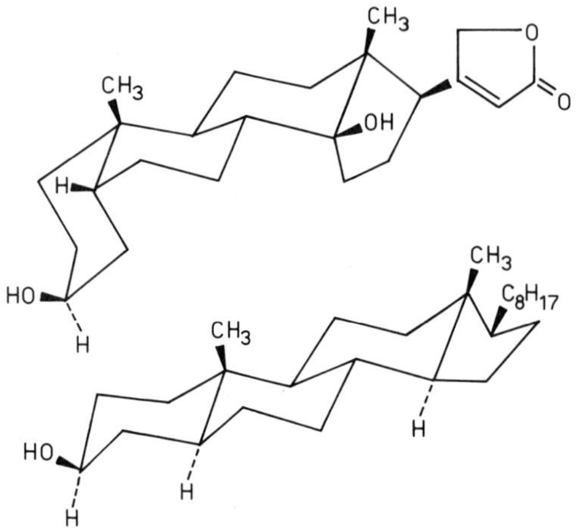

Fig. 38.12 Stereochemistry of digitoxigenin (top) and cholestanol (bottom). The ring junctions of digitoxigenin are cis/trans/cis, whereas those of cholestanol are all trans.

function and are cleaved with varying degrees of ease by acid-catalyzed hydrolysis. Some important reactions of genins are shown in Fig. 38.13.

3.1.4 SUGARS. When the sugars are cleaved from the genins, biological activity is retained by the latter but is absent in the free sugars. In spite of this, the sugars play a key role in modulating the activity of the glycoside to such an extent that the genins are quite unsatisfactory as therapeutic agents. The reasons for this are examined below.

The number of sugar units in cardiac glycosides varies from one to four. Digoxin, for example, contains three digitoxose units. The sugars are invariably in the pyranose form and the attachment to the

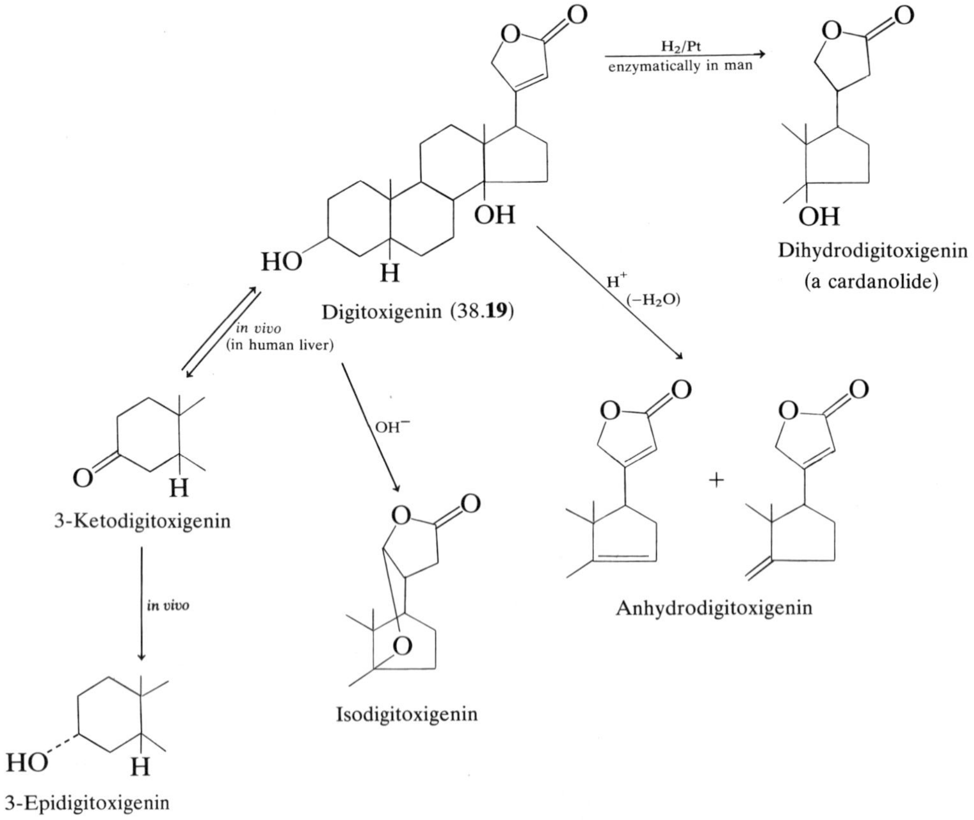

Fig. 38.13 Chemistry of digitoxigenin.

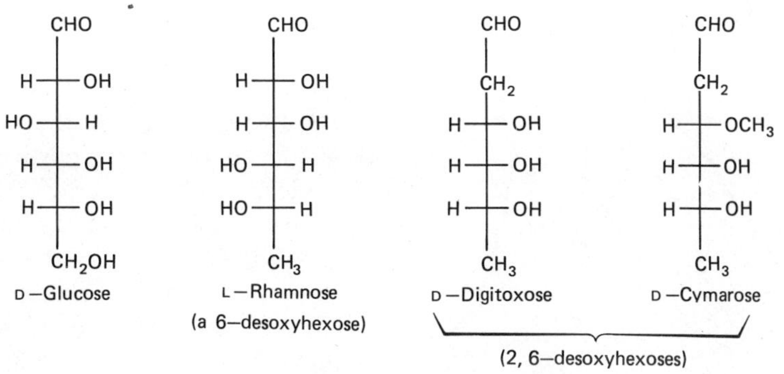

```
      CHO                CHO                CHO                CHO
       |                  |                  |                  |
  H —— OH            H —— OH             CH₂                CH₂
       |                  |                  |                  |
 HO —— H             H —— OH            H —— OH            H —— OCH₃
       |                  |                  |                  |
  H —— OH            HO —— H            H —— OH            H —— OH
       |                  |                  |                  |
  H —— OH            HO —— H            H —— OH            H —— OH
       |                  |                  |                  |
     CH₂OH              CH₃                CH₃                CH₃
   D –Glucose        L –Rhamnose        D –Digitoxose       D –Cymarose
                   (a 6–desoxyhexose)
                                      _____    _____/
                                                   (2, 6–desoxyhexoses)
```

Fig. 38.14 Selection of sugar components of naturally occurring cardiac glycosides. Among the large range of such sugars are fully oxygenated sugars such as glucose; monodesoxy sugars such as rhamnose; bisdesoxy sugars such as digitoxose and cymarose; and methylated sugars such as cymarose. Sugars of both D and L series are found, and amino sugars have been recently reported. The sugars usually occur in the pyranose form.

genin is β for D sugars. A selection of sugars found in cardiac glycosides is shown in Fig. 38.14.

3.2 Biological Activity

3.2.1 NATURE OF THE INOTROPIC RESPONSE. In this and subsequent sections, the term digitalis is used in a generic sense to encompass all cardiotonic agents that act as the digitalis glycosides do. The pharmacology of digitalis involves a complex set of interactions between the direct and indirect effects of the drug and the pathophysiology of the patient. Such considerations are beyond the scope of this article and the reader is referred to textbooks of pharmacology (e.g., Ref. 21) for an account of the spectrum of effects of digitalis on the normal and failing heart. Some accounts of the clinical pharmacology of digitalis are given in Refs. 22–36. The reader is cautioned that many of the practical aspects of digitalis use are being redefined; the problem is discussed in Ref. 35. A good account of the indications and contraindications for digitalis therapy is given by Duca and Brest (32).

Digitalis acts directly on the myocardium to produce an increase in contractility (positive inotropic effect). In the failing di-lated heart this leads to a decrease in size and an increase in cardiac output. The efficiency of the failing heart is increased as a result of an improvement in the force–length relationship as defined by the Starling curve. The inotropic effect of digitalis is manifested in both normal and failing hearts, although in the former, increased output may be offset by physiological compensation. Digitalis also causes an increase in myocardial excitability and automaticity resulting in the development of arrhythmias. Digitalis can increase the refractory period of the myocardium; such effects in the atrioventricular node may protect the ventricles from excessive stimuli in atrial tachyarrhythmias but may also lead to excessive bradycardia and even complete heart block. Highly toxic doses of digitalis produce a paradoxical electrophysiological effect in which there is a decrease in excitability, leading to block, and a decrease in refractory period, allowing re-entry phenomena and thus the development of highly dangerous arrhythmias including fibrillation. Finally, digitalis increases vagal activity leading to a decrease in the atrial refractory period, a delay in atrioventricular conduction, and bradycardia. In the failing heart, digitalis also induces a reflex mediated reduction in rate as a consequence of improved output. In summary, the

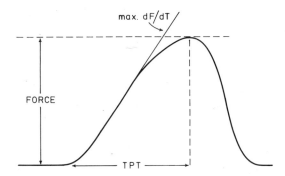

Fig. 38.15 Facsimile of a recorder tracing of a single isometric twitch of cardiac muscle. Developed force or tension (represented by the height of the tracing) is a function of the intensity of the active state and the time to peak tension (TPT). The intensity of the active state is directly proportional to the maximum first derivative of the rate of tension development (max dF/dt). Digitalis-like compounds increase dF/dt but reduce TPT; that is, force develops at a faster rate but for a shorter duration.

main therapeutic property of digitalis is its inotropic action. Other responses such as increase in cardiac output, decrease in cardiac enlargement, reduction in heart rate, fall in venous pressure, and improvement in renal function are consequent to the positive inotropic effect. An inotropic effect can arise by increasing either the duration or the intensity of the active state. This is shown diagrammatically in Fig. 38.15. Digitalis shortens the duration of the active state and if this alone occurred it would produce a negative inotropic effect. However, digitalis also increases the intensity of the active state (dF/dt), and it is this property that leads to its inotropic action. Any hypothesis for the mechanism of digitalis activity must explain this effect.

3.2.2 BIOCHEMICAL PHARMACOLOGY. The mode of action of digitalis has been the subject of intensive study. Some recent reviews of this work are given in Refs. 37–43. In spite of significant progress, there remains much conflicting evidence and many uncertainties about the mode of action of digitalis. There is also a major conceptual problem: are the toxic effects of digitalis an extension of the therapeutic effects or are they mediated by some different mechanism? If the latter is the case, then the question of whether a particular biochemical effect is related to the therapeutic or to the toxic effects of digitalis becomes crucial. Likewise, in the design of experiments, the question of what is a therapeutic level and what is a toxic level is extremely important. Unfortunately, many investigators have disregarded the complex pharmacokinetics of digitalis, have worked with doses that are too high, and have not allowed sufficient time for both pharmacokinetic and pharmacodynamic equilibration to occur.

Although digitalis increases the efficiency of the failing heart, it appears to have no direct effects on mitochondria or on the uptake of energy yielding substrates. Nor does it have any direct effects on the contractile elements within the sarcomere. Digitalis does not appear to reverse any biochemical "defect" associated with heart failure. There is reasonable evidence indicating that low output heart failure may be associated with decreased actomyosin ATPase activity but digitalis does not affect this enzyme. Other suggested abnormalities include defects in the sarcoplasmic reticulum Ca^{2+} pump, reduction in the levels of high energy phosphate compounds, and abnormalities in the membrane action potential. The evidence connecting these defects with congestive heart failure is not consistent, and, in any event, their reversal cannot be related to digitalis action. There is a fair body of evidence that indicates that digitalis acts on the extracellular face of the cell membrane. Digitoxin–albumin conjugates, for example, were found to be inotropic, and this would indicate that penetration into the cell was not necessary for biological activity. Digoxin antibodies were found to reverse both the inotropic and the toxic effects of digoxin, the antibody being bound to the cell membrane. Cytochemical studies, though far from reliable, confirm that little or no glycoside enters the cell. It should be pointed out that a minority of workers believe that the glycosides act intracellularly and that small amounts are carried into the cell by active transport.

The bulk of evidence supports the view that both the toxic and the therapeutic effects of digitalis are mediated through an effect on the cell membrane. This would infer an effect on either excitation or on the mechanism that links excitation with contraction.

From a consideration of the issues raised in Section 2, and inasmuch as digitalis does not affect the actual contractile elements within the sarcomere, the most likely mechanism for the inotropic effects of digitalis is an increase in the level of activator Ca^{2+}. Increasing levels of free intracellular Ca^{2+} (Fig. 38.6) produce a positive inotropic effect that is identical to that produced by digitalis (Fig. 38.15). Calcium and digitalis have synergistic effects that suggest a common action. Although the measurement of ion fluxes in the myocardium is difficult, there is a substantial body of evidence to suggest that therapeutic levels of digitalis produce an increase in the rate of Ca^{2+} uptake (13). Of considerable significance are observations that show that the inotropic effects of digitalis are not manifested under conditions in which intracellular Ca^{2+} availability is maximum (9).

Most workers in the field agree that digitalis produces its characteristic inotropic effect by increasing the levels of activator Ca^{2+}. The various stores and fluxes of Ca^{2+} depicted in Fig. 38.8 suggest a variety of mechanisms whereby digitalis could increase the levels of free intracellular Ca^{2+}. Most of these mechanisms have been postulated in one form or another, and a few are considered here. The most common but by no means the only starting point is the known effect of digitalis on the Na^+,K^+ pump (Na^+,K^+-ATPase) (see Fig. 38.1 and Section 2.1). The interaction of digitalis with this enzyme is discussed in more detail

in Section 3.3.3. For the moment it need only be stated that this enzyme is located in the plasma membrane and that digitalis binds to its external face. This results in inhibition of the active transport of Na^+ and K^+. Therapeutic doses of digitalis are believed to inhibit a moderate percentage of total pump units so that the *rate* at which Na^+ and K^+ are restored to steady-state levels following repolarization is slowed (Fig. 38.1). This effect has been linked with increased levels of activator Ca^{2+} in a number of ways. Langer (41) and several other investigators have suggested that Ca^{2+} influx is increased by increasing levels of intracellular Na^+. Schön et al. (44) have suggested that Na^+,K^+-ATPase actively transports Ca^{2+} out of the cell. Inhibition of the enzyme would therefore lead to inhibition of Ca^{2+} efflux and hence to higher intracellular levels of Ca^{2+}. By means of lanthanum displacement, Nayler (45) has demonstrated that ouabain increases the amount of Ca^{2+} stored on the outer face of the plasma membrane. Gervais et al. (46) have published findings suggesting that the phospholipid component of Na^+,K^+-ATPase binds Ca^{2+} and that ouabain can alter the Ca^{2+} binding constant in various ways. There is also evidence that digitalis may interact with Na^+,K^+-ATPase so as to stabilize a form which promotes a Ca^{2+} influx/K^+ efflux exchange. It should also be pointed out that the sarcolemma invaginates in many cardiac cells to form T-tubes (Fig. 38.7). This locates many membrane-associated phenomena deep within the fiber. The various cisternae shown in Fig. 38.7 may well contain the principal store of activator Ca^{2+}. The close association of these cisternae with the plasma membrane suggests the possibility that plasma membrane components in the region of the cisternae may execute a specialized function in initiating a Ca^{2+} release process.

In summary, it seems that the inotropic effects of digitalis result from an increase in the levels of activator Ca^{2+}, resulting from a mechanism yet to be established, but in which Na^+,K^+-ATPase is strongly implicated. The toxic effects of digitalis could result from either excessive influx of Ca^{2+} or excessive loss of K^+, or both.

3.2.3 NA^+,K^+-ATPASE: THE DIGITALIS RECEPTOR?.

Na^+, K^+-ATPase has already been defined (Section 2) as a membrane-bound, Mg^{2+}-dependent ATPase that is activated by certain concentrations of Na^+ and K^+ and is specifically inhibited by digitalis. This enzyme appears to exist in the plasma membranes of all animal cells where it plays a key role in maintaining the high K^+/Na^+ ratio that is characteristic of the intracellular fluid. It is particularly abundant in kidney and excitable tissue. Regardless of whether it mediates the effects of digitalis on contractility there is no doubt that Na^+,K^+-ATPase binds digitalis under both *in vivo* and *in vitro* conditions and that the binding site meets the criteria for a specific drug receptor. Since very few authentic drug receptors have been isolated, the properties of Na^+,K^+-ATPase are of considerable interest to the medicinal chemist.

The enzyme was first isolated by Skou (47) in 1957 and since then has been the subject of several thousand publications. Comprehensive reviews are given in Refs. 40 and 48–50. Na^+,K^+-ATPase probably evolved very early in the history of life to serve the primitive function of maintaining osmotic equilibrium. Subsequently, evolving species utilized the uneven distribution of Na^+ and K^+ across the cell membrane to carry out several specialized functions such as the conduction of impulses along nerve and muscle membranes. Because of its involvement in so many processes, it has been estimated that up to 30% of the energy of resting respiration is devoted to the Na^+,K^+ pump.

Although purified Na^+,K^+-ATPase has yet to be obtained from myocardium (52), the purified enzyme has been obtained from other tissues and shown to contain two catalytic subunits, each with a molecular weight of about 95,000 plus a glycoprotein subunit with a molecular weight of 55,000. The amino acid content for the above proteins has been determined and shown to be remarkably constant for a variety of quite different species suggesting that no drastic changes have been made to these proteins throughout evolution. Purified Na^+,K^+-ATPase contains about one-third by weight of phospholipid. The main phospholipids are phosphatidyl choline, phosphatidyl ethanolamine, and phosphatidyl serine. It is clear that phospholipids are required for Na^+,K^+-ATPase activity because activity is lost when the phospholipids are removed and can be restored by adding back the phospholipids.

In summary, Na^+,K^+-ATPase appears to consist of two large polypeptides which have catalytic (i.e., ATP splitting) activity plus one smaller glycoprotein unit, whose role has yet to be defined, and a block of supporting phospholipids. The whole system constitutes the Na^+,K^+ pump and extends across the full width of the plasma membrane. It has been established that the pump is spatially oriented so that the site for splitting ATP and for subsequent phosphorylization of the enzyme is on the inner face of the membrane and the site for binding digitalis is on the outer face. The inner face also contains binding sites with high affinity for Na^+ and Ca^{2+} and the outer face contains binding sites with high affinity for K^+. Although the role of the glycoprotein has not been determined, it has been suggested that it may serve to orient the enzyme in the membrane bilayer. In those tissues in which it is easy to study ion fluxes, the stoichiometry of the pump has been clearly established as three Na^+ out to two K^+ in, giving a net loss of cations to the intracellular fluid. There is mounting evidence that this ratio, or something close to it, applies to all tissues.

There has been much study of the kinetics of Na^+,K^+-ATPase and this can be summarized by the following series of reactions:

$$E_1 + Mg.ATP \xrightleftharpoons{Na_i^+} (E_1P) - Na + ADP \tag{38.1}$$

$$(E_1P) - Na \xrightleftharpoons{(Mg^{2+})?} (E_2P) + Na_o^+ \tag{38.2}$$

$$H_2O + (E_2P) \xrightleftharpoons{K_o^+} (E_2K) + P_i \tag{38.3}$$

$$E_2K \rightleftharpoons E_2 + K_i^+ \tag{38.4}$$

$$E_2 \xrightarrow{ATP} E_1 \tag{38.5}$$

E_1 and E_2 represent different states of the enzyme, Na_i, K_i, Na_o, and K_o represent intracellular and extracellular Na^+ and K^+, and P_i represents inorganic phosphate. The model suggests that the binding of various ligands induces major conformational changes in the enzyme which result in the outward transport of Na^+ and the inward transport of K^+. Direct evidence that the pump elements undergo major conformational changes has been obtained. Digitalis inhibits this system apparently by binding to the E_2P form of the enzyme. The model predicts that the proportion of the enzyme in the E_2P state is increased by Na^+ and decreased by K^+.

The increase in rate of digitalis binding by Na^+ and decrease by K^+ support the suggestion that the digitalis receptor is associated with the E_2P state (48). It also explains the clinical observation that the effects of digitalis are enhanced by Na^+ and antagonized by K^+. Studies of the key amino acids of the catalytic site have indicated that serine, threonine, aspartic acid, lysine, and cysteine are involved in binding ATP to the enzyme (50). The involvement of these amino acids is shown in Fig. 38.16. This figure also shows the digitalis receptor as being on the outer face of the high molecular weight subunit of the pump. This

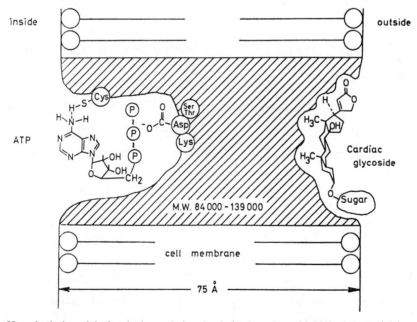

Fig. 38.16 Hypothetical model of a single catalytic subunit (mol wt about 90,000) of the Na^+, K^+ pump. Shown are receptors for ATP on the inner face of the subunit and for digitalis on the outer face. (From W. Schoner, H. Pauls, and R. Patzelt-Wenczler, in *Myocardial Failure*, G. Riecker, A. Weber, and J. Goodwin, Eds., Springer-Verlag, Berlin–Heidelberg, 1977, p. 107. Used with permission.)

location for the digitalis receptor has been assumed for several years but has now been confirmed using purified reconstituted enzyme.

Earlier, it was mentioned that Na^+,K^+-ATPase contains two high molecular weight proteins plus one glycoprotein. Recent evidence from several laboratories has established that these units appear to work in a coordinated fashion. Schoner and co-workers (51) have proposed the oscillating system shown in Fig. 38.17 in which $E_1 - E_2$ converts to $E_2 - E_1$. As described for equations 38.1–38.5, E_1 has high affinity for ATP and low affinity for digitalis, whereas the reverse applies to E_2. It is suggested that each time the system interconverts from $E_1 - E_2$ to $E_2 - E_1$, a channel is opened and Na^+ and K^+ are transported. Once digitalis is bound, the system is frozen; no more oscillations can occur and hence no more ion transport can take place. It is interesting that all pore and transport proteins consist of at least two protein subunits, suggesting the presence of a water-filled channel which opens and shuts in accord with changes in the conformations of the transport proteins.

There is no doubt about the existence of a digitalis receptor on Na^+,K^+-ATPase. There is dispute as to whether this is the receptor that mediates the effects of digitalis on contractility. The proposition that the contractility effects of digitalis are mediated by inhibition of myocardial Na^+,K^+-ATPase was first suggested by Repke in 1961 (53). The hypothesis has remained controversial and the evidence for and against has been summarized by Schwartz (42) and, more recently, by Akera (54) and Akera and Brody (55). In support of the proposal is a large body of circumstantial evidence (summarized in Table 38.1) which shows a fairly consistent parallelism between the inotropic effects of digitalis and its ability to inhibit Na^+,K^+-ATPase. This parallelism applies to species differences, structure–activity relationships, time-dependent factors, and the effects of other ligands that modify digitalis action. In addition, inotropic doses of digitalis have been shown to produce *in vivo* inhibition of Na^+,K^+-ATPase. The theory is supported by evidence (previously discussed) that the contractility effects of digitalis appear to result from an effect on the external face of

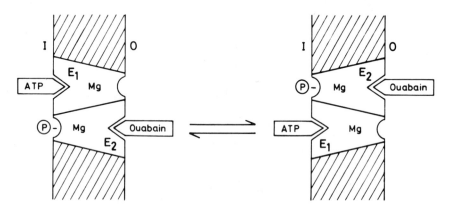

Fig. 38.17 Possible coordinated conformational changes in the catalytic subunits of the Na^+,K^+ pump. It is suggested that when one monomer is in the E_1 conformation, the other monomer must, of necessity, take the E_2 conformation. Coordinated changes from the $E_1 - E_2$ to the $E_2 - E_1$ arrangement open a pore through which Na^+ and K^+ are transported. Digitalis, by binding to a receptor found only on the E_2 conformation, "freezes" the system so that further conformational changes are prevented and, consequently, the transport pore remains closed. (From W. Schoner, H. Pauls, and R. Patzelt-Wenczler, in *Myocardial Failure*, G. Riecker, A. Weber, and J. Goodwin, Eds., Springer-Verlag, Berlin–Heidelberg, 1977, p. 115. Used with permission.)

the cell membrane and by evidence which supports a link between inhibition of Na^+,K^+-ATPase and transient increases in the levels of free intracellular Ca^{2+}. Even so, it must be recognized that the weak point in this theory is that definitive evidence of a link between Na^+,K^+-ATPase inhibition and the release of activator Ca^{2+} has not been obtained. The arguments against the proposal have centered mainly on the question of whether therapeutic levels of digitalis produce significant inhibition of the enzyme *in vivo* or, if they do, whether there is a cause and effect relationship. It is clear that the therapeutic and toxic manifestations of digitalis overlap and it is argued that the inhibition of Na^+,K^+-ATPase associated with therapeutic doses of digitalis is really a subphysiological manifestation of toxicity and is unrelated to inotropy. It should also be pointed out that the dose of digitalis used in man is much lower than what is customarily used in experimental animals. Therapeutic effects of digoxin in man are associated with plasma drug levels of the order of $1–2 \times 10^{-9}\,M$ and toxic effects with drug levels only twice as high. At such low levels of drug, it takes several days for the subject to become digitalized.

3.3 Structure–Activity Relationships

The structural formulas of most of the naturally occurring cardiac glycosides were determined during the first six decades of this century, although published investigations into the chemical nature of these substances go back to 1808, and work is still in progress. The first laboratory synthesis of a cardiotonic genin was achieved in 1962 by Sondheimer (20), thereby culminating almost 30 years of continuous endeavor by various groups. This gives some idea of the difficult nature of cardiac glycoside chemistry and explains why the classical structure–activity relationship (SAR) studies were limited to natural products and a few of their simple derivatives. These studies (56a, 56b) established the idea that significant digitalis-like activity is to be found only with 14β-OH steroids substituted, in the 17β position, with a lactone of the butenolide or pentadienolide type. The unique stereochemistry of this class of compound is illustrated by digitoxigenin (Fig. 38.12). These features were still being described (19) as "essential for cardiac activity" as late as 1969 in spite of the known digitalis-like activity of the erythrophleum alkaloids such as cassaine (38.7) and the

Table 38.1 Relationship between Binding of Digitalis to Na^+,K^+-ATPase *in vitro* and Positive Inotropic Action[a]

Parameter	Binding *in vitro*	Inotropic Action
Onset rate	Slow	Slow
	Inhibited by K^+	Delayed by K^+
	Stimulated by Na^+	Facilitated by Na^+
	Dependent on intracellular Na^+	Dependent on depolarizations
	No species difference	No species difference
Equilibrium	Glycosides: slightly decreased by K^+	Glycosides: slightly decreased by K^+
	Aglycones: markedly decreased by K^+	Aglycones: markedly decreased by K^+
	Marked species difference	Marked species difference
Offset rate	Dependent on chemical structure	Dependent on chemical structure
	Delayed by K^+	Delayed by K^+
	Marked species difference	Marked species difference

[a] From T. Akera, *Science*, **198,** 569 (1977).

report in 1964 that bisguanylhydrazones such as 38.**9** have pronounced digitalis-like activity (57, 58). There now exists a large body of work dealing with synthetic and semisynthetic digitalis analogs. Thomas et al. (43) have reviewed the literature on this subject up till 1974.

The objectives for synthesizing new digitalis-like substances should be stated. They are as follows.

1. To produce a less toxic compound. Digitalis is one of the most toxic compounds in common use (59). It is responsible for one of the highest rates of drug-induced death and one of the highest rates of drug-induced hospital admission.

2. To define the nature of the digitalis receptor and to develop tools for studying various biological processes such as the control of transmembrane ion fluxes and the nature of the link between excitation and contraction in the heart.

3. To develop new categories of drug activity. This possibility arises because of the universal distribution of Na^+,K^+-ATPase in body tissues. Selective effects on nerve, brain, kidney, and smooth muscle, for example, may give rise to new therapeutic agents.

A few of the major developments in synthetic digitalis analogs are now discussed. Claims have been made for improvement in therapeutic ratio for some of these compounds; it is my opinion that these claims, though possibly correct, are based on inadequate testing procedures and may reflect differential *rates* of distribution within the myocardium. Therapeutic ratios are meaningful only if measurements are taken *after* tissue distribution and equilibration are complete. This is a long and complex procedure in the intact animal.

Various possible mechanisms could form the basis of a partial or complete separation of the toxic and therapeutic effects of dig-

italis. These include (1) mediation of these effects by different mechanisms (so far there is no firm evidence for accepting this proposition); (2) achievement of a *selective* reduction in steady-state levels of drug in the ventricular conducting tissue (this being the site of origin of most of the clinical manifestations of digitalis toxicity); (3) reduction in the extracardiac activity which contributes to digitalis toxicity in the heart (effects of digitalis on peripheral and central nervous systems).

In 1972, Thomas and co-workers developed procedures for replacing the lactone of digitoxigenin with open chain structures to produce a series of compounds with a wide range of biological activity extending from compounds with inotropic activity comparable to the parent compound, digitoxigenin, to compounds that were inactive or had a negative inotropic effect (reviewed in Ref. 43). The structures and biological activity of a selection of these compounds are shown in Fig. 38.18. Neglecting for the moment the guanylhydrazone (38.**35**), it seems that the essential requirement for the isosteric replacement of the lactone is the following coplanar arrangement of atoms: $-CH{=}CH-C(R){=}A$, where A is a hetero atom. Activity falls if R is larger than OCH_3 (for example, 38.**33**), suggesting that the receptor may lie within a cleft or that R extends into a hydrophilic region. Neither the R group nor the ester is essential, as shown by the high activity of the nitrile (38.**34**). As with the lactone, activity is lost if the olefinic group is reduced (38.**30**), which could infer that the resonance-induced fractional positive charge on the β carbon atom is important. Activity is almost abolished if the conjugated system is extended (38.**32**) confirming the importance of the $-CH{=}CH-C(R){=}A$ system. From considerations such as these, a model was proposed to describe that portion of the digitalis receptor that accommodates the C-17 side chain (Fig. 38.19). The essential features

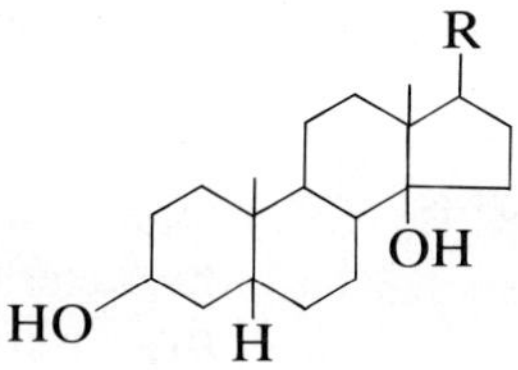

| | | Biological Activity (60) (Relative Potency) | |
No.	R	Positive Inotropic Effects	Inhibition of Na^+,K^+-ATPase
38.**19**	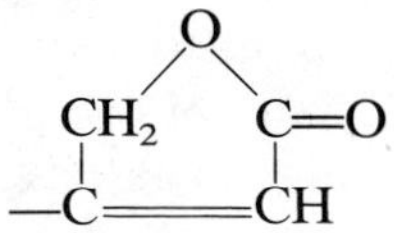 (digitoxigenin)	100	100
38.**29**	$-CH=CH-C=O$ (with OCH_3), β, α	50	130
38.**30**	$-CH_2-CH_2-C=O$ (with OCH_3)	Inactive	Inactive
38.**31**	$-CH=CH-C=O$ (with OH)	Inactive	Inactive
38.**32**	$-CH=CH-CH=CH-C=O$ (with OCH_3)	0.4	3
38.**33**	$-CH=CH-C=O$ (with OCH_2CH_3)	3	9
38.**34**	$-CH=CH-C\equiv N$	70	110
38.**35**	$-CH=N-NH-C=NH$ (with NH_2)	20	14
38.**36**	$-CH=N-NH-C=O$ (with NH_2)	Inactive	Inactive

Fig. 38.18 Replacement of the lactone of digitoxigen with open chain moieties of varying steric and electronic resemblance to the lactone. (From Thomas et al., Ref. 58.)

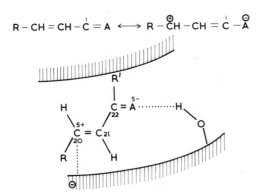

Fig. 38.19 Proposed interaction of the C-17 side chain of active cardenolide analogs with the "digitalis" receptor. The side chain is shown as lying within a cleft on the enzyme surface. Binding is depicted as involving two points on the side chain, the electron-rich hetero atom (A) and the electron-deficient C-20. The origin of the charge distribution in the side chain is shown by the resonance structures drawn above the receptor model. The scheme is compatible with SAR analyses based on both inhibition of Na^+,K^+-ATPase and positive inotropic effects. (From R. Thomas, J. Boutagy, and A. Gelbart, *J. Pharm. Sci.*, **63**, 1649 (1974). Used with permission.)

of this model are a two-point attachment involving electrostatic interactions between the side chain and the receptor, together with certain steric restraints limiting the width of the side chain.

A nucleophilic site, possibly a full negative charge, is postulated for the receptor surface, partly to explain the apparent importance of the fractional positive charge on the side chain but also to account for the activity of the acid (38.**31**) and the guanylhydrazone (38.**35**). The acid has the necessary —CH=CH—C(R)=A system but is completely inactive. Since the acid is ionized at biologic pH, its negative charge would be repelled by the negative charge proposed for the receptor. On the other hand, the guanylhydrazone (38.**35**) is biologically active although it lacks the side chain common to other active members of the series. However, the guanylhydrazone is a strong base and exists as a cation. It is therefore capable of undergoing a strong ion-pair association with the proposed

anionic site on the receptor. This reasoning can be extended to explain the powerful digitalis-like activity of the bisguanylhydrazones such as prednisolone bisguanylhydrazone (38.**9**) shown in Fig. 38.9. Although these compounds do not possess the steroid system thought to be essential by earlier investigators (refer to Fig. 38.12), they possess two powerful electrophilic groups at each end of the molecule. The group at C-17 would interact with the anionic group in the proposed model (Fig. 38.19) and there is reason to believe that a reactive nucleophilic group exists in the region of the receptor that would bind the C-3 guanylhydrazone moiety (61). Thus the digitalis-like activity of compounds such as prednisolone bisguanylhydrazone may be explained in terms of two powerful interactions at binding sites at each end of the receptor. This would infer that the nature of the steroid system for such compounds would not be critical, and this has been confirmed (62).

The model shown in Fig. 38.19 is also compatible with the established SAR for the erythrophleum alkaloids (reviewed in Ref. 43). Cassaine (38.**7**) and its active analogs possess the required $>$C=CH— C(R)=A grouping (in this case —C(R)=A is an ester). As with the compounds shown in Fig. 38.18, activity is lost when the ester is hydrolyzed to give the free acid or when the double bond is reduced. Beard et al. (63) have shown that it is possible to replace the C-17 lactone of digitoxigenin with the amino-ester side chain of cassaine (—CH=CH—COOCH$_2$CH$_2$N(CH$_3$)$_2$) to yield an analog with high digitalis-like activity and an apparent improvement in therapeutic ratio.

The interactions depicted in Fig. 38.19 are not sufficient to account for the high potency and specific biological activity of digitalis-like substances. Simple ring systems bearing a butenolide substituent are inactive (16). There is ample evidence to indicate that both the steroid and the C-3 sugar substituents are involved in the drug–receptor interactions of cardiac glycosides. Though the sugars *per se* are inactive, their attachment to the steroid contributes greatly to both the pharmacodynamic and pharmacokinetic characteristics of the cardiac glycosides. With respect to pharmacokinetics, the free genins are more rapidly absorbed and more widely distributed than the corresponding glycoside showing, for example, a greatly increased tendency to accumulate in the CNS. Most importantly, the genins are rapidly metabolized to give less active 3-epimers and rapidly excreted sulfates and glucuronides, conjugated through the 3-OH group (see Section 3.4). The genins are therefore quite unsuitable as therapeutic agents. Pharmacodynamically, the genins are usually less potent than the glycosides and, in contrast to the latter, show rapid onset and

reversal of receptor interaction. The glycosides usually form very stable complexes with Na⁺,K⁺-ATPase, a property described by Schwartz as pseudo-irreversibility (40). Digoxigenin and digitoxigenin have very rapid onset and reversal of action (64). It is important to emphasize that the pharmacodynamic differences between genins and glycosides are applicable to effects on contractility as well as to inhibition of Na⁺,K⁺-ATPase. It is clear, then, that the sugars can play an important role in the drug–receptor interactions of cardiac glycosides as well as contributing greatly to their pharmacokinetic characteristics.

Taking into account all known SAR data for both inhibition of Na⁺,K⁺-ATPase and effects on contractility, it is possible to propose a model for the complete digitalis receptor (Fig. 38.20). Digitalis inhibits

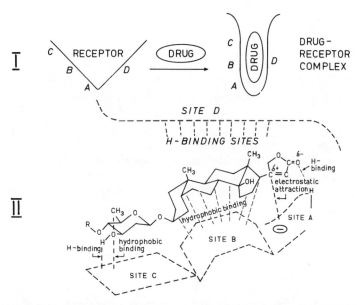

Fig. 38.20   A model for the digitalis receptor. Interaction is initiated by long-range attraction between the lactone and site A. This leads to a two-point attachment of the lactone to the receptor (see Fig. 38.17). The steroid then undergoes short-range interactions of the van der Waals and/or hydrophobic type with site B. This is reinforced by interactions above the molecule resulting from a rearrangement of the receptor cleft as shown in part I. The interaction of the sugar residue with site C greatly increases the stability of the complex, giving it the property of pseudo-irreversibility. Only one sugar is shown since it is the sugar residue closest to the genin that is chiefly involved in binding. SAR data indicate the presence of nucleophilic groups in sites A and C. Rearrangement of the receptor cleft as shown in part I produces an allosteric effect that mediates biological activity. The model is compatible with data for inhibition of Na⁺,K⁺-ATPase and effects on myocardial contractility.

Na$^+$,K$^+$-ATPase by a long-range allosteric mechanism and hence must induce a conformational change or "freeze" a particular conformation associated with the pump cycle (Section 3.3.3, equations 38.1–38.5). This is depicted in part I of Fig. 38.20 and in Fig. 38.17. There also appear to be three binding sites (designated A, B, and C), which are complementary to the α or "under" side of the digitalis molecule, and at least one region which lies above the molecule and is capable of multiple interactions with β-directed hydroxy substituents. Space does not permit a complete discussion of all supporting evidence but some recent data are cited. The nature of the binding interactions with site A have already been discussed. The classical SAR studies (55, 56) established that the optimal stereochemistry for the steroid system is the cis/trans/cis arrangement shown in Fig. 38.20. These studies also showed, as recently confirmed and extended by Haustein (65, 66), that activity is greatly decreased by α-directed hydroxyl groups, whereas β-OH groups usually increase activity. In most cases, acetylation of β-OH groups decreases activity. This has been shown for the 3β-, 12β-, and 19(β)-OH groups (65). A notable exception is the 16β-OH of gitoxin, where acetylation increases activity. The role of the 14β-OH group has been the subject of much speculation as to whether it is involved in binding or whether its presence is important simply as a reflection of the *cis* geometry of the C/D ring junction. Shigei et al. (67) have prepared the 14β-H analog of digitoxigenin and shown it to be one-tenth as active as the parent molecule. Hence both the C/D ring geometry and the 14β-OH are important. All this evidence infers an interaction between certain β-OH groups and a binding region above the molecule.

In summary, there is excellent evidence in support of the idea that the α face of the steroid is involved in some form of shape-specific "hydrophobic-type" interaction with the receptor. There is also evidence which indicates that at least some β-OH substituents contribute to binding, and this infers a binding region above the molecule.

A number of studies (reviewed in Ref. 40) have clearly established that the sugars of cardiac glycosides can contribute greatly to the stability of the drug–receptor complex, and several investigations have been undertaken to define the optimum characteristics of the sugar moiety. It seems that the principal binding interactions involve the sugar unit closest to the steroid and that hydrogen bonding plays a key role in the drug receptor interaction (65, 68, 69). The 3-OH group and the 5-CH$_3$ group seem to be the principal binding groups in 2,6-desoxy sugars (69).

Replacement of the sugar residues with nitrogen-containing side chains gives potent digitalis-like compounds (61, 70). Of particular interest is the N-(4'-amino-n-butyl)-3-aminoacetyl derivative of strophanthidin, which forms a complex with Na$^+$,K$^+$-ATPase with an affinity constant 60 times greater than that of the parent genin (61). Highly significant is the recent work of Caldwell and Nash (71) in which a substantial increase in therapeutic ratio was reported for the amino sugar cardenolide AS1-222 (38.**37**).

A very substantial increase in therapeutic ratio was reported (72) for Actodigin® (AY22241) (38.**38**). This compound contains an isomeric lactone at C-17 and a glucose moiety at C-3. A compound with similar properties is 16α-gitoxin. Like Actodigin, this compound has been described as having an increased therapeutic ratio, low potency, and rapid onset and reversal of activity (65, 66). Thomas et al. (73) have explained the low potency and rapid onset and reversal of Actodigin in terms of the receptor model shown in Fig. 38.20: once the lactone has interacted with site A, it is not possible, for structural reasons, for the sugar to approach site C. The compound therefore behaves as a genin.

Prigent et al. (74) have produced an extensive series of nonsteroidal digitalis analogs of the type shown in structure 38.**39**. These compounds were less active than ouabain but showed a marked increase in therapeutic ratio. Unlike ouabain, they inhibited both Na^+,K^+-ATPase and Mg^{2+}-ATPase.

Thomas and Gelbart (75) have prepared guanylhydrazone derivatives from a series of 17β-formyl androstanes of the type shown in structure 38.**40**. These compounds, like those produced by Prigent et al., inhibited both Na^+,K^+-ATPase and Mg^{2+}-ATPase, but unlike other analogs they showed negative inotropic activity when applied in small increments over the dose range 10^{-8}–10^{-4} M. This would seem to negate the theory that inhibition of Na^+,K^+-ATPase results in positive ino-

tropic activity. However, further work showed that these compounds inhibited mitochondrial respiration, which would explain their negative inotropy. In fact, when a single high dose of these compounds was added to isolated atria, there was an immediate positive inotropic effect followed much later by negative inotropy, indicating that the receptor for positive inotropy was very accessible (64).

In summary, it is possible to explain the diversity of compounds with digitalis-like activity (Fig. 38.9) in terms of the receptor model shown in Fig. 38.20. This applies to both inhibition of Na^+,K^+-ATPase and positive inotropic activity. Even so, a particular compound may show marked differences in potency with respect to inhibition of Na^+,K^+-ATPase and inotropic activity (for example, see Fig. 38.18). This may

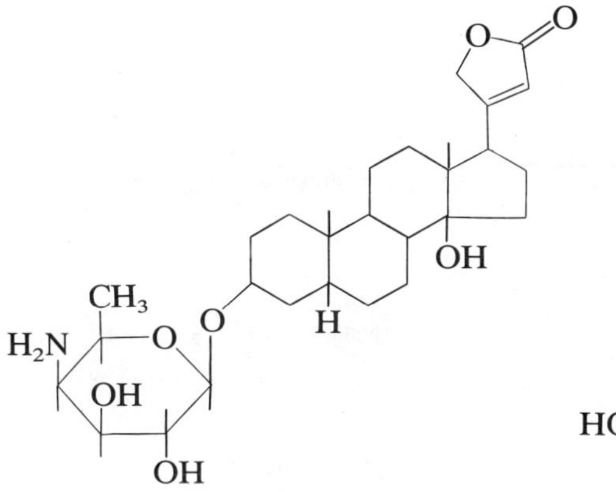

38.**37** ASI-222

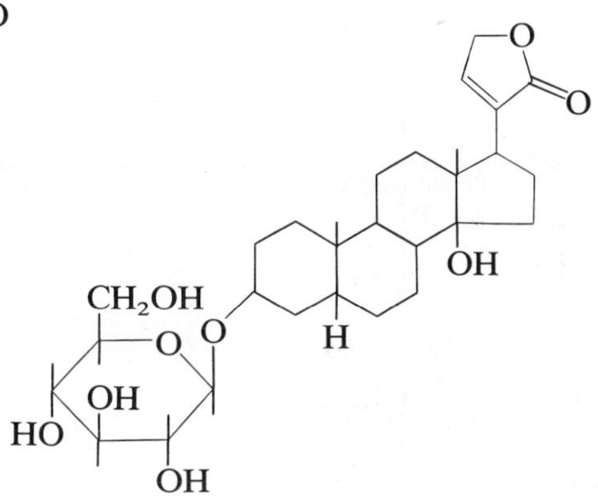

38.**38** AY22241

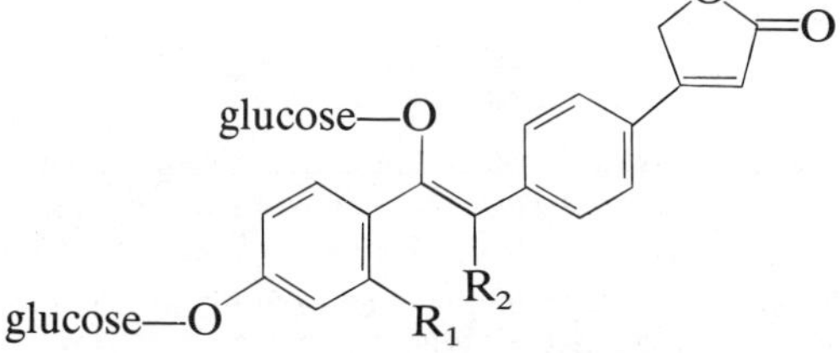

38.**39**

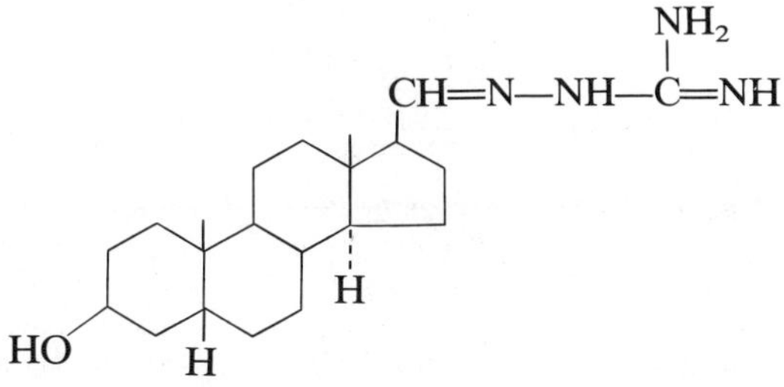

38.**40**

infer that the receptor mediating inotropic activity is similar to but different from that mediating inhibition of Na$^+$,K$^+$-ATPase.

3.4 Biotransformation

The pathways for the biotransformation of the digitalis gylcosides (Fig. 38.21) were established mainly by Repke and co-workers (53). The extent of metabolism varies with species and the lipid solubility of the glycoside. It was generally agreed until recently that in man digoxin is ex-creted largely unchanged, whereas the more lipid-soluble digitoxin is excreted mainly as metabolites. This belief led to the suggestion that digitoxin may be the prefer-red glycoside in renal failure (21). Al-though there is no doubt that digitoxin is metabolized more extensively than digoxin, workers in this field now report that dig-oxin is metabolized to a greater degree than previously admitted, whereas dig-itoxin, in some patients at least, is less extensively metabolized than previously be-lieved. The confusion about digoxin arose because investigators, using solvents such

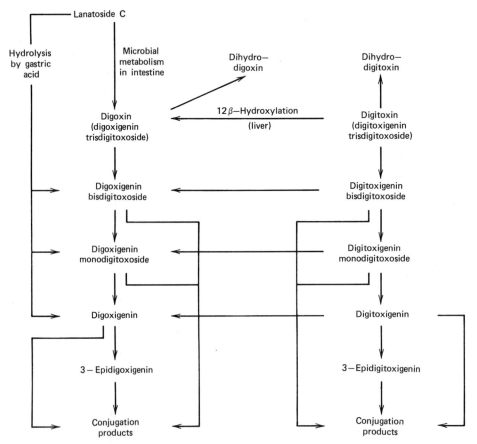

Fig. 38.21 Metabolic pathways for lanatoside C, digoxin, and digitoxin. 3-Epimerization, conjugation, and 20,22-reduction (to give dihydro compounds) are the detoxification steps. 12β-Hydroxylation of digitoxin to give digoxin and digoxin metabolites is extensive in some species (e.g., the rat) but occurs only to the extent of about 8% in man. Lanatoside C given orally is largely converted to digoxin and digoxin metabolites in the gut before absorption. The extent to which cardiac glycosides are metabolized and the nature of the metabolites formed vary greatly with different subjects.

as chloroform, recovered only 50–60% of the drug from plasma and urine and found that most of the *recovered* drug was unchanged digoxin. The nature of the nonrecovered drug was ignored or else assumed to be the same as the recovered drug. It has now been reported that most of the nonrecovered drug (or "water-soluble" fraction) is not digoxin (Ref. 76, p. 36). There is an important lesson here for the student, and the point can be made no better than in the words of Dr. T. Smith of Boston, who stated recently: "I think there has been a kind of 'emperor's new clothes' syndrome for some time in that we have continued to teach that digoxin is essentially quantitatively excreted unchanged in the urine of patients with normal renal function, despite the fact that our own studies—and I think nearly everyone else's—have consistently demonstrated recovery of about 40–50% of administered doses either in single dose or steady-state studies" (Ref. 76, p. 50).

The metabolism and other aspects of the pharmacokinetics of cardiac glycosides were the subject of an international symposium in 1977, and the reader is referred to the proceedings of this symposium (76) for an account of this subject. It is not possible to summarize here the 426 pages of these proceedings. Suffice it to say that there is much difference of opinion about the extent and nature of digitalis metabolism but at least it is now recognized that digoxin undergoes a significant degree of metabolism in man. The occurrence of 20,22-reduction (to give dihydro compounds) has been confirmed, although the amount of dihydro compound formed varies greatly between subjects. The metabolic pattern of digoxin and other cardiac glycosides seems to be time-dependent, which may infer a first-pass effect. The metabolic pattern also, seems to be different for maintenance therapy as compared with single dose treatment. Among the polar metabolites reported are digoxigenic

acid (formed by opening the lactone ring) and conjugates (glucuronides and sulfates) of the genin, epigenin, and the mono- and bisdigitoxosides (see Fig. 38.21). The cardiac glycosides and their metabolites can also undergo enterohepatic cycling, the extent of which is inversely proportional to lipid solubility (77). Enterohepatic cycling is not a significant factor in the pharmacokinetics of digoxin in man under conditions of normal renal function (78) but excretion via the bile can be an important route for the elimination of polar glycosides and glycoside metabolites (79).

3.5 Absorption and Bioavailability

The cardiac glycosides are neutral molecules that appear to be absorbed by a passive nonsaturable process at rates that are proportional to their lipid solubility. Highly polar molecules such as ouabain are so poorly absorbed from the gastrointestinal tract that they are administered only by the intravenous route. Likewise lanatoside C is too polar to be absorbed in significant amounts from the gastrointestinal tract. Following oral administration of ^{3}H-lanatoside C, only ^{3}H-digoxin and its metabolites were detected by Aldous and Thomas (80) in the plasma and urine of most patients studied. Apparently, lanatoside C is converted to digoxin and digoxin metabolites in the GI tract, partly by the action of gastric acid and partly by metabolism by intestinal microorganisms.

Since a 50% change in the therapeutic steady-state levels of plasma digoxin can result in either subtherapeutic or toxic levels of digoxin, factors controlling the bioavailability and pharmacokinetics of the cardiac glycosides have received great attention over the last few years. Improved analytical and control procedures, introduced at the end of the 1960s, greatly reduced the wide variations in digoxin content of digoxin tablets commercially available in the United States, Canada, and the

United Kingdom. The development of the radioimmunoassay (81,82) capable of measuring serum digoxin in subnanogram quantities established that many lots of digoxin tablets showed wide variation in digoxin bioavailability, even among tablets that conformed to digoxin-content specifications (83). Several studies established that variations in digoxin bioavailability correlated with dissolution rate, which in turn was related to particle size (84). As a consequence, regulatory bodies in the United States (in 1973) and the United Kingdom (in 1975) established specifications to ensure high and uniform bioavailability of digoxin tablets. These new dissolution rate requirements are now incorporated in the USP XIX. The problem of digoxin bioavailability has been extensively reviewed (85–88). It is now possible to formulate rapidly dissolving digoxin tablets having dissolution rates of 85% or more in 1 hr (86). Such tablets give high and uniform bioavailability approaching the 80–85% absorption achieved when digoxin is given in aqueous alcoholic solution. An interesting consequence of these endeavors to improve the formulation of oral digoxin preparations was the development of a soft gelatin capsule formulation that increased the bioavailability of digoxin to 97% (89).

Following dissolution, digoxin is efficiently absorbed from the intestine (90), although it is poorly absorbed from the stomach (91). The rate and extent of digoxin dissolution and absorption can be modified by many factors (reviewed by Greenblatt et al. Ref. 86). Digoxin absorption is reduced in certain malabsorption syndromes and by the coadministration of adsorbants such as kaolin, aluminum hydroxide, cholestyramine, and activated charcoal. Coadministration of digoxin tablets with food reduces the rate but not the extent of digoxin absorption. The older, more slowly dissolving forms of digoxin were sensitive to changes in gastrointestinal motility. The bioavailability of such preparations was reduced by agents that increase motility (for example, metoclopramide) and increased by agents that reduce motility (for example, propantheline). This may be explained in terms of the time available for dissolution. As already mentioned, this is not a problem with the newer, rapidly dissolving preparations of digoxin.

Chemical modification has also been used to modify the bioavailability and pharmacokinetic properties of cardiac glycosides. An example of this type of modification is pentaacetylgitoxin (see Ref. 92 for a review of the development of this compound). Gitoxin (38.**18**) is the 16-OH derivative of digitoxin and is of therapeutic interest because it is claimed to have low CNS toxicity. However, it shows low water solubility and low lipid solubility, having one-quarter the water solubility of digitoxin and one-fifth its lipid solubility. This means that it shows both poor dissolution and poor absorption—so much so that it cannot be given orally. In fact, it cannot be given intravenously because it is not sufficiently soluble in any injectable vehicle. By contrast, pentaacetylgitoxin (pengitoxin) has four times the water solubility of gitoxin and 20 times its lipid solubility; however, its biological activity is reduced to a few percent of that of gitoxin. Because of its changed solubilities, pengitoxin shows good bioavailability when given orally and, following absorption, undergoes rapid deacetylation to produce a potent cardiotonic drug. Pengitoxin thus acts as a prodrug. Haustein and co-workers (93) studied the fate of ^{3}H-pengitoxin in man. They found that the principal metabolite was 16-acetylgitoxin (formed by the loss of the four sugar acetyl groups) and that serum radioactivity declined with a half-life of about 60 hr. The duration of action of pengitoxin is thus intermediate between digoxin and digitoxin.

Other examples of prodrugs among the cardiac glycosides include β-acetyldigoxin

(4‴-acetyldigoxin) and diacetylcymarol. Boutagy and Thomas (94) showed that although diacetylcymarol was rapidly absorbed, it was also converted rapidly to polar metabolites which were eliminated in the bile at a rate that could not sustain adequate therapeutic levels.

Another digitalis analog that has been the subject of much clinical study is β-methyldigoxin (95–97). Like pengitoxin, β-methyl digoxin shows higher water solubility than might be expected on simple chemical considerations. However, as with many compounds, the stability of the crystal lattice is a major factor in controlling solubility. The solubilities of some cardiac glycosides are shown below (from Ref. 95).

	Water Solubility, mg/l	Apolarity
Digitoxin	13	10.9
β-Methyldigoxin	460	6.0
Digoxin	40	2.1
Lanatoside C	86	—

β-Methyldigoxin is claimed to have better bioavilability than digoxin, but as Garrett has pointed out (96), the evidence in the literature is equivocal and it could well be that new-formulation digoxin gives better bioavailability than β-methyldigoxin in spite of the latter's greater lipid solubility.

There is also lack of agreement on the pharmacokinetic parameters of β-methyldigoxin, but it does seem that the drug has a longer half-life than digoxin and a greater tendency to accumulate in the CNS.

3.6 Pharmacokinetics of Digoxin

The pharmacokinetics of digoxin have been studied extensively (see Refs. 23–25, 35, 36, 98–102 for reviews of the literature). It has been established that in individual patients there exists a linear relationship between steady-state plasma levels and digoxin dose. About 20–30% of plasma digoxin is protein bound. Plasma protein binding is not saturable in the concentration range met with in clinical practice. In fact, nonlinear processes do not appear to apply to any aspect of digoxin pharmacokinetics (102). Enterohepatic circulation does not appear to make a significant contribution to digoxin pharmacokinetics in normal subjects. The renal clearance of digoxin is complex and involves glomerular filtration, tubular secretion, and tubular reabsorption. The total renal excretion approximates the glomerular filtration rate and correlates well (in most cases) with creatinine clearance. Estimates of the half-life of digoxin in patients with normal renal function have ranged from 35 to 55 hr (102). The volume of distribution is in the range of 400–500 l (depending on calculation assumptions).

The pharmacokinetics of digoxin fit an open three-compartment model comprising a central (plasma) compartment, a shallow compartment, and a deep compartment, with all rate constants including absorption and elimination showing first-order kinetics (99). The observable pharmacodynamic effects of digoxin take 2–6 hr (depending on parameter measured) to reach maximum intensity following intravenous administration (103). Kinetic changes in the central compartment do not correlate with pharmacodynamic effects until at least 8 hr after oral administration. This represents the time required for a constant relationship to develop between tissue and plasma levels of drug. It is for this reason that plasma digoxin measurements are somewhat meaningless as an index of therapeutic or toxic effects if taken less than 8 hr following the last oral dose. The relationship between pharmacodynamics and pharmacokinetics is further complicated by the variation in rate of onset of effects for different regions of the heart. Deutscher et al. (104) found for the open chest dog preparation that the

Table 38.2   Clinically Important Drug Interactions that May Influence Response to Digoxin and Digitoxin[a]

Interacting Drug	Mech-anism[b]	Possible Effect/Action[c]
Antacids (nonabsorbable) Antidiarrheals (adsorbent-type)	DA	Decreased bioavailability of digoxin. More likely to be a potential problem with slowly dissolving tablets
Anticholinergic drugs	IA	Increased risk of digoxin toxicity if bio availability significantly increased. A problem only with slowly dissolving tablets
Calcium	PD	Avoid intravenous calcium. If essential, do not give rapidly or in large amounts
Cholestyramine Colestipol	DA	Decreased digoxin bioavailability (give drugs about 2 h apart)
	DA+IE	Decreased bioavailability of digitoxin (give drugs about 2 h apart)
Diuretics Carbenoxolone Amphotericin B	PD	Increased risk of toxicity owing to electrolyte abnormalities—hypokalemia, hypomagnesemia Replenish potassium stores in those on daily diuretics. Avoid carbenoxolone
Neomycin	DA	Digoxin toxicity when prolonged neomycin therapy withdrawn
Phenobarbitone Phenylbutazone Phenytoin (diphenylhydantoin)	AM	Accelerated metabolism of digitoxin. Two fold decrease in plasma levels induced by pheno-barbitone. If necessary, increase dose of digitoxin or use a substitute for pheno-barbitone (e.g., diazepam) or phenylbutazone (e.g., indomethacin). Other enzyme-inducing agents also likely to have same effect. Carefully watch for signs of toxicity if enzyme-inducing agents withdrawn from stable digitoxin regimen
Rauwolfia	PD	? Possible increased risk of toxicity. Best to avoid large parenteral doses of reserpine
Suxamethonium (succinyl choline)	PD	Increased risk of toxicity due to release of potassium, especially in patients with trauma, burns, wounds, or muscular disorders
Sympathomimetic drugs	PD	Increased risk of toxicity. Use these drugs with caution

inotropic effects of digoxin peaked at 60 min in the left ventricle and at 180 min in the right ventricle.

For most individuals, the therapeutic range of digoxin corresponds to steady-state plasma digoxin concentrations of 1–2 ng/ml, above which toxic effects are likely to occur. (Note: the radioimmunoassay used for measurement of plasma digoxin levels measures both free and protein-bound digoxin). It has been shown that the high incidence of digitalis toxicity can be significantly reduced by monitoring serum concentrations of drug and by the use of pharmacokinetic principles to devise dosage regimes (31). The main pharmacokinetic factors to be considered in predicting digoxin dosage are, in order of correlation with actual serum concentration: renal function (as measured by creatinine clearance), lean body weight, and serum albumin concentration (100). This assumes the use of a dosage form with a high and reliable bioavailability. Nomograms for predicting digoxin dosage have been devised by several authors. That produced by Jelliffe and Brooker (105) assumes that renal function and weight are the major determinants of serum digoxin concentration. Such procedures are likely to produce plasma levels within the predicted range in 70–80% of patients, although there have been reports of unacceptably large errors (discussed in Refs. 98 and 100). Finally, for patients whose plasma levels of digoxin fall within the "therapeutic" range, a number of other variables can lead to either therapeutic failure or toxicity. These factors are discussed in Refs. 25 and 35. In particular, digoxin toxicity is increased in

hypokalemia and hypothyroidism, whereas higher doses are usually required in thyrotoxic patients. Digoxin therapy should be stopped or lowered at least 3 days before cardiac operations or cardioversion in order to avoid precipitation of arrhythmias. The effects of possible drug interactions are summarized in Table 38.2. It should be noted that interaction with K^+-depleting diuretics is the most important and likely problem. Other interactions that have been reported are far less well documented. (See Ref. 148 for a review of drug interactions involving digitalis glycosides.)

Recently it has been shown that co-administration of quinidine significantly increases the plasma levels of digoxin (149). Displacement from binding sites and reduced renal clearance seem to be involved.

4 ANTIARRHYTHMIC DRUGS

4.1 Molecular Basis of Cardiac Arrhythmia

In order for the heart to function as an efficient pump, the various contractile units must operate in a coordinated or rhythmic fashion. Since the contractile units (sarcomeres) are subdivisions of subcellular units (Fig. 38.2) it is apparent that the heart needs an extremely efficient telegraph system in order to signal to this vast multitude of contractile units in such a way that coordinated contraction is achieved. In addition, for the heart to function automatically, a signal generator (pacemaker) is required. Finally, since the atria must contract and empty their contents before the ventricles commence contraction, the atria

---

[a] From J. G. Sloman, "Cardiovascular Diseases," in *Drug Treatment*, G. S. Avery, Ed., Adis Press, Sydney, 1976, Chap. 16. (Used with permission).

[b] Mechanism known or thought to be most likely. Digoxin and digitoxin have different pharmacokinetic properties. DA = Decreased absorption; IA = increased absorption; IE = inhibition of enterohepatic recirculation; AM = accelerated hepatic metabolism; PD = pharmacodynamic action (influence on tissue response).

[c] Diuretics are by far the most important and likely problem. The possibility of interaction with other compounds has been suggested by a few case reports or studies.

and ventricles must be separated from each other by a layer of tissue that is nonconducting except for one small region that conducts slowly and functions as a delay circuit. This region is called the atrioventricular (AV) node. Once the signal has passed through the AV node it is picked up and propagated rapidly by fast-conducting fibers (His and Purkinje fibers) to all regions of the ventricles. The myocardium is thus a nonhomogeneous tissue showing varying capacity to generate and conduct an electrical impulse. These properties are expressed by the different types of action potential recorded for the various regions of the heart (Fig. 38.22).

All the variations shown in Fig. 38.22 are the result of differences in the nature of the various transmembrane ion fluxes and, to quote Morgan and Mathison (3), "every disturbance in heart rhythm, normal or abnormal, can ultimately be traced to changes in the ratios of intracellular to extracellular ionic concentrations which are mediated by changes in the permeability of the cell membrane." The antiarrhythmic drugs, which correct abnormalities in impulse generation and conduction, act because they directly or indirectly modify the macromolecules that control transmembrane ion fluxes. Antiarrhythmic drugs are classified according to the phase (0 to 4; see Fig. 38.1) of the action potential that they are believed to affect.

The heart owes its property of automaticity to certain cells that automatically depolarize during phase 4. This occurs as a result of a steady decrease in K^+ efflux associated with a small but constant Na^+ influx. This causes the transmembrane potential to fall until the threshold value (T.P.) is reached, at which point certain molecular "gates" open and an action potential is generated as described in Section 2. The action potentials of automatic cells are shown in Fig. 38.22; A and C. Normally the automatic cells of the sinoatrial (SA) node depolarize first and hence the SA node is the pacemaker (or signal generator) for the whole heart. Automatic cells are also found in the AV node and in the specialized conducting fibers of atrial and ventricular tissue (Fig. 38.22, C). If, for any reason, the signal from the SA node is slowed or blocked, other automatic cells (called latent pacemakers) take over as the signal generator of the heart. The means whereby the signal is propagated may be described in simple terms as follows. When any particular segment of membrane is depolarized, the *inner* face of that section of membrane becomes positive with respect to adjoining regions of the *inner* face. Charges then flow from the adjoining region into the depolarized region causing the transmembrane potential of the adjoining region to fall to its threshold value, thereby triggering an action potential. Thus an action potential, once generated, leads to depolarization of an adjoining segment of

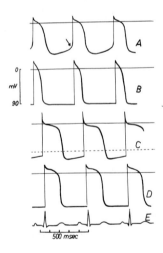

Fig. 38.22 Transmembrane action potentials recorded from cells of (A) sinoatrial node, (B) atrial muscle, (C) Purkinje system, and (D) ventricular muscle; on the same time axis is the ECG (E). Note differences in diastolic depolarization and level of threshold potential in rows A and C. The different cell types and the delays in atrioventricular conduction are indicated by the delay in upstroke between B and C. [From W. Trautwein, *Pharmacol. Rev.*, **15**, 279 (1963), Williams & Wilkins, Baltimore Md. Used with permission.]

membrane and this, in turn, leads to depolarization of a further membrane segment, and so on, in domino fashion, until the wave of depolarization has spread throughout the entire myocardium, passing from cell to cell via the nexus of the intercalated disk. The rate at which the action potential is propagated depends on many factors such as the capacitance of the membrane, the speed and magnitude of the depolarization current (phase 0), and the diameter of the fiber.

The spontaneous discharge rate of automatic cells depends on (1) the slope of phase 4, (2) the magnitude of the threshold potential, and (3) the magnitude of the maximum diastolic potential. Changes in all these parameters can occur in disease states or as a consequence of drug action. Adrenergic drugs increase heart rate by increasing the slope of phase 4 of pacemaker cells. Cholinergic drugs slow the heart by decreasing the slope of phase 4. On the other hand, drugs such as atropine that block the parasympathetic nervous system increase heart rate, whereas drugs that block the sympathetic nervous system slow the heart (See Ref. 106 for a more rigorous discussion of the generation and propagation of action potentials in the heart).

The etiology, classification, and treatment of cardiac arrhythmias have been largely empirical although advances over the last few years (reviewed in Refs. 107–109) have now laid the basis for a rational approach (110) to the use of antiarrhythmic drugs. The complex and detailed treatment that this subject requires is beyond the scope of this text. However, a simplified discussion of the genesis of arrhythmia is given as a basis for classifying the various groups of antiarrhythmic drugs.

Cardiac arrhythmias arise from abnormalities in impulse formation and conduction. Abnormalities in impulse formation (automaticity) give rise to changes in heart rate and to the development of ectopic beats originating in latent pacemaker cells,

either or both of which may occur in the one patient. Such abnormalities are thought to be due to changes in the rate of spontaneous diastolic depolarization (slope of phase 4) in automatic cells. Disturbances in conduction can be partial or complete (delay or block), can be unidirectional or bidirectional, and can occur with or without re-entry or circus movement. The latter (described in Fig. 38.23) is invoked to explain flutter and fibrillation. As discussed in Section 2.1, the upstroke of the action potential (phase 0) results from the opening of either fast Na^+ channels or of moderately fast Na^+ and Ca^{2+} channels. The latter are

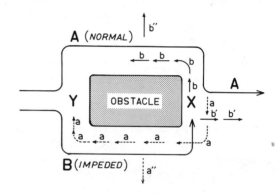

Fig. 38.23 Model for circus or re-entrant activity. A depolarization impulse approaches an "obstacle" (or nonconducting region of the heart). The impulse traverses two pathways (A and B) to circumvent the obstacle. If pathway B is partially or completely impeded, the following events may occur. (1) If impulse B is slowed and arrives at X after the absolute refractory period of cells depolarized by A, the impulse may continue around the obstacle as shown by path b and/or follow A along path b′. (2) If pathway B shows unidirectional block, impulse A may continue around the obstacle in the direction a. If the obstacle is large enough so that the cells in the region of Y are repolarized before the return of a or b, then a circus movement may be established that may also propagate impulses in other directios (a″ and b″). These phenomena can give rise to coupled beats and, in the extreme situation, to fibrillation. The obstacle can be any anatomic or pathological feature of the heart, but the most relevant example is that of an infarcted area with an associated region of depressed myocardium; the infarct is the obstacle and the depressed myocardium is pathway B.

associated with SA and AV cells and con- duct at a much slower rate than fast re- sponse fibers. There is now good evidence (111) that most, if not all, conducting ab- normalities arise as a result of the conver- sion of fast response fibers to slow response fibers. This, as we have seen, is a function of transmembrane ion fluxes, which in turn are controlled by the movement of mac- romolecules within the membrane in accor- dance with the charge distribution on the membrane (Section 2.1). Although changes in automaticity and conduction have been related to changes in phases 4 and 0 of the action potential, respectively, the absolute and effective refractory periods (controlled by phases 1–3) also contribute significantly to the final expression of the arrhythmia.

4.2   Chemistry and Classification of Antiarrhythmic Drugs

The major antiarrhythmic drugs were intro- duced into medicine as either antimalarials, anticonvulsants, or local anesthetics, and it was only by chance that their antiarrhyth- mic properties were discovered. The struc- tures and names of established and new or experimental antiarrhythmic agents are shown in Figs. 38.24 and 38.25. Apart from phenytoin (38.**45**), which is a weak acid, all antiarrhythmic drugs contain basic or quaternary nitrogen and are therefore capable of existing as cations and forming salts. The antiarrhythmic drugs may be di- vided into two broad groups: (1) those that act specifically by interacting with a recep- tor (e.g., β-adrenergic blocking agents such as propranolol) and (2) those that act non- specifically by accumulation in membranes (includes quinidine and the local anesthe- tics).

Attempts to classify antiarrhythmic drugs in terms of their effects on the elec- trophysiology of the heart have met with disagreement, partly because the phar- macological effects of the drugs vary in different subjects and with different dose levels and partly because of the difficulty in correlating clinical effects with effects on the action potential. The problem is further complicated by the fact that most drugs have more than one effect. For example, quinidine normally slows the rate of con- duction but in low doses it may exert a vagolytic effect leading to increased con- duction. Thus, in spite of many published schemes (111–113) for classifying the effects of antiarrythmic drugs, there are only two parameters of *practical* signifi- cance:

1. Effects on ectopic pacemakers.
2. Effects on AV conduction.

Apart from bretylium, all antiarrhythmic drugs in clinical use depress automaticity in ectopic pacemakers. This effect correlates with reduction in the slope of phase 4 of the action potential.

Drugs that prolong AV conduction include procainamide, quinidine, β- adrenergic blocking agents, verapamil, and disopyramide. This effect correlates with a decrease in the rate of rise of phase 0 of the action potential. Drugs that in usual dosage do not prolong AV conduction include lig- nocaine and phenytoin.

4.3   Mechanism of Action of Nonspecific Antiarrhythmic Drugs

The problems that apply to the classifica- tion of antiarrhythmic drugs also apply to the study of their mode of action: the drugs exert a spectrum of pharmacological effects which vary for different regions of the heart and there is also great difficulty in correlat- ing events at the cellular level with events at the clinical or physiological level. The problem is further complicated by the poor correlation that exists between effects in laboratory animals with model arrhythmias and effects in patients. In spite of this there

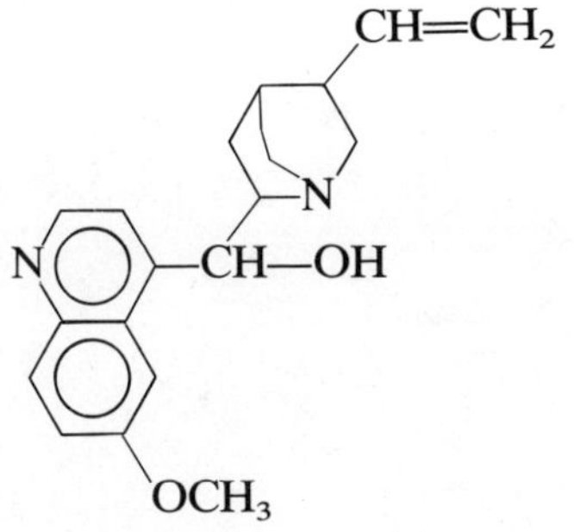

38.**41** Quinidine

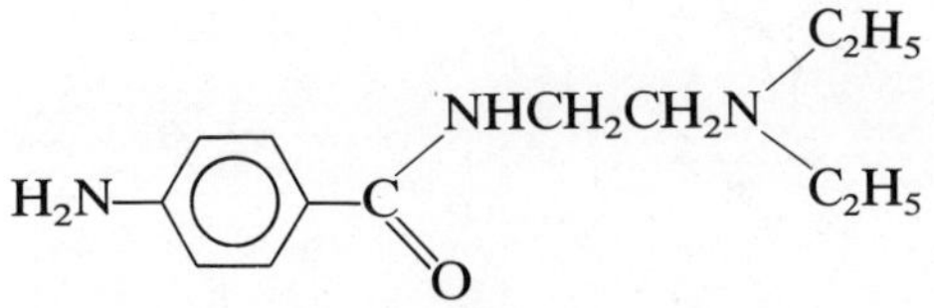

38.**42** Procainamide

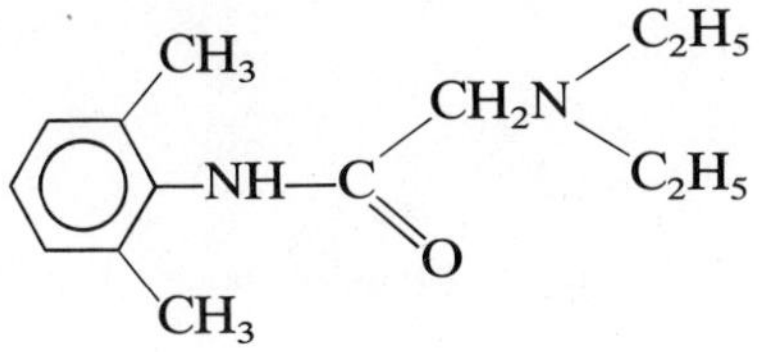

38.**43** Lidocaine

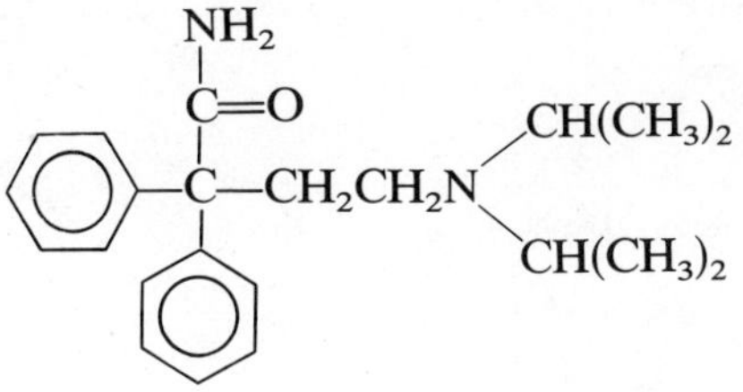

38.**44** Disopyramide

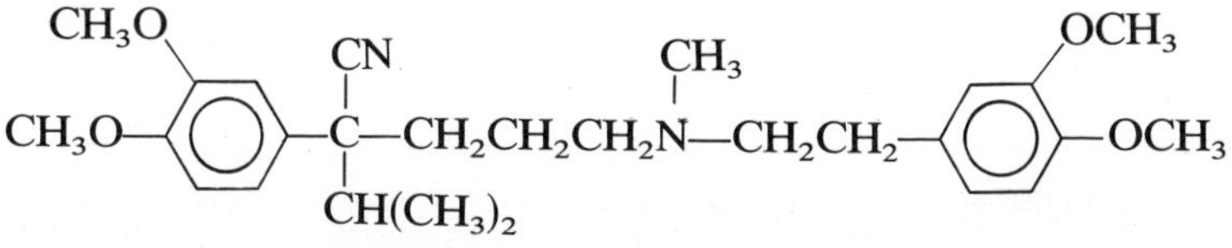

38.**2** Verapamil

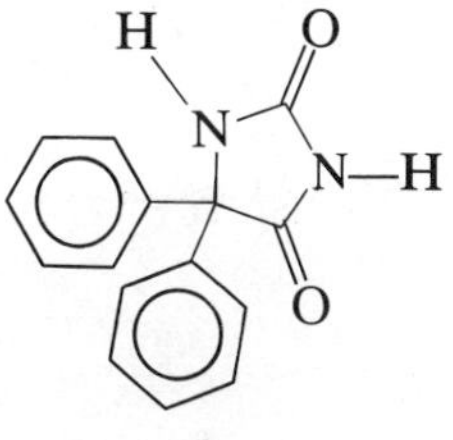

38.**45** Phenytoin

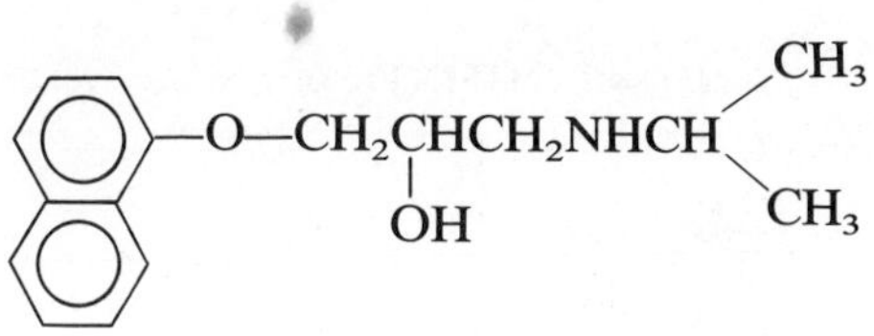

38.**46** Propranolol

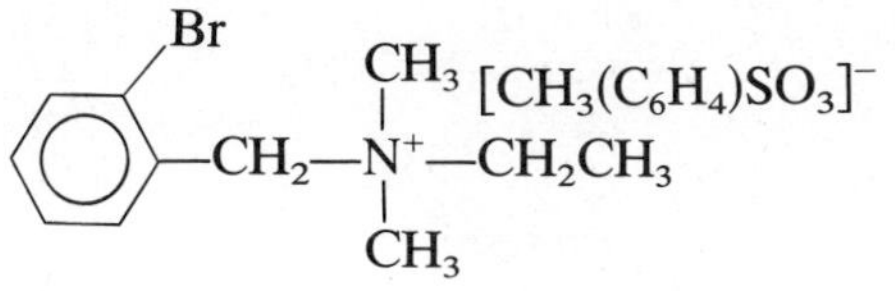

38.**47** Bretylium tosylate

Fig. 38.24 Antiarrhythmic drugs in regular use.

is general agreement that antiarrhythmic drugs, apart from those that affect the autonomic nervous system, act by a non-specific mechanism. It is thought that the drugs act by accumulating in certain regions of the plasma membrane where their action may be correlated with an increase in membrane surface pressure. The presence of the drug in the membrane compresses the normal membrane components so that their biological function is inhibited. Although this effect is *non-specific*, that is, it does not involve stereospecific interaction with a receptor, the effects are selective since only certain membrane activities are depressed. Na^+,K^+-ATPase, for example, is

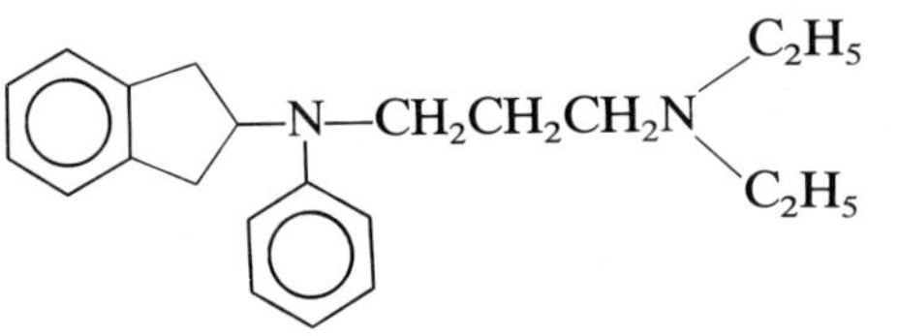

38.**48** Aprindine

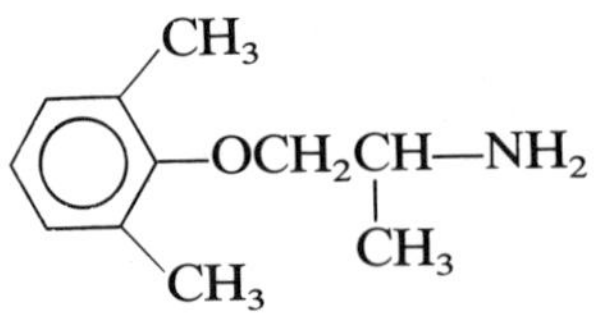

38.**49** Mexiletine

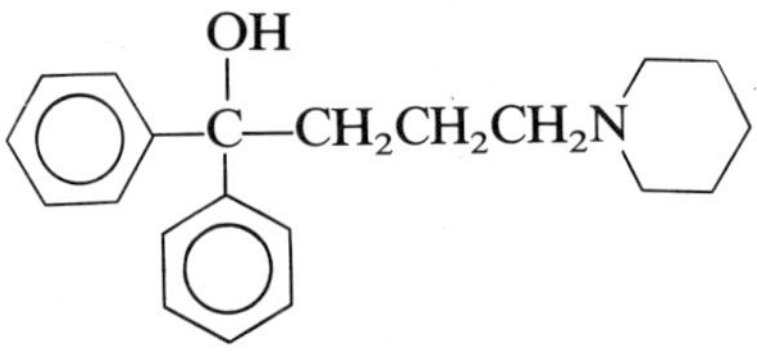

38.**50** Diphenidol

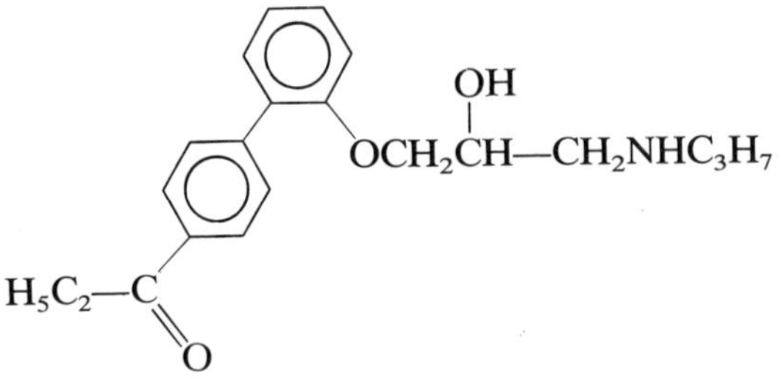

38.**51** Propafenone

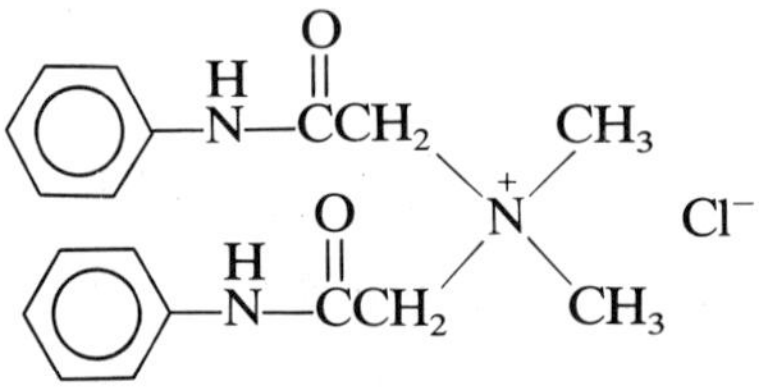

38.**52**

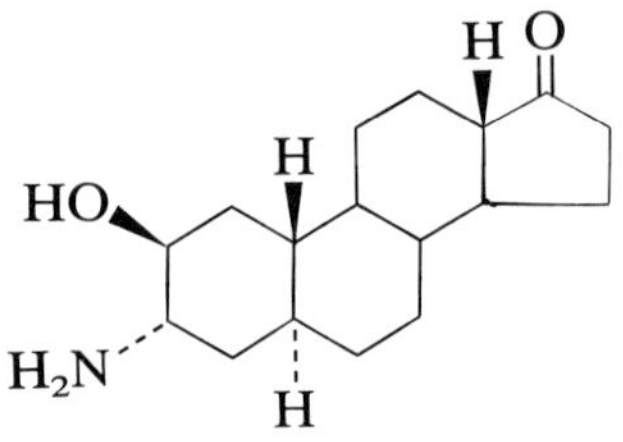

38.**53**

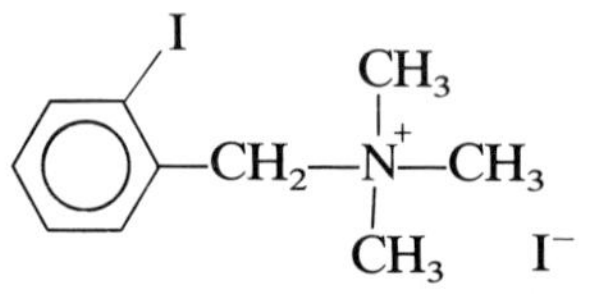

38.**54**

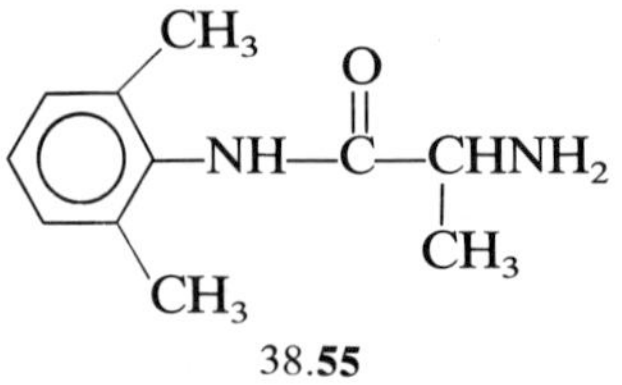

38.**55**

Fig. 38.25 New and experimental antiarrhythmic drugs.

not affected by therapeutic levels of antiarrhythmic agents. The drugs decrease membrane permeability with respect to certain types of ion transport, presumably because they block certain ion channels or prevent the conformational changes in proteins associated with the movement of ion "carriers" or the opening of "molecular gates." This type of action is called "membrane stabilization," and is depicted in Fig. 38.26.

4.4 Structure–Activity Relationships

The chemical features that seem to be essential for nonspecific antiarrhythmic activity are shown in Fig. 38.27. These same

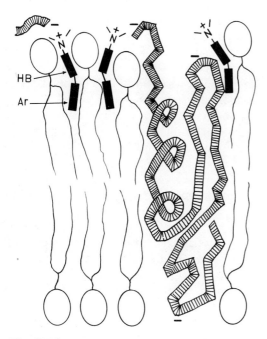

Fig. 38.26 Model depicting the accumulation of an anti-arrhythmic drug in cell membranes. The aromatic portion of the molecule (Ar) interacts with the alkyl chains of membrane phospholipids. The ionized amino group interacts with anionic groups in the phospholipid head or in protein components of the membrane. The interconnecting alkyl chain (HB) hydrogen bonds with polar groups in the head of the phospholipid molecule.

centrations exert a nonspecific, quinidine-like antiarrhythmic effect.

According to the model shown in Fig. 38.26, nonspecific antiarrhythmic agents interact with three regions of the membrane: (1) the aromatic ring (or ring system) intercalates between the alkyl chains of membrane phospholipids; (2) the amino group (as a cation) associates with an anionic group of a membrane polypeptide; and (3) the polar substituents on the interconnecting alkyl chain hydrogen bond with the polar heads of the membrane phospholipids. These properties result in the *selective* accumulation of the drug in certain regions of the membrane. The physical presence of sufficient numbers of drug molecules in a particular region of the membrane compresses the membrane components, resulting in *nonspecific* inhibition of certain categories of membrane function.

Phenytoin (38.**45**) is a weak acid and hence does not fit the specifications given in Fig. 38.26. However, it possesses the necessary aromatic system and is capable of hydrogen bonding. A compound that is less readily reconciled with the proposed model is the steroid 38.**53**. This compound lacks both local anesthetic activity and β-adrenergic blocking properties, yet it is an extremely potent antiarrhythmic agent, being seven times more potent and five times less toxic than lidocaine in the treatment of aconitine-induced arrhythmias in rats (114).

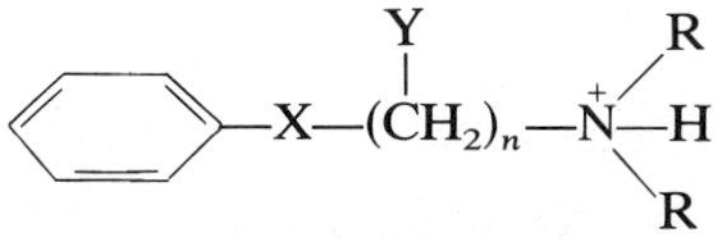

features are associated with local anesthetic activity (Chapter 51) and with β-adrenergic blocking activity (Chapter 42). It is interesting to note that β-adrenergic blocking agents (which act by combining with a stereoselective receptor) can at higher con-

$$\text{Ar}-X-(CH_2)_n-\overset{+}{N}\overset{Y}{\underset{R}{\overset{R}{|}}}H$$

| Lipophilic aromatic group capable of intercalating between the alkyl chains of phospholipids | Interconnecting alkyl chain bearing substituents (X and Y), capable of hydrogen bonding | Amino group ionized at biological pH (pK_a 8–9) |

Fig. **38.27** Molecular features that seem essential for nonspecific antiarrhythmic activity.

Structure–activity relationships for the nonspecific antiarrhythmic drugs have been extensively reviewed by Morgan and Mathison (3) and Szekeres and Papp (115). The effects of chemical modification can be interpreted in terms of changes in the physical properties that control the pharmacokinetics and the selective accumulation of the drugs in membranes. In general, chemical modifications that increase the potency of nonspecific antiarrhythmic agents correlate with increased lipid solubility (oil–water partition coefficient) determined directly or by the Hansch method (116, 117). The nonspecific antiarrhythmic activity of β-adrenergic blocking agents may also be related to hydrophobicity. Hansch analysis of a series of these compounds showed a parabolic relationship between log potency versus log P (118). The hydrophobicity of the compounds was varied by substitution on the aromatic ring, but the nature and position of the substituent did not influence the relationship between potency and hydrophobicity.

Scatchard plot analysis for the plasma-protein binding of a series of 20 disopyramide derivatives showed that only one primary binding site was involved (119). The evidence indicated that binding involved principally the aromatic ring, which was postulated to intercalate into a hydrophobic region of the protein helix. This type of evidence provides indirect support for the model suggested in Fig. 38.26. The antiarrhythmic activities of an extensive series of quinidine analogs showed good correlation between antiarrhythmic activity and lipophilicity as measured by the partition coefficient in an octanol/pH 7.4 buffer (reviewed in Ref. 3). An interesting feature of this work is that the series included a large number of cis and trans isomers, but activity correlated with lipophilicity and not with stereochemistry. However, where isomeric pairs had nearly equal lipophilicity, the more planar trans isomer was the more potent, which may indicate greater ease in ability to intercalate between hydrophobic molecules. These results do not infer a stereoselective receptor since where the cis isomer was more lipophilic, it was also more potent.

N-Dealkylation is associated with a reduction in antiarrhythmic potency. The experimental drug tocainide (38.**55**) is a primary amine analog of lidocaine. Studies in laboratory animals indicate that this drug may have clinical indications similar to those for lidocaine. The interesting SAR feature of this drug is the effect of the primary amine structure on its pharmacokinetics in man (120). Although less potent than lidocaine, tocainide is not subject to variable first-pass N-de-ethylation (the main reason why lidocaine is ineffective by mouth). In normal subjects, tocainide is rapidly absorbed with a bioavailability approaching 100%. The elimination half-life is several times greater than that of lidocaine or procainamide. Preliminary evidence (120) suggests that the oral dosage interval may be three to four times longer than the 3 hr recommended for procainamide.

Quaternization appears to abolish β-blocking activity and reduces local anesthetic activity but does not reduce antiarrhythmic activity. Toxic effects on the CNS are also abolished by quaternization. Most of the changes associated with quaternization are explicable in terms of changes in distribution. Thus the antiarrhythmic effects on the heart are not greatly affected by quaternization because the plasma membrane of myocardial cells is readily accessible (forms part of the central compartment), whereas local anesthetic activity and CNS effects are abolished or greatly reduced because the permanently charged cation cannot reach the target membrane. A number of quaternary antiarrhythmic drugs (such as 38.**52**) are at present being clinically evaluated (121) and appear to have rapid onset and long duration of action, as well as having reduced incidence of side effects. The N-acetyl derivative of pro-cainamide has been shown to be an effective antiarrhythmic compound (122) with an elimination half-life of about 6 hr compared with an average of 3.5 hr for procainamide. N-Acetylprocainamide occurs as a metabolite of procainamide in man and an increased tendency to produce this metabolite may explain why some individuals require less frequent dosage with procainamide.

The antiarrythmic drugs available now are far from satisfactory and the development of safe long-acting agents, preferably with high oral bioavailability, is a matter of considerable urgency. Unfortunately, the SAR studies that have so far been carried out for nonspecific acting antiarrhythmic agents offer few guidelines for the separation of toxic and therapeutic effects. This is in contrast to the β-adrenergic blocking agents where SAR studies have proved far

more effective in developing cardioselective drugs useful as antiarrhythmic agents (discussed in Chapter 42).

4.5   Pharmacokinetics

Some pharmacokinetic properties of antiarrhythmic drugs are shown in Table 38.3. These values are useful only as a rough guide to the development of dose regimens since the pharmacokinetic properties of antiarrhythmic drugs vary greatly even for normal individuals. In heart failure, the pharmacokinetics of antiarrhythmic drugs in particular (but of all drugs in general) may be radically altered. Reduced tissue perfusion in heart failure leads to increased levels of drug in the central compartment and, as far as antiarrhythmic drugs are concerned, the central compartment includes the myocardial membranes where these

Table 38.3   Some Pharmacokinetic Properties of Commonly Used Antiarrhythmic Agents[a]

Drug	Peak plasma level,[b] hr	Half-Life (Normals), hr	Plasma Protein Binding, %	Hepatic Metabolism, %	Urinary Excretion,[c] %
Quinidine	1.5–2	3–16	80%	50–90	10–50%
Procainamide	1–2	2.2–4	15	35–55[d]	45–65
Lidocaine (lignocaine)	—	1–2	80%	90–95%	5–10
Phenytoin (diphenylhydantoin)	3–12	10–40[e]	90	95	≤5
Propranolol	1–2	2–4 (iv) 3.5–6 (oral)	90–96	Extensive[f]	negligible
Practolol	1–2	9–12	<10	Nil	85–100

[a] Adapted from J. G. Sloman, "Cardiovascular Diseases," in *Drug Treatment*, G. S. Avery, Ed., Adis Press, Sydney, 1976, Chap. 16. (Used with permission.)
[b] Time taken in most subjects to attain peak level after oral administration.
[c] Urinary excretion of unchanged drug.
[d] A metabolite, N-acetylprocainamide is potentially active and appears to accumulate in uremia.
[e] Plasma half-life of phenytoin depends on dosage.
[f] Subject to extensive hepatic first-pass metabolism after oral administration. A metabolite, 4-hydroxypropranolol, is formed after oral but not intravenous administration. It is present in plasma at approximately the same concentration as parent drug and has about the same β-adrenoreceptor blocking activity.

drugs act. In heart failure patients, the steady-state levels of lidocaine, following bolus injection and then infusion, can be five to eight times higher than the levels found in normal subjects receiving the same dosage per kilogram (123). (refer to Fig. 38.28.). To quote Greenblatt et al. (124); "the use of pharmacokinetic principles to guide lidocaine therapy may enhance the likelihood of effectiveness and nontoxicity, but it cannot substitute for clinical judgement." This comment applies to all other drugs affecting the heart. In addition to profound effects on pharmacokinetics, cardiac disease can also change the pharmacodynamic characteristics of cardiac drugs by inducing changes in cardiac responsiveness and alterations in the environment of the biophase. The influence of these factors had been reviewed by Thomson (125).

Unlike the cardiac glycosides, the nonspecific-acting antiarrhythmic drugs undergo rapid association and dissociation from the biophase. This difference is an expected consequence of their respective modes of action. Because of their rapid rate

of equilibration, the initial tissue distribution of the nonspecific-acting antiarrhythmic drugs is proportional to the regional distribution of blood flow. Thus the drugs accumulate first in tissues, such as the heart, that are well-perfused and then redistribute more uniformly throughout the body as recirculating blood carries the drug to less well-perfused tissues, (refer to Fig. 38.29.). In general, the pharmacokinetics of the nonspecific-acting antiarrhythmic drugs may be described in terms of a two-compartment open model.

4.5.1 QUINIDINE. Quinidine is absorbed almost completely following oral administration. Maximum effects are seen at about 2 hr and parallel peak plasma levels. The elimination half-life averages about 5 hr but shows wide variation between individuals. Approximately 60–80% of total plasma quinidine in the therapeutic range is bound to plasma protein. Quinidine is metabolized by the liver to give products with little or no biological activity. The extent of metabolism varies greatly between individuals, and this probably accounts for the

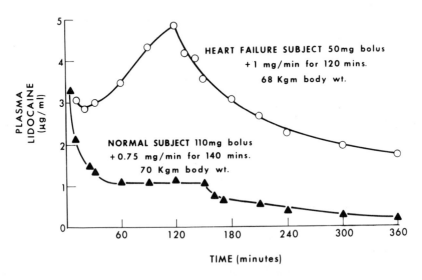

Fig. 38.28 Plasma levels of lidocaine after intravenous bolus and infusion of lidocaine in normal and heart failure patients of comparable weight. [From P. D. Thomas, M. Rowland, and K. L. Melmon, *Am. Heart J.*, **82**, 417 (1971). Used with permission.]

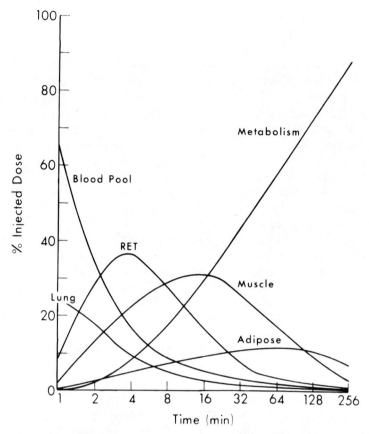

Fig. 38.29   Perfusion model for simulated lidocaine content in various tissues following an intravenous injection of lidocaine (1 mg/kg) into a 70 kg man. Rapidly equilibrating tissue (RET) includes heart and kidney. (From N. L. Benowitz, in *Cardiovascular Drug Therapy*, K. L. Melmon and A. N. Brest, Eds., F. A. Davis, Philadelphia, 1974, p. 78. Used with permission.)

wide variations in elimination half-lives. Unchanged drug and metabolites are eliminated via the kidney. Extensive tubular reabsorption of unchanged drug occurs in alkaline urine and quinidine toxicity has been induced by coadministration of agents such as absorbable antacids that alkalinize the urine. Quinidine dosage should be reduced in kidney and liver disease and conditions such as low output heart failure that reduce glomerular filtration. Quinidine sulfate (1% soluble in water) is usually the form given orally, whereas quinidine gluconate (10% soluble in water) is recommended for intravenous injection. The injection is diluted with 5% glucose solution and injected slowly.

4.5.2   PROCAINAMIDE. The absorption of procainamide is rapid and almost complete when given orally to normal fasting subjects but is much less reliable under the clinical conditions in which the drug is used. In acute myocardial infarction, peak plasma levels may not be reached until 5 hr and bioavailability may be reduced by as much as 50%. In therapeutic concentrations only about 15% of the plasma content is protein bound. The drug is extensively bound in tissues. The apparent volume of distribution in normal subjects ranges from about 1.7 to 2.2 l/kg and is independent of body weight and build. In patients with depressed circulatory function, apparent volumes of distribution may be as low as

1.4 l/kg. The distribution half-life of procainamide is about 5 min and the elimination half-life ranges from 2 to 4 hr. The therapeutic effects of procainamide are associated with steady-state plasma levels of 4–10 μg/ml of drug. Both renal excretion of unchanged drug and hepatic metabolism are significant in the elimination of the drug. Renal clearance of procainamide usually exceeds glomerular filtration rate which infers rapid diffusion of the lipid-soluble drug across renal tubular membranes followed by ion trapping in the normally acid urine. As the pH of the urine rises the extent of tubular reabsorption increases and renal clearance becomes less than the glomerular filtration rate when the urine is alkaline. The elimination half-life of procainamide can rise from an average of 3 hr in normal patients to up to 8 hr in patients with renal disease or conditions such as heart failure, in which renal perfusion is decreased. In normal subjects, biotransformation is less important than renal clearance of unchanged drug but assumes greater significance in renal insufficiency. The principal metabolite of procainamide is the acetyl derivative of the aromatic nitrogen (N-acetylprocainamide). This metabolite, although less active than procainamide, still retains antiarrhythmic activity (see Section 4.4) and has an elimination half-life twice as long as procainamide. Since acetylprocainamide is more polar than procainamide it has less tendency to enter the tubules by passive diffusion, and this may explain the longer half-life. The activity of N-acetyltransferase shows a genetically linked biphasic distribution and conversion to the less active but longer-acting acetyl derivative is obviously slower in "slow acetylators." The pharmacokinetics, dosage schedules, and clinical applications of procainamide have been reviewed by Koch-Weser (126).

4.5.3 LIDOCAINE. Because of extensive and variable first-pass metabolism by the liver, lidocaine cannot be given by the oral route. On an average, two-thirds of the drug is N-dealkylated in one pass through the liver. Lidocaine is administered intravenously as a bolus followed by continuous infusion to maintain a steady-state plasma level of 1–4 μg/ml. At this concentration lidocaine is about 70–80% protein bound, but the proportion bound falls as the plasma levels rise above 4 μg/ml. Lidocaine shows its greatest affinity for lung and spleen. Its partition coefficient with respect to lung is more than three times greater than for heart. The lung therefore sequesters a large amount of drug in the first few moments following administration and has the effect of converting a bolus into an elongated bolus (Fig. 38.29). If pulmonary shunting occurs (for example, in lung disease or following myocardial infarction), the damping effect of the lung is reduced and high peak levels occur in brain (the main site of toxicity) and in heart. This increases the risk of toxicity and may, for example, precipitate convulsions. The apparent volume of distribution of lidocaine following tissue equilibrium is about 1.3 l/kg, but would be very much larger if calculated on the basis of unbound drug in the plasma. The elimination half-life is about 1–2 hr. Lidocaine is eliminated mainly by oxidative N-de-ethylation in the liver and, as already mentioned, the liver is normally capable of metabolizing about two-thirds of the drug that passes through the liver in one passage. Lidocaine elimination is therefore controlled largely by the perfusion rate of the liver: a 50% reduction in cardiac output more than halves the rate of plasma clearance of lidocaine. Patients with advanced liver disease also show a marked reduction in lidocaine clearance. Drugs that induce hepatic metabolism significantly accelerate lidocaine clearance. Renal excretion of unchanged drug amounts to 5–10% of total lidocaine clearance. Thus renal disease and changes in urinary pH have no significant effects on the overall pharmacokinetics of lidocaine even though they have profound effects on the excretion of unchanged drug. The pharmacokinetics, dosage schedules, and clinical applications of lidocaine have been reviewed by Benowitz (127).

4.5.4 PHENYTOIN. Phenytoin is a poorly soluble weak acid and is used as the sodium salt. However, the pK_a of the acid is so low (8.3) that it exists largely as the free acid even in the intestine. This leads to slow and variable oral absorption and consequently peak plasma levels occur over an extended period (3–12 hr). The problem has been compounded by significant differences in the bioavailability of oral preparations (128).Phenytoin sodium given intramuscularly precipitates at the site of injection giving rise to a depot effect. About 90% of plasma phenytoin is protein bound. The apparent volume of distribution is about 0.7 1/kg but, as with lidocaine, this value would be much larger if calculated on the basis of free drug. Phenytoin is eliminated largely by hepatic metabolism, the major metabolites being the p-hydroxyphenyl derivative and its glucuronide conjugate, which are excreted in both bile and urine. Metabolites excreted in the bile undergo enterohepatic circulation and most material is eventually excreted in the urine. The amount of unchanged drug excreted in the urine is less than 5% of the total dose. Elimination shows first-order kinetics at plasma concentrations below 10 μg/ml. Above this level, the elimination rate decreases, presumably because of saturation or product-inhibition of metabolism. The elimination half-life of phenytoin varies greatly (10–40 hr) and depends on the ability of the individual to metabolize the drug. The metabolism of phenytoin can be inhibited by other drugs including isoniazid, aminosalicyclic acid, chlorpromazine, prochlorperazine, chlordiazepoxide, estrogens, disulfiram, and warfarin. Since phenytoin is an acid and is strongly bound to albumin it may displace other acidic drugs such as bishydroxycoumarin from its albumin-binding sites. Finally, the metabolism of phenytoin may be induced by agents such as phenobarbitone resulting in greatly diminished pharmacological effects. The pharmacokinetics, dosage schedules, and antiarrhythmic properties of phenytoin have been reviewed by Cohen (129).

4.5.5 DISOPYRAMIDE. Disopyramide (38.**44**) is a recently introduced antiarrhythmic compound. Its electrophysiological and hemodynamic effects are similar to those of quinidine and procainamide. Its efficacy is reported to be similar to that of quinidine and the incidence of its side effects are claimed to be very much lower. The drug shows high bioavailability from the oral route and does not undergo significant first-pass hepatic metabolism. In fact, the drug is excreted 50–60% unchanged.

N-Dealkylation is the main metabolic pathway. The extent of protein binding depends on concentration and shows wide interpatient variation ranging from 5 to 65% of total plasma concentration (although one study put the range at 50–90%). The elimination half-life has been reported as 4-8 hr in healthy subjects, 7–12 hr in patients with recent infarction, and 8–43 hr in patients with severe renal failure. Dosage should be reduced in renal failure in accordance with creatinine clearance values. Therapeutic plasma levels of disopyramide are probably in the range 3–6 μg/ml. The pharmacology, pharmacokinetics, and clinical evaluation of disopyramide have been reviewed by Heel at al. (130).

5 ANTIANGINAL DRUGS

5.1 Pathophysiology of Angina—the Basis for Drug Design

Angina occurs when the blood supply to the heart is unable to meet the metabolic demands of the heart for oxygen. The result is acute, reversible left ventricular failure with consequent increase in left ventricular end-diastolic volume. Since the heart normally extracts almost all the available oxygen from blood it cannot, in contrast to skeletal muscle, increase its oxygen uptake by further extraction of oxygen, and its capacity for anaerobic metabolism is very limited. The heart must therefore meet its metabolic demands for oxygen by increasing the rate of coronary blood flow. Angina is caused by coronary vessel constriction which prevents the increase in blood flow needed to meet the oxygen demands associated with exercise or stress. The most common cause of coronary vessel constriction is atherosclerosis, but there is increasing evidence that a significant number of angina patients have no demonstrable coronary atherosclerotic lesions and normal coronary angiograms have been found in 9-36% of anginal patients (131). There is evidence that reflex coronary spasm may be a cause of angina in some patients (132).

The first effective drug for the treatment of angina was amyl nitrite, which was introduced into medicine by Brunton in 1867. It was long believed that this drug and the related nitrates and nitrites relieved angina by dilating the coronary vessels. This view, now known to be substantially incorrect, stimulated a large body of fruitless research involving the synthesis and testing of many new drugs that dilated coronary vessels in test animals. There is an obvious message here for the medicinal chemist: do not accept a particular model for drug action simply because it seems plausible, particularly if the pathophysiology of the disease cannot be simulated in a test animal—as is the case with angina.

The pathophysiology of angina involves a "vicious circle" which tends to increase and prolong the ischemia even after the initial stimulus has ceased. The therapeutic objective in treating an anginal attack is to break this cycle. The normal response to exercise is an increase in cardiac output consequent to an increase in heart rate and venous return. This increase in work promotes a metabolite-induced dilation of the coronary vessels which leads to increased coronary flow and increased available oxygen. Patients with coronary vessel constriction can make this response only to a limited degree. Insufficient oxygen is available to enable the left ventricle to expel the increased venous return and the heart dilates as end-diastolic volume increases. Subsequently, the heart enters acute left ventricular failure, causing a reflex increase in peripheral resistance and venous return, which further increases heart rate and end-diastolic volume and promotes an even greater demand for oxygen. This cycle can be broken by (1) decreasing venous return with drugs such as nitroglycerin; (2) decreasing demand for oxygen with β-blockers; or (3) increasing cardiac output with cardiac stimulants. The pathophysiology and treatment of angina are reviewed in Refs. 132–135.

5.2 Nitrites and Nitrates

A selection of nitrites and nitrates is shown in Fig. 38.30. Of these compounds, nitroglycerin (38.**58**), one of the first to be developed, remains the drug of choice. Although the nitrates are more potent than the nitrites, there is good evidence that the nitrite is the active form of the drug and that nitrates are reduced to nitrites by sulfhydryl groups at the site of action (136, 137). Tolerance to nitrates develops when tissue levels of sulfhydryl groups are depleted (137). Presumably the greater potency of the nitrates is due to more effective uptake by the target tissues.

The pharmacology of nitroglycerin is complex and the reader is referred to Refs. 132–135 for an account of this subject. Very briefly, the nitrates and nitrites are general vasodilators but their actual effects depend on the state of the vessel and the degree of reflex sympathetic override. The major effect is to increase the venous capacitance and thereby break the cycle of

NITRITES

NaONO

38.**56** Sodium nitrite

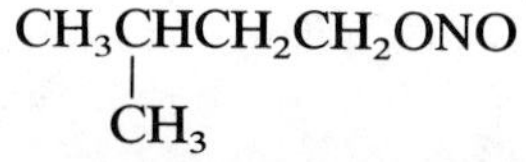

$$CH_3CHCH_2CH_2ONO$$
$$|$$
$$CH_3$$

38.**57** Amyl nitrite

NITRATES

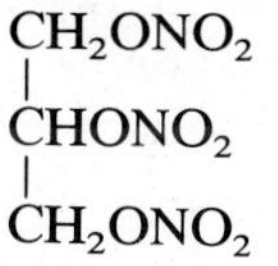

$$CH_2ONO_2$$
$$|$$
$$CHONO_2$$
$$|$$
$$CH_2ONO_2$$

38.**58** Nitroglycerin

$$CH_2ONO_2$$
$$|$$
$$CHONO_2$$
$$|$$
$$CHONO_2$$
$$|$$
$$CH_2ONO_2$$

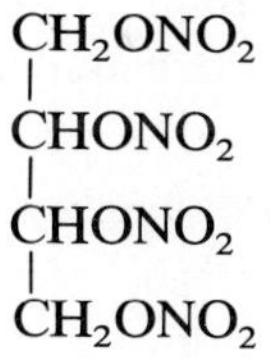

38.**59** Erythritol tetranitrate

$$CH_2ONO_2$$
$$|$$
$$O_2NOCH_2-C-CH_2ONO_2$$
$$|$$
$$CH_2ONO_2$$

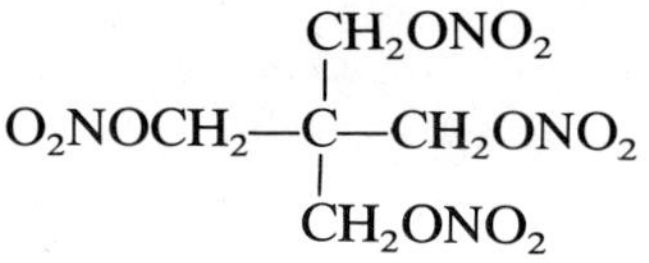

38.**60** Pentaerythritol tetranitrate

$$CH_2ONO_2$$
$$|$$
$$O_2NOCH$$
$$|$$
$$O_2NOCH$$
$$|$$
$$CHONO_2$$
$$|$$
$$CHONO_2$$
$$|$$
$$CH_2ONO_2$$

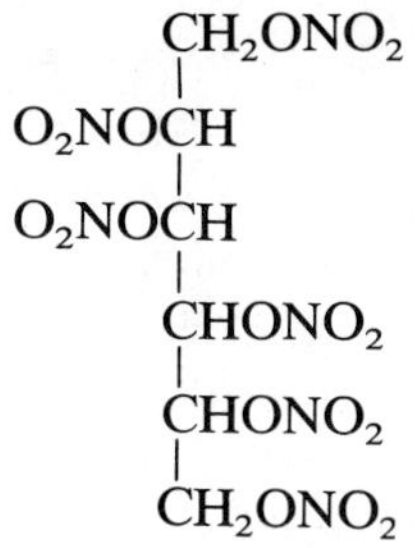

38.**61** Mannitol hexanitrate

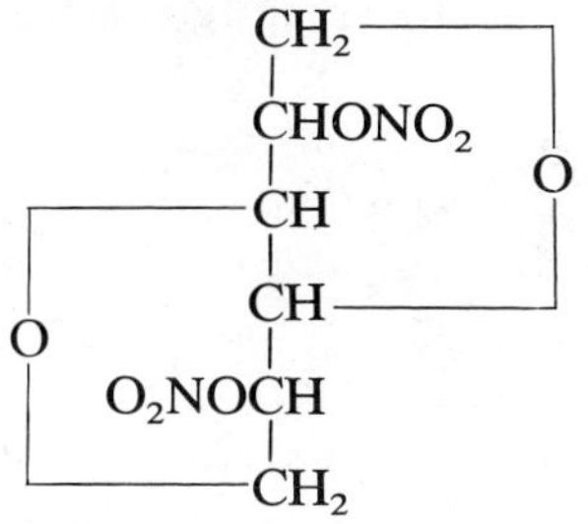

38.**62** Isosorbide dinitrate

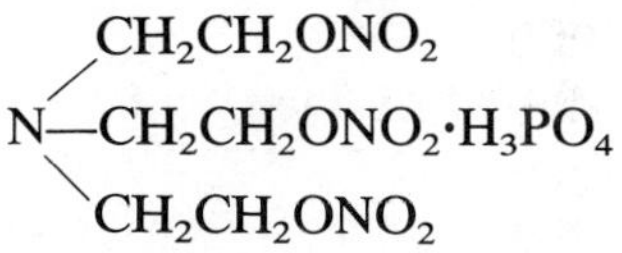

$$CH_2CH_2ONO_2$$
$$N-CH_2CH_2ONO_2 \cdot H_3PO_4$$
$$CH_2CH_2ONO_2$$

38.**63** Trolnitrate phosphate

Fig. 38.30 Nitrites and nitrates used as antianginal agents.

increasing ischemia by reducing cardiac return (see Section 5.1). The drugs also dilate systemic arterioles leading to a fall in peripheral vascular resistance. Effects on coronary vessels are minimal since, within the limits imposed by atherosclerosis, these vessels make a near-to-maximum vasodilatory response to ischemia and there is little or no margin left for a further response to drugs. Although the drugs have no significant effects on overall coronary blood flow, there is evidence that they may induce a redistribution of coronary flow in favor of the ischemic areas. This would supplement the effects of reduced venous return and reduced peripheral resistance in reducing the gap between work load and available oxygen.

The nitrates and nitrites tend to be extensively degraded during one pass through the liver and consequently absorption from the gastrointestinal tract is often low and variable. The drugs are therefore best given by the sublingual route where absorption is rapid and extensive. Certain nitrates, for example, 38.**59**–38.**63**, are claimed to be "long-acting," with duration of effects ranging from 3 to 6 hr. Some evidence suggests that there is no basis for this claim since equieffective doses are said to be eliminated over approximately the same time period (138). However, more recent evidence has confirmed that some nitrates such as pentaerythritol tetranitrate (139) and isosorbide dinitrate (140) have effects that persist for 4–5 hr. Another approach to the problem of achieving a long-acting form of nitrate for prophylaxis of angina, is the development of new routes of administration and new methods of formulation. Reichek et al. (141) have shown that an "old-fashioned" preparation of nitroglycerin—nitroglycerin ointment—appears to be effective in angina prophylaxis. Nitroglycerin ointment rubbed into the skin of the chest produces effects that last for about 3 hr compared with about 30 min following sublingual nitroglycerin. A sustained-release oral preparation of glyceryl trinitrate has also been developed (142). Nitroglycerin is a volatile substance and must be stored in well-closed amber glass containers at all times. Improvements in tablet formulation have decreased the problem of volatilization of nitroglycerin, but patients should still be instructed to store reserve supplies in the refrigerator and not to transfer the tablets to plastic vials or any other type of nonglass container. Modern tablets in a mannitol base retain their activity for at least 2 years if stored in an airtight container, protected from light, and kept in a cool place.

5.3   Beta-Adrenergic Blocking Agents

The introduction of β-adrenergic blocking agents for prophylaxis of angina was a great advance in the treatment of severe angina. Although a number of β-blockers are now available, it is still too early to conclude that any of the newer drugs have significant advantages over propranolol except that practolol should not be used because of its occasional severe side effects (143) and a cardioselective agent should be used in patients subject to bronchospasm. Dosage should be increased slowly and, likewise, when the drug is withdrawn, dosage should be reduced slowly to avoid precipitation of severe and sometimes fatal angina. The medicinal chemistry of β-adrenergic blocking agents is discussed elsewhere in this text (Chapter 41 and 42). It is appropriate to point out that the action of β-blockers on the heart seems to include effects additional to β-blockade, and these should be noted by the medicinal chemist as pointers in the search for new drugs.

The first response to exercise is parasympathetic withdrawal. If this does not provide the required increase in cardiac output, it is followed by activation of the sympathetic nervous system. The release of catecholamines in response to exercise or stress of any type is the major factor that determines the frequency and severity of angina attacks. Not only do catecholamines increase oxygen demand by increasing myocardial activity, but also they produce what is known as an "oxygen wasting" effect by increasing metabolic production of heat over and above the increase in heat production associated with increased contractility. Beta-blockade with agents such as propranolol (38.**46**), alprenolol, oxprenolol, and pindolol reduces or inhibits the sympathetic-induced demand for oxygen and, at the same time, permits the patient to exercise for longer periods and to achieve a greater work load. This increased capacity for exercise may be due in part to improved perfusion of the deeper (and usually more ischemic) regions of the left ventricular wall (144) as well as to a reduction in the affinity of hemoglobin for oxygen at low oxygen tension (145), producing a greater release of oxygen in ischemic tissues. These properties may also be of value in limiting the effects of infarction. In 1975 the results of an extensive double-blind trial of the long-term effects of β-blockade using practolol in postinfarction patients was published (143). Although the trial had to be terminated because of the side effects of the drug, it was nevertheless established that the practolol-treated group showed a significant reduction in overall mortality and sudden deaths, and there was a highly significant reduction for "all cardiac events." Thus for the first time a statistically significant advantage was shown for a postinfarction intervention.

6 VASODILATORS IN HEART FAILURE

The most important recent advance in the treatment of heart failure has been the introduction of unloading agents or vasodilators (146). These drugs decrease both preload and afterload by increasing the size of the vascular bed. This improves myocardial function without increasing myocardial energy demands. This is a particularly useful property in heart failure associated with ischemic myocardial disease.

All recent literature referring to the use of vasodilators in heart failure makes extensive reference to the terms preload and afterload. Preload is a measure of the extent to which heart muscle fibers are stretched just prior to contraction. For a particular heart, this is a function of the volume of blood in the ventricle just prior to contraction (the end-diastolic volume). The main factors that contribute to preload include venous return, degree of ventricular

emptying during systole, and diastolic ventricular compliance. Venous return is controlled by the total volume of blood and the capacitance of the systemic venous system. Venous capacitance refers to the volume of blood held in the venous system. When capacitance is increased, more blood remains in the veins and less returns to the heart. Certain vasodilators decrease the load on the heart by increasing venous capacitance.

Cardiac afterload is the tension that the ventricles must develop in order to eject the stroke volume. The principal factors that contribute to afterload are ventricular radius and systolic impedance. Impedance is a measure of the pressure needed to achieve a particular blood flow from the ventricle. Factors that contribute to impedance include the compliance (ability to dilate) of the major arteries and the vascular resistance, which is controlled mainly by the tone (tension) of the arterioles. Blood viscosity and arterial blood volume are also important contributing factors to impedance. Although many factors contribute to afterload, the most significant clinically is vascular resistance and it is this factor that is altered by vasodilators.

Vasodilator drugs act by reducing the tone in vascular smooth muscle with consequent dilation of the arteries and veins. Vasodilators act either by direct action on the vascular smooth muscle or by blockade of α-adrenoceptors or stimulation of β-adrenoceptors. Many vasodilators act by several mechanisms, and drugs such as phentolamine, tolazoline, and prazosin, which are often classified as α-adrenoceptor blockers, act mainly by direct action on smooth muscle. Vasodilators usually act on all blood vessels, although the relative effects on the various vascular beds varies considerably with different drugs.

The effects of vasodilator drugs on cardiac performance depends on which type of vessel (vein or artery) is most affected and on the hemodynamic status of the patient. The optimum setting for the use of vasodilator drugs and the vasodilator of choice are still very much under investigation but, clearly, blood pressure and ventricular filling pressure must be adequate for vasodilator therapy to be used; otherwise the patient is liable to hypotension, which is the major hazard in vasodilator therapy.

6.1 Nitrates

The nitrates and nitrites act mainly on the venous capacitance vessels. They therefore reduce preload. (See Section 5.2.)

6.2 Phentolamine and Tolazoline

These drugs have an array of different categories of effect, depending on the organ system studied. On the cardiovascular system, they show α-adrenoceptor blocking activity as well as a direct vasodilator effect. In the doses used, their direct effect is the main component of their activity. This effect is shown mainly in the arterioles and capillaries. These drugs reduce preload by increasing venous capacitance (mainly as a consequence of α-adrenoceptor blockade) and decrease afterload by reducing peripheral arterial resistance (mainly as a result of direct vasodilator activity). The effects on afterload are greater than their effects on preload.

6.3 Sodium Nitroprusside

Sodium nitroprusside is a general vasodilator that produces a balanced reduction in both preload and afterload. It is an extremely powerful hypotensive agent and its effects appear within seconds of commencing infusion. It must be given under close supervision. It is used in the treatment of hypertensive crises and in treating acute cardiac failure where there is a normal or elevated blood pressure plus reduced cardiac output associated with high preload and afterload. Infusion solutions are prepared immediately before use by dissolving the sterile solid in dextrose injection.

6.4 Prazosin and Hydralazine

The activity of prazosin resembles somewhat that of phentolamine and tolazoline in that it shows both α-adrenoceptor blocking activity and direct vasodilator activity. However, its range of uses is closer to that of hydralazine, which is virtually a purely direct acting vasodilator with little or no significant α-blocking activity.

Prazosin and hydralazine are given orally and produce vasodilation lasting 3–5 hr. Prazosin reduces both venous and arterial tone and thus reduces both preload and afterload. Hydralazine acts mainly on arterioles to reduce afterload. It may be given with a nitrate to produce balanced reduction in preload and afterload. See Ref. 147 for a list of references relating to the use of unloading agents in the treatment of heart failure.

REFERENCES

1. A. J. Brady, "Electrophysiology of Cardiac Muscle," in *The Mammalian Myocardium*, G. A. Langer and A. J. Brady, Eds., Wiley, New York–London–Sydney–Toronto, 1974, pp. 163–192.
2. H. A. Fozzard and W. R. Gibbons, *Am. J. Cardiol.*, **31**, 182 (1973).
3. P. H. Morgan and I. W. Mathison, *J. Pharm. Sci.*, **65**, 467 (1976).
4. M. Vassalle, "Electrophysiology of the Heart Cells," in *Cardiac Physiology for the Clinician*, M. Vassalle, Ed., Academic, New York–San Francisco–London, 1976, pp. 1–26.
5. B. C. Pressman and N. T. de Guzman, *Ann. N.Y. Acad. Sci.*, **227**, 380 (1974).
6. J. M. Murray and A. Weber, *Sci. Am.* **230,** 58 (1974).

7. Symposium "Na-Ca Interaction as a Pharmacological Trigger," in *Brain, Nerves and Synapses,* Vol. 4 of *Proceedings of the Fifth International Congress on Pharmacology,* F. E. Bloom and G. H. Acheson, Eds., S. Karger, Basel–Munich–Paris–London–New York–Sydney, 1973, pp. 344–371.

8. S. Hajdu and E. J. Leonard, *Life Sci.* **17,** 1527 (1975).

9. W. G. Nayler, J. Dunnett, and A. Sullivan, "Drug-Induced Changes in the Superficially Located Stores of Calcium in Heart Sarcolemma," in *The Sarcolemma,* P. Roy and N. S. Dhalla, Eds., University Park Press, Baltimore–London–Tokyo, 1976, pp. 53–70.

10. G. Inesi and N. Malan, *Life Sci.* **18,** 773 (1976).

11. A. Schwartz, *Fed. Proc.,* **35,** 1279 (1976).

12. G. A. Langer, *Fed. Proc.,* **35,** 1274 (1976).

13. G. A. Langer, "Ionic Movements and the Control of Contraction," in *The Mammalian Myocardium,* G. A. Langer and A. J. Brady, Eds., Wiley, New York–London–Sydney–Toronto, 1974, pp. 193–218.

14. M. Cattell and H. Gold, *J. Pharmacol. Exp. Ther.,* **62,** 116 (1938).

15. R. B. Turner, *Chem. Rev.,* **43,** 1 (1948).

16. L. F. Fieser and M. Fieser, *Steroids,* Reinhold, New York, 1959, Chap. 20.

17. R. Reichstein, *Angew. Chem.,* **63,** 412 (1951).

18. C. Tamm, *Progr. Org. Chem. Nat. Prod.* **13,** 137 (1956); **14,** 71 (1957).

19. F. G. Henderson, "Chemistry and Biological Activity of the Cardiac Glycosides," in *Digitalis,* C. Fisch and B. Surawicz, Eds., Grune and Stratton, New York–London, 1969, pp. 3–12.

20. F. Sondheimer, *Chem. Brit.,* **1,** 454 (1965).

21. G. K. Moe and A. E. Farah, "Digitalis and Allied Cardiac Glycosides, in *The Pharmacological Basis of Therapeutics,*" L. S. Goodman and A. Gilman, Eds., 5th Ed., Macmillan, New York, 1975, pp. 653–682.

22. B. H. Marks and A. M. Weissler, Eds., *Basic and Clinical Pharmacology of Digitalis,* Charles C Thomas, Springfield, Ill., 1972.

23. T. W. Smith, *New Engl. J. Med.,* **288,** 719 (1973).

24. *Ibid.,* 942 (1973).

25. J. E. Doherty, *Ann. Intern. Med.,* **79,** 229 (1973).

26. D. T. Mason, R. Zelis, G. Lee, J. L. Hughes, J. F. Spann, and E. A. Amsterdam, *Amer. J. Cardiol.,* **27,** 546 (1971).

27. L. F. Soyka, *Pediatr. Clin. North Am.,* **19,** 241 (1972).

28. C. Fisch, *J. Am. Med. Assoc.,* **216,** 1770 (1971).

29. J. T. Bigger and H. C. Strauss, *Semin. Drug Treat.,* **2,** 147 (1972).

30. R. A. Massumi, E. A. Amsterdam, R. Zelis, and D. T. Mason, *Semin. Drug Treat.,* **2,** 221 (1972).

31. R. W. Jelliffe, J. Buell, and R. Kalaba, *Ann. Intern. Med.,* **77,** 891 (1972).

32. P. Duca and A. N. Brest, "Indications, Contraindications and Nonindications for Digitalis Therapy," in *Cardiovascular Drug Therapy,* K. L. Melmon and A. N. Brest, Eds., F. A. Davis, Philadelphia, 1974, pp. 131–140.

33. G. A. Ewy, F. I. Marcus, S. J. Fillmore, and N. P. Mathews, "Digitalis Intoxication—Diagnosis, Management and Prevention," in *Cardiovascular Drug Therapy,* K. L. Melman and A. N. Brest, Eds., F. A. Davis, Philadelphia, 1974, pp. 153–174.

34. D. H. Huffman, *Am. J. Hosp. Pharm.,* **33,** 179 (1976).

35. J. K. Aronson and D. G. Grahame-Smith, *Brit. J. Clin. Pharm.* **3,** 639 (1976).

36. D. J. Greenblatt and T. W. Smith, *Postgrad. Med.* **59,** 134 (1976).

37. W. Wilbrandt and P. Lindgren, Eds., Symposium "New Aspects of Cardiac Glycosides," in *Proceedings of the First International Pharmacological Meeting,* Vol. 3, Pergamon, Oxford–London–New York–Paris, 1963.

38. M. Vassalle and E. Musso, "Therapeutic and Toxic Actions of Digitalis," in *Cardiac Physiology for the Clinician,* M. Vassalle, Ed., Academic, New York–San-Francisco–London, 1976, pp. 204–240.

39. K. S. Lee and W. Klaus, *Pharm. Rev.,* **23,** 193 (1971).

40. A. Schwartz, G. Lindenmayer, and J. C. Allen, *Pharm. Rev.,* **27,** 3 (1975).

41. G. A. Langer, *Ann. Rev. Physiol.,* **35,** 55 (1973).

42. A. Schwartz, *Circ. Res.,* **39,** 2 (1976).

43. R. Thomas, J. Boutagy, and A. Gelbart, *J. Pharm. Sci.,* **63,** 1649 (1974).

44. R. Schön, W. Schönfeld, K-H. Menke, K. R. H. Repke, *Acta Biol. Med. Germ.,* **29,** 643 (1972).

45. W. G. Nayler, *J. Mol. Cell. Cardiol.,* **5,** 101 (1973).

46. A. Gervais, L. K. Lane, B. M. Anner, G. E. Lindenmayer, and A. Schwartz, *Circ. Res.,* **40,** 8 (1977).

47. J. C. Skou, *Biochim. Biophys. Acta,* **23,** 394 (1957).

48. A. Schwartz, G. E. Lindenmayer, and J. C. Allen, "The Na⁺,K⁺-ATPase membrane transport system: importance in cellular function," in

Current Topics in Membranes and Transport, F. Bonner and A. Kleinzeller, Eds., Vol. 3, Academic, New York, 1972, pp. 1–82.

49. A. Askari, Ed., "Properties and Functions of $(Na^+ + K^+)$-Activated Adenosine-triphosphatase," *Ann. N.Y. Acad. Sci.,* **242,** 1–741 (1974).

50. R. W. Albers, "The (Sodium plus Potassium)—Transport ATPase," in *The Enzymes of Biological Membranes,* Vol. 3, A. Martonosi, Ed., Plenum, New York, 1976, pp. 283–301.

51. W. Schoner, H. Pauls, and R. Patzelt-Wenczler, "Biochemical Characteristics of the Sodium Pump: Indications for a Half-of-Sites Reactivity of $(Na^+ + K^+)$-ATPase," in *Myocardial Failure,* G. Riecker, A. Weber, and J. Goodwin, Eds. Springer-Verlag, Berlin–Heidelberg, 1977, pp. 104–117.

52. B. J. R. Pitts and A. Schwartz, *Biochim. Biophys. Acta,* **401,** 184 (1975).

53. K. H. R. Repke, "Metabolism of Cardiac Glycosides," in Ref. 37, pp. 47–73.

54. T. Akera, *Science,* **198,** 569 (1977).

55. T. Akera and T. Brody, *Pharmacol. Rev.* **29,** 187, 1978.

56a. C. Tamm, "The Stereochemistry of the Glycosides in Relation to Biological Activity," in Ref. 37, pp. 11–26.

56b. K. K. Chen, "Possibilities of Further Developments in the Glycoside Field by Modifying the Glycoside Structure," in Ref. 37, pp. 27–41.

57. G. Kroneberg, K. H. Meyer, E. Schraufstätter, S. Schütz, and K. Stoepel, *Naturwissenschaften,* **51,** 192 (1964).

58. G. Kroneberg and K. Stoepel, *Arch. Exp. Pathol. Pharmakol.,* **249,** 393 (1964).

59. G. A. Beller, T. W. Smith, W. H. Abelmann, E. Haber, and W. B. Hood, Jr., *New Engl. J. Med.,* **284,** 989 (1971).

60. R. Thomas, J. Boutagy, and A. Gelbart, *J. Pharmacol. Exp. Ther.,* **191,** 219 (1974).

61. J. Kyte, *J. Biol. Chem.,* **247,** 7634 (1972).

62. S. Schütz, K. Meyer, and H. Krätzer, *Arzneim.-Forsch.,* **19,** 69 (1969).

63. N. A. Beard, W. Rouse, and A. R. Sommerville, *Brit. J. Pharm.,* **54,** 65 (1975).

64. R. Thomas, L. Brown, J. Boutagy, and A. Gelbart, *Circ. Res.* (in press).

65. K. O. Haustein, *Pharmacology,* **11,** 117 (1974).

66. K. O. Haustein and J. Hauptmann, *Pharmacology,* **11,** 129 (1974).

67. T. Shigei, H. Tsuru, Y. Saito, and M. Okada, *Experientia,* **29,** 449 (1973).

68. A. Yoda nad S. Yoda, *Mol. Pharmacol.,* **11,** 653 (1975).

69. A. Yoda, *Mol. Pharmacol.,* **9,** 51 (1972).

70. K. Meyer (to Hoffmann-La Roche), Swiss Pat. 559, 219; through *Chem. Abstr.,* **83,** 28459 (1975).

71. R. W. Caldwell and C. B. Nash, *J. Pharmacol. Exp. Ther.,* **197,** 19 (1976).

72. R. Mendez, G. Pastelin, and E. Kabela, *J. Pharmacol. Exp. Ther.,* **188,** 189 (1974).

73. R. Thomas, J. Allen, B. Pitts, and A. Schwartz, *Eur. J. Pharmacol.* **53,** 227 (1979).

74. A-F. Prigent, M. Roche, and H. Pacheco, *Eur. J. Med. Chem.,* **10,** 498 (1975).

75. R. Thomas and A. Gelbert, *J. Med. Chem.,* **21,** 284 (1978).

76. G. Bodem and H. J. Dengler, Eds., *Cardiac Glycosides,* Springer-Verlag, Berlin–Heidelberg, 1978.

77. G. T. Okita, "Distribution, Disposition and Excretion of Digitalis Glycosides," in *Digitalis,* C. Fisch and B. Surawicz, Eds., Grune and Stratton, New York–London, 1969, pp. 13–26.

78. J. E. Doherty, W. J. Flanigan, M. L. Murphy, R. T. Bulloch, G. L. Dalrymple, O. W. Beard, and W. H. Perkins, *Circulation,* **42,** 867 (1970).

79. J. Boutagy and R. Thomas, *Xenobiotica,* **7,** 267 (1977).

80. S. Aldous and R. Thomas, *Clin. Pharmacol. Ther.,* **21,** 647 (1977).

81. T. W. Smith and E. Haber, *Pharmacol. Rev.,* **25,** 219 (1973).

82. V. P. Butler, "Evaluation of Different Methods of Determining Serum Concentrations of Cardiac Glycosides," in *Cardiac Glycosides,* G. Bodem and H. J. Dengler, Eds., Springer-Verlag, Berlin–Heidelberg, 1978 pp. 1–21.

83. F. I. Marcus, *Am. J. Med.,* **58,** 452 (1975).

84. E. J. Fraser, R. H. Leach, J. W. Poston, A. M. Bold, L. S. Culank, and A. B. Lipede, *J. Pharm. Pharmacol.,* **25,** 968 (1973).

85. S. K. Sim, *Am. J. Hosp. Pharm.,* **33,** 44 (1976).

86. D. J. Greenblatt, T. W. Smith, and J. Koch-Weser, *Clin. Pharmacokinet.* **1,** 36 (1976).

87. T. R. D. Shaw, "Bioavailability Studies: Their Influence on the Clinical Use of Digitalis," in *Cardiac Glycosides,* G. Bodem and H. J. Dengler, Eds., Springer-Verlag, Berlin–Heidelberg, pp. 187–198 (1978).

88. F. Keller and N. Rietbrock, *Int. J. Clin. Pharmacol.,* **15,** 549 (1977).

89. B. F. Johnson, C. Bye, G. Jones, and G. A. Sabey, *Clin. Pharmacol. Ther.,* **19,** 746 (1976).

90. B. Beerman, K. Hellström, and A. Rosén, *Clin. Sci.,* **43,** 507 (1972).

91. W. H. Hall and J. E. Doherty, *Am. J. Dig. Dis.,* **16,** 903 (1971).

92. R. Megges, H. J. Portius, and K. R. H. Repke, *Pharmazie*, **32,** 665 (1977).

93. K.-O. Haustein, C. Pachaly, and D. Murawski, *Int. J. Clin. Pharmacol.*, **16,** 285 (1978).

94. J. Boutagy and R. Thomas, *Xenobiotica*, **7,** 267 (1977).

95. W. Schaumann, "β-Methyl-Digoxin, a new Lipophilic Digoxin Derivative," in *Cardiac Glycosides*, G. Bodem and H. J. Dengler, Eds., Springer-Verlag, Berlin–Heidelberg, 1978, pp. 93–108.

96. Garrett et al., *J. Pharm. Sci.*, **66,** 242, 314, 326, 806 (1977).

97. K. Dietmann, E. Hrstka, and W. Schaumann, *Arch Pharmacol.*, **302,** 87 (1978).

98. W. J. Jusko, S. J. Szefler, and A. L. Goldfarb, *J. Clin. Pharm.* **14,** 525 (1974).

99. D. J. Sumner, A. J. Russell, and B. Whiting, *Brit. J. Clin. Pharm.*, **3,** 221 (1976).

100. S. M. Dobbs, G. E. Mawer, E. M. Rodgers, B. G. Woodcock, and S. B. Lucus, *Brit. J. Clin. Pharm.*, **3,** 231 (1976).

101. P. F. Binnion, "Comparative Pharmacokinetics of Various Digoxin Preparations in Man," in *Cardiac Glycosides*, G. Bodem and H. J. Dengler, Eds., Springer-Verlag, Berlin–Heidelberg, 1978, pp. 199–210.

102. H. J. Dengler, G. Bodem, and H. J. Gilfrich, "Digoxin Pharmacokinetics and their Relation to Clinical Dosage Parameters," in *Cardiac Glycosides*, G. Bodem and H. J. Dengler, Eds., Springer-Verlag, Berlin–Heidelberg, 1978, p. 211–225.

103. A. M. Weissler, R. P. Lewis, R. F. Leighton, and C. A. Bush, "Comparative responses to the digitalis glycosides in man," in *Basic and Clinical Pharmacology of Digitalis*, B. H. Marks and A. M. Weissler, Eds., Charles C Thomas, Springfield, Ill., 1972, pp. 260–280.

104. R. N. Deutscher, D. C. Harrison, and R. H. Goldman, *Am. J. Cardiol.*, **29,** 47 (1972).

105. R. W. Jelliffe and G. Brooker, *Am. J. Med.*, **57,** 63 (1974).

106. M. Vassalle, Ed., *Cardiac Physiology for the Clinician*, Academic, New York–San Francisco–London, 1976, Chaps. 2–5.

107. L. S. Dreifus and W. A. Likoff, Eds., *Cardiac Arrhythmias; the Twenty-Fifth Hahnemann Symposium*, Grune and Stratton, New York, 1973.

108. S. Bellet, *Clinical Disorders of the Heart Beat*, 3rd ed., Lea and Febiger, Philadelphia, 1971, Chaps. 43–47.

109. J. T. Bigger and F. M. Weld, "Arrhythmias and Antiarrhythmic Drugs," in *Cardiac Physiology for the Clinician*, M. Vassalle, Ed., Academic, New York–San Francisco–London, 1976, pp. 141–171.

110. J. T. Bigger and E. G. V. Giardina, "Rational Use of Antiarrhythmic Drugs Alone and in Combination in *Cardiovascular Drug Therapy*, K. L. Melmon and A. N. Brest, Eds., F. A. Davis, Philadelphia, 1974, pp. 103–117.

111. P. F. Cranefield, *The conduction of the Cardiac Impulse—the Slow Response and Cardiac Arrhythmias*, Futura, Mt. Kisco, N. Y., 1975.

112. E. M. Vaughan Williams, in *Symposium on Cardiac Arrhythmias*, E. Sandoe, E. Flensted-Jensen, and K. M. Olsen, Eds., A. B. Astra, Södertälje, Sweden, 1970, pp. 449–472.

113. B. F. Hoffman, A. L. Wit, and M. R. Rosen, *Am. Heart J.*, **88,** 95 (1974).

114. W. R. Buckett, F. A. Marwick, and B. B. Vargaftig, *Brit. J. Pharmacol.*, **54,** 3 (1975).

115. L. Szekeres and G. J. Papp, *Experimental Cardiac Arrhythmias and Antiarrhythmic Drugs*, Akadémiai Kiadó, Budapest, 1971.

116. C. Hansch and W. J. Dunn, *J. Pharm. Sci.*, **61,** 1 (1972).

117. M. S. Tute, *Advan. Drug. Res.*, **6,** 1 (1971).

118. C. Hansch and J. M. Clayton, *J. Pharm. Sci.*, **62,** 1 (1973).

119. Y. W. Chien, H. J. Lambert, and T. K. Lin, *J. Pharm. Sci.*, **64,** 961 (1975).

120. D. Lalka, M. B. Meyer, B. R. Duce, and A. T. Elvin, *Clin. Pharmacol. Ther.*, **19,** 757 (1976).

121. L. Rydén, B. Olsson, and J. Kvasnička, *Cardiovasc. Res.*, **9,** 81 (1975).

122. W-K. Lee, J. M. Strong, R. F. Kehoe, J. S. Dutcher, and A. J. Atkinson, *Clin. Pharmacol. Ther.*, **19,** 508 (1976).

123. P. D. Thomson, M. Rowland, and K. L. Melmon, *Am. Heart J.*, **82,** 417 (1971).

124. D. J. Greenblatt, V. Bolognini, J. Koch-Weser, and J. S. Harmatz, *J. Am. Med. Assoc.*, **236,** 273 (1976).

125. P. D. Thomson, "Alteration in Pharmacologic Response Induced by Cardiovascular Disease," in *Cardiovascular Drug Therapy*, K. L. Melmon, and A. N. Brest, Eds., F. A. Davis, Philadelphia, 1974, pp. 55–61.

126. J. Koch-Weser, "Clinical Application of the Pharmaco-kinetics of Procainamide," in *Cardiovascular, Drug Therapy*, K. L. Melmon and A. N. Brest, Eds., F. A. Davis, Philadelphia, 1974, pp. 63–75.

127. N. L. Benowitz, "Clinical Applications of the Pharmaco-kinetics of Lidocaine," in *Cardiovascular Drug Therapy*, K. L. Melmon and A. N.

Brest, Eds., F. A. Davis, Philadelphia, 1974, pp. 77–101.

128. A. J. Glazko, *Pharmacology*, **8**, 163 (1972).

129. L. S. Cohen, "Diphenylhydantoin Sodium (Dilantin)," in *Drugs in Cardiology*, Vol. I, part 1, E. Donoso, Ed., Stratton Intercontinental Medical Book Corporation, New York, 1975, pp. 49–79.

130. R. C. Heel, R. N. Brogden, T. M. Speight, and G. S. Avery, *Drugs*, **15**, 331 (1978).

131. W. S. Aronow, *Am. Heart J.*, **85**, 132 (1973).

132. J. R. Parratt, "Pharmacological Approaches to the Therapy of Angina," in *Advances in Drug Research*, Vol. 9, N. J. Harper and A. B. Simmonds, Eds., Academic, London–New York–San Francisco, 1974, pp. 103–134.

133. B. F. Robinson, "Mechanisms in Angina Pectoris in Relation to Drug Therapy," in *Advances in Drug Research*, Vol. 10, Academic, London–New York–San Francicso, 1975, pp. 93–100.

134. R. Zelis, D. T. Mason, E. A. Amsterdam, and J. F. Green, "Current Concepts in the Drug Management of Angina Pectoris," in *Cardiovascular Drug Therapy*, K. L. Melmon and A. N. Brest, Eds., F. A. Davis, Philadelphia, 1974, pp. 239–253.

135. M. Nickerson, "Vasodilator Drugs", in *The Pharmacological Basis of Therapeutics*, 5th ed., L. S. Goodman and A. Gilman, Eds., Macmillan, New York, 1975, pp. 727–743.

136. P. Needleman, D. J. Blehm, and K. S. Rostkoff, *J. Pharmacol. Exp. Ther.*, **165**, 286 (1969).

137. P. Needleman and E. M. Johnson, *J. Pharmacol. Exp. Ther.*, **184**, 709 (1973).

138. R. E. Goldstein and S. E. Epstein, *Circulation*, **48**, 917 (1973).

139. R. C. Klein, E. A. Amsterdam, C. Pratt, L. Laslett, M. Miller, G. Lee, A. N. DeMaria, and D. T. Mason, *Clin. Res.* **26**, 243A (1978).

140. D. O. Williams, W. J. Bommer, R. R. Miller, E. A. Amsterdam, and D. T. Mason, *Am. J. Cardiol.*, **39**, 84 (1977).

141. N. Reichek, R. E. Goldstein, M. Nagel, and S. E. Epstein, *Am. J. Cardiol.*, **31**, 153 (1972).

142. E. A. Amsterdam, J. E. Price, A. N. DeMaria, M. J. Tonkin, N. A. Awan, G. Hamilton, R. R. Miller, and D. T. Mason, *Clin. Res.* **25**, 204A (1977).

143. Multicentre International Study, *Brit. Med. J.*, **3**, 735 (1975).

144. N. J. Fortuin, S. Kaihara, L. C. Becker, and B. Pitt, *Cardiovasc. Res.*, **5**, 331 (1971).

145. J. D. Schrumpf, D. S. Sheps, S. Wolfson, and A. L. Aronson, *Am. J. Cardiol.*, **33**, 170 (1974).

146. J. N. Cohn and J. A. Franciosa, *New Engl. J. Med.*, **297**, 27 and 254 (1977).

147. L. Lemberg, *Arch. Intern. Med.*, **138**, 451 (1978).

148. P. F. Binnion, *Drugs*, **15**, 369 (1978).

149. W. D. Hager, P. Fenster, M. Mayersohn, D. Perrier, P. Graves, F. Marcus and S. Goldman, *N. Engl. J. Med.*, **300**, 1238 (1979).

CHAPTER THIRTY-NINE

Thyromimetic and Antithyroid Drugs

EUGENE C. JORGENSEN

Department of Pharmaceutical Chemistry
School of Pharmacy
University of California
San Francisco, California 94143, USA

CONTENTS

1 INTRODUCTION AND THYROID-RELATED DISEASES

The primary thyroid hormones are two closely related amino acids that vary only in their degree of iodination. These are thyroxine (L-3,5,3′,5′-tetraiodothyronine, T_4, **39.1**) and L-3,5,3′-triiodothyronine (T_3, **39.2**). Both hormones are formed in the thyroid gland and released into the general circulation where deiodination of T_4 leads to further production of T_3. The primary thyroid-related diseases are associated with low (hypothyroidism) or high (hyperthyroidism) levels of circulating hormones. In rare instances these disorders are derived from hypo- or hypersensitivity of tissues to normal levels of available hormones.

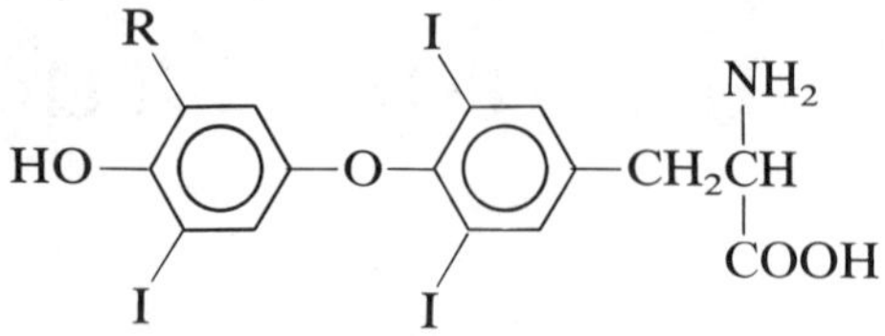

39.1   R=I: thyroxine, T_4
39.2   R = H: 3,5,3′-triiodothyronine, T_3

1.1 Hypothyroidism

Human life can exist in the absence of the thyroid hormones, but that life is of minimal quality. Hormonal effects are important in both the developing fetus and in adult life. A well developed thyroid gland is formed by the seventh week of gestation, and by 11–12 weeks hormone synthesis can be demonstrated (1). Effects on tissue differentiation and development predominate early in life, whereas effects on metabolic function are primary later. Adequate fetal thyroid hormone secretion is of major importance for development of the central nervous system and for skeletal maturation. Hypothyroidism beginning *in utero* and present at birth results in *cretinism*. In severe cases of prenatal hormone deprivation, dwarfism, mental dullness, and neurological defects, including deafness and seizures, are common. The incidence of respiratory-distress syndrome has been correlated with premature birth and with low thyroid activity at birth (2), and it appears likely that the thyroid hormones are important in human fetal lung development.

There is presently no method available for diagnosis of fetal hypothyroidism. The placenta is impermeable to the thyroid hormones, owing to their strong associations with plasma proteins in the maternal blood, so replacement therapy *in utero* is not possible by administration of the hormones via the maternal circulation. Early postnatal replacement therapy results in satisfactory bone and intellectual development. However, despite early thyroid hormone treatment of cretins, such children generally show significant psychomotor retardation, indicating the importance of the hormones in prenatal tissue differentiation and development. If treatment of cretinism is not initiated within the first 6 months of life, the damage is largely irreversible.

Postnatal hypothyroidism, also called *myxedema* from the common accumulation of mucopolysaccharides and fluid in the skin (Greek *myxa*, mucus; *oidema*, swelling), causing the characteristic swollen lips, thickened nose, and puffy eyelids, can develop at any age. Symptoms of weakness, tiredness, dry and cool skin, coarse hair, and mental and physical lethargy are common to juvenile and adult, but retardation of physical development is superimposed in the juvenile. Treatment by oral administration of synthetic T_4 or T_3 or of desiccated thyroid gland or extracts from pork or beef thyroid glands is highly successful in treatment of juvenile or adult-onset hypothyroidism.

1.2   Hyperthyroidism

When the amount of thyroactive substances delivered to the cells of the body exceeds the needs of those cells, a condition of hyperthyroidism or thyrotoxicosis results. Excessive thyroid hormone may be produced by a diffusely enlarged or goitrous thyroid gland (Graves' disease) or one with hyperfunctional nodules (Plummer's disease). In the more common Graves' disease a protein that behaves as a long-acting thyroid stimulator (LATS) is present in the blood, although its causative role in the

disease is controversial (3). LATS has been identified as an immunoglobulin which is an integral part of a gamma globulin component of serum protein. This supports the concept that Graves' disease may be initiated by an autoimmune process.

Increased thyroid hormone secretion leads to enhancement of most of the body's metabolic processes, resulting in weight loss, warm and moist skin, and increased nervous system activity that produces insomnia, anxiety, nervousness, and hyperactive tendon reflexes. Sensitivity to the sympathetic amines of cardiac muscle and most other organs is increased in hyperthyroidism, and tachycardia, palpitations, and systolic hypertension frequently occur. Hyperthyroidism is alleviated by antithyroid drugs by lowering the rate of synthesis and release of hormone from the thyroid gland. When these drugs are ineffective, thyroid tissue may be destroyed by administration of radioactive iodide ion, or the gland may be removed surgically, either partially or totally. Replacement therapy is commonly required following thyroidectomy.

2   HISTORICAL DEVELOPMENTS

2.1   Identification of Thyroxine and Other Iodothyronines

2.1.1   PRESENCE OF IODINE IN THE THYROID GLAND.   Recognition in the 1880s that cretinism and myxedema were associated with loss of function of the thyroid gland led in the early 1890s to feeding of fresh sheep thyroid glands in the effective treatment of myxedema (4). Eugen Baumann, professor of chemistry on the medical faculty of the University of Freiburg, working on the isolation of the active principle from sheep thyroid, found in 1895 that a material effective in relieving the symptoms of myxedema in man and animals was obtained by hydrolysis of the gland with 10% sulfuric acid (5). During studies to characterize this material Baumann fused a sample with sodium hydroxide and potassium nitrate. He dissolved the melt in water, and observed violet fumes of iodine when by chance he acidified the warm solution with nitric acid rather than the more usual sulfuric acid. Baumann recognized the uniqueness of this observation and carefully established that the biologically active material from the thyroid gland, which collaborators from Bayer laboratories named iodothyrin (*Thyrojodin*), contained iodine in organically bound form. In public lectures in Freiburg he displayed crystals of sublimed iodine produced from hydrolysates of the thyroid glands of humans and of sheep (6). Baumann was in an ideal position to further purify and characterize the thyroid hormone. He had the cooperation of Bayer laboratories in which large quantities of sheep thyroids were processed, he was experienced in isolating amino acids from natural sources, and he had the active collaboration of a colleague, Dr. E. Roos, in carrying out biological testing of active fractions. However, his death of a chronic heart condition in 1896 at the age of 49 (7), within a year of his discovery of iodothyrin, led to a delay of almost 20 years in the isolation and characterization of the primary thyroid hormone.

2.1.2 ISOLATION AND CHARACTERIZATION OF THYROXINE. In 1910, at the research laboratory of Parke, Davis and Co. in Detroit, Michigan, Edward Kendall was assigned the problem of isolating the hormone of the thyroid gland (8). Kendall, supported by funds and provided with processed animal thyroid glands by Parke, Davis, continued these studies at the Mayo Clinic at Rochester, Minnesota. On Christmas Day, 1914, he isolated the first crystals of thyroxine. From an erroneously estimated molecular weight of the sulfate salt, and the elemental analysis of the *N*-acetyl derivative, Kendall and Osterberg (9) calculated the empirical formula of the parent compound as $C_{11}H_{10}I_3NO_3$. A pine splint test following NaOH treatment, and other

39.3

color reactions, were interpreted to indicate the presence of an indole nucleus, and Kendall assigned the structure as 4,5,6-*trihydro*-4,5,6-triiodo-2-*oxy*-β-*in*dolepropionic acid (39.**3**), from which the name thyroxyindole, later shortened to *thyroxin*, was derived (10). Kendall selected this name, which recognized the origin from thyroid gland and its assigned chemical structure, rather than one that emphasized the unusual iodine content of the molecule, because he felt that the hormonal activity resided in the organic nucleus to which the iodine was attached, rather in any unique biological role for iodine (10).

During a postdoctoral year in 1922, which included a project with H. D. Dakin at the Rockefeller Institute in New York, Charles Harington became convinced on chemical grounds that Kendall had assigned an erroneous structure to thyroxine (11). Harington proposed a chemically more reasonable iodinated phenylpyrrolidone-carboxylic acid structure and, encouraged by Dakin, during his first year as lecturer in chemical pathology at University College Hospital Medical School, London, initiated studies on the thyroid hormone by the synthesis of this compound (12). Its inactivity in dogs and in normal and hypothyroid humans convinced Harington that this "shot in the dark" approach was futile and that it was necessary to isolate amounts of thyroxine sufficient to carry out systematic chemical degradation studies (13). He devised an improved isolation procedure using dilute barium hydroxide hydrolysis of fresh thyroid glands. This produced in good yield an insoluble barium salt from which thyroxine could be generated by treatment with an alkaline solution of sodium sulfate. A large-scale isolation by the British Drug Houses, Ltd., subsidized by a research grant from the medical school, made it possible for Harington to carry out the analytical and degradation reactions from which he established the correct structure for thyroxine (14). His elemental analysis best fit an empirical formula of $C_{15}H_{11}I_4NO_4$. Catalytic hydrogenation yielded desiodothyroxine (thyronine), $C_{15}H_{15}NO_4$, which gave color reactions characteristic of a phenolic amino acid. Degradation reactions of the desiodo compound yielded fragments that indicated a phenolic hydroxyl group, a three-carbon amino acid side chain, two benzene rings, and an unreactive oxygen atom: $HO(C_{12}H_8O)CH_2CH(NH_2)COOH$. Harington proposed from these data that the thyronine structure was the most likely candidate, and he established its structure as the p-hydroxyphenyl ether of tyrosine by synthesis (14). Characteristic color reactions of thyroxine with nitrous acid and ammonia were shown to be general for o-diiodophenols such as 3,5-diiodotyrosine. Harington concluded that it was highly likely that thyroxine was formed in the thyroid gland from two molecules of 3,5-diiodotyrosine, from which he proposed the 3,5,3′,5′-iodination pattern of the thyronine nucleus (15). This structure of thyroxine as α-amino-β-[3, 5-diiodo-4-(3′,5′-diiodo-4′-hydroxyphenoxy)phenyl]propionic acid was confirmed by degradation of the isolated hormone, and synthesis of both DL- and L-thyroxine (15). Dakin had established the same structure for thyroxine at the same time as Harington but, apparently in a generous gesture toward his young and unknown former associate, withdrew his pending publication in the *Journal of Biological Chemistry* when he learned of Harington's work (15). Harington's research on thyroxine, and his subsequent success as the administrative head of the British National Institute for Medical Re-

search, where he encouraged further basic studies on the thyroid, led to his receiving the British knighthood. The original name proposed by Kendall, thyroxin, was modified by Harington to the now generally accepted name, *thyroxine*, the terminal "e" being added to recognize its identity as an amino acid and its relationship to tyrosine and alanine, for example.

2.1.3   3,5,3′-TRIIODOTHYRONINE. Thyroxine, following its identification as a tetraiodinated thyronine in 1926, was considered to be the only thyroid hormone until the availability of ^{131}I and the newly developed technique of paper chromatography provided more sensitive methods for studying other iodinated compounds in the thyroid. In 1951, Gross and Leblond (16) showed the presence of ^{131}I-containing compounds different from thyroxine and the iodinated tyrosines in the thyroid glands of rats treated with [131]I. Gross and Pitt-Rivers (17), working at the British National Institute for Medical Research near London, showed that one of these substances was present in the plasma of patients treated with radioiodine. The unknown compound was shown to be different from a number of thyroxine analogs prepared by Harington that contained altered side chains, and to closely resemble thyroxine in its chromatographic characteristics. Gross and Pitt-Rivers concluded that a partially iodinated thyronine was the most likely candidate, so they prepared 3,5,3′-L-triiodothyronine (T_3), and in 1953 showed this to be chromatographically identical with the unknown substance (18). They completed the characterization of this second thyroid hormone, which was shown shortly thereafter to be the more biologically potent (19), by its isolation from ox thyroid and identity with the synthetic material. Roche and co-workers (20) simultaneously reported the synthesis of 3,5,3′-triiodo-DL-thyronine and its chromatographic detection in the hydrolysates of rat thyroids following administration of [131]I.

2.1.4 3,3',5'-TRIIODOTHYRONINE AND 3,3'-DIIODOTHYRONINE. Other partially iodinated thyronines have been prepared (21, 22) and have been detected in animal thyroid glands with the aid of radioactive iodine and chromatography (23). Following early studies on impure preparations of 3,3'-diiodothyronine and 3,3',5'-triiodothyronine, which indicated activity (24), the lack of significant hormonal activity established for pure samples in classical bioassay studies (25, 26) initially resulted in these partially iodinated thyronines being rejected as hormones, or considered of no biological significance. More recently it has been shown by Chopra et al. (27) that 3,3',5'-triiodothyronine (reverse-T_3, r-T_3, 3,3',5'-T_3) is present in high concentrations in the serum of the developing human fetus and of the human newborn; r-T_3 concentrations fall to those of the normal adult by 9–11 days of neonatal life. During this time T_4 levels remain fairly constant, while T_3 levels, which are very low in the fetus, rise to adult levels shortly after birth. Whether r-T_3 serves only as an inactive deiodination product of T_4, with this metabolic event moderating fetal levels of active hormone, or whether it plays a more positive role during development has not been established. Reciprocal changes in serum concentrations of reverse-T_3 and of T_3 have also been shown to occur in systemic illnesses, such as hepatic cirrhosis, chronic renal failure, and acute febrile conditions (28). This suggests that the metabolism of T_4 may be altered so that the 5-deiodination reaction is increased with the generation of poorly calorigenic r-T_3 at the expense of the normally occurring 5'-deiodination that forms the highly active T_3.

3 FORMATION, DISTRIBUTION, AND METABOLISM OF THE THYROID HORMONES

The thyroid hormones are formed in the thyroid gland by a process of active accumulation of iodide ion, oxidation of the ion, and rapid iodination of the tyrosine residues of the glycoprotein, thyroglobulin (Tgb). Neighbouring residues of diiodotyrosine (DIT) couple to form thyroglobulin-bound thyroxine (Tgb–T_4). Smaller amounts of monoiodotyrosine (MIT) condense with DIT to form Tgb-bound 3,5,3'-triiodothyronine (Tgb–T_3). The thyroglobulin is hydrolyzed by proteases to liberate T_4 and T_3, and these are secreted into the circulation where they are solubilized and transported by associations with specific plasma proteins. Small amounts of free T_4 and of T_3 in equilibrium with protein-bound material enter cells where their interactions with cellular components initiate events leading to the observable hormonal responses. The free hormones also undergo enzymatically mediated metabolic reactions, the most important being deiodination. Inorganic iodide ion is excreted in urine, whereas the iodine lost in feces is almost entirely organically bound. The following sections describe these processes in greater detail.

3.1 Biosynthesis of the Thyroid Hormones

3.1.1 CONCENTRATION OF IODIDE BY THE THYROID GLAND. Iodine is a trace element; this low abundance and the uneven distribution of iodine in the environment and in the diet make it essential that organisms requiring the element possess a mechanism for its concentration. Iodine, ingested either in organically bound form or as iodide ion, is absorbed primarily in the small intestine. Deiodination of organic iodo compounds takes place primarily in the liver. In normal man an active transport system of the thyroid gland maintains a concentration of iodide ion some thirty–fortyfold higher in the gland than in the general circulation. Other univalent ions that are spherical or tetrahedral in shape, and that approximate iodide ion in size, are also concentrated by the thyroid gland. These ions include astadide (At⁻), bromide (Br⁻), perchlorate (ClO₄⁻), and fluoroborate (BF₄⁻). These ions act as competitive inhibitors of thyroidal uptake of iodide ion, and may be used an antithyroid agents (see Section 9.1.1). Some linear pseudohalides of a similar partial molal ionic volume, such as thiocyanate (SCN⁻) and selenocyanate (SeCN⁻), are not themselves transported but act as competitive inhibitors of iodide uptake.

The pituitary glycoprotein thyrotropin (TSH) is the most important endogenous factor for stimulation of the mechanisms of iodide transport in the thyroid (29). Reduced levels of circulating thyroid hormones produce enhanced secretion of TSH, which in turn stimulates many reactions leading to increased thyroid hormone synthesis, including a marked increase in thyroidal uptake of iodide ion.

3.1.2 IODINATION OF TYROSINE RESIDUES.

Within the thyroid gland iodide is oxidized to the oxidation level of iodine by a membrane-bound hemoprotein enzyme, thyroid peroxidase. The reactive iodinating species formed is not known, but free iodine has not been detected. The reactive iodine may be stored as a protein-bound sulfenyl iodide (E–SI), since the cysteine residues of proteins have been shown to react with iodine to form stable, but highly reactive, sulfenyl iodides (30, 31). Alternatively, it has been proposed that the iodine may exist as an enzyme-bound radical (E–İ). In the latter case, it is suggested that a separate site on the peroxidase enzyme may oxidize tyrosyl residues of the large glycoprotein thyroglobulin to form tyrosyl radicals, with iodotyrosine formation taking place by reaction of the iodine and tyrosyl radicals (32). There are approximately 120 tyrosine residues present in human thyroglobulin, and a range of 10–50 iodine atoms are normally incorporated

into the protein. Iodination occurs ortho to the phenolic hydroxyl group to yield protein-bound 3-iodotyrosine (MIT) and 3,5-diiodotyrosine (DIT). In this state the iodotyrosines act as a nondiffusible reservoir of iodine and serve as immediate precursors of the thyroid hormones. Other residues, such as histidine, are iodinated to a minor extent, but about 50% of the iodine in thyroglobulin is present as 3,5-diiodotyrosine with about 20% as 3-iodotyrosine. In the presence of excess iodine the relative amount of diiodotyrosine increases.

3.1.3 COUPLING OF IODOTYROSINE RESIDUES.

Although the sequence and spatial arrangements of the amino acids in thyroglobulin are unknown, it is likely that some iodotyrosine residues are spatially positioned to permit their ready interaction. The same thyroid peroxidase enzyme that oxidizes iodide ions to a reactive iodine state is also responsible for the oxidative coupling of iodotyrosine residues to form the iodothyronines. Thyroglobulin is uniquely constituted to form T_4 at relatively low levels of iodination, since it has been shown that the tyrosine residues that are first iodinated are also those that are most readily converted to T_4 (33).

A free-radical coupling mechanism was originally proposed in terms of free 3,5-diiodotyrosine (DIT) (34, 35). This has been modified as shown in Fig. 39.1 to occur within the matrix of the protein. DIT free radicals are formed by the action of thyroid peroxidase. The reactive resonance forms, with the unpaired electron shown localized on the phenolic oxygen atom or on the C-1 carbon atom, couple to form an unstable quinol ether (not shown). The reaction is driven by formation of the stable aromatic ring of T_4, one former DIT residue being converted to a dehydroalanine residue. This may hydrate to form a serine residue, or cleave via the tautomeric imine to form pyruvic acid and peptide fragments. Quinol

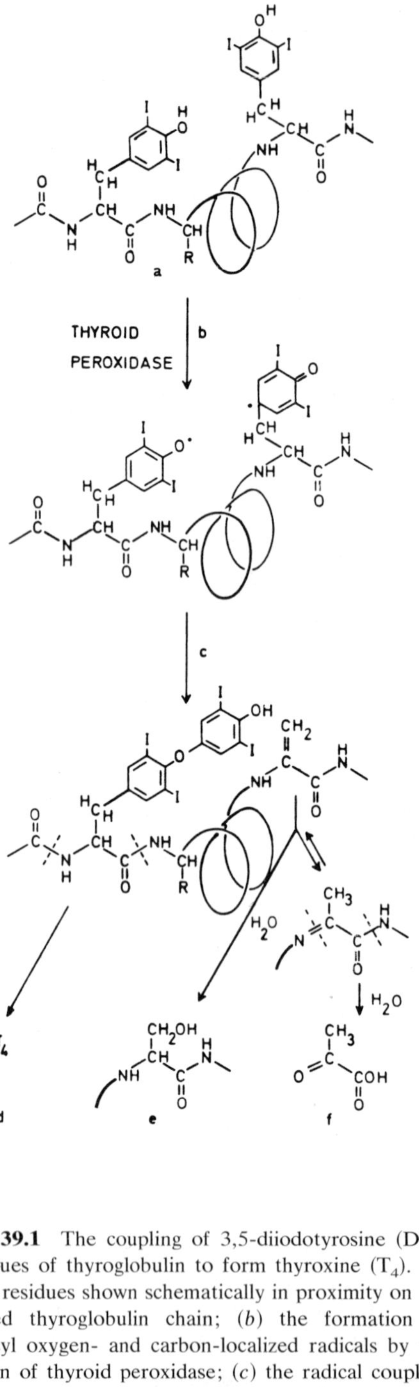

Fig. 39.1 The coupling of 3,5-diiodotyrosine (DIT) residues of thyroglobulin to form thyroxine (T_4). (a) DIT residues shown schematically in proximity on the folded thyroglobulin chain; (b) the formation of tyrosyl oxygen- and carbon-localized radicals by the action of thyroid peroxidase; (c) the radical coupling reaction to form thyroglobulin-bound T_4 and dehydroalanine; and proteolytic and hydrolytic reactions yielding (d) free T_4, (e) a serine residue, and (f) pyruvic acid.

ethers related to the postulated intermediate have been isolated in model reactions (36, 37) and pyruvic acid was identified in model reactions with DIT (34).

Formation of T_3 may be visualized to occur by a similar reaction involving MIT and DIT. The molar ratio of T_4 to T_3 in human thyroglobulin is approximately 20 : 1 (38). This scheme is consistent with the formation of relatively larger amounts of T_3 in iodine deficiency, a condition in which the MIT/DIT ratio in thyroglobulin is increased.

Although other partially iodinated thyronines would be expected to be formed in iodine deficiency, only trace amounts of 3,3′,5′-triiodothyronine (reverse-T_3) and the diiodothyronines have been found in the thyroid gland. These substances are hormonally inactive.

3.1.4 RELEASE AND DISTRIBUTION OF THYROID HORMONES. Thyroglobulin acts not only as a site of hormone synthesis, but as a poorly diffusible storage site for hormone and iodine in its usual extracellular location in the lumen of thyroid follicles. This storage process acts as a buffer to the highly variable supply of iodine in the diet. As hormone is required there is a daily uptake by thyroid cells of less than 1% of the stored thyroglobulin. The colloid droplets containing thyroglobulin fuse with cellular lysozymes. Proteolytic enzymes digest the thyroglobulin, and iodotyrosines and iodothyronines are released. Free MIT and DIT are almost completely deiodinated within the cell and most of the iodide ion is conserved and mixed with that entering from the circulation. Free T_4 and T_3 are resistant to intracellular deiodinase enzymes and are largely released unchanged into the general circulation. The hormones are poorly soluble and are immediately bound by specific proteins in the plasma which act as transport vehicles. About 99.9% of circulating T_4 is normally bound to serum carrier proteins. The differences in onset, magnitudes, and duration of action of the thyroid hormones are in large part due to their differences in strengths of transport protein binding and the rate at which they are metabolized.

The circulating thyroid hormones are principally bound to a protein that migrates to the inter α-globulin zone on filter paper electrophoresis—hence the name thyroxine-binding globulin (TBG). Although present in the low concentration of about 2 mg/100 ml of human plasma, TBG has a high binding affinity for T_4 (K_a *ca.* 10^{10}) and carries about 65% of the total 900 μg of circulating T_4. TBG is an acidic glycoprotein of *ca.* mol. wt 63,000. It appears to be composed of a single polypeptide chain (39) with one high-affinity T_4 binding site per molecule. The amino acid sequence of TBG has not yet been reported. T_3 is bound to TBG with about one-tenth the affinity of T_4 [$K_a(T_3)$ *ca.* 10^9].

The second most important carrier protein of T_4 migrates in a zone anodal to albumin on electrophoresis, hence the name thyroxine-binding prealbumin (TBPA). TBPA has a binding affinity for T_4 only about 1% that of TBG ($K_a \sim 10^8$), but its higher concentration in plasma (25–30 mg/100 ml) results in its carrying about 30% of the circulating T_4. TBPA is a simple (nonglycosidic) protein of mol wt 54,980. It has been crystallized, its complete amino acid sequence has been determined (40), and the three-dimensional orientation of most of its residues has been established at a resolution of 1.8 Å (41). TBPA is made up of four identical subunits, each containing 127 amino acids. There are no disulfide bridges. The subunit peptides associate through hydrogen bonding and hydrophobic interactions to form an olive-shaped protein with dimensions of $70 \times 55 \times 50$ Å, with an open channel passing completely through the protein along its long axis. X-Ray crystallographic studies

at the low resolution of 6 Å (42) and affinity labeling studies with an alkylating analog of T_4 (43) have localized the binding site for T_4 within the channel in the approximate region shown schematically in Fig. 39.2. Symmetry elements create two equivalent binding sites. Occupancy of one binding site by T_4 reduces affinity for the second site 100-fold. This is an example of "negative cooperation."

In addition to carrying T_4 within its core, TBPA exists in plasma as a protein–protein complex, associated independently with retinol-binding protein (mol wt 21,000) on its surface. This protein binds retinol (Vitamin A alcohol) and is responsible for the relatively slow metabolism and excretion of the vitamin (44).

TBPA is an excellent model for studying the specific nature of the interaction of a hormone and a biologically important protein. The structure of TBPA is also intriguing owing to the presence of two identical folds on its surface which are complementary in size and shape to a region of the α-helical backbone of DNA, and rich in

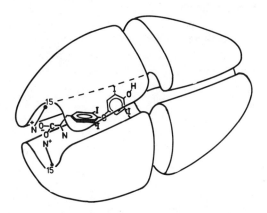

Fig. 39.2 A schematic drawing of the four identical subunits of thyroxine-binding prealbumin (TBPA) associated to form a central channel. T_4 is shown in the channel with the carboxylate ion of its alanine side chain forming ion-paired associations with the ε-ammonium groups of paired lysine residues of TBPA. Drawn from the X-ray data of Blake et al. (41).

ionic side chains that could interact with DNA. It has been suggested by Blake and Oatley (45) that TBPA may serve as a model for, or be structurally related to, the nuclear receptor protein (NRP) that is associated with DNA in the chromatin region of the cell nucleus. A specific mechanism has been advanced by which binding of the T_4 phenolate ion with serine residue 117 in the central channel of TBPA could be transmitted to the "DNA binding region" by intervening hydrogen-bonded tyrosine-116 and glutamate-92 residues. TBPA, TBG, and NRP are of approximately the same size and molecular weight. Section 8.2 discusses similarities and differences in the binding affinities of hormone analogs to these proteins.

The thyroid hormones are also bound weakly to human serum albumin. T_4 binds to albumin with a K_a of *ca.* 10^6 (46, 47). The high concentration of circulating albumin (*ca.* 4.5 g/100 ml) causes it to be a minor carrier of T_3 and of T_4.

3.2   Metabolism and Excretion of Thyroid hormones

The small amounts of T_4 (0.03%) and of T_3 (0.3%) that are unbound in the circulation are available for metabolic transformation reactions and for interactions with the hormone receptors. The diphenyl ether bond is metabolically stable *in vivo* as indicated by experiments in normal man with ^{14}C and ^3H doubly labeled thyroxine (48). The most important metabolic reaction is deiodination. About 85% of the T_4 produced daily is monodeiodinated in either the 5' or 5 position to form approximately equal amounts of T_3 and r-T_3 (49, 50). Since T_3 has some three to seven times the overall metabolic potency of T_4, much of the hormonal activity of T_4 may be expressed as T_3. The r-T_3 formed is hormonally inactive. Further deiodinations of T_3 and of r-T_3 occur, and most of the resulting hormonally

inactive iodothyronines have been identified in low concentrations in the plasma (51, 52). Some of the iodide ion formed is excreted in the urine. About 85% of the iodide passing into the glomerular filtrate is conserved by tubular reabsorption. In the liver, T_4 and other iodinated thyronines are partially conjugated with sulfuric and glucuronic acids through the phenolic hydroxyl group. The conjugates are secreted with bile into the duodenum and are poorly reabsorbed. The conjugates are hydrolyzed in the lower intestine and the iodothyronines are excreted in the feces in the unbound form. To a minor extent the alanine side chains of T_4 and of T_3 are metabolically deaminated and oxidized to the acetic acid side chain analogs 3,5,3',5'-tetraiodothyroacetic acid (tetrac) and 3,5,3'-triiodothyroacetic acid (triac). Tetrac and triac show low hormonal activities *in vivo* owing to their rapid further metabolism and excretion (53). Studies with ^{14}C-labeled thyroxine in man show the presence of the totally deiodinated compounds, thyronine and thyroacetic acid, in urine (54).

4   THEORIES OF MECHANISMS OF THYROID HORMONE ACTION

The overall effects of the thyroid hormones are well-known. Major among these are stimulation of oxygen consumption, heat production, and early development and growth. Dramatic progress is currently being made in identifying the fundamental reactions that initiate these and other hormonal effects.

Early studies were guided by the hypothesis that metabolic stimulation was produced by a direct involvement of the hormone in the energy-producing reactions. Niemann (55) postulated the reversible oxidation of thyroxine to a quinoid form coupled with electron transfer to a substrate involved in energy-generating metabolism (Fig. 39.3). Szent-Györgyi (56)

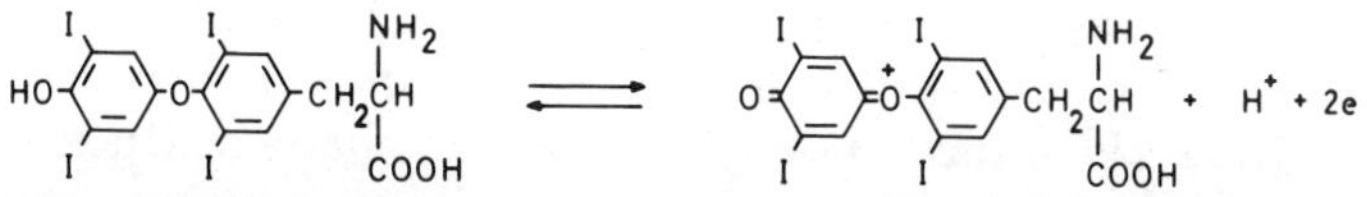

Fig. 39.3 The Niemann hypothesis of thyroid hormone action in which T_4 transmits electrons by reversible oxidation to the quinoid state.

proposed that thyroxine serves as a carrier for iodine, and that the unique heavy atom properties of this element provide for the generation and transmittal of energy by way of the excited triplet state of iodine. Green (57) suggested the direct interaction of hormone and enzymes. The pronounced calorigenic effects of the thyroid hormones directed studies to the enzymes of mitochondria, the major site of energy metabolism of the cell. Transitional hypotheses that have not survived extensive studies include that of uncoupling of mitochondrial oxidation and phosphorylation reactions (58), and related effects on mitochondrial membrane permeability (59). It gradually became clear through the lag period in stimulation of mitochondrial function and the blockade of hormonal effects by inhibitors of protein synthesis that the major effects of the thyroid hormones are expressed as a consequence of the enhancement of protein synthesis. For example, much of the calorgenic effect of the thyroid hormones is explained by stimulation of the synthesis of the mitochondrial enzyme, sodium- and potassium-requiring adenosine triphosphatase (Na^+, K^+-ATPase). Increased hydrolysis of adenosine triphosphate (ATP) at the sodium pump site stimulates mitochondrial oxidative phosphorylation. Increased energy expenditure for transmembrane active Na^+ transport would account for a significant fraction of the heat production by the thyroid hormones (60). Thyroid hormone-mediated increases in enzymes are striking, such as the twentyfold or greater increase in mitochondrial α-glycerophosphate dehydrogenase (61).

In the 1970s, led by successful studies on steroid hormones, emphasis shifted to a search for receptors among specific thyroid hormone-binding components of hormone-responsive cells. In 1972 Oppenheimer et al. (62) reported the binding of T_3 to nuclei of rat liver and kidney cells following *in vivo* administration of labeled hormone. This association was of high affinity ($K_a \sim 5 \times 10^{11} M^{-1}$) and of limited capacity, and the binding component was identified as an extractable acidic protein of an apparent mol wt of about 60,000–70,000 (63). The relative concentrations of these specific T_3 nuclear binding sites in various rat tissues were found to parallel the level of tissue responsiveness as measured by hormone-induced increases in α-glycerophosphate dehydrogenase activity and oxygen consumption (64). Soluble forms of this nuclear receptor protein (NRP) have been extracted by $0.4 M$ KCl from pituitary cell cultures and from rat liver (65, 66). Cell nuclei and soluble NRP show about a tenfold higher association with the more biologically active T_3 than with T_4. Soluble NRP preparations show equilibrium association constant values for T_3 ranging from K_a $10^8 M^{-1}$ to $10^{10} M^{-1}$, whereas most of the data obtained *in vivo* show a K_a of $\sim 10^{11} M^{-1}$. However, the same relative order of affinity for T_3, T_4, and for a variety of hormone analogs is displayed in *in vivo* and *in vitro* studies. As discussed in Section 8.3, an excellent correlation has been observed between hormonal activities *in vivo* and the relative binding affinities of hormone structural analogs to the T_3 binding site of cell nuclei and to the solubilized nuclear receptor protein (67, 68).

The NRP is closely associated with chromatin deoxyribonucleic acid (DNA) in the cell nucleus (63, 69). The protein–DNA complex appears to be involved in DNA transcription, and the earliest event detected after thyroid hormone injection is an augmentation of ribonucleic acid synthesis (70). These facts have supported the proposal (Fig. 39.4) that the binding of T_3 (or T_4) to the nuclear receptor protein transmits a signal to a specific DNA template, which in turn stimulates the synthesis and release of specific messenger ribonucleic acids (mRNA). The mRNA stimulate the increased synthesis of proteins, including those used for structural or functional purposes during growth and development, and those enzymes that mediate the physiological expressions of the hormones.

In addition to the NRP, additional high-affinity low-capacity binding sites (in rat liver) are found in the cytosol, plasma membrane, microsomes, and inner mitochondrial membranes (71, 72). It is not yet clear whether these interactions mediate direct hormonal effects on cellular structures that supplement or complement the effects initiated by binding to nuclear receptor protein. Sterling and Milch (73) have presented evidence supporting a direct hormone action on mitochondria, and Goldfine et al. (74) have shown a direct and rapid stimulation of cellular uptake of amino acids by isolated rat thymocytes, independent of protein synthesis.

5 CONFORMATIONAL CHARACTERISTICS OF THE THYROID HORMONES

The planar nature of the benzene rings, the coplanarity of the atoms attached directly to a ring, and the symmetrical shape of the iodine substituents all serve to limit the conformations accessible to the thyroid hormones. Studies of functionally modified and conformationally constrained analogs indicate that the relative spatial positions of substituents are important in determining biological activities (see Section 8.1.4).

5.1 Diphenyl Ether Orientations

The atoms of 3,5,3'-triiodo-L-thyronine labeled as suggested by Cody (75) are shown in Fig. 39.5. X-Ray crystallographic data on T_3 and T_4 show that the diphenyl ether link (C-4—O-4—C-1') is angled at about 120° (76, 77). The diphenyl ether conformation is further defined by the torsion angles ϕ (C-5—C-4—O-4—C-1') and ϕ' (C-4—O-4—C-1'—C-6') (75). X-Ray crystallographic studies (75–78), molecular orbital calculations (79), and NMR studies at low temperatures (80) indicate the preferred low energy conformation shown in Figure 39.5 in which the planes of the rings are mutually perpendicular ($\phi = 90°$, $\phi' = 0°$). X-Ray data (75) also show that those analogs which crystallize with a slight "twist" in the ϕ' bond (±30°) tend to compensate with a slight "swing" in the ϕ bond

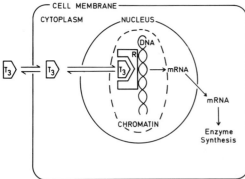

Fig. 39.4 A schematic representation of the early events proposed in thyroid hormone action. T_3 = 3,5,3'-Triiodothyronine. R = Nuclear receptor protein (NRP) associated with chromatin deoxyribonucleic acid (DNA). mRNA = Messenger ribonucleic acid.

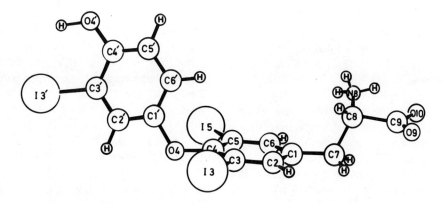

Fig. 39.5   L-3,5,3'-triiodothyronine (L-T$_3$) showing the numbering of the atoms. L-T$_3$ is shown with the aromatic rings in the "skewed" conformation, $\phi = 90°$, $\phi' = 0°$, and with the alanine side chain in the cisoid conformation, $\chi^2 = 90°$. The carboxylate residue is most distant from the aromatic ring, $\chi^1 = -60°$, and coplanar with the NH atoms, $\psi^1 = 0°$.

($\pm 20°$). The resulting conformations are described as either "skewed" ($\phi = 90°$, $\phi' = 0°$) or as "twist-skewed" ($\phi = 108°$, $\phi' = -28°$; $\phi = -108°$, $\phi' = 28°$). Some typical ϕ and ϕ' angles determined by X-ray crystallography are listed in Table 39.1.

5.2   Side Chain Conformations

The conformations of the side chain of an aromatic amino acid are established by rotations of three bonds. The torsion angles are defined as χ^2 (C-2—C-1—C-7—C-8), χ^1 (C-1—C-7—C-8—N-8), and ψ^1 (N-8—C-8—C-9—O-10) (75, 81). Values of χ^2 close to $+90°$ are seen in the crystal state for a wide variety of aromatic amino acid derivatives (82). The thyroid hormones show χ^2 values close to $+90°$ or $-90°$ corresponding to a cisoid or transoid orientation relative to the position of the phenolic ("outer") ring and the plane of the non-phenolic ("inner") ring. Compounds with

Table 39.1   Conformational Parameters (in Degrees) for Thyroxine Analogs[a]

Compound	ϕ[b]	ϕ'[c]	χ^{2}[d]	χ^{1}[e]	ψ^{1}[f]	ψ^{2}[g]	Ref.
3,5,3'-Triiodothyroacetic acid[h]	92	−1	78			33	83
3,5,3',5'-Tetraiodothyroacetic acid[h]	−95	−4	129			−8	75
3,5,3'-Triiodo-L-thyronine	116	−21	76	−164	8		77
3,5,3'-Triiodo-L-thyronine methyl ester	−108	33	121	−54	8		84
3,5,3'-Triiodo-L-thyronine hydrochloride	90	−11	98	56	8		76
L-Thyroxine[h]	108	−30	152	−170	−41		75
L-Thyroxine	−112	33	87	−160	49		75
L-Thyroxine hydrochloride	105	−34	98	67	−39		76

[a] From Cody et al. (75). The signs of the torsion angles are determined as recommended by the IUPAC–IUB Commission on Biochemical Nomenclature (81).
[b] $\phi = $ (C-5—C-4—O-4—C-1').
[c] $\phi' = $ (C-4—O-4—C-1'—C-6').
[d] $\chi^2 = $ (C-2—C-1—C-7—C-8).
[e] $\chi^1 = $ (C-1—C-7—C-8—N-8).
[f] $\psi^1 = $ (N-8—C-8—C-9—O-10).
[g] $\psi^2 = $ (C-1—C-7—C-8—O-8).
[h] N-Diethanolamine (1 : 1) complex.

$\phi = +90°$, $\chi^2 = +90°$ (or the identical $\phi = -90$, $\chi^2 = -90°$) are cisoid. Figure 39.5 shows T_3 in the cisoid conformation. Compounds are transoid if their torsional angles approximate $\phi = +90°$, $\chi^2 = -90°$ (or the identical $\phi = -90°$, $\chi^2 = +90°$).

In the crystalline state 48 aromatic amino acids and derivatives are divisible into three major classes of rotamers representing the staggered positions of χ^1 (C-1—C-7—C-8—N-8) (82). The most energetically favored is the rotamer $\chi^1 = -60°$ in which the carboxylate residue is most distant from the aromatic ring as in Fig. 39.5. There are also examples of the less favored conformation $\chi^1 = 180°$ (NH_3^+ most distant from C-1) and of the least favored $\chi^1 = +60°$ (COO^- and NH_3^+ folded towards C-1). In a series of 48 aromatic amino acids the frequency of occurrence of χ^1 is $+60°$ (46%), $+180°$, (31%), $-60°$ (23%). Table 39.1 from Cody et al. (75) lists the conformational parameters for side chains of thyroxine analogs. In this limited thyronine series a folded side chain ($\chi^1 \sim +60°$) is favored for the amine hydrochloride, an extended NH_4^+ group ($\chi^1 \sim \pm 180°$) for free amino acids or for the diethanolamine complex, and an extended CO_2R group ($\chi^1 \sim -60°$) for the more bulky methyl ester. It is clear that all staggered rotamers of χ^1 are accessible to the thyroid hormones.

There is a strong intramolecular attraction between the O-10 (or equivalent O-9) oxygen atom of the carboxylate group and the NH of the ammonium group. This results in ψ^1 (N-8—C-8—C-9—O-10) values always being close to 0° (±10°). This leads to an approximately coplanar orientation of the N-8—C-8—C-9—O-10 and N–H atoms as shown in Fig. 39.5.

In addition to the five rotations described above, a coplanar orientation with the aromatic ring is energetically favored for the phenolic 4'-OH group (83). The weak hydrogen bond to the 3'-I is shown in Fig. 39.5.

The distance between the phenolic O-4'

and the carboxylate O-10 of the thyroid hormones may be varied from a minimum of about 8.5 Å for the cisoid-folded side chain to a maximum of about 13.5 Å for the transoid-extended side chain conformation.

5.3 Distal versus Proximal Orientation of the 3' Substituent

In 1959 it was proposed by Zenker and Jorgensen (84) that a perpendicular orientation of the planes of the aromatic rings of 3,5-diiodothyronines would be favored, in order to provide minimal interactions between the bulky 3,5 iodines and the 2',6' hydrogens. In this ϕ, ϕ'; 90°, 0° conformation the 3' and 5' positions are not equivalent, and the 3' iodine of T_3 could be oriented either distal or proximal to the inner (alanine-bearing) ring (Fig. 39.6). Both 3'-distal and 3'-proximal conformations of 3,5-diiodo-3'-substituted thyronines have been observed by X-ray crystallography, depending on the conditions of crystallization (75–78, 85–88). These results are reinforced by molecular orbital calculations (79) and by low temperature NMR studies (80) that estimate a rotational barrier about the diphenyl ether linkage of about 8.5–11 kcal/mol. This low barrier would permit rotation of the rings at ordinary temperatures and would provide access by 3,5,3'-trisubstituted analogs to the essentially equi-energetic 3'-distal and 3'-proximal conformations. The 3'-distal conformation of L-T_3 is shown in Fig. 39.5.

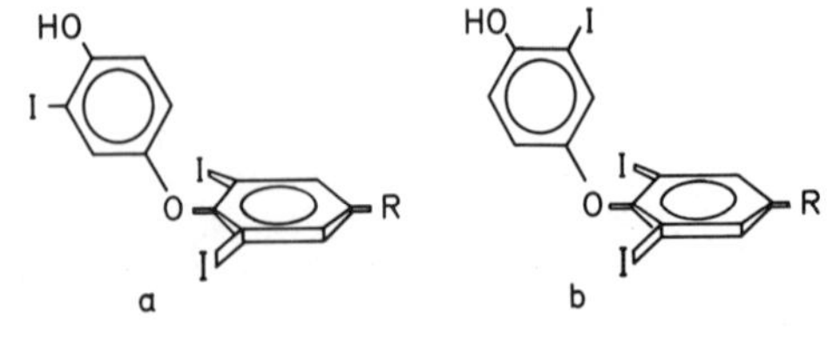

Fig. 39.6 The minimum energy (a) distal and (b) proximal conformers of T_3; $R = CH_2CH(NH_2)COOH$.

This is presumed to be the hormonally active conformation based on studies of conformationally constrained 3'-distal and 3'-proximal substituted analogs (see Section 8.1.4).

6 BIOLOGICAL TEST SYSTEMS

Recent studies have provided strong evidence for the hypothesis that the major expressions of hormonal effects are initiated by the associations of hormones with receptor proteins of the cell nucleus. Complementary effects may be produced by interactions of hormones with other cell components, such as the cell membrane and mitochondrial proteins, but these have been little studied. The onset, duration, and intensity of expression of activites *in vivo* are further influenced by the binding affinities to transport proteins and susceptibilities to metabolic modification of hormones and analogs. Several *in vivo* and *in vitro* test symptoms have been used to measure relative hormonal activities. Comparisons of the data from different test methods provide insight into the relative importance of individual biological processes in influencing the expressions of activity *in vivo*.

6.1 Biological Tests *in vivo*

The *rat antigoiter* assay has been the method most often used in determining activity *in vivo* (89). Oral or parenteral administration of an antithyroid drug such as thiouracil or propylthiouracil inhibits formation of the thyroid hormones. The decrease in levels of circulating hormone stimulates release of pituitary thyrotropin (TSH), which in 10 days effects a three- to six-fold increase in thyroid weight and size (goiter). Activity is estimated by the amount of analog required to suppress TSH release and goiter formation as compared

with standard doses of L-T_4 (2.5 μg) or of L-T_3 (0.5 μg) per 100 g of body weight administered subcutaneously and daily for 10 days.

The *amphibian metamorphosis test* measures the thyroid hormone-induced changes in form and function that adapt the aquatic life stage for transition to the terrestrial environment. Shrinkage of the tadpole tail is the effect most often measured. The salientian (frog) tadpole is immersed for 24–48 hr in a solution of test compound, then transferred to plain water for observation over several days. Activity is estimated by the concentration of test compound required to produce either the same decrease in tail width (90) or tail length (91) as reference concentrations of T_4 or T_3. Injection of the test compound eliminates artifactually high activities for lipophilic aliphatic carboxylic acid side chain analogs owing to their greater uptake and concentration from the test solution than that of the more polar alanine side chain reference compounds (92).

More limited studies *in vivo* have measured increases in *oxygen consumption* and in *heart rate* (93), reductions in *serum and organ cholesterol levels* (94), and increases in specific enzyme levels, such as kidney *transamidinase* (95), or liver or kidney α-glycerophosphate dehydrogenase (96) in the rat.

6.2 Biological Tests *in vitro*

6.2.1 BINDING TO TRANSPORT PROTEINS. The strength of association of a thyroid hormone or analog to the hormone-specific transport proteins of plasma influences its accessibility to hormone receptors and to metabolizing enzymes. Radioiodinated T_4 is bound to the purified protein, thyroxine-binding globulin (97), thyroxine-binding prealbumin (98), or albumin (99). Varying concentrations of nonlabeled L-T_4 or of analogs are added and the free ^{125}I-T_4 or

^{131}I-T$_4$ is determined following its separation from protein-bound hormone by electrophoresis or equilibrium dialysis. Displacement of fluorescent binding probes has also been used (100). Relative binding affinity is usually determined by comparing the relative concentrations of analog and of hormone standard required to displace 50% of the radioactive or fluorescent compound.

6.2.2 BINDING TO CELL NUCLEAR RECEPTORS. ^{125}I-T$_3$ is bound to intact cell nuclei (67) or to the solubilized protein from cell nuclei of rat liver (68). The relative binding affinities of analogs are determined by the relative concentrations required to displace the ^{125}I-T$_3$. The slow off-rate of the hormone permits protein-bound ^{125}I-T$_3$ to be separated from free ^{125}I-T$_3$ by rapid gel filtration at low temperature.

7   CURRENT THYROID HORMONE DRUGS

Desiccated, defatted porcine, bovine, or ovine thyroid glands, designated *thyroid USP*, and the partially purified iodinated protein of thyroid gland, *thyroglobulin*, are used in hormone replacement therapy. The synthetic hormones, L-thyroxine and L-3,5,3′-triiodothyronine, are distributed as their sodium salts, *levothyroxine sodium* USP and *liothyronine sodium* USP. A combination of the synthetic sodium salts of L-T$_4$:L-T$_3$ in a 4:1 ratio by weight is distributed as *liotrix*. Equivalent daily doses for oral therapy are as follows: thyroid or thyroglobulin, 65 mg; levothyroxine sodium, 0.1 mg; liothyronine sodium, 25 μg; liotrix, 50 μg T$_4$, 12.5 μg T$_3$.

The synthetic optical isomer of L-T$_4$, dextrothyroxine sodium NF is used for lowering plasma lipid and cholesterol levels. Methods of synthesis and physical properties of the thyroid hormones and of analogs have been described by Jorgensen (101).

8   STRUCTURE–ACTIVITY RELATIONSHIPS FOR THYROID HORMONAL ACTIVITIES

8.1   Activities *in vivo*

Comprehensive lists of thyroxine analogs and their biological activities *in vivo* have been presented (102–105). Only compounds with the appropriately substituted phenyl-X-phenyl nucleus of structure 39.**4** have shown significant thyroid hormonal activities *in vivo*. Single ring compounds such as 3,5-diiodotyrosine and a variety of its aliphatic and alicyclic ethers showed no T$_4$-like activity in the rat antigoiter test (106). Structural requirements are discussed in relation to the five regions of structure 39.**4**, *a–e*.

8.1.1   REGIONS *a*: ALIPHATIC SIDE CHAIN. Table 39.2 presents the biological activity of selected side chain analogs in the rat and tadpole. The L-alanine group in the 1 position of the inner ring provides maximal hormonal activity *in vivo* in all tests reported in mammals. The D isomer (*b, d*) is always less active than the corresponding L isomer (*a, c*). D-T$_4$ (dextrothyroxine) is used clinically for lowering blood cholesterol although there is no absolute separation of the undesirable effects of enhanced calorigenesis and heart rate (108).

The carboxylate ion and the number of atoms connecting it to the inner ring are more important for activity than is the presence of the ammonium ion. As shown in Table 39.2, compounds *e–l*, activity in the carboxylate series is low for the one-carbon formic acid residue (*e, f*), rises to a maximum with the two-carbon acetic acid side chain (*g, h*), and falls slightly for the three-

39.**4**

Table 39.2 Relative Biologic Activities *in vivo* of Side Chain Analogs of Thyroxine and Triiodothyronine[a]

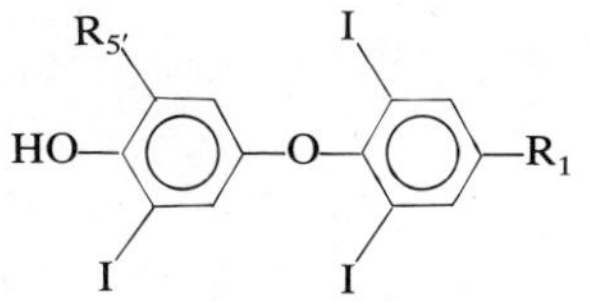

No.	Abbreviation	R_1	$R_{5'}$	Rat Anti-goiter	Rat O_2 Consumption	Tadpole Metamorphosis Immersion	Tadpole Metamorphosis Injection[b]
a	L-T$_4$	L-Alanine	I	100	100	100	100
b	D-T$_4$	D-Alanine	I	17	17	50	30
c	L-T$_3$	L-Alanine	H	550	500	317	1000
d	D-T$_3$	D-Alanine	H	41	125	110	500
e	T$_4$Fo	COOH	I	0.1	3	15	—
f	T$_3$Fo	COOH	H	0.4	0	100	—
g	Tetrac	CH$_2$COOH	I	50	10	840	300
h	Triac	CH$_2$COOH	H	36	25	1680	700
i	Tetraprop	(CH$_2$)$_2$COOH	I	15	7	6860	300
j	Triprop	(CH$_2$)$_2$COOH	H	20	35	21460	700
k	T$_4$Bu	(CH$_2$)$_3$COOH	I	4	5	1050	—
l	T$_3$Bu	(CH$_2$)$_3$COOH	H	5	7	920	—
m	Thyroxamine	(CH$_2$)$_2$NH$_2$	I	0.6	10	900	—
n	Triiodothyronamine	(CH$_2$)$_2$NH$_2$	H	6	10	3600	—

[a] See Refs. 102–105. Activities are average literature values standardized on a molar basis. L-T$_4$ = 100 = reference compound.
[b] See Refs. 92, 107. Values changed to a molar basis.

carbon propionic acid side chain (*i, j*). Activity in the rat is much lower for the butyric acid side chain (*k, l*). Analogs of T$_3$ and T$_4$ with the ethylamine side chain (*m, n*) are less active in the rat than are the corresponding acetic and propionic acid analogs.

Activities in the immersed tadpole metamorphosis test are strikingly high for aliphatic carboxylic acids and amines (Table 39.2, *e–n*). This is in part due to the lipophilic character of these groups as compared with the zwitterionic alanine side chain. Such lipophilic compounds are ab-

sorbed and concentrated from the test solution through the tadpole's gills and skin. Activities of analogs determined following injection are closer to mammalian results. High values in the injected tadpole may be due to slower loss of the lipophilic compounds relative to T$_3$ or T$_4$ into the aqueous environment.

Structural variations intended to slow the rate of metabolic degradation of the alanine side chain, such as α-methyl-DL-thyroxine (39.**5**)(109) and a *trans*-cyclopropylamine acid (39.**6**)(110) showed very low T$_4$-like activities *in vivo*.

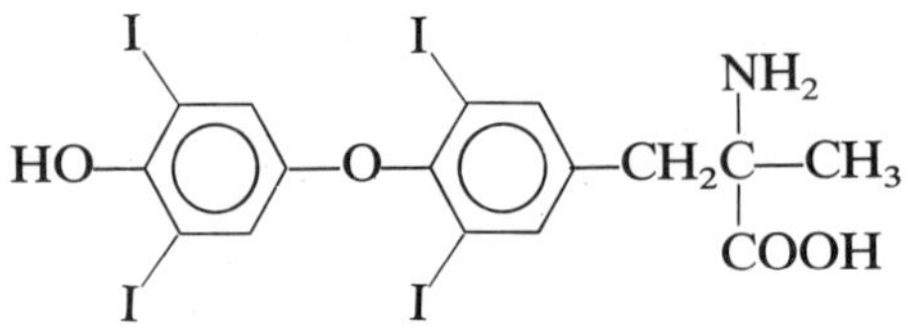

39.**5**

Isomers of L-T$_3$ in which the alanine side chain occupies position 2 or 3 of the inner ring were inactive in rat antigoiter tests (111).

8.1.2 REGION b: INNER RING SUBSTITU-ENTS. Table 39.3 presents relative T$_4$-like activities in the rat antigoiter assay for thyronines variously substituted in the 3 and 5 positions of the inner ring. In addi-tion, these analogs carry activity-enhancing substituents in the 3' or 3', 5' positions of the outer ring (see Section 8.1.4). As shown in Table 39.3, a–f, replacement in T$_4$ or T$_3$ of one or both of the inner ring iodine atoms by hydrogen atoms leads to essential loss of activity *in vivo*. These partially iodi-nated thyronines are major metabolites of T$_4$ in man (49–52).

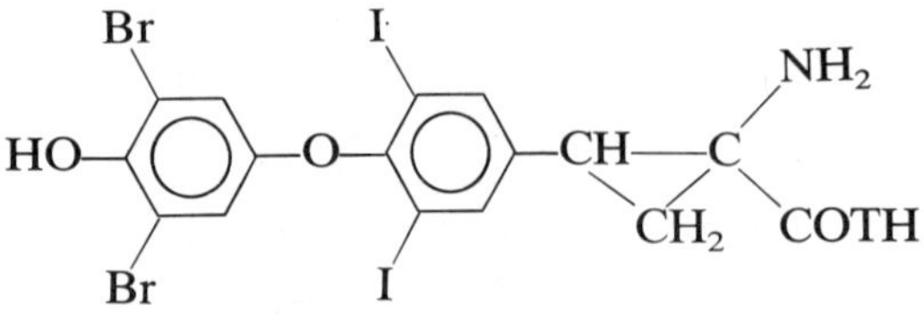

39.**6**

Table 39.3   Relative Biologic Activities *in vivo* of Analogs Substituted in the Inner Ring of Thyronine[a]

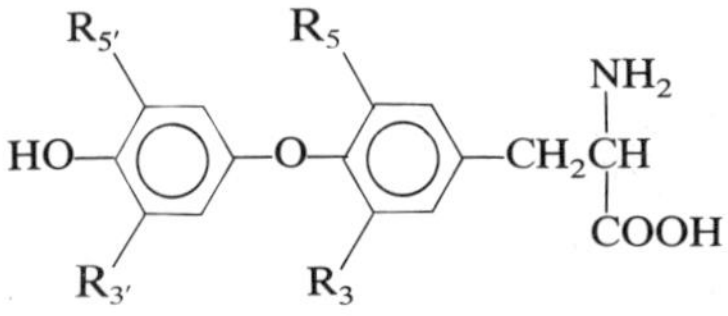

No.	Abbreviation	R$_3$	R$_5$	R$_{3'}$	R$_{5'}$	Activity, % L-T$_4$ or DL-T$_4$ (*)— Rat Antigoiter
a	L-T$_4$	I	I	I	I	100
b	L-T$_3$	I	I	I	H	550
c	L-3'-T$_1$	H	H	I	H	<0.01
d	L-3',5'-T$_2$	H	H	I	I	<0.01
e	L-3,3'-T$_2$	I	H	I	H	0.5
f	L-3,3',5'-T$_3$	I	H	I	I	<0.2
g	DL-Br$_2$I	Br	Br	I	H	93*
h	L-Br$_2$iPr	Br	Br	iPr	H	166
i	L-Me$_2$I	Me	Me	I	H	5
j	L-Me$_3$	Me	Me	Me	H	3
k	L-Me$_4$	Me	Me	Me	Me	2
l	L-Me$_2$iPr	Me	Me	iPr	H	20
m	DL-IMeI	I	Me	I	H	20
n	DL-iPr$_2$I	iPr	iPr	I	H	0
o	DL-sBu$_2$I	sBu	sBu	I	H	0

[a] See Refs. 104 and 105. Activities are average literature values standardized on a molar basis. L-T$_4$ = 100 or (*) DL-T$_4$ = 100 as reference compounds.

Replacement of the 3 and 5 iodine atoms with the less bulky bromine atoms (g, h) results in good retention of activity. The high activity of L-3,5-dibromo-3'-isopropyl-thyronine (h) in a variety of tests (112) shows that iodine does not play a unique role in thyroid hormone action. Methyl groups will also replace the 3,5 iodine atoms with retention of moderate levels of activity (i–l). The broad spectrum of hormone activities displayed *in vivo* by completely halogen-free analogs such as j–l shows that the presence of a halogen atom is not essential for activity (113–116). L-3,5-Dimethyl-3'-isopropylthyronine (39.**7**, DIMIT) crosses the placental barrier in experimental animals, and is hormonally active in the developing fetus when administered to the mother (117–119). Since T_3 and T_4 do not appreciably cross the placenta, DIMIT, or an analog with similar properties, could prove useful in treating fetal thyroid hormone deficiencies or in stimulating lung development immediately before premature birth (120).

Among known analogs, iodine atoms in the 3 and 5 positions impart maximal activities. The hybrid analog, DL-3,3'-diiodo-5-methylthyronine (Table 39.3, m), shows activity intermediate to that of L-3,5-dimethyl-3'-iodothyronine (i) and L-T_3 (b). Substitutions in the 3 and 5 positions by alkyl groups significantly larger and less symmetrical than methyl groups, such as isopropyl $[CH(CH_3)_2]$ and secondary butyl $[CH(C_2H_5)CH_3]$ residues, produce inactive analogs (Table 39.3, n, o). Analogs containing the intermediate-sized 3,5-diethyl substituents have not been reported.

A variety of more polar groups [nitro (121), amino, carboxy, cyano (122)] or more bulky lipophilic groups [thioethyl, thiophenyl (123)] in the 3 and 5 positions have produced inactive analogs.

8.1.3 REGION *c*: THE BRIDGING ATOM. Table 39.4 lists activities in the rat and tadpole for analogs in which the ether oxygen bridging the aromatic rings has been removed or replaced by other atoms. As shown by the biphenyl analogs b–d activity is essentially lost if the aromatic rings are linked directly. This structure introduces drastic changes in the distance and bond angle between the rings. The 120° angle of a diphenyl ether is changed to a 180° (linear) orientation in a biphenyl. Replacement of the bridging oxygen atom by sulfur (124) (e, f) or by a methylene group (g, h) produces highly active analogs. These invoke minimal changes in ring orientations from the natural hormones. However, the —S— and —CH_2— groups would not participate in the quinoid oxidation and electron transfer reactions proposed by Niemann (55) (see Section 4) as a possible mode of hormone action. The high activity of the sulfur-bridged and methylene-bridged analogs indicates the importance of the three-dimensional structure and receptor fit of the hormones, rather than a role as reaction intermediates.

Attempts to prepare bridged —NH— analogs (diphenylamines) have been unsuccessful (125–127).

8.1.4 REGION *d*: OUTER RING SUBSTITUENTS. The 3' or 3',5'-substituted thyronines of Table 39.5 illustrate the major effects on biological activity of substituent variations in the outer ring. The unsubstituted core structure of this series, L-3,5-diiodothyronine (a), shows low activity. As the size of a halogen atom in the 3' position increases, activity increases in the order F < Cl < Br < I (b–e). The smallest alkyl group in the 3' position (f) produces a

39.**7**

Table 39.4   Relative Biologic Activities *in vivo* of Analogs with Variations in the Bridging Atom[a]

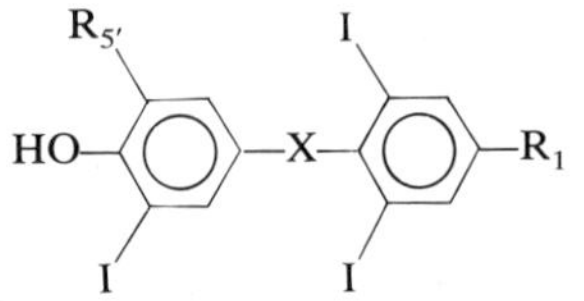

No.	Abbreviation	$R_{5'}$	X	R	Rat Anti-goiter	Tadpole Meta-Morphosis	Rat Heart Rate[b]
a	L-T$_4$	I	O	L-Ala	100	100	100
b	DL-BPT$_4$	I	—	DL-Ala	0[c]	—	—
c	BP-triac	H	—	CH$_2$COOH	—	—	0.14
d	BP-tetrac	I	—	CH$_2$COOH	—	—	0.14
e	DL-SBT$_3$	H	S	DL-Ala	132[d]	—	—
f	DL-SBT$_4$	I	S	DL-Ala	1.2[d]	20[e]	—
g	DL-MBT$_3$	H	CH$_2$	DL-Ala	300[f]	1200[g]	—
h	MB-tetrac	I	CH$_2$	CH$_2$COOH	—	150[g]	—

[a] All literature values were converted to a molar basis.
[b] Ref. 93.
[c] Jorgensen, unpublished data.
[d] Ref. 89 compared with DL-T$_4$ = 100.
[e] Ref. 124.
[f] Ref. 114.
[g] Ref. 115.

sixteen-fold enhancement of activity. Activity is further enhanced by 3'-ethyl (*g*) or 3'-isopropyl (*h*) substitution. L-3,5-Diiodo-3'-isopropylthyronine is the most potent analog known, being about 1.4 times as active as L-T$_3$. The *n*-propyl substituent (*i*) is only about one-fourth as effective as isopropyl, apparently due to its less compact shape. Activity falls as the 3'-alkyl series is ascended. 3'-Butyl groups (*j–l*) show highest activity if they possess a —C(CH$_3$) structural element like that of isopropyl next to the aromatic ring. For example, *sec*-butyl [—CH(CH$_3$)C$_2$H$_5$] > *t*-butyl [C(CH$_3$)$_3$] > isobutyl [—CH$_2$CH(CH$_3$)]. Activity is further reduced for the more bulky 3'-phenyl substituent (*m*). Highly polar substituents such as hydroxyl (*n*) and nitro (*o*) reduce activity relative to the unsubstituted compound. An analog with the same atom or group substituted in *both* the 3' and 5' positions (*p–s*) always shows lower activity *in vivo* than the corresponding 3'-monosubstituted analog. In the case of the 3',5'-dihalogen analogs (*p–r*) this decrease in activity has been attributed to the increase in ionization of the phenolic hydroxyl group and the resulting increase in binding to transport proteins (see Section 8.2.1). This is not the sole factor, however, as shown by the decreased activity of 3',5'-dialkyl analogs such as 3,5-diiodo-3',5'-dimethylthyronine (*s*) compared with the more active 3'-methyl derivative (*f*). The alkyl group does not increase acidity of the ortho phenolic group, and both the 3'-alkyl and 3',5'-alkylthyronines are very weakly bound to transport proteins. A more important feature appears to be the size-related effect of the 5' substituent in interfering with binding to the hormone receptor (see Section 8.2.2).

The proper spatial orientation of the 3' substituent is also important for its ability

Table 39.5   Relative Biologic Activities *in vivo* of 3′,5′-Substituent Variations on 3,5-Diiodothyronine[a]

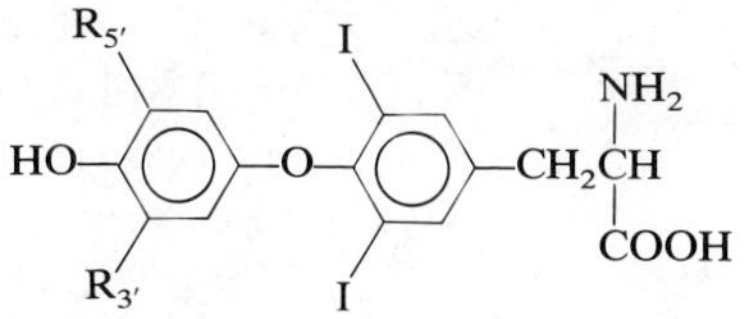

No.	Abbreviation	DL Form	$R_{3'}$	$R_{5'}$	Rat Antigoiter
a	T_2	L	H	H	5
b	T_2F	DL	F	H	6[b]
c	T_2Cl	L	Cl	H	27
d	T_2Br	DL	Br	H	132[b]
e	T_3	L	I	H	550
f	T_2Me	L	Me	H	80
g	T_2Et	L	Et	H	517
h	T_2iPr	L	iPr	H	786
i	T_2nPr	L	nPr	H	200
j	T_2sBu	L	sBu	H	442
k	T_2tBu	L	tBu	H	120
l	T_2iBu	L	iBu	H	43
m	T_2Phe	DL	C_6H_5	H	11
n	T_2OH	L	OH	H	1.5
o	T_2NO_2	L	NO_2	H	<1
p	T_2F_2	DL	F	F	2.3[b]
q	T_2Cl_2	L	Cl	Cl	21
r	T_4	L	I	I	100
s	T_2Me_2	L	Me	Me	50

[a] See Refs. 102–105. Activities are average literature values standardized on a molar basis. L-T_4 = 100.
[b] DL-T_4 = 100.

to enhance hormonal activity. As described in Section 5.3, the 3′ iodine atom may occupy a position in space either distal or proximal to the inner ring. The aromatic rings of T_3 and of other 3,5-diiodo-3′-substituted thyronines rotate rapidly at ordinary temperatures. The active 3,5,3′-substituted analogs are therefore able to position the 3′ substituent in either the proximal or distal orientation as needed for the most effective transport protein binding or receptor interaction. Sterically con-

strained analogs, 3,5-diiodo-2′,3′-dimethyl-thyronine (Fig. 39.7a) and the corresponding 2′,5′-dimethylthyronine (Fig. 39.7b), have been used to establish the active conformation. The 2′-methyl group is forced to occupy a position distal in space to the inner ring, and ring rotation is prevented by steric interaction of the 2′-methyl group and bulky 3,5-iodine atoms. The 3′-methyl group must also be in the distal orientation, and any 5′ substituent, para to the orienting 2′-methyl group, must occupy the proximal

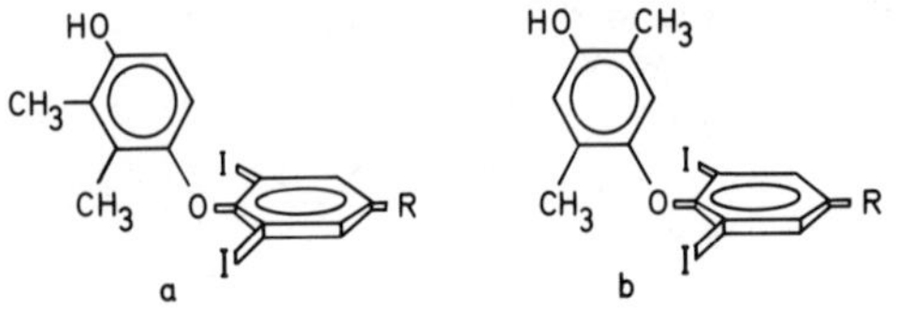

Fig. 39.7 Analogs of 3,5-diiodothyronine in which the 2'-methyl group constrains a second methyl group in the (a) 3'-methyl distal or the (b) 5'-methyl proximal orientation. $R = CH_2CH(NH_2)COOH$.

spatial position. 3,5-Diiodo-2',3'-dimethylthyronine (Fig. 39.7a) in which the activating 3'-methyl group is in the distal position, is 50% as active as L-T_4, whereas the corresponding 2',5'-dimethyl analog (Fig. 39.7b), in which the 5'-methyl group is in the proximal position, is only 1% as potent. Several other examples of highly active distally oriented 3' substituents and of the deactivating effects of the proximal 5' substituent have been presented (128).

8.1.5 REGION e: THE 4'-PHENOLIC HYDROXYL GROUP. Table 39.6 shows representative examples of the effects of replacement of the 4'-OH group of 3,5-diiodothyronines on T_4-like activities in the rat. 4'-Amino analogs (b, c) show weak activity, if otherwise properly substituted. The decrease in activity relative to the corresponding hydroxyl analog may be due to the weak hydrogen bonding ability of an aromatic amino group. 4'-Deoxy-3'-substituted 3,5-diiodothyronines (d–f) show high activities *in vivo* which parallel the activities of the corresponding 4'-hydroxy compounds. It appears that metabolic 4'-hydroxylation occurs as an activating step (129). Introduction of a methyl group in the 4' position blocks metabolic hydroxylation and produces an inactive analog such as g. 4'-Methyl ethers of active analogs are themselves highly active (h, i) owing to the ready metabolic cleavage of such alkyl ethers. Isomers of

Table 39.6   Relative Biologic Activities *in vivo* of 4'-Substituent Variations of 3,5-Diiodo-3'(5')-Substituted Thyronines[a]

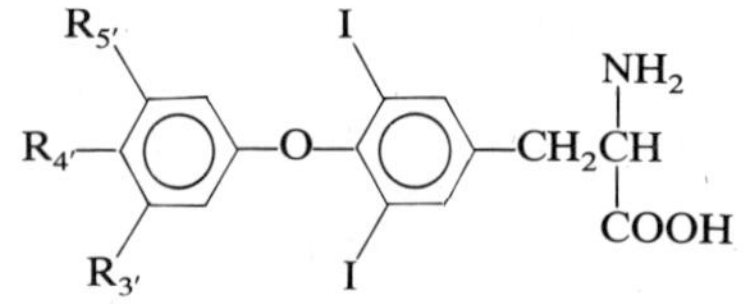

No.	Abbreviation	DL Form	$R_{4'}$	$R_{3'}$	$R_{5'}$	Rat Anti-goiter	Rat O_2 Consumption
a	T_4	L	OH	I	I	100	100
b	NH_2-T_3	L	NH_2	I	H	<1.5	17.3
c	NH_2-T_3Me_2	L	NH_2	CH_3	CH_3	0.7	0.5
d	4'H-T_2Me	DL	H	CH_3	H	15	8.1
e	4'H-T_2CF_3	DL	H	CF_3	H	75	20
f	4'H-T_3	DL	H	I	H	>150	—
g	4'Me-T_2Me	DL	CH_3	CH_3	H	0	0
h	4'MeO-T_3	L	CH_3O	I	H	225	250[b]
i	4'MeO-T_2iPr	L	CH_3O	iPr	H	105	—

[a] See Refs. 102–105. Activities are average literature values standardized on a molar basis.
[b] DL-T_4 = 100.

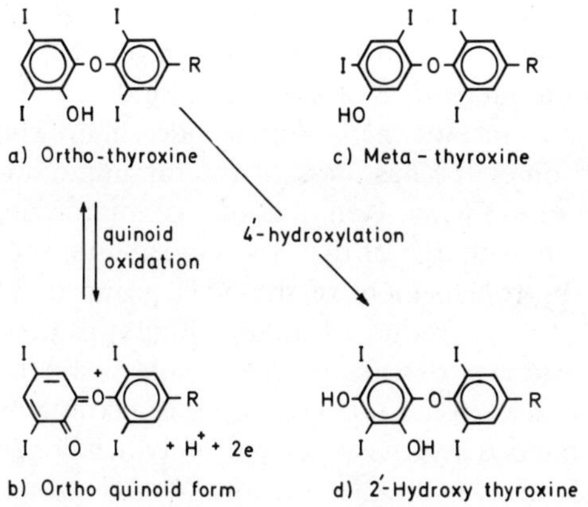

Fig. 39.8 Phenolic ring isomers of T_4 and their potential metabolic oxidation products. $R =$ $CH_2CH(NH_2)COOH$. (*a*) 3,5-Diiodo-4-(2-hydroxy-3,5-diiodophenoxy)phenylalanine $= o$-T_4. (*b*) The postulated *o*-quinoid oxidation product of (*a*). (*c*) 3,5-Diiodo-4-(2,4-diiodo-5-hydroxyphenoxy)-*phenylal-anine* $= m$-T_4. (*d*) The postulated 4′-hydroxylation product of (*a*). 2′-OH-T_4.

L-T_4 have been prepared in which the 4′-hydroxyl group has been moved to alternate positions on the outer ring (130). The weak activity of *o*-T_4 (Fig. 39.8*a*) was ascribed to its potential for metabolic 4′-hydroxylation to form 2′-OH-T_4 (Fig. 39.8*d*), rather than acting as a substrate for oxidation to an *o*-quinoid form (Fig. 39.8*b*). The inactivity of *m*-T_4 (Fig. 39.8*c*) is likely due to the 4′-iodine atom blocking requisite metabolic 4′-hydroxylation.

8.1.6 QUANTITATIVE STRUCTURE–ACTIVITY RELATIONSHIPS FOR ACTIVITIES *in vivo.* In the earliest attempts to express biological activity in a quantitative mathematical expression, Bruice and his associates (131) in 1956 developed an empirical correlation of thyroid hormone activities in the rat and the tadpole comprising additive values for $3, 5, 3′, 4′,$ and $5′$ substituents on the thyronine nucleus. Hansch and Fujita (132), in one of the early applications of the Hansch approach to quantitative structure–activity relationships (QSAR), developed equation (39.1) containing π

(lipophilic substituent constants) and σ (electronic substituent constants) as descriptors of the roles of the 3′- and 5′-halogen atoms in nine halogenated thyronines.

$$\log A = -1.134\,\pi^2 + 7.435\,\pi$$
$$-16.323\,\sigma - 0.287 \quad (39.1)$$

This equation suggests the importance of an electron-donating moderately lipophilic 3′ substituent, and Hansch and Fujita accurately predicted the effectiveness of propyl and butyl groups in this position. Subsequent QSAR studies which correlate activities of T_4 analogs *in vivo* have been reported in 1975 by Jorgensen and associates (133), in 1976 by Kubinyi (134) and Kubinyi and Kehrhahn (135), and in 1977 by Dietrich and associates (136). Each study added insight and new analog data.

Dietrich and associates (136) reported a QSAR study of the rat antigoiter activities of 36 3, 5, 3′, 5′-substituted thyronines and their 4′-*O*-methyl ethers. Activity (A) was expressed in the terms of equation 39.2:

$$\log A$$
$$= 1.354\pi_{35} + 1.344\pi_{3′} - 1.324(3′\,\text{size} > I)$$
$$-0.359\pi_{5′} - 0.658\sigma_{3′5′}$$
$$-0.890(4′ - OCH_3) - 2.836$$
$$n = 36, \ r = 0.938, \ s = 0.304 \quad (39.2)$$

On the basis of equation 39.2 it was concluded:

1. Activity is enhanced by bulky and lipophilic 3 and 5 substituents ($\pi_{35} = \sum \pi$ for 3 and 5 substituents). This is consistent with the role of 3 and 5 substituents in defining ring conformations, and with 3 and 5 substituents providing a hydrophobic binding contribution in receptor interaction.

2. The 3′-substituent contribution is directly related to its lipophilicity ($\pi_{3′}$).

However, activity is decreased if this lipophilic bulk extends from the 3′ position further than iodine (3′ size > I). This collection of terms describes hydrophobic binding of the 3′ substituent to a size-limited cavity in the hormone receptor.

3. Activity is enhanced by electron-donating 3′ and 5′ substituents ($\sigma_{3'5'} = \Sigma\sigma$ for 3′ and 5′ substituents).

4. Activity is decreased by 5′-substituent lipophilicity ($\pi_{5'}$). The almost quantitative parallelism between lipophilicity and bulk in the series studied permits use of either descriptor.

5. Activity correlates well with an indicator variable [I(4′-OCH$_3$)] = 1 for 4′-O-methyl ethers. This is consistent with metabolic conversion *in vivo* to the more active 4′-OH compound.

6. Within the series studied there is no parabolic dependence of activity on lipophilicity (no π^2 term). Therefore, substituent effects on overall partition behavior are of little importance as compared with their roles in interacting with specific transport and receptor proteins.

8.2 Activities *in vitro*

Two major kinds of *in vitro* activities are considered: binding to specific transport proteins and binding to the cell nuclear receptor.

8.2.1 BINDING TO TRANSPORT PROTEINS

8.2.1.1 *Thyroxine-binding Globulin.* As described in Section 3.1.4, thyroxine-binding globulin (TBG) is the primary carrier of the thyroid hormones in human plasma. Table 39.7 presents selected data from Snyder et al. (137), who measured the relative binding affinities of analogs to TBG using equilibrium dialysis at pH 7.4 in diluted human serum. Barbital buffer was

present to prevent competitive binding with thyroxine-binding prealbumin (TBPA). Compounds *a–e* of Table 39.7 indicate the importance of the L-alanine side chain. The D-isomer (*b*) has 54% of the binding affinity of L-T$_4$ (*a*). Removal of the ammonium positive charge of L-T$_4$ by *N*-acetylation (*c*) or by replacement of the NH$_3^+$ group by H (*d*) further reduces binding affinity, as does shortening of the propionic side chain by one carbon atom (*e*). Binding is also highly enhanced by the presence of two halogen atoms *ortho* to the phenolic 4′-OH group. This substitution increases the acidity (ionization) of the phenolic group. Successive removal of the 5′-iodine atom of T$_4$ (pK_a 6.73) to form T$_3$ (pK_a 8.45) and of the 3′-iodine atom to form 3,5-diiodothyronine (T$_2$; pK_a 6.73) (138) produces tenfold and thousandfold decreases in binding affinities. The outer ring (3′, 5′) iodine atoms contribute more to binding to TBG than do the inner ring (3, 5) iodine atoms, as shown by the relative binding affinities of the partially iodinated and noniodinated thyronines (*f–m*). The bromothyronines follow a similar pattern of binding (*n–q*). Bromine in the outer ring contributes less than iodine does to TBG binding, but is more effective in the inner ring. DL-3,5-Dibromo-3′,5′-diiodothyronine (*q*), with a binding affinity 1.6 times that of L-T$_4$, shows the highest binding affinity of a compound to TBG yet measured.

Compounds *r–t* of Table 39.7 show that 3′ or 3′,5′-alkyl substitution contributes only weakly to binding as compared with the unsubstituted 3,5-diiodothyronine (T$_2$, *g*). Analogs with alkyl groups on both inner and outer rings (*u, v*) are very weakly bound to TBG. The weak but significant enhancement of binding by 3′ alkyl groups has permitted evaluation of the relative importance of methyl groups in the 3′-distal or 3′-proximal conformations. Using the sterically constrained 3,5-diiodo-2′,3′-dimethyl- and 2′,5′-dimethylthyronines (Fig. 39.7), both Schussler (139) and

Table 39.7   Relative Binding Affinities of Thyroxine Analogs to Thyroxine-Binding Globulin (TBG)[a]

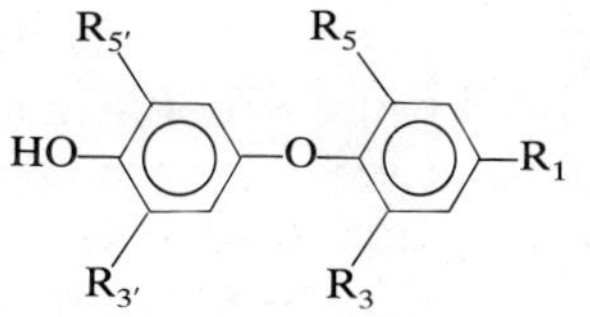

No.	Abbreviation	R_1	R_3	R_5	$R_{3'}$	$R_{5'}$	Binding Affinity to TBG
a	T_4	L-Ala[b]	I	I	I	I	100
b	D-T_4	D-Ala	I	I	I	I	54
c	AcT$_4$	L-AcAla[c]	I	I	I	I	25
d	T_4Pr	(CH)$_2$COOH	I	I	I	I	3.6
e	T_4Ac	CH$_2$COOH	I	I	I	I	1.7
f	T_3	L-Ala	I	I	I	H	9
g	T_2	L-Ala	I	I	H	H	0.07
h	T_1	L-Ala	I	H	H	H	0.05
i	3,3',5'-T_3	L-Ala	I	H	I	I	38
j	3,3'-T_2	L-Ala	I	H	I	H	1.3
k	3',5'-T_2	DL-Ala	H	H	I	I	0.1
l	3'-T_1	L-Ala	H	H	I	H	0.023
m	T_0	L-Ala	H	H	H	H	<0.005
n	Br$_4$	DL-Ala	Br	Br	Br	Br	40
o	Br$_3$	DL-Ala	Br	Br	Br	H	6.2
p	3,3',5'-Br$_3$	DL-Ala	Br	H	Br	Br	6.5
q	Br$_2$I$_2$	DL-Ala	Br	Br	I	I	161
r	I$_2$Me	L-Ala	I	I	Me	H	0.28
s	I$_2$Me$_2$	L-Ala	I	I	Me	Me	0.29
t	I$_2$iPr	L-Ala	I	I	iPr	H	3.53
u	Me$_4$	L-Ala	Me	Me	Me	Me	0.29
v	Me$_2$iPr	L-Ala	Me	Me	iPr	H	0.05

[a] Snyder et al. (137). K_a(L-T_4) = 2.5×10^9 M^{-1}.
[b] L-Alanine [CH$_2$CH(NH$_2$)COOH].
[c] N-Acetyl-L-alanine [CH$_2$CH(NHCOCH$_3$)COOH].

Snyder et al. (137) found the distally oriented 2',3'-dimethyl analog (Fig. 39.7a) to bind more firmly than the proximally oriented 2',5'-dimethyl analog (Fig. 39.7b). These results indicate that the direct hydrophobic binding effect of a 3'-methyl group is most effective in the distal conformation, although it is clear that TBG can accommodate both 3' and 5' substituents as large as methyl or iodine.

Dietrich et al. (136) used a selected group of 3,5-diiodothyronines from the data of Snyder et al. (137) to develop a QSAR equation describing contributions of 3' and 5' substituents in binding to TBG.

$$\log A = 0.563\pi_{3'5'} - 1.100 \, (3' \, \text{size} > \text{I})$$
$$+ 2.366\sigma_{3'5'} - 0.098$$
$$n = 10, \, r = 0.962, \, s = 0.355 \quad (39.3)$$

Equation 39.3 shows that a size-limited (3' size > I) hydrophobic association by 3' and 5' substituents ($\pi_{3'5'}$) contributes only moderately to binding. Of greater importance is apparent binding by the phenoxide ion, as indicated by the large positive regression coefficient for the electronic term $\sigma_{3'5'}$.

8.2.1.2 Thyroxine-binding Prealbumin.
Thyroxine-binding prealbumin (TBPA) is the secondary carrier of the thyroid hormones in human plasma. Table 39.8 presents data from Andrea (140), who measured relative binding affinities of analogs to

pure TBPA at pH 8.0 by equilibrium dialysis. Compounds a–i of Table 39.8 show the importance of the asymmetry and ionic character of the L-alanine side chain. D-T$_4$ (b) and D-T$_3$ (i) both show about 3% of the binding affinity of the corresponding L isomer. The carboxylate ion is the feature of the side chain primarily responsible for binding to TBPA whereas the α-ammonium group inhibits binding. All the homologous carboxylic acids of Table 39.8 (c–f) bind more firmly than L-T$_4$, with maximum affinity for the acetic acid analog, tetrac (d). Removal of the carboxylate ion from T$_4$ to form thyroxamine (g) results in very low binding affinity. Binding is

Table 39.8 Relative Binding Affinities of Thyroxine Analogs to Thyroxine-Binding Prealbumin (TBPA)[a]

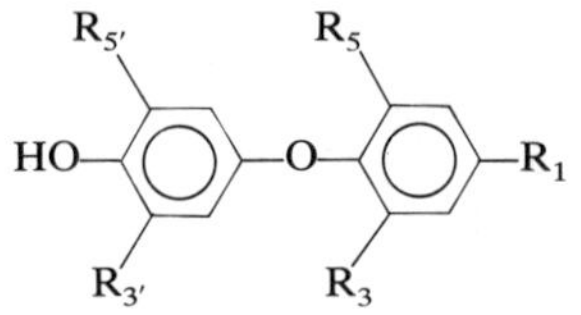

No.	Abbreviation	R$_1$	R$_3$	R$_5$	R$_{3'}$	R$_{5'}$	Binding Affinity to TBPA
a	T$_4$	L-Ala[b]	I	I	I	I	100
b	D-T$_4$	D-Ala	I	I	I	I	2.7
c	T$_4$Fo	COOH	I	I	I	I	225
d	T$_4$Ac	CH$_2$COOH	I	I	I	I	275
e	T$_4$Pr	(CH$_2$)$_2$COOH	I	I	I	I	205
f	T$_4$Bu	(CH$_2$)$_3$COOH	I	I	I	I	175
g	T$_4$Ea	(CH$_2$)$_2$NH$_2$	I	I	I	I	0.23
h	T$_3$	L-Ala	I	I	I	H	4.8
i	D-T$_3$	D-Ala	I	I	I	H	0.15
j	T$_2$	L-Ala	I	I	H	H	0.12
k	T$_1$	L-Ala	I	H	H	H	0.009
i	3,3',5'-T$_3$	L-Ala	I	H	I	I	8.0
m	3,3'-T$_2$	L-Ala	I	H	I	H	0.7
n	3',5'-T$_2$	DL-Ala	H	H	I	I	2.3
o	3'-T$_1$	DL-Ala	H	H	I	H	0.03
p	T$_0$	L-Ala	H	H	H	H	<0.005

[a] Andrea (140). K_a (L-T$_4$) = $4.9 \times 10^7 \, M^{-1}$.
[b] L-Alanine [CH$_2$CH(NH$_2$)COOH].

strongly enhanced by the presence of two iodine atoms ortho to the phenolic hydroxyl group. Successive removal of the 5'-iodine atom of T_4 to form T_3 (h) and of the 3'-iodine atom to form T_2 (j) result in twenty- and thousandfold decreases in binding affinities. Similar ten- and thousandfold decreases in binding affinities are seen for successive removals of the 3'- and 5'-iodine atoms of 3, 3', 5'-T_3 (l) to form 3,3'-T_2 (m) and T_1 (k).

These data are consistent with studies of affinity labeling of TBPA with dansyl chloride and with N-bromoacetyl-T_4 (141, 43), which indicate proximity of the α-ammonium groups of one or more lysine residues (Lys 9, Lys 15) in the entrance of the binding channel of TBPA (Fig. 39.2). Andrea (140) has pointed out that the addition of a positively charged α-ammonium group to T_4Pr (Table 39.8, e) to form T_4 (a) would introduce an electrostatic repulsion to the carboxylate–lysine ammonium

ion pair, and would decrease binding, as observed. Blake and Oatley (45) have noted that association of the paired Lys 15 residues of two subunits of TBPA with the carboxylate ion of T_4 would position the 4'-phenolate ion of T_4 in close proximity to a cluster of paired hydroxyl groups (Ser 115, Ser 117, Thr 119) near the center of the binding channel. The intervening space between the polar serine and threonine residues and the ionic lysine residues is made up of primarily hydrophobic amino acid side chains which extend into the channel from the opposed β-sheet surfaces of the protein. These residues form hydrophobic pockets, lined with the side chains of Leu 17 and Leu 110, and with the methyl groups of Thr 106, Ala 108, Val 121, and with the β- and γ-methylenes of Lys 15, into which the iodine atoms of T_4 could fit. Figure 39.9 presents a schematic representation of this proposed T_4-binding region of TBPA. The associations pictured

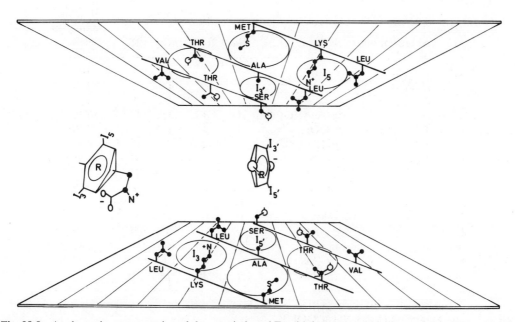

Fig. 39.9 A schematic representation of the association of T_4 with its proposed binding region in TBPA. The T_4 molecule is shown in two parts. The diiodophenylalanine structure (inner ring) on the left should be pictured as attached as R to the oxygen of the outer ring at the center of the binding region. I_3, I_5, $I_{3'}$, $I_{5'}$, within circled regions of the protein represent the pockets into which the designated iodine atoms are proposed to fit.

with T_4 are slight modifications of the proposal of Blake and Oatley (45).

8.2.1.3 *Human Serum Albumin.* The thyroid hormones are weakly bound to human serum albumin (HSA), but the high concentration of the protein results in its acting as carrier of about 10–15% of the circulating T_4. Table 39.9 lists analog binding affinities as measured at pH 7.4 by Tabachnick and Giorgio (142) using purified HSA and equilibrium dialysis. As shown in Table 39.9, compounds $a-f$, HSA is insensitive to the nature of the side chain.

L and D isomers bind with equal affinity, as do analogs which remove one or both charges from the side chain (c, d). The formic and propionic acid side chain analogs (e, f) bind somewhat more strongly than T_4, reflecting the attraction to albumin of negatively charged lipophilic molecules, such as the free fatty acids. Data on partially iodinated thyronines $(g-l)$, bromo- and chlorothyronines (m, n), and 3′,5′-dialkylthyronines indicate that the primay binding feature is the 3′,5′-o-dihalophenol which is largely in the phenolate ion form at pH 7.4. The intact thyronine nucleus is not required for bind-

Table 39.9   Relative Binding Affinities of Thyroxine Analogs to Human Serum Albumin (HSA)[a]

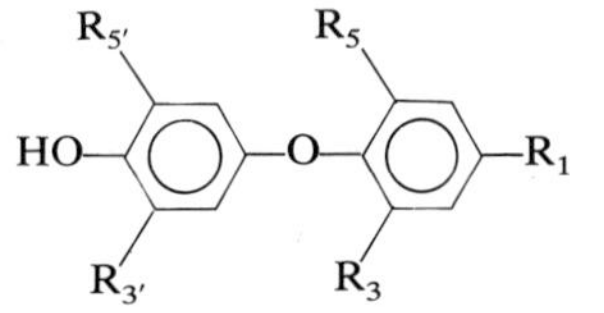

No.	Abbreviation	R_1	R_3	R_5	$R_{3'}$	$R_{5'}$	Binding Affinity to HSA
a	T_4	L-Ala[b]	I	I	I	I	100
b	D-T_4	D-Ala	I	I	I	I	100
c	AcT_4	L-AcAla[c]	I	I	I	I	110
d	AcT_4OEt	L-AcAlaOEt[d]	I	I	I	I	120
e	T_4Fo	COOH	I	I	I	I	140
f	T_4Pr	$(CH_2)_2COOH$	I	I	I	I	135
g	T_3	L-Ala	I	I	I	H	55
h	T_2	DL-Ala	I	I	H	H	30
i	3,3′,5′-T_3	DL-Ala	I	H	I	I	100
j	3′,5′-T_2	DL-Ala	H	H	I	I	85
k	3′-T_1	DL-Ala	H	H	I	H	15
l	T_0	DL-Ala	H	H	H	H	0
m	Br_4	L-Ala	Br	Br	Br	Br	85
n	Cl_4	DL-Ala	Cl	Cl	Cl	Cl	65
o	I_2Me_2	D-Ala	I	I	Me	Me	15

[a] Tabachnick and Giorgio (142). K_a (L-T_4) = 1.5×10^6 M^{-1}.
[b] L-Alanine [$CH_2CH(NH_2)COOH$].
[c] N-Acetyl-L-alanine [$CH_2CH(NHCOCH_3)COOH$].
[d] N-Acetyl-L-alanine ethyl ester [$CH_2CH(NHCOCH_3)COOC_2H_5$].

ing to HSA. Tabachnick et al. (143) have shown that many single-ring compounds bind as strongly as T_4, and that binding by a simple phenol is enhanced by substituents in the order alkyl $<NO_2$, $Cl < Br$, I.

8.2.1.4 *Summary and Comparison of Structural Requirements for Binding to Transport Proteins.*

The thyroid hormones bind to TBG with high affinity because this protein associates with both the carboxylate and ammonium groups of the alanine side chain. Paired lysine residues of TBPA bind primarily to the side chain carboxylate ion of the hormone, whereas the α-ammonium group of the side chain weakens this binding association. TBPA is highly sensitive, TBG is moderately sensitive, and HSA is insensitive to the stereochemistry of the side chain.

The *o*-diiodophenolic structure is very important to all three transport proteins, and this is the sole major binding feature for HSA. In TBPA this binding association is proposed to involve formation of a hydrogen bond between the 4'-phenolate ion and a cluster of serine and threonine hydroxyl groups, perhaps through bridging water molecules. The intact diphenyl ether nucleus, assisted by steric constraints on the rings and hydrophobic associations of iodine atoms with the side chains of the protein, is important for binding to TBG and TBPA, but not for HSA.

A more detailed knowledge of structural requirements for binding to transport proteins, as well as those features most susceptible to metabolism, will aid in the selection or design of hormone analogs with useful properties of onset, duration, and sites of action. The specific structural requirements and high binding affinities of hormones and analogs to TBG and to TBPA make these proteins useful as models in studies of the nature and structural requirements for binding interactions with the less accessible receptor proteins.

8.2.2   BINDING TO CELL NUCLEAR RECEPTORS AND CORRELATIONS OF RECEPTOR BINDING AFFINITIES *in vitro* WITH HORMONAL ACTIVITY *in vivo.*

The presence of cell nuclear binding sites with high affinity and low capacity for the thyroid hormones has been well demonstrated (Sections 4 and 6.2.2). The importance of these sites as hormone receptors has been tested by examining the relative binding affinities *in vitro* of a wide variety of structural analogs, and comparing these binding affinities with the hormonal activities observed *in vivo*. It is recognized that some analogs could differ in their susceptibilities to competing biological processes *in vivo*, such as binding to transport proteins, and ease of penetration of cell membranes (distribution), metabolism, and excretion. Such differences would introduce deviations from a linear correlation with intrinsic activities at the receptor level. However, a general parallelism between binding affinities and hormonal activities would be expected if the cell nuclear binding event is directly coupled with expression of the observed hormonal responses.

Table 39.10 collects data on the relative binding affinities of 25 analogs to intact nuclei from rat liver cells for a wide variety of structural types of thyroxine analogs (67). This table also shows the relative binding affinities of 34 analogs, more limited in their types of structural variations, to the solubilized receptor preparation from rat liver cell nuclei (68). Hormonal activities *in vivo* in the rat antigoiter assay are reported for 40 analogs.

8.2.2.1   *Relative Binding Affinities to Cell Nuclear Receptors.*

For the series of analogs listed in Table 39.10, all of which contain the alanine side chain, there is a strong similarity in binding affinities to intact nuclei and to the soluble receptor preparation. The following qualitative description refers to both test systems.

The binding affinities of the analogs of

Table 39.10 Antigoiter Activities and Binding Affinities to Intact Nuclei and to Soluble Receptor from Rat Hepatic Nuclei for Thyroid Hormone Analogs[a]

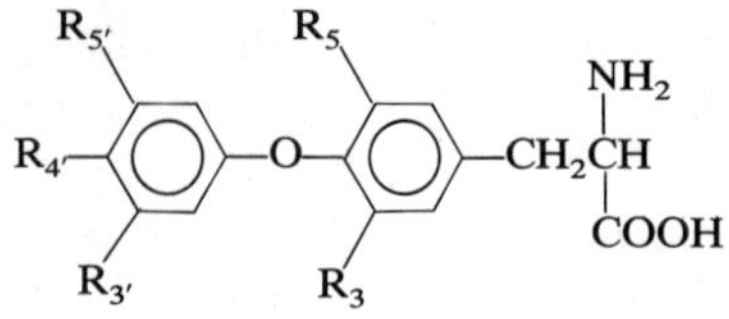

No.	Abbreviation	$R_3 = R_5$	$R_{4'}$	$R_{3'}$	$R_{5'}$	In Vivo Rat Anti-goiter (A)	In Vitro, Rat Liver Cell Relative Binding Affinity Intact Nuclei[b] (BN)	Soluble Receptor[c] (BS)
a	T_3	I	OH	I	H	100	100	100
b	T_2	I	OH	H	H	0.81	0.30	0.08
c	T_2Me	I	OH	Me	H	14.47	13.5	3.30
d	T_2Et	I	OH	Et	H	40.8	21.0	—
e	T_2iPr	I	OH	iPr	H	142.1	104.0	89.15
f	T_2nPr	I	OH	nPr	H	39.5	—	23.97
g	T_2sBu	I	OH	sBu	H	79.9	—	78.29
h	T_2tBu	I	OH	tBu	H	21.7	38.5	8.45
i	T_2iBu	I	OH	iBu	H	7.74	20.0	—
j	T_2Phe	I	OH	Phe	H	2.03	2.0	—
k	T_2cHex	I	OH	cHex	H	—	1.4	—
l	T_2F	I	OH	F	H	0.65	—	0.16
m	T_2Cl	I	OH	Cl	H	4.88	6.2	3.73
n	T_2Br	I	OH	Br	H	23.78	—	15.89
o	T_2NO_2	I	OH	NO_2	H	0.18	—	0.23
p	T_2Cl_2	I	OH	Cl	Cl	3.80	4.5	3.71
q	T_2Br_2	I	OH	Br	Br	1.58	—	5.07
r	T_4	I	OH	I	I	18.1	12.5	13.85
s	T_2Me_2	I	OH	Me	Me	9.04	6.2	0.85
t	T_2iPr_2	I	OH	iPr	iPr	Inact.	1.4	1.10
u	T_2iPrCl	I	OH	iPr	Cl	—	—	52.56
v	T_2iPrBr	I	OH	iPr	Br	—	—	21.95
w	T_2iPrI	I	OH	iPr	I	—	—	12.41
x	Br_2iPr	Br	OH	iPr	H	30.0	36.0	—
y	Me_3	Me	Oh	Me	H	0.54	0.1	—
z	Me_4	Me	OH	Me	Me	0.36	0.1	—
a'	Me_2iPr	Me	OH	iPr	H	3.60	0.7	—
b'	iPr_2I	iPr	OH	I	H	Inact.	0.2	—
c'	$3,3'-T_2$	I[d]	OH	I	H	0.25	0.5	0.69
d'	$3,3',5'-T_3$	I[d]	OH	I	I	0.125	0.1	0.09
e'	$4'H-T_2$	I	H	H	H	1.24	—	0.01
f'	$4'H-T_3$	I	H	I	H	27.12	0.4	0.23
g'	$4'H-T_2Br$	I	H	Br	H	18.0	—	0.24
h'	$4'H-T_2Cl$	I	H	Cl	H	7.78	—	0.12

Table 39.10 (Continued)

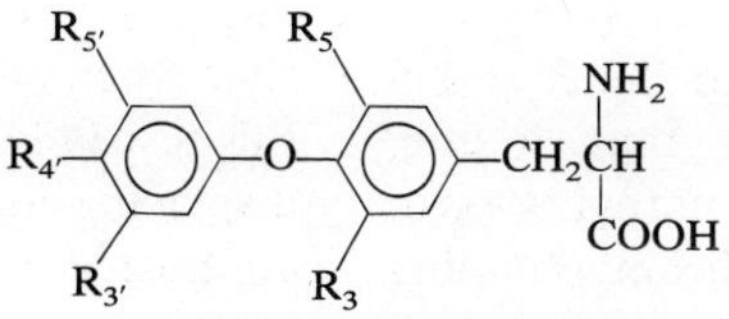

No.	Abbreviation	$R_3 = R_5$	$R_{4'}$	$R_{3'}$	$R_{5'}$	In Vivo Rat Anti-goiter (A)	In Vitro, Rat Liver Cell Relative Binding Affinity Intact Nuclei[b] (BN)	Soluble Receptor[c] (BS)
i'	4'H-T$_2$F	I	H	F	H	1.39	—	0.01
j'	4'H-T$_2$Me	I	H	Me	H	2.71	0.2	0.23
k'	4'H-T$_2$tBu	I	H	tBu	H	—	—	0.34
l'	4'H-T$_2$CF$_3$	I	H	CF$_3$	H	13.6	0.2	—
m'	4'-OMe-T$_3$	I	OMe	I	H	11.25	—	1.29
n'	4'OMe-T$_2$iPr	I	OMe	iPr	H	19.0	—	16.82
o'	4'OMe-T$_2$tBu	I	OMe	tBu	H	2.35	—	0.27
p'	4'NH$_2$-T$_2$	I	NH$_2$	H	H	0.04	—	0.003
q'	4'NH$_2$-T$_3$	I	NH$_2$	I	H	0.27	0.76	—
r'	4'NH$_2$-T$_2$Me	I	NH$_2$	CH$_3$	H	0.036	—	0.03
s'	4'NH$_2$-T$_2$Me$_2$	I	NH$_2$	CH$_3$	CH$_3$	0.13	—	0.04

[a]   Dietrich et al. (136). On a molar basis relative to L-T$_3$ = 100. No correction for DL isomers.
[b]   Koerner et al. (67).
[c]   Jorgensen et al. (68) and unpublished data.
[d]   R$_3$ = I, R$_5$ = H.

the homologous series of 3'-alkyl-3,5-diiodothyronines of Table 39.10 (b–i) increase in the order hydrogen, methyl, ethyl, reaching a maximum equal to that of T$_3$ (a) with the 3'-isopropyl substituent (e). 3,5-Diiodothyronines with 3' aliphatic, aromatic, or alicyclic substituents larger than isopropyl (f–k), show decreasing binding affinities as the size of the 3' residue increases. The 3' sec-butyl group, which imparts higher affinity than does the 3' n-propyl group, possesses a shorter extended size and a closer similarity to the isopropyl substituent in the partial structure of its side chain [—CH(CH$_3$)—] than does the 3' n-propyl group (—CH$_2$CH$_2$CH$_3$).

The 3'-halogen analogs (l–n, a) show increasing binding affinities as the halogen increases in size: F < Cl < Br < I. A 3'-alkyl group [e.g., ethyl (d)] contributes more to binding affinity than does a 3'-halogen atom of about the same size [e.g., chlorine (m)]. The 3'-nitro substituent (o) does not contribute to binding. 3',5'-Disubstituted 3,5-diiodothyronines, whether of the 3',5'-dialkyl (s, t), 3',5'-dihalo (p–r), or 3'-alkyl-5'-halo (u–w) types, show lower binding affinities than do the corresponding 3'-monosubstituted analogs. Binding affinities decrease as the size of the 5' substituent increases, if the 3' position is assigned to the substituent that promotes the highest binding affinity when present alone (e.g., 3'-isopropyl-5'-chloro, not 3'-chloro-5'-isopropyl for u).

Symmetrical substituents in the 3 and 5 positions which are smaller than iodine, such as bromine (x) and methyl ($y-a'$), produce lower but significant binding affinities. The unsymmetrical and larger 3,5-diisopropyl substitution (b') produces a low binding affinity. Removal of one inner ring iodine atom from T_3 to form $3,3'-T_2$ (c') or from T_4 to form $3,3',5'-T_3$ (d') leads to low binding affinities. Removal of a bulky 3 (and/or 5) iodine atom removes the steric constraint of T_3 and T_4 ($\phi = 90°$, $\phi' = 0°$; see Fig. 39.5 and Section 5.1). A reasonable alternate minimum energy conformation for $3,3',5'-T_3$ near $\phi = 0°$, $\phi' = 90°$ is shown in Fig. 39.10. Like the 3,5-disubstituted analogs, the 3',5'-diiodo outer ring of (d') is associated with an analog of lower affinity than one containing the 3'-monoiodo substitution (c').

Compounds lacking the 4'-hydroxyl group ($e'-l'$) show very low binding affinities relative to the corresponding 4'-hydroxy analog. Because these 4'-deoxy analogs are relatively active *in vivo*, and because there is evidence for their

metabolic 4'-hydroxylation (129), Koerner et al. (67) tested the ability of $4'H-T_3$ (f') to displace $^{125}I-T_3$ from liver nuclear binding sites when administered to the intact rat. In this test *in vivo*, $4'H-T_3$ showed 10% of the displacing activity of nonradioactive T_3 as contrasted with 0.2–0.4% *in vitro* where metabolism does not occur.

4'-Methoxy derivatives of 3'-substituted 3,5-diiodothyronines ($m'-o'$) show lower binding affinities than do the corresponding free 4'-OH compounds. Replacement of the 4'-OH group with the 4'-NH$_2$ group ($p'-s'$) results in analogs with very low binding affinities, the strongest binder of the group being the 4'-amino analog of T_3 (q').

In addition to the data of Table 39.10 Koerner et al. (67) showed that analogs with 3'-alkyl or 3'-aryl substituents sterically positioned in the 3'-distal orientation, such as the 2',3'-dimethyl derivative of T_2 (Fig. 39.7a), showed much higher binding affinities than did analogs with substituents in the 5'-proximal orientation, such as the 2',5'-dimethyl derivatives of T_2 (Fig. 39.7b).

The data from Koerner et al. (67) shown in Table 39.10 were used by Dietrich et al.

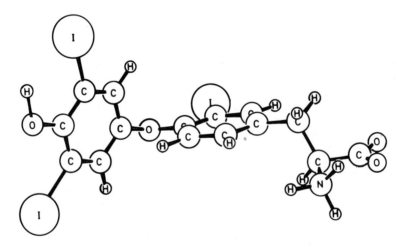

Fig. 39.10   L-3,3',5'-Triiodothyronine shown in a minimum energy conformation for the aromatic rings, $\phi = 0°$, $\phi' = 90°$.

(136) to formulate equation 39.4, which correlates relative binding affinities to the T_3 receptor site of intact rat liver nuclei with physical parameters of substituents on the thyronine or 4'-deoxy thyronine nucleus.

$$\log (BN)$$
$$= 1.680\pi_{35} + 1.147\pi_{3'} - 1.218 \, (3' \text{ size} > I)$$
$$- 0.873\pi_{5'} - 2.049 I(4'H) - 3.292$$
$$n = 25, \; r = 0.969, \; s = 0.280 \quad (39.4)$$

where (BN) = Binding affinity to rat liver nuclei relative to L-T_3 = 100

$\pi_{35} = \Sigma\pi$ [Hansch et al. (144) lipophilic parameter for substituents in the 3,5 positions

$\pi_{3'}, \pi_{5'} = \pi$ values for substituents in the 3' and 5' positions

(3' size > I) = Average distance a substituent extends further than iodine from the 3' position

I(4' − H) = Indicator variable that equals 1.0 for a 4' hydrogen and equals 0 for a 4'-OH group

The parameters of equation 39.4 show that binding to intact nuclei is enhanced by bulky lipophilic 3,5 substituents (π_{35}) and decreased by 5' substituent size or lipophilicity (estimated by $\pi_{5'}$). The 3' substituent binds in the distal orientation in a hydrophobic pocket ($\pi_{3'}$) approximately the size of iodine (3' size > I). The emergence of the same lipophilicity, size, and stereochemistry parameters in equation 39.2 describing *in vivo* activities and in equation 39.4 describing binding affinities suggests that these structural features correlate receptor binding directly with activity. The large negative coefficient for the indicator variable [I(4'—H)] shows the importance of the 4'-OH group in binding. Electronic effects (σ) of 3' and 5' substituents are not significant in describing receptor binding affinities in this series. This is in contrast to the importance of this

term in equation 39.2 for describing activities *in vivo*, and in equation 39.3 for describing binding to the transport protein TBG.

The data from Jorgensen et al. (68) of Table 39.10 were used by Dietrich et al. (136) to develop equation 39.5, which correlates relative binding affinities to soluble receptor preparations of rat liver cell nuclei with physical parameters of 3', 4', and 5' substituents on the 3,5-diiodothyronine nucleus.

$$\log (BS)$$
$$= 1.546\pi_{3'} - 1.904(3' \text{ size} > I) - 0.780\pi_{5'}$$
$$- 1.553 I(4'\text{-H})$$
$$- 1.323 I(4'\text{-OCH}_3) + 1.306\sigma_{3'5'}$$
$$- 0.114(\text{Interact}_{3'}) - 0.222$$
$$n = 31, \; r = 0.960, \; s = 0.364 \quad (39.5)$$

In addition to the same substituent parameters as used in equation 39.4, $\pi_{3'}$, $\pi_{5'}$, (3' size > I), and I(4'-H), the following new factors were introduced in equation 39.5:

BS = Binding affinity to rat hepatic soluble nuclear receptor relative to L-T_3 = 100

I(4'-OCH$_3$) = Indicator variable that equals 1.0 for a 4'-methoxy group and equals 0 for the 4'-OH group

$\sigma_{3'5'}$ = Sum of electronic σ_p values from Hansch et al. (144) for substituents in the 3' and 5' positions

(Interact$_{3'}$) = estimate of the free energy change in kilocalories per mole for orientation of the 4'-OH from cis to the 3' (distal) substituent to cis to the 5' (proximal) substituent

The parameters of equation (39.5), like those of equation 39.4, show that the 3' substituent binds in a size-limited hydrophobic pocket, that any 5' substituent bulk or lipophilicity decreases binding, and that the free 4'-OH group is important for binding. In addition, this series of analogs, more varied in the 3' and 5' positions, shows that binding is moderately enhanced by electron-withdrawing substituents in the 3' and 5' positions ($\sigma_{3'5'}$); the (Interact$_{3'}$) term describes a favorable effect by substituents that orient the 4'-OH group with its hydrogen atom close to the 5' (proximal) position. These data suggest that the 4'-OH group binds to the receptor by proton donation in hydrogen bond formation with an element of the receptor that is near the 5' position. This further supports the concept that the 5' substituent is detrimental to receptor binding because of its interference with the 4'-OH hydrogen bonds with the receptor, and/or because of its direct and unfavorable steric interaction with the receptor surface.

8.2.2.2 *Correlations of Receptor Binding Affinities in vitro with Hormonal Activities in vivo.* The binding affinities of thyroxine analogs to rat liver nuclei (BN) and to soluble nuclear receptor (BS) listed in Table 39.10, together with the hormonal activities *in vivo* in the rat antigoiter assay (A), have been used by Dietrich et al. (136) to develop the very similar equations 39.6 and 39.7 which correlate receptor binding affinities with hormonal activities.

$$\log (A) = 0.730 \log (BN) + 1.116I(4'\text{-H})$$
$$+ 0.241$$
$$n = 29, r = 0.917, s = 0.371 \quad (39.6)$$

$$\log (A) = 0.757 \log (BS) + 1.159I(4'\text{-H})$$
$$+ 0.623I(4'\text{-OCH}_3) + 0.274$$
$$n = 26, r = 0.937, s = 0.402 \quad (39.7)$$

Equations 39.6 and 39.7 show that binding affinities measured *in vitro* are excellent predictors of hormonal activities *in vivo*, as long as factors are included to account for

the metabolic transformations *in vivo* of the poorly binding 4'-deoxy and 4'-methoxy analogs into the stronger binding and more active 4'-hydroxy metabolites. This correlation between *in vivo* activities and *in vitro* affinities supports the assignment of an important role to the nuclear binding event in the initiation of hormonal effects.

8.3 Summary of Structural Requirements for Thyroid Hormonal Activity

The qualitative and quantitative descriptions in the preceding sections of structural requirements for binding to transport proteins, for metabolic activation and deactivation of analogs, for binding affinities to nuclear receptor preparations, and for activities *in vivo*, provide the perspective for the following summary of structural requirements for the expression of thyroid hormonal activities *in vivo*:

1. A central lipophilic core of two aromatic rings, insulated from each other electronically by a connecting oxygen, sulfur, or carbon atom which establishes an inter-ring bond angle of about 120°.

2. Nonpolar groups, thus far limited to halogen and methyl, in the 3 and 5 positions of the inner (alanine-bearing) ring. These groups establish minimum energy conformations of the aromatic rings in which the planes of the rings are approximately mutually perpendicular. The 3 and 5 substituents also contribute by size-limited hydrophobic associations with the receptor.

3. An α-amino acid or anionic side chain, preferably the length of two or three carbon atoms, attached para to the bridging atom at the 1 position of the inner aromatic ring. Side chains that are metabolized to form the amino acid or an anionic group also contribute to activity. The carboxylate ion of an acetic

or propionic acid side chain contributes maximal binding to the nuclear receptor. The additional presence of an L-α-amino group (e.g., L-alanine) reduces receptor binding affinity but enhances activity *in vivo* by increasing access to the receptor and by retarding metabolism and excretion.

4. A phenolic hydroxyl group in the 4′ position of the outer ring. The 4′-OH group contributes a proton to a hydrogen-bonding site near the 5′ (proximal) position of the hormone. The 4′-phenolate ion is the structural feature responsible for strong association with transport proteins. An unsubstituted 4′ position, or one occupied by a phenolic ether or ester group, may be converted to the active 4′-OH metabolite *in vivo*. An isosteric group, such as the 4′ amino, may impart a low level of activity.

5. Activity of a core structure of the type described in 1–4 above (e.g., 3,5-diiodothyronine or 3,5-dimethylthyroacetic acid) is enhanced by a lipophilic halogen, alkyl, or aryl substituent adjacent to the 4′-OH group. High activity is imparted by an iodine atom or by an alkyl group that approximates iodine in

size (e.g., isopropyl). The 3′-isopropyl group provides maximal activity because of its weak associations with transport proteins, its strong association to the nuclear receptor, and its resistance to metabolic modification. The 3′ substituent expresses its activating effect when oriented in space distal to the inner ring.

6. A second lipophilic substituent adjacent to the 4′-OH group (5′ position) reduces activity in direct relationship to its size. This effect may be caused by interference with the 4′-OH hydrogen bond with the receptor and/or by direct steric interference with the hormone–receptor interaction.

The general functional and steric features of the hormone–receptor interaction, as presented in this summary, are shown schematically in Fig. 39.11. The carboxylate ion of the hormone side chain is shown forming an ion pair with a positive region of the hormone receptor. In the model system of the transport protein, thyroxine-binding prealbumin (TBPA), this positive site appears to be formed by the two ε-ammonium groups of paired lysine residues

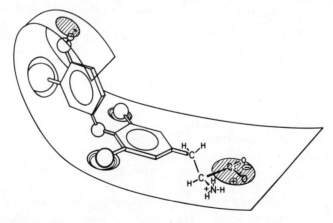

Fig. 39.11 A schematic representation of the functional and steric features of a hormonally active 3,5,3′-trisubstituted thyronine binding to the receptor of the cell nucleus. (From E. C. Jorgensen and T. A. Andrea, "The Nature of the Thyroid Receptor," in *Thyroid Research*, J. Robbins and L. E. Braverman, Eds., Excerpta Medica, Amsterdam, 1976, p. 306, with permission of the publishers.)

at the entrance of a hydrophobic binding channel. The aromatic rings of the hormone are skewed, and the 3, 5, and 3′ substituents are shown in size-limited hydrophobic associations with complementary lipophilic pockets of the hormone receptor. The 4′-hydroxyl group is shown contributing a proton to a hydrogen bond with the receptor on the proximal side of the outer ring. Steric constraint, by which the bulk of the 5′ substituent reduces activity, is shown by the close approach of the receptor surface to the 5′ proximal side of the hormone.

The summation of highly specific multiple binding contacts between the hormone and its receptor are facilitated by the semirigid core structure of the hormone and the resulting highly defined relative spatial locations of its functional groups. As a receptor model, TBPA provides a similar semirigid and highly structured cluster of specific amino acid side chains which provide a preordered complementary binding site for the thyroid hormones. It is a consequence of the structurally specific binding interaction between hormone and receptor that hormonal activity is expressed, rather than any reaction in which the hormone reacts as a chemical intermediate.

A thyroid hormone may be described in general terms as a three-dimensional matrix, with a spatial array of substituents constituting a coded message. This message is transmitted by specific carriers, the plasma transport proteins, and is delivered to and read by a group of specific hormone receptors. One biologically important receptor is an acidic protein associated with the deoxyribonucleic acid (DNA) of the cell nuclear chromatin. It is reasonable, based on the time course of subsequent events, that the hormone–receptor interaction brings about a conformational perturbation of the receptor that results in transmission of a second message to the closely coupled DNA. This message is amplified and broadened in its scope by generation of a spectrum of specific messenger ribonucleic acids

(mRNA) which stimulate the synthesis of a variety of proteins, including the enzymes that mediate the growth, developmental, and metabolic expressions of hormonal activity (see Fig. 39.4).

9 ANTITHYROID DRUGS

The term *antithyroid drug* is most generally used to describe those drugs that act within the thyroid gland to block the biosynthesis of the thyroid hormones (*intrathyroidal inhibitors*). Reduction in circulating hormone stimulates pituitary secretion of thyrotropin (TSH), which in turn stimulates circulation and tissue development of the thyroid gland. The resulting enlarged gland, in which hormone synthesis is inhibited, is called a goiter. Because of this action the intrathyroidal inhibitors are often called goitrogens.

Some of the same drugs that act as intrathyroidal inhibitors as well as other drugs act outside the thyroid gland by various mechanisms to reduce the expressions of activity by the circulating hormones. Although they are classed as antithyroid drugs, these *peripheral antagonists* do not often produce goiters.

The history, nature, and mechanisms of action of the antithyroid drugs have been reviewed (145–147), as has their use in treatment of hyperthyroidism (148).

9.1 Intrathyroidal Inhibitors

9.1.1 IODIDE ION AND INORGANIC ANIONS. Large doses of iodide ion cause a transient inhibition of the synthesis and release of the thyroid hormones (Wolff–Chaikoff effect). In man there is rapid adaptation to high intrathyroid iodide levels and normal thyroid synthesis resumes in 1–2 days, in spite of continued administration of iodide ion.

The selective concentration of iodide ion by the thyroid gland has been the basis for the use of radioactive iodine as an alternative to surgery in treatment of hyperthyroidism. The isotope currently used in therapy is ^{131}I, half-life 8 days, although use of ^{125}I, half-life 60 days, is under investigation. The high energy beta particles of ^{131}I are absorbed within 2 mm of their origin, producing selective destruction of thyroid cells without injury to other nearby organs or tissues. Most of the γ-ray emission of ^{131}I is of sufficiently high energy to pass through the thyroid gland unabsorbed, and to be detected by external scanning devices.

Several inorganic monovalent anions whose partial molal ionic volumes are similar to that of iodide ion are concentrated by the active transport mechanism of the thyroid gland. These anions competitively inhibit the active transport of iodide and are active in the order:

$$TcO_4^- \gg ClO_4^- > ReO_4^- > BF_4^- > I^-$$

Sodium or potassium perchlorate ($NaClO_4$, $KClO_4$) are used to a limited extent in treatment of hyperthyroidism. Their use is restricted by a high incidence of gastric irritation and occasional serious toxic reactions such as nephrosis and aplastic anemia. Tracer doses of TcO_4^- labeled with the short-lived (half-life 6 h) technetium-99 m (^{99m}Tc) are useful for assessing the activity of the iodide transport mechanism in man. The isotope emits readily measured gamma rays but no beta emissions, and the pertechnetate ion does not undergo metabolic transformation in the gland.

Thiocyanate ion (SCN^-) blocks the iodide concentrating mechanisms, and by acting as a substrate for thyroid peroxidase, inhibits iodination of the tyrosine residues of thyroglobulin. The toxicity of thiocyanate prevents its use in therapy, and its excessive formation in body fluids may be responsible for some cases of endemic goiter. The starchy material (cassava) from the

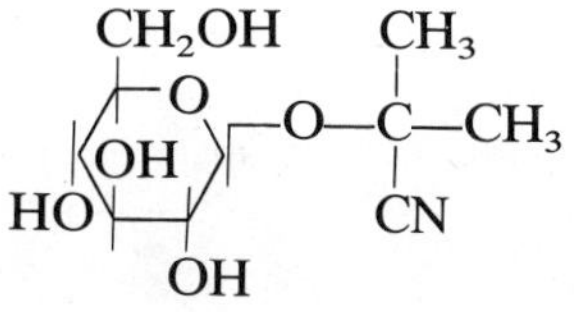

39.**8**

fleshy roots of the cassava plant (also manioc or tapioca plant) is a principal item of diet in central Africa. Cassava contains a cyanogenic glucoside, linamarin (39.**8**). Upon ingestion, hydrolysis yields cyanide ion (CN^-), which is metabolically detoxified to form thiocyanate ion (SCN^-). In regions where iodide ion intake is low the plasma concentration of thiocyanate is sufficient to block adequate thyroid hormone synthesis, leading to hypothyroidism, goiter, and even cretinism in a significant percentage of the population (149). A similar report from Sicily describes a local dietary regime leading to high thiocyanate and low iodide blood levels, and a high incidence of goiter and cretinism (150).

9.1.2 THIONAMIDES. A family of compounds containing the common structural feature of the thionamide group (39.**9**) are the most widely used drugs in the treatment of hyperthyroidism. The most potent of the class contain the thiourea nucleus (39.**10a,b**); they are also called thioureylenes. This structure may exist in the thioketo (39.**10a**) or thioenol (39.**10b**) tautomeric forms. These agents inhibit the peroxidase enzymes responsible for iodination of tyrosine residues of thyroglobulin and the coupling of the iodotyrosine residues to form iodothyronines (151) (see Sections 3.1.2 and 3.1.3). The coupling step

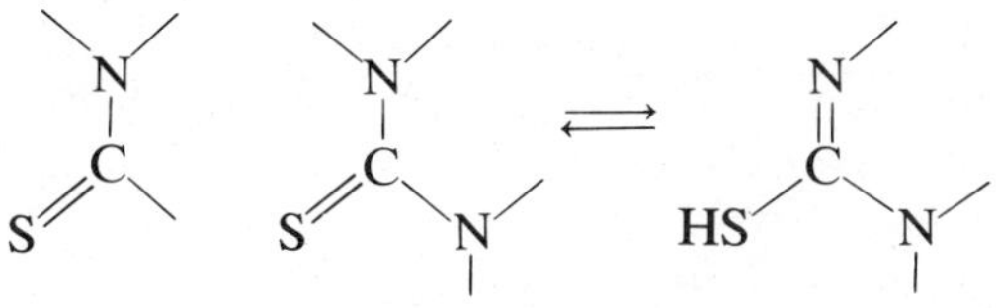

39.9   39.**10a**   39.**10b**

Table 39.11   Thioureylene Antithyroid Drugs in Current Clinical Use

Generic and Chemical Names	Structure
Methylthiouracil NF, 6-methyl-2-thiouracil (39.**11a**, R = CH₃)	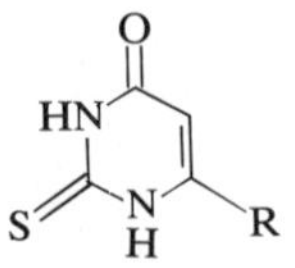 39.**11**
Propylthiouracil USP, 6-propyl-2-thiouracil (39.**11b**, R = CH₂CH₂CH₃)	
Methimazole USP, 1-methyl-2-mercaptoimidazole (39.**12**)	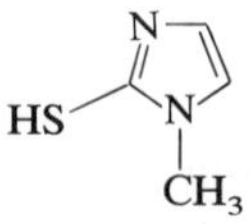 39.**12**
Carbimazole, 1-methyl-3-carbethoxy-2-mercaptoimidazole (39.**13**)	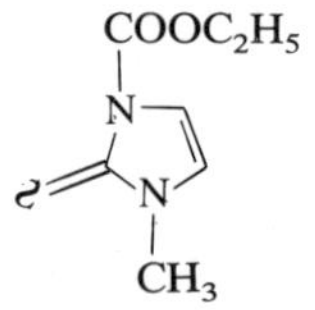 39.**13**

in thyroid hormone biosynthesis is the most susceptible to the thionamide drugs.

The thioureylene antithyroid drugs in current use are collected in Table 39.11. The thiouracil derivatives methylthiouracil (39.**11a**) and propylthiouracil (39.**11b**), with daily oral maintenance doses of 50–200 mg, are about one-tenth as potent as the imidazole derivatives, methimazole (39.**12**) and carbimazole (39.**13**), which require daily oral doses of 5–20 mg. Carbimazole is a prodrug derivative of methimazole, developed to mask the bitter taste of the parent compound.

The presence of the thionamide or thiourea moiety in a structure imparts the potential for that compound to act as an antithyroid agent. Thiobarbiturates, such as thiopental, are cyclic thiourea derivatives and are widely used as hypnotic–sedative drugs and for the production of anesthesia when administered by injection. Their antithyroid activity makes invalid any test of thyroid function for several days after their use.

Antithyroid substances of the thionamide type are also found in some foods. Goitrin (39.**14**), (S)-5-vinyl-2-oxazolidinethione, was shown by Astwood et al. (152) to be the active goitrogen in turnips, rutabaga,

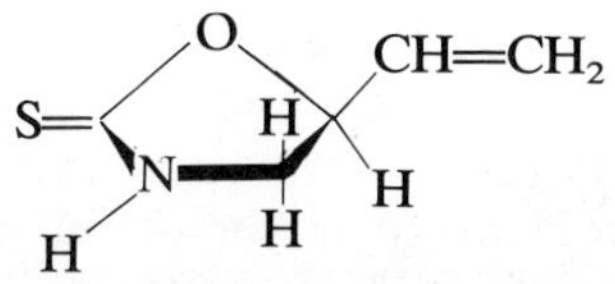

39.**14** Goitrin

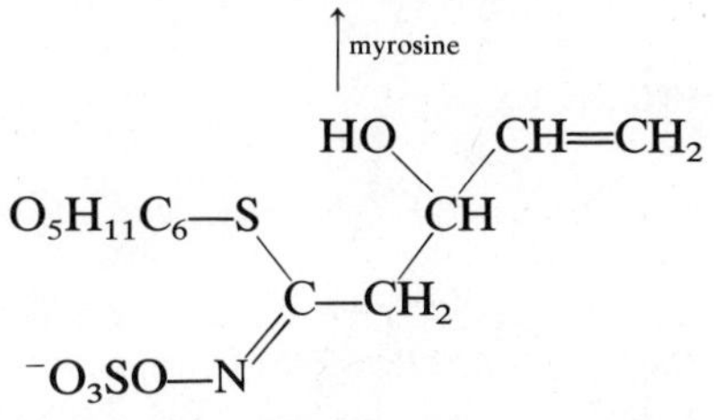

39.**15** Progoitrin

and other species of plants of the mustard family (genus *Brassicae*). The stereochemistry of goitrin as determined by Kjaer et al. (153) is shown in 39.**14**. Goitrin is present in the plant as an inactive thioamide, progoitrin (39.**15**), which is conjugated with sulfuric acid and glucose (154). Hydrolysis by the plant enzyme myrosin, or following ingestion by related bacterial enzymes in the intestine, releases the free thioamide. This undergoes a Lossen rearrangement to the isothiocyanate and cyclization to form the active thiooxazolidinone, goitrin. Ingestion of large amounts of goitrogen-containing foods does not by itself produce goiter. However, when such foods are a common part of the diet of a region where moderate iodine deficiency also exists, such as central Europe, the result is endemic goiter.

9.1.3 AROMATIC AMINES AND PHENOLS. Extensive studies of aromatic compounds with antithyroid activities have shown that a free aromatic amine or aromatic hydroxyl group is required for maximal goitrogenic activity. These compounds are not used as antithyroid drugs, but their goitrogenic properties are frequently exhibited as side effects to their other uses. Sulfaguanidine [p-$H_2NC_6H_5SO_2NHC(NH_2)$=NH], in addition to its antibacterial properties, was the first aromatic amine in which

goitrogenic activity was recognized (155). p-Aminosalicylic acid (p-H_2N-o-$HOC_6H_3CO_2H$), which is used in high doses for long periods in the treatment of tuberculosis, sometimes causes goiters, as did the obsolete oral hypoglycemic agent, carbutamide (p-$H_2NC_6H_4SO_2$-$NHCONHC_4H_9$). Many phenolic compounds show antithyroid activity. The most potent possess the 1,3-dihydroxy substitution pattern of resorcinol [$1,3$-$(HO)_2C_6H_4$] or of phloroglucinol [$1,3,5$-$(HO)_3C_6H_3$]. The aromatic amines and phenols are inhibitors of peroxidases. They produce their goitrogenic effects by the intrathyroidal inhibition of the iodination of thyroglobulin, and the coupling of iodotyrosines, thus suppressing synthesis of the thyroid hormones.

9.1.4 LITHIUM SALTS. In the course of the widespread use of lithium carbonate in the treatment of psychotic states, occasional production of hypothyroidism and of goiter has been observed (156). Lithium ion inhibits adenyl cyclase, which forms cyclic adenosine monophosphate (cAMP). This "second messenger" is formed in response to TSH, and is a stimulator of the processes involved in thyroid hormone release from the thyroid gland. Inhibition of hormone release by lithium ion has proved a useful adjunct to the more classical methods of treating hyperthyroidism (157).

9.2 Peripheral Antagonists

9.2.1 INHIBITORS OF HORMONE DEIODINATION. In addition to their intrathyroidal inhibition of thyroid hormone formation, methythiouracil (39.**11a**) and propylthiouracil (39.**11b**) inhibit the extrathyroidal metabolic conversion of T_4 to T_3 (158). This action of the thiouracils results in a rapid fall in serum T_3 concentration and, since T_3 is the more potent hormone, in a rapid lowering of the thyrotoxic state. In contrast, methimazole (39.**12**) inhibits only intrathyroidal hormone synthesis and has no effect on peripheral deiodination reactions.

The compound n-butyl 3,5-diiodo-4-hydroxybenzoate ($3,5\text{-}I_2\text{-}4\text{-}HO\text{-}C_6H_2CO_2\text{-}C_4H_9$) also inhibits peripheral deiodination of the thyroid hormones and reduces the calorigenic effects of T_4. However, its primary effect as a peripherally acting antithyroid drug is attributed to its stimulation of T_4 and T_3 conjugation, biliary excretion, and loss in the feces. This effect is caused by displacement of the thyroid hormones from transport proteins (159).

9.2.2 INHIBITORS OF HORMONE ACTION. A large number of analogs of the thyroid hormones have been tested for their abilities to block actions of the circulating hormones. $3,3',5'$-Triiodothyronine ($3,3',5'\text{-}T_3$, Fig. 39.10), $3,3'$-diiodothyronine ($3,3'\text{-}T_2$), and their propionic acid side chain analogs decreased the oxygen consumption of T_4-maintained thyroidectomized rats in molar ratios of analog : T_4 of 50–200 : 1. Antagonistic effects were also demonstrated in man (160). As discussed in Section 9.2.1 the effects of T_4 are reduced by agents that inhibit the T_4 to T_3 conversion, and $3,3',5'\text{-}T_3$ has been shown to inhibit this reaction *in vitro* (161). The low binding affinities of $3,3',5'\text{-}T_3$ and of $3,3'\text{-}T_2$ to nuclear receptors (Section 8.2.2) make it unlikely that they inhibit thyroid hormone actions at the nuclear receptor level. To date, there are no well demonstrated and potent peripheral antagonists among thyroid hormone analogs.

Many of the cardiovascular and metabolic manifestations of the hyperthyroid state are the result of excessive adrenergic stimulation. Therefore, adrenergic blocking agents such as reserpine and guanethidine were used with some success in decreasing the tachycardia and related cardiovascular effects of thyrotoxicosis. The side effects of these drugs have led to the current use of propranolol, the specific β-adrenergic receptor antagonist in the early management of acutely ill thyrotoxic patients (162), in preparation for thyroid surgery (163), and in combination with antithyroid drugs in long-term management of hyperthyroidism (164).

REFERENCES

1. T. H. Shepard, *J. Clin. Endocrinol. Metab.*, **27,** 945 (1967).

2. R. A. Cuestas, A. Lindall, and R. R. Engal, *New Engl. J. Med.*, **295,** 297 (1976).

3. J. M. McKenzie, in *Handbook of Physiology*, Section 7: *Endocrinology*, Vol. 3, R. O. Greep and E. B. Astwood, Eds., *Thyroid*, American Physiological Society, Washington, D.C., 1974, p. 285.

4. H. W. G. Mackenzie, *Brit. Med. J.*, **1892 II,** 940.

5. E. Baumann, *Hoppe–Seyler's Z. Physiol. Chem.*, **21,** 319 (1895).

6. E. Baumann, *Muench. Med. Wochenschr.*, **43,** 309 (1896).

7. A. Kossel, *Hoppe–Seyler's Z. Physiol. Chem.*, **23,** 1 (1897).

8. E. C. Kendall, *Proc. Mayo Clinic*, **39,** 548 (1964).

9. E. C. Kendall and A. E. Osterberg, *J. Biol. Chem.* **40,** 265 (1919).

10. E. C. Kendall, *Thyroxine*, American Chemical Society Monograph Series No. 47, Chemical Catalog Company, New York, 1929.

11. H. Himsworth and R. Pitt-Rivers, *Biog. Mem. Fellows R. S.*, **18,** 267 (1972).

12. C. R. Harington, *J. Biol. Chem.*, **64,** 29 (1925).

13. C. R. Harington, *Biochem. J.*, **20,** 293 (1926).

14. C. R. Harington, *Biochem. J.*, **20,** 300 (1926).

15. C. R. Harington and G. Barger, *Biochem. J.*, **21,** 169 (1927).

16. J. Gross and C. P. Leblond, *Endocrinology*, **48,** 714 (1951).

17. J. Gross and R. Pitt-Rivers, *Lancet*, **1952 I,** 439.

18. J. Gross and R. Pitt-Rivers, *Biochem. J.*, **53,** 645 (1953).

19. J. Gross and R. Pitt-Rivers, *Biochem. J.*, **53,** 652 (1953).

20. J. Roche, S. Lissitzky, and R. Michel, *C. R. Hebd. Seances Acad. Sci. Paris*, **234,** 997, 1228 (1952).

21. J. Roche, R. Michel, and W. Wolf, *Bull. Soc. Chim. Fr.*, **1957,** 464.

22. J. S. Varcoe and W. K. Warburton, *J. Chem. Soc.*, **1960,** 2711.

23. J. Roche, R. Michel, J. Nunez, and W. Wolf, *Biochim. Biophys. Acta,* **18,** 149 (1955).

24. J. Roche, R. Michel, W. Wolf, and N. Etling, *C. R. Seances Soc. Biol.,* **148,** 1738 (1954).

25. N. R. Stasilli, R. L. Kroc, and R. I. Meltzer, *Endocrinology,* **64,** 62 (1959).

26. E. G. Tomich, E. A. Woollett, and M. A. Pratt, *J. Endocrinol.,* **20,** 65 (1960).

27. I. J. Chopra, J. Sack, and D. A. Fisher, *J. Clin. Invest.,* **55,** 1137 (1975).

28. I. J. Chopra, U. Chopra, S. R. Smith, M. Reza, and D. H. Solomon, *J. Clin. Endocrinol. Metab.,* **41,** 1043 (1975).

29. W. Tong, *Pharm. Ther.* B, **1,** 769 (1975).

30. L. Jirousek and E. T. Pritchard, *Biochim. Biophys. Acta,* **243,** 230 (1971).

31. L. Field and J. E. White, *Proc. Natl. Acad. Sci. U.S.,* **70,** 328 (1973).

32. J. Nunez and J. Pommier, *Eur. J. Biochem.,* **7,** 286 (1969).

33. L. Lamas, A. Taurog, G. Salvatore, and H. Edelhoch, *J. Biol. Chem.,* **249,** 2732 (1974).

34. T. B. Johnson and L. B. Tewkesbury, Jr., *Proc. Natl. Acad. Sci. U.S.,* **28,** 73 (1942).

35. C. R. Harington, *J. Chem. Soc.,* **1944,** 193.

36. T. Matsuura and H. J. Cahnmann, *J. Am. Chem. Soc.,* **82,** 2055 (1960).

37. T. Matsuura and A. Nishinaga, *J. Org. Chem.,* **27,** 3072 (1962).

38. I. J. Chopra, D. A. Fisher, D. H. Solomon, and G. N. Beall, *J. Clin. Endocrinol. Metab.,* **36,** 311 (1973).

39. M. C. Gershengorn, S.-Y. Cheng, R. E. Lippoldt, R. S. Lord, and J. Robbins, *J. Biol. Chem.,* **252,** 8713 (1977).

40. Y. Kanda, D. S. Goodman, R. E. Canfield, and F. J. Morgan, *J. Biol. Chem.,* **249,** 6796 (1974).

41. C. C. F. Blake, M. J. Geisow, S. J. Oatley, B. Rérat, and C. Rérat, *J. Mol. Biol.,* **121,** 339 (1978).

42. C. C. F. Blake, I. D. A. Swan, C. Rérat, J. Berthou, A. Laurent, and B. Rérat, *J. Mol. Biol.,* **61,** 217 (1971).

43. S.-Y. Cheng, M. Wilcheck, H. J. Cahnmann, and J. Robbins, *J. Biol. Chem.,* **252,** 6076 (1977).

44. M. Kanai, A. Raz, and D. S. Goodman, *J. Clin. Invest.,* **47,** 2025 (1968).

45. C. C. F. Blake and S. J. Oatley, *Nature,* **268,** 115 (1977).

46. R. F. Steiner, J. Roth, and J. Robbins, *J. Biol. Chem.,* **241,** 560 (1966).

47. M. Tabachnick, *J. Biol. Chem.,* **242,** 1646 (1967).

48. C. S. Pittman, V. H. Read, J. B. Chambers, Jr., and H. Nakafuji, *J. Clin. Invest.,* **49,** 373 (1970).

49. I. J. Chopra, *J. Clin. Invest.,* **58,** 32 (1976).

50. L. Gavin, J. Castle, F. McMahon, P. Martin, M. Hammond, and R. R. Cavalieri, *J. Clin. Endocrinol. Metab.,* **44,** 733 (1977).

51. L. A. Gavin, M. E. Hammon, J. N. Castle, and R. R. Cavalieri, *J. Clin. Invest.,* **61,** 1276 (1978).

52. T. Sakurada, M. Rudolph, S. L. L. Fang, A. G. Vagenakis, L. E. Braverman, and S. H. Ingbar, *J. Clin. Endocrinol. Metab.,* **46,** 916 (1978).

53. B. Goslings, H. L. Schwartz, W. Dillman, M. I. Surks, and J. H. Oppenheimer, *Endocrinology,* **98,** 666 (1976).

54. C. S. Pittman, M. W. Buck, and J. B. Chambers, Jr., *J. Clin. Invest.,* **51,** 1759 (1972).

55. C. Niemann, *Fort. Chem. Org. Naturst.,* **7,** 167 (1950).

56. A. Szent-Györgyi, *Bioenergetics,* Academic, New York, 1957, pp. 24, 29, 112–114.

57. D. E. Green, *Advan. Enzymol.,* **1,** 177 (1941).

58. F. L. Hoch and F. L. Lipman, *Proc. Natl. Acad. Sci. U.S.,* **40,** 909 (1954).

59. D. F. Tapley, *J. Biol. Chem.,* **222,** 325 (1956).

60. F. Ismail-Beigi and I. S. Edelman, *J. Gen. Physiol.,* **57,** 710 (1971).

61. Y. P. Lee, A. E. Takemori, and H. Lardy, *J. Biol. Chem.,* **234,** 3051 (1959).

62. J. H. Oppenheimer, D. Koerner, H. J. Schwartz, and M. I. Surks, *J. Clin. Endocrinol. Metab.,* **35,** 330 (1972).

63. M. I. Surks, D. Koerner, W. Dillman, and J. H. Oppenheimer, *J. Biol. Chem.,* **248,** 7066 (1973).

64. J. H. Oppenheimer, H. L. Schwartz, and M. I. Surks, *Endocrinology,* **95,** 897 (1974).

65. H. H. Samuels, J. S. Tsai, J. Casanova, and F. Stanley, *J. Clin. Invest.,* **54,** 853 (1974).

66. K. R. Latham, J. Ring, and J. D. Baxter, *J. Biol. Chem.,* **251,** 7388 (1976).

67. D. Koerner, H. L. Schwartz, M. I. Surks, J. H. Oppenheimer, and E. C. Jorgensen, *J. Biol. Chem.,* **250,** 6417 (1975).

68. E. C. Jorgensen, M. B. Bolger, and S. W. Dietrich, "Thyroid Hormone Analogs: Correlations Between Structure Nuclear Binding and Hormonal Activity," in *Proceedings of the Fifth International Congress of Endocrinology, Hamburg, July, 1976,* Vol. 1, V. H. T. James, Ed., Excerpta Medica, Amsterdam, 1977.

69. B. J. Spindler, K. M. MacLeod, J. Ring, and J. D. Baxter, *J. Biol. Chem.,* **250,** 4113 (1975).

70. J. Tata and C. C. Widnell, *Biochem. J.,* **98,** 604 (1966).

71. J. R. Tata, *Nature,* **257,** 18 (1975).

72. K. Sterling and P. O. Milch, *Proc. Natl. Acad. Sci U.S.,* **72,** 3225 (1975).

73. K. Sterling, P. O. Milch, M. A. Brenner, and J. H. Lazarus, *Science*, **197**, 996 (1977).

74. I. D. Goldfine, C. G. Simons, G. J. Smith, and S. H. Ingbar, *Endocrinology*, **96**, 1030 (1975).

75. V. Cody, J. Hazel, D. A. Langs, and W. L. Duax, *J. Med. Chem.*, **20**, 1628 (1977).

76. A. Camerman and N. Camerman, *Acta Crystallogr.*, **B30**, 1832 (1974).

77. V. Cody, *J. Am. Chem. Soc.*, **96**, 6720 (1974).

78. N. Camerman, J. K. Fawcett, and A. Camerman, "Conformational Studies of Thryoid Hormones and Analogues," in *Molecular and Quantum Pharmacology*, E. D. Bergmann and B. Pullman, Eds., D. Reidel, Dordrecht, Holland, 1974, p. 413.

79. P. A. Kollman, W. J. Murray, M. E. Nuss, E. C. Jorgensen, and S. Rothenberg, *J. Am. Chem. Soc.*, **95**, 8518 (1973).

80. J. C. Emmett and E. S. Pepper, *Nature*, **257**, 334 (1975).

81. IUPAC-IUB Commission on Biochemical Nomenclature, *Biochem. J.*, **121**, 577 (1971).

82. V. Cody, W. L. Duax, and H. Hauptmann, *Int. J. Protein Res.*, **5**, 297 (1973).

83. S. W. Dietrich, E. C. Jorgensen, P. A. Kollman, and S. Rothenberg, *J. Am. Chem. Soc.*, **98**, 8310 (1976).

84. N. Zenker and E. C. Jorgensen, *J. Am. Chem. Soc.*, **81**, 4643 (1959).

85. V. Cody, and W. L. Duax, *Biochem. Biophys. Res. Commun.*, **52**, 430 (1973).

86. V. Cody, *J. Med. Chem.*, **18**, 126 (1975).

87. J. K. Fawcett, N. Camerman, and A. Camerman, *J. Am. Chem. Soc.*, **98**, 587 (1976).

88. V. Cody and W. L. Duax, *Science*, **181**, 758 (1973).

89. M. V. Mussett and R. Pitt-Rivers, *Metab. Clin. Exp.*, **6**, 18 (1957).

90. T. C. Bruice, R. J. Winzler, and N. Kharasch, *J. Biol. Chem.*, **210**, 1 (1954).

91. A. Wahlborg, C. Bright, and E. Frieden, *Endocrinology*, **75**, 561 (1964).

92. E. Frieden and G. W. Westmark, *Science*, **133**, 1487 (1961).

93. S. B. Barker, M. Shimada, and M. Makiuchi, *Endocrinology*, **76**, 115 (1965).

94. K. G. Hermann, C. C. Lee, and R. Parker, *Arch. Int. Pharmacodyn. Ther.*, **83**, 284 (1961).

95. J. F. Van Pilsum, M. Carlson, J. R. Boen, D. Taylor, and B. Zakis, *Endocrinology*, **87**, 1237 (1970).

96. W. W. Westerfield, D. A. Richert, and W. R. Ruegamer, *Endocrinology*, **77**, 802 (1965).

97. Y.-L. Hao and M. Tabachnick, *Endocrinology*, **88**, 81 (1971).

98. R. A. Pages, J. Robbins, and H. Edelhoch, *Biochemistry*, **12**, 2773 (1973).

99. K. Sterling, *J. Clin. Invest.*, **43**, 1721 (1964).

100. S.-Y. Cheng, R. A. Pages, H. A. Saroff, H. Edelhoch, and J. Robbins, *Biochemistry*, **16**, 3707 (1977).

101. E. C. Jorgensen, "Thyroid Hormones and Analogs. I. Synthesis, Physical Properties and Theoretical Calculations," in *Hormonal Proteins and Peptides*, Vol. 6, *Thyroid Hormones*, C. H. Li, Ed., Academic, New York, 1978.

102. H. A. Selenkow and S. P. Asper, Jr., *Physiol. Rev.*, **35**, 426 (1955).

103. C. S. Pittman and J. A. Pittman, in *Handbook of Physiology*, Section 7: *Endocrinology*, Vol. 3, R. O. Greep and E. B. Astwood, Eds., *Thyroid*, American Physiological Society, Washington, D.C., 1974, p. 233.

104. E. C. Jorgensen, *Pharm. Ther. B*, **2**, 661 (1976).

105. E. C. Jorgensen, "Thyroid Hormones and Analogs. II. Structure-Activity Relationships," in *Hormonal Proteins and Peptides*, Vol. 6, *Thyroid Hormones*, C. H. Li, Ed., Academic, New York, 1978, p. 108.

106. E. C. Jorgensen and P. A. Lehman, *J. Org. Chem.*, **26**, 894 (1961).

107. H. Ashley, P. Katti, and E. Frieden, *Dev. Biol.*, **17**, 293 (1968).

108. G. S. Boyd and M. F. Oliver, *J. Endocrinol.*, **21**, 33 (1960).

109. B. Blank, E. G. Rice, F. R. Pfeiffer, and C. M. Greenberg, *J. Med. Chem.*, **9**, 10 (1966).

110. R. A. Pages and A. Burger, *J. Med. Chem.*, **10**, 435 (1967).

111. E. C. Jorgensen and J. A. W. Reid, *J. Med. Chem.*, **7**, 701 (1964).

112. R. E. Taylor, Jr., T. Tu, S. B. Barker, and E. C. Jorgensen, *Endocrinology*, **80**, 1143 (1967).

113. J. A. Pittman, R. J. Beschi, P. Block, Jr., and R. H. Lindsay, *Endocrinology*, **93**, 201 (1973).

114. E. C. Jorgensen, W. J. Murray, and P. Block Jr., *J. Med. Chem.*, **17**, 434 (1974).

115. E. Frieden and K. Yoshizato, *Endocrinology*, **95**, 188 (1974).

116. E. I. Tamagna, J. M. Hershman, and E. C. Jorgensen, *J. Clin. Endocrinol. Metab.*, **48**, 196 (1979).

117. F. Comite, G. N. Burrow, and E. C. Jorgensen, *Endocrinology*, **102**, 1670 (1978).

118. B. M. Kriz, A. L. Jones, and E. C. Jorgensen, *Endocrinology*, **102**, 712 (1978).

119. M. C. Benson, J. P. Liu, Y. P. Huang, A. Burger, and R. S. Rivlin, *Endocrinology*, **102,** 562 (1978).

120. P. L. Ballard, A. Brehier, B. J. Benson, B. M. Kriz, and E. C. Jorgensen, *Pediatr. Res.,* **12,** 1164 (1978).

121. H. A. Selenkow, C. A. Plamondon, J. G. Wiswell, and S. P. Asper, Jr., *Bull. Johns Hopkins Hosp.,* **102,** 94 (1958).

122. E. C. Jorgensen and R. A. Wiley, *J. Med. Chem.,* **6,** 459 (1963).

123. E. C. Jorgensen, R. O. Muhlhauser, and R. A. Wiley, *J. Med. Chem.,* **12,** 689 (1969).

124. C. R. Harington, *Biochem. J.,* **43,** 434 (1948).

125. R. C. Cookson, *J. Chem. Soc.,* **1953,** 643.

126. E. Van Heyningen, *J. Org. Chem.,* **26,** 5005 (1961).

127. R. Mukherjee and P. Block, Jr., *J. Chem. Soc.,* (C) **1971,** 1596.

128. E. C. Jorgensen, *Mayo Clin. Proc.,* **39,** 560 (1964).

129. S. B. Barker and M. Shimada, *Mayo Clin. Proc.,* **39,** 609 (1964).

130. E. C. Jorgensen and P. A. Berteau, *J. Med. Chem.,* **14,** 1199 (1971).

131. T. C. Bruice, N. Kharasch, and R. J. Winzler, *Arch. Biochem. Biophys.,* **62,** 305 (1956).

132. C. Hansch and T. Fujita, *J. Am. Chem. Soc.,* **86,** 1616 (1964).

133. E. C. Jorgensen, S. W. Dietrich, D. Koerner, M. I. Surks, and J. H. Oppenheimer, *Proc. West. Pharmacol. Soc.,* **18,** 389 (1975).

134. H. Kubinyi, *J. Med. Chem.,* **19,** 587 (1976).

135. H. Kubinyi and O.-H. Kehrhahn, *J. Med. Chem.,* **19,** 578 (1976).

136. S. W. Dietrich, M. B. Bolger, P. A. Kollman, and E. C. Jorgensen, *J. Med. Chem.,* **20,** 863 (1977).

137. S. M. Snyder, R. R. Cavalieri, I. D. Goldfine, S. H. Ingbar, and E. C. Jorgensen, *J. Biol. Chem.,* **251,** 6489 (1976).

138. C. L. Gemmill, *Arch. Biochem. Biophys.,* **54,** 359 (1955).

139. G. C. Schussler, *Science,* **178,** 172 (1972).

140. T. Andrea, Ph.D. dissertation, University of California, San Francisco, 1977.

141. S.-Y. Cheng, H. J. Cahnmann, M. Wilchek, and R. N. Ferguson, *Biochemistry,* **14,** 4132 (1975).

142. M. Tabachnick and N. A. Giorgio, Jr., *Arch. Biochem. Biophys.,* **105,** 563 (1964).

143. M. Tabachnick, F. J. Downs, and N. A. Giorgio, Jr., *Arch. Biochem. Biophys.,* **136,** 467 (1970).

144. C. Hansch, A. Leo, S. H. Unger, K. H. Kim, D. Nitaitani, and E. J. Lien, *J. Med. Chem.,* **16,** 1207 (1973).

145. T. Yamada, A. Kijihara, Y. Takemura, and T. Onaya, "Antithyroid Compounds," in *Handbook of Physiology,* Section 7: *Endocrinology,* Vol. 3, *Thyroid,* R. O. Greep and E. B. Astwood, Eds., American Physiological Society, Washington, D.C., 1974, p. 345.

146. P. Langer and M. A. Greer, *Antithyroid Substances and Naturally Occurring Goitrogens,* S. Karger, A. G., Basel, 1977.

147. W. L. Green, "Mechanisms of Action of Antithyroid Compounds," in *The Thyroid,* S. C. Werner and S. H. Ingbar, Eds., Harper and Row, Hagerstown, M., 1978, p. 77.

148. D. H. Solomon, "Antithyroid Drugs," in *The Thyroid,* S. C. Werner and S. H. Ingbar, Eds., Harper and Row, Hagerstown, M., 1978, p. 814.

149. P. Bourdoux, F. Delange, M. Gerard, M. Mafuta, A. Hanson, and E. M. Ermans, *J. Clin. Endocrinol. Metab.,* **46,** 613 (1978).

150. F. Delange, R. Vigneri, F. Trimarchi, S. Filetti, V. Pezzino, P. Polosa, and E. M. Ermans, *Ann. Endocrinol.* (Paris), **38,** 80A (1977).

151. A. Taurog, *Endocrinology,* **98,** 1031 (1976).

152. E. B. Astwood, M. A. Greer, and M. G. Ettlinger, *J. Biol. Chem.,* **181,** 121 (1949).

153. A. Kjaer, B. W. Christensen, and S. E. Hansen, *Acta Chem Scand.,* **13,** 144 (1959).

154. M. A. Greer, *Recent Progr. Horm. Res.,* **18,** 187 (1962).

155. J. B. MacKenzie, C. G. MacKenzie, and E. V. McCollum, *Science,* **94,** 518 (1941).

156. S. C. Berens, R. S. Bernstein, J. Robbins, and J. Wolff, *J. Clin. Invest.,* **49,** 1357 (1970).

157. R. Templer, M. Berman, J. Robbins, and J. Wolff, *J. Clin. Invest.,* **51,** 2746 (1972).

158. J. H. Oppenheimer, H. L. Schwartz, and M. I. Surks, *J. Clin. Invest.,* **51,** 2493 (1972).

159. F. Escobar del Rey and G. Morreale de Escobar, *Acta Endocrinol.,* **40,** 1 (1962).

160. S. B. Barker, C. S. Pittman, J. A. Pittman, Jr., and S. R. Hill, Jr., *Ann. N.Y. Acad Sci.,* **86,** 545 (1960).

161. F. C. Larson and E. C. Albright, *J. Clin. Invest.,* **40,** 1132 (1961).

162. R. G. Shanks, D. R. Hadden, D. C. Lowe, D. G. McDevitt, and D. A. D. Montgomery, *Lancet,* **1969-I,** 993.

163. A. I. Vinik, B. L. Pimstone, and R. Hoffenberg, *J. Clin. Endocrinol. Metab.,* **28,** 725 (1968).

164. J. F. Mackin, J. J. Canary, and C. S. Pittman, *New Engl. J. Med.,* **291,** 1396 (1974).

CHAPTER FORTY

Diuretic and Uricosuric Agents

LINCOLN H. WERNER

Pharmaceuticals Division
CIBA-GEIGY Corporation
Summit, New Jersey 07901, USA

CONTENTS

1   INTRODUCTION

Diuretics are generally defined as drugs that increase the flow of urine; uricosuric agents are drugs that enhance the excretion of uric acid. Recently compounds have been found that combine both properties, however, diuretics may cause uric acid retention and uricosuric agents may be devoid of diuretic activity.

Diuretic drugs represent a major and indispensable group of therapeutic agents. In 1976 diuretics represented 4.3% of all ethical drugs prescribed. The diuretic effect of certain compounds has been known for many years; actually Paracelsus adminis-

tered calomel (mercurous chloride) as a diuretic in the sixteenth century. Numerous safe and effective diuretics have been developed in the past 30 years encompassing compounds of widely differing structures.

2   RENAL PHYSIOLOGY AND PHARMACOLOGY

2.1   Renal Physiology (1, 2)

It is generally accepted that diuretics exert their effect mainly in the kidneys. These two organs, responsible for the regulation of body fluids in man, weigh together about 300 g and directly control the volume of extracellular fluid and indirectly also affect the intracellular fluid. This regulatory function is fulfilled so successfully that over a wide range of water and solute intake the composition of fluids in the body is held remarkably stable. The unit of structure and function in the kidney is the nephron; each kidney contains between 1 and 2 million such units with its associated blood supply. Urine is formed in the nephrons and total renal function can be considered as a summation of all of these units. A nephron (Fig. 40.1) is composed of two major sections, a glomerulus and a tubule. The tubule begins at the glomerulus, undergoes several convolutions, then straightens out and descends in a straight line toward the medulla. The convoluted tubule and the first part of the descending tubule constitute the proximal tubule. The walls of the tubule in the lower descending portion become exceedingly thin. This is the thin segment of the loop of Henle. After a sharp hairpin turn, the tubule travels back to its glomerulus. Along this ascending limb the walls thicken again, forming the thick segment of the ascending limb of Henle (TALH). The tubule, now called the distal tubule, undergoes several more convolutions and then empties into the system of collecting ducts. These ducts travel in

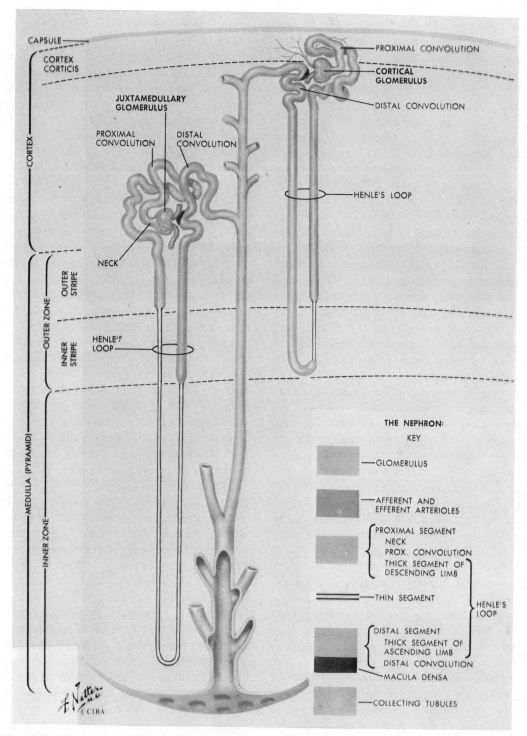

Fig. 40.1 The nephron. Copyright © 1973 by CIBA Pharmaceutical Company, Division of CIBA–GEIGY Corporation. Reproduced with permission from The CIBA Collection of Medical Illustrations by Frank H. Netter, M.D. All rights reserved.

straight lines through the medulla, accepting fluid from several nephrons, coalesce, and then enter the renal papillae. Nephrons with glomerula in the upper part of the cortex have a somewhat different structure, as can be seen in Fig. 40.1. The quantity of blood entering the kidney every minute represents $\frac{1}{4}-\frac{1}{5}$ of the resting cardiac output and corresponds to 1–1.5 l of blood per minute. This is equivalent to an average renal blood plasma flow of 600–655 ml/min.

Two roles are played by the blood that enters the kidney: it must supply oxygen and metabolites to enable the kidney to function and it must also supply the water and solute material that the kidney processes. The main activity of the kidney is to transport solute materials and water across tubular cells, either from the bloodstream into the lumen of the tubule (secretion) or from the tubule into the peritubular capillaries (reabsorption). The transport of most physiologically important solutes is active; this requires a pump and a relatively impermeable membrane that will prevent rapid diffusion of material back to the site from which it came. As the blood flows through the glomerular capillaries about $\frac{1}{5}$ of the plasma water (an average of 118–127 ml/min passes through the membranes of the capillaries and of the glomerulus to enter the proximal portion of the renal tubule. The blood remaining in the vascular system perfuses the tubules via the peritubular arteries. The plasma water removed from the blood by glomerular filtration is called the glomerular filtrate. It is an ultrafiltrate and normally contains no erythrocytes and little or no plasma protein. Other molecules which are in true solution pass freely through the glomerular membranes, e.g., glucose, amino acids, urea, and major ions, and appear in the glomerular filtrate in about the same concentration as in plasma.

In Fig. 40.2 a schematic representation of salt and water transport along the nephron is shown (3). Under normal circumstances 50–60% of salt and water reabsorption occurs in the proximal tubule. The proximal tubule reabsorbs physiologically important solutes and secretes organic substances that are destined for excretion. The filtered glucose and amino acids are reabsorbed, as are most of the filtered Na^+, HCO_3^+, and phosphate ions. As solutes are removed by active transport processes, resulting in an osmotic gradient, reabsorption of water also occurs. The reabsorption of HCO_3^+, which depends on intracellular carbonic anhydrase, leads to a corresponding increase in chloride concentration in the tubular fluid. Since much of the water and solute contained in the glomerular filtrate are reabsorbed in the proximal tubule, the flow rate of the tubular fluid in the distal tubule is relatively small. Thus normally about 40% of the glomerular filtrate, still isoosmotic to plasma but with major changes in composition, enters the thin descending limb of Henle's loop. It has been show that the thin descending limb of Henle lacks active sodium chloride transport and has low permeability to sodium and high osmotic permeability to water (4). These properties enable the descending limb to play an important passive role in the countercurrent system by allowing water removal and osmotic equilibration with the hypertonic interstitium. Hypertonic fluid, mostly due to sodium chloride, thus enters the thin ascending limb of Henle. This thin ascending limb is relatively impermeable to water, highly permeable to sodium and chloride, and less permeable to urea. Sodium chloride appears to be passively reabsorbed in this segment; thus the absolute quantity and concentration of sodium chloride gradually decreases as the fluid enters the thick ascending limb of Henle. It now appears that the thick ascending limb actively reabsorbs sodium chloride by active chloride reabsorption

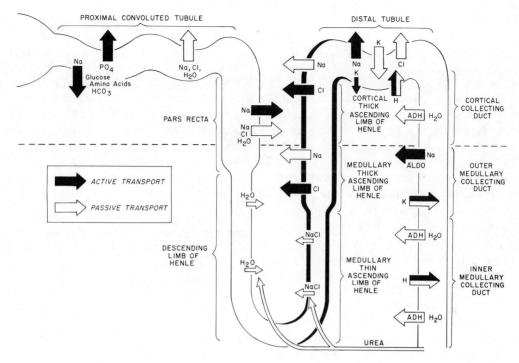

Fig. 40.2   Major transport processes influencing net transport of solute and/or water out of various nephron segments. Reproduced with permission from H. R. Jacobson and J. P. Kokko, *Ann. Rev. Pharmacol. Toxicol.*, **16,** 201 (1976). Copyright © 1976 by Annual Reviews Inc. All rights reserved.

(5, 6). It is relatively impermeable to water even in the presence of antidiuretic hormone (ADH). As a consequence of active chloride reabsorption with subsequent passive sodium reabsorption combined with water impermeability, the thick ascending limb can complete two most important functions. It generates hypotonic luminal fluid that moves into the distal convoluted tubule and adds osmotically active sodium chloride to the medullary interstitium. The medullary section is the active force behind the generation of the sodium chloride component of the hypertonic medullary interstitium; owing to its water impermeability and active transport of sodium chloride, the cortical portion is the main diluting segment of the nephron.

The distal convoluted tubule actively reabsorbs sodium; potassium secretion in this segment is essentially passive. Although under normal circumstances potassium is secreted in mammalian distal tubules, this segment also appears to be able to actively reabsorb potassium under conditions of potassium depletion (7). Recent *in vitro* microperfusion experiments suggest that the distal tubule is impermeable to water even in the presence of ADH (8).

The fluid leaves the distal tubule and enters the collecting duct system. This segment also has been shown to actively reabsorb sodium dependent on the presence of the mineral corticoid aldosterone (8). Potassium secretion appears to depend on the same passive driving forces as in the distal tubule (9–11). In the absence of

ADH the collecting ducts are impermeable to water, but in its presence they are the important segments responsible for free water reabsorption and final concentration of the urine (8, 12–14).

The papillary portion of the collecting duct is important for the recirculation of urea. It appears to be the only segment distal to the thin ascending limb with any degree of permeability to urea. Thus urea can diffuse out of the papillary portion of the collecting duct into the interstitium and the thin ascending limb. It is thus kept in the papillary interstitium where it can exert its osmotic effect.

The human kidney can produce urine that is 4-5 times more concentrated or 7–10 times less concentrated than blood as measured by its osmolality (2). In a normal adult with a glomerular filtration rate of 125 ml/min, 180 l of filtrate containing 25,000 meq of sodium is formed daily. Under normal conditions only 1–2 l of urine containing approximately 100 meq. of sodium is voided; this means that more than 99% of the filtered sodium is reabsorbed and that only a small reduction in the amount of reabsorbed sodium and water need be made to induce a considerable diuresis.

2.2 Renal Pharmacology

2.2.1 CLASSES OF DIURETIC SUBSTANCES. The most important classes of diuretics are those that act by inhibition of renal tubular transport mechanisms. These include organomercurials, xanthines, pyrimidines, triazines, carbonic anhydrase inhibitors, aromatic sulfonamides, thiazides and related sulfonamide derivatives, aldosterone antagonists, acylphenoxyacetic acids and related compounds, pteridines, and pyrazines. In an alternate classification (5), certain members of the class of aromatic sulfonamides and the acylphenoxyacetic acid derivatives have been grouped together as high ceiling diuretics. This term describes a group of highly potent drugs with relatively steep dose response relationships and includes agents such as furosemide and ethacrynic acid. Steroidal aldosterone antagonists, pteridines, and pyrazines have been grouped together as potassium-sparing diuretics. This group includes spironolactone, triamterene, and amiloride. Other classes of diuretics of less interest are the osmotic diuretics and the acid-forming salts.

2.2.2 PHARMACOLOGICAL EVALUATION OF DIURETICS. The following three statements or generalizations are direct quotes from a paper by K. H. Beyer (16) and refer to the pharmacological evaluation of new drugs in general and to diuretics in particular:

The more closely one can approximate under controlled laboratory conditions the physiological correlates of clinically defined disease, the more likely one will be able to modulate it effectively.

In vitro experiments are apt to be inadequate and hence misleading when employed solely to anticipate the physiological correlates of complex clinical situations.

Often aberrations in function we call toxicity, relate more to changes a compound induces physiologically than to a direct, inherent, destructive effect of the agent, per se, on tissues.

Newer testing procedures have been designed with these generalizations in mind. Diuretics are generally evaluated in two species, the rat and the dog. The rat is used, as a rule, in initial screening for convenience and economy. However, many compounds exhibit diuretic activity in the rat, e.g., antihistamines such as tripelennamine, but are inactive in the dog and in man. On the other hand, mercurial diuretics and ethacrynic acid are inactive in the rat; furosemide exhibits diuretic activity in the rat only at doses several times higher than those effective in the dog. Various modifications of the experimental procedure of Lipschitz et al. (17) are frequently used. Lipschitz measured urine volumes following administration of the drug to saline loaded rats and compared the response to that obtained with a standard. i.e., urea. More recent modifications (18) measure urine volume, Na^+, K^+, and Cl^- excretion; e.g., male rats, fasted for 18 h, are given 5 ml of 0.2% NaCl solution/100 g body weight by stomach tube. The diuretic drugs are given by stomach tube at the time of fluid loading. The rats are placed in metabolism cages and urine volumes measured at 30 min intervals over a 3 hr period. Total amounts of Na^+ and K^+ excreted over the 3 hr period are determined by flame photometry; chloride can be determined in the Technicon Autoanalyzer using Skegg's modification of Zall's method (19).

The diuretic activity in dogs has been evaluated according to one procedure (20) as follows: at the start of each experiment, six carefully selected mongrel dogs are given the drug by capsule followed immediately by a subcutaneous injection of 100 ml of 0.9% saline. The urinary bladder is emptied by catheterization at the onset and at 2, 4, and 6 hr after administration of the test compound. The dogs are kept in metabolism cages and urine volume measured; urine aliquots are analyzed for Na^+, K^+, and Cl^- content as described for the rat assay procedure. The colony of dogs is used repeatedly and only for diuretic tests. A control test with placebo is given prior to each test run.

Results obtained with diuretic agents in dogs are more predictive of the response in man than those obtained in the rat.

A number of standard diuretics have also been tested in the mouse (64). In this animal, ethyacrynic acid is a potent diuretic in contrast to the very low diuretic activity seen with this compound in the rat.

The chimpanzee (21) has also been used to evaluate certain diuretics. In this animal, the effect of the compound on uric acid excretion can also be studied, because these great apes, like man, are devoid of hepatic uricase and therefore maintain a relatively high level of circulating serum urate (22).

The evaluation of a new diuretic requires more than an assessment of its ability to increase salt and water excretion; its effect on potassium excretion, uric acid blood levels, and blood glucose levels should also be considered. The effect of a diuretic on Na^+, K^+, Cl^-, and water excretion can be studied readily in rats and dogs. The effect on uric acid blood levels cannot be determined in these animals because uric acid is rapidly metabolized by hepatic uricase in all mammals except the primates and man. Chimpanzees have been used in the study of uricosuric agents (21) but tests with such large animals obviously present numerous problems. Attempts have also been made to block the enzyme uricase in rats by administering potassium oxonate and thus to obtain higher serum uric acid levels (23).

Considerable evidence is available that demonstrates the tendency of certain benzothiadiazine diuretics to elevate blood glucose values in seemingly normal, as well as diabetic or prediabetic, individuals (24). A method using high doses of the compounds injected intraperitoneally into rats and determining blood glucose levels as compared to control values has been used to estimate a possible hyperglycemic effect of diuretics (25).

2.2.3 CLINICAL ASPECTS OF DIURETICS. In a healthy human subject, changes in dietary intake or variations in the extrarenal loss of fluid and electrolytes are followed relatively rapidly by adjustments in the rate of renal excretion, thus maintaining the normal volume and composition of extracellular fluid in the body. Edema is an increase in extracellular fluid volume. In almost every case of edema encountered in clinical medicine, the underlying abnormality involves a decreased rate of renal excretion.

One of the factors influencing the normal relationship between the volumes of interstitial fluid and the circulating plasma is the pressure within the small blood vessels. In diseases of hepatic origin, e.g., cirrhosis, the pressure relationships are disturbed primarily within the portal circulation and ascites results. In congestive heart failure pressure–flow relationships may be disturbed more in the pulmonary or systemic circulation and edema may be localized accordingly.

There is overwhelming evidence to indicate that the primary disturbance of the kidney is in its ability to regulate sodium excretion which underlies the pathogenesis of edema. Three approaches are available when edema fluid accumulates owing to excessive reabsorption of sodium and other electrolytes by the renal tubules. First, one can attempt to correct the primary disease if possible: second one can reduce renal reabsorption of electrolytes by the use of drugs; and third, one can restrict sodium intake to a level that corresponds to the diminished renal capacity for sodium excretion. Cardiac decompensation is one of the most common causes of edema. Treatment consists of full digitalization which should be considered the primary therapeutic agent. Diuretic drugs must be considered to have a secondary though very important role, for it has been shown that by blocking excessive electrolyte reabsorption in the renal tubule not only are the symptoms of cardiac failure alleviated, but also an improvement in cardiac function is observed. Chronic administration of sulfonamide diuretics, because of their variable kaluretic effect, may lead to hypokalemia. To minimize this effect, combinations with potassium-sparing diuretics are frequently used. Dietary potassium supplements may also be prescribed.

The use of highly potent diuretics can lead to complications resulting from fluid and electrolyte imbalance due to excessively rapid mobilization of edema fluid and intense diuresis. Discussion of these conditions is beyond the scope of this chapter.

Diuretics are also used in the treatment of hypertension. This aspect is discussed in Chapter 42. Currently used and more thoroughly studied diuretic agents are listed in Tables 40.1 to 40.24.

3 OSMOTIC DIURETICS

Mannitol (Table 40.1, 40.2) is the prototype of the osmotic diuretics and has been studied most extensively. The compound is poorly absorbed following oral administration and is therefore administered by intravenous infusion. It is freely filtered at the glomerulus and tubular reabsorption is quite limited. The usual diuretic dose is 50–100 g given as a 25% solution. The glomerular filtrate is isosmotic with plasma, and normally sodium and the accompanying anion represent almost the entire osmotically active solute in the tubules. In the presence of mannitol the proximal tubular fluid remains isosomotic with plasma and the concentration of sodium is lowered. Normally, about 60–70% of the proximal tubular fluid is reabsorbed owing to the active reabsorption of sodium and the passive diffusion of water. When sodium is replaced by a nonreabsorbable substance, such as mannitol, the tubule is unable to reabsorb the remaining small amount of sodium. An increased load of mannitol, unreabsorbable sodium, and an osmotically equivalent amount of fluid are delivered to the distal tubule and collecting ducts, which are unable to reabsorb the excess water. From recent studies (26, 27) it would appear that mannitol and similar osmotic diuretic agents have multiple sites and mechanisms of action; their major component probably is a decrease in medullary solute content resulting in less water reabsorption from the thin descending loop of Henle and collecting duct and less NaCl reabsorption in the ascending limb of Henle.

One of the most important indications for the use of mannitol is the prophylaxis of acute renal failure. Following cardiovascular operations or severe traumatic injury,

Table 40.1 Osmotic Diuretics

No.	Generic Name	Trade Name	Structure
40.1	Ammonium chloride		NH_4Cl
40.2	Mannitol USP		$HOCH_2\overset{\overset{H}{\underset{}{|}}}{\underset{\underset{O}{|}}{\underset{H}{}}}C$ ... CH_2OH
40.3	Urea	Ureaphil, Urevert	NH_2CONH_2

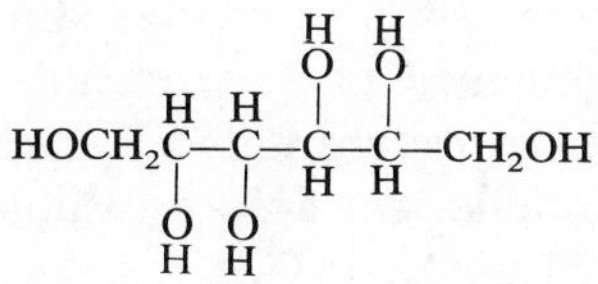

for instance, a precipitous fall in urine flow may be anticipated. Administered mannitol, under such conditions, exerts an osmotic effect within the tubular fluid inhibiting water reabsorption. A reasonable flow of urine can thus be maintained and the kidney protected from damage.

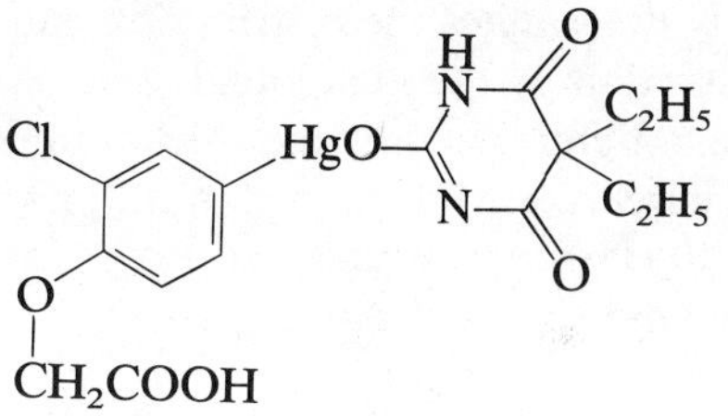

40.4

4 MERCURIAL DIURETICS

For a period of approximately 30 years, mercurial diuretics were the most important diuretic agents. Since the introduction of orally active, potent, nonmercurial diuretics, beginning in 1950 with acetazolamide, their use has greatly declined. Today they represent only a small fraction of the injectable diuretics used, and injectable diuretics in turn are only a small portion of the total diuretic market.

4.1 Historical

Calomel was used by Paracelsus in the sixteenth century as a diuretic and again as an ingredient of the famous Guy's Hospital pill (calomel, squill, and digitalis) in the nineteenth century. Calomel exerted a cathartic effect and its absorption from the intestine was unpredictable. In 1919 Vogl (28) discovered the diuretic effect of merbaphen (40.4) following parenteral administration of this antisyphilitic agent. General use of the drug as a diuretic was

short-lived because of its toxicity. It did, however, lead to the synthesis of a large number of organomercurials between 1920 and 1950.

4.2 Structure–Activity Relationships

The active form of mercurial diuretics has been a controversial subject. Evidence now suggests that the diuretic response is due to the release of mercuric ion in the kidney, by rupture of the carbon–mercury bond (29–31). With the drugs commonly employed this occurs in only a small fraction of the dose administered. Most mercurial diuretics have the general structure 40.5, in which Y is usually CH_3 and R is a complex organic moiety, usually incorporating an amide function or a urea grouping. All diuretic organic mercurials thus

$$R—CH_2—CH—CH_2HgX$$
$$|$$
$$OY$$

40.5

$$R—CH_2CH_2Hg^+$$

40.**6**

far examined are acid-labile *in vitro*. The rupture of the carbon mercury bond is catalyzed by thiols. It is interesting to note that compounds of the related structure 40.**6** with an unsubstituted β-carbon atom are acid stable and do not exhibit diuretic activity. Formula 40.**7** shows the structure characteristic of a mercurial diuretic. The more important mercurial diuretics are shown in Table 40.2. The R substituent largely determines the distribution and rate of excretion of the compound. The Y substituent, determined by the solvent in which the mercuration is carried out, generally has little effect on the properties of the compound (32, 33). Among others, Y substituents such as H, CH_3, CH_2CH_2OH, and $CH_2CH_2OCH_3$ have been studied.

The nature of the X substituent affects the toxicity of the compound, irritation at the site of injection, and rate of absorption (32, 33). Theophylline has been used commonly as an X substituent (34). When X is a thiol such as mercaptoacetic acid or thiosorbitol, cardiac toxicity and local irritation are reduced (35, 36). Diglucomethoxane (Mersoben®) (43), 40.**12**, should perhaps be cited as a well tolerated, potent mercurial diuretic that does not conform to the general structure 40.**7**. Generally, mercurial diuretics are administered parenterally; chlormerodrin (Table 40.2, 40.**8**), which lacks a carboxylic acid group, is orally effective but gastric irritation precludes its widespread use (37).

$$
\begin{array}{ccc}
CH_2—CONHCONH\!-\!CH_2CH—CH_2Hg—\text{theophylline} \\
CH_2—COOH \qquad\quad OCH_3 \\
R \qqu\qquad\qquad Y \qquad\qquad X
\end{array}
$$

40.**7**

Table 40.2 Mercurial Diuretics

No.	Generic Name	Trade Name	Structure
40.**8**	Chloromerodrin	Neohydrin	$NH_2CONH—CH_2CH—CH_2HgCl$ $\quad\quad\quad\quad\quad OCH_3$
40.**9**	Meralluride USP	Mercuhydrin	$HOOCCH_2CH_2CONHCONHCH_2CH—CH_2Hg—R$ $\quad\quad\quad\quad\quad\quad\quad\quad\quad OCH_3$ R = theophylline
40.**10**	Sodium mercaptomerin	Thiomerin	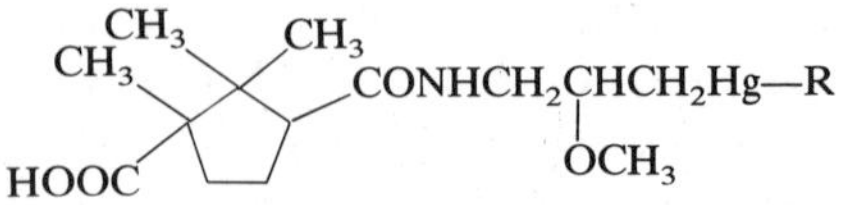 (structure) $CONHCH_2CHCH_2Hg—R$ OCH_3 R = SCH_2COONa
40.**11**	Mercurophylline NF XII	Mercupurin, Novurit	R = theophylline

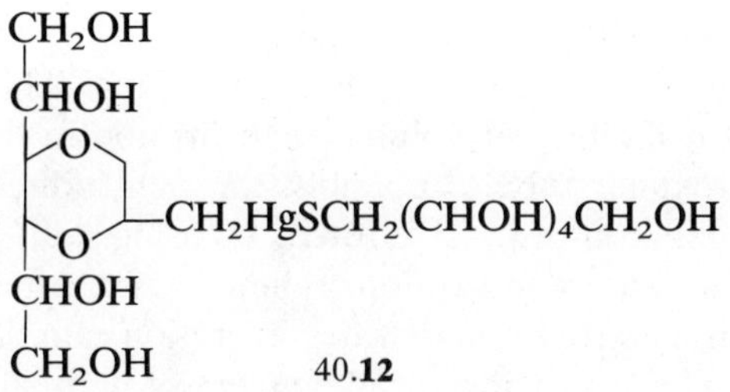

CH$_2$OH
|
CHOH

—O
| —CH$_2$HgSCH$_2$(CHOH)$_4$CH$_2$OH
—O

CHOH
|
CH$_2$OH   40.**12**

4.3 Pharmacology

Before the development of the loop diuretics, the organomercurials were the most potent diuretics abailable. Most recent studies have consistently found that the major effect of organomercurials appears to be in the ascending limb of Henle (38–40). During diuresis, the urine contains a high concentration of chloride anion matched by almost equivalent amounts of sodium (41). The effects of the mercurial diuretics on potassium excretion are complex. They depress the tubular secretion of potassium and for this reason the diuresis is accompanied by significantly less potassium loss than occurs with other diuretics that do not inhibit the secretory mechanism. However, mercurials can have a paradoxical effect in increasing slightly potassium excretion when initial excretory rates are low. Inhibition of organic acid secretion is seen in man but not in the dog. In the chimpanzee and to a lesser extent in man, mercurials, e.g., mersalyl, have an intense uricosuric action (42).

In summary, the organomercurials inhibit active chloride reabsorption in the thick ascending limb of Henle and under appropriate circumstances inhibit distal potassium secretion. The molecular basis of these effects and the precise role of pH on the degree of diuretic response are unresolved (3).

4.4 Clinical Application

Organomercurials are generally given intramuscularly. The usual dose is 1 ml solution corresponding to 40 mg Hg. In a responsive, edematous patient, an increase in urine flow is evident in 1–2 hr and may persist up to 12 hr. A loss of about 2.5% of body weight represents an average response (41).

5 CARBONIC ANHYDRASE INHIBITORS

Carbonic anhydrase, first identified in red blood cells, has subsequently been found in many sites, including the renal cortex, gastric mucosa, pancreas, eye, and central nervous system. This enzyme catalyzes the reversible hydration of carbon dioxide to carbonic acid:

$$CO_2 + H_2O \leftrightharpoons H_2CO_3 \leftrightharpoons H^+ + HCO_3^-$$

The noncatalyzed hydration or dehydration reaction can, of course, occur in the absence of the enzyme. However, the quantitative relationship between the two reaction rates depends on many factors. Normally the enzyme is present in tissues in high excess.

Hydrogen ion secretion takes place in the proximal tubule, the distal tubule, and the collecting duct. The driving force for H^+ secretion in the distal portions is the transtubular negative potential. In the proximal tubule H^+ is actively secreted in exchange for reabsorbed Na^+ (44). The source of the cellular hydrogen ions is the hydration of CO_2 within proximal tubular cells to produce cellular H^+ and HCO_3^-. The hydrogen ion is secreted into the tubular lumen and the reabsorbed Na^+ enters the peritubular blood as $NaHCO_3$. In the proximal tubule the secreted H^+ combines with HCO_3^- to form H_2CO_3, which is then dehydrated to $CO_2 + H_2O$. This reaction is catalyzed by the enzyme carbonic anhydrase located on the luminal border of proximal tubular cells (1). The carbon dioxide diffuses back into the cell, where it is again hydrated and used as the source of hydrogen ions to be secreted into the tubule (Fig. 40.3). The secreted hydrogen ions provide for the reabsorption of filtered bicarbonate ions and for the excretion of titratable acid and ammonium ions.

The administration of an inhibitor of carbonic anhydrase promptly leads to an increase in urine volume, the normally acidic urine becomes alkaline, and the urinary concentrations of HCO_3^-, Na^+, and K^+ increase. The concentration of chloride ion drops. In addition there is a fall in titratable acid and ammonium excretion. Recent studies (45, 46) have led to the conclusion that carbonic anhydrase inhibitors inhibit the enzyme via the intermediary step of adenyl cyclase stimulation (3). Carbonic anhydrase inhibitors cause a significant kaliuresis which can be attributed to passive forces in the distal tubule, i.e., increased lumen electronegativity and increased flow of luminal fluid.

In summary, inhibitors of carbonic anhydrase decrease bicarbonate reabsorption in the proximal tubule by decreasing the secretion of H^+ into the lumen. They also inhibit net volume reabsorption in the proximal tubule, possibly through indirect inhibition of passive forces favoring sodium chloride reabsorption. Their major effect on electrolyte and water excretion may be explained by increased delivery of nonreabsorbable $NaHCO_3$ to the thick ascending limb of Henle and the distal tubule.

5.1 History

Building on earlier work by Strauss and Southworth in 1937 (47), Mann and Keilin (48), and Davenport and Wilhelmi (49), Pitts and Alexander in 1945 (50) proposed that the normal acidification of the urine results from the secretion of hydrogen ions by tubular cells. They confirmed that in dogs sulfanilamide renders the urine alkaline, perhaps because of reduction of the availability of H^+ for secretion brought about by inhibition of the enzyme carbonic anhydrase. The resulting increase in Na^+ and HCO_3^- excretion suggested to Schwartz (51) the diuretic potential of sulfanilamide, which, however, was of no practical significance because of the very high doses required for diuresis.

5.2 Structure–Activity Relationships

Following the discovery of the carbonic anhydrase inhibitory activity of sulfanilamide, a variety of aromatic sulfonamides were found to exhibit the same type of activity (52). Aliphatic sulfonamides were much less active; substitution of the sulfonamide nitrogen in aromatic sulfonamides eliminated the activity. Roblin and co-workers (53, 54), stimulated by the work of Schwartz (51), decided to investigate a series of heterocyclic sulfonamides. Compounds that were up to 800 times more active *in vitro* than sulfanilamide as carbonic anhydrase inhibitors were found

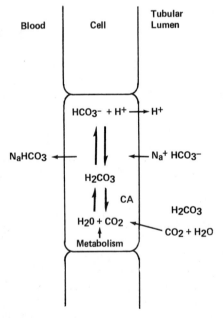

Fig. 40.3 Diagram of normal renal reabsorption of $NaHCO_3$ after Anderton and Kincaid-Smith (65a).

Table 40.3 Carbonic Anhydrase Inhibitors

No.	Generic Name	Trade Name	Structure	Ref.
40.**13**	Acetazolamide USP	Diamox	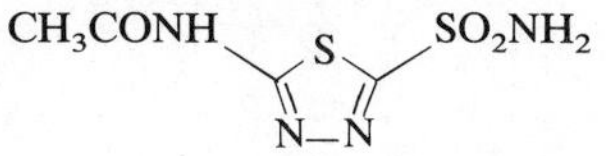 CH_3CONH—thiadiazole—SO_2NH_2	57
40.**14**	Dichlorphenamide USP	Daranide, Oratrol	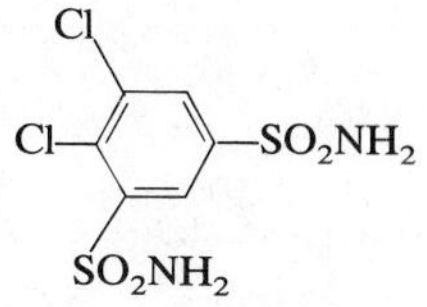 Cl, Cl—benzene—SO_2NH_2, SO_2NH_2	56
40.**15**	Ethoxzolamide USP	Cardrase, Ethamide	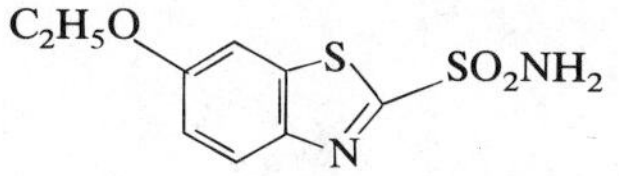 C_2H_5O—benzothiazole—SO_2NH_2	63
40.**16**	Methazolamide USP	Neptazane	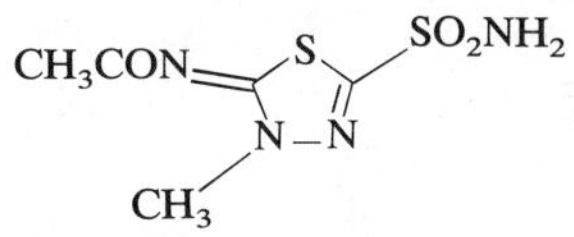 CH_3CON=thiadiazole—SO_2NH_2, CH_3	
40.**17**	Benzolamide		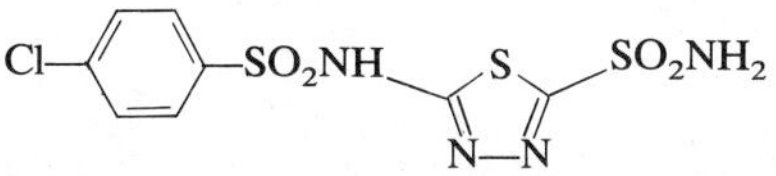 Cl—benzene—SO_2NH—thiadiazole—SO_2NH_2	61

(Table 40.3). An attempt to correlate pK_a values and *in vitro* carbonic anhydrase inhibitory activity in a series of closely related, 1,3,4-thiadiazole-2-sulfonamides (40.**18**) was not successful (55). The relationship between *in vitro* enzyme inhibition and *in vivo* diuretic potency is not very predictable owing to variation in drug distribution, binding, and metabolism (56) (Table 40.4), especially when different types of aromatic or heterocyclic sulfonamides are compared.

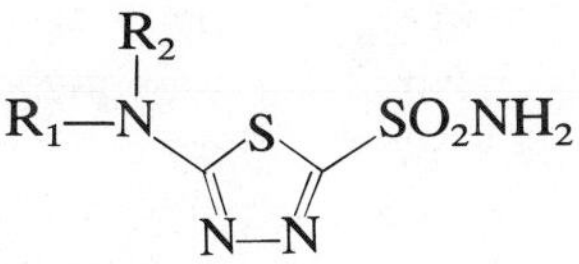

R_1—N(—R_2)—thiadiazole—SO_2NH_2

40.**18** R_1 = lower alkyl, C_6H_5
R_2 = H, CH_3CO

Certain derivatives of 1,3,4-thiadiazole-sulfonamides were among the most active *in vitro* inhibitors of carbonic anhydrase with potencies several hundred time that of sulfanilamide (53, 54). One of these, 5-acetylamino-1,3,4-thiadiazole-2-sulfonamide (acetazolamide, Tables 40.3 and 40.4, 40.13), was studied pharmacologically in detail by Maren et al. (57) and became the first clinically effective and useful diuretic of the carbonic anhydrase inhibitor class. A number of structural modifications of acetazolamide have been studied. An increase of the number of carbons in the acyl group is accompanied by retention of *in vitro* enzyme inhibitor activity and diuretic activity, but side effects become more pronounced. Removal of the acyl group leads to a markedly lower activity *in vitro* (58,

Table 40.4 Dissociation of Carbonic Anhydrase Inhibitory Activity *in Vitro* from Renal Electrolyte Effects in the Dog (56)

No.	Structure	Concn. causing 50% Inhibition of carbonic Anhydrase, M	Dose (i.v.),[a] mg/kg	Urinary Excretion rate, μeq/min			
				Na	K	Cl	pH
40.**20**	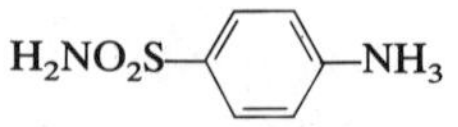 H_2NO_2S—⟨⟩—NH_3 (sulfanilamide)	1.3×10^{-5}	C	14	14	3	6.8
			25	51	25	13	6.9
40.**21**	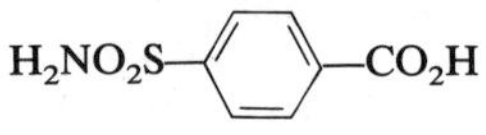 H_2NO_2S—⟨⟩—CO_2H	4.4×10^{-6}	C	26	53	7	6.6
			25	102	136	32	7.7
40.**22**	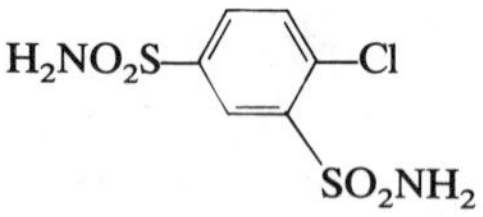 H_2NO_2S—⟨⟩—Cl, SO_2NH_2	1.4×10^{-7}	C	42	24	15	5.9
			2.5	468	101	303	7.4
40.**14**	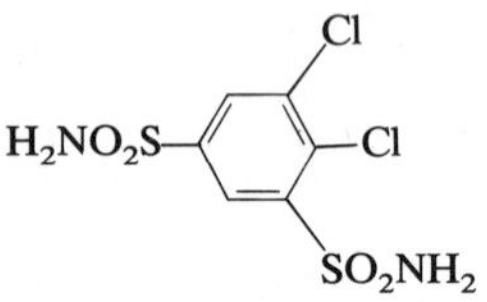 H_2NO_2S—⟨⟩—Cl, Cl, SO_2NH_2	7.5×10^{-6}	C	23	37	21	5.9
			2.5	188	110	64	7.7
40.**13**	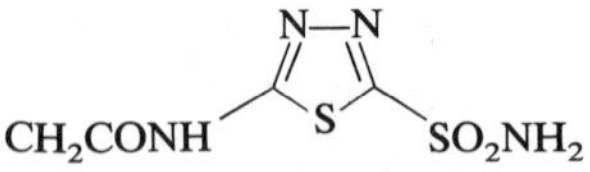 CH_2CONH—⟨N–N / S⟩—SO_2NH_2 (acetazolamide)	7.2×10^{-8}	C	43	22	21	6.3
			2.5	186	128	53	8.0
40.**23**	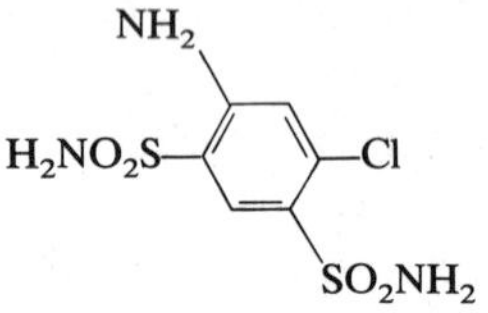 NH_2, H_2NO_2S—⟨⟩—Cl, SO_2NH_2	3.8×10^{-6}	C	5	20	19	5.5
			0.05	14	46	63	5.4
			0.25	54	57	96	5.5
40.**24**	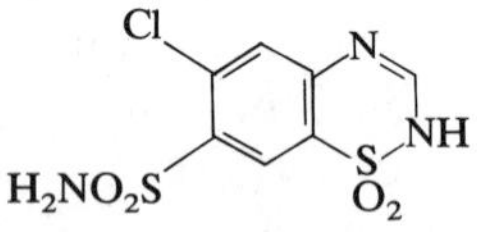 Cl, H_2NO_2S—⟨benzothiadiazine⟩ (chlorothiazide)	1.7×10^{-6}	C	11	11	7	6.1
			0.05	20	24	7	6.6
			0.25	115	38	80	6.7
			1.25	308	65	236	6.9
40.**25**	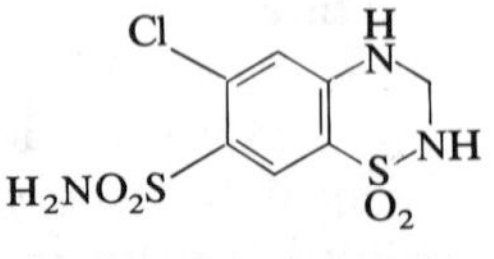 Cl, H_2NO_2S—⟨benzothiadiazine⟩ (hydrochlorothiazide)	2.3×10^{-5}	C	62	34	43	6.5
			0.01	126	32	122	5.9
			0.05	265	33	291	5.5
			0.25	414	39	427	5.9

[a] C = Control phase (no drug), average of two or three 10 min clearances.

59). Substitution on the sulfonamide nitrogen abolishes the enzyme inhibitory activity *in vitro*, but diuretic activity in animals is still present if the substituent is removable by metabolism (60). Two isomeric products 40.**19** and 40.**16** (methazolamide) are obtained on methylation of acetazolamide (55). Both these compounds are somewhat more active *in vitro* than acetazolamide but offer no advantages as diuretics over the parent compound.

A related sulfamoylthiadiazolesulfonamide, benzolamide (40.**17**, Table 40.3), is about five times more active than acetazolamide. Clinical studies showed that at 3 mg/kg p.o. it produces a full bicarbonate diuresis with increased excretion of sodium and potassium (61, 62). Ethoxzolamide, a benzothiazole derivative, (Table 40.3, 40.**15**) ia a clinically effective diuretic carbonic anhydrase inhibitor (63). The compound lacking the ethoxy group is inactive as a diuretic when given orally to dogs although it is a potent carbonic anhydrase inhibitor *in vitro* (64).

Dichlorphenamide (Tables 40.**3** and 40.**4**, 40.**14**) a benzenedisulfonamide derivative is, *in vitro*, as active as acetazolamide as a carbonic anhydrase inhibitor and equally active as diuretic (56).

A large number of benzenedisulfonamide derivatives have been prepared and studied as diuretics. Some of these are very active as diuretics, although they are weak carbonic anhydrase inhibitors. In contrast to the compounds just discussed $Na^+HCO_3^-$ excretion is not increased; instead an approximately equal amount of chloride ion accompanies the sodium. These are described in the section on aromatic sulfonamides.

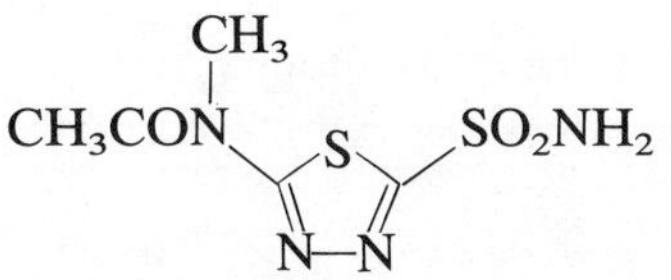

5.3 Clinical Application

Acetazolamide is the prototype of the carbonic anhydrase inhibitor and is a safe, orally effective diuretic. It is rapidly absorbed from the stomach, reaches a peak plasma level within 2 hr and is eliminated unchanged in the urine within 8–12 hr. The dose is 250 mg–1 g daily. During continuous administration of acetazolamide, the excretion of HCO_3^- leads to the development of metabolic acidosis and because under acidotic conditions the diuretic effect of carbonic anhydrase inhibition is much reduced or completely absent, the effect of the drug is self-limiting (65). This is due to the fall in level of plasma and filtered bicarbonate as bicarbonate is lost in the urine. A state of equilibrium is reached when the small amount of hydrogen ion that is secreted in spite of carbonic anhydrase blockade is sufficient to reabsorb the reduced amount of filtered bicarbonate ion. The present use of acetazolamide is restricted to cases of mild edema and to the treatment of glaucoma to reduce intraocular pressure. Methazolamide is preferred for the latter indication. Carbonic anhydrase inhibitors also have some anticonvulsant activity in grand mal and especially petit mal epilepsy, but they have not gained wide acceptance for either of these indications (41).

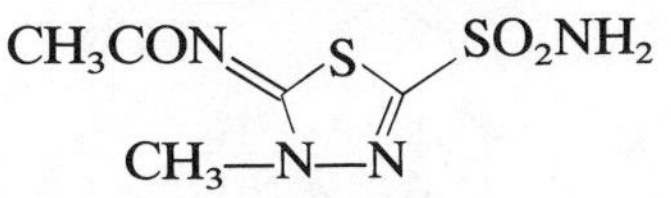

6 AROMATIC SULFONAMIDES

6.1 Introduction

Beyer and Baer (66), in a paper published in 1975, discussed their early findings on the natriuretic and chloruretic activity of *p*-carboxybenzenesulfonamide (40.**21**, Table

$$CH_3CON \underset{N-N}{\overset{\underset{\displaystyle CH_3}{|}}{\bigvee_{S}}} SO_2NH_2$$

40.**19**

$$CH_3CON \underset{CH_3-N-N}{\bigvee_{S}} SO_2NH_2$$

40.**16**

40.4). Although the compound is considerably less active as a carbonic anhydrase inhibitor than acetazolamide, the way the kidney handles the carboxybenzene-sulfonamide was considered by them to be more important and served to define the saluretic properties sought and ultimately found in chlorothiazide (40.**24**, Table 40.4).

A key discovery by Sprague (67) was that the introduction of a second sulfamoyl group meta to the first can markedly increase not only the natriuretic effect but also the chloruretic action of the compound. This is evident when the data for compounds 40.**20** or 40.**21** are compared with compound 40.**22**, Table 40.4. Interestingly, the introduction of a second chlorine substituent as in compound 40.**14** (Table 40.3), dichlorphenamide, produces a compound that is considerably less chloruretic with an excretion pattern typical of a carbonic anhydrase inhibitor.

The activity of 6-chlorobenzene-1,3-disulfonamide (40.**22**, Table 40.4) is further enhanced by the introduction of an amino group ortho to the second sulfonamide group as in 40.**23** (Table 40.4). Thus 4-amino-6-chloro-1,3-benzenedisulfonamide (40.**23**) is an effective diuretic agent with a more favorable electrolyte excretion pattern than 40.**22**. Chloride is the major anion excreted, and HCO_3^- excretion is low, since the urinary pH does not increase. The carbonic anhydrase inhibitory activity of 40.**23** is only about three times that of sulfanilamide (40.**20**). The chlorine in the 6 position of 40.**23** can be replaced by bromine, trifluoromethyl, and nitro without much change in activity, whereas a fluoro, amino, methyl, or methoxy group is less effective (68).

Substitution on the nitrogen atoms of 4-amino-6-chloro-1,3-benzenedisulfonamide gives compounds 40.**26**. Methyl or allyl substitution of the aromatic amino group yields compounds with reduced oral activity. Acylation of the anilino group leads to an increase in activity when R_4 is a simple

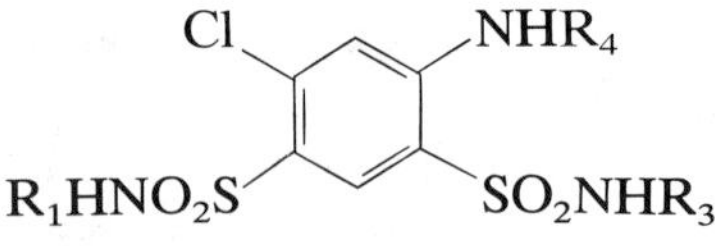

40.**26** $R_1 = R_3 = H$, $R_4 = CH_3$ or $CH_2CH{=}CH_2$
$R_1 = R_3 = H$, $R_4 = CO(CH_2)_{2-4}CH_3$
$R_1 = R_3 = R_4 = CH_3CO$
$R_1 = R_3 = CH_3$ or C_2H_5, $R_4 = H$

aliphatic acyl radical and reaches a maximum at four to six carbon atoms. Aromatic acyl derivatives are less active. Acylation with formic acid results in a cyclized product, 6-chloro-1,2,4-benzothiadiazine-7-sulfonamide 1,1-dioxide, chlorothiazide (Table 40.4, 40.**24**) (69). This compound was the starting point for the development of the thiazide diuretics, one of the most important groups of diuretics, which are discussed in Section 7. Complete acetylation ($R_1 = R_3 = R_4 = CH_3CO$) lowers the activity (68). Methylation of both sulfonamide groups ($R_1 = R_3 = CH_3$ or C_2H_5; $R_4 = H$) gives a compound that has diuretic activity in the rat, but the observed activity is attributable to *in vivo* dealkylation of the sulfonamide function (70).

6.2 Mefruside

Horstmann and co-workers (71) at a later date realized that 6-chloro-1,3-benzene-disulfonamide (40.**22**, Table 40.4) had shown an excretion pattern combining Na^+, HCO_3^-, and a substantial amount of chloride ions even though it is an active carbonic anhydrase inhibitor. Investigation

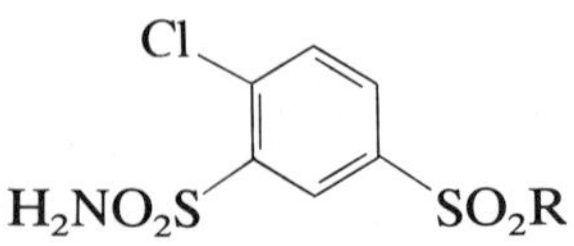

40.**22**   R = NH₂
40.**27**   R = NHCH₃
40.**28**   R = N(CH₃)₂

of derivatives substituted on the sulfonamide nitrogen para to the chloro substituent led to compounds with high diuretic activity. Introduction of a single methyl group (40.**27**) does not reduce the HCO_3^- excretion as compared to 40.**22**, but disubstitution as in 40.**28** leads to a substantially lower excretion of HCO_3^- and an improved Na/Cl ratio owing to less carbonic anhydrase activity. a large number of *N*-substituted benzenesulfonamide derivatives were prepared; the *N*-disubstituted compounds were of more interest because they exhibited primarily a saluretic effect. A selected number of these compounds are shown in Table 40.5. The threshold dose levels and the increase in sodium excretion over control values in the rat are also given. These compounds are relatively weak carbonic anhydrase inhibitors with little effect on HCO_3^-, excretion, particularily those that are disubstituted on the sulfonamide nitrogen. A particularly favorable type of substituent is the tetrahydrofurfuryl group (Table 40.5, 40.**33**–40.**36**). Activity is enhanced when the tetrahydrofuran ring bears a methyl substituent in the 2 position. A diuretic effect in rats is obtained with this compound (40.**35**, mefruside) at the low dose of 0.04 mg/kg. This compound has an asymmetric carbon atom; however, the difference in diuretic activity between the more active l form and the racemate is not of practical significance. The action of mefruside is characterized by a prolonged increase in the rate of excretion of NaCl and water (73). the corresponding pyrrolidine derivatives are also active diuretics (Table 40.5, 40.**37** and 40.**38**).

Studies with ^{14}C labeled mefruside have shown that the compound is almost completely metabolized *in vivo* to the lactone (Table 40.5, 40.**36**) (72). This lactone has about the same diuretic activity as the parent compound and may be responsible for much of the observed activity of mefruside (71). Mefruside has been compared with chlorothiazide in the dog and the findings

suggest that mefruside has a mechanism of action similar to the thiazide diuretics without any unique features (138). Mefruside has also been studied in man at doses of 25 and 100 mg. In volunteers undergoing water diuresis the drug caused natriuresis and chloruresis extending for 20 h with only insignificant increases in potassium excretion acutely. Bicarbonate excretion was increased; *in vivo* carbonic anhydrase studies revealed 50% inhibition at 7.3×10^{-7} *M* concentration (chlorothiazide: $1.7 \times 10^{-6} M$). The potency of mefruside and its effect on renal concentrating and diluting mechanisms suggest that its action is similar to that of the thiazide diuretics (74, 139). Studies in hypertensive patients also showed a close correlation with the thiazide diuretics in terms of both desirable and undesirable effects (140, 141).

7   THIAZIDES AND HYDROTHIAZIDES

7.1   Thiazides

This very important group of diuretics developed from the work of Novello and Sprague on benzenesulfonamides in general and on 4-acylamino-6-chloro-1,3-benzenedisulfonamides in particular. Research in this area was based on the conviction of Beyer (16) that it should be possible to find a sulfonamide derivative that is saluretic, that increases Na^+ and Cl^- excretion in approximately equal quantities—in other words, a compound that does not act as a classical carbonic anhydrase inhibitor, which increases water, Na^+, and HCO_3^- elimination. A saluretic diuretic should permit a substantial reduction of edema without affecting the normal acid–base balance. Treatment of 4-amino-6-chlorobenzene-1,3-disulfonamide with formic acid resulted in the formation of the cyclic benzothiadiazine derivative, chlorothiazide (Table 40.4, 40.**24**) (69). This compound was the first orally active, potent diuretic

Table 40.5 Diuretic Activity in Rats of some 4-Chloro-3-sulfamoyl-N-substituted Benzenesulfonamides (71)

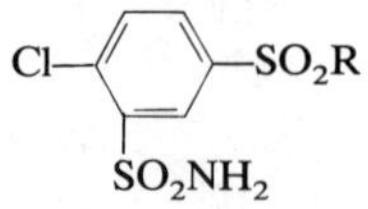

Cl—⟨benzene ring⟩—SO$_2$R
SO$_2$NH$_2$

No.	R	Threshold dose, mg/kg p.o.	Increase in Na$^+$ Excretion at 80 mg/kg p.o., μeq/kg/6 hr (Rat)
40.29	NHCH$_2$CH(CH$_3$)$_2$	2.4	4615
40.30	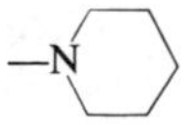 —N⟨piperidine⟩	2.1	3000
40.31	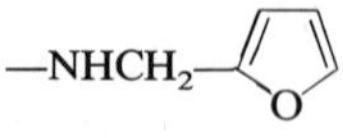 —NHCH$_2$—⟨furan⟩	6	3910
40.32	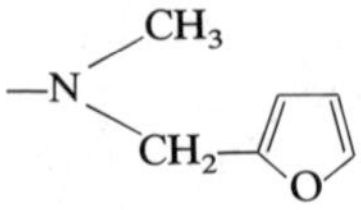 —N(CH$_3$)CH$_2$—⟨furan⟩	18	2900
40.33	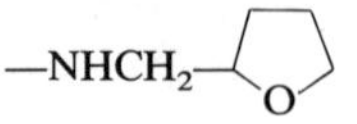 —NHCH$_2$—⟨tetrahydrofuran⟩	0.9	3150
40.34	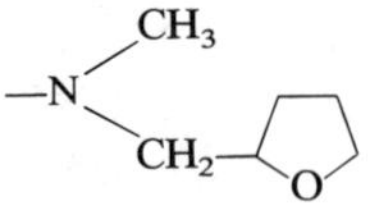 —N(CH$_3$)CH$_2$—⟨tetrahydrofuran⟩	1.0	3000
40.35	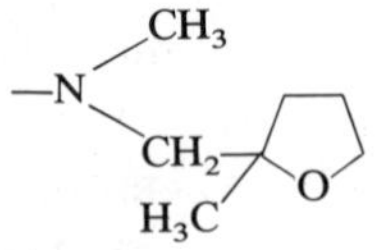 —N(CH$_3$)CH$_2$—⟨(H$_3$C)tetrahydrofuran⟩	0.04	4100
40.36	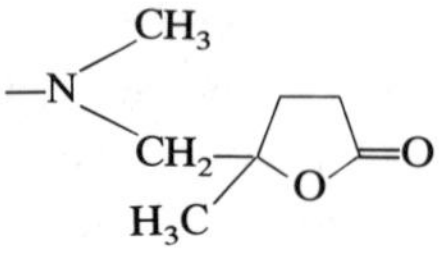 —N(CH$_3$)CH$_2$—⟨(H$_3$C)lactone (=O)⟩	0.04 i.v. 0.15 p.o	3700 i.v. 3000 p.o.
40.37	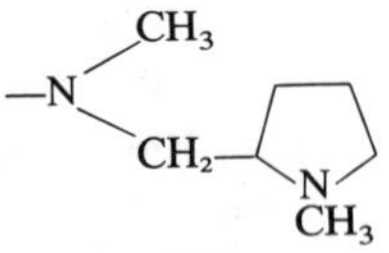 —N(CH$_3$)CH$_2$—⟨N-CH$_3$ pyrrolidine⟩	0.15	3300
40.38	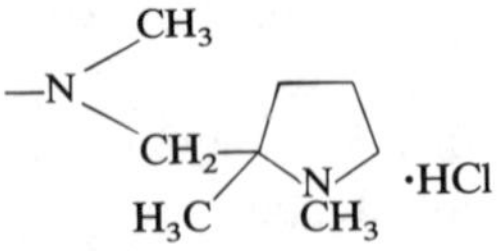 —N(CH$_3$)CH$_2$—⟨H$_3$C, N-CH$_3$ pyrrolidine⟩ ·HCl	0.3	2515
40.39	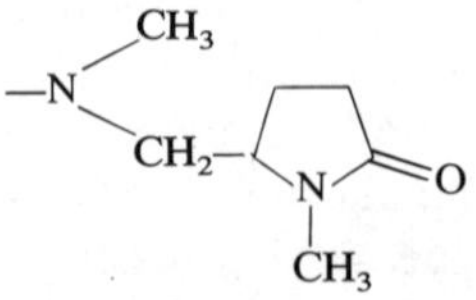 —N(CH$_3$)CH$_2$—⟨N-CH$_3$ pyrrolidinone (=O)⟩	0.04	3000

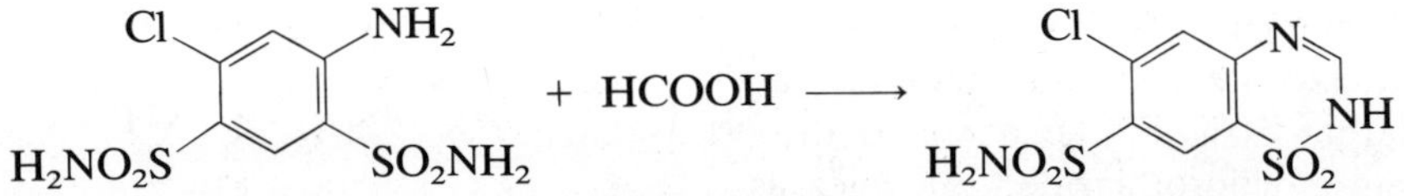

$$\text{40.23} \quad + \text{ HCOOH} \longrightarrow \quad \text{40.24}$$

that could be used to the full extent of its functional capacity as a natriuretic agent without upsetting the normal acid–base balance. Chlorothiazide is a saluretic with minimal side effects and fulfilled a clinical need.

Structure–activity relationships have been developed for the thiazides. The effect of varying the 3 and 6 substituents is shown in Table 40.6. Interestingly, compound 40.**40**, $R_6 = H$, has very little diuretic activity, whereas compounds where $R_6 = Cl$, Br, or CF_3 are highly active; an alkyl group in

the 3 position decreases the activity slightly. The 3-oxo derivative of chlorothiazide also has weak diuretic activity (67). Interchanging the chlorine and sulfamoyl group at positions 6 and 7 in chlorothiazide lowers the activity. Replacement of the 7-sulfamoyl group by CH_3SO_2 or H gives compounds with little activity (68).

The degree of activity observed with compounds bearing an acyl or alkyl group on the 7-sulfamoyl group is in accord with the hypothesis that metabolic cleavage of the N-substituent occurs to yield the free

Table 40.6 Comparative Effects of 3- and 6-substituted Thiazides on Electrolyte Excretion in the Dog (67)

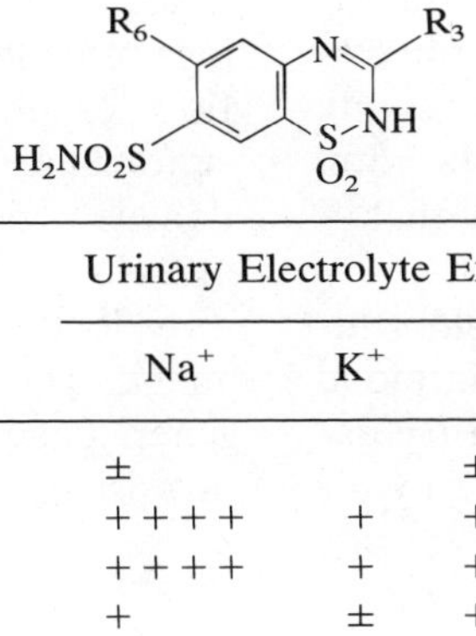

No.	R_6	R_3	Na$^+$	K$^+$	Cl$^-$	Ref.
40.**40**	H	H	±		±	
40.**24**	Cl	H	+ + + +	+	+ + + +	Chlorothiazide
40.**41**	Br	H	+ + + +	+	+ + + +	
40.**42**	CH$_3$	H	+	±	+	
40.**43**	OCH$_3$	H	+ +	±	+ +	
40.**44**	NO$_2$	H	+ + +	±	+ + +	
40.**45**	NH$_2$	H	±		±	
40.**46**	Cl	CH$_3$	+ + +	±	+ + +	
40.**47**	Cl	n-C$_3$H$_7$	+ + +	±	+ + +	
40.**48**	Cl	n-C$_5$H$_{11}$	+ + +	±	+ + +	
40.**49**	Cl	C$_6$H$_5$	±	±	± ±	
40.**50**	CF$_3$	H	+ + + +		+ + +	Flumethiazide (75
40.**51**	Cl	CH$_2$SCH$_2$C$_6$H$_5$	+ + + +	+	+ + + +	Benzthiazide (78, 79)
40.**52**	Cl	CHCl$_2$	+ + + +	+	+ + + +	80
40.**53**	Cl	CH$_2$– 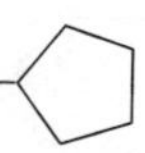 (cyclopentyl)	+ + + +	+	+ + + +	80

The header row for Urinary Electrolyte Excretion^a spans Na$^+$, K$^+$, Cl$^-$.

^{a} Compounds administered p.o.

sulfamoyl function (75, 76). In the case of N^7-caproylchlorothiazide, urinary bioassay indicated that 50% of the excreted drug was present as chlorothiazide (56), whereas the N^7-acetyl derivative showed only weak saluretic activity with no detectable cleavage of the acetyl group (77). Substitution of the ring nitrogen atoms at position 2 or 4 with methyl reduces the activity and makes the heterocyclic ring more vulnerable to hydrolytic cleavage (68). The introduction of a more complex substituent in the 3 position, e.g., $R_3 = CH_2SCH_2C_6H_5$ (40.**51**, Table 40.6) led to a compound which was 8–10 times more potent on a weight basis than chlorothiazide (78, 79). Similarily, the dichloromethyl and cyclopentylmethyl analogs (40.**52** and 40.**53**, Table 40.6) were 10–20 times more potent, respectively, than chlorothiazide on a weight basis when tested in experimental animals (80). A number of "aza" analogs of chlorothiazide, derived from 2-amino-pyridine-3,5-disulfonamide and 4-aminopyridine-3,5-disulfonamide, have been prepared (40.**54**–40.**61**, Table 40.7). In general, the activity of each compound was comparable with, although somewhat less potent than, that of its 1,2,4-benzothiadiazine analog (81).

In addition to diuretic activity, chlorothiazide and its congeners exert a mild blood pressure lowering effect in hypertensive patients and are frequently used clinically for

40.**62**

this action. Initially the antihypertensive effect was thought to be a consequence of the diuretic action. It was subsequently found, however, that removal of the 7-sulfonamide group from compounds of the chlorothiazide class eliminated the diuretic effect, but not the antihypertensive action (82, 83). A compound of this type, diazoxide (40.**62**), is a much more effective antihypertensive agent. Surprisingly, salt and water retention has been observed with this compound (83).

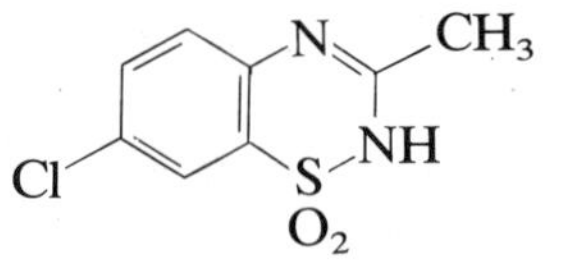

7.2 Hydrothiazides

A new phase in the development of the thiazide diuretics was opened by the findings of deStevens et al. (84) that condensation of 4-amino-6-chloro-1,3-benzenedisulfonamide (40.**23**) with 1 mol of formaldehyde gives 6-chloro-3,4-dihydro-2H-1,2,4-benzothiadiazine-7-sulfonamide 1,1-dioxide (40.**25**), a stable crystalline compound. This compound has been given the generic name hydrochlorothiazide. It was surprising that saturation of the 3,4 double

Table 40.7   Pyrido-1,2,4-thiadiazines 1,1-Dioxides (81)

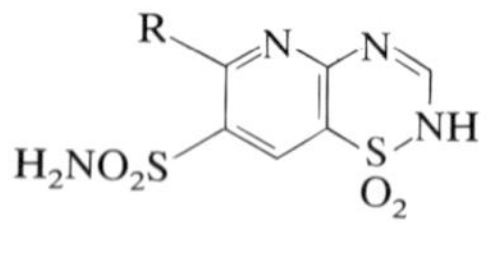

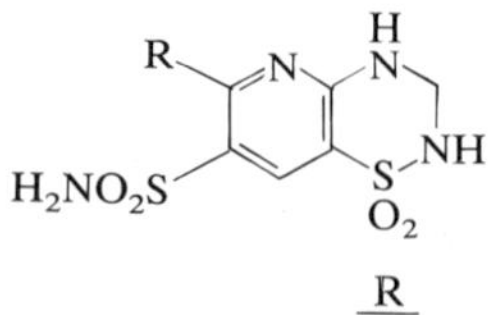

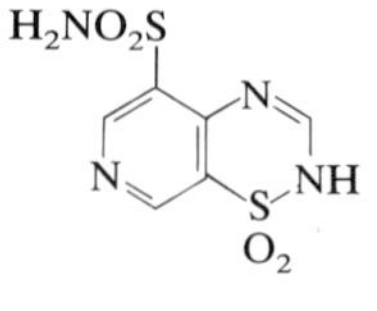

40.**54** R = H	40.**56** H	40.**61**
40.**55** R = CH$_3$	40.**57** CH$_3$	
	40.**58** NH$_2$	
	40.**59** OH	
	40.**60** Cl	

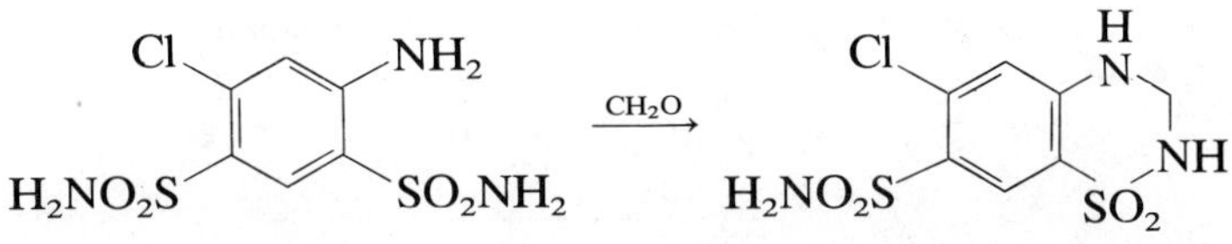

40.**23**   40.**25**

bond in chlorothiazide leads to a compound that is 10 times more active in the dog (84–86) and in man (87–89) as a diuretic. Hydrochlorothiazide (40.**25**) has less than $\frac{1}{10}$ the carbonic anhydrase inhibiting activity of chlorothiazide (40.**24**, Table 40.4). Like chlorothiazide it also exerts a mild anti-hypertensive effect in hypertensive subjects (90).

7.2.1 STRUCTURE–ACTIVITY RELATIONSHIPS. Structure-activity relationships have been extensively investigated by various groups (68, 91–106). Substitution in the 6 position of hydrochlorothiazide follows the same rules as found for chlorothiazide; i.e., compounds of approximately equal activity result when the substituent in the 6 position is Cl, Br, or CF_3. Compounds where $R_6 = H$ or NH_2 are only weakly active. Substitution in the 3 position of hydrochlorothiazide has a pronounced effect on the diuretic potency and compounds that are more than 100 times as active as hydrochlorothiazide on a weight basis have been obtained. It should be noted, however, that the maximal diuretic and saluretic effect that can be achieved with any of the thiazide diuretics is of the same magnitude, although the dose required may vary considerably.

Substituents in the 3 position of hydro-chlorothiazide having the most favorable effect on activity were alkyl, cycloalkyl, haloalkyl, and aralkyl, all of which may be classified as hydrophobic in character. This is illustrated in Table 40.8 where the structures of derivatives of hydrochlorothiazide and the respective diuretic response in the dog are shown. Table 40.9 lists the commercially available thiazide diuretics and

the respective optimally effective dose per day in man. Beyer and Baer (66) have studied four thiazides covering a thousand-fold increase in saluretic activity on a log-stepwise basis from chlorothiazide to hy-drochlorothiazide, to trichlormethiazide, to cyclopenthiazide. This increase in activity appears to correlate with their lipid solubil-ity (in terms of their ether/phosphate buffer partition coefficient), rather than their car-bonic anhydrase inhibitory effect (Table 40.8).

7.2.2 PHARMACOLOGY AND MECHANISM OF ACTION. Chlorothiazide and hydrochloro-thiazide are the prototypes of a group of related heterocyclic sulfonamides that differ among themselves mainly in regard to the dosage required for natriuretic activ-ity and duration of activity. Examples of these compounds are shown in Tables 40.8 and 40.9. The unique property of these drugs is their ability to produce a much larger chloruresis associated with a greater natriuretic potency than the carbonic anhydrase inhibitor acetazolamide and its congeners.

Following oral administration to normal subjects, hydrochlorothiazide is rapidly ab-sorbed. Peak plasma levels are reached after 2.6 ± 0.8 hr and the drug is still detect-able after 9 h. Approximately 70% of a 65 mg dose was accounted for in the urine after 48 hr (107). Hydrochlorothiazide and other benzothiadiazine diuretics are ex-creted by the kidneys both through glomerular filtration and tubular secretion. The latter is shared with other organic acids and is specifically inhibited by probenecid. Concurrent administration of hydrochlor-othiazide and probenecid did not modify

Table 40.8   Hydrochlorothiazide Derivatives—Structure–Activity Relationships of Canine Studies

No.	Structure	Dose p.o., μg/kg	Average Excretion per Dog over 6 hr			Natriuretic activity, Approx.	Partition Coefficient (66) Ether/Water
			Urine, ml	Na$^+$,meq	K$^+$,meq		
Control average		0	42.5–53.2	7.1–10.0	4.75		
40.**24**	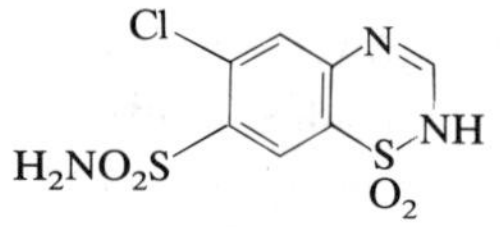	1250	102	18.5	6.5	1	0.08
	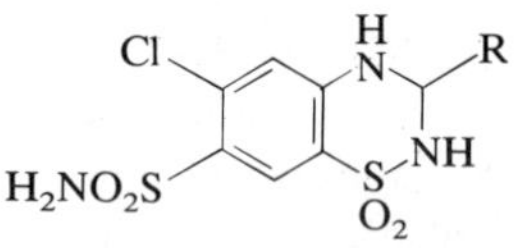						
40.**25**	R = H	20	69	12.1	4.35		
		310	100	20.3	6.0	10	0.37
		1250	125	26.1	8.6		
40.**63**	R = CH$_2$CH(CH$_3$)$_2$	1.3	59	13.8	4.3		
		20	100	20.7	6.8		
40.**64**	R = CH$_2$Cl	20	83	17.2	4.0		
		310	131	30.6	6.1		
40.**65**	R = CHCl$_2$	1.3	65	11.6	5.1	100	1.53
		20	113	22.5	6.5		
40.**66**	R = CH$_2$C$_6$H$_5$	1.3	74	18.6	4.0		
40.**67**	R = CH$_2$– 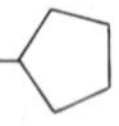	1.3	95	22.7	4.9	1000	10.2

the effects of hydrochlorothiazide on the urinary excretion of calcium, magnesium, and citrate. This combined therapy also prevented or abolished the increased serum uric acid levels associated with the use of thaizide diuretics (108). Although the thiazides are excreted by an active process located in the proximal segment, one cannot infer a direct action in the proximal tubule. Clearance studies suggest that the thiazides have no effect on the medullary segment of the loop of Henle and that their major site of action is the cortical thick ascending limb of Henle, where they inhibit active chloride transport and reabsorption of the attendant sodium ion (15, 65). The organomercurials and high ceiling loop diuretics also inhibit active chloride reabsorption in this segment of the nephron (3).

As a class, the thiazides have an important action on potassium excretion. In most patients a satisfactory chloruretic and natriuretic response is accompanied by significant kaliuresis also seen in dog diuretic studies (see Table 40.8) (109, 110). At low doses, with some selected thiazides, a separation of natriuretic and kaliuretic effects has been observed but at higher doses and repeated administration these differences disappear. The kaliuresis, although enhanced by the carbonic anhydrase activity of many of these compounds, is probably a consequence of increased delivery of sodium and fluid to the distal segment of

Table 40.9 Benzothiadiazine Diuretics

No.	Generic Name (Clinical Dose, mg p.o.)	Trade Name	Structure	Ref.
40.**68**	Bendroflumethiazide NF (2–5)	Bristuron, Naturetin	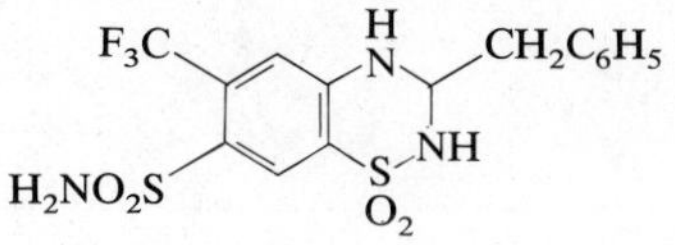	101
40.**51**	Benzthiazide NF (25–50)	Aquatag, Exna	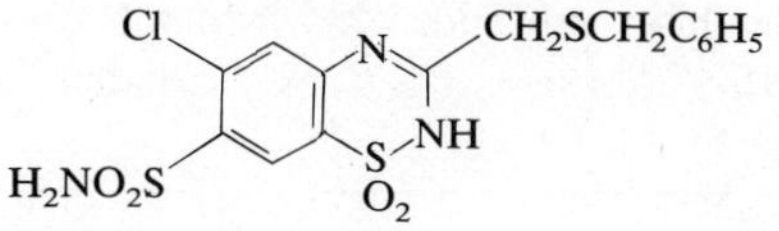	78, 79
40.**63**	Buthiazide (thiabutazide)	Saltucin, Eunephran	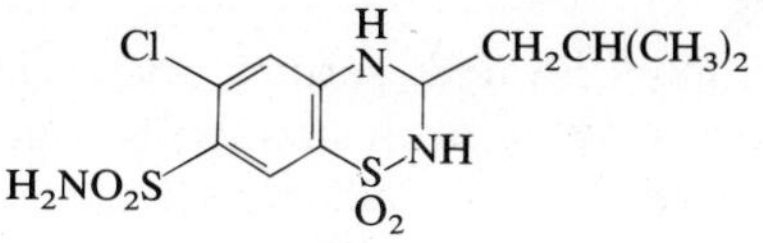	91, 93
40.**24**	Chlorothiazide NF (500–2000)	Diuril	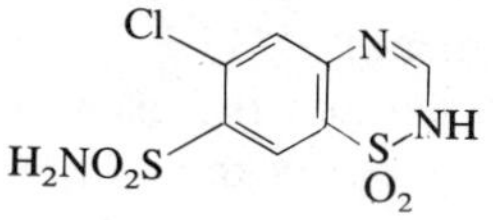	68
40.**67**	Cyclopenthiazide (0.5–1.5)	Navidrix	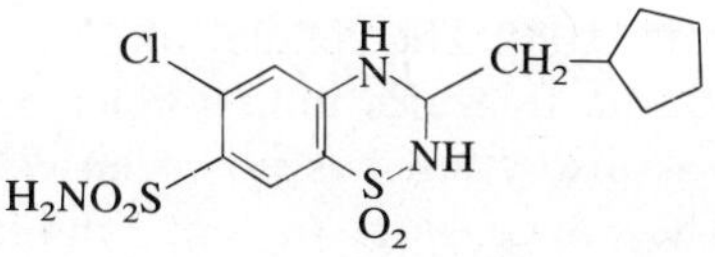	104, 111
40.**69**	Cyclothiazide NF (1–6)	Anhydron	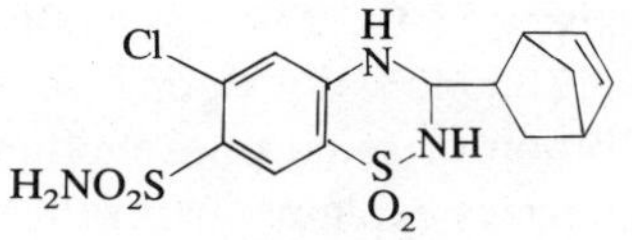	104
40.**25**	Hydrochlorothiazide USP (25–100)	Esidrix, HydroDiuril, Oretic	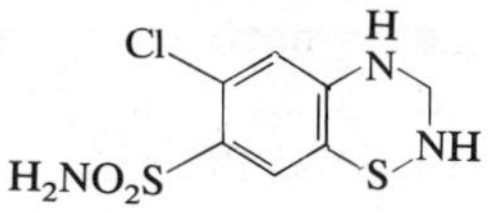	84,91
40.**70**	Hydroflumethiazide NF (25–50)	Saluron	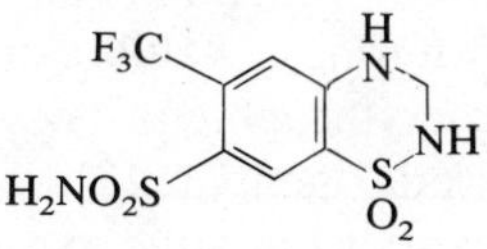	101
40.**71**	Methyclothiazide NF (5–10)	Enduron	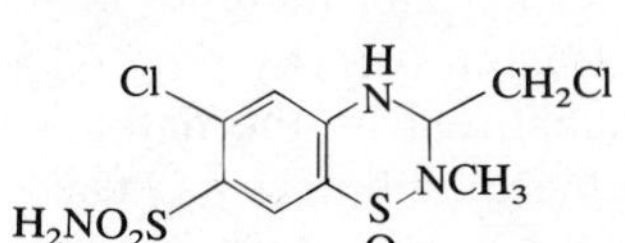	98

Table 40.9 (Continued)

No.	Generic Name (Clinical Dose, mg p.o.)	Trade Name	Structure	Ref.
40.**72**	Polythiazide NF (4–8)	Renese	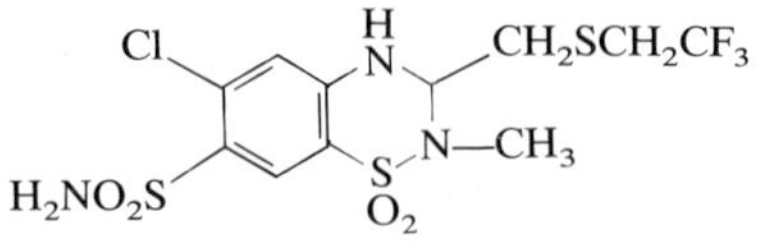	103, 112
40.**65**	Trichlormethiazide NF (4–8)	Metahydrin, Naqua	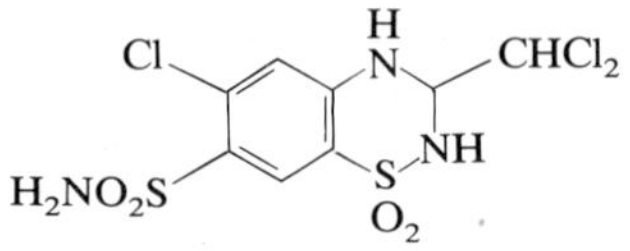	113, 114

the nephron. Elevated serum uric acid levels, which may be associated with gout, owing to decreased uric acid excretion during chronic thiazide administration, have been well documented (110). Calcium excretion is decreased and the excretion of magnesium is enhanced by the administration of thiazide diuretics in normal subjects and in patients (108). The cellular mechanism by which the thiazides inhibit chloride and sodium reabsorption has not been established. They apparently do not inhibit Na^+K^+-dependent ATPase, an enzyme present in high activity in the thick ascending limb of Henle (110, 115), nor does it seem likely that inhibition of renal phosphodiesterase by the thiazides explains their saluretic activity (116).

Recent investigations have examined the possible role played by the renal prostaglandins (PGE_2, PGA_2, and $PGF_{2\alpha}$) in renal function and in their relationship with other regulators of kidney function, i.e., renin–angiotensin–aldosterone, kallikrein–kinin, vasopressin, and erythropoietin, as well as with various diuretic agents (117).

The hypothesis that the antihypertensive and natriuretic effects of diuretics might be mediated, at least in part, by prostaglandin synthesis is supported by the findings that when indomethacin, a potent prostaglandin synthetase inhibitor, was given in combination with furosemide to patients or normal subjects, the antihypertensive and natriuretic effects were diminished or obviated (118).

7.2.3 CLINICAL APPLICATION. The thiazide diuretics have their greatest usefulness in the managment of edema of chronic cardiac decompensation. In hypertensive disease, with or without overt edema, the thiazides have a mild antihypertensive effect. They should be used with caution in patients with significantly impaired renal function. In some patients with nephrosis they have been effective, but their therapeutic usefulness in such cases has been unpredictable. Clinical toxicity is relatively rare and usually results from unexpected hypersensitivity. The thiazide diuretics are available as tablets; the wide range of dosages of the individual preparations is shown in Table 40.9. To minimize the possibility of potassium depletion, fixed combinations with potassium-sparing diuretics have been made available, e.g., hydrochlorothiazide–spironolactone, hydrochlorothiazide–triamterene, and hydrochlorothiazide–amiloride.

Since 1957 the use of the thiazide diuretics has increased to a point where they represent the most commonly used diuretic agents. This is a reflection of their efficacy, safety, and ease of application.

8   OTHER SULFONAMIDE DIURETICS

This group of diuretics includes compounds that produce a pharmacological response similar to that seen with the thiazide diuretics; i.e., they are saluretics and the maximally attainable level of urinary sodium excretion is in the same range as hydrochlorothiazide.

The compounds in this group differ considerably in chemical structure; however, most of them are derivatives of *m*-sulfamoylbenzoic acid.

8.1   Chlorthalidone

An interesting class of compounds was developed from certain substituted benzophenones (119). Optimum diuretic properties were found in 3-(4-chloro-3-sulfamoylphenyl)-3-hydroxy-1-oxoisoindoline (40.**74**, chlorthalidone, Table 40.10), which is the tautomeric form of an ortho-substituted benzophenone. The related compounds 40.**80** and 40.**81** are more potent carbonic anhydrase inhibitors than chlorthalidone but are less active as diuretics and have a shorter duration of action.

Chlorthalidone has shown good diuretic activity in dogs (120), characterized by an unusually long duration of action. It is about 70 times as active as hydrochlorothiazide as a carbonic anhydrase inhibitor *in vitro* and, although it induces primarily a saluresis, there is an increased

output of K^+ and HCO_3^- at higher doses (56). Clinical studies have substantiated the pharmacological properties (121–124). As with the thiazide diuretics, a mild antihypertensive effect was seen (125). The recommended clinical dosage is 50–200 mg daily or every other day.

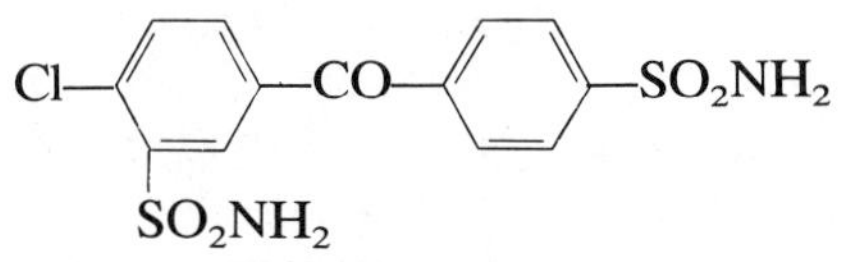

8.2   Hydrazides of *m*-Sulfamoylbenzoic Acids

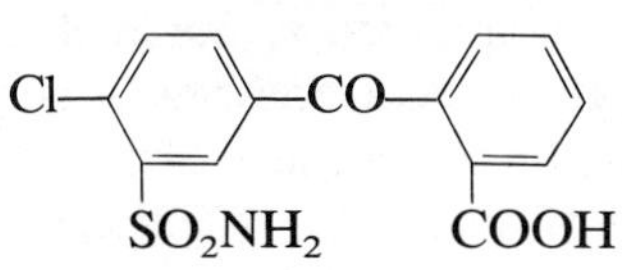

The diuretic properties of a large series of compounds derived from 2-chlorobenzene-sulfonamide, with a wide variety of functional groups in the 5 position (40.**82**), have been studied in the rat and in the dog (126). The R group includes such functional groups as substituted amines, hydrazines, pyrazoles, ketones, ester groups, substituted carboxamides, and hydrazides. The hydrazides are the most active group of compounds. One of these, *cis-N*-(2,6-dimethyl-1-piperidyl)-3-sulfamoyl-4-chlorobenzamide, clopamide (40.**75**, Table 40.10), has been studied in greater detail (126–128).

A dose-related diuretic response was seen in rats at doses of 0.01–1 mg/kg. In unanesthetized dogs a diuretic response was seen with doses as low as 2 μg/kg given orally. In anesthetized dogs the natriuretic response observed was dose related between 0.01 and 1 mg/kg administered i.v. The drug produced a prompt increase in urine flow and excretion of sodium, potassium, and chloride. A small increase in bicarbonate excretion that did not significantly alter plasma or urinary pH was noted. During maximal diuresis produced by hydrochlorothiazide, administration of clopamide had no effect on sodium excretion.

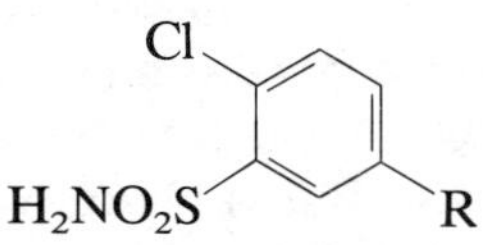

40.**80**

40.**81**

40.**82**

Table 40.10   Other Sulfonamide Diuretics

No.	Generic Name (Clinical Dose, mg p.o.)	Trade Name	Structure	Ref.
40.73	Alipamide (20–80)		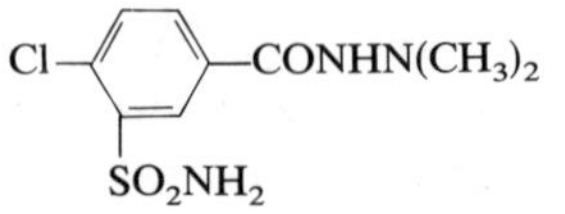	129
40.74	Chlorthalidone (50–200)	Hygroton	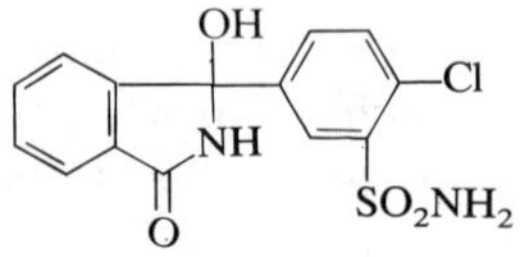	119
40.75	Clopamide (10–40)	Aquex, Brinaldix	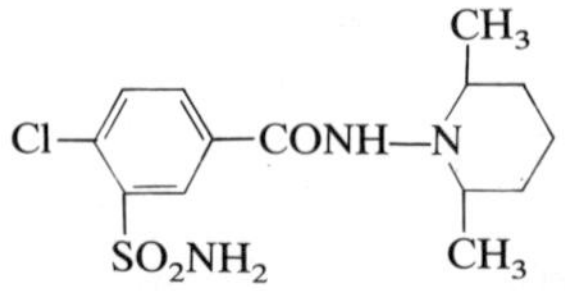	126
40.76	Clorexolone (25–100)	Flonatril, Nefrolan	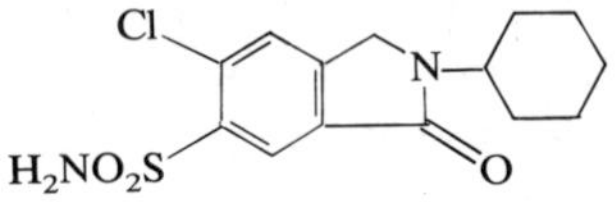	133
40.77	Diapamide (500)	Vectren	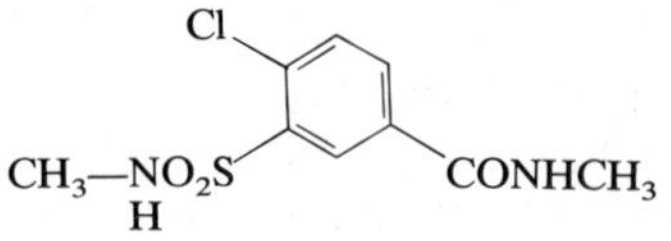	131
40.35	Mefruside (25–100)	Baycaron	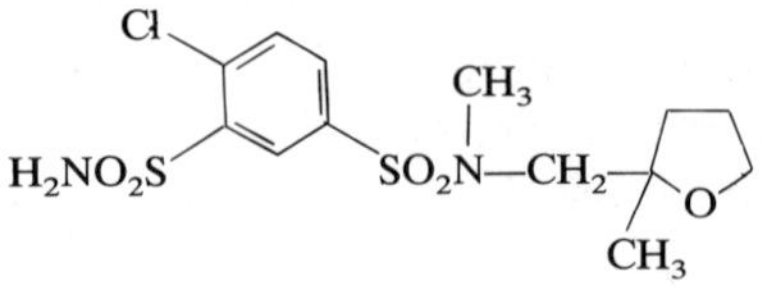	71
40.78	Metolazone (2.5–20)	Zaroxolyn	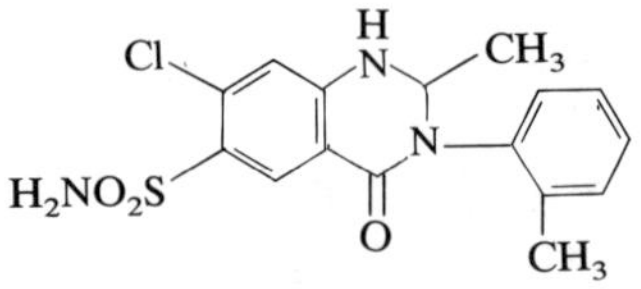	144
40.79	Quinethazone (50–200)	Hydromox	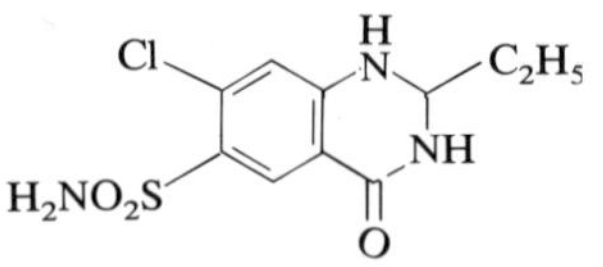	142

Conversely, after a maximally effective dose of clopamide, hydrochlorothiazide was without effect, although in both cases, an additional response to furosemide and spironolactone was observed. This suggests that although clopamide is not a thiazide diuretic its natriuretic action closely resembles that of the thiazides. The recommended clinical dose is 10–40 mg/day.

A related hydrazide, alipamide (40.**73**,

Table 40.10) is an effective diuretic agent in rats, dogs, monkeys, and man (129). The suitable therapeutic dosage in man probably lies between 20 and 80 mg/day. Alipamide exhibits primarily a saluretic action; carbonic anhydrase inhibition becomes an important factor only at high dose levels. A structure–activity study, done in rats in connection with alipamide, showed that a hydroxamic acid moiety could replace a hydrazide group without loss of activity (130).

Similarly, diapamide (40.**77**, Table 40.10) is an effective saluretic agent in rats, dogs, and monkeys (131). In man, the compound is comparable to the thiazides in terms of urine volume and electrolyte excretion (132). Elevated plasma urate and glucose levels accompany chronic administration. The clincally effective dose is 500 mg/day.

8.3   1-Oxoisoindolines

Interesting results have come from studies on a series of 4-chloro-5-sulfamoyl-N-substituted phthalimidines (40.**83**). Maximum activity, about six times that of chlorothiazide on a weight basis, was seen when the N-substituent R was a saturated ring containing six to eight carbons. Compounds in which R represented a smaller or larger ring were less active. For R = lower alkyl, decreased activity was also found. Reduction of one of the carbonyl groups to yield the corresponding 3-hydroxy-1-oxoisoindoline (40.**84**, R = cyclohexyl) resulted in a tenfold increase in

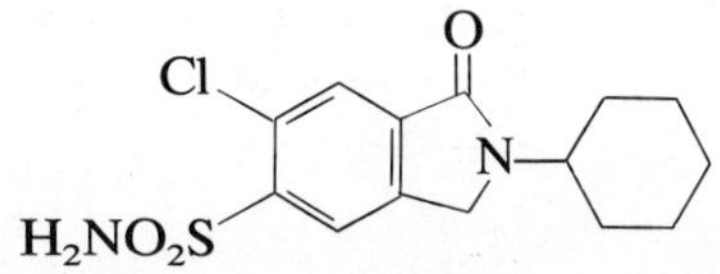

40.**85**

potency. Complete reduction of the carbonyl function to methylene yielded clorexolone (40.**76**, Table 40.10, R = cyclohexyl), which was 300 times as active as chlorothiazide on a weight basis when tested in the rat (133).

Interestingly, reduction of the other oxo group to yield the isomeric 6-chloro-5-sulfamoyl-1-oxoisoindoline 40.**85** results in complete loss of activity. Structure–activity relationships for a number of 2-substituted 1-oxoisoindolines are shown in Table 40.11 (133).

Methylation or acetylation of the sulfamoyl group of clorexolone decreases the activity by at least a factor of 10.

In man, clorexolone is a potent diuretic. The clinical dose is in the range of 25–100 mg/day; the pattern of water and electrolyte excretion is similar to that caused by the benzothiadiazine diuretics. Urinary pH and HCO_3^- excretion remain unchanged after administration of clorexolone, indicating that there is no significant *in vivo* involvement of renal carbonic anhydrase inhibition. As is the case with the thiazide diuretics, elevated serum uric acid levels are seen, but there may be less propensity for hyperglycemia (134–136). In man and in dogs, in contrast to the thiazide diuretics, insignificant amounts of the drug are excreted unchanged. The metabolites are

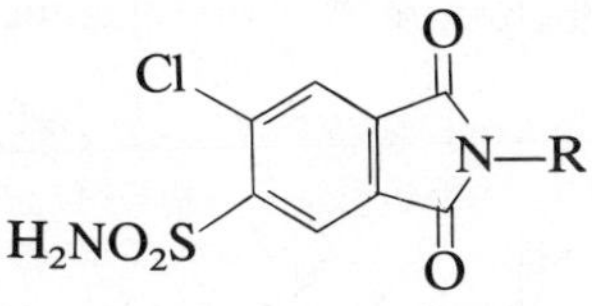

40.**83**   R = alkyl, cycloalkyl 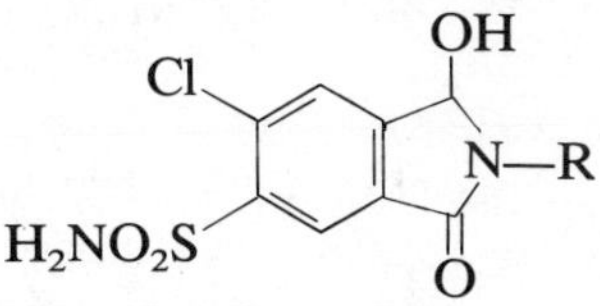   40.**84** 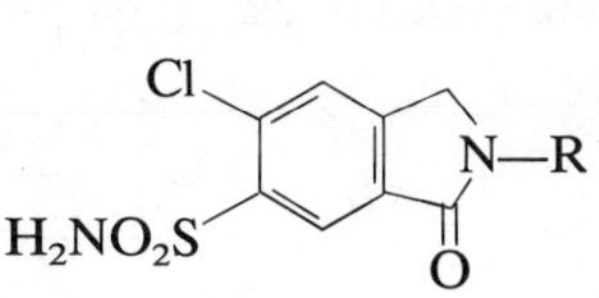   40.**76**

Table 40.11 Diuretic Activity in Rats of 2-Substituted 1-Oxoisoindolines (133)

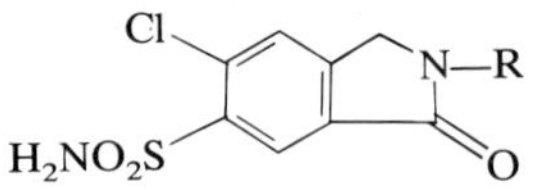

No.	R	Diuretic Activity (Chlorothiazide = 1)
40.**86**	Isobutyl	75–100
40.**87**	Cyclopentyl	100
40.**76**	Cyclohexyl	300
40.**88**	4-Methylcyclohexyl	100
40.**89**	3-Methylcyclohexyl	100
40.**90**	3,4-Dimethylcyclohexyl	200
40.**91**	Cycloheptyl	50–100
40.**92**	Cyclooctyl	100
40.**93**	Norborn-2-yl	100
40.**94**	Cyclohexylmethyl	200

compounds monohydroxylated in the cyclohexane ring. Neither the compound nor its metabolites are stored in body tissues (137).

8.4 Quinazolinone Sulfonamides

Replacement of the ring sulfone group in the thiazides by carbonyl yields quinazolinones and dihydroquinazolinones (40.**95**, 40.**96**), respectively. These compounds produce nearly the same diuretic response as the parent thiazide derivatives, the dihydroderivatives again being more active on a dose/kilogram basis. Substitution at R_3 by alkyl is disadvantageous in that it reverses the favorable Cl^- and K^+ excretion patterns seen in the few examples studied (142). The preferred member of the series was quinethazone (40.**79**, Table 40.10; 40.**96**,

$R_2 = C_2H_5$, $R_3 = H$), which in man has the same order of potency as hydrochlorothiazide with a high Na^+/K^+ excretion ratio. The duration of activity appears to be about 24 hr (143). The recommended clinical dose is 50–200 mg/day.

Extensive studies in a series of dihydroquinazolinones substituted in the 3 position, structure 40.**96**, R_3 = aryl and aralkyl, showed that some of these compounds were highly active diuretics. All the more active derivatives have at least one hydrogen in the 2 position, a primary SO_2NH_2 group in the 6 position, and an ortho or para lower alkyl or CF_3-substituted aromatic ring in the 3 position of the quinazoline nucleus. The most interesting member of the series is metolazone (40.**78**, Table 40.10; 40.**96**, $R_2 = CH_3$, $R_3 = o$—CH_3—C_6H_4) (144). Studies in normal volunteers led to the conclusion that metolazone ex-

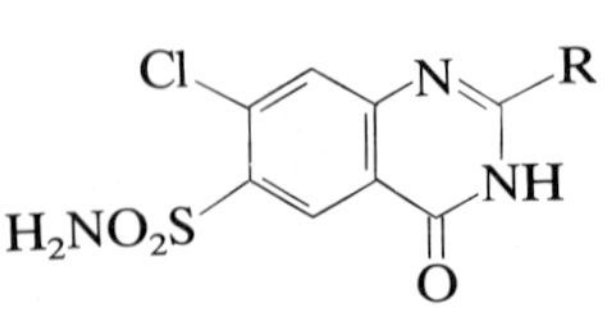

40.**95**

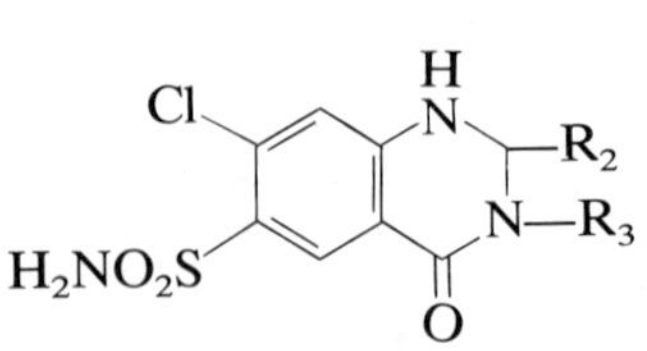

40.**96**

erts its effect in the proximal tubule and in the cortical segment of the ascending limb of Henle or early distal convoluted tubule. The absence of significant bicarbonatriuria is evidence against carbonic anhydrase inhibition. Metolazone did not impair the ability to acidify normally the urine in response to an oral load of NH_4Cl; it was concluded therefore that metolazone has no effect on the distal H^+ secretory mechanism (145–147). In dogs, metolazone was found to be excreted by glomerular filtration and renal tubular secretion; although the secretory mechanism was antagonized by probenecid, this did not affect the diuretic action of metolazone (149). Metolazone at 10–15 mg was approximately equivalent to 50 mg hydrochlorothiazide. The time course of diuretic action was similar to hydrochlorothiazide. No acute elevation of urate or glucose or signs of toxicity were seen in a short-term study (148). The recommended clinical dose is 5–20 mg/day. In a double-blind study in hypertensive patients comparing a dose of 50 mg of hydrochlorothiazide with 2.5 mg and 5.0 mg of metolazone, similar effects on blood pressure were observed. The effects on other parameters, e.g., body weight, electrolytes, serum uric acid, and blood sugar levels, were also comparable (150). In a study in patients with nonedematous, stable chronic renal failure, high dosage of metolazone (20–150 mg) increased urine flow significantly. Its activity was greater than that of the thiazides which are ineffective at glomerular filtration rates of less than 15–20 ml/min, but less than that of furosemide (151).

9 HIGH CEILING DIURETICS

9.1 Introduction

The term high ceiling diuretics has been used to denote a group of diuretics that have a distinctive action on renal tubular function. These drugs produce a peak diuresis far greater than that observed with other diuretic agents. The chemical structure of these agents differs considerably; however, they are alike in the most important aspect underlying their potency, in their site of action in the medullary and cortical thick ascending limb of Henle (3).

The discovery of the countercurrent multiplier system of the nephron as the mechanism responsible for the concentration and dilution of the urine has provided a framework for the identification of the site of action of diuretic drugs. Compounds that act at a single anatomical site in the nephron can be expected to alter the pattern of urine flow in a predictable way. A drug that acts solely in the proximal convoluted tubule by inhibiting reabsorption of water and solutes resulting in an increased delivery of glomerular filtrate to the loop of Henle and the distal convolution, would augment the clearance of solute-free water (C_{H_2O}) during water diuresis and augment the reabsorption of solute-free water (TC_{H_2O}) during water restriction. Drugs that inhibit sodium reabsorption in Henle's loop would impair both C_{H_2O} and TC_{H_2O}. Finally, drugs that act only in the distal tubule would reduce C_{H_2O} but not TC_{H_2O}.

The high ceiling or loop diuretics now in use or currently being studied are shown in Table 40.12. They are discussed in the approximate chronological order of their development.

9.2 Ethacrynic Acid

Soon after the introduction of organomercurials as diuretics, the idea arose that their biological activity resulted from the blockade of essential sulfhydryl groups. From these considerations, several series of highly active diuretics were developed that were designed to react selectively with functionally important sulfhydryl groups, or possibly other nucleophilic groups, that are essential for sodium transport in the nephron. These compounds generally contain

Table 40.12   High Ceiling Diuretics

No.	Generic Name (Clinical dose, mg p.o.)	Trade Name	Structure	Ref.
40.**117**	Bumetanide (1–5)	Burinex, Lunetron	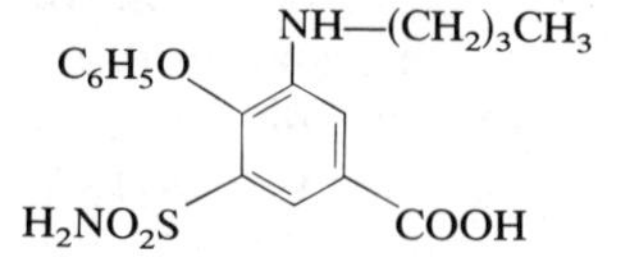	179, 195
40.**103**	Ethacrynic acid (50–200)	Edecrin	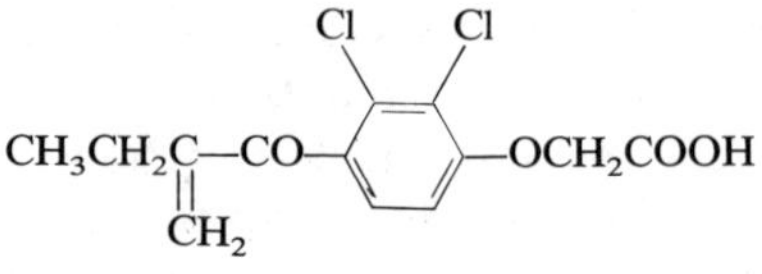	152
40.**108**	Furosemide	Lasix	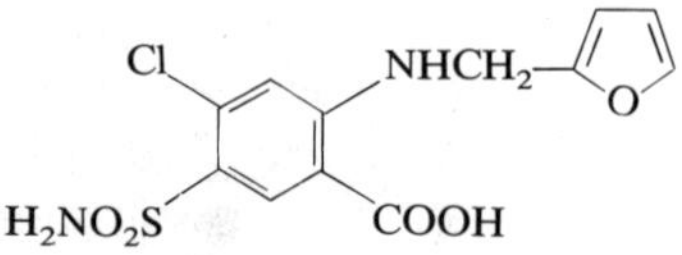	159
40.**138**	Indapamide (2.5–15)	Fludex, Natrilix	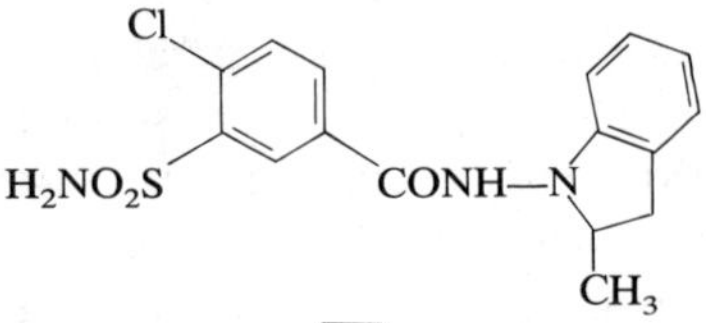	196
40.**139**	Piretanide		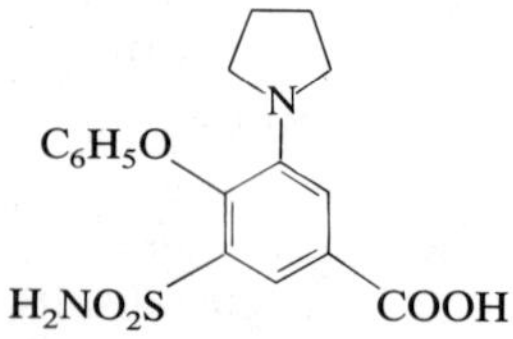	203
40.**140**	Triflocin (1000)		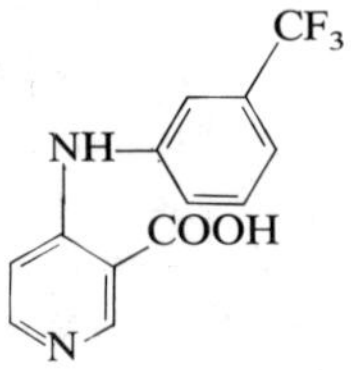	204
40.**141**	Xipamide (40–80)	Aquaphor	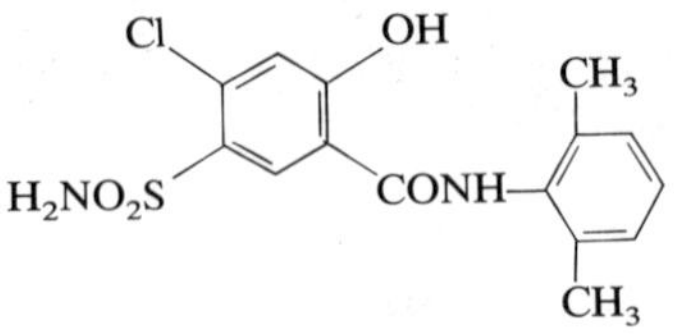	209
40.**151**	Muzolimine (Bay g 2821)		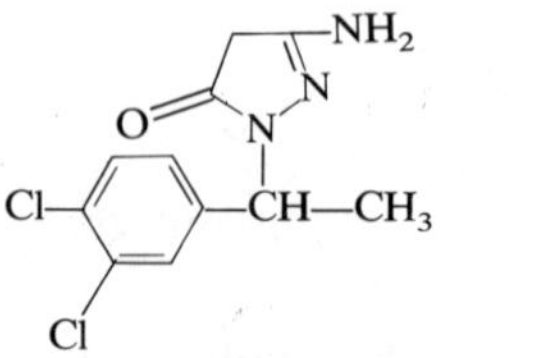	218

176

Table 40.12   *(Continued)*

No.	Generic Name (Clinical dose, mg p.o.)	Trade Name	Structure	Ref.
40.**153**	MK 447		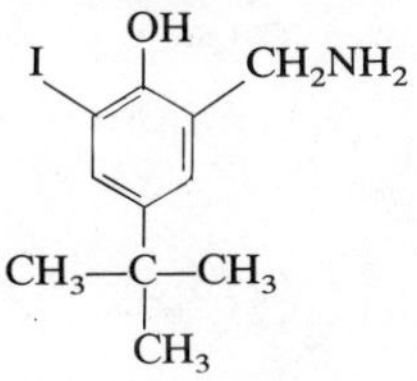	225

an activated double bond attached to a moiety containing a carboxylic acid group of a type expected to assist transport into, or excretion by, the kidney. The general structure of these compounds is exemplified by formulas 40.**97** and 40.**98**. They are highly active in the dog when administered orally or parenterally, but are inactive in the rat.

A marked increase in diuretic activity was observed when chlorine was introduced ortho to the carbonyl group of the aryl side chain. Not only was the diuretic activity increased, but also the rate at which chemical addition of sulfhydryl compounds across the double bond in an *in vitro* system occurred. The presence of two chlorines in positions 2 and 3 of the phenoxyacetic acid further increased the activity. A number of compounds corresponding to structures 40.**97** and 40.**98** and their diuretic activity

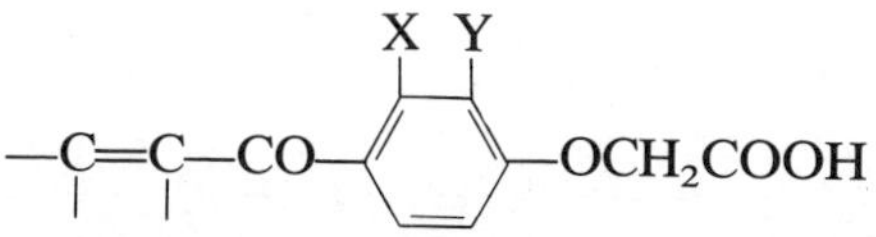

40.**97**

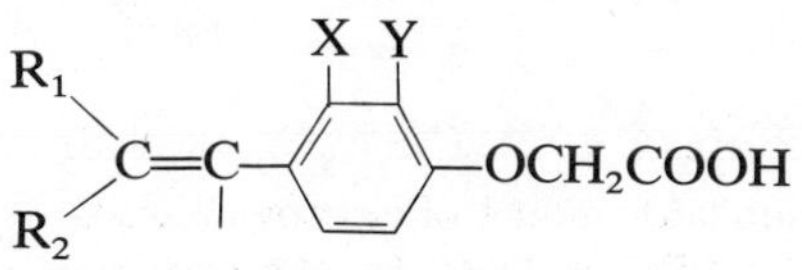

40.**98**   X, Y = H, Cl; R_1, R_2 = CH_3CO, NO_2, CN, alkyl

in dogs are shown in Table 40.13 (152, 153). Ethacrynic acid 40.**103**, Table 40.12 and 40.13, is the most interesting compound of this series and has been studied extensively. A more recent report on (diacylvinylaryloxy) acetic acids has shown that compound 40.**105**, Table 40.13, is approximately three times as active as ethacrynic acid (154). The corresponding (acylvinylaryloxy) acetic acids are less active, e.g., 40.**107** (Table 40.13) (156). The 4-(2-nitropropenylphenoxyacetic acid derivatives (40.**106**, Table 40.13) are also three to five times as active as ethacrynic acid (166).

It can be seen from these examples that the presence of the double bond activated toward nucleophilic attack is critical to the high potency of these compounds. Interestingly, the cysteine adduct of ethacrynic acid is still a highly potent diuretic; however, only those sulfhydryl (or other nucleophilic) adducts are diuretic that also show *in vitro* a ready exchange for other sulfhydryl reagents, e.g., mercaptoacetic acid.

Ethacrynic acid is characterized by excellent oral absorption and rapid onset of action when administered orally or intravenously (157). Excretion by both glomerular filtration and tubular secretion is rapid and the duration of action short. The drug recovered from the urine is about equally divided into three fractions, the parent compound, a cysteine adduct, and an unstable metabolite of undetermined nature (157).

Table 40.13 Structure–Activity Relationships of Ethacrynic Acid Analogs

No.	Structure	Diuretic Activity (dog i.v.)	$T_{1/2}$,[a] min	Ref.
40.**99**	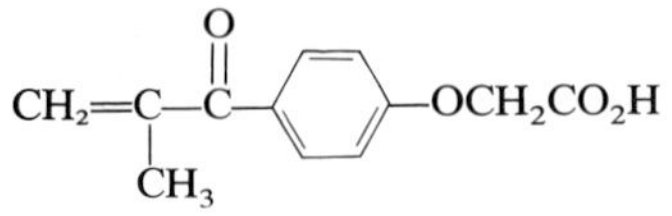 CH$_2$=C(CH$_3$)–C(=O)–⟨C$_6$H$_4$⟩–OCH$_2$CO$_2$H	±	90	153
40.**100**	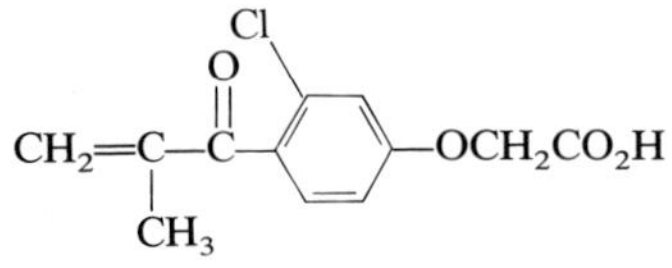 CH$_2$=C(CH$_3$)–C(=O)–⟨C$_6$H$_3$(Cl)⟩–OCH$_2$CO$_2$H	+2	11	153
40.**101**	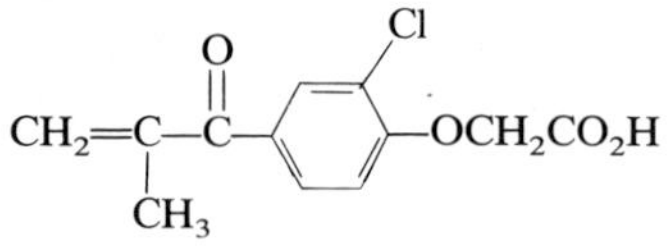 CH$_2$=C(CH$_3$)–C(=O)–⟨C$_6$H$_3$(Cl)⟩–OCH$_2$CO$_2$H	+1	27	153
40.**102**	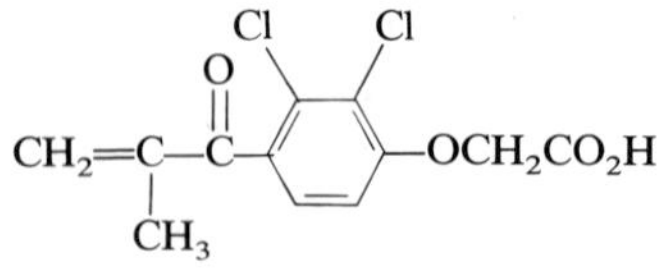 CH$_2$=C(CH$_3$)–C(=O)–⟨C$_6$H$_2$(Cl)(Cl)⟩–OCH$_2$CO$_2$H	+3	1	153
40.**103**	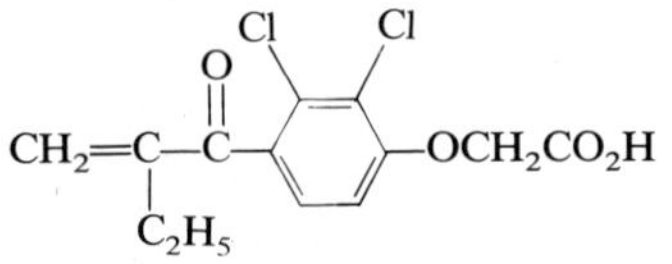 CH$_2$=C(C$_2$H$_5$)–C(=O)–⟨C$_6$H$_2$(Cl)(Cl)⟩–OCH$_2$CO$_2$H ethacrynic acid	+6	<1	153
40.**104**	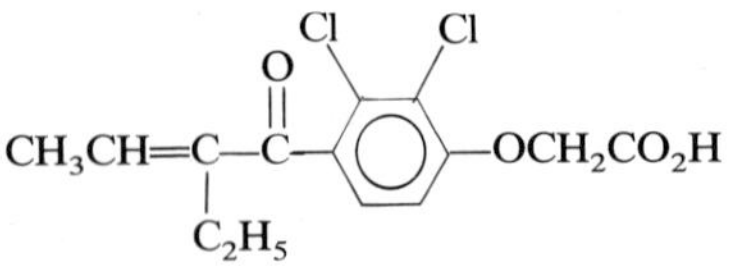 CH$_3$CH=C(C$_2$H$_5$)–C(=O)–⟨C$_6$H$_2$(Cl)(Cl)⟩–OCH$_2$CO$_2$H	+5	(210)	153
40.**105**	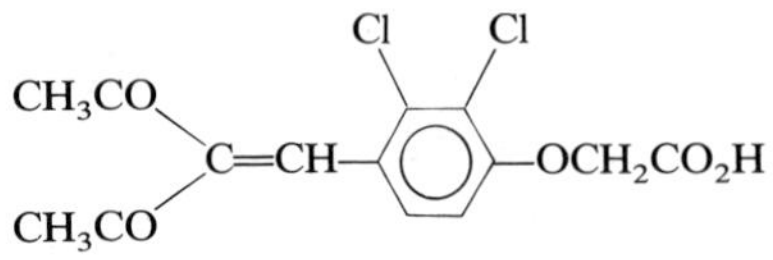 (CH$_3$CO)$_2$C=CH–⟨C$_6$H$_2$(Cl)(Cl)⟩–OCH$_2$CO$_2$H	(+7)	2	153, 154
40.**106**	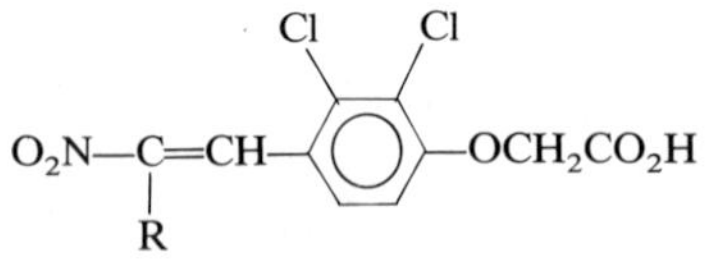 O$_2$N–C(R)=CH–⟨C$_6$H$_2$(Cl)(Cl)⟩–OCH$_2$CO$_2$H R = CH$_3$, C$_2$H$_5$	+6	2	153
40.**107**	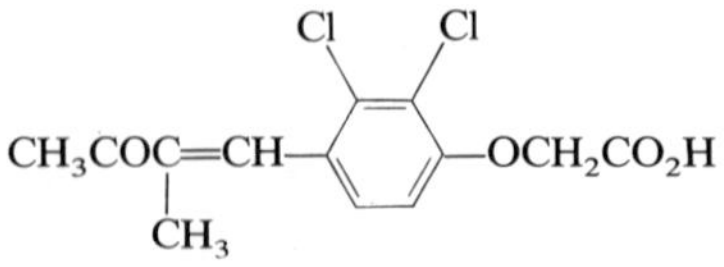 CH$_3$COC(CH$_3$)=CH–⟨C$_6$H$_2$(Cl)(Cl)⟩–OCH$_2$CO$_2$H			156

[a] $T_{1/2}$ = Time in minutes required for one-half of a standard amount of test compound to react with excess mercaptoacetic acid at pH 7.4 and 25°C in DMF–phosphate buffer analogous to the procedure of Duggan and Noll (155).

Ethacrynic acid does not inhibit carbonic anhydrase *in vitro*. It has a steeper dose–response curve than hydrochlorothiazide and the magnitude of its maximum saluretic effect is several times that of hydrochlorothiazide (157). The renal corticomedullary electrolyte gradient, after administration of ethacrynic acid and other high ceiling diuretics, is virtually eliminated as a result of nearly total inhibition of Na^+ transport in the ascending limb of Henle (158). The clinical dose lies between 50 and 200 mg/day. In a long-term study, the antihypertensive effects of 100 mg ethacrynic acid were similar to 50 mg hydrochlorothiazide in patients with mild hypertension (167). Ethacrynic acid as well as furosemide continue to be effective diuretics even at very low glomerular filtration rates and are therefore useful in the treatment of patients with chronic renal failure (168). Ototoxicity has been reported; this manifests itself as transient deafness (168). Permanent deafness has also been observed after treatment with high doses of ethacrynic acid in renal failure (169).

9.3   Furosemide

At the time work on ethacrynic acid was proceeding at Merck, Sharp and Dohme, furosemide was being developed in the Hoechst laboratories in Germany. Investigation of a series of 5-sulfamoylanthranilic acids, 40.**108**, substituted on the aromatic amino group showed that these compounds were effective diuretics. The isomeric series (40.**109**) did not show saluretic properties (154, 160).

More than 100 variously substituted derivatives were studied pharmacologically, but only those that corresponded to the general structure 40.**108** exhibited outstanding saluretic activity. The most active was furosemide 40.**108** (R = 2-methylfurfuryl) (Table 40.12). In contrast to the dihydrobenzothiadiazine diuretics, where the substituent in the 3 position of the heterocyclic ring can be varied to a considerable degree, the requirements for high activity in the 5-sulfamoylanthranilic acid series are much more stringent. On parenteral and oral administration to different species and to man, the degree of diuretic effect elicited, as measured by urine flow and Na^+ and Cl^- excretion, was several times that obtainable with the thiazide diuretics (161, 162).

In a study undertaken to explore the effect of furosemide on water excretion during hydration and hydropenia in dogs it was found that as much as 38% of filtered sodium was excreted during furosemide diuresis and both C_{H_2O} and TC_{H_2O} were inhibited, indicating a marked effect in the ascending loop of Henle. During antidiuresis as much as 38% of the glomerular filtrate was excreted, strongly suggesting that furosemide also acts in the proximal tubule (15, 162). To a large extent furosemide is excreted unchanged in the urine, but a metabolite, 4-chloro-5-sulfamoylanthranilic acid, has been identified (164, 165). Studies by Hook et al. (170) and Ludens et al. (171) indicate that furosemide reduces renal vascular resistance and therby enhances total renal blood flow in dogs.

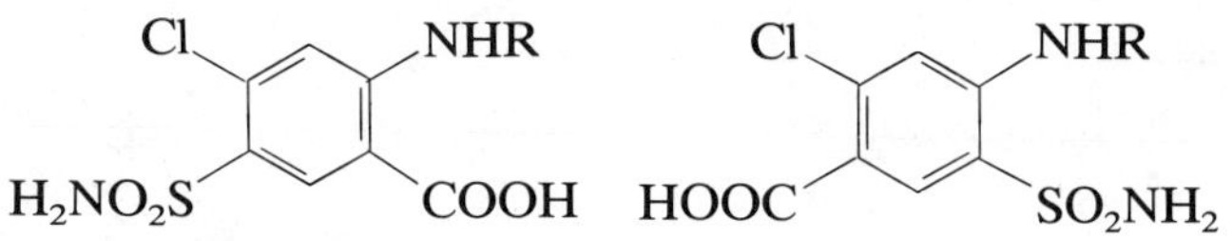

40.**108**

40.**109**

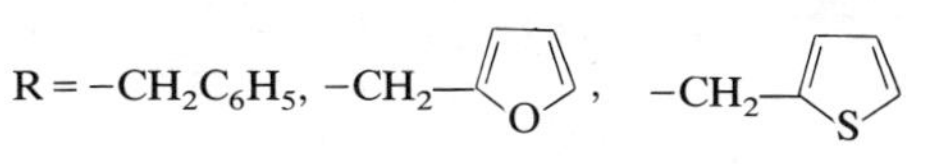

$R = -CH_2C_6H_5, -CH_2-\!\!\!\overset{O}{\diagdown}\,, -CH_2-\!\!\!\overset{S}{\diagdown}$

Clinical studies in normal subjects and in patients with edema of various etiologies have clearly shown that furossmide is an extremely potent saluretic drug (172, 173).

The antihypertensive effects of furosemide were shown to be qualitatively and quantitatively similar to chlorothiazide in nonedematous patients with essential hypertension (174). Furosemide has been reported to produce a moderate diuretic response in patients with renal disease and resistant edematous states, when other diuretics e.g., thiazides, mercurials, triamterene, spironolactone, have failed. Doses up to 1.4 g/day may be required (175, 176). Ototoxicity has also been reported following large doses of furosemide (177).

9.4 Bumetanide

In a series of papers starting in 1970, Feit and co-workers in Denmark investigated the diuretic activity of derivatives of 3-amino-5-sulfamoylbenzoic acid 40.**110**. In the initial series R_2 was chlorine, and R_1 was varied widely from alkyl to substituted benzyl. The most interesting compound was 40.**111**, 3-butylamino-4-chloro-5-sulfamoylbenzoic acid, which approached the activity of furosemide when given i.v. (10 mg/kg in NaOH solution) to dogs. Interestingly, whereas in the anthranilic acid–furosemide series the N-2-methylfurfuryl substituent afforded outstanding activity, this was not the case in this series (178).

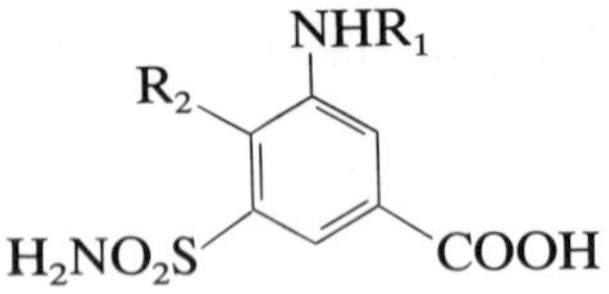

Further investigation showed that compounds in which $R_2 = -OC_6H_5$, $-NHC_6H_5$, or $-SC_6H_5$ (40.**110**) are much more active diuretics; the structure and saluretic activity in dogs of the more active derivatives are shown in Table 40.14.

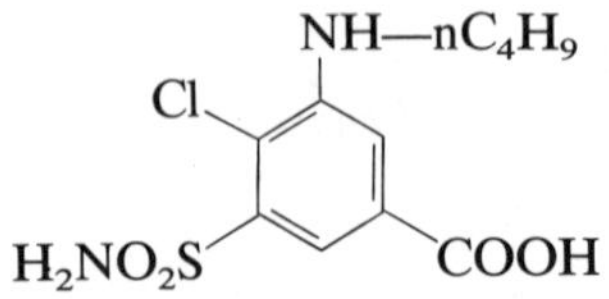

Compound 40.**117**, Table 40.14, bumetanide was the most interesting and has been studied extensively (179). Further structure–activity studies uncovered related compounds with equally high diuretic potency; compounds 40.**119**–40.**134**, Table 40.15, are representative of the series studied. It was found that a phenoxy group in the 4 position enhances activity in the anthranilic acid series as well as in the 3-amino-5-sulfamoylbenzoic acid series, e.g., compound 40.**119** (180). The phenoxy group could be replaced by C_6H_5CO, $C_6H_5CH_2$ (181), and even a directly bonded C_6H_5 group (184), e.g., compounds 40.**120**, 40.**121**, and 40.**127** (Table 40.15).

Interestingly, an equilibrium appears to exist between the benzisothiazole 40.**120** and the corresponding benzoyl derivative 40.**136**. In the case of compound 40.**136** dehydration occurred and only the benzisothiazole derivative was isolated. It is postulated, however, that at physiological pH in the body the compound is present as the open ring benzoyl derivative 40.**136**. Compounds 40.**130** and 40.**131**, Table 40.15, which do not have an amino substituent attached to the benzene ring of the sulfamoylbenzoic acid, were more stable and only cyclodehydrated on heating (184).

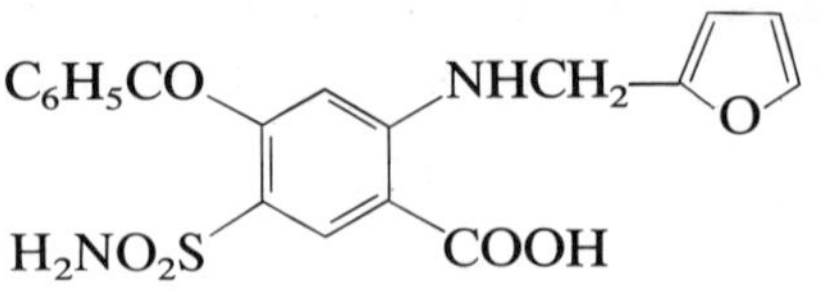

40.**110**

40.**111**

40.**136**

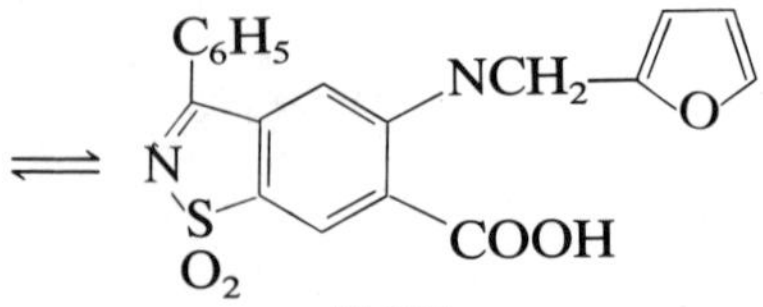

40.**120**

Table 40.14 Compounds Related to Bumetanide (179)

No.	Structure	Dose, mg/kg p.o.	Volume, ml/kg Urine	Urinary Excretion per 6 hr (Dog), meq/kg		
				Na$^+$	K$^+$	Cl$^-$
40.**112**	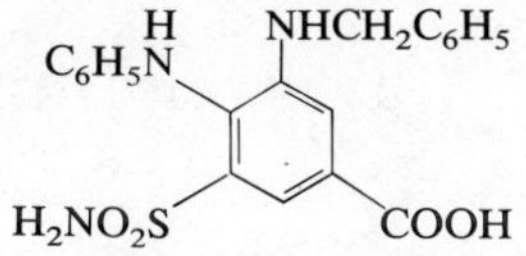 C$_6$H$_5$NH, NHCH$_2$C$_6$H$_5$, H$_2$NO$_2$S, COOH	0.1	39	3.7	0.6	4.8
40.**113**	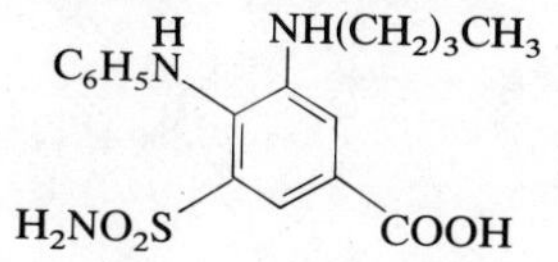 C$_6$H$_5$NH, NH(CH$_2$)$_3$CH$_3$, H$_2$NO$_2$S, COOH	0.1	31	3.2	0.9	4.5
40.**114**	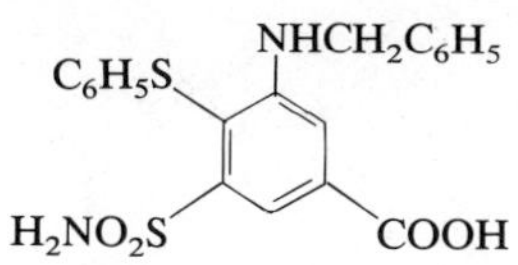 C$_6$H$_5$S, NHCH$_2$C$_6$H$_5$, H$_2$NO$_2$S, COOH	0.1	38	3.1	0.9	5.0
40.**115**	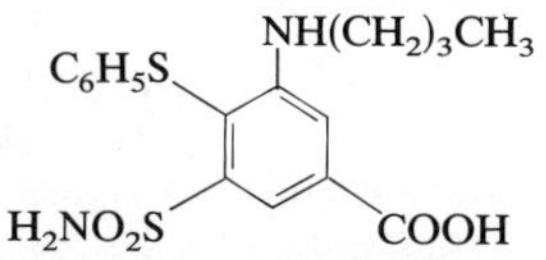 C$_6$H$_5$S, NH(CH$_2$)$_3$CH$_3$, H$_2$NO$_2$S, COOH	0.25	40	4.0	1.1	5.7
40.**116**	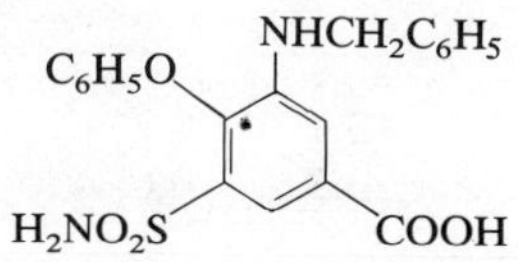 C$_6$H$_5$O, NHCH$_2$C$_6$H$_5$, H$_2$NO$_2$S, COOH	0.1	36	4.0	2.1	5.9
40.**117**	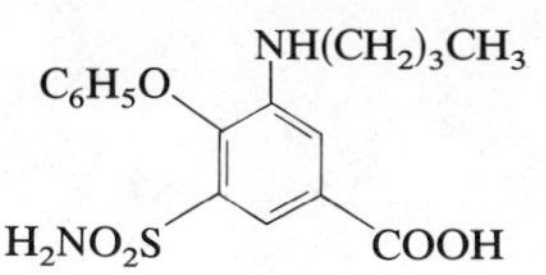 C$_6$H$_5$O, NH(CH$_2$)$_3$CH$_3$, H$_2$NO$_2$S, COOH, bumetanide	0.25	51	4.8	1.0	7.0
		0.1	31	3.3	0.49	4.5
		0.01	13	1.2	0.3	1.4
		0.25 i.v.	39	4.0	0.84	5.7
40.**118**	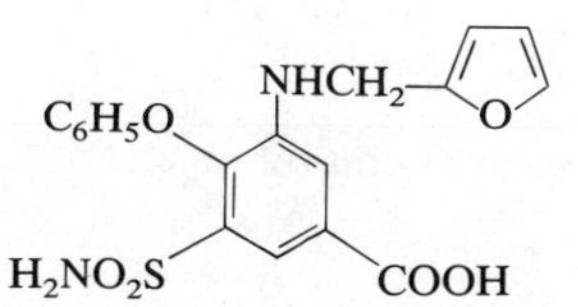 C$_6$H$_5$O, NHCH$_2$-furyl, H$_2$NO$_2$S, COOH	0.05	27	3.2	0.6	3.9
40.**108**	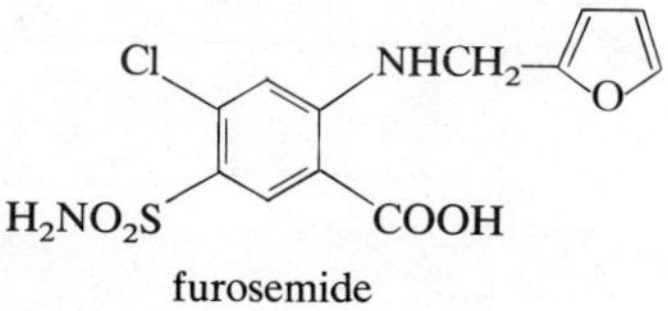 Cl, NHCH$_2$-furyl, H$_2$NO$_2$S, COOH, furosemide	0.5	8	1.5	0.2	1.8

Table 40.15 Compounds Related to Bumetanide

No.	Structure	dose, mg/kg i.v.	Volume, Urine, ml/kg	Urinary Excretion per 3 hr, meq/kg			Ref.
				Na$^+$	K$^+$	Cl$^-$	
40.**119**		1.0 0.1	43 25	5.0 2.9	0.8 0.45	6.4 3.8	180
40.**120**		1.0 0.1	44 26	4.8 2.7	0.7 0.8	5.9 3.3	181
40.**121**	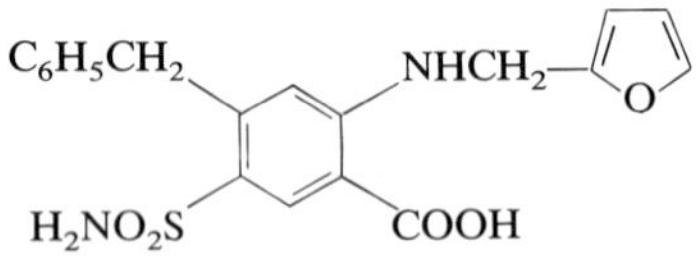	0.25	19	2.1	0.4	2.7	181
40.**122**	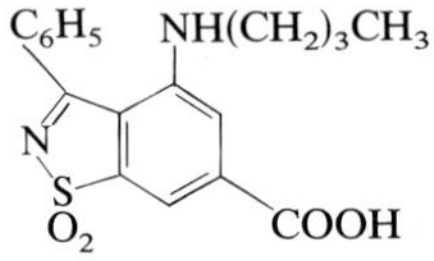	0.25	18	2.4	0.4	2.9	182
40.**123**	 besunide	0.25 0.25 p.o.	28 29	3.1 3.3	0.7 0.6	4.2 4.1	182
40.**124**		0.1 0.1 p.o.	25.7 29.8	2.5 3.3	0.57 0.69	3.5 3.8	183
40.**125**	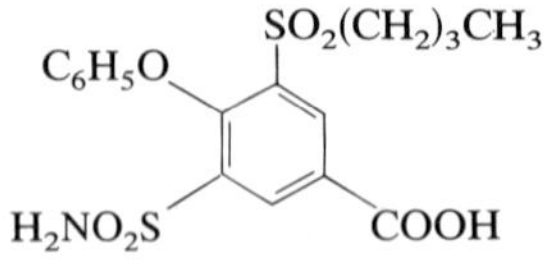	1.0	Same as control				183
40.**126**	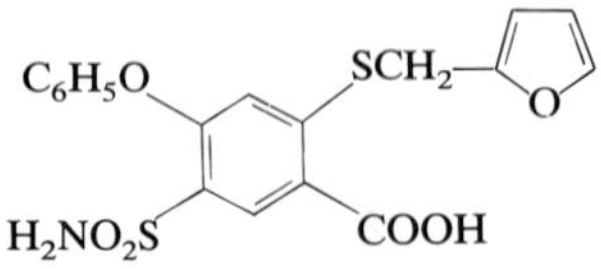	1.0	8	0.8	0.3	0.8	183

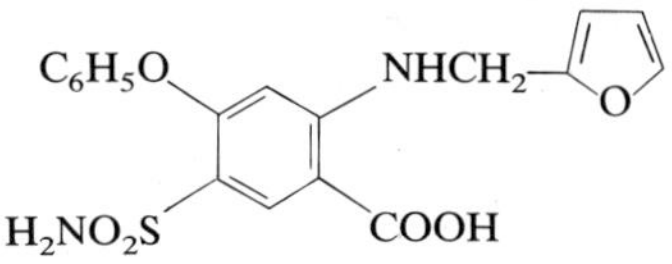

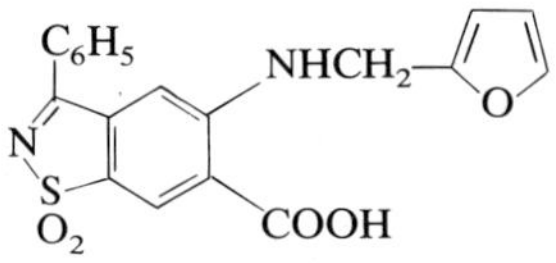

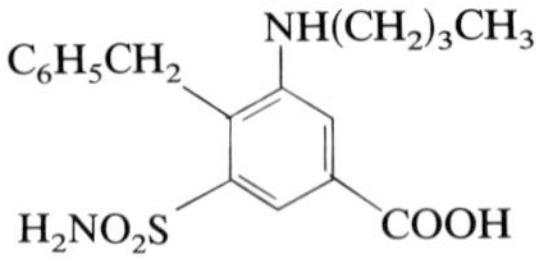

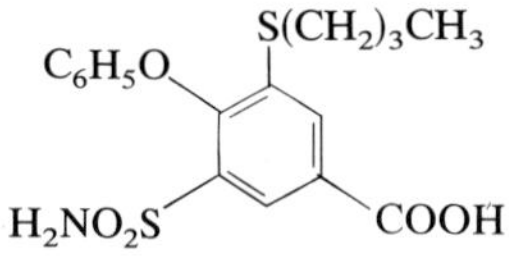

182

Table 40.15 (*Continued*)

No.	Structure	dose, mg/kg i.v.	Volume, Urine, ml/kg	Urinary Excretion per 3 hr, meq/kg			Ref.
				Na$^+$	K$^+$	Cl$^-$	
40.**127**	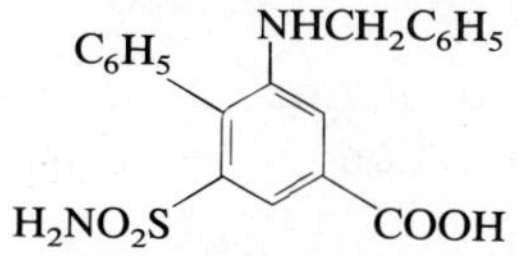 C_6H_5, NHCH$_2$C$_6$H$_5$, H$_2$NO$_2$S, COOH	1	23	3.3	0.81	3.4	184
40.**128**	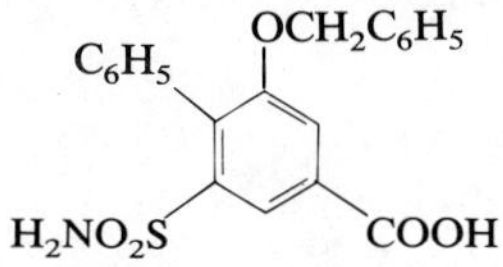 C_6H_5, OCH$_2$C$_6$H$_5$, H$_2$NO$_2$S, COOH	1	28	3.2	0.64	4.1	184
40.**129**	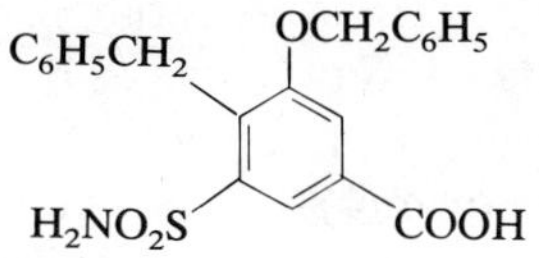 C$_6$H$_5$CH$_2$, OCH$_2$C$_6$H$_5$, H$_2$NO$_2$S, COOH	0.1	26	3.0	0.59	4.1	184
40.**130**	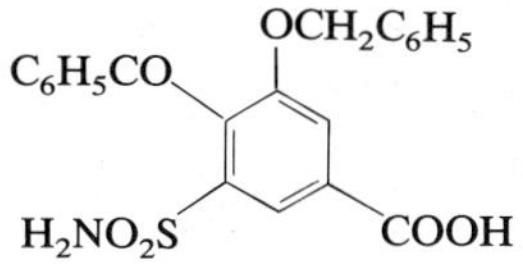 C$_6$H$_5$CO, OCH$_2$C$_6$H$_5$, H$_2$NO$_2$S, COOH	0.25 / 0.1	33 / 12	3.6 / 1.0	0.89 / 0.42	4.4 / 2.0	184
40.**131**	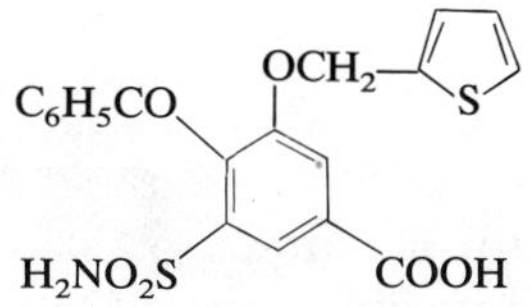 C$_6$H$_5$CO, OCH$_2$-thienyl, H$_2$NO$_2$S, COOH	0.1 / 0.01	38 / 23	4.4 / 2.5	0.97 / 0.53	4.9 / 3.5	184
40.**132**	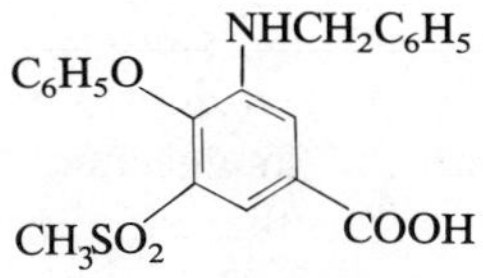 C$_6$H$_5$O, NHCH$_2$C$_6$H$_5$, CH$_3$SO$_2$, COOH	1	31	4.8	0.98	5.1	185
40.**133**	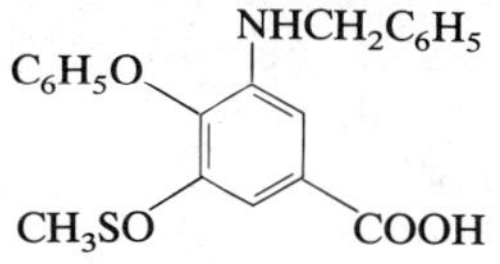 C$_6$H$_5$O, NHCH$_2$C$_6$H$_5$, CH$_3$SO, COOH	1	7	0.9	0.17	1.1	185
40.**134**	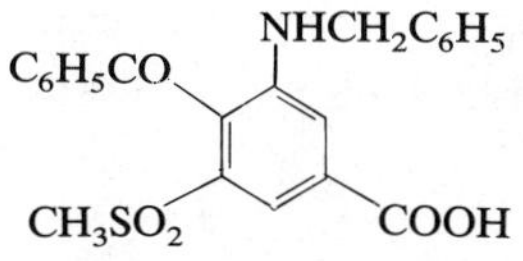 C$_6$H$_5$CO, NHCH$_2$C$_6$H$_5$, CH$_3$SO$_2$, COOH	1 p.o.	33	3.9	0.64	4.7	185
40.**135**	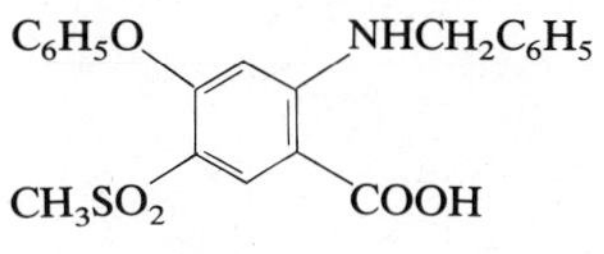 C$_6$H$_5$O, NHCH$_2$C$_6$H$_5$, CH$_3$SO$_2$, COOH	10	Same as control				185

In the 3-amino-5-sulfamoylbenzoic acid series the 3-amino substituent can be replaced by an OR or SR group (40.**124**, 40.**128**, 40.**131**, Table 40.15) (183, 184); however, oxidation of the SR group to SO_2R (40.**125**, Table 40.15) eliminates the diuretic activity (183). Compound 40.**131**, Table 40.15, is one of the most potent benzoic acid diuretics ever reported. It shows significant diuretic activity in dogs at 1 μg/kg, which represents a potency approximately five times as high as bumetanide (184). In the anthranilic acid series the structural requirements are more exacting and the thiosalicyclic acid analog (40.**126**, Table 40.15) is only weakly active (183).

A series of compounds in which the sulfamoyl group is replaced by a methylsulfonyl group was also investigated (185). Many of the 5-methylsulfonylbenzoic acid derivatives showed considerable diuretic activity, e.g., 40.**132** and 40.**134**, Table 40.15. The diuretic patterns of these compounds resembled those of previously discussed corresponding sulfamoylbenzoic acids. However, substitution of the sulfamoyl group by the spatially and sterically similar methylsulfonyl group generally led to decreased potency. Substitution of methylthio or methylsulfinyl for the methylsulfonyl group reduced the potency considerably. e.g., 40.**133**, Table 40.15. The anthranilic acid analog (40.**135**, Table 40.15) of the highly active 3,4-substituted methylsulfonylbenzoic acid derivative 40.**132**, Table 40.15, was inactive at the dose tested, again confirming that the structural requirements in the anthranilic acid series are more demanding.

Interestingly, replacement of the chloro group in hydrochlorothiazide, by a C_6H_5S

group (40.**137**) eliminated the diuretic activity (186). Similar results were found in the case of quinethazone and clopamide (40.**79**, 40.**75**, Table 40.10) (186).

9.4.1 PHARMACOLOGY. Bumetanide is a potent diuretic in dogs after both oral and i.v. administration. It is comparable to furosemide in its type of action and its maximum effect, but when given orally bumetanide is approximately 100 times more active. In dogs the drug is excreted extremely rapidly by glomerular filtration and tubular secretion. No metabolites were detected in dogs (187). A parallelism between bumetanide excretion and saluretic action in man over the total period of response has been shown (188). The drug is a highly potent diuretic in patients with congestive heart failure (189, 190) and in subjects with liver cirrhosis (191). Studies in man indicate a major site of action in the ascending limb of the loop of Henle; a significant phosphaturia induced during the period of maximum diuresis suggests an additional action on the proximal tubule (192, 193). Bumetanide produces a rapid diuretic response with a pattern of salt and water excretion resembling that of furosemide. At the time of maximal diuresis 13–23% of the filtered load of sodium is excreted; urinary calcium and magnesium are also increased. As with other sulfonamide diuretics, hyperuricemia is seen following prolonged therapy. There is no evidence of significant metabolism of bumetanide in man (195). Microperfusion studies of isolated renal tubular fragments from rabbits and rats confirmed the findings that the thick ascending limb of the loop of Henle is the major site of action of bumetanide (194).

The recommended clinical dose is 1–5 mg/day.

9.5 Indapamide

Indapamide (40.**138**, Table 40.12) is a high ceiling diuretic similar to furosemide and bumetanide, but lacks a free carboxyl

40.**137**

40.**138**

group (196). In a study in normal subjects given a single oral dose of 40 mg, pronounced diuresis was found starting 3 hr after ingestion and continuing for a total of 36 hr. A drop in systolic blood pressure occurred 24 hr after ingestion, coincident with the period of maximum dehydration. Free water clearance (C_{H_2O}) rose, which may indicate inhibition of proximal tubular reabsorption of sodium. No change in plasma HCO_3^- was seen at the time of a transient urinary alkalinization. In animals indapamide does not inhibit carbonic anhydrase. The prolonged activity of the drug can be correlated with its comparatively slow elimination and long biologic half-life. The slow elimination of indapamide may be explained by the greater lipid solubility of the molecule. Interestingly, only 4.4% of the ingested dose was excreted unchanged in the urine over a 48 hr period. Preliminary data indicate that indapamide is extensively metabolized in man (197).

Using ^{14}C labeled indapamide it was shown that following oral administration the drug is rapidly absorbed into plasma, enters the red blood cells, and is bound reversibly to the carbonic anhydrase fraction, producing concentrations four times higher than those found in plasma (198). Radioactivity was slowly eliminated into urine (60%) and feces (20% of the dose) over 8 days. Less than 5% of the dose was excreted in the urine unchanged (198).

The antihypertensive effect of indapamide has been studied in cats, dogs, and rats. The drug exerted an antihypertensive effect in experimental hypertensive animals and after a 10 day pretreatment period also markedly reduced the cardiovascular reac-

tivity to various pressor agents. Since after similar pretreatment with hydrochlorothiazide, no changes in cardiovascular reactivity were observed, indapamide may have a novel mode of action as an antihypertensive agent (199, 200).

Satisfactory control of blood pressure in patients with mild to moderate hypertension was achieved with doses of 5–15 mg daily. Potassium supplements are recommended (201, 202).

9.6   Piretanide

Piretanide, HOE 118 (40.**139**, Table 40.12) is a new high ceiling diuretic related to bumetanide. Studies in rats indicated that it is an effective saluretic at doses as low as 1–2 mg/kg in rats with a favorable Na/K ratio (203). Studies in other species and in the clinic must be considered before the role of this new diuretic can be assessed.

9.7   Triflocin

The discovery of triflocin (40.**140**, Table 40.12) resulted from a study of derivatives of flufenamic acid for possible antiinflammatory activity. Compounds incorporating a nicotinic acid moiety unexpectedly exhibited diuretic activity. Triflocin is a structurally novel and highly efficacious diuretic agent capable of promoting the excretion of as much as 30% of the sodium chloride filtered at the glomerulus. It was effective in the rat, rabbit, guinea pig, dog, and monkey. Triflocin was characterized by excellent oral absorption, rapid onset of action, and short duration of effect. The magnitude of diuresis produced by the compound is similar to that seen with furosemide and ethacrynic acid. The renal sites of action are interpreted to be the proximal tubule and the ascending limb of Henle (204, 205). Interestingly, a study of rats and dogs indicated that triflocin has no propensity for evoking hyperglycemia

(206). The drug was studied in normal volunteers and found to be a markedly potent natriuretic agent; free water clearance (C_{H_2O}) was inhibited during water diuresis and solute-free water reabsorption TC_{H_2O} reduced during hydropenia, indicating a major site of action in the ascending limb of Henle. In addition a fall in glomerular filtration rate of 10–15% was found at doses of 1 g given orally (207). Long-term toxicity studies revealed adverse effects; clinical studies were therefore discontinued (208).

9.8 Xipamide

Xipamide (40.**141**, Table 40.12) is a derivative of 5-sulfamoyl salicyclic acid (209); 4-chloro-5-sulfamoylsalicyclic acid itself had previously been reported by Feit and co-workers (186) to be a high ceiling diuretic. Investigation of esters, aliphatic, cycloaliphatic, aromatic and heterocyclic amides, ureides, and hydrazides of 4-chloro-5-sulfamoylsalicyclic acid showed that 4-chloro-2',6'-dimethyl-5-sulfamoyl-salicylanilide is the most active derivative. Replacement of the Cl group by Br, F, or CF_3 led to compounds with lower activity. The effects of modification of the anilide group are shown in Table 40.16 (209). Compounds methylated on oxygen and/or nitrogen are less active.

The hydrazide (40.**149**, Table 40.16) corresponding to xipamide was also only weakly active. Interestingly, the 2,6-dimethylpiperidino derivative (40.**150**, Table 40.16) related to clopamide (40.**75**) is inactive (209).

Xipamide is active in rats and dogs following oral or i.v. administration. Application of 0.2 mg/kg i.v. in the dog accompanied by a continuous infusion of 5% mannitol solution led to a diuretic effect starting 40 min postinjection. After 2 hr a diuretic effect could still be detected. An antihypertensive effect in spontaneous

Table 40.16 Analogs of Xipamide (209)

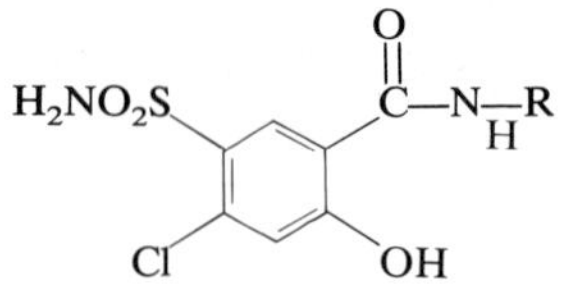

No.	R	Urine Volume in rats, ml/kg	
		Dose 1 mg/kg	Dose 100 mg/kg
Controls		4–5	
40.**141**	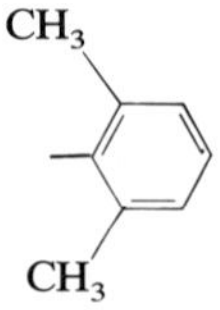	22.0	41.6
40.**142**	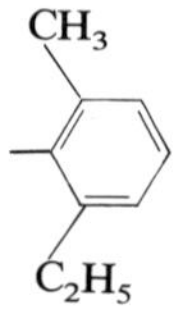	8.1	16.4
40.**143**	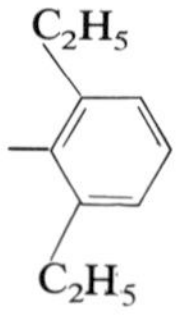	3.2	11.1
40.**144**	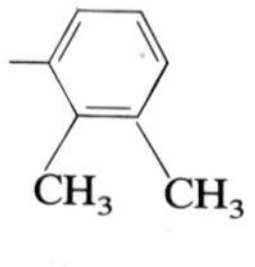	>10[a]	11.4
40.**145**	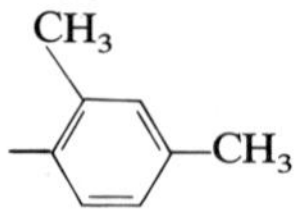	0.56[a]	13.8
40.**146**	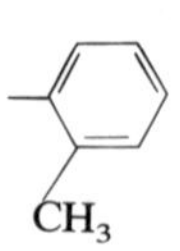	0.60[a]	31.2
40.**147**	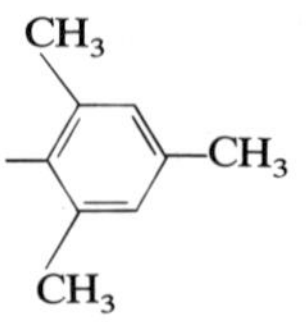	0.74[a]	17.8

Table 40.16 (*Continued*)

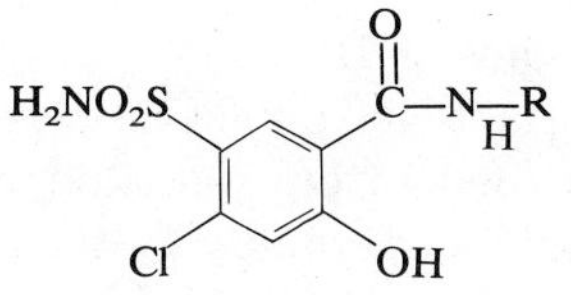

No.	R	Urine Volume in rats, ml/kg	
		Dose 1 mg/kg	Dose 100 mg/kg
Controls		4–5	
40.**148**	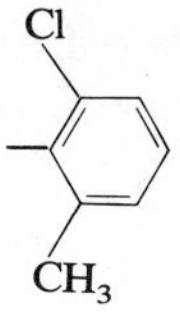	*ca.* 5[a]	19.6
40.**149**	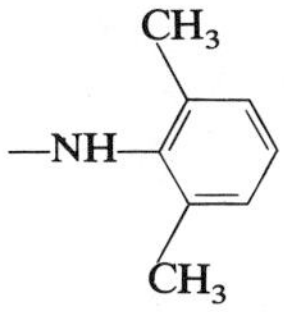	1.1	11.5
40.**150**	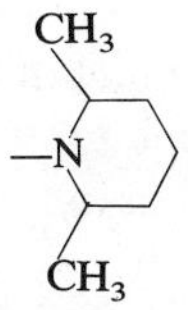	—	0

[a] Dose in mg/kg which increases 5 hr urine volume by 50%.

hypertensive rats was observed following 1 mg/kg p.o. (210). Xipamide is a weak carbonic anhydrase inhibitor, $ED_{50} = 1.1 \times 10^{-5} M$, comparable to sulfanilamide $ED_{50} = 1.3 \times 10^{-5} M$ or hydrochlorothiazide $ED_{50} = 2.3 \times 10^{-5} M$ (Table 40.4) (211). At its therapeutic plasma level, xipamide is bound to 99% to plasma proteins (212). In normal volunteers doses of 0.5 mg/kg p.o. of xipamide were more effective than 0.5 mg/kg chlorthalidone or furosemide. The diuretic effect lasted 24 hr with the maximum occurring during the first 12 hr (213). In an evaluation in patients with edema of cardiac origin

xipamide was found to be an effective diuretic at 40 mg/day p.o. Serum potassium levels were slightly lowered (214). In rats, serum potassium depletion could be avoided and an equilibrated potassium balance achieved in a 13 day study by combining xipamide with triamterene (215).

Although ototoxicity has been seen with salicyclic acid and with furosemide, studies with xipamide in guinea pigs did not reveal any ototoxicological properties (216).

9.9 Muzolimine

Investigation of a series of 1-substituted pyrazol-5-ones disclosed that some of the compounds were highly active diuretics (217). Muzolimine, Bay g 2821 (40.**151**, Table 40.12), was selected for further study (218).

The structure of this compound differs considerably from that of other high ceiling diuretics since it contains neither a sulfonamide nor a carboxyl group. Clearance studies in dogs indicated that muzolimine does not increase the glomerular filtration rate, but has a saluretic effect similar to furosemide, induced by inhibition of tubular reabsorption in the ascending limb of Henle's loop (219).

Micropuncture studies in rat kidneys showed that muzolimine was effective only when given as a peritubular perfusion and not when administered intraluminally, in contrast to furosemide and bumetanide, which were effective when applied either peritubularly or intraluminally (219). Renal Na,K-ATP activity *in vitro* is inhibited only at high concentrations; Mg-ATPase activity was not affected (220).

Preliminary studies with muzolimine in patients showed that the drug is a high ceiling diuretic with an onset of action and a peak diuresis similar to that of furosemide. The duration of action was 6–8 hr as compared to 3–5 hr after furosemide; 40 mg of muzolimine was more potent than 40 mg furosemide in all parameters investigated (221). In normal volunteers the threshold dose was 10 mg and the dose–response curve for sodium was practically linear for doses up to 80 mg (222). Acute water diuresis and hydropenic studies carried out in 7 normal volunteers suggested that muzolimine acts in the proximal tubule and in the medullary portion of the ascending limb of the loop of Henle (223).

9.10   MK 447

By screening procedures, 2-aminomethyl-3,4,6-trichlorophenol (40.**152**) was found to display significant saluretic–diuretic properties. Exploration of structure–activity relationships showed that alkyl substituents, preferably α-branched, in position 4 and halo substituents in position 6 resulted in greatly enhanced activity. Optimal activity was displayed by 2-aminomethyl-4-(1,1-dimethylethyl)-6-iodo-phenol, MK 447 (224) (40.**153**, Table 40.12).

The saluretic effects of MK 447 in rats and dogs were generally superior, both qualitatively and quantitatively, to those of earlier high ceiling loop diuretics. A study in normal volunteers confirmed the high potency of the compound. Despite copious diuresis and natriuresis, no significant change in the elimination rate of potassium was observed (225). MK 447 may act by stimulating prostaglandin PGE_2 biosynthesis; the compound has earlier been described as an anti-inflammatory agent which facilitates the conversion of prostag-

landin endoperoxide PGG_2 to PGH_2. Recent studies have indicated that the primary prostaglandins PGE_2 and $PGF_{2\alpha}$ are not the important inflammation-inducing agents obtained from arachidonic acid. Rather the endoperoxide PGG_2 itself, or a nonprostaglandin product derived from it, seems to be the major inflammatory agent (226). Recently, definite evidence has been obtained that low levels of PGE_2 and $PGF_{2\alpha}$ are present in human urine and that these prostaglandins may originate from the kidney (227). The prostaglandins can facilitate salt and water excretion, largely through effects on physical forces in proximal peritubular capillaries as evidenced by augmented renal blood flow (228). The role of renal prostaglandins has recently been reviewed (228, 229); their full significance is yet to be determined, however.

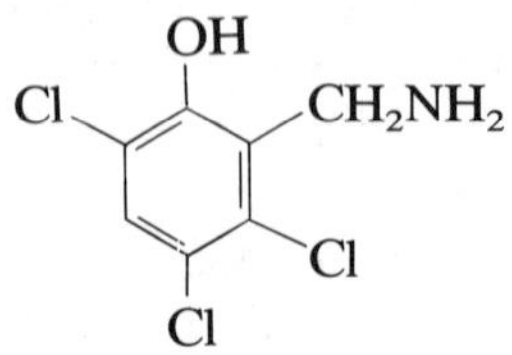

9.11   Etozolin

During the investigation of a series of 4-thiazolidones, some of which had choleretic properties (363), a number of compounds with high diuretic activity were found (364). Compound 40.**230** piprozoline is a choleretic compound without diuretic activity; compound 40.**231**, etozolin, is a highly active diuretic with weak choleretic properties. Minor deviations from structure 40.**231** led to a loss of diuretic activity. The different pharmacodynamic properties of 40.**230** and 40.**231** could not be traced to thermodynamic factors but rather must be related to closely defined receptor interactions (364).

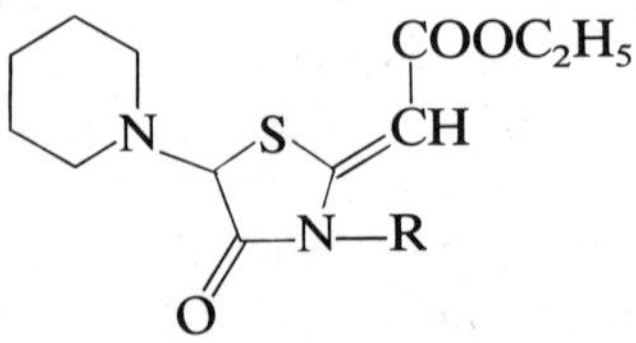

40.**152**

40.**230**   R = C_2H_5
40.**231**   R = CH_3

Long-term toxicity studies in rats and dogs have shown that etozolin is well tolerated and that it has a wide margin of safety (365). Studies in rats and dogs indicated that the compound is a potent saluretic with a relatively slow onset of action and prolonged activity. The maximal diuretic effect of etozolin lies between that of the thiazides and furosemide. Antihypertensive effects were seen in the spontaneous hypertensive rat, DOCA, and Goldblatt rat. Etozolin does not appear to influence glucose tolerance in rats and dogs; these results are of particular interest because the tests were carried out in animals that had been treated with high doses of drug for 18 and 12 months, respectively (366).

Clearance and micropuncture studies have shown that an initial dose of 50 mg/kg i.v. followed by 50 mg/kg/hr i.v. result in a markedly increased urinary flow and sodium excretion combined with a decreased glomerular filtration rate. Reabsorption in the proximal tubule was not affected significantly; however, fluid and electrolyte reabsorption in the loop of Henle were definitely decreased. Although etozolin differs chemically from furosemide and ethacrynic acid, it appears to share the same site of action in the nephron (367).

Absorption and metabolic studies with ^{14}C etozolin in the rat, dog, and man indicated that at least 90% is absorbed following oral administration in man. In the rat, blood levels could be described with a two-compartment body model, the absorption half-life being 0.6 hr and the elimination half-life approximately 6 hr. In man the elimination half-life was 8.5 hr; the blood levels followed with high probability a one-compartment body model (370).

The main metabolite of etozolin is the free acid formed by enzymatic cleavage of the ester group and its glucuronide. Other metabolites have also been detected (368, 369). The main metabolite appears to have the same pharmacokinetic properties as the parent compound (370).

Etozolin has been studied in normal volunteers and in patients. In normal volunteers a dose of 400 mg of etozoline was equipotent to 75 mg of a thiazide diuretic; 1200 mg was 2.8 times more effective than the 75 mg dose of the thiazide. Diuresis starts within 1–2 hr after dosing, reaches a peak after 2–4 hr, and then gradually decreases over the next 6 hr (371). Owing to the long-lasting effect of etozolin, the compound would seem indicated for the treatment of cardiac and renal edema as well as for the treatment of hypertension (372). No significant diuretic effect was observed in patients with moderate (glomerular filtration rate, 20–80 ml/min) or chronic (GFR < 20 ml/min) renal insufficiently (373). The drug was introduced in 1977 as Elkapin.

10   STEROIDAL ALDOSTERONE ANTAGONISTS

Renal conservation of Na^+ is a complex process. Among the humoral factors known to affect rates of urinary Na^+ excretion, aldosterone (40.**154**), a hormone of the adrenal cortex, is the most potent of the steroidal regulators. The sites of action of aldosterone have been studied by micropuncture techniques and found to be the distal tubule and the collecting ducts (230, 231). More recent studies have localized the site of action to the collecting duct (3).

In some edematous conditions there is increased tubular reabsorption of Na^+, brought about by an excessive secretion of aldosterone. It is possible to counteract this

40.**154**

in two ways: (1) by blocking the action of aldosterone at the renal tubular site, and (2) by inhibiting the biosynthesis of aldosterone.

During the late 1950s Cella, Kagawa, and associates reported (232–236) on the synthesis and structure–activity relationships of a series of steroidal spirolactones with aldosterone blocking activity. This type of biological activity was established because the compounds had no action in adrenalectomized animals unless aldosterone or another mineralocorticoid was administered prior to the spirolactone (233), and because the spirolactones produced the same effect as impaired aldosterone synthesis (237).

The first compound of interest was 3-(3-oxo-17β-hydroxy-4-androsten-17α-yl)propanoic acid lactone (40.**155**), which showed aldosterone-blocking activity when administered subcutaneously to rats. Studies on related compounds established the importance, for activity, of both the five-membered spirolactone and the 3-keto-Δ^4 function in ring A. An isomer of 40.**155** with the opposite configuration at C-17 was devoid of activity (238). However, the 19-nor analog, 40.**156**, was somewhat more active than 40.**155** in rats.

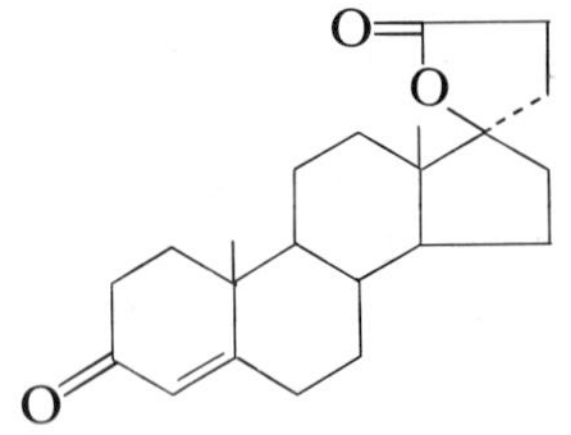

Rats maintained on a low-sodium diet and treated with 40.**156**, with consequent renal loss of Na^+, compensated by increasing aldosterone secretion (239). Likewise, sodium diuresis was accompanied clinically by increased aldosterone excretion in the urine (240). The compound has been used clinically with success in primary aldosteronism (241), in cases of nephrotic edema (242, 243), and in hepatic cirrhosis (243, 244), but patients with cardiac failure did not respond well (243). The effect of 40.**156** is determined by the degree to which sodium reabsorption is controlled by aldosterone, and thus it is ineffective in patients with untreated Addison's disease (245) and in normal subjects with a low-sodium diet (246). Because the compound blocks the effect of aldosterone on the kidney, Na^+ and Cl^- excretion are increased whereas K^+, H^+, and NH_4^+ excretion are decreased. This represents a different electrolyte excretion pattern from most other diuretics, which increase K^+ excretion to some extent.

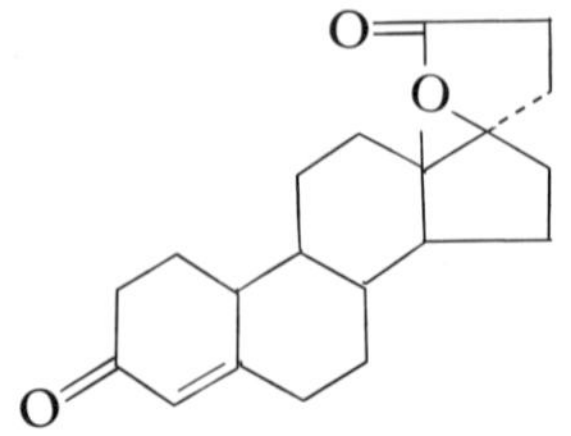

Both 40.**155** and 40.**156** showed much better activity after parenteral administration than when given orally, and therefore new compounds were sought with improved absorption characteristics. Some degree of success was achieved by the introduction of additional double bonds into 40.**155** at positions 1 and 6 to give 40.**157**, 40.**158**, and 40.**159**, all of which showed increased oral activity compared to the parent compound (235). Enhancement of oral activity was also noted with substitution of an acetylthio grouping at position 1α (40.**160**), and even better results were obtained with this substituent at position 7 (40.**161**). The latter compound, 3-(3-oxo-7α-acetylthio-17β-hydroxy-4-androsten-17α-yl)propanoic acid lactone (spironolactone), has undergone extensive pharmacological and clinical studies. It is interesting that in spite of markedly increased oral activity, both 40.**160** and 40.**161** were less active by the parental route than the

40.**155**

40.**156**

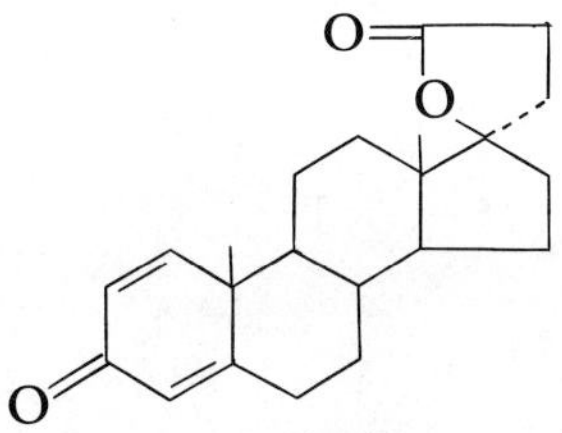

40.**157** 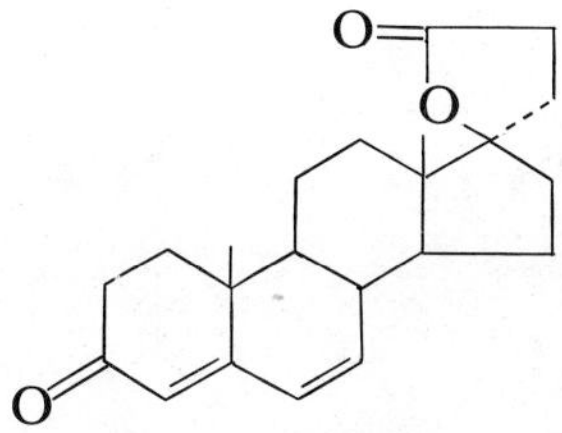   40.**158** 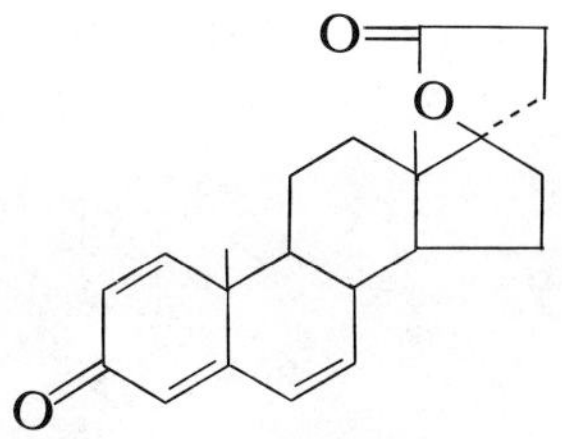   40.**159**

parent compound 40.**155**. In further synthetic work on related structures inversion of the 7-acetylthio group in spironolactone reduced both the oral and parenteral activity by 90%, whereas 6-methylation did not change the activity significantly (247). Other structural modifications of 40.**155**, such as introduction of methyl groups at 2, 4, 6, 7, or 16, keto or hydroxyl substituents at position 11, or a fluoro substituent at position 9, did not impart to the resulting compounds properties superior to 40.**161** (248, 249). The spirolactams 40.**162** and 40.**163**, corresponding to 40.**155** and

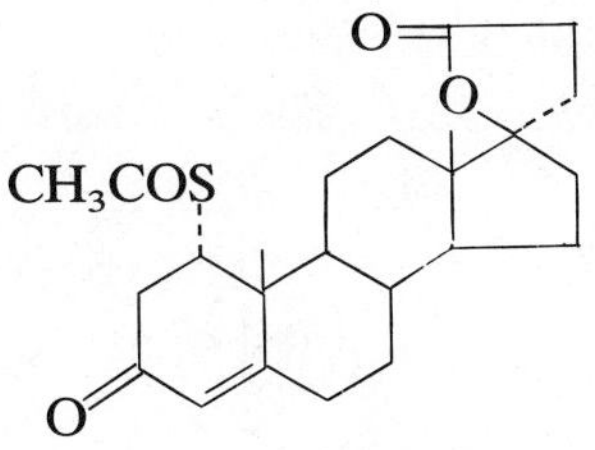

Several metabolites of spironolactone (40.**164**–40.**168**) have been isolated from the urine of normal subjects (253, 254).

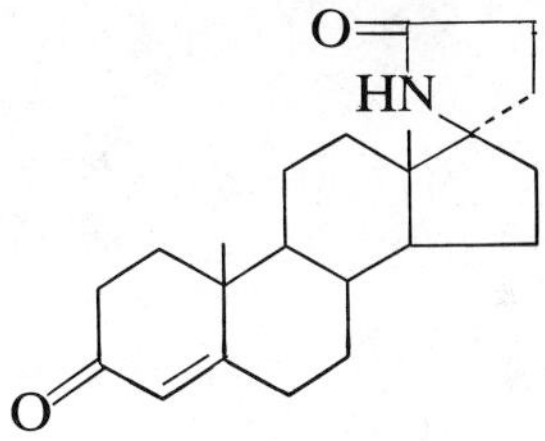

40.**162**

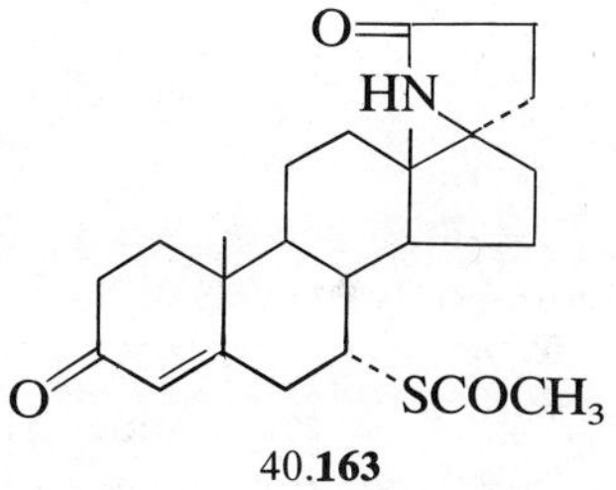

40.**163**

In earlier investigations (255) postasium 3-(3-oxo-17β-hydroxyl-4,6-androstadien-17α-yl)propanoate (40.**169**), a water-soluble, open lactone salt was obtained from saponification of 40.**158**. The compound was equally effective orally and parenterally, and was approximately

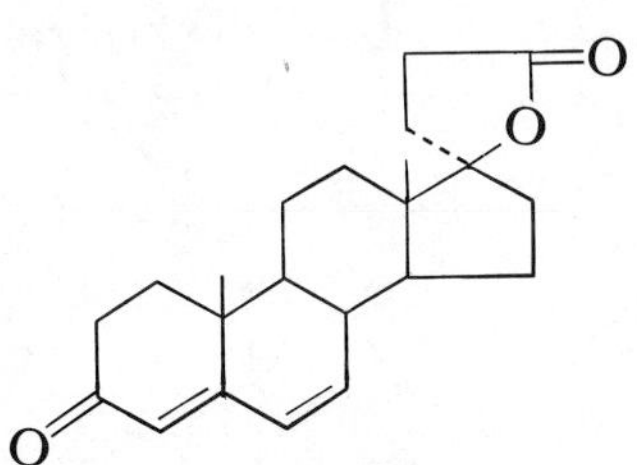

40.**160**

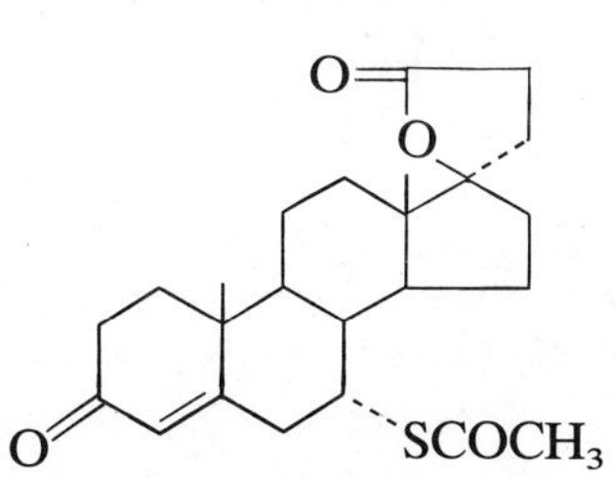

40.**161**

spironolactone (40.**161**), respectively, have been synthesized (250, 251), but have no significant aldosterone-blocking activity (252).

40.**164**

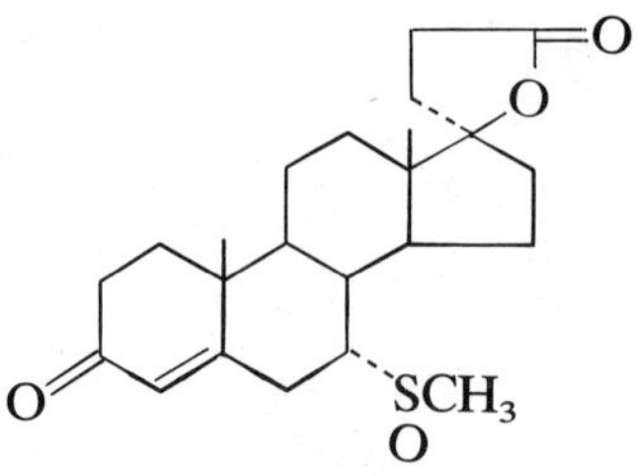

40.**165**

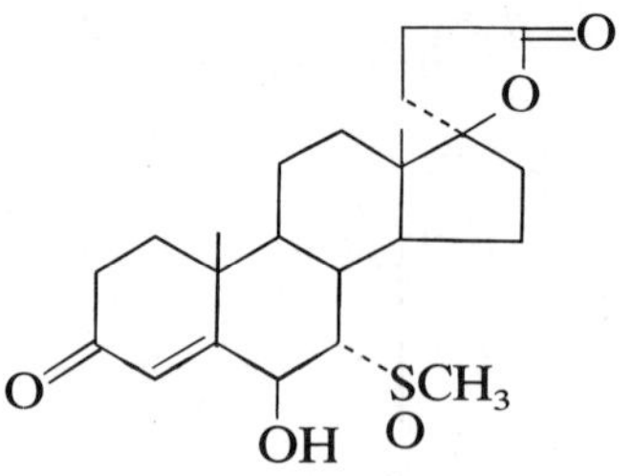

40.**166**

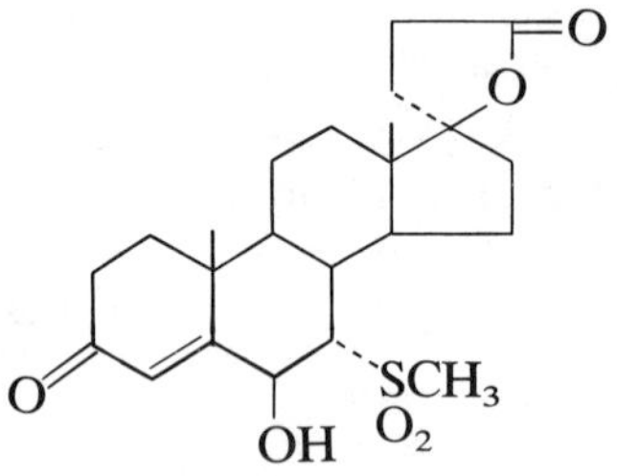

40.**167**

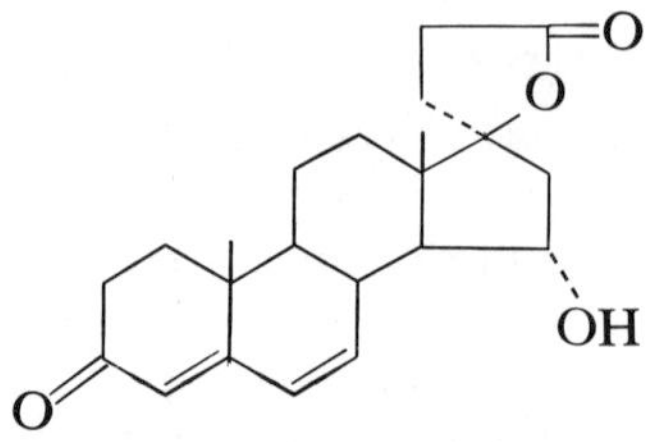

40.**168**

equipotent with spironolactone. It was relatively ineffective in the absence of mineralocorticoids. Potassium canrenoate (40.**169**, Table 40.17) is a specific antagonist of mineralocorticoids with pharmacodynamic properties like those of spironolactone.

Continued search for new steroidal aldosterone antagonists led to potassium prorenoate (40.**170**, Table 40.17). Potassium prorenoate is a water-soluble steroidal compound with the ability to antagonize the sodium-retaining and, when apparent, the potassium-dissipating effects of mineralocorticoids (256). In the aldosterone-treated dog, the compound had three times the potency of spironolactone. Prorenoate is relatively inactive at the renal level in adrenalectomized rats without

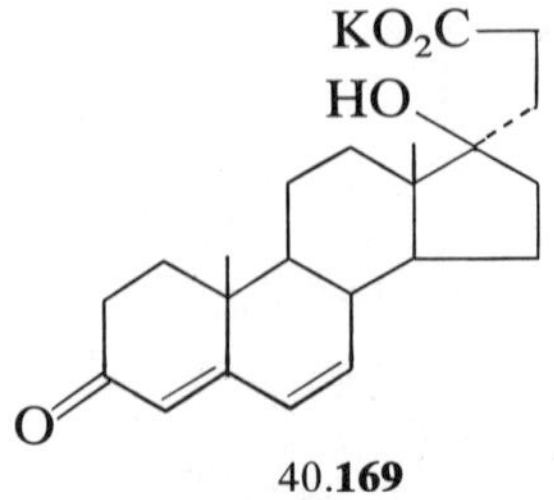

mineralocorticoid replacement. The compound possesses no more than 2% of the natriuretic activity of hydrochlorothiazide in the intact animal. Clearance studies in dogs indicated a direct renal tubular site of interaction between prorenoate and aldosterone (256). The relative potency of prorenoate and spironolactone was compared

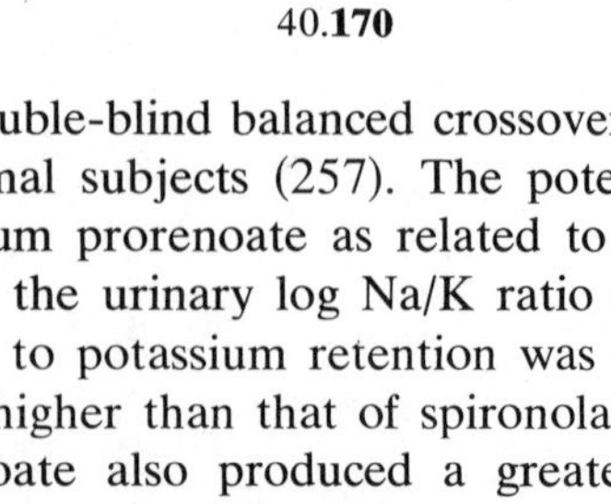

40.**170**

in a double-blind balanced crossover study in normal subjects (257). The potency of potassium prorenoate as related to elevation of the urinary log Na/K ratio and as related to potassium retention was significantly higher than that of spironolactones. Prorenoate also produced a greater natriuresis, but the difference was not significant. In *in vivo* experiments it was found that prorenoate is converted to the corresponding spirolactone (258).

40.**169**

A new series of steroidal aldosterone antagonists was prepared based on the finding
that introduction of a carbalkoxy function
in the 7α position of steroidal spirolactones
enhances the activity. The most interesting
compound in this series was potassium
mexrenoate 40.**171**, Table 40.17 (259).
The oral activity of the hydroxycarboxylic
acid, 40.**171**, was superior to that of the
corresponding spirolactone, 40.**172**. Potassium mexrenoate is a water-soluble compound. Dose-related natriuretic responses,
indexed as a reversal (increases) in the
aldosterone-depressed urinary $\log Na/K$

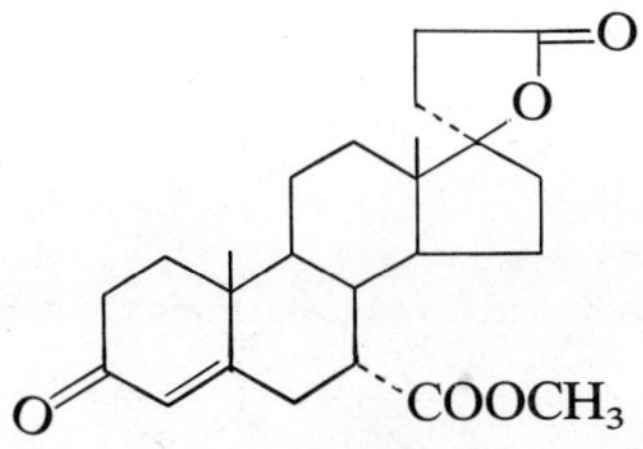

40.**172**

ratio indicated that mexrenoate was between 2.1 (dog) and 4.5 (rat) times as potent as spironalactone. Based on sodium
output, in intact rats, mexrenoate was
essentially inactive as a diuretic. Diuretic

Table 40.17 Steroidal Aldosterone Antagonists

No.	Generic Name	Trade Name	Structure	Ref.
40.**161**	Spironolactone USP (24–75 mg)	Aldactone	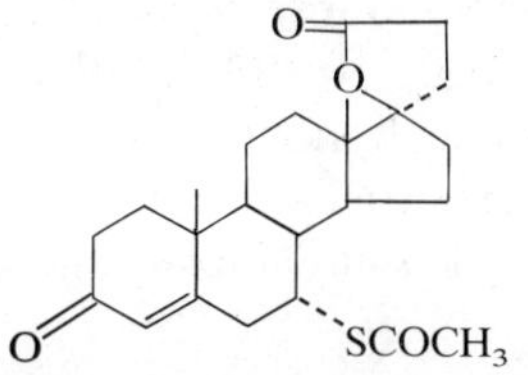	235
40.**169**	Potassium canrenoate	Soldactone	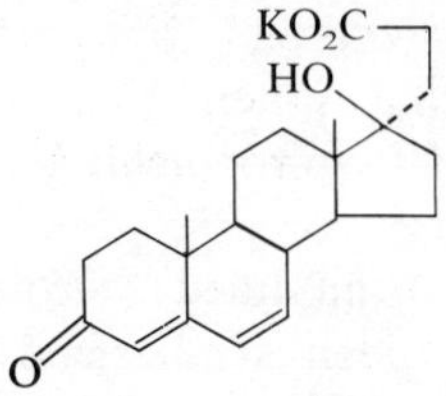	255
40.**170**	Potassium prorenoate		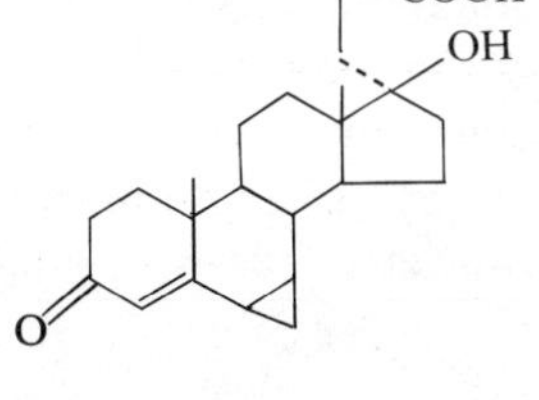	256
40.**171**	Potassium mexrenoate		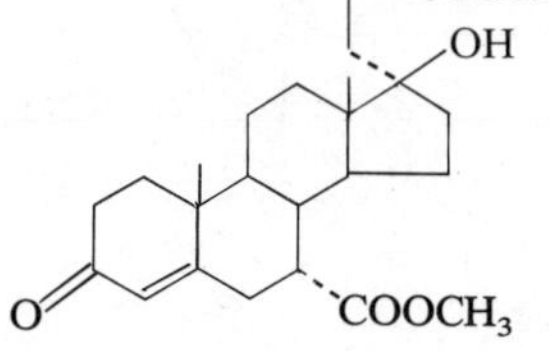	258

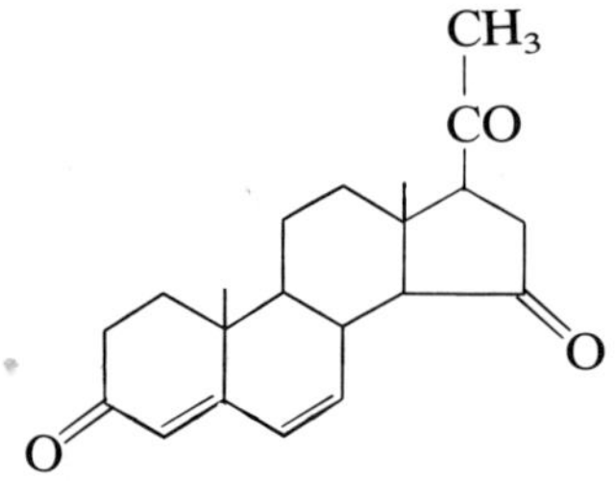

40.**173**

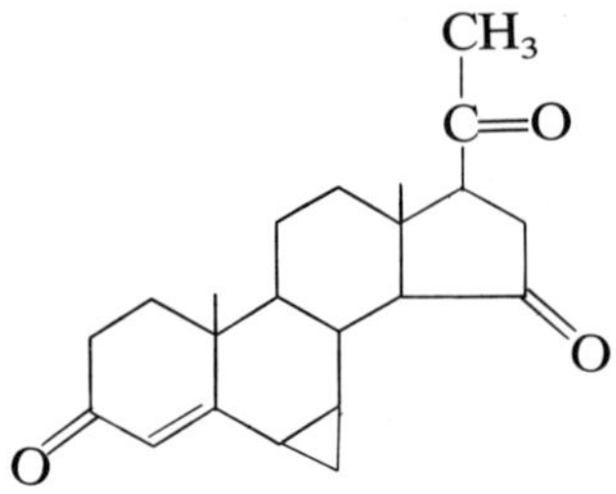

40.**174**

potency, however, was not indicative of antihypertensive activity. In dogs with established hypertension (Page model) both mexrenoate and spironolactone exhibited equivalent antihypertensive responses (260).

Progesterone has been reported to block aldosterone at high doses. This effect is enhanced by the introduction of an oxygen function at C-15 and insertion of a Δ^1 or Δ^6 double bond, e.g., 40.**173**. Methylenation of the Δ^6 double bond to yield 15-keto-6β,7β-methyleneprogesterone, 40.**174**, resulted in decreased antialdosterone activity (261).

A 16β-hydroxyspirolactone 40.**175** has also been prepared but the antimineralocarticoid potency is less than 14% of that of spironolactone, 40.**161** (262).

A number of modified steroidal type structures have been synthesized and examined for mineralocorticoid-blocking activity. An analog of 40.**155** lacking ring A (40.**176**) blocks the sodium-retaining activity of the mineralocorticoids to some extent (263). In more extensive modifications of the steroid nucleus some 2-naphthyl-

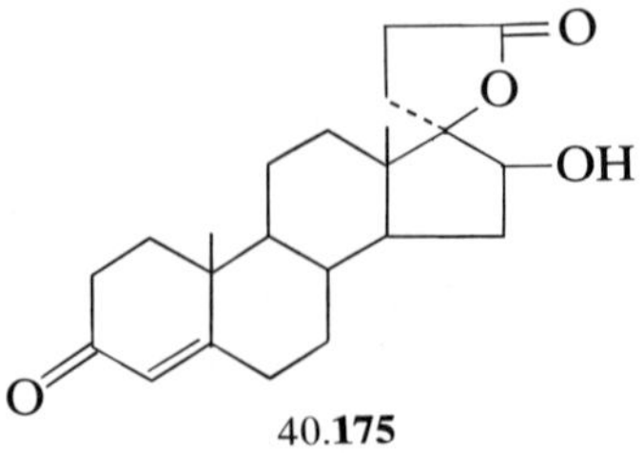

cyclopentanol ketones (40.**177**) were synthesized and evaluated for blocking activity (264). The hydroxymethyl ketone 40.**177** (X = OH) showed the best properties in the series, being effective when administered by both the subcutaneous and oral routes. With X = F or Cl activity is reduced.

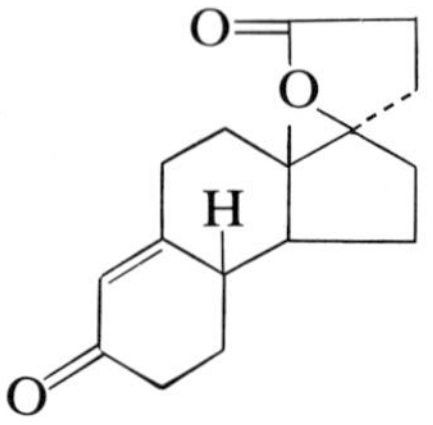

40.**176**

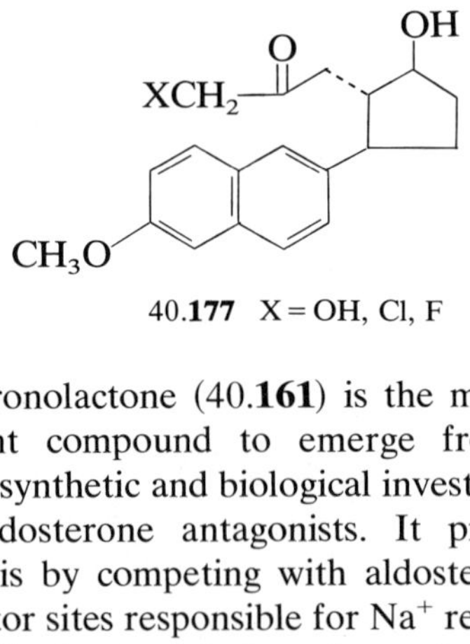

40.**177**   X = OH, Cl, F

Spironolactone (40.**161**) is the most important compound to emerge from the many synthetic and biological investigations on aldosterone antagonists. It promotes diuresis by competing with aldosterone at receptor sites responsible for Na$^+$ reabsorption. The best results have been obtained in patients with cirrhosis and the nephrotic syndrome, in whom the aldosterone secretion rate is very high. It has been much less impressive in patients with congestive heart failure, in whom aldosterone secretion is not normally raised. Spironolactone causes

40.**175**

Na$^+$ diuresis without K$^+$ secretion, leading to particular interest in using the drug in the treatment of cirrhosis with ascites, a condition in which most other diuretics would cause excretion of excessive amounts of K$^+$.

The usual dose of spironolactone is 25 mg four times daily, but as much as 300 mg/day may be administered safely, either alone or in combination with other diuretics. The compound has no anti-inflammatory or other glucocorticosteroid activity, and no estrogenic, progestational, or androgenic properties have been noted. There appears to be no depression of adrenal or pituitary function.

Spironolactone, when administered for several weeks to hypertensive patients, has a modest antihypertensive action, but no effect on blood pressure is seen in normotensive subjects. The drug also increases the antihypertensive effect of chlorthalidone and other diuretics. This effect may be due to an alteration of the extracellular–intracellular sodium gradient (265).

Recently spironolactone was found to be a tumorigen in chronic toxicity studies in rats at high doses (266).

11   ALDOSTERONE INHIBITORS

Compounds that inhibit the synthesis of aldosterone by the adrenal cortex theoretically have potential diuretic activity, but these are not of practical usefulness.

Metyrapone 40.**178** exemplifies this type of compound (267). Metyrapone has undergone considerable biological and clinical study. In moderate doses it blocks 11β-hydroxylation and so inhibits the production and secretion of hydrocortisone, corticosterone, and aldosterone. However, compensatory secretion of 11-deoxycorticosterone, a potent salt-retaining hormone, negates the effects of reduced aldosterone levels.

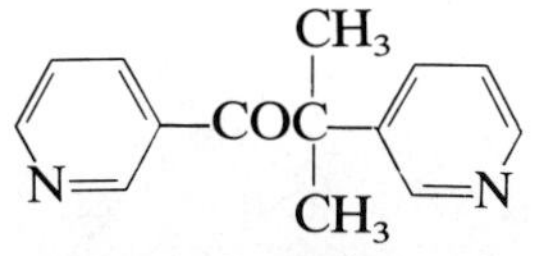

40.**178**

12   CYCLIC POLYNITROGEN COMPOUNDS

12.1   Xanthines

The use of xanthines as diuretics in the form of extracts of tea and coffee has been known for centuries. Of the xanthines, theophylline has the greatest action on the kidney. Theophylline is used mainly in the form of a double compound with ethylenediamine, i.e., aminophylline (40.**179**, Table 40.18). Numerous attempts were made to improve the diuretic properties and to reduce CNS stimulation of theophylline by modification of the xanthine structure but were not successful (268).

The xanthines exert their diuretic effect by decreasing tubular electrolyte reabsorption and by increasing the glomerular filtration rate. The increase in glomerular filtration rate, however, is not essential to the diuretic response. Administration of xanthines during water diuresis causes a rise in the concentrations of Na$^+$ and Cl$^-$ in the urine, providing good evidence of an effect on the tubular transport of these ions. The transport systems for other ions apparently are unaffected by xanthines, and the observed increase in K$^+$ excretion is probably nonspecific (269).

Sixty years ago the xanthines were employed widely for their diuretic properties.

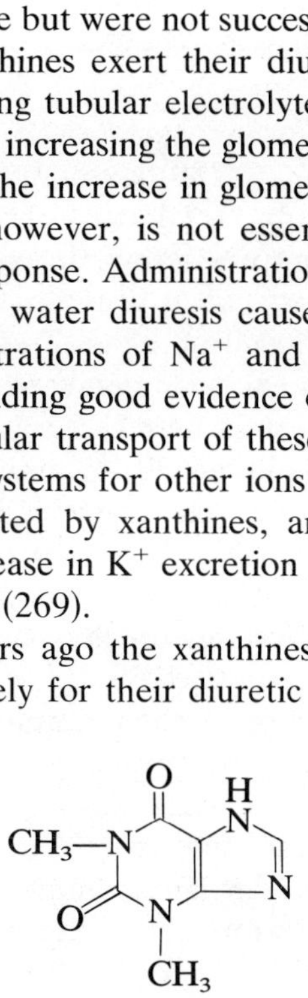

40.**179**

Since then their use for this purpose has steadily declined as better agents have become available, and they now have little therapeutic value as diuretics. Aminophylline is used mainly to relax bronchial smooth muscle and to stimulate the myocardium.

12.2   Aminouracils

During an extensive study of compounds related to the xanthines, the observation was made that certain of the intermediate substituted 6-aminouracils administered orally showed considerable diuretic activity in animals (270).

40.**180**

The 1,3-disubstituted derivatives of 6-aminouracil (40.**180**) are diuretics, whereas the monosubstituted compounds are not. The 1-n-propyl-3-ethyl derivative, which was the most potent diuretic in the series, was unsuitable for clinical use owing to gastrointestinal side effects. The compounds that were used clinically are 1-allyl-3-ethyl-6-aminouracil, aminometradine (40.**181**), and the 1-methallyl-3-methyl analog (40.**182**, Table 40.18). Clinical studies in edematous subjects indicated that mercurial diuretics usually have a greater and more reliable effect (271).

At the time of their development they represented some advance over the xanthines, but they were displaced by more effective oral diuretics within a relatively short time. Aminometradine is currently not available for general use in the United States.

12.3   Triazines

Recognition of the triazines as a class of diuretic agents stemmed from the work of Lipschitz and Hadidian (272), who tested a group of compounds of this type in rats, among them melamine (40.**183**) and formoguanamine (40.**184**). Formoguanamine was effective orally as a diuretic in man (273), but subsequent clinical studies revealed side effects such as crystalluria (274) and poor Na^+ excretion (275), which precluded its further use. A structural variant, prepared in an attempt to overcome the side effects, was diacetylformoguanamine (40.**185**), which was potent as an oral diuretic in dogs (276) but still caused crystalluria and inadequate Na^+ excretion. Unfortunately the extraordinary potency of the triazines in rats does not carry over into the dog and the compounds are only moderately active in man.

Among other derivatives of formoguanamine, those with one substituted amino group had a particularly favorable diuretic effect in rats (277). The most potent compounds in the series were 2-amino-4-anilino-s-triazine (40.**186**) (amanozine) and 2-amino-4-(p-chloroanilino)-s-triazine (40.**187**) (chlorazanil). The diuretic activity of the last two compounds was confirmed in dogs (278, 279) and also in man (280, 281). The m-chloro isomer of chlorazanil, 2-amino-4-(m-chloroanilino)-s-triazine, was a potent, orally effective diuretic in rats, dogs, and man (282, 283) and may be significantly more active than chlorazanil, with an enhanced saluretic

40.**183** $R_1 = NH_2$, $R_2 = R_3 = H$
40.**184** $R_1 = R_2 = R_3 = H$
40.**185** $R_1 = H$, $R_2 = R_3 = Ac$

Table 40.18 Cyclic Polynitrogen Compounds

No.	Generic Name	Trade Name	Structure	Ref.
40.**189**	Amiloride	Collectril		323
40.**181**	Aminometradine	Mictine		270
40.**182**	Amisometradine	Rolicton		270
40.**187**	Chlorazanil	Daquin, Diurazine, Orpizin		277
40.**198**	Clazolimine			327
40.**179**	Theophylline (aminophylline)		(Combination with $NH_2CH_2CH_2NH_2$ Ratio 2:1)	269
40.**188**	Triamterene	Dyrenium		296

40.**186** R = H
40.**187** R = Cl

effect. 2-Amino-4-(p-fluoroanilino)-s-tria-
zine was twice as active as chlorazanil
(279). Replacement of the halogen in
chlorazanil with acetyl, carbethoxy, or sulfamoyl groups reduced activity (284), but
replacement with methylmercapto and
some other alkylmercapto groups led to a
twofold increase in activity (285). Both the
incidence and degree of crystalluria in dogs
were greater with the alkylmercapto compounds than with chlorazanil, but oral toxicity in mice was reduced (285).

The only triazine to achieve any degree
of clinical use is chlorazanil. It has a more
pronounced effect on water excretion than
on Na^+ and Cl^- (281) and has little effect
on K^+ excretion, which is probably linked
to a lack of marked enhancement of Na^+
excretion. Since diuresis is not accompanied by changes in glomerular filtration
rate (286), the drug probably exerts its
action through inhibition of tubular reabsorption. The effects of deoxycorticosterone and chlorazanil on Na^+ and K^+
excretion are mutually antagonistic, which
may mean that the natriuretic and diuretic
properties of the drug are due to inhibition
of Na^+ reabsorption in the distal segment
(287).

The triazines, in particular chlorazanil,
have been employed clinically mainly in
Europe. Interest in this type of compound
declined with the advent of the more effective thiazide diuretics.

12.4 Potassium-Sparing Diuretics

12.4.1 INTRODUCTION. Three potassium-
sparing diuretics are currently in clinical
use: spironolactone (40.**161**, Table 40.17),
a steroidal aldosterone inhibitor discussed
in Section 10; triamterene; and amiloride
(40.**188**, 40.**189**, Table 40.18). The last two
compounds are basic, cyclic polynitrogen
compounds.

The sodium ion is the most important ion
in the body if one considers the composition of only plasma, extracellular fluid, and
ultrafiltrates. Nevertheless, the body as a
whole contains approximately 140 g potassium (K^+) and only 105 g sodium (Na^+). A
calculation shows that 98% of the K^+ is intracellular and only 2% is in the extracellular compartment. Therefore removal or addition of a small amount of K^+ to this
extracellular pool will be very evident
(288).

Triamterene and amiloride are potassium-sparing, not dependent on aldosterone, and have mild natriuretic activity
(289–291). Some years ago (1961) it was
shown that in the dog the filtered K^+ is
almost completely reabsorbed in the proximal segment and that the K^+ which appears
in the urine is introduced into the lumen of
the nephron at a more distal site (292).

The details of the processes by which K^+
enters the lumen in the distal segment have
been the subject of additional studies.
Sodium (Na^+) passively diffuses into the
cells of the tubule from the lumen; the Na^+
is pumped from the cells into the interstitium in exchange for K^+. This provides a
net electrical gradient across the cell of
about 45 mV and also maintains a high
concentration of K^+ within the cell. K^+ can
thus move passively into the lumen down
an electrical and chemical gradient. Therefore there is no need to assume an active
transport of K^+ at the lumen (293).

In the case of amiloride (40.**189**) experimental studies in rat kidneys by a free flow
micropuncture technique have established
that in drug-treated animals the transtubular potential is sharply reduced. Thus the
potential along which K^+ can move from
the cell into the lumen is reduced. At the

same time Na$^+$ influx from the lumen into the cells is decreased. The overall effect therefore is a mild natriuretic action accompanied by a decrease in passive K$^+$ secretion (294).

12.4.2 TRIAMTERENE. Pteridines in general have shown a rather diverse potential for influencing biological events. The observation that xanthopterin (40.**190**) was capable of affecting renal tissue led Wiebelhaus, Weinstock, and associates to test a series of pteridines in a simple rat diuretic screening procedure (295). One compound, 2,4-diamino-6,7-dimethyl-pteridine (40.**191**), showed sufficient diuretic activity to encourage further investigation of the diuretic potential of the pteridines. A number of related 2,4-diaminopteridines were studied but only 40.**191** showed good activity in both the saline-loaded and saline-deficient rat. Changes in the 2,4-diamino part of the molecule resulted in a marked decrease in diuretic activity (296).

Another class of related pteridines, of which 4,7-diamino-2-phenyl-6-pteridine-carboxamide (40.**192**) is the prototype, has been investigated. This derivative is active in both the saline-loaded and sodium-deficient rat, but in contrast to 40.**191**, it causes substantial K$^+$ loss in the sodium-deficient rat. In structure–activity studies particular attention was directed toward modification of the carboxamide function (296–298).

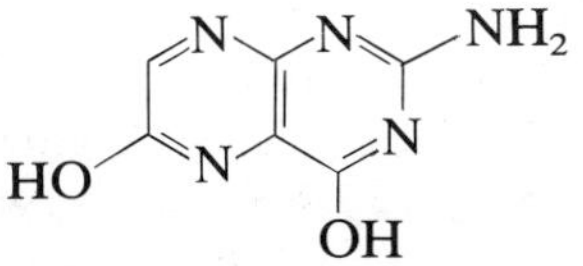

40.**190**

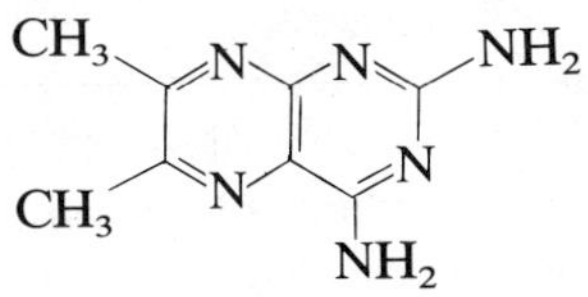

40.**191**

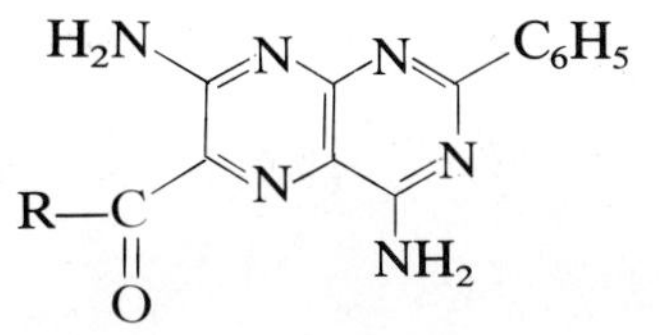

40.**192**   R = NH$_2$
40.**193**   R = NHCH$_2$CH$_2$N⟨   ⟩O

One of the more interesting compounds was 4,7-diamino-N-(2-morpholinoethyl)-2-phenyl-6-pteridinecarboxamide (40.**193**). In pharmacological investigations (299) this compound was an orally active diuretic agent, generating about the same maximum degree of response in dogs as hydrochlorothiazide. The urinary excretion of Na$^+$ and Cl$^-$ was markedly enhanced, with minimal augmentation of K$^+$ excretion and little effect on urine pH. Onset of action was rapid, with the greater saluretic effect occurring within 2 hr of oral administration to saline-loaded dogs. The compound showed diuretic activity in both normal and adrenalectomized rats, which, together with the absence of K$^+$ retention, indicated that aldosterone antagonism is not a major component of its saluretic activity.

A consideration of the structural features of 2,4-diamino 6,7-dimethylpteridine (40.**191**) and 4,7-diamino-2-phenyl-6-pteridinecarboxamide (40.**192**) led to the investigation of 2,4,7-triamino-6-phenylpteridine, triamterene (40.**188**), as a potential diuretic agent (296).

This compound was very potent in the saline-loaded rat, and in the sodium-deficient rat it not only caused a marked excretion of sodium but simultaneously decreased K$^+$ excretion. In structure–activity studies of compounds related to triamterene, replacement of one of the primary amino groups by lower alkylamino groups led to compounds that retained triamterene-like diuretic activity. More extensive changes generally led to substantially less active compounds. Table 40.19 lists the

Table 40.19   2,4,7-Triamino-6-substituted Pteridines (296)

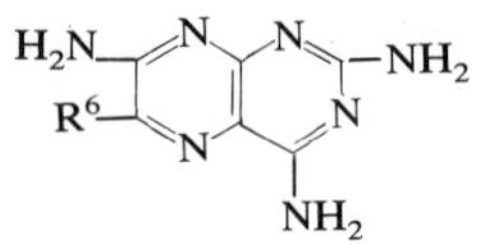

R^6	Diuretic Activity in Saline-Loaded Rat[a]	R^6	Diuretic Activity in Saline-Loaded Rat
C_6H_5 (triamterene)	$3(3)^b$	3-Thienyl	1(2)
2-$CH_3C_6H_4$	2(1)	4-Thiazolyl	0
3-$CH_3C_6H_4$	1(1)	2-Pyridyl	0
4-$CH_3C_6H_4$	2(1)	3-Pyridyl	0
2-FC_6H_4	2	4-Pyridyl	0
4-FC_6H_4	1	H	2(3)
4-$CH_3OC_6H_4$	1	CH_3	3(2)
4-$C_6H_5C_6H_4$	0	$CH(CH_3)_2$	1
2-Furyl	0(1)	$(CH_2)_3CH_3$	2(2)
3-Furyl	1(2)	Δ^3-Cyclohexenyl	1
2-Thienyl	2(2)	$CH_2C_6H_5$	2(2)

[a] Rating scheme for saline-loaded rat assay: maximum response at any dose, in volume per cent of urine, compared to volume of 0.9% saline load, less that of untreated control. $<22\% = 0$, $22–45\% = 1$, $46–69\% = 2$, and $>69\% = 3$. Rating scheme for sodium-deficient rat assay: maximum response at any dose, in milligrams of sodium excreted in the urine per rat. $<3\,mg = 0$, $3–6\,mg = 2$, and $>9\,mg = 3$.

[b] Numbers in parentheses refer to sodium-deficient rata data.

activities of some 2,4,7-triamino-6-substituted pteridines. In substitution of the phenyl group of triamterene only small changes are possible if diuretic activity is to be retained. The p-tolyl compound, for example, is only about half as active as triamterene. In general, ortho isomers seem to be more active than the other isomers. The p-hydroxy analog of triamterene, a metabolite of the latter, is essentially inactive. In an attempt to increase activity by reducing rate of metabolism, the 4-deutero analog of triamterene was prepared, but its activity is very similar to that of the parent compound. When the phenyl group of triamterene is replaced by a heterocyclic nucleus the size of the group again appears to be important, and high activity is seen only in the case of small, nonbasic groups.

The low activity of compounds containing basic centers in this position, such as thiazole and pyridine, may be rationalized by assuming that the basic centers are highly solvated and are, in effect, large substituents. The 6-alkyl analogs are active diuretics; however, size is important, because although good activity is seen in the 6-n-butyl homolog, the isopropyl and cyclohexenyl derivatives have only modest activity. Isomers of triamterene were also studied; the 7-phenyl isomer was one of the most potent K^+ blockers found in the pteridines even though it is only a weak natriuretic agent. The 2-phenyl isomer is very similar in its biological properties to triamterene. Among pyrimidopyrimidines related to triamterene, 2,4,7-triamino-5-phenylpyrimido[4,5-d]pyrimidine (40.**194**)

H$_2$N $\quad$ N $\quad$ N $\quad$ NH$_2$

N $\qquad\qquad$ N

C$_6$H$_5$ NH$_2$

40.**194**

was investigated in some detail. It resembled 40.**192** in not blocking K$^+$ excretion in the sodium-deficient rat.

The structure–activity relationships of pteridine diuretics may be rationalized by assuming that the pteridines bind to some active site at two points (296). The more important site involves a basic center of the drug, which in triamterene may be N-1, N-8, or both. Groups that decrease the base strength of the pteridine nucleus reduce activity. The other site probably involves the phenyl substituent of triamterene and may be hydrophobic in nature. There appear to be critical size limitations at this site, as shown by the change in activity in relation to methyl substitution. Because compounds such as 2,4,7-triaminopteridine are active, the phenyl group is not a primary requirement for activity and apparently acts in a reinforcing capacity, such as increasing the degree of binding and establishing the correct orientation of the molecule at the receptor site.

Triamterene (40.**188**) is a potent, orally effective diuretic in both the saline-loaded and sodium-deficient rat, with no increase in K$^+$ excretion. Also, the effects of aldosterone on the excretion of electrolytes in the adrenalectomized rat are completely antagonized by triamterene. Similar results were obtained in dogs, and it appeared that the compound might be functioning as an aldosterone antagonist (300). Initial clinical studies (301, 302) established the natriuretic properties of triamterene in man in cases when aldosterone excretion might be at an elevated level, and evidence was obtained for inhibition of the nephrotropic effect of aldosterone. However, triamterene possessed natriuretic activity in adrenalec-

tomized dogs and rats (303–305) and in an adrenalectromized patient (306), which was inconsistent with an aldosterone antagonism mechanism. Thus although triamterene reverses the end results of aldosterone, its activity does not depend on the displacement of aldosterone. The compound appears to act directly on a renal transport system for Na$^+$, including the system involved in Na$^+$/K$^+$ exchange (295). Stopflow studies in dogs pointed to an effect on the distal site on Na$^+$/K$^+$ exchange, and no evidence was found for a proximal renal tubular effect (307).

The overall effect of triamterene on electrolytes is to increase moderately the excretion of Na$^+$ and, to a lesser extent, of Cl$^-$ and HCO$_3^-$, and to reduce K$^+$ and NH$_4^+$ excretion (302, 308, 309). Triamterene is a more active natriuretic agent than spironolactone and is well absorbed following administration of single oral doses of 50–300 mg/day (301, 302). The duration of action of the drug in man is about 16 hr (310). After an oral dose some 20–30% is excreted in the urine in 24 hr (311, 312), although excretion may continue for 5–7 days (313). In addition to unchanged drug, four metabolites have been found in the urine: 2,4,7-triamino-6-p-hydroxyphenyl-pteridine, the corresponding sulfuric acid ester, an N-glucuronide of triamterene, and an unknown metabolite (314). A pteridine nucleotide has been isolated from the kidney tissue of triamterene-treated rats (315).

An increased diuresis ensued when triamterene was administered to patients who were receiving the aldosterone antagonist spironolactone (316, 317), thus further emphasizing the fundamental difference in the mechanism of action of these two drugs. Triamterene potentiates the natriuretic action of the thiazides while reducing their kaliuretic effect (316), and other clinical studies with this combination showed that normal serum potassium levels could be maintained without potassium supplements (317). The natriuretic potency of triamterene does not approach that of the thiazide diuretics, and the main value of the drug would appear to be its use in combination with thiazides in clinical situations in which K^+ loss is a problem.

12.4.3 OTHER BICYCLIC POLYAZA DIURETICS. A group of workers at the Takeda laboratories in Japan synthesized and studied the diuretic activity of a large series of polynitrogen heterocycles (318). The ring systems investigated are shown in Table 40.20, documenting the extensive effort made in this investigation. Of the 219 compounds studied in this series, two compounds, DS 210 (40.**195**) and DS 511 (40.**196**), were selected for more extensive evaluation.

The compounds were initially screened in rats; hydrochlorothiazide was used as a reference compound. DS 210 produces a maximal natriuretic effect similar to hydrochlorothiazide in rats without affecting potassium excretion. It shows additive activity with hydrochlorothiazide, acetazolamide, amiloride, and furosemide. Potassium excretion induced by other diuretics is not modified by DS 210. The diuretic effect is lost in adrenalectomized rats and restored by cortisol treatment (319). DS 511 (40.**196**) has shown diuretic activity comparable to hydrochlorothiazide in rats, dogs, and man, and seems to have a unique mode and site of action in the nephron (320).

12.4.4 AMILORIDE. An empirical approach was taken by a group at Merck, Sharp and Dohme seeking compounds with no or minimal kaluretic effects. Screening procedures indicated that *N*-amidino-3-amino-6-bromopyrazinecarboxamide (40.**197**), a compound available through previous work in the folic acid series, was of interest. The introduction of an amino group in the 5 position markedly increased the sodium and chloride excretion without affecting potassium excretion: *N*-amidino-3,5-diamino-6-chloropyrazine-

Table 40.20 Polyaza Heterocyclic Systems Studied as Diuretics (318)

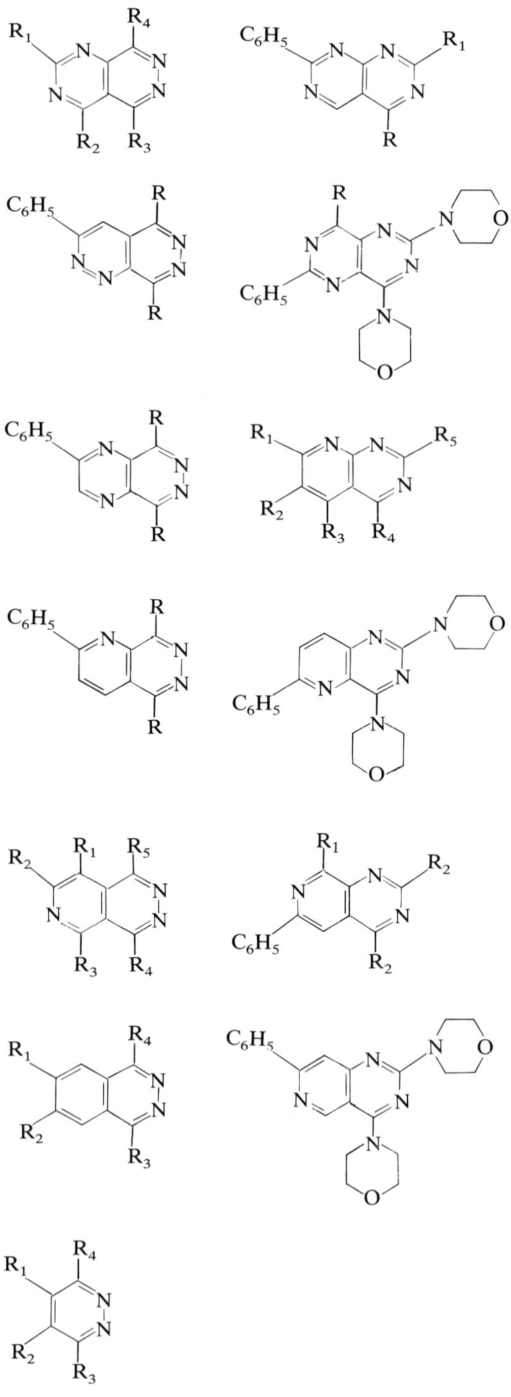

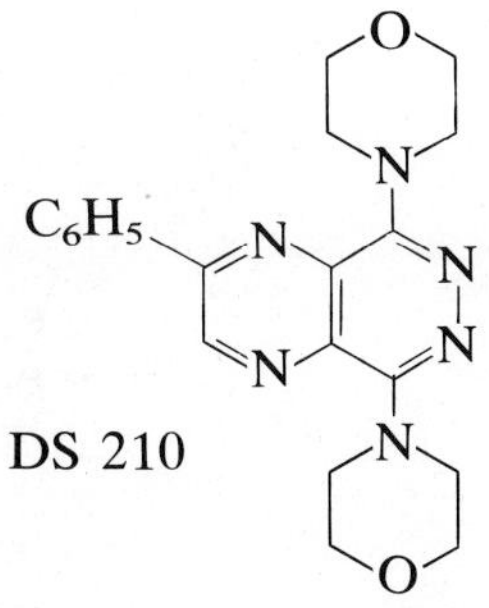

DS 210

40.**195**

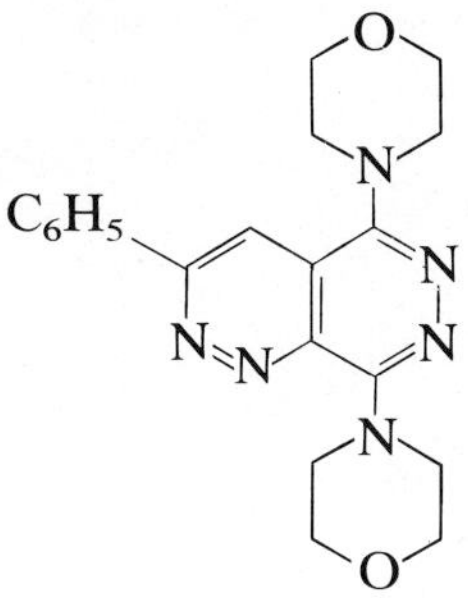

DS 511

40.**196**

carboxamide, amiloride (40.**189**), was among the most promising in animals and man (153). Its saluretic activity is, however, less than that of other diuretics. When amiloride is coadministered with a kaluretic diuretic such as hydrochlorothiazide, there is enhanced natriuresis with conservation of potassium (153). The N-amidinopyrazinecarboximides produce a pronounced diuresis in normal rats while leaving unaffected or repressing K^+ excretion. In the adrenalectomized rat they antagonize the renal actions of exogenous aldosterone, DOCA, or hydrocortisone. In dogs, the compounds are less potent, but the relative activities in the series are the same as those in rats.

Structure–activity relationships in this

series have been investigated in considerable detail and some representative compounds from these studies are listed in Table 40.21. The activities of the compounds were determined on the basis of their DOCA inhibitory activity, although these closely paralleled the diuretic activity in intact rats and dogs (321, 323–325).

The related nature of the structure of amiloride and triamterene (40.**189** and 40.**188**, Table 40.18) and their similar bioligical actions have raised the question of whether the pteridines are, in fact, closed ring versions of the N-amidinopyrazinecarboxamides. The open chain analogs of triamterene and the bicyclic analogs of amiloride have been studied and are generally less active than the drugs themselves. Triamterene is a weaker base (pK 6.2) than amiloride (pK 8.67). Amiloride as the hydrochloride is readily water-soluble, whereas triamterene is slightly soluble. Furthermore, triamterene is metabolized, mainly to a p-hydroxyphenyl derivative, whereas amiloride is excreted unchanged. Thus the resemblance between the two series may be more apparent than real (153, 288).

In the usual dosage amiloride has no important pharmacological actions except those related to the renal tubular transport of electrolytes. Clinically it is used extensively in combination with hydrochlorothiazide (e.g., Moduretic: 5 mg amiloride + 50 mg hydrochlorothiazide).

12.4.5 CLAZOLIMINE. A series of imidazolones was studied by a group at the Lederle Laboratories in their search for a nonsteroidal antagonist of the renal effects of mineralocorticoids.

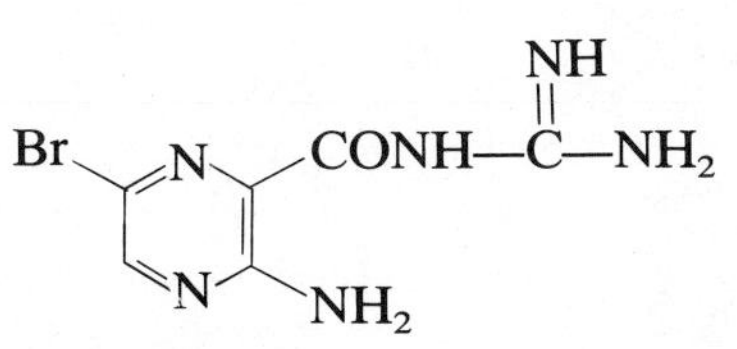

40.**197**

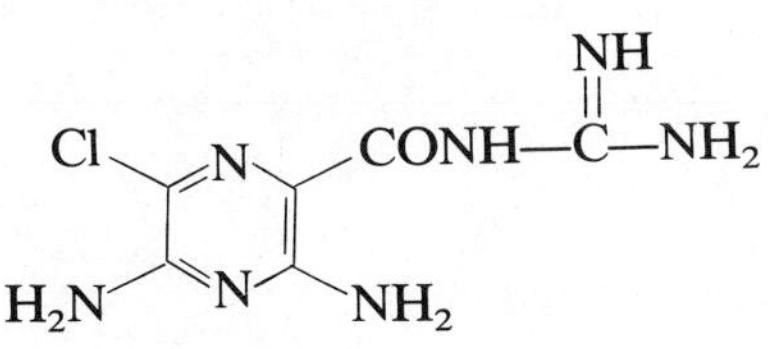

40.**189**

Table 40.21 DOCA Inhibitory Activity in Adrenalectomized Rats of Some N-Amidino-3-aminopyrazinecarboxamides (321, 323–325)

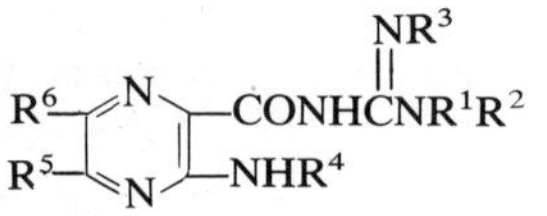

$$\begin{array}{c} NR^3 \\ \| \\ R^6 - N - CONHCNR^1R^2 \\ R^5 - N - NHR^4 \end{array}$$

No.	R^1	R^2	R^3	R^4	R^5	R^6	DOCA Inhibition Score[a]
1	H	H	H	H	H	Cl	+ + +
2	H	H	H	H	H	Br	+ +
3	H	H	H	H	H	I	+
4	CH_3	CH_3	H	H	H	Cl	+ + +
5	CH_3	H	H	H	H	Cl	+
6	H	H	H	H	H	H	O
7	H	H	H	H	H	CF_3	±
8	H	H	H	H	H	CH_3	+ +
9	H	H	H	H	CH_3	H	+
10	H	H	H	H	H	C_6H_5	+
11	H	H	H	H	NH_2	Cl	+ + + +
12	H	H	H	H	CH_3NH	Cl	+ + +
13	H	H	H	H	$(CH_3)CHCH_2NH$	Cl	+
14	H	H	H	H	$(CH_3)_3CNH$	Cl	±
15	H	H	H	H	$(CH_3)_2N$	Cl	+ +
16	H	H	H	H	C_6H_5NH	Cl	+ +
17	CH_3	H	H	H	NH_2	Cl	+ + + +
18	CH_3	CH_3	H	H	NH_2	Cl	+ + + +
19	$3,4\text{-}Cl_2C_6H_3CH_2$	H	H	H	NH_2	Cl	+ + +
20	H	H	H	H	NH_2	Br	+ + +
21	H	H	H	H	Cl	Cl	0
22	H	H	H	H	OH	Cl	±
23	H	H	H	H	OCH_3	Cl	±
24	H	H	H	H	SH	Cl	±
25	H	H	H	H	CH_3S	Cl	+
26	H	H	H	H	CH_3S	Cl	+
27	CH_3CO	H	H	CH_3CO	H	Cl	±
28	H	H	H	H	H	CH_3S	±
				Aldosterone			±
				Triamterene			+ +

[a] This score is related to the dose of each compound that produces a 50% reversal of the electrolyte effect from the administration of 12 μg of DOCA to adrenalectomized rats, as follows:

Dose Producing 50% Reversal of DOCA Na^+/K^+ Effects in Rats, μg	DOCA Inhibition Score
<10	+ + + +
10–50	+ + +
51–100	+ +
101–800	+
>800	±

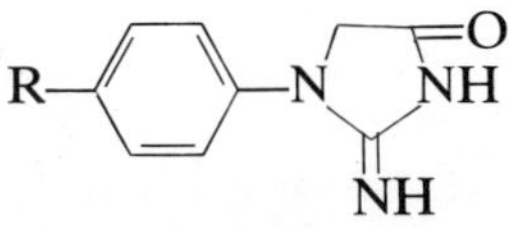

R = H, Cl

40.**198**

Azolimine (40.**198**, R = H) and clazolimine (40.**198**, R = Cl) were the most interesting in this series. Azolimine antagonized the effects of mineralocorticoids on renal electrolyte excretion in several animal models. Large doses of azolimine produced natriuresis in adrenalectomized rats in the absence of exogeneous mineralocorticoid, but its effectiveness was greater in the presence of a steroid agonist. In conscious dogs azolimine was effective only when deoxycorticosterone was administered. Azolimine significantly improved the urinary Na/K ratio when used in combination with thiazides and other classical diuretics in both adrenalectomized, deoxycorticosterone-treated rats and sodium-deficient rats (326). Similar effects were found for clazolimine (327). The compound may be useful in combination with the classical diuretics as an aldosterone antagonist diuretic in humans.

13   URICOSURIC AGENTS AND URICOSURIC DIURETICS

13.1   Introduction

In man, one product of catabolism of purines is uric acid, implicated in several human diseases, e.g., gout. Guanine and adenine are both converted to xanthine (40.**199**); oxidation catalyzed by xanthine oxidase yields uric acid (40.**200**). In man uric acid is the excretory product; most of it is excreted by the kidney. In most mammals, uric acid is further hydrolyzed by uricase to allantoin (40.**201**), a more soluble excretory product. Allantoin, in turn, is further degraded to allantoic acid (40.**202**) by allantoinase, and then to urea and glyoxylic acid (40.**203**) by allantoicase.

Uric acid is not the major pathway of nitrogen excretion in man. Instead, the ammonia nitrogen of most amino acids, the major nitrogen source, is shunted into the urea cycle. Uric acid is rather insoluble in acidic solutions, although alkalinity increases its solubility. At the pH of blood (pH 7.44) uric acid is present as the monosodium salt, which is also very slightly soluble but tends to form supersaturated solutions.

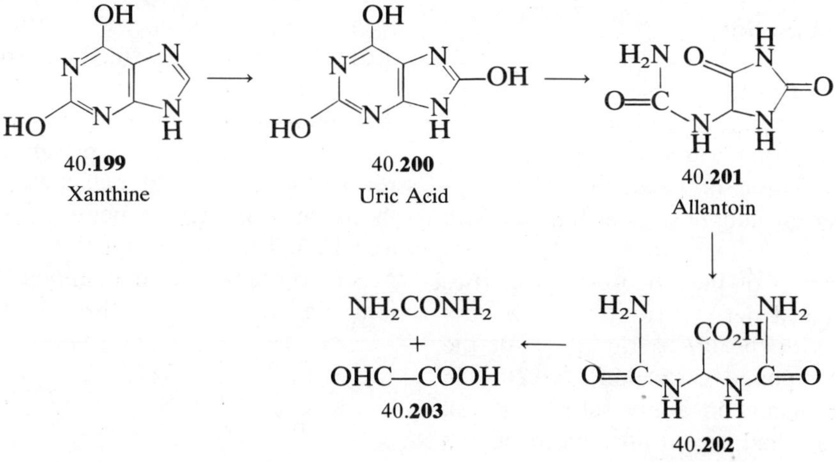

40.**199**
Xanthine

40.**200**
Uric Acid

40.**201**
Allantoin

NH$_2$CONH$_2$
+
OHC—COOH

40.**203**

40.**202**
Allantoic acid

Uric acid is formed from purines, which are liberated as a result of enzymatic degradation of tissue and dietary nucleoproteins and nucleotides, but it is also formed by purine synthesis (328). When the level of monosodium urate in the serum exceeds the point of maximum solubility, urate crystals may form, particularly in the joints and connective tissues. These crystal deposits are responsible for the manifestations of gout. Serum urate levels can be lowered by decreasing the rate of production of uric acid or increasing its rate of elimination. The most common method of reducing uric acid levels is to administer uricosuric drugs which increase the rate of elimination of uric acid by the kidneys.

13.2   Sodium Salicylate

The uricosuric properties of sodium salicylate (40.**204**, Table 40.22) were noted before 1890, and its use continued through 1950. As late as 1955 sodium salicylate was used for the long-term treatment of gout (329). For adequate uricosuric activity, however, salicylate must be administered in doses greater than 5 g/day, often resulting in serious side effects, so that its usage has gradually declined.

13.3   Probenecid

Probenecid (40.**205**, Table 40.22) was developed as a result of a planned search for a compound that would depress the renal tubular secretion of penicillin (330) at a time when the supply of penicillin was still limited.

Recognition of the uricosuric properties of probenecid derived from the prior experience with the uricosuric effects of the related compound carinamide (40.**206**) in normal man and in gouty subjects (332). Carinamide had been introduced as an agent for increasing penicillin blood levels

$$C_6H_5CH_2SO_2\overset{H}{N}-\!\!\!\left\langle\;\right\rangle\!\!\!-COOH$$

40.**206**

by blocking rapid excretion via the kidney. Its biological half-life was relatively short and the search for compounds with a longer half-life that would not have to be administered so frequently led to probenecid.

In a study of series of N-dialkylsulfamoylbenzoates (40.**207**), Beyer (331) found that as the length of the N-alkyl groups increased, the renal clearance of the compounds decreased. This is most likely due to the enhanced lipid solubility imparted by the longer alkyl groups, which would account for their more complete back-diffusion in acid urine. Optimal activity was found in probenecid, the N-dipropyl derivative. The structure–activity relationship of probenecid congeners and that of other uricosuric agents has been reviewed in detail by Gutman (332).

Normally a high percentage of the uric acid filtered by the glomerulus is reabsorbed by an active transport process in the proximal tubule. It is now clear that the human proximal tubule also secretes uric acid, as does the proximal tubule of many lower animals. Small doses of probenecid depress the excretion of uric acid by blocking tubular secretion, whereas high doses lead to greatly enhanced excretion of uric acid by depressing proximal reabsorption of uric acid (333).

Probenecid is completely absorbed after oral administration; peak plasma levels are reached in 2–4 hr. The half-life of the drug in plasma for most patients is between 6 and 12 h. The drug is bound to 85–95% to plasma protein. The small unbound portion is filtered at the glomerulus; a much larger

$$\begin{array}{c}R\\\diagdown\\N O_2 S-\!\!\!\left\langle\;\right\rangle\!\!\!-COOH\\\diagup\\R\end{array}$$

40.**207**   R = H, CH_3, C_2H_5, C_3H_7

Table 40.22   Uricosuric Agents and Uricosuric Diuretics

No.	Generic Name	Trade Name	Structure	Ref.
40.**204**	Salicyclic acid		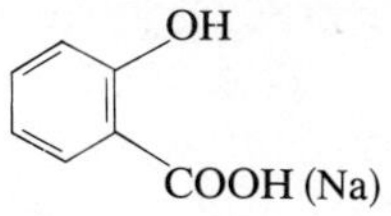	329
40.**205**	Probenecid USP	Benemid	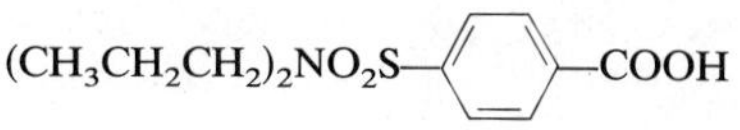 $(CH_3CH_2CH_2)_2NO_2S$—⟨ ⟩—COOH	332
40.**210**	Sulfinpyrazone USP	Anturane	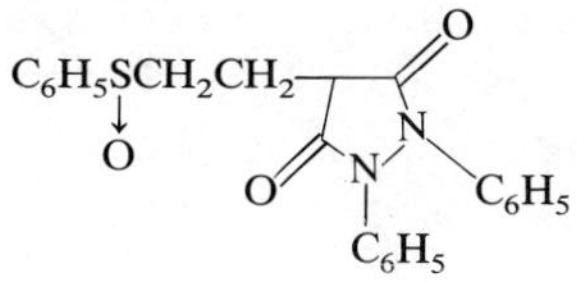	334
40.**213**	Allopurinol	Zyloprim	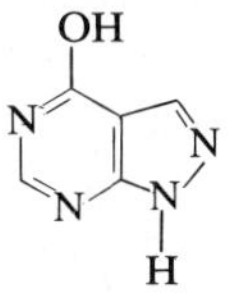	341
40.**215**	Tienilic acid	Ticrynafen	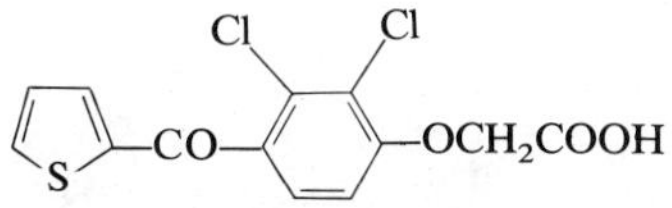	347
40.**228e**	MK 196		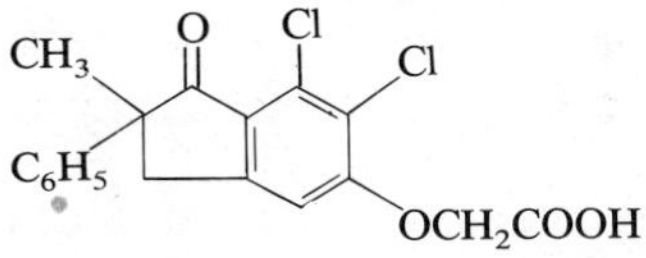	354, 355

portion is actively secreted by the proximal tubule. The high lipid solubility of the undissociated form results in virtually complete reabsorption by back-diffusion unless the urine is markedly alkaline.

Probenecid is insoluble is water, but the sodium salt is freely soluble. In the treatment of chronic gout, a single daily dose of 250 mg is given for 1 week, followed by 500 mg administered twice daily. A daily dose of up to 2 g may be required.

13.4   Sulfinpyrazone

Despite the therapeutic efficacy of phenylbutazone (40.**208**) as an anti-inflammatory and uricosuric agent, its side effects were severe enough to preclude its continuous use in the treatment of chronic gout. Evaluation of a number of chemical congeners indicated that the phenylthioethyl analog of phenylbutazone (40.**209**) had promising anti-inflammatory and uricosuric activity

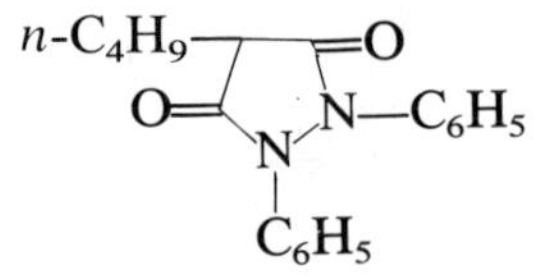

40.**208**

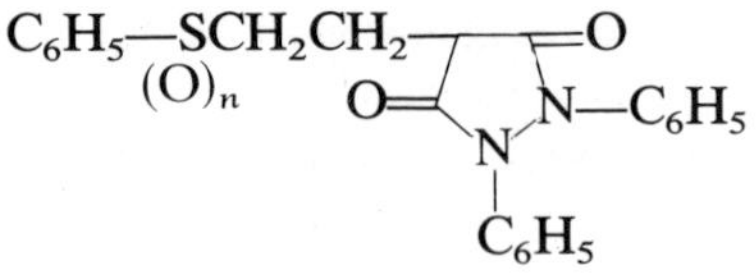

40.**209** $n = 0$
40.**210** $n = 1$
40.**211** $n = 2$

(334). A metabolite, the sulfoxide sulfin-pyrazone (40.**210**), exhibited enhanced uricosuric activity (335, 336). Interestingly, the corresponding sulfone (40.**211**) appar-ently is not a metabolite (334). Sulfinpyr-azone lacks the clinically striking anti-inflammatory and analgesic properties of phenylbutazone.

Sulfinpyrazone is a strong acid (pK_a 2.8) and readily forms soluble salts. Evaluation of a number of congeners indicated that a low pK_a and polar side chain substituents favor uricosuric activity (337) and increase the rate of renal excretion (340). The in-verse relationship between uricosuric po-tency and pK_a has also been confirmed in a number of 2-substituted analogs of prob-enecid (40.**212**). All three compounds were considerably stronger acids than prob-enecid. Evaluation in the *Cebus albifrons* monkey indicated that these compounds were about 10 times as potent as prob-enecid when compared on the basis of con-centration of drug in plasma (338).

In small doses, as seen with other uricosuric agents, sulfinpyrazone may re-duce the excretion of uric acid, presumably by inhibiting secretion but not tubular reabsorption. Its uricosuric action is addi-tive to that of probenecid and phenyl-butazone but antagonizes that of the salicy-lates. Sulfinpyrazone can displace, to an unusual degree, other organic anions that are bound extensively to plasma protein (e.g., sulfonamides, salicylates), thus alter-ing their tissue distribution and renal excre-tion (333, 339). Depending on concomitant medication, this may be a clinical asset or liability.

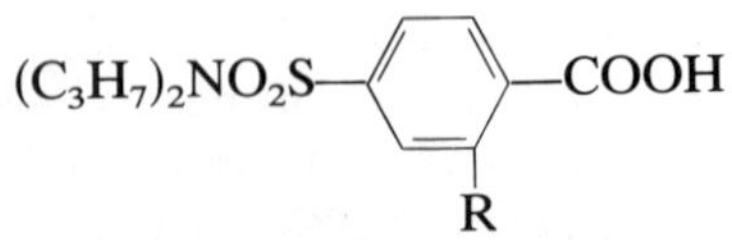

For the treatment of chronic gout, the initial dosage is 100–200 mg/day. After the first week the dose may be increased up to 400 mg/day until a satisfactory lowering of plasma uric acid is achieved.

The effect of sulfinpyrazone on platelet aggregation is discussed in Chapter 39.

13.5 Allopurinol

Allopurinol (40.**213**) is not a uricosuric agent in that it reduces serum uric acid levels by increasing renal uric acid excre-tion; instead it lowers plasma urate levels by inhibiting the final steps in uric acid biosynthesis.

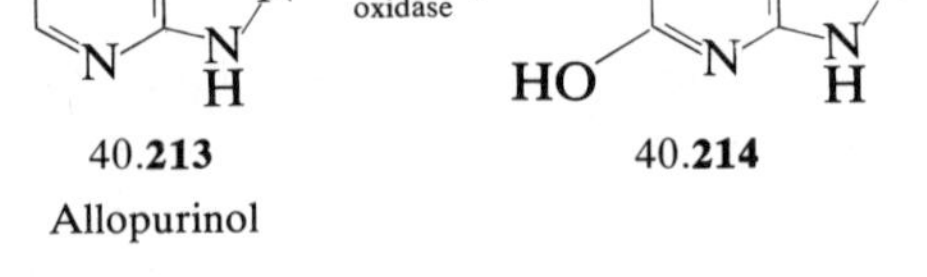

40.**213**
Allopurinol

40.**214**

Uric acid in man is primarily formed by the xanthine oxidase catalyzed oxidation of hypoxanthine and xanthine (40.**199**) to uric acid (40.**200**). Allopurinol (40.**213**) and its primary metabolite alloxanthine (40.**214**) are inhibitors of xanthine oxidase.

$(C_3H_7)_2NO_2S$—⟨ ⟩—COOH

R

40.**212** R = OH, Cl, NO_2

Inhibition of the last two steps in uric acid biosynthesis by blocking xanthine oxidase reduces the plasma concentration and urinary excretion of uric acid and increases the plasma levels and renal excretion of the more soluble oxypurine precursors. Normally, in man the urinary purine content is almost solely uric acid; treatment with allopurinol results in the urinary excretion of hypoxanthine, xanthine, and uric acid each with its independent solubility. By lowering the uric acid concentration in plasma below its limit of solubility, the dissolution of uric acid deposits is facilitated. The effectiveness of allopurinol in the treatment of gout and hyperuricemia resulting from hematological disorders or antineoplastic therapy has been demonstrated (341–343).

For the control of hyperuricemia in gout an initial daily dose of 100 mg is increased at weekly intervals by 100 mg. The usual daily maintenance dose for adults is 300 mg.

13.6   Uricosuric Diuretics

Chronic administration of thiazide diuretics, ethacrynic acid, or furosemide leads to an increase in serum uric acid; however, gouty arthritis is rarely seen as a consequence (344, 345). A possible explanation for the hyperuricemia is a decreased renal clearance of uric acid due to the sharing of a common secretory pathway with the diuretic. The risk of gouty arthritis is proportionate to the degree and duration of the hyperuricemia. This risk is negligible at serum urate concentrations below 7 mg/100 ml; however, at concentrations between 7 and 8 mg/100 ml there is at least a 7%/year chance. This rises to more than 20% at urate concentrations greater than 8 mg/100 ml serum. Normal serum values for uric acid lie between 2.5 and 8 mg/100 ml (346). Recently, compounds have been found that combine diuretic, antihypertensive, and uricosuric activity. This

type of compound would thus not have the potential for causing gouty arthritis.

13.6.1 TIENILIC ACID. Examination of the structure of ethacrynic acid (40.**103**) reveals the presence of a 2,3-dichlorophenoxyacetic acid group responsible for transporting the compound to the kidney and an α,β-unsaturated acyl group with selective affinity to sulfhydryl groups similar to the mercurial diuretics. A group of workers in France decided to study heterocyclic acyl derivatives of 2,3-dichlorophenoxyacetic acid.

The structure of these new compounds does not include a reactive unsaturated acyl group of other similarly activated double bond, nor do these compounds appear to act by the same mechanism as the mercurial diuretics or ethacrynic acid (347).

Among the compounds prepared in this series (40.**215**, Table 40.22), tienilic acid was the most interesting. Not only did the compound show good diuretic activity, but in addition, the compound exhibited a strong uricosuric effect. The structure of tienilic acid and related compounds prepared in this series, as well as their diuretic and uricosuric properties, are shown in Table 40.23. Interestingly, none of the compounds that lacked diuretic activity exhibited uricosuric activity. Reduction of the carbonyl group to a secondary alcohol group (Compound 40.**225**) reduced the diuretic activity and eliminated the uricosuric effect. Reduction to a CH_2 group greatly reduced both the diuretic and uricosuric effect (Compound 40.**226**) (347).

A study in normal volunteers during sustained water diuresis and hydropenia indicated that tienilic acid was a potent diuretic in man with a major site of action in the

$$C_2H_5\underset{\underset{CH_2}{\overset{\|}{C}}}{}-CO-\underset{Cl\;Cl}{\bigcirc}-OCH_2COOH$$

40.**103**

$$R-\underset{\text{(Cl, Cl)}}{\boxed{}}-OCH_2COOH$$

No.	R	LD_{50}	Urine Volume	Na^+	K^+	Uric Acid
40.215	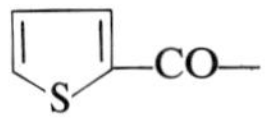 thiophene-2-yl—CO—	1275	2.7[b]	2.86[b]	1.52	1.98[b]
40.216	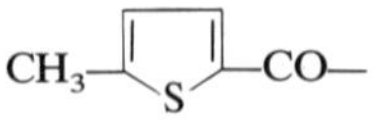 5-CH$_3$-thiophene-2-yl—CO—	MLD[c] > 1000	1.2	1.75	1.06	0.98
40.217	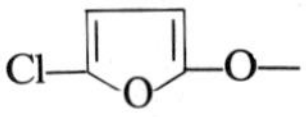 5-Cl-furan-2-yl—O—	787	0.8	0.74	0.61	0.88
40.218	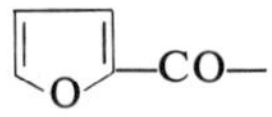 furan-2-yl—CO—	MLD > 1000	1.8[b]	5.35[b]	1.53[b]	1.10
40.219	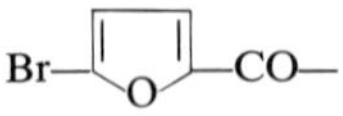 5-Br-furan-2-yl—CO—	MLD > 500	1.1	1.38	0.82	1.09
40.220	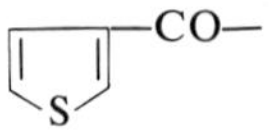 thiophene-3-yl—CO—	900	2.7[b]	2.20[b]	1.88[b]	1.55[b]
40.221	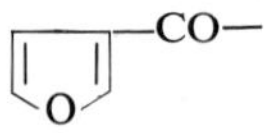 furan-3-yl—CO—		1.6[b]	1.98[b]	0.11	0.92
40.222	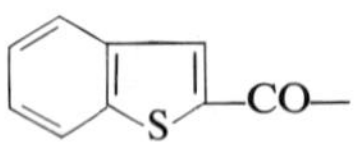 benzothiophene-2-yl—CO—	MLD > 1000	1.2	1.18	0.91	1.05
40.223	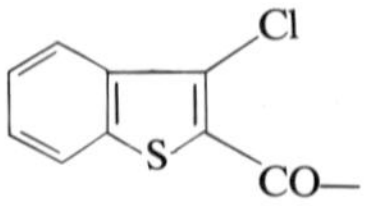 3-Cl-benzothiophene-2-yl—CO—	< 1000	1.3	1.29	1.17	1.26
40.224	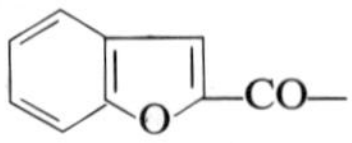 benzofuran-2-yl—CO—	< 1000	1.3	1.52[b]	1.74[b]	1.56[b]

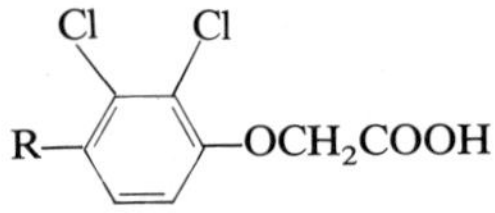

Urinary Excretion,[a] Dose 100 mg/kg p.o.

Table 40.23   (Continued)

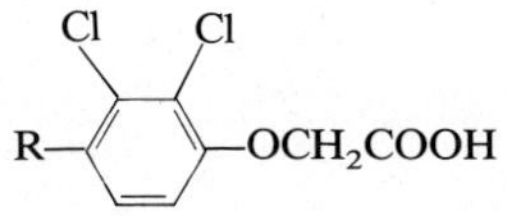

$$R \overset{Cl \quad Cl}{\underset{}{\bigcirc}} OCH_2COOH$$

No.	R	LD_{50}	Urinary Excretion,[a] Dose 100 mg/kg p.o.			
			Urine Volume	Na^+	K^+	Uric Acid
40.**225**	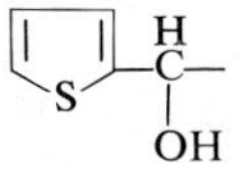 (thiophene ring)-$\overset{H}{\underset{OH}{C}}$-	1000	1.6	1.95	1.12	0.93
40.**226**	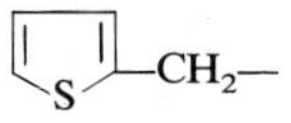 (thiophene ring)-CH_2-	1000	1.2	1.32	1.33	1.16
40.**103**	Ethacrynic acid[d]	600	2.4	2.76[b]	1.48	1.27
40.**108**	Furosemide[d]	1125	3.0[b]	4.28[b]	1.51	1.34

[a] Coefficient = excretion treated animals/excretion controls at time of peak activity.
[b] $p < 0.05$.
[c] MLD = mimimum lethal dose.
[d] Dose 20 mg/kg p.o.

distal nephron beyond the loop of Henle (348). Renal clearance methods during water diuresis following oral administration of tienilic acid, pyrazinamide, and probenecid indicated that the potent uricosuric effect of tienilic acid is due to inhibition of a high capacity urate reabsorption system distal to the site of urate secretion (349).

In a double-blind comparison of tienilic acid and probenecid in patients with hyperuricemia, 125–250 mg/day of tienilic acid reduced the average serum uric acid from 9.7 ± 0.36 to 6.49 ± 0.37 mg/100 ml serum. Doses of 500–1000 mg/day of probenecid were slightly less effective (350).

In an additional clinical study, tienilic acid was compared with hydrochlorothiazide in hypertensive patients. Blood pressure was significantly reduced with both medications, although most patients required 250 mg of tienilic acid twice daily, compared to 50 mg hydrochlorothiazide given once or twice daily. Whereas the serum uric acid level rose moderately in the hydrochlorothiazide-treated patients, it fell strikingly to less than half of the pretreatment levels in patients treated with tienilic acid. Body weight decreased slightly in both groups, as did serum potassium levels. Tienilic acid thus appears to be a useful new antihypertensive agent because of its desirable combination of diuretic, antihypertensive, and hypouricemic effects (351, 352).

13.6.2 (1-OXO-INDANYLOXY)ACETIC ACIDS, MK 196. The mercurial diuretics, particularly the phenoxyacetic acids, e.g., merbaphen (40.**4**) and mersalyl, because of their many desirable pharmacodynamic properties, including saluresis, proper urinary Na^+/Cl^- balance, and uricosuric activity, served as a model for the development of ethacrynic acid and related compounds.

Ethacrynic acid and the mercurial diuretics have some properties in common, e.g., potent saluretic activity with proper Na^+/Cl^- balance and sulfhydryl-binding activity; however, in contrast to the mercurials, ethacrynic acid causes uric acid retention.

It was observed that hydrogenation of the double bond in ethacrynic acid to yield 40.**227** resulted in a compound that retained significant saluretic activity even though the sulfhydryl binding activity had been eliminated. This led to the investigation of a series of (1-oxo-5-indanyloxy)acetic acids substituted in the 2 position (40.**228a–e**). These compounds are inert to reaction with sulfhydryl-containing compounds and exhibit marked saluresis in several species, i.e., chimpanzees, dogs,

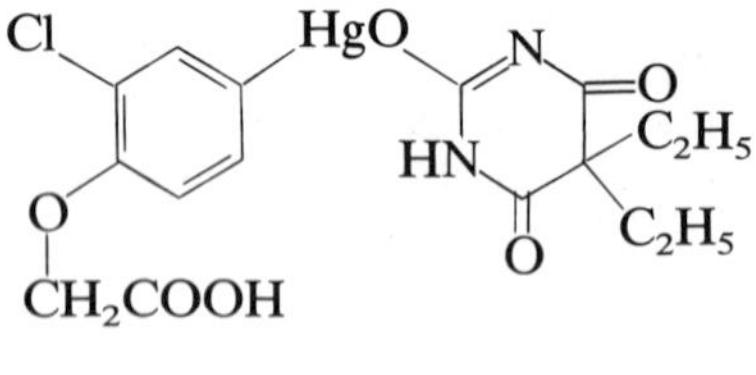

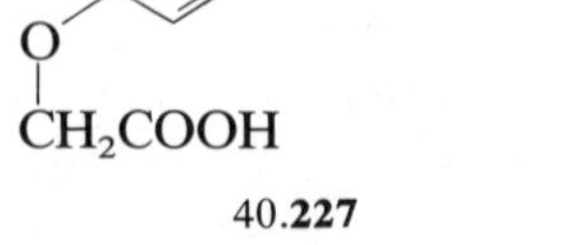

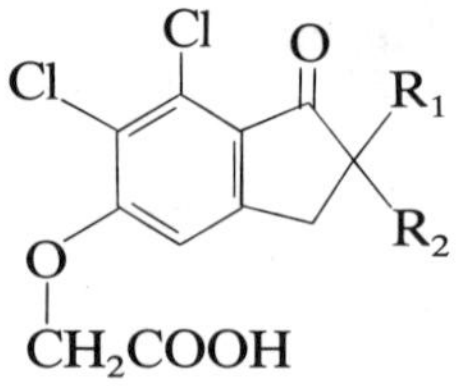

	R_1	R_2	
40.**228a**	$CH(CH_3)_2$	H	
40.**228b**	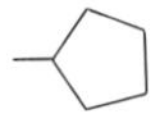	H	
40.**228c**	$CH(CH_3)_2$	CH_3	
40.**228d**	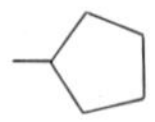	CH_3	
40.**228e**	C_6H_5	CH_3	(MK 196)

and, surprisingly, rats. Even more unexpected was the finding that these compounds possess significant uricosuric activity in chimpanzees. The significance of sulfhydryl binding in the mechanism of action of the known phenoxyacetic acid diuretics would therefore appear to be secondary in this series (353). The nature of R_1 and R_2 in structure 40.**228** is important for both saluretic and uricosuric activity; the introduction of a second substituent such as $R_2 = CH_3$ enhanced the activity. Resolution of three racemic pairs (40.**228b–d**) showed some differences in the relative activities of the enantiomorphs. The diuretic and uricosuric data obtained with compounds 40.**228a–e** as well as with the corresponding enantiomers are given in Table 40.24. The values obtained with furosemide, hydrochlorothiazide, and probenecid are given for reference.

Further investigation indicated that compound 40.**228e** (MK 196) is a highly active uricosuric saluretic; the threshold dose in chimpanzees was about 0.03 mg/kg p.o., and in conscious dogs about 0.625 mg/kg p.o. At 20 mg/kg p.o. in the dog, Na^+ and Cl^- responses were increased approximately sixfold above placebo (354, 355). Clearance studies in the rat indicated that

40.**227**

Table 40.24   (2-Substituted 1-Oxo-5-indanyloxy)acetic Acids (353, 355)—Diuretic and Uricosuric Data Obtained in Chimpanzees[a]

No.	Isomer	Dose, mg/kg p.o.	ΔUrine Volume, ml/min	$\Delta C_{urate}/C_{inulin}$	Δμeq/min		
					Na^+	K^+	Cl^-
40.228a	±	5	6.2	0.18	649	146	748
40.228b	±	5	1.6	0.18	123	51	326
		10	4.6	0.26	568	131	715
	+	5	3.1	0.26	300	102	370
	−	5	2.9	0.10	292	74	365
40.228c	±	5	5.5	0.02	506	84	612
	+	5	10.9	0.41	1593	156	1906
	−	5	8.3	0.06	992	145	1271
40.228d	±	0.25	1.4	0.01	225	21	331
		5	2.5	0.20	425	64	367
		10	4.6	0.36	735	133	985
	+	5	0.3	0.10	325	110	477
	−	5	1.4	0.17	268	44	308
40.228e	±	5	3.6	0.33	411	83	554
Furosemide		5	8.8	−0.02	1035	55	1073
Hydrochloro-thiazide		5	1.0	−0.02	144	73	198
Probenecid		5	0.1	0.05			
		10		0.29			

[a] Fasted, male chimpanzees weighing 21–77 kg were immobilized with phencyclidine (which was shown not to affect the results) (1.0–1.5 mg/kg i.m. plus 0.25 mg/kg i.v. as needed) and were prepared by catheterization for standard renal clearance studies using routine clinical aseptic procedures. Pyrogen-free inulin (i.v.) was used to measure glomerular filtration rate. Clearance of inulin, urate, and the excretion rates of Na^+, K^+, and Cl^- was determined by standard Autoanalyzer techniques. (Inulin and urate in chimpanzee plasma are freely filterable.) Average control clearances were calculated from three 20 min consecutive periods. Drug-response values were derived as the average of eight 15–20 min clearance periods after oral administration of an aqueous solution of the compound through an indwelling nasal catheter. All data are reported as the difference between (average) treatment and control values obtained from single experiments.

MK 196 is a potent diuretic acting in the ascending limb of Henle, which results in significant increases in urinary excretion of sodium, calcium, magnesium, water (356), and uric acid (359).

The physiological disposition of ^{14}C-labeled MK 196 was studied in rat, dog, monkey, and chimpanzee. The drug was well absorbed and showed minimal metabolism in rat, dog, and monkey. Triphasic rates of elimination of drug and radioactivity were observed in these three species. In the dog the terminal half-life was estimated to be about 68 h; in the monkey a longer terminal half-life of approximately 105 h was found. The long terminal half-life of this compound may be due in part to binding to plasma proteins. The major route of radioactivity elimination is via the feces for the rat (~94%) and dog (~80%). In contrast, the monkey and the chimpanzee eliminate the majority of the dose via the urine. Minimal metabolism of MK 196 was observed in the rat, dog, and monkey; however, in man and in the chimpanzee extensive biotransformation was found. The major metabolite resulted from para hydroxylation of the phenyl group to yield [6,7-dichloro-2-(4-hydroxyphenyl)-2-methyl-1-oxo-5-indanyloxy]-acetic acid (40.**229**). This metabolite accounted for more than 40% of the 0–48 hr urinary radioactivity; about 20% of the radioactivity was accounted for as unchanged drug (357, 358).

In clinical studies in healthy subjects consuming a standard diet, 10 mg of MK 196 produced a slightly smaller diuresis than 40 mg of furosemide, and did not influence uric acid excretion or 24 h urate clearance. A single dose of 40 mg of furosemide caused uric acid retention with a significant decrease of 24 h urate clearance; prolonged administration caused a statistically significant increase in plasma uric acid levels. Prolonged administration of MK 196 did not increase plasma uric acid levels and the ratio of urate–creatinine clearance was indistinguishable from the values found in the placebo group. MK 196 thus appears to be a diuretic without uric acid-retaining properties (360).

In a comparison of the diuretic effects of MK 196 and furosemide in normal volunteers receiving the drug every day for 14 days, it was found that at an oral dose of 10 mg MK 196 caused a gradual diuretic and saluretic response resulting in a maximal plateau during the period 4–7 hr after drug administration, followed by a slow return to base line during the next 16–18 h. Although at the doses studied (10 and 20 mg MK 196), the maximum response to furosemide (40 mg) was always higher than

the maximal response to MK 196; the total 24 h saluresis following 10 mg MK 196 was equivalent to that produced by furosemide and after 20 mg MK 196 the 24 h response was greater than that seen with furosemide (361). A double-blind pilot study was conducted to compare the antihypertensive efficacy of two doses of MK 196 (10 and 15 mg) with 50 mg hydrochlorothiazide in patients with mild to moderate hypertension. Both doses of MK 196 lowered blood pressure as much as or more than 50 mg hydrochlorothiazide during the 24 h period following drug administration (362).

Initial clinical results thus indicate that MK 196 is a highly active diuretic with a gradual onset of action which reaches a plateau that persists for 4–7 h, then gradually returns to base-line values over the next 16–18 h. This is probably due to the long half-life of this compound as observed in animals. The antihypertensive effect is comparable to that observed with hydrochlorothiazide. MK 196 did not exhibit uricosuric activity in man, but it did not cause uric acid retention and no changes in urate clearance were observed. The drug would therefore appear to be indicated for the treatment of edema and hypertension in patients with high plasma uric acid levels.

14 CONCLUSION

In the past 50 years continuous progress has been made toward the development of safe and effective diuretics. Between 1920 and 1950 a large number of organic mercurials were prepared and evaluated as diuretics. Lack of oral activity and potential toxicity provided the stimulus for the search for nomercurial, orally effective diuretics. The carbonic anhydrase inhibitors, developed in 1950 and later years, were orally active but upset the acid–base balance and could only be given intermittently. The thiazide diuretics, developed in

40.**229**

1957 and later, represented a true advance in the treatment of edema. They were remarkably nontoxic and effective in most cases. It very soon became apparent that not only were they effective diuretics, but that they were also useful in the treatment of hypertension by themselves and in combination with other antihypertensive drugs.

Three side effects were noticed following the widespread and prolonged use of the thiazide diuretics:

1. Potassium depletion.
2. Uric acid retention.
3. Hyperglycemia.

Potassium depletion has been encountered most frequently. The kaliuretic effect of the thiazides can be compensated for by supplementary dietary potassium; nevertheless research was directed toward the development of potassium-sparing diuretics. Amiloride (1965), spironolactone (1959), and triamterene (1965) were discovered as a result of this effort; these compounds are weak diuretics, however, and are generally used in combination with other diuretics, e.g., hydrochlorothiazide.

The next step was the discovery of the high ceiling diuretics, e.g., ethacrynic acid (1962), furosemide (1963), and bumetanide (1971), shorter acting and more potent than the thiazide diuretics. They too have the same potential side effects as the thiazides. One advantage of the high ceiling diuretics is their efficacy in chronic renal insufficiency, particularly in cases with low glomerular filtration rates.

Recent developments include high ceiling diuretics of new structural types, e.g., MK 447 (1976), reported to have very little effect on potassium excretion in man, and muzolimine, an aminopyrazolone (1977). Two other new diuretics, tienilic acid (1974) and MK 196 (1975), may well eliminate the problem of uric acid retention. Tienilic acid has been reported to significantly lower plasma urate levels below pre-

treatment levels and treatment with MK 196 has not led to any increase in plasma urate levels.

Almost all diuretics in current use have at some time been reported to cause diabetes. There are no grounds at this time for a definite conclusion that any of them is free from this effect, and no such claim is made for any of the compounds currently being developed.

Diuretics are amongst the most widely used drugs, and considering that they are often used daily for indefinite periods, side effects are few. We most likely can expect diuretics to become available with less effect on potassium, plasma urate levels, or glucose tolerance so that a drug can be selected to suit the individual requirements of the patient.

15 ADDENDUM

Since this chapter was written, the proceedings of a symposium on diuretic agents, sponsored by the Division of Medicinal Chemistry of the American Chemical Society in 1977, has been published (374). Recent advances in the medicinal chemistry of diuretics are described in some detail.

It was shown that the roles of the renal hormones, prostaglandin, and the kallikrein-kinin system are extremely complex but are of such importance that they must be considered by scientists involved in renal research. Some additional subjects from the symposium are discussed briefly below.

15.1 Structure Activity Relations in the Bumetanide Series

Structural modifications of bumetanide (Table 40.14, 40.**117**) were further explored by Nielsen and Feit (375). It was found that the carboxy group in the 1-position of bumetanide could be replaced by a sulfinic or sulfonic acid group or even converted to an aminomethyl group (376) (40.**232** to 40.**234**) with retention of diuretic activity.

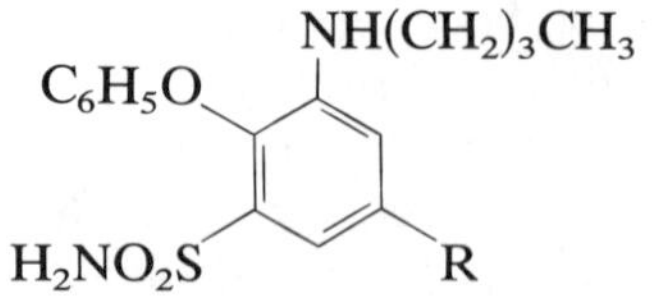

40.**232** R = SO$_2$H
40.**233** R = SO$_3$H
40.**234** R = NHCH$_2$C$_6$H$_5$

In a further modification the sulfamoyl group in the 5-position was replaced by formamido group (377) (40.**235**); this compound was found to have approximately one-tenth the activity of bumetanide. The electrolyte excretion pattern was still similar to that of bumetanide.

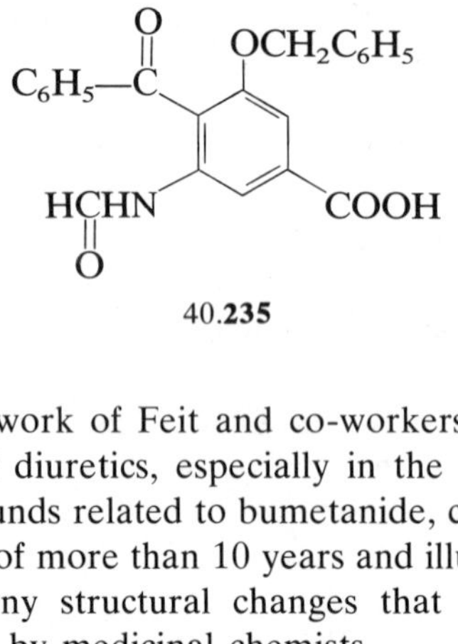

40.**235**

The work of Feit and co-workers in the field of diuretics, especially in the area of compounds related to bumetanide, covers a period of more than 10 years and illustrates the many structural changes that can be studied by medicinal chemists.

15.2   Tizolemide

A new structural type sulfonamide diuretic has recently been developed by Lang and co-workers at Hoechst (378). Hoe 740 or Tizolemide (40.**236**) was selected from a series of compounds for further investigation. Optimal activity was associated with an unsubstituted sulfamoyl group. In dogs the diuretic activity was similar to that of

hydrochlorothiazide. Interestingly, tizolemide lowered serum uric acid levels in the cebus monkey, indicating a possible uricosuric effect.

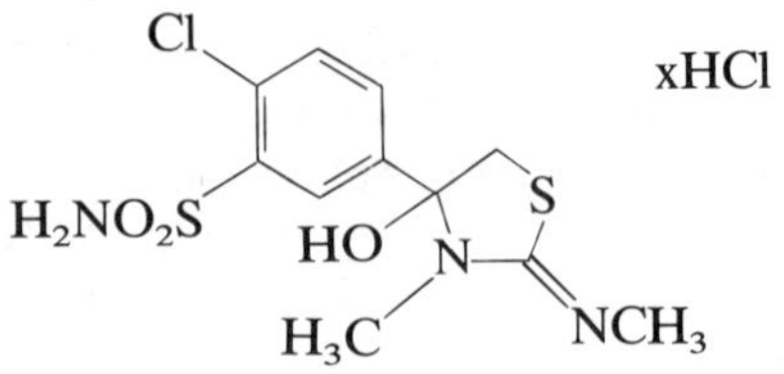

40.**236**   Tizolemide

15.3   Quincarbate

Quincarbate (40.**237**) is a representative of a new class of diuretics with 1,4-dioxino[2,3-g]quinolone structure developed by van Dijk and co-workers (379, 380). It was the most active compound to emerge from this series. The diuretic activity was absent in the mouse and hamster, slight in the rhesus monkey. In nonsaline loaded beagles the natriuretic effect was comparable to furosemide. Quincarbate is not a carbonic anhydrase inhibitor and dose not act by aldosterone antagonism. In man doses of 10–20 mg given orally showed natriuretic effects comparable to those of 100 mg of hydrochlorothiazole or 40 mg of furosemide. With 80 mg of furosemide greater natriuresis and diuresis could be achieved than with quincarbate.

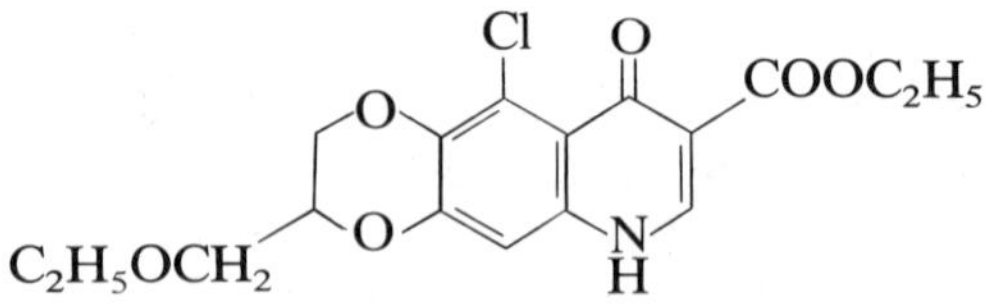

40.**237**   Quincarbate

REFERENCES

1. A. Koch, in *Physiology and Biophysics*, Vol. II, 20th ed., Section IV, T. C. Ruch and H. D. Patton, Eds., Saunders, Philadelphia, 1973, p. 417

2. W. Berliner, in *Best and Taylor's Physiological Basis of Medical Practice*, ed. 9th, J. R. Brobeck, Section 5, Williams and Wilkins, Baltimore, 1973.

3. H. R. Jacobson and J. P. Kokko, *Ann. Rev. Pharmacol. Toxicol.*, **16**, 201 (1976).

4. J. P. Kokko, *J. Clin. Invest.*, **49**, 1838 (1970).

5. M. Burg, L. Stoner, J. Cardinal, and N. Green, *Am. J. Physiol.*, **225**, 119 (1973).

6. A. S. Rocha and J. P. Kokko, *J. Clin. Invest.*, **52**, 612 (1973).

7. G. Malnic, R. M. Klose, and G. Giebisch, *Am. J. Physiol.*, **206**, 674 (1964).

8. J. B. Gross, M. Imai, and J. P. Kokko, *J. Clin. Invest.*, **55**, 1284 (1975).

9. G. Malnic, R. M. Klose, and G. Giebisch, *Am. J. Physiol.*, **211**, 529 (1966).

10. R. N. Khuri, M. Wiederholt, N. Strieder, and G. Giebisch, *Am. J. Physiol.*, **228**, 1249 (1975).

11. F. S. Wright, *Am. J. Physiol.*, **220**, 624 (1971).

12. J. A. Schafer and T. E. Andreoli, *J. Clin. Invest.*, **51**, 1264 (1972).

13. J. J. Grantham and J. Orloff, *J. Clin. Invest.*, **47**, 1154 (1968).

14. J. J. Grantham and M. B. Burg, *Am. J. Physiol.*, **211**, 255 (1966).

15. W. N. Suki, G. Eknoyan, and M. Martinez-Maldonado, *Ann. Rev. Pharmacol*, **13**, 91 (1973).

16. K. H. Beyer, Jr., *Perspect. Biol. Med.*, **19**, 500 (1976).

17. W. L. Lipschitz, Z. Hadidian, and A. Kerpcsar, *J. Pharmacol. Exp. Ther.*, **79**, 97 (1943).

18. A. A. Renzi, J. J. Chart, and R. Gaunt, *Toxicol. Appl. Pharmacol.*, **1**, 406 (1959).

19. D. M. Zall, D. Fisher, and M. Q. Garner, *Anal. Chem.*, **28**, 1665 (1956).

20. W. E. Barrett, R. A. Rutledge, H. Sheppard, and A. J. Plummer, *Toxicol. Appl. Pharmacol.*, **1**, 333 (1959).

21 G. M. Fanelli, Jr., D. L. Bohn, A. Scriabine, and K. H. Beyer, Jr., *J. Pharmacol. Exp. Ther.*, **200**, 402 (1977).

22. G. M. Fanelli, D. L. Bohn, and H. F. Russo, *Comp. Biochem. Physiol.*, **33**, 459 (1970).

23. B. Stavric, W. J. Johnson, and H. C. Grice, *Proc. Soc. Exp. Biol. Med.*, **130**, 512 (1969); B. Stavric, E. A. Nera, W. J. Johnson, and F. A. Salem, *Invest. Urol.*, **11**, 3 (1973).

24. F. W. Wolff, W. W. Parmley, K. White, and R. Okun, *J. Am. Med. Assoc.*, **185**, 568 (1963).

25. I. I. A. Tabachnick, A. Gulbenkian, and A. Yannell, *Life Sci.*, **4**, 1931 (1965).

26. J. F. Seely and J. H. Dirks, *J. Clin. Invest.*, **48**, 2330 (1969).

27. R. C. Blantz, *J. Clin. Invest.*, **54**, 1135 (1974).

28. A. Vogl, *Am. Heart J.*, **39**, 881 (1950).

29. I. M. Weiner, R. I. Levy, and G. H. Mudge, *J. Pharmacol. Exp. Ther.*, **138**, 96 (1962).

30. T. W. Clarkson and J. J. Vostal, in *Modern Diuretic Therapy in the Treatment of Cardiovascular and Renal Disease*, Excerpta Medica, Amsterdam, 1973, pp. 229–240.

31. E. J. Cafruny, K. C. Cho, V. Nigrovic, and A. Small, in *Modern Diuretic Therapy in the Treatment of Cardiovascular and Renal Diseases*, Excerpta Medica, Amsterdam 1973, pp. 124–134.

32. G. deStevens, *Diuretics: Chemistry and Pharmacology*, Academic, New York, 1963, p. 38.

33. R. H. Kessler, R. Lozano, and R. F. Pitts, *J. Clin. Invest.*, **36**, 656 (1957).

34. R. C. Batterman, D. Unterman, and A. C. DeGraff, *J. Am. Med. Assoc.*, **140**, 1268 (1949).

35. W. Modell, *Am. J. Med. Sci.*, **231**, 564 (1956).

36. L. H. Werner and C. R. Scholz, *J. Am. Chem. Soc.*, **76**, 2453 (1954).

37. J. Moyer, S. Kinard, and R. Herschberger, *Antibiot. Med. Clin. Ther.*, **3**, 179 (1956).

38. R. W. Berliner, J. H. Dirks, and W. J. Cirksena, *Ann. N. Y. Acad. Sci.*, **139**, 424 (1966).

39. J. R. Clapp and R. R. Robinson, *Am. J. Physiol.*, **215**, 228 (1968).

40. R. L. Evanson, E. A. Lockhart, and J. H. Dirks, *Am. J. Physiol.*, **222**, 282 (1972).

41. G. H. Mudge, in the *Pharmacological Basis of Therapeutics*, 5th ed., L. S. Goodman and A. Gilman, Eds., Section VIII, Macmillan, New York, 1975, p. 809.

42. G. M. Fanelli, Jr., D. L. Bohn, S. S. Reilly, and I. M. Weiner, *Am. J. Physiol.*, **224**, 985 (1973).

43. R. H. Chaney and R. F. Maronde, *Am. J. Med. Sci.*, **231**, 26 (1956).

44. F. C. Rector, N. W. Carter, and D. W. Seldin, *J. Clin. Invest.*, **44**, 278 (1965).

45. H. J. Rodriguez, J. Wallss, J. Yates, and S. Klahr, *J. Clin. Invest.*, **53**, 122 (1974).

46. N. Beck, K. S. Kim, M. Wolak, and B. B. Davis, *J. Clin. Invest.*, **55**, 149 (1975).

47. M. B. Strauss and H. Southworth, *Bull. Johns Hopkins Hosp.*, **63**, 41 (1938).

48. T. Mann and D. Keilin, *Nature* (London), **146**, 164 (1940).

49. H. W. Davenport and A. E. Wilhelmi, *Proc. Soc. Exp. Biol. Med.*, **48**, 53 (1941).

50. R. F. Pitts and R. S. Alexander, *Am. J. Physiol.*, **144**, 239 (1945).

51. W. B. Schwartz, *New Engl. J. Med.*, **240,** 173 (1949).

52. H. A. Krebs, *Biochem. J.*, **43,** 525 (1948).

53. R. O. Roblin, Jr., and J. W. Clapp, *J. Am. Chem. Soc.*, **72,** 4890 (1950).

54. W. H. Miller, A. M. Dessert, and R. O. Roblin, Jr., *J. Am. Chem. Soc.*, **72,** 4893 (1950).

55. R. W. Young, K. H. Wood, J. A. Eichler, J. R. Vaughan, Jr., and G. W. Anderson, *J. Am. Chem. Soc.*, **78,** 4649 (1956).

56. K. H. Beyer and J. E. Baer, *Pharmacol. Rev.*, **13,** 517 (1961).

57. T. H. Maren, E. Mayer, and B. C. Wadsworth, *Bull. Johns Hopkins Hosp.*, **95,** 199 (1954).

58. R. V. Ford, C. L. Spurr, and J. H. Moyer, *Circulation*, **16,** 394 (1957).

59. J. R. Vaughan, Jr., J. A. Eichler, and G. W. Anderson, *J. Org. Chem.*, **21,** 700 (1956).

60. T. H. Maren, *J. Pharmacol. Exp. Ther.*, **117,** 385 (1956).

61. D. M. Travis, *J. Pharmacol. Exp. Ther.*, **167,** 253 (1969).

62. R. T. Kunan, Jr., *J. Clin. Invest.*, **51,** 294 (1972).

63. A. Posner, *Am. J. Ophthalmol.* **45,** 225 (1958).

64. T. W. K. Hill and P. J. Randall. *J. Pharm. Pharmacol.*, **28,** 552 (1976).

65. T. H. Maren, *Bull. Johns Hopkins Hosp.*, **98,** 159 (1956). T. H. Maren, in *Handbook of Experimental Pharmacology*, Vol. 24, *Diuretics*, H. Herken, Ed., Springer, Berlin–Heidelberg–New York, 1969, p. 195.

65a. J. L. Anderton and P. Kincaid-Smith, *Drugs*, **1,** 54 (1971).

66. K. H. Beyer, Jr., and J. E. Baer, *Med. Clin. North Am.*, **59,** 735 (1975).

67. J. M. Sprague, *Ann. N. Y. Acad. Sci.*, **71**:4, 328 (1958).

68. F. C. Novello, S. C. Bell, E. L. A. Abrams, C. Ziegler, and J. M. Sprague, *J. Org. Chem.*, **25,** 965–970 (1960).

69. F. C. Novello and J. M. Sprague, *J. Am. Chem. Soc.*, **79,** 2028 (1957).

70. F. J. Lund and W. Kobinger, *Acta Pharmacol. Toxicol.*, **16,** 297 (1960).

71. H. Horstmann, H. Wollweber, and K. Meng, *Arzneim.-Forsch.*, **17,** 653 (1967).

72. B. Duhm, W. Maul, H. Medenwald, K. Patzchke, and L. A. Wegner, *Arzneim.-Forsch.*, **17,** 672 (1967).

73. K. Meng and G. Kroneberg, *Arzneim.-Forsch.*, **17,** 659 (1967).

74. R. J. Santos, V. Paz-Martinez, J. K. Lee, and J. H. Nodine, *Int. J. Clin. Pharmacol.*, **3,** 14 (1970).

75. F. J. Lund and W. Kobinger, *Acta Pharmacol. Toxicol.*, **16,** 297 (1960).

76. E. H. Wiseman, E. C. Schreiber, and R. Pinson, Jr., *Biochem. Pharmacol.*, **11,** 881 (1962).

77. T. H. Maren and C. E. Wiley, *J. Pharmacol. Exp. Ther.*, **143,** 230 (1964).

78. R. L. Hauman and J. M. Weller, *Clin. Pharmacol. Ther.*, **1,** 175 (1960).

79. S. Y. P'An, A. Scriabine, D. E. McKersie, and W. M. McLamore, *J. Pharmacol. Exp. Ther.*, **128,** 122 (1960).

80. G. deStevens, *Diuretics: Chemistry and Pharmacology*, Academic, New York, 1963, p. 100.

81. E. J. Cragoe, Jr., J. A. Nicholson, and J. M. Sprague, *J. Med. Pharm. Chem.*, **4,** 369 (1961).

82. J. G. Topliss, M. H. Sherlock, H. Reimann, L. M. Konzelman, E. P. Shapiro, B. W. Pettersen, H. Schneider, and N. Sperber, *J. Med. Chem.*, **6,** 122 (1963).

83. A. A. Rubin, F. E. Roth, R. M. Taylor, and H. Rosenkilde, *J. Pharmacol. Exp. Ther.*, **136,** 344 (1962).

84. G. deStevens, L. H. Werner, A. Halamandaris, and S. Ricca, Jr., *Experientia*, **14,** 463 (1958).

85. W. E. Barrett, R. A. Rutledge, and A. J. Plummer, *Toxicol. Appl. Pharmacol.*, **1,** 333 (1959).

86. J. E. Baer, H. F. Russo, and K. H. Beyer, *Proc. Soc. Exp. Biol. Med.*, **100,** 442 (1959).

87. A. F. Esch, I. M. Wilson, and E. D. Freis, *Med. Ann. Dist. Columbia*, **28,** 9 (1959).

88. C. W. H. Havard and J. C. B. Fenton, *Brit. Med. J.*, **1,** 1560 (1959).

89. H. Losse, H. Wehmeyer, W. Strobel, and H. Wesselkock, *Muench. Med. Wochenschr.*, **101,** 677 (1959).

90. W. Hollander, A. V. Chobanian, and R. W. Wilkins, in *Hypertension*, J. H. Moyer, Ed., Saunders, Philadelphia, 1959, p. 570.

91. L. H. Werner, A. Halamandaris, S. Ricca, Jr., L. Dorfman, and G. deStevens, *J. Am. Chem. Soc.*, **82,** 1161 (1960).

92. E. J. Cragoe, Jr., O. W. Woltersdorf, Jr., J. E. Baer, and J. M. Sprague, *J. Med. Chem.*, **5,** 896 (1962).

93. J. G. Topliss, M. H. Sherlock, F. H. Clarke, M. C. Daly, B. W. Pettersen, J. Lipski, and N. Sperber, *J. Org. Chem.*, **26,** 3842 (1961).

94. J. Klosa and H. Voigt, *J. Prakt. Chem.*, **16,** 264 (1962).

95. J. Klosa, *J. Prakt. Chem.*, **18,** 225 (1962).

96. J. Klosa, *J. Prakt. Chem.*, **33,** 298 (1966).

97. J. Klosa, *J. Prakt. Chem.*, **21,** 176 (1963).

98. W. J. Close, L. R. Swett, L. E. Brady, J. H. Short, and M. Vernsten, *J. Am. Chem. Soc.*, **82,** 1132 (1960).

99. J. H. Short and U. Biermacher, *J. Am. Chem. Soc.*, **82,** 1135 (1960).

100. J. H. Short and L. R. Swett, *J. Org. Chem.*, **26,** 3428 (1961).

101. C. T. Holdrege, R. B. Babel, and L. C. Cheney, *J. Am. Chem. Soc.*, **81,** 4807 (1959).

102. W. M. McLamore and G. D. Laubach, U.S. Pat. 3,111,517 (Nov. 19, 1963).

103. J. M. McManns, U.S. Pat. 3,009,911 (Nov. 21, 1961).

104. C. W. Whitehead, J. J. Traverso, H. R. Sullivan, and F. J. Marshall, *J. Org. Chem.*, **26,** 2814 (1961).

105. C. W. Whitehead and J. J. Traverso, *J. Org. Chem.*, **27,** 951 (1962).

106. F. J. Lund and W. Kobinger, *Acta Pharmacol. Toxicol.*, **16,** 297 (1960).

107. B. Beermann, M. Groschinsky-Grind, and B. Lindstrom, *Eur. J. Clin. Pharmacol.*, **11,** 203 (1977).

108. D. A. Garcia and E. R. Yendt, *C. M. A. J.*, **103,** 473 (1970).

109. M. Hohenegger, *Advances Clin. Pharmacol.*, **9,** 1 (1975).

110. M. Goldberg, "The renal Physiology of Diuretics," in *Handbook of Physiology*, Section 8, J. Orloff and R. W. Berliner, Eds., American Physiology Society, Washington, D.C., 1973, pp. 1003–1031.

111. V. L. Dettli, P. Spring, and M. Baur, *Arzneim.-Forsch.*, **12,** 289 (1962).

112. R. V. Ford, *Curr. Ther. Res.*, **3,** 320 (1961).

113. G. deStevens, L. H. Werner, W. E. Barrett, J. J. Chart, and A. H. Renzi, *Experientia*, **16,** 113 (1960).

114. M. H. Sherlock, N. Sperber, and J. G. Topliss, *Experientia*, **16,** 184 (1960).

115. J. C. Skou, *Physiol. Rev.* **45,** 596 (1965).

116. G. R. Zins, *Ann. Rep. Med. Chem.* **8,** 83 (1973).

117. R. L. Smith, O. W. Waltersdorf, Jr., and E. J. Cragoe, Jr., *Ann. Rep. Med. Chem.*, **11,** 71 (1976).

118. R. V. Patak, B. K. Mookerjee, C. J. Bentzel, P. E. Hysert, M. Babej, and J. B. Lee, *Prostaglandins*, **10,** 649 (1975).

119. W. Graf, E. Girod, E. Schmid, and W. G. Stoll, *Helv. Chim. Acta*, **42,** 1085 (1959).

120. E. G. Stenger, H. Wirz, and R. Pulver, *Schweiz Med. Wochenschr.*, **89,** 126, 1130 (1959).

121. R. Veyrat, E. F. Arnold, and A. Duckert, *Schweiz Med. Wochenschr.*, **89,** 1133 (1959).

122. F. Reutter and F. Schaub, *Schweiz Med. Wochenschr.*, **89,** 1158 (1959).

123. W. Leppla, H. Büch, and G. A. Jutzler, *Ger. Med. Monthly*, **5,** 402 (1960).

124. M. Fuchs, B. E. Newman, S. Irie, R. Maranoff, E. Lippman, and J. H. Moyer, *Curr. Ther. Res.*, **2,** 11 (1960).

125. W. E. Bowlus and H. G. Langford, *Clin. Pharmacol. Ther.*, **5,** 708 (1964).

126. E. Jucker, A. Lindenmann, E. Schenker, E. Fluckiger, and M. Taeschler, *Arzneim.-Forsch.* **13,** 269 (1963).

127. B. Terry and J. B. Hook, *J. Pharmacol. Exp. Ther.*, **160,** 367 (1968).

128. V. Parsons and R. Kemball Price, *Practitioner*, **195,** 648 (1965).

129. D. H. Kaump, R. L. Fransway, L. T. Blouin, and D. Williams, *J. New Drugs*, **4,** 21 (1964).

130. M. L. Hoefle, L. T. Blouin, H. A. DeWald, A. Holmes, and D. Williams, *J. Med. Chem.*, **11,** 970 (1968).

131. L. T. Blouin, D. H. Kaump, R. L. Fransway, and D. Williams, *J. New Drugs*, **3,** 302 (1963).

132. E. V. Mackay and S. K. Khoo, *Med. J. Aust.*, **1,** 607 (1969).

133. E. J. Cornish, G. E. Lee, and W. R. Wragg, *J. Pharm. Pharmacol.*, **18,** 65 (1966).

134. A. F. Lant, W. I. Baba, and G. M. Wilson, *Clin. Pharmacol. Ther.*, **7,** 196 (1966).

135. W.I. Baba, A. F. Lant, and G. M. Wilson, *Clin. Pharmacol. Ther.*, **7,** 212 (1966).

136. J. L. Verbov, D. S. Tunstall-Pedoe, and T. J. C. Cooke, *Brit. J. Clin. Pract.*, **20,** 351 (1966).

137. K. Corbett, S. A. Edwards, G. E. Lee, and T. L. Threlfall, *Nature*, **208,** 286 (1965).

138. C. B. Wilson and W. M. Kirkendall, *J. Pharmacol. Exp. Ther.*, **173,** 422 (1970).

139. C. B. Wilson and W. M. Kirkendall, *J. Pharmacol. Exp. Ther.*, **171,** 288 (1970).

140 W. H. R. Auld and W. R. Murdoch, *Brit. Med. J.*, **4,** 786 (1971).

141. S. J. Jachuck, *Brit. Med. J.*, **3,** 590 (1972).

142. E. Cohen, B. Klarberg, and J. R. Vaughan, Jr., *J. Am. Chem. Soc.*, **82,** 2731 (1960).

143. R. H. Seller, M. Fuchs, G. Onesti, C. Swartz, A. N. Brest, and J. H. Moyer, *Clin. Pharmacol. Ther.*, **3,** 180 (1962).

144. B. V. Shetty, L. A. Campanella, T. L. Thomas, M. Fedorchuk, T. A. Davidson, L. Michelson, H. Volz, and S. E. Zimmerman, *J. Med. Chem.*, **13,** 886 (1970).

145. W. N. Suki, F. Dawoud, G. Eknoyan, and M. Martinez-Maldonado, *J. Pharmacol. Exp. Ther.*, **180,** 6 (1972).

146. J. W. Smiley, G. Onesti, and C. Swartz, *Clin. Pharmacol. Ther.*, **13**, 336 (1972).

147. M. F. Michelis, F. DeRubertis, N. P. Beck, R. H. McDonald, Jr., and B. B. Davis, *Clin. Pharmacol. Ther.*, **11**, 821 (1970).

148. B. J. Materson, J. L. Hotchkiss, J. S. Barkin, B. H. Rietberg, K. Bailey, and E. C. Perez-Stable, *Curr. Ther. Res.*, **14**, 545 (1972).

149. E. J. Belair, A. I. Cohen, and J. Yelnoski, *Brit. J. Pharm.*, **45**, 476 (1972).

150. R. M. Pilewski, E. T. Scheib, J. R. Misage, E. Kessler, E. Krifcher, and A. P. Shapiro, *Clin. Pharmacol. Ther.*, **12**, 843, (1971).

151. H. J. Dargie, M. E. M. Allison, A. C. Kennedy, and M. J. B. Gray, *Brit. Med. J.*, **4**, 196 (1972).

152. E. M. Schultz, E. J. Cragoe, Jr., J. B. Bicking, W. A. Bolhofer, and J. M. Sprague, *J. Med. Chem.*, **5**, 660 (1962).

153. J. M. Sprague, *Ann. Rep. Med. Chem.*, **5**, XI, (1970).

154. J. B. Bicking, W. J. Holtz, L. S. Watson, and E. J. Cragoe, Jr., *J. Med. Chem.*, **19**, 530 (1976).

155. D. E. Duggan and R. M. Noll, *Arch. Biochem. Biophys.*, **109**, 388 (1965).

156. J. B. Bicking, C. M. Robb, L. S. Watson, and E. J. Cragoe, Jr., *J. Med. Chem.*, **19**, 544 (1976).

157. K. H. Beyer, J. E. Baer, J. K. Michaelson, and H. F. Russo, *J. Pharmacol. Exp. Ther.*, **147**, 1 (1965).

158. M. Goldberg, *Ann. N.Y. Acad. Sci.*, **139**, 443 (1966).

159. K. Sturm, W. Siedel, R. Weyer, and H. Ruschig, *Chem. Ber.*, **99**, 328 (1966).

160. W. Siedel, K. Sturm, and W. Scheurich, *Chem. Ber.*, **99**, 345 (1966).

161. R. J. Timmerman, F. R. Springman, and R. K. Thoms, *Curr. Ther. Res.*, **6**, 88 (1964).

162. R. Muschaweck and P. Hajdu, *Arzneim.-Forsch.*, **14**, 46 (1964).

163. W. Suki, F. C. Rector, Jr., and D. W. Seldin, *J. Clin. Invest.*, **44**, 1458 (1965).

164. A. Häussler and P. Hajdu, *Arzneim.-Forsch.*, **14**, 710 (1964).

165. A. Häussler and H. Wicha, *Arzneim.-Forsch.*, **15**, 81 (1965).

166. E. M. Schultz, J. B. Bicking, A. A. Deana, N. P. Gould, T. P. Strobaugh, L. S. Watson, and E. J. Cragoe, Jr., *J. Med. Chem.*, **19**, 783 (1976).

167. C. T. Dollery, E. H. O. Parry, and D. S. Young, *Lancet*, **1**, 947 (1964).

168. J. F. Maher and G. E. Schreiner, *Ann. Intern. Med.*, **62**, 15 (1965).

169. V. K. G. Pillay, F. D. Schwartz, K. Aimi, and R. M. Kark, *Lancet*, **1969-I**, 77.

170. J. B. Hook, A. H. Blatt, M. J. Brody, and H. E. Williamson, *J. Pharmacol. Exp. Ther.*, **154**, 667 (1966).

171. J. H. Ludens. J. B. Hook, M. J. Brody, and H. E. Williamson, *J. Pharmacol. Exp. Ther.*, **163**, 456 (1968).

172. W. Stokes and L. C. A. Nunn, *Brit. Med. J.*, **2**, 910 (1964).

173. W. M. Kirkendall and J. H. Stein, *Am. J. Cardiol.*, **22**, 162 (1968).

174. C. R. Bariso, I. B. Hanenson, and T. E. Gaffney, *Curr. Ther. Res.*, **12**, 333 (1970).

175. R. G. Muth, *J. Am. Med. Assoc.*, **195**, 1066 (1966).

176. D. S. Silverberg, R. A. Ulan, M. A. Baltzan, and R. B. Baltzan, *Can. Med. Assoc. J.*, **103**, 129 (1970).

177. O. H. Morelli, L. I. Moledo, E. Alanis, O. L. Gaston, and O. Terzaghi, *Postgrad. Med. J.*, **47**: April Suppl., 29 (1971).

178. P. W. Feit, H. Bruun, and C. K. Nielsen, *J. Med. Chem.*, **13**, 1071 (1970).

179. P. W. Feit, *J. Med. Chem.*, **14**, 432 (1971).

180. P. W. Feit and O. B. Tvaermose Nielsen, *J. Med. Chem.*, **15**, 79 (1972).

181. P. W. Feit, O. B. Tvaermose Nielsen, and N. Rastrup-Andersen, *J. Med. Chem.*, **16**, 127 (1973).

182. O. B. Tvaermose Nielsen, C. K. Nielsen, and P. W. Feit, *J. Med. Chem.* **16**, 1170 (1973).

183. P. W. Feit, O. B. Tvaermose Nielsen, and H. Bruun, *J. Med. Chem.*, **17**, 572 (1974).

184. O. B. Tvaermose Nielsen, H. Bruun, C. Bretting, and P. W. Feit, *J. Med. Chem.*, **18**, 41 (1975).

185. P. W. Feit and O. B. Tvaermose Nielsen, *J. Med. Chem.*, **19**, 402 (1976).

186. P. W. Feit, P. B. Tvaermose Nielsen, and H. Brunn, *J. Med. Chem.*, **15**, 437 (1972).

187. E. H. Østergaard, M. P. Magnussen, C. Kaergaard Nielsen, E. Eilertsen, and H. H. Frey, *Arzneim.-Forsch.*, **22**, 66 (1972).

188. P. W. Feit, K. Roholt, and H. Sørensen, *J. Pharm. Sci.*, **62**, 375 (1973).

189. M. J. Asbury, P. B. B. Gatenby, S. O'Sullivan, and E. Bourke, *Brit. Med. J.*, **1**, 211 (1972).

190. K. H. Olesen, B. Sigurd, E. Steiness, and A. Leth, *Acta Med. Scand.*, **193**, 119 (1973).

191. K. H. Olesen, B. Sigurd, E. Steiness, and A. Leth, "Modern Diuretic Therapy in the Treatment of Cardiovascular and Renal Disease," in *Excerpta Medica*, A. F. Lant and G. M. Wilson, Eds., Amsterdam, 1973, p. 155.

192. E. Bourke, M. J. A. Asbury, S. O'Sullivan, and P. B. Ꝺ. Gatenby, *Eur. J. Pharmacol.*, **23,** 283 (1973).

193. S. Carrière and R. Dandavino, *Clin. Pharmacol. Ther.* **20,** 428 (1976).

194. M. Imai, *Eur. J. Pharmacol.*, **41,** 409 (1977).

195. D. L. Davies, A. F. Lant, N. R. Millard, A. J. Smith, J. W. Ward, and G. M. Wilson, *Clin. Pharmacol. Ther.*, **15,** 141 (1974).

196. W. P. Leary, A. C. Asmal, and P. Samuel, *Curr. Ther. Res.*, **15,** 571 (1973).

197. D. B. Campbell and E. M. Phillips, *Eur. J. Clin. Pharmacol.*, **7,** 407 (1974).

198. D. B. Campbell, A. R. Taylor, and R. Moore, *Brit. J. Clin. Pharmacol.*, **3,** 971P (1976).

199. J. Kyncl, K. Oheim, T. Seki, and A. Solles, *Arzneim.-Forsch.*, **25,** 1491 (1975).

200. L. Finch and P. E. Hicks, *Brit. J. Pharmacol.*, **58,** 282P (1976).

201. Y. K. Seedat and J. Reddy, *Curr. Ther. Res.*, **16,** 275 (1974).

202. S. Witchitz, J. F. Giudicelli, H. El Guedri, A. Kamoun, and P. Chiche, *Therapie*, **29,** 109 (1974).

203. W. Merkel, D. Bormann, D. Mania, R. Muschaweck, and M. Hropot, *Eur. J. Med. Chem.*, **11,** 399 (1976).

204. R. Z. Gussin, J. R. Cummings, E. H. Stokey, and M. A. Ronsberg, *J. Pharmacol. Exp. Ther.*, **167,** 194 (1969).

205. E. A. Lockhart, J. H. Dirks, and S. Carrière, *Am. J. Physiol.*, **223,** 89 (1972).

206. R. Z. Gussin and M. A. Ronsberg, *Proc. Soc. Exp. Biol. Med.*, **131,** 1258 (1969).

207. Z. S. Agus and M. Goldberg, *J. Lab. Clin. Med.*, **76,** 280 (1970).

208. *FDC Rep.* **36**: 39, A6 (Sept. 30, 1974).

209. W. Liebenow and F. Leuschner, *Arzneim.-Forsch.*, **25,** 240 (1975).

210. F. Leuschner, W. Neumann, and H. Barhmann, *Arzneim.-Forsch.*, **25,** 245 (1975).

211 F. W. Hempelmann, *Arzneim.-Forsch.*, **25,** 259 (1975).

212. F. W. Hempelmann, *Arzneim.-Forsch.*, **25,** 258 (1975).

213. F. W. Hempelmann, F. Leuschner, and W. Liebenow, *Arzneim. -Forsch.*, **25,** 252 (1975).

214. G. Voltz, *Arzneim.-Forsch.*, **25,** 256 (1975).

215. M. Hohenegger and F. Holzer, *Int. J. Clin. Pharmacol.*, **13,** 298 (1976).

216. P. Federspil and H. Mausen, *Int. J. Clin. Pharmacol.*, **9,** 326 (1974).

217. Bayer AG, Belg. Pats. 813–746 to 813–748 (1973).

218. E. Möller, H. Horstmann, K. Meng, and D. Loew, *Experientia*, **33,** 382 (1977).

219. D. Loew and K. Meng, *Pharmatherapeutica*, **1,** 333 (1977).

220. H. J. Kramer, *Pharmatherapeutica*, **1,** 353 (1977).

221. K. J. Berg, S. Jørstad, and A. Tromsdal, *Pharmatherapeutica*, **1,** 319 (1976).

222. D. Loew, *Curr. Med. Res. Opin.*, **4,** 455 (1977).

223. M. Mussche and N. Lameire, *Curr. Med. Res. Opin.*, **4,** 462 (1977).

224. R. L. Smith, G. E. Stokker, and E. J. Cragoe, Jr., *J. Med. Chem.*, in press.

225. M. B. Affrime, D. T. Lowenthal, G. Onesti, P. Busby, C. Swartz, and B. Lei, *Clin. Pharmacol. Ther.*, **21,** 97 (1977).

226. F. A. Kuehl, Jr., J. L. Humes, R. W. Egan, E. A. Ham, G. C. Beveridge, and C. G. Van Arman, *Nature*, **265,** 170 (1977).

227. J. C. Frölich, T. W. Wilson, B. J. Sweetman, M. Smigel, A. S. Nies, K. Carr, J. T. Watson, and J. A. Oates, *J. Clin. Invest.*, **55,** 763 (1975).

228. G. R. Zins, *Am. J. Med.*, **58,** 14 (1975).

229. R. L. Smith, O. W. Woltersdorf, Jr., and E. J. Cragoe, Jr., in *Ann. Rep. Med. Chem.*, **11,** 71 (1976).

230. M. Wiederholt, H. Stolte, J. P. Brecht, and K. Hierholzer, *Pflügers Arch.*, **292,** 316 (1966).

231. E. Uhlich, C. A. Baldamus, and K. J. Ullrich, *Pflügers Arch.*, **308.**, 111 (1969).

232. J. A. Cella and C. M. Kagawa, *J. Am. Chem. Soc.*, **79,** 4808 (1957).

233. C. M. Kagawa, J. A. Cella, and C. G. Van Arman, *Science*, **126,** 1015 (1957).

234. J. A. Cella, E. A. Brown, and R. R. Burtner, *J. Org. Chem.*, **24,** 743 (1959).

235. J. A. Cella and R. C. Tweit, *J. Org. Chem.*, **24,** 1109 (1959).

236. E. A. Brown, R. D. Muir, and J. A. Cella, *J. Org. Chem.*, **25,** 96 (1960).

237. G. W. Liddle, in *The Clinical Use of Aldosterone Antagonists*, F. C. Barter, Ed., Charles C Thomas, Springfield, Ill., 1960, p. 14.

238. H. J. Hess, *J. Org. Chem.*, **27,** 1096 (1962).

239. B. Singer, *Endrocrinology*, **65,** 512 (1959),

240. E. Bolte, M. Verdy, J. Marc-Aurele, J. Brouillet, P. Beauregard, and J. Genest, *Can. Med. Assoc. J.*, **79,** 881 (1958).

241. R. M. Salassa, V. R. Mattox, and M. H. Power, *J. Clin. Endrocrinol. Metab.*, **18,** 787 (1958).

242. G. W. Liddle, *Arch. Intern. Med.*, **102,** 998 (1958).

243. J. D. H. Slater, A. Moxham, R. Hurter, and J. D. N. Nabarro, *Lancet*, **1958-II,** 931.

244. D. N. S. Kerr, A. E. Read, R. M. Haslam, and S. Sherlock, *Lancet*, **1959-II,** 1084.

245. G. W. Liddle, *Science*, **126,** 1016 (1957).

246. E. J. Ross and J. E. Bethune, *Lancet*, **1959-I,** 127.

247. R. C. Tweit, F. B. Colton, N. L. McNiven, and W. Klyne, *J. Org. Chem.*, **27,** 3325 (1962).

248. J. A. Cella, in *Edema*, J. H. Moyer and M. Fuchs, Eds., Saunders, Philadelphia, 1960, p. 303.

249. N. W. Atwater, R. H. Bible, Jr., E. A. Brown, R. R. Burtner, J. S. Mihina, L. N. Nysted, and P. B. Sollman, *J. Org. Chem.* **26,** 3077 (1961).

250. L. N. Nysted and R. R. Burtner, *J. Org. Chem.* **27,** 3175 (1962).

251. A. A. Patchett, F. Hoffman, F. F. Giarrusso, H. Schwam, and G. E. Arth, *J. Org. Chem.*, **27,** 3822 (1962).

252. G. deStevens, *Diuretics: Chemistry and Pharmacology*, Academic, New York, 1963, p. 130.

253. A. Karim and E. A. Brown, *Steroids*, **20,** 41 (1972). L. J. Chinn, E. A. Brown, S. S. Mizuba, and A. Karim, *J. Med. Chem.*, **20,** 352 (1977).

254. U. Abshagen, H. Rennekamp, K. Koch, M. Senn, and W. Steingross, *Steroids*, **28,** 467 (1976).

255. C. M. Kagawa, D. J. Bouska, M. L. Anderson, and W. F. Krol, *Arch. Int. Pharmacodyn.*, **149,** 8 (1964).

256. L. M. Hofmann, L. J. Chinn, H. A. Pedrera, M. I. Krupnick, and O. D. Suleymanov, *J. Pharmacol. Exp. Ther.*, **194,** 450 (1975).

257. L. Ramsay, I. Harrison, J. Shelton, and M. Tidd, *Clin. Pharmacol. Ther.*, **18,** 391 (1975).

258. J. W. Funder, J. Mercer, and J. Hood, *Clin. Sci. Mol. Med.*, **51,** Suppl. 3, 333 (1976).

259. R. M. Weier and L. M. Hofmann, *J. Med. Chem.* **18,** 817 (1975).

260. L. M. Hofmann, R. M. Weier, O. D. Suleymanov, and H. A. Pedrera, *J. Pharmacol. Exp. Ther.*, **201,** 762 (1977).

261. L. J. Chinn and B. N. Desai, *J. Med. Chem.*, **18,** 268 (1975).

262. L. J. Chinn and L. M. Hofmann, *J. Med. Chem.*, **16,** 839 (1973).

263. L. J. Chinn, H. L. Dryden, Jr., and R. R. Burtner, *J. Org. Chem.*, **26,** 3910 (1961).

264. L. J. Chinn, *J. Org. Chem.*, **27,** 1741 (1962).

265. E. J. Ross, *Clin. Pharmacol. Ther.*, **6,** 65 (1965).

266. *Physicians Desk Reference*, 31st ed., Medical Economics Co., Oradell, N.J., 1977 p. 1444.

267. W. L. Bencze and M. J. Allen, *J. Am. Chem. Soc.*, **81,** 4015 (1959).

268. G. deStevens, *Diuretics, Chemistry and Pharmacology*, Academic, New York, 1963, p. 16.

269. K. H. Beyer and J. F. Baer, in *Progress in Drug Research*, Vol. 2, E. Jucker, Ed., Birkhäuser, Basle-Stuttgart, 1960. p. 21.

270. V. Papesch and E. F. Schroeder, *J. Org. Chem.*, **16,** 1879 (1951).

271. A. Kattus, T. M. Arrington, and E. V. Newman, *Am. J. Med.*, **12,** 319 (1952).

272. W. L. Lipschitz and Z. Hadidian, *J. Pharmacol. Exp. Ther.*, **81,** 84 (1944).

273. H. Ludwig, *Schweiz. Med. Wochenschr.*, **76,** 822 (1946).

274. V. Papesch and E. F. Schroeder, in *Medicinal Chemistry*, Vol. III, F. F. Blicke and R. H. Cox, Eds., Wiley, New York, 1956, p. 175.

275. A. Turchetti, *Riforma Med.*, **64,** 405 (1950).

276. E. V. Newman, J. Franklin, and J. Genest, *Bull. Johns Hopkins Hosp.*, **82,** 409 (1948).

277. O. Clauder and G. Bulcsu, *Magy. Kem. Foly*, **57,** 68 (1951); *Chem. Abstr.*, **46,** 4023 (1952).

278. G. Szabo, O. Clauder, and Z. Magyar, *Magy. Belorv. Arch.*, **6,** 156 (1953).

279. C. M. Kagawa and C. G. Van Arman, *J. Pharmacol. Exp. Ther.*, **124,** 318 (1958).

280. D. V. Miller and R. V. Ford, *Am. J. Med. Sci.*, **236,** 32 (1958).

281. R. V. Ford, J. B. Rochelle, A. C. Bullock, C. L. Spurr, C. Handley, and J. H. Moyer, *Am. J. Cardiol.*, **3,** 148 (1959).

282. M. H. Sha, M. Y. Mhasalkar, and C. V. Deliwala, *J. Sci. Ind. Res.* (India), **19c,** 282 (1960); D. J. Mehta, U. K. Sheth, and C. V. Deliwala, *Nature* (London), **187,** 1034 (1960).

283. K. N. Modi, C. V. Deliwala, and U. K. Sheth, *Arch. Int. Pharmacodyn.* **151,** 13 (1964).

284. L. Szabo, L. Szporny, and O. Clauder, *Acta Pharm. Hung.*, **31,** 163 (1961); through *Chem. Abstr.*, **55,** 24780i (1961).

285. W. B. McKeon, Jr., *Arch. Int. Pharmacodyn.*, **151,** 225 (1964).

286. D. A. LeSher and F. E. Shideman, *J. Pharmacol. Exp. Ther.*, **116,** 38 (1956).

287. H. E. Williamson, F. E. Shideman, and D. A. LeSher, *J. Pharmacol. Exp. Ther.*, **126,** 82 (1959).

288. J. E. Baer, in *Modern Diuretic Therapy*, A. F. Lant and G. M. Wilson, Eds., Excerpta Medica, Amsterdam, 1973, p. 148.

289. W. I. Baba, G. R. Tudhope, and G. M. Wilson, *Clin. Sci.*, **27,** 181 (1964).

290. W. I. Baba, A. F. Lant, A. J. Smith, M. M. Townshend, and G. M. Wilson, *Clin. Pharmacol. Ther.*, **9,** 318 (1968).

291. J. E. Baer, C. B. Jones, S. A. Spitzer, and H. F. Russo, *J. Pharmacol. Exp. Ther.*, **157,** 472 (1967).

292. R. W. Berliner, *Harvey Lect.*, **55,** 141 (1960).

293. G. Giebisch, E. L. Boulpaep, and G. Whittembury, *Phil. Trans. R. Soc. London Ser. B*, **262,** 175 (1971).

294. C. G. Duarte, F. Chomety, and G. Giebisch, *Am. J. Physiol.*, **221,** 632 (1971).

295. V. D. Wiebelhaus, J. Weinstock, A. R. Maass, F. T. Brennan, G. Sosnowski, and T. Larsen, *J. Pharmacol. Exp. Ther.*, **149,** 397 (1965).

296. J. Weinstock, J. W. Wilson, V. D. Wiebelhaus, A. R. Maass, F. T. Brennan, and G. Sosnowski, *J. Med. Chem.*, **11,** 573 (1968).

297. T. S. Osdene, A. A. Santilli, L. E. McCardle, and M. E. Rosenthale, *J. Med. Chem.*, **9,** 697 (1966).

298. T. S. Osdene, A. A. Santilli, L. E. McCardle, and M. E. Rosenthale, *J. Med. Chem.*, **10,** 165 (1967).

299. M. E. Rosenthale and C. G. Van Arman, *J. Pharmacol. Exp. Ther.* **142,** 111 (1963).

300. V. D. Wiebelhaus, J. Weinstock, F. T. Brennan, G. Sosnowski, and T. J. Larsen, *Fed. Proc.*, **20,** 409 (1961).

301. A. P. Crosley, Jr., L. Ronquillo, and F. Alexander, *Fed. Proc.* **20,** 410 (1961).

302. J. H. Laragh, E. B. Reilly, T. B. Stites, and M. Angers, *Fed. Proc.* **20,** 410 (1961).

303. V. D. Wiebelhaus, J. Weinstock, F. T. Brennan, G. Sosnowski, T. Larsen, and K. Gahagan, *Pharmacologist*, **3**:2, **59** (1961).

304. W. Schaumann, *Klin. Wochenschr.*, **40,** 756 (1962).

305. W. I. Baba, G. R. Tudhope, and G. M. Wilson, *Brit. Med. J.*, **2,** 756 (1962).

306. G. W. Liddle, *Metab. Clin. Exp.*, **10,** 1021 (1961).

307. G. M. Ball and J. A. Greene, Jr., *Proc. Soc. Exp. Biol. Med.*, **113,** 326 (1963).

308. A. P. Crosley, Jr., L. Ronquillo, W. S. Strickland, and F. Alexander, *Ann. Intern. Med.*, **56,** 241 (1962).

309. D. J. Ginsberg, A. Saad, and G. J. Gabuzda, *New Engl. J. Med.*, **271,** 1229 (1964).

310. P. Baume, F. J. Radcliffe, and C. R. Corry, *Am. J. Med. Sci.*, **245,** 668 (1963).

311. A. Badinand, R. Mallein, J. Rondelet, J. J. Vallon, and O. Chappuis, *C. R. Soc. Biol.*, **157,** 1629 (1963).

312. J. B. Lassen and O. E. Nielsen, *Acta Pharmacol. Toxicol.*, **20,** 309 (1963).

313. A. Gerard, F. Guerrin, C. Clacys, and J. Lescut, *Therapie* **19,** 585 (1964).

314. K. Lehmann, *Arzneim.-Forsch.*, **15,** 812 (1965).

315. H. Herken, V. Neuhoff, and G. Senft, *Klin. Wochenschr.*, **43,** 960 (1965).

316. W. R. Cattell and C. W. H. Havard, *Brit. Med. J.*, **2,** 1362 (1962).

317. R. A. Thompson and M. F. Crowley, *Postgrad. Med. J.* (Oxford), **41,** 706 (1965).

318. K. Nishikawa, H. Shimakawa, Y. Inada, Y. Shibouta, S. Kikuchi, S. Yurugi, and Y. Oka, *Chem. Pharm. Bull.* (Tokyo), **24,** 2057 (1976).

319. K. Nishikawa and S. Kikuchi, *Jap. J. Pharmacol.*, **22**:Suppl., 103 (1972); Y. Nakai, Y. Shirakawa, and T. Fujita, *ibid.*, 102 (1972).

320. H. Kawaki, R. Tsukuda, K. Nishikawa, S. Kikuchi, and T. Hirano, *J. Takeda Res. Labs*, **32,** 299 (1973); Y. Inada, K. Nishikawa, A. Nagaoka, and S. Kikuchi, *Arzneim.-Forsch.*, **27,** 1663 (1977).

321. J. B. Bicking, J. W. Mason, O. W. Woltersdorf, Jr., J. H. Jones, S. F. Kwong, C. M. Robb, and E. J. Cragoe, Jr., *J. Med. Chem.*, **8,** 638 (1965).

322. M. S. Glitzer and S. L. Steelman, *Proc. Soc. Exp. Biol. Med.*, **120,** 364 (1965).

323. E. J. Cragoe, Jr., O. W. Woltersdorf, Jr., J. B. Bicking, S. F. Kwong, and J. H. Jones, *J. Med. Chem.*, **10,** 66 (1967).

324. J. B. Bicking, C. M. Robb, S. F. Kwong, and E. J. Cragoe, Jr., *J. Med. Chem.*, **10,** 598 (1967).

325. J. H. Jones, J. B. Bicking, and E. J. Cragoe, Jr., *J. Med. Chem.*, **10,** 899 (1967).

326. R. Z. Gussin, M. A. Ronsberg, E. H. Stokey, and J. R. Cummings, *J. Pharmacol. Exp. Ther.*, **195,** 8 (1975).

327. M. A. Ronsberg, R. Z. Gussin, E. H. Stokey, and P. S. Chan, *Pharmacologist*, **18,** 150 (1976).

328. R. Walter and P. L. Hoffman, in *Best and Taylor's Physiological Basis of Medical Practice*, ed. 9th, Section 1, (6), J. R. Brobeck, Ed., Williams and Wilkins, Baltimore, 1973.

329. F. G. W. Marson, *Lancet*, **1955-II,** 360.

330. K. H. Beyer, H. F. Russo, E. K. Tillson, A. K. Miller, W. F. Verwey, and S. R. Gass, *Am. J. Physiol.*, **166,** 625 (1951).

331. K. H. Beyer, *Arch. Int. Pharmacodyn.*, **98,** 97 (1954).

332. A. B. Gutman, *Advan. Pharmacol.*, **4,** 91 (1966).

333. P. Brazeau, in *The Pharmacological Basis of Therapeutics*, 5th ed. Section VIII, L. S. Goodman and A. Gilman, Eds., Macmillan, New York, 1975, p. 860.

334. R. Pfister and F. Häfliger, *Helv. Chim. Acta*, **44,** 232 (1961).

335. J. J. Burns, T. F. Yü, A. Ritterband, J. M. Perel, A. B. Gutman, and B. B. Brodie, *J. Pharmacol. Exp. Ther.*, **119,** 418 (1957).

336. T. F. Yü, J. J. Burns, and A. B. Gutman, *Arth. Rheum.*, **1,** 352 (1958).

337. J. J. Burns, T. F. Yü, P. Dayton, L. Berger, A. B. Gutman, and B. B. Brodie, *Nature* **182,** 1162 (1958).

338. K. C. Blanchard, D. Maroske, D. G. May, and I. M. Weiner, *J. Pharmacol. Exp. Ther.*, **180,** 397 (1972).

339. A. H. Anton, *J. Pharmacol. Exp. Ther.*, **134,** 291 (1961).

340. A. B. Gutman, P. G. Dayton, T. F. Yü, L. Berger, W. Chen, L. E. Sicam, and J. J. Burns, *Am. J. Med.*, **29,** 1017 (1960).

341. T. F. Yü and A. B. Gutman, *Am. J. Med.*, **37,** 885 (1964).

342. R. W. Rundles, E. N. Metz, and H. R. Silberman, *Ann. Intern. Med.*, **64,** 229 (1966).

343. D. M. Woodbury and E. Fingl, in *The Pharmacological Basis of Therapeutics*, 5th ed. Section II, L. S. Goodman and A. Gilman, Eds., Macmillan, New York, 1975, p. 352.

344. J. M. Bryant, T. F. Yü, L. Burger, N. Schwartz, S. Torosdag, L. Fletcher, H. Fertig, M. S. Schwartz, and R. B. F. Quan, *Am. J. Med.*, **33,** 408 (1962).

345. K. E. Kim, G. Onesti, J. H. Moyer, and C. Swartz, *Am. J. Cardiol.*, **27,** 407 (1971).

346. B. T. Emmerson, *Drugs,* **9,** 141 (1975).

347. G. Thuillier, J. Laforest, B. Cariou, P. Bessin, J. Bonnet, and J. Thuillier, *Eur. J. Med. Chem.*, **9,** 625 (1974).

348. K. Lau, M. Goldberg, R. Stote, and Z. S. Agus, *Clin. Res.*, **24,** 405*A* (1976).

349. K. Lau, R. Stote, M. Goldberg, and Z. S. Agus, *Clin. Res.*, **24,** 405 (1976).

350. A. K. Jain, F. G. McMahon, R. Vargas, and J. R. Ryan, *Clin. Pharmacol. Ther.*, **21,** 107 (1977).

351. R. Vargas, A. Jain, J. Ryan, and F. G. McMahon, *Clin. Pharmacol. Ther.*, **21,** 119 (1977).

352. M. Nemati, M. C. Kyle, and E. D. Freis, *J. Am. Med. Assoc.*, **237,** 652 (1977).

353. E. J. Cragoe, Jr., E. M. Schultz, J. D. Schneeberg, G. E. Stokker, O. W. Woltersdorf, Jr., G. M. Fanelli, Jr., and L. S. Watson, *J. Med. Chem.*, **18,** 225 (1975).

354. L. S. Watson and G. M. Fanelli, *Fed. Proc.* **34,** 802 (1975), Abstract 3294.

355. G. M. Fanelli, Jr., D. L. Bohn, A. Scriabine, and K. H. Beyer, Jr., *J. Pharmacol. Exp. Ther.*, **200,** 402 (1977).

356. R. McKenzie, T. Knight, and E. J. Weinman, *Proc. Soc. Exp. Biol. Med.*, **153,** 202 (1976).

357. A. G. Zacchei, T. I. Wishousky, B. H. Arison, and G. M. Fanelli, Jr., *Drug Metab. Dispos.*, **4,** 479 (1976).

358. A. G. Zacchei and T. I. Wishousky, *Drug Metab. Dispos.*, **4,** 490 (1976).

359. E. J. Weinman, T. Knight, R. McKenzie, and G. Eknoyan, *Clin. Res.*, **24,** 416A (1976).

360. Z. E. Dziewanowska, K. F. Tempero, F. Perret, G. Hitzenberger, and G. H. Besselaar, *Clin. Res.*, **24,** 253A (1976).

361. K. F. Tempero, G. Hitzenberger, Z. E. Dziewanowska, and H. Halkin, *Clin. Pharmacol. Ther.*, **19,** 116 (1976).

362. K. F. Tempero, J. A. Vedin, C. E. Wilhelmsson, P. Lund-Johansen, C. Vorburger, C. Moerlin, H. Aaberg, W. Enenkel, J. Bolognese, and Z. E. Dziewanowska, *Clin. Pharmacol. Ther.*, **21,** 97 (1977).

363. G. Satzinger, *Arzneim.-Forsch.*, **27,** 466 (1977).

364. G. Satzinger, *Arzneim.-Forsch.*, **27,** 1742 (1977).

365. M. Herrmann, J. Wiegleb, and F. Leuschner, *Arzneim.-Forsch.*, **27,** 1758 (1977).

366. M. Herrmann, H. Bahrmann, E. Berkenmayer, V. Ganser, W. Heldt, and W. Steinbrecher, *Arzneim.-Forsch.*, **27,** 1745 (1977).

367. J. Greven and O. Heidenreich, *Arzneim.-Forsch.*, **27,** 1755 (1977).

368. K. O. Vollmer, A. v. Hodenberg, A. Poissson, V. Gladigau, and H. Hengy, *Arzneim.-Forsch.*, **27,** 1767 (1977).

369. A. v. Hodenberg, K. O. Vollmer, W. Klemisch, and B. Liedtke, *Arzneim.-Forsch.* **27,** 1776 (1977).

370. V. Gladigau and K. O. Vollmer, *Arzneim.-Forsch.*, **27,** 1786 (1977).

371. G. Biamino, *Arzneim.-Forsch.*, **27,** 1814 (1977).

372. E. Scheitza, *Arzneim.-Forsch.*, **27,** 1804 (1977).

373. E. Scheitza, *Arzneim.-Forsch.*, **27,** 1807 (1977).

374. Diuretic Agents, E. J. Cragoe, ed., ACS Symposium Series 83, American Chemical Society, Washington, DC, 1978.

375. O. B. Tvaermose-Nielsen and P. W. Feit, Ref. 374, p. 12.

376. P. W. Feit, O. B. T. Nielsen, C. Bretting, and H. Bruun, U. S. Patent 4,082,851 (1978).

377. P. W. Feit and O. B. T. Nielsen, *J. Med. Chem.*, **20,** 1687 (1977).

378. H. J. Lang, B. Knabe, R. Muschaweck, M. Hropot, and E. Lindner, Ref. 374, p. 24.

379. J. van Dijk, J. Hartog, and Th. A. C. Boschman, *J. Med. Chem.*, **19,** 982 (1976).

380. Th. A. C. Boschman, J. van Dijk, J. Hartog, and J. N. Walop, Ref. 374, p. 140.

CHAPTER FORTY-ONE

Adrenergics: Catecholamines and Related Agents

D. J. TRIGGLE

Department of Biochemical Pharmacology
School of Pharmacy
State University of New York
Buffalo, New York 14260, USA

CONTENTS

1 DISCOVERY, LOCALIZATION, AND DISTRIBUTION OF THE CATECHOLAMINE TRANSMITTERS

In 1895, Oliver and Schaefer (1) found that extracts of the adrenal gland produced a pressor response and a generally stimulant effect on smooth muscle. They could not identify the active constituent but presumed it to be of physiological importance. Some four years later the active principle, epinephrine (41.**1**), was isolated by Abel (2) and Takamine (3), and, almost simultaneously, Langley (4) commented on the similarities between the effects of adrenal gland extracts and those of sympathetic stimulation. The first syntheses of epinephrine [adrenaline, 2-(*N*-methylamino)-1-(3,4-dihydroxyphenyl)ethanol] were reported almost simultaneously by Stolz (5) and Dakin (6).

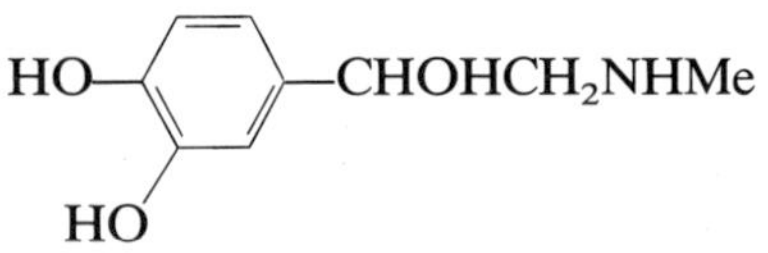

HO—⟨benzene ring⟩—CHOHCH₂NHMe

HO

41.**1**

Struck by the similarities between the effects of administered epinephrine and those of sympathetic nerve stimulation, Elliot (7) suggested that epinephrine was liberated in response to nerve stimulation:

. . . the point at which the stimulus of the chemical excitant is received and transformed into what may cause the change of tension of the muscle fibre, is perhaps a mechanism developed out of the muscle cell in response to its union with the synapsing sympathetic fibre, the function of which is to receive and transform the nervous impulses. Adrenaline might then be the chemical stimulant liberated on each occasion when the impulse arrives at the periphery.

Although epinephrine was to be accepted quite generally as the transmitter at sympathetic neuroeffector junctions for the next 40 years—a view strengthened by its apparent liberation from, and presence in,

sympathetically innervated tissues—a number of observations were recognized as not readily consistent with this view. The greater pressor potency of norepinephrine was recognized early (5, 6) and, more particularly, Dale (8, 9) observed that the ability of ergot alkaloids to reverse the motor effects of epinephrine was much more pronounced than with sympathetic stimulation (see Section 7). In their classic paper of 1910 Barger and Dale (10) noted very specifically important differences between the effects of sympathetic stimulation and those of administered epinephrine:

The conception of sympathetic nerve-impulses as acting by liberation of adrenine seems to us unsatisfactory for another reason. It involves the assumption of a stricter parallel between the two actions than actually exists. The inhibitor effects of these methylamino-bases are relatively prominent not only as compared with those of homologous bases, in particular the amino-bases, but also in comparison with those of sympathetic nerves.

However, it was not recognized that norepinephrine, rather than epinephrine, is the principal transmitter at sympathetic synapses until the 1940s, when von Euler (11–14) was able to demonstrate that the principal catecholamine stored and released in bovine cardiac and nerve tissues is norepinephrine. Subsequent work has used delicate fluorescent, electron microscopic, and autoradiographic observations to map pathways for norepinephrine (41.**2**) and dopamine (41.**3**) in both the peripheral and central nervous systems (15–17).

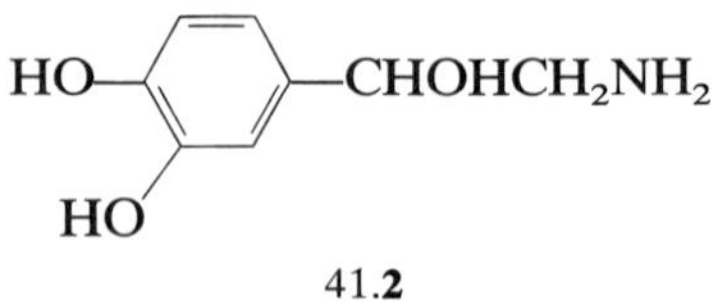

HO—⟨benzene ring⟩—CHOHCH₂NH₂

HO

41.**2**

HO—⟨benzene ring⟩—CH₂CH₂NH₂

HO

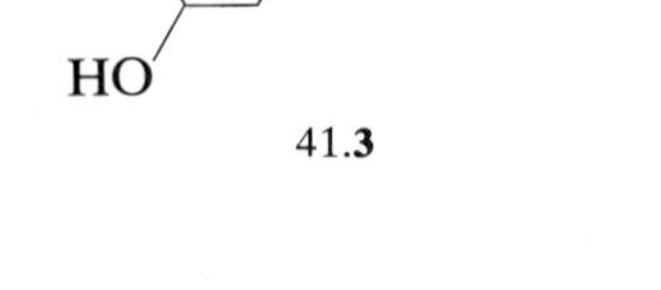

41.**3**

Epinephrine, which can be regarded as the original adrenergic agent, is useful for the general therapeutic application of adrenergic activation. Nonetheless, a great deal of chemical and pharmacological experience has gone into the search for analogs of epinephrine—sympathomimetic agents—that may have increased pharmacological or therapeutic utility by virtue of, for example, increased selectivity or increased duration of action. At present there are a number of such agents available and a summary of the names, structures, and uses of the more important of these is given in Table 41.1. Further details can be found in standard pharmacology texts.

2   OCCURRENCE AND DISTRIBUTION OF CATECHOLAMINES

The three most commonly occurring catecholamines are $(-)$-norepinephrine, $(-)$-epinephrine, and dopamine. They are remarkably widespread throughout animal phyla. Fairly extensive compilations of their distribution are available (18–20).

Catecholamines have been found in virtually all invertebrates examined including protozoa, coelenterates, mollusks, and insects (18, 20, 21). From the data thus far available, dopamine appears to be the dominant catecholamine, present in higher concentrations than norepinephrine, with epinephrine often present only in very low concentrations. There is considerable evidence that dopamine plays a transmitter role in molluscan ganglia (21–24). From the evolutionary standpoint it is of the utmost interest that catecholamine-containing neurones are found in platyhelminthes (flatworms), the first invertebrate phylum to show centralization of the nervous system. Apparently, the role of the catecholamines as transmitter molecules is of considerable antiquity.

Interesting variations in the amounts of the three major catecholamines are found

in vertebrates. In cyclostomes, teleosts, and amphibians the major catecholamine is epinephrine, whereas in elasmobranchs, reptiles, birds, and mammals norepinephrine dominates. Dopamine measurements are rare in nonmammalian systems but dopamine is found in the brain of the lamprey and dogfish, suggestive of its early association with vertebrate central nervous system function.

In the mammalian nervous system, with which the remainder of this chapter is largely concerned, norepinephrine functions as the transmitter at the peripheral neuroeffector junctions of the sympathetic nervous system (heart, smooth muscle, glands, Table 41.2) and dopamine has a peripheral role thus far identified in the renal vasculature and ganglionic transmission. Both norepinephrine and epinephrine are liberated from the adrenal medulla but epinephrine is the dominant catecholamine ($\sim 80\%$) in man.

Fluorescence and electron microscopic observations have greatly facilitated the difficult task of localizing catecholamine pathways in the central nervous system (15–17) and the discrete character of the norepinephrine and dopamine pathways is now well recognized (Fig. 41.1). The norepinephrine pathways are quite diffuse and appear to be concerned with many generalized CNS functions including sleep, emotion, temperature regulation, neuroendocrine functions, appetite control, and vasomotor function. The dopamine pathways are more discretely localized, the nigro-neostriatal system being largely involved in motor control, hypothalamic–pituitary control, and mental function (Section 4.1).

3   ORGANIZATION OF ADRENERGIC AND DOPAMINERGIC SYNAPSES

A schematic view of catecholamine-utilizing synapses is shown in Fig. 41.2. The

Table 41.1 Structures and Therapeutic Uses of Some Sympathomimetic Amines

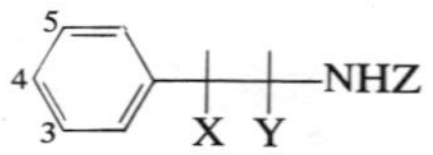

Generic structure: benzene ring (positions 3, 4, 5 indicated) bearing the side chain —C(X)(Y)—NHZ.

Amine	X	Y	Z	α Pressor	α Local Vaso-constriction	α Allergy	α Nasal Decon-gestion	α Broncho dilation	β Cardio accelera-tion	β Muscle Vessel Dilation	CNS Anorexia (Appetite Control)	CNS Stimulant
Dopamine, 3-OH, 4-OH	H	H	H	✓								
Norepinephrine, 3-OH, 4-OH	OH	H	H	✓								
Epinephrine, 3-OH, 4-OH	OH	H	Me	✓	✓	✓		✓	✓			
Isoproterenol, 3-OH, 4-OH	OH	H	CH(Me)$_2$					✓	✓			
Metaproterenol, 3-OH, 5-OH	OH	H	CH(Me)$_2$					✓				
Terbutaline, 3-OH, 5-OH	OH	H	C(Me)$_3$					✓				
Salbutamol, 3-CH$_2$OH, 4-OH	OH	H	C(Me)$_3$					✓				
Soterenol, 3-MeSO$_2$NH, 4-OH	OH	H	CH(Me)$_2$					✓				
Metaraminol, 3-OH	OH	Me	H	✓								
Hydroxyamphetamine, 4-OH	OH	Me	H	✓			✓					
Methoxamine, 2-MeO, 5-MeO	OH	Me	H	✓								
Amphetamine	H	Me	H				✓				✓	✓
Methamphetamine	H	Me	Me				✓				✓	✓
Ephedrine	OH	Me	Me	✓				✓	✓			
Phenylpropanolamine	OH	Me	H									
Mephentermine	H	—C(Me)$_2$—	Me									
Fenfluramin, 3-CF$_3$	H	Me	Et								✓	
Nylidrin, 4-OH	OH	Me	CH(Me)CH$_2$CH$_2$Ph							✓		
Tuaminoheptane, C$_4$H$_9$CH$_2$CHMeNH$_2$							✓					
Propylhexedrine, C$_5$H$_9$CH$_2$CHMeNHMe							✓					
Naphazoline, (41.23)							✓					
Tetrahydrozoline, (41.25)							✓					

Table 41.2 Some Effector Responses to Adrenergic Stimuli

Effector	Response	Receptor Type	
Heart			
Atria	Increased contractility		β
Ventricles	Increased contractility		β
SA node	Increased firing rate		β
AV node	Increased automaticity		β
Arteries, skeletal muscle	Constriction, dilatation	α	β
Coronary	Constriction, dilatation	α	β
Skin	Constriction, dilatation	α	
Viscera	Constriction, dilatation	α	β
Veins	Constriction	α	
Lung (bronchial muscle)	Relaxation		β
Intestine			
Motility and tone	Decrease	α	β
Sphincter muscles	Contraction	α	
Eye			
Radial muscle	Contraction (mydriasis)	α	
Ciliary muscle	Relaxation (far vision)		β
Skin			
Pilomotor muscle	Contraction	α	
Spleen capsule	Contraction, relaxation	α	β
Bladder			
Fundus	Relaxation		β
Trigone and sphincter	Contraction	α	
Fat cells	Lipolysis		β
Salivary glands	Water, amylase secretion	α	β
Pancreatic β cells	Increased, decreased secretion	α	β
Liver	Glycogenolysis		β

general features include the presynaptic biosynthetic machinery which utilizes L-tyrosine as the starting material for dopamine, norepinephrine, and epinephrine, (Section 4.1). The catecholamines are stored largely in vesicular form in the nerve terminal. However, since the biosynthetic pathway does not exhibit absolute specificity, nonphysiological substrates can also be utilized and give rise to neurotransmitter analogs, "false transmitters." The arrival of the nerve impulse at the nerve terminal stimulates the Ca^{2+}-dependent release of catecholamine, which then diffuses across the synaptic gap or, in the case of the adrenal medulla, enters the general circulation. The geometry of the synapse varies widely from close junctions in the rat and mouse vas deferens (~ 200 Å) to extremely loose junctions ($\sim 10,000$ Å) in some vascular tissues. Such considerations of synapse geometry are important in determining the concentrations of neurotransmitter achieved at the postsynaptic receptors, the rates of onset and offset of response, and the importance of different routes of inactivation of the transmitter (17).

The receptors determining the response of the effector cell, neurone, smooth muscle, cardiac muscle, or gland cell, are located on the postsynaptic surface and are

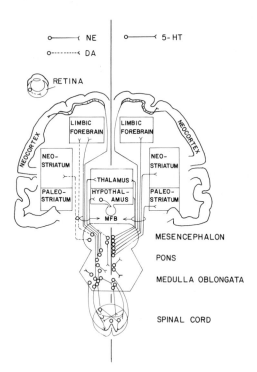

Fig. 41.1 Pathways of norepinephrine, dopamine, and 5-hydroxytryptamine tracts in the central nervous system. [Reproduced with permission from Anden, Dahlström, Fuxe, Larsson, Olson, and Ungerstedt, *Acta Physiol. Scand.*, **67**, 313 (1966).]

classified primarily according to the structure–activity relationships of agonist and antagonist ligands (Section 7.1). Thus the receptors for dopamine and norepinephrine are clearly distinguishable and the receptors for norepinephrine are subdivided into two major categories, α and β, which generally mediate opposing responses (Table 41.2).

Although there are degradative enzymes, monoamine oxidase (MAO) and catechol 0-methyltransferase (COMT), that inactivate catecholamines, the major inactivation pathway is through active transport into the nerve terminal (Section 6.1), and, as with the receptors, a clear distinction is also possible in this regard between dopamine- and norepinephrine-utilizing synapses. The discovery of these neuronal uptake processes has proved to be of the utmost signifi-

cance to the understanding of the structure–activity relationship of sympathomimetic amines, for many of these agents actually produce their pharmacological responses by releasing norepinephrine from sympathetic nerve terminals (Section 6.4).

The synapse must not, however, be regarded as a mechanism for processing a strictly unidirectional information flow, for there exist presynaptic receptors that respond to dopamine and norepinephrine and that serve to inhibit the transmitter release process (Section 6.2). Additionally, the presynaptic surface possesses receptors for the prostaglandins, PGE_2 and $PGF_{2\alpha}$, which appear to exert inhibitory and facilitatory effects, respectively, on adrenergic transmission processes, probably through modulation of the Ca^{2+}-dependent release process (25,26). Evidence also indicates the existence of presynaptic acetylcholine (muscarinic) receptors that serve to inhibit norepinephrine release (27). Hence synaptic transmission represents a finely regulated process at which the interactions of distinct classes of drugs serve to control quite closely the flow of neuronal traffic.

An appreciation of these general principles of synapse construction and function is vital to any understanding of drug action in adrenergic and dopaminergic systems since the observed actions of a given agent may well depend on its simultaneous interaction at and modulation by several sites within the synapse.

4   BIOSYNTHESIS, STORAGE, AND RELEASE OF CATECHOLAMINES

4.1   Biosynthetic Pathways for Dopamine, Norepinephrine, and Epinephrine

The major biosynthetic pathway to dopamine, norepinephrine, and epinephrine (Fig. 41.3) was proposed by Blaschko

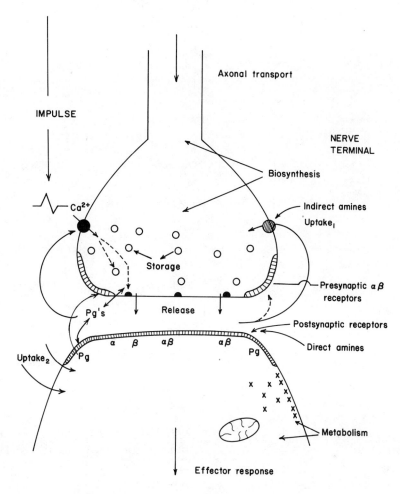

Fig. 41.2 Schematic representation of adrenergic synapse.

in 1939 (28) and substantial discussion of this pathway is available (16, 17, 29–32).

Tyrosine hydroxylase (L-tyrosine tetrahydropteridine oxygen oxidoreductase, 3-hydroxylating), the first enzyme in the pathway, is a predominantly soluble enzyme requiring oxygen and tetrahydrobiopterin as cofactors. The hydroxylation of tyrosine represents the rate-limiting step in the overall pathway and inhibition of this step only, by such agents as α-methyltyrosine (41.**4**), is effective in reducing catecholamine levels.

Dopa decarboxylase, which catalyzes the decarboxylation of dihydroxyphenylala-

nine, is widely distributed in tissues (kidney, liver, etc.) and is associated with all catecholamine-utilizing neurons. It is a soluble enzyme requiring pyridoxal as a cofactor and is without absolute substrate specificity; it is often referred to as aromatic amino acid decarboxylase.

Dopamine β-hydroxylase (dopamine β-monooxygenase) catalyzes the final stage of norepinephrine biosynthesis. It is a copper-containing enzyme functioning by coupling

$$\text{HO}\!-\!\!\underset{}{\bigcirc}\!\!-\!\text{CH}_2\text{CMe(NH}_2)\text{COOH}$$

41.**4**

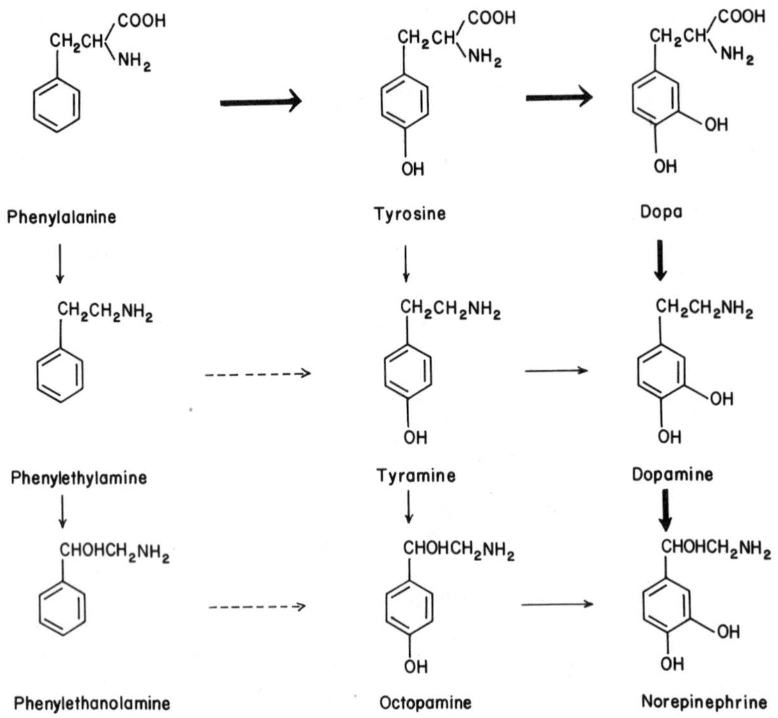

Fig. 41.3 Major and minor pathways to the biosynthesis of dopamine and norepinephrine. The major pathway is shown in bold arrows, and alternative pathways as thin (*in vivo*) and dashed (*in vitro*) arrows.

the oxidation of ascorbate to the hydroxylation of dopamine:

$$\text{dopamine} + \text{ascorbate} + O_2 \rightarrow$$

$$\text{norepinephrine} +$$

$$\text{dehydroascorbate} + H_2O$$

Dopamine β-hydroxylase is associated with norepinephrine and epinephrine (but not dopamine) storage vesicles and thus the presence of these organelles is essential for norepinephrine and epinephrine biosynthesis.

Phenylethanolamine N-methyltransferase (S-adenosylmethionine : phenylethanolamine N-methyltransferase) has a dominant localization in the adrenal medulla and catalyzes the transfer reaction:

$$\text{norepinephrine} + S\text{-adenosylmethionine} \rightarrow$$

$$\text{epinephrine} + S\text{-adenosyl-}$$

$$\text{homocysteine} + H^+$$

It has, however, also been localized in other tissues including the central nervous system (lower brain stem, locus coeruleus, and hypothalamus), indicating that epinephrine, like dopamine and norepinephrine, may also have a central transmitter function.

It is of great importance to the understanding of the mechanism and structure–function relationships of sympathomimetic amines that the enzymes in this biosynthetic pathway do not exhibit absolute substrate specificity. Thus other agents may serve as precursors for alternate pathways (shown as dashed lines in Fig. 41.3) or enter the biosynthetic pathway and be converted and stored as "false" transmitters. Thus α-methyldopa is converted and stored as α-methylnorepinephrine and α-methyl-*m*-tyrosine is converted to metaraminol.

Under physiological conditions the concentrations of tissue catecholamines remain sensibly constant because of the existence of trans-synaptic regulatory mechanisms that serve to modify the rate of catecholamine biosynthesis (17, 30–34). Thus catecholamines serve as end product inhibitors of tyrosine hydroxylase acting through competition with the pteridine cofactor. During sympathetic nerve activity there is an increased rate of synthesis of catecholamines. The response to short-term increases in sympathetic stimulation may arise from relief of end product inhibition of tyrosine hydroxylase or, more probably, from allosteric activation of the enzyme caused by nerve impulse traffic possibly mediated through changes in ionic environment or degree of polymerization of the enzyme. With longer term increases in sympathetic activity there is, however, a net increase in the level of tyrosine hydroxylase apparently mediated through an increase in cyclic adenosine 3′,5′-monophosphate (cAMP, Section 9.1).

4.2 Catecholamine Storage and Release Processes

The catecholamines, like other transmitters, are stored in nerve terminals packaged in specialized subcellular particles, vesicles, which contain the transmitter stored within a limiting outer membrane. In the case of norepinephrine the vesicle also represents the locus of action of dopamine- β-hydroxylase (16, 17, 29, 32). Considerable evidence indicates that the release of the transmitters involves an increase in the permeability of the nerve terminal membrane to Ca^{2+}, the influx of which is the major stimulus for the release process. The release of catecholamines from the chromaffin cells of the adrenal medulla is believed to be a process of exocytosis in which the contents of the vesicle, including transmitter, the ATP which is a major component of adrenergic vesicles, and various proteins are discharged following vesicle fusion with the nerve terminal membrane (35). It is less certain, however, that trans-

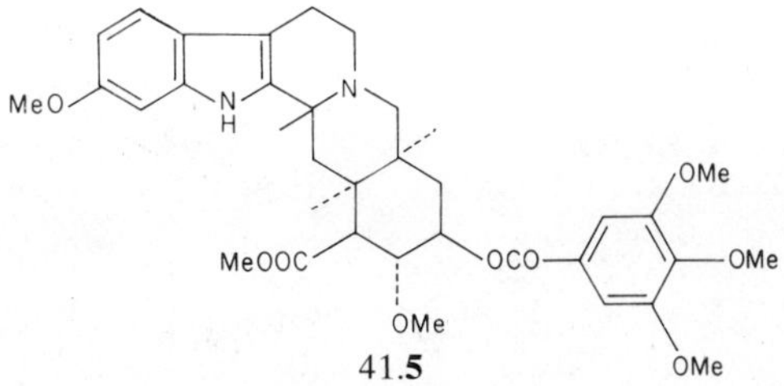

mitter release from adrenergic or dopaminergic terminals occurs exclusively by this mechanism (36, 37); a detailed examination lies outside the scope of this chapter. The storage vesicles represent a site of action of the hypotensive agents reserpine (41.5), guanethidine (41.6), and bretylium (41.7), which serve to inhibit catecholamine vesicular uptake and thus cause a depletion of catecholamine stores (Chapter 42).

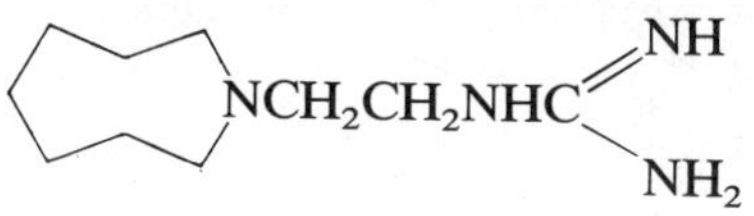

41.5

41.6

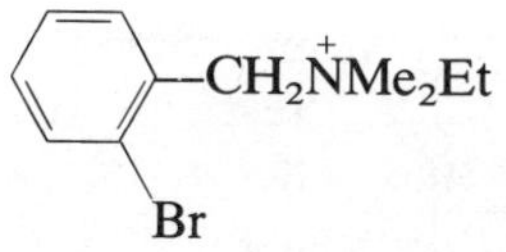

41.7

5 METABOLISM OF CATECHOLAMINES

The two enzymes of importance in the metabolism of catecholamines are monoamine oxidase (MAO) and catechol O-methyltransferase (COMT) (16, 17, 32, 38). The metabolic sequences are shown in Fig. 41.4). Monoamine oxidase is widely distributed and occurs both intraneuronally and extraneuronally, very high concentrations being found in the liver. Catechol O-methyltransferase is a widespread cytoplasmic enzyme and substantial amounts are found in liver, kidney, and sympathetically innervated tissues. Neither enzyme has particularly stringent specificity, MAO deaminating a wide variety of phenylethylamine structures and COMT methylating a

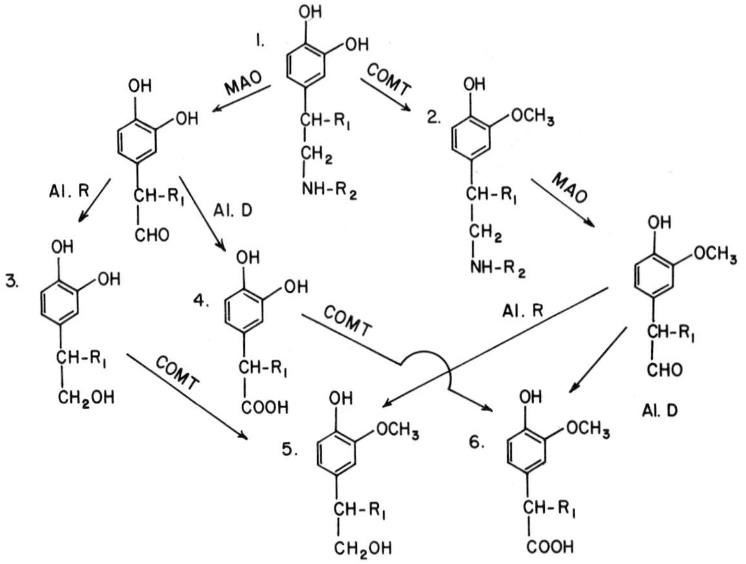

Fig. 41.4 Metabolic pathways for catecholamines. MAO monoamine oxidase; COMT, catechol O-methyltrans-ferase; Al.D, aldehyde dehydrogenase; Al.R, aldehyde reductase.

large number of catechols. Since, however, inhibition of neither MAO nor COMT by such agents as pargyline (41.**8**) and tropolone (41.**9**), respectively, markedly potentiates the effects of sympathetic stimulation it is generally agreed that these enzymes do not represent the primary mode of inactivation of catecholamines re-leased at nerve terminals. However, MAO does serve to inactivate neuronal catechol-amines not protected by intracellular stor-age and COMT does serve to inactivate extraneuronal catecholamines (Fig. 41.2).

For norepinephrine, epinephrine, and dopamine the major mechanism of removal

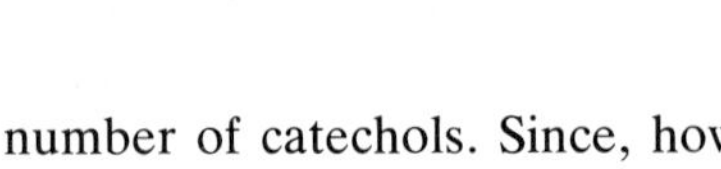

is by active transport (uptake) into the pre-synaptic nerve terminals where the major-ity of the transmitter is repackaged. This transport process is extremely efficient and represents a major site of action of drugs that activate or antagonize adrenergic and dopaminergic transmission.

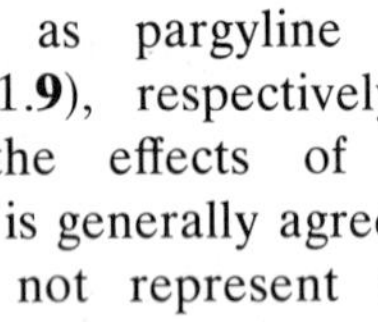

6 CATECHOLAMINE UPTAKE PROCESSES

J.H. Burn in 1932 proposed that cat-echolamines might be taken up into peripheral storage sites, and with the avail-ability of ^{3}H-labeled catecholamines this process has been documented rather thoroughly (39–45). The physiological role of neuronal uptake for norepinephrine and dopamine is indicated by the specificity of the process and by the distinctions that can be made between neuronal uptake of norepinephrine and dopamine. There is a correlation between norepinephrine uptake and endogenous norepinephrine content so that uptake is greatest in tissues with a rich

$$-CH_2NMeCH_2C{\equiv}CH$$

41.**8**

41.**9**

sympathetic innervation, such as the heart (46, 47); after destruction of sympathetic innervation, uptake and retention of exogenous norepinephrine are markedly reduced (48–50). Fluorescence histochemical methods, which allow the optical visualization of tissue catecholamines, have shown that uptake of exogenous norepinephrine is confined to adrenergic nerve terminals and that after catecholamine depletion by reserpine exogenous norepinephrine can restore the fluorescent pattern characteristic of adrenergic innervation (17, 51–53).

The properties of the neuronal catecholamine uptake process (uptake$_1$) appear to be very similar in a variety of tissues both peripheral and central, and it is of no little interest that similar neuronal uptake processes occur for other transmitters such as 5-hydroxytryptamine and amino acids, although not for acetylcholine (54). The uptake process is saturable and appears to be mediated by an energy-dependent membrane carrier and can generate a considerable catecholamine concentration gradient, 1000:1 or more. Uptake$_1$ has strict ionic requirements, being virtually completely dependent on the presence of Na$^+$ (and low K$^+$) in the external medium (55–57). These ionic requirements of catecholamine uptake are very similar to those of a number of other active transport processes including intestinal amino acid and sugar transport (58). Thus catecholamine uptake is inhibited by ouabain which inhibits the Na$^+$, K$^+$-ATPase (sodium pump) presumably because catecholamine transport utilizes energy generated by the downhill transport of Na$^+$, the operation of the sodium pump being required to maintain the transmembrane Na$^+$ gradient.

Catecholamine uptake by this process exhibits stereochemical selectivity in favor of (−)-norepinephrine (Table 41.3). The data of Table 41.3 also reveal the distinction in the uptake processes for catecholamines at adrenergic and dopaminergic neurones. Thus in rat striatum, neuronal uptake shows higher affinity for dopamine and shows no stereoselectivity toward the enantiomers of norepinephrine (59–60). (Further distinctions between these two processes are shown by antagonist action, Table 41.11.) Additional evidence for the stereoselectivity of the adrenergic neuronal uptake process is shown by the effects of cocaine, an inhibitor of uptake, on tissue responses to the isomers of sympathomimetic amines (64, 65; Table 41.4A), which reveal greater potentiation of the effects of the (−) isomers.

Table 41.3   Kinetic Constants for Catecholamine Uptake in Rat

| | K_M, μM | | | | |
| | Norepinephrine Terminals | | | | Striatum (Dopamine Terminals) |
Amine	Heart	Iris	Vas deferens	Hypo-thalamus	
(±)-Norepinephrine	0.67	1.40	1.90	0.40	1.8
(−)-Norepinephrine	0.27	—	—	0.20	2.0
(+)-Norepinephrine	1.39	—	—	0.80	1.90
(±)-Epinephrine	1.40	—	—	—	—
Dopamine	0.69	—	—	—	0.31

[a] Data from Refs. 39, 59, and 61–63.

Table 41.4   Effects of Cocaine on Responses to Sympathomimetic Amines in the Cat

A.   Cat Blood Pressure Preparation (65)

Amine	ED_{90}, μg/kg		Ratio before/after Cocaine
	Before Cocaine	After Cocaine	
(−)-Norepinephrine	3.3	0.58	5.7
(+)-Norepinephrine	134	173	<1
(−)-Epinephrine	2.6	0.81	3.2
(+)-Epinephrine	74.3	49.6	1.5
(−)-Nordefrine	4.3	1.1	3.8
(+)-Nordefrine	153	569	<1
(−)-Phenylephrine	48.9	43.7	1.1
(+)-Phenylephrine	826	2377	<1

B.   Cat Nictitating Membrane Preparation (64)

Amine	ED_{50} in Denervated Preparation, μg/kg	Ratio ED_{50}s' with and without Cocaine
(−)-Norepinephrine	1.2	40.0
(−)-Phenylephrine	6.2	7.0
(±)-Metaraminol	82.5	4.9
m-Tyramine	244.0	1.4
(−)-Ephedrine	474.0	0.8

However, the extent to which inhibition of neuronal uptake potentiates the effects of directly acting amines and antagonizes the effects of indirectly acting agents (Section 6.4) depends very much on the affinity of the amine for both the uptake and receptor sites and on the density of adrenergic innervation of the effector tissue (45, 63, 66, 67). In tissues with sparse adrenergic innervation or in which the distance between nerve terminal and effector cell surface is long, potentiating effects are small or nonexistent (Fig. 41.5; 68). For weakly active agonists saturation of the uptake mechanism may occur at the concentrations needed to stimulate receptors, and hence no potentiation occurs. Even if the amine has a low affinity for both receptors and uptake sites little potentiation is found on inhibition of uptake because at high substrate concentrations the rate of uptake is insufficient to alter significantly the agonist concentration in the biophase adjacent to the receptors. The data of Table 41.4B show that as agonist potency decreases there is less potentiation of response following inhibition of neuronal uptake. Such considerations are clearly of substantial importance in the formulation of quantitative structure–activity relationships for ligands active at dopaminergic and adrenergic synapses.

Although norepinephrine is the physiological substrate for neuronal uptake in adrenergic neurones a large number of phenylethylamines can serve as substrate or antagonists and the actual specificity of the uptake process is rather low. However,

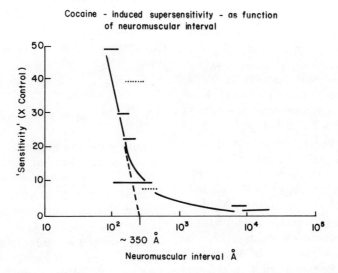

Fig. 41.5 Correlation of the potentiation of norepinephrine response by cocaine and the neuromuscular interval in smooth muscles. (Reproduced with permission from M. A. Verity, in *Physiology and Pharmacology of Vascular Neuroeffector Systems*, J. A. Bevan, R. F. Furchgott, R. A. Maxwell, and A. P. Somlyo, Eds., Karger, Basel, 1971.)

with increasing structural deviation from norepinephrine the ability of the amine to serve as a substrate is increasingly impaired. Thus increasing *N*-substitution (isopropylnorepinephrine is not a substrate), removal of phenolic hydroxyl groups (amphetamine is not a substrate), and introduction of methoxy groups (normetanephrine, 3-*0*-methyl derivative of norepinephrine, is not a substrate) are all detrimental to the ability of a phenylethylamine to act as a substrate for the uptake process. A qualitative summary of the structural specificity for uptake is given in Table 41.5. In addition to the listed phenylethylamine derivatives other less closely related agents can also utilize the neuronal uptake process including the antihyper-

Table 41.5   Structural Specificity of Catecholamine Uptake

Amines Accumulated by a Cocaine-, Desipramine-, or Ouabain-Sensitive Mechanism	Amines not Accumulated by a Cocaine-, Desipramine-, or Ouabain-Sensitive Mechanism
Norepinephrine	Isoprenaline
Epinephrine	Normetanephrine
Metaraminol	Amphetamine
Dopamine	Phenylethanolamine
α-Methyltyramine	Norephedrine
α-Methylnorepinephrine	
α-Methylepinephrine	
p-Tyramine	
m-Tyramine	
5-Hydroxytryptamine	
6,7-Dihydroxytetrahydroisoquinoline	

tensive neurone-blocking agents (Chapter 42), bretylium (41.**7**) and guanethidine (41.**6**) (40, 69–72).

The norepinephrine neuronal uptake process is of enormous importance in the delineation of the structure–activity relationships of sympathomimetic amines. It was early recognized that important differences exist between many sympathomimetic amines and norepinephrine or epinephrine. Thus the actions of epinephrine but not of p-hydroxy-2-phenylethylamine (tyramine, 41.**10**) or 2-(N-Methylamino)-1-phenyl-1-propanol) (ephedrine, 41.**11**) are potentiated by cocaine (73, 74). Similarly, the supersensitivity of denervated structures to norepinephrine and epinephrine is not seen with a number of sympathomimetic amines (75). Such findings form the basis for the classification by Fleckenstein (76, 77) of sympathomimetic amines into the direct-acting agents, the indirect-acting agents which serve to displace norepinephrine from nerve terminal storage sites, and the mixed-acting amines which can share both mechanisms of action. As representatives of these three classes of agents may be cited norepinephrine, tyramine, and ephedrine, respectively. The basis of this classification was confirmed by Burn and Rand (78, 79), who showed that indirect-acting amines were ineffective in tissues depleted of catecholamines by reserpine and that the response to indirect-acting amines could be restored temporarily by norepinephrine treatment. Table 41.4 presents a classification of sympathomimetic amines, but it should be noted that the classification is not absolute and that, in

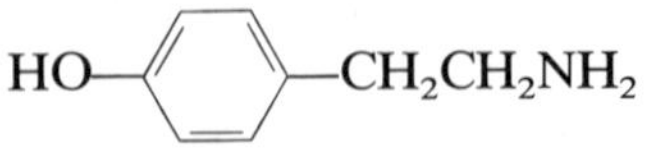

particular, the amount of activity exhibited by an indirect-acting amine depends on the tissue innervation pattern, which is reduced in sparsely innervated systems.

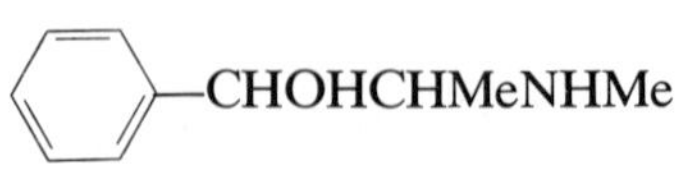

6.1 Inhibitors of Catecholamine Uptake

A large number of agents have been shown to act as inhibitors of norepinephrine uptake into adrenergic neurones including cocaine and the tricyclic antidepressants imipramine, amitriptyline, and their derivatives Tables 41.5, 41.6 Chapter 58), a number of the α-adrenergic antagonistic 2-haloethylamines (Chapter 42), and a miscellany of other agents including antihistamines and monoamine oxidase inhibitors (41, 80).

Extensive studies have been undertaken of the inhibitory effects of phenylethylamines on the norepinephrine uptake process by determining the amine concentration required to block norepinephrine uptake by 50% into rat heart and brain (39). This method gives an approximation to the K_I value but does not, of course, distinguish between competitive inhibitors and competitive substrates of the uptake process. The broad conclusions concerning the structural demands of the norepinephrine uptake process may be summarized as follows. In the basic phenylethylamine pattern:

1. Phenolic hydroxyl groups increase affinity for the uptake site (Table 41.7; part 1).
2. N-Alkylation decreases affinity for the uptake site (Table 41.7; part 2).
3. α-Methylation increases affinity for the uptake site (Table 41.7; part 3).
4. Methylation of phenolic OH groups decreases affinity for the uptake site (Table 41.7; part 4).
5. β-Hydroxylation decreases affinity for the uptake site (Table 41.7; part 5).

HO—⟨benzene ring⟩—CH₂CH₂NH₂

41.**10**

⟨benzene ring⟩—CHOHCHMeNHMe

41.**11**

Table 41.6   Inhibition of Norepinephrine Uptake in Isolated Rat Heart (81)

Compound	Structure	IC_{50}, μM
Imipramine	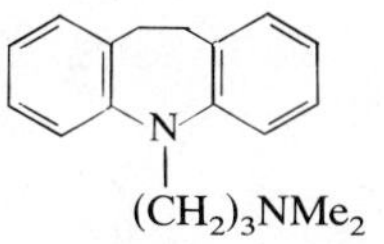 $(CH_2)_3NMe_2$	0.041
Desipramine (desmethylimipramine)	$(CH_2)_3NHMe$	0.007
Amitriptyline	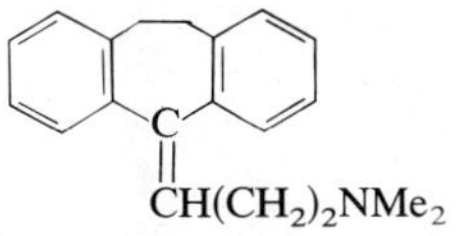 $CH(CH_2)_2NMe_2$	0.110
Nortriptyline	$CH(CH_2)_2NMe$	0.024
Cocaine	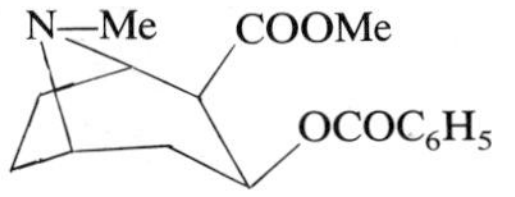 N—Me COOMe OCOC$_6$H$_5$	0.38
Phenoxybenzamine	$PhOCH_2CH(Me)N(CH_2Ph)CH_2CH_2Cl,HCl$	0.75

Despite the many agents studied as substrates and inhibitors of the neuronal uptake system little is known of the conformational aspects of the phenylethylamine interaction (a discussion of conformational requirements of catecholamine–receptor interaction is presented in Section 7.5). Maxwell and his colleagues (80, 82–85) have argued that the high potency of a number of tricyclic compounds as competitive inhibitors of norepinephrine uptake (Table 41.8) is best rationalized on the basis that these agents are, in part, superimposable on the planar antiperiplanar (trans) phenylethylamine conformation, which is thus assumed to represent the conformation of amines at the uptake site. Figure 41.6 depicts phenylethylamine in the planar, trans conformation and the binding of desmethylimipramine (DMI) showing the correspondence of one phenyl ring and the protonated side chain nitrogens. The sec-

ond phenyl ring of desmethylimipramine is held above the plane of the phenylethylamine, and it would be predicted that planar tricycles, such as carbazoles (Table 41.7), would be very much less potent because the second ring can sterically hinder binding of the side chain nitrogen. Additionally, there must also be some rather specific interaction of the N-methyl substituent since the sequence of inhibitory activities is clearly $NHMe \gg NMe_2 > NH_2$, and this contrasts with the phenylethylamines where the sequence is $NH_2 > NHMe$. The trans conformation of phenylethylamines is also suggested by the very much higher activity of the trans isomer of 2-phenylcyclopropylamine (Table 41.9) as an inhibitor of norepinephrine uptake (88), although this compound does not exhibit the planar conformation advocated by Maxwell. Further insight into the conformations of phenylethylamines adopted at

Table 41.7 Inhibition of Norepinephrine Uptake by Sympathomimetic Amines (86, 87)

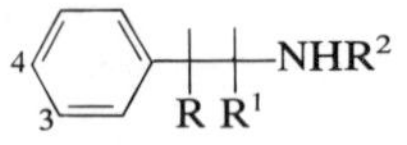

$$\text{(ring positions 4,3)}\!\!-\!\!\underset{R\ R^1}{\mid\mid}\!\!-NHR^2$$

Amine	4	3	R	R^1	R^2	Heart	Hypothalamus
						IC$_{50}$, μM	

Amine	4	3	R	R^1	R^2	Heart	Hypothalamus
1. Effects of Phenolic OH Groups							
Phenylethylamine	H	H	H	H	H	1.10	5.2
Tyramine	OH	H	H	H	H	0.45	1.0
Dopamine	OH	OH	H	H	H	0.17	0.08
(±)-Phenylethanolamine	H	H	OH	H	H	4.80	130.0
(±)-Norsynephrine	OH	H	OH	H	H	1.30	50.0
(±)-Norepinephrine	OH	OH	OH	H	H	0.67	0.41
2. Effects of N-Alkyl Groups							
(−)-Norepinephrine	OH	OH	OH	H	H	0.27	—
(−)-Epinephrine	OH	OH	OH	H	Me	1.00	—
(±)-N-Ethylnorepinephrine	OH	OH	OH	H	Et	3.20	—
(±)-N-Isopropylnorepinephrine	OH	OH	OH	H	iPr	25	—
3. Effects of α-Methylation							
Phenylethylamine	H	H	H	H	H	1.10	5.2
(±)-Amphetamine	H	H	H	Me	H	0.46	0.92
(−)-Norepinephrine	OH	OH	OH	H	H	0.27	—
(−)-α-Methylnorepinephrine	OH	OH	OH	Me	H	0.20	—
Tyramine	OH	H	H	H	H	0.45	1.0
p-Hydroxyamphetamine	OH	H	H	Me	H	0.18	0.84
4. Effects of 0-Methylation							
(±)-Norepinephrine	OH	OH	H	H	H	0.67	0.41
(±)-Normetanephrine	OH	OMe	H	H	H	200	740.0
Tyramine	OH	H	H	H	H	0.45	1.0
p-Methoxyphenylethylamine	OMe	H	H	H	H	10.0	240
5. Effects of β-Hydroxylation							
Phenylethylamine	H	H	H	H	H	1.10	5.2
(±)-β-Hydroxyphenylethylamine	H	H	OH	H	H	4.8	130.0
Tyramine	OH	H	H	H	H	0.45	1.0
(±)-Octopamine (norsynephrine)	OH	H	OH	H	H	50.0	5.3
(±)-Amphetamine	H	H	H	Me	H	0.46	0.92
(±)-Norpseudoephedrine (phenyl-propanolamine)	H	H	OH	Me	H	2.0	6.2

Table 41.8 Inhibition of Norepinephrine Uptake Into Rabbit Aorta Neurones (80)

			Relative Potency		
	Dihydro-dibenzazepines 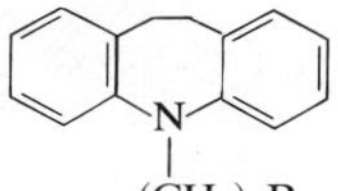 $(CH_2)_3R$	Dibenzocycla-heptadienes 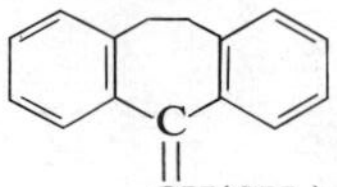 $CH(CH_2)_2R$	Dibenzocyclo-heptatrienes 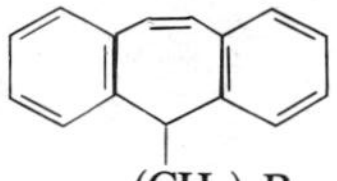 $(CH_2)_3R$	Diphenylmethyl-idenes 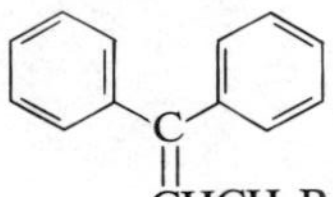 $=CHCH_2R$	Carbazoles 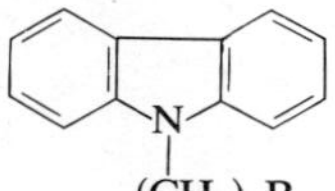 $(CH_2)_3R$
R					
NMe_2	38 (Imipramine)	16 (Amitriptyline)	20	1.0^a	0.5
NHM_e	3000 (DMI)	120 (Nortriptyline)	280 (Protriptyline)	82	1.1
NH_2	24	10	12	5.0	0.2

[a] Standard compound, $ID_{50} = 4.0 \times 10^{-6}$ M.

241

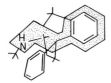

Fig. 41.6 Representation of the molecular overlap between phenylethylamine and desmethylimipramine. [Reproduced from Maxwell, Chaplin, Eckhardt, Soares, and Hite, *J. Pharmacol. Exp. Ther.*, **173,** 158 (1970), with permission of Williams & Wilkins, Baltimore, MD.]

the uptake site is provided by the finding that *o*-hydroxyphenylethanolamines have very low affinity whereas *o*-hydroxyphenyl-ethylamines have significant inhibitory activity and are transported (Table 41.10; 89). These findings may suggest that a syncl-inal conformation of phenylethylamines (stabilized by $-OH \cdots \overset{+}{N}H_3$ interaction, Fig. 41.7) is permitted in the uptake process but is not permitted for the corresponding phenylethanolamines which therefore likely adopt the antiperiplanar conformation (Fig. 41.7).

6.2 Mechanism of Indirect Sympathomimetic Activity

There is no complete agreement as to the mechanisms by which indirectly acting sympathomimetic amines produce their

Table 41.9   Activities of Amphetamine and Analogs as Inhibitors of Norepinephrine and Dopamine Uptake (88)

	ID_{50}, M	
Compound	Hypothalamus (Norepineph-rine)	Striatum (Dopamine)
(+)-*trans*-2-Phenyl cyclopropylamine (tranylcypromine)	1.2×10^{-6}	1.7×10^{-6}
(+)-*cis*-2-Phenyl cyclopropylamine	7.2×10^{-4}	5.5×10^{-6}
(±)-Amphetamine	9.2×10^{-7}	4.0×10^{-7}
Phenylethylamine	5.2×10^{-6}	1.4×10^{-6}

Table 41.10   Inhibition of Norepinephrine Uptake into Mouse Heart by Phenylethylamines and Phenylethanolamines

	ED_{50}, μmol/kg	
Aromatic Substitution	Phenylethyl-amine	Phenyleth-anolamine
H	3.8	9.2
2-OH	13.8	137.2
3-OH	0.35	0.40
4-OH	0.69	0.82
2,5-(OH)$_2$	2.48	116.8
2,4,5-(OH)$_3$	0.73	Inactive
2,3,4-(OH)$_3$	0.63	—
2,3,5-(OH)$_3$	1.20	—

pharmacological effects. This is probably because several different mechanisms operate, the relative importance of which depends on the agent in question. One obviously important mechanism is through inhibition of norepinephrine uptake at the neuronal membrane, thus potentiating the effects of norepinephrine released through leakage or physiological stimulus. This mechanism may be assumed to be of greatest importance for amines such as amphetamine which are inhibitors, but not substrates, of the uptake process (Table 41.7). However, amphetamine and related amines are relatively lipophilic and are known to be accumulated by nonspecific processes (90–92), indicating that they may

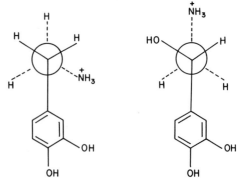

Fig. 41.7 Conformational views of phenylethyl-amines and phenylethanolamines.

also affect intracellular storage and release processes. Although amines that enter the adrenergic neurone may serve to release norepinephrine it is clear that the releasing action of such indirect sympathomimetics is quite unlike physiological release and involves a Ca^{2+}-independent nonexocytotic mechanism (36, 39, 93) promoting release from a relatively small cytoplasmic pool (45, 94, 95). Neuronally accumulated sympathomimetic amines may serve to block incorporation of norepinephrine into the storage vesicles or, more commonly, to enter the stores and to displace norepinephrine (96, 97). Additionally, the resistance of many indirect-acting amines to monoamine oxidase action further increases their ability to interfere with vesicle storage. Finally, the amine may be metabolized to give agents that more closely resemble direct-acting sympathomimetic agents, that are actually stored in place of norepinephrine, and that can be released on subsequent stimulus ("false transmitters").

It may be presumed that all the above mechanisms contribute in some degree to the pharmacological effectiveness of the indirect sympathomimetic agents but since their individual importance is likely to be determined by compound, tissue, and species, the quantitative relationship between structure and activity is of substantial complexity.

6.3   Extraneuronal Uptake

In addition to the neuronal uptake process for catecholamines there exists a second uptake process (extraneuronal uptake, or uptake$_2$) that occurs in cardiac muscle, smooth muscle, and glands and that is quite distinct from the neuronal uptake process (Table 41.11). Extraneuronal uptake has a lower affinity for norepinephrine and epinephrine than neuronal uptake, is not stereoselective, and is not inhibited by cocaine and desipramine, the potent in-

hibitors of the neuronal uptake process (39, 98). Additionally, the structure–activity relationship for phenylethylamine inhibition of extraneuronal uptake is quite distinct, inhibitory activity being increased by N-substitution and o-methylation and decreased by phenolic hydroxylation and α-methylation (41, 86, 99, 100). Despite the low K_m values of norepinephrine and epinephrine for this process the high V_{max} values (relative to neuronal uptake, Table 41.11) indicate that significant amounts of catecholamines can be removed by this process. However, at low catecholamine levels very little cellular accumulation can be detected because the catecholamines are rapidly metabolized by monoamine oxidase and catechol O-methyltransferase (40, 41, 100–102). Thus extraneuronal uptake can be regarded as transport-and-metabolism and neuronal uptake as transport-and-retention.

6.4   Physiological, Pharmacological, and Therapeutic Relevance of Norepinephrine Uptake Processes

There can be little doubt that neuronal uptake, rather than enzymatic destruction, represents the most important mechanism for the termination of norepinephrine action in densely adrenergically innervated tissues. However, extraneuronal uptake and metabolism will be of greater importance in adrenergically innervated tissues where the density of innervation is low and where the diffusion distance from nerve terminal to effector cell surface is long (i.e., large arteries). Extraneuronal uptake is also likely to be of significance in removing circulating (adrenal medulla released) norepinephrine and epinephrine (63, 67). It is of interest that extraneuronal uptake is potently blocked by various steroids (Table 41.12), posing the possibility that steroid–catecholamine interactions may be important in generating certain hypertensive states.

Table 41.11 A Comparative Summary of Neuronal and Extraneuronal Catecholamine Transport Processes

| | Norepinephrine | | | | Dopamine— | |
| | Neuronal Uptake (Rat Heart) | | Extraneuronal Uptake (Rat Heart) | | Neuronal Uptake (Rat Corpus Striatum) | |
Amine	K_m, μM	V_{max}, nmol/ min/g	K_m, μM	V_{max}, nmol/ min/g	K_m, μM	V_{max}, nmol/ min/g
(−)-Norepinephrine	0.27	0.20	252	100	2.0	2.34
(+)-Norepinephrine	1.39	0.29	252	100	1.9	2.80
(±)-Epinephrine	1.40	0.19	52.0	64.4	—	—
(±)-Isopropylnorepi-nephrine	—	—	23.0	15.5	—	—
Dopamine	0.69	1.45	590	140	0.31	—

	Inhibitors (K_I, μM)		
	Desipramine (0.01)	Desipramine (ineffective)	Benztropine (0.12)
	Cocaine (0.38)	Cocaine (ineffective)	(−)-Amphetamine (0.1)
	(−)-Amphetamine (3.7)	(±)-Amphetamine (110)	(+)-Amphetamine (0.1)
	(+)-Amphetamine (0.2)	(−)-Metaraminol (>500)	Desipramine (50.0)
	(−)-Metaraminol (0.08)	Phenoxybenzamine (2.8)	
	Phenoxybenzamine (0.78)		

There is substantial pharmacological significance to these uptake mechanisms. Thus the pharmacological effects of the tricyclic antidepressants (Chapter 58) are likely related to their ability to inhibit neuronal norepinephrine uptake, and it is of interest that they are significantly less effective in inhibiting neuronal dopamine uptake (Table 41.11). The selective properties of neuronal uptake probably provide a basis for the antihypertensive actions of bretylium and guanethidine, (Chapter 42) which are accumulated in adrenergic neurones, and for the chemical sympathectomy produced by 6-hydroxydopamine, which is similarly selectively accumulated (103).

The uptake of 6-hydroxydopamine has

Table 41.12 Inhibition of Extraneuronal Uptake by Steroids in Rat Heart (98, 109)

Steroid	ID_{50}, μM
17-β-Estradiol	2.0
Corticosterone	2.7
Testosterone	3.6
Deoxycorticosterase	4.5
Cholesterol	18.1

proved to be very useful in studies of sympathetic neurone pathways and function (103, 103a). Once accumulated the 6-hydroxydopamine is converted to the reactive 4,6,7-trihydroxyindoline, which then reacts with nucleophilic groups to form stable condensation products with concomitant loss of sympathetic neurone functions both centrally and peripherally. Noradrenergic neurones are more sensitive than dopaminergic neurones and although some effect is also seen at serotonergic neurones other synapses appear to be unaffected. There are marked differences in tissue sensitivity with cardiac neurones being the most sensitive and the adrenal gland being insensitive. The chemical sympathectomy produced by 6-hydroxydopamine is essentially irreversible if produced during the neuronal developmental stage, but in the adult the sympathectomy is reversible. In addition, the neuronal uptake process makes possible the generation of false adrenergic transmitters derived from amines which are taken up, metabolized, and stored, and which are then released on physiological demand. Such false transmitters include α-methylnorepinephrine (from α-methyldopa), octopamine (from tyramine), α-methyloctopamine (from amphetamine), and metaraminol (from α-methyl-m-tyramine) (36, 104–108). It seems probable that the hypotensive actions of such agents as α-methyldopa arise from their conversion to the false transmitter and the subsequent action of this agent probably in the CNS centers concerned with vasomotor control (36, 104–108; Chapter 42).

7 STRUCTURE–ACTIVITY RELATIONSHIPS OF AMINES ACTIVE AT NOREPINEPHRINE RECEPTORS

It was early recognized that a large number of agents structurally related to norepinephrine possess sympathomimetic activity

(10), yet until comparatively recently such studies had not led to conclusions significantly more advanced than that drawn by Barger and Dale, who noted in their classic study of 1910 (10, 110),

In a general way it can be stated, that approximation to adrenine (epinephrine) in structure is attended by increase of sympathomimetic activity.

Significant progress in structure–activity analyses, has been possible, however, since the discovery of the indirect basis of action of many sympathomimetic amines (Section 6.2) and since the realization that there exists more than a single type of receptor for the directly acting sympathomimetic amines.

A very important distinction between the actions of norepinephrine and epinephrine was made in 1905 by Dale (8), who noted that the normal pressor effect of epinephrine was converted to a depressor effect in the ergot-treated cat; in 1910 Barger and Dale (10), commenting on the abilities of catecholamines to produce excitatory or inhibitory effects, suggested that,

... it seems impossible at present to summarize the known facts in this direction, without having recourse to a more complicated and morphological conception such as that of Elliot, and further regarding his myoneural function as multiple or composite, the receptive substances, or solvents, in the portions concerned with inhibition and motor activity respectively, not being identical.

It remained, however, for Ahlquist in 1948 (111) to actually propose the concept of two distinct receptors based on the observation that in a series of six catecholamines, there were two distinct sequences of activities in a variety of smooth and cardiac muscle preparations:

1. (−)-Epinephrine > (±)-epinephrine > norepinephrine > α-methylnorepinephrine > α-methylepinephrine > isoproterenol.

2. Isoproterenol > (±)-epinephrine > α-methylepinehprine > (±)-epinephrine > α-methylnorepinephrine > norepinephrine.

Responses following sequence 1 were considered to be mediated through α-receptors and responses following sequence 2 through β-receptors. Some quantitative comparisons of norepinephrine, epinephrine, and isoproterenol are shown in Table 41.13. Powerful support for this classification is provided by examination of receptor antagonists. Classic adrenergic blocking agents such as Dibenamine (41.**12**), phentolamine (41.**13**), and dihydroergokryptine (an ergot derivative, 41.**14**) block α-receptor-mediated responses, whereas agents such as propranolol (41.**15**) and practolol (41.**16**) block responses mediated through β-receptors. Actually many adrenergically innervated tissues contain both α- and β-receptors and the use of one antagonist can reveal the effects of an agonist on the other (unblocked) receptor system. Hence the pressor effects of epinephrine (dominant α-excitation) are converted to depressor (dominant β-excitation) following α-receptor blockade.

Although much effort has been devoted to analyzing structure–activity relationships of sympathomimetic amines considerable caution may be necessary in the interpretation of the available data. The complexity of the adrenergic synapse indicates that the response produced by a given agonist is determined by many competing processes including uptake, metabolism, and interaction with receptor systems other than the one under investigation (112).

7.1 Stereoselectivity of Agonist Activity

The absolute configurations of a number of catecholamines have been established (113), the more active levorotatory isomers having the $R(\text{D})$ configuration. Isomer activity differences for norepinephrine in a number of α-receptor preparations are listed in Table 41.14. The essential constancy of stereoselectivity between tissues suggests a basic identity of the stereochemical demands of α-receptors. However, comparison of the stereoselectivity of

Table 41.13 Comparative Activities of Norepinephrine, Epinephrine, and Isopropylnorepinephrine

Animal	Tissue	Relative Activity			Receptor Type
		NE	E	ISO	
Rabbit	Aorta	1	65	130	β
Rabbit	Aorta	1	0.8	0.01	α
Rabbit	Stomach muscle	1	1.2	2.5	β
Rabbit	Stomach muscle	1	1	0.001	α
Rabbit	Uterus	1	2	0.002	α
Cat	Spleen	1	1.2	0.03	α
Guinea pig	Trachea	1	12	47	β
Guinea pig	Atria	1	0.5	3	β
Rabbit	Duodenum	1	0.2	1.5	β
Frog	Chromatophore	1	0.25	35	β

$(PhCH_2)_2NCH_2CH_2Cl$

41.**12**

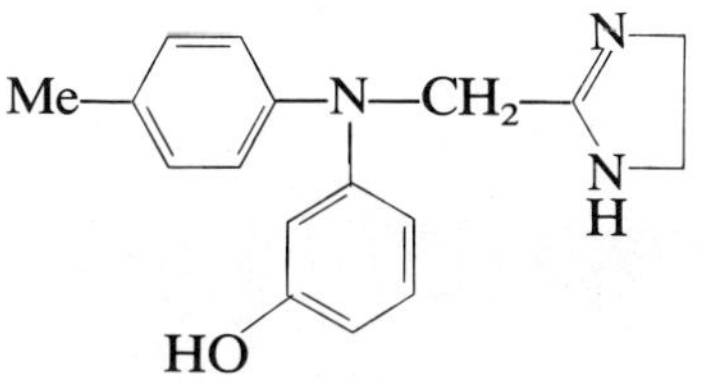

41.**13**

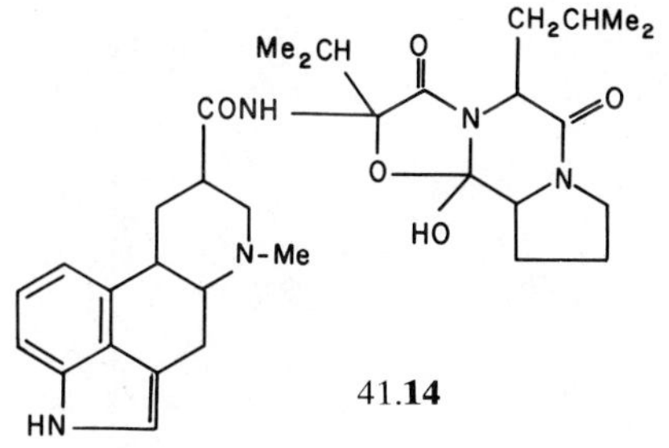

41.**14**

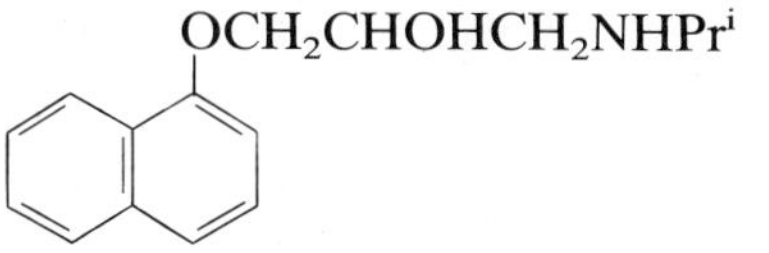

$OCH_2CHOHCH_2NHPr^i$

41.**15**

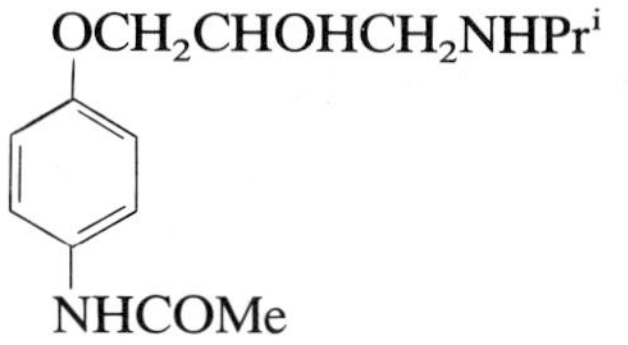

$OCH_2CHOHCH_2NHPr^i$

NHCOMe

41.**16**

norepinephrine in β-receptor preparations does reveal significant differences (Table 41.14). The data in Table 41.14 were obtained in the presence of cocaine and tropolone, to inhibit neuronal uptake and catechol o-methyltransferase activity, respectively, and with either sotalol (β-antagonist) or phentolamine (α-antagonist) present to eliminate opposing receptor activities. In the absence of such precautions measured stereoselectivities may be substantially erroneous (Fig. 41.8). (R) Stereoselectivity is seen with other β-agonists (Table 41.15) and β-antagonists (116, 117, 119–123; Table 41.32), consistent with a common locus of agonist and antagonist binding at the β-receptor.

Early attention was drawn to the stereoselectivity of catecholamine action by Easson and Stedman (124), who proposed a three-point interaction of the catechol, β-hydroxyl, and amino groups (Fig. 41.9).

According to this view it would be anticipated that the less active (S) enantiomers where binding of the β-hydroxyl group is absent should have the same activity as the corresponding phenylethylamines, which indulge only in two-point binding. This has been found to be true in both α- and β-receptor preparations (Table 41.16), but primarily where only direct sympathomimetic activity is being measured. This is clearly seen in a comparison of the data from the rat vas deferens in untreated and reserpine-treated (norepinephrine-depleted) situations.

Although the evidence thus far indicates that a β-hydroxyl group of the appropriate configuration is very important for generating optimum agonist activity at both α- and β-receptors it may not be an indispensible molecular feature, for clearly deoxy derivatives do possess activity, albeit at a reduced level. Of greater significance, however, is

Table 41.14 Stereoselectivity of Norepinephrine in α-and β-Receptor Preparations (114–116)

α-Receptors[a]

Tissue	pD$_2$		(R)/(S) Ratio
	(R)-(–)-NE	(S)-(+)-NE	
Rabbit spleen	6.59	4.16	274
Rabbit vena cava	6.37	3.96	251
Rabbit ileum	6.08	3.68	319
Rat vas deferens	6.62	4.14	302
Rat seminal vesicle	6.07	3.63	275
Rabbit aorta	8.18	5.71	293
Rat aorta	8.93	6.70	170
Cat aorta	6.74	4.52	166
Guinea pig aorta	6.34	3.95	251

β-Receptors[b]

Tissue	pD$_2$		(R)/(S) Ratio
	(R)-(–)-NE	(S)-(+)-NE	
Rat atria	8.89	5.42	3000
Guinea pig atria	7.50	5.00	320
Rabbit atria	7.28	4.63	400
Guinea pig trachea	6.67	4.52	178
Rabbit aorta	7.28	4.63	441
Bovine iris sphincter	6.50	5.67	7

[a] Preparation treated with cocaine, tropolone, and sotalol.
[b] Preparation treated with cocaine, tropolone, and phentolamine.

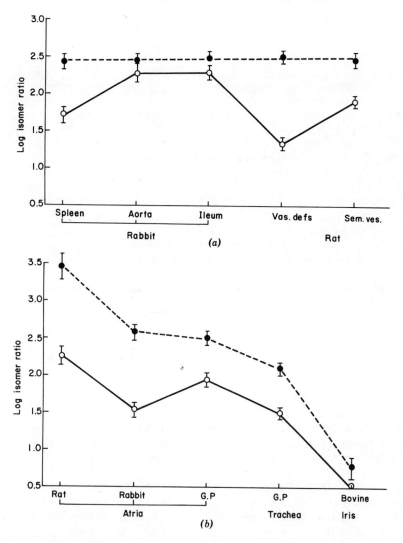

Fig. 41.8   (*a*) Stereoselectivity of interaction of (−) and (+)-norepinephrine in α-receptor preparations in untreated (O—O) and treated (cocaine, sotalol, tropolone, ●−−−●) cases. (*b*) Stereoselectivity of interaction of (−)- and (+)-norepinephrine in β-receptor preparations in untreated (O—O) and treated (cocaine, phentolamine, tropolone, ●−−−●) cases. [Reproduced from P. N. Patil, D. G. Patel, and R. D. Krell, *J. Pharmacol. Exp. Ther.*, **176,** 622 (1971), with permission of Williams & Wilkins, Baltimore, MD.]

the finding that 1-(3,4,5-trimethoxybenzyl)-6,7-dihydroxytetrahydroisoquinoline (41.**17**; trimetoquinol) is approximately equivalent in activity to isoproterenol in some β-receptor preparations (118–126) even though it lacks the β-hydroxyl group. Since, however, activity at β-receptors tends to increase with increasing size of N-substitution it is likely that the absence

of the β-hydroxyl group is compensated by the presence of the 3,4,5-trimethoxybenzyl substituent.

Of very considerable interest is that although isopropylnorepinephrine shows (*R*) stereoselectivity in β-receptor preparations it has been found that for lowering intra-ocular pressure the (*S*)-(+) isomer is more potent (127).

Table 41.15 Stereoselectivity of β-Agonist Action (114, 116, 118)

Compound	Guinea Pig Atria[a]		Guinea Pig Trachea[a]	
	pD_2	Ratio $(R)/(S)$	pD_2	Ratio $(R)/(S)$
(R)-$(-)$-Norepinephrine	7.50	320	6.67	200
(S)-$(+)$-Norepinephrine	5.00		4.52	
(R)-$(-)$-Epinephrine	7.83	30	7.83	30
(S)-$(+)$-Epinephrine	6.36		6.36	
(R)-$(-)$-Isopropylnorepinephrine	8.65	1000	8.50	600
(S)-$(+)$-Isopropylnorepinephrine	5.66		5.77	
(R)-$(-)$-Soterenol	7.78	75	8.30	150
(S)-$(+)$-Soterenol	5.92		6.10	
(R)-$(-)$-Salbutamol	7.70	200	8.44	300
(S)-$(+)$-Salbutamol	5.42		5.97	

[a] Preparation treated with cocaine, tropolone, and phentolamine.

Table 41.16 Stereoselectivities of Norepinephrine Analogs in α- and β-Receptor Preparations (125, 126)

Compound	Rat Vas Deferens Preparation (α-Receptor)			
	Normal		Reserpine Treated	
	pD_2	% Max. Effect	pD_2	% Max. Effect
$(-)$-3,4-$(HO)_2C_6H_3CHOHCH_2NH_2$ (norepinephrine)	5.23	100	4.80	100
$(+)$-3,4-$(HO)_2C_6H_3CHOHCH_2CH_2$	4.51	107	4.08	78
3,4-$(HO)_2C_6H_3CH_2CH_2NH_2$ (dopamine)	4.64	107	3.95	67
$(-)$-3,4-$(HO)_2C_6H_3CHOHCH_2NHMe$ (epinephrine)	5.78	84	5.39	91
$(+)$-3,4-$(HO)_2C_6H_3CHOHCH_2NHMe$	4.51	106	3.96	70
3,4-$(HO)_2C_6H_3CH_2CH_2NHMe$ (epinine)	4.77	100	4.07	84
$(-)$-3,4-$(HO)_2C_6H_3CHOHCHMeNH_2$ (corbasil)	4.96	104	4.80	61
$(+)$-3,4-$(HO)_2C_6H_3CHOHCHMeNH_2$	4.42	40	—	10
3,4-$(HO)_2C_6H_3CH_2CHMeNH_2$	4.86	89	3.94	32
$(-)$-3-$HOC_6H_4CHOHCH_2NHMe$ (phenylephrine)	5.05	109	5.19	91
$(+)$-3-$HOC_6H_4CHOHCH_2NHMe$	4.16	84	—	7
3-$HOC_6H_4CH_2CH_2NHMe$	4.71	100	—	6

Compound	Rat Fat Cell (β-Receptor)	
	pD_2	% Max. Effect
$(-)$-3,4-$(HO)_2C_6H_3CHOHCH_2NH_2$	5.8	100
$(+)$-3,4-$(HO)_2C_6H_3CHOHCH_2NH_2$	3.8	100
3,4-$(HO)_2C_6H_3CH_2CH_2NH_2$	3.5	43
$(-)$-3,4-$(HO)_2C_6H_3CHOHCH_2NHPr^i$	6.7	100
$(+)$-3,4-$(HO)_2C_6H_3CHOHCH_2NHPr^i$	4.2	100
3,4-$(HO)_2C_6H_3CH_2CH_2NHPr^i$	4.2	57

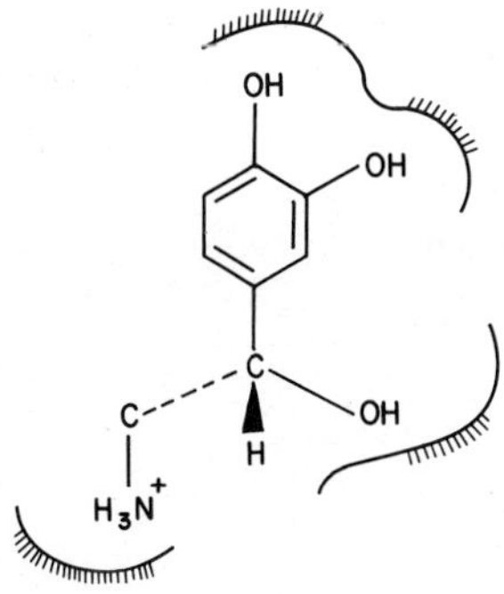

Fig. 41.9 Representation of stereoselective three-point binding of norepinephrine.

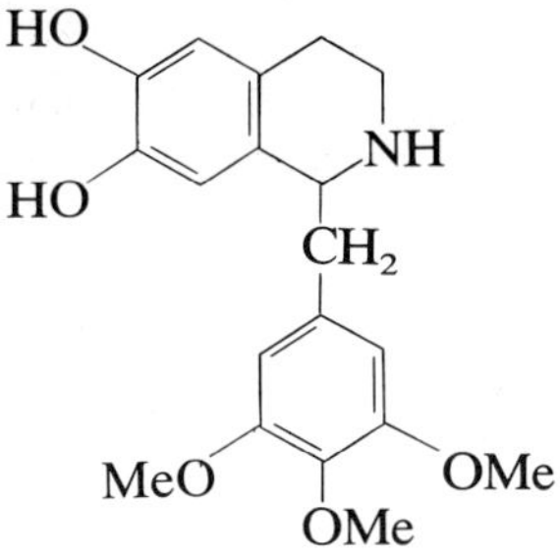

41.**17**

7.2   The Effects of N-Substitution

In their study of phenylethylamines related to epinephrine Barger and Dale (10) examined the N-n-propyl homolog, but because of its very low pressor activity they did not extend their work to other homologs. These compounds were not examined until 1942, when Konzett (128) observed the powerful depressor and bronchodilator effects of N-isopropylnorepinephrine. In an extension of this work Lands and co-workers reported (129–132) the vasodepressor activities of N-alkylnorepinephrines to be in the following order:

t-butyl $>$ isopropyl $>$ sec-butyl

$>$ ethyl $>$ n-butyl

The effects of N-substitution have been quantitated in both α- and β-receptor sys-

tems, and the data of Table 41.17 are typical, showing the decreasing α-activity and increasing β-activity with increased size of the N-substituent. The presence of the ammonium cation appears very important for activity since carbon isosteres of catecholamines have drastically reduced activity (134). Furthermore, optimum activity is associated with primary and secondary amines and conversion to tertiary or quaternary amines is highly detrimental. Hence, although norepinephrine and its N-alkyl analogs exist almost completely in the protonated form at physiological pH (133, 135), this being the active form (136, 137) it is unlikely that a simple ionic interaction alone determines the role of the ammonium function. Extensive discussions of the N-substitution pattern in β-agonist activity (138, 139) indicate that the N-isopropyl or N-t-butyl substituent confer optimum activity and, quite generally, in a variety of N-substitution patterns the presence of the —CMe_2— function adjacent to the nitrogen is very important for high activity (Table 41.18). Addition of further hydrocarbon bulk alone does not increase activity (nos. 7, 9, Table 41.18) but apparently bridging can eventually occur to a

Table 41.17   Effects of N-Substitution in DL-Norepinephrine (133)

	α-Receptors (Rat Vas Deferens)			β-Receptors (Calf Trachea)	
	\multicolumn{3}{c}{}			

$3,4$-$(HO)_2C_6H_3CHOHCH_2NHR$

R	i.a.	pD$_2$	pA$_2$	i.a.	pD$_2$
H	1	5.4		1	5.8
CH_3	1	5.9		1	6.7
C_2H_5	0.9	5.2		1	7.2
C_3H_7	0.3	3.3		—	—
$C_3H_7{}^i$	0.6	3.0		1	7.5
$C_4H_9{}^t$	0		3.0	1	7.6
$CHMeCH_2Ph$	0		4.4		
CMe_2CH_2Ph	0		5.9		

Table 41.18 Effects of N-Substitution on β-Receptor Stimulant Activity of Norepinephrine (138)

No.	R	Relative Bronchodilator Activity
	$3,4\text{-}(HO)_2C_6H_3CHOHCH_2NHR$	
1	CH_3	40
2	CH_2CH_3	25
3	$CH(CH_3)_2$	100
4	$C(CH_3)_3$	170
5	$CH_2(CH_2)_3CH_3$	25
6	Cyclopentyl	70
7	$CH_2CH_2C_6H_5$	10
8	$CH_2CH_2C_6H_4{-}OH(4)$	50
9	$CH(Me)CH_2C_6H_5$	100
10	$CH(Me)CH_2C_6H_4{-}OH(4)$	800
11	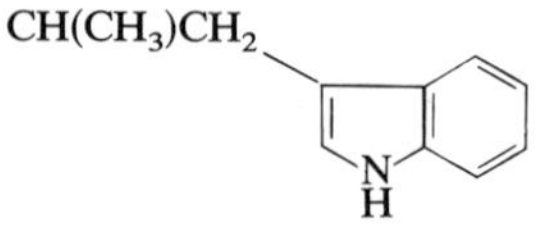	750

$CH(CH_3)CH_2$— (indole structure)

Table 41.19 Ratio of Molecular Volumes of N-Alkyl Substituents (140)

Substituent α	β	E (α/β)
—C⫶C		0.75
C⫶C—C		0.42
—C⫶C (with C above)		1.49
—C⫶C—C—C		0.30
—C⫶C—C (with C above)		0.30
—C⫶C—C (with C above)		0.85
—C⫶C (with C above and below)		2.24

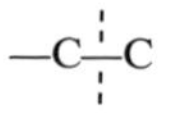

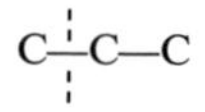

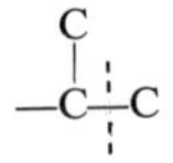

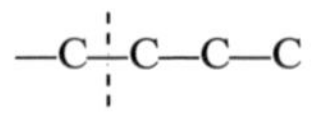

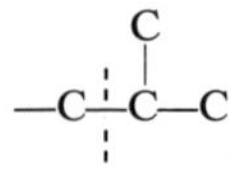

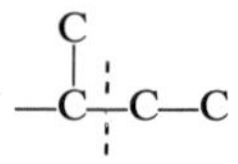

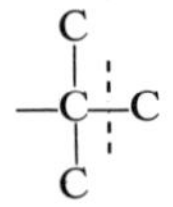

polar area (compare nos. 7 and 8, 9 and 10, Table 41.18; see also Table 41.26).

It seems probable that both nonpolar and ionic interactions are important in determining the N-substituent interaction at the receptor site. It may well be that the ionic interaction represents a constant contribution to both α- and β-agonist activity and that the presence of an appropriately located nonpolar binding site at the β-receptor is responsible for the progressive transition from α- to β-activity. The validity of this conclusion is strengthened by the work of Pratesi (140), who has calculated the ratio of the molecular volumes of the C_α and C_β components of the N-substituents (Table 41.19) and has shown an excellent correlation between this ratio and the apparent affinity of the catecholamine in two β-receptor systems (Fig. 41.10). Clearly, there is an optimum size of N-alkyl substituent that can be accommodated at the β-receptor, and furthermore,

this optimum appears to be significantly different for the β-receptors of guinea pig atria and calf trachea (Section 7.6).

7.3 Effects of Modification of The Catechol Group

Many investigations have been concerned with the effects on sympathomimetic activity of replacing or modifying the catechol group of norepinephrine and its analogs. Unfortunately, many of the earlier data do not make any distinction between the direct and indirect components of sympathomimetic activity and are thus not useful in the formulation of quantitative structure–activity relationships.

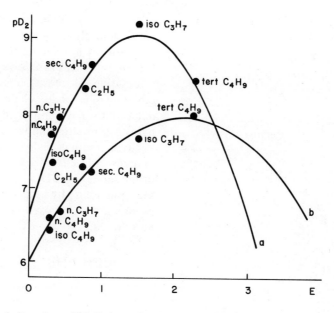

Figure 41.10 Plot of pD$_2$ values of N-alkylnorepinephrine vs. E (Table 41.19) for β-mimetic activity in (a) atria and (b) trachea. [Reproduced with permission from P. Pratesi, L. Villa, and E. Grana, *Farm. Ed. Sci.*, **30**, 1315 (1951).]

Table 41.20 shows that deletion of the p-phenolic group of norepinephrine or epinephrine results in a very considerable drop in activity in both α- and β-receptor preparations. There are indications that the catechol nucleus may be more critical for β-receptor than for α-receptor activation since compound 4 retains approximately 35% of the activity of compound 2 as an α-receptor stimulant, but less than 1% as a β-receptor stimulant. Further support for this conclusion is derived from the data of Table 41.21, which show that deletion of either phenolic group from isopropylnorepinephrine or its analogs leads to compounds with negligible activity at β-receptors.

Although the catechol group has received major attention as a critical determinant of direct activity, the phenolic groups can be successfully replaced by other substituents to maintain agonist activity.

Important work has been concerned with the substitution of the alkyl- or arylsul-fonamide function into the benzene ring of phenylethanolamines (145, 146), the rationale being the similarity in pK_a and geometry of the NH and OH groups. In a

Table 41.20 Influence of the Catechol Function on Sympathomimetic Amine Activity (141)

$$4\text{—}\!\!\underset{3}{\underbrace{}}\!\!\text{—CHONCH}_2\text{NHR}$$

			Relative Activity[a]	
			Blood Pressure	Heart Rate
No.	4	3	R	α-Receptor	β-Receptor
1	HO	HO	H	100	100
2	HO	HO	CH$_3$	14	170
3	H	HO	H	3.0	1.2
4	H	HO	CH$_3$	5.0	0.9
5	HO	H	H	Inactive	0.6
6	HO	H	CH$_3$	0.3	0.3

[a] Reserpine-treated cat preparations.

Table 41.21   Influence of Catechol Function on β-Agonist Activity (138, 142–144)

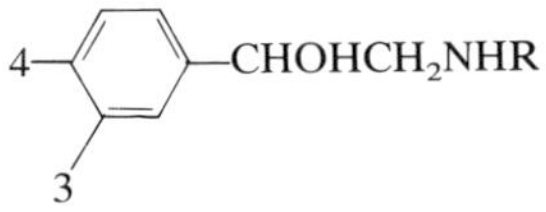

$$4-\!\!\!\bigcirc\!\!\!-CHOHCH_2NHR$$
$$3$$

			Relative Activity	
No.	4	3	R	Vaso-depressor	Bron-chodilator
1	HO	HO	$C_3H_7^i$	100	100
2	H	HO	$C_3H_7^i$	1.3	1.2
3	HO	H	$C_3H_7^i$	0.1	Very weak
4	HO	HO	C_2H_5	50	—
5	H	HO	C_2H_5	Inactive	—
6	HO	H	C_2H_5	Inactive	—
7	HO	HO	C_3H_5	20	—
8	H	HO	C_3H_7	Inactive	—
9	HO	H	C_3H_7	Inactive	—

series of 3- and 4-(2-amino-1-hydroxy-ethyl)methanesulfonanilides (41.**18** and 41.**19**), the 3-substituted derivatives show α- or β-receptor stimulant activity, dependent on the N-substituent (Table 41.22). In particular, the high activity of compound 2 is noteworthy and departure from this structure results in the loss of α-agonist activity and with increasing N-alkyl substitution the appearance of α-antagonism, β-stimulant, and β-blocking activity. In contrast the dominant activity of the 4-substituted derivatives (41.**19**) is that of β-receptor blockade. In a related series of

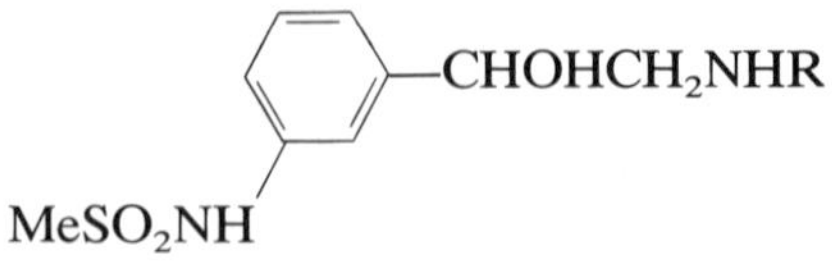

$$\bigcirc\!\!\!-CHOHCH_2NHR$$
$$MeSO_2NH$$
41.**18**

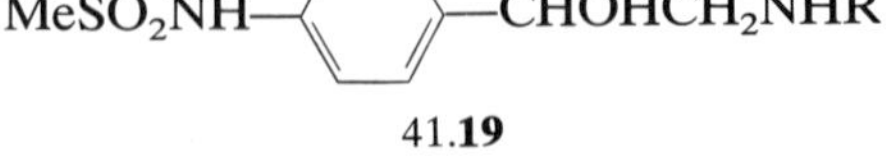

$$MeSO_2NH-\!\!\!\bigcirc\!\!\!-CHOHCH_2NHR$$
41.**19**

compounds containing both the sulfon-amide and phenolic hydroxyl groups in the aromatic ring of phenylethanolamines (41.**10** and 41.**21**) the effect of the relative orientation of these substituents and the ethanolamine side chain becomes very marked with α- and β-receptor stimulant being essentially confined to the 5-(2-amino-1-hydroxyethyl(-2-hydroxyalkane-sulfon-anilides (41.**20**; Table 41.23). In the other series (41.**21**) where the positions of the phenolic hydroxy and sulfonamide groups are transposed stimulant activity is absent.

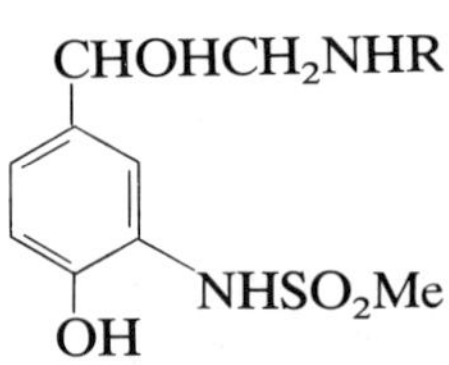

$$CHOHCH_2NHR$$
$$\bigcirc\quad NHSO_2Me$$
$$OH$$
41.**20**

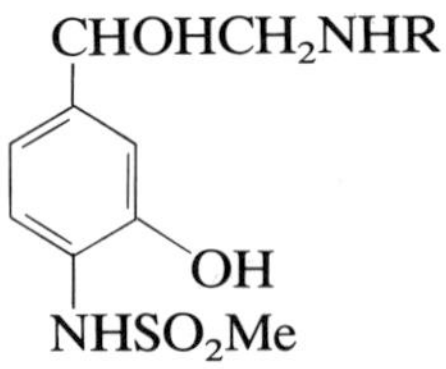

$$CHOHCH_2NHR$$
$$\bigcirc\quad OH$$
$$NHSO_2Me$$
41.**21**

A rationalization of these findings holds that the binding of the more acidic sul-fonamide substituent is determinant and so orients the rest of the molecule. Thus in the active meta series (41.**18** and 41.**20**) it might be assumed that the sulfonamide group interacts with a receptor function normally responsible for binding the *m*-phenolic group of catecholamines and this produces a "productive" binding, whereas similar binding of the *p*-sulfonamide group orients the ethanolamine side chain in a "nonproductive" mode (Fig. 41.11). This attractive speculation is, however, difficult to reconcile with the finding that the active saligenin derivative carries the more acidic group in the para position and the reversed isomers are inactive (Table 41.24). Actually, a variety of substituents can replace the *m*-phenolic group of catecholamines to retain high agonist activity, including $MeSO_2NH-$, $HOCH_2-$, $HO(CH_2)_2-$, $MeSO_2NHCH_2-$, and several amino functions (147; Table 41.25). Since such meta substitution encompasses acidic, basic, and

Table 41.22 α- and β-Receptor Activities of 3- and 4-Methanesulfonamidophenylethanolamines (145)

$$\text{xMeSO}_2\text{NH}\!-\!\langle\!\bigcirc\!\rangle\!-\text{CHOHCH}_2\text{NHR}$$

No.	R	X	α-Receptors (Rat Seminal Vesicle)		β-Receptors (Rat Uterus)	
			Stimulant ED$_{50}$, μg/ml^a	Blocker ID$_{50}$, μg/ml^b	Stimulant ED$_{50}$, μg/ml^c	Blocker $\times$DCI^d
1	H	3	320	—	60	0.07
2	Me	3	2.8	—	0.4	0.1
3	CH(Me)$_2$	3	—	100	0.01	1.0
4	CH(Me)CH$_2$OC$_6$H$_5$	3	—	2.0	0.003	0.03
5	H	4	—	—	350	0.2
6	Me	4	—	—	1800	0.2
7	CH(Me)$_2$	4	—	—	900	6.0
8	C(Me)$_3$	4	—	—	1600	24.2
9	CH(Me)CH$_2$OC$_6$H$_5$	4	—	—	195	4.0

^{a} Concentration required to produce contractions of the rat seminal vesicle 50% as intense as those produced by (−)-epinephrine (2.0 μg/ml).
^{b} Concentration required to reduce by 50% the contraction of the rat seminal vesicle produced by (−)-epinephrine (4.0 μg/ml).
^{c} Concentration required to reduce by 50% the spontaneous contractions of the rat uterus.
^{d} β-Blocking activity relative to DCI = 1 (dichloroisopreterenol)

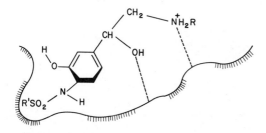

Fig. 41.11 Schematic representation of binding of sulfonamido analogs of catecholamines showing productive (top) and nonproductive (bottom) binding.

neutral substituents emphasis is directed towards the *p*-phenolic substituent as the more important acidic group of the catechol nucleus (148); however, since 3,5-dihydroxyphenylethanolamines are also highly active (Table 41.26) it is not clear that a single rationalization can be offered for the effects of aryl substitution in determining receptor stimulant activity.

7.4 Effects of Modification of the Side Chain

Alkyl substitution in the ethanolamine side chain decreases direct stimulant activity at both α- and β-receptors. Of particular interest is the influence of the α-methyl group in norepinephrine and epinephrine

Table 41.23 Adrenergic Activity of Alkanesulfonamidohydroxyphenylethanolamines (146)

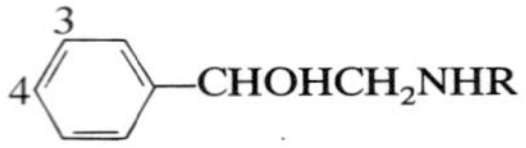

CHOHCH$_2$NHR (positions 3, 4 on ring)

4	3	R	Relative Activity[a]			
			α-Receptors		β-Receptors	
			Stimulant (Rat Seminal Vesicle)	Blocker	Stimulant (Rat Uterus)	Stimulant (Guinea Pig Trachea)
HO	CH$_3$SO$_2$NH	H	7.8	—	0.003	0.005
HO	CH$_3$SO$_2$NH	CH$_3$	12.0	—	0.001	0.03
HO	CH$_3$SO$_2$NH	(CH$_3$)$_2$CH	0.01	—	1.2	1.0
HO	CH$_3$SO$_2$NH	(CH$_3$)$_3$C	—	0.001	0.2	1.4
HO	CH$_3$SO$_2$NH	3,4(CH$_2$O$_2$)C$_6$H$_3$CH$_2$CH$_2$CH(CH$_3$)	—	0.04	4.0	4.0
CH$_3$SO$_2$NH	HO	H	Inactive	—	0.00001	Inactive
CH$_3$SO$_2$NH	HO	CH$_3$	Inactive	—	Inactive	Inactive
CH$_3$SO$_2$NH	HO	(CH$_3$)$_2$CH	Inactive	—	Inactive	Inactive
		Norepinephrine	1.0	—	0.001	0.02
		Epinephrine	3.3	—	0.2	0.15
		Isopropylnorepinephrine	—	—	1.0	1.0
		Phentolamine	—	1.0	—	—

[a] Calculated as bases (molar).

Table 41.24 Relative Activities of Saligenin Derivatives as Bronchial Relaxants (139)

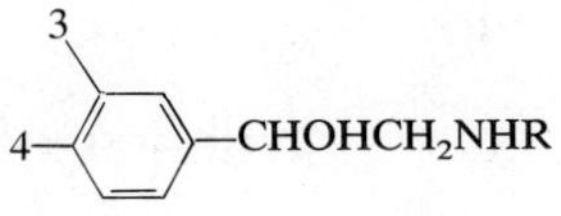

3	4	R	Relative Activity[a]
HO	HO	CHMe$_2$	1.0
CH$_2$OH	HO	CHMe$_2$	2.5
CH$_2$OH	HO	CMe$_3$	1.1
CH$_2$OH	HO	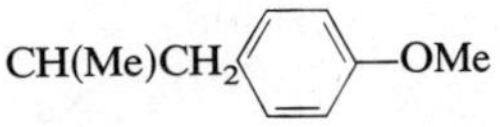 CH(Me)CH$_2$⟨C$_6$H$_4$⟩—OMe	0.67
CH$_2$OH	HO	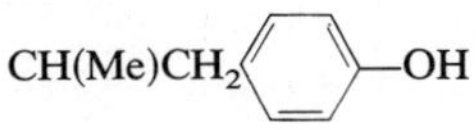 CH(Me)CH$_2$⟨C$_6$H$_4$⟩—OH	0.33
HO	CH$_2$OH	CHMe$_2$	Inactive
HO	CH$_2$OH	CMe$_3$	Inactive

[a] Activity relative to isopropylnorepinephrine = 1.

Table 41.25 β-Receptor Stimulant Activities of *m*-Aminophenylethanolamines (147)

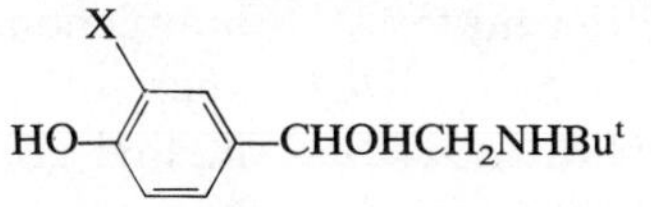

X	ED$_{50}$, M Guinea Pig Trachea	ED$_{50}$, M Guinea Pig Atria	i.a. (Atria)	Ratio ED$_{50a}$/ED$_{50t}$
H$_2$N	2.1×10^{-8}	1.1×10^{-7}	1.0	5.2
MeNH	1.0×10^{-10}	9.2×10^{-9}	1.0	92
Me$_2$N	1.2×10^{-7}	2.9×10^{-5}	0.3	242
HCONH	1.1×10^{-9}	1.7×10^{-8}	0.9	15
MeCONH	2.8×10^{-8}	1.4×10^{-6}	0.5	50
H$_2$NCONH(−)	6.7×10^{-9}	1.3×10^{-7}	0.4	18
H$_2$NCONH(+)	2.7×10^{-6}	9.4×10^{-5}	0.3	35
MeNHCONH	1.8×10^{-7}	6.5×10^{-6}	0.4	36
MeOCONH	9.6×10^{-9}	1.2×10^{-7}	0.7	125
HO (*t*-butylnorepinephrine)	1.3×10^{-9}	7.1×10^{-9}	1.0	5.5
MeSO$_2$NH(soterenol)	2.6×10^{-8}	7.6×10^{-8}	0.7	3.0

Table 41.26 β-Receptor Stimulant Activities of Resorcinol (Orciprenaline) Derivatives (149)

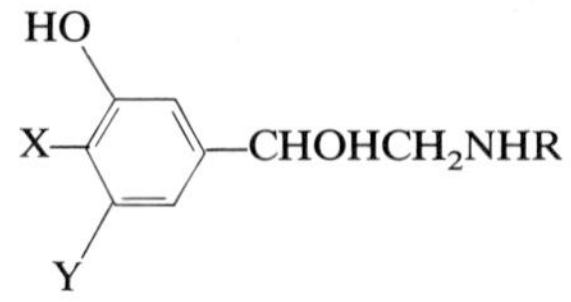

HO

X⟩⟨⟩—CHOHCH₂NHR

Y

X	Y	R	Guinea Pig Trachea	Guinea Pig Atria
			pD₂	
HO	H	CH(Me)₂	8.26	8.61
H	HO (orciprenaline)	CH(Me)₂	7.03	6.56
HO	H	C(Me)₃	8.93	7.92
H	HO (terbutaline)	C(Me)₃	7.09	5.43
HO	H	CH(Me)CH₂Ph	7.93	8.00
H	HO	CH(Me)CH₂Ph	7.03	6.07
HO	H	CH(Me)CH₂C₆H₄OH-4	9.76	9.04
H	HO	CH(Me)CH₂C₆H₄OH-4	8.65	7.28

because of the probable occurrence of the α-methyl derivatives as "false transmitters" derived from α-methyldopa. (2S)-(−)-α-Methyldopa is converted to (1R, 2S)-(−)-α-methylnorepinephrine (erythro) which is stored in nerve terminals (116, 153–155). Direct activity is found with the erythro but not with the three isomers of ephedrine, α-methylnorepinephrine (cobefrin), α-methylepinephrine (N-methylcobefrin), and metaraminol (41.**22a–d**). From the data in Table 41.27 it is also clear that the presence of two asymmetric centers within the molecule has a significant influence upon activity. Thus only (1R, 2S)-ephedrine has direct α-agonist activity and the (1S,2R) isomer is indirectly acting. Similarly, in the α-methylnorepinephrine isomers activity is confined to the (1R,2S) enantiomer. Apparently, the configuration at the carbon atom adjacent to the β-hydroxyl group is of considerable impor-

tance in determining the agonist–receptor interaction. This may involve steric hindrance of β-hydroxyl binding by the α-methyl group perhaps coupled with an influence of the methyl group on the solution conformation of the phenylethylamine (Section 7.5). However, it is interesting to note that the tracheal β-receptor system is considerably less restrictive in its acceptance of α-methyl-substituted compounds (Table 41.27). Similar effects of α-methyl substitution are seen also with the sulfonamide series of compounds (Table 41.28), thus further suggesting similarity of binding of the catecholamine and sulfonamide series.

The evidence thus far discussed indicates that optimum direct activity at α- and β-receptors is provided essentially by the 3,4-dihydroxyphenylethanolamine structure and that relatively limited deviation from this causes progressive loss of activity. An

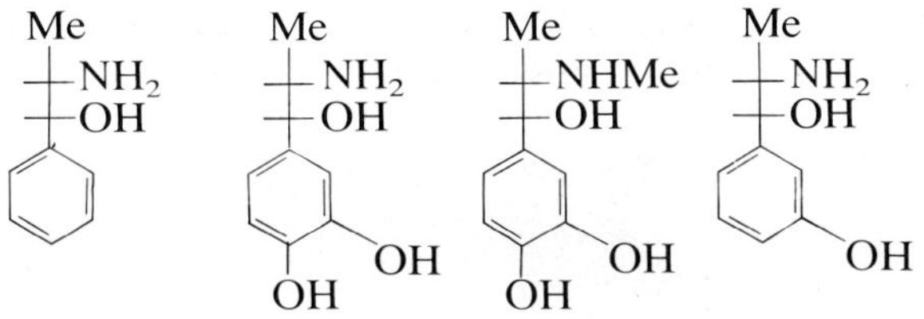

| 41.**22a** | 41.**22b** | 41.**22c** | 41.**22d** |

exception to the previously discussed structural generalizations appears to be provided by the potent sympathomimetic activities of imidazolines. The series includes 2-(1-naphthylmethyl)imidazoline (41.**23**; naphazoline), 2-2,6-dimethyl-3 hydroxy-4-t-butylbenzyl)imidazoline (41.**24**; oxymetazoline), and (1,2,3,4-tetrahydro-1-naphthyl)-2-imidazoline (41.**25**; tetrahydrozoline), and the activity of these and related imidazolines (154) is potent and direct at α-receptors without significant β-receptor stimulant properties (157). Table 41.29 presents a summary of their α-receptor stimulant activity in both central and peripheral systems. The activity of the imidazolines (2–5, Table 41.29) and the 2-aminoimidazolines (7–10, Table 41.29) as

peripheral α-receptor stimulants increases with increasing pK_a (159):

$$pD_2 = 2.088 + 0.362\,pK_a, \qquad r = 0.837,$$
$$s = 0.242$$

with a further improvement resulting from addition of a term for molar volume (MV):

$$pD_2 = 0.870 + 1.876 \log MV + 0.299\,pK_a,$$
$$r = 0.888,\ s = 0.216$$

However, there are probably two separate structure–activity relationships revealed for the imidazolines in the data of Table 41.29. Although it is more difficult to define quantitative relationships for compounds acting in the central nervous system, those imidazolines that have potent

Table 41.27   Effects of α-Methyl Substitution on α- and β-Receptor Activities (150–152)

	Rat Vas Deferens[a]		Guinea Pig Trachea[a]	
	pD_2	% Max. Response	pD_2	% Max. Response
(1R)-(−)-Epinephrine	5.78	100	—	—
(1R,2S)-Ephedrine (D(−)-*erythro*)	4.73	60	4.45	77
(1R,2R)-Pseudoephedrine (D(−)-*threo*)	—[b]	30	3.87	84
(1S,2R)-Ephedrine (L(+)-*erythro*)	—[b]	30	3.22	59
(1S,2S)-Pseudoephedrine (L(+)-*threo*)	—[b]	30	3.74	44
(1R,2S)-Cobefrin (D(−)-*erythro*)	4.80	60	5.52	100
(1S,2R)-Cobefrin (L(+)-*erythro*)	—[b]	10	—	—
(±)-Cobefrin (*threo*)	—[b]	6	4.80	100
(±)-N-Methylcobefrin (*erythro*)	4.47	88	5.67	100
(±)-N-Methylcobefrin (*threo*)	—[b]	21	5.96	100

[a] Reserpine treated.
[b] Response too small to measure ED_{50} accurately.

Table 41.28 Effects of α-Methyl Substitution on α- and β-Receptor Activities of 5-(2-Amino-1-hydroxyethyl)-2-hydroxyalkanesulfonanilides (146)

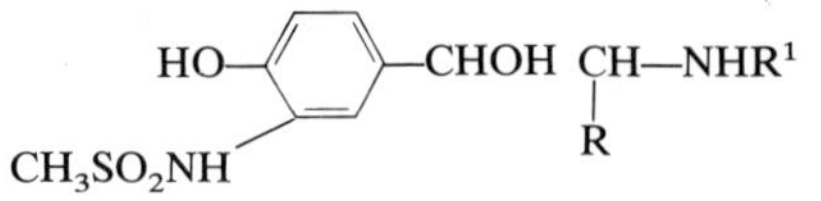

$$\text{HO}\!-\!\!\langle\ \rangle\!-\!\text{CHOH}\ \underset{\underset{\text{R}}{|}}{\text{CH}}\!-\!\text{NHR}^1$$

$$\text{CH}_3\text{SO}_2\text{NH}$$

		Relative Stimulant Activities		
		α-Receptor	β-Receptor	
		Rat	Rat	Guinea Pig
R	R¹	Seminal Vesicle	Uterus	Trachea
H	H	7.8	0.003	0.005
Me	H[a]	1.9	0.002	0.001
H	Me	12	0.001	0.03
Me	Me[a]	1.0	0.005	0.02
H	CH(Me)CH₂C₆H₃(O₂CH₂)-3,4	—	4.0	4.0
Me	CH(Me)CH₂C₆H₃(O₂CH₂)-3,4[a]	—	0.04	0.04
Norepinephrine		1.0		
Isopropylnorepinephrine			1.0	1.0

[a] Erythro racemates.

peripheral sympathomimetic activity have weak central α-receptor activity (peripheral vasodilation and bradycardia) and vice versa. This is clearly seen with clonidine and its 2,6-dibromo analog which are potent α-receptor activators in the central vasomotor control center (160–164). Among the imidazolines it appears that the presence of a nitrogen atom between the phenyl and imidazoline rings is important in determining this difference (compare 6 and 7, Table 41.29).

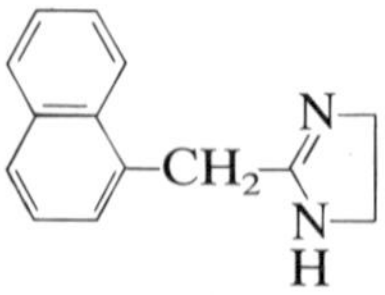

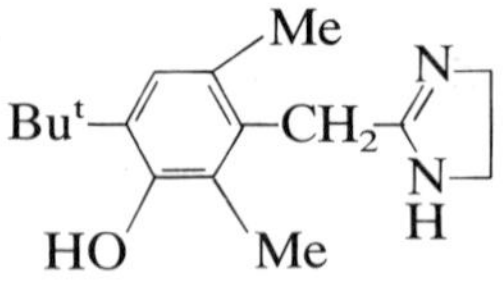

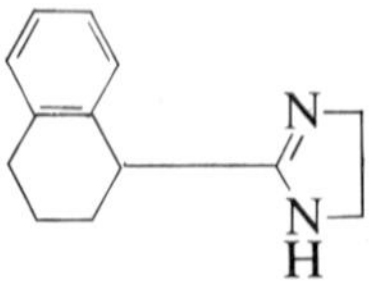

Similarly, it is interesting to note the distinction between (−)-norepinephrine and

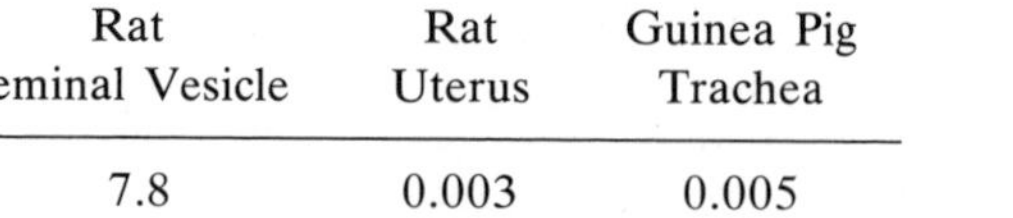

41.**26a**   41.**26b**

(−)-α-methylnorepinephrine since norepinephrine is more potent at peripheral α-receptors and α-methylnorepinephrine more potent at central α-receptors (108, 164). Apparently, differences may exist between central and peripheral α-receptors (Section 7.6).

A major distinction between the imidazolines and the 2-aminoimidazolines is that the latter exist in the imino form (41.**26a, b**), and it has been suggested (165) that in clonidine the perpendicular conformation (41.**27b**) is preferred over the conformation (41.**27a**), where the phenyl and

41.**23**

41.**24**

41.**25**

Table 41.29   α-Receptor Stimulant Properties of Imidazolines (158, 159)

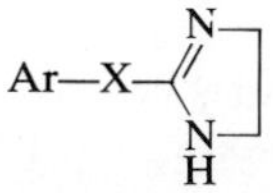

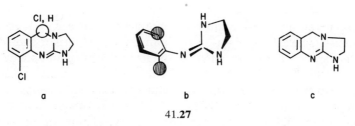

No.	Ar	X	Rabbit Intenstine pD$_2$	Rabbit Intenstine i.a.	BP Inc., Rel. Pot.	BP Dec.,[a] mm Hg (nmols)	H.R. dec.,[a] nmol— Dose to Produce 40 b/m ↓	pK$_a$
			Peripheral Effects			Central Effects		
1.	(−)-Norepinephrine		6.8	1.0	100	15 (40)	20	—
2.	1-C$_{10}$H$_7$(naphazoline)	CH$_2$	6.1	1.0	2	—	>100	10.35
3.	2,6-(Me)$_2$, 3-OH, 4-Bu^{t}C$_6$H$_2$ (oxymetazoline)	CH$_2$	8.8	1.0	30	0 (100)	>100	—
4.	1-C$_{10}$H$_{11}$(tetrahydrozoline)		5.6	1.0	0.3	—	60	10.51
5.	2,6-Cl$_2$C$_6$H$_3$	CH$_2$	5.6	0.3	—	—	>50	9.96
6.	2,4,6-Me$_3$C$_6$H$_2$	CH$_2$	5.7	0.6	—	—	>100	10.7
7.	2,6-Cl$_2$C$_6$H$_3$(clonidine)	NH	5.2	0.4	2	20 (4)	7	8.05
8.	2,6-Br$_2$C$_6$H$_3$	NH	4.9	0.2	—	—	12	8.13
9.	3,4-(HO)$_2$C$_6$H$_3$	NH	5.8	1.0	—	—	3	—
10.	2-Me, 5-FC$_6$H$_3$	NH	5.4	0.5	0.5	27 (4)	50	9.98
11.	(−)-α-Methylnorepinephrine		6.2	1.0	—	—	5	—

[a] Injection into anterior hypothalamus of rat.

41.**27**

imidazoline rings are coplanar and interact sterically. That the planar conformation may not be important biologically is suggested by the finding that the rigid analog, 41.**27c**, does not exert its anti-hypertensive effect at a central location (166). The role of the imino form as the centrally active species of 2-amino-imidazolines is supported by the activity of 2,6-dichlorobenzylidene aminoguanidine (41.**28**; 167). Whether the α-agonistic imidazolines and catecholamines interact at the same or different sites remains to be determined, but it is of interest that the 2-(3,4-dihydroxyphenylamino)imidazoline (no.

9, Table 41.29), containing a catechol nucleus, is more potent than clonidine.

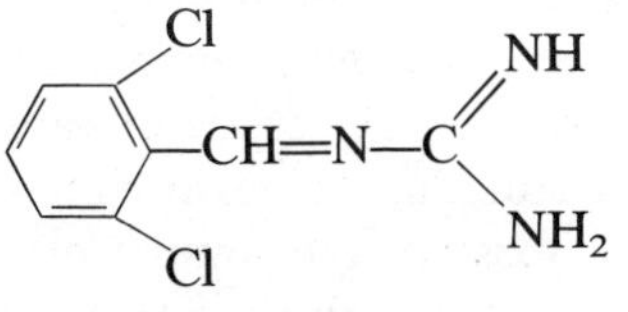

41.**28**

7.5   Conformational Requirements For Sympathomimetic Activity

A question of importance in the analysis of any drug–receptor interaction is that of the conformation of the receptor-bound drug

Table 41.30   Conformations of Sympathomimetic Molecules

Compound	Torsion angle,[a] X-Ray (168) τ_1	τ_2	Conformational Population[b] PMR (169) P_I	P_{II}	P_{III}	MO (170) P_I	P_{II}	P_{III}
Norepinephrine	−97	176	0.14	0.76	0.10	0	0.76	0.24
Epinephrine	−3	−179	0.17	0.77	0.06	0	0.96	0.04
Isopropylnorepinephrine			0.11	0.83	0.06			
Dopamine	−99	174		0.57		0.35	0.35	0.30
Phenylethylamine	−72	171		0.44		0.29	0.40	0.29
Phenylethanolamine				0.16				

[a] τ_1 measures ⟨Ar⟩–C—C—N; τ_2 measures ⟨Ar⟩—C—C—N.

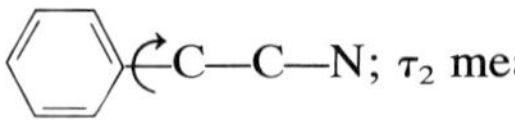

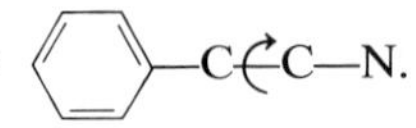

[b] P_I, P_{II}, and P_{III} represent the following three conformational populations:

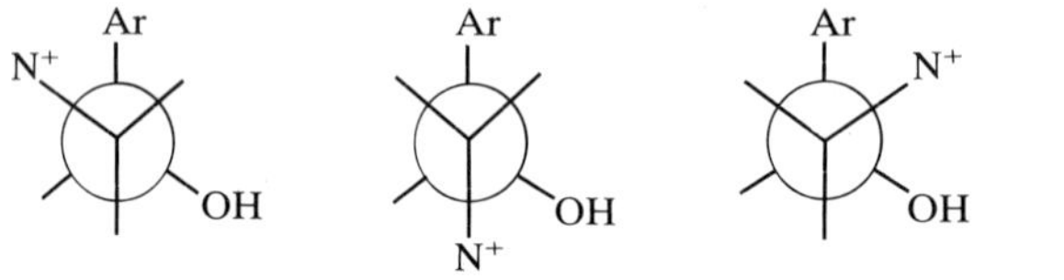

molecule. The general structural requirements for agonist activity at α-or β-receptors are similar, but there are differences, notably in the effects of N-alkyl substitution and, to a lesser extent, α-methyl substitution (Section 7.2). Such differences may reflect different receptor binding surfaces and also the demands of α- and β-receptors for different catecholamine conformations.

Solid-state and solution conformations of a number of phenylethylamines have been determined. X-Ray crystallography indicates that norepinephrine, epinephrine, and dopamine exist in the antiperiplanar conformation where the phenyl and ammonium groups are trans (Table 41.30). The dominance of this conformation is also revealed in solution by PMR analysis, although this is not an exclusive preference (Table 41.30).

It is also clear that a determinant of the antiperiplanar conformation selection is the interaction between $\overset{+}{N}H_3$ and β-OH (compare norepinephrine and dopamine and phenylethylamine and phenylethanolamine, Table 41.30). Quantum calculations also support this conformational preference.

It must be emphasized that there is no necessary relationship between the conformation of a molecule in the solution or crystalline state and that adopted when bound to the receptor. However, the results shown in Table 41.30 are of interest in that they indicate that the energy barriers for interconversion of conformers are small and are therefore unlikely to contribute significantly to the energetics of the drug–receptor interaction. Furthermore, the data reveal no major differences between α- or β-agonists or, for that matter, between direct and indirect acting sympathomimetic agents.

A further approach to the analysis of conformational requirements for drug activity has been in the design of rigid analogs

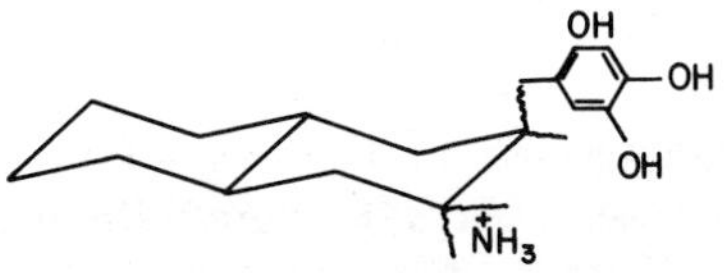

41.**29** 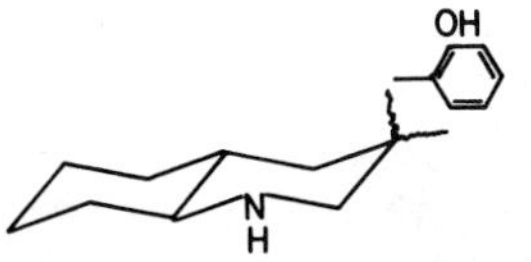   41.**30** 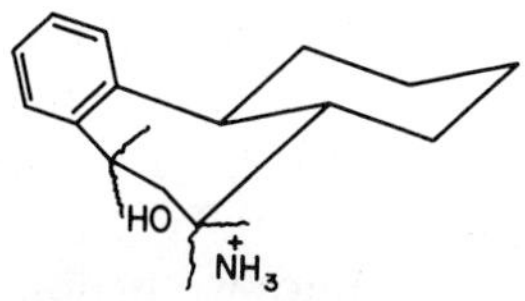   41.**31**

that duplicate one or another presumed conformation of the flexible molecule. This approach has been quite successful in some areas, notably with acetylcholine analogs (Chapter 44), but has not been particularly helpful for sympathomimetic agents. Among the rigid analogs synthesized are the 3-amino-2-(3,4-dihydroxyphenyl)-*trans*-2-decalols (41.**29**; 171), the 3-phenyl-3-hydroxy-*trans*-decahydroquinolines (41.**30**; 172) and the 9-hydroxy-10-amino-1,2,3,4,4α,9,10,10α-(*trans*-4α, 10 α)-octa-hydrophenanthrenes (41.**31**; 173). However, all these agents have rather low activity and it is not possible to conclude whether this is because they present the wrong conformations or because the presence of the added hydrocarbon skeleton reduces activity.

7.6   Subclassification of Receptors

The primary division of adrenergic receptors into the α- and β-types is well accepted, but the question arises as to whether α- or β-receptors are necessarily identical in different tissues or species. There are a number of difficulties in any simple approach to this question. Thus a mere comparison of the relative activities of agonists or antagonists in different tissues may be grossly misleading if such factors as diffusion barriers, synapse geometry, uptake, and metabolism are not considered or controlled, since these factors may differ widely between tissues. Patil and his colleagues (114–116) have suggested that stereoselectivity may be used as a criterion of receptor classification, similar stereoselectivities being generated by similar receptors in different tissues. The differing

stereoselectivity of norepinephrine in a number of tissues is shown in Fig. 41.8; however, a constant stereoselectivity of norepinephrine action at α-receptors is found when uptake, catechol o-methyltransferase, and β-receptor functions are minimized by cocaine, tropolone, and sotalol (Fig. 41.8*a*). According to the stereoselectivity index the α-receptors in the listed tissues are identical. Despite these findings a remarkable apparent difference between the α-receptors of vascular and nonvascular tissue is revealed in the activity of imidazolines (174, 175; Table 41.31).

Evidence for the subclassification of β-receptors is derived from a comparison of the activities of norepinephrine, epinephrine, and isopropylnorepinephrine in a variety of mammalian tissues (Table 41-3; 112, 176). Two distinct sequences are observed, ISO > E ≫ NE (aorta, trachea) and ISO > NE > E (gut, atria). significant differences in agonist stereoselectivity are also seen with β-receptors (Fig. 41-8*b*). A major subclassification of β-receptors has been advanced (178), based on a comparison of the activities of 15 sympathomimetic amines in four β-receptor systems—lipolysis, cardioacceleration, bronchodilation, and vascular relaxation. Since es-

Table 41.31 α-Receptor Activities of Imidazolines (174, 175)

Compound	Tissue	i.a.	pD_2	pA_2
Naphazoline	Rabbit aorta	0.82	7.95	—
Oxymetazoline	Rabbit aorta	0.82	8.43	—
Phentolamine	Rabbit aorta	—	—	8.0
Naphazoline	Rat vas deferens	0.8	3.3	5.5
Oxymetazoline	Rat vas deferens	0.1	3.7	6.0
Phentolamine	Rat vas deferens	—	—	6.5

sentially identical activity sequences are found for lipolysis–cardioacceleration ($r = 0.96$) and for bronchodilation–vascular relaxation ($r = 0.95$) a distinction of β-receptors into two major subtypes has been made: β_1 (heart, fat cells) and β_2 (bronchi, vascular smooth muscle). However, this widely accepted classification differs from that advanced on the basis of stereoselectivity of agonist (Fig. 41-8b) or antagonist (Table 41-32) action. It may well be that the stereoselectivity index, quite aside from the very practical question that small changes in stereochemical purity may exert (116), is an imperfect criterion of receptor subclassification.

Several lines of evidence continue to support the β_1,β_2 subclassification. A number of agonists are known that appear to exhibit substantial selectivity for the β_2-receptor. Such selective agonists include salbutamol (41.**32**), soterenol (41.**33**), and trimetoquinol (41.**17**) which are more effective in tracheal than in atrial preparations (118, 139; Table 41.33). This distinction by agonists is paralleled by the actions of a number of antagonists including prac-

tolol (41.**16**) described as a selective β_1-antagonist, butoxamine (41.**34**) as a selective β_2-antagonist, and propranolol (41.**15**) and alprenolol (41.**35**) as nonselective β-antagonists (122, 174, 177). Further evidence for the β-receptor subclassification stems from observations that similar ligand discrimination is exhibited toward adenylate cyclase, activation of which is believed to be an integral component of β-receptor activation (Section 9). Thus the β_2 selective agonists salbutamol, soterenol, and terbutaline (41.**36**) are more effective in stimulating lung than heart adenylate cyclase, and the β_1- and β_2-selective antagonists practolol and butoxamine also show appropriate selectivity (184, 185).

Although major emphasis has been placed on the subclassification of peripheral postsynaptic α- and β-receptors, it appears likely that differences may also exist between peripheral and central receptors. The structure–activity relationships of the imidazolines appear to demonstrate different structural requirements for peripheral and central α-receptor stimulation (Table 41.29), and this is paralleled by the action

Table 41.32 Stereoselectivity of Antagonist Action in β-Receptor Preparations (118, 179)

Guinea Pig Tissue	Antagonist	pA$_2$	Slope[a]	Stereo Selectivity
Atria	(R)-$(-)$-Sotalol	6.77	0.99	48
	(S)-$(+)$-Sotalol	5.09	1.00	
Trachea	$(-)$-Sotalol	7.73	0.65	39
	$(+)$-Sotalol	6.13	0.57	
Atria	$(-)$-INPEA	6.81	1.02	23
	$(+)$-INPEA	5.44	0.60	
Trachea	$(-)$-INPEA	7.12	0.65	251
	$(+)$-INPEA	4.72	0.86	
Atria	$(-)$-Alprenolol	9.40	0.91	204
	$(+)$-Alprenolol	7.09	0.89	
Trachea	$(-)$-Alprenolol	9.63	0.64	65
	$(+)$-Alprenolol	7.84	0.72	

[a] Slope of dose–ratio (Schild) plot: pure competitive antagonism generates unit slope.

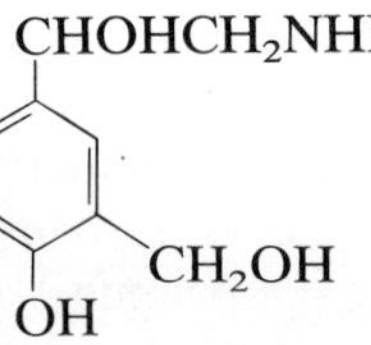

CHOHCH$_2$NHPr^i

CH$_2$OH

OH

41.**32**

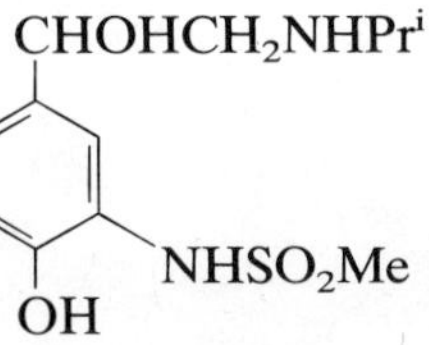

CHOHCH$_2$NHPr^i

NHSO$_2$Me

OH

41.**33**

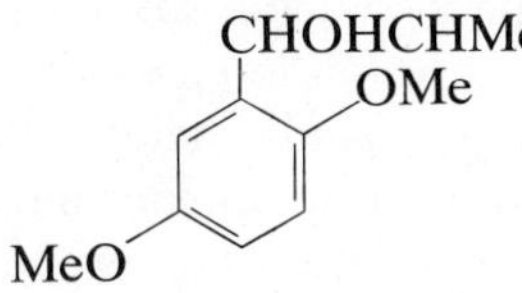

CHOHCHMeNHBu^t

OMe

MeO

41.**34**

OCH$_2$CHOHCH$_2$NHPr^i

CH$_2$CH=CH$_2$

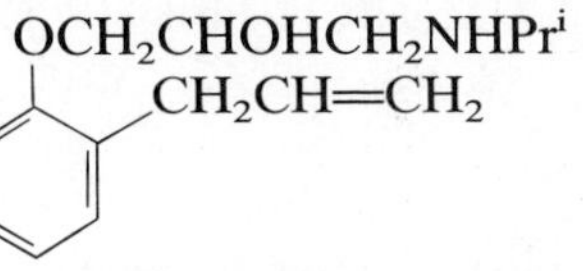

41.**35**

of α-methylnorepinephrine, which is less potent than norepinephrine peripherally but more active centrally. It is likely that differences also exist between pre- and postsynaptic α-receptors, the former being responsible for regulation of norepinephrine release (Section 6.4). Distinctions between pre- and postsynaptic receptors have been based upon essentially the same criteria as discussed previously for postsynaptic receptors. The stereoselectivity of presynaptic receptors appears to be higher than for postsynaptic receptors (186) and a series of agonists can be classified into distinct sequences according to their relative affinities for pre- or postsynaptic receptors (187).

1. Preferentially postsynaptic—methoxamine, phenylephrine.
2. No preference—norepinephrine, epinephrine, naphazoline.
3. Preferentially presynaptic—oxymetazoline, clonidine, α-methylnorepinephrine.

Phenoxybenzamine (41.**37**), an irreversible α-receptor antagonist, has a higher affinity for postsynaptic α-receptors (188).

Table 41.33   Activities of Selective β-agonists (139, 180–183)

		Relative Activities	(Dose Ratios for 50% Change in Response, Isopropyl norepinephrine = 1)	
	Receptor Class	Salbutamol (41.**32**)	Soterenol (41.**33**)	Trimetoquinol (41.**17**)
Guinea pig trachea	β_2	5	5	2
Guinea pig atria	β_1			
Force		2500^{a,b}	>10,000^a	>10,000^{a,d}
Rate		500^{a,c}	3.3	>10,000^{a,d}

[a] Partial agonist.
[b] pd$_2$ 5.96, i.a. 0.35 (isopropylnorepinephrine, pD$_2$ 8.19, i.a. 1.0).
[c] pD$_2$ 5.90, i.a. 0.50 (isopropylnorepinephrine, pD$_2$ 8.53, i.a. 1.0).
[d] i.a. 0.3.

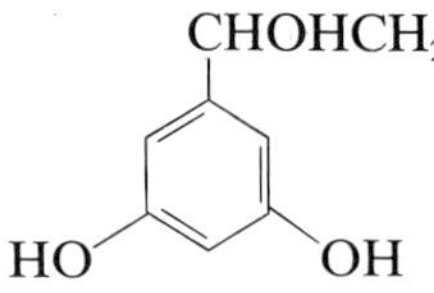

CHOHCH$_2$NHBu^t

HO · OH

41.**36**

PhOCH$_2$CHMeN(CH$_2$Ph)CH$_2$CH$_2$Br

41.**37**

Clearly, much remains to be learned of the details and significance of any subclassification of adrenergic receptors. It is probable, however, that distinct differences do exist and that these contribute powerfully to any observed selectivity of agonist and antagonist action.

8 STRUCTURE–ACTIVITY RELATIONSHIPS OF AMINES ACTIVE AT DOPAMINE RECEPTORS

Knowledge of structural requirements for activation of dopamine receptors is, by comparison with norepinephrine receptors, relatively meager. This deficiency arises because of the relatively recent discovery of the dopamine-utilizing pathways and because of the few convenient tissue systems available for quantitative determinations of structure–activity relationships. Because of the close structural resemblance between dopamine and norepinephrine it is, of course, particularly important to determine that the actions of dopamine are not exerted, partially or totally, at norepinephrine receptors. This has not always proved to be easy.

Dopamine-induced relaxation of some peripheral blood vessels, including mesenteric, renal, and coronary arteries, appears to be mediated through specific dopamine receptors (189, 190). The structural requirements appear to be remarkably strict since in a large series of phenylethylamines only dopamine, N-methyldopamine (epi-

nine), and at a reduced level, apomorphine (41.**38**), are effective in producing canine renal vasodilation after administration of phenoxybenzamine and propranolol. Dopamine behaves like norepinephrine in producing contractions of the rat vas deferens. However, the two agents appear to act at specific receptors as judged by the differences in activity of phentolamine and haloperidol (Table 41.34) and because apomorphine, a partial agonist, potentiates the response to norepinephrine and inhibits the response to dopamine (191).

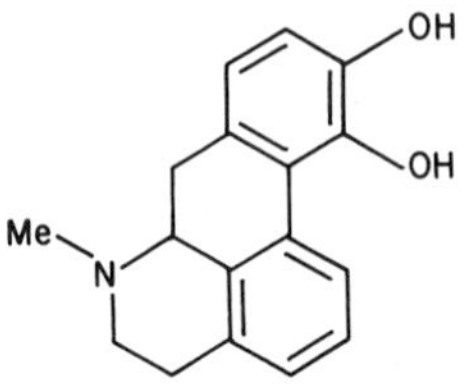

41.**38**

Dopamine is an important vertebrate central transmitter and structural requirements for striatal dopaminergic activation have been determined by the measurement of behavioral effects including rotational and stereotyped behavior (192, 193). Thus in the rat, amphetamine increases spontaneous locomotor activity and produces stereotyped responses, such as compulsive sniffing and gnawing, and apomorphine behaves similarly. The actions of amphetamine and apomorphine likely represent indirect (action at dopamine uptake site) and direct (receptor) actions, respectively.

Table 41.34 Rat Vas Deferens Sensitivity to Norepinephrine and Dopamine Antagonists (191)

Antagonist	pA$_2$ vs. Agonist	
	Norepinephrine	Dopamine
Phentolamine	7.1	8.0
Haloperidol	6.5	7.3

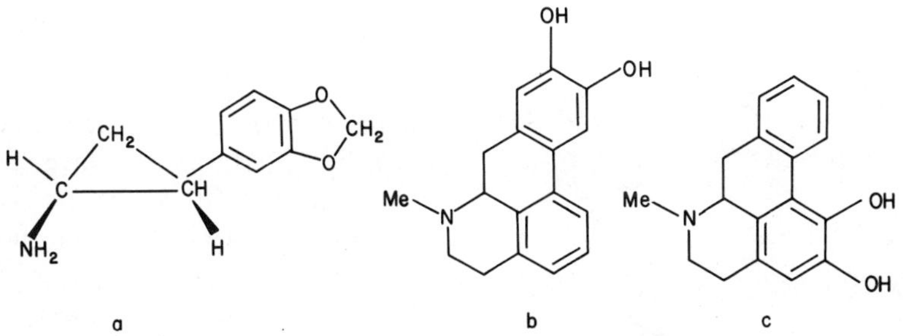

Fig. 41.12   Formulas of (*a*) *trans*-2-(3,4-methylenedioxyphenyl)cyclopropylamine; (*b*) isoapomorphine; and (*c*) 1,2-dihydroxyapomorphine.

Structural requirements for striatal dopamine activity have been determined by intracerebral administration to avoid peripheral metabolism and distribution and general distribution within the CNS (193). The structure–activity relationship thus determined is qualitatively similar to that found for peripheral vertebrate preparations. Thus among phenylethylamines optimum activity is found with dopamine; *N*-substitution reduces activity but epinine is still active. The catechol nucleus is clearly important since monophenolic amines (tyramine and *m*-tyramine) are inactive and 3,4-methylenedioxyphenylethylamine is only feebly active. Modification of the ethylamine side chain by OH and Me substitution decreases activity and thus serves to distinguish quite clearly the dopamine receptor from the norepinephrine receptor.

From the X-ray coordinates for dopamine and apomorphine the distance of the nitrogen atom to the center of the catechol ring is ~5.1 Å, a distance that may be important in the design of both agonists and antagonist species (194). Some definition of the conformational requirements for dopamine receptor activation is provided by the analysis of rigid analogs. Apomorphine corresponds to the antiperiplanar conformation of dopamine or epinine, and the importance of this conformation is indicated by the activity of *trans*-2-(3, 4-methylenedioxyphenyl)cyclopropylamine

and the inactivity of the cis isomer (Fig. 41.12*a*). Furthermore, 1,2-dihydroxyapomorphine (Fig. 41.12*c*), which approximates a synclinal dopamine conformation, is inactive and the reduced activity of isoapomorphine relative to apomorphine also indicates the apparent requirement for an antiperiplanar dopamine conformation (Fig. 41.12*b*). 2-Amino-6,7-dihydroxy-1,2,3,4-tetrahydronapthalene (41.**39**) simulates the antiperiplanar conformation of dopamine and is active in both behavioral assay (195) and as a stimulant of brain adenylate cyclase (Section 9.1).

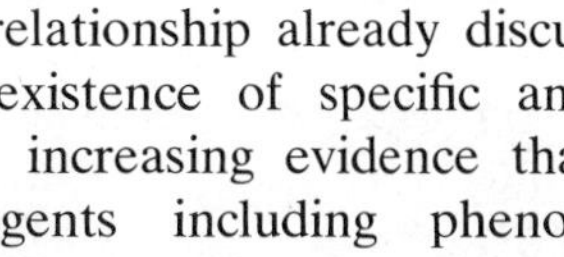

41.**39**

Dopamine and norepinephrine receptors are distinguished by the agonist structure–activity relationship already discussed and by the existence of specific antagonists. There is increasing evidence that neuroleptic agents including phenothiazines, thioxanthenes, and butyrophenones (Fig. 41.13) serve as dopamine antagonists since they block the peripheral and central effects of dopamine receptor activation, inhibit the activation of dopamine-sensitive adenylate cyclase (Section 9.1), increase dopamine synthesis and turnover, and pro-

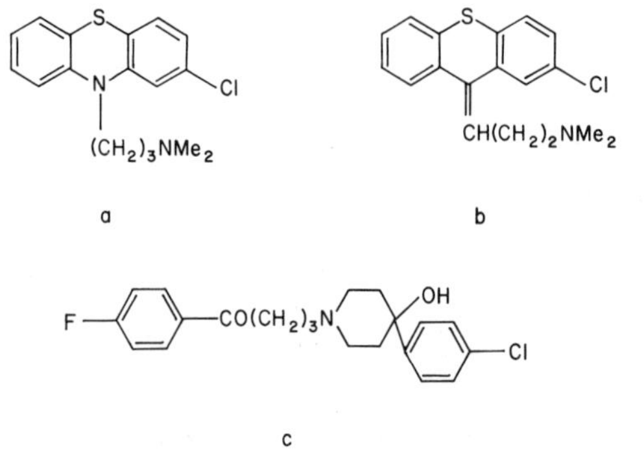

Fig. 41.13 Structural formulas of neuroleptic agents: (*a*) a phenothiazine (chlorpromazine); (*b*) a thioxanthene (chlorprothixene); (*c*) a butyrophenone (haloperidol).

duce extrapyrimidal effects of the Parkinson type (196–199; Chapters 45, 46).

Although an initial comparison of dopamine and neuroleptic structures may suggest little obvious similarity, a more thorough comparison of dopamine and the tricyclic agents reveals within the latter an interesting degree of molecular complementarity to the dopamine, epinine, and apomorphine structures. Thus dopamine is superimposable on a portion of the chlorpromazine structure such that ring A of chlorpromazine and the catechol ring of dopamine overlap, together with overlap of the ammonium group of dopamine and the side chain dimethylamine group of chlorpromazine (200–201; Fig. 41.14). The most potent of the tricyclic agents generally have an electron-withdrawing substituent

(Cl, CF$_3$, etc.) in the 2 position (a more detailed structure–activity analysis is presented in Chapter 56) and the importance of this substituent in determining activity is seen in rigid agents such as the thioxanthenes (41.**40**) where the cis isomers are very much more active than the trans isomers. Similarly, the dibenzodiazepine HF-2046 (41.**41a**) is much more potent than its positional isomer clozapine (41.**41b**); furthermore, the position of the Cl atom is critical and its substitution elsewhere results in abolition of activity (202). Additionally, it is necessary that the tricyclic nucleus be nonplanar since incorporation of activity conferring features (nuclear substituent and amino side chains) into planar aromatic systems, such as anthracene and acridine, does not produce activity. These differences in activity are seen both *in vivo*

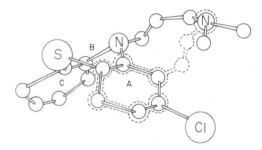

Fig. 41.14 Superimposed view of chlorpromazine and dopamine showing side chain of dopamine tilted toward A ring of chlorpromazine [Reproduced with permission from A. P. Feinberg and S. H. Snyder, *Proc. Natl. Acad. Sci. U.S.*, **72**, 1899 (1975).]

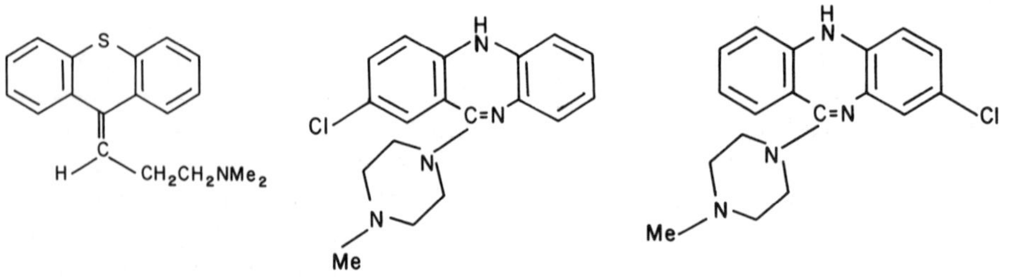

41.**40**   a   41.**41**   b

Table 41.35   Distances of Side Chain Nitrogen from Benzene Ring Centers in Dopamine Antagonists (203)

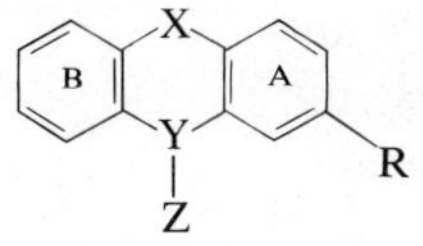

Name	X	Y	Z	R	Distance, Å $A \rightarrow N_1$	Distance, Å $B \rightarrow N_1$
Chlorpromazine	S	N	$(CH_2)_3NMe_2$	Cl	5.12	6.81
Triflupromazine	S	N	$(CH_2)_3\overset{+}{N}Me_2H$	CF_3	6.28	7.28
α-Flupenthixol (cis)	S	C=	$=C(CH_2)_2$	CF_3	5.82	7.46

$$-N_1 \diagup \diagdown NCH_2CH_2OH$$

Name	X	Y	Z	R	$A \rightarrow N_1$	$B \rightarrow N_1$
β-Flupenthixol (trans, weak activity)	S	C=	$=C(CH_2)_2$	CF_3	6.09	6.45

$$-N_1 \diagup \diagdown NCH_2CH_2OH$$

Name	X	Y	Z	R	$A \rightarrow N_1$	$B \rightarrow N_1$
α-Chloroprothixene (cis)	S	C=	$=C(CH_2)_2NMe_2$	Cl	6.24	7.43
Thiethylperazine (weak activity)	S	N	$(CH_2)_3$	SEt	5.93	6.42

$$-N_1 \diagup \diagdown NCH_2CH_2OH$$

Name	X	Y	Z	R	$A \rightarrow N_1$	$B \rightarrow N_1$
Promethazine (weak activity)	S	N	$CH_2CH(Me)NMe_2$	—	6.04	5.36
2-Methoxypromazine	S	N	$(CH_2)_3NMe_2$	OMe	6.35	6.64

(behavioral) and *in vitro* (adenylate cyclase, Section 9.1).

Clearly, the ability of the tricyclic agents to interact at the dopamine receptor depends on a conformationally asymmetric molecule in which the amino group of the side chain is located asymmetrically with respect to the geometric centers of the two benzene rings (Table 41.35, 203). Apparently, a difference in these two distances of ~1.5 Å confers optimum activity. This rationalization of the dopamine–antagonist activity of the tricyclic neuroleptic agents is,

however, not so easy to extend to the butyrophenone systems which may serve as antagonists by interacting at a site other than the dopamine-binding site. In any event it is worth noting that many of the neuroleptic agents are significantly active in other pharmacological systems, including antagonism at cholinergic muscarinic receptors (204).

Differences may exist, however, between dopamine receptors in vertebrates. Thus dopamine is involved in mediating the slow inhibitory response in peripheral ganglionic transmission (205, 206) but this dopamine-mediated response is insensitive to the neuroleptic agents, although it is antagonized by the classical α-adrenergic antagonists (207). In certain respects the structural requirements for dopamine action at invertebrate neurones appear quite similar to those already discussed for vertebrate preparations. Thus in the snail (*Helix aspersa*) inhibitory activity requires the presence of the catechol function, is reduced by N-substitution larger than Me, and is reduced by β-hydroxyl substitution. However, apomorphine is inactive as an agonist and the antagonist selectivity resembles that of the vertebrate peripheral ganglion, since chlorpromazine and haloperidol are inactive and α-antagonists do inhibit dopamine responses (208–210). These findings may suggest that there exist several distinct types of dopamine receptors.

It is of considerable interest that lysergic acid derivatives including ergometrine

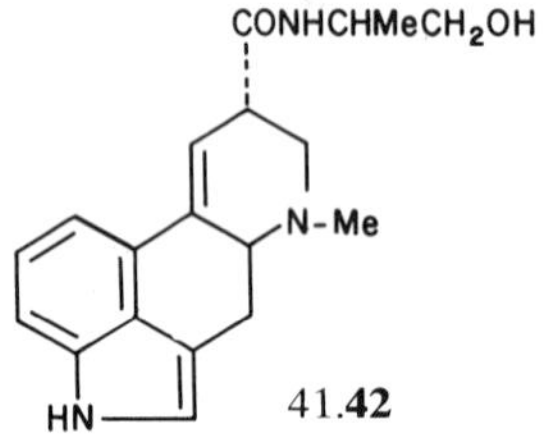

CONHCHMeCH₂OH

41.42

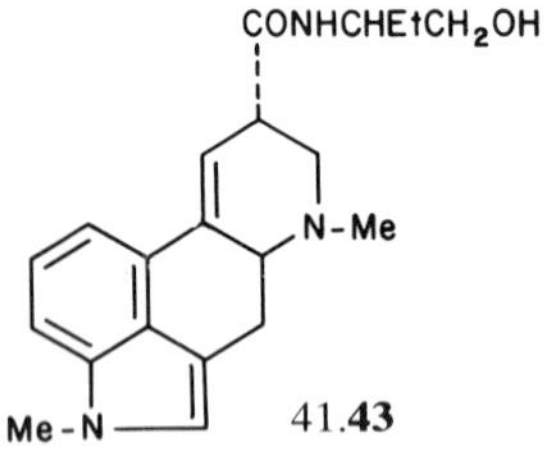

CONHCHEtCH₂OH

41.43

CONEt₂

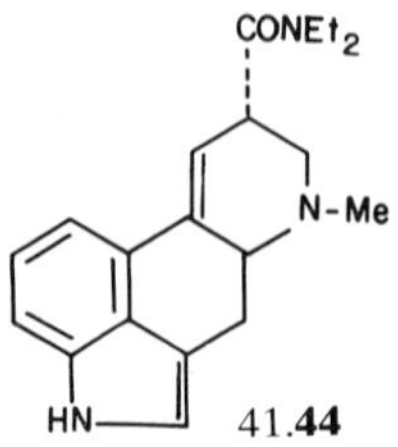

41.44

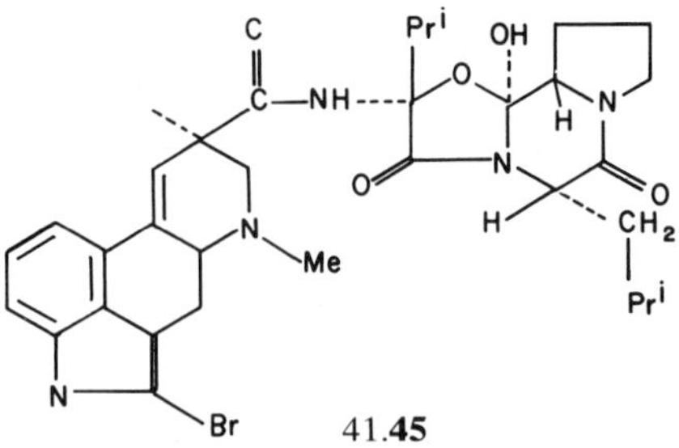

41.45

(41.**42**), methylsergide (41.**43**), and LSD (41.**44**) antagonize dopamine in invertebrate preparations (208, 210–212). These, and related agents, are usually thought of as 5-hydroxytryptamine antagonists (Chapter 58) but there is increasing evidence in mammalian systems for behavioral (213, 214), adenylate cyclase (215), and receptor binding (216, 217) studies that these agents also act with high affinity at dopamine receptors. Indeed, the ergot derivative 2-bromo-α-ergocriptine (41.**45**) is used clinically in the treatment of parkinsonism (218). Apparently, there may exist intriguing similarities between dopamine and 5-hydroxytryptamine receptors.

Dopamine receptor analysis in invertebrates is complicated by the existence of both inhibitory and excitatory responses to dopamine. In *Helix* neurons the receptors mediating the excitatory response appear to resemble more closely those of the mammalian central nervous system since the effects of dopamine are mimiced by apomorphine and antagonized by haloperidol (212). The complexity of invertebrate responses is further illustrated by a particularly intriguing excitatory dopamine response, found in *Aplysia* and *Planorbis* (water snail) neurones, which is antagonized by tubocurarine, classically known as an acetylcholine antagonist in skeletal muscle (211, 219).

9 RECEPTOR FUNCTION

The specific receptors with which catecholamines and their analogs interact

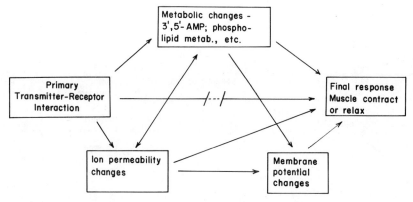

Fig. 41.15 Schematic view of the various events that may interpose between the primary drug–receptor interaction and the final response.

to initiate the biologic stimuli are defined by the structure–activity relationships outlined in the preceding sections. Definition of mechanisms and pathways by which such receptor interactions lead to the observed biologic response is a central problem in neurobiology. It is clear that the sequence of events initiated at catecholamine receptors is a more or less complex pathway including biochemical, ion permeability, membrane conductance, and potential changes, and that the causal interrelationships between these various events are currently not very clear (17; Figs. 41.15). However, an increasing weight of evidence does suggest that certain of the events outlined in Fig. 41.15 may be of general importance. A detailed examination of receptor activation processes is beyond the scope of this chapter and other texts should be consulted (17, 220). However, the processes of dopamine receptor and β-adrenoreceptor activation appear to be clearly linked to the function of adenylate cyclase, and this aspect of receptor activation is briefly discussed.

9.1 Receptors and Adenylate Cyclase

The enzyme adenylate cyclase is stimulated by catecholamines in virtually every tissue believed to contain pharmacologically defined β-receptors (221, 222). The activation of adenylate cyclase by catecholamines is just one example of the ubiquitous involvement of this enzyme in hormone-mediated processes, which has given rise to the general concept of cAMP as a "second messenger" whereby the hormone receptor is viewed as a regulatory site of the enzyme (Fig. 41.16). The detailed organization of this enzyme is not well defined. However, there is little doubt that the receptor is a membrane component in view of the rapidity of catecholamine mediated electrical events (17, 223); the activity of catecholamines covalently attached to glass beads (222, 224), and the inactivity of intracellularly applied norepinephrine (225). Whether the catecholamine recognition site and the enzyme active site are components of the same protein is not known, and some evidence indicates that they may be carried on separate proteins (226, 227).

That the β-receptor and adenylate cyclase are intimately associated is well supported by both qualitative and quantitative indexes (17, 222, 228–231) including temporal and causal associations between cAMP changes and biological events. Furthermore, the order of potency of catecholamines in activating adenylate cyclase is typically that of β-receptors, catecholamine stimulation of the enzyme is competitively antagonized by β-antagonists

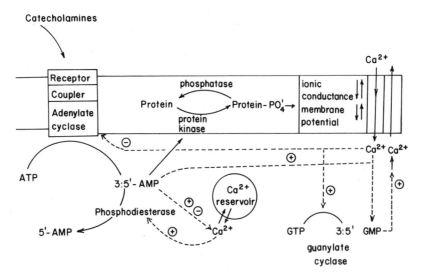

Fig. 41.16   General view of adenylate cyclase activation. 3′,5′-cAMP is shown as controlling phosphorylation of a membrane protein which in turn may control membrane ionic conductance. Also shown are potential inter-relationships to Ca^{2+} and to guanylate cyclase. An increased membrane permeability to Ca^{2+} may cause inhibition of adenylate cyclase and activation of guanylate cyclase. 3′,5′-cAMP may serve to activate Ca^{2+} channels and also to control intracellular Ca^{2+} stores.

but not by α-antagonists, and the marked stereoselectivity of β-agonists and antagonists is also observed with adenylate cyclase activation. Additionally, the β_1,β_2 receptor subdivision us paralleled by a corresponding ligand specificity of the adenylate cyclase from the same tissues (Section 10). Quantitative confirmation of this intimate association is derived from the excellent agreement of the abilities of β-antagonists to inhibit β-receptor processes, adenylate cyclase, and β-antagonist binding (Table 41.36).

A similarly intimate link appears to exist between adenylate cyclase and dopamine receptors. Dopamine-sensitive adenylate cyclase appears to be associated with pharmacologically defined vertebrate dopamine receptors in the renal vasculature (234), sympathetic ganglia (235, 236), and central nervous system tracts (198). The structural requirements for agonists as measured through pharmacological responses or through dopamine-sensitive adenylate cyc-

lase appear to be very similar (237, 238; Table 41.37). The dopamine-sensitive activity is readily distinguished from the β-receptor sensitive adenylate cyclase activity through antagonist action, the latter activity being sensitive to the β-adrenergic antagonist propranolol (239, 240), whereas dopamine-stimulated activity is sensitive to inhibition by the neuroleptic agents (Section 8; 196, 241, 242). Furthermore, there is a generally good correlation between the abilities of these agents to act as inhibitors of dopamine-sensitive adenylate cyclase, their abilities to act as dopamine antagonists in blockade of stereotyped behavior, and their clinical effectiveness as antipsychotic agents (196, 198, 242; Table 41.38). However, an extremely good correlation also exists between the clinical dosage of these compounds and their activity in preventing presynaptic dopamine release (243). Thus the activities of dopamine antagonists may not be confined to a single site.

Table 41.36 Affinities of β-Adrenergic Antagonists for Adenylate Cyclase, Biological Response, and Binding (232, 233)

| Compound | K_I, M | | | Tissue |
	Adenylate Cyclase	Chronotropic Action	Binding	
Dichloroisoproterenol	1.7×10^{-8}	1.2×10^{-8}		Kitten atria
1-$C_{10}H_7OCH_2CHOHCH_2NHPr^i$ (propranolol)	2.8×10^{-9}	3.2×10^{-9}		Kitten atria
$2MeC_6H_4OCH_2CHOCH_2NHPr^i$				
$(-)$ (KL 255)	4.1×10^{-10}	2.3×10^{-10}		Kitten atria
$(+)$	4.4×10^{-8}	2.7×10^{-8}		Kitten atria
2-$CH_2{=}CHCH_2OC_6H_4OCH_2CHOHCH_2NHPr^i$				
$(-)$ Oxprenolol	1.3×10^{-9}	7.4×10^{-10}		Kitten atria
$(+)$ Oxprenolol	5.6×10^{-8}	2.2×10^{-8}		Kitten atria
Propranolol				
$(-)$	1.1×10^{-9}		2.1×10^{-9}	Turkey erythrocyte
$(+)$	2.7×10^{-7}		3.7×10^{-7}	Turkey erythrocyte
$(-)$-Oxprenolol	2.3×10^{-9}		1.4×10^{-9}	Turkey erythrocyte
2-$C_{10}H_7CHOHCH_2NHPr^i$ (pronethalol)	1.4×10^{-7}		2.1×10^{-7}	Turkey erythrocyte
Hydroxybenzylpindolol	2.5×10^{-11}		7.5×10^{-11}	Turkey erythrocyte

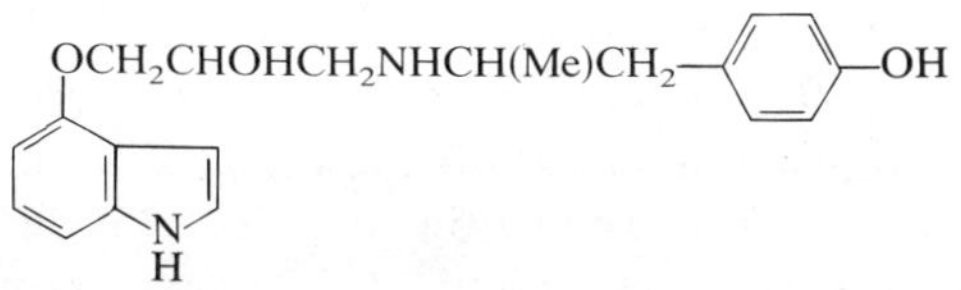

Table 41.37 Effect of Dopamine Analogs on Cyclic AMP Production in Rat Striatal Homogenates (237)

Compound	EC_{50}, M	Max. Stimulation, %
Dopamine	2×10^{-6}	100
Epinine	1.5×10^{-6}	100
N,N-Dimethyldopamine	2×10^{-5}	48
$(-)$-Norepinephrine[a]	4×10^{-5}	97
Apomorphine (41.**38**)	2×10^{-6}	45
6,7-Dihydroxytetra hydroisoquinoline	2×10^{-5}	48
2-Amino-6,7-dihydroxy-1,2,3,4-tetrahydronaphthalene (41.**39**)	4×10^{-6}	115

[a] A number of other phenylethylamines including tyramine, amphetamine, and $(+)$-norepinephrine were all inactive at concentrations up to 10^{-3} M.

Table 41.38 Comparison of Biochemical and Pharmacological Effects of Neuroleptic Agents (242)

Agent	IC_{50}, M Inhibition of Adenylate Cyclase	ED_{50}, mg/kg Antagonism of Stereotypy in Rats	
		Apomorphine	Amphetamine
α-Flupenthixol	2.2×10^{-8}	0.3	0.07
β-Flupenthixol	$>10^{-4}$	>80	>160
α-Clopenthixol[a]	3.3×10^{-7}	30	0.2
α-Chlorprothixene	7.8×10^{-7}	45	0.5
Fluphenazine[b]	9.2×10^{-8}	0.2	0.08
Chlorpromazine	1.0×10^{-6}	59	0.6

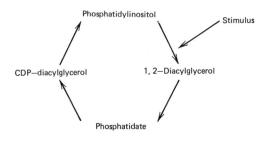

Although activation of adenylate cyclase and an increase in cAMP levels appear to be quite generally associated with events initiated by β-adrenoreceptors and dopamine receptors the linkage remains to be established (17). Thus β-receptor activation leads to an increase in cardiac contractility, to smooth muscle relaxation and hyperpolarization, and to inhibition (hyperpolarization) of norepinephrine-sensitive central neurones whereas dopamine relaxes renal vasculature and mediates a hyperpolarizing ganglionic response (17). These and other diverse events apparently initiated through the common intermediacy of cAMP may actually enjoy a common basis according to which the function of cAMP is to regulate the activity of a class of enzymes, the protein kinases (244, 236). Activation of protein kinases leads to the phosphorylation of a wide variety of protein substrates and the specificity of the cAMP action (physiological response) is then interpreted in terms of the specificities of the protein kinase and the substrate (phosphorylated) protein. The specific cAMP-mediated actions of neurotransmitters on postsynaptic membranes

may involve the phosphorylation of membrane proteins associated with ion channels, which in turn leads to selective increases in ion conductance (Na^+, K^+, Ca^{2+}, etc.) and membrane potential changes (236, 245, 246: Fig. 41.16).

At present no comparable unifying hypothesis is available for the process of α-adrenoreceptor activation. There are indications for a few tissues that activation of adenylate cyclase (247, 248) or guanylate cyclase (249, 250) occurs but the generality of such changes is not established. However, a biochemical event that appears linked to α-adrenoreceptor activation is the increased phosphatidylinositol turnover (Fig. 41.17) that has been demonstrated in

Fig. 41.17 The phosphatidylinositol pathway.

a number of tissues (251, 252). Since activation of adenylate or guanylate cyclases or acceleration of phosphatidylinositol breakdown may all lead to changes in membrane phosphorylation, it is possible that such reactions provide the underlying basis for the membrane changes initiated at the α-adrenoreceptor.

10 RECEPTOR-RELATED EVENTS

The discussion thus far has carried the implicit assumption that, within a given category, the contribution of the receptor to the observed biological response is a constant factor. It is becoming increasingly apparent, however, that the properties of the receptor are subject to a number of important regulatory influences.

The concentration of the transmitter (or hormone) itself plays a very important role in determining the concentration of receptors. Quite generally increases or decreases in the concentration of the interacting ligand produce decreases and increases, respectively, in the concentration of the receptor (253). This has been directly observed for β-adrenoreceptors by measuring the binding of the potent β-receptor antagonist ^{3}H-dihydroalprenolol (254). Thus prolonged exposure of frog erythrocytes to isopropylnorepinephrine results in a decrease in both adenylate cyclase activity and the β-receptor concentration (255; Fig. 41.18). Of particular interest in this regard are the β-receptors of the pineal gland where there exists a circadian rhythm in the production of the pigment melatonin that is under β-receptor control (256). During dark exposure there is an increase in norepinephrine output and an increase in melatonin synthesis whereas during light exposure norepinephrine output falls. This day to night rhythm in norepinephrine output is accompanied by increases and decreases, respectively, in receptor sensitivity, which are apparently determined by corres-

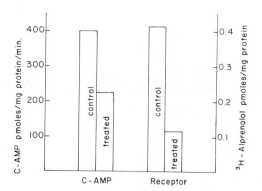

Fig. 41.18 Effect of preincubation of frog erythrocytes treated with (−)-isopropylnorepinephrine (10^{-5} M, >5 hr) on adenylate cyclase activity and receptor binding (^{3}H-alprenolol binding) compared to control. [Data from J. V. Mickey, R. Tate, D. Mullikin, and R. J. Lefkowitz, *Mol. Pharmacol.*, **12**, 409 (1976).]

ponding changes in the β-adrenoreceptor concentration (257; Fig. 41.19). Increases in effector cell sensitivity are well known to occur after denervation or other interference with sympathetic nerve output (258, 259), and it seems likely that the postsynaptic component of such supersensitivity involves an increase in receptor concentration.

In addition to changes in receptor concentration it is also possible that receptor type is under regulatory influence. Thus temperature and thyroid state have been shown in a variety of tissues to modify the sensitivities of α- and β-adrenoreceptors (260–263). These effects are seen quite dramatically in the frog heart, where at low temperatures (18°C) α-receptors dominate and at high temperatures (18–27°C) β-receptors dominate (260). These effects of temperature are seen not only with the order of activities of catecholamines (18°C, NE > E > ISO; 27°C, ISO > E > NE) but also with antagonist action, α-antagonists being effective at low temperature and β-antagonist at high temperature. Furthermore, treatment with the irreversible α-receptor antagonist at low temperatures prevented the appearance of β-receptor activity at high temperatures. Such

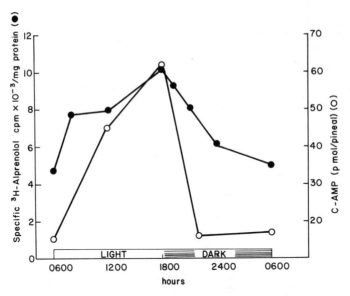

Fig. 41.19 Diurnal variation in the accumulation of cAMP (○) in the rat pineal gland after administration of (−)-isopropylnorepinephrine and the variation in ³H-alprenolol binding (●). [Reproduced with permission from J. A. Romero, M. Katz, J. W. Kebabian, and J. Axelrod, *Nature*, **258**, 435 (1975).]

changes in receptor sensitivity with temperature are seen also in mammalian species and an expression of α-receptor activity in rat atrium is seen at low temperatures (261). Thyroid state may also play a role similar to that of temperature in determining receptor expression since α-receptor expression dominates in atria from hypothyroid rats whereas in hypothyroid rats treated with thyroxine β-receptor expression dominates (261–263). These apparent interconversions of receptor type are of considerable interest and have led to the suggestion that there may exist a single pool of adrenoreceptors, the ligand recognition characteristics of which are subject to modification by metabolic and other regulatory influences.

In addition to regulatory influences on receptor concentration and (possibly) receptor type it is likely that there also exists regulation of the linkage between the receptor recognition site and the subsequent biological signal. One such example of a regulatory influence can be seen very

clearly in the influence of guanine nucleotides on β-adrenoreceptor systems. The guanine nucleotides serve to increase hormone-sensitive adenylate cyclase activity in a number of systems (264). The influence of guanylylimidodiphosphate (Gpp (NH)p, a stable analog of GTP) on the β-adrenoreceptor system of turkey erythrocytes is to increase the apparent affinity of β-agonists, as measured by adenylate cyclase activation, without increasing the actual affinity as measured by binding (265; Fig. 41.20). Thus the effect of the guanyl nucleotides is to produce superimposition of the binding and effect curves so that a 1 : 1 relationship is expressed. In the absence of such regulatory influence receptor binding is not accompanied by an equivalent amount of adenylate cyclase activation. Furthermore, the guanine nucleotides also convert a number of agents including some β-antagonists and α-agonists into weak β-stimulants with partial agonist character.

The preceding considerations make it

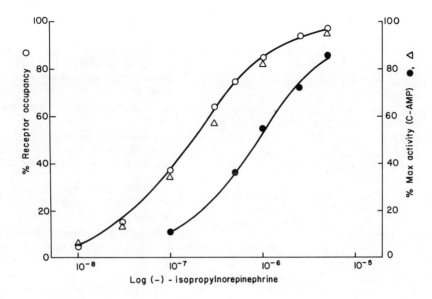

Fig. 41.20 Relationship between receptor occupancy and adenylate cyclase activation in turkey erythrocyte membranes. Receptor occupancy (○) was measured as specific ^{131}I-hydroxybenzylpindolol binding and adenylate cyclase activity (biological response) was measured in the presence of $10^{-6} M$ Gpp (NH)p (●) or $10^{-5} M$ GPP (NH)p (Δ). [Data from E. M. Brown, S. A. Fedak, C. J. Woodard, G. D. Aurbach, and D. Rodbard, *J. Biol. Chem.*, **251**, 1239 (1976).]

quite clear that the interpretation of structure–activity relationships for agonist action at catecholamine receptors is a formidable task. The overall view of such receptors must be, in harmony with increasingly expressed views for receptors in general, that they are composed of at least three functions, recognition site, amplification (e.g., catalytic site, ion channel), and a coupling or linkage process. Structure–activity relationships are the expression of ligand interaction at the recognition site, but this expression may not be constant and is likely subject to a variety of membrane regulatory influences. Similarly, the biological effect mediated through the activation of the amplification site is also regulated by the membrane environment. The analysis of structure–activity relationships must therefore be viewed from the perspective of mobility of receptor structure and function.

REFERENCES

1. G. Oliver and E. A. Schaefer, *J. Physiol.* (London), **18**, 230 (1895).
2. J. J. Abel, *Z. Physiol. Chem.*, **28**, 318 (1899).
3. J. Takamine, *Am. J. Pharm.*, **73**, 523 (1901).
4. J. N. Langley, *J. Physiol.* (London), **27**, 237 (1901).
5. L. Stolz, *Chem. Ber.*, **37**, 4149 (1904).
6. H. D. Dakin, *Proc. Roy. Soc.* (London), **76**, 491 (1905).
7. T. R. Elliott, *J. Physiol.* (London), **31**, XXP (1904).
8. H. H. Dale, *J. Physiol.* (London), **34**, 163 (1906).
9. H. H. Dale, *Adventures in Physiology*, Pergamon, London, 1953.
10. G. Barger and H. H. Dale, *J. Physiol.* (London), **41**, 19 (1910).
11. U. S. von Euler, *Acta Physiol. Scand.*, **11**, 168 (1946).
12. U. S. von Euler, *Pharmacol. Rev.*, **6**, 15 (1954).

13. U. S. von Euler, *Pharmacol. Rev.*, **18,** 29 (1966).

14. U. S. von Euler, *Noradrenaline*, Charles C Thomas, Springfield, Ill., 1956.

15. B. G. Livett, *Brit. Med. Bull.*, **29,** 93 (1973).

16. J. R. Cooper, F. E. Bloom, and R. H. Roth, *The Biochemical Basis of Neuropharmacology*, 2nd ed., Oxford University Press, Oxford, 1974.

17. D. J. Triggle and C. R. Triggle, *Chemical Pharmacology of The Synapse,*, Academic, London. and New York, 1976.

18. J. H. Welsh, in *Handbook of Experimental Pharmacology*, Vol. 33 *The Catecholamines*, H. Blaschko and E. Muscholl, Eds., Springer-Verlag, Berlin, 1972.

19. M. Holzbauer and D. F. Sharman, in *Handbook of Experimental Pharmacology*, Vol. 33, *The Catecholamines*, H. Blaschko and E. Muscholl, Eds., Springer-Verlag, Berlin, 1972.

20. R. Fänge and A. Hanson, in *Comparative Pharmacology*, Vol. I, M. J. Michelson, Ed., Pergamon, Oxford, 1973.

21. G. A. Kerkut, *Brit. Med. Bull.*, **29,** 100 (1973).

22. G. N. Woodruff, *Comp. Gen. Pharmacol.*, **2,** 439 (1971).

23. P. Ascher, *J. Physiol.* (London), **225,** 173 (1972).

24. M. S. Berry and G. A. Cottrell, *J. Physiol.* (London), **244,** 589 (1975).

25. P. Hedqvist, in *The Prostaglandins*, P. W. Ramwell, Ed., Plenum, New York, 1973.

26. P. J. Kadowitz, P. D. Joiner, and A. L. Hyman, *Ann. Rev. Pharmacol.*, **15,** 285 (1975).

27. M. J. Rand, M. W. McCulloch, and D. F. Story, in *Central Action of Drugs in Blood Pressure Regulation*, D. S. Davies and J. L. Reid, Eds., University Park Press, Baltimore, Md., 1975.

28. H. Blaschko, *J. Physiol.* (London), **96,** 50P (1939).

29. U. S. V. Euler, in *Handbook of Experimental Pharmacology* Vol. 33, *The Catecholamines*, H. Blaschko and E. Muscholl, Eds., Springer-Verlag, Berlin, 1972.

30. A. J. Mandell, Ed., *New concepts in Neurotransmitter Regulation*, Plenum, New York, 1973.

31. E. Costa and J. L. Meek, *Ann. Rev. Pharmacol.*, **14,** 491 (1974).

32. J. M. Musacchio, in *Handbook of Psychopharmacology*, Vol. 3, L. L. Iversen, S. D. Iversen, and S. H. Snyder, Eds., Plenum, New York, 1975.

33. N. Weiner, G. Cloutier, R. Bjur, and R. I. Pfeffer, *Pharmacol. Rev.*, **24,** 203 (1972).

34. H. Thoenen, in *Handbook of Psychopharmacology*, Vol. 3, L. L. Iversen, S. D. Iversen, and S. H. Snyder, Eds., Plenum, New York, 1975.

35. W. W. Douglas, *Brit. J. Pharmacol.*, **34,** 451 (1968).

36. R. J. Baldessarini, in *Handbook of Psychopharmacology*, Vol. 3, L. L. Iversen, S. D. Iversen, and S. H. Snyder, Eds., Plenum, New York, 1975.

37. L. Stjärne, in *Handbook of Psychopharmacology*, Vol. 6, L. L. Iversen, S. D. Iversen, and S. H. Snyder, Eds., Plenum, New York, 1975.

38. I. J. Kopin, in *Handbook of Pharmacology*, Vol. 33, *The Catecholamines*, H. Blaschko and E. Muscholl, Eds., Springer-Verlag, Berlin, 1972.

39. L. L. Iversen, *The Uptake and Storage of Noradrenaline in Sympathetic Nerves*, Cambridge University Press, Cambridge, 1967.

40. L. L. Iversen, *Brit. Med. Bull.*, **29,** 130 (1973).

41. L. L. Iversen, in *Handbook of Psychopharmacology*, Vol. 3, L. L. Iversen, S. D. Iversen, and S. H. Snyder, Eds., Plenum, New York, 1975.

42. S. B. Ross, in *The Mechanism of Neuronal and Extraneuronal Transport of Catecholamines*, D. M. Paton, Ed., Raven Press, New York, 1976.

43. D. M. Paton, Ed. *The Mechanism of Neuronal and Extraneuronal Transport of Catecholamines*, Raven Press, New York, 1976.

44. U. S. von Euler, in *Handbook of Experimental Pharmacology* Vol. 33, *The Catecholamines*, H. Blaschko and E. Muscholl, Eds., Springer–Verlag, Berlin, 1972.

45. U. Trendelenburg, in *Handbook of Experimental Pharmacology* Vol. 33, *The Catecholamines*, H. Blaschko and E. Muscholl, Eds., Springer-Verlag, Berlin, 1972.

46. L. G. Whitby, J. Axelrod, and H. Weil-Malherbe, *J. Pharmacol. Exp. Ther.*, **132,** 193 (1961).

47. I. J. Kopin, E. K. Gordon, and W. D. Horst, *Biochem. Pharmacol.*, **14,** 753 (1965).

48. G. Hertting and T. Schiefthaler, *Int. J. Neuropharmacol.*, **3,** 65 (1964).

49. L. L. Iversen, J. Glowinski, and J. Axelrod, *J. Pharmacol. Exp. Ther.*, **151,** 273 (1966).

50. N. J. Uretsky and L. L. Iversen, *J. Neurochem.*, **17,** 269 (1970).

51. B. Hamberger, T. Malmfors, K. A. Norberg,

and C. Sachs, *Biochem. Pharmacol.*, **13,** 841 (1964).

52. B. Hamberger, *Acta Physiol. Scand. Suppl.*, **295** (1967).

53. C. Sachs, *Acta Physiol. Scand. Suppl.*, **341,** (1970).

54. L. L. Iversen, in *Drugs and Transport Processes*, B. A. Callingham, Ed., University Park Press, Baltimore, Md., 1974.

55. D. F. Bogdanski and B. B. Brodie, *Life Sci.*, **5,** 1563 (1966).

56. D. F. Bogdanski and B. B. Brodie, *J. Pharmacol. Exp. Ther.*, **165,** 181 (1969).

57. D. M. Paton, Ed., *The Mechanism of Neuronal and Extraneuronal Transport of Catecholamines*, Raven Press, New York, 1976.

58. H. N. Christensen, *Biological Transport*, 2nd ed., Benjamin, New York, 1975.

59. J. T. Coyle and S. H. Snyder, *J. Pharmacol. Exp. Ther.*, **170,** 221 (1969).

60. S. H. Snyder and J. T. Coyle, *J. Pharmacol. Exp. Ther.*, **165,** 78 (1969).

61. G. Hellman, G. Hertting, and B. Peskar, *Brit. J. Pharmacol.*, **41,** 256 (1971).

62. L. L. Iversen, B. Jarrott, and M. A. Simmonds, *Brit. J. Pharmacol.*, **43,** 845 (1971).

63. L. L. Iversen, *Brit. J. Pharmacol.*, **41,** 571 (1971b).

64. U. Trendelenburg, *J. Pharmacol. Exp. Ther.*, **148,** 329 (1965).

65. A. Tye, P. N. Patil, and J. B. LaPidus, *J. Pharmacol. Exp. Ther.*, **155,** 24 (1967).

66. S. Z. Langer and U. Trendelenburg, *J. Pharmacol. Exp. Ther.*, **167,** 117 (1969).

67. L. L. Iversen, in *Biogenic Amines and Physiological Membranes in Drug Therapy*, J. H. Biel and L. G. Abood, Eds., Dekker, New York, 1971.

68. M. A. Verity, in *Physiology and Pharmacology of Vascular Neuroeffector Systems*, J. A. Bevan, R. F. Furchgott, R. A. Maxwell, and A. P. Somlyo, Eds., Karger, Basel, 1971.

69. M. D. Day, *Brit. J. Pharmacol.*, **18,** 421 (1962).

70. C. A. Stone, C. C. Porter, J. M. Stavorski, C. T. Ludden, and J. A. Totaro, *J. Pharmacol. Exp. Ther.*, **144,** 196 (1964).

71. J. A. Oates, J. R. Mitchell, O. T. Feagin, J. S. Kaufmann, and D. G. Shand, *Ann. N.Y. Acad. Sci.*, **179,** 302 (1971).

72. S. B. Ross and T. Gosztonyi, *Naunyn-Schmiedebergs Arch. Pharmacol.*, **288,** 283 (1975).

73. M. L. Tainter and D. K. Chang, *J. Pharmacol. Exp. Ther.*, **30,** 193 (1927).

74. M. L. Tainter, *J. Pharmacol. Exp. Ther.*, **36,** 569 (1929).

75. J. H. Burn and M. L. Tainter, *J. Physiol.* (London), **71,** 169 (1931).

76. A. Fleckenstein and J. H. Burn, *Brit. J. Pharmacol.*, **8,** 69 (1953).

77. A. Fleckenstein, *Verh. Deut. Ges. Inn. Med.*, 17 (1953).

78. J. H. Burn and M. J. Rand, *J. Physiol.* (London), **144,** 314 (1958).

79. U. Trendelenburg, *Pharmacol. Rev.*, **18,** 629 (1966).

80. R. A. Maxwell, R. M. Ferris, and J. E. Burscu, in *The Mechanisms of Neuronal and Extraneuronal Transport of Catecholamines*, D. M. Paton, Ed., Raven Press, New York, 1976.

81. B. A. Gallingham, in *First International Symposium on Antidepressant Drugs*, 35, *Excerpta Medica International Congress Series*, No. 122, Excerpta Medica, Amsterdam, 1967.

82. R. A. Maxwell, P. D. Keenan, E. Chaplin, B. Roth, and S. B. Eckhardt, *J. Pharmacol. Exp. Ther.*, **166,** 320 (1969).

83. R. A. Maxwell, E. Chaplin, S. B. Eckhardt, J. R. Soares, and G. Hite, *J. Pharmacol. Exp. Ther.*, **173,** 158 (1970).

84. R. A. Maxwell, S. B. Eckhardt, E. Chaplin, and J. Burscu, in *Proceedings Symposium Physiol. Pharmacol. Vasc. Neuroeffector Systems*, J. A. Bevan, R. F. Furchgott, R. A. Maxwell, and A. P. Somlyo, Eds., Karger, Basel, 1971.

85. R. A. Maxwell, R. M. Ferris, J. Burscu, E. C. Woodward, D. Tang, and K. Williard, *J. Pharmacol. Exp. Ther.*, **191,** 418 (1974).

86. A. S. V. Burgen and L. L. Iversen, *Brit. J. Pharmacol. Chemother.*, **25,** 34 (1965).

87. A. S. Horn, *Brit. J. Pharmacol.*, **47,** 332 (1973).

88. A. S. Horn and S. H. Snyder, *J. Pharmacol. Exp. Ther.*, **180,** 523 (1972).

89. A. Rotman, J. Lundstrom, E. McNeal, J. Daly, and C. R. Creveling, *J. Med. Chem.*, **18,** 138 (1975).

90. S. B. Ross and A. L. Renyi, *Acta Pharm. Toxicol.*, **24,** 297 (1966).

91. H. Thoenen, A. Hürlimann, and W. Haefely, *J. Pharm. Pharmacol.*, **20,** 1 (1968).

92. P. N. Patil, K. Shimada, D. R. Feller, and L. Malspeis, *J. Pharmacol. Exp. Ther.*, **188,** 342 (1974).

93. I. Chubb, W. DePotter, and A. DeSchaep-
    dryver, *Naunyn-Schmiedebergs Arch. Phar-
    macol.*, **274,** 281 (1972).

94. U. Trendelenburg and J. R. Crout, *J. Phar-
    macol. Exp. Ther.*, **145,** 151 (1964).

95. L. L. Iversen, J. Glowinski, and J. Axelrod, *J.
    Pharmacol. Exp. Ther.*, **150,** 173 (1965).

96. U. S. von Euler and F. Lishajko, *Acta Physiol.
    Scand.*, **73,** 78 (1968).

97. A. Philippu, in *The Mechanism of Neuronal and
    Extraneuronal Transport of Catecholamines*, D.
    M. Paton, Ed., Raven Press, New York (1976).

98. P. J. Salt, *Eur. J. Pharmacol.*, **20,** 329 (1972).

99. B. A. Callingham and A. S. V. Burgen, *Mol.
    Pharmacol.*, **2,** 37 (1966).

100. J. S. Gillespie, *Brit. Med. Bull.*, **29,** 136 (1973).

101. S. L. Lightman and L. L. Iversen, *Brit. J. Phar-
     macol.*, **37,** 638 (1969).

102. U. Trendelenburg, in *The Mechanism of
     Neuronal and Extraneuronal Transport of
     Catecholamines*, D. M. Paton, Ed., Raven
     Press, New York, 1976.

103. H. Thoenen and J. P. Tranzer, *Ann. Rev. Phar-
     macol.*, **13,** 169 (1973).

103a. R. M. Kostrzewa and D. M. Jacobowitz, *Phar-
      macol. Rev.*, **26,** 199 (1974).

104. M. D. Day and M. J. Rand, *J. Pharm. Phar-
     macol.*, **15,** 221 (1963).

105. J. Crout, H. Alpers, E. Tatum, and P. Shore,
     Science, **145,** 828 (1964).

106. J. Fischer, W. D. Horst, and I. J. Kopin, *Brit. J.
     Pharmacol.*, **24,** 477 (1965).

107. M. D. Day, A. G. Roach, and R. L. Whiting,
     Eur. J. Pharmacol., **21,** 271 (1973).

108. M. Henning, in *Central Action of Drugs in
     Blood Pressure Regulation*, D. S. Davies and J.
     L. Reid, Eds., University Park Press, Balti-
     more, 1975.

109. L. L. Iversen and P. J. Salt, *Brit. J. Pharmacol.*,
     40, 528 (1970).

110. W. H. Hartung, *Chem. Rev.*, **9,** 389 (1931).

111. R. P. Ahlquist, *Am. J. Physiol.*, **153,** 586
     (1948).

112. R. F. Furchgott, in *Handbook of Experimental
     Pharmacology*, Vol. 33, *The Catecholamines*, H.
     Blaschko and E. Muscholl, Eds., Springer-
     Verlag, Berlin, 1972.

113. P. Pratesi, *Pure Appl. Chem.*, **6,** 435 (1963).

114. P. N. Patil, D. G. Patel, and R. D. Krell, *J.
     Pharmacol. Exp. Ther.*, **176,** 622 (1971).

115. P. N. Patil, K. Fudge, and D. Jacobowitz, *Eur.
     J. Pharmacol.*, **19,** 79 (1972).

116. P. N. Patil, D. D. Miller, and U. Trendelen-
     burg, *Pharmacol. Rev.*, **26,** 323 (1975).

117. C. K. Buckner and P. N. Patil, *J. Pharmacol.
     Exp. Ther.*, **176,** 634 (1971).

118. C. K. Buckner and P. Abel, *J. Pharmacol. Exp.
     Ther.*, **189,** 616 (1974).

119. R. Howe and S. B. Rao, *J. Med. Chem.*, **11,**
     1118 (1968).

120. P. N. Patil, *J. Pharmacol. Exp. Ther.*, **160,** 308
     (1968).

121. M. Dukes and L. H. Smith, *J. Med. Chem.*, **14,**
     326 (1971).

122. D. J. Triggle and C. R. Triggle, *Chemical Phar-
     macology of The Synapse*, Chapter III,
     Academic, London, 1976.

123. L. M. Weinstock, D. M. Mulvey, and R. Tull, *J.
     Org. Chem.*, **41,** 3121 (1976).

124. L. H. Easson and E. Stedman, *Biochem. J.*, **27,**
     1257 (1933).

125. P. N. Patil, J. B. LaPidus, D. Campbell, and A.
     Tye, *J. Pharmacol. Exp. Ther.*, **155,** 13 (1967).

126. R. F. Schonk, D. D. Miller, and D. R. Feller,
     Biochem. Pharmacol., **20,** 3403 (1971).

127. R. J. Seidehamel, K. W. Dungan, and T. E.
     Hickey, *Am. J. Ophthal.*, **79,** 1018 (1975).

128. H. Konzett, *Naunyn-Schmeid. Arch. Exp.
     Pathol. Pharmakol.*, **197,** 27, 41 (1940).

129. A. M. Lands, V. L. Nash, H. M. McCarthy, H.
     R. Granger, and B. L. Dertinger, *J. Pharmacol.
     Exp. Ther.*, **90,** 110 (1947).

130. L. Dertinger, H. R. Granger, and H. M.
     McCarthy, *J. Pharmacol. Exp. Ther.*, **92,** 369
     (1948).

131. A. M. Lands, *Am. J. Physiol.*, **169,** 11 (1952).

132. A. M. Lands, G. E. Groblewski, and T. G.
     Brown, *Arch. Int. Pharmacodyn.*, **161,** 68
     (1966).

133. P. Pratesi and E. Grana, *Advan. Drug. Res.*, **2,**
     127 (1965).

134. P. Pratesi, E. Grana, and L. Villa, *Jl. Farm. Ed.
     Sci.*, **26,** 379 (1971).

135. G. P. Lewis, *Brit. J. Pharmacol.*, **9,** 488 (1954).

136. H. F. Hardman and R. C. Reynolds, *J. Phar-
     macol. Exp. Ther.*, **149,** 219 (1965).

137. R. C. Reynolds and H. F. Hardman, *Eur. J.
     Pharmacol.*, **20,** 249 (1972).

138. A. M. Lands and T. G. Brown, in *Drugs Affect-
     ing The Peripheral Nervous System*, A. Burger,
     Ed., Dekker, New York, 1967.

139. R. T. Brittain, D. Jack, and A. C. Ritchie,
     Advan. Drug Res., **5,** 197 (1970).

140. P. Pratesi, L. Villa, and E. Grana, *Il Farm. Ed. Sci.*, **30,** 315 (1975).

141. U. Trendelenburg, A. Muskus, W. W. Fleming, and B. G. A. de la Sierra, *J. Pharmacol. Exp. Ther.*, **138,** 170 (1962).

142. A. M. Lands and M. L. Tainter, *Naunyn-Schmiedebergs Arch. Exp. Pathol. Pharmakol.*, **219,** 76 (1953).

143. A. M. Lands, E. E. Rickards, V. L. Nash, and K. Z. Hooper, *J. Pharmacol. Exp. Ther.*, **89,** 297 (1947).

144. K. Unna, *Naunyn-Schmiedebergs Arch. Exp. Pathol. Pharmakol.*, **213,** 207 (1951.)

145. R. H. Uloth, J. R. Kirk, W. A. Gould, and A. A. Larsen, *J. Med. Chem.*, **9,** 88 (1966).

146. A. A. Larsen, W. A. Gould, H. R. Roth, W. T. Comer, R. H. Uloth, K. W. Dungan, and P. M. Lish, *J. Med. Chem.*, **10,** 462 (1967).

147. C. Kaiser, D. F. Colella, M. S. Schwartz, E. Garvey, and J. R. Wardell, *J. Med. Chem.*, **17,** 49 (1974).

148. A. A. Larsen, *Nature* (London), **224,** 25 (1969).

149. S. R. O'Donnell and J. C. Wanstall, *Brit. J. Pharmacol.*, **52,** 407 (1974).

150. P. N. Patil, J. B. LaPidus, and A. Tye, *J. Pharmacol. Exp. Ther.*, **155,** 1 (1967).

151. A. Tye, R. Baldsberger, J. B. LaPidus, and P. N. Patil, *J. Pharmacol. Exp. Ther.*, **157,** 356 (1967).

152. P. N. Patil and D. Jacobowitz, *J. Pharmacol. Exp. Ther.*, **161,** 279 (1968).

153. E. Muscholl, in *Handbook of Experimental Pharmacology*, Vol. 33, *The Catecholamines*, H. Blaschko and E. Muscholl, Eds., Springer-Verlag, Berlin, 1972.

154. H. Kilbinger, R. Lindmar, K. Löffelholz, E. Muscholl, and P. N. Patil, *Naunyn-Schmiedebergs Arch. Pharmakol.*, **271,** 234 (1971).

155. K. S. Marshall and N. Castagnoli, *J. Med. Chem.*, **16,** 266 (1973).

156. M. Hartmann and H. Isler, *Naunyn-Schmiedebergs Arch. Exp. Path. Pharmakol.*, **192,** 141 (1939).

157. M. Mujic and J. M. van Rossum, *Arch. Int. Pharmacodyn.*, **155,** 432 (1965).

158. H. S. Boudier, G. Smeets, G. Brouwer, and J. van Rossum, *Life Sci.*, **15,** 887 (1974).

159. H. S. Boudier, J. de Boer, G. Smeets, E. J. Lien, and J. van Rossum, *Life Sci.*, **17,** 377 (1975).

160. P. A. Van Zwieten, *J. Pharm. Pharmacol.*, **25,** 89 (1973).

161. G. Haeusler, *Naunyn-Schmiedebergs Arch. Pharmacol.*, **278,** 231 (1973).

162. P. J. Chalmers, in *Central Actions of Drugs in Blood Pressure Regulation*, D. S. Davies and J. L. Reid, Eds., University Park Press, Baltimore, 1975.

163. W. Kobinger, in *Central Actions of Drugs in Blood Pressure Regulation*, D. S. Davies and J. L. Reid, Eds., University Park Press, Baltimore, 1975.

164. A. Scriabine, B. V. Clineschmidt, and C. S. Sineet, *Ann. Rev. Pharmacol.*, **16,** 113 (1976).

165. L. M. Jackman and T. Jen, *J. Am. Chem. Soc.*, **97,** 2811 (1975).

166. T. Jen, B. Dienel, H. Bowman, J. Petta, A. Helt, and B. Loev, *J. Med. Chem.*, **15,** 727 (1972).

167. P. Holme, H. Corrodi, and K. Fuxe, *Eur. J. Pharmacol.*, **23,** 175 (1973).

168. D. Carlstrom, R. Bergin, and G. Falkenberg, *Quart. Rev. Biophys.*, **6,** 257 (1973).

169. R. R. Ison, P. Partington, and G. C. K. Roberts, *Mol. Pharmacol.*, **9,** 756 (1973).

170. B. Pullman, J.-L. Coubeils, P. Courriere, and J.-P. Gervois, *J. Med. Chem.*, **15,** 17 (1972).

171. E. E. Smissman and R. T. Borchardt, *J. Med. Chem.*, **14,** 377 (1971).

172. E. E. Smissman and G. S. Chappell, *J. Med. Chem.*, **12,** 429 (1969).

173. W. L. Nelson and D. D. Miller, *J. Med. Chem.*, **13,** 807 (1970).

174. J. Sanders, D. D. Miller, and P. N. Patil, *J. Pharmacol. Exp. Ther.*, **195,** 362 (1975).

175. W. Kobinger and L. Pichler, *Eur. J. Pharmacol.*, **40,** 311 (1976).

176. S. E. Taylor and R. S. Teague, *J. Pharmacol. Exp. Ther.*, **199,** 222 (1976).

177. H. H. Harms, *J. Pharmacol. Exp. Ther.*, **199,** 329 (1976).

178. A. Arnold, *Il. Farm. Ed. Sci.*, **27,** 79 (1972).

179. P. N. Patil, *J. Pharmacol. Exp. Ther.*, **160,** 308 (1968).

180. V. A. Cullum, J. B. Farmer, D. Jack, and G. P. Levy, *Brit. J. Pharmacol.*, **35,** 141 (1969).

181. J. B. Farmer, I. Kennedy, G. P. Levy, and R. J. Marshall, *J. Pharm. Pharmacol.*, **22,** 63 (1970).

182. J. B. Farmer, G. P. Levy, and R. J. Marshall, *J. Pharm. Pharmacol.*, **22,** 945 (1970).

183. C. Raper and E. Malta, *J. Pharm. Pharmacol.*, **25,** 661 (1973).

184. R. A. Burges and K. J. Blackburn, *Nature New Biol.*, **235,** 249 (1972).

185. V. Vulliemoz, M. Verosky, and L. Triner, *J. Pharmacol. Exp. Ther.*, **195,** 549 (1975).

186. L. Stjärne, *Acta Physiol. Scand.*, **90,** 286 (1974).

187. K. Starke, T. Endo, and H. D. Taube, *Naunyn-Schmiedebergs Arch. Pharmacol.*, **291,** 55 (1975).

188. M. Dubovich and S. Z. Langer, *J. Physiol.* (London), **237,** 505 (1974).

189. L. I. Goldberg, *Biochem. Pharmacol.*, **24,** 651 (1975).

190. L. I. Goldberg, P. F. Sonneville, and J. L. McNay, *J. Pharmacol. Exp. Ther.*, **163,** 188 (1968).

191. A. Simon and E. F. van Maanen, *Arch. Int. Pharmacodyn.*, **222,** 4 (1976).

192. B. Costall, R. J. Naylor, and T. Wright, *Arzneim.-Forsch.*, **22,** 178 (1972).

193. B. Costall, R. J. Naylor, and R. M. Pinder, *J. Pharm. Pharmacol.*, **26,** 753 (1974).

194. A. S. Horn, M. L. Post, and O. Kennard, *J. Pharm. Pharmacol.*, **27,** 553 (1975).

195. G. N. Woodruff, A. O. Elkhawad, and R. M. Pinder, *Eur. J. Pharmacol.*, **25,** 80 (1974).

196. L. L. Iversen, *Neurosci. Res.*, **13:** Suppl., 29 (1974).

197. S. H. Snyder, S. P. Banerjee, H. I. Yamamura, and D. Greenberg, *Science*, **184,** 1243 (1974).

198. L. L. Iversen, *Science*, **188,** 1084 (1975).

199. A. S. Horn, in *Handbook of Psychopharmacology*, L. L. Iversen, S. D. Iversen, and S. H. Snyder, Eds., Vol., 2, Plenum, New York, 1975.

200. A. S. Horn and S. H. Snyder, *Proc. Natl. Acad. Sci. U.S.*, **68,** 2325 (1971).

201. A. P. Feinberg and S. H. Snyder, *Proc. Natl. Acad. Sci., U.S.*, **72,** 1899 (1975).

202. H. R. Burki, W. Ruch, H. Asper, M. Baggiolini, and G. Stille, *Eur. J. Pharmacol.*, **27,** 180 (1974).

203. A. S. Horn, M. L. Post, and O. Kennard, *J. Pharm. Pharmacol.*, **27,** 553 (1975).

204. R. J. Miller and C. R. Hiley, *Nature*, **248,** 596 (1974).

205. B. Libet, *Fed. Proc.*, **29,** 1945 (1970).

206. B. Libet and Ch. Owman, *J. Physiol.* (London), **237,** 635 (1974).

207. P. Kalix, D. A. McAfee, M. Schorderet, and P. Greengard, *J. Pharmacol. Exp. Ther.*, **188,** 676 (1974).

208. R. J. Walker, G. N. Woodruff, B. Glaizner, C. B. Sedden, and G. A. Kerkut, *Comp. Biochem. Physiol.*, **24,** 455 (1968).

209. G. N. Woodruff and R. J. Walker, *Int. J. Neuropharmacol.*, **8,** 279 (1969).

210. G. N. Woodruff, *Comp. Gen. Pharmacol.*, **2,** 439 (1971).

211. P. Ascher. *J. Physiol.* (London), **225,** 173 (1972).

212. H. A. S. Boudier, W. Gielen, A. R. Cools, and J. M. van Rossum, *Arch. Int. Pharmacodyn.*, **209,** 324 (1974).

213. A. J. J. Pijnenburg, G. N. Woodruff, and J. M. van Rossum, *Brain Res.*, **59,** 289 (1973).

214. G. N. Woodruff, A. O. Elkhawad, and A. R. Crossman, *J. Pharm. Pharmacol.*, **26,** 455 (1974).

215. K. von Hungen, S. Roberts, and D. F. Hill, *Brain Res.*, **94,** 67 (1975).

216. D. R. Burt, I. Creese, and S. H. Snyder, *Mol. Pharmacol.*, **12,** 631 (1976).

217. D. R. Burt, I. Creese, and S. H. Snyder, *Mol. Pharmacol.*, **12,** 800 (1976).

218. A. M. Johnson, D. M. Loew, and J. M. Vigouret, *Brit. J. Pharmacol.*, **56,** 59 (1976).

219. M. S. Berry and G. A. Cottrell, *J. Physiol.* (London), **244,** 589 (1975).

220. S. W. Kuffler and J. G. Nicholls, *From Neuron to Brain*, Sinauer, Sunderland, Mass., 1976.

221. G. A. Robison, R. W. Butcher, and E. W. Sutherland, *Cyclic AMP*, Academic, New York, 1971.

222. R. J. Lefkowitz, L. E. Limbird, C. Mukherjee, and M. G. Caron, *Biochim. Biophys. Acta*, **457,** 1 (1976).

223. D. H. Jenkinson, *Brit. Med. Bull.*, **29,** 142 (1973).

224. J. C. Venter, L. J. Arnold, and N. O. Kaplan, *Mol. Pharmacol.*, **11,** 1 (1975).

225. H. Reuter, *J. Physiol.* (London), **242,** 429 (1974).

226. P. Cuatrecasas and M. Hollenberg, *Advan. Protein Chem.*, **30,** 252 (1976).

227. P. A. Insel, M. E. Maguire, A. G. Gilman, H. R. Bourne, P. Coffino, and K. L. Melmon, *Mol. Pharmacol.*, **12,** 1062 (1976).

228. R. G. G. Andersson, *Acta Physiol. Scand. Suppl.*, 382, (1972).

229. M. L. Entman, *Advan. Cyclic Nucleotide Res.*, **4,** 163 (1974).

230. M. J. Berridge, *Advan. Cyclic Nucleotide Res.*, **6,** 1 (1975).

231. W. R. Kukovetz, G. Pöch, and A. Wurm, *Advan. Cyclic Nucleotide Res.*, **5,** 395 (1975).

232. A. J. Kaumann and L. Birnbaumer, *J. Biol. Chem.*, **249,** 7874 (1974).

233. E. M. Brown, S. A. Fedak, C. J. Woodard, G. D. Aurbach, and D. Rodbard, *J. Biol. Chem.*, **251,** 1239 (1976).

234. V. V. Murthy, J. C. Gilbert, L. Goldberg, and J. F. Kuo, *J. Pharm. Pharmacol.*, **28,** 567 (1976).

235. J. W. Kebabian and P. Greengard, *Science*, **174,** 1346 (1971).

236. P. Greengard, *Nature*, **260,** 101 (1976).

237. R. Miller, A. Horn, L. L. Iversen, and R. M. Pinder, *Nature*, **250,** 338 (1974).

238. J. W. Kebabian, G. L. Petzold, and P. Greengard, *Proc. Natl. Acad. Sci. U.S.*, **69,** 2145 (1972).

239. K. von Hungen and S. Roberts, *Eur. J. Biochem.*, **36,** 391 (1973).

240. J. Forn, B. K. Krueger, and P. Greengard, *Science*, **186,** 1118 (1974).

241. Y. C. Clement-Cormier, J. W. Kebabian, G. L. Petzold, and P. Greengard, *Proc. Natl. Acad. Sci. U.S.*, **71,** 1113 (1974).

242. R. J. Miller, A. S. Horn, and L. L. Iversen, *Mol. Pharmacol.*, **10,** 759 (1974).

243. P. Seeman and T. Lee, *Science*, **188,** 1217 (1975).

244. T. A. Langar, *Advan. Cyclic Nucleotide Res.*, **3,** 99 (1973).

245. P. Greengard, D. A. McAfee, and J. W. Kebabian, *Advan. Cyclic Nucleotide Res.*, **1,** 337 (1972).

246. J. L. Marx, *Science*, **178,** 1188 (1972).

247. P. Skolnick and J. W. Daly, *Mol. Pharmacol.*, **11,** 545 (1975).

248. P. Skolnick and J. W. Daly, *Eur. J. Pharmacol.*, **39,** 11 (1976).

249. G. Schultz, J. G. Hardman, K. Schultz, J. W. Davis, and E. W. Sutherland, *Proc. Natl. Acad. Sci. U.S.*, **70,** 1721 (1973).

250. R. F. O'Dea and M. Zatz, *Proc. Natl. Acad. Sci. U.S.*, **73,** 3398 (1976).

251. R. H. Michell, *Biochim. Biophys. Acta*, **415,** 81 (1975).

252. A. A. Abdel-Latif, M. P. Owen, and J. L. Matheny, *Biochem. Pharmacol.*, **25,** 461 (1976).

253. M. Raff, *Nature*, **259,** 265 (1976).

254. R. J. Lefkowitz, L. E. Limbird, C. Mukherjee, and M. G. Caron, *Biochim. Biophys. Acta*, **457,** 1 (1976).

255. J. V. Mickey, R. Tate, D. Mullikin, and R. J. Leflowitz, *Mol. Pharmacol.*, **12,** 409 (1976).

256. J. Axelrod, *Science*, **184,** 1341 (1974).

257. J. A. Romero, M. Zatz, J. W. Kebabian, and J. Axelrod, *Nature*, **258,** 435 (1975).

258. W. W. Fleming, J. J. McPhillips, and D. P. Westfall, *Ergeb. Physiol.*, **68,** 56 (1973).

259. R. K. Dismukes and J. W. Daly, *J. Cyclic Nucleotide Res.*, **2,** 321 (1976).

260. G. Kunos and M. Nickerson, *J. Physiol.* (London), **256,** 23 (1976).

261. B. G. Benfey, G. Kunos, and M. Nickerson, *Brit. J. Pharmacol.*, **51,** 253 (1974).

262. G. Kunos, L. Mucci, and V. Jaeger, *Life Sci.*, **19,** 1597 (1976).

263. G. Kunos, I. Vermes-Kunos, and M. Nickerson, *Nature*, **250,** 779 (1974).

264. M. Rodbell, M. C. Lin, Y. Salomon, C. Londos, J. P. Harwood, B. R. Martin, M. Rendell, and M. Berman, *Advan. Cyclic Nucleotide Res.*, **5,** 3 (1975).

265. E. M. Brown, S. A. Fedak, C. J. Woodard, G. D. Aurbach, and D. Rodbard, *J. Biol. Chem.*, **251,** 1239 (1976).

CHAPTER FORTY-TWO

Antihypertensive Agents

WILLIAM T. COMER

W. LESLEY MATIER

Mead Johnson Pharmaceuticals
Evansville, Indiana 47721, USA

and

M. SAMIR AMER

International Division
Bristol-Myers & Co.
New York, New York 10022, USA

CONTENTS

1   INTRODUCTION

Hypertension is a pathologically elevated systemic arterial pressure. It is the most common cardiovascular disease; as many as 23 million Americans have this largely asymptomatic condition. Hypertension is a major risk factor in cardiovascular mortality and may be a precursor of coronary and cerebral atherosclerosis (1, 2). Antihypertensive therapy has certainly contributed to the recently observed reduction in morbidity and mortality from cerebral hemorrhage, kidney failure, and heart failure. The striking increase in the use of antihypertensive agents during the past 15 years has been largely due to the availability of safe and chronically effective drugs, the widespread efforts to identify and treat patients with elevated blood pressure, and the important demonstration that reduction of blood pressure in moderate to severe hypertensives is associated with a significant reduction in cardiovascular mortality.

Higher blood pressure is considered to be a normal result of aging, and the mortality ratio increases with every increment of blood pressure (3). It is difficult to determine a specific pressure at which hypertension begins—it may be useful to consider normal systolic/diastolic blood pressures to be 120/75–85, borderline hypertensives (40%) to be 140/90–95, *mild* hypertensives (35%) to be 140–160/95–105, *moderate* hypertensives (20%) to be >140/105–120, and *severe* hypertensives (5%) to be >140/>120. From 7 to 15% of the adult population have a diastolic pressure of >95 mm Hg. Systolic blood pressures are better predictors of the long-term consequences of hypertension, but they are so variable that diastolic blood pressures are more frequently used to define hypertension and to follow the progress of treatment.

Some 5–15% of all hypertension is secondary to definable causes, such as renal artery stenosis, a pheochromocytoma, or an endocrine disorder, and is referred to as *secondary* hypertension (4). In the remaining cases, the cause of elevated blood pressure cannot be clearly defined, and they are classified as *essential hypertension.* They frequently differ in the relative contribution of increased cardiac output, expanded plasma volume, elevated renin levels, or other factors to their elevated blood pressure (see Fig. 42.1).

The efficacy of antihypertensive drugs for prolonging life has been well established among moderate and severe hypertensives (5,6), but the difference between treated and control groups with diastolic pressure

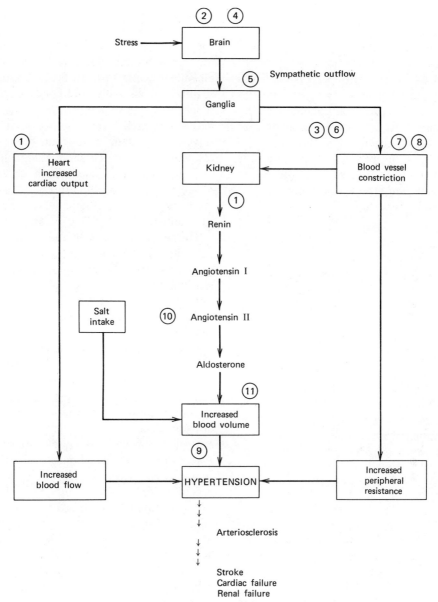

Fig. 42.1 Major action sites and mechanisms of antihypertensive agents. (1) β-Adrenergic blockers; (2) methyldopa; (3) reserpine; (4) clonidine; (5) ganglion blockers; (6) guanethidine; (7) vasodilators; (8) prazosin; (9) thiazide diuretics; (10) angiotensin inhibitors; (11) spironolactone.

<105 is not convincing. Data from various studies indicate that antihypertensive drug therapy reduces short interval deaths such as renal failure, left ventricular heart failure, and intracranial hemorrhage, but mortalities among mild hypertensives tend to be of the long interval type, such as from atherosclerosis or coronary artery disease, that are not significantly affected by available agents. Although the average survival time of hypertensive patients has been increased by antihypertensive drugs, their longevity is still less than normal. The incidence of arteriosclerosis and conditions

secondary to atherosclerosis as a cause of death remains higher among treated hypertensives than normotensives. Unless the extensive demographic studies now in progress indicate that antihypertensive drugs contribute to a decrease in myocardial infarction, the major component of cardiovascular mortality, or to a significant increase in longevity by treating mild hypertensives, the benefits of drug therapy versus the risks of adverse drug effects will become an important consideration for treating mild hypertensives.

1.1 Etiology

There may never be a simple explanation for essential hypertension because patients may have the same elevated blood pressures but derived from different biochemistries or pathophysiologies. In fact, Page's mosaic theory of hypertension (4, 7) embodies most conceivable factors or known defects, singly or collectively, as contributing to the etiology of the disease but does not rule out a common mechanism for the sustained maintenance of high blood pressure (8). The principal etiologic factors are discussed in some detail because of their bearing on preferred treatment approaches.

1.1.1 NEURAL FACTORS. Excessive sympathetic nerve discharge, probably triggered by stress or emotionality early in the development of hypertension, is thought to play a major role in the etiology of this disease. Increased sympathetic outflow from the brain promotes an increased cardiac output and elevated peripheral resistance. These hemodynamic effects characterize labile hypertension which generally proceeds to the irreversible chronic form of the disease. Prolonged high peripheral resistance causes a reduced venous return to the heart with a resulting decrease in cardiac output. Established hypertension therefore is characterized by almost normal cardiac output in the presence of an elevated peripheral resistance.

Adaptation of baroreceptors to higher levels of arterial pressure has been suggested as a primary factor in maintaining essential hypertension (9, 10). When elevated blood pressure is chronically maintained, as with continued stress or a biochemical malfunction, the carotid sinus and aortic arch baroreceptors reset themselves to maintain rather than suppress the elevated pressure. This is accomplished via sustained increases in sympathetic outflow which may underlie the utility of drugs that interfere with sympathetic nerve function in the control of high blood pressure.

The involvement of increased sympathetic tone or elevated levels of circulating catecholamines in stable essential hypertension continues to be debated (11, 12) but cannot alone explain the sustained elevated blood pressures. Peripheral arterial tone may be influenced not only by the extent of nerve discharge but also by the overproduction or incomplete destruction of pressor amines. Norepinephrine is the principal nerve transmitter both centrally and peripherally, but abnormal serotonin, dopamine, or epinephrine levels may play a critical role in the etiology of hypertension. Agents lowering peripheral levels of these pressor amines or blocking their effects on receptors or centrally mimicking the adrenergic stimulation all lower blood pressure, as discussed below.

1.1.2 HORMONAL FACTORS. The renin–angiotensin-aldosterone system has been established as an important blood pressure regulatory mechanism during the past five years largely through the work of Laragh (13). Renin, excreted by the kidney in response to lowered perfusion pressure and sodium load, catalyzes the formation of angiotensin I, a decapeptide with the sequence Asp-Arg-Val-Tyr-Ile-His-Pro-Phe-His-Leu (14). Angiotensin I is rapidly converted in the plasma by a chloride-activated enzyme (primarily in the lungs) to angiotensin II, an octapeptide lacking the His-Leu terminal of its precursor. Angiotensin II is the most potent vasoconstrictor known. It plays an important role in the control of arterial pressure via three mechanisms: (1) it rapidly constricts the arterial bed to increase peripheral resistance; (2) it slowly stimulates the release of aldosterone which increases sodium retention and plasma volume; and (3) it releases catecholamines from the adrenal medulla and possibly from peripheral sympathetic nerves. The catecholamines in turn stimulate renin release and provoke an increase in cardiac output. The net effect of the three mechanisms is to increase sodium load and perfusion pressure to the kidney which tends to inhibit renin release. The three hormones of this humoral feedback system work in parallel to regulate salt balance over a wide range of dietary intakes. It can be seen in Fig. 42.1 that an increase in activity from this humoral axis affects all three primary factors for elevating blood pressure—blood vessel constriction, increased blood volume, and increased cardiac output.

Severe hypertension is often accompanied by high renin levels, but it is not clear whether this is a cause or an effect of renal damage. Plasma renin levels are frequently measured today to aid in the understanding of pathophysiology as well as the treatment of patients. Elevated renin–angiotensin levels appear to play a critical role in a group of young, high-renin hypertensives which constitute 10–15% of the essential hypertension population. All the antiadrenergic drugs inhibit renin secretion, with β-blockers being the most effective; whereas sulfonamide diuretics, direct vasodilators, and aldosterone antagonists all stimulate renin secretion. The advocacy of renin suppressors as sole therapy for hypertension has some flaws: (1) renin levels do not always correlate well with the response to therapy; (2) effective therapy can be achieved by some combinations of agents that do not alter renin levels; and (3) renin levels vary almost to the same degree in normal subjects as in hypertensives. With an improved understanding of the role that the renin–angiotensin–aldosterone system

plays in the disease process, we suspect the knowledge of patient renin levels will be more useful for knowing etiology and selecting the therapeutic agent than for predicting the response to therapy. The routine acquisition of renin levels for diagnostic purposes has been questioned. Nevertheless, β-blockers are quite effective for high-renin patients, moderately effective for normal renins, and less effective for low-renin patients; conversely, sulfonamide diuretics or spironolactone are effective alone for most low-renin patients, who are probably volume expanded.

Other hormones and vasopressor substances have also been implicated in the etiology or maintenance of essential hypertension. Prostaglandins (15) and related arachidonic acid metabolites, notably the ratio of thromboxanes to prostacyclins (16), may be crucial to the vasoconstricting processes in vascular tissues. Corticoids (17), the kinins (18), vasopressin (19), and some yet unidentified hormones have been discussed for a possible role in the regulation of blood pressure.

1.1.3 ELECTROLYTE FACTORS. The inability of the kidney to excrete an adequate daily amount of salt and water is believed by Guyton and associates (20, 21) to be the main cause of elevated arterial pressures. In fact, Freis has suggested (22) that controlling salt intake below 2 g/day would permit the prevention of essential hypertension and its disappearance as a major health problem. This emphasizes the fundamental value of diuretics in treating hypertension. Abnormal retention of salt and water increases the blood volume, which increases the work load on the heart by increasing blood flow (see Fig. 42.1). Volume-dependent hypertensives have been estimated at 20–30% of the total essential hypertension population. Just as renin levels vary considerably among normal and hypertensive subjects, there is no simple relationship between the amount of sodium or fluid volume excreted per day and blood pressure levels since salt balance is largely regulated by the renin–angiotensin–aldosterone system.

Potassium balance is largely regulated by the renin axis also, but daily excretion rates fluctuate less than sodium rates with changes in renin or blood pressure. Hence potassium levels are less implicated in the etiology of hypertension than are sodium levels. Selenium intake has been implicated to play an etiologic role in hypertension (23), along with other dietary and environmental factors (24).

1.1.4 VESSEL WALL FACTORS. Folkow et al. (25) suggested that intermittent increases in cardiac output induce wall thickening and hypertrophy of the vasculature as an adaptive response to increased perfusion pressure. The smaller lumen-to-wall ratio of resistance vessels helps maintain the chronic elevation of peripheral resistance that characterizes essential hypertension. These structural changes could at least partly explain the increased sensitivity of vascular smooth muscles to contractile stimuli observed in hypertensive animals (26), and support the value of direct-acting vasodilators in hypertension.

1.1.5 GENETIC FACTORS. The involvement of hereditary factors in hypertension is widely accepted (27). Parents and siblings of individuals with essential hypertension are generally affected by the same condition. Siblings of hypertensives develop an abnormal increase in blood pressure during middle age.

The development of several hypertensive animal models, solely by selective inbreeding, that parallel human hypertension in their response to therapeutic agents adds further support. Whether or not genetic factors underlie the increased sensitivity of vascular smooth muscle to vasoconstrictors in hypertension, the increased susceptibility of hypertensives to stress, or their reduced ability to excrete an adequate amount of salt, will continue to spur investigation.

1.2 Hemodynamic Profile in Established Hypertension

Irrespective of the differing etiologic factors that may be involved in the development of essential hypertension, most patients with established hypertension have a similar hemodynamic profile (28) characterized by elevated peripheral vascular resistance with nearly normal cardiac output and plasma volume.

Blood pressure is the product of the blood flow and the resistance to that flow. Blood flow is determined completely by the cardiac output, which depends on how fast the heart beats and the volume of blood ejected with each beat. This stroke volume in turn depends on the capacity of the heart, its strength of contraction, and the total blood volume in the body. The peripheral resistance to flow is primarily influenced by the diameter of the smaller arterial vessels or arterioles and, to a much lesser extent, blood viscosity. It becomes important, therefore, that antihypertensive drugs should decrease peripheral resistance by direct or indirect dilation of the arterioles. Although some agents reduce cardiac output (β-blockers) and diuretics decrease blood volume, all widely used antihypertensive drugs cause a significant decrease in peripheral resistance by dilating the arterioles. The myocardial baroreceptors apparently can accommodate increased resistance and pressure to maintain a normal cardiac output in the hypertensive state. But the vascular contractile mechanism loses its sensitivity to neurotransmitters with time, and vessel walls hypertrophy and become clogged with atherosclerotic plaques; yet there seems to be no compensatory mechanism for restoring vascular compliance or for clearing congested arterioles. Therefore, the well established hypertensive patient must depend on the effectiveness of therapeutic agents to decrease his peripheral resistance regardless of the blood pressure level or pathophysiologic etiology.

Attempts to classify essential hypertension into well defined subgroups based on renin levels, volume versus vasoconstriction hypertension (13), or other etiologic factors (29) have met with limited success. But the rapidly expanding awareness of pathophysiological considerations, as well as the increasing understanding of their role in essential hypertension, suggests that such knowledge will increasingly be used as a basis for the rational selection of specific therapeutic agents. The goal of antihypertensive therapy will continue to be the chronic reduction of arterial pressure to reduce cardiovascular mortality with minimal risks to the patient. But the level to which arterial pressure should be lowered (30) and the need for aggressive therapy in the elderly will require further study and discussion.

2 AGENTS FOR TREATING HYPERTENSION

A large number of drugs having a variety of pharmacological actions are presently used for the treatment of hypertension. Since uncomplicated hypertension is largely an asymptomatic condition, the management of hypertension is often dictated by the drug side effects. Side effects such as daytime drowsiness and exercise hypotension may be tolerated acutely but are considered a nuisance chronically. One of the big challenges for new antihypertensive agents is to be free from chronic nuisance effects as well as toxic effects. Patient compliance is poor for treatment over the rest of a patient's life if there are nuisance effects or if the dosage schedule is inconvenient, and noncompliance quickly reduces the effectiveness of any therapy. The mechanism of drug action is at least as significant for the side effect profile as it is

for efficacy in lowering blood pressure, and a pharmacokinetic pattern allowing once-a-day dosing is becoming increasingly important. Physician compliance also is low if each patient must be carefully titrated to establish a safe and effective dose. The concerns for nuisance effects, patient compliance, and physician compliance are especially critical for assessing the risk/benefit ratio in treating mild hypertensives.

The site and mechanisms by which drugs lower blood pressure greatly determine their usefulness as well as their side effects. The potency and side effects of neuronal blocking agents are roughly similar, as they are for β-blocking agents, sulfonamide diuretics, central adrenergic agents, and vasodilators. Many of the side effects can be expected from their pharmacological action. It is rare, however, that only one site or mechanism is involved for a drug. In order to encourage the rational selection of antihypertensive agents based on their mechanisms and site of action, matched with an understanding of patient pathophysiology, the agents presently used or being clinically investigated are discussed according to their primary mechanism. Combinations are discussed throughout this section since they are frequently used to minimize side effects by counteracting undesired mechanisms as well as to extend the effectiveness of blood pressure lowering.

The challenge for medicinal chemists and pharmacologists in developing new antihypertensive drugs today is to identify agents with a mechanism and site of action unique to the control of blood pressure so as to avoid side effects. This ideal agent also should be orally effective with an absorption and excretion pattern that supports continued action from a single daily dose and with minimal drug metabolism. This singular function is difficult to achieve for adrenergic blockers, agents acting in the central nervous system, agents acting on renal function or the renin axis, and agents reducing cardiac output, but may be possible for agents acting strictly on the vascular contractile mechanism to reduce peripheral resistance.

2.1   Neural Mechanisms

2.1.1   MODULATION OF AFFERENT NERVE IMPULSES. The *Veratrum* alkaloids are the only agents known to lower arterial blood pressure by reflexly stimulating medullary vasomotor centers. By initially increasing the excitability of the afferent vagal fibers in the coronary sinus, left ventricle, and carotid sinus of the heart, a falsely exaggerated nerve impulse reaches the central nervous system via the ninth and tenth cranial nerves. This is interpreted centrally as a higher level of blood pressure than really exists, so the brain responds by sending a decreased sympathetic signal to the periphery which reduces the arterial pressure (31). Sustained hypotension is attributed to resetting the baroreceptors in the carotid sinus (32), the homeostatic pressure control mechanism. Blood pressure is lowered proportionate to the dose of *Veratrum* alkaloids regardless of the initial pressure.

Although the mechanism of the *Veratrum* alkaloids is quite desirable because its primary effect is vasomotor depression with a small decrease in heart rate, the duration of action is short and the margin between hypotensive and emetic doses of these alkaloids is minimal. The *Veratrum* alkaloids are readily absorbed orally, are slowly metabolized, and tolerance does not develop. They are still used somewhat in hypertensive crises, but extensive chemical modifications have not shown a significant separation of the severe nausea and vomiting or bradycardia from the hypotensive action. The bradycardia in man is blocked by atropine whereas the hypotensive and emetic effects are not changed.

More than 20 ester *Veratrum* alkaloids have been isolated, but all are derived from one of four alkamines. It is not commercially worthwhile to isolate and use single alkaloids because their isolation or synthesis is too tedious and costly, and they all still provoke severe vomiting. The isolation and characterization of these alkaloids was largely carried out in the early 1950s. The chemistry of these materials has not changed appreciably since previous reviews (33, 34) and is not detailed here owing to their presently insignificant role in the treatment of hypertension. The four most potent esters are all derived from germine, 42.**1**, and differ by the acyl groups at C-3 and C-15; three of them have an acetyl at C-7. Synthetic esters of germine have not resulted in an increase of potency or a relative decrease in emesis. Because of the desirable mechanism on the vasomotor center, several research groups are pursuing the synthesis of *Veratrum* fragments in hopes of retaining the hypotensive capacity but eliminating the emesis that is probably the result of stimulating the vomiting center in the medulla.

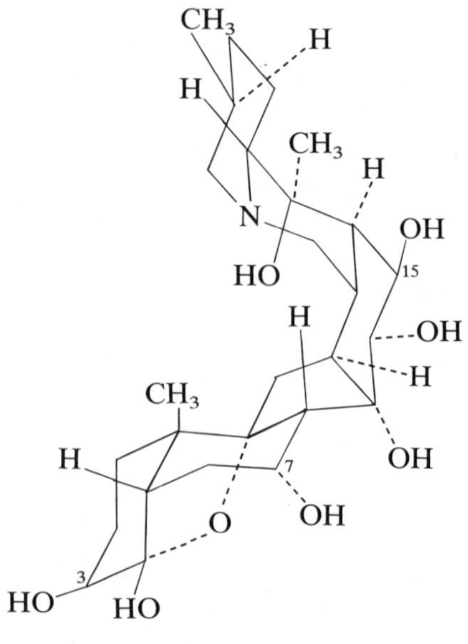

42.**1**

2.1.2   ACTION IN THE CENTRAL NERVOUS SYSTEM.   Drugs acting directly on the central nervous system have long been used for lowering high blood pressure, especially sedatives and tranquilizers. Barbiturates depress cortical function, thus reducing its influence on sympathetic centers located in the subcortex. Phenothiazines, meprobamate, and its homolog mebutamate act directly at subcortical levels. Although the sedative or tranquilizing action of these agents may contribute some benefit, psychic depression and autonomic effects severely limit their usefulness. The results of several clinical studies with these agents on hypertensives have been neither consistent nor convincing (35, 36).

A significant component of reserpine's hypotensive action is on the central control over sympathetic function, and α-methyldopa is recognized to exert its primary effect via a metabolite, α-methylnorepinephrine, on central adrenergic receptors. Nevertheless, the strongest interest in developing new agents that act on the central nervous system followed the more recent discovery and use of clonidine. This compound directly stimulates α-adrenergic receptors in the midbrain and hypothalamus especially, which decreases the sympathetic outflow and causes vasomotor relaxation. Aside from the sedation and drowsiness generally found with agents acting directly on the central nervous system, they do not provoke postural hypotension or poor tolerance to exercise.

The most severe liability, however, may be a variable incidence of withdrawal hypertension found with clonidine, which is further aggravated by β-adrenergic blockers. The increasing use of combination therapy and the early use of propranolol or other β-blockers in many regimens will continue to highlight this problem for compliance. Also, many of the centrally acting antihypertensive agents have peripheral actions as well. Peripheral α-adrenergic stimulation produces an increase in blood pressure that may antagonize the central action or cause a biphasic response. The antihypertensive effect of any drug is the sum of all its actions, so further work in this area requires a quest for better drug distribution to the brain or a more centrally selective α-stimulation.

2.1.2.1   *Clonidine.*   This anilinoimidazoline, 42.**2**, was developed in Germany from a large number of guanidine analogs and has been chemically available for almost a decade. It is an extremely potent antihypertensive agent with a sustained effect. Its central sympathetic depression correlates with its α-adrenergic stimulant potency and its partition coefficient, an indication of its ability to cross the blood–brain barrier (37). From a large series of analogs it has been shown that at least one *o*-Cl, Br, or CH$_3$ group is essential but two *ortho* groups are clearly preferred (38). The antihypertensive activity in anesthetized rabbits does not have a simple correlation with electronic, steric, or lipophilic properties of the phenyl substituents. This is well illustrated by the 2,6-diethyl analog, 42.**3**, which is 2.6 times more potent as a peripheral α-stimulant but has $P = 0.06$ compared with $P = 3.0$ for clonidine (39). This diethyl and most other 2,6-disubstituted analogs of clonidine are comparably hypotensive when administered intracisternally but not intravenously to anesthetized rabbits. Although many of these analogs are comparable in α-adrenergic activity, only those that are readily accessible to α-receptors in the

42.**2**   Clonidine, X=Cl, Y = 6 − Cl
42.**3**   ST-91, X = Et, Y = 6 − Et
42.**4**   Flutonidine, X = CH$_3$, Y = 5 − F
42.**5**   Tolonidine, X = CH$_3$, Y = 4 − Cl

medullary vasomotor center are potent hypotensives. Therefore, lipid solubility, as indicated by the partition coefficient, is a most critical parameter for hypotensive activity as well as minimal peripheral effects (37, 39). The 2,6-dichlorophenyl substituent is optimal for this purpose.

Clonidine acts primarily on α-adrenergic receptor sites in the medullary vasomotor center of the brainstem, especially the nucleus solitarius where the input from the carotid sinus and aortic arch baroreceptors synapse. This brain center integrates and regulates the cardiovascular system via modulation of sympathetic outflow. Clonidine acts on this center in the same way as does norepinephrine (40), and clonidine's effects are completely abolished by central α-adrenergic blockade. Other central sites of action and an action on afferent input have also been suggested for clonidine (41). Peripherally, clonidine stimulates presynaptic α-receptors mediating the inhibition of norepinephrine release as well as peripheral postsynaptic α-receptors, but this mechanism probably contributes little to its effects on blood pressure (42). In considering the balance of pressor effects from peripheral α-stimulation, especially when administered intravenously, and depressor effects from central α-stimulation, it is important to recognize that only blood pressure lowering is observed in humans by oral administration. This means the centrally mediated effects are clearly dominant and reflect the facile distribution of clonidine to the brain following oral administration.

Unfortunately, the sedation and inhibition of salivation observed with clonidine administration also depend on central α-adrenergic stimulation (39). In addition to these two side effects, severe withdrawal hypertension owing to excessive sympathetic outflow and excessive available norepinephrine has been a serious complication to clonidine therapy (43). Postural hypotension is not a problem, and renal blood flow and glomerular filtration are not seriously affected during chronic clonidine administration. The occasional fluid and sodium retention sometimes observed during clonidine administration are easily correctable by diuretics. Some interference with clonidine's antihypertensive effects has been noted with propranolol and tricyclic antidepressants (44).

2.1.2.2 Drugs Related to Clonidine.

A plethora of agents with some structural resemblance to clonidine have been reported during the past decade (45). Many of these have retained the lipophilic and steric properties of the anilino portion and the pK_a of the guanidine system but have different spacer groups to achieve a comparable distance from the cationic center to the center of the aromatic ring (5.0–5.1 Å) and from the cationic center to the plane of the aromatic ring (1.28–1.36 Å) and to be patentably distinct. A major objective in developing an alternative drug to clonidine is to retain the central α-adrenergic mechanism while eliminating the sedation and decreasing salivation. Sedation and salivary secretion inhibition are relatively weaker for flutonidine, 42.**4**, than for clonidine (46). However, flutonidine is a less potent antihypertensive agent clinically. It is antihypertensive in humans with a longer duration of action (8–12 hr) and with milder side effects than clonidine (47). For flutonidine or tolonidine, 42.**5**, a clinical dose 4–10 times relative to clonidine is required for useful antihypertensive effects. It remains to be shown that a clinically meaningful advantage in reduced sedation or salivary inhibition can be demonstrated for either of these clonidine analogs.

Another interesting aspect of the structure–activity relationship is the critical size of the imidazoline ring. Extension of the ring to six members (three CH_2 groups) causes a 300-fold decrease in hypotensive activity. Other ring annelations or substituents in the imidazoline ring reduce activity considerably. No substituted heterocycle has replaced the dichloroanilino moiety and imparted comparable antihypertensive potency (45). It should be recalled that other aralkyl imidazolines, such as naphazoline (42.**6**) and tetrahydrozoline (42.**7**), are useful nasal decongestants because of their direct α-adrenergic actions. In fact, they are more potent α-agonists than norepinephrine or α-methylnorepinephrine and cause blood pressure and heart rate to fall after an initial increase in anesthetized dogs, but they are not appreciably distributed to the CNS. In fact, clonidine was first synthesized as a nasal decongestant.

One of the first agents of this type to exhibit strong hypotensive and central α-sympathomimetic properties was xylazine, 42.**8**. The influence of central α-adrenergic receptors on blood pressure regulation and their possible causal relationship has been established with xylazine (48). Xylazine lowered the blood pressure significantly when perfused through the cat cerebral ventricles but produced only a modest reduction when infused intravenously. Further, this agent induced a long-lasting pressure increase in spinal cats after a single i.v. injection, and this increase was blocked by α-blocking agents. By intraventricular infusion, the centrally mediated hypotensive effects of xylazine, norepinephrine, α-methylnorepinephrine,

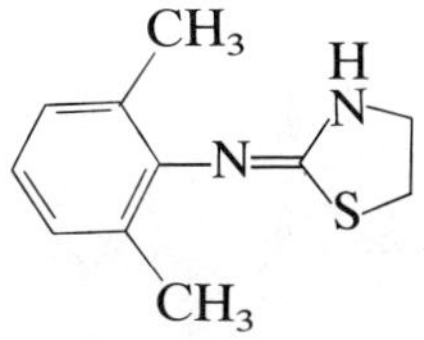

42.**8**

and tyramine are inhibited by phentolamine. Local vasoconstriction was ruled out as a cause for the depressor effect because angiotensin II perfusion induced a dose-dependent increase in pressure. Perfusion with isoproterenol or propranolol had no effect on blood pressure suggesting minimal β-adrenergic control in the hypotensive response to central adrenergic stimulation. Stimulation of dopaminergic receptors within the CNS lowers the blood pressure—this effect is blocked by haloperidol or pimozide but not by phentolamine, whereas the hypotensive effect of norepinephrine is blocked by phentolamine and not by pimozide. This offers preliminary support that central α-adrenergic and dopaminergic receptors may mediate hypotensive responses to clonidine and analogs. This gives further basis to the belief that the centrally mediated hypotensive action and unwanted central effects can be separated.

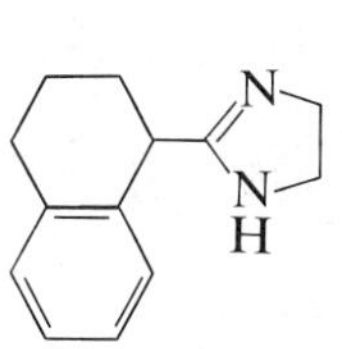

Xylazine has strong analgesic, hypnotic, central muscle relaxant, antisecretory, and antihypertensive effects (49). It also inhibits postganglionic adrenergic and cholinergic nerve stimulation. For significant hypotensive potency, compounds of this structural type should have substituents in the ortho positions and a pK_a close to that of clonidine (~8.0) (50). In hypertensive patients, xylazine lowers systolic and diastolic pressure for more than 5 hr after single 10–20 mg oral doses. However, it causes drowsiness and tiredness, and was not pursued as an antihypertensive agent but was found useful as a veterinary analgesic.

A common variant of the clonidine structure is a replacement of the benzenoid

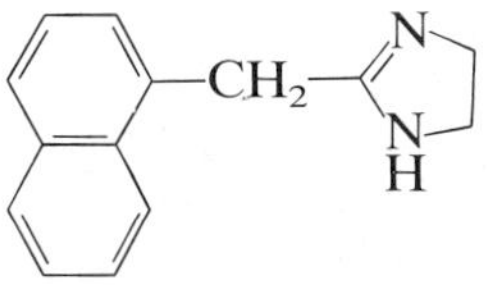

42.**6** Naphazoline

42.**7** Tetrahydrozoline

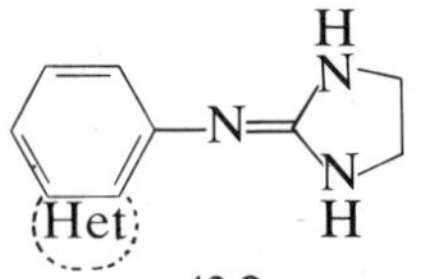

42.**9**

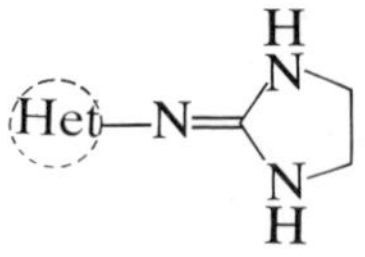

42.**10**

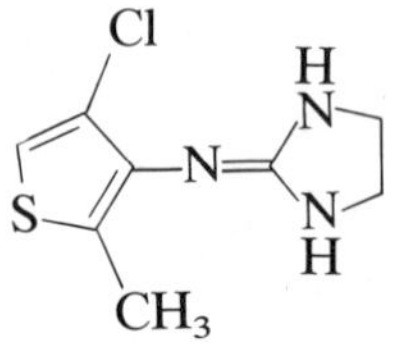

42.**11**

ring by heterocyclic systems. Various quinolines, quinoxalines, benzothiophenes, and indazoles of type 42.**9** as well as thiophenes, isoxazoles, and pyrroles of type 42.**10** have been patented as potent antihypertensives in animals, but tiamenidine, 42.**11**, is the most studied of this class (51). Tiamenidine also inhibits sympathetic nerve activity via central α-adrenergic receptor stimulation. It is one-third as potent as clonidine in renal hypertensive rats and produces relatively less sedation (42). In human studies its side effects are quite similar to clonidine at equal hypotensive doses (53).

Potent, centrally mediated antihypertensive activity has been shown for several clonidine analogs in which the guanidine moiety is varied. One such compound is guanabenz, 42.**12**, a potent antihypertensive agent in animals (54) and man (55). In animals, guanabenz blocks sympathetic impulses centrally. It also appears to have a peripheral neuronal blocking action. Its hypotensive effect, however, appears to be largely due to its central action (56). In hypertensive patients, guanabenz causes significant reductions in blood pressure at 16–32 mg/day orally. It induces drowsiness in some patients as does clonidine, but does not cause the postural hypotension, diarrhea, or suppression of ejaculation which is seen with most peripherally acting

sympathetic inhibitors. This indicates that the hypotensive activity at these doses is largely the result of central α-adrenergic stimulation. Guanabenz does not cause sodium and fluid retention during chronic administration, in contrast to most other antihypertensive agents acting via similar mechanisms.

Insertion of the —CH$_2$CO— grouping between the ring and guanidine fragments produced a potent antihypertensive compound, guanfacine, 42.**13**, which has central and peripheral α-adrenergic stimulant activity. It causes a centrally mediated drop in blood pressure but very little sedation in animals (57). At oral doses of 1–5 mg/kg, a dose-related marked hypotension and bradycardia are seen in rats and dogs. The site of central action may be somewhat different from that for clonidine since guanfasine does not stimulate central dopaminergic receptors nor does it induce a depressor effect when infused directly into the ventricles of the cat medulla in contrast to clonidine. Clinical studies with this drug demonstrated good blood pressure reductions without drowsiness in more than 70% of patients treated with a few mg/day orally (58). Other studies showed hypotensive effectiveness equal to that of clonidine at a 10-fold higher dose. However, tiredness and dry mouth occurred as frequently and as

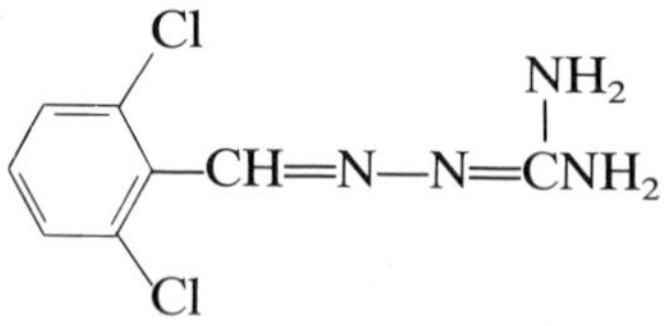

42.**12**

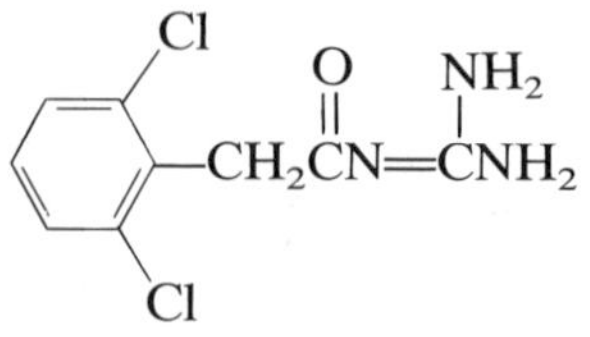

42.**13**

intensely as with clonidine (59, 60). Detailed structure–activity studies on guanfacine analogs illustrate the 2,6-dichlorophenyl requirement, no substitution of the amide nitrogen suggesting the conjugated acylimino form as an active species, only small alkyl groups are tolerated on terminal nitrogens, and no substitution on the methylene group in order to retain potent hypotensive activity (61).

A thiazoloimidazoline, 42.**14**, represents a modification of clonidine in which an unsubstituted nitrogen is not required for hypotensive activity. However, the activity is quite sensitive to structural changes. This agent produces a clonidine-like central α-adrenergic stimulation and hypotensive effect (62) but is slightly less potent than clonidine on oral administration to hypertensive rats.

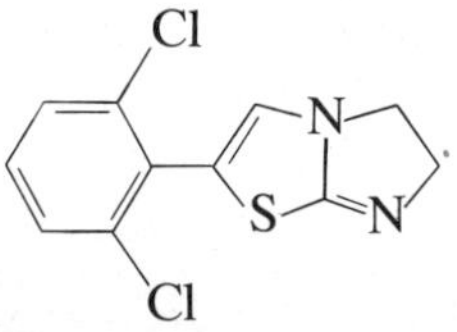

42.**14**

2.1.2.3 R-28,935.

A new type of centrally acting antihypertensive agent has been discovered in R-28,935, 42.**15**, chemically related to pimozide. Pimozide is a neuroleptic agent and a specific dopaminergic blocking agent; whereas R-28,935 is a much more potent hypotensive agent than pimozide or haloperidol and has much less neuroleptic or sedative activity (63). Its structure contains the benzodioxan–ethanolamine moiety found in potent β-adrenergic blockers and some α-blockers plus the 4-piperidylbenzimidazolinone moiety found in pimozide. Its hypotensive activity is found largely in the erythro isomer.

R-28,935 induces a long-lasting hypotensive effect and a slight bradycardia when administered orally or parenterally to

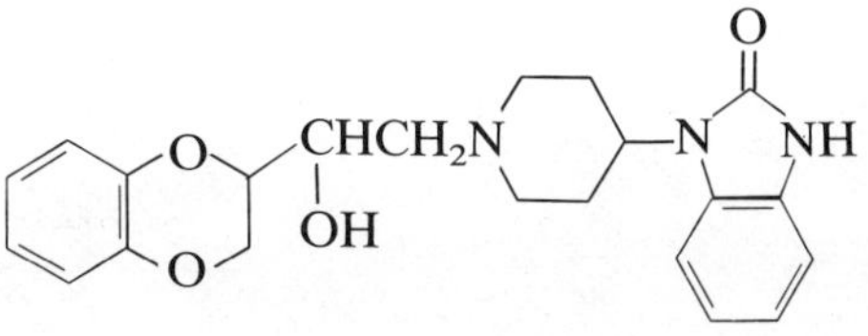

42.**15**

hypertensive animals (64). Yet administration of this agent directly into the CNS of dogs or cats causes dose-related and prolonged blood pressure reductions at much lower doses than required by i.v. administration (65, 66). This action is not blocked by centrally administered α-blockers, so its mechanism appears different from that of clonidine. Its inhibition of norepinephrine and isoproterenol effects occurs only at much higher doses than required for blood pressure lowering, so its mode of action could be on central dopaminergic receptors. This agent causes a prompt, centrally mediated reduction in peripheral vascular resistance along with the blood pressure reduction. Because this drug shows a separation of central hypotensive and central depressant effects, a major potential advantage over clonidine, it likely will be the prototype of a useful new class of centrally acting drugs. Further elucidation of its central mechanism and evidence of clinical usefulness are being pursued, although vestibular disturbances in man have been reported and may prevent its further development.

2.1.3 DRUGS AFFECTING THE NOREPINEPHRINE PATHWAY.

The sympathetic nervous system neurotransmitter, norepinephrine, 42.**20**, is intimately involved in the control of blood pressure by its actions on the heart and blood vessels. Many compounds can alter neurohumoral function by affecting the biosynthesis, storage, metabolism, and release of catecholamines at the postganglionic presynaptic nerve terminals. Several compounds that reduce the amount of norepinephrine released at the sympathetic

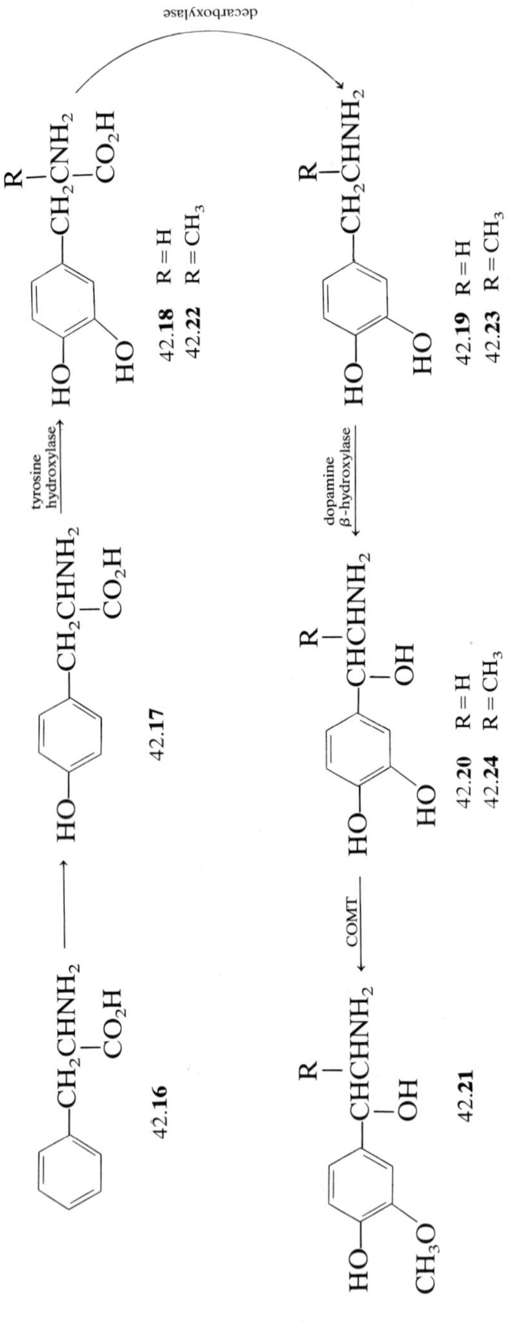

42.16

CH_2CHNH_2
CO_2H

42.17

HO—⬡—CH_2CHNH_2
CO_2H

tyrosine hydroxylase →

42.18 R = H
42.22 R = CH₃ (R = CH_3)

R
CH_2CHNH_2
CO_2H
HO—⬡
HO

decarboxylase

42.19 R = H
42.23 R = CH_3

R
CH_2CHNH_2
HO—⬡
HO

dopamine β-hydroxylase →

42.20 R = H
42.24 R = CH_3

R
$CHCHNH_2$
OH
HO—⬡
HO

COMT →

42.21

R
$CHCHNH_2$
OH
HO—⬡
CH_3O

nerve endings have been investigated and used as antihypertensive agents. The natural amino acids phenylalanine, 42.**16**, and L-tyrosine, 42.**17**, are the precursors of norepinephrine. They are converted to L-dopa, 42.**18**, within the neurones by tyrosine hydroxylase, then to dopamine, 42.**19**, by aromatic amino acid decarboxylase, and finally hydroxylated by dopamine β-hydroxylase to norepinephrine, which is retained in storage granules in the nerve endings. Nerve stimulation causes release of norepinephrine which acts on receptors of the target organ and is deactivated by reuptake into the nerve terminal, by catechol O-methyltransferase conversion to 42.**21**, or by monoamine oxidase degradation of the side chain. Norepinephrine also may undergo N-methylation to epinephrine by phenethanolamine N-methyltransferase.

Hypotensive agents that act at each of these steps of the norepinephrine pathway have been described, but the relationships between the biochemical intervention and the blood pressure lowering have usually not been established. Only those classes of drugs that include clinically active agents are discussed.

2.1.3.1 *Methyldopa*. The wide use of α-methyldopa, 42.**22**, in the therapy of hypertension is largely due to the relative absence of unpleasant side effects with its chronic use. It acts primarily centrally to reduce arterial blood pressure. It is absorbed orally and readily crosses the blood–brain barrier. In the brain it is metabolized to a-methyldopamine, 42.**23**, and α-methylnorepinephrine, 42.**24**. The latter is a potent central α-adrenoceptor stimulant and accounts for most of the antihypertensive action of α-methyldopa. When α-methylnorepinephrine is formed from α-methyldopa peripherally, it is a weaker agonist and therefore acts as a false transmitter, resulting in decreased receptor stimulation. Both central and peripheral effects of α-methyldopa are additive, to

cause the inhibition of sympathetic tone at all levels of the cardiovascular system.

Methyldopa is modestly absorbed orally; peak blood levels occur within 4 hr but maximal lowering of blood pressure appears by the second day. In man it produces a decrease in arterial pressure associated with a decrease in cardiac output. Effects on heart rate and total peripheral resistance vary initially, but peripheral resistance is consistently reduced with continued treatment. Methyldopa therapy is associated with some side effects, notably sedation and somnolence, some orthostatic hypotension, sexual dysfunction, occasional drug fever, and abnormal liver function tests (67). Methyldopa is a very useful agent for moderate to severe essential hypertension; tolerance does not develop, and its effects may be potentiated by thiazide diuretics.

The development of α-methyldopa is an interesting story. The recognition of its competitive inhibition of the enzyme dopa decarboxylase *in vitro* (68) and in humans (60) and its significant antihypertensive activity in animals and humans permitted the assumption of a causal relationship. It was thought that excessive norepinephrine may be released at sympathetic nerve endings of arteriolar smooth muscle in hypertension and that inhibition of the decarboxylase would reduce the norepinephrine available for release. Intensive research into the mode of action of α-methyldopa (70) resulted in the realization that decarboxylase inhibition might have very little influence on the norepinephrine content of sympathetic neurons. Decarboxylation is not the rate-limiting step in norepinephrine biosynthesis but is a very efficient process. Further evidence that norepinephrine synthesis is not appreciably influenced by α-methyldopa came with the observation that the urinary excretion of norepinephrine metabolites is not significantly altered following treatment of hypertensive patients with α-methyldopa. The ability of

α-methyldopa to actually serve as a substrate for the decarboxylase enzymes and be effectively converted to α-methylnorepinephrine is now generally believed to account for its hypotensive properties.

Methyldopa is the only decarboxylase inhibitor that is useful for the treatment of hypertension. Several other compounds, such as 4-bromo-3-hydroxybenzyloxyamine and α-methyldopa hydrazine, are much more potent decarboxylase inhibitors than α-methyldopa but they do not lower the blood pressure of hypertensive patients (70). Stringent structural requirements among methyldopa analogs must be met for antihypertensive activity. Even the closely related α-ethyldopa (71) and the indan 42.**25** are not very effective antihypertensives and are not good substrates for dopa decarboxylase. Ring-methylated derivatives of methyldopa also show no antihypertensive activity.

2.1.3.2. *False Neurotransmitters.* Although methyldopa and α-methylnorepinephrine are no longer thought to be antihypertensive because they are false peripheral transmitters for norepinephrine, this mechanism appears valid for some α-methyl derivatives of physiological amines and their metabolic precursor amino acids. These related phenethanolamines are formed and stored along with norepinephrine in the nerve endings, then are released by nerve impulses. These agents cause less receptor stimulation than norepinephrine and are longer acting because they are not as rapidly metabolized by monoamine oxidase.

The best studied false transmitter is metaraminol, 42.**26**, which is a potent pressor agent when administered intravenously

42.**26**

and has been used in the treatment of shock. It causes a gradual lowering of blood pressure when given orally owing to its replacement of norepinephrine in sympathetic neurones. It is formed metabolically from α-methyl-*m*-tyrosine (α-MMT) via α-methyl-*m*-tyramine. The relative antihypertensive activities of metaraminol and α-MMT are greater than methyldopa and parallel their ability to deplete norepinephrine stores. However, the rate of norepinephrine release into the circulation is unchanged following α-MMT or metaraminol (72). It remains difficult to prove that release of false neurotransmitters causes reduced sympathetic transmission because their effects are difficult to study in the presence of norepinephrine. Just as the α-methylnorepinephrine biosynthesized from L-α-methyldopa is levorotatory, only the ($-$) erythro (1R, 2S) isomer of metaraminol shows appreciable antihypertensive and norepinephrine-depleting activity (73). Nevertheless, the use of this agent is not recommended for hypertension because it sometimes causes dangerous, acute pressor responses (74). The acute pressor effects of metaraminol may be avoided by administering the *m*-chlorobenzyl ether prodrug, which is slowly dealkylated to metaraminol *in vivo*.

Another false transmitter is α-methyloctopamine, the para isomer of metaraminol. It lowered arterial blood pressure in hypertensive patients without postural hypotension or CNS side effects and with only a transient pressor response (75). Chronic administration of *p*-hydroxyamphetamine, a metabolic precursor of α-methyloctopamine, lowers standing blood pressure in hypertensive patients but has little effect in the supine position.

42.**25**

2.1.3.3. *Tyrosine Hydroxylase Inhibitors*. The amino acid precursor of α-methyl-octopamine, α-methyl-*p*-tyrosine, 42.**27**, is effective in hypertensive patients with malignant pheochromocytoma whose elevated blood pressure is directly related to increased norepinephrine synthesis and release but not in essential hypertensives. It decreases the rate of catecholamine synthesis by 50–80% (76), and its hypotensive action is undoubtedly related to its inhibition of tyrosine hydroxylase, the rate-limiting step in norepinephrine biosynthesis. Several other analogs of *p*-tyrosine are potent tyrosine hydroxylase inhibitors *in vitro*, but few are active inhibitors *in vivo*. Only the *m*-ethyl derivative, 42.**28**, is known to be antihypertensive in rats (77).

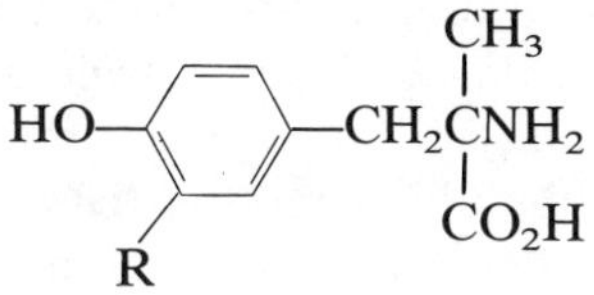

42.**27** R = H
42.**28** R = CH₃CH₂

Oudenone, 42.**29**, is a tyrosine hydroxylase inhibitor which has a potent blood pressure lowering action in hypertensive rats (78) and may be acting in the hydrated form 42.**30**. The structurally related pyratrione, 42.**31**, was active in hypertensive patients (79).

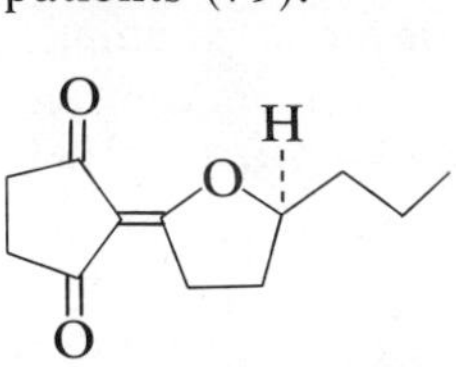

42.**29** 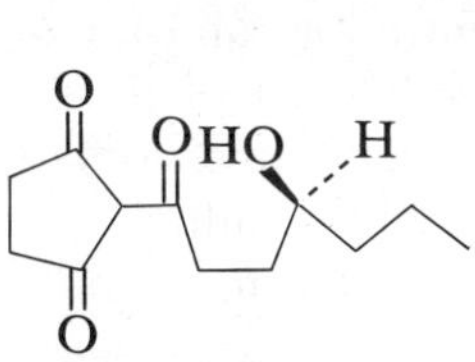   42.**30**

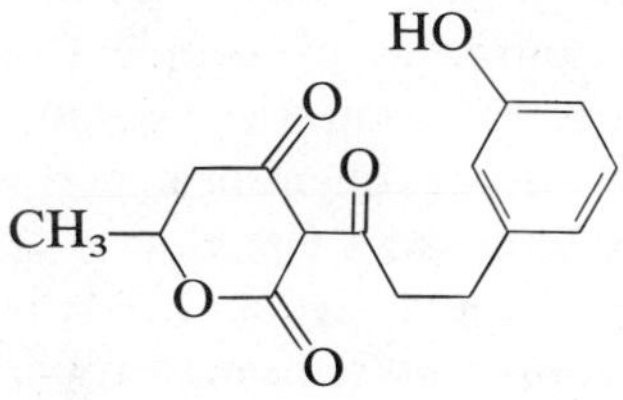

42.**31**

2.1.3.4 *Dopamine β-hydroxylase*. Various agents are known to inhibit dopamine β-hydroxylase, the enzyme that converts dopamine to norepinephrine, resulting in decreased norepinephrine synthesis. However, few such agents are effective antihypertensives. Fusaric acid, 42.**32**, was isolated from microbial cultures and inhibits dopamine β-hydroxylase. This compound lowers blood pressure and decreases tissue norepinephrine and increases dopamine levels significantly in animals (80). In humans, the calcium salt of fusaric acid decreases blood pressure without postural effects. Since the compound does not modulate sympathetic nerve function but does decrease peripheral vascular resistance, it may act by direct vasodilatation (81). Bupicomide, 42.**33**, which is metabolized to fusaric acid *in vivo* (82), causes hemodynamic changes similar to hydralazine in humans (83). Other derivatives

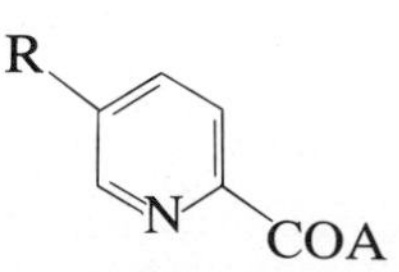

42.**32** R = CH₃(CH₂)₃–, A = OH
42.**33** R = CH₃(CH₂)₃–, A = NH₂
42.**34** R = Cl(CH₂)₄–, A = OH
42.**35** R = BrCH₂CH(CH₂)₂–, A = OH
         |
         Br
42.**36** R = (CH₃)₂NCCH₂–, A = OH
            ‖
            S

42.**37** R = HO—⟨ ⟩—CH₂–, A = OH

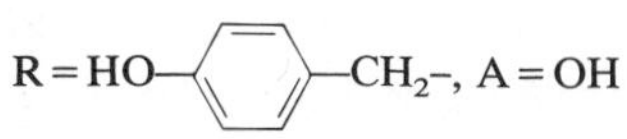

of fusaric acid, such as chlorofusaric acid, 42.**34** (84), dibromofusaric acid, 42.**35**, YP-279, 42.**36** (85), and phenopicolinic acid, 42.**37** (86), differ only in the 5 substituent and are claimed to be more potent agents. The importance of dopamine β-hydroxylase inhibition for the antihypertensive action of these agents and their place in the treatment of hypertension remain to be established.

2.1.3.5 *Monoamine Oxidase Inhibitors.* Monoamine oxidases are enzymes that deaminate amines to aldehydes and rapidly metabolize norepinephrine intracellularly. Inhibition of these oxidases prolongs the level and action of intracellular norepinephrine which would be expected to increase blood pressure. Paradoxically, several of these agents are antihypertensives. MAO inhibitors, such as tranylcypromine, phenelzine, iproniazid, and nialamide are clinically useful antidepressants with postural hypotension as a major side effect, but only pargyline, 42.**38**, has been useful in essential hypertension (87).

$$\text{CH}_2\text{NCH}_2\text{C}{\equiv}\text{CH}$$
$$|$$
$$\text{CH}_3$$

42.**38**

The antihypertensive action of pargyline is due to diminished sympathetic nerve activity. This may be caused by a negative feedback on norepinephrine synthesis or by accumulation of false transmitter amines peripherally. Central inhibition of MAO increases central α-adrenoceptor stimulation, which decreases sympathetic outflow similar to the action of clonidine and methyldopa. The therapeutic effect of pargyline develops slowly and persists for about 1 week after the drug is discontinued. It has been used for moderate to severe hypertension, but side effects and interference by other drugs and foods has limited its clinical usefulness for hypertension.

2.1.4 PERIPHERAL ACTING AGENTS. There is no convincing evidence that sustained elevation of sympathetic tone is involved in maintaining the elevated arterial pressure in hypertension. Yet agents that interfere with peripheral sympathetic function include several of the important classes of antihypertensive agents—centrally acting agents, ganglionic blockers, neuronal blockers, and adrenergic receptor blockers that interfere with sympathetic tone (See Fig. 42.2). Most sympathetic inhibitors show similar pharmacological actions, beneficial effects, and side effects. They all cause some postural hypotension, sexual dysfunction, and gastrointestinal effects, and generally have a long duration of action.

2.1.4.1 *Ganglionic Blockers.* The use of quaternary salts and hindered tertiary amines that block nerve impulses to the peripheral nervous system by inhibition of acetylcholine transmission at ganglionic synapses are no longer important in the treatment of hypertension. Tetraethylammonium chloride and hexamethonium chloride were among the first agents used for severe hypertension. The more potent and longer-lasting quaternaries, chlorisondamine chloride and trimethidinium methosulfate, are not well absorbed orally, whereas the hindered tertiary amines, mecamylamine and pempidine, are well absorbed but have a short duration of action and several nuisance side effects.

Ganglionic blockers generally lack specificity for the sympathetic ganglia; the interruption of parasympathetic pathways causes side effects such as constipation, dryness of mouth and skin, blurred vision, and impotence. This class of agents also produces excessive postural hypotension and a decrease in renal flow and glomerular filtration, and tolerance develops gradually with most of them. Their antihypertensive effect is due primarily to decreased cardiac output resulting from decreased venous return due to venous pooling.

2.1.4.2 *Reserpine.* Materials from the *Rauwolfia* genus of plants were used for medicinal purposes by people from India and Asia several centuries ago but first reported for the treatment of hypertension in 1918. Three decades ago clinical confirmation of the hypotensive and sedative properties of *Rauwolfia serpentina* roots prompted the isolation, characterization, and

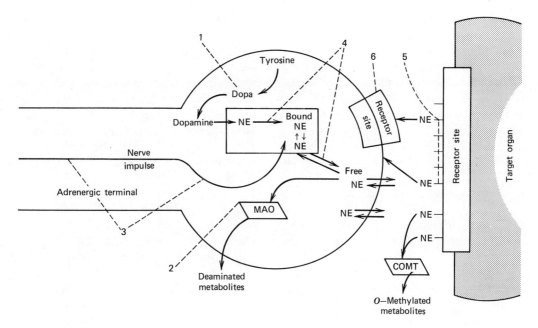

Fig. 42.2 Sites of action of drugs at the adrenergic nerve terminal. Drugs influence sympathetic transmission by (1) decreasing synthesis of norepinephrine by acting as a preferential substrate (methyldopa); (2) decreasing metabolism of free norepinephrine through inhibition of monoamine oxidase (pargyline); (3) inhibition of the release of norepinephrine in the postganglionic adrenergic terminal (bretylium) or of nerve impulse transmission at sympathetic ganglia (ganglionic blocking agents); (4) inhibition of the transmitter storage mechanism and/or reentry of transmitter into storage sites (guanethidine, reserpine); (5) antagonism of released transmitter at postsynaptic receptor sites (α- and β-blocking agents); (6) action at presynaptic α- or β-receptors (clonidine and β-blockers).

biological evaluation of more than 60 alkaloids (88). In 1952, Swiss chemists succeeded in isolating reserpine which is now recognized as the major active constituent of *Rauwolfia*. The alkaloids isolated from various *Rauwolfia* species have been reviewed (89). Reserpine, 42.**39**, is the most ubiquitous of this alkaloid family and is the only one widely used today as an antihypertensive agent.

Following intensive studies by several groups, the structural elucidation of reserpine was completed in 1955; within a year, Woodward and co-workers achieved its

42.**39**

total synthesis (90). The E ring was constructed with substituents having the desired stereochemistry, then reacted with 6-methoxytryptamine, and subsequently cyclized. The 3β-configuration had to be established by isomerization, and the ester functions at positions 16 and 18 were established at the final step; so Woodward's sequence allowed ready access to several reserpine isomers as well as related derivatives. Although reserpine is one of 64 possible stereoisomers, the other stereoisomers made by isomerizations all have the cis-fused D/E ring system. None of the other isomers showed significant pharmacological activity so the β configuration at positions 3, 16, and 18 plus 17α configuration is essential for the hypotensive and sedative activity.

The pharmacology of reserpine has been reviewed (89, 36, 91). It produces autonomic suppression as evidenced by a decrease in blood pressure, bradycardia, and miosis in addition to a depressant effect on the central nervous system which is characterized by calmness, sedation, and depression. The sedative and hypotensive effects of reserpine probably do not result from a single pharmacological mechanism or site. Some reserpine analogs possess only one of reserpine's effects. The action of reserpine appears to be primarily due to depletion of norepinephrine and serotonin stores in peripheral and central sympathetic neurones. Whether the sedative action of reserpine results predominantly from decreased brain levels of norepinephrine or serotonin has not been completely resolved. Sympathetic blockade caused by peripheral depletion of norepinephrine and central inhibition resulting in the lowering or peripheral resistance with very little change in cardiac output contribute to the hypotensive action of reserpine. The lack of orthostatic hypotension indicates a central site in its blood pressure effects since peripheral sympathetic blockers in general produce orthostatic hypotension.

The principal biochemical effect of reserpine is its inhibition of the active transport of neurohumoral amines into tissue storage sites. The ATP–Mg^{2+}-dependent transport of these amines, norepinephrine, epinephrine, dopamine, and serotonin, into specialized intracellular granules is specifically attenuated. The unbound amines are then rapidly inactivated by intraneuronal monoamine oxidase (92) which results in their rapid depletion from nerve endings. Exogenous norepinephrine is likewise denied transport to the storage granules and is oxidized. Not allowing the depleted stores to be refilled with norepinephrine results in a postganglionic sympathetic inhibition.

Species variations in the response to reserpine prevents clear agreement on the predicted functional changes. A decrease of norepinephrine concentrations in tissues, a decrease in peripheral vascular resistance, and a fall in blood pressure are invariably observed following the administration of reserpine in man. Reserpine produces prolonged dilation of peripheral blood vessels in man and does not interfere with sympathetic reflex responses. The onset of blood pressure reduction is characteristically delayed following i.v. or oral administration to animals or man with 2–6 weeks required to attain maximum effectiveness. Renal and cerebral blood flows in man are unaltered following reserpine.

The endocrine glands are influenced by reserpine in a variety of ways (89). Its action on pituitary function is largely independent of neural involvement; reserpine lowers pituitary prolactin content and thereby induces lactation. Owing to the increased lactation following administration of reserpine, just as with bromocriptine, an association between reserpine and breast cancer has been made, although this relationship has not been supported in recent studies (93).

Deserpidine lacks the 11-OCH_3 group of reserpine but produces the same degree of hypotensive activity, central depression, and norepinephrine depletion; so the aromatic OCH_3 function is not essential for biological activity. On the other hand, naturally occurring alkaloids differing from reserpine or deserpidine in their C-17 or C-18 functionalities exhibit reduced antihypertensive activity or are inactive. A 17α-OH group renders the molecule inactive, but the 17α-CH_3 derivatives are hypotensive. Free acids in the 16 position are inactive, an ester moiety in the 18 position appears essential, and unsaturation in the C, D, or E rings eliminates activity. Various ester groups at position 18 have been evaluated—none are more potent antihypertensive agents than reserpine, but syrosingopine and methoxyphenoserpine produce less sedation and less norepinephrine depletion at equal antihypertensive doses. Modifications in the indole moiety, retaining the C, D, and E rings like reserpine, have permitted compounds with considerable antihypertensive activity and minimal sedation. The 10-OCH_3, 12-OCH_3, and 12-SCH_3 analogs show a good separation of activities; but mediodespidine, a methylenedioxydespyrrolodeserpidine, 42.**40**, is equipotent with reserpine as a hypotensive agent and produces no sedation (94, 95). Mediodespidine also causes minimal depletion of brain norepinephrine and serotonin and represents the most peripherally selective antihypertensive agent among reserpine analogs. No significant new agents of this structural class have been developed since the preceding edition (34, 96).

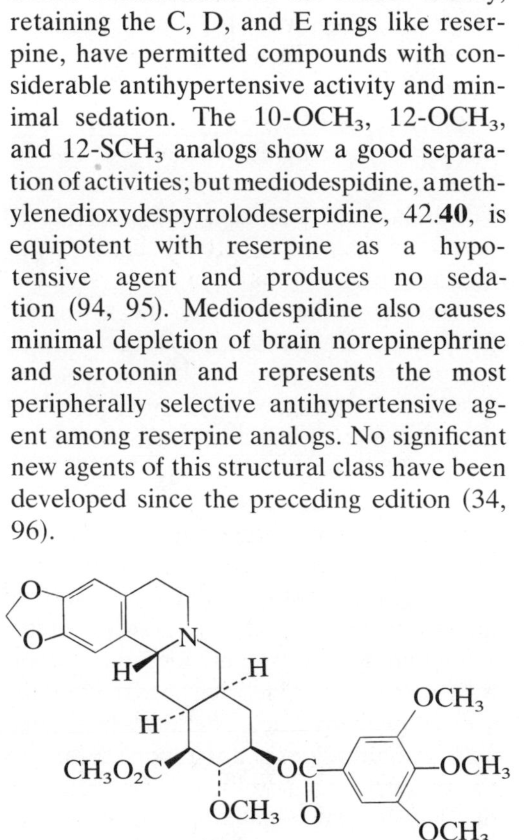

42.**40**

2.1.4.3 *Adrenergic Neurone Blockers.* In addition to the classes of drugs described above which act via a neural mechanism, a large group of guanidines and benzylammonium compounds block sympathetic nerve transmission by their action at nerve

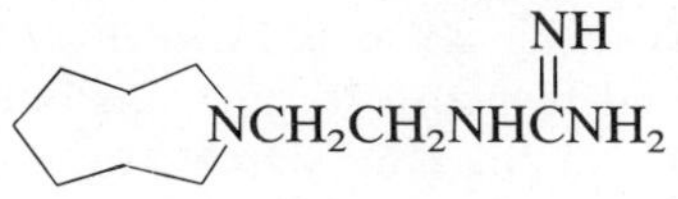

42.**41**

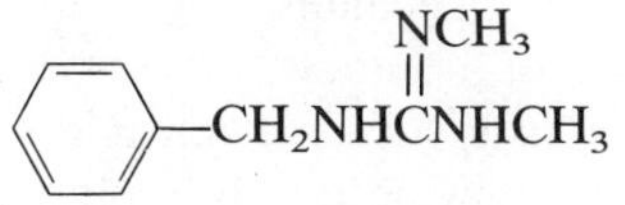

42.**42**

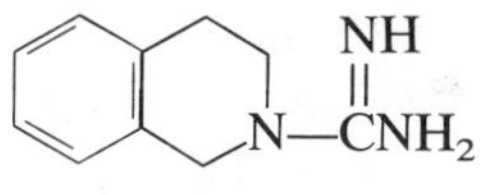

42.**43**

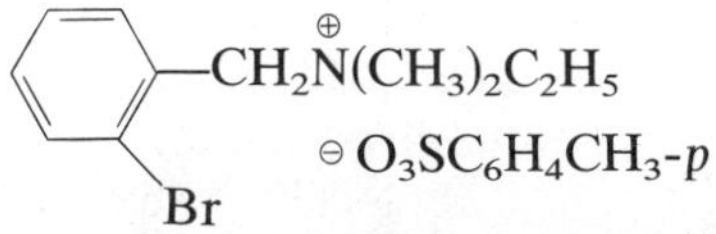

42.**44**

endings. The most important drugs in this class are guanethidine, 42.**41**, bethanidine, 42.**42**, debrisoquin, 42.**43**, and bretylium, 42.**44**. These drugs suppress responses to sympathetic postganglionic nervous stimulation without antagonizing responses to circulating catecholamines. They all lower standing blood pressure and cause varying degrees of postural hypotension and sexual dysfunction. They do not cross the blood–brain barrier and do not produce central depressant effects. Of these four drugs, only guanethidine causes significant depletion of norepinephrine stores which may account for its long duration of action and such side effects as diarrhea.

Bretylium was the most potent, longest acting, and least toxic agent of an extensive series of benzylammonium salts (97). The *o*-halogen substituent is essential to avoid muscarinic effects. The pharmacology of bretylium has been reviewed (98). Its initial effects are sympathomimetic, probably due to an induced release of norepinephrine, which are followed by a prolonged blockade. The blockade is characterized by a decreased response to postganglionic sympathetic stimulation similar to that produced by sympathectomy. Bretylium specifically affects catecholamine storage and release mechanisms, resulting in an inhibition of norepinephrine release from nerve endings. Initial clinical results were favorable, showing that bretylium produces selective antiadrenergic and antihypertensive effects in man. Its usefulness is hampered by poor oral absorption and by a rapid development of tolerance. Bretylium has been replaced largely by guanidines when a powerful antihypertensive agent is required.

The introduction of guanethidine sulfate in 1960 permitted the effective management of essential hypertension with an adrenergic neuronal blocking agent (99). Like bretylium, guanethidine prevents the release of norepinephrine from nerve terminals but it also depletes tissue stores of norepinephrine. Although at least four related compounds are being tested currently in man (100), guanethidine remains the only neuronal blocker approved in the United States for the treatment of moderate and severe hypertension. The initial pressor effect is associated with an increase in cardiac rate and output and is probably related to the released norepinephrine. The subsequent hypotensive phase is primarily the result of a reduction in heart rate and cardiac output and is probably related to reduced sympathetic tone. With the fall in blood pressure, cerebral blood flow is moderately decreased, renal flow is decreased parallel to cardiac output, and hepatic flow decreases markedly (97, 98). Orthostatic hypotension usually occurs, probably as a

result of decreased venous return and reduced vascular reflexes. In addition to these postural effects which may result in dizziness and weakness, bronchial asthma may be exacerbated and inhibition of ejaculation due to the sympathetic blockade is observed. Guanethidine also causes bradycardia and diarrhea. These clinical problems associated with the use of guanethidine have restricted its use to the more severe cases of hypertension.

Many medicinal chemists participated in the exhaustive synthesis of guanidines in search of a separation of neuronal blockade from norepinephrine depletion and a separation of the antihypertensive property from the clinical side effects of guanethidine. In addition to a variety of aminoethylguanidines (101, 97), benzylguanidines such as bethanidine, 42.**42** (102), debrisoquin, 42.**43** (103), and MJ 10459, 42.**45** (104, 105) plus phenoxyethylguanidines such as guanoxan, 42.**46** (106), guanoclor, 42.**47** (107, 108), and guanadrel, 42.**48** (109) are clinically effective antihypertensives. Bethanidine and debrisoquin do not cause rapid depletion of catecholamines but are potent neuronal blockers, whereas MJ 10459 causes some neuronal blockade but significant reduction in norepinephrine levels of the heart and peripheral vasculature. Yet all these agents cause a rapid and prolonged reduction in sympathetic function; clinically, none of these agents is greatly distinguished from guanethidine. At comparably effective antihypertensive doses, all sympathetic blockers cause some bradycardia, orthostatic hypotension, impaired ejaculation, and reduced renal blood flow. In spite of quantitative clinical differences from guanethidine, no sympathetic inhibitor yet is free from the side effects that limit the use of guanethidine. The diarrhea found with guanethidine is not reported for debrisoquin or guanadrel which may relate to the lack of intestinal norepinephrine depletion reported for these two agents. In

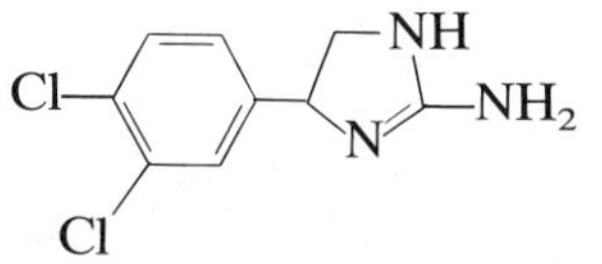

42.**45**

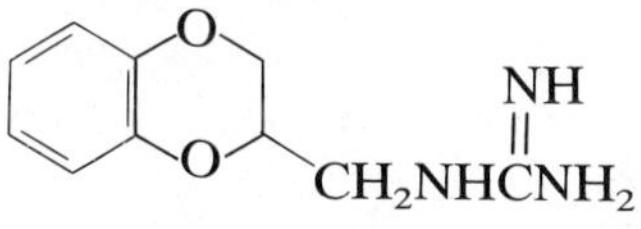

42.**46**

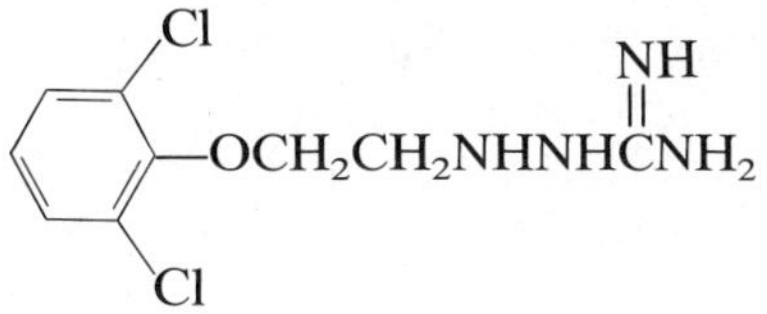

42.**47**

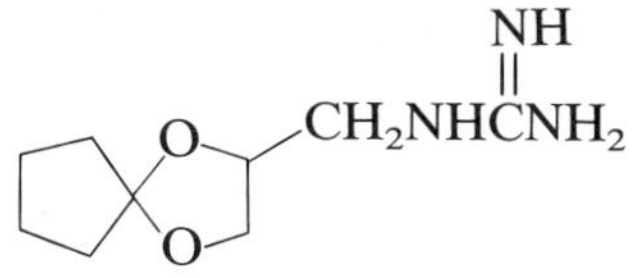

42.**48**

spite of these nuisance effects for patients, sympathetic inhibitors are predictably rapid and effective antihypertensives for mild to severe cases.

Sympathetic blockade can therefore be achieved with a variety of structural types. Neuronal receptor binding, in general, appears enhanced by a lipophilic and π-electron rich benzene ring, an ammonium moiety which may be a quaternary or highly ionized and delocalized guanidinium ($pK_a \sim 12$–14), and an appropriate conformation of the ammonium and π-electron sites. For neuronal blockers, α-receptor blockers, and β-receptor blockers, two main structural classes exist in which the cationic site and benzenoid ring are separated by linking units differing by OCH_2 (34). An explanation of comparable conformations has been given (110). Differences in biological effects from optical isomers of the asymmetric neuronal blockers—MJ 10459, guanoxan, and guanadrel—further support the conformational requirements.

2.2 Vascular Mechanisms

Relaxation of peripheral arterioles permits a very desirable reduction in peripheral resistance (See Fig. 42.1) and lowering of blood pressure. The moderation of vascular constriction or actual relaxation can be achieved by postsynaptic blockade of sympathetic nerve transmission or direct vasodilation.

2.2.1 RECEPTOR BLOCKERS. Agents that block the transmission of sympathetic impulses at the postsynaptic receptor sites of effector organs (see Fig. 42.2) are frequently called adrenolytics. They inhibit responses to the sympathomimetic amines and were originally intended to modulate the vascular contractile mechanisms. Ahlquist (111, 112) has differentiated the adrenergic responses into α and β; α responses are generally excitatory except for intestinal relaxation, and β responses are inhibitory except for myocardial stimulation. Several comprehensive reviews are available on agents affecting these receptors (113). Since the subject is covered in more detail in Chapter 41, this section is confined primarily to their antihypertensive usefulness.

2.2.1.1 *α-Blockers.* α-Adrenergic receptor blocking agents were among the first drugs tried for the treatment of hypertension. Since these drugs block the vasoconstrictor effects of norepinephrine and epinephrine at receptors on vascular smooth muscle, they were logical choices for use in hypertension. However, the use of these agents in patients was disappointing owing to poor efficacy and severe side effects such as postural hypotension, sexual dysfunction, tachycardia, and CNS effects. A blockade of only α-receptors permits compensatory increases in cardiac output causing incomplete lowering of blood pressure. Phentolamine, 43.**49**, is used clinically to diagnose patients with primary hypertension due to pheochromocytoma, an adrenal

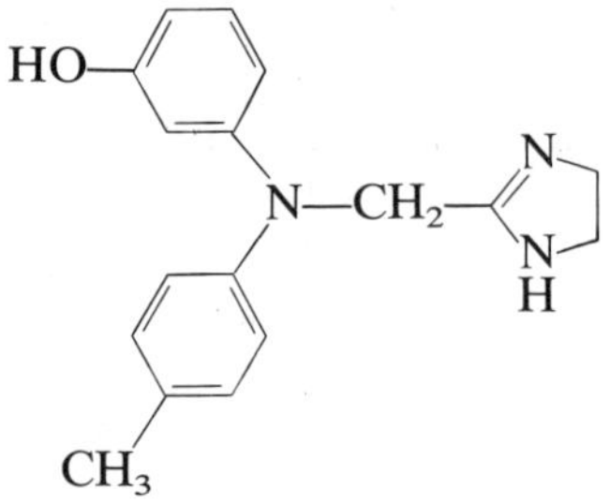

42.**49**

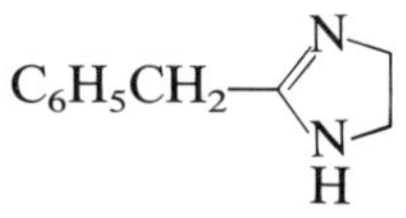

42.**50**

$$C_6H_5OCH_2\overset{|}{C}HCH_3$$
$$C_6H_5CH_2NCH_2CH_2Cl$$

42.**51**

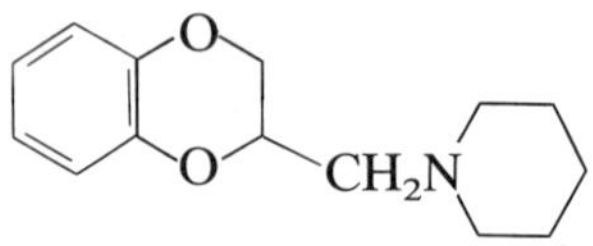

42.**52**

tumor which produces excessive amounts of norepinephrine. Other agents, such as tolazoline, 42.**50**, and the irreversible α-receptor blocker phenoxybenzamine, 42.**51**, are used in the treatment of peripheral vascular diseases characterized by high α-adrenergic tone in cutaneous blood vessels, such as frostbite, Raynaud's disease, thrombophlebitis, and spastic peripheral vascular disorders.

Although many imidazolinylmethyl compounds were patterned after tolazoline and phentolamine, they all provoke a variety of autonomic side effects and frequently show additional histaminergic and cholinergic effects. Benzodioxanes such as piperoxan, 42.**52**, and 1-alkyl-4-arylpiperazines have also served as useful prototypes for many reversible α-blockers (114). Considerable work has been required to separate the

hypotensive property from psychosedative and antianxiety effects.

β-Haloethylamines have been studied extensively as potent and irreversible α-blockers. Dibenamine, 42.**53**, first recognized as an adrenolytic by Nickerson and Goodman (115), served as a prototype for others such as phenoxybenzamine, 42.**51**, which differs by an OCH_2 unit, and the orally effective cyclic analog, 42.**54** (116). Optimum activity is found with β-haloalkyl tertiary amines having at least one benzyl or phenoxyethyl group. The halogen may be Cl, Br, I, or a sulfonate ester; these agents have been shown to cyclize to the aziridinium species in physiologic solutions. In fact, the degree of adrenergic blockade is proportional to the aziridinium ion concentration, but steric requirements also exist in many structural series. The initial phase of adrenergic blockade is competitive, but this is followed by a prolonged irreversible blockade due to alkylation of sulfhydryl and amino groups by the aziridinium ion or open chain carbonium ion. Such α-receptor alkylations have been used to label the receptors selectively and estimate 10^{12} receptors per milligram of tissue, dry weight (117). These irreversible α-blockers block the excitatory effects of adrenergic stimulation but not inhibitory responses such as intestinal relaxation and bronchodilation.

Several types of α-blockers have been introduced recently for the treatment of hypertension, the most prominent being prazosin, 42.**55**. This drug, which is approved for the treatment of hypertension in

$$(C_6H_5CH_2)_2NCH_2CH_2Cl$$
42.**53**

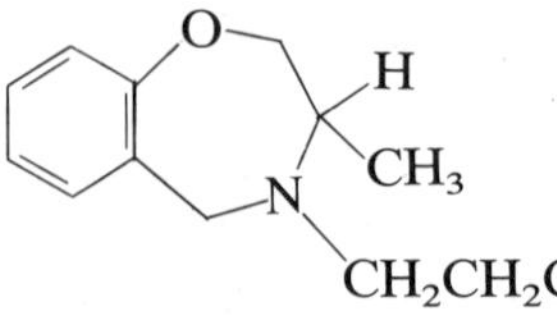

42.**54**

many countries including the United States, lowers blood pressure by decreasing peripheral resistance through α-blockade and direct vascular smooth muscle relaxation in animals and man. (118). Although prazosin was designed as a direct vasodilator based on cyclic nucleotide mechanisms, its predominant action appears to be α-blockade, although an inhibition of adrenergic transmission distal to the α-receptor has also been proposed. Theoretically, this would allow the blockade to be overcome under stressful conditions and normal physiological reflexes could operate. Prazosin does differ significantly from classical α-blockers and direct vasodilators since its blood pressure lowering is not associated with tachycardia or increased renin release (119). Prazosin is effective in a high percentage of hypertensive patients and lowers blood pressure more in the erect than supine position. Side effects, such as dizziness, palpitations, and weakness, have been severe in some studies and are probably associated with the α-blocking properties (120). The major limiting effect is the sudden loss of consciousness or syncope that occurs in 2–10% of patients, usually following the initial dose. Therapy is often initiated with subtherapeutic doses (less than 0.5 mg) to avoid the syncope since subsequent doses do not generally cause collapse, but this effect still makes initiation of therapy hazardous (121). Its lack of significant cardiostimulation by reflex or direct mechanisms is a distinct advantage over other α-blockers and vasodilators. This intrinsic myocardial inhibition is possibly a result of prazosin-induced elevation of cyclic GMP in the heart.

Prazosin was selected for clinical use from a series of several hundred 4-quinazolinones and 4-aminoquinazolines. In both series, 6,7-dimethoxy substitution is critical for potent activity, and the 2-NEt_2 is a preferred substituent (122). The 4-aminoquinazolines are generally more

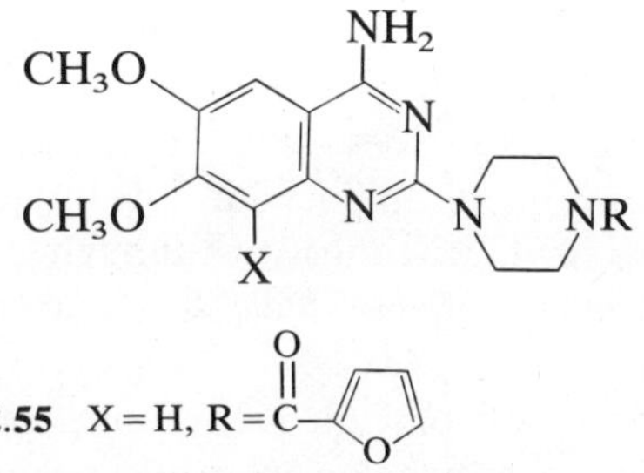

42.55   X = H, R = C(O)-furanyl

42.56   X = H, R = $CH_2CH=CH_2$
42.57   X = H, R = $CO_2CH_2CH(CH_3)_2$
42.58   X = CH_3O, R = $CO_2CH_2C(CH_3)_2OH$

potent and longer acting than the quinazolinones. In addition to the NEt_2 analog, 42.56 and 42.57 are as potent antihypertensives in animals as prazosin and do not affect heart rate (123). Trimazosin, 42.58, directly inhibits vascular smooth muscle contraction in humans and is devoid of adrenergic blocking activity in animals. But in clinical trials, much higher doses of trimazosin were required than for prazosin. to demonstrate an antihypertensive effect (124).

A series of indolethylpiperidines has also been studied for α-blocking, antihistamine, and local anesthetic activities; indoramine, 42.59, being the most extensively studied in man (125). It causes a sustained blood pressure reduction in animals after oral doses of 20–40 mg/kg owing to a decreased peripheral vascular resistance resulting from α-adrenergic blockade and cardioinhibitory actions (126). Like prazosin, the cardioinhibitory properties of indoramine eliminate the tachycardia generally observed with α-blockers and direct vasodilators and actually confer antiarrhythmic properties. A central action also may contribute to the hypotensive and bradycardic

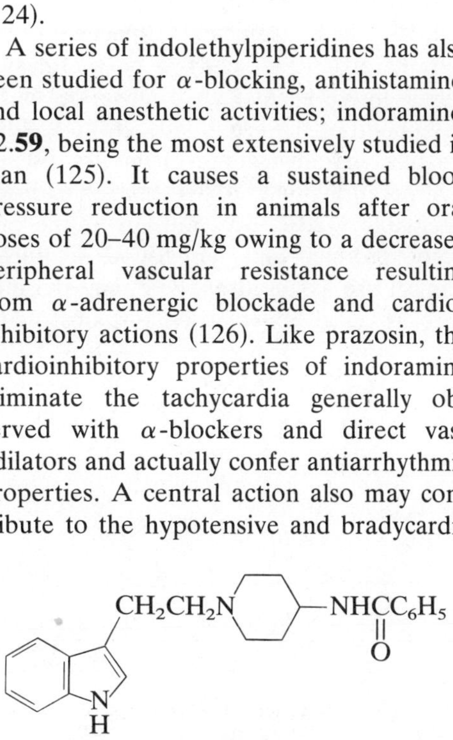

42.59

effects (127). Indoramine is equally effective clinically in the upright and supine positions and does not cause postural hypotension. Its major side effects are sedation and tiredness, although other troublesome effects have been reported (128).

Several analogs of indoramine possess the same pharmacological properties in animals. The indole moiety may be replaced by aryl and even cyclohexyl, but other heterocyclic systems are less effective for antihypertensive activity. Changes in the ethylene bridge cause no change in antihypertensive potency, but the benzamido group is more critical. The antihypertensive activity of these derivatives does not correlate well with α-blocking or antihistamine properties (125).

Sir Henry Dale's observation in 1906 that ergot blocked responses to circulating epinephrine and to sympathetic nerve stimulation was the first recognition of an adrenolytic agent. Pure crystalline ergot alkaloids lack sufficient specificity for peripheral vascular beds to be useful antihypertensive agents. Hydrogenation of the 9,10 bond of the ergotoxine group yields a mixture of dihydroergocornine, 42.**60**, dihydroergocryptine, 42.**61**, and dihydroergocristine, 42.**62**. This mixture is the only ergot product that has found significant clinical use as an adrenolytic, and the mixture is used extensively for obstructive

peripheral vascular diseases and cerebral vascular diseases as a performance enhancer among geriatrics rather than for hypertension. Its capacity and general predictability for maintaining a lower blood pressure is simply not great enough (129).

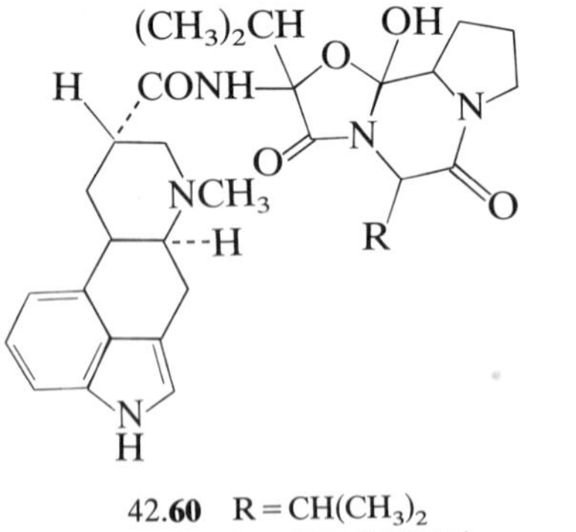

The drug nicergoline, 42.**63**, is an α-blocker which has recently been used to treat essential hypertension as well as peripheral vascular diseases (130). Another α-blocker, methylapogalanthamine, 42.**64**, has been recommended for clinical use in the Soviet Union (131).

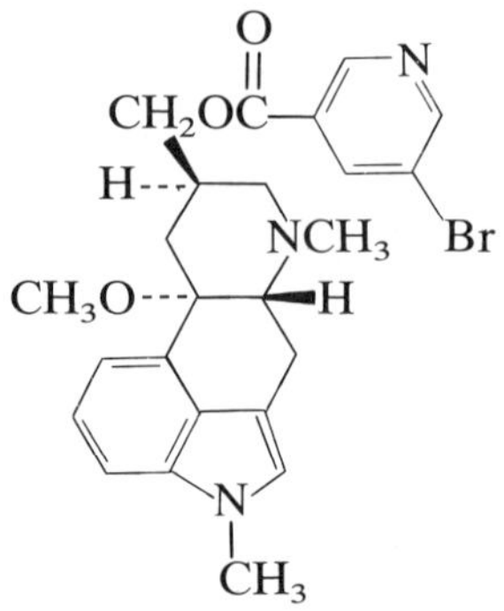

42.**63**

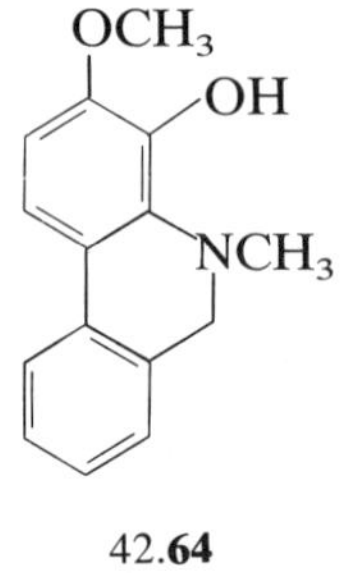

42.**64**

2.2.1.2 *β-Blockers.* It was a decade after Ahlquist first proposed classification of α- and β-adrenergic receptors, and only two decades ago when the first agent, DCI, 42.**65**, was described. DCI blocked the myocardial stimulant and vasodilator properties of epinephrine and isoproterenol (132) and became the first recognized β-adrenoceptor blocker. Subsequently, many new agents were prepared that are potent β-receptor antagonists, and their effects on

42.**60** R = CH(CH$_3$)$_2$
42.**61** R = CH$_2$CH(CH$_3$)$_2$
42.**62** R = CH$_2$C$_6$H$_5$

isolated tissues, cardiac function, and hemodynamics were widely studied (133). A considerable amount of work has been devoted to establishing which effects result strictly from antagonism of β-adrenergic receptors and which actions are not related to β-blockade.

The β-blockers have many structural features in common, but they vary in their potency and ancillary biological effects. Nearly all β-blockers with significant potency have a structural resemblance to epinephrine and isoproterenol (134). There are two general classes, the arylethanolamines and the aryloxypropanolamines, again a difference in the critical pharmacophore side chain of an OCH_2 unit. Many of the structural features permitting optimum activity were first developed in the arylethanolamines, but only sotalol (42.66) of this class is a widely used drug today, even through pronethalol (42.67) and INPEA (42.68) have been widely studied. The aryloxypropanolamines in general have greater potency by an order of magnitude and comprise most of the clinically useful β-blockers.

Substitution on the methylene carbon with alkyl groups generally causes a reduction of β-blocking potency proportional to the size of the alkyl group, although some metabolic selectivity is achieved with methyl or ethyl groups in the erythro configuration (135, 136). Replacement of the secondary alcohol group by anything that does not readily hydrolyze or metabolize to

the OH group generally eliminates β-blocking activity. Replacement of the ethereal oxygen in aryloxypropanolamines with S, CH_2, or NCH_3 is detrimental to β-blocking activity, but a tissue-selective β-blocker has been obtained with an NH substituted for the oxygen. Most chemical modifications of these two structural classes which have been aimed at improved β-blocking potency or selectivity have been aromatic ring substituents or, more recently, amine substituents (137, 138). The most commonly employed amine substituents have been isopropyl or t-butyl. Longer alkyl chains are less effective but arylethyl substituents are suitable, providing the carbon adjacent to the amine nitrogen has one or two additional methyl groups resembling the t-butyl in immediate environment around the nitrogen. The steric hindrance afforded by the t-butyl group may give optimum basicity or nucleophilicity to the amine group for receptor affinity, but it was previously stated that the methylene carbon should not be further substituted for optimum potency and the amine must be secondary for good β-blocking activity. The t-butyl group may allow optimum receptor affinity because it offers optimum steric interaction with the OH group according to Newman's rule of six.

The steric requirements for good β-adrenergic receptor affinity and antihypertensive potency are quite strict. β-Blocking activity resides chiefly in the D(−) absolute configuration for both structural classes. With α-alkyl phenethanolamine derivatives, the erythro (RS) configuration is best. The dextro isomer more closely resembles the deoxy derivative than the levo isomer and generally shows no significant antihypertensive activity. The strict requirements for these side chains have been rationalized into a single model, 42.69 (110), which is useful for envisioning drug–receptor interactions and for planning new drug syntheses. The two structures in 42.69

X—⟨benzene ring⟩—
$$CHCH_2NHCH(CH_3)_2$$
OH   ·HCl

42.65 X = 3, 4 − Cl_2
42.66 X = 4 − CH_3SO_2NH: sotalol

42.67 X = 3, 4 −⟨ring⟩

42.68 X = 4 − NO_2

42.**69**

may be superimposed at the phenyl ring, bond of attachment to side chain, and the ammonium group such that the distance between the ammonium nitrogen and the p-phenyl position is 6.4 Å in both structures. When this is done, the oxygen atoms of the aliphatic hydroxyl groups are about 2.0 Å apart. This may indicate that the hydroxyl group need not be critically oriented for adrenergic activity, but it may account for the β_1-adrenergic selectivity (myocardial) in aryloxypropanolamines compared to arylethanolamines—agonists and antagonists. The rigid 6–5 bicyclic doubly intra-hydrogen-bonded conformation for the aryloxypropanolamines is quite stable in solution, according to NMR, and does indeed represent strict structural requirements.

β-Blocking drugs are rapidly gaining acceptance as primary agents for the treatment of hypertension, a trend that has rapidly accelerated over the past few years and is likely to continue (139). They are presently being used as the initial antihypertensive agent for about half of the patients of some countries (140) and are being advocated for a similar role in the United States (141, 142). The general alternative for primary therapy is a diuretic. β-Blockers are especially suited for the chronic treatment of hypertension because of (1) their relative freedom from the troublesome side effects associated with CNS agents or sympathetic inhibitors (e.g., postural hypotension, sedation, and sexual dysfunction) (143), (2) their smoothness of effect and onset, and (3) the ease with which they combine and complement other types of antihypertensive drugs. For example, β-blockers antagonize the hyper-reninemia and reflex cardiostimulation produced by direct vasodilating antihypertensives (144) and the hypokalemia associated with many of the diuretics, whereas the antihypertensive effects are additive.

Although β-adrenergic blocking drugs are now recognized as effective antihypertensive agents, this has been true only during the past decade, and none of the hypotheses to explain their mechanism for lowering blood pressure is entirely satisfactory. On strict pharmacological grounds, these agents could be expected to raise rather than lower arterial pressure by blocking the vasodilation-mediating vascular β-receptors. In many animal models of hypertension, β-blockers are devoid of antihypertensive activity and are, in fact, hypertensive in certain groups of patients (145). The excellent antihypertensive profile of these agents in the majority of hypertensive patients, however, continues to stimulate the search for mechanistic explanations of their effects. Presently, postulated mechanisms include (1) inhibition of renin release (146), (2) inhibition of cardiac output, (3) inhibition of sympathetic outflow by central action or by reducing afferent input, (4) regression of cardiac hypertrophy (147), (5) restoration of vascular relaxation response (148), and (6) inhibition of synaptic norepinephrine release (149). Of course, several or all of these mechanisms may be operant.

Pharmacologically, all β-blockers are not the same although clinically they are similar (150). In addition to β-adrenergic antagonism, most β-blockers have several ancillary pharmacological activities that can add or detract from their profiles (see Table 42.1).

Table 42.1 β-Adrenergic Blocking Agents of Clinical Importance

Name	Antihypertensive Dose Range, mg/day	Cardioselectivity	Sympathomimetic Activity
Propranolol	240–480	−	−
Pindolol	15–45	−	+
Alprenolol	400–800	−	+
Oxprenolol	480–960	−	+
Bunitrolol	60–240	−	+
Tolamolol	300–900	+	−
Practolol	600–1200	+	+
Atenolol	100–200	+	−
Metoprolol	150–300	+	−
Acebutolol	400–1200	(+)	+
Nadolol	60–160	−	−
Timolol	30–60	−	−
Sotalol	160–320	−	−

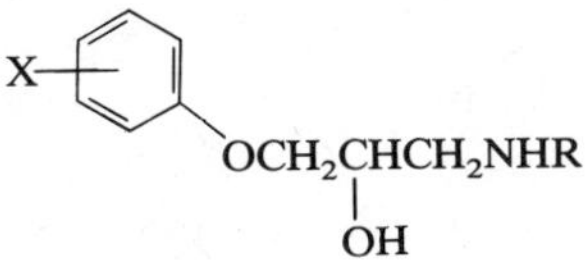

$$X \overline{} \text{phenyl} - OCH_2CHCH_2NHR$$
$$\underset{OH}{|}$$

No.	X	R	Name
42.**70**	2,3– 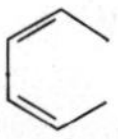 (fused ring)	iPr	Propranolol
42.**71**	2,3– 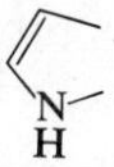 (indole ring, N—H)	iPr	Pindolol
42.**72**	2—$CH_2{=}CHCH_2$	iPr	Alprenolol
42.**73**	2—$CH_2{=}CHCH_2O$	iPr	Oxprenolol
42.**74**	2—CN	tBu	Bunitrolol
42.**75**	2—CH_3	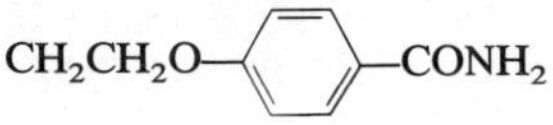 CH_2CH_2O—phenyl—$CONH_2$	Tolamolol
42.**76**	2,3– 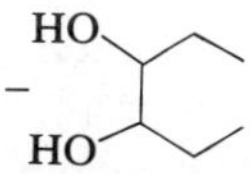 (HO, HO substituted ring)	tBu	Nadolol
42.**77**	4—CH_3CONH	iPr	Practolol
42.**78**	4—H_2NCOCH_2	iPr	Atenolol
42.**79**	4—$CH_3OCH_2CH_2$	iPr	Metoprolol
42.**80**	4—C_3H_7CONH, 2—CH_3CO	iPr	Acebutolol
42.**81**	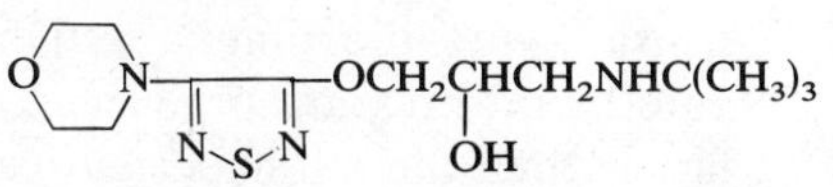 (morpholino-thiadiazole)—$OCH_2CHCH_2NHC(CH_3)_3$, OH		Timolol

The first important property to consider is cardioselectivity. Some of these agents block cardiac β-receptors (β_1) at lower doses than required to block bronchial or vascular β-receptors (β_2). This is not an absolute specificity since vascular and bronchial receptors are blocked at higher doses. This selectivity may be due to unequal distribution of the drugs in various tissues or inability to reach receptor sites since no receptor selectivity has been observed in cell-free systems (15). The cardioselective β-blockers are generally hydrophilic, having $P < 1.0$. Cardioselectivity has been claimed to reduce the asthmagenic potential of β-blockers by reducing their antagonism to the bronchodilating receptors. However, direct support for the contribution of cardioselectivity to the reduction of asthma attacks or their severity is weak, and β-blockers with or without cardioselectivity are contraindicated in asthma (152). Cardioselective β-block has been speculated to reduce peripheral vasoconstriction and thus prevent the increase in ventricular afterload.

On the other hand, cardioselectivity may detract from the antihypertensive profile since cardioselective β-blockers are generally less potent antihypertensives (153, 154). Cardioselective β-blockers often have flat dose–response curves so that little additional effect can be achieved by increasing the dose. Cardioselective β-blockers, such as atenolol or metoprolol, are not good inhibitors of renin release since this effect appears to be primarily under control of β_2-receptors. The possibility of developing congestive heart failure is theoretically greater with cardioselective agents since venous return is not reduced in the face of negative inotropic and chronotropic effects (155). Since the majority of experts feel the antihypertensive effects of β-blockers are due to a reduction of peripheral resistance (156), cardioselectivity may be of questionable importance to the clinical antihypertensive profile of these

agents. The cardioselective agents may lower pressure primarily via decreased cardiac output since no lowering of peripheral resistance could be demonstrated for atenolol (157). Decreasing cardiac output is certainly not desired in hypertensive patients with already compromised cardiac function. Some cardioselective agents also produce undesirable metabolic effects (elevated free fatty acids and cholesterol levels) that could counterbalance their desirable antihypertensive effects in the long run. This could be due to their relatively lower ability to antagonize the metabolic effects of epinephrine (β_2). It is not clear to what extent these effects are common to all cardioselective agents. It should be noted that most β-blockers including propranolol are vasculoselective.

The second important ancillary property is intrinsic sympathomimetic activity. Some β-blockers stimulate the same receptors they block. They have some intrinsic activity for β-receptors as well as affinity for blocking these receptors to catecholamine stimulation. This intrinsic activity should reduce the risk of heart failure, myocardial depression (158), and bronchoconstriction most importantly (159), yet agents with this property produce some of these effects. Intrinsic sympathomimetic effects may attenuate the excessive slowing of the heart produced by most β-blockers (160). Sympathomimetic activity may be important in patients whose sympathetic tone represents a necessary compensatory mechanism for maintaining cardiac function, and it may permit a quicker onset for blood pressure lowering via direct peripheral vasodilation. However, intrinsic sympathomimetic activity may attenuate the inhibition of renin release, flatten the dose–response curve, and generally weaken the desired β-blocking effects (16). β-blockers with intrinsic sympathomimetic activity can elevate blood pressure if given in doses much larger than the antihypertensive ones.

Another   important   pharmacological

parameter is membrane stabilizing activity, which could contribute to the antiarrhythmic effects of β-blockers, but appears to have little significant clinical importance because 10–100 times the dose would be required than is needed for maximal β-blockade (162). This activity correlates well with lipophilicity, so agents having this property are more likely to cross the blood–brain barrier and provoke central depressant effects and bizarre dreams. More important, this effect is correlated with the inhibition of myocardial contractility which may predispose the patient to heart failure. Propranolol has P 3.60 and pindolol has P 1.75, both show membrane stabilization, myocardial depression, and central effects. Atenolol has P 0.23; it exhibits no membrane stabilization but is cardioselective.

From a clinical standpoint, none of these ancillary pharmacologic properties contributes significantly to the antihypertensive capability found with all β-blockers, but they do contribute to the total drug effect and hence to the selection among available β-blockers for a given patient. Table 42.1 lists the major clinically used β-blockers with ancillary pharmacological characteristics. There are significant differences among these agents in absorption, serum binding, and half-life of unchanged drug—sotalol, practolol, and nadolol having the greatest duration. But nearly all β-blockers are effective long-term with twice-daily dosing, so patient compliance is good with these drugs.

It is important to note here that an important factor in the development of β-blockers for hypertension in the United States is the role played by the Food and Drug Administration with respect to carcinogenicity testing. Propranolol was approved for the treatment of arrhythmias in 1967 and not for hypertension for nearly another decade. The delay in approval of other β-blockers is due to an assumed potential for carcinogenicity in the class as

well as a desire for clinical differences from propranolol. Pronethalol caused an increased incidence of sarcomas in mice as did practolol, and alprenolol caused an increased incidence of thymic lymphosarcomas. The entire class is not considered tumorigenic, but differentiation cannot be made between arylethanolamines and aryloxypropanolamines or cardioselective β-blockers. Tolamolol caused mammary adenocarcinoma and hepatocellular carcinoma in rats, and pamatolol caused hepatocellular carcinoma in rats. Bunolol has caused an increased incidence of uterine leiomyomata in mice and liver adenomas in rats—benign lesions. The significance of these long-term high dose animal findings to humans at antihypertensive doses needs further study and interpretation.

With the achievement of β-blockers that are safe and effective long-term antihypertensives, are cardioselective, and have desirable absorption and half-life characteristics, the next challenge for medicinal chemists appears to be to combine several desirable mechanisms and clinical features into one molecule. For example, labetalol, 42.**82** (136), has α-blocking as well as β-blocking properties. This combination of mechanisms allows a quicker onset of antihypertensive effect than β-blockade alone and may also have a reduced tendency to cause bronchospasm. However, labetalol does produce some postural hypotension as would be expected for an α-blocker, so the optimum balance between α- and β-blockade is important. Another compound, 42.**83** (164), has direct vasodilating effects in addition to β-blockade which may also

42.**82**

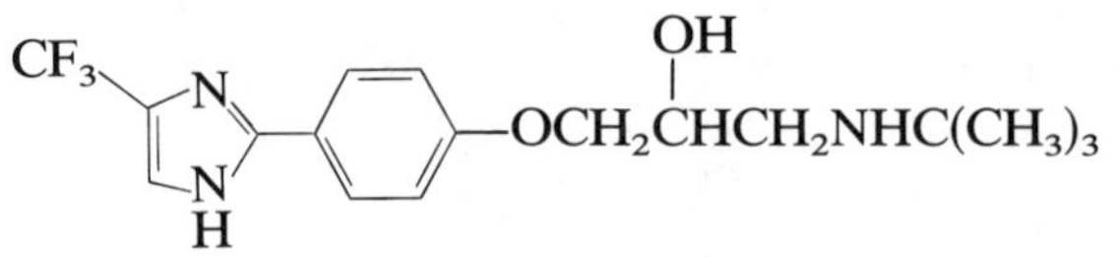

$$CF_3 \overset{N}{\underset{\underset{H}{N}}{\diagup}} \quad \text{—} \quad \text{—OCH}_2\overset{\overset{\text{OH}}{|}}{\text{CH}}\text{CH}_2\text{NHC(CH}_3)_3$$

42.**83**

offer rapid onset, minimal inhibition of myocardial contractility, and desirable hemodynamics with a reduced peripheral resistance. The use of β-blockers with vasodilators such as minoxidil and hydralazine has produced good clinical results, so these single agents with several complementary mechanisms may prove to be clinically quite useful.

2.2.2 DIRECT-ACTING VASODILATORS. This class of drugs represents the most logical approach for the treatment of hypertension. They act by inducing vascular smooth muscle relaxation and a consequent decrease of peripheral resistance without significant effects on the sympathetic nervous system. An elevated peripheral resistance is the most consistent hemodynamic parameter in hypertension.

Agents as diverse as sodium nitroprusside, thiazides, and hydralazine promote dilation of the arterioles by a direct relaxation of the vascular smooth muscle or by inhibition of the physiological vasoconstricting mechanisms. However, these agents suffer from two major disadvantages that limit their usefulness as antihypertensive agents: cardiostimulation and renin release. The cardiostimulation is probably due to increased venous return since most of the agents, except sodium nitroprusside, relax predominantly arterial smooth muscle. Renin release is primarily due to a reflex increase in sympathetic tone. High levels of plasma renin activity underlie the salt and water retention generally associated with these agents and probably contribute to an increased risk of cerebrovascular and cardiovascular mishaps. Both these effects can be controlled by

β-blockers, hence the value of the combination.

2.2.2.1 *Sodium Nitroprusside.* $Na_2Fe(CN)_5$-NO as a photosensitive aqueous solution and diazoxide, 42.**84**, are reserved for the intravenous control of severe hypertension. They are particularly suited for severe and emergency episodes because they produce an immediate lowering of blood pressure, and sodium nitroprusside does not cause cardiostimulation. The rapid action of the nitroprusside is probably due to the nitroso group. Its effect ends when the infusion is stopped owing to its rapid conversion to thiocyanate. The hypotensive effect is augmented by ganglionic blocking agents. Sodium nitroprusside infusions must be accompanied by continuous monitoring of blood pressure. Oral antihypertensive therapy could be initiated simultaneously with no adverse interactions.

2.2.2.2 *Diazoxide.* This drug is reserved for the treatment of hypertensive crises and is given intravenously in bolus doses of 300 mg or more. It directly relaxes vascular smooth muscle and its use is associated with cardiostimulation and fluid retention The concomitant use of a diuretic is desirable if prolonged use of diazoxide is required. In contrast to sodium nitroprusside, the reduction in blood pressure from diazoxide is more gradual in onset and persists with continued administration, but it is not orthostatic in nature.

By deleting the sulfamoyl substituent from the thiazide diuretics, it was found that diazoxide is hypotensive but not diuretic (165). Methylation of either ring nitrogen

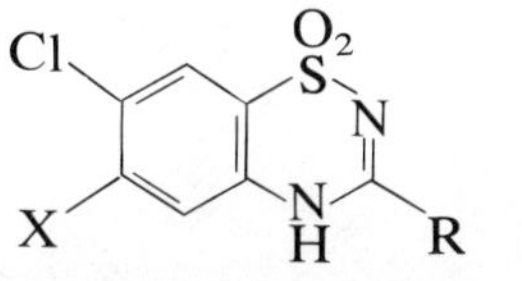

42.**84** X = H, R = CH$_3$

42.**85** X = Cl, R =

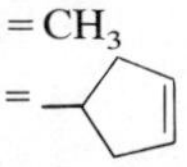

42.**86** X = H, R = NHCH$_2$CH$_3$

42.**87** X = H, R =

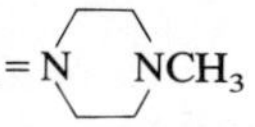

reduced hypotensive activity. Considerable variations in the 3, 6, and 7 positions were investigated and a QSAR analysis for antihypertensive activity was performed (166). A broad range of potencies is correlated by equations based on the π values of substituents in these three critical positions. Requirements for maximum activity are (1) highly lipophilic substituents at positions 6 and/or 7, (2) a group at position 3 with a specific lipophilicity that depends on the biological test system, and (3) a p$K_a > 8.0$ to minimize ionization. Pazoxide, 42.**85**, was predicted to be the optimum compound by the QSAR study and it did show the highest antihypertensive potency in hypertensive rats. Another benzothiadiazine, 42.**86** (167), has been clinically evaluated as an antihypertensive agent, and a related derivative, 42.**87**, has been investigated (168). In fact, hypotensive activity is retained with the arylthiadiazine system,

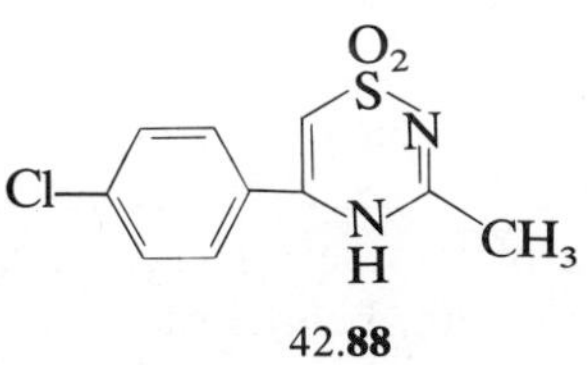

42.**88**

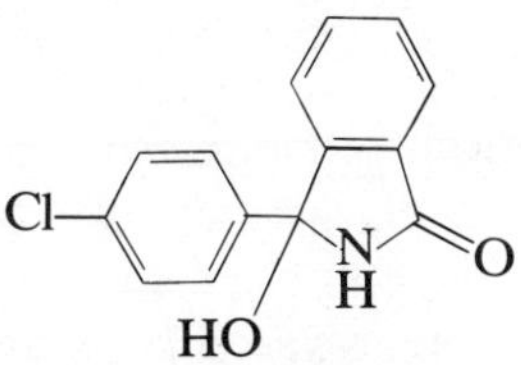

42.**89**

42.**88** (169), and the desulfamoyl analog, 42.**89**, of chlorthalidone (170). Unfortunately, not enough is yet known about the molecular mechanism by which diazoxide affects contractile system of vascular smooth muscle to extend the physical and structural properties to molecules that would be devoid of fluid retention and cardiostimulating properties.

2.2.2.3 *Hydralazine.* The complex and unique actions of hydrazinophthalazines on the cardiovascular system were first reported in 1950. Since that time many modifications have been made and structural requirements for good hypotensive activity have been elucidated (171). Hydralazine, 42.**90**, produces direct peripheral vasodilation in addition to a suppression of vasoconstrictor impulses originating in the central nervous system. Some confusion about site and mechanism of action existed because hydralazine's depression of the vasomotor center in the midbrain of animals is not prevalent in man. The increase of blood flow in regions devoid of sympathetic innervation supports a mechanism of direct peripheral vasodilation. It dilates precapillary resistance vessels much more than postcapillary capacitance vessels. Vascular resistance in coronary, cerebral, and renal circulations decreases more than in muscle or skin (172). The peripheral vasodilation results from a direct action on smooth muscle of the arteriolar bed, probably involving metal chelation and cyclic AMP phosphodiesterase inhibition (173). In fact, hydralazine has a special affinity for smooth muscle which permits a longer antihypertensive action than its plasma half-life would suggest (174).

The use of hydralazine is not associated with postural hypotension or sexual dysfunction. Its increase of cardiac output is mainly reflex to the reduced peripheral resistance, but this tends to reduce its antihypertensive effect. Hydralazine generally increases sodium and water retention via stimulation of the renin–angiotensin system. Both the increase in cardiac output and fluid retention may be counteracted by concomitant use of β-blockers. Acetylation represents a major hepatic pathway for the detoxication of hydralazine, and variations in acetylating capability probably account for the variation in response of different patients (175). The chronic administration of hydralazine causes a condition resembling lupus erythematosus (176) in 10–20% of patients treated with at least 400 mg/day. However, it rarely develops in patients receiving less than 200 mg/day, and hydralazine is very useful with minimal side effects when combined with β-blockers and diuretics (177).

The clinically useful analogs of hydralazine are closely related phthalazines and pyridazines. Phthalazines such as dihydralazine, 42.**91**, escarazine, 42.**93**, and picodralazine, 42.**92**, are used in Europe but do not have significant advantages over hydralazine. One hydrazone, 42.**94**, has much less cardiac stimulation at equieffective antihypertensive doses in hypertensive rats (178).

Although the only marketed hydrazinopyridazine is hydracarbazine, 42.**95**,

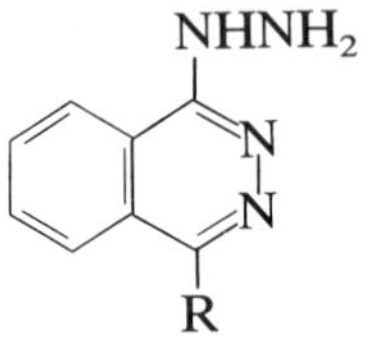

NHNH$_2$

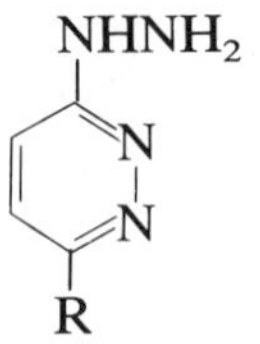

42.**95**   R = CONH$_2$
42.**96**   R = N(CH$_2$CH$_2$OH)$_2$
42.**97**   R = NCH$_2$CHOH
                    | |
                   CH$_3$ CH$_3$

two amino derivatives are being clinically investigated as hypotensive vasodilators, 42.**96** (179) and 42.**97** (180), which are very similar to hydralazine in their profile but are more potent with lower toxicity (181). In a related series of 6-aryl-3-hydrazinopyridazines, hypotensive activity was quantitatively correlated with π of the aromatic substituents (182).

A related series of dihydropyridazinones show potent hypotensive properties in animals even though lacking the hydrazine function (183, 184). One of these compounds, 42.**98**, has been clinically studied

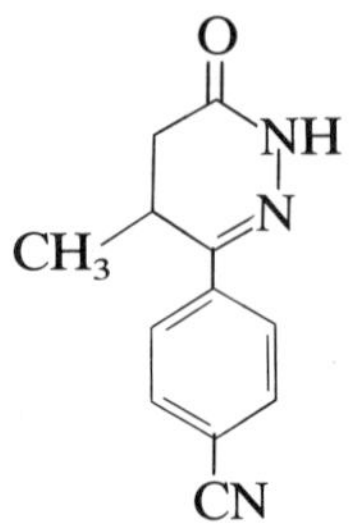

42.**98**

as an antihypertensive agent, and its activity is largely due to vasodilation. Active members of this series cause hemorrhagic patches in the hearts of several animal species.

2.2.2.4 *Minoxidil.* The discovery that the long-lasting hypotensive effect of the triazine, 42.**99**, in animals is due to its N-oxide metabolite led to development of the very potent vasodilator antihypertensive agent, minoxidil, 42.**100**. It is generally

NHNH$_2$

42.**90**   R = H
42.**91**   R = NHNH$_2$

42.**92**   R = CH$_2$—[pyridine]

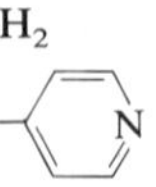

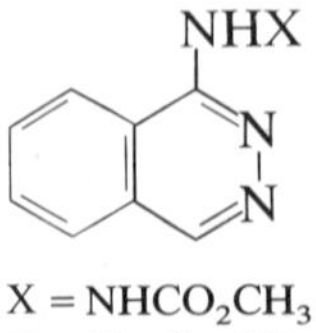

NHX

42.**93**   X = NHCO$_2$CH$_3$
42.**94**   X = N=C—CH=C(CH$_3$)$_2$
                    |
                   CH$_3$

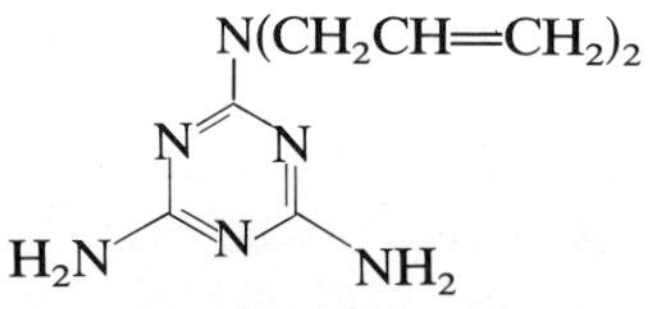

N(CH₂CH=CH₂)₂ structure

42.99

piperidine-substituted pyrimidine structure with H₂N, NH, OH

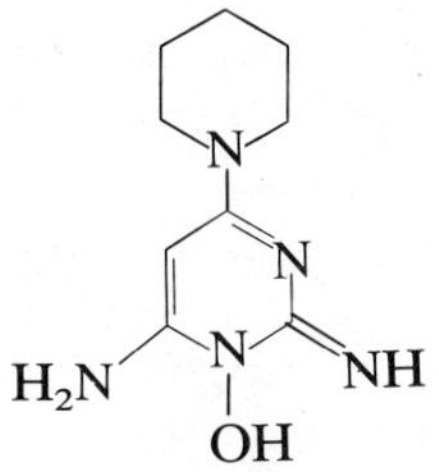

42.100

reserved for use in resistant hypertension. Minoxidil produces reflex cardiac stimulation (185), fluid retention, and hypertrichosis which makes it unsuitable for chronic use. Prolonged administration in dogs resulted in a degenerative lesion of the right atrium that caused some concern about the safety of minoxidil, but no similar lesion has been observed in other animal species or in man. Like hydralazine, minoxidil should be used in combination with a β-blocker, a diuretic, or both (186).

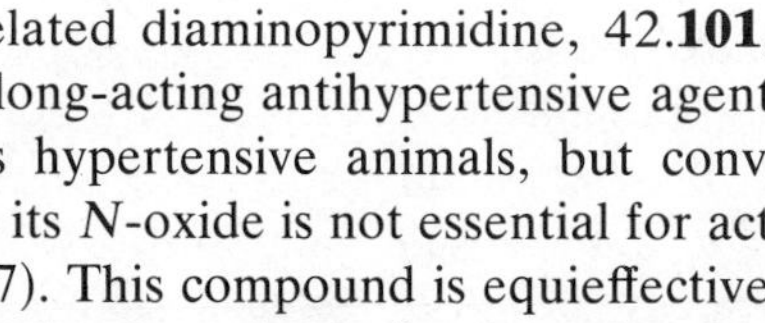

OCH₂CH₂CH₂N(CH₃)₂ pyrimidine structure with H₂N, NH₂

42.101

A related diaminopyrimidine, 42.**101**, is also a long-acting antihypertensive agent in various hypertensive animals, but conversion to its *N*-oxide is not essential for activity (187). This compound is equieffective to hydralazine in animals for lowering blood pressure and causes less tachycardia. It also acts by a direct relaxation of vascular smooth muscle.

2.2.2.5 *Dihydropyridines.* Several groups of investigators independently discovered that dihydropyridines from the Hantzsch reaction are potent vasodilator hypotensives (188). Nifedipine, 42.**102**, is used as an antianginal and coronary dilator (189). It dilates only resistance vessels, and its tachycardia can be prevented by concurrent use of a β-blocker. The related compound, 42.**103**, SKF 24260, is being clinically evaluated in hypertension (190). It also lowers blood pressure by selectively dilating resistance vessels and causes tachycardia that may be prevented by propranolol. It lowers blood pressure at doses as low as 5 mg but the duration is less than 3 hr. Electrocardiographic changes with these agents are similar to those observed with other vasodilator hypotensives. The direct effect on vascular smooth muscle from these dihydropyridines is probably by inhibiting cellular membrane calcium transport.

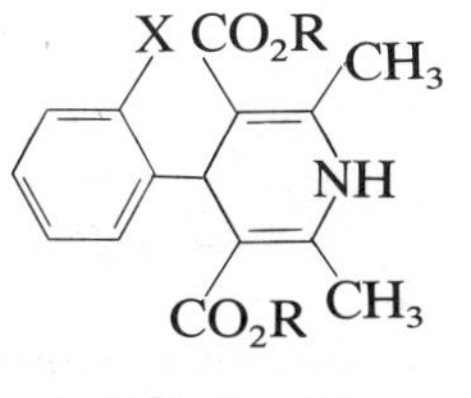

dihydropyridine structure with X, CO₂R, CH₃, NH, CO₂R, CH₃

42.102   X = NO₂, R = CH₃
42.103   X = CF₃, R = CH₂CH₃

The structure–activity relationships of these agents shows that an ortho-substituted aryl is critical in the 4 position, as is the unsubstituted nitrogen; 2,6-dimethyl is important, and carbalkoxy groups are preferred to other electron-withdrawing groups in the 3,5 positions. The aromatic pyridine derivatives have little activity and the dihydropyridines are rapidly metabolized by dehydrogenation to the pyridines.

Other structural types have also been found clinically to lower blood pressure by a direct action on vascular smooth muscle. Guancydine, 42.**104**, has a potency less

CH$_3$ NCN

CH$_3$CH$_2$CNHCNH$_2$

CH$_3$

42.**104**

42.**105**

than hydralazine but a similar profile including cardiac stimulation and sodium accumulation (185). It is useful when combined with β-blockers or diuretics but does not offer good prospects when used alone.

Certain 3-aminosydnones cause a pronounced lowering of blood pressure in animals with hemodynamic effects similar to nitroglycerin (191, 192). Molsidomine, 42.**105**, is clinically effective in gradually lowering blood pressure. It increases pulse rate, but shows no signs of fluid retention (193) or excessive orthostatic hypotension. It is a coronary dilator with no peripheral dilation and no vascular steal. It improves collateral blood flow, reduces myocardial wall tension and extravascular resistance, causing a reduction of ventricular work, and a fall in myocardial oxygen consumption. These sydnones are metabolized to a ring-opened structure which releases nitrite, possibly the hypotensive species.

None of the direct vasodilators currently under investigation appear to correct the fundamental shortcomings of those in current use—primarily cardiac stimulation plus sodium and fluid accumulation. To avoid concurrent use of a β-blocker or diuretic, the development of a new vasodilator should include a combination of these properties in a single agent.

2.2.3 CYCLIC NUCLEOTIDES (see also Chapter 34). The role of cyclic nucleotides in hypertension has been investigated in ani-

mals (194) and man (195). In general, the cyclic nucleotide levels in plasma or urine reflect the level of prevailing sympathetic activity. A basic biochemical lesion in hypertensive animals causes less cyclic AMP synthesis in response to hormonal stimulation in the vasculature and heart (196). A similar lesion may also exist in human essential hypertension (197). An elevated cyclic GMP/cyclic AMP ratio in vascular tissue, primarily due to decreased cyclic AMP synthesis, may underlie the increased vascular muscle tone associated with the increased peripheral resistance in hypertension.

The development of selective inhibitors of phosphodiesterase (PDE), the enzyme that catalyzes cyclic nucleotide hydrolysis, should furnish useful therapeutic agents for restoring normal cyclic nucleotide levels in hypertensives. The structure–activity relationship of two PDE inhibitors, papaverine and theophylline, contributed to the development of prazosin (198). Although the dominant mechanism of prazosin may be its α-adrenergic blockade, it is an interesting PDE inhibitor and vasodilator because it demonstrates some selectivity for cyclic AMP–PDE in the vasculature and for cyclic GMP–PDE in the heart. This tissue selectivity may be responsible for the absence of reflex cardiostimulation with prazosin. The development of other selective PDE inhibitors without adrenergic inhibitory properties is certainly a worthwhile objective.

2.2.4 PROSTAGLANDINS (see also Chapter 33). The interplay between prostaglandins and both the renin–angiotensin and kallikrein–kinin systems may be important to the renal control of normal blood pressure. Further, some forms of chronic hypertension may result from a prostaglandin deficiency because reduced activity from these counteracting hormones results in overactivity of the renin–angiotensin‹ or other systems. Prostaglandin synthesis within resistance vessel walls, as well as within the kidney, participates in blood pressure regulation (199). Both vascular and renal actions of endogenous prostaglandins contribute to their antihypertensive effects. However, the antihypertensive effect may be largely due to intrarenal vasodilation by PGE_2 rather than to general vascular circulation, since the more stable PGA_2 is not readily biosynthesized in the mammalian kidney or extrarenal tissues (16). An increased renal production of vasodilating prostaglandins may, in fact, be a response to an elevated systemic blood pressure (200).

It is important for the development of new antihypertensive agents to recognize that prostaglandins have their effects at or near the site of synthesis (201). Prostaglandins synthesized in the walls of major resistance vessels modify the vasoconstrictor responses to other hormonal and neural stimuli and thereby reduce peripheral resistance. This suggests that exogenous prostaglandins are not useful antihypertensive agents, especially since they are not very stable when taken orally. But agents that affect the balance of prostaglandins by increasing the synthesis of vasodilating prostaglandins within the kidney or vessel walls should be extremely selective and useful antihypertensive agents. Such modulators of prostaglandin synthesis should be rather tissue selective but need not be closely related to the prostaglandins in structure. Although prostaglandin synthetase inhibitors of varied structures have played a major role in the elucidation of the physiological functions of prostaglandins (202), selective stimulators of prostaglandin synthesis or inhibitors of PGE_2 degradation are yet to be developed.

2.3 Diuretics (see also Chapter 40)

Use of thiazide-type diuretics in less than maximal doses is recommended as the first step or cornerstone of therapy for mild and moderate hypertension (203). Their antihypertensive effect is primarily due to the reduction of extracellular fluid volume and sodium which is associated with a decrease in cardiac output (204). However, blood pressure and peripheral resistance remain decreased after plasma volume and cardiac output have returned to control levels, and the persistent deficit in exchangeable sodium reflecting an outward movement of sodium from vascular smooth muscle may be the explanation (205). About 20 g of salt per day completely abolishes the antihypertensive effect of previously administered thiazides, whereas expansion of plasma volume in hypertensive patients does not abolish the effect of thiazide therapy. Dietary restriction of sodium is recommended when thiazide therapy is initiated for hypertension. In addition, thiazides counteract the fluid and sodium retention produced by other agents, such as vasodilators, and therefore are generally useful and even a necessary component of combination therapy.

The thiazides and thiazide-related diuretics are all similar in their profile, mechanism, and side effects. They differ mainly in their effective dosage and their duration of action. Chlorothiazide and flumethiazide require 250–500 mg twice daily, hydrochlorothiazide requires 25–50 mg twice daily, and hydroflumethiazide requires 50–100 mg daily. Benzthiazide, bendroflumethiazide, trichlormethiazide, methyclothiazide, cyclothiazide, and polythiazide are listed in order of increasing potency and duration such that a 1–2 mg dose will last at least 24 hr. Other thiazide-related sulfonamide derivative diuretics, such as chlorthalidone, quinethazone, metolazone, xipamide, and indapamide (see Chapter 40 for structures) require from 2.5 to 50 mg/day in a single dose. When effective blood levels of thiazide diuretics decline, compensatory mechanisms cause retention of sodium that leads to an increase in blood volume and an elevated blood pressure. To maintain a decreased blood pressure, sodium must be excreted consistently throughout each 24 hr period. A twice-daily dosing of hydrochlorothiazide is required to maintain 24 hr control of sodium resorption, whereas chlorthalidone with a duration of 2–3 days produces good control with once-daily dosing (206). Patient compliance may be slightly greater with once-daily dosing.

The major side effects of thiazide diuretics are a decrease in serum potassium, azotemia, and an increase in serum uric acid and glucose. Although hypokalemia and hyperuricemia may be greater for hydrochlorothiazide than for an equally antihypertensive dose of chlorthalidone or some of the newer sulfonamide derivatives, all these agents produce some degree of these same side affects. Whereas laboratory-reported hypokalemia (<3.5 mEq/l) occurs in 23% of patients on thiazide therapy, clinical hypokalemia (<3.0 mEq/l) occurs in only about 6% of patients (207). Clinical hypokalemia is frequently associated with leg cramps, cardiac abnormalities, and generalized weakness. It can be treated with potassium supplements, including dietary supplementation, or adjunctive use of potassium-sparing agents. Although hyperuricemia is a common side effect of diuretics and may increase the patient's risk for cardiovascular disease, it seldom results in frank gout and there is disagreement on whether it should be treated. The carbohydrate intolerance resulting in hyperglycemia is generally mild and a serious problem only in diabetic hypertensives. An increase in serum cholesterol and triglycerides following thiazide therapy has been cited as a possible major side effect also (208).

The more potent diuretics that act proximally on the loop of Henle, such as furosemide and ethacrynic acid, are not generally used as first-step therapy for hypertension. They have the same side effects but to a greater extent than thiazides, including massive sodium and potassium loss. They require at least twice-daily dosing. Hypovolemia may lead to cardiovascular problems and even to a myocardial infarct in congestive heart failure patients. These loop diuretics are especially useful, though, in pulmonary edema, renal insufficiency, and resistant or severe cases.

There are two widely used potassium-sparing diuretics, triamterene and spironolactone. Triamterene requires less frequent dosage, costs less, and provokes fewer side effects than spironolactone. These are also not used alone as initial therapy because they cause hyperkalemia and some nausea, and may provoke renal failure while producing only a modest reduction of blood volume. But the combination of a potassium-sparing diuretic with a thiazide produces a very desirable balance of properties. The volume diuresis of the two agents is at least additive when combined, but very little change in serum potassium is noted with a significant depletion of serum sodium. These diuretic combinations have become preferred agents for initial antihypertensive therapy because they avoid the risk of hypokalemia or the need for potassium supplementation. They cause minimal side effects and encourage patient compliance with once daily dosing.

2.4 Humoral Mechanisms

2.4.1 RENIN–ANGIOTENSIN SYSTEM. Since the discovery in 1898 that injections of saline kidney extracts produce an increase in arterial blood pressure (209), the role of renin in the control of blood pressure and in the etiology of hypertension has been vigorously investigated. Renin is a proteolytic enzyme released primarily from the kidneys in response to decreased perfusion pressure, decreased sodium or increased potassium load, or sympathetic stimulation. Stimulation of β-adrenergic receptors causes a release of renin primarily from the kidneys, whereas α-adrenergic stimulation inhibits renin release (210). Renin in turn acts on circulating angiotensinogen, a 14-amino acid α-2-globulin manufactured in the liver, to produce angiotensin I (42.**106**), a weak vasoconstrictor decapeptide. The original discovery that angiotensin was formed in the plasma prompted the suggestion that it may be responsible for an increase in blood pressure and perhaps play an etiologic role in hypertension (211). Angiotensin I is rapidly changed in the plasma to an octapeptide, angiotensin II (42.**107**), by chloride-activated converting enzymes. These converting enzymes are primarily located in the lungs but are also present in other tissues (212). They can also produce the heptapeptide, angiotensin III (42.**108**) (213). Angiotensin II has been isolated from human materials and its exact sequence confirmed by independent synthesis (14). The terminal phenylalanine, the phenolic group of tyrosine, proline in the penultimate position, and a specific three-dimensional configuration have been established as critical to the pressor activity.

Angiotensin II is the most potent direct vasoconstrictor known. It also elevates arterial pressure via a central action which results from a net increase in sympathetic outflow via release of catecholamines from the adrenal medulla. Angiotensin II additionally stimulates the release of aldosterone from the adrenal medulla, which promotes sodium and volume expansion, and this effect is also produced by angiotensin III. Angiotensin II even evokes a positive inotropic effect on the heart. Thus the net result of increased renin release is an elevated arterial pressure, sodium, and

volume load. These effects in turn inhibit renin release and through a negative feedback they initiate an autoregulation of peripheral blood flow, a reduction in cardiac output, maintenance of a high peripheral resistance, and thereby an increase in blood pressure. Later in the course of established hypertension, this suppressed renin release is reflected by normal or subnormal levels of plasma renin activity (214).

Although there may be some controversy concerning the role of the renin–angiotensin system in the regulation of normal blood pressure, there is little disagreement about its important role in high-renin hypertension, in the blood pressure response to postural changes or to sodium depletion, and in renovascular hypertension (215). The renin–angiotensin system is involved in the action of nearly all major classes of antihypertensive agents (216), and its control is important to the success of any antihypertensive therapy (217). It is a well supported opinion that elevated renin levels themselves are an important risk factor in the incidence of cerebrovascular accidents (218). The determination of plasma renin activity can have important diagnostic value in hypertension, particularly when sodium intake is strictly controlled and the assays are done properly (219). Determination of plasma renin activity can give important clues to the type of treatment that should best control a given hypertensive patient (220), but interpretation of the results is not simple and such determinations will probably not become routine in all initial diagnoses. In many cases, the step approach is used initially

Asp-Arg-Val-Tyr-Ile-His-Pro-Phe-His-Leu   42.**106**

Asp-Arg-Val-Tyr-Ile-His-Pro-Phe   42.**107**

Arg-Val-Tyr-Ile-His-Pro-Phe   42.**108**

5-oxoPro-Trp-Pro-Arg-Pro-Gln-Ile-Pro-Pro   42.**109**

and, if it is successful, plasma renin assays are not done.

Drugs can affect the renin–angiotensin sequence at a number of sites.

2.4.1.1 *Inhibition of Renin Release.* As discussed previously, renin release is partially controlled by the sympathetic–adrenal system. Agents interfering with sympathetic tone or effects, such as β-blockers, centrally acting antihypertensives, and neuronal blockers, all inhibit renin release. The extent of the contribution of this mechanism to the overall antihypertensive effect varies with the prevailing sympathetic tone. Aldosterone and other mineralocorticoids also may inhibit renin release directly rather than just via their effects on sodium and water excretion. Renin release caused by sodium depletion or by the use of diuretics is less sensitive to modulation by sympathetic inhibitors (221).

Agents inhibiting renin release lower arterial pressure primarily in renin-dependent hypertension, which includes renovascular and young high-renin hypertensives. These agents complement the antihypertensive effects of diuretics and vasodilating agents that cause renin release. A lowering of plasma renin activity is associated also with an increase in age.

2.4.1.2 *Inhibition of Angiotensin Converting Enzyme.* Inhibition of the converting enzyme prevents formation of angiotensin II from angiotensin I, thus aborting the effects of renin. Such converting enzyme inhibitors presently are used only as an emergency treatment for malignant hypertension (222) and as a diagnostic tool to identify those patients with renin-dependent hypertension (223). In these patients, infusion of a converting enzyme inhibitor produces a significant fall in blood pressure, which might indicate the amount of contribution of the renin–angiotensin system to the elevated arterial pressure.

Until recently, specific converting enzyme inhibition was limited to peptides structurally related to angiotensin I—notably teprotide (SQ 20,881), 42.**109** (223). Although useful as diagnostic tools (224), the peptides are not suitable for oral administration so this mechanistic approach has not been well developed for general therapy. However, a simple cysteinyl proline derivative, 42.**110**, captopril, now has been designed from the presumed active sites on the peptides (225) and is indeed antihypertensive in man as a converting enzyme inhibitor (226). The sulfhydryl group is apparently essential to chelate the zinc ions in the active center of the converting enzymes. One concern for this agent, and a significant challenge for further research, is its concomitant inhibition of bradykinin (42. **111**) decay. In addition to augmenting the vasodepressor effect of bradykinin, a biphasic hypotensive–hypertensive response is obtained because of epinephrine released from the adrenal glands (227). Agents of this type cause an increased accumulation of angiotensin I, which may result in excessive angiotensin II levels if dosage of the drug is interrupted. Converting enzyme inhibitors also interrupt the negative feedback effect on renin release, which depends on angiotensin II formation. Whether these increased plasma levels of renin and angiotensin I cause significant hypertension on withdrawal of treatment remains to be seen (228). From the preliminary human studies, captopril is effective regardless of pretreatment plasma renin levels. It remains to be determined whether the drug-induced pulse rate increase or plasma potassium increase is a clinical problem (226), and the lack of correlation with plasma renin activity is a puzzle at this time.

2.4.1.3 *Angiotensin II Antagonists.* Antagonism of angiotensin II activity, perhaps by receptor blockade, has been limited to peptide analogs of the angiotensins. Saralasin, 42.**112**, a specific and competitive inhibitor of angiotensin II, has been used

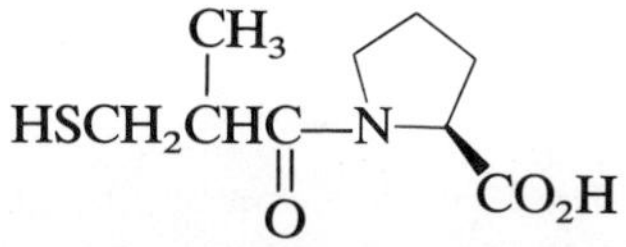

42.**110**

Arg-Pro-Pro-Gly-Phe-Ser-Pro-Phe-Arg   42.**111**

Sar-Arg-Val-Tyr-Ile-His-Pro-Ala   42.**112**

clinically as a diagnostic tool to identify renin-mediated hypertensives (229)—renovascular hypertension or high-renin essential hypertension. A 10 mg bolus of saralasin gives a rapid, brief, and marked depressor response in renin-dependent hypertensives. In hypertensive patients with normal or low plasma renin activity, no depressor response is obtained. Saralasin has been used also for hypertensive emergencies (230). It may be less desirable than converting enzyme inhibitors because it possesses some angiotensin II-like activity. This can produce a further rise in blood pressure that can be substantial and dangerous, especially in low-renin patients.

2.4.1.4 *Aldosterone Antagonists.* Spironolactone, 42.**113**, and other aldosterone antagonists find primary use in the treatment of hyperaldosteronism (231), and are frequently useful in the treatment of low-renin hypertension (232). Spironolactone has been a useful component in combination with a thiazide diuretic because it minimizes hypokalemia. The use of spironolactone has been associated with side effects such as breast tenderness and possible carcinogenesis (233). This has stimulated an effort to produce safer aldosterone antagonists with prorenoate, 42.**114** (234), and canrenoate, 42.**115** (235), being clinically investigated agents.

2.4.2 OTHER HORMONAL MECHANISMS. Peptide hormones other than those in the renin–angiotensin system could also be involved in the etiology or control of hyper-

tension. Bradykinin and related kinins such as kallidin, 42.**116**, are found in plasma and produce a direct vasodilation and increased capillary permeability. It has been previously mentioned that kinins are inactivated by the same or similar enzymes as those converting angiotensin I to II. Very potent vasodilating peptides, such as eledoisin, physalaemin, and substance P, are clinically

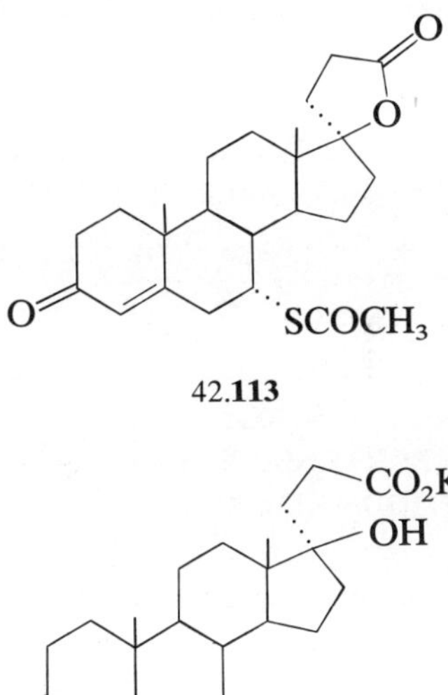

42.**113**

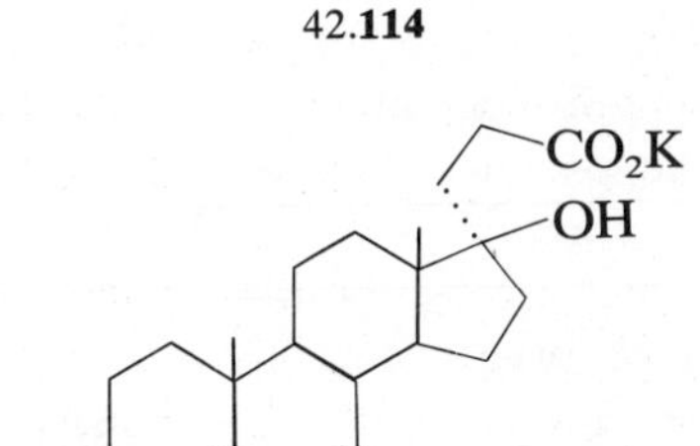

42.**114**

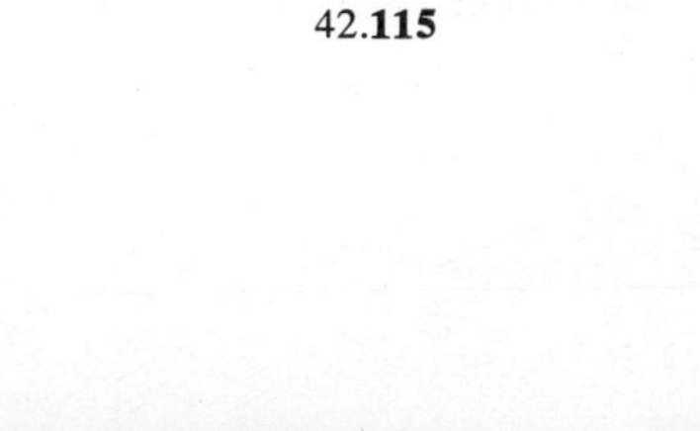

42.**115**

Lys-Arg-Pro-Pro-Gly-Phe-Ser-Pro-Phe-Arg   42.**116**

hypotensive (236), but most of these produce a secondary hypertensive response mediated via epinephrine released from the adrenal glands. Owing to the brief duration of these peptides administered parenterally and to their rapid inactivation following oral administration, they are not widely used antihypertensive agents.

Estrogens are thought to play a role in the susceptibility of females to hypertension, and perhaps in their resistance to the cardiovascular mortality resulting from long-term hypertension. But estrogens are not effective antihypertensive agents and have too many side effects for useful chronic therapy (see Chapter 29). Estrogen-containing oral contraceptives produce hypertension in up to 20% of women taking them, about 50% of whom develop a sustained hypertension with a slow onset. The pathogenesis of this hypertension may be due to their threefold increase in plasma renin activity, followed by aldosterone increases, then salt and water retention (237).

3   CHOICE AMONG ANTIHYPERTENSIVE AGENTS AND COMBINATIONS

The degree of success in treating hypertension depends on the extent of reduction in the elevated arterial pressure. Maintaining a blood pressure close to normal can, in addition to increasing survival time and reducing the incidence of vascular accidents, lead to improvement in symptoms such as headache, dyspnea, spasms, and angina that sometimes accompany hypertension.

Hygienic intervention is generally the most appropriate, responsible, and cost-effective initial approach, especially for mild hypertension. This includes weight reduction to reduce adiposity (238), moderate salt restriction (70 meq/day), smoking cessation, a reasonable physical exercise program, and an effort to remove stressful conditions or to improve coping with stress. Antihypertension drug therapy should be used initially for the moderate hypertensive patient to promptly reduce strain on the heart and arteries, but the value of treating mild hypertensives is less clear. At this time there are inadequate data on the benefits of treating mild hypertension versus the chronic risks and patient acceptance of drug side effects. The lack of symptoms from mild hypertension compared with the side effects of most drugs results in low patient compliance, and a significant number of people do not regard high blood pressure as a serious problem (239). It may be appropriate to defer drug therapy for mild hypertensives until a progressive blood pressure rise or ECG changes are seen, but data from well controlled trials are needed. Several long-term, double-blind, placebo-controlled, multicenter studies on mild hypertension are planned or underway (240–242), but it may require 5–10 years to assess any difference in the end points of death, myocardial infarction, and stroke in addition to blood pressure reductions between the treated and untreated groups.

The clinical availability of a large variety of antihypertensive agents with different profiles and side effects presents the physician with a selection problem. Although the selection should be custom fitted to each patient, some useful guidelines are applicable to the majority of patients with uncomplicated essential hypertension. The concept of a stepped-care approach has been recommended by the Joint National Committee on Detection, Evaluation, and Treatment of High Blood Pressure (203). This approach to therapy involves a small initial dose, then increasing the dose of that drug, then adding other drugs one at a time as needed. Periodic evaluations, stepping down the drug dose whenever possible, and optimizing patient convenience with minimal adverse reactions are all considered. Tranquilizers and sedatives are not recommended because they are not effective in lowering blood pressure. The important feature of this report for medicinal chemists is the specific recommendations for certain types of agents.

For patients with diastolic pressures <105 mm Hg, the first step should be a thiazide-type diuretic at a less than maximal dose. Dietary or potassium supplements or potassium-sparing diuretics should be used to manage hypokalemia when below 3.2 mEq/1. The therapeutic goal is to maintain diastolic pressure at <90 mm Hg with minimal adverse effects. If the therapeutic goal is not reached with a thiazide alone, the second step involves addition of propranolol, methyldopa, or reserpine to the regimen. Any of these drugs may be effective in some patients and ineffective in others. Reserpine offers once-a-day administration, low cost, and high efficacy versus possible depression and lethargy. The drowsiness, fatigue, and possible impotence from methyldopa may limit its use (243), and fatigue or aggravation of a heart condition or asthma may limit propranolol. Tolerance to any of these three may indicate fluid retention and a need to increase the diuretic dose. Clonidine or prazosin may be substituted as a step 2 drug even though there is less clinical experience with them. Dry mouth and drowsiness are common with clonidine, whereas postural dizziness, weakness, or sudden collapse may be limiting for prazosin. There is no reason to use simultaneously two drugs of the same type, such as two thiazides or two β-blockers (244). If the therapeutic goal is still not reached, hydralazine may be added as step 3, but should be used in combination with a diuretic and β-blocker. If the first three steps still fail to achieve

the therapeutic goal, and other causes for unresponsiveness have been investigated, guanethidine may be added as step 4. Even though guanethidine is potent and often effective in refractory cases, patients require more supervision owing to the incidence of postural dizziness, diarrhea, and ejaculatory failure. The stepped-care approach is also advocated for patients with diastolic pressures of 105–129 mm Hg, but treatment may be initiated with a full dose of thiazide and other drugs added more rapidly to achieve blood pressure control sooner. Patients with diastolic pressures >130 mm Hg may require urgent treatment with several drugs simultaneously. At low doses the drugs mentioned for step 2, 3, or 4 each normalize blood pressure for mild hypertensives about as well as thiazides, but the stepped approach accommodates the lifelong need to manage blood pressure as close to normal as possible with minimal adverse effects for patient compliance. This approach offers convenient guidelines to the physician who may not be close·to a hypertension clinic in order to initially investigate pathophysiologic causes of the high blood pressure, and it will most likely have a profound effect on prescribing practices. Clearly this tells the medicinal chemist that he should seek new agents with minimal adverse side effects and minimal ancillary pharmacological or compensatory effects on cardiac output or extracellular fluid volume, not just agents that lower blood pressure.

In the treatment of severe hypertension, intravenous sodium nitroprusside or diazoxide are generally used to produce an immediate lowering of blood pressure. Minoxidil may be valuable for the acute oral maintenance of such patients. A combination of a diuretic, vasodilator, β-blocker, neuronal blocker, and a centrally acting agent may be needed for adequate chronic blood pressure control of resistant patients—no one type of agent is usually sufficient.

An alternate to the stepped-care approach is used in some of the hypertension clinics. Patients, especially those with >105 mm Hg diastolic pressures, are thoroughly examined and tested to ascertain an etiologic or pathophysiological cause when possible. Plasma renin profiles (245), several renal function tests, sodium balance, cardiac performance, and sometimes serum catecholamines are determined. From a more extensive diagnosis, a rational therapeutic regimen can be selected that may recognize a specific cause and more effectively or rapidly achieve the therapeutic goal (246). Whether the extra time and cost to achieve this approach are justified or desired depends on individual circumstances. Fewer drugs may be required to achieve the therapeutic goal by individualized therapy than by automatically adding agents by the stepped approach. This rational approach may underlie the trend towards selection of β-blockers as the initial agent for treating hypertension (140). The thiazide diuretics are not recommended for high-renin hypertension, and their side effects do detract somewhat from their value in chronic use (208). Although the chronic impact of β-blocker use may be less severe, they have not been as widely used alone. β-Blockers are additonally useful in angina and cardiac arrhythmias, which are often associated with hypertension.

We have discussed the mechanisms and side effects of each agent individually and mentioned the advantages of some rational combinations. Several fixed combinations are designed to minimize the adverse and compensatory effects of single agents, to require lower doses of each drug in the combination than when used alone, and to more effectively achieve the therapeutic goal by affecting several mechanisms at once. This can be achieved not only by the stepped approach but also by use of fixed combinations.

The use of potassium-sparing diuretics combined with thiazide diuretics is widespread for reasons previously mentioned.

Vasodilators like hydralazine produce reflex cardiostimulation, renin release, and fluid retention. Hence fixed combinations of vasodilators with thiazide diuretics or β-blockers are becoming popular. The vasodilator and β-blocker offset each other's side effects except fluid retention. The vasodilator and diuretic offset each other's side effects except tachycardia, leading to increased cardiac output. Fixed combinations of β-blockers with thiazide diuretics are now being used with some reduction of the hypokalemia and hyperuricemia at equieffective doses. Sympathetic inhibitors may also moderate the reflex cardiostimulation and renin release due to vasodilators. It is expected that use of such fixed combinations may also allow step 3 or 4 drugs to be used sooner and more widely in combination than alone. This may permit a more rapid achievement of the therapeutic goal. Fixed combinations are more convenient for the patient, which should improve compliance although they lack the flexibility of titrating the patient to his optimum combination dosage. Certainly the pharmacokinetics of each drug should be considered in establishing fixed dosage combinations.

The combination of several desired mechanisms into a single agent has been achieved with prazosin and labetalol as previously discussed. Now the combination of direct vasodilation with β-blockade is in the development stage, but combining diuretic properties with β-blockade, vasodilation, or sympathetic inhibition awaits the ingenuity of medicinal chemists. An improved understanding of prostaglandin functions in vascular and renal tissue, plus an improved knowledge of the renin–angiotensin system, will certainly aid this search at least conceptually.

4 MODELS FOR TESTING ANTIHYPERTENSIVE AGENTS

Animal models of hypertension useful in the screening and evaluation of antihypertensive drug candidates are generally developed utilizing genetic, neural, stress, renal, and salt factors either singly or in combination. These models generally respond to most classes of antihypertensive drugs; they only reflect isolated aspects of what is probably a multifactoral human disease. No available animal model of hypertension responds to two main classes of antihypertensive agents—the diuretics and β-adrenoceptor blockers—with a consistent fall in blood pressure that duplicates the human response. Direct tests for diuretic activity and β-blocking actions have to a large degree obviated the need for animal models of hypertension that respond to these two classes of drugs. In this section, the major animal models of hypertension are briefly discussed.

4.1 Genetic Models of Hypertension

4.1.1 SPONTANEOUSLY HYPERTENSIVE RATS. The most widely used antihypertensive animal model is a strain of spontaneously hypertensive rats (SHR), generally referred to as the Okamoto–Aoki strain (247); it is perhaps the closest animal model to human essential hypertension (248). This model is particularly sensitive to those antihypertensive agents that interfere with sympathetic function. It is not consistently sensitive acutely to the antihypertensive effects of diuretics or β-blockers.

SHR appear to reflect a nonspecific genetic defect since disorders in other hormonal systems related to the thyroid and unrelated to hypertension exist in these animals. Such disorders are not generally associated with human essential hypertension. Genetically there is no good normotensive control for this model, and inadequate approximations of controls are consistently and unjustifiably used.

4.1.2 GENETICALLY HYPERTENSIVE RATS. This rat strain (GHR) differs in a number of respects from the Japanese strain (249) and is also sensitive to the anti-

hypertensive effects of most classes of antihypertensive agents (250). Furthermore, GHR appear to respond to β-blockers with a lowering of blood pressure similar in profile to their effects in human essential hypertension (251). The problem with normotensive controls is similar to that with the SHR.

4.1.3 MILAN HYPERTENSIVE RATS. The defect underlying hypertension in this strain, developed by Bianchi and associates (252), appears to be an inability to excrete sodium. Thus this is basically a volume-dependent type hypertension brought about by physical defects in the filtration membranes of the kidney (253). Since a similar etiology is not widely found in human essential hypertension, the predictive value of this model is yet to be determined.

4.1.4 SPONTANEOUS HYPERTENSION IN OTHER SPECIES. Studies have been published using dogs (254) and monkeys (255) with spontaneously elevated blood pressure. The isolation of a genetically hypertensive strain of large animals would be helpful since it would allow better study of the hemodynamic profiles of new antihypertensive agents where manipulation that is difficult or impossible in rats can be carried out with greater ease.

4.2 Renal Models of Hypertension

The demonstration by Goldblatt (256) that renal artery constriction in dogs can lead to chronic hypertension pioneered the way for development of a variety of renal hypertensive models, not only in dogs but also in other species. Involvement of the renin–angiotensin system is the major focus, although other factors may be more important in the maintenance of the elevated arterial pressure in some of these models (257).

4.2.1 TWO KIDNEY GOLDBLATT HYPERTENSION. In this model, which can be done in a number of species including rat, dog, and rabbit, the renal artery is constricted to one kidney whereas the other kidney is left intact. This form of hypertension is totally renin-dependent and is exquisitely sensitive to agents that interfere with the renin–angiotensin system such as angiotensin II inhibitors or β-blockers (258). This may not be true for rabbits (259) or dogs (260), however. This model also responds to antihypertensive agents acting directly on the vascular smooth muscle or interfering with sympathetic outflow.

4.2.2 ONE KIDNEY GOLDBLATT HYPERTENSION. This type of hypertension can be produced in rats, dogs, and other species. In this model, one renal artery is constricted and the other kidney is removed. In its initial stages, this model of hypertension is renin-dependent (261, 262). Later, renin release is suppressed due to excessive accumulation of salt and water, and the hypertension becomes volume dependent. There appears to be no involvement of the sympathetic nervous system in the development or maintenance of this type of hypertension (263).

4.2.3 KIDNEY-STRESS MODELS. Ways other than renal artery constriction were developed to stress the kidney and a variety of models have been developed in a number of species. These include cellophane wrap in rats and dogs (264, 265) and figure 8 ligature in rats and dogs. In general, these models differ little from the renal artery constriction models and present similar biochemical and hemodynamic profiles depending on whether one or both kidneys are involved.

4.3 Excess Salt Models of Hypertension

Dahl (266) isolated a genetic strain of rats that were particularly sensitive to salt and easily developed hypertension on saltwater. The administration of salt-retaining steroids strongly facilitates the development of salt hypertension in rats and dogs (267), although chronic salt administration alone is effective. Man and rat respond similarly to excessive salt with very similar vascular changes in the renal arteries and arterioles. Furthermore, excessive salt administration can increase the severity of hypertension in other hypertensive animal models and increase the incidence of mortality and cerebro- or cardiovascular accidents (268). DOCA (deoxycorticosterone acetate) hypertensive rats, with or without unilateral nephrectomy, are used extensively as a screening model for antihypertensive agents, primarily because of the ease of their preparation and their sensitivity to diuretics and other classes of antihypertensive agents. Only the β-adrenergic blockers fail to produce consistent antihypertensive responses following oral administration in this model. It should be emphasized that this model is characterized by excessive sympathetic tone (269) in addition to blood volume factors, hence its value for a wider variety of antihypertensive agents.

4.4 Neurogenic Hypertension Models

Neurogenically produced hypertension has been established with a variety of techniques.

4.4.1 NTS-LESIONED HYPERTENSIVE ANIMALS. Producing a lesion in the nucleus tractus solitarius eliminates pressure signals going to the sympathetic nerve control center of the brain and causes acute elevations of blood pressure in rats that are fatal in the first day (270). In the cat, similar lesions produce hypertension (271). The elevated blood pressure is due almost entirely to elevated sympathetic tone. It is valuable as a mechanistic tool to isolate the sympathetic effects of candidate drugs.

4.4.2 STRESS HYPERTENSIVE RATS. Several models of hypertension produced by neurogenic stress have been developed in rats (272–274). These models are considered to closely represent hypertension associated with stressful industrialized societies. The animals generally develop moderately elevated levels of arterial pressure that become independent of the stress for at least several weeks. These animals respond well to the various classes of antihypertensive agents and may represent a model sensitive to the antihypertensive effects of β-blockers (275).

4.5 Other Animal Models of Hypertension

Several other models of hypertension based on a variety of factors have been developed (276–278). These models have only limited utility based primarily on the etiologic factors involved.

The use of several animal models of hypertension, based on multiple etiologic factors, ensures greater confidence in the applicability of the results obtained to human essential hypertension, since the latter is generally believed to be a multifactoral disease. Reliance on a single animal model of hypertension could bias the interpretation of the antihypertensive activity of a particular compound or class of compounds. Each of the above-mentioned models is more sensitive to particular classes of antihypertensive agents but less sensitive or insensitive to others. Care must be exercised in the interpretation of the data obtained with any one model in relation to the etiologic factors involved in its development.

REFERENCES

1. W. C. Roberts, *Am. J. Med.*, **59,** 523 (1975).

2. W. B. Kannel, *Angiology*, **26,** 1 (1975).

3. H. D. Itskovitz, in *New Antihypertensive Drugs*, A. Scriabine and C. S. Sweet, Eds., Spectrum Publications, New York, 1976, pp. 3–12.

4. I. H. Page, *Arch. Intern. Med.*, **111,** 103 (1963).

5. Veterans Administration Cooperative Study, *J. Am. Med. Assoc.*, **202,** 1028–1034 (1967).

6. Veterans Administration Cooperative Study, *J. Am. Med. Assoc.*, **213,** 1143–1152 (1970).

7. I. H. Page, *J. Am. Med. Assoc.*, **140,** 451 (1949).

8. M. Mendlowitz, *Am. Heart J.*, **73,** 121 (1967).

9. D. T. Horrobin, *Lancet*, **1966 I,** 574.

10. H. Aars, *Scand. J. Clin. Lab. Invest.*, **35,** 97 (1975).

11. W. S. Peart, *Pharmacol. Rev.*, **18,** 667 (1966).

12. M. Mendlowitz and N. D. Vlachakis, *Am. Heart J.*, **91,** 378 (1976).

13. J. H. Laragh, in *New Antihypertensive Drugs*, A. Scriabine and C. S. Sweet, Eds., Spectrum Publications, New York, 1976, pp. 167–178.

14. H. Aoyagi, K. Arakawa, and N. Izumiya, *Bull. Chem. Soc. Jap.*, **41,** 433 (1968).

15. S. Bergstrom, *Science*, **157,** 382 (1967).

16. J. R. Vane and J. C. McGiff, *Circ. Res.*, **36–37**:Suppl. I, I-68 (1975).

17. J. I. S. Robertson, *Brit. J. Hosp. Med.*, **11,** 707 (1974).

18. H. S. Margolin, D. Horwitz, J. J. Pisano, and H. R. Keiser, *Fed. Proc.*, **35,** 203 (1976).

19. J. Möhring, B. Möhring, M. Petri, and D. Haack, *Lancet*, **1976-I,** 170.

20. A. C. Guyton, T. G. Coleman, A. W. Cowley, R. D. Manning, Jr., R. A. Norman, Jr., and J. D. Ferguson, *Circ. Res.*, **35,** 159 (1974).

21. A. C. Guyton, D. B. Young, J. W. DeClue, J. D. Ferguson, R. E. McCaa, A. Gevise, N. C. Trippado, and J. E. Hall, "The Role of the Kidney in Hypertension," in *Pathophysiology and Management of Arterial Hypertension*, G. Berglund, L. Hansson, and L. Werkö, Eds., Astra Pharmaceuticals A. B., Sweden, 1975, pp. 78.

22. E. D. Freis, *Circulation*, **53,** 589 (1976).

23. S. C. Glauser, C. T. Bello, and E. M. Glauser, *Lancet*, **1976-I,** 717.

24. L. B. Page, *Am. Heart J.*, **91,** 527 (1976).

25. B. Folkow, M. Hallbäck, Y. Lundgren, R. Sivertsson, R. S. and L. Weiss, *Circ. Res.*, **32**:Suppl. I, I-2 (1973).

26. B. Folkow, "Vascular Changes in Hypertension-Review and Recent Animal Studies," in *Pathophysiology and Management of Arterial Hypertension*, G. Berglund, L. Hansson, and L. Werkö, Eds., Astra Pharmaceuticals A. B., Sweden, 1975, pp. 95.

27. E. A. Murphy, *Circ. Res.*, **32–33**: Suppl. I, I-129 (1973).

28. E. D. Frohlich, *Hosp. Pract.* **9,** 59 (1974).

29. E. Iisalo and A. Lehtonen, *Ann. Clin. Res.,* **7,** 71 (1975).

30. E. D. Freis, *J. Am. Med. Assoc.,* **232,** 1017 (1975).

31. E. D. Freis and J. R. Stanton, *Am. Heart J.,* **36,** 723 (1948).

32. H. L. Borison, V. F. Fairbanks, and C. A. White, *Arch. Int. Pharmacodyn. Ther.,* **101,** 189 (1955).

33. S. M. Kupchan, *J. Pharm. Sci.,* **50,** 273 (1961).

34. W. T. Comer and A. W. Gomoll, in *Medicinal Chemistry,* A. Burger, Ed., 3rd ed. Wiley, New York, 1970, pp. 1019–1064.

35. W. I. Cranston, in *Antihypertensive Therapy,* F. Gross, Ed., Springer-Verlag, Berlin, 1966, p. 184.

36. A. D. Bender, in *Topics in Medicinal Chemistry,* J. L. Rabinowitz and R. M. Myerson, Eds., Wiley-Interscience, New York, 1967, pp. 177–239.

37. W. Hoefke, W. Kobinger, and A. Walland, *Arzneim.-Forsch.,* **25,** 786–793 (1975).

38. W. Hoefke, in *Antihypertensive Agents,* E. L. Engelhardt, Ed., American Chemical Society, Washington, D. C., 1976, pp. 27–54.

39. W. Hoefke, in *New Antihypertensive Drugs,* A. Scriabine and C. S. Sweet, Eds., Spectrum Publications, New York, 1976, pp. 441–459.

40. H. Schmitt and H. Schmitt, *Eur. J. Pharmacol.,* **6,** 8 (1969).

41. A. Walland, W. Kobinger, and A. Csongrady, *Eur. J. Pharmacol.,* **26,** 184 (1974).

42. G. Haeusler, *Naunyn-Schmiedebergs Arch. Pharmakol.,* **295,** 191 (1976).

43. L. Hansson, S. N. Hunyor, S. Julius, and S. W. Hoobler, *Am. Heart J.,* **85,** 605 (1973).

44. R. H. Briant, J. L. Reid, and C. T. Dollery, *Brit. Med. J. I.* **1973,** 522.

45. H. Stähle, in *Medicinal Chemistry,* J. Maas, Ed., Elsevier, Amsterdam, 1974, pp. 75–105.

46. R. Laverty, *Eur. J. Pharmacol.,* **9,** 163 (1969).

47. T. L. Kho, M. A. D. H. Schalekamp, G. A. Zaal, A. Wester, and W. H. Birkenhäger, *Arch. Int. Pharmacodyn. Ther.,* **217,** 162 (1975).

48. A. Heise, in *New Antihypertensive Drugs,* A. Scriabine and C. S. Sweet, Eds., Spectrum Publications, New York, 1976, pp. 135–145.

49. G. Kroneberg, A. Oberdorf, F. Hoffmeister, and W. Wirth, *Naunyn-Schmiedebergs Arch. Pharmakol. Exp. Pathol.,* **256,** 257 (1967).

50. T. Jen, H. Van Hoeven, W. Groves, R. A. McLean, and B. Loev, *J. Med. Chem.,* **18,** 90 (1975).

51. E. Linder and J. Kaiser, *Arch. Int. Pharmacodyn. Ther.,* **211,** 305 (1974).

52. P. Simon, R. Chermat, and J-R. Boissier, *Therapie,* **30,** 855 (1975).

53. F. Kersting, *Arzneim.-Forsch.,* **23,** 1657 (1973).

54. T. Baum, A. T. Shropshire, G. Rowles, R. Van Pelt, S. P. Fernandez, D. K. Eckfeld, and M. I. Gluckman, *J. Pharmacol. Exp. Ther.,* **171,** 276 (1970).

55. P. Bosanac, J. Dubb, B. Walker, M. Goldberg, and Z. S. Agus, *J. Clin. Pharmacol.,* **16,** 631 (1976).

56. T. Baum and A. T. Shropshire, *Eur. J. Pharmacol.,* **37,** 31 (1976).

57. G. Scholtysik, H. Lauener, E. Eichenberger, H. Bürki, R. Salzmann, E. Müller-Schweinitzer, and R. Waite, *Arzneim.-Forsch.,* **25,** 1483 (1975).

58. A. S. Turner, *XII World Congr. Cardiol., Buenos Aires,* 1974, abstr. no. 336.

59. A. Jaattela, *Eur. J. Clin. Pharmacol.,* **10,** 69, 73 (1976).

60. I. Esch, *Int. J. Clin. Pharmacol. Ther. Toxicol.,* **14,** 109 (1976).

61. J. B. Bream, H. Lauener, C. W. Picard, G. Scholtysik, and T. G. White, *Arzneim.-Forsch.,* **25,** 1477 (1975).

62. P. A. van Zwieten, *Pharmacology,* **13,** 352 (1975).

63. P. A. van Zwieten, *Arch. Int. Pharmacodyn. Ther.,* **215,** 104 (1975).

64. D. Wellens, L. Snoeckx, R. DeReese, R. Kruger, A. Van de Water, L. Wouters, and R. S. Reneman, *Arch. Int. Pharmacodyn. Ther,* **215,** 119 (1975).

65. L. Finch, *Eur. J. Pharmacol.,* **33,** 409 (1975).

66. D. Wellens, J. M. Van Nueten, and P. A. J. Janssen, *Arch. Int. Pharmacodyn. Ther.,* **213,** 334 (1975).

67. Editorial: Side Effects of Methyldopa, *Brit. Med. J.,* **1,** 646 (1975).

68. T. L. Sourkes, *Arch. Biochem. Biophys.,* **51,** 444 (1954).

69. J. A. Oates, L. Gillespie, Jr., S. Udenfriend, and A. Sjoerdsma, *Science,* **131,** 1890 (1960).

70. T. L. Sourkes and H. R. Rodriguez, in *Antihypertensive Agents,* E. Schlittler, Ed., Academic, New York, 1967, pp. 151–189.

71. R. J. Levine and A. Sjoerdsma, *J. Pharmacol. Exp. Ther.,* **146,** 42 (1964).

72. E. Muscholl, *Ann. Rev. Pharmacol.,* **6,** 107 (1966).

73. N. F. Albertson, F. C. McKay, H. E. Lape, J. O. Hoppe, W. H. Selberis, and A. Arnold, *J. Med. Chem.,* **13,** 132 (1970).

74. W. S. Saari, A. W. Raab, W. H. Staas, M. L. Torchiana, C. C. Porter, and C. A. Stone, *J. Med. Chem.*, **13**, 1057 (1970).

75. R. E. Rangno, J. S. Kaufmann, J. H. Cavanaugh, D. Island, J. T. Watson, and J. Oates, *J. Clin. Invest.*, **52**, 952 (1973).

76. K. Engelman, D. Horwitz, E. Jéquier, and A. Sjoerdsma, *J. Clin. Invest.*, **47**, 577 (1968).

77. A. H. El Masry, S. E. El Masry, L. E. Hane, and R. E. Counsell, *J. Med. Chem.*, **18**, 16 (1975).

78. M. Ohno, M. Okamoto, N. Kawabe, H. Umezawa, T. Takeuchi, H. Inuma, and S. Takahashi, *J. Am. Chem. Soc.*, **93**, 1285 (1971).

79. T. Kimura, E. Takahashi, M. Ozawa, S. Uchiyama, S. Maekawa, O. Yashima, and M. Sato, *Clin. Sci. Mol. Med.*, **48**, 1755 (1975).

80. T. Nagatsu, H. Hidaka, H. Kuzuya, K. Takeya, H. Umezawa, T. Takeuchi, and H. Suda, *Biochem. Pharmacol.*, **19**, 35 (1970).

81. F. Terazawa, L. H. Ying, T. Suzuki, and H. Hidaka, *Jap. Circ. J.*, **40**, 1033 (1976).

82. S. Symchowicz and M. Staub, *J. Pharmacol. Exp. Ther.*, **191**, 324 (1974).

83. S. G. Chrysant, P. Adamopoulos, M. Tsuchiya, and E. D. Frohlich, *Am. Heart J.*, **92**, 335 (1976).

84. Y. Ishii, C. Mimura, and M. Homma, *J. Pharmacol. Exp. Ther.*, **198**, 589 (1976).

85. H. Hidaka, F. Shoka, Y. Hashizume, N. Takemoto, and M. Yamamoto, *Jap. J. Pharmacol.*, **25**, 515 (1975).

86. T. Nakamura, H. Yasuda, A. Obayashi, O. Tanabe, S. Matsumura, F. Ueda, and K. Ohata, *J. Antibiot.*, **28**, 277 (1975).

87. L. B. Page and J. J. Sidd, *N. Engl. J. Med.*, **287**, 1074 (1976).

88. R. A. Lucas, *Progr. Med. Chem.*, **3**, 146 (1963).

89. E. Schlittler and H. J. Bein, in *Antihypertensive Agents*, E. Schlittler, Ed., Academic, New York, 1967, pp. 191–221.

90. R. B. Woodward, F. E. Bader, H. Bickel, A. J. Frey, and R. W. Kierstead, *J. Am. Chem. Soc.*, **78**, 2023, 2657 (1956).

91. A. F. Green, *Advan. Pharmacol.*, **1**, 161 (1962).

92. L. L. Iversen, J. Glowinski, and J. Axelrod, *J. Pharmacol. Exp. Ther.*, **150**, 173 (1965).

93. T. M. Mack, B. E. Henderson, V. R. Gerkins, M. Arthur, J. Baptista, and M. C. Pike, *N. Engl. J. Med.*, **292**, 1366 (1975).

94. V. Trcka, A. Dlabac, and M. Vanecek, *Life Sci.*, **4**, 2257 (1965).

95. V. Trcka and A. Carlsson, *Life Sci.*, **4**, 2263 (1965).

96. B. S. Jandkyala, D. E. Clarke, and J. P. Buckley, *J. Pharm. Sci.*, **63**, 1497 (1974).

97. R. P. Mull and R. A. Maxwell, in *Antihypertensive Agents*, E. Schlittler, Ed., Academic, New York, 1967, pp. 115–149.

98. A. L. Boura and A. F. Green, *Ann. Rev. Pharmacol.*, **5**, 183 (1965).

99. I. H. Page and H. P. Dustan, *J. Am. Med. Assoc.*, **170**, 1265 (1959).

100. T. P. Pruss, in *New Antihypertensive Drugs*, A. Scriabine and C. S. Sweet, Eds., Spectrum Publications, New York, 1976, pp. 347–357.

101. E. Schlittler, J. Druey, and A. Marxer, *Progr. Drug Res.*, **4**, 341 (1962).

102. A. L. A. Boura, T. C. Copp, A. F. Green, H. F. Hodson, G. K. Ruffell, M. R. Sim, E. Walton, and E. M. Grivsky, *Nature*, **191**, 1312 (1961).

103. M. Blechman, C. Sokol, and M. Moser, *Curr. Ther. Res.*, **11**, 71 (1969).

104. W. L. Matier, D. A. Owens, W. T. Comer, D. Deitchman, H. C. Ferguson, R. J. Seidehamel, and J. R. Young, *J. Med. Chem.*, **16**, 901 (1973).

105. D. Deitchman, J. L. Perhach, and G. R. McKinney, in *New Antihypertensive Drugs*, A. Scriabine and C. S. Sweet, Eds., Spectrum Publications, New York, 1976, pp. 387–408.

106. J. Ruedy and R. O. Davies, *Clin. Pharmacol. Ther.*, **8**, 38 (1967).

107. T. D. V. Lawrie, A. R. Lorimer, S. G. McAlpine, and H. Reinert, *Brit. Med. J.*, **1**, 402 (1964).

108. J. Augstein, S. M. Green, A. M. Monro, T. I. Wrigley, A. R. Katritzky, and G. J. T. Tiddy, *J. Med. Chem.*, **10**, 391 (1967).

109. L. Hansson, A. Pascual, and S. Julius, *Clin. Pharmacol. Ther.*, **14**, 204 (1973).

110. T. Jen and C. Kaiser, *J. Med. Chem.*, **20**, 693 (1977).

111. R. P. Ahlquist, *Am. J. Physiol.*, **153**, 586 (1948).

112. R. P. Ahlquist, *J. Pharm. Sci.*, **55**, 359 (1966).

113. D. J. Triggle, in *Chemical Aspects of the Autonomic Nervous System*, Academic, New York, 1965, pp. 198–266.

114. L. H. Werner and W. E. Barrett, in *Antihypertensive Agents*, E. Schlittler, Ed., Academic, New York, 1967, pp. 331–392.

115. M. Nickerson and L. S. Goodman, *J. Pharmacol. Exp. Ther.*, **89**, 167 (1947).

116. N. B. Chapman and J. D. P. Graham, in *Drugs Affecting the Peripheral Nervous System*, A. Burger, Ed., Vol. 1, Dekker, New York, 1967, pp. 496–511.

117. J. F. Moran, M. May, H. Kimelberg, and D. J. Triggle, *Mol. Pharmacol.*, **3**, 15, 28 (1967).

118. J. W. Constantine, in *Prazosin—Evaluation of a New Antihypertensive Agent*, D. W. K. Cotten, Ed., American Elsevier, New York, 1974, pp. 16–33.

119. R. Massingham and M. L. Hayden, *Eur. J. Pharmacol.*, **30,** 121 (1975).

120. M. E. Kosman, *J. Am. Med. Assoc.*, **238,** 157 (1977).

121. R. M. Graham, I. R. Thornell, J. M. Gain, C. Bagnoli, H. F. Oates, and G. S. Stokes, *Brit. Med. J.*, **2,** 1293 (1976).

122. H-J. Hess, T. H. Cronin, and A. Scriabine, *J. Med. Chem.*, **11,** 130 (1968).

123. A. Scriabine, J. W. Constantine, H-J. Hess, and W. K. McShane, *Experientia*, **24,** 1150 (1968).

124. N. D. Vlachakis, M. Mendlowitz, and D. DeG. DeGuzman, *Curr. Ther. Res.*, **17,** 564 (1975).

125. J. L. Archibald, P. Fairbrother, and J. L. Jackson, *J. Med. Chem.*, **17,** 739 (1974).

126. T. Baum, A. T. Shropshire, D. K. Eckfeld, N. Metz, J. L. Dinish, J. R. Peters, F. Butz, and M. S. Gluckman, *Arch. Int. Pharmacodyn. Ther.*, **204,** 390 (1973).

127. T. Baum and A. T. Shropshire, *Eur. J. Pharmacol.*, **32,** 30 (1975).

128. J. Ramirez, *Curr. Med. Res. Opin.*, **4,** 177 (1976).

129. S. W. Hoobler and A. S. Dontas, *Pharmacol. Rev.*, **5,** 135 (1953).

130. E. Pogliani, A. Della Volpe, R. Ferrari, P. Recalcati, and C. Praga, *Farm. Ed. Prat.*, **30,** 630 (1975).

131. V. B. Zakirov, *Farmakol. Toksikol.*, **35,** 708 (1972).

132. C. E. Powell and I. H. Slater, *J. Pharmacol. Exp. Ther.*, **122,** 480 (1958).

133. *Ann. N.Y. Acad. Sci.*, **139,** 549–1009 (1967).

134. M. S. K. Ghouri and T. J. Haley, *J. Pharm. Sci.*, **58,** 511 (1969).

135. P. N. Patil, A. Tye, and J. B. La Pidus, *J. Pharmacol. Exp. Ther.*, **156,** 445 (1967).

136. D. A. Riggle, W. T. Comer, and H. R. Roth, *Proc. Soc. Exp. Biol. & Med.*, **140,** 667 (1972).

137. J. Augstein, D. A. Cox, A. L. Ham, P. R. Leeming, and M. Snarey, *J. Med. Chem.*, **16,** 1245 (1973).

138. M. L. Hoefle, S. G. Hastings, R. F. Meyer, R. M. Corey, A. Holmes, and C. D. Stratton, *J. Med. Chem.*, **18,** 148 (1975).

139. P. Kincaid-Smith, I. M. MacDonald, A. Hua, M. C. Laver, and P. Fang, *Med. J. Aust.*, **1,** 327 (1975).

140. F. O. Simpson, *Drugs*, **11**:Suppl. 1, 45–47 (1976).

141. F. R. Bühler, J. H. Laragh, E. D. Vaughan, Jr., H. R. Brunner, H. Gavras, and L. Baer, *Am. J. Cardiol.*, **32,** 511 (1973).

142. J. H. Laragh, *Am. J. Med.*, **61,** 797 (1976).

143. F. J. Zacharias, *Postgrad. Med.*, **52**:Suppl. 4, 87 (1976).

144. W. A. Pettinger and H. C. Mitchell, *Aust. N. Z. J. Med.*, **6**:Suppl. 3, 76 (1976).

145. J. I. Drayer, H. J. Keim, M. A. Weber, D. B. Case, and J. H. Laragh, *Am. J. Med.*, **60,** 897 (1976).

146. F. R. Bühler, J. H. Laragh, L. Baer, E. D. Vaughan, Jr., and H. R. Brunner, *N. Engl. J. Med.*, **287,** 1209 (1975).

147. J. D. Fitzgerald, in *Pathophysiology and Management of Arterial Hypertension*, G. Berghend, L. Hansson, and L. Werkö, Eds., Astra Pharmaceuticals A. B., Sweden, 1975, pp. 211.

148. M. S. Amer, *Biochem. Pharmacol.*, **26,** 171 (1977).

149. M. Weinstock, *Life Sci.*, **19,** 1453 (1976).

150. C. Davidson, U. Thadani, W. Singleton, and S. H. Taylor, *Brit. Med. J.*, **2,** 7 (1976).

151. R. Clarkson, *ACS Symp. Ser.*, **27,** 1 (1976).

152. H. J. Waal-Manning and F. O. Simpson, *Lancet*, **1971-II,** 1264

153. B. N. C. Prichard, A. J. Boakes, and G. Day, *Postgrad. Med. J.*, **47**:Suppl. 84 (1971).

154. F. O. Simpson, *Drugs*, **7,** 85–105 (1974).

155. F. H. H. Leenen, in *β-Adrenoceptor Blocking Agents*, P. R. Saxena and R. P. Forsyth, Eds., North-Holland, Amsterdam, 1976.

156. R. C. Tarazi, H. P. Dustan, and E. L. Bravo, *Postgrad. Med. J.*, **52**:Suppl. 4, 92 (1976).

157. A. Amery, L. Billiet, A. Boel, R. Fagard, T. Reybrouck, and J. Willems, *Am. Heart J.*, **91,** 634 (1976).

158. J. F. Giudicelli, F. Lhoste, and J. R. Bossier, *Eur. J. Pharmacol.*, **31,** 216 (1975).

159. V. M. S. Oh, C. M. Kaye, S. J. Warrington, E. A. Taylor, and J. Wadsworth, *Brit. J. Clin. Pharm.*, **5,** 107 (1978).

160. I. Amende, in *β-Adrenoceptor Blocking Agents*, P. R. Saxena and R. P. Forsyth, Eds., North Holland Publishing Co., Amsterdam, 1976.

161. R. G. Shanks, *Postgrad. Med. J.*, **52**:Suppl. 4, 14 (1976).

162. M. E. Connolly, F. Kersting, and C. T. Dollery, *Progr. Cardiovasc. Dis.*, **19,** 203 (1976).

163. R. T. Brittain and G. P. Levy, *Brit. J. Clin. Pharmacol.*, **3**:Suppl. 3, 681 (1976).

164. J. J. Baldwin, R. Hirschmann, P. K. Lumma, W. C. Lumma, Jr., G. S. Ponticello, C. S. Sweet, and A. Scriabine, *J. Med. Chem.*, **20,** 1024 (1977).

165. J. G. Topliss, M. H. Sherlock, H. Reimann, L. M. Konzelman, E. P. Shapiro, B. W. Petterson, H. Schneider, and N. Sperber, *J. Med. Chem.*, **6**, 122 (1963).

166. J. G. Topliss and M. D. Yudis, *J. Med. Chem.*, **15**, 394 (1972).

167. L. Raffa, L. Lilla, and E. Grana, *Farm. Ed. Sci.*, **29**, 411 (1974).

168. M. Shimizu, K. Yoshida, T. Kadokawa, N. Hatano, J. Kuwashima, K. Nakatsuji, I. Nose, and M. Kobayashi, *Experientia*, **33**, 55 (1977).

169. W. L. Matier and W. T. Comer, *J. Med. Chem.*, **17**, 549 (1974).

170. J. G. Topliss, L. M. Konzelman, N. Sperber, and F. E. Roth, *J. Med. Chem.*, **7**, 453 (1964).

171. J. Druey and J. Tripod, in *Antihypertensive Agents*, E. Schlittler, Ed., Academic, New York, 1967, pp. 223–262.

172. B. Ablad and G. Johnson, *Acta Pharmacol. Toxicol.*, **20**, 1 (1963).

173. M. S. Amer and W. E. Kreighbaum, *J. Pharm. Sci.*, **64**, 1 (1975).

174. J. Koch-Weser, *Am. Heart J.*, **95**, 1 (1978).

175. R. Zacest and J. Koch-Weser, *Clin. Pharmacol. Ther.*, **13**, 420 (1972).

176. H. M. Perry, Jr., *Am. J. Med.*, **54**, 58 (1973).

177. J. Koch-Weser, *N. Engl. J. Med.*, **295**, 320 (1976).

178. A. Akashi, T. Chiba, and A. Kasahara, *Eur. J. Pharmacol.*, **29**, 161 (1974).

179. C. DePonti, U. Bardi, and M. Marchetti, *Arzneim.-Forsch.*, **26**, 2089 (1976).

180. G. Pifferi, F. Parravicini, C. Carpi, and L. Dorigotti, *J. Med. Chem.*, **18**, 741 (1975).

181. L. Dorigotti, R. Rolandi, and C. Carpi, *Pharmacol. Res. Comm.*, **8**, 295 (1976).

182. G. Leclerc, C-G. Wermuth, F. Miesch, and J. Schwartz, *Eur. J. Med. Chem.*, **11**, 107 (1976).

183. W. C. Curran and A. Ross, *J. Med. Chem.*, **17**, 273 (1974).

184. F. J. McEvoy and G. R. Allen, Jr., *J. Med. Chem.*, **17**, 281 (1974).

185. J. Koch-Weser, *Arch. Intern. Med.*, **133**, 1017 (1974).

186. C. A. Chidsey, *Clin. Sci. Mol.*, **45**, 1715 (1973).

187. S. J. Ehrreich, J. E. Henngslake, F. R. Warner, J. Weinstock, and R. E. Tedeschi, *Arch. Int. Pharmacodyn.*, **179**, 284 (1969).

188. B. Loev, M. M. Goodman, K. M. Snader, R. Tedeschi, and E. Macko, *J. Med. Chem.*, **17**, 956 (1974).

189. M. Muramaki, E. Murakami, N. Takekoshi, M. Tsuchiya, T. Kin, T. Onoe, N. Takeuchi, T. Funatsu, S. Hara, S. Ishise, J. Mifune, and M. Maeda, *Jap. Heart J.*, **13**, 128 (1972).

190. R. Fielden, D. A. A. Owen, and E. M. Taylor, *Brit. J. Pharmacol.*, **52**, 323 (1974).

191. F. Takenaka, N. Takeya, T. Ishihara, S. Inove, E. Tsutusumi, T. Nakamura, Y. Mitsufuji, and M. Sumie, *Jap. J. Pharmacol.*, **20**, 253 (1970).

192. M. Götz, K. Grozinger, and J. R. Oliver, *J. Med. Chem.*, **16**, 671 (1973).

193. H. P. Blumenthal, J. R. Ryan, and F. G. McMahon, *Eur. J. Clin. Pharmacol.*, **8**, 409 (1975).

194. M. S. Amer, *Life Sci.*, **17**, 1021 (1975).

195. P. Hamet, O. Kuchel, J. Fraysse, and J. Genest, *CMA J.*, **111**, 323 (1974).

196. M. S. Amer, A. W. Gomoll, J. L. Perhach, H. C. Ferguson, and G. R. McKinney, *Proc. Natl. Acad. Sci. U.S.*, **71**, 4930 (1974).

197. F. H. Messerli, O. Kuchel, P. Hamet, G. Tolis, G. P. Guthrie, Jr., J. Fraysse, W. Nowaczynski, and J. Genest, *Circ. Res.*, **38**:Suppl. II, II-42 (1976).

198. H-J. Hess, *Postgrad. Med.—Prazosin Clin. Sym. Proc.*, Suppl. I, 9 pp. (1975).

199. J. C. McGiff, *Hosp. Pract.*, **10**, 101 (1975).

200. J. B. Lee and B. K. Mookerjee, *Cardiovasc. Med.*, **1**, 320 (1976).

201. P. Y-K. Wong, J. C. McGiff, and A. Terragno, in *Prostaglandins and Thromboxanes*, F. Berti, B. Samuelsson, and G. P. Velo, Eds., Plenum, New York, 1977, pp. 251–264.

202. J. C. McGiff, N. A. Terragno, and H. D. Itskovitz, in *Prostaglandin Synthetase Inhibitors*, H. J. Robinson and J. R. Vane, Eds., Raven Press, New York, 1974, p. 259.

203. Report of the Joint National Committee on Detection, Evaluation and Treatment of High Blood Pressure. A Cooperative Study, *J. Am. Med. Assoc.*, **237**, 255 (1977).

204. H. P. Dustan, G. R. Cumming, A. C. Corcoran, and I. H. Page, *Circulation*, **19**, 360 (1959).

205. B. M. Winer, *Circulation*, **23**, 211 (1961).

206. N. Kakaviatos and F. A. Finnerty, Jr., *Am. J. Cardiol.*, **10**, 570 (1962).

207. Veterans Administration Cooperative Study Group on Antihypertensive Agents, *Circulation*, **45**, 991 (1972).

208. R. P. Ames and P. Hill, *Am. J. Med.*, **61**, 748 (1976).

209. R. Tigerstedt and P. G. Bergman, *Skand. Arch. Physiol.*, **8**, 223 (1898).

210. W. A. Pettinger, T. K. Keeton, W. B. Campbell, and D. C. Harper, *Circ. Res.*, **38**, 338 (1976).

211. E. Braun-Menéndez and I. H. Page, *Science*, **127**, 242 (1958).

212. H. Thurston and J. D. Swales, *Circ. Res.*, **35**, 325 (1974).

213. J. O. Davis and R. H. Freeman, *Biochem. Pharmacol.*, **26**, 93 (1977).

214. F. R. Bühler, F. Burkart, B. E. Lütold, M. Küng, G. Marbet, and M. Pfisterer, *Am. J. Cardiol.*, **36**, 653 (1975).

215. E. Haber, *Circulation*, **54**, 849 (1976).

216. C. I. Johnston, *Drugs*, **12**, 274 (1976).

217. G. P. Guthrie, Jr., J. Genest, and O. Kuchel, *Ann. Rev. Pharmacol. Toxicol.*, **16**, 287 (1976).

218. H. Gavras, G. R. Brunner, and J. H. Laragh, *Progr. Cardiovasc. Dis.*, **17**, 39 (1974).

219. H. R. Brunner and H. Gavras, *J. Am. Med. Assoc.*, **233**, 1091 (1975).

220. J. H. Laragh, *Johns Hopkins Med. J.*, **137**, 184 (1975).

221. P. Omvik, E. Enger, and I. Eide, *Am. J. Med.*, **61**, 608 (1976).

222. E. E. Muirhead, B. Brooks, and K. K. Arora, *Lab. Invest.*, **30**, 129 (1974).

223. H. Gavras, H. R. Brunner, J. H. Laragh, J. E. Sealey, I. Gavras, and R. A. Vukovich, *N. Engl. J. Med.*, **291**, 817 (1974).

224. R. Re, R. Novelline, M-T. Escourrou, C. Athanasoulis, J. Burton, and E. Haber, *N. Engl. J. Med.*, **298**, 582 (1978).

225. M. A. Ondetti, B. Rubin, and D. Cushman, *Science*, **196**, 441 (1977).

226. H. Gavras, H. R. Brunner, G. A. Turini, G. R. Kershaw, C. P. Tifft, S. Cuttelod, I. Gavras, R. A. Vukovich, and D. N. McKinstry, *N. Engl. J. Med.*, **298**, 991 (1978).

227. E. G. Erdös, *Advan. Pharmacol.*, **4**, 1 (1966).

228. R. A. Vukovich, D. A. Willard, and L. J. Brannick, *J. Int. Med. Res.*, **5**, 1 (1977).

229. L. S. Marks, M. H. Maxwell, and J. J. Kaufman, *Lancet*, **1975-II**, 784.

230. H. R. Brunner, H. Gavras, J. H. Laragh, and R. Keenan, *Circ. Res.*, **34–35**:Suppl. I, I-35 (1974).

231. J. Genest, W. Nowaczynski, O. Kuchel, R. Boucher, and J. M. Rojo-Ortega, *Mayo Clin. Proc.*, **52**, 291 (1977).

232. J. G. Douglas, J. W. Hollifield, and G. W. Liddle, *J. Am. Med. Assoc.*, **227**, 518 (1974).

233. S. D. Loube and R. A. Quirk, *Lancet*, **1975-I**, 1428.

234. L. M. Hofman, *J. Pharmacol. Exp. Ther.*, **194**, 450 (1975).

235. L. Ramsay, M. Asbury, J. Shelton, and I. Harrison, *Clin. Pharmacol. Ther.*, **21**, 602 (1977).

236. E. G. Erdös, N. Back, and F. Sicuteri, Eds., Springer, Berlin, 1966.

237. G. S. Stokes, *Drugs*, **12**, 222 (1976).

238. E. Reisin, R. Abel, M. Modan, D. S. Silberberg, H. E. Eliahou, and B. Modan, *N. Engl. J. Med.*, **298**, 1 (1978).

239. Medical News, *J. Am. Med. Assoc.*, **238**, 109 (1977).

240. H. M. Perry, *Circ. Res.*, **40**, 180 (1977).

241. Hypertension Detection and Follow-up Program Cooperative Group, *Circ. Res.*, **40**, 106 (1977).

242. W. M. Smith, *Circ. Res.*, **40**, 98 (1977).

243. Editorial: Side Effects of Methyldopa, *Brit. Med. J.*, I, **1975**, 646.

244. A. J. Zweifler and M. D. Esler, *Postgrad. Med.*, **60**, *81* (July 1976).

245. W. A. Pettinger, *Arch. Intern. Med.*, **137**, 679 (1977).

246. C. T. Dollery, *Ann. Rev. Pharmacol. Toxicol.*, **17**, 311 (1977).

247. K. Okamoto and K. Aoki, *Jap. Circ. J.*, **27**, 282 (1963).

248. *Spontaneous Hypertension: Its Pathogenesis and Complications—Proc. Second Int. Symp. on the Spontaneously Hypertensive Rat*, National Institutes of Health, DHEW Publication No. (NIH) 77-1179, 1977.

249. E. L. Phelan, *N. Z. Med. J.*, **67**, 334 (1968).

250. E. L. Phelan, D. R. Lee, A. J. Wood, and F. O. Simpson, *Clin. Exp. Pharmacol. Physiol. Suppl.*, **2**, 137 (1975).

251. D. R. Lee, E. L. Phelan, and F. O. Simpson, "Effect of Propranolol in Genetically Hypertensive Rats," in *Spontaneous Hypertension: Its Pathogenesis and Complications—Proc. Second Int. Symp. on the Spontaneously Hypertensive Rat*, National Institutes of Health, DHEW Publication No. (NIH) 77–1179, p. 340 (1977).

252. G. Bianchi, U. Fox, and E. Imbasciati, *Life Sci.*, **14**, 339 (1974).

253. G. Bianchi, P. Baer, U. Fox, L. Duzzi, D. Pagetti, and A. M. Giovannetti, *Circ. Res.*, **36–37**: Suppl. I, I-153 (1975).

254. G. J. Kelliher and S. P. Shanor, *J. Pharm. Sci.*, **62**, 1425 (1973).

255. K. K. Modi and R. N. Chakravarti, *Wochenschr.*, **53**, 363 (1975).

256. H. Goldblatt, J. Lynch, R. F. Hanzel, and W. W. Summerville, *J. Exp. Med.*, **59**, 347 (1934).

257. C. M. Ferrario and J. W. McCubbin, *Hosp. Pract.* **9**, 71 (1974).

258. H. R. Brunner, J. D. Kirshman, J. E. Sealey, and J. H. Laragh, *Science*, **174**, 1344 (1971).

259. J. A. Johnson, J. O. Davis, and B. Braverman, *Am. J. Physiol.*, **228**, 11 (1975).

260. B. E. Watkins, J. O. Davis, R. C. Hanson, T. E.

Lohmeier, and R. H. Freeman, *Am. J. Physiol.*, **231,** 954 (1976).

261. J. S. Hutchinson, P. G. Matthews, E. Dax, and C. I. Johnston, *Clin. Exp. Pharmacol. Physiol. Suppl.*, **2,** 83 (1975).

262. E. D. Miller, Jr., A. I. Samuels, E. Haber, and A. C. Barger, *Am. J. Physiol.*, **228,** 448 (1975).

263. J. R. Douglas, E. M. Johnson, Jr., J. F. Heist, G. R. Marshall, and P. Needleman, *J. Pharmacol. Exp. Ther.*, **196,** 35 (1976).

264. I. H. Page, *J. Am. Med. Assoc.*, **113,** 2046 (1939).

265. C. M. Ferrario, *Am. J. Physiol.*, **226,** 711 (1974).

266. L. K. Dahl, K. D. Knudsen, M. Heine, and G. Leitl, *J. Exp. Med.*, **126,** 687 (1967).

267. P. E. Wisenbaugh, G. V. Bogarty, and R. W. Hill, *Lab. Invest.*, **14,** 2140 (1965).

268. L. S. Dahl and R. Tuthill, *J. Exp. Med.*, **139,** 617 (1974).

269. J. L. Reid, J. A. Ziven, and I. J. Kopin, *Circ. Res.*, **37,** 569 (1975).

270. N. Doba and D. J. Reis, *Circ. Res.*, **32,** 584 (1973).

271. M. A. Nathan and D. J. Reis, *Circ. Res.*, **40,** 72 (1977).

272. J. A. Rosecrans, N. Watzman, and J. P. Buckley, *Biochem. Pharmacol.*, **15,** 1707 (1966).

273. J. F. Marwood and M. F. Lockett, *J. Pharm. Pharmacol.*, **25,** 42 (1973).

274. E. J. Farris, E. H. Yeakel, and H. S. Medoff, *Am. J. Physiol.*, **144,** 331 (1945).

275. J. L. Perhach, Jr., H. C. Ferguson, and G. R. McKinney, *Life Sci.*, **16,** 1731 (1975).

276. M. Fernandes, M., G. Onesti, A. Weder, R. Dykyj, A. B. Gould, K. E. Kim, and C. Swartz, *J. Lab. Clin. Med.*, **87,** 561 (1976).

277. C. E. Hall, S. Ayachi, and O. Hall, *Endocrinology*, **94,** 355 (1974).

278. C. E. Hall, S. Ayachi, and O. Hall, *Endocrinology*, **95,** 1268 (1974).

CHAPTER FORTY-THREE

Cholinergics

JOSEPH G. CANNON

College of Pharmacy
University of Iowa
Iowa City, Iowa 52242, USA

CONTENTS

1   INTRODUCTION

The transmission of impulses throughout the cholinergic nervous system is mediated by acetylcholine (43.**1**), and compounds that produce their pharmacological effect by mimicking or substituting for acetylcholine are called cholinergics or parasympathomimetics. Compounds that inhibit or inactivate the body's normal hydrolysis of acetylcholine by acetylcholinesterase are called anticholinesterases. The gross observable pharmacological effects of both types of compounds are quite similar.

$$CH_3COOCH_2CH_2\overset{+}{N}(CH_3)_3$$

43.1

Although many nerve impulses transmitted to the striated muscles result from conscious demands of the living animal, other impulses necessary to life are transmitted continuously from higher centers to smooth and sometimes to striated muscles without dependence on the conscious will of the animal. These impulses include those that regulate circulation, respiration, the secretory glands, peristalsis, the urinary bladder, and contraction and dilatation of the pupils of the eyes, and they are carried by the autonomic nervous system from the brain and the spinal cord through a network of nerves to the muscles that exert the response to the stimulus. Such nerve pathways end in synapses in which the dendrites or nerve endings of one nerve do not contact nor form a contiguous system with the next nerve. Acetylcholine is liberated at the synapse and, acting as a chemical mediator, it transmits the impulse across the anatomic gap to the next nerve segment. A critical role for calcium ions in acetylcholine release is now generally accepted, but there is no agreement on how or where calcium acts (1), although Ticku and Triggle (2) have described roles for calcium at the cholinergic receptor. At the effector muscle, the nerve endings do not make direct contact with the muscle, and again a chemical mediator is necessary to translate the nerve impulse into a muscle response. At these sites, either acetylcholine or norepinephrine is synthesized and stored near the nerve endings, to be released upon receipt of the nerve impulse. Knowledge of some details of nerve impulse transmission has permitted the design of synthetic compounds that have a more prolonged effect and frequently have a more specific action than the natural neurotransmitter.

The complex mechanism by which acetylcholine acts as a neurohormone involves reaction of the molecule with a macromolecular receptor in or near the nervous tissue involved. The result of this reaction is an alteration of the nerve's action potential, which derives from the movement of ions (Na^+, K^+, Cl^-) in and out of the interior of the nerve membrane. For an orderly flow of impulses to occur from autonomic nerve to nerve or from nerve to muscle or gland, the chemical mediator must be destroyed after reaction with its receptor and subsequent dissociation of the agonist–receptor complex. In the case of acetylcholine, the enzyme acetylcholinesterase effects the hydrolysis to acetic acid and choline, which may later be reesterified by reaction with acetyl coenzyme A [under the catalytic action of choline acetylase (3)]. This deactivation mechanism, which normally proceeds at an extremely rapid rate, offers another opportunity to affect the activity of the system innervated by cholinergic nerves, employing anticholinesterases. In such cases there is an accumulation of free acetylcholine at the nerve endings or at the motor end plate, which reacts with the receptor and provides a prolonged stimulation of organ systems innervated by cholinergic nerves.

The effects of stimulation of the cholinergic nervous system by acetylcholine, its analogs, or anticholinesterases may be divided somewhat artificially into two types of physiological actions:

1. *Muscarinic actions*: at postganglionic parasympathetic neuroeffector sites, primarily smooth muscle and secretory glands.

2. *Nicotinic actions*: at neuromuscular junctions and at autonomic ganglia. Muscarinic actions include cardiac inhibition; peripheral vasodilatation; contraction of the pupils of the eyes; increased flow of most secretory glands; and contractions and/or peristaltic motion in the gastrointestinal tract and urinary tract. These physiological responses are similar to those produced by

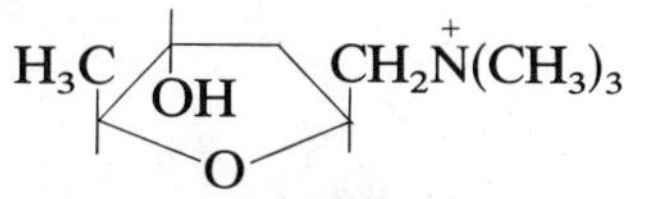

43.2

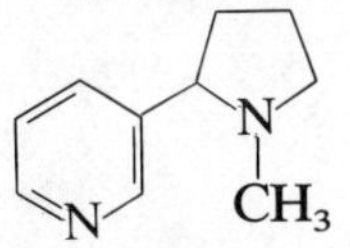

43.3

the alkaloid muscarine (43.**2**). The nicotinic activity of acetylcholine appears to parallel the pharmacological activity of the alkaloid nicotine (43.**3**) and is involved in the stimulation and then blockade of end plates of autonomic ganglia and of skeletal muscles. Natural (−)-nicotine is only about eight times more potent a nicotinic agent than its (+)-enantiomer (4). Structure–activity studies and comparison of nicotinic and muscarinic actions are complicated by the likelihood that many nicotinic agents including nicotine itself act indirectly through release of endogenous acetylcholine (5). It is widely accepted that acetylcholine muscarinic and nicotinic receptors differ chemically and sterically as well as physiologically. Purves (6) noted marked kinetic differences between nicotinic and muscarinic receptors, and he proposed that muscarinic receptors are specialized to allow temporal summation and thus continuity of action, whereas nicotinic receptors are specialized to prevent it.

Therapeutic indications for cholinergics and/or anticholinesterases in contemporary practice include the following. (1) Relief of postoperative atony of the gut and the urinary tract and bladder: in such conditions cholinergics or anticholinesterases may relieve the stasis by stimulating peristaltic movements of the intestine and ureters and constriction of the bladder. (2) Reduction of intraocular pressure in glaucoma, by increasing the drainage of intraocular fluid through the canal of Schlemm; this is accompanied by constriction of the pupils of the eyes. (3) Relief of muscular weakness in myasthenia gravis: this muscular weakness reflects a failure of an appropriate amount of acetylcholine to reach cholinoceptive sites of the post myoneural junctional membrane following rapidly repetitive nerve impulses. The reduced level of acetylcholine may result from excessive enzyme-catalyzed hydrolysis of it, or from diminished production or release. However, the etiology of the disease remains obscure.

2 ACETYLCHOLINE AND ANALOGS

Although serving admirably its physiological role in the body, acetylcholine is a poor therapeutic agent. Its rapid rate of hydrolysis in the gastrointestinal tract precludes oral administration, and a similarly rapid hydrolysis via the esterases in the blood and acetylcholinesterase catalysis in the tissues limits its usefulness by injection. By parenteral administration, its action is fleeting and many of the effects of cholinergic nerve stimulation are not discernible. Clinical use of acetylcholine seems limited to topical application in the eye to produce rapid, brief miosis (7).

The need for therapeutically satisfactory cholinergic agents and the simple and easily synthesized structures necessary for cholinergic activity have stimulated preparation and biological examination of a host of derivatives, analogs, and congeners of acetylcholine. Molecular modifications have included the following structural variations:

1. Alteration of the quaternary ammonium head.
2. Replacement of the acetyl group by other acyl groups.
3. Alteration of the alkyl chain connecting the quaternary ammonium and the ester groups.

4. Substitution of another group for, or elimination of, the ester moiety. Synthesis of compounds and examination of their biological activities have supplied considerable information on structural requirements for cholinergic activity, but these data must be interpreted with care. Not only are they subject to the usual errors in biological testing, but they have been obtained from a variety of testing procedures in a variety of animal species. Often, different biological properties associated with stimulation of the cholinergic nervous system have been measured. Furthermore, the observed effectiveness of a cholinergic agent in producing a biological response is the result of its inherent potency and the rate at which it is hydrolyzed by acetylcholinesterase and by blood esterases. Usually, these individual factors have not been separately and individually assessed. Therefore, in the following discussion of the relationship of chemical structure to cholinergic activity, only generalized statements can be made, and these are usually based on a composite of the various cholinergic activities for which the compound was tested.

2.1 Variations of the Quaternary Ammonium Group

Two types of structural alterations of the quaternary head have been studied: replacement of the nitrogen atom by other atoms; and replacement of the N-methyl groups by alkyl, hydrogen, or oxygen.

Acetylphosphonocholine (43.**4**) (8), acetylarsenocholine (43.**5**) (8), and acetylsulfonocholine (43.**6**) (9) exhibit muscarinic effects, but they are considerably less active than acetylcholine. Ing (8) has presented a rationalization for these data. The carbon isostere (43.**7**) of acetylcholine exhibits no cholinergic activity, but it is a substrate for acetylcholinesterase (10). Studies of the

$$CH_3COOCH_2CH_2R$$

43.**4** $R = \overset{+}{P}(CH_3)_3$

43.**5** $R = \overset{+}{As}(CH_3)_3$

43.**6** $R = \overset{+}{S}(CH_3)_2$

43.**7** $R = C(CH_3)_3$

effect of substitution of the N-methyl groups by hydrogen strongly indicate that optimum activity is achieved with trimethylammonium. The acetate esters of N,N-dimethylethanolamine, N-methylethanolamine, and ethanolamine lack the nicotinic activity of acetylcholine and possess only a small fraction of its muscarinic activity (11). The tertiary amine congener of carbachol (Table 43.1, no. 18) exhibits greatly diminished nicotinic and muscarinic effects compared with the N-trimethyl quaternary compound (11a). These observations seem valid for cholinergic agents having, like acetylcholine, a high degree of molecular flexibility (12). In contrast, in certain heterocyclic systems in which the elements of acetylcholine are incorporated into a rigid cyclic framework, tertiary amine salts are more potent muscarinics than their methchloride derivatives (12). For such a comparison to be meaningful, it must be assumed that the tertiary amino compounds are protonated at their *in vivo* sites of action.

Replacement of one N-methyl group of acetylcholine by ethyl permits retention of most of the cholinergic activity, but as more N-methyl groups are replaced by ethyl, there is a progressive loss of cholinergic effect (13). When one N-methyl is replaced by n-propyl or n-butyl, the resulting systems display almost no cholinergic action (9). Acetylpyrrolidinecholine (43.**8**) is $\frac{1}{3}-\frac{1}{5}$ as potent as acetylcholine (14); this compound is considered to be a cyclic congener of acetyl "diethylcholine" and it is decidedly more potent than the diethylcholine ester. However, in general, incorporation of the choline moiety into a heterocyclic

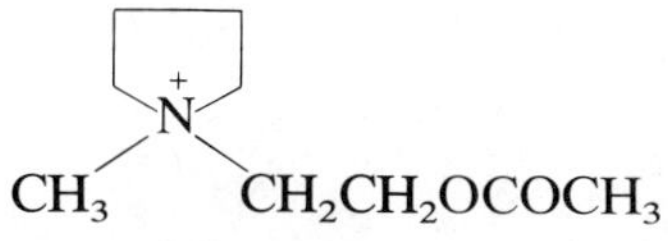

$$CH_3 \qquad CH_2CH_2OCOCH_3$$
43.8

ring markedly lowers potency compared with acetylcholine (15).

Replacement of one *N*-methyl by methoxyl in acetylcholine and in three congeners (43.**9a–d**) permits retention of some cholinergic effects, and in certain compounds, nicotinic or muscarinic activities are enhanced over the parent *N*-trimethyl system (16). Amine oxide analogs of cholinergic agonists (43.**10a–d**) exhibit little or no cholinergic effect, and they are not substrates for cholinesterases (17).

The observed biological effects of several variations of the quaternary head of acetylcholine and its congeners may be explainable by invoking the conclusion [based on molecular orbital calculations (18)], that in both muscarine and acetylcholine, the nitrogen atom is nearly neutral and a large part (70%) of the formal charge is distributed among the three attached methyl groups, which form a large ball of spreading positive charge. Furthermore, Kimura

et al. (19) determined that extension of one alkyl chain of tetramethylammonium produces a great decrease in the charge density on the nitrogen, and they proposed that cholinergic agonist activity for a quaternary ammonium compound requires a minimum level of charge density on the nitrogen.

2.2   Variations of the Acyl Group

Although choline itself possesses residual amounts of some of the nicotinic and muscarinic properties of acetylcholine, esterification of its alcohol function usually increases potency. However, homologation of the acetate methyl group of acetylcholine produces compounds that are less potent than acetylcholine (Table 43.1). Polar groups such as OH (no. 16) and NH_2 (no. 3, Table 43.1) markedly decrease muscarinic potency, but a C=O group (no. 15) permits retention of considerable activity.

$$RCOOCHCH_2\overset{\overset{CH_3}{+|}}{N}OCH_3$$
$$\underset{R'}{|} \quad \underset{CH_3}{|}$$

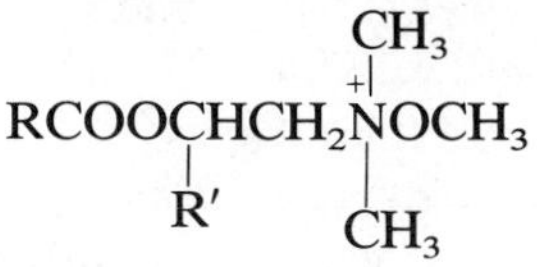

43.**9a**   R = CH$_3$, R′ = H
43.**9b**   R = R′ = CH$_3$
43.**9c**   R = H$_2$N, R′ = H
43.**9d**   R = H$_2$N, R′ = CH$_3$

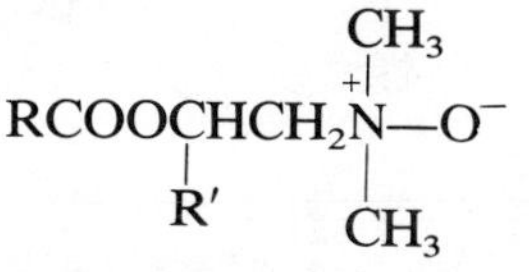

$$RCOOCHCH_2\overset{\overset{CH_3}{+|}}{N}-O^-$$
$$\underset{R'}{|} \quad \underset{CH_3}{|}$$

43.**10a**   R = CH$_3$, R′ = H
43.**10b**   R = R′ = CH$_3$
43.**10c**   R = H$_2$N, R′ = H
43.**10d**   R = H$_2$N, R′ = CH$_3$

Table 43.1   Representative Esters of Choline

	$ROCH_2CH_2\overset{+}{N}(CH_3)_3$	
No.	R	Ref.
1	HCO	20
2	C$_2$H$_5$CO	20, 21
3	H$_2$NCH$_2$CO	22
4	n-C$_3$H$_7$CO	20, 21
5	i-C$_3$H$_7$CO	21
6	n-C$_4$H$_9$CO	20, 21
7	C$_6$H$_5$CO	21
8	C$_6$H$_5$CH$_2$CO	21
9	C$_6$H$_5$CH=CHCO	21
10	(C$_6$H$_5$)$_2$C(OH)CO	23
11	CH$_3$(CH$_2$)$_{10}$CO	24
12	CH$_3$(CH$_2$)$_{14}$CO	24
13	HOCH$_2$CO	20
14	CH$_2$=CHCO	25
15	CH$_3$COCO	20
16	CH$_3$CHOHCO	26
17	O$_2$N	27
18	H$_2$NCO	28, 29
19	(CH$_3$O)$_2$PO	30

Acrylylcholine (no. 14) has relatively high cholinergic activity; this compound is of some interest in that it has been isolated from tissues of a marine gastropod. Higher fatty acid esters (nos. 11, 12) were prepared for testing as hemolytic agents, but their cholinergic properties have apparently never been reported.

Carbamate esters of choline and its analogs and congeners have provided interesting and useful pharmacological ·agents. In general, these esters are more potent and more toxic than the corresponding acetates (31). The carbamate ester of choline, carbachol (Table 43.1, no. 18), is a potent muscarinic agent and has a markedly greater nicotinic effect than acetylcholine, but because of its toxicity (attributable to the high nicotinic action) it is obsolete for many clinical uses (32a). This compound and carbamate esters of C-methyl choline analogs are less easily hydrolyzed by esterases than is acetylcholine, and most of the carbamate esters may be administered orally as well as by injection. Their action is of longer duration.

The nitrate ester (Table 43.1, no. 17) has pronounced nicotinic and muscarinic effects and, in addition, an intense paralyzing nicotine action. The dimethylphosphate ester (no. 19) displays little muscarinic but powerful nicotinic action. Bromoacetylcholine, a direct nicotinic and muscarinic agonist, binds irreversibly to nicotinic but not to muscarinic receptors. On the basis that some neuroblastoma cells contain cholinergic receptors, the compound has been proposed to have potential antitumor activity (33).

Acetylthiocholine (43.**11**) and acetylselenocholine (43.**12**) exert acetylcholine-like effects on the guinea pig ileum and the frog rectus abdominis, but both are somewhat less potent than acetylcholine (34). Unesterified thiocholine and selenocholine systems display a relatively high degree of acetylcholine-like activity compared to their acetate esters. Contradictory earlier

$$CH_3CO—X—CH_2CH_2\overset{+}{N}(CH_3)_3$$

43.**11** X = S
43.**12** X = Se
43.**13** X = NH

accounts ascribed the biological effects of these unesterified thiols and selenols to their air oxidation to disulfide and diselenide derivatives (34). The amide congener (43.**13**) of acetylcholine has little or no cholinergic activity (28). Acetylthionocholine, in which the carbonyl oxygen of acetylcholine is replaced by sulfur, displays some acetylcholine-like effects in an electroplax preparation (35).

2.3 Alterations of the Ethylene Bridge

The distance between the ester and the cationic groups of acetylcholine seems to be critical. Acetyl-γ-homocholine (43.**14**) is decidedly less active than acetylcholine (36); 4-acetoxybutyltrimethylammonium (43.**15**) exhibits extremely low muscarinic and nicotinic effects (37). Replacement of one or more of the hydrogen atoms of the ethylene bridge with alkyl groups produces marked changes in activity. Acetyl-β-methylcholine (43.**16**) is a more potent muscarinic agent than acetylcholine, but it has a much weaker nicotinic action (32a). Acetyl-α-methylcholine (43.**17**) is a more potent nicotinic than a muscarinic, but both effects are decidedly less than for acetylcholine (38). A factor in the observed potency of acetyl-β-methylcholine is its

$$CH_3COO(CH_2)_n\overset{+}{N}(CH_3)_3$$

43.**14** $n = 3$
43.**15** $n = 4$

$$CH_3COOCHCH\overset{+}{N}(CH_3)_3$$
$$\overset{|}{R'}\ \overset{|}{R}$$

43.**16** R = H, R' = CH$_3$
43.**17** R = CH$_3$, R' = H
43.**18** R = R' = CH$_3$

slower rate of hydrolysis by acetylcholine-sterase (38), which has been ascribed to a poor affinity of the compound for the enzyme's catalytic site (39), and to its extremely high resistance to hydrolysis by nonspecific serum cholinesterases. The acetate ester (methacholine) and the carbamate ester (bethanechol) of $(\pm)$-β-methylcholine are useful therapeutic agents.

The muscarinic effect of acetyl β-methylcholine resides in the (S)-$(+)$ isomer; the (R)-$(-)$ isomer is 1/240 as active as acetylcholine (38, 40). Acetyl-(S)-$(+)$-β-methylcholine is hydrolyzed by acetylcholine-sterase at about half the rate of acetylcholine, but its (R) enantiomer is a weak inhibitor of the enzyme (38). Both acetyl-α-methylcholine enantiomers show a low order of potency and a lower degree of stereoselectivity of effect than does acetyl-β-methylcholine (38). The (S)-$(+)$ enantiomer is more active in most but not in all assays (41). $(\pm)$-*erythro*-Acetyl-α,β-dimethylcholine (43.**18**) exhibits 14% of the muscarinic potency of acetylcholine and is almost completely resistant to acetyl-cholinesterase; the $(\pm)$-*threo* isomer is inert as a cholinergic but is a poor substrate for acetylcholinesterase (42). *gem*-Dimethyl substitution of acetylcholine, either on the α,α or the β,β positions, markedly reduces but does not abolish muscarinic activity (43). Replacement of C-methyl groups in the ethylene bridge by longer chains causes an increase in toxicity and a reduction in muscarinic activity, for example, the acetate esters of β-n-propyl- and β-n-butylcholines (44, 45).

2.4   Substitution of the Ester Group by Other Functional Groups

The ester moiety does not appear to be essential to cholinergic activity. In general, alkyl ethers of choline and of thiocholine are less active than acetylcholine (15). Aromatic choline ethers display marked nicotinic activity, but are muscarinically inactive (46). Contrary to some prior literature reports, the vinyl ether of choline is not a more potent muscarinic agent than the ethyl ether (47), but it is a better nicotinic, displaying higher potency than acetylcholine. α-Methyl substitution of choline in its ethyl and vinyl ethers greatly diminishes muscarinic potencies; β-methyl substitution also results in diminution of activity in both ethers, but to a much smaller extent. In ethyl and vinyl ethers, nicotinic effect is influenced by α- and β-methylation, parallel to acetylcholine itself. A series of open chain congeners of muscarine, typified by 43.**19**, exhibit low muscarinic potency, which has been ascribed by Friedman (15) to the compounds' lack of stereochemical homogeneity. An open chain analog of desmethylmuscarine (43.**20**) lacking chiral centers exhibits extremely low muscarinic activity (48). Ketonic systems, carbon isosteres of the ester moiety (43.**21**), display weak activities and are more nicotinic than muscarinic (15); the alcohol analogs of these ketones are even weaker (49).

Ing's "five atom rule" (8) states that, for maximum muscarinic activity, there should be attached to the nitrogen atom, in addition to three methyl groups, a fourth group with a chain of five atoms, as illustrated for acetylcholine: C—C—O—C—C—N. This

43.**19**

43.**20**

$$\text{RCO-alkylene-}\overset{+}{N}(CH_3)_3$$

43.**21**

empirical observation has been found to hold for a large number of molecules, regardless of the precise nature of the five atoms involved.

3 CHOLINERGICS NOT CLOSELY RELATED STRUCTURALLY TO ACETYLCHOLINE

3.1 Muscarine and Related Compounds

The structure and absolute configuration of naturally occurring L-(+)-muscarine (43.**22**) has been established (50) and confirmed by stereospecific synthesis (51). This compound provides a semirigid molecule with known stereochemistry which can be employed in assessment of structural requirements for muscarinic activity. The muscarine molecule exhibits a high degree of stereospecificity of pharmacological effects; the enantiomer of L (+)-muscarine is almost inert, as are its three diastereomers (epimuscarine, allomuscarine, and epiallomuscarine) (52). The oxidation product of L(+)-muscarine, L(+)-muscarone (43.**23**), is an active muscarinic agent but it also exhibits a nicotinic component of activity not possessed by muscarine. In contrast to the high stereospecificity of action in the muscarine series, the enantiomers and diastereomers of muscarone show a low degree of stereoselectivity toward the muscarinic receptor (38), and D(−)-muscarone is a somewhat more potent muscarinic than is the L(+)-isomer. The absolute configuration of this D(−)-muscarone (2R, 5R) corresponds to that of

the almost inactive D(−)-muscarine. Beckett et al. (53) have presented evidence suggesting that the approximate equivalence of muscarinic action shown by enantiomers of muscarone and by 4,5-dehydromuscarone (43.**24**) may be related to enolization phenomena. It was concluded that the keto tautomer of muscarone is active at muscarinic receptors, and that enolization occurs before the drug reaches the receptor.

Incorporation of the elements of muscarine structure into an aromatic ring has produced some potent systems, such as 43.**25** (52). Activity was lowered by changing the C-2 methyl to ethyl (54). (±)-4,5-Dehydromuscarines (43.**26**) retain considerable activity (52).

Muscarinic activity of 2-methyl-4-trimethylammoniummethyl-1,3-dioxolane systems (43.**27**) resides in the cis isomer (55); stereospecific synthesis of the two enantiomers of this cis isomer revealed that the L(+)-enantiomer (C-4 = R) is more than 100 times more potent than the D(−) isomer (C-4 = S), and is approximately six times as potent as acetylcholine in the guinea pig ileum. This compound has been described as the most potent and selective muscarinic agonist known (2). It is related configurationally to the most potent muscarine isomer, although it should be noted that several authors improperly assign the (S) absolute configuration to position 4 of L(+)-cis-43.**27**, apparently through misapplication of priority rules. 2,2-Dialkyl analogs of these dioxolanes are much weaker muscarinic agonists than the parent systems (43.**27**) and the difference in

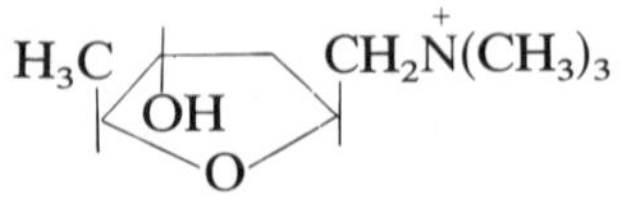

43.**22**

(2S,3R,5S)-(+)-Muscarine

L(+)-Muscarine

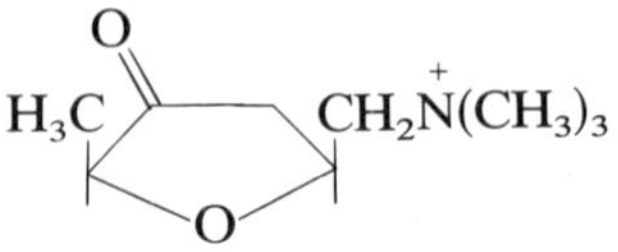

43.**23**

(2S,5S)-(+)-Muscarone

L(+)-Muscarone

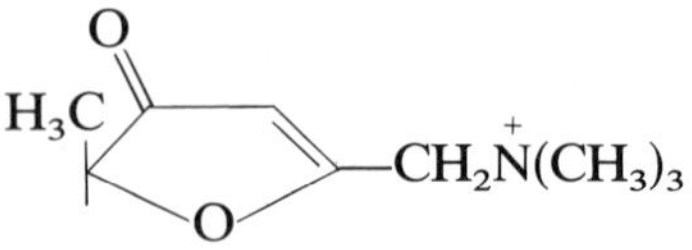

43.**24**

$$CH_3\text{---}\underset{O}{\overbrace{}}\text{---}CH_2\overset{+}{N}(CH_3)_3$$

43.**25**

$$\underset{O}{\overset{H_3C}{\overbrace{OH}}}\text{---}CH_2\overset{+}{N}(CH_3)_3$$

43.**26**

$$CH_3\underset{O}{\overbrace{}}CH_2\overset{+}{N}(CH_3)_3$$

43.**27**

potency between the C-4 (*R*) and (*S*) enantiomers diminishes sharply with increasing size of substituents at C-2 (56). A thio analog (43.**28**) of the dioxolane, consisting of a mixture of cis and trans isomers, had high muscarinic activity and also had some nicotinic effect (57). Dioxolane congeners, again consisting of mixed cis and trans isomers, bearing sulfur, phosphorus, or arsenic cationic heads (43.**29**), display lower muscarinic effects than the corresponding nitrogen system (58).

The *cis*-1- and *cis*-3-desether dioxolane systems 43.**29a** and 43.**29b** in general exhibit only a slight drop in muscarinic activity compared to the "supermuscarinic" dioxolane, *cis*-43.**27** (58a). It has been suggested (58a) that occupation of only one of the two receptor sites proposed to be reacting with the ring oxygens of the *cis*-dioxolane 43.**27** is sufficient to induce cholinergic activity.

The moderately high potency (1/10 acetylcholine) of a rigid spirodioxolane derivative (43.**30**) as compared with low muscarinic action of a more flexible isomeric system (43.**31**) (1/300 acetylcholine) led Ridley and co-workers (59) to speculate that the rigid molecule may approximate the conformation of the *cis*-dioxolane 43.**27** bound at the muscarinic receptor.

A carbocyclic muscarine analog, (±)-desethermuscarine (43.**32**) exhibits striking muscarinic effects (60), although the compound is considerably less potent than was originally reported (61). The other three optical isomers of desethermuscarine (epi-, allo-, and epiallodesethermuscarine) are weaker cholinergic agents (61a, 61b). Two attempts to obtain (±)-desethermuscarone (43.**33**) resulted in inseparable mixtures of cis and trans isomers (60, 62), which were reported to be equipotent to acetylcholine in muscarinic and nicotinic assays (60). The high potencies of 43.**32** amd 43.**33** suggest the necessity for a critical reexamination of theories of muscarinic drug–receptor interaction in which the ring oxygen of muscarine or muscarone is assigned a crucial role. These findings on desethermuscarine and desethermuscarone tend to support previously cited proposals (53) for the prime importance of the keto group of muscarone (as compared to the ring oxygen) in interaction with the muscarinic receptor. Cyclohexane analogs of desethermuscarine and of desethermuscarone show greatly diminished muscarinic activity (62a). In contrast, simple, nonoxygenated cyclohexane quaternary systems, typified by 43.**33a**, retain some degree of muscarinic effect, which seems to confirm Triggle's

$$CH_3\underset{O}{\overset{S\text{---}CH_2\overset{+}{N}(CH_3)_3}{\overbrace{}}}$$

43.**28**

$$CH_3\underset{O}{\overset{O\text{---}CH_2\text{---}X}{\overbrace{}}}$$

43.**29**   X = $\overset{+}{S}(CH_3)_2$, $\overset{+}{P}(CH_3)_3$, $\overset{+}{As}(CH_3)_3$

$$\underset{H_3C\quad\quad CH_2\overset{+}{N}(CH_3)_3}{\overset{O\text{---}}{\overbrace{}}}$$

43.**29a**

$$\underset{H_3C\quad O\quad CH_2\overset{+}{N}(CH_3)_3}{\overbrace{}}$$

43.**29b**

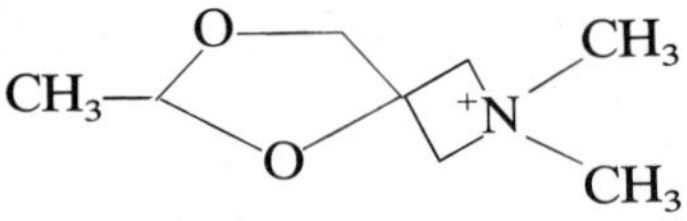

43.30

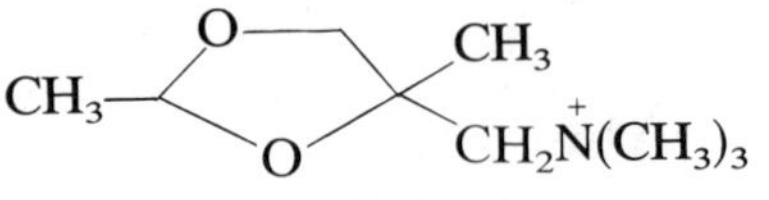

43.31

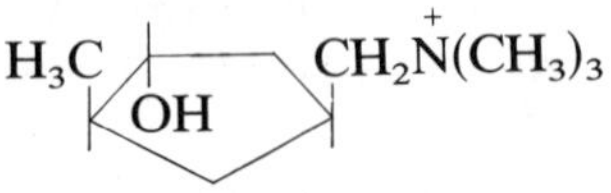

43.32

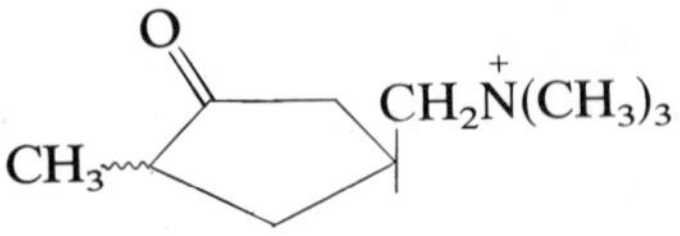

43.33

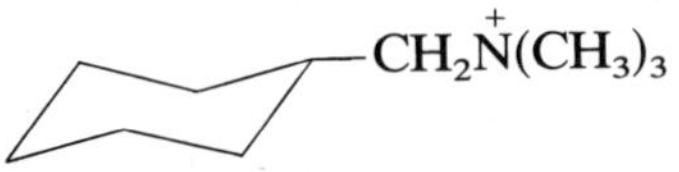

43.33a

statement (62b) that cholinergic compounds lacking an oxygenated function interact at the receptor level with an accessory receptor site of reduced polarity. Desmethyldesethermuscarine, epidesmethyldesethermuscarine, and desmethyldesethermuscarone are less potent muscarinics than their *C*-methyl homologs, further demonstrating the importance of the *C*-methyl group. For nicotinic activity, the *C*-methyl seems less critical (63).

3.2   Miscellaneous Structures

The natural products pilocarpine (43.**34**) and arecoline (43.**35**) have as their principal action the stimulation of the same autonomic effector cells as those acted upon by cholinergic postganglionic nerve impulses (32b). Although these agents act primarily at muscarinic receptors, their observed effects are complicated by other sites of action. Their structures are distinguished by the absence of a quaternary ammonium head; it is presumed that a nitrogen-protonated form of the molecule is the biologically active species.

Tremorine (43.**36**) is metabolized to the lactam oxotremorine (43.**37**), which is approximately equipotent to acetylcholine as a muscarinic agent (64). The carbonyl

group of oxotremorine is essential for activity, as is the acetylenic group. Increase in the size of the lactam ring results in a change from agonist to antagonist (65a). An allenic oxotremorine analog (43.**37a**),

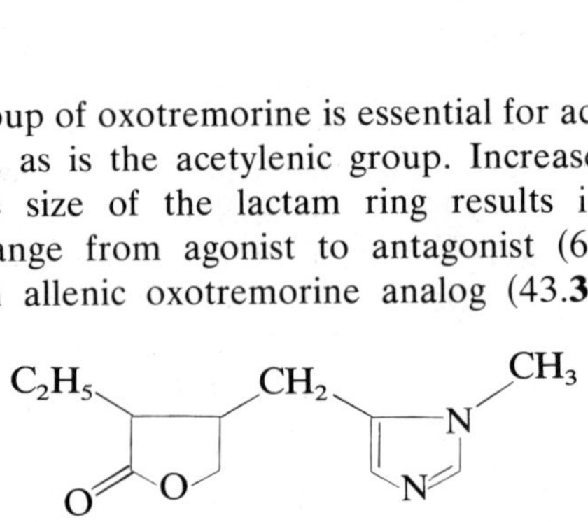

43.34

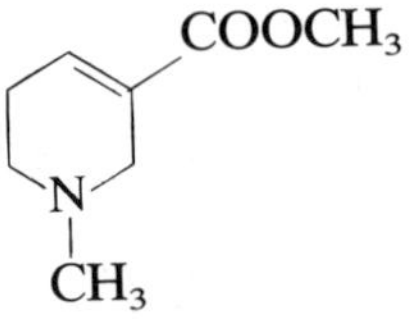

43.35

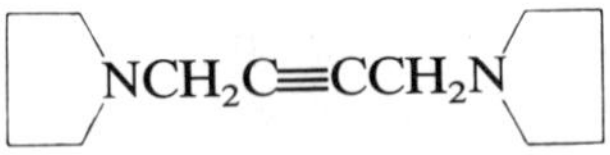

43.36

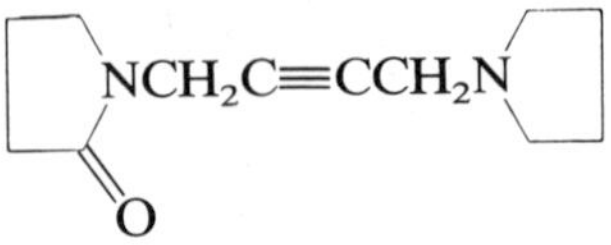

43.37

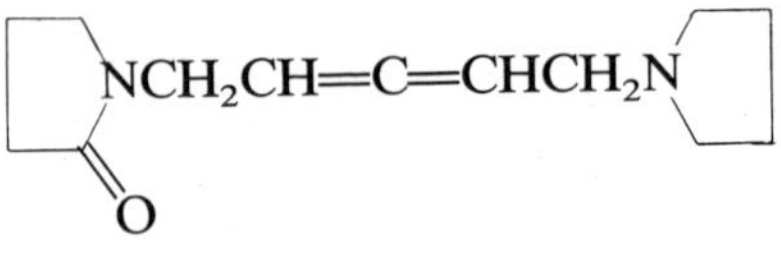

43.37a

with the heterocyclic rings separated by a five-carbon chain, was inert as an agonist or an antagonist in mice (66a).

4 STEREOCHEMISTRY–ACTIVITY RELATIONSHIPS

Casy (5) has advanced four questions to which stereochemical studies of cholinergic agonists must be directed:

1. Does the "active" conformation of a cholinergic ligand correspond to its preferred stereochemistry, or is an energetically less favored form bound to the receptor?
2. Is there a unique mode of ligand binding to cholinergic receptors, or do multiple modes exist?
3. May the dual effects (nicotinic and muscarinic) of acetylcholine be explained in terms of conformational isomerism?
4. Do agonist and antagonist ligands occupy the same or different binding sites (with one or more features common to both)?

The large body of chemical and biological work in the field has not yet produced adequate answers to these challenging questions.

The three-dimensional steric disposition of acetylcholine and its congeners is defined on the basis of torsion angle τ. In a system

X–C–C–Y, τ is defined as the angle between the plane containing the C–C and C–X bonds and the plane containing the C–C and C–Y bonds, and is illustrated with Newman projections (66) in Fig. 43.1. The smaller rotation needed to make the front ligand eclipsed with the rear one is the torsion angle τ. If this rotation is clockwise, it is assigned a + sign, if counterclockwise, a − sign (66). Casy (5) has concluded that evaluation of magnitude of torsion angles by NMR solution studies in general complements the results of X-ray studies in the crystalline state.

The torsion angles τ_2 and τ_3 are useful in defining significant conformations for acetylcholine (43.**38**) and related molecules. From X-ray studies, Baker et al. (67) noted that, in most cases, τ_3 values fall in the range $180 \pm 36°$ (*antiplanar*), placing the quaternary head and the acetyl group far apart, and the τ_2 angle commonly has a value of 73–94°, so that the N and O functions are approximately *synclinal* (*gauche*). Many compounds with the O–C–C–N$^+$ moiety where the oxygen function is hydroxy or acyloxy prefer the τ_2 synclinal (gauche) N/O disposition in the solid state: L($+$)-muscarine iodide (43.**22**); the (4R)-($+$)-*cis*-dioxolane (43.**27**); and the furan derivative (43.**25**). However, there are many exceptions: the potent muscarinic agonists carbamoylcholine (Table 43.1, no. 18) and ($+$)-*trans*-ACTM (43.**48**) (67) in the crystal state prefer the τ_2 anticlinal τ_3 antiplanar conformations, as do the weakly

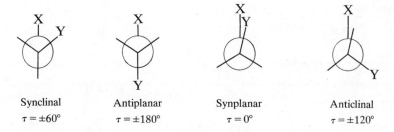

Synclinal	Antiplanar	Synplanar	Anticlinal
$\tau = \pm 60°$	$\tau = \pm 180°$	$\tau = 0°$	$\tau = \pm 120°$

Fig. 43.1 Torsion angle (τ). From Ref. 66.

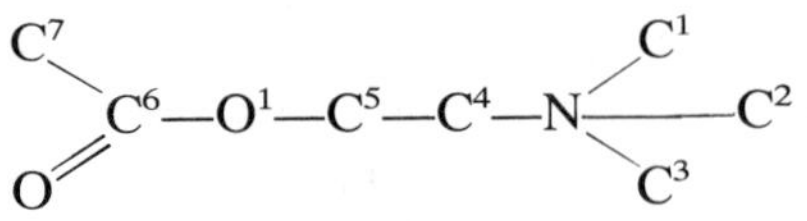

$$C^7$$
$$\diagdown C^6 - O^1 - C^5 - C^4 - N \diagdown \diagup C^2$$
$$O \diagup \qquad\qquad\qquad C^3$$

43.**38**

$$\tau_1 \quad C^5 - C^4 - N - C^3$$
$$\tau_2 \quad O^1 - C^5 - C^4 - N$$
$$\tau_3 \quad C^6 - O^1 - C^5 - C^4$$
$$\tau_4 \quad C^7 - C^6 - O^1 - C^5$$

active thio and seleno analogs of acetylcholine (43.**11** and 43.**12**). L(+)-Muscarone (43.**23**) exhibits a τ_2 that is antiplanar (68).

The crystal structures of certain nicotinic agents, for example, acetyl-α-methylcholine (43.**17**) and lactoylcholine (Table 43.1, no. 16) have torsion angle (τ_2 and τ_3) features similar to most muscarinic agents (100). In contrast, some cyclic analogs of aryl choline ethers exhibit maximum nicotinic effects when the τ_2 is *transoid* (antiplanar) (69).

However, there is no assurance that any of the preferred conformations determined by X-ray or solution NMR methods represent the geometry of the agonist at cholinergic receptors; barriers to rotation in molecules such as acetylcholine are low (70, 71), and there is considerable rotational freedom in the muscarine and muscarone systems (5). An alternative strategy is the study of conformationally restrained analogs with the quaternary head and the ester functions in relatively "frozen" positions. This approach presents the limitation of requiring molecules larger than the parent, with reduced receptor affinity and different solvent partition characteristics a likely consequence. Schueler (72), in proposing the possibility that muscarinic and nicotinic effects of acetylcholine are mediated by different conformers of the flexible molecule, evaluated 43.**39** and 43.**40** as conformational extremes. Both exhibit only feeble effects, and the difference in activity between the two compounds is not great. The *trans*-sulfur isostere (43.**39a**) of the 3-acetoxypiperidinium system 43.**39** is a potent muscarinic agonist ($\frac{1}{10}-\frac{1}{15}$ as active as acetylcholine), but the cis isomer (43.**39b**) is virtually inert (72a). In contrast, both the cis and the trans isomers (43.**39b** and 43.**39a**) display nicotinic action; the cis isomer is approximately $\frac{1}{5}$ as active as acetylcholine and is approximately seven times as potent as the trans. In the trans system (43.**39a**), the τ_2 angle (S–C–C–O) is described as anticlinal–antiplanar (72a), on the basis that the chair conformer has an axial S-methyl and an equatorial acetoxy.

Quaternary tropyl acetates (43.**41**, 43.**42**), in which a greater degree of molecular rigidity is imposed, are extremely weak muscarinics, and both exhibit potent

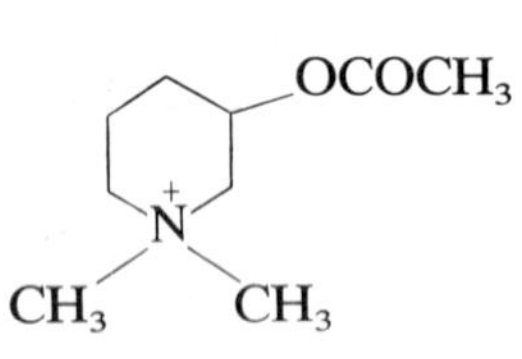

43.**39**

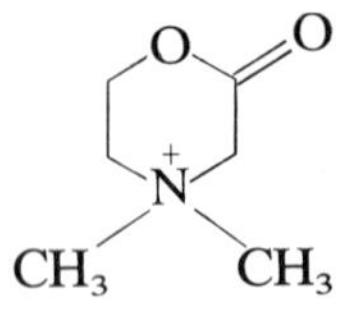

43.**40**

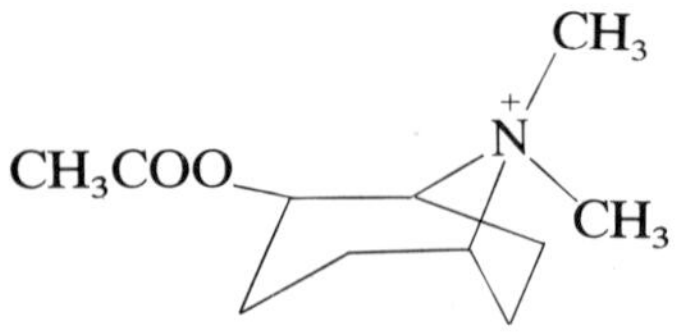

43.**41**

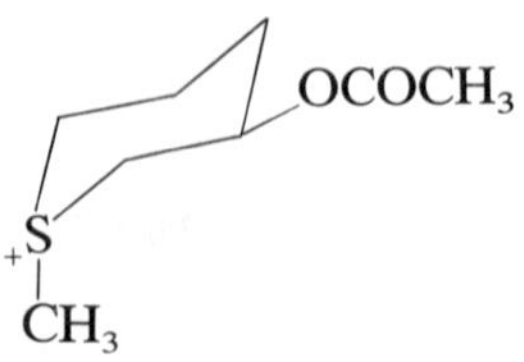

43.**39a**   trans

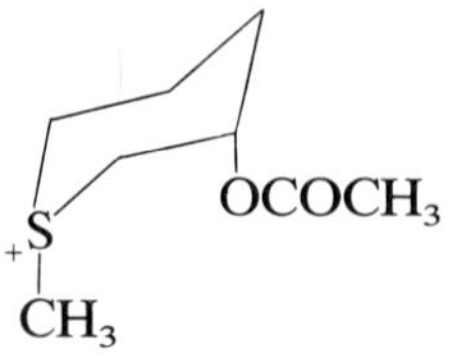

43.**39b**   cis

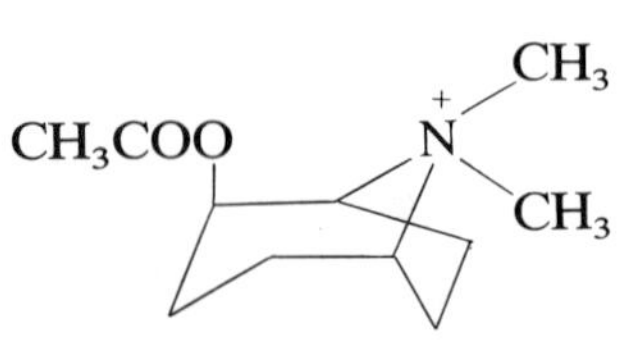

43.**42**

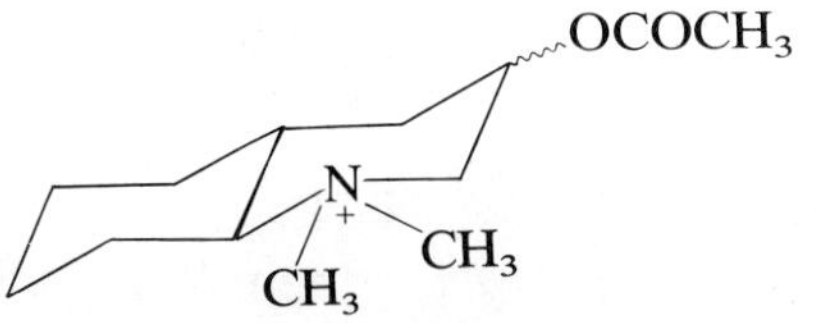

43.**43**

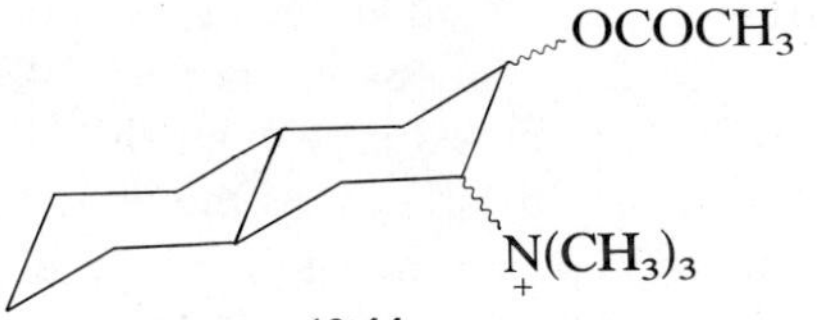

43.**44**

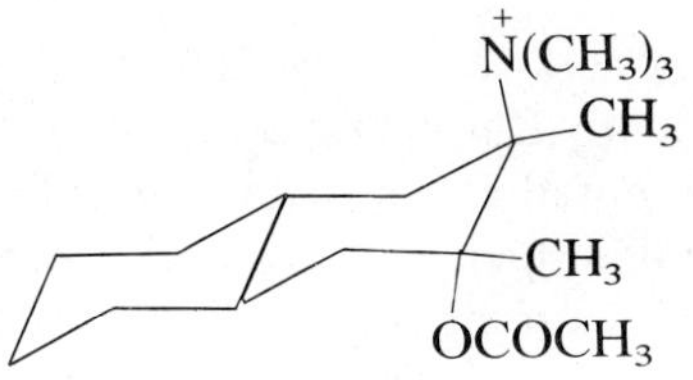

43.**45**

nicotinic effects (73). Stereoisomers of the *trans*-decahydroquinoline (43.**43**) (74) and *trans*-decalin (43.**44**) (42) display extremely low orders of muscarinic effect, with the 2,3-trans-diaxial isomer of 43.**44** being the most active of the four stereoisomers of this structure (0.06% the activity of acetylcholine). In a series of *C*-methylated *trans*-decalins, the 2,3-dimethyl compound 43.**45** is the most potent muscarinic, but it is only $\frac{1}{50}$ as active as acetylcholine (75). It has been concluded (5) that data on these decalins and decahydroquinolines are inconclusive, although it is noted that all of the active decalin-derived systems have antiplanar τ_2 dispositions.

In the series of cyclohexane-derived compounds (43.**46**), the (1*R*, 2*R*)-(−)-trans system is a weak muscarinic ($\frac{1}{400}$–$\frac{1}{1000}$ as active as acetylcholine), and the (±)-cis isomer is completely inert (76). Casy (5)

43.**46**

43.**47**

suggested that an unfavored trans-diaxial conformer (antiplanar τ_2) for 43.**46** may be the biologically active form of the molecule. However, inclusion of a *t*-butyl group into the cyclohexane system to freeze the 1,2-trans-diaxial geometry does not lead to a greatly increased muscarinic effect (77). The cis and trans cyclopentane systems (43.**47**) have been described (5) as feeble spasmogenics with τ_2 angle near anticlinal. A series of congeners of acetyl-γ-homocholine (43.**14**) and 4-acetoxybutyl-trimethylammonium (43.**15**) (78, 79), in which the amino alcohol entity is a part of cyclopropane or cyclobutane ring systems, exhibits feeble muscarinic and appreciable nicotinic effects, and these compounds provide little insight into active conformations for acetylcholine. The cyclopropane ring has been exploited as the smallest system capable of conferring conformational rigidity on an acetylcholine analog (80, 81); (+)-*trans*-ACTM (43.**48**) equals or surpasses acetylcholine muscarinic potency in two test systems. The (−)-trans enantiomer is several hundred times less active, and the racemic cis system (43.**49**) is almost inert. All isomers are feeble nicotinics.

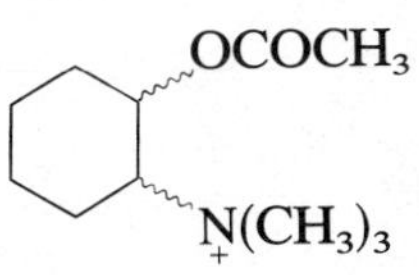

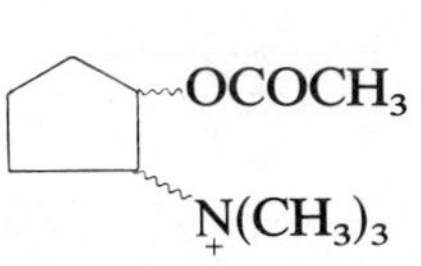

X-Ray analysis of (+)-*trans*-ACTM (82) established the τ_2 angle as 137° (which is within the anticlinal range), and because of the rigidity of the cyclopropane ring, this value probably closely approaches the solute conformation. The (1*S*, 2*S*) configuration of (+)-*trans*-ACTM superimposes on the equivalent centers in the potent muscarinic agonists (*S*)-(+)-acetyl-β-methylcholine and (2*S*, 3*R*, 5*S*)-(+)-muscarine (83). A (±)-cyclobutane analog (43.**50**) of *trans*-ACTM is decidedly less potent than (±)-ACTM (84). No conformational study has been reported on 43.**50**, and inspection of molecular models does not reveal convincing structural differences between the cyclopropane and the cyclobutane systems.

Pauling and co-workers have defined the following molecular parameters for acetylcholine congeners (based on structure

$(CH_3)_3\overset{+}{N}$ | OCOCH₃
43.**48**

$(CH_3)_3\underset{+}{N}$ OCOCH₃
43.**49**

OCOCH₃
$\underset{+}{N}(CH_3)_3$
43.**50**

43.**48**) for potent muscarinic activity: $\tau_1 = 180°$, $\tau_2 = +73$ to $+137°$; $\tau_3 = 180 \pm 35°$; $\tau_4 = 180°$ or $-137°$. Interatomic distances are defined as $N^+-O^1 = 360$; $N^+-C^6 = 450$; and $N^+-C^7 = 540$ pm. Low potency or inactivity of certain acetylcholine derivatives is attributed to deviations from one or more of these parameters. However, Casy (5) has cited deviations from these values in which potent agonist activity is manifested.

It has not been possible to demonstrate unequivocally that acetylcholine assumes different conformations at nicotinic and at muscarinic receptors; neither has this theory been disproved by the body of chemical and biological data. Chothia (85) has proposed that the conformations of acetylcholine relevant to the nicotinic and the muscarinic receptors are the same, but that different sides of the molecule react with nicotinic and muscarinic receptors, the "methyl side" activating muscarinic, and the "carbonyl side" activating nicotinic receptors. This concept has been used to explain specificity of action of several cholinergic agonists. Several groups have criticized this theory, from experimental as well as theoretical considerations (5, 86). The absence of nicotinic properties in almost all the conformationally restricted congeners of acetylcholine has impeded definition of specific geometry with respect to nicotinic effects. It must be concluded that the relationship of acetylcholine's molecular geometry to its physiological roles is still largely unknown.

5 THE MUSCARINIC RECEPTOR

On the basis of classical structure–activity studies, Beckett (38) defined the muscarinic receptor as illustrated in Fig. 43.2. This diagram has been modified as a result of further studies on oxotremorine (43.**37**) and extended Hückel molecular orbital calculations (65b) to present as the dimensions of the receptor the following: $1 \rightarrow 3$, 5.6 ± 0.2 Å; $1 \rightarrow 2$, 3.2 ± 0.2 Å; $2 \rightarrow 3$, 2.8 ± 0.6 Å.

A model of the cholinergic receptor proposed by Karlin and co-workers (87, 88) is represented as a protein dimer transversing the lipid bilayer of the nerve membrane (Fig. 43.3). For a further discussion see Chapter 46. The binding site for acetylcholine is visualized as being a slot on the outer surface of the protein. Close to one end of the slot is an anionic subsite, and at the other end are a reducible disulfide group, a hydrogen that is available for hydrogen bonding to C=O, and a variety of other sites involved in hydrophobic bonding to CH_3. Karlin proposed that acetylcholine induces a conformational change around the anionic subsite such that the distance between the anionic subsite and the S–S region (where the hydrogen bonding moiety and the hydrophobic bonding moieties are located) is shortened. The consequence of the change in conformation of

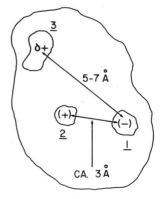

Fig. 43.2 Dimensions of the muscarinic receptor (adapted from Beckett, Ref. 38).

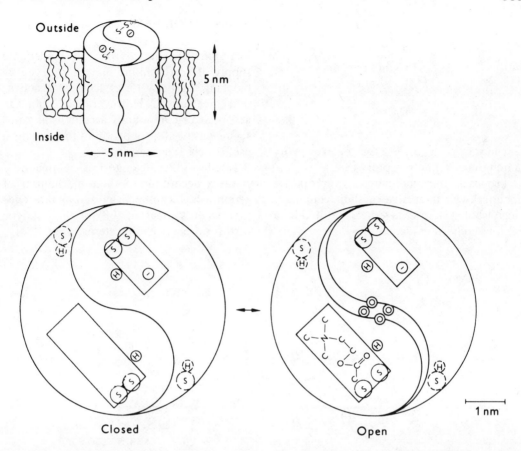

Fig. 43.3   The cholinergic receptor as proposed by Karlin, Ref. 87. (Reproduced by permission of Macmillan, London and Basingstoke.)

the protein in the region of the slot is that the two molecules forming the dimeric protein are forced apart, forming a channel that runs through the membrane into the inner part of the nerve cell, through which ions migrate to generate the nerve impulse.

On the basis of studies of reductive alkylation of neural membranes with N-ethylmaleimide, Aronstam et al. (88a) concluded that conformational states of the muscarinic receptor differ only with respect to their affinities for agonists, not for antagonists. Moreover, these workers stated that it seems likely that muscarinic agonist and antagonist binding sites partially overlap. The results of this study were concluded to be supportive of a theoretical

model for the muscarinic receptor proposed by Birdsall and Hulme (88b).

Ticku and Triggle (2) suggested that the muscarinic receptor is composed of two components: a *recognition component* (determining ligand specificity) and an associated *amplification* or *catalytic component*. The acetylcholine recognition site is linked to a Ca^{2+} channel and upon activation, membrane-bound Ca^{2+} is translocated to generate the response.

A proposal (88c) that there are differences in muscarinic receptors in different tissues has been supported by description of subtle differences in receptor specificity toward a spiro dioxolane quinuclidine muscarinic agonist (43.**50a**). This compound is

CH$_3$

43.50a

advanced as a probe for heterogeneity among muscarinic receptors (88d).

Proposals that cholinergic receptors are identical with the active catalytic centers of acetylcholinesterase have been refuted by a sizable body of evidence (89).

6   ANTICHOLINESTERASES

Symptoms resulting from an inadequate supply of acetylcholine may be relieved by blocking the body's acetylcholine deactivation mechanism. However, the attention accorded to compounds accomplishing this seems out of all proportion to their medical use, which is limited (65c).

Koelle (32c) categorizes anticholinesterases according to their mechanism of action, which can be visualized by reference to Beckett's diagram (38) of the catalytic surface of acetylcholinesterase (Fig. 43.4).

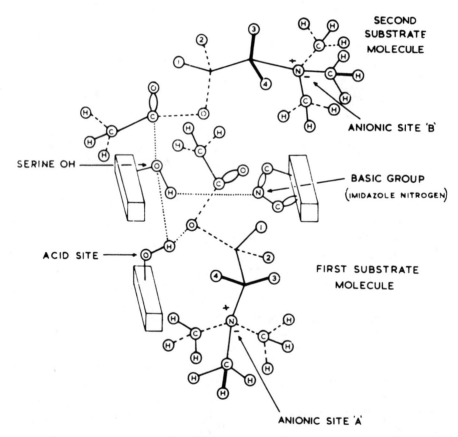

Fig. 43.4 The catalytic surface of acetylcholinesterase (38). (Reproduced by permission of The New York Academy of Sciences.)

6.1   Reversible Inhibitors

Simple quaternary compounds such as tetramethylammonium combine only with the anionic site of the active catalytic surface of acetylcholinesterase, and deny access to this site to acetylcholine. Cohen and Oosterbaan (90) tabulated a comprehensive list of tetraalkyl quaternary ammonium acetylcholinesterase inhibitors and described the kinetic studies on which the designation of "reversibility" for these types of compounds was based. Homologation of the methyl groups on the tetramethylammonium molecule tends to increase activity (Table 43.2) (91). Attempts to correlate biological test data with the calculated diameter of the unhydrated quaternary head seem inconclusive.

Belleau (92) calculated enthalpies and entropies of binding for a homologous series of alkyltrimethylammonium compounds (43.**51**) and provided a rationalization for observed relative biological potencies in the series, based on hydrophobic bonding phenomena and ability of the alkyl chain in 43.**51** to displace ordered water from the acetylcholinesterase surface.

Edrophonium (43.**52**) combines a quaternary head for interaction with the anionic site with a phenolic OH which hydrogen bonds to a portion of the esteratic

$$R\overset{+}{N}(CH_3)_3$$

43.**51**   R=CH$_3$ through n-C$_{12}$H$_{15}$

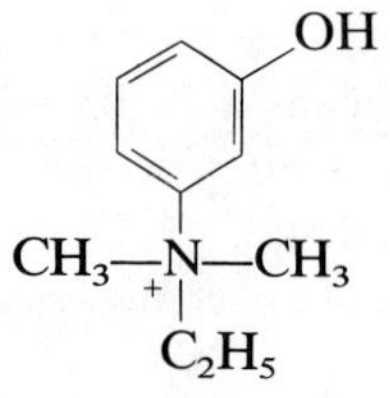

43.**52**

area of acetylcholinesterase (Fig. 43.4), thus increasing overall binding strength of the drug and producing higher potency. However, even this compound displays a rapidly reversible inhibition of the enzyme, and its duration of action is short (22c).

6.2   Inhibitors that Form a Covalent Bond with the Catalytic Site of Acetylcholinesterase

The prototypical carbamate-type acetylcholinesterase inhibitor is physostigmine (43.**53**). At the pH of the body fluids, a significant proportion of physostigmine molecules is protonated at N^1 (43.**53**) and this cationic species forms a complex with the catalytic surface of acetylcholinesterase (Fig. 43.4), following which cleavage of the

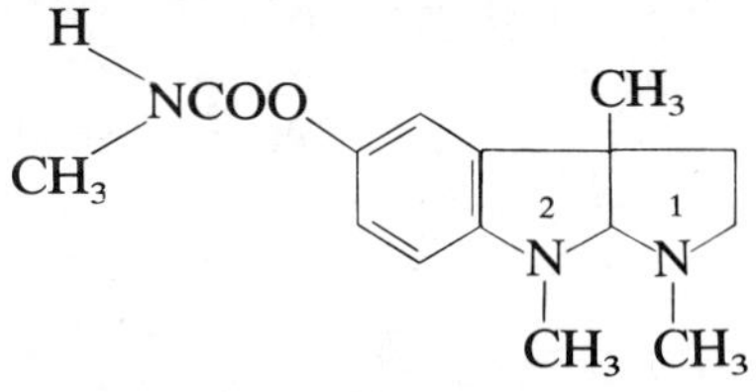

Table 43.2   Inhibition of Acetylcholinesterase by Quaternary Ammonium Ions[a]

Ion	Relative Anticholinesterase Potency
$(CH_3)_4N^+$	1
$(C_2H_5)_4N^+$	5
$(n\text{-}C_3H_7)_4N^+$	100
$(n\text{-}C_4H_9)_4N^+$	50
$n\text{-}C_3H_7\overset{+}{N}(CH_3)_3$	5
$n\text{-}C_4H_9\overset{+}{N}(CH_3)_3$	7.5
$n\text{-}C_5H_{11}\overset{+}{N}(CH_3)_3$	10
$n\text{-}C_7H_{15}\overset{+}{N}(CH_3)_3$	25

[a] Adapted from Ref. 91.

43.**53**

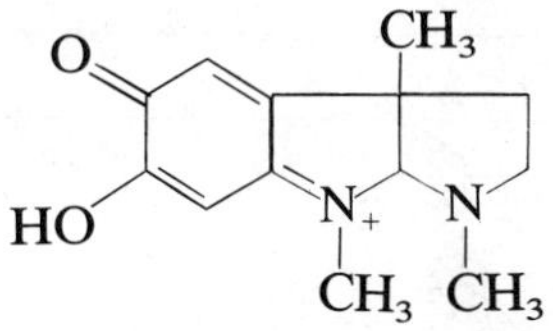

43.**54**

carbamate ester moiety proceeds in a manner analogous to that for the ester group of acetylcholine. The net effect is a transfer of the *N*-methylcarbamoyl moiety from the inhibitor molecule to a nucleophilic entity on the esteratic site, presumably the OH of serine. The half-life of dimethylcarbamoyl acetylcholinesterase is more than 40 million times greater than that of the acetylated enzyme (93). Rubreserine (43.**54**), an oxidation product of the ester-cleaved physostigmine molecule, is approximately 1/250 as active as physostigmine as an acetylcholinesterase inhibitor (94). Koelle (32d) has designated physostigmine and synthetic carbamate anti-acetylcholinesterases as "competitive substrates" or "acid-transferring inhibitors."

Watts and Wilkinson (94a) have developed a kinetic scheme which is offered as a more adequate explanation for carbamate–acetylcholinesterase reactions, and which explains the observed catalysis of decarbamoylation of carbamoylated acetylcholinesterase by excess carbamate.

In compounds of type 43.**55**, meta-substituted systems frequently exhibit high miotic action (which is taken as a reflection of anticholinesterase activity), whereas ortho- and para-substituted systems are inert (94). Foldes et al., (95) concluded that the optimum N^+—C=O interatomic distance for compounds of the type 43.**55** is 4.7 Å. The meta isomers of these compounds meet this requirement, as does pyridostigmine (43.**56**), which is employed clinically. Molecular models demonstrate that the active *m*-quaternary ammonium

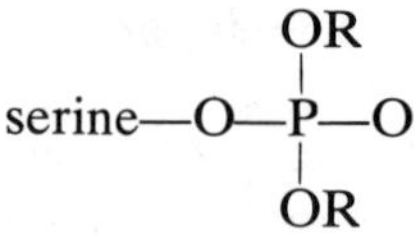

$$\text{serine—O—P—O} \quad \begin{array}{c} OR \\ | \\ | \\ OR \end{array}$$

43.**58**

phenylcarbamate systems can assume reasonable conformations in which their cationic heads and C=O groups coincide with similar groups in acetylcholine. Long (94) has reported that 43.**57** is a potent acetylcholinesterase inhibitor, whereas the meta and para isomers are much less active. This molecule (43.**57**) conforms to the 4.7 Å N^+–C=O distance requirement, but the meta and para isomers do not.

Among the most powerful anticholinesterases are the phosphorus-containing compounds. Certain of these are extremely toxic, and much of the developmental work in the field was done with the object of preparing chemical warfare agents ("nerve gases"). Compounds of these types are potent and useful insecticides. The reaction between acetylcholinesterase and most organophosphorus inhibitors occurs only at the esteratic site of the enzyme (32d), and the reaction here is comparable to that involving the carbamate esters and acetylcholinesterase. The resulting serine-phosphorylated enzyme is extremely stable; if the R groups attached to the phosphorus (43.**58**) are methyl or ethyl, regeneration of the enzyme by hydrolytic cleavage requires several hours. If the R groups are isopropyl, essentially *no* hydrolysis occurs and reestablishment of enzyme activity can

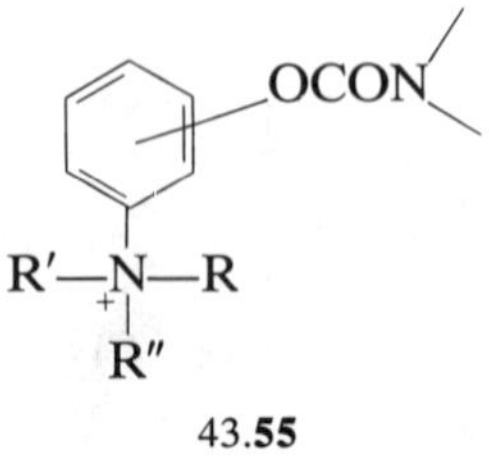

43.**55**

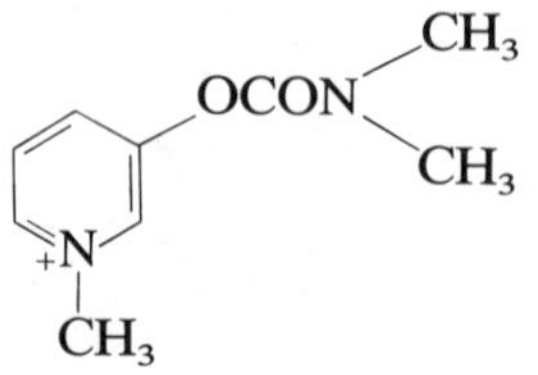

43.**56**

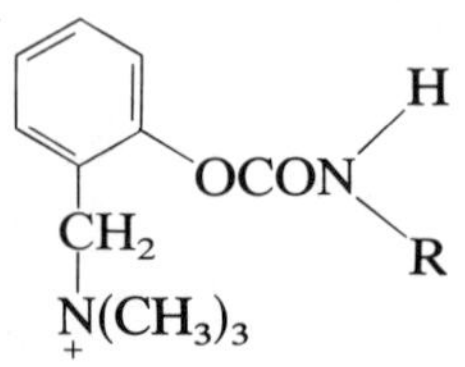

43.**57**

occur only after *de novo* synthesis of the enzyme, which may require months (32d). A characteristic structural feature of the anticholinesterase phosphorus compounds is the grouping P–Z, where Z is an electronegative moiety, a good leaving group, and the cleavage of the P–Z bond is accompanied by liberation of a large amount of energy. The P–Z bond is eminently susceptible to attack by nucleophiles, such as the serine OH of the esteratic site of acetylcholinesterase. The potency of the organophosphorus compounds parallels the ease of nucleophilic attack on the phosphorus atom.

Compounds in this category include ester and amide derivatives of orthophosphoryl halides, pyrophosphate esters and amides, alkyl and aryl phosphonic acid derivatives, and thiophosphoric acid derivatives. Holmsted (96, 97) has surveyed, tabulated, and classified organophosphorus acetylcholinesterase inhibitors. Representative compounds are shown in Table 43.3.

Table 43.3 Some Phosphorus-Containing Acetylcholinesterase Inhibitors

No.	Structure	Chemical, Proprietary, or Generic Names
1	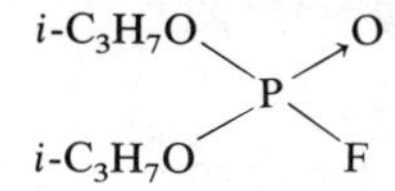	DFP, diisopropyl fluorophosphate, diisopropyl phosphofluoridate
2	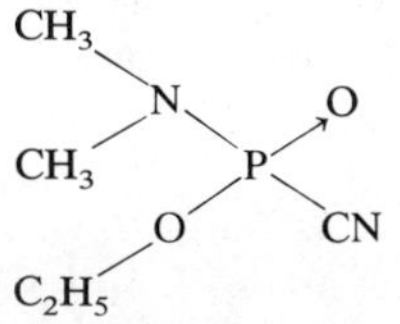	Tabun
3	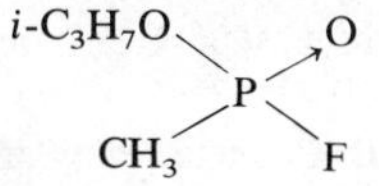	Sarin, isopropyl methyl phosphonofluoridate
4	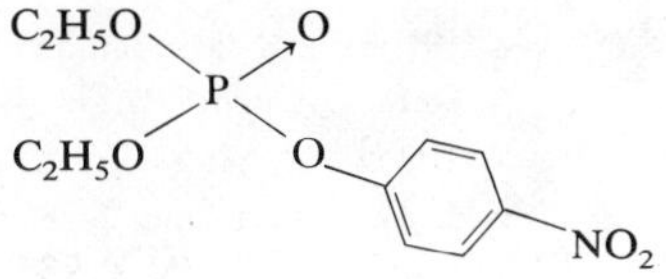	Diethyl *p*-nitrophenylphosphate, E-600, Mintacol
5	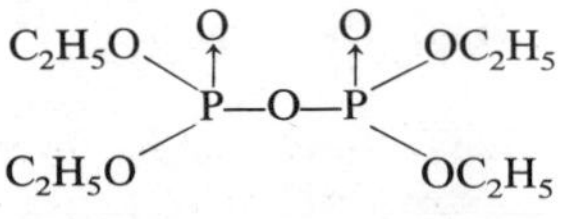	Tetraethyl pyrophosphate, TEPP
6	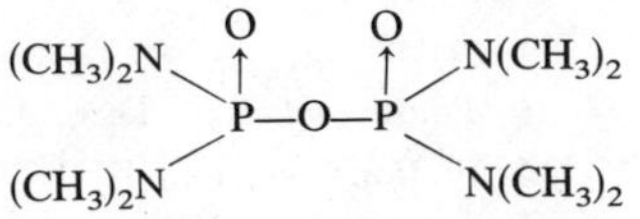	Octamethylpyrophosphoramide, OMPA
7	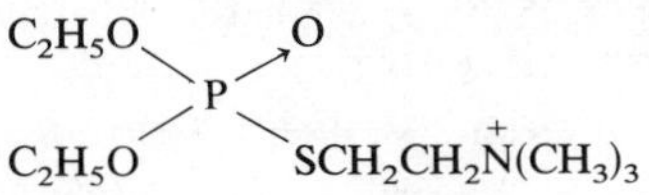	Echothiophate, diethoxyphosphinylthiocholine

43.**59**   43.**60**

Tabun and Sarin (nos. 2 and 3, Table 43.3) are among the most toxic war gases known. OMPA (no. 6) is inert as such, but it is metabolized to an *N*-oxide derivative which is the biologically active entity (98). Echothiophate (no. 7) is representative of inhibitors that bind initially to the anionic site of acetylcholinesterase as well as to the esteratic area. This compound is used clinically.

An α-chloro-β-phenethylamine (43.**59**) irreversibly inactivates acetylcholinesterase (99); the active pharmacophoric species is the aziridinium cation 43.**60**. The quaternary ion nature of the aziridinium cation allows for reversible addition complex formation with the anionic site of the enzyme, and this precedes slow alkylation of the nucleophilic site. Tetramethylammonium retards the irreversible inactivation of the enzyme by this compound.

REFERENCES

1. E. S. Vizi, "Release Mechanisms of Acetylcholine and the Role of Na^+–K^+–Activated ATPase," in *Cholinergic Mechanisms*, P. G. Waser, Ed., Raven Press, New York, 1975, pp. 199–211.

2. M. K. Ticku and D. J. Triggle, *Gen. Pharmacol.*, **7**, 133 (1976).

3. D. Nachmansohn and M. Berman, *J. Biol. Chem.*, **165**, 551 (1946).

4. R. B. Barlow, in *Wenner Gren Center International Symposium on Tobacco Alkaloids and Related Compounds*, Pergamon, Oxford, 1964, p. 277.

5. A. F. Casy, *Progr. Med. Chem.*, **11**, 1 (1975).

6. R. D. Purves, *Nature*, **261**, 149 (1976).

7. A. B. Rizzuti, *Am. J. Ophthal.*, **63**, 484 (1967).

8. H. R. Ing, *Science*, **109**, 264 (1949).

9. H. R. Ing, P. Kordik, and D. P. H. Tudor Williams, *Brit. J. Pharmacol.*, **7**, 103 (1952).

10. J. Bannister and V. P. Whittaker, *Nature*, **167**, 605 (1951).

11. R. L. Stehle, K. I. Melville, and F. K. Oldham, *J. Pharmacol. Exp. Ther.*, **56**, 473 (1936).

11a. J. Trzeciakowski and C. Y. Chiou, *J. Pharm. Sci.*, **67**, 531 (1978).

12. A. K. Cho, D. J. Jenden, and S. I. Lamb, *J. Med. Chem.*, **15**, 391 (1972).

13. P. Holton and H. R. Ing, *Brit. J. Pharmacol.*, **4**, 190 (1949).

14. H. Kilbinger, A. Wagner, and R. Zerban, *Naunyn-Schmiedebergs Arch. Pharmakol. Exp. Pathol.*, **295**, 81 (1976).

15. H. L. Friedman, "Postganglionic Parasympathetic Stimulants (Muscarinic Drugs)," in *Medicinal Research Series*, Vol. 1, A. Burger, Ed., Dekker, New York, 1967, pp. 79–131.

16. L. L. Darko, J. G. Cannon, J. P. Long, and T. F. Burks, *J. Med. Chem.*, **8**, 841 (1965).

17. J. G. Cannon, R. V. Smith, G. A. Fisher, J. P. Long, and F. W. Benz, *J. Med. Chem.*, **14**, 66 (1971).

18. B. Pullman, Ph. Courrière, and J. L. Coubeils, *Mol. Pharmacol.*, **7**, 397 (1971).

19. I. Kimura, I. Morishima, T. Yonezawa, and M. Kimura, *Chem. Pharm. Bull.* (Tokyo), **22**, 429 (1974).

20. H. C. Chang and J. H. Gaddum, *J. Physiol.* (London), **79**, 255 (1933).

21. R. Hunt and R. de M. Taveau, *Brit. Med. J.*, 1788 (1906).

22. D. Bovet and F. Bovet-Nitti, *Médicaments du Système Nerveux Végétatif*, S. Karger, Basel, 1948.

23. H. R. Ing, G. S. Dawes, and L. Wajda, *J. Pharmacol. Exp. Ther.*, **85**, 85 (1945).

24. E. Fourneau and H. J. Pye, *Bull. Soc. Chim. Fr.*, **15**, 544 (1949).

25. V. P. Whittaker, *Biochem. Pharmacol.*, **1**, 342 (1959).

26. B. V. Rama Sastry, C. C. Pfeiffer, and A. Lasslo, *J. Pharmacol. Exp. Ther.*, **130**, 346 (1960).

27. R. Hunt and R. R. Renshaw, *J. Pharmacol. Exp. Ther.*, **25**, 315 (1925).

28. J. M. Van Rossum and E. J. Ariëns, *Arch. Int. Pharmacodyn. Ther.*, **118**, 418 (1959).

29. R. T. Major and H. T. Bonnet, U.S. Pat. 2, 347, 367 (1945); through *Chem. Abstr.*, **39**, 4721 (1945).

30. R. R. Renshaw and C. Y. Hopkins, *J. Am. Chem. Soc.*, **51**, 953 (1929).

31. A. Ercoli, *Ann. Chim. Appl.*, **25**, 263 (1935).

32. G. B. Koelle in L. S. Goodman and A. Gilman, Eds., *The Pharmacologic Basis of Therapeutics*, 5th ed., Macmillan, New York, 1975, (a) pp. 468, 471. (b) p. 472. (c) p. 466. (d) p. 447.

33. C. Y. Chiou, *J. Pharm. Sci.*, **64**, 469 (1975).

34. K. A. Scott and H. G. Mautner, *Biochem. Pharmacol.*, **13**, 907 (1964).

35. H. G. Mautner, *Ann. Rep. Med. Chem.*, 230 (1969).

36. A. Blankart, in *Festschrift Emil C. Barell*, 1936, p. 284; through *Chem. Abstr.*, **31**, 2675 (1937).

37. A. M. Lands and C. J. Cavallito, *J. Pharmacol. Exp. Ther.*, **110**, 369 (1954).

38. A. H. Beckett, *Ann N.Y. Acad. Sci.*, **144**, 675 (1967).

39. M. M.-L. Chan and J. B. Robinson, *J. Med. Chem.*, **17**, 1057 (1974).

40. B. W. Ellenbroek and J. M. Van Rossum, *Arch. Int. Pharmacodyn. Ther.*, **125**, 216 (1960).

41. E. Lesser, *Brit. J. Pharmacol.*, **25**, 213 (1965).

42. E. E. Smissman, W. L. Nelson, J. LaPidus, and J. L. Day, *J. Med. Chem.*, **9**, 458 (1966).

43. G. H. Cocolas, E. C. Robinson, and W. L. Dewey, *J. Med. Chem.*, **13**, 299 (1970).

44. A. Simonart, *Arch. Int. Pharmacodyn. Ther.*, **48**, 328 (1934).

45. R. Hunt and R. de M. Taveau, *J. Pharmacol. Exp. Ther.*, **1**, 303 (1909).

46. P. Hey, *Brit. J. Pharmacol.*, **7**, 117 (1952).

47. J. G. Cannon, A. Gangjee, J. P. Long, and A. J. Allen, *J. Med. Chem.*, **19**, 934 (1976).

48. J. G. Cannon, P. J. Mulligan, J. P. Long, and S. Heintz, *J. Pharm. Sci.*, **62**, 830 (1973).

49. J. H. Welsh and R. Taub, *J. Pharmacol. Exp. Ther.*, **103**, 62 (1951).

50. F. Kögl, C. A. Salemink, H. Schouter, and F. Jellinek, *Rec. Trav. Chim. Pays-Bas*, **76**, 109 (1957).

51. E. Hardegger and F. Lohse, *Helv. Chim. Acta*, **40**, 2383 (1957).

52. P. G. Waser, *Pharmacol. Rev.*, **13**, 465 (1961).

53. A. H. Beckett, B. H. Warrington, R. Griffiths, E. S. Pepper, and K. Bowden, *J. Pharm. Pharmacol.*, **28**, 728 (1976).

54. A. K. Armitage and H. R. Ing, *Brit. J. Pharmacol.*, **9**, 376 (1954).

55. B. Belleau and J. Puranen, *J. Med. Chem.*, **6**, 325 (1963).

56. K. J. Chang, R. C. Deth, and D. J. Triggle, *J. Med. Chem.*, **15**, 243 (1972).

57. J. G. R. Elferink and C. A. Salemink, *Arzneim.-Forsch.*, **25**, 1702 (1975).

58. J. G. R. Elferink and C. A. Salemink, *Arzneim.-Forsch.*, **25**, 1858 (1975).

58a. C. Melchiorre, P. Angeli, M. Gianella, F. Gualtieri, M. Pigini, M. L. Cingolani, G. Gamba, L. Leone, P. Pigini, and L. Re, *Eur. J. Med. Chem.*, **13**, 357 (1978).

59. H. F. Ridley, S. S. Chatterjee, J. F. Moran, and D. J. Triggle, *J. Med. Chem.*, **12**, 931 (1969).

60. R. S. Givens and D. R. Rademacher, *J. Med. Chem.*, **17**, 457 (1974).

61. K. G. R. Sundelin, R. A. Wiley, R. S. Givens, and D. R. Rademacher, *J. Med. Chem.*, **16**, 235 (1973).

61a. F. Gualtieri, M. Gianella, C. Melchiorre, M. Pigini, M. L. Cingolani, G. Gamba, P. Pigini, and L. Rossini, *Farm. Ed. Sc.*, **30**, 223 (1975).

61b. C. Melchiorre, P. Angeli, M. Gianella, M. Pigini, M. L. Cingolani, G. Gamba, and P. Pigini, *Farm. Ed. Sc.*, **32**, 25 (1977).

62. F. Gaultieri, M. Gianella, C. Melchiorre, and M. Pigini, *J. Med. Chem.*, **17**, 455 (1974).

62a. P. Angeli, C. Melchiorre, M. Gianella, M. Pigini, and M. L. Cingolani, *J. Med. Chem.*, **20**, 398 (1977).

62b. D. J. Triggle, *Neurotransmitter–Receptor Interactions*, Academic, New York, 1971, Chap. IV.

63. C. Melchiorre, F. Gaultieri, M. Gianella, M. Pigini, M. L. Cingolani, G. Gamba, P. Pigini, and L. Rossini, *Farm. Ed. Sci.*, **30**, 287 (1975).

64. A. K. Cho, W. L. Haslett, and D. J. Jenden, *J. Pharmacol. Exp. Ther.*, **138**, 249 (1962).

65. R. W. Brimblecomb, *Drug Actions on Cholinergic Systems*, University Park Press, Baltimore, 1974, (a) p. 26. (b) pp. 24–30. (c) p. 63.

66. IUPAC Tentative Rules, *J. Org. Chem.*, **35**, 2849 (1970).

66a. A. Claesson, A. Asell, S. Bjorkman, and L.-I. Olsson, *Acta Pharm. Suec.*, **15**, 105 (1978).

67. R. W. Baker, C. H. Chothia, P. Pauling, and T. J. Petcher, *Nature*, **230**, 439 (1971).

68. P. Pauling and T. J. Petcher, *Nature New Biol.*, **236**, 112 (1972).

69. E. R. Clark, I. E. Hughes, and C. F. C. Smith, *J. Med. Chem.*, **19,** 692 (1976).

70. A. F. Casy, *Ann. Rep. Progr. Chem.*, Sect. B, 477 (1974).

71. D. Lichtenberg, P. A. Kroon, and S. I. Chan, *J. Am. Chem. Soc.*, **96,** 5934 (1974).

72. F. W. Schueler, *J. Am. Pharm. Assoc., Sci. Ed.*, **45,** 197 (1956).

72a. G. Lambrecht, *Eur. J. Med. Chem.*, **12,** 41 (1977).

73. S. Archer, A. M. Lands, and T. R. Lewis, *J. Med. Pharm. Chem.*, **5,** 423 (1962).

74. E. E. Smissman and G. S. Chappell, *J. Med. Chem.*, **12,** 432 (1969).

75. E. E. Smissman and G. R. Parker, *J. Med. Chem.*, **16,** 23 (1973).

76. J. B. Kay, J. B. Robinson, B. Cox, and D. Polkonjak, *J. Pharm. Pharmacol.*, **22,** 214 (1970).

77. A. F. Casy, E. S. C. Wu, and B. D. Whelton, *Can. J. Chem.*, **50,** 3998 (1972).

78. J. G. Cannon, A. B. Rege, T. L. Gruen, and J. P. Long, *J. Med. Chem.*, **15,** 71 (1972).

79. J. G. Cannon, Y. Lin, and J. P. Long, *J. Med. Chem.*, **16,** 27 (1973).

80. P. D. Armstrong, J. G. Cannon, and J. P. Long, *Nature*, **220,** 65 (1968).

81. C. Y. Chiou, J. P. Long, J. G. Cannon, and P. D. Armstrong, *J. Pharmacol. Exp. Ther.*, **166,** 243 (1969).

82. C. Chothia and P. Pauling, *Nature*, **226,** 541 (1970).

83. P. D. Armstrong and J. G. Cannon, *J. Med. Chem.*, **13,** 1037 (1970).

84. J. G. Cannon, T. Lee, V. Sankaran, and J. P. Long, *J. Med. Chem.*, **18,** 1027 (1975).

85. C. Chothia, *Nature*, **225,** 36 (1970).

86. E. Shefter and D. J. Triggle, *Nature*, **227,** 1354 (1970).

87. A. Karlin, D. A. Cowburn, and M. J. Reiter, in *Drug Receptors*, H. P. Rang, Ed., University Park Press, Baltimore, Md., 1973, pp. 193–209.

88. A. Karlin, *Fed. Proc.*, **32,** 1847 (1973).

88a. R. S. Aronstam, W. Hoss, and L. G. Abood, *Eur. J. Pharmacol.*, **46,** 279 (1977).

88b. N. J. M. Birdsall and E. C. Hulme, *J. Neurochem.*, **27,** 7 (1976).

88c. A. Fisher, M. Weinstock, and S. Cohen, *Israel J. Med. Sci.*, **11,** 861 (1975).

88d. A. Fisher, M. Weinstock, S. Gitter, and S. Cohen, *Eur. J. Pharmacol.*, **37,** 329 (1976).

89. J. S. Bindra, *Ann. Rep. Med. Chem.*, **8,** 269 (1973).

90. J. A. Cohen and R. A. Oosterbaan, in *Cholinesterases and Anticholinesterase Agents, Handbuch Exp. Pharmakol.*, Vol. 15, G. B. Koelle, Ed., Springer-Verlag, Berlin, 1963, p. 299.

91. F. Bergmann and A. Shimoni, *Biochim. Biophys. Acta*, **10,** 49 (1953).

92. B. Belleau, *Ann. N.Y. Acad. Sci.*, **144,** 705 (1967).

93. I. B. Wilson and M. A. Harrison, *J. Biol. Chem.*, **236,** 2292 (1961).

94. J. P. Long, in *Cholinesterases and Anticholinesterase Agents, Handbuch Exp. Pharmakol.*, Vol. 15, G. B. Koelle, Ed., Springer-Verlag, Berlin, 1963, p. 374.

94a. P. Watts and R. G. Wilkinson, *Biochem. Pharmacol.*, **26,** 757 (1977).

95. F. F. Foldes, E. G. Erdos, N. Baart, J. Zwart, and E. K. Zsigmond, *Arch. Int. Pharmacodyn. Ther.*, **120,** 286 (1959).

96. B. Holmsted, *Pharmacol. Rev.*, **11,** 567 (1959).

97. B. Holmsted, in Ref. 90, pp. 428–485.

98. J. E. Casida, T. C. Allen, and M. A. Stahmann, *J. Biol. Chem.*, **210,** 607 (1954).

99. B. Belleau and H. Tani, *Mol. Pharmacol.*, **2,** 411 (1966).

100. C. Chothia and P. Pauling, *Proc. Natl. Acad. Sci. U.S.*, **65,** 477 (1970).

CHAPTER FORTY-FOUR

Anticholinergics: Antispasmodic and Antiulcer Drugs

B. V. RAMA SASTRY

Department of Pharmacology
School of Medicine
Vanderbilt University
Nashville, Tennessee 37232, USA

CONTENTS

361

1 INTRODUCTION

The role of acetylcholine as a parasympathetic neurotransmitter and its effects on smooth muscle and glands are reviewed in Chapter 43. Typical parasympathetic effects, in addition to cardiac inhibition and vasodilation in certain areas, are miosis and increased gastrointestinal motion and secretion. It is believed that acetylcholine is the common factor in many of these processes. Electrical stimulation of parasympathetic nerves causes the appearance of acetylcholine at the neuromuscular junction; presumably acetylcholine appears regularly during the spontaneous functioning of the postganglionic fibers of the parasympathetic nerves, and is regularly kept from accumulating by hydrolysis with acetylcholinesterase (Chapter 43). Spontaneous release of acetylcholine at the parasympathetic nerve endings results in the involuntary contraction or spasm of the muscle. Therefore, the contractions of the stomach, intestinal tract, heart, certain blood vessels, and many other structures in various pathological situations are often attributed to the amounts of acetylcholine in excess of normal requirements. Gastric secretion, salivation, micturition, lacrimation, sweating, and miosis are influenced by

acetylcholine. The rates of these activities can be controlled by certain anticholinergic drugs.

Anticholinergic drugs interfere with physiological functions that depend on cholinergic nerve transmission. These drugs do not prevent acetylcholine from being released at nerve endings, but they may compete with the liberated neurohormone for cholinergic receptor sites. Acetylcholine is the chemical transmitter at the postganglionic parasympathetic nerve endings, as well as at autonomic ganglia and somatic neuromuscular junctions. Different types of anticholinergic drugs antagonize the actions of acetylcholine at these three types of synapses. Anticholinergic drugs which block somatic neuromuscular junction (curareform drugs) and autonomic ganglia (ganglionic blocking drugs) are described in Chapters 42 and 46. The pharmacological actions of anticholinergic drugs discussed in this chapter mimic the effects of cutting the parasympathetic nerve supply to various organs; therefore they are designated as parasympatholytics. Muscarine mimics the actions of acetylcholine on the structures innervated by parasympathetic nerves; it is relatively inactive at autonomic ganglia and somatic neuromuscular junction. Parasympatholytics that antagonize the actions of muscarine are also known as antimuscarinic agents.

The classical parasympatholytic agent is atropine, and therefore anticholinergic drugs used to be referred to as atropinic agents. Typical effects produced by atropine are mydriasis, tachycardia, decreased gastrointestinal peristalsis, and diminished secretions of gastric juice, saliva, and sweat. A large number of anticholinergic agents has been synthesized that have specific actions and uses. Although all anticholinergics could be considered as antispasmodics to different degrees, for convenience they are divided into three categories: (1) antispasmodics, which are specifically used to relieve spasms of the bowel (e.g., irritable colon, spastic colitis), (2) antiulcer agents which reduce gastric secretion, and (3) mydriatics and cycloplegics which relax the sphincter of the iris and the ciliary muscles.

1.1 Types and Selectivity of Antispasmodics

Substances patterned on atropine are widely used as antispasmodics of the gastrointestinal tract. Theoretically any such substance that relaxes the acetylcholine-induced spasm of the smooth muscles in suitable doses can be termed an antispasmodic. In practice, not every anticholinergic agent can be used as an antispasmodic. The reason is that in addition to their spasmolytic action, anticholinergics influence the functions of other organs including heart, sweat and salivary glands, and iritic and ciliary muscles, producing side effects. Moreover, a number of them in small doses cause undesirable disorders in the central nervous system. The same antispasmodic is not suitable for the spastic states of all organs. Further, there are differences in the *in vitro* and *in vivo* efficacies of antispasmodics. Atropine abolishes the acetylcholine-induced spasm of guinea pig ileum completely; however, it is a familiar clinical experience that atropine does not antagonize completely the spasm caused by increased tone of the intestinal vagus nerve.

A number of agents cause spasm of the gastrointestinal tract. The spasm may be induced not only by acetylcholine, but also by histamine, 5-hydroxytryptamine, or barium chloride. Atropine and other anticholinergics are effective mostly against acetylcholine-induced spasm, and less against the remaining three spasmogens. Against a spasm induced by acetylcholine, atropine is effective at the lowest concentrations, e.g., 10^{-9} g/ml. Higher concentrations are necessary to antagonize 5-hydroxytryptamine spasm (10^{-7}), histamine spasm (10^{-6}), and Ba^{2+} spasm (10^{-5}). Thus atropine is a highly specific anticholinergic neurotropic spasmolytic.

Barium ion acts on all smooth muscles regardless of innervation and is called a musculotropic spasmogen. Drugs that relieve the spasm produced by barium ions are called musculotropic spasmolytics. Papaverine and nitrites are typical members of this class. However, various drugs that resemble atropine manifest both kinds of spasmolytic action in widely varying situations.

The ideal atropine-like antispasmodic should be specific for the spasmogen, should have selectivity for smooth muscles, and should abolish completely the spasm induced by the stimulation of the parasympathetic nerve to the organ. None of the available antispasmodics satisfy all these requirements. However, a great many compounds have been synthesized with the hope of developing drugs that will exhibit more selective antispasmodic action and have fewer side effects than atropine.

1.2 Gastric Secretion, Peptic Ulcer, and Anticholinergics as Antiulcer Agents

The pathophysiology of peptic ulcer is not fully known, and in the present state of knowledge it is not possible to present the pertinent normal physiology briefly. For a detailed discussion on the physiology and chemistry of gastric secretion and the pathologic physiology of peptic ulcer, reference should be made to reviews on the subject (1–5). The following is a brief summary of the gastric secretion and its relationship to peptic ulcer, a knowledge of which is necessary to understand the problems of developing antiulcer agents.

Gastric juice contains a mixture of water, inorganic ions, hydrochloric acid, pepsinogens, mucus, various polypeptides, and the intrinsic factor. Pepsinogens are precursors of the proteolytic enzymes, pepsins. They are readily converted into the corresponding pepsins by either acid or pepsin itself. Conversion by acid is instantaneous at pH 2.0. In man, gastric juice contains hydrochloric acid during the period of interdigestive secretion as well as during the period of digestive secretion. Although the mechanisms of interdigestive secretion are not known, they depend partly on the tonic activity of the vagus. The gastric secretory activity during the period of digestive secretion may be divided into three phases, cephalic, gastric, and intestinal. Each phase is named to denote the region in which the stimuli act to induce gastric secretion.

In the cephalic phase the stimuli are initiated in the central nervous system. The stimuli are the sight, smell, taste, and thought of food, which act through conditioned and unconditioned reflexes. The final efferent path is the vagus nerve. The impulses in the vagus nerve stimulate the secretory cells in the gastric glands. Acetylcholine which is released from the postganglionic nerve endings exerts a direct action on the secretory cells. Administration of atropine abolishes this phase. The secretion is high in acid and pepsinogens, and its concentration of mucus is lower than that of the basal secretion; mucus output rises 8–10 times as volume increases.

The gastric phase of secretion begins copiously as soon as the food enters the stomach; and it may continue 3–4 hr with a total volume of 600 ml or more of strongly acid juice containing a high concentration of pepsinogens. The gastric phase of secretion is caused by local and vagal responses to distension and by the hormone, gastrin, released by the mucosa of the pyloric gland area. The local nerves of the pyloric area are confined to the mucosa and are cholinergic. Irrigation of the pyloric gland area with acetylcholine releases gastrin, and this liberation of gastrin is abolished by atropinization. There is a synergism between gastrin and acetylcholine at the target cells; the effect of injected gastrin on both acid and pepsinogen secretion is increased two to eight by subthreshold parasympathometic stimuli, and it is strongly inhibited by atropinization.

The intestinal phase which begins when chyme passes from the stomach to intestine, contributes about 10% of the total response to a test meal. Protein and its digestion products, milk, dilute alcohol, and acid itself are effective stimulants. Although there may be a nervous component, the intestinal phase includes humoral stimulation of secretion by unknown agents. Gastrin released from the small intestine may be involved. The response to whatever humoral agent comes from the intestine is greatly increased when subthreshold doses of cholinergic drugs are given.

A number of humoral inhibitors of gastric secretion arise in the small intestine. They are termed as enterogastrones. An enterogastrone is present in the jejunum and duodenal mucosa. It is released in the presence of fat and it inhibits gastric secretion and motility. The hormone, secretin, which stimulates pancreatic secretion, is an enterogastrone. It is produced in the proximal duodenum and it inhibits gastric secretion in the presence of acids. Cholicystokinin, which is the same as pancreozymin, and gastrin share the same terminal tetrapeptide. Given alone, cholicystokinin is only a mild stimulant of gastric acid secretion. It is a competitive inhibitor of the receptor for gastrin, which is a powerful stimulant of gastric acid secretion. Therefore, in the presence of gastrin, cholicystokinin decreases the total output of acid. Glucagon (and possibly enteroglucagon) reduces the gastrin-induced acid secretion by noncompetitive inhibition of the receptors to gastrin. A gastric inhibitory polypeptide (GIP) that is present in duodenal mucosa inhibits histamine- as well as gastrin-induced acid secretion. A vasoactive intestinal peptide (VIP), which has been isolated from small intestinal mucosa, inhibits histamine-induced acid secretion. GIP and VIP are two possible enterogastrones whose significance has yet to be established.

Histamine, the exact role of which is not clearly understood, stimulates secretion of gastric juice that is rich in hydrochloric acid. Recently, histamine receptors have been divided into two types, H1 and H2 (Chapter 48). Stimulation of H2 receptors by histamine results in increased gastric acid secretion. H2 receptor antagonists (burinamide, metiamide, cimetidine, Chapter 48) inhibit histamine-induced gastric acid secretion in man and animals. In man, H2 antagonists inhibit not only histamine- but also pentagastrin (a synthetic analog of gastrin)-stimulated gastric acid secretion. This suggests that, at least in man, gastrin acts partially via histamine (3). Blockage of acetylcholine receptors by atropine and histamine receptors by H2 antagonists results in reduction of the effectiveness of gastrin to induce acid secretion. Therefore, there seems to be a complex interaction among the three receptors, acetylcholine receptors, H2 receptors, and gastrin receptors involved in the acid secretion by parietal cells.

Among local hormones and messengers, prostaglandins (PGE_1, PGA_1, Chapter 33) cyclic adenosine $3',5'$-monophosphate (cyclic AMP, cAMP, Chapter 34) inhibit both pentagastrin- and histamine-stimulated gastric secretion. According to present evidence, all hormones that reduce gastric acid secretion increase both adenylcyclase and intracellular cAMP activity. Conversely, all hormones that primarily stimulate gastric acid secretion reduce intracellular cAMP levels. Therefore, cAMP is involved in the final links of gastric acid secretion (3).

The interplay among various neuronal and hormonal factors in the gastric acid secretion by the parietal cell during cephalic, gastric, and intestinal phases are schematically shown in Fig. 44.1. In addi-

tion to being inhibited by atropine-like agents and enterogastrones shown in Fig. 44.1, the acid secretion is inhibited by gastrone in the mucus of human stomach, by urogastrone isolated from the urine of men and dogs, by strongly acid solutions in the duodenum, and by stimulation of the sympathetic nervous system.

Peptic ulcer occurs in the pyloric region of the stomach or the first few centimeters of the intestine. The gastroduodenal mucosa is exposed constantly to mechanical, physical, and chemical insults, some of which have already been described. A peptic ulcer does not develop without the presence of a pepsin-containing juice of such low pH that it can exert a peptic influence on the gastric wall itself. The extent of this insult is determined by the number of acid- and pepsinogen-producing cells, their irritability, and/or the magnitude of the stimuli which reach them. These stimuli are partly nervous (vagal) and partly hormonal (gastrin, corticosteroids).

The healthy stomach does not digest itself. Counteracting the aggression are defensive factors such as buffering and dilution by food, inhibition of the secretion of gastric juice, and drainage of gastric contents. In addition, however, the local condition of the mucosa (the mucosal resistance) is also of importance. Some of the determinants of mucosal resistance are the mucous barrier, the local circulation, and the healing capacity of the mucosa. A peptic ulcer forms when the insult is more powerful than the defense. In the case of duodenal ulcers, the powerful irritation is often the important factor; in gastric ulcers it is the insufficient defense.

The ideal agent for the treatment of the peptic ulcer would be one that selectively inactivates pepsin or inhibits the output of hydrochloric acid so as to maintain the pH of the gastric contents at about 4.5 for long periods after its oral ingestion. It should produce no, or only minimal, side effects, induce no tolerance, and be inexpensive. It

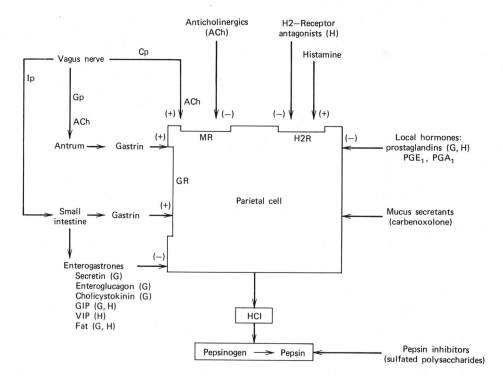

Fig. 44.1 Interactions among neuronal and hormonal factors and pharmacological agents during cephalic (Cp), gastric (Gp), and intestinal (Ip) phases of gastric acid secretion by parietal cell. ACh, acetylcholine; GIP, gastric inhibitory peptide; VIP, vasoactive intestinal peptide; MR, muscarinic receptor; H2R, histamine H2 receptor; GR, gastrin receptor; (+), stimulation of acid secretion; (−), inhibition of acid secretion. In parentheses, next to the inhibitory agents, is indicated the blocked stimulant agent (ACh, acetylcholine, H, histamine, G, gastrin).

should be effective during all periods and phases of gastric secretion and prevent the formation of ulcers.

Atropine-like anticholinergics do not satisfy all requirements of an antiulcer agent. They block acetylcholine action at the neuroeffector junction of the vagus. They give relief to patients with a peptic ulcer by their antisecretory and antispasmodic effects. They decrease the basal hydrochloric acid and pepsin secretion, thereby allowing the healing of ulcers. The antispasmodic effects of atropine-like agents are as consistent as their antisecretory effects. Motor activity is closely related to

ulcer pain, and the pain-relieving action of anticholinergic agents seems to be related to their effect on depressing motor activity (antispasmodic effect).

An "effective" atropine-like anticholinergic drug is capable of favorably influencing the excessive gastric secretion under certain conditions. It exerts a significant effect on acid secretion during the basal and interdigestive night secretion to the point of abolishing it completely for many hours (6). Its effect on secretion during the feeding of milk and cream is significant (7, 8). However, anticholinergic drugs do not effectively perform a "medical vagotomy" and they do not effectively reduce gastric acidity to the extent of achlorhydria when patients are fed (8, 9).

1.3 Anticholinergics as Mydriatics and Cycloplegics

The size of the pupil is determined by the balance of forces exerted by the dilator muscle fibers (sympathetically innervated and radially arranged) and the constrictor muscle fibers (parasympathetically innervated and circularly arranged) of the iris. Normally both sets of muscle fibers have a constant degree of tonus and act reciprocally to dilate or constrict the pupil. Any substance that paralyzes the constrictor muscle fibers (parasympatholytic) allows the unopposed tone of dilator muscle fibers to widen the pupil.

Acetylcholine is the transmitter between the constrictor muscle fibers and the parasympathetic nerve which innervates them. Therefore acetylcholine and its congeners stimulate the constrictor muscle fibers of the iris, and constrict the pupil. Atropine and related compounds paralyze the constrictor muscle fibers and cause widening or dilatation of the pupil.

The ciliary muscle is innervated by the parasympathetic nerve, and acts to decrease the tone on the supporting muscle fibers of the lens, and thus increases the accommodative power of the eye. Acetylcholine and its congeners constrict the ciliary muscle fibers; and atropine and related compounds paralyze the ciliary muscle.

Mydriatics are drugs that dilate the pupil, but have minimal effect on the ciliary muscle and thus on accommodation. Cycloplegics are drugs that partially or completely paralyze accommodation. Most of the anticholinergics have both properties to varying degrees.

For mydriatics other than anticholinergics and for drugs that constrict the pupil (miotics) Chapter 41 should be consulted.

Mydriatics and cycloplegics are special types of antispasmodics. In clinical practice mydriasis is produced by local instillation of the chosen drug into the conjunctival sac. This enables one to produce the desired effects on the eye with minimal systemic effects. However, such compounds should possess properties that allow them to penetrate the cornea in effective concentrations.

2 BIOCOMPARATIVE ASSAY OF ANTICHOLINERGICS

Many of the methods of obtaining experimental evidence for the antispasmodic, antiulcer, and mydriatic activities do not measure precisely and selectively only one type of pharmacological activity. However, the techniques that are available (10, 11), if used with an understanding of their scope and limitations, can provide useful information in the development of anticholinergic agents and their structure–activity relationships.

2.1 Antispasmodic Activity

In studying drugs more or less like atropine, it is customary to test their antispasmodic action on smooth muscles, such as the isolated guinea pig ileum, duodenum, or jejenum of rabbit or rat intestine. Acetylcholine or any one of the cholinergics may be used as a spasmogen, and the ability of the antispasmodic to inhibit or abolish the cholinergic-induced spasm may be measured. The antagonistic activities may be expressed as affinity constants or relative molar activities in relation to a standard antagonist. The selectivity of the antispasmodic activity may be determined by using different spasmogens, e.g., histamine, 5-hydroxytryptamine, nicotine, and barium chloride.

Thiry-Vella fistulas (10), prepared at various levels of the gastrointestinal tract, have been used in the conscious dog for determining motility by (1) placing an indigestible bolus in the oral end of the fistula and determining the traverse time before and after treatment with drugs (2) placing a balloon containing water and attached to a kymographic recording system in the fistula and recording the pressure waves and their alterations by the action of drugs, (3) placing a French catheter in the aboral end of the fistula, connecting it to a suitable recording system, and thus making a record of normal pressures and those occurring after treatment.

Other qualitative and quantitative methods to study the antispasmodics have been described (10). These include (1) the fluroscopic study of the gastrointestinal motility and (2) the use of an ingestible pressure-sensitive radio-telemetering capsule (Transensor) for measuring the pressure in the gastrointestinal tract.

2.2 Antiulcer Activity

The problems encountered in testing drugs for antiulcer activity result in part from a lack of complete understanding of the physiological and biochemical mechanisms involved in the formation of ulcers, and in part from the testing of drugs for activity on normal or quasi-normal animal preparations though they are ultimately applied to abnormal or pathological human states. The various methods differ in producing ulcers in experimental animals (10).

A preparation developed by Shay et al. (12) has been used to test for antiulcer activity on an all-or-none basis. The ligation of the pylorus of rats, previously fasted for 48–72 hr, leads to the accumulation of acid gastric contents and ulceration of the stomach 17–19 hr after the operation. The antiulcer agents are given subcutaneously or intraduodenally at the time of ligation of the pylorus, or orally 1 hr before. The animals are killed 17–19 hr after pyloric ligation and the stomach contents are collected for examination. The stomach is opened along the greater curvature and the ulcers are examined and scored by a suitable scheme such as 0 = normal, 1 = scattered hemorrhagic spots, 2 = deeper hemorrhagic spots and some ulcers, 3 = hemorrhagic spots and ulcers, and 4 = perforation. Variable results have been reported by investigators using this technique.

Production of chronic experimental peptic ulcers in dogs (or rats) by the Mann–Williamson procedure (13) has become a standard method. The gastric juice is diverted into the intestine some distance from the pancreatic and biliary secretions. The objective is achieved by isolating the duodenum from the pylorus and the jejunum. The oral end of the duodenum is closed and its distal end is anastomosed with a loop of ileum, so as to discharge the pancreatic and biliary secretions into the lower portion of the bowel. The cut end of the jejunum is then anastomosed to the pylorus. About 95% of dogs so prepared develop typical chronic peptic ulcers just distal to the gastric anastomosis with the jejunum. With similar operative procedures 85% of rats develop gastric, marginal, or jejunal ulcers.

The complete reversal of the duodenum in dogs produces chronic peptic ulcers in about 6 months (10). These animals maintain their weight until the development of ulcerations and might become a useful preparation for detecting and comparing antiulcer activity.

Stress produces ulcers in the rats, which could be used to test antiulcer activity of drugs (14). Rats fasted for 48 hr and immobilized in a galvanized screen cage under light ether anesthesia develop ulcers in the glandular region of the stomach after 4 hr of restraint. The estimate of severity can be all or none or may be coded in the same way as the Shay preparation.

One of the side effects of adrenocorticotropic hormone (ACTH) and corticoid therapy in man is the development or reactivation of gastroduodenal ulcers. Daily subcutaneous administration of cortisol or Δ^1-cortisol to rats for 4 days results in the regular development of gastric ulcers (15). This procedure has been adapted to testing antiulcer activity (16). There are certain differences between steroid ulcers and "natural" ulcers in localization, rate of development, and severity (17).

The antisecretory activities of anticholinergics are as important as their antiulcer activities for their therapeutic usefulness. The Pavlov gastric pouch (18) with intact vagal and sympathetic nerve supply and a modified Heidenhain pouch (19), which is essentially denervated, are prepared from dog stomach and have been used for determining the action of drugs on gastric secretion. Histamine or a test meal is usually used as a stimulus. Similar methods for the preparation and use of chronic total gastric fistulas and chronic denervated gastric pouches have been described for determining drug action on gastric secretion in rats (20–22).

There are a significant number of reports in which antisecretory and antimobility effects of anticholinergic drugs have been evaluated in ulcer patients (9, 23). The antisecretory potency can be measured best in the duodenal ulcer patient in whom the acid output is already high. Ability of the drug to abolish or diminish acid output under histamine stimulation is a stringent test of activity, but the test has limited physiological relevance. The effect of the drug on the amount of acid secreted under ordinary clinical conditions is the most pertinent of all tests in relation to therapeutic application. In clinical comparison, not only the degree of effects but also the duration of the antisecretory effects should be compared.

2.3   Mydriatic and Cycloplegic Activities

A simple and relatively accurate test for mydriatic activity has been described (24). The method requires mice and a binocular microscope magnifying about 10 times and provided with a scale in the eyepiece with which to examine and measure the diameter of the pupil of the mouse. A strong light shining into the eye of the mouse must be attached to the microscope. The diameter of the pupil is measured at the peak effect after administration of the anticholinergic agent by intraperitoneal injection. The duration of the effect is also important since one of the most characteristic and valuable properties of atropine and analogous compounds is the prolonged effect which they produce in the eye.

Entopic pupillometry is an accurate and practical method for measuring the size of the pupil in human beings (25). With a Cogan entopic pupillometer, the normal size of the pupil and the near and far points before and after instillation of the drug in the conjunctival sac can be measured at different time intervals. The amount of light entering the eye is quite small and the movements of the eye during the measurement do not interfere with the test.

2.4   Miscellaneous Anticholinergic Activities

A number of other methods are available for comparing the activities of anticholinergic agents, of which the antitremor and antisalivary effects are widely used. Arecoline or pilocarpine may be used to induce tremor or salivation in a suitable species which can be blocked by an anticholinergic agent. There seems to be good correlation between anticholinergic and antitremor effects (26). Recovery of the salivary gland from cholinergic block may conceivably precede that of the gastric glands and the two effects may therefore not necessarily parallel each other in duration (9).

3 SOLANACEOUS ALKALOIDS

The older anticholinergic drugs are the various galenical preparations of belladonna, hyoscyamus, and stamonium, all of which are derived from plants of the potato family, the Solanaceae. The species used as drugs include *Atropa belladonna*, one of several plants known colloquially as "deadly nightshade," *Hyoscymus niger* (black henbane), and *Datura stramonium* (jimsonweed, jamestown weed, or thorn apple). The active principles in all these plants consist mostly of (−)-hyoscyamine, with smaller variable amounts of (−)-scopolamine (hyoscine). Atropine is (±)-hyoscyamine.

3.1 History

The poisonous nature of solanaceous alkaloids has been known for many centuries (27). The toxic properties of deadly nightshade are evident when children eat the black berries which look attractive in a fall hedgerow in England. The children become delirious, and their eyes have widely dilated pupils. The deadly nightshade was used by the poisoners of the Middle Ages to induce obscure and often delayed poisoning. Therefore, Linné in 1753 named the shrub *Atropa belladonna*, after *Atropos*, the oldest of the Three Fates, who cuts the thread of life. "Belladonna" does not refer to *Atropos*, who is considered as a grim and awesome female, but to the Italian name ("handsome women") of the plant, which was used by Venetian ladies to give them dilated pupils ("sparkling eyes").

Datura has an ancient history, for it is said to have been used at the oracular shrine of Apollo in his temple at Delphi. Here the priestess of the god, Pythia, sat on a tripod uttering incoherent words in a divine ecstacy, in reply to the questions which were asked. Pythia was intoxicated by the fumes from burning datura leaves; her replies were interpreted by a priest in the form of a verse. The more common uses of datura were for robbery or conspiracy. Indian courtesans were known to place datura in their visitors' wine, so that they could be robbed without interference. As recently as 1908, there was a plan to poison the European garrison in Hanoi in Vietnam using datura. Those in the conspiracy intended to stupefy the soliders, and then to kill them.

The pharmacological actions of atropine and related alkaloids are intimately connected with our knowledge of the organization and function of the autonomic nervous system. Schmiedeberg and Koppe (28) were the first in 1869 to focus attention on the similarity between a drug effect and electrical stimulation, when they pointed out that muscarine and vagus stimulation affected the heart in the same fashion and the actions of both were antagonized by atropine. Further, they recommended atropine as an antidote for mushroom poisoning. As early as 1887, Kobert and Sohrt (29) provided experimental proof for both similarities and dissimilarities between atropine and scopolamine.

Atropine was isolated by Mein in 1831 (30) and since then the synthesis of both atropine and scopolamine has been achieved (31, 32). A biogenetic scheme for the synthesis of atropine alkaloids in datura species starting from ornithine has been described (33).

3.2 Chemical Structure

All the solanaceous alkaloids are esters of the dicyclic amino alcohol 3-tropanol (tropine, 44.**1**). Atropine is an ester of tropic acid and tropine. In scopolamine the organic base is scopine. Scopine differs

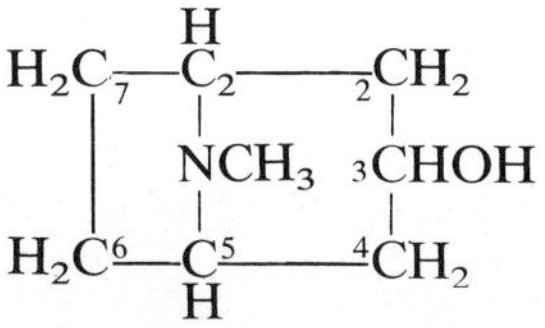

$$H_2C_{\,7}\!\!-\!\!\underset{\displaystyle |}{\overset{\displaystyle H}{C_2}}\!\!-\!\!_2CH_2$$

NCH₃ ₃CHOH

$$H_2C^6\!\!-\!\!\underset{\displaystyle H}{C^5}\!\!-\!\!^4CH_2$$

44.**1**

from tropine in having an oxygen bridge between C-6 and C-7. There are some other alkaloids that are members of the solanaceous alkaloids (e.g., apoatropine, noratropine, belladonnine) but they are not of sufficient therapeutic value to be discussed in this context.

The carbon α to the carboxyl group of tropic acid is asymmetric and is easily racemized during the isolation of the solanaceous alkaloids. Atropine and atroscine are racemic forms. The corresponding levo isomers, (−)-hyoscyamine and (−)-scopolamine (hyoscine) occur naturally in the solanaceous plants.

The absolute configuration of (−)-tropic acid has been established by its correlation with (−)-alanine (34). According to the Cahn–Ingold–Prelog convention (35), natural (−)-tropic acid possesses the (S) configuration. Accordingly (−)-hyoscyamine and (−)-hyoscine have an (S) configuration (36) (Chapters 6 and 9).

The piperidine ring system can exist in two principal conformations. Its chair form has the lowest energy requirement. However, the alternate boat form can also exist, because the energy barrier is not great. The formula of 3-hydroxytropine (44.**1**) indicates that, even though there is no optical activity because of the plane of symmetry, two stereoisomeric forms, tropine (44.**2**) and pseudotropine (44.**3**), can exist because of the rigidity imparted to the molecule through the ethane chain across the 1,5 positions (37a). In tropine, the axially oriented hydroxyl group, trans to the nitrogen bridge, is designated as α or anti, and the alternate, equatorially oriented hydroxyl group as β or syn. It is generally

considered that cycloheptane is fixed through an —N(CH₃)— bridge in the structures of tropine and pseudotropine. Therefore, a chair conformation is ascribed to the piperidine ring system in tropine and pseudotropine. However, there is only a seeming difference between the two conformations of tropane derivatives (38). The tropane system can be considered with equal justification as a piperidine twisted through the —CH₂CH₂— bridge, or as a cycloheptane fixed through an —N(CH₃)— bridge. When the tropane system is structured by the chair form of piperidine, it represents also the boat form of cycloheptane. Similarly, the boat form of piperidine is at the same time a chair form of cycloheptane ring. Therefore, it may be assumed that both forms are present in a state of equilibrium (37a). Based on the conformations of the tropane system, the structure of atropine (44.**4**) can be represented by 44.**5** and 44.**6**, of which 44.**5** is more generally accepted.

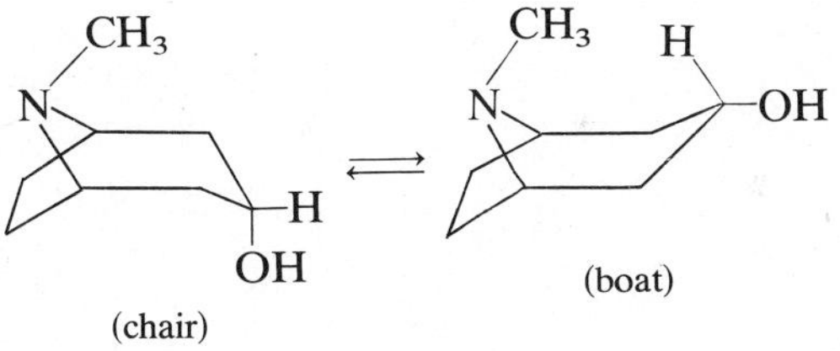

(chair)   (boat)

44.**2**

(boat)

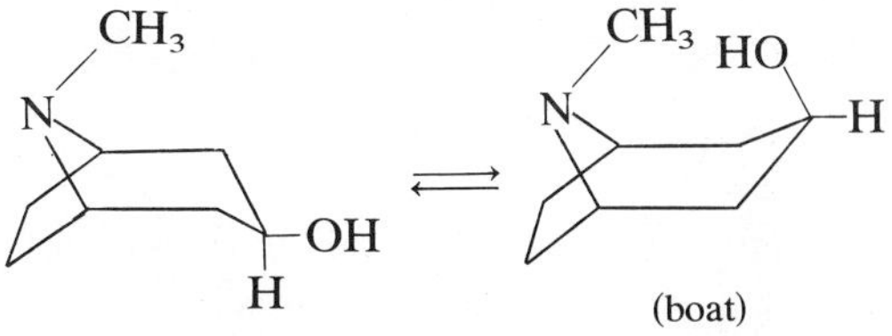

44.**3**

The amino alcohol derived from scopolamine (44.**7**), that is, scopine (44.**8**), has the axial orientation of the 3-OH group but in addition has a β-oriented epoxy group bridged across the 6,7 positions.

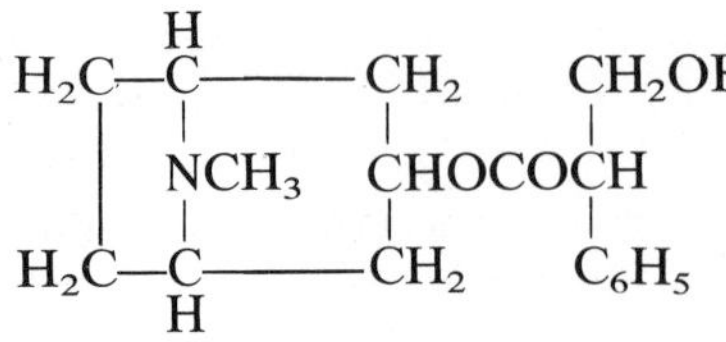

44.4

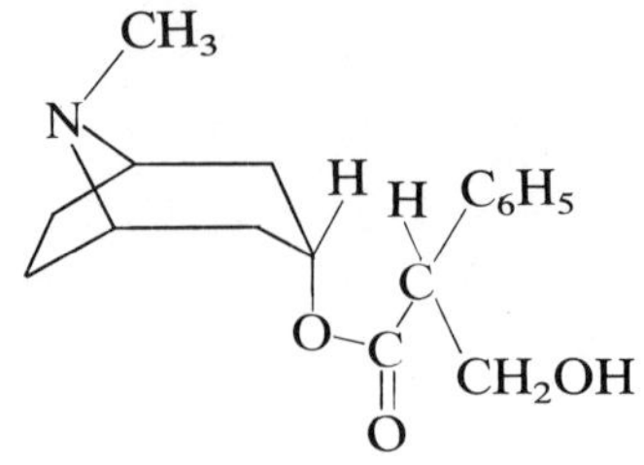

44.5

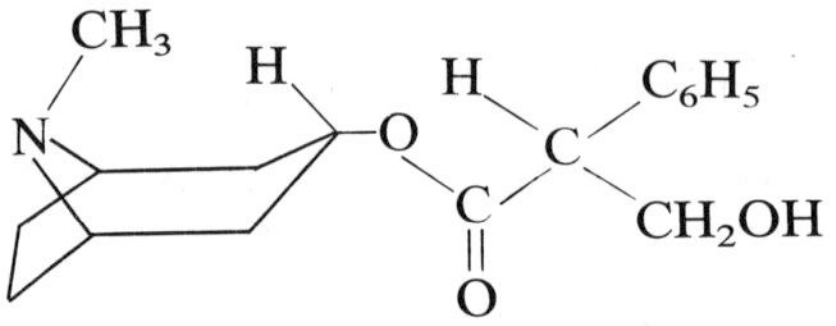

44.6

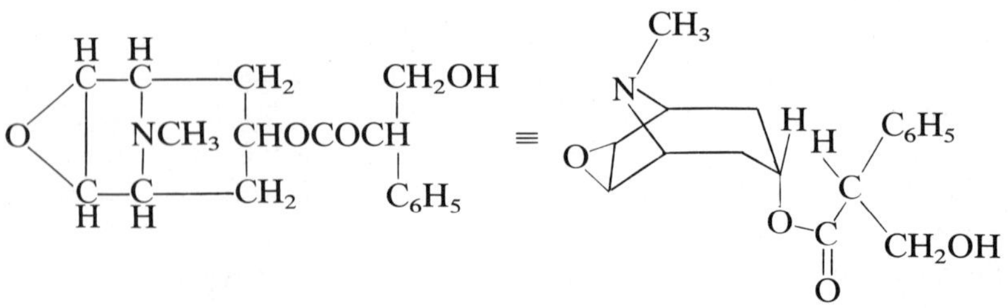

44.7

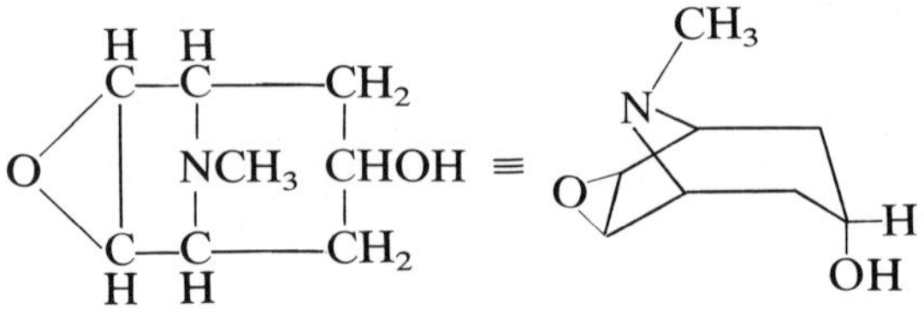

44.8

3.3 Preparative Methods

Conventional methods of alkaloid isolation are used to obtain a crude mixture of atropine and (−)-hyoscyamine from the plant products. This crude mixture of alkaloids is racemized to atropine by refluxing in chloroform or by treatment with cold dilute alkali (39).

Atropine can be synthesized from tropinone and tropic acid as starting materials. Tropinone can be prepared by Robin-

son's synthesis (40) and reduced under proper conditions to tropine. (±)-Tropic acid can be prepared from ethyl phenyl-acetate (41, 42) or acetophenone (43). The acetyl derivative of tropyl chloride is condensed with tropine hydrochloride to yield the O-acetyl derivative of atropine hydrochloride, from which the acetyl group is split spontaneously in aqueous solution (44).

One of the commercial sources for (−)-hyoscyamine is Egyptian henbane (*Hyos-*

cyamus muticus), in which it occurs to the extent of 0.5%. Another method for extraction of the alkaloid uses *Duboisia* species. It is prepared from the crude plant material in a manner similar to that used for atropine and is purified as the oxalate. (±)-Tropic acid can be resolved through its quinine salt and the separate enantiomorphs can be converted into (+) and (−)-hyoscyamines.

(−)-Scopolamine (hyoscine) is isolated from the mother liquor remaining after the isolation of hyoscyamine, and is marketed as its hydrobromide. Scopolamine is readily racemized to atroscine, when subjected to treatment with dilute alkali.

The synthesis of scopolamine differs from that of atropine in the synthesis of the amino alcohol scopine portion of the molecule. Fodór and co-workers (32, 45, 46) have synthesized scopine starting from 6-β-hydroxy-3-tropanone. Esterification of scopine with acetyltropyl chloride and mild hydrolysis of the acetylscopolamine give scopolamine.

3.4   Molecular Factors in the Absorption, Fate, and Excretion of Atropine and Related Compounds

The belladonna alkaloids are absorbed rapidly after oral administration (47). They enter the circulation when applied locally to the mucosal surfaces of the body. Atropine absorbed from inhaled smoke of medicated cigarettes can abolish the effects of intravenous infusion of methacholine in man. The transconjunctival absorption of atropine is considerable. About 95% of radioactive atropine is absorbed and excreted following subconjunctival injection in the rabbit. The total absorption of quaternary ammonium derivatives (Section 3.5) of the alkaloids after an oral dose is only about 25%. The liver, kidney, lung, and pancreas are the most important organs that take up the labeled atropine. The liver

probably excretes metabolic products of atropine via bile into the intestine (in mice and rats).

Because most of the synthetic antispasmodic and antiulcer agents are administered orally, their absorption through the gastrointestinal tract limits their therapeutic usefulness. There are striking differences in the absorption of tertiary amines and quaternary ammonium compounds (48–50). The tertiary amines (e.g., noroxyphenonium, mepiperphenidol, Section 4) are absorbed completely from rat intestinal loops. The maximal absorption of the corresponding quaternary ammonium compounds is about $\frac{1}{5}$ of the total dose. The poor absorption of quaternary ammonium compounds may be partly due to the positive charge which promotes the formation of a nonabsorbable complex with mucin. The ready absorption of tertiary amines may be explained partly by their permeability through lipid membranes (51). The existence of a special carrier-mediated transport mechanism for the intestinal absorption of amines and quaternary ammonium compounds is yet to be investigated.

Considerable species variations have been reported for the metabolic detoxification of atropine in mammals (52–63). These differences seem to be more quantitative than qualitative. At least four types of molecular modifications occur for the urinary excretion of atropine (Fig. 44.2). Cleavage of the ester bond takes place in the rabbit and the guinea pig (56), whereas para and meta hydroxylation of the benzene ring of tropic acid occurs in the mouse and the rat (52, 54). The tropine moiety of atropine is also chemically modified for excretion in man and mouse and, though unidentified, "tropine-modified atropines" are excreted in man and mouse (55). Tropic acid itself does not undergo metabolic alteration for urinary excretion in all species mentioned above. The metabolic conversions of tropine itself are not known. However, demethylation of atropine-N-$^{14}CH_3$

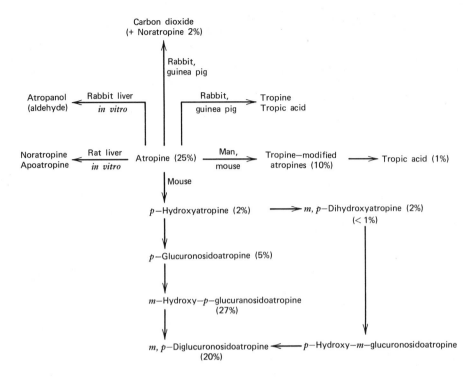

Fig. 44.2 Metabolism of atropine.

(or tropine-N-$^{14}CH_3$) has been reported in a number of species with exhalation of $^{14}CO_2$ (62). The possible metabolic changes of atropine are schematically represented in Fig. 44.2.

After intravenous injection of atropine, approximately 25% of the dose is excreted in the mouse urine as atropine, more than 50% as conjugates with glucuronic acid, and the remaining 20–25% as intermediate oxidation products (probably p-hydroxy-atropine and 3,4-dihydroxyatropine) and "tropine-modified atropines." Rats are known to metabolize atropine in a manner similar to mice. In man, about 50% of the administered dose of atropine is excreted unchanged in the urine and about 33% as unknown metabolites which are esters of tropic acid. Neither hydroxylation of the

tropic acid moiety nor glucuronide formation has been demonstrated in man (55). Only less than 2% appears as tropic acid in urine.

It has been known for more than a century that rabbits can tolerate large quantities of atropine (56, 57). The cause of this observation is the ability of the serum of some, but not all, rabbits to hydrolyze atropine into tropic acid and tropine. The hydrolysis is due to an enzyme, atropinesterase, which is found in most other tissues as well as the serum of these rabbits. The highest activities are found in the liver and intestinal mucosa; only the brain and aqueous humor of the eye contain no enzyme. The enzyme is also found in the liver of the guinea pig and accounts for the appearance of tropic acid in the urine of the rabbit or the guinea pig, but not other animals, following the administration of atropine.

The presence of atropinesterase in rabbits is inherited through an incompletely dominant gene (56). This gene is associated with another gene which influences the color of the fur, causing "extension of black pigment in the fur."

Atropinesterase can also hydrolyze homatropine and scopolamine. This enzyme is stereospecific for (S)-$(-)$-hyoscamine which is split; the more inert (R)-$(+)$ isomer is not readily hydrolyzed (56).

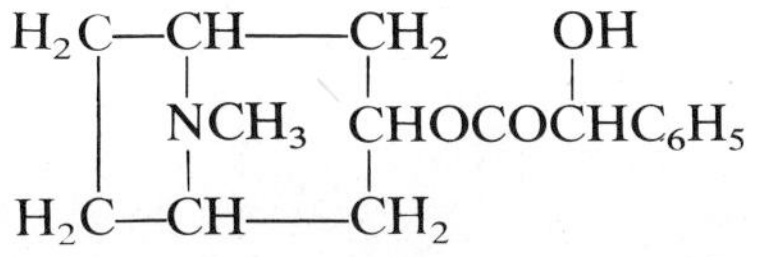

3.5   Semisynthetic Derivatives of Solanaceous Alkaloids

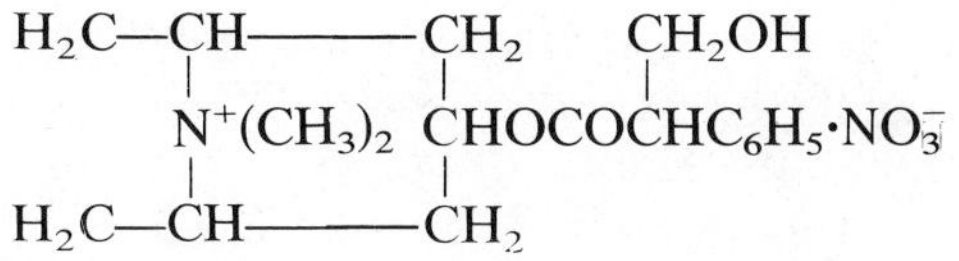

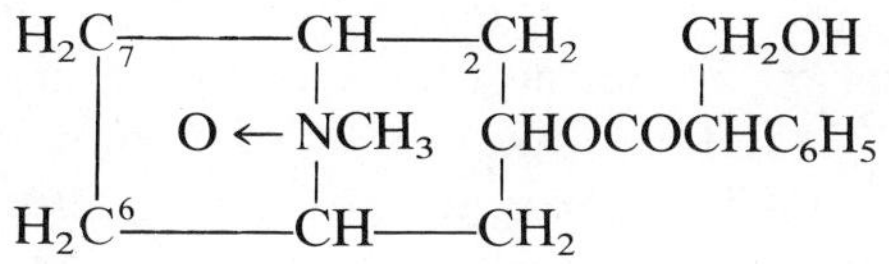

Early attempts to modify the atropine molecule (44.**4**) were aimed at converting the solanaceous alkaloids containing the tertiary nitrogen into quaternary ammonium compounds and N-oxides. Later developments have been to retain the tropine (or scopine) portion of the molecule and substitute various acids for tropic acid. In this way a series of tropeines have been synthesized, among which a number of active compounds have been found (64). Of the tropeines, mandelyl tropeine (44.**9**, homatropine), has survived as a therapeutic agent to the present.

Methylatropine nitrate (44.**10**) (or bromide) is a synthetic quaternary derivative of atropine. Atropine oxide (atropine N-oxide) is known as a genatropine (44.**11**) and may be prepared by oxidation of the alkaloid with hydrogen peroxide.

The derivatives of scopolamine (44.**7**) prepared by similar methods are available commercially. These include methscopolamine bromide (44.**12**), methscopolamine nitrate, and genoscopolamine (scopolamine N-oxide, 44.**13**).

Homatropine (44.**9**) is prepared by evaporating tropine with mandelic and hydrochloric acids. Homatropine methyl-

bromide (44.**14**) may be prepared from homatropine by treating it with methyl bromide.

Quaternization may or may not increase all types of anticholinergic activity significantly. However, there are certain practical advantages to quaternization. The quaternary ammonium derivatives usually penetrate the central nervous system less readily than the corresponding tertiary amine

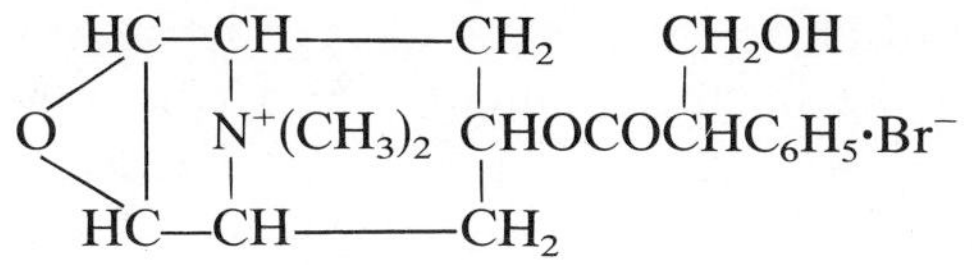

44.**9**

44.**10**

44.**11**

44.**12**

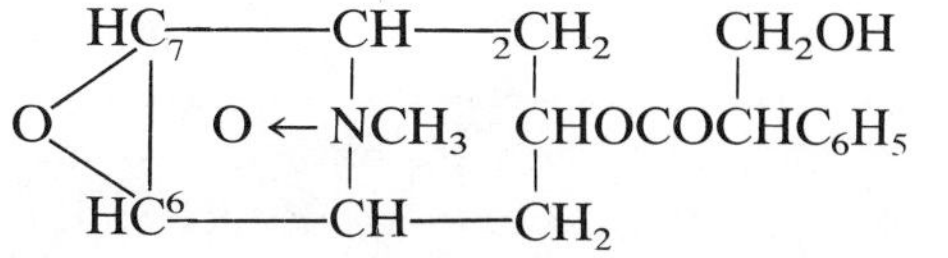

44.**13**

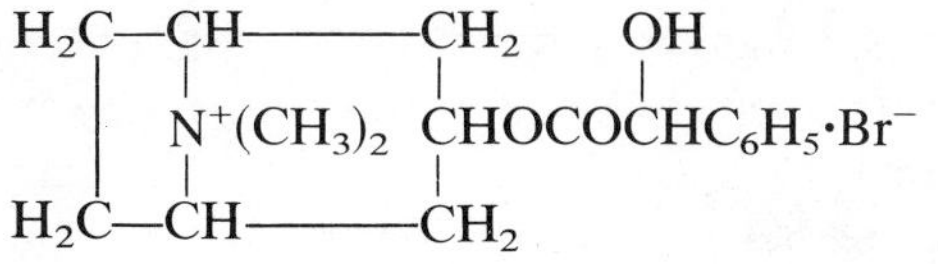

44.**14**

analogs. Therefore, quaternization serves as a useful technique to avoid or minimize the side effects caused by the stimulation of the central nervous system by the tertiary amines when the drugs are used for their peripheral actions. When a tertiary alkaloidal base is converted to the quaternary form, the latter is also less readily absorbed through the intestinal wall (65, 66; Section 3.2). This is not a disadvantage when the drug is used for its effects in the gastrointestinal tract. However, if the drug is used for its systemic or central actions the effect becomes erratic and unpredictable because the absorption is poor after oral administration. The tertiary amines are preferred for ophthalmic use, because they penetrate the cornea better than their quaternary ammonium derivatives. However, when a drug (e.g., atropine) has a long-lasting mydriatic effect, its recovery period can be shortened by quaternization. Therefore, the selection of the type of the derivative (Table 44.1) depends on the specific purpose for which it is used, the mode of its administration, and the duration of the desired effect.

The N-oxides are converted to the corresponding tertiary bases *in vivo*. Atropine N-oxide and scopolamine N-oxide are slowly reduced to atropine and scopolamine in the animal body. Therefore, N-oxidation is a convenient technique for prolonging the duration of the action of the alkaloidal bases. The N-oxides are said to be less toxic.

Solanaceous alkaloids have a wide and variable spectrum of anticholinergic activities and are widely used in therapeutics. The various derivatives of atropine, scopolamine, and homatropine are listed in Table 44.1. Because of their chemical differences and the resulting biological interactions, different derivatives are preferred for antispasmodic, antisecretory, mydriatic, or central effects. Scopolamine produces the same type of depression of the parasympathetic nervous system as does atropine and homatropine, but it differs markedly from atropine in its action in the central nervous system. Whereas atropine stimulates the CNS, causing restlessness, scopolamine acts as a narcotic and sedative. It also causes temporary amnesia ("twilight sleep") when used along with morphine in obstetric and gynecologic procedures. For a detailed discussion of the anticholinergic activities of solanaceous alkaloids and their related compounds, the standard textbooks or reviews in pharmacology should be consulted (47, 67–69).

4 SYNTHETIC ANTICHOLINERGICS

Although atropine and its related alkaloids are potent anticholinergics they have a wide spectrum of pharmacological activities. Therefore, therapeutic administration of these alkaloids to elicit a particular desired activity invariably results in some undesirable side effects. For this reason, the search for compounds possessing one or another of the specific desirable actions has been an active field of investigation in medicinal chemistry. The ideal specificity of action has not been attained in these attempts; perfect atropine substitutes with predominantly antispasmodic, antisecretory, or cycloplegic actions have yet to be synthesized.

The synthetic anticholinergic drugs can be considered as analogs of atropine or antagonists of acetylcholine. Most of these compounds were designed using broad principles of molecular modification such as (1) scission of the atropine molecule into simpler molecules containing the essential pharmacodynamic groups; (2) molecular modification by introducing "blocking" moieties into cholinergics; and (3) changes in other anticholinergics using principles of bioisosterism.

The structure of atropine has been the basis for a large number of synthetic anticholinergic agents. However, no significant changes have been made to effect the

Table 44.1 Derivatives of Solanaceous Alkaloids and Their Semisynthetic Substitutes[a]

Generic Name	Trade Names	Dose or Preparation	Advantage, if any, of Molecular Modification	Therapeutic Use
Atropine sulfate USP		0.5 mg (oral i.v. or s.c.); 0.5–1.0% ophthalmic solution		Mydriatic with long recovery period; preanesthetic medication to decrease secretions, treatment of Parkinsonism, and anti-ChE poisoning
Atropine tannate	Atratran	1–2 mg (tablet)	Slow absorption with sustained release of the alkaloid	Antispasmodic in ureteral and renal colic
Atropine N-oxide hydrochloride	X-tro Gena-tropine	0.5–1.0 mg (capsule)	Slow release of the alkaloid	Same as atropine for oral use
Hyoscyamine hydrobromide		0.25–1.0 mg	Possibly fewer central effects than atropine owing to small doses administered	Same as atropine for oral use
Methylatropine bromide	Mydriasine	0.5–2% solution	Mydriatic with short recovery period	Mydriatic
Methylatropine nitrate	Metropine	1–5% solution	Same as above	Mydriatic
Scopolamine hydrobromide USP		0.6 mg (oral, (s.c.); 0.2% solution	"Central depressant" (twilight sleep)	As a sedative during pre- or postoperative gynecologic care
Genescopolamine hydrobromide		1–2 mg	Gradual release of alkaloid	Same as above
Methscopolamine bromide NF	Pamine Lescopine	2.5–5.0 mg (oral); 0.25–1.0 mg (s.c. or i.m.)	Parasympatholytic without central effects	Antisecretory and anti-spasmodic in peptic ulcer
Methscopolamine nitrate NND	Skopolate Skopyl	2–4 mg (oral) 0.25–0.5 mg (s.c. or i.m.)	Same as above	Same as above
Homatropine hydro-bromide USP		1–2% solution	Mydriatic with recovery period less than that of atropine (see Table 44.14)	Mydriatic
Homatropine methyl bromide NF	Novatro-pine Mesopin	5 mg (oral)	Parasympatholytic without central effects	Antisecretory and antispasmodic
Anisotropine methylbromide[b]	Valpin Endo	10 mg (oral)	Parasympatholytic without central effects	Antisecretory and antispasmodic

[a] For details of the preparations and their uses standard references (47, 67, 68) in pharmacology should be consulted.

[b] 8-methyl-3-(2-propylpentonoyloxy)tropinium bromide, octatropine bromide.

377

"ester-complex" grouping because its presence has been regarded as essential for manifestations of atropine-like properties. Another probable consideration is that it is far simpler to synthesize a fairly complex molecule from two halves by esterification than by any other method. Therefore, many esters of amino alcohols and carboxylic acids have been synthesized as atropine substitutes, in which the structures of either one or both halves have been changed. For example, in homatropine, the tropic acid moiety has been replaced by mandelic acid. The complex and massive amino alcohol moiety (tropine, 44.**1**) of atropine has afforded unusually rich opportunities for the synthesis of anticholinergics (Fig. 44.3). Scission of its piperidine ring at point X gives the derivatives of hydroxyalkylpyrrolidines (44.**15**), and scission of its pyrrolidine ring at point Y makes it possible to proceed to derivatives of 4-hydroxypiperidine (44.**16**). The scission of both rings at Z leads to dialkylaminoalkanol derivatives (44.**17**). Further, simplification and alteration of these three groups of

amino alcohols has resulted in the synthesis of esters containing structural features more or less similar to atropine.

Antagonists of acetylcholine often have chemical structures resembling that of acetylcholine, although they differ from it by greater complexity of the molecule and higher molecular weight. Acetylcholine is a quaternary ammonium compound; atropine and tropine contain a tertiary nitrogen. Therefore, a number of atropine-like compounds having quaternary nitrogen atoms have been synthesized. In some of them, the acetyl group of ACh has been replaced by acid moieties containing blocking groups (e.g., diphenylacetic acid).

The principles used in the design of antimetabolites have been applied to synthesize atropine-like compounds. The ester group in atropine-like compounds has been replaced by a thioester, an amide, an ether group, or a chain of methylene carbons (Table 44.2).

All synthetic anticholinergic agents have some structural features in common. In most, the molecule has bulky "blocking

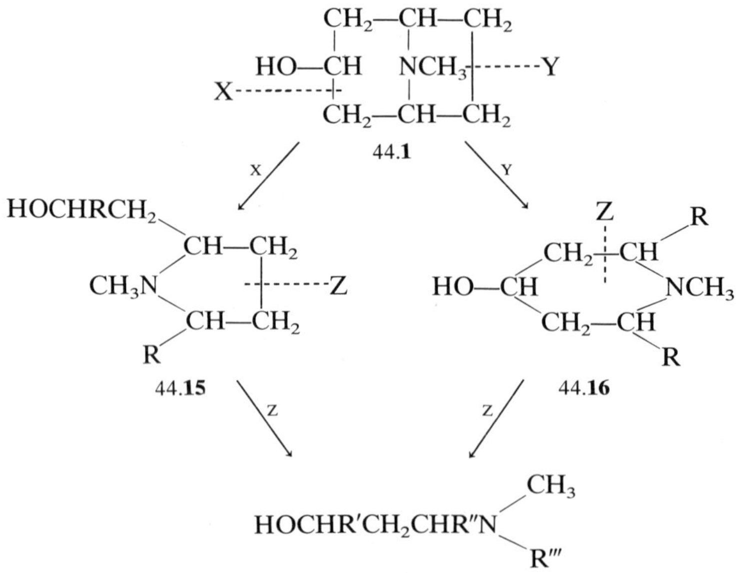

Fig. 44.3 "Scissions" of tropane ring.

Table 44.2 Classification of Synthetic Anticholinergics

Group	Characteristic Group in the Main Chain	Atoms in the Chain[a]	Additional Pharmacophoric Groups that may be Present
1	Ester	C—C(=O)—O—C	-OH
2	Thioester	C—C(=O)—S—C	-OH
3	Amide	—C(=O)—N(H)—C	-OH
4	Carbamate	>N—C(=O)—O—C	
5	Alkane	—C—C—C—	
	(a) Amino alcohols		-OH
	(b) Amides		—$CONH_2$
6	Alkene	—C=C—	

[a] A large number of compounds have been synthesized containing an ether link in the main chain. These compounds are useful as antiparkinsonian drugs (Chapter 45) and antihistaminic agents (Chapter 49). For specific examples see Table 44.3.

moieties," often cyclic radicals, linked by a chain of atoms of limited length, to a positively charged amine nitrogen (Fig. 44.4). The length and structure of the main chain have considerable influence on the anticholinergic activity of the substance. At the same time the chemical nature of the main chain determines the class of organic substances to which a given substance belongs. Therefore, the classification of synthetic anticholinergics in Table 44.2 is based on the structure of the main chain of the molecule, taking into consideration wherever necessary the presence or absence of any additional pharmacophoric groups (OH, $CONH_2$). It is beyond the scope of this text to consider all compounds that belong to each group. However, examples from drugs used as therapeutics are listed in Table 44.3. These compounds may be classified differently, and the same compound may be placed in more than one group. Each one of them may be considered as an agent with optimum anticholinergic activities among a series of structurally related compounds whose structure–activity relationships have been evaluated for different types of pharmacological effects.

5 STRUCTURE–ACTIVITY RELATIONSHIPS

Although atropine-like agents are antagonists of acetylcholine at one type of cholinergic receptor (muscarinic receptor) which is specific for activation by L(+)-muscarine,

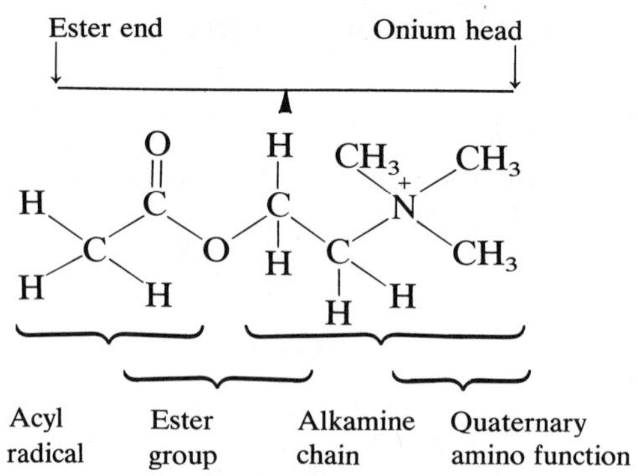

Fig. 44.4 Structural features of acetylcholine and atropine.

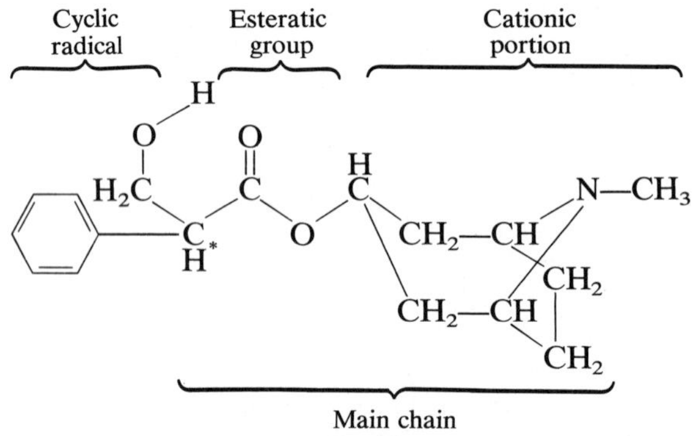

they may demonstrate many other pharmacological properties (ganglionic blocking, neuromuscular blocking, musculotropic, central stimulant, or depressant activities). The following discussion of the relationships of structure to activity is limited to their inhibitory actions at the muscarinic receptors. Certain structural features are common in many anticholinergic agents that have been synthesized and evaluated pharmacologically (Fig. 44.4). Some of these features appear in cholinergics also (44.**18**). A typical atropine-like anticholinergic agent (44.**19**) contains a cationic head and a heavy blocking moiety (cyclic groups) which are connected by a chain of atoms of definite length. Their molecules include essential constituent groups (cationic head, cyclic radicals) as

well as nonessential but contributing anchoring groups (e.g., hydroxyl). The steric factors that are related to the essential groups influence the anticholinergic activity significantly.

5.1 Cationic Head

The cationic head is an essential group in a large number of anticholinergic and cholinergic compounds. Ordinarily, this is a substituted ammonium group or, less frequently, a sulfonium or a phosphonium group. The mechanism of the cholinergic or anticholinergic action of substances has long been linked to such cationic groups (112–118). It is reasonable to assume that the cationic head with its positive charge is

Table 44.3   Synthetic Anticholinergics

Nonproprietary Name	Selected Proprietary Names	Chemical Name of Salt	Structure of Base	Reference for Synthetic Procedures
		Tertiary Amines—Characteristic Group in the Main Chain: Ester		
Adiphenine	Trasentine	2-Diethylaminoethyldiphenyl-acetate hydrochloride	$(C_6H_5)_2CHCO_2CH_2CH_2N(C_2H_5)_2$	70, 71
Amprotropine	Syntropan	3-Diethylamino-2,2-dimethyl-propyl tropate phosphate	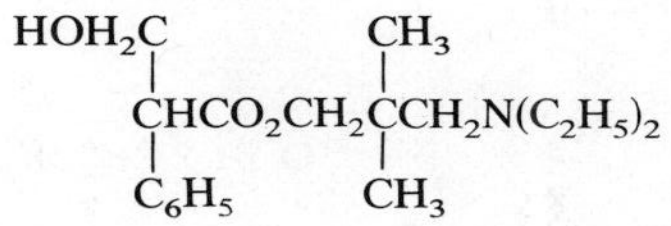 HOH_2C—$CHCO_2CH_2C(CH_3)_2CH_2N(C_2H_5)_2$ (with C_6H_5 and CH_3, CH_3 substituents)	72, 73
Amino-carbofluorene	Pavatrine	2-Diethylaminoethyl-9-fluorene-carboxylate hydrochloride	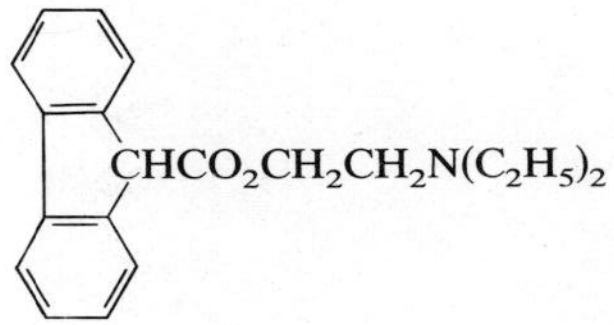 fluorene, 9-$CHCO_2CH_2CH_2N(C_2H_5)_2$	74
Cyclopentolate USP	Cyclogyl	β-Dimethylaminoethyl (1-hydroxycyclopentyl)-phenylacetate hydrochloride	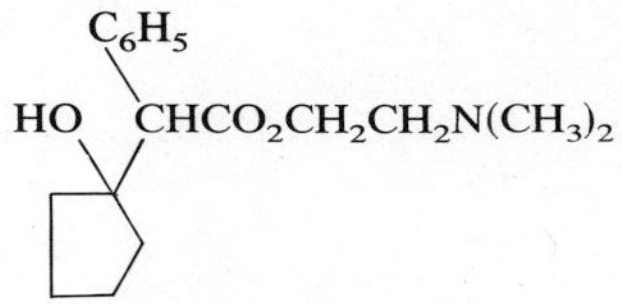 cyclopentyl(HO)—$CHCO_2CH_2CH_2N((CH_3)_2)$, C_6H_5	75
Dicyclomine NND	Bentyl	2-Diethylaminoethyl bicyclo-hexyl-1-carboxylate hydrochloride	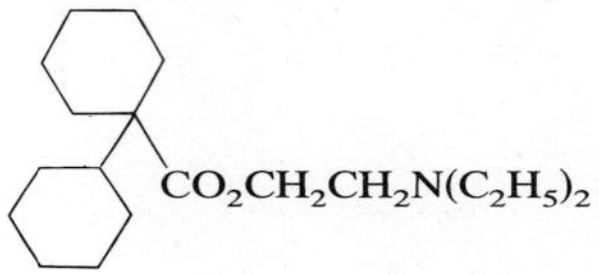 bicyclohexyl—$CO_2CH_2CH_2N(C_2H_5)_2$	76

381

Table 44.3 **Synthetic Anticholinergics** (*Continued*)

Nonproprietary Name	Selected Proprietary Names	Chemical Name of Salt	Structure of Base	Reference for Synthetic Procedures
Eucatropine	Euphthalmine	4-(1,2,2,6-Tetramethyl-piperidyl) mandelate hydrochloride	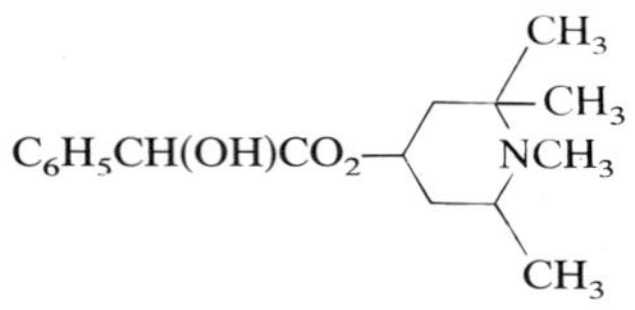	77, 78
Oxyphencyclimine ND	Daricon, Vio-Thene	1-Methyl-1,4,5,6-tetrahydro-2-pyrimdylmethyl α-cyclo-hexyl-α-phenylglycolate hydrochloride	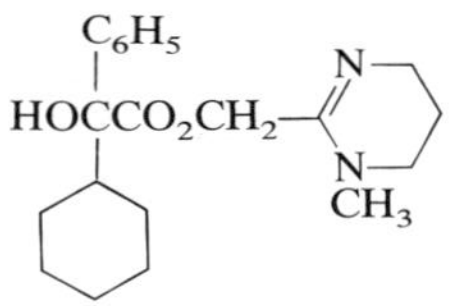	79
Piperidolate NND	Dactil	1-Ethyl-3-piperidyl diphenyl-acetate hydrochloride	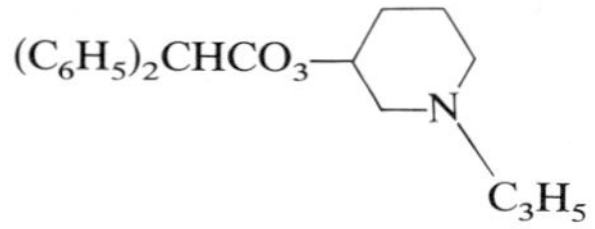	80
Pipethanate	Sycotrol	2-(1-Piperidino)ethyl benzilate hydrochloride	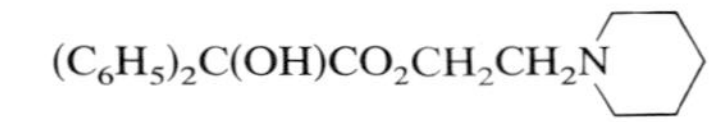 $(C_6H_5)_2C(OH)CO_2CH_2CH_2N$	81
		Quaternary Ammonium Compounds—Characteristic Group in the Main Chain: Ester		
Glycopyrrolate ND	Robinul	3-Hydroxy-1,1-dimethyl-pyrrolidinium bromide α-cyclopentylmandelate	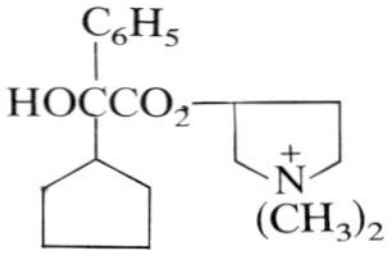	82

Generic name	Trade name	Chemical name	Structure	References
Mepenzolate ND	Cantil	N-Methyl-3-piperidyl benzilate methylbromide	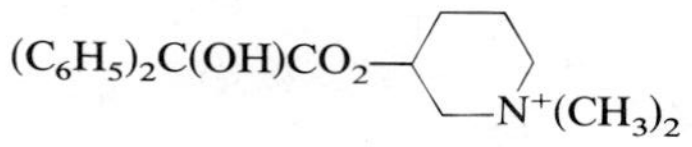 $(C_6H_5)_2C(OH)CO_2$— (3-piperidyl) $N^+(CH_3)_2$	83, 84
Methantheline NF	Banthine	β-Diethylaminoethyl 9-xanthenecarboxylate methobromide	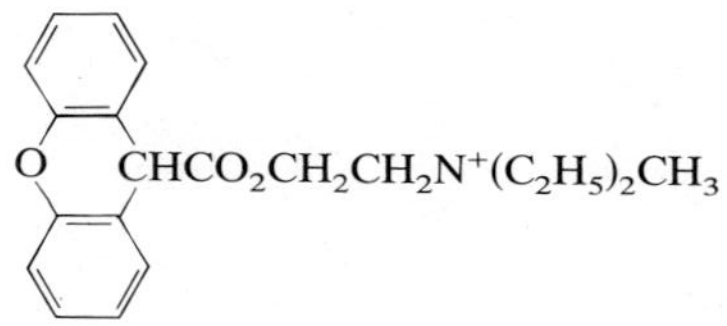 (xanthene) $CHCO_2CH_2CH_2N^+(C_2H_5)_2CH_3$	74
Oxyphenonium NND	Antrenyl	Diethyl(2-hydroxyethyl)-methylammonium-α-phenyl-α-cyclohexylglycolate bromide	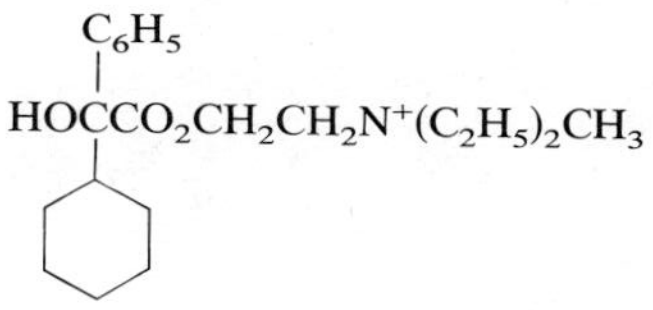 C_6H_5 / (cyclohexyl) C $HOCCO_2CH_2CH_2N^+(C_2H_5)_2CH_3$	85
Penthienate NF	Monodral	2-Diethylaminoethyl α-cyclopentyl-2-thiophene-glycolate methobromide	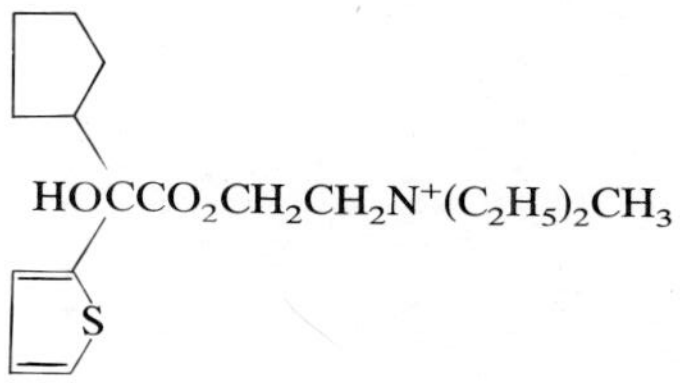 (cyclopentyl) / (thiophene) $HOCCO_2CH_2CH_2N^+(C_2H_5)_2CH_3$	86, 87
Pipenzolate NND	Piptal	N-Ethyl-3-piperidyl benzilate methobromide	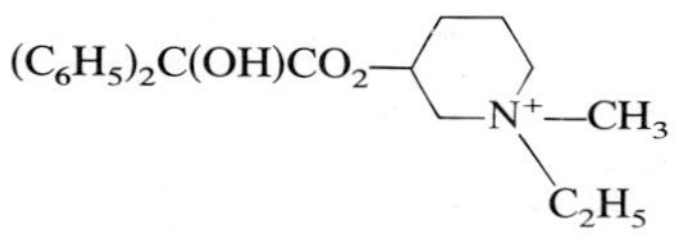 $(C_6H_5)_2C(OH)CO_2$— (3-piperidyl) N^+—CH_3 / C_2H_5	80

Table 44.3 Synthetic Anticholinergics (*Continued*)

Nonproprietary Name	Selected Proprietary Names	Chemical Name of Salt	Structure of Base	Reference for Synthetic Procedures
Poldine	Nacton	2-Hydroxymethyl-1,1-di-methylpyrrolidinium methyl-sulfate benzilate	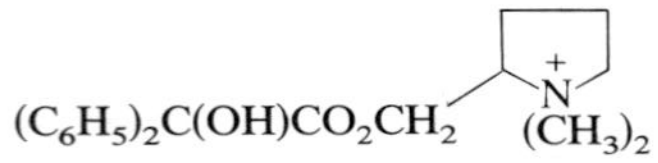 $(C_6H_5)_2C(OH)CO_2CH_2$ pyrrolidinium $N^+(CH_3)_2$	88
Propantheline USP	Pro-Banthine	β-Diisopropylmethylaminoethyl 9-xanthenecarboxylate bromide	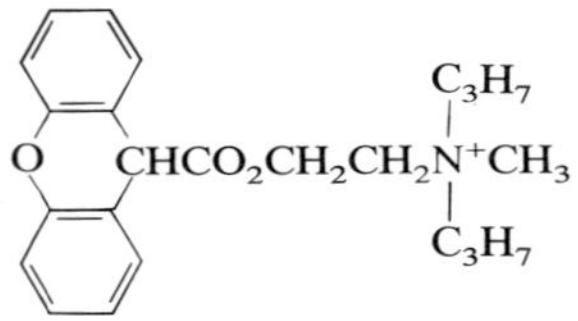 xanthene $CHCO_2CH_2CH_2N^+CH_3$, C_3H_7, C_3H_7	74
Valethamate ND	Murel	2-Diethylaminoethyl-3-methyl-2-phenylvalerate methobromide	$CH_3CHCHCO_2(CH_2)_2N^+(C_2H_5)_2CH_3$, C_2H_5, C_6H_5	89, 90
Characteristic Groups in the Main Chain: Thioester, Amide, or Carbamate				
Thioesters				
Thiphenamil	Trocinate	β-Diethylaminoethyldiphenyl-thiolacetate hydrochloride	$(C_6H_5)_2CHCOSCH_2CH_2N(C_2H_5)_2$	91–94
Amides				
Tropicamide ND	Mydriacyl	N-Ethyl-2-phenyl-N-(4-pyridylmethyl)hydracryl-amide	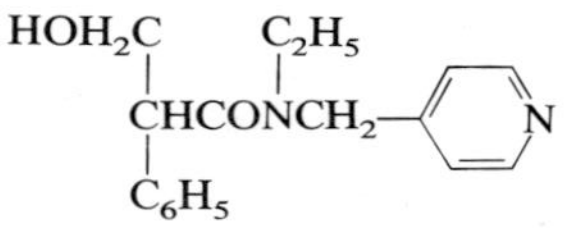 HOH_2C, C_2H_5, $CHCONCH_2-$ pyridine, C_6H_5	95

			Structure	Ref.
Carbamates				
Dibutoline NND	Dibuline	Bis[dibutylcarbamate of ethyl-(2-hydroxyethyl)-dimethylammonium]sulfate	$\begin{array}{c} C_4H_9 \\ \quad\diagdown \\ \qquad NCO_2CH_2CH_2N^+(CH_3)_2C_2H_5 \\ \quad\diagup \\ C_4H_9 \end{array}$	96, 97

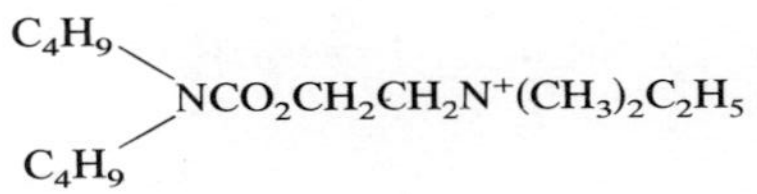

Characteristic Groups in the Main Chain; Alkane

			Structure	Ref.
Amino alcohols containing quaternary nitrogen ND				
Hexocyclium ND	Tral	N-(β-Cyclohexyl-β-hydroxy-β-phenylethyl)-N'-methyl-piperazine methylsulfate	C_6H_5 $HOCCH_2N$ ... $N^+(CH_3)_2$ (cyclohexyl)	98
Mepiperphenidol	Darstine	5-Methyl-4-phenyl-1-(1-methylpiperidinium)-3-hexanol bromide	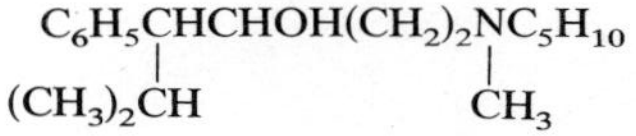 $C_6H_5CHCHOH(CH_2)_2NC_5H_{10}$ CH_3 $(CH_3)_2CH$	99
Tricyclamol NND	Elorine, Tricoloid	1-Cyclohexyl-1-phenyl-3-pyrrolidino-1-propanol methochloride	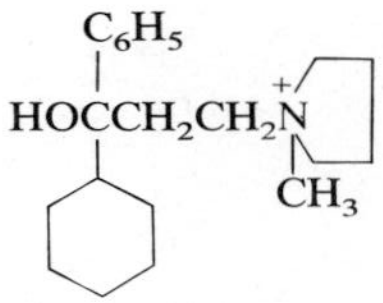 C_6H_5 $HOCCH_2CH_2N^+$ CH_3 (cyclohexyl)	100–102
Tridihexethyl NF	Pathilon	3-Diethylamino-1-phenyl-1-cyclohexyl-1-propanol ethiodide	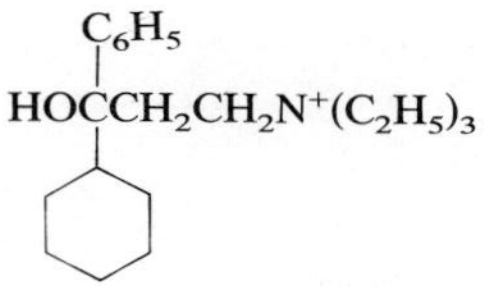 C_6H_5 $HOCCH_2CH_2N^+(C_2H_5)_3$ (cyclohexyl)	103–104

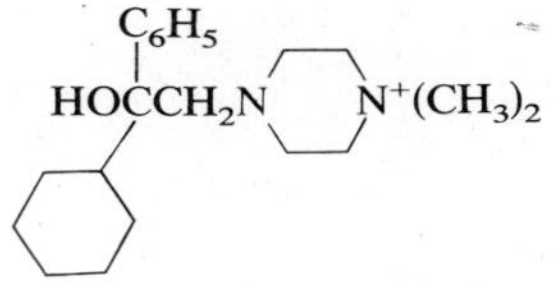

Table 44.3 Synthetic Anticholinergics (*Continued*)

Nonproprietary Name	Selected Proprietary Names	Chemical Name of Salt	Structure of Base	Reference for Synthetic Procedures
Amino alcohols containing tertiary nitrogen Procyclidine	Kemadrin	1-Cyclohexyl-1-phenyl-3-pyrrolidino-1-propanol hydrochloride	$\text{HOCCH}_2\text{CH}_2\text{N}$ with C_6H_5 and cyclohexyl substituents; pyrrolidine ring	100–102
Amino amides containing quaternary nitrogen ND Isopropamide	Darbid	(3-Carbamoyl-3,3-diphenylpropyl)diisopropylmethyl-ammonium iodide	$\text{H}_2\text{NCOCCH}_2\text{CH}_2\overset{+}{\text{N}}(\text{C}_3\text{H}_7)(\text{CH}_3)(\text{C}_3\text{H}_7)$ with two C_6H_5	105
Amino amides containing tertiary nitrogen Aminopentamide	Centrine	α,α-Diphenyl-γ-dimethylaminovaleramide	$\text{H}_2\text{NCOCCH}_2\text{CH}(\text{CH}_3)\text{N}(\text{CH}_3)_2$ with two C_6H_5	106–109
Miscellaneous Methixene ND Trest	Trest	1-Methyl-3-(thioxanthen-9-ylmethyl)piperidine hydrochloride hydrate	thioxanthene with CH_2 link to N-CH_3 piperidine	110
		Characteristic Group in the Main Chain: Alkene		
Diphemanil NF	Prantal	4-Diphenylmethylene-1,1-dimethylpiperidinium methylsulfate	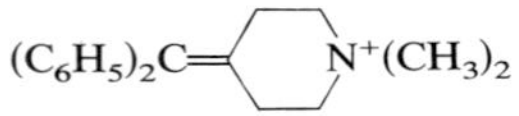 $(\text{C}_6\text{H}_5)_2\text{C}=$ piperidine $\text{N}^+(\text{CH}_3)_2$	111

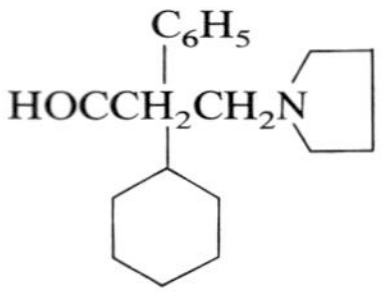

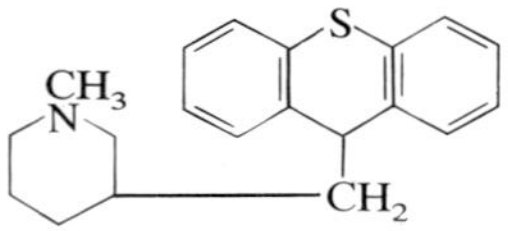

attracted by the negatively charged field (anionic center) of the muscarinic receptor. Thus the cationic head seemingly starts the process of the adsorption of the substance at the receptor. Following the attraction of the oppositely charged groups, the weaker dipole–dipole, hydrophobic, and van der Walls forces go into action; if there are many of them, especially in the case of anticholinergics, they contribute to the stability of the drug–receptor complex. In such an interaction not only the charge of the cation head but also its size and shape are of vital importance.

The basicity of different amino derivatives, and consequently the degree of their ionization at physiological pH, varies over a broad range. The more ions of the anticholinergic ammonium compound or amine in solution, the greater the probability of their interaction with the anionic center of the muscarinic receptor to form the drug–receptor complex. In addition, the stability of the drug–receptor complex that has formed should depend on the basicity, inasmuch as rate of hydrolysis of salts is inversely proportional to the base strength.

Thus high basicity should favor the anticholinergic activity of a substance. Although the logic of this conclusion is simple, its proof involves great difficulties. In a series of anticholinergics, transition from one derivative to another is associated with stepwise changes in basicity, as well as steric factors. In this respect the N-oxides, which are obtained through the oxidation of the corresponding tertiary amines, have lower basicities and also lower anticholinergic activities (109, 119, 120). The N-oxides are closer to the corresponding quaternary ammonium compounds than to the tertiary ammonium ions in steric respect and partition between aqueous and organic phases. Alkylation converts the N-oxides into typical quaternary ammonium compounds. By this procedure, both the basicity and anticholinergic activity (Table 44.4) of the substance increase sharply (37b).

The influence of a steric factor is more evident among compounds in which the size of the substituents at the nitrogen atom is varied both in the series of anticholinergic and cholinergic compounds. Progressive replacement of the N-methyl groups of

Table 44.4 Basicity and Anticholinergic Activity of Substituted Aminoethyl Esters of Benzilic Acid

$$(C_6H_5)_2C(OH)COOCH_2CH_2\overset{+}{N}(CH_3)_2R$$

R	Basicity, pK_a	Van der Waals Radius[a] of N–R (Å)	Dose[b] Required to Eliminate the Effects of Arecoline in Mice, $\mu mol/kg$	
			Salivation	Tremor
H	8.08	2.25	5.0	6.8 (6.7)
CH_3	10.87	3.09	0.48	—
OH	4.68	3.01	94.8	284.5
OCH_3	10.18	4.37	4.5	—

[a] The Van der Waals' radius of N–R bond gives an estimate of the steric volume and, therefore, steric hindrance for the interaction of the cationic head at the muscarinic receptor.

[b] Doses are calculated from the values reported by Kuznetsov and Golikov (37b).

acetylcholine with ethyl groups leads to a stepwise reduction in muscarinic activity (121). Likewise, maximal anticholinergic or blocking activity (Table 44.5) is obtained by replacing the N-methyl groups of β-dimethylaminoethyl benzilate methyl chloride with ethyl groups (113). Further increases in size to butyl or larger alkyl groups reduce or abolish the activity (113, 122–126). Therefore, it seems that for stimulant activity the small cationic head must fit into a definite space and must aid the neutralization of the charge of the anionic site of the receptor. The inhibitory action is obtained when large enough groups are substituted on the cationic portion to prevent close contact with the receptor and hence the neutralization of the charge (127, 128). Thus the cationic portion of the blocking agents provides the electrostatic forces necessary to orient the molecules toward the receptor and hold them in place.

The anticholinergic activity depends not only on the number and the molecular weight of the alkyl radicals which are con-

Table 44.5   Influence of the Number, Size, and Structure of Alkyl Groups in the Cationic Head on the Anticholinergic Activity

Compound Pair	Name or Structure of Compound[a]		Test System	Activity Ratio[b] B/A	Ref.
	Series A	Series B			
1	$RN(CH_3)_2$	$RN(C_2H_5)_2$	Cat: salivation	1.63	113
			Cat: blood pressure	2.09	
			Mouse: mydriasis	0.45	
2	$R\overset{+}{N}(CH_3)_2nC_3H_7$	$R\overset{+}{N}(CH_3)_2isoC_3H_7$	Cat: salivation	2.00	113
			Cat: blood pressure	2.38	
			Mouse: mydriasis	4.09	
3	$R\overset{+}{N}(CH_3)_2nC_3H_7$	$R\overset{+}{N}(CH_3)_2nC_4H_9$	Cat: salivation	0.49	113
			Cat: blood pressure	0.52	
			Mouse: mydriasis	0.63	
4	$R\overset{+}{N}(CH_3)_2C_2H_5$	$R\overset{+}{N}CH_3(C_2H_5)_2$	Cat: salivation	1.06	
			Cat: blood pressure	1.31	
	(lachesine)		Mouse: mydriasis	0.60	
5	$R\overset{+}{N}CH_3(C_2H_5)_2$	$R\overset{+}{N}(C_2H_5)_3$	Cat: salivation	1.00	113
			Cat: blood pressure	0.79	
			Mouse: mydriasis	1.33	
6	Atropine (>NCH_3)	N-Ethylnoratropine	Cat: blood pressure	0.04	133
7	Homatropine	N-Isopropylnor-homatropine	Cat: blood pressure	0.12	133
8	Atropine	N-Allylnora-tropine	Cat: blood pressure	0.04	134
			Rat: mydriasis	0.13	

[a] $R = (C_6H_5)_2C(OH)CO_2CH_2CH_2$-
[b] In Tables 44.5–44.7, 44.9, and 44.11, the influence of the molecular modification on the pharmacological activity is expressed as activity ratios. An activity ratio represents the ratio of the relative molar activities of two substances, whose activities are compared with a standard substance. A ratio of 1.0 indicates that the molecular modification which converts the compound in series A to the corresponding compound in series B does not change the pharmacological activity. An activity ratio of greater than unity indicates that the molecular modification has increased the activity; when it is less than unity the molecular modification has decreased the activity.

Table 44.6 Differences Between the Anticholinergic Activities of Tertiary and Quaternary Ammonium Compounds and Atropine-like Agents

Compound Pair	Series A: Tertiary Ammonium Compounds	Series B: Quaternary Ammonium Compounds	Test System	Activity Ratio B/A	Ref.
1	Atropine	Methylatropine	Guinea pig: ileum	2.10	113
			Mouse: mydriasis	2.30	116
2	(−)-Hyoscyamine	(−)-Methylhyoscyamine	Mouse: mydriasis	2.70	117
3	(−)-Scopolamine	(−)-Methscopolamine	Guinea pig: ileum	7.60	137–139
			Mouse: mydriasis	1.00	
4[a]	Tertiary analog of methantheline $XN(C_2H_5)_2$	Methantheline $X\overset{+}{N}(C_2H_5)_2CH_3$	Rabbit: intestine	2.83	140, 141
5[b]	Tertiary analog of penthienate $XN(C_2H_5)_2$	Penthienate $X\overset{+}{N}(C_2H_5)_2CH_3$	Rabbit: ileum	1.24	116
			Rabbit: salivation	30.80	
6	(±)-Procyclidine	(±)-Tricyclamol	Guinea pig: ileum	18.3	142, 143
			Mouse: mydriasis	13.5	
7	(±)-Benzhexol[c]	Methyl analog of (±)-benzhexol	Guinea pig: ileum	2.64	144
			Mouse: mydriasis	8.89	
8[d]	$RN(CH_3)_2$	$R\overset{+}{N}(CH_3)_3$	Cat: salivation	17.9	113
			Cat: blood pressure	10.3	
			Mouse: mydriasis	2.41	
9[d]	$RN(C_2H_5)_2$	$R\overset{+}{N}(CH_5)_2$	Cat: Salivation	15.1	113
			Cat: blood pressure	9.06	
			Mouse mydriasis	14.2	

[a] For complete structures see Table 44.3.
[b] For complete structures see Table 44.3.
[c] 1-Piperidino-3-phenyl-3-cyclohexyl-propan-1-ol.
[d] $R = (C_6H_5)_2C(OH)CO_2CH_2CH_2{}^-$.

nected to the nitrogen atom but also on their structure. In contrast to di-*n*-propylamino derivatives, diisopropylamino derivatives have an anticholinergic activity close to or higher than the activity of diethylamino derivatives (81, 129–132). The close correlation of the activities of the diethyl and diisopropyl derivatives could be related with the equal linear lengths (from the nitrogen atom) of these radicals.

In the case of cyclic amino alcohols where nitrogen enters into the composition of the cycle, the optimal anticholinergic effect is produced not by the *N*-ethyl, *N*-isopropyl, or *N*-allyl, but by *N*-methyl radical, as is apparent from a comparison of the esters of tropine (Table 44.9). It may be that the elements of the cyclic structure occupy a sufficiently large space besides the nitrogen atom.

As a general rule, quaternization with a small alkyl group increases activity (Table 44.6), although a few exceptions have been reported (135, 136).

Besides the charge on the cationic head of anticholinergics (and cholinergics), other factors seem to contribute to the interaction between the muscarinic receptor and the anticholinergics. The substituents at the nitrogen atom apparently participate actively in the process. This is evident from the anticholinergic action of the 3,3-dimethylbutyl ester of benzilic acid, $(C_6H_5)_2C(OH)CO_2CH_2CH_2C(CH_3)_3$, which contains no nitrogen and consequently is not ionized but which has in the corresponding position a t-butyl radical which sterically imitates the trimethylammonium group (145). A similar replacement of a trimethylammonium group with a t-butyl radical in acetylcholine leads to its "carbon analog," $CH_3CO_2CH_2CH_2C(CH_3)_3$, which is similar to acetylcholine in its behavior toward cholinesterase (146).

5.2 Cyclic Moieties

The introduction of two phenyl groups into a molecule of acetylcholine or a cholinergic substance [i.e., $CH_3CO_2(CH_2)_2\overset{+}{N}(CH_3)_3$ or $CH_3(CH_2)_4\overset{+}{N}(CH_3)_3$] changes the compound to an anticholinergic agent

[$(C_6H_5)_2CHCO_2(CH_2)\overset{+}{N}(CH_3)_3$ and $(C_6H_5)_2CH(CH_2)_4N(CH_3)_3$, respectively].

Anticholinergics contain varied cyclic structures, the phenyl group being the most common (37c). Very often one encounters cyclohexyl and cyclopentyl radicals and the corresponding unsaturated groups (cyclohexenyl, cyclopentenyl). Substances containing α-, or, less frequently, β-thienyl radicals may possess high anticholinergic activity. Often unbranched (methyl, ethyl) or branched (isobutyl, isoamyl) groups are located at the same carbon atom together with one or two cyclic groups. The anticholinergic activities of substances that contain only aliphatic radicals are lower than those of the corresponding compounds with cyclic substituents.

The most common and, as a rule, the most active anticholinergics contain two cyclic substituents as blocking groups at the same carbon atom (Table 44.7) but a third cyclic substituent lowers the anticholinergic activity (147). When these cyclic groups are too large, such as biphenyl and naphthyl, the compounds have low anticholinergic activities. A sufficiently large number of anticholinergics that contain only one cyclic group on carbon are known; however,

Table 44.7 The Influence of Cyclic Radicals on Anticholinergic Activity (Test System: Rabbit Intestine)

Compound Pair	Name or Structure of Compound[a]		Activity Ratio[b] B/A	Ref.
	Series A	Series B		
1	$C_6H_5CH_2R$	$(C_6H_5)_2CHR$ (adiphenine[c])	6.7	147
2	$C_6H_5CH_2R$	$(C_6H_5)_3CR$	0.7	147
3	$CH_2(OH)R$	$C_6H_5CH(OH)R$	23.3	147
4	$C_6H_5CH(OH)R$	$(C_6H_5)_2C(OH)R$	114	147
5	Adiphenine (transentine)	$(C_6H_5)CH(C_6H_{11})R$ (transentine-H)	3.3	148, 149
6	Adiphenine	Dicyclomine	10.0	150

[a] $R = CO_2CH_2CH_2N(C_2H_5)_2$.
[b] For explanation see Table 44.5.
[c] For structure see Table 44.3.

there is usually also an aliphatic radical or, even better, a hydroxyl group present in such a case. Examples of such compounds are the esters of tropic acid. The introduction of a second phenyl into the α-carbon of tropic acid lowers the anticholinergic activity of its aminoalkyl esters (37c).

It is difficult to assess which cyclic substituents contribute the most for the anticholinergic activity. It could be that the effect of one or another moiety depends on the substituents already present and on other characteristics of the substance. An overwhelming majority of the therapeutically most active anticholinergics contain at least one phenyl group (Table 44.3). The second cyclic group, where there is one, need not be a phenyl. It is even better if, for example, it is cyclohexyl, cyclopentyl, or any other cyclic structure. Such unsymmetrical doubly substituted compounds have higher anticholinergic activities and lower toxicities (37, 148, 149). This is a situation similar to that in 5,5-disubstituted barbituric acid hypnotics and anticonvulsants.

A question might arise whether the aromatic (flat surface) nature of one of the cyclic radicals is essential for anticholinergic activity, because such a large number of anticholinergics contain a phenyl group. The sufficiently high activity of compounds in which both substituents are alicyclic (e.g., cyclohexyl or cyclopentyl) provides a basis for asserting that the aromatic nature of the substituents is not essential in anticholinergics (37c).

Not only the number and the character of the cyclic group but also the mode of linking of the substituents are important for anticholinergic activity. Two phenyl nuclei are linked differently in 2-diethylamino-ethyl esters of diphenylacetic acid (44.**20**), fluorene-9-carboxylic acid (44.**21**), and p-biphenylacetic acid (44.**22**). Of these, the diphenylacetic acid derivatives have the highest anticholinergic activity (147).

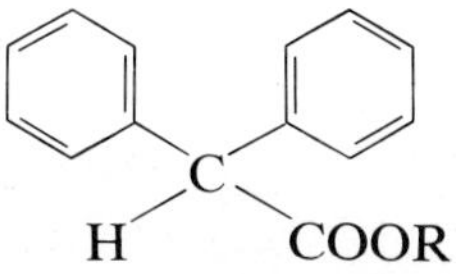

The importance of the cyclic nature of

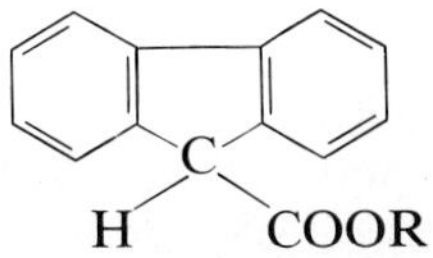

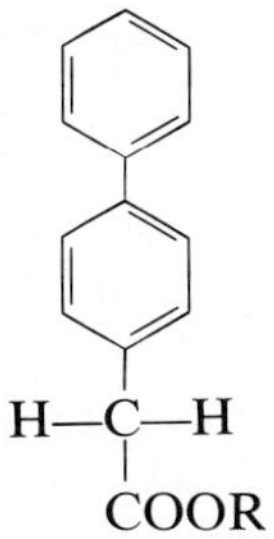

44.**20**

44.**21**

44.**22**

the substituent and not simply of its mass is evident from the comparison of the anticholinergic activities of 1-cyclohexyl-1-phenyl-3-piperidino-1-propanol (44.**23**) and 1-(n-hexyl)-1-phenyl-3-piperidino-1-propanol (44.**24**), of which 44.**23** is an active anticholinergic whereas 44.**24** is not effective (128).

As far as the contribution of cyclic structures to anticholinergic activity is concerned, the introduction of cyclic groups

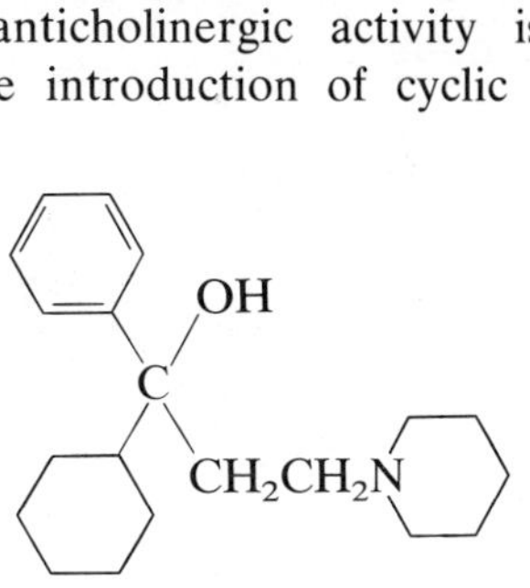

44.**23**

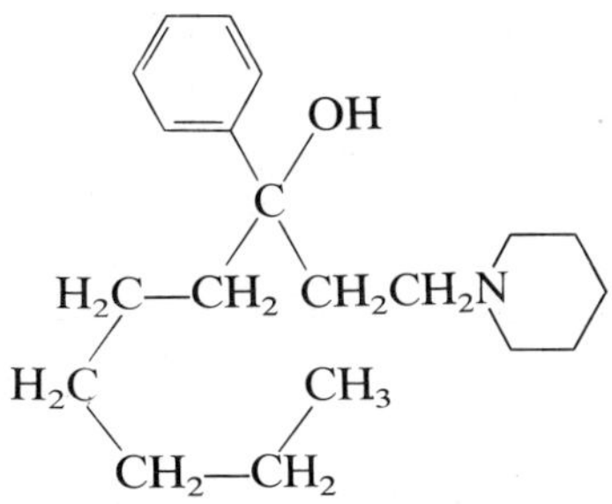

44.**24**

into acetylcholine or a cholinergic compound leads to a change in the pharmacological properties which, without lowering and possibly even strengthening its affinity for the muscarinic receptor, abolishes or blocks the action of the chemical transmitter. This phenomenon is similar to the transition from a metabolite to an antimetabolite. It has been suggested that the cyclic groups of the anticholinergic agent form an additional contact with the muscarinic receptor by hydrophobic or van der Walls forces; as a result this contact is strengthened and the muscarinic receptors are protected from approaching molecules of acetylcholine (128, 151). Cyclic groups of substantial size can create a kind of protective screen which sterically hinders the approach of molecules of acetylcholine not only to the given active site but also to the vicinity of the active sites of the receptor.

5.3   Length of the Main Chain Connecting the Cationic Head and the Cyclic Groups

The presence of the cationic head and of cyclic groups is not sufficient for optimal anticholinergic activity of a compound. The activity depends on the mutual distribution of these groups. This establishes the basic requirements for a chain of atoms which connects the cationic head and the cyclic moieties; these apply to the length and form of the chain, lateral branching, and functional groups in the chain, if any.

A considerable number of the anticholinergics belong to the group of aminoalkyl esters of substituted acetic acids. In an overwhelming majority of cases, the substituted esters of β-aminoethanol are more active as anticholinergics than the corresponding derivatives of γ-aminopropanol (113, 124, 129, 152). Further increase of the chain length of the amino alcohol leads to a decrease or disappearance of the anti-

cholinergic activity. The aminoalkyl esters of diphenylacetic acid are more active anticholinergics than the corresponding aminoalkyl esters of β,β-diphenylpropionic acid (153). Therefore, in all these esters with high anticholinergic activity the main chain connecting the cyclic moieties and the cationic head contains five atoms (Table 44.8, series 1–3). In an homologous series of compounds in which the ester group is replaced by a chain of carbon atoms (Table 44.8, series 4–9), there are three atoms in the main chain in compounds with maximal anticholinergic activity. To explain the differences in the anticholinergic activities of different series of compounds the ability of their structures to exist in different spatial conformations has to be taken into account.

Acetylcholine and related esters can exist in two conformations (Fig. 44.5), the skewed and extended forms (154) (e.g., 44.**25** and 44.**26**, respectively, for acetylcholine). The skewed form (44.**25**) of acetylcholine is closely related to the structure of muscarine (44.**27**) (154). Similarly the substituted aminoethyl esters, which are anticholinergics, may exist in two conformations. The skewed forms of acetylcholine (44.**25**), muscarine (44.**27**), the skewed form of aminoethyl esters (44.**28**), and the extended form of aminopropane derivatives (44.**29**) all interact at the same muscarinic receptors. In the former two compounds the interatomic distance between the quaternary nitrogen and the ether oxygen atom is nearly the same, and both of them are agonists. In 44.**28** and 44.**29** the interatomic distance between the quaternary nitrogen and the carbon atom to which the cyclic radicals are attached is the same, and both of them are antagonists (37d). Thus anticholinergic activity depends not only on the length of the main chain of the molecule but also on its ability to adopt a certain conformation that is favorable for the interaction of the substance with the receptor.

Table 44.8   The Chain Length Between Cationic Head and Cyclic Radicals Among Anticholinergics

No.	Series	Value of 'n' for High Anticholinergic Activity	Total Number of Atoms in the Chain	Test System	Ref.
1	$(C_6H_5)_2C(OH)CO_2(CH_2)_nNC_5H_{10}\cdot HCl$	2^a	5	Rabbit: mydriasis	152
2	$(C_6H_5)_2C(OH)CO_2(CH_2)_n\overset{+}{N}C_5H_{10}\cdot CH_3Br$	2^a	5	Rabbit: mydriasis	152
3	$(C_6H_5)_2C(OH)CO_2(CH_2)_n\overset{+}{N}(C_2H_5)(CH_3)\cdot$ CH$_3$Cl	2^a	5	Mouse: mydriasis	113
4	$(C_6H_5)(C_2H_5)C(OH)(CH_2)_nN(C_2H_5)_2\cdot$ HCl	2	3	Rabbit: ileum	103
5	$(C_6H_5)(C_2H_5)C(OH)(CH_2)_nNC_5H_{10}\cdot$ HCl	2	3	Rabbit: ileum	103
6	$(C_6H_5)_2C(OH)(CH_2)_nNC_5H_{10}\cdot HCl$	2	3	Rabbit: ileum	103
7	$(C_6H_5)_2CH(CH_2)_nN(C_2H_5)_2\cdot CH_3I$	2	3	Mouse: salivation	37d
8	$(C_6H_5)_2C(OH)(CH_2)_nN(C_2H_5)_2\cdot HCl$	2	3	Mouse: salivation Mouse: tremor	37d
9	$(C_6H_5)_2C(OH)(CH_2)_nN(C_2H_5)_2\cdot CH_3I$	2	3	Mouse: salivation	37d

^{a} No exact values are available for esters with $n-1$.

There is less information about the influence of branching of the main chain on the anticholinergic activity. Esters with a methyl group α to the ester oxygen in the amino alcohol part are less active than compounds without the methyl group (129, 152, 155). Similarly, the derivatives of 1,3-aminopropanol, aminopropane, and γ-aminobutyronitrile (156, 157) that contain a branch at the carbon atom β to the nitrogen are less active anticholinergics than the compounds without the branching.

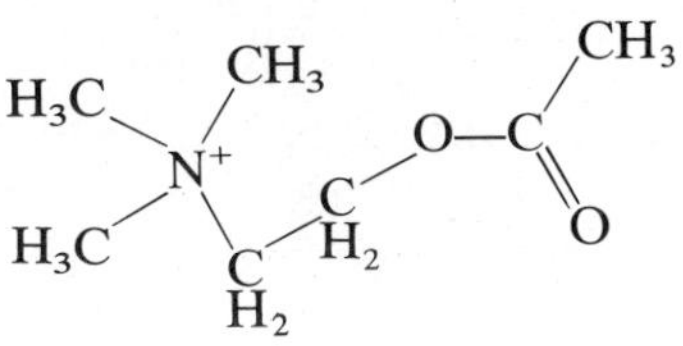

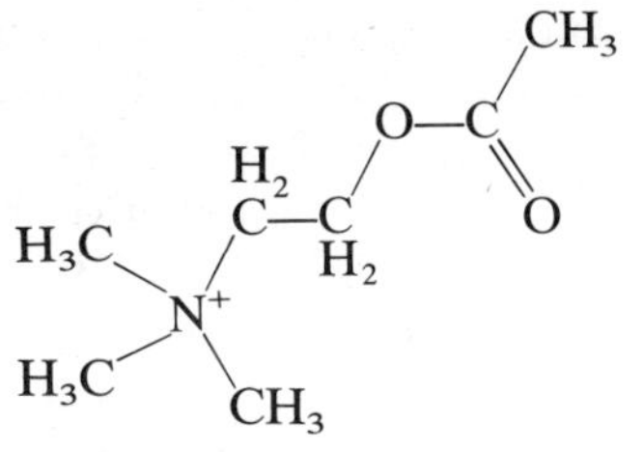

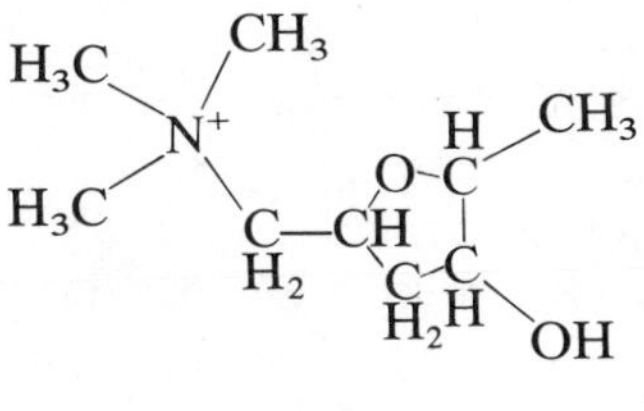

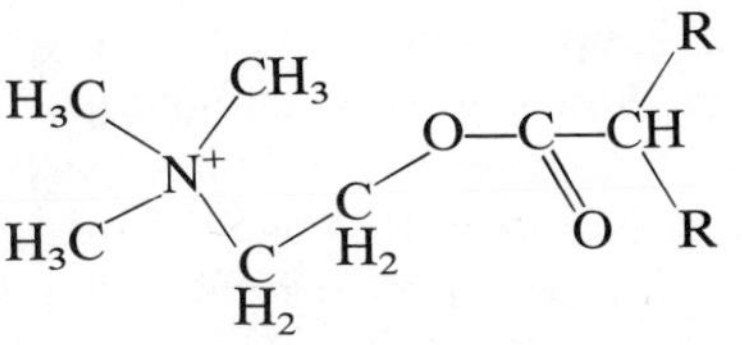

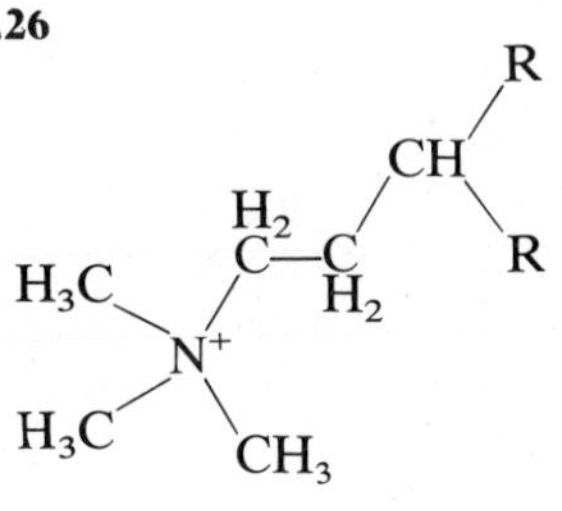

Fig. 44.5   Conformations of cholinergics and anticholinergics.

The negative influence of such a side chain has been explained by steric hindrance at the receptor (128).

The inclusion in the main chain of optimum length of other atoms such as oxygen, sulfur, nitrogen, and other functional groups changes any anticholinergic activity (37). However, such compounds are considerably potent (see Section 5.4).

5.4 Esteratic Linkage

The question of the importance of complex ester grouping in anticholinergics, and even more of its role, has not been cleared up sufficiently. Although very great importance was attached to the complex esters in the initial period of the search for atropine-like substances, when active compounds were known only among the esters of amino alcohols and carboxylic acids, there is no question that the presence of this grouping is not necessary for the manifestation of anticholinergic activity. Presently a large number of substances are known that belong to different chemical structures and that possess high anticholinergic activity (Table 44.3).

The influence of an ester link can be assessed by comparing similar compounds that do not contain pharmacophoric groups other than the anchoring groups (amino nitrogen, cyclic radicals). Comparative data on the anticholinergic activities of the 2-diethylaminoethyl ester of diphenylacetic acid $[(C_6H_5)_2CHCO_2CH_2CH_2N(C_2H_5)_2]$ and 1,1-diphenyl-5-diethylaminopentane $[(C_6H_5)_2CHCH_2CH_2CH_2CH_2N(C_2H_5)_2]$ indicate that they are equally active (37d). Thus the complex ester group is not essential for anticholinergic activity; however, it may contribute to optimal activity when it is present in atropine-like compounds (117). It may influence the conformation of a molecule that in turn determines the effectiveness of the interaction of the essential anchoring groups, the cationic head and the cyclic radicals (37d), with the muscarinic receptor.

5.5 Hydroxyl Group

The anticholinergic compounds that contain a hydroxyl group in a certain position of a molecule possess considerably higher activity than similar compounds without the hydroxyl. That position is of great importance. For esters of amino alcohols and hydroxycarboxylic acids, maximum activity is achieved if the hydroxyl is β to carboxyl. Atropine is about 10 times more active than homatropine. However, esters with an α-hydroxyl also possess considerable anticholinergic activity. In anticholinergic amino alcohols the hydroxyl on the third carbon atom from the nitrogen gives optimal activity (Table 44.3). The location of the hydroxyl group in relation to the cyclic radicals is also of vital importance. In the great majority of anticholinergics they are located at the same carbon atom or at adjacent carbons.

The hydroxyl group in anticholinergics can be replaced by CN and $CONH_2$ groups while preserving some degree of activity. However, replacement of the hydroxyl by methoxy or an acetoxy group lowers the activity (158, 159).

The hydroxyl group may interact by hydrogen bonding with a site on the muscarinic receptor which is rich in electrons. In support of this statement (37e), hydroxylated anticholinergics form complexes in solution with substances such as amines which contain electron donor atoms. In a series of structurally related compounds the anticholinergic activity was proportional to their capacity for molecular association by way of the hydroxyl group. There is a direct relationship between the anticholinergic activity and the mobility of the hydrogen atom of the hydroxyl group as determined by the rate of acetylation. The contribution of the hydroxyl group to the free energy of adsorption is quite high, of the order of 2 kcal; it is apparently independent of the number of methyl groups attached to the cationic head (160).

Although a hydroxyl group increases the activity of an anticholinergic, it does not convert a cholinergic substance into an anticholinergic. Propionyl-, α-hydroxypropionyl-, and α,β-dihydroxypropionylcholines possess cholinergic properties (161). α-Hydroxy substitution decreases the original muscarinic activity to about $\frac{1}{3}$, whereas the introduction of both α- and β-OH functions decreases the muscarinic activity to about $\frac{1}{10}$.

The introduction of a hydroxyl group into 2-diethylaminoethyl phenylacetate approximately doubles its activity (Table 44.9), whereas the same structural change in the corresponding ester of diphenylacetic acid increases its activity about 140 times. The positive influence of the hydroxyl group has been observed in a large number of anticholinergics (Table 44.3). The exceptions are those cases in which the cyclic groups are too large or are connected in such a way that they can sterically prevent the interaction of the hydroxyl with the surface of the muscarinic receptor.

5.6 Epoxy Group

The presence of an epoxy group seems to increase the mydriatic activity (Table 44.9). However, scopolamine (44.**7**) which contains an epoxy group, is a central depressant, as indicated by drowsiness, euphoria, amnesia, and dreamless sleep. Atropine (44.**4**), which does not contain an epoxy group, stimulates the medulla and higher cerebral centers. In clinical doses (0.5–1.0 mg), this effect is usually confined to mild vagal excitation. Toxic doses of atropine cause restlessness, disorientation, hallucinations, and delirium.

5.7 Stereoisomerism and Anticholinergic Activity

5.7.1 OPTICAL ISOMERISM. Atropine (44.**4**–44.**6**) is the racemic form of hyoscyamine, which is the (S)-$(-)$-tropyl ester of 3α-tropanol (44.**2**). The carbon α to the carbonyl group is asymmetric. (S)-$(-)$-Hyoscyamine is more active than (R)-$(+)$-hyoscyamine as an anticholinergic (Table 44.10). The alkaloid scopolamine (44.**7**) is the (S)-$(-)$-tropyl ester of scopine (44.**8**); again the (S)-$(-)$ isomer is more active than (R)-$(+)$ isomer in its anticholinergic activities.

Table 44.9   The Influence of the Hydroxyl and Epoxy Groups on Anticholinergic Activity

Group	Name or Structure of Compound		Test System	Activity Ratio[a] B/A	Ref.
	Series A	Series B			
Hydroxyl	$C_6H_5CH_2CO_2CH_2CH_2N(C_2H_5)_2$	$C_6H_5CH(OH)CO_2CH_2CH_2N(C_2H_5)_2$	Rabbit: intestine	2.3	147
	$(C_6H_5)_2CHCO_2CH_2CH_2N(C_2H_5)_2$	$(C_6H_5)_2C(OH)CO_2CH_2CH_2N(C_2H_5)_2$	Rabbit: intestine	143	147
Epoxy	$(-)$-Hyoscyamine	$(-)$-Scopolamine	Guinea pig: ileum	0.24	162
			Mouse: eye	2.70	
			Cat: eye	5.80	
			Cat: blood pressure	0.64	
			Cat: salivation	0.77	
	$(-)$-Methylhyoscamine	$(-)$-Methylscopolamine	Mouse: eye	1.00	162
			Cat: eye	3.33	
			Cat: blood pressure	0.80	
			Cat: salivation	0.80	

[a] For explanation see Table 44.5.

Table 44.10 Optical Isomerism and Anticholinergic Activity

No.	Compounds whose (+) and (−) Isomers are tested	Test System	Position of the Asymmetric Carbon	Active Isomer	Isomeric Ratio[a]	Ref.
1	Hyoscyamine	Dog: salivation		(−)	30	162
		Cat: salivation	α-carbon to	(−)	20	162
		Cat: blood pressure	the carbonyl	(−)	23	162
		Guinea pig: ileum	group	(−)	32	162
		Rabbit: ileum		(−)	110	162
2	Scopolamine	Dog: salivation	α-carbon to	(−)	17	162
		Rabbit: intestine	the carbonyl group	(−)	15	
3	Tricyclamol	Guinea pig: ileum	Carbon with cyclic radical	(−)	160	163
				(−)	62	
4	Benzhexol	Guinea pig: ileum	Carbon with	(−)	10	163
		Rabbit: intestine	cyclic radical	(−)	160	117
		Mice: mydriasis		(−)	5	163
5	Procyclidine	Guinea pig: ileum	Carbon with	(−)	49	163
		Mice: mydriasis	cyclic radical	(−)	18	163
6	1,1-Diphenyl-3-piperidino-1-butanol hydrochloride	Rabbit: intestine	α to N	(+)	84	164 165
7	Methiodide of no. 6	Rabbit: intestine	α to N	(+)	3	164 165
8	Diphenylacetate of 3-quinuclidinol	Rabbit: intestine	β to N	(−)	24	166

[a] Activity ratio between the enantiomers.

A considerable number of synthetic anticholinergic agents patterned after the structure of atropine contain an asymmetric carbon atom corresponding to the position of the asymmetric carbon in atropine. In all compounds examined, the asymmetric carbon is located in the acyl moiety and is connected with the cyclic and the hydroxyl groups (directly or through a methylene group). The absolute configurations of all these substances are not known, and hence no definite conclusions concerning the stereospecificity of the muscarinic receptor can be drawn. However, (−) isomers are often more active than (+) isomers (Table 44.10), indicating some apparent stereospecificity with respect to the carbon atom α to the carbonyl group of atropine.

The atropine-like activities of some compounds in which the asymmetric carbon atom is considerably closer to the amino group have been described. In 1,1-diphenyl-3-piperidino-1-butanol, the carbon α to the nitrogen is asymmetric. In this case the (+) isomer seems to be more active than the (−) isomer. In 3-quinuclidinyl diphenylacetate, the carbon atom β to the nitrogen is asymmetric; the (−) isomer has more atropine-like activity than the (+) isomer.

5.7.2 DERIVATIVES OF TROPINE AND PSEUDO-TROPINE. The configuration of the 3-OH group in the tropine part of the molecule has significant influence on the activity at the muscarinic receptor (Table 44.11). The

Table 44.11   Relative Anticholinergic Activities of the Esters of Tropine and Pseudotropine

Iso-mer Pair	Pair of Structural Isomers		Test System	Activity Ratio[a] A/B	Ref.
	A	B			
1	Atropine	Tropyl-ψ-tropine	Cat (?): blood pressure	2	167
2	Benzoyl-tropine HCl	Benzoyl-ψ-tropine	Rabbit or Guinea pig: intestine	3	168
3	CH_3I of no. 2	CH_3I of no. 2	Guinea pig: intestine	13	168
4	C_2H_5Br of no. 2	C_2H_5Br of no. 2	Guinea pig: intestine	4	168

[a] For explanation see Table 44.5.

derivatives of ψ-tropine (pseudotropine, 44.**3**) are less active; the activity ratio for the ψ compound relative to the isomeric tropine varies from 2 to 13, but more information is needed on this point.

5.7.3   STEREOCHEMICAL   CONFIGURATION. The acetylcholine-like cholinergics and atropine-like anticholinergics contain similar pharmacodynamic groups. In various hypotheses, it has been assumed that both stimulant and blocking drugs interact with the muscarinic receptor through the essential pharmacodynamic groups. The tropic acid portion of atropine contains an asymmetric carbon, and the muscarinic receptor is stereospecific for the carbon α to the carbonyl group in anticholinergics. Acetylcholine does not contain such an asymmetric carbon atom. Lactoylcholine is an agonist which contains an asymmetric carbon (161), and the muscarinic receptor is stereospecific for the carbon α to carbonyl group among lactoylcholine-like cholinergics (169). Owing to the structural similarities in tropic and lactic acids, it has even been suggested that a lactoylcholine-like parasympathetic neurohormone may occur in animal tissues (161, 170). However, this has not been corroborated.

5.7.4   DISSOCIATION CONSTANTS OF CHOLINERGICS AND ANTICHOLINERGICS.   The absolute

configuration [(R) and (S)] is self-consistent for a molecule in question and cannot be used to relate a series of compounds. The configuration in relation to a standard substance (D and L) is very useful to compare a series of compounds. For example, the pharmacological parameters of all D compounds in a series can be compared with those of the L compounds, provided each one of the compounds contains a single asymmetric carbon (171).

In a number of studies on structure–activity relationships, the pharmacological activities are expressed in terms of potencies or relative molar activities, which are derivatives of their ED_{50}s. The reciprocals of ED_{50}s do not give exact measures of affinities (172), which are required to make valid conclusions on the stereoisomer–receptor interactions and the nature of receptor surfaces. The differences in the potencies of a pair of stereoisomers may be due to the differences in their affinities or intrinsic efficacies. For these reasons, the following information is necessary to make definite conclusions for delineating receptor surfaces using stereoisomer–receptor interactions (171): (1) the dissociation constant of agonists (K_A) and antagonists (K_B) that act at the same receptors, (2) the absolute configuration of the compounds, and (3) the interrelationships between the configurations of agonists and antagonists acting at the same receptors.

The dissociation constants of very few cholinergic agonists and antagonists have been determined (Table 44.12). D(+)- and L(+)-lactoylcholines are agonists at muscarinic receptors and there is no significant difference in their intrinsic efficacies. The K_A of D(+)-lactoylcholine is lower than the K_A of the L(−) isomer at the muscarinic receptor. Therefore, the D(+) isomer has a higher affinity to the muscarinic receptor than the L(−) isomer (173). Mandeloyl- and tropinoylcholines are competitive antagonists of acetylcholine and lactoylcholine at the muscarinic receptors (174–176). Among these anticholinergics, the D isomer has a higher affinity ($1/K_B$) than the corresponding L isomer. The above anticholinergics did not exhibit sig-

nificant intrinsic efficacies at the muscarinic receptors. The carbon α to the carbonyl carbon of the ester group is asymmetric in agonists (lactoylcholines) and their competitive antagonists (mandeloylcholines and tropinoylcholines). Therefore, the D isomers have the preferred relative configuration which comes into definite spatial position with the muscarinic receptor. Similarly, D(−)-hyoscamine has higher affinity to the muscarinic receptor than the L(+) isomer and has the preferred configuration (177).

5.8   Compounds with Dual Action: Cholinergic and Anticholinergic Activities

In several groups of atropine-like agents, derived from acetylcholine-like compounds, agonist activity is replaced by par-

Table 44.12   Dissociation Constants and Intrinsic Efficacies of Cholinergic and Anticholinergic Agents

Cholinergic or Anticholinergic and Configuration	Type of Receptor[a] (Test System)	Activity		Ref.
		Dissociation Constant[b] (K_A or K_B)	Relative Intrinsic Efficacy	
Acetylcholine	Muscarinic	1.08×10^{-6}	1.00	173
	Nicotinic	2.17×10^{-6}	1.00	173
(R)−D(+)-Lactoylcholine	Muscarinic	7.3×10^{-5}	0.52	173
	Nicotinic	1.85×10^{-5}	1.07	173
(S)-L-(−)-Lactoylcholine	Muscarinic	3.02×10^{-4}	0.30	173
	Nicotinic	8.08×10^{-5}	1.15	173
(R)-D-(−)-Acetyl-β-methylcholine	Muscarinic	Inactive	—	178
(S)-L-(+)-Acetyl-β-methylcholine	Muscarinic (active isomer)	1.24×10^{-6}	—	178
(R)-D-(−)-Mandeloylcholine	Muscarinic	3.00×10^{-6}	NS[c]	174, 175
(S)-L-(+)-Mandeloylcholine	Muscarinic	5.22×10^{-6}	NS	174, 175
(S)-D-(−)-Tropinoylcholine	Muscarinic	2.15×10^{-8}	NS	174, 176
(R)-L-(+)-Tropinoylcholine	Muscarinic	3.26×10^{-7}	NS	174, 176
(S)-D-(−)-Hyoscyamine	Muscarinic	4.47×10^{-10}	NS	177
(R)-L-(+)-Hyoscyamine	Muscarinic	1.41×10^{-8}	NS	177

[a] Muscarinic activities are tested on the guinea pig longitudinal ileal muscle in all cases except acetyl-β-methylcholine, which is tested on the circular muscle from fundus of rabbit stomach. Nicotinic activities are tested on the frog rectus abdominis muscle.
[b] Moles/liter.
[c] Not significant.

Table 44.13 Cholinergic and Anticholinergic Activities of Choline Esters

$$RCO_2CH_2CH_2\overset{+}{N}(CH_3)_3 \cdot I^-$$

R	Intrinsic Activity α	pD_2	pA_2	Test System	Ref.
H	1	5.2		Rat: intestine	179, 180
CH_3	1	7.0		Rat: intestine	179, 180
CH_3CH_2	1	5.3		Rat: intestine	179, 180
$CH_3(CH_2)_2$	0.5	5.1		Rat: intestine	179, 180
$CH_3(CH_2)_3$	0	—	4.7	Rat: intestine	179, 180
$CH_3(CH_2)_5$	—	—	4.7	Guinea pig: ileum	181
$CH_3(CH_2)_6$	—	—	4.7	Guinea pig: ileum	181
$CH_3(CH_2)_7$	—	—	5.0	Guinea pig: ileum	181
$CH_3(CH_2)_8$	—	—	5.5	Guinea pig: ileum	181
$CH_3(CH_2)_9$	—	—	6.0	Guinea pig: ileum	181
$CH_3(CH_2)_{10}$	—	—	6.5	Guinea pig: ileum	181
	0	—	5.4	Rat: intestine	179, 180

tial agonist activity and eventually antagonist activity with increasing substitution (178–181). For example, a transition between cholinergic and anticholinergic properties occurs when the acyl group of acetylcholine is progressively lengthened. Cholinergic activity decreases from formylcholine to butyrylcholine, and the higher members of the series are anticholinergics (Table 44.13). More recently it has been demonstrated that hyoscyamine and atropine at small dose levels exhibit cholinergic properties (182, 183).

6 INTERACTION OF ANTICHOLINERGICS AT THE MUSCARINIC RECEPTORS

It is generally accepted that acetylcholine and atropine interact with the same postganglionic muscarinic receptors. Whereas acetylcholine stimulates these receptors, atropine blocks them. Although considerable progress has been made in understanding these interactions of stimulant and blocking drugs, many aspects of drug–receptor interaction are not clear. For detailed discussions of cholinergic and anticholinergic

drugs at the muscarinic receptors see original papers and reviews on the subject (37, 129, 162, 175–177, 184–190).

6.1 Kinetic Basis for the Mechanism of Action of Anticholinergics

The major action of a number of anticholinergics is a competitive antagonism to acetylcholine and other cholinergic agents. The antagonism can therefore be overcome by increasing the concentration of acetylcholine at receptor sites of the effector organs. Thus anticholinesterases partially reverse the antagonism of anticholinergics by sparing acetylcholine at the receptor sites. The anticholinergics can inhibit all muscarinic actions of acetylcholine and other choline esters. Responses to postganglionic cholinergic nerve stimulation may also be inhibited, but less readily than responses to administered choline esters. The differences in the ability of anticholinergics to block the effects of exogenous choline esters and the effects of endogenous acetylcholine liberated by the postganglionic parasympathetic nerves may be due to the release of the chemical transmitter by the nerve at the receptors in relatively inaccessible sites where diffusion limits the concentration of the antagonist.

6.2   Specificity of Antagonism

Atropine is a highly selective antagonist of acetylcholine, muscarine, and other cholinergic agents on the smooth and cardiac muscles and glands. This antagonism is so selective for cholinergic agents that atropine blockade of the actions of other types of drugs has been taken as evidence for their actions through cholinergic mechanisms. For example, the smooth muscle of guinea pig ileum is stimulated by muscarine, 5-hydroxytryptamine, histamine, and barium chloride. Atropine is more specific in blocking the stimulant effects of muscarine and acetylcholine at lower dose levels than those of the other three stimulant agents.

6.3   Molecular Basis for the Interaction of Acetylcholine and Anticholinergics at the Muscarinic Receptors

Structure–activity relationships among muscarinic agents (or cholinergics) indicate the existence on the receptor of two active sites separated by a distance 3.2 ± 0.2 Å (173, 191–193). One of them is an anionic site with which the quaternary ammonium group interacts to induce stimulant or blocking actions. The ether oxygen of muscarine and the ester oxygen of acetylcholine interact with the second site. There are some similarities between the active sites on acetylcholinesterase and the muscarinic receptor (Chapters 7 and 9). The amine portion of anticholinergics interacts at the same anionic site as the quaternary group of acetylcholine and atropine. Although every detail of acetylcholine–atropine antagonism is not clear, some facets of this

antagonism are well known: (1) one molecule of atropine blocks one molecule of acetylcholine. Atropine is a larger molecule than acetylcholine and either mechanically or electrostatically inactivates receptors engaged by it. (2) Atropine has greater affinity than acetylcholine for the receptor. Its intrinsic activity is not significant, whereas acetylcholine has high intrinsic activity. Substances with intermediate intrinsic activities behave either as cholinergics or as anticholinergics depending on the nature of their influence on the receptor. Among such substances are partial agonists with "dual action"; cholinergic activity precedes the anticholinergic activity. The partial agonists can be detected in a homologous series by gradually proceeding from agonists to antagonists with increasing molecular weight. (3) Besides the cationic head, bulky cyclic groups are essential constituents of compounds with anticholinergic activity. It seems clear that the van der Waals or hydrophobid binding of the planar cyclic groups together with the binding of the amine group produce a strong drug–receptor complex which effectively blocks the close approach of acetylcholine to the receptor. (4) Acetylcholine increases potassium efflux and causes depolarization of the membrane, both of which effects are blocked by atropine. (5) The receptor proteins on the membrane may undergo molecular disorientation during the interaction of acetylcholine with the cholinergic receptor, and this change in the receptor proteins may be prevented by a suitable blocking agent (194).

7   THERAPEUTIC USES OF ANTICHOLINERGICS

The chief use of most of the antispasmodic agents is as an adjunct in the management of the peptic ulcer; this group of drugs includes adiphenine, aminopentamide, amprotropine, dibutoline, diphemanil, glycopyrrolate, hexocyclium, homoatropine methylbromide, methscopolamine bromide, methscopolamine nitrate, oxyphencyclimine, oxyphenonium, penthienate, pipenzolate, piperidolate, pipethonate, propanthelin, tricyclamol, and trihexethyl (195).

The anticholinergic agents that are useful as adjuvants in the management of the functional disorders of the bowel (e.g., irritable colon, spastic colitis, ulcerative colitis, and diverticulitis) include dicyclomine, hexocyclium, mepenzolate, and valethamate.

The mydriatic and cycloplegic activities of anticholinergics in man are listed in Table 44.14. Atropine is recommended in situations requiring complete and prolonged relaxation of the sphincter of iris and the ciliary muscle. Mydriatics, like cyclopentolate, eucatropine, and homatropine bromide, with a shorter duration of action, are usually preferred for measuring refractive errors because of the relative rapidity with which their cycloplegic effects are terminated.

Atropine and scopolamine are used for premedication prior to the administration of some inhalation anesthetics to reduce excessive salivary and bronchial secretions. Atropine and related agents have been used in the treatment of renal colic and hyperhidrosis, and to control sweating that may aggravate certain dermatologic disorders. Atropine also may be used to counteract the toxicity of certain cholinergic drugs and anticholinesterase agents.

Certain drugs with anticholinergic effects are used for the symptomatic treatment of Parkinson's disease (paralysis agitans) and related syndromes of the extrapyramidal tracts (see Chapter 45). (Of the presently available drugs, none are useful in all cases of Parkinsonism.) Despite claims of superiority for newly introduced synthetic agents, none possess outstanding efficacy and freedom from adverse side effects when compared clinically with atropine and scopolamine (195).

Table 44.14   Mydriatic and Cycloplegic Activities of Anticholinergics in Man[a]

No.	Drug[b]	Strength of Solution, %	Mydriasis		Cycloplegia	
			Maximal, min	Recovery, days	Maximal, hr	Recovery, days
1	Atropine sulfate	1.0	30–40	7–10	1–3	8–12
2	Oxyphenonium bromide	1.0	30–40	7–10	1–3	8–12
3	Scopolamine hydrobromide	0.5	20–30	3–5	$\frac{1}{2}$–1	1–2
4	Atropine methyl nitrate	1.0–5	30	2	1	2
5	Homatropine bromide	1.0	10–30	$\frac{1}{4}$–4	$\frac{1}{2}$–1$\frac{1}{2}$	$\frac{1}{2}$–2
6	Cyclopentolate hydrochloride	0.5–1.0	30–60	1	$\frac{1}{2}$–1	1
7	Dibutoline sulfate	5.0–7.5	60	$\frac{1}{4}$–$\frac{1}{2}$	1	$\frac{1}{4}$–$\frac{1}{2}$
8	Tropicamide[c]	1.0	20–35	$\frac{1}{4}$	$\frac{1}{2}$	2–6 hr
9	Eucatropine hydrochloride	5–10	30	$\frac{1}{4}$–$\frac{1}{2}$	None	—

[a] For details see Refs. 37, 47, 68, and 195–198. The values should be considered approximate.
[b] One instillation of one drop unless otherwise specified.
[c] Two drops at 5 min intervals.

8 MOLECULAR BASIS FOR THE SIDE EFFECTS OF ANTICHOLINERGICS

The most widely used mode of approach in the design of anticholinergics is based upon the use of tropine alkaloids as models of prototypes, from which congeners or homologs or analogs have been designed. Tropine alkaloids have many pharmacological activities and interact at many cholinergic sites. In drug design the main purpose is to increase one pharmacological action at one particular site of action while suppressing other pharmacological activities at other sites. It is not always possible to abolish all pharmacological effects other than the desired activity by molecular modification. Though the desired activity is useful in its therapeutic applications, other pharmacological activities manifest themselves as side effects. For example, atropine, scopolamine, and cocaine are structurally related, each having a tropine nucleus. They differ in some of their pharmacological activities. Atropine stimulates the central nervous system, scopolamine depresses the central nervous system, and cocaine is a local anesthetic and CNS stimulant.

By molecular modification, it has been possible to produce a series of anticholinergics having qualitative effects resembling those produced by parasympathectomy to a particular organ. Although these drugs exert specific therapeutic effects at one organ, they exert side effects at other organs.

The untoward effects associated with the use of anticholinergics are manifestations of their pharmacological actions, and usually occur on excessive dosage. The effects include dryness of mouth, blurred vision, difficulty in urination, increased intraocular tension, tachycardia, and constipation. Most of these side effects are lessened when the quaternary anticholinergics are administered orally in the treatment of peptic ulcer because of lower absorption into the systemic circulation. In the case of tertiary amines the central side effects of euphoria, dizziness, and delirium may be observed because the drugs can cross the blood–brain barrier.

Many synthetic quaternary ammonium compounds may block acetylcholine at ganglia at high doses (see Chapter 42). Ganglionic blocking agents cause impotence as a side effect. High doses of methantheline may also cause impotence, an effect rarely produced by pure antimuscarinic drugs and indicating ganglionic blockade. Toxic doses of quaternary ammonium compounds (e.g., menthantheline, propantheline, and oxyphenonium) block acetylcholine at the somatic neuromuscular junction and paralyze respiration.

Adiphenine and amprotropine have local anesthetic activities, and anesthesia of the oral mucosa results when tablets of these drugs are chewed. It should be remembered that local anesthetic esters and amides exert their action by anticholinergic mechanisms, probably essentially at the nodes of Ranvier.

The central side effects have appeared among children even when cyclopentolate, tropicamide, and other anticholinergics are used as mydriatics. All anticholinergics increase intraocular pressure in most patients with simple glucoma.

Some of the cyclic groups in anticholinergics are pharmacophoric moieties for other types of activities. For example, the compounds containing a phenothiazine nucleus exhibit central depressing and antihistaminic side effects. These side effects are of advantage in the treatment of Parkinson's syndrome. The side effects of certain drugs which result from their anticholinergic activities are prominent among some analgesics (e.g., meperidine), antihistamines (e.g., promethazine), psychosedatives (e.g., benactizine), and psychotomimetics (e.g., dexoxodrol).

9 PROFILE OF ANTICHOLINERGIC ACTIVITIES OF VARIOUS AGENTS

The relative anticholinergic activities of the well-known therapeutic compounds are listed in Table 44.15. Although it is very difficult to justify collecting the results of a wide variety of experiments, it seems likely that the Table gives some idea of their relative antisecretory, antispasmodic, and mydriatic activities relative to atropine. Ratios less than unity indicate that they are more active than atropine.

Atropine itself is a very active substance in all three types of activities. (−)-Methscopolamine seems to be the most active of all compounds; it is about five times as active as atropine. None of the synthetic compounds are more active than (−)-methscopolamine, and very few of them are more active than atropine. The compounds with high antisecretory activities also exhibit high antispasmodic and mydriatic activities. Therefore, there is no dissociation between the three types of anticholinergic activities. Compounds with only one type of anticholinergic activity have yet to be synthesized. Only among very weak compounds is there any dissociation between the antispasmodic and the mydriatic activities (e.g., propivane). However, this difference may be related to the mode of administration. Mydriatic activities are measured after instillation into the eye, whereas antispasmodic and antisecretory activities are measured after parenteral administration to the animal or on *in vitro* preparations. To establish a claim that one compound has only one type of anticholinergic activity, two types of data should be available: (1) all types of activities should be measured in the same animal after the drug is administered by the same route; (2) the exact concentrations of the drugs at the sites of their action should be known. Such information is not available for most compounds in published literature.

For their antispasmodic and antisecretory activities in man, the drugs are administered orally. A comparison of their oral doses (micromoles) indicates that atropine is the most active compound. In clinical experience all three types of anticholinergic activities are exhibited by all compounds. The principal advantage of the available quaternary ammonium compounds lies in the fact that they are relatively free of any of the CNS effects that may be seen with atropine. This may permit the administration of sufficient quantities of the compounds to achieve a more fully effective peripheral anticholinergic action.

10 NONANTICHOLINERGICS AS ANTIULCER AGENTS

The interplay of various neuronal, hormonal, and other factors in gastric acid secretion are shown in Fig. 44.1. Pharmacological agents can be used to decrease gastric acid secretion by their action at different sites. So far, the principal medications other than anticholinergics and antacids to treat peptic ulcer are limited (69). Experimental and clinical investigations are in progress on a number of agents that can decrease the volume and acidity of gastric secretion through mechanisms other than blockade of the cholinergic nervous system (217–227). These include (1) histamine H2-receptor antagonists (Chapter 48; 221), (2) gastrin inhibitors (Chapter 27; 218), (3) pepsin inactivators (218), (4) mucus producers (69), (5) prostaglandin analogs (Chapter 33; 69), (6) enterogastone and its analogs (218, 222), and (7) noncholinergic antispasmodics (69, 217).

Recently, histamine H2 receptor antagonists have become popular for the treatment of peptic ulcer (Chapter 48,

Table 44.15   Relative Activities of Anticholinergics[a]

No.	Drug[b]	Equipotent Molar Ratios Relative to Atropine[c]			Total Dose per day in Man[f]		Ref.
		Antise-cretory[d]	Antispas-modic[e]	Mydria-tic	mg	μmol	

Solanaceous Alkaloids and Semisynthetic Substitutes

No.	Drug	Antisecretory	Antispasmodic	Mydriatic	mg	μmol	Ref.
1	Atropine sulfate	1.0	1.0	1.0	0.8–2.0	2.3–5.8	196
2	Methylatropine	0.48c 3.02r,a	0.47g	0.44m			162
3	(−)-Hyoscyamine	0.56c	0.31g	0.54m			162
4	(+.)-Hyoscyamine	11.0c	10.0g				162
5	(−)-Methylhyoscyamine	0.25c	—	0.20m			162
6	(−)-Scopolamine	0.73c	1.3g	0.20m			162
7	(−)-Methscopolamine	0.29c	0.17g	0.21m	5–10	13–25	162
8	(±)-Homatropine	0.44r,a 30d	8.5g	7.7c			199
9	(±)-Methylhomatropine	1.8rb	7.2rb	2.4m			200

Synthetic Anticholinergics: Esters, Quaternary

No.	Drug	Antisecretory	Antispasmodic	Mydriatic	mg	μmol	Ref.
10	Glycopyrrolate	0.9r,a	1.0g	1.0m	2–6	5–15	201
11	Lachesine	0.39c	0.96rb	0.96m			113
12	Mepenzolate	—	—	—	100	238	
13	Methantheline	0.37c	0.48g	3.0m	400	952	202
14	Methyleucatropine	1.6c	—	36m			113, 139
15	Oxyphenonium	1.0rb 1.0d,a	1.0g	1.0rb	40	93	203, 204
16	Penthionate	0.26rb	0.39rb		20–40	48–95	116
17	Pipenzolate		1.0g		20–25	46–58	205
18	Poldine methyl sulfate	1.0c	1.0g	1.0m	8–48	18–106	206
19	Propantheline	0.26c	0.40g	1.6m	75–240	167–536	202
20	Valethamate				30–80	78–207	

Esters, Tertiary

No.	Drug	Antisecretory	Antispasmodic	Mydriatic	mg	μmol	Ref.
21	Adiphenine		42rb		300–600	865–1729	150, 207
22	Amprotropine phosphate	20rb	55rb	20	200–400	494–988	162, 207
23	Benactyzine	5.6c	3.5rb	17m	3–9	8.3–24.8	113
24	Carbofluorene	100d	7.5rb		500	1449	150, 208
25	Cyclopentolate	—	—	—	See Table 44.14		
26	Dicyclomine	60r,a	8.0rb	8.8r	60–80	173–231	150
27	Eucatropine	29c		250m	See Table 44.14		113, 139
28	Oxyphencyclimine				20–50	53–132	
29	Piperidolate				200	557	
30	Propivane	40rb	29rb	5000c	400	1274	140, 207 208

Table 44.15 (*Continued*)

No.	Drug[b]	Equipotent Molar Ratios Relative to Atropine			Total Dose per day in Man[f]		Ref.
		Antise-cretory[d]	Antispas-modic[e]	Mydria-tic	mg	μmol	

Thioesters, Tertiary

No.	Drug[b]	Antise-cretory[d]	Antispas-modic[e]	Mydria-tic	mg	μmol	Ref.
31	Triphenamil		6.0rb		800	2204	37d,209

Carbamates, Quaternary

| 32 | Dibutoline sulfate | 10.8d,a | | 7.7h | 75–100 | | 210 |
| | | 43h,a | | | | 233–311 | |

Main Chain: Alkane, Quaternary

33	Hexocyclium methyl sulfate				100	234	
34	Isopropamide iodide		0.85rb		10	21	211
35	Mepiperphenidol	0.37c	0.48g		200–500	541–1351	212, 213
36	Tricyclamol chloride		1.2g	2.3m	200–300	593–890	163
37	Trihexethyl chloride	1.0r,a	2.17rb		75–200	212–567	214

Main Chain: Alkane, Tertiary

38	Aminopentamide		2.1rb		2	6.8	215
39	Benzhexol		3.7g	16m			163
40	Procyclidine		22g	31m	20	62	163
41	Methixene				3–6	8–16	196

Main Chain: Alkene, Quaternary

| 42 | Diphemanil methyl sulfate | 0.74 | 8.0g | | 400–600 | 1026–1538 | 216 |

[a] No comparative studies of all anticholinergics in the same animal species or on the same test system are available. The above data were assembled or cross-calculated from information reported in a number of sources; therefore the activities are relative and approximate. However, the information is useful to compare the available anticholinergic agents.

[b] All quaternary salts are bromides, and all tertiary amines are listed as hydrochlorides unless otherwise specified.

[c] The compounds were tested in different species. The following abbreviations are used to indicate the species: c, cat; d, dog; h, human; g, guinea pig; m, mouse; r, rat; rb, rabbit. Values less than unity indicate that they are more active than atropine.

[d] Antisecretory activities are on salivation unless otherwise indicated. "a" after the species indicates inhibition of acid secretion.

[e] All antispasmodic activities are inhibition of the contraction of intestine using cholinomimetic as spasmogen.

[f] The total dose includes the initial dose, as well as maintenance dose used orally (except dibutoline, which is administered subcutaneously) in man.

221). A single dose of cimitidine, an H2 receptor antagonist, has a maximum effect on nocturnal acid output in man, and no further effect is obtained by adding poldine, an anticholinergic agent, to cimitidine (221c). Cimitidine is also an effective drug in healing gastric and duodenal ulcers. Anticholinergic drugs and antacids help to control symptoms, but they do not accelerate healing.

Promethazine, an antihistaminic (Chapters 11 and 49) inhibits the release of gastrin in the dog and man (218). The definitive studies to clarify this intriguing pharmacological action have yet to be performed.

Pepsin inhibitors, sulfated amylopectin (Depepsin), and carrageenin decrease acid secretion in experimental animals and protect animals against histamine-induced ulcers (218). They have not been studied adequately to ascertain their therapeutic usefulness.

Carbenoxolone and cimetidine are complementary in their contribution to the healing of peptic ulcers, and the use of both may be better than either singly for some patients. Carbenoxolone accelerates healing by helping the defense mechanisms of the body. It stimulates extramucus secretion and prolongs cell life in the gastric epithelium. Cimetidine reduces gastric acid secretion. It would be interesting to know if anticholinergic drugs are more effective for the treatment of peptic ulcer in the presence of carbenoxolone.

Carbenoxolone (Biogastrone, Duogastrone) is the disodium salt of glycyrrhetinic acid hemisuccinate. It is prepared by hydrolysis of glycyrrhizic acid, a glycoside in licorice root. It increases the secretion of mucus and accelerates the healing of gastric ulcers. This drug is now under clinical investigation in the United States.

Pharmacological doses of several prostaglandins and their analogs inhibit gastric acid secretion. 15-(R)-Methyl-PGE$_2$, in small doses (100–200 μg, oral), reduces gastric acid secretion and output in man and animals, and it is currently being studied in the treatment of peptic ulcer.

Among the nonanticholinergic antispasmodics, alverine citrate (Spacolin) and isometheptene (octin) hydrochloride or mucate are available on the market. They relax smooth muscle by nonspecific actions. They exert little effect on gastric acid secretion. They are most useful in the symptomatic treatment of gastrointestinal disorders characterized by hypermotility and spasm.

ACKNOWLEDGMENTS

The author is supported by USPHS-NIH Research Grants HD-08561, HD-10607, HL-25358, AG-02077 and The Council for Tobacco Research, U.S.A., Inc.

REFERENCES

1. J. B. Kirsner, *Gastroenterology*, **49,** 79 (1965).
2. B. I. Hirschowitz, in *Functions of the Stomach and Intestine*, M. F. F. Friedman, Ed., University Park Press, Baltimore, Md., 1975, pp. 145–166.
3. K. J. Ivey, *Am. J. Med.*, **58,** 389 (1975).
4. K. J. Ivey, *Gastroenterology*, **68,** 154 (1975).
5. A. M. Ebeid and J. E. Fischer, *Surg. Clin. North Am.*, **56,** 1249 (1976).
6. D. C. H. Sun, H. Shay, and J. L. Ciminera, *J. Am. Med. Assoc.*, **158,** 713 (1955).
7. D. C. H. Sun, and H. Shay, *Arch. Intern. Med.*, **97,** 442 (1956).
8. J. E. Lennard-Jones, *Brit. Med. J.*, **5232,** 1071 (1961).
9. W. H. Bachrach, *Am. J. Dig. Dis.*, **3,** 743 (1958).
10. D. D. Bonnycastle, in *Evaluation of Drug Activities: Pharmacometrics*, Vol. 2, D. R. Laurence and A. L. Bacharach, Eds., Academic, New York, 1964, pp. 507–520.
11. E. G. Vernier, in *Evaluation of Drug Activities: Pharmacometrics*, Vol. 1, D. R. Laurence and A. L. Bacharach, Eds., Academic, New York, 1964, pp. 301–311.

12. H. Shay, S. A. Komarov, S. S. Fels, D. Meranze, M. Gruenstein, and H. Siplet, *Gastroenterology*, **5,** 43 (1945).

13. F. C. Mann and C. S. Williamson, *Ann. Surg.*, **77,** 409 (1923).

14. H. M. Hanson and D. A. Brodie, *J. Appl. Physiol.*, **15,** 291 (1960).

15. A. Robert and J. E. Nezamis, *Proc. Soc., Exp. Biol. med.*, **99,** 443 (1958).

16. T. A. Lynch, W. L. Highley, and A. G. Worton, *J. Pharm. Sci.*, **51,** 529 (1962).

17. O. J. T. Thije, in *Drug Induced Diseases*, L. Meyler and H. M. Peck, Eds. Excerpta Medica Foundation, Leyden, 1965, pp. 30–34.

18. J. Markowitz, J. Archibald, and H. G. Downie, *Experimental Surgery*, Williams and Wilkins, Baltimore, Md., 1959.

19. R. A. Gregory, *J. Physiol.*, **144,** 123 (1958).

20. R. S. Alphin and T. M. Lin, *Am. J. Physiol.*, **197,** 257 (1959).

21. T. M. Lin, R. S. Alphin, and K. K. Chen, *J. Pharmacol. Exp. Ther.*, **125,** 66 (1959).

22. S. A. Komarov, S. P. Bralow, and E. Boyd, *Proc. Soc. Exp. Biol. Med.*, **112,** 451 (1963).

23. G. Dotevall, G. Schroder, and A. Walon, *Acta Med. Scand.*, **177,** 169 (1965).

24. P. Pulewka, *Arch. Exp. Path. Pharmakol.*, **168,** 307 (1932).

25. D. G. Cogan, *Am. J. Opthalmol.*, **24,** 1431 (1941).

26. A. Ahmad and P. B. Marshall, *Brit. J. Pharmacol.*, **18,** 247 (1962).

27. H. Burn, *Drugs, Medicines and Man*, Scribner, New York, 1962, pp. 225–232.

28. O. Schmiedeberg and R. Koppe, *Das Muscarin Das Giftige Alkaloid des Fliegenpilzes*, Vogel, Leipzig, 1869, pp. 27–29.

29. R. Kobert and A. Sohrt, *Arch. Exp. Path. Pharmakol.*, **22,** 396 (1887).

30. Mein, *Annalen*, **6,** 67 (1833).

31. K. W. Bentley, *The Alkaloids*, Vol. 1, Wiley-Interscience, New York–London, 1957, pp. 10–24.

32. G. Fodór, J. Toth, I. Koczor, and I. Vincze, *Chem. Ind.*, **1955,** 1260.

33. E. Leete, in *Biogenesis of Natural Compounds*, P. Bernfeld, Ed., Pergamon Press, New York, 1963, pp. 745–746.

34. G. Fodór and G. Csepreghy, *Tetrahedron Lett.* **1959**: 7, 16.

35. R. S. Cahn, C. K. Ingold, and V. Prelog, *Experientia*, **12,** 81, 1956.

36. G. Fodór and G. Csepreghy, *J. Chem. Soc.* (London), **1961,** 3222.

37. S. G. Kuznetsov and S. N. Golikov, *Synthetic Atropine-like Substances* [in Russian], State Publishing House of Medical Literature, Leningrad, 1962; Engl. Transl. OTS: 63–22078, U.S. Government Printing Office, Washington, D.C., 1965, (a) p. 121. (b) p. 291. (c) p. 302. (d) p. 310. (e). p. 332.

38. G. Fodór, *Experientia*, **11,** 129 (1955).

39. W. Will, *Chem. Ber.*, **21,** 1717 (1888).

40. R. Robinson, *J. Chem. Soc.* (London), **111,** 762 (1917).

41. E. Müller, *Chem. Ber.*, **51,** 252 (1918).

42. W. Wislicenus and E. A. Bilhüber, *Chem. Ber.*, **51,** 1237 (1918).

43. A. McKenzie and J. K. Wood, *J. Chem. Soc.* (London), **115,** 828 (1919).

44. R. Wolffenstein and L. Mamlock, *Chem. Ber.*, **41,** 723 (1908).

45. G. Fodór, J. Tóth, I. Koczor, and I. Vincze, *Chem. Ind.*, **1956,** 764.

46. G. Fodór, J. Tóth, A. Romeike, I. Vincze, P. Dobó and G. Janzsó, *Angew. Chem.*, **69,** 678 (1957).

47. I. R. Innes and M. Nickerson, in *The Pharmacological Basis of Therapeutics*, L. S. Goodman and A. Gilman, Eds., A. G. Gilman and G. B. Koelle, Assoc. Eds., Macmillan, New York, 1975, pp. 514–532.

48. R. M. Levine, M. R. Blair, and B. B. Clark, *J. Pharmacol. Exp. Ther.*, **114,** 78 (1955).

49. R. M. Levine and B. B. Clark, *J. Pharmacol. Exp. Ther.*, **121,** 63 (1957).

50. R. M. Levine and E. M. Pelikan, *J. Pharmacol. Exp. Ther.*, **131,** 319 (1961).

51. T. H. Wilson, *Intestinal Absorption*, Saunders, Philadelphia, 1962, pp. 241–254.

52. R. E. Gosselin, J. D. Gabourel, S. C. Kalser, and J. H. Wills, *J. Pharmacol. Exp. Ther.*, **115,** 217 (1955).

53. S. C. Kalser, J. H. Wills, J. D. Gabourel, R. E. Gosselin, and C. F. Epes, *J. Pharmacol. Exp. Ther.*, **121,** 449 (1957).

54. J. D. Gabourel and R. E. Gosselin, *Arch. Int. Pharmacodyn.*, **115,** 416 (1958).

55. R. E. Gosselin, J. D. Gabourel, and J. H. Wills, *Clin. Pharmacol. Ther.*, **1,** 597 (1960).

56. W. Kalow, *Pharmacogenetics*, Saunders Philadelphia, 1956, pp. 54–56.

57. G. Werner and R. Wurker, *Naturwissenschaften*, **22,** 627 (1959).

58. V. Evertsbusch and E. M. K. Geiling, *Arch. Int. Pharmacodyn.*, **105,** 175 (1956).

59. H. L. Schmidt and G. Werner, *Proc. Meet. Coll. Int. Neuro-Psychopharmacol., 3rd Munich*, 1962, 427–432 (1964); through *Chem. Abstr.*, **65**, 7818 (1966).

60. K. Matsuda, *Niigata Igakkai Zasshi*, **80**: (2), 53, (1966); through *Chem. Abstr.*, **65**, 1265 (1966).

61. G. Werner, P. C. Bosque, and J. C. Quevedo, *Abh. Deut. Akad. Wiss Berlin*, *K1. Chem., Geol. Biol.*, **1966**: 3, 541–544, 629–636; through *Chem. Abstr.* **66**, 7885 (1967).

62. G. Werner, *Planta Med.*, **9**, 293 (1961); through *Chem. Abstr.*, **57**, 6543 (1962).

63. R. Truhaut and J. Yonger, *C. R. Acad. Sci., Paris, Ser. D*, **264**: 21, 2526 (1967); through *Chem. Abstr.*, **67**, 4904 (1967).

64. W. F. Von Oettingen, *The Therapeutic Agents of the Pyrrole and Pyridine Group*, Edwards, Ann Arbor, 1936, p. 130.

65. B. B. Brodie and C. A. M. Hogben, *J. Pharm. Pharmacol.*, **9**, 345 (1957).

66. L. S. Schanker, *J. Med. Pharm. Chem.*, **2**, 343 (1960).

67. H. Collumbine, in *Drills' Pharmacology in Medicine*, J. R. Dipalma, Ed., McGraw-Hill, New York, 1971, pp. 608–626.

68. H. Collumbine, in *Physiological Pharmacology*, Vol. III, W. S. Root and F. G. Hofman, Eds., Academic, New York-London, 1967, pp. 323–362.

69. American Medical Association—Department of Drugs, *AMA Drug Evaluations*, Publishing Sciences Group, Inc., Acton, Mass. 1977.

70. Swiss Pat. 190, 541 (1937); through *Chem. Abstr.*, **32**, 589 (1938).

71. Ger. Pat. 653,778 (1937); through *Chem. Abstr.*, **32**, 2956 (1938).

72. H. Horenstein and H. Pählicke, *Chem. Ber.*, **71**, 1644 (1938).

73. A. Blankart, (to Hoffman-LaRoche Inc.) U.S. Pat., 1,987,546 (1935); *Chem. Abstr.*, **29**, 1432 (1935).

74. R. R. Burtner and J. W. Cusic, *J. Am. Chem. Soc.*, **65**, 1582 (1943).

75. G. R. Treves and F. C. Testa, *J. Am. Chem. Soc.*, **74**, 46 (1952).

76. C. H. Tilford, M. G. Van Campen, Jr., and R. S. Shelton, *J. Am. Chem. Soc.*, **69**, 2902 (1947).

77. C. Harries, *Ann. Chem.*, **296**, 341 (1897).

78. C. Harries, *Chem. Ber.*, **31**, 665 (1898).

79. J. A. Faust, A. Mori, and M. Sahyun, *J. Am. Chem. Soc.*, **81**, 2214 (1959).

80. J. H. Biel, H. L. Friedman, H. A. Leiser, and E. P. Sprengeler, *J. Am. Chem. Soc.*, **74**, 1485 (1952).

81. A. H. Ford-Moore and H. R. Ing, *J. Chem. Soc.* (London), **1947,** 55.

82. B. V. Franko and C. D. Lumford, *J. Med. Pharm. Chem.*, **2**, 523 (1960).

83. J. H. Biel, E. P. Sprengeler, H. A. Leiser, J. Horner, A. Drukker, and H. L. Friedman, *J. Am. Chem. Soc.*, **77**, 2250 (1955).

84. J. P. Long and H. K. Keasling, *J. Am. Pharm. Assoc. Sci. Ed.*, **43**, 616 (1954).

85. Ciba, Swiss Pat. 259,958 (1949); through *Chem. Abstr.*, **44**, 5910 (1950).

86. F. F. Blick and M. U. Tsao, *J. Am. Chem. Soc.*, **66**, 1645 (1944).

87. F. F. Blicke, (to Regents, Univ. of Michigan) U.S. Pat. 2,541,634 (1951); through *Chem. Abstr.*, **46**, 538 (1952).

88. F. P. Doyle, M. D. Mehta, G. S. Sach, and J. L. Pearson, *J. Chem. Soc.* (London) **1958**, 4458.

89. D. Krause and D. Schmidtke-Ruhnau, *Arzneim-Forsch.*, **5**, 599 (1955).

90. D. Krause and S. Schmidtke-Ruhnau, *Arch. Exp. Path. Pharmakol.*, **229**, 258 (1956).

91. H. G. Kolloff, J. H. Hunter, E. H. Woodruff, and R. B. J. Moffett, *J. Am. Chem. Soc.*, **71**, 3988 (1949).

92. F. Leonard and L. J. Simet, *J. Am. Chem. Soc.*, **77**, 2855 (1955).

93. E. H. Woodrugg (to Upjohn Co.) U.S. Pat. 2,488,253 (1949); through *Chem. Abstr.*, **44**, 1534, (1950).

94. R. O. Clinton and V. J. Salvador, *J. Am. Chem. Soc.*, **68**, 2076 (1946).

95. Roche Products, Brit. Pat. 728,579 (1955); through *Chem. Abstr.*, **50**, 5773 (1956).

96. K. C. Swan and N. G. White, U.S. Pat. 2,408,893; through *Chem. Abstr.*, **41**, 775 (1947).

97. K. C. Swan and N. G. White, U.S. Pat. 2,432,049 (1947); through *Chem. Abstr.*, **42**, 1962 (1948).

98. A. W. Weston (to Abbott Laboratories) U.S. Pat. 2,907,765 (1959); through *Chem. Abstr.*, **54**, 7746 (1960).

99. E. M. Schultz (to Merck & Co.) U.S. Pat. 2,665,278 (1954); through *Chem. Abstr.*, **49**, 5525 (1955).

100. D. W. Adamson (to Burroughs Wellcome Inc.) U.S. Pat. 2,891,890 (1959); through *Chem. Abstr.*, **54**, 1546 (1960).

101. E. M. Bottorff (to Eli Lilly & Co.) U.S. Pat., 2,826,590 (1958); through *Chem. Abstr.*, **52**, 11124 (1958).

102. D. W. Adamson, P. A. Barrett, and S. Wilkinson, *J. Chem. Soc.* (London), **1951,** 52.

103. J. J. Denton and V. A. Lawson, *J. Am. Chem. Soc.*, **72,** 3279 (1950).

104. D. W. Adamson (to Burroughs Wellcome Inc.) U.S. Pat., 2,698,325 (1954); through *Chem. Abstr.*, **50,** 1919 (1956).

105. P. Janssen, D. Zivkovic, P. Demoen, D. K. De Jongh, and E. G. van Proosdij-Hartzema, *Arch. Int. Pharmacodyn.*, **103,** 82 (1955).

106. L. C. Cheney, W. B. Wheatley, M. E. Speeter, W. M. Byrd, W. E. Fitzgibbon, W. F. Minor, and S. B. Binkley, *J. Org. Chem.*, **17,** 770 (1952).

107. M. E. Speeter (to Bristol Laboratories) U.S. Pat., 2,647,926 (1953); through *Chem. Abstr.*, **48,** 9405 (1954)

108. W. B. Wheatley, W. F. Minor, W. M. Byrd, W. E. Fitzgibbon, Jr., M. E. Speeter, L. C. Cheney, and S. B. Brinkley, *J. Org. Chem.*, **19,** 794 (1954).

109. R. B. Moffett and B. D. Aspergren, *J. Am. Chem. Soc.*, **79,** 4451 (1957).

110. J. Schmutz (to Dr. A. Wander, A.-G.), Swiss Pat. 358,081 (1961); through *Chem. Abstr.*, **57,** 13731 (1962).

111. N. Sperber, F. J. Villani, M. Sherlock, and D. Papa, *J. Am. Chem. Soc.*, **73,** 5010 (1951).

112. C. C. Pfeiffer, *Science*, **107,** 94 (1948).

113. H. R. Ing, G. S. Dawes, and J. J. Wajda, *J. Pharmacol. Exp. Ther.*, **85,** 85 (1945).

114. H. R. Ing, *Science*, **109,** 264 (1949).

115. A. M. Lands, *J. Pharmacol. Exp. Ther.*, **102,** 219 (1951).

116. F. P. Luduena and A. M. Lands, *J. Pharmacol. Exp. Ther.*, **110,** 282 (1954).

117. J. P. Long, F. P. Luduena, B. F. Tuller, and A. M. Lands, *J. Pharmacol. Exp. Ther.*, **117,** 29 (1956).

118. F. W. Schueler, *Arch. Int. Pharmacodyn.*, **93,** 417 (1953).

119. R. B. Moffett and B. D. Aspergren, *J. Am. Chem. Soc.*, **78,** 3448 (1956).

120. J. P. Long and A. M. Lands, *J. Pharmacol. Exp. Ther.*, **120,** 46 (1957).

121. P. Holton and H. R. Ing., *Brit. J. Pharmacol.*, **4,** 190 (1949).

122. R. Meier and K. Hoffman, *Helv. Med. Acta* **7:** Suppl. 6, 106 (1941).

123. A. M. Lands, V. L. Nash, and K. Z. Hooper, *J. Pharmacol. Exp. Ther.*, **86,** 129 (1946).

124. R. R. Burtner and J. W. Cusic, *J. Am. Chem. Soc.*, **65,** 262 (1943).

125. D. K. de Jongh, E. G. van Proosdij-Hartzema, and P. Janssen., *Arch. Int. Pharmacodyn.*, **103,** 120 (1955).

126. M. H. Ehrenberg, J. A. Ramp, E. W. Blanchard, and G. R. Treves, *J. Pharmacol. Exp. Ther.*, **106,** 141 (1952).

127. A. M. Lands and C. J. Cavalitto, *J. Pharmacol. Exp. Ther.*, **110,** 369 (1954).

128. A. M. Lands and F. P. Luduena, *J. Pharmacol. Exp. Ther.*, **116,** 177 (1956).

129. J. G. Cannon and J. P. Long, in *Drugs Affecting the Peripheral Nervous System* A. Burger, Ed., Dekker, New York, 1967, p. 133.

130. J. W. Cusic and R. A. Robinson, *J. Org. Chem.*, **16,** 1921 (1951).

131. R. F. Feldkamp and J. A. Faust, *J. Am. Chem. Soc.*, **71,** 4012 (1949).

132. J. Krapcho, C. F. Turk, and E. J. Pribil, *J. Am. Chem. Soc.*, **77,** 3632 (1955).

133. L. Gyorgy, M. Doda, and K. Nador, *Acta Physiol. Hung.*, **17,** 473 (1960); through *Chem. Abstr.*, **55,** 13672 (1961).

134. K. Nador, L. Gyorgy, and M. Doda, *J. Med. Pharm. Chem.*, **3,** 183 (1961).

135. R. Foster, P. J. Goodford, and H. R. Ing, *J. Chem. Soc.* (London), **1957,** 3575.

136. L. H. Strenbach and F. Kaiser, *J. Am. Chem. Soc.*, **75,** 6068 (1953).

137. E. Nyman, *Acta Med. Scand.*, **118,** 466 (1944).

138. P. B. Marshall, *Brit. J. Pharmacol.*, **10,** 354 (1955).

139. E. Büllbring and G. S. Dawes, *J. Pharmacol. Exp. Ther.*, **84,** 177 (1945).

140. G. Lehmann and P. K. Knoeffel, *J. Pharmacol. Exp. Ther.*, **80,** 335 (1944).

141. W. E. Hambouger, D. L. Cook, M. M. Winbury, and H. B. Freese, *J. Pharmacol. Exp. Ther.*, **99,** 245 (1950).

142. Montuschi, J. Phillips, F. Prescott, and A. F. Green, *Lancet*, **1,** 583 (1952).

143. H. M. Lee, W. Gibson, W. G. Dinwiddle, and J. Mills, *J. Am. Pharm. Assoc. Sci. Ed.*, **43,** 408 (1954).

144. R. W. Cunningham, B. K. Harned, M. C. Clark, R. R. Cosgrove, N. S. Daughterty, C. H. Hine, R. E. Vessey, and N. N. Yuda, *J. Pharmacol. Exp. Ther.*, **96,** 151 (1949).

145. A. B. Funke and R. F. Rekker, *Arzneim.-Forsch.*, **9,** 539 (1959).

146. L. A. Mounter and V. P. Whittaker, *Biochem. J.*, **47,** 525 (1950).

147. A. M. Lands, J. O. Hoppe, J. R. Lewis, and E. Ananenko, *J. Pharmacol. Exp. ther.*, **100,** 19 (1950).

148. J. D. P. Graham and S. Lazarus, *J. Pharmacol. Exp. Ther.* **69,** 331 (1940).

149. J. D. P. Graham and S. Lazarus, *J. Pharmacol. Exp. Ther.*, **70,** 165 (1940).

150. B. B. Brown, C. R. Thompson, G. R. Klahm, and H. W. Werner, *J. Am. Pharm. Assoc. Sci. Ed.*, **39,** 305 (1950).

151. A. M. Lands and F. P. Luduena, *J. Pharmacol. Exp. Ther.*, **117,** 331 (1956).

152. F. F. Blicke and C. E. Maxwell, *J. Am. Chem. Soc.*, **64,** 428 (1942).

153. A. A. Goldberg and A. H. Wragg, *J. Chem. Soc.* (London), **1957,** 4823.

154. F. Jellinek, *Acta Crystallogr.*, **10,** 277 (1957).

155. H. G. Kolloff, J. H. Hunter, and R. B. Moffett, *J. Am. Chem. Soc.*, **72,** 1650 (1950).

156. A. W. Ruddy and J. S. Buckley, *J. Am. Chem. Soc.* **72,** 718 (1950).

157. J. J. Denton, V. A. Lawson, W. B. Neier, and R. J. Turner, *J. Am. Chem. Soc.*, **71,** 2050 (1949).

158. K. Fromherz, *Arch. Exp. Path. Pharmakol.*, **173,** 86 (1933).

159. F. F. Blicke and C. E. Maxwell, *J. Am. Chem. Soc.*, **64,** 431 (1942).

160. R. B. Barlow, K. A. Scott, and R. P. Stephenson, *Brit. J. Pharmacol.*, **21,** 509 (1963).

161. B. V. R. Sastry, C. C. Pfeiffer, and A. Lasslo, *J. Pharmacol. Exp. Ther.*, **130,** 346 (1960).

162. R. B. Barlow, *Introduction to Chemical Pharmacology*, Wiley, New York, 1964, p. 211.

163. W. M. Duffin and A. F. Green, *Brit. J. Pharmacol.*, **10,** 383 (1955).

164. Y. Kasuya, *Chem. Pharm. Bull* (Japan), **6**:, 147 (1958); through *Chem. Abstr.*, **53,** 4553 (1959).

165. Y. Kasuya, *J. Pharm. Soc.* (Japan) **78,** 509 (1958); through *Chem. Abstr.*, **52,** 17196 (1958).

166. L. O. Randall, W. M. Benson, and P. L. Stefko, *J. Pharmacol. Exp. Ther.*, **104,** 284 (1952).

167. C. Liebermann and L. Limpach, *Chem. Ber.*, **25,** 927 (1892).

168. L. Gyermek, *Nature*, **171,** 788 (1953).

169. B. V. R. Sastry and J. V. Auditore, *Proc. First Int. Pharmacol. Congr.*, **7,** 323 (1963).

170. C. C. Pfeiffer, *Int. Rev. Neurobiol.*, **1,** 195 (1959).

171. B. V. R. Sastry, *Am. Rev. Pharmacol.*, **13,** 253 (1973).

172. R. F. Furchgott, Advan. Drug Res., **3,** 21 (1966).

173. B. V. R. Sastry and H. C. Cheng, *J. Pharmacol. Exp. Ther.*, **180,** 326 (1972).

174. B. V. R. Sastry and H. C. Cheng, *Toxicol. Appl. Pharmacol.*, **19,** 367 (1971).

175. H. C. Cheng and B. V. R. Sastry, *Arch. Int. Pharmacodyn. Ther.*, **223,** 246 (1976).

176. B. V. R. Sastry and H. C. Cheng, *J. Pharmacol. Exp. Ther.*, **201,** 105 (1977).

177. P. B. Marshall, *Brit. J. Pharmacol.*, **10,** 270 (1955).

178. R. F. Furchgott and P. Bursztyn, *Ann. N.Y. Acad. Sci.*, **144,** 882 (1967).

179. J. M. van Rossum and J. A. Th.M. Hurkmans, *Acta Physiol. Pharmacol. Neerl.*, **11,** 173 (1962).

180. E. J. Ariens and A. M. Simonis, *Acta Physiol. Pharmacol. Neerl.*, **11,** 151 (1962).

181. R. Schneider and A. R. Timms, *Brit. J. Pharmacol.*, **12,** 30 (1957).

182. A. Teitel, *Nature*, **190,** 814 (1961).

183. A. Ashford, G. B. Penn, and J. W. Ross, *Nature*, **193,** 1082 (1962).

184. A. Bebbington and R. W. Brimblecombe, *Advan. Drug. Res.*, **2,** 143 (1965).

185. D. J. Triggle, *Chemical Aspects of the Autonomic Nervous System*, Academic, New York, 1965, pp. 108–159.

186. E. J. Ariens, A. M. Simonis, and J. M. Van Rossum, in *Molecular Pharmacology*, Vol. I, E. J. Ariens, Ed., Academic, New York-London, 1964, pp. 156–169.

187. W. D. M. Paton and H. P. Rang, *Proc. Roy. Soc.*, **163B,** 488 (1966).

188. H. P. Rang, *Ann N.Y. Acad. Sci.*, **144,** 756 (1967).

189. C. D. Thron, *J. Pharmacol. Exp. Ther.*, **181,** 529, (1972).

190. R. W. Brimblecombe, *Drug Actions on Cholinergic Systems*, University Park Press, Baltimore, Md., 1974, pp. 19–42.

191. L. B. Kier, *Mol. Pharmacol.* **3,** 487 (1967).

192. C. Y. Chiou and B. V. R. Sastry, *Arch. Int. Pharmacodyn. Ther.*, **181,** 94 (1969).

193. C. Y. Chiou and B. V. R. Sastry, *J. Pharmacol. Exp. Ther.*, **172,** 351 (1970).

194. B. Csillik, *Functional Structure of the Post-Synaptic Membrane in the Myoneural Junction*, Publishing House of the Hungarian Academy of Sciences, Budapest, 1965, pp. 95–112.

195. R. G. Janes and J. F. Stiles, *Arch. Opthalmol.*, **62,** 69 (1959).

196. AMA Council on Drugs, *New Drugs*, American Medical Association, Chicago, Ill. 1967, p. 441.

197. W. H. Havener, *Ocular Pharmacology*, C. V. Mosby, St. Louis, Mo., 1966, pp. 177–267.

198. H. L. Williams, *Mod. Hosp.*, **78**: 2, 102 (1952).

199. A. R. Cushny, *J. Pharmacol. Exp. Ther.*, **15,** 105 (1920).

200. R. L. Cahen and K. Tvede, *J. Exp. Pharmacol. Ther.*, **105,** 166 (1952).

201. B. V. Franko, R. S. Alphin, J. W. Ward, and C. D. Lunsford, *Ann. N.Y. Acad. Sci.*, **99,** 131 (1962).

202. E. A. Johnson and D. R. Wood, *Brit. J. Pharmacol.*, **9**, 218 (1954).

203. A. J. Plummer, W. E. Barrett, R. Rutledge, and F. F. Yonkman, *J. Pharmacol. Exp. Ther.*, **108**, 292 (1953).

204. D. M. Brown and R. M. Quinton, *Brit. J. Pharmacol.*, **12**, 53 (1957).

205. J. Y. P. Chen and H. Beckman, *J. Pharmacol. Exp. Ther.*, **104**, 269 (1952).

206. P. Acred, E. M. Atkins, J. G. Bainbridge, D. M. Brown, R. M. Quinton, and D. Turner, *Brit. J. Pharmacol.*, **12**, 447 (1957).

207. G. Lehmann and P. K. Knoefel, *J. Pharmacol. Exp. Ther.*, **74**, 217, 274 (1942).

208. B. N. Halpern, *Arch. Int. Pharmacodyn.*, **59**, 149 (1938).

209. H. Ramsey and A. G. Richardson, *J. Pharmacol. Exp. Ther.*, **89**, 131 (1947).

210. K. C. Swan and N. G. White, *Arch. Opthalmol.*, **33**, 16 (1945).

211. A. Jageneau and P. Janssen, *Arch. Int. Pharmacodyn.*, **106**, 199 (1956).

212. S. C. McManus, J. M. Bochey, and K. H. Beyer, *J. Pharmacol. Exp. Ther.*, **108**, 364 (1953).

213. J. D. McCarthy, S. O. Evans, H. Ragins, and L. R. Dragstedt, *J. Pharmacol. Exp. Ther.*, **108**, 246 (1953).

214. A. C. Osterberg and W. D. Gray, *Arch. Int. Pharmacodyn.*, **137**, 250 (1962).

215. J. B. Hoekstra and H. L. Dickison, *J. Pharmacol. Exp. Ther.*, **98**, 14 (1950).

216. S. Margolin, M. Doyle, J. Giblin, A. Markovsky, M. T. Spoerlein, I. Stephens, H. Berchtold, G. Belloff, and R. Tislow, *Proc. Soc. Exp. Biol. Med.*, **78**, 576 (1951).

217. D. E. Butler, R. A. Purdon, and P. Bass, *Am. J. Dig. Dis.*, **15**, 157 (1970).

218. P. Bass, *Advan. Drug. Res.*, **8**, 205 (1974).

219. R. F. Barreras, *Surg. Clin. North. Am.*, **56**, 1243 (1976).

220. R. R. Dozois and K. A. Kelley, *Surg. Clin. North. Am.*, **56**, 1267 (1956).

221. W. L. Burland and M. A. Simkins, Eds., *Cimetidine: Proceedings of the Sec. Int. Symp.* on Histamine H2-Receptor Antagonists, Excerpta Medica, Amsterdam and Oxford, 1977, (a) G. J. Durant, J. C. Emmett, and C. R. Ganellin, pp. 1–12. (b) G. O. Barbezat and S. Bank, pp. 110–121. (c) R. E. Pounder, J. G. Williams, R. H. Hunt, S. H. Vincent, G. J. Milton-Thompson, and J. J. Misiewicz, pp. 189–204. (d) E. Aadland, A. Berstad, and L. S. Semb, pp. 87–97. (e) W. S. Blackwood and T. C. Northfield, pp. 124–130.

222. I. E. Gillespie, *Disease-a-Month*, **1971**: August, 1–41.

CHAPTER FORTY-FIVE

Antiparkinsonism Drugs

VERNON G. VERNIER

Pharmaceuticals Division
E. I. du Pont de Nemours & Co., Inc.
Newark, Delaware 19711, USA

CONTENTS

1   INTRODUCTION

Which accepted drugs control the tremor, rigidity, and akinesia of Parkinson's disease and drug-induced extrapyramidal reactions to major tranquilizer treatment? How can such drugs be found? What is their mechanism of action? What new agents have shown efficacy in patients? What new chemical entities have shown promising activity in laboratory experiments? What consequently are the most fruitful directions for medicinal chemistry effort? We consider these questions in the light of the considerable neurochemical and clinical progress that has been made in the last 20 years.

This chapter brings up to date the previous edition of this series (1) and the review by Vernier (2).

2 THE DISEASE

Parkinson's disease is a clinical neurological entity with a classical symptom triad of tremor, rigidity, and akinesia. Patients often display other symptoms including autonomic disturbances, posture and gait abnormalities, and cognitive, perceptual, and memory deficits. The cause of the syndrome described by James Parkinson in 1817 is not known. The generic term parkinsonism is applied to several forms of the symptom complex, and is called idiopathic when the original description fits. The postencephalitic type (von Economo) follows influenza A encephalitis (encephalitis lethargica). Drug-induced parkinsonism often accompanies major tranquilizer administration (presumably due to dopamine receptor blockade in the basal ganglia).

Idiopathic parkinsonism is a slowly progressive degenerative disease leading to total disability and death with an onset in older adults usually over 50 years of age. The biochemical basis is a deficiency of dopamine in the basal ganglia due to loss of pigmented cells in the substantia nigra of the midbrain. These cells synthesize dopamine, which is essential to extrapyramidal motor control of primitive coordinated movements. Dopamine is carried by axonal transport from the A8 and A9 neurons in the substantia nigra in the rat brain to the striatum (caudate nucleus, putamen, and globus pallidum) shown in Fig. 45.1 from Moore and Kelly (3). It is an inhibitory neurotransmitter (4) which is liberated from nerve endings in the striatum by neural impulses and maintains balance with acetylcholine, the excitatory transmitter.

The biochemical relationships of dopamine to its precursors and norepinephrine, another neurohumoral transmitter derived from it, are outlined in Fig. 45.2. The enzymes involved are also indicated. Other important metabolic transformations, mainly O-methylation (by catechol O-methyltransferase) and amine oxidation (by

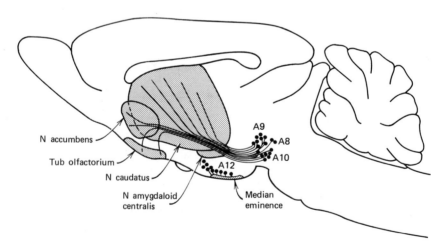

Fig. 45.1 Sagittal projections of nigrostriatal, mesolimbic, and tuberoinfundibular pathways in rat brain. Cells A8 and A9 in the substantia nigra synthesize dopamine, which is axonally transported forward to caudate nucleus and the rest of the striatum. (Reproduced with permission from K. E. Moore and P. H. Kelly, "Biochemical Pharmacology of Mesolimbic and Mesocortical Dopaminergic Neurons," in *Psychopharmacology: A Generation of Progress*, M. A. Lipton, A. DiMascio, and K. F. Killam, Eds., Raven Press, New York, 1978, p. 221.)

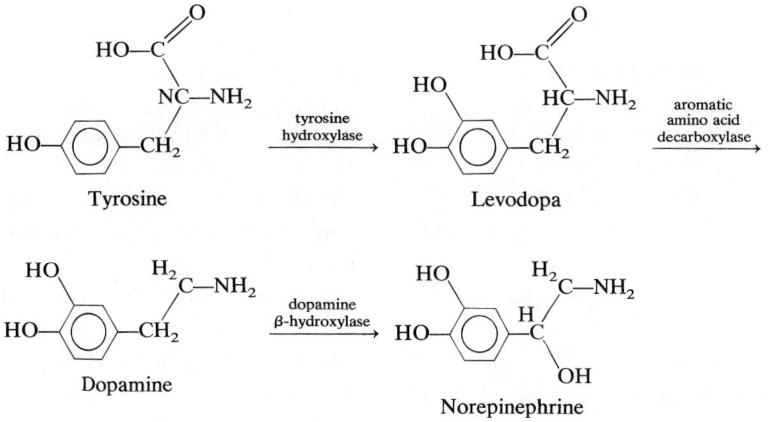

Fig. 45.2 Neurohumoral transmitter chemical pathways.

monoamine oxidase), have not been included in the interest of simplicity, but can be found in standard texts.

Parkinson's disease is one of the leading causes of neurological disability in persons over 60 years of age; it occurs throughout the world with similar incidence in both sexes. There are about an estimated 200,000–400,000 cases in the United States with about 40,000 new cases annually (5).

The discovery that Parkinson's disease patients suffer a marked deficiency of dopamine in the basal ganglia has led to an understanding of how the important newer drugs act. They can be placed into three groups: dopamine replacements, dopamine releasers, and dopamine receptor stimulants. Within this highly simplified framework, the therapeutic and other actions of the newer and older drugs to be discussed can be understood. These drugs also have other actions that complicate classification, and the mechanism of action in man can usually be inferred only from indirect evidence.

3 TEST METHODS

The antagonism of oxotremorine-induced tremor (45.**1**) in mice (6, 7) is a convenient predictor of central anticholinergic efficacy,

but should be coupled with other tests of skeletal muscular function to rule out sedative and other actions. However, research emphasis has now overwhelmingly shifted to tests that measure dopaminergic activity of the extrapyramidal nervous system. Stereotyped behavior in rodents (8) is an indicator of dopaminergic receptor stimulation. Drug-induced rotatory behavior or restoration of function following electrolytic, suction, or chemical lesions (6-hydroxy-dopamine, etc.) (9) and alteration of function caused by electrical stimulation (10) are now being extensively employed. Antagonism of the catalepsy caused by major tranquilizer-induced dopamine blockade is convenient and useful (11, 12). Additionally the operant behavioral changes induced by major tranquilizers may be antagonized by some dopaminergic agents (13, 14). Biochemical measurements of local changes in dopamine and other neurotransmitters and changes in their release, turnover, and metabolism (homovanillic acid, for example) may yield clues to the action of newer compounds (15).

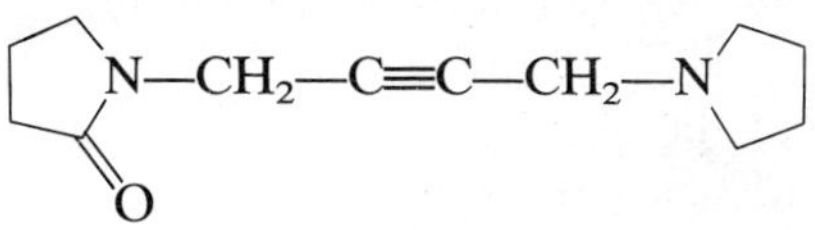

45.**1**

4 CLASSIFICATION AND STRUCTURES OF DRUGS TESTED FOR ANTIPARKINSONISM EFFECT

Antiparkinsonism drugs, accepted or prospective, can be classified into groups by mechanism of action as shown in Table 45.1

5 STATUS OF ANTIPARKINSONISM DRUGS

5.1 Dopamine Replacements

Levodopa has revolutionized the treatment of Parkinson's disease because it possesses greater intrinsic activity than any of the previous therapeutic agents that have been employed (2). It reaches to the heart of the biochemical defect in these patients. Levodopa is absorbed from the gastrointestinal tract, crosses the blood–brain barrier, and is converted in the brain to dopamine to replenish the supply of missing neurohumoral transmitter in the basal ganglia. Although it is able to reverse the major symptoms of parkinsonism, levodopa causes both peripheral side effects (nausea, emesis, cardiac arrhythmias, and hypotension) and serious central nervous side effects (abnormal involuntary movements, psychotic episodes, and "on–off" phenomena). The "on–off" effect seen during levodopa therapy is a sudden, brief (few minutes to 2 hr) loss of therapeutic effect occurring unpredictably, usually after 1–2 years of drug treatment (16). The peripheral signs can be markedly reduced by coadministration of carbidopa, a decarboxylase inhibitor that does not penetrate into the brain and that also reduces by five times the required dose of levodopa, minimizing the cost of treatment to the patient (2). Benserazide yields similar advantages (2). These two agents selectively reduce the activity of the enzyme aromatic amino acid decarboxylase shown in Fig. 45.2. This blocks the peripheral conversion

of levodopa to dopamine, which is responsible for most of the gastrointestinal and cardiovascular side effects. However, the central side effects of levodopa, abnormal involuntary movements, and psychiatric difficulties persist, whereas the "on–off" phenomenon is diminished by administration of decarboxylase inhibitors and other agents (17).

Many structural modifications of levodopa have been made, tested, and found inactive (18). Other amino acids have been administered and D-phenylalanine has been reported active (19). L-Metatyrosine has been suggested for study since it is a precursor of levodopa (20). Although early trials met with mixed success (21), it is essentially ineffective, possibly due to deficiency of the enzyme tyrosine hydroxylase.

Levodopa chelated with copper or zinc showed twice the brain levodopa concentration of unchelated drug following intraperitoneal dosing in rats (22).

Most approaches to Parkinson's disease therapy now test the ability of other agents to improve the maximal effects of levodopa, the most effective agent, lower its dose and decrease the incidence of its side effects, and minimize the "on–off" phenomenon.

5.2 Dopamine Releasers

Amantadine, an organic cage amine that is useful in preventing and treating influenza A, is more effective and less toxic than the classical anticholinergics in rapidly diminishing the symptoms of Parkinson's disease (2, 23). The amantadine mechanism of action is not entirely clear but evidence points to release of dopamine from basal ganglia neurons with some possibility of direct receptor activation (24, 25).

Amantadine glucuronide (gludantane) has been reported effective in 33 parkinsonism patients at a daily dose of 600 mg,

Table 45.1   Antiparkinsonism Drugs Classified by Major Type of Action

Nonproprietary Name or Code	Structure

Dopamine Replacements

Levodopa

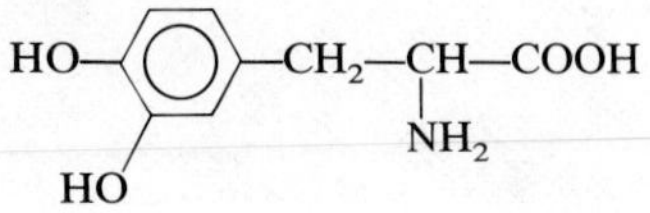

Carbidopa

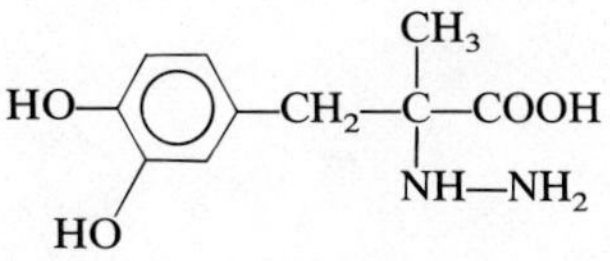

Benserazide

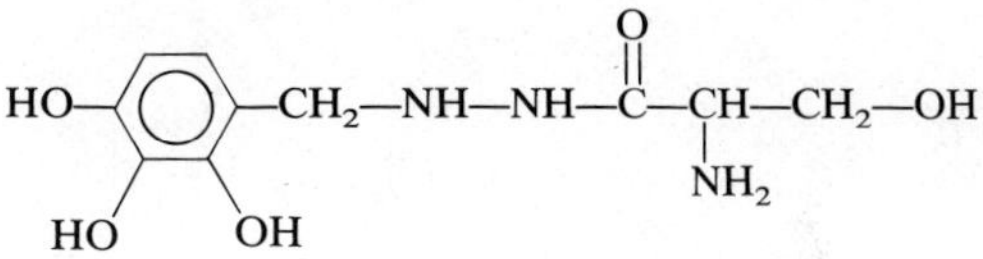

Phenylalanine

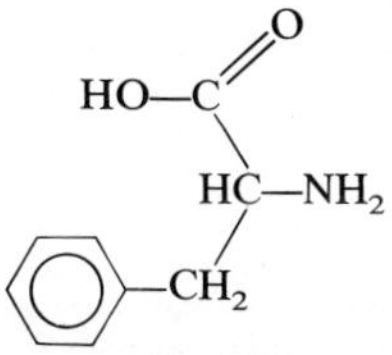

Metatyrosine

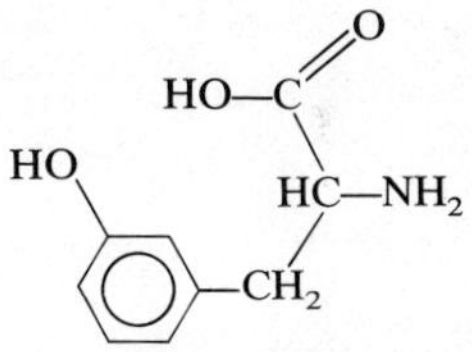

Levodopa metal chelates

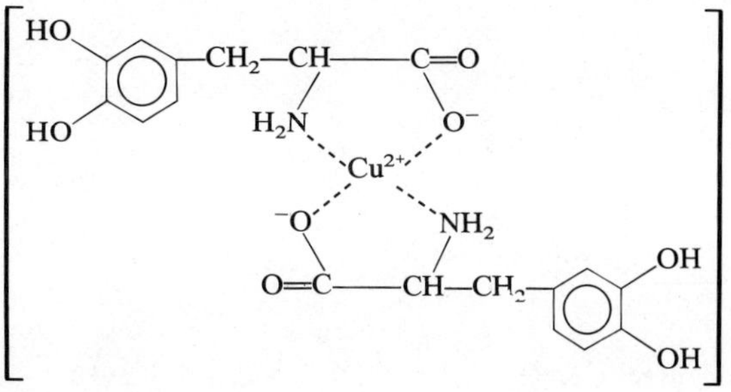

Dopamine Releasers

Amantadine

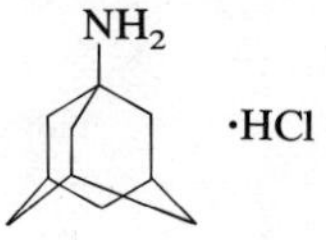

417

Table 45.1   Antiparkinsonism Drugs (*Continued*)

Nonproprietary Name or Code	Structure

Gludantane

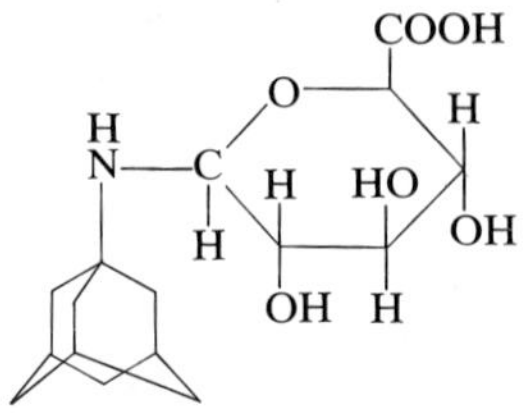

Rimantadine

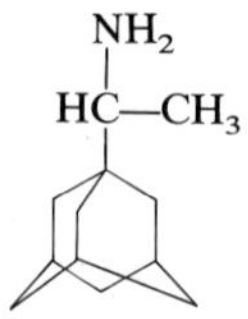

Memantine

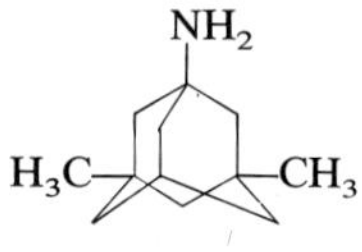

Carmantadine

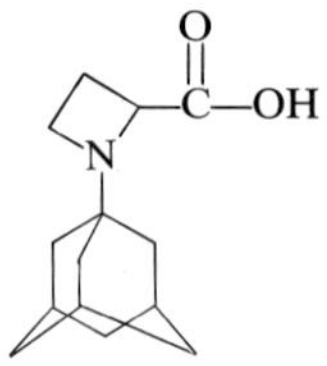

Dopamantine

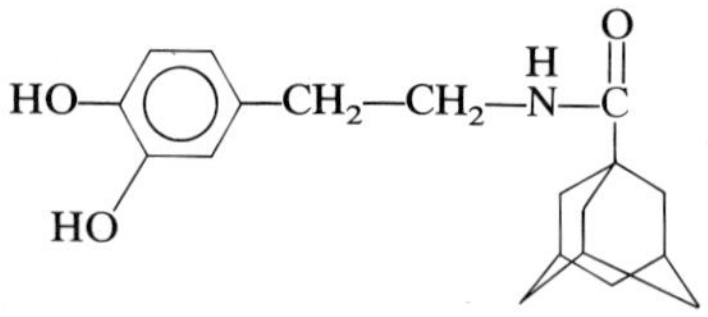

Amphetamine

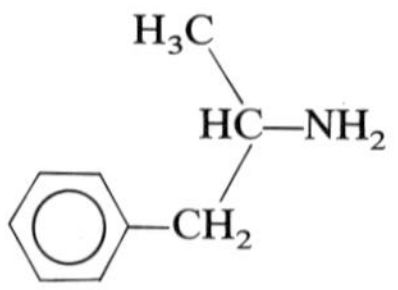

Amineptine

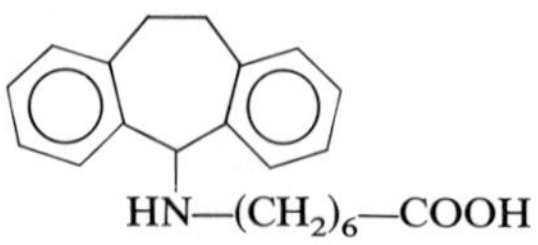

Table 45.1 Antiparkinsonism Drugs (*Continued*)

Nonproprietary Name or Code	Structure

Dopamine Receptor Stimulants

Apomorphine

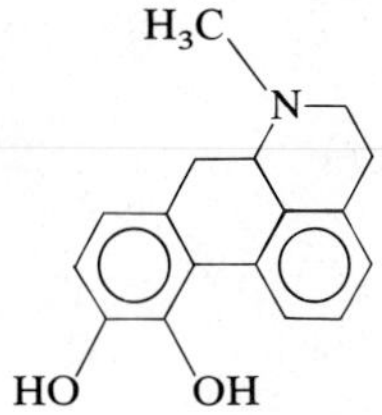

N-Propylnoraporphine

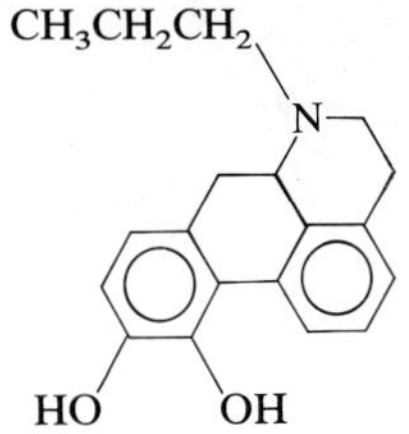

Piribedil

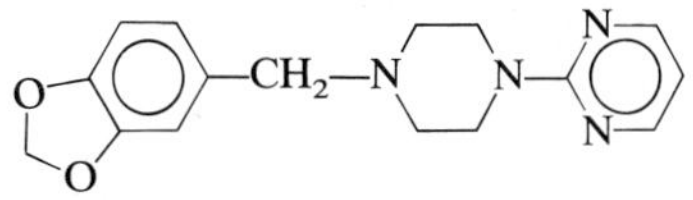

Bromocriptine

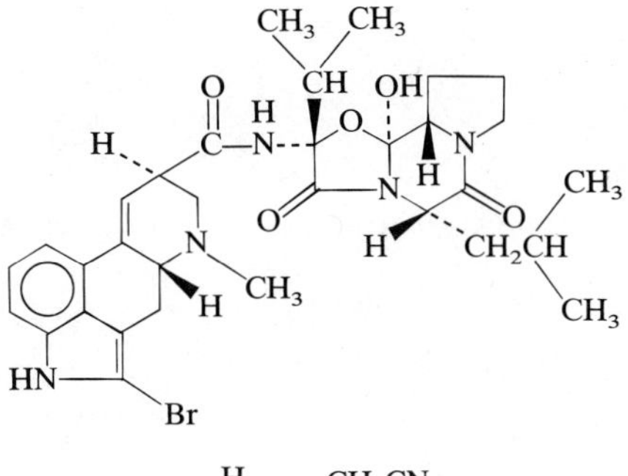

Lergotrile

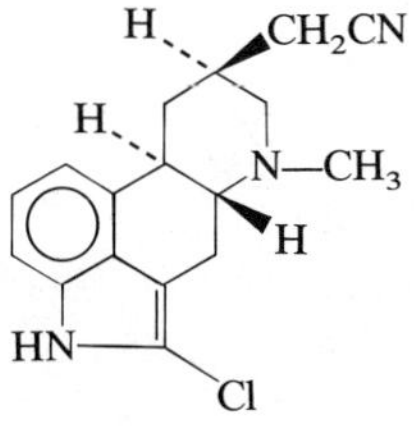

Ergoline (CF 25–397)

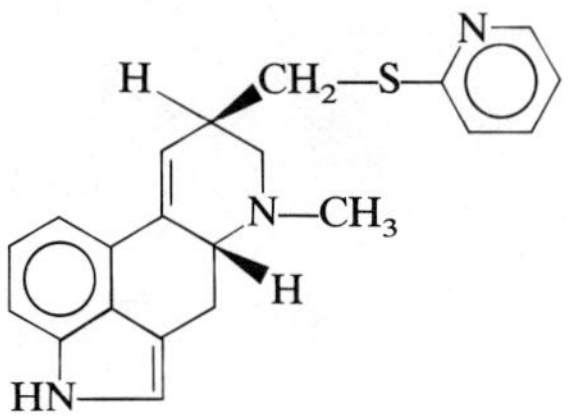

Table 45.1 Antiparkinsonism Drugs (*Continued*)

Nonproprietary Name or Code	Structure

Tetrahydropapaveroline

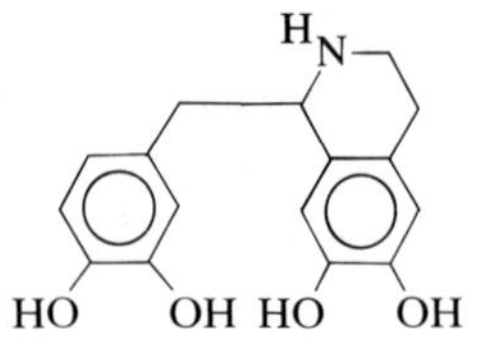

NBTI

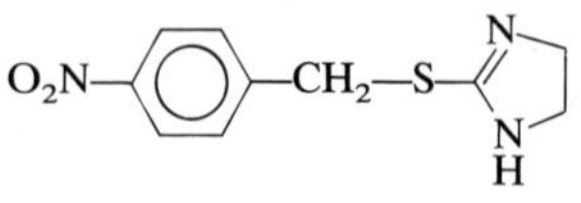

Anticholinergics—Old

Atropine

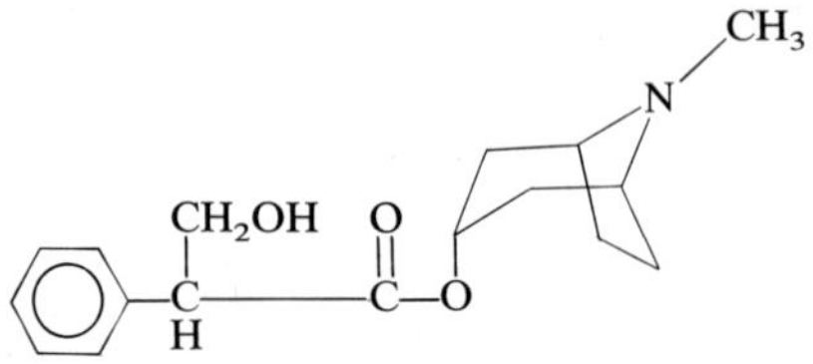

Scopolamine

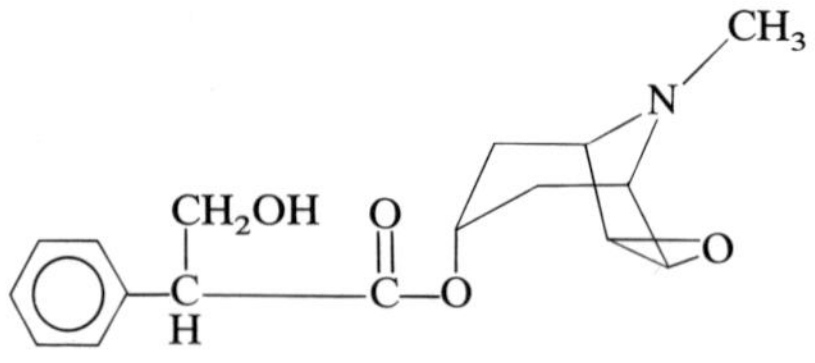

Benztropine

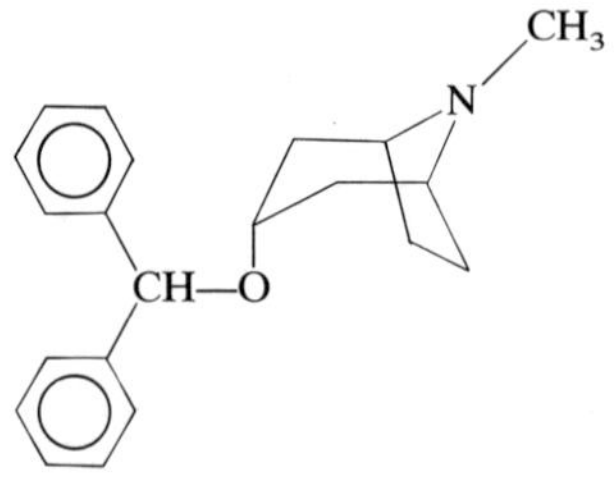

Trihexyphenidyl

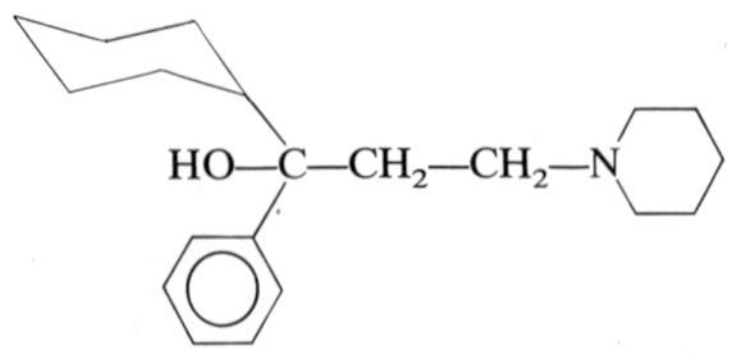

Biperiden

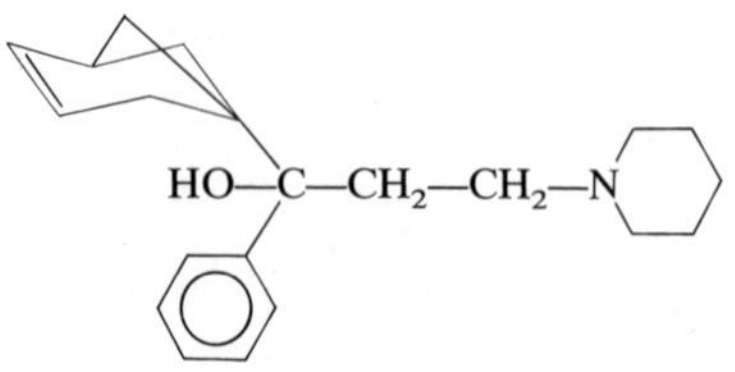

420

Table 45.1 **Antiparkinsonism Drugs** (*Continued*)

Nonproprietary Name or Code	Structure

Procyclidine

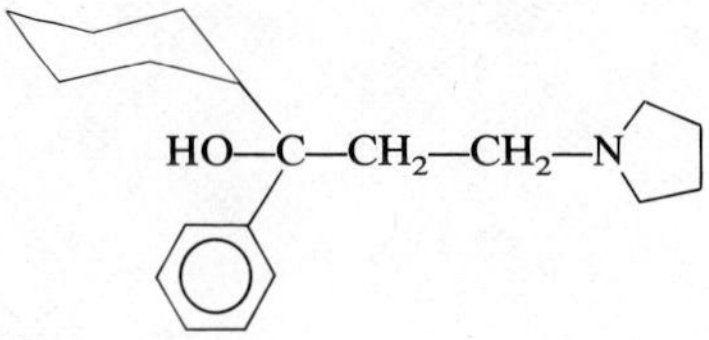

Cycrimine

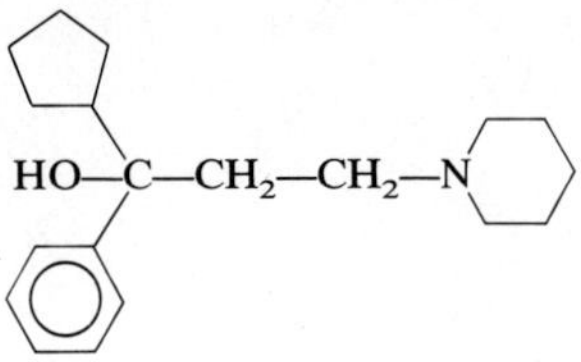

Orphenadrine

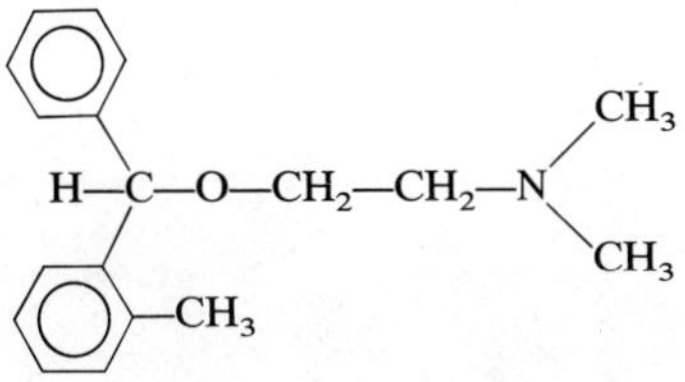

Chlorphenoxamine

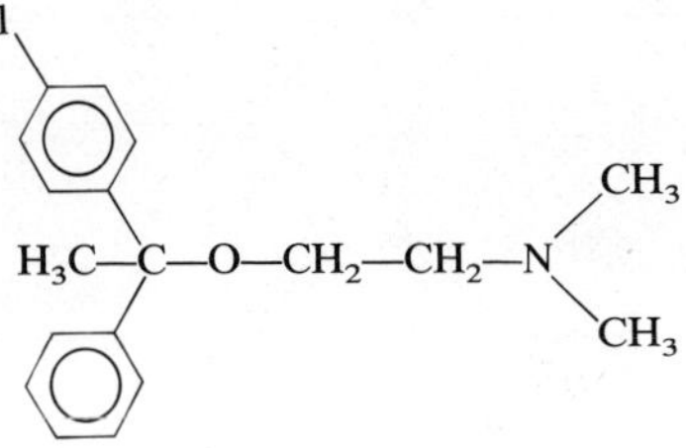

Caramiphen

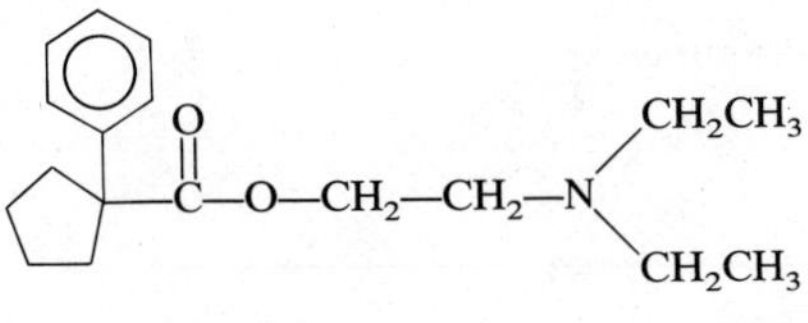

Ethopropazine

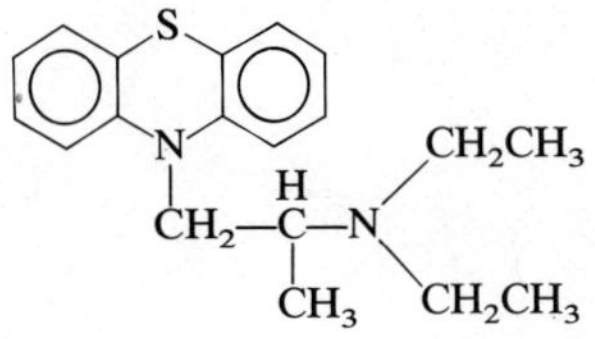

421

Table 45.1 **Antiparkinsonism Drugs** (*Continued*)

Nonproprietary Name or Code	Structure

Anticholinergics—New

Benapryzine

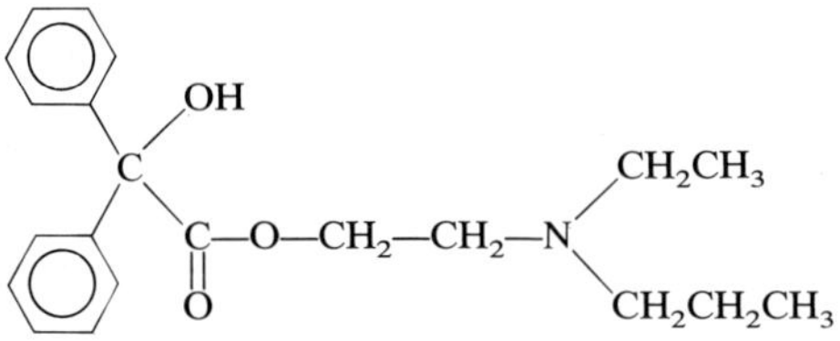

Elantrine

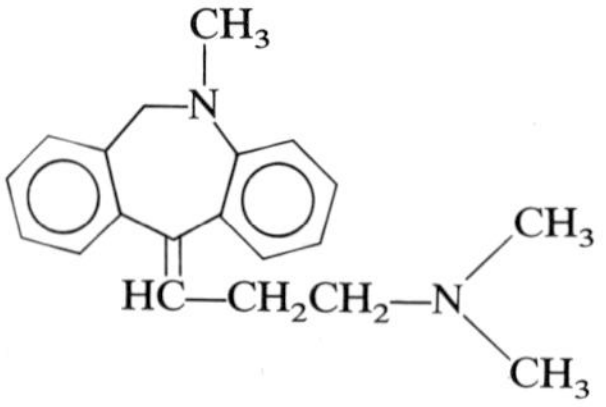

Dexetimide

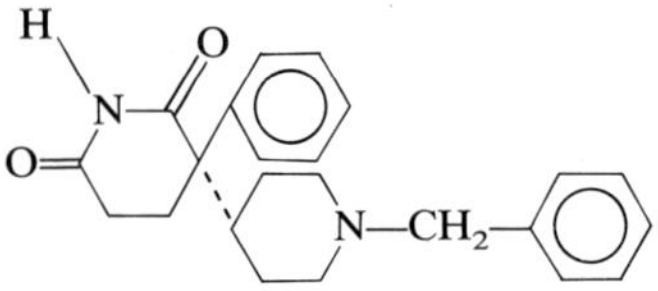

KR 339

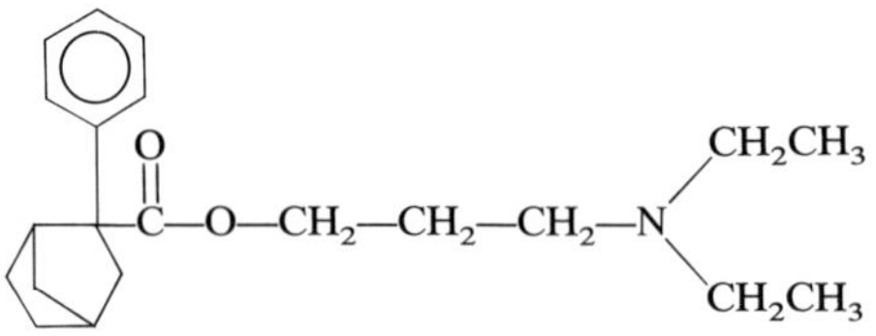

Antihistamines

Diphenhydramine

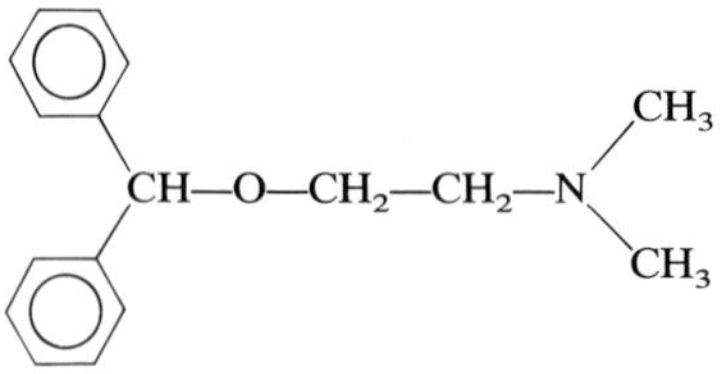

Promethazine

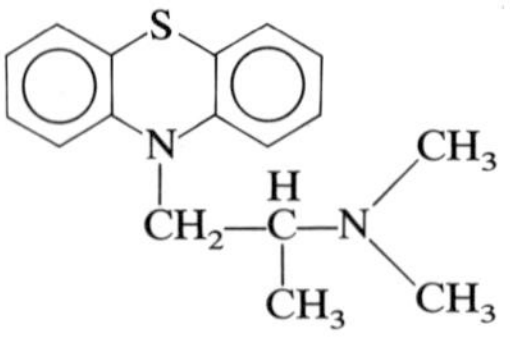

Table 45.1 Antiparkinsonism Drugs (*Continued*)

Nonproprietary Name or Code	Structure

Antidepressants—Tricyclics

Amitriptyline

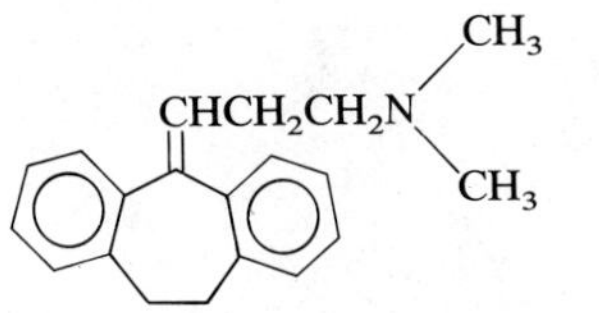

Desipramine

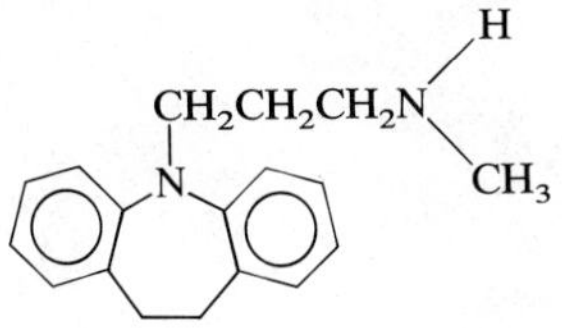

Imipramine

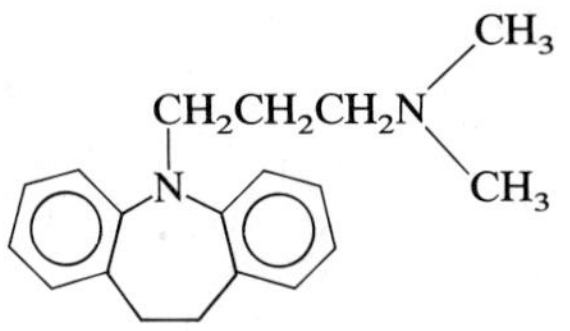

G 31406

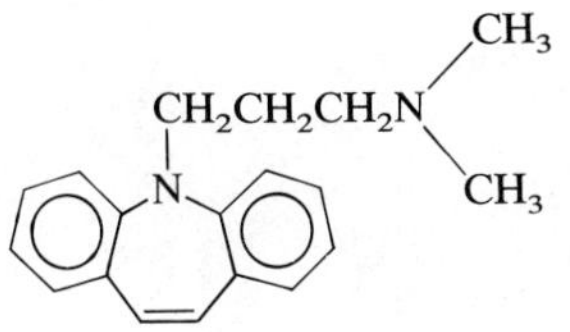

Nomifensine

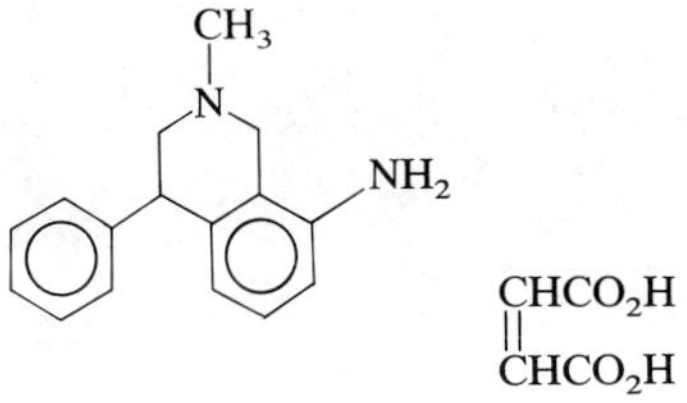

Cyclobenzaprine

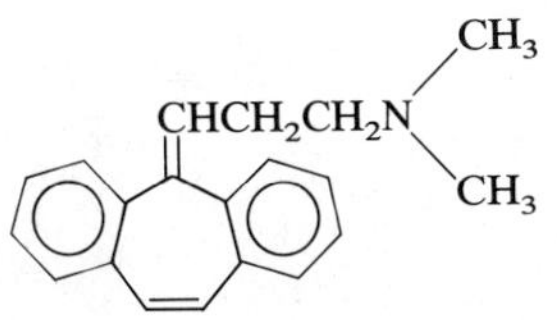

Antidepressants—Monoamine Oxidase, Inhibitors

Phenelzine

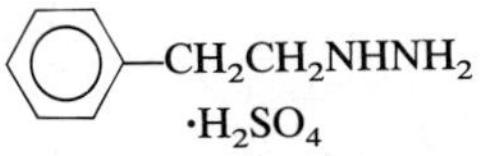

Table 45.1 Antiparkinsonism Drugs (*Continued*)

Nonproprietary Name or Code	Structure
Tranylcypromine	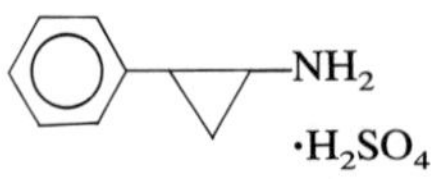
Isocarboxazide	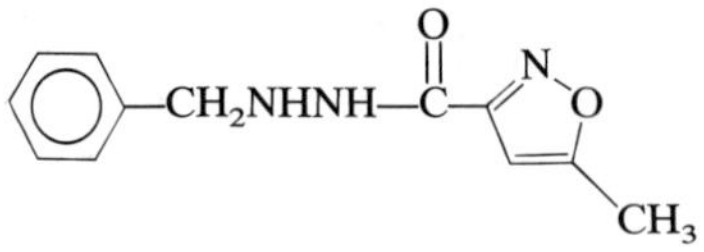
Deprenil	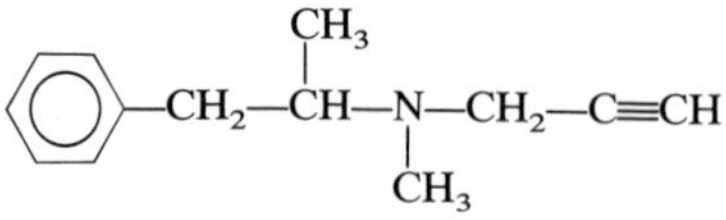

Others

Melanocyte-stimulating hormone inhibitory factor (MIF-I, MRIF-I), L-prolyl-L-leucylglycine amide (PLG)	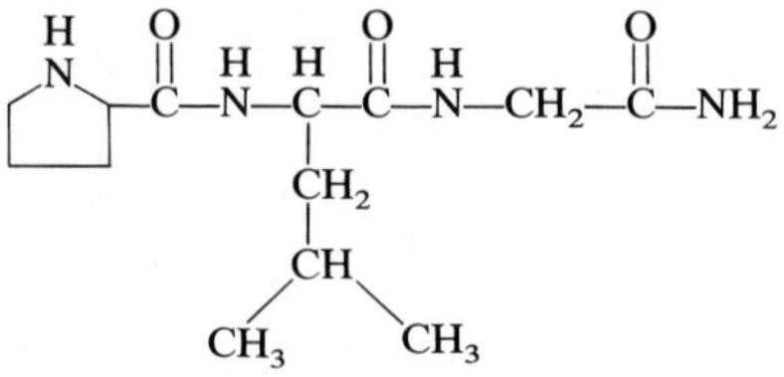
Somatostatin (growth hormone releasing inhibitory factor, GH-RIF), somatotrophin releasing inhibitory factor (SRIF)	Ala-Gly-Cys-Lys-Asn-Phe-Phe-Trp Cys-Ser-Thr-Phe-Thr-Lys
Melatonin	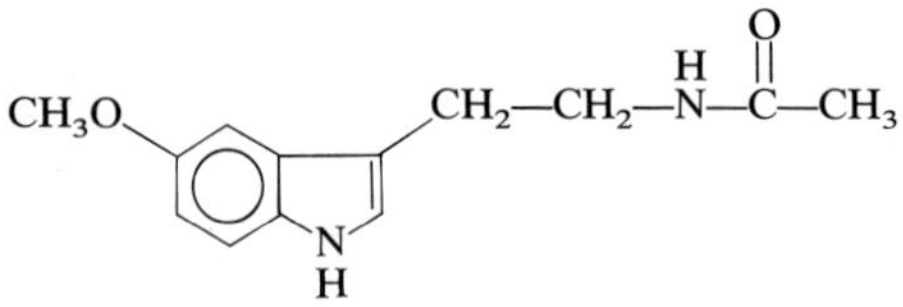
Fusaric acid	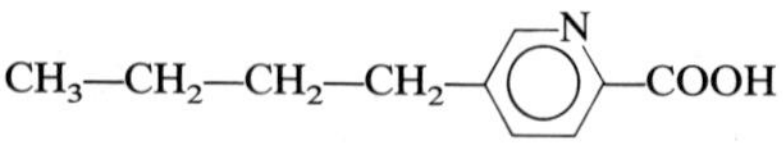
Disulfiram	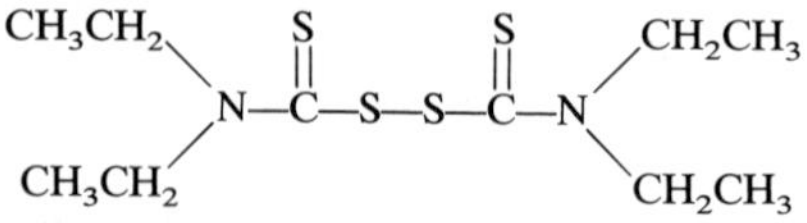
Methyldopa	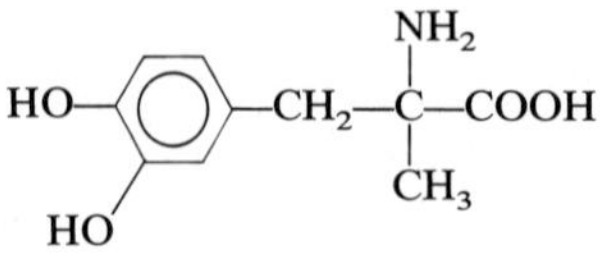

Table 45.1 Antiparkinsonism Drugs (*Continued*)

Nonproprietary Name or Code	Structure
Clonidine	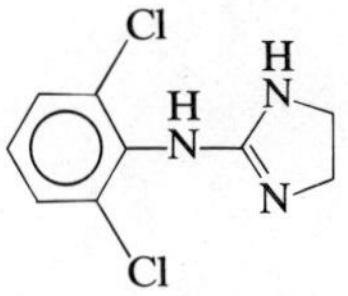
Propranolol	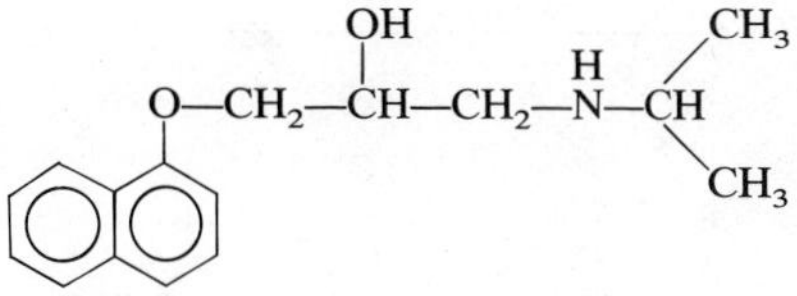
Oxprenolol	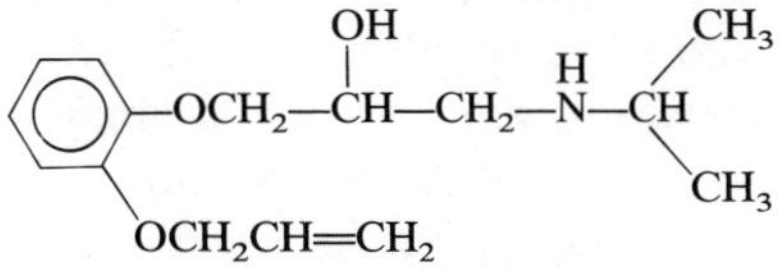
Deanol	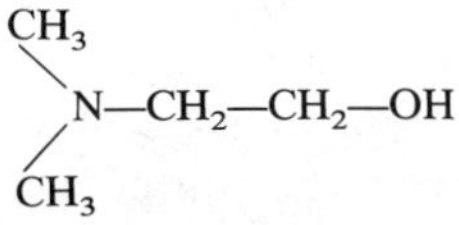
Fenclonine (PCPA)	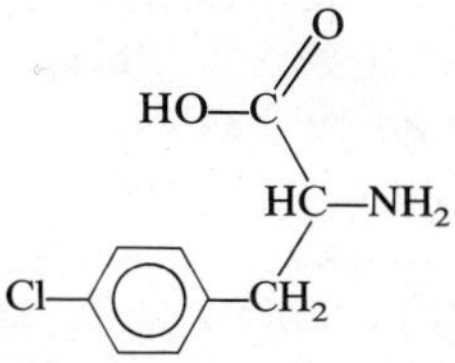
5-Hydroxytryptophan (5HTP)	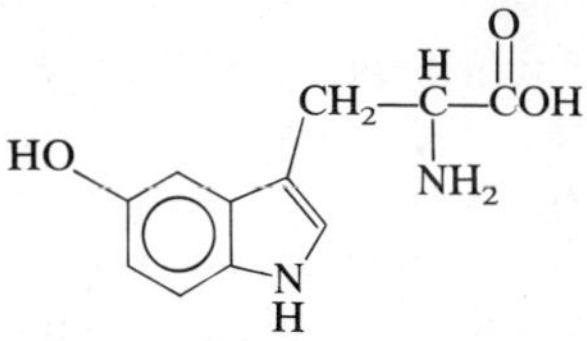
Baclofen	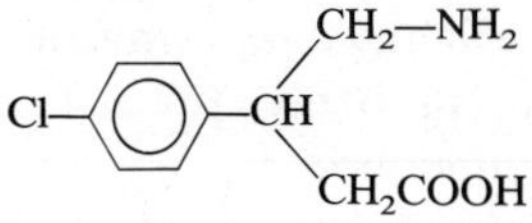
Metoclopramide	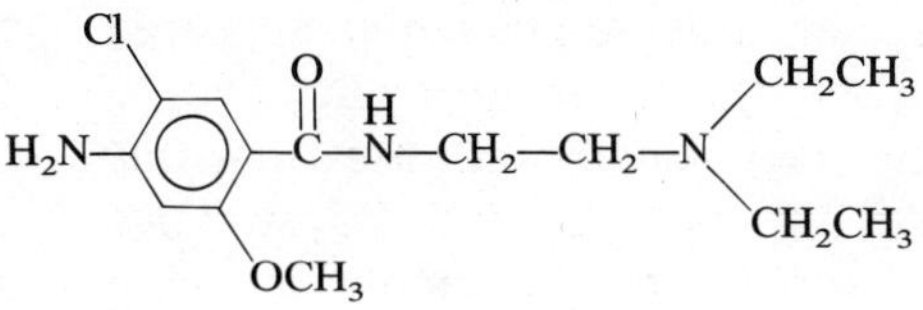

Table 45.1   Antiparkinsonism Drugs (*Continued*)

Nonproprietary Name or Code	Structure
Sulpiride	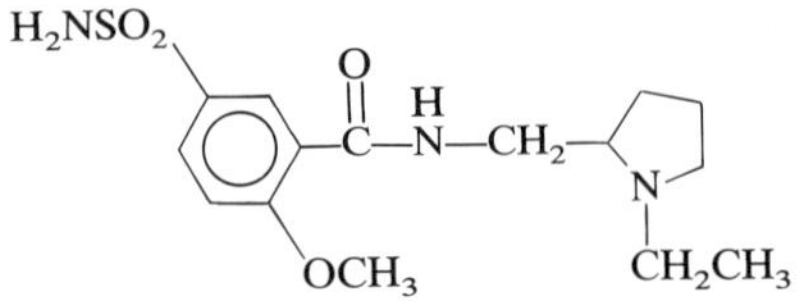 H_2NSO_2 — (benzene ring with OCH_3) — $\overset{O}{\overset{\|}{C}}$—N(H)—$CH_2$— (pyrrolidine, N—$CH_2CH_3$)

twice that of amantadine, to which it may be cleaved (26). Rimantadine, an effective anti-influenza agent, does not share amantadine's actions in central nervous system studies and was ineffective in Parkinson's disease patients (27). Intravenous administration of memantine, a related compound which laboratory reports suggest may act by a similar mechanism, caused favorable effects in 12 patients on tremor, rigidity, and akinesia (28–30). Oral efficacy compared with amantadine has not been reported. Other amantadine derivatives have been synthesized and are being tested, but no reports of action in patients are yet available for carmantadine (31) and dopamantine (32).

Levoamphetamine and dextroamphetamine have been reexamined for the efficacy in parkinsonism that was reported 40 years ago (33). Somnolent postencephalitic parkinsonism patients probably profited most from the alerting effect. The two isomers slightly but significantly reduced disability, probably to a lesser extent than anticholinergics.

In rats and cats with lesions of the entopeduncular nucleus, amineptine appeared to increase striatal homovanillic acid, a dopamine metabolite, and thus possibly dopamine turnover, enhanced ipsiversive circling like levodopa, apomorphine, and amphetamine, and was thought suitable for trial as a dopamine-releasing agent (34).

5.3   Dopamine Receptor Stimulants

Apomorphine effectively controls Parkinson's disease symptoms but is only effective parenterally for brief periods and causes nausea and vomiting at or near effective doses (35). It acts by stimulating dopamine receptors in the central nervous system and also has peripheral, renal, and other actions. High oral doses of apomorphine have been effective but prerenal azotemia prevents its further use (36–38).

Piribedil has similar characteristics but is only moderately effective orally, and although it has a better margin between the therapeutic dose and side effects, it still leaves much to be desired with respect to gastrointestinal and psychiatric side effect incidence (39, 40).

Bromocriptine, an ergot derivative developed to inhibit prolactin release, has been reported by several groups to have clinical efficacy in Parkinson's disease patients (41–43). Another ergot derivative, lergotrile, has been reported to control Parkinson's disease symptoms probably by the same mechanism of dopamine receptor stimulation (44). The intrinsic efficacy of these two agents is probably only modest. Ergoline (CF 25–397), a related compound, although effective in a number of animal tests was ineffective in patients and in fact made them worse (45).

N-Propylnoraporphine has been reported by Cotzias to be useful in controlling Parkinson's disease symptoms in short-term trials (38) without the renal effects of apomorphine.

Tetrahydropapaveroline, an alkaloid metabolite of dopamine and a possible precursor of apomorphine, given intravenously caused tachycardia, did not alter rigidity and akinesia, and worsened tremor (46). Nitrobenzylthioimidazoline (NBTI) stimulates dopamine receptors in laboratory experiments and has been suggested for trial in man (47).

5.4 Anticholinergics

5.4.1 OLD. Classically atropine and scopolamine have been used successfully for nearly a hundred years, but the peripheral actions occur at the effective dose causing dry mouth, pupil dilation, and gastrointestinal signs. They also have only moderate intrinsic activity, and tolerance develops so that the dose must be escalated. Newer but established anticholinergic agents include benztropine, trihexyphenidyl, biperiden, procyclidine, cyrimine, orphenadrine, chlorphenoxamine, caramiphen, and ethopropazine; these are predominantly anticholinergic in action. Some of these drugs, which have some antihistaminic activity, may also block reuptake of dopamine, contributing to their Parkinson's disease efficacy (48).

5.4.2 NEW. Several newer agents that act predominantly by an anticholinergic mechanism and have been in early human trials include benapryzine (49, 50), elantrine (51, 52), dexetimide (53), and KR 339 (54). The anticholinergic approach is much less promising than the possibilities availa-

ble by modification of the dopamine system which lies closer to the heart of the etiologic defect.

5.5 Antihistamines

Diphenhydramine has been used in Parkinson's disease for many years with modest success, again probably as a result of its anticholinergic and depressant potential, but reuptake block may contribute to its efficacy. Promethazine has also been used but with only minimal response. Other antihistamines have also been tried with limited success, but those with a significant dopamine reuptake blocking component have been suggested for reconsideration (48).

5.6 Antidepressants

5.6.1 TRICYCLIC. Amitriptyline and other tricyclic antidepressants have been used in Parkinson's disease therapy to deal with the depressed mental state of the patients, but their usefulness may also be attributed to their anticholinergic activity and also possibly to their effects in causing catecholamine reuptake block. Desipramine and imipramine have been tried with some efficacy. G 31406, the 10,11-unsaturated congener of imipramine, was effective combined with levodopa in two trials (55, 56). Nomifensine is a new antidepressant that has been tried as an antiparkinsonism agent with modest success (59, 60). Cyclobenzaprine is less effective in Parkinson's disease than as a skeletal muscle relaxant in spastic states (57, 58).

5.6.2 MONOAMINE OXIDASE INHIBITORS. Several monoamine oxidase inhibitors have been studied, including phenelzine, tranylcypromine and isocarboxazide, but their potential for toxicity has been a drawback (61). Recently, deprenil, described as a selective monoamine oxidase inhibitor of the B isoenzyme, has been reported to have some promise when combined with levodopa and a decarboxylase inhibitor (62), but inhibitors of monoamine oxidase A isoenzyme (tranylcypromine and nialamide) are less effective and more toxic.

5.7 Others

A group of miscellaneous agents with various mechanisms of action have been tested and are discussed below. In most cases success has been moderate or worse and the mechanisms of action are not well understood.

Melanocyte-stimulating hormone inhibitory factor (MIF-I, L-prolyl-L-leucylglycine amide, PLG) is a tripeptide and although reported effective intravenously, was not orally effective in a 4 month double-blind trial in 20 Parkinson's disease patients (63, 64). The failure may be attributable to poor oral absorption and a short biological half-life. Animal studies suggest that it probably does not interact with brain dopamine systems, unlike levodopa, apomorphine, amantadine, and amphetamine (65).

Somatostatin, the somatotrophic (growth) hormone releasing inhibitory factor, has been suggested for investigation of efficacy on the basis of observations of growth hormone blood level increases induced by levodopa and N-propylnoraporphine (66, 36).

Melatonin, a pineal hormone which controls pigmentation, was well tolerated but inactive (21).

Fusaric acid, a dopamine β-hydroxylase inhibitor, in doses of 300–500 mg daily markedly reduced the abnormal involuntary movements of six patients on levodopa (67). This implicates excess norepinephrine formation as a possible factor and suggests an approach to the control of abnormal involuntary movements. Another group found that fusaric acid treatment alone was

not helpful, but that in combination it reduced the optimal levodopa dose and decreased side effects when given in a range of 200–700 mg daily (68). Disulfiram, which is useful as a deterrent in alcoholism and also has dopamine β-hydroxylase inhibitory activity, has been tried in Parkinson's disease with levodopa without success (69, 70).

Methyldopa, widely used as an antihypertensive, has been reported to be effective in parkinsonism both alone (71) and with levodopa (72), but there are also divergent clinical reports and uncertainty about the probable modes of action (70). It may act by decarboxylase inhibition, by the formation of false catecholamine neurotransmitters, and possibly by other mechanisms. Clonidine at blood pressure lowering doses decreased the efficacy of levodopa and piribedil (73). The β-adrenergic blocking agents, propranolol and oxprenolol, did not alter or improve the levodopa effect in parkinsonian patients (74, 75).

Deanol, which may relieve cholinergic deficit by serving as an acetylcholine precursor, has been claimed to be active in dystonias, but was not effective in treating levodopa-induced dyskinesias (76). Manipulations of the serotonin system in patients showed that fenclonine (PCPA), which depletes serotonin, did not improve signs (77, 78). 5-Hydroxytryptophan, which is a precursor for serotonin and which raises serotonin levels, did not improve signs and in fact made akinesia and rigidity worse (78).

Baclofen, a muscle relaxant that is a γ amino butyric acid antagonist, was not efficacious in Parkinson's disease (79, 80).

Metoclopramide blocks levodopa-induced nausea and vomiting without worsening parkinsonism signs or levodopa-induced abnormal involuntary movements (81, 82). Promethazine can be used similarly, but pimozide exacerbates extrapyramidal symptoms. Metoclopramide raises human prolactin levels and, like sulpiride, blocks certain CNS dopaminergic receptors in a manner differing from chlorpromazine and other major tranquilizers (83–85).

ACKNOWLEDGMENTS

Mrs. S. L. Zehnder contributed thorough literature searches and Mrs. B. L. Fitzgerald skillfully prepared this manuscript.

REFERENCES

1. E. L. Engelhardt and C. A. Stone, "Antiparkinsonism Drugs," in *Medicinal Chemistry*, 3rd ed., Part III, A. Burger, Ed., Wiley-Interscience, New York–London, 1970, p. 1538.

2. V. G. Vernier, *Ann. Rep. Med. Chem.*, **9**, 19 (1974).

3. K. E. Moore and P. H. Kelly, "Biochemical Pharmacology of Mesolimbic and Mesocortical Dopaminergic Neurons," in *Psychopharmacology: A Generation of Progress*, M. A. Lipton, A. DiMascio, and K. F. Killam, Eds., Raven Press, New York, 1978, p. 221.

4. G. R. Siggins, "Electrophysiological Role of Dopamine in Striatum: Excitatory or Inhibitory?," in *Psychopharmacology: A Generation of Progress*, M. A. Lipton, A. DiMascio, and K. F. Killam, Eds., Raven Press, New York, 1978, p. 143.

5. M. D. Yahr, *Clin. Ther.*, **1**, 95 (1977).

6. A. Ahmed and P. Marshall, *Brit. J. Pharmacol.*, **18**, 247 (1962).

7. C. Bianchi and L. Tomasi, *Pharmacol.*, **10**, 226 (1973).

8. H. Schnieden and B. Cox, *Eur. J. Pharmacol.*, **39**, 133 (1976).

9. S. D. Glick, T. P. Jerussi, and L. N. Fleisher, *Life Sci.*, **18**, 889 (1976).

10. A. Barnett and J. Goldstein, *J. Pharmacol. Exp. Ther.*, **194**, 296 (1975).

11. G. Zetler, *Naunyn-Schmiedebergs Arch. Pharmakol.*, **266**, 276 (1970).

12. P. Simon, J. Malatray, and J. R. Boissier, *J. Pharm. Pharmacol.*, **22**, 546 (1970).

13. J. A. Davies, B. Jackson, and P. H. Redfern, *Neuropharmacol.*, **12**, 735 (1973).

14. J. J. Szekely, Z. Dunai-Kovacs, and J. Borsy, *Pharmacol.*, **14**, 240 (1976).

15. P. F. Von Voigtlander and K. E. Moore, *J. Pharmacol. Exp. Ther.*, **184**, 542 (1973).

16. A. R. Damasio, A. Castro-Caldas, and A. Levy, *Advan. Neurol.*, **3**, 11 (1973).

17. R. D. Sweet, F. H. McDowell, C. G. Wasterlain, and P. H. Stern, *Arch. Neurol.*, **32**, 560 (1975).

18. A. Brossi, W. Pool, H. Sheppard, J. J. Burns, A. Kaiser, R. Bigler, G. Bartholini, and A. Pletscher, *Advan. Neurol.*, **5**, 291 (1974).

19. B. Heller, E. Fischer, and R. Martin, *Arzneim.-Forsch.*, **26**, 577 (1976).

20. U. Ungerstedt, K. Fuxe, M. Goldstein, A. Battista, M. Ogawa, and B. Anagnoste, *Eur. J. Pharmacol.*, **21**, 230 (1973).

21. K. M. Shaw, G. M. Stern, and M. Sandler, *Advan. Neurol.*, **3**, 115 (1973).

22. K. A. Rajan, A. A. Manian, J. M. Davis, and H. Dekirmenjian, *Brain Res.*, **107**, 317 (1976).

23. J. D. Parkes, "Amantadine," in *Advances in Drug Research*, Academic, New York, 1974, p. 11.

24. P. F. Von Voigtlander and K. E. Moore, *Science*, **174**, 408 (1971).

25. E. V. Bailey and T. W. Stone, *Arch. Int. Pharmacodyn.*, **216**, 246 (1975).

26. I. M. Kamyanov and R. A. Andrezinya, *Zh. Nevropatol. Psikhiatr.*, **75**, 910 (1975).

27. R. S. Schwab, D. C. Poskanzer, and A. C. England, paper given at *Am. Acad. Neurol.*, *Bal Harbour, Florida, April 29, 1970*.

28. B. Costall and R. J. Naylor, *Psychopharmacologia*, **43**, 53 (1975).

29. M. Smialowska, *Pol. J. Pharmacol. Pharm.*, **28**, 259 (1976).

30. P. A. Fischer, P. Jacobi, E. Schneider, and B. Schonberger, *Arzneim.-Forsch.*, **27**, 1487 (1977).

31. A. Barnett, J. Goldstein, and E. Fiedler, *Fed. Proc.*, **33**, 293 (1974).

32. *J. Am. Med. Assoc.*, **228**, 1162 (1974).

33. J. D. Parkes, D. Tarsy, C. D. Marsden, K. T. Bovill, J. A. Phipps, P. Rose, and P. Asselman, *J. Neurol., Neurosurg. Psychiatr.*, **38**, 232 (1975).

34. J. Dankova, R. Boucher, and L. J. Poirier, *Eur. J. Pharmacol.*, **42**, 113 (1977).

35. G. C. Cotzias, P. S. Papavasiliou, C. Fehling, B. Kaufman, and I. Mena, *New Engl. J. Med.*, **282**, 31 (1970).

36. G. C. Cotzias, P. S. Papavasiliou, and J. Z. Ginos, *Assoc. Res. Nerv. Ment. Dis.*, **55**, 305 (1976).

37. G. C. Cotzias and P. S. Papavasiliou, E. S. Tolosa, J. S. Mendez, and M. Bell-Midura, *New Engl. J. Med.*, **294**, 567 (1976).

38. G. C. Cotzias, P. S. Papavasiliou, E. Tolosa, M.

A. Bell-Midura, and J. Z. Ginos, *Trans. Am. Neurol. Assoc.*, **100,** 178 (1975).

39. J. S. Feigenson, R. D. Sweet, and F. H. McDowell, *Neurol.*, **26,** 430 (1976).

40. J. Engel, A.-K. Granerus, and A. Svanborg, *Eur. J. Clin. Pharmacol.*, **8,** 233 (1975).

41. J. D. Parkes, A. G. Debono, and C. D. Marsden, *J. Neurol. Neurosurg. Psychiatr.*, **39,** 1101 (1976).

42. A. Lieberman, M. Kupersmith, E. Estey, and M. Goldstein, *New Engl. J. Med.*, **295,** 1400 (1976).

43. R. Kartzinel, P. Teychenne, M. M. Gillespie, M. Perlow, A. C. Gielen, D. A. Sadowsky, and D. B. Calne, *Lancet*, **1976-II, 2,** 272.

44. A. Lieberman, T. Miyamoto, A. F. Battista, and M. Goldstein, *Neurology*, **25,** 459 (1975).

45. P. F. Teychenne, R. Pfeiffer, S. M. Bern, and D. B. Calne, *Neurology*, **27,** 1140 (1977).

46. G. Dordain, M.-A. Goujet, and P. Simon, *Therapie*, **29,** 429 (1974).

47. M. K. Menon, W. G. Clark, and D. Aures, *Eur. J. Pharmacol.*, **19,** 43 (1972).

48. J. P. Coyle and S. H. Snyder, *Science*, **166,** 899 (1969).

49. D. M. Brown, B. O. Hughes, C. D. Marsden, J. C. Meadows, and B. Spicer, *Brit. J. Pharmacol.*, **47,** 476 (1973).

50. S. Lamid and R. B. Jenkins, *J. Clin. Pharmacol.*, **15,** 622 (1975).

51. E. R. Blonsky, A. D. Ericsson, A. S. McKinney, A. Rix, R. I. Wang, and A. A. Rimm, *Clin. Pharmacol. Ther.*, **15,** 46 (1974).

52. H. Freeman and I. S. Mehta, *Curr. Ther. Res.*, **14,** 470 (1972).

53. H. Hakkarainen and M. Viukari, *Duodecin.*, **89,** 1473 (1973).

54. M. Iivanainen, *Acta Neurol. Scand.*, **50,** 469 (1974).

55. J. Deze and G. W. Völler, *Med. Welt*, **26,** 1457 (1975).

56. B. Couto, C. Oliveira, J. P. Mattos, and M. R. Freitas, *Neurol. Neurocir. Psiquiatr.*, **17,** 285 (1976).

57. P. Molina-Negro and R. A. Illingworth, *Union Med. Can.*, **102,** 303 (1973).

58. *Med. Lett.*, **20,** 12 (1978).

59. P. F. Teychenne, D. M. Park, L. J. Findley, F. C. Rose, and D. B. Calne, *J. Neurol. Neurosurg. Psychiatr.*, **39,** 1219 (1976).

60. B. Costall, D. M. Kelly, and R. J. Naylor, *Psychopharmacologia*, **41,** 153 (1975).

61. P. F. Teychenne, D. B. Calne, P. F. Lewis, and L. F. Findley, *Clin. Pharmacol. Ther.*, **18,** 273

(1975).

62. W. Birkmayer, P. Riederer, and L. Ambrozi, *Lancet*, **1977-I:** 8009, 439.

63. A. J. Kastin, A. Barbeau, R. H. Ehrensing, N. P. Plotnikoff, and A. V. Schally, *Advan. Neurol.*, **5,** 225 (1974).

64. A. Barbeau, M. Roy and A. J. Kastin, *Can. Med. Assoc. J.*, **114,** 120 (1976).

65. B. Cox, A. J. Kastin, and H. Schnieden, *Eur. J. Pharmacol.*, **36,** 141 (1976).

66. G. C. Cotzias and P. S. Papavasiliou, *New Engl. J. Med.*, **294,** 398 (1976).

67. I. Mena, J. Court, and G. C. Cotzias, *J. Am. Med. Assoc.*, **218,** 1829 (1971).

68. E. Herskovits and G. E. Figueroa, *Medicina* (Buenos Aires), **33,** 51 (1973).

69. P. A. Serrano and M. Irigoyen, *Prensa Med. Mex.*, **37,** 246 (1972).

70. R. D. Duvoisin and C. D. Marsden, *Brain Res.*, **71,** 178 (1974).

71. D. O. Marsh, H. Schneiden, and J. Marshall, *J. Neurol., Neurosurg. Psychiatr.*, **26,** 505 (1963).

72. R. D. Sweet, J. E. Lee, and F. H. McDowell, *Clin. Pharm. Ther.*, **13,** 23 (1972).

73. I. Shoulson and T. N. Chase, *Neuropharmacol.*, **15,** 25 (1976).

74. C. D. Marsden, J. D. Parkes, and J. E. Rees, *Lancet*, **1974-II,** 410.

75. M. Sandler, L. E. Fellows, D. B. Calne, and L. J. Findley, *Lancet*, **1975-I:** 7899, 168.

76. H. L. Klawans, J. L. Topel, and D. Bergen, *Neurology*, **25,** 290 (1975).

77. M. H. Van Woert, L. M. Ambani, and R. J. Devine, *Dis. Nerv. System*, **33,** 777 (1972).

78. T. N. Chase, *Advan. Neurol.*, **5,** 31 (1974).

79. Statement by Chairman, Medical Practice, *Med. J. Aust.*, **1,** 322 (1976).

80. R. N. Brogden, T. M. Speight, and G. S. Avery, *Drugs*, **8,** 1 (1974).

81. D. Tarsy, J. D. Parkes, and C. D. Marsden, *Lancet*, **1975-I:** 7918, 1244.

82. D. Tarsy, J. D. Parkes, and C. D. Marsden, *J. Neurol., Neurosurg. Psychiatr.*, **38,** 331 (1975).

83. R. W. McCallum, J. R. Sowers, J. M. Hershman, and R. A. Sturdevant, *J. Clin. Endocrin. Metal.*, **42,** 1148 (1976).

84. P. N. C. Elliott, P. Jenner, G. Hutzing, C. D. Marsden, and R. Miller, *Neuropharmacology*, **16,** 333 (1977).

85. G. U. Corsini, M. Del Zompo, C. Cianchetti, and A. Mangoni, *Psychopharmacologia*, **47,** 169 (1976).

CHAPTER FORTY-SIX

Neuromuscular Blocking Agents

JOHN B. STENLAKE

Department of Pharmaceutical Chemistry
University of Strathclyde
Glasgow G1 1XW, Scotland

CONTENTS

1   INTRODUCTION

The term neuromuscular blockade is applied generally to describe any mechanism that results in the inhibition of nervous transmission at motor nerve endings in skeletal muscle. Neuromuscular blockade, therefore, causes muscle relaxation, which is useful clinically if suitably controlled. It is widely used as an adjunct to surgical anesthesia, mainly for the relaxation of skeletal muscles in abdominal surgery (1, 2) and also in ophthalmic surgery (3). Short-acting muscle relaxants are also used to facilitate intubation procedures (4) and in orthopedics for the manipulation of fractured or dislocated bones (5). Other uses of neuromuscular blocking agents include the control of convulsions in tetanus (6) and in electroconvulsive therapy of psychiatric disorders (7) to prevent muscle and bone damage.

All neuromuscular blocking agents in clinical use act either by depolarization of the motor end plate or by competition with the chemical transmitter, acetylcholine, at the neuromuscular junction. Various other ways of achieving neuromuscular blockade by interfering with the synthesis and availability of acetylcholine are known, but so far no clinically useful drug acting by such a mechanism has been evolved. However, in order to understand the action of the drugs in use, and also to appreciate fully the potential for new drug development in this field, it is necessary to consider not only the function of acetylcholine at the neuromuscular junction but also the innervation of skeletal muscle and the biosynthesis and storage of acetylcholine.

2   INNERVATION OF SKELETAL MUSCLE

2.1   Motoneurons

Skeletal muscles are innervated by fast-conducting myelinated motor nerves that have their origins in either the motor nuclei within the brainstem or in the anterior horns of the spinal cord. These fibers are described as *lower motoneurons* to distinguish them from the upper motoneurons, with which they synapse, that have their origins in the frontal lobes of the cerebral cortex. Together the upper and lower motoneurons provide the pathways for central control of skeletal support and movement.

The axons of peripheral motoneurons are protected by a lipoprotein (myelin) sheath, which is developed from the surface membranes of the associated Schwann cells. These are multiply coiled about the axon to form a protective layer. This, however, is not continuous throughout the length of the axon, but is constricted at intervals between one Schwann cell and the next, at what are known as nodes of Ranvier.

The axons of the lower motoneurons branch extensively at the terminal nodes of Ranvier in contact with the muscles, so that each axon innervates a large number of individual muscle fibers. Axon and innervated muscle fibers together make up a single functional unit known as a *motor unit*. However, although the individual muscle fibers of each motor unit are of the same type (fast white, fast red, or slow intermediate) they do not usually form a distinct bundle, but instead are scattered throughout the muscle.

2.2   Neuromuscular Junction

At the axon terminal, each nerve branch subdivides into a number of short twigs which lie in channels in the muscle fiber membrane known as the junctional clefts. The surface of the clefts is multiply folded so that a large area of the muscle fiber membrane is exposed to the nerve terminal (Fig. 46.1). At their narrowest, the junctional folds leave a gap of about 50 nm wide between the nerve terminal and muscle fiber membrane. The junctional clefts contain mucopolysaccharide material and

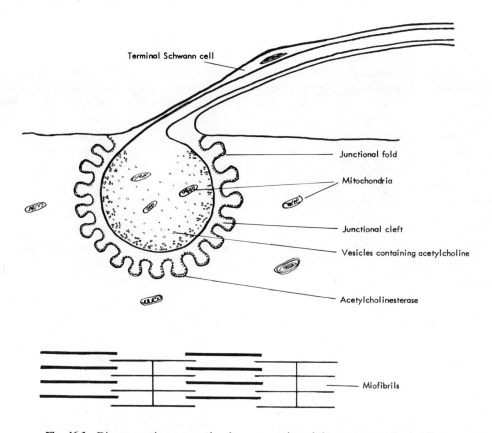

Terminal Schwann cell

Junctional fold

Mitochondria

Junctional cleft

Vesicles containing acetylcholine

Acetylcholinesterase

Miofibrils

Fig. 46.1 Diagrammatic cross-sectional representation of the neuromuscular junction.

are enclosed by fusion of the terminal Schwann cell of the axon branch with the sarcolemma.

The nerve terminals contain large numbers of synaptic vesicles, which are the storage sites for acetylcholine. The enzyme, acetylcholinesterase, that is responsible for the hydrolysis of acetylcholine and termination of its action is concentrated in the region of the junctional folds on the surface of the postsynaptic membrane.

2.3 Focally and Multiply Innervated Muscle Fibers

Muscle fibers receive their innervation either *focally* at a single or at most two or three sites or, alternatively, *multiply* from numerous nerve endings spread over the entire membrane. The fibers of most mammalian muscles are focally innervated, whereas multiply innervated fibers are more common in birds and amphibians. Exceptionally in man, however, the extraocular muscles, the internal ear muscle, and the striated muscles of the upper esophagus contain a proportion of multiply innervated fibers.

All focally innervated muscles are innervated by fast-conducting axons, irrespective of the muscle type. The rate of response, however, is determined not by the axon type, but by the end plate characteristics. Thus the terminals of fast white fibers are characterized by *en plaque* end plates composed of several junctional clefts all with numerous, heavily creased junctional folds. End plates on fast red fibers, however, are much simpler with fewer junctional folds, and slow intermediate fibers terminate in end plates with intermediate characteristics. In contrast, axon terminals in multiply innervated muscle fibers appear as groups of small swellings resembling a bunch of grapes. They are known as *en grappe* end plates and have smooth junctional clefts.

Differences in response to neuromuscular blocking agents between species and between muscles in the same species, which are often quite marked, reflect these differences in muscle and end plate characteristics.

3 BIOSYNTHESIS, STORAGE, AND RELEASE OF ACETYLCHOLINE

It has long been realized that the electric currents generated in the transmission of nervous impulses along nerve trunks are themselves too small to effect direct excitation of the muscle fibers which they innervate. It is now firmly established that the contraction of skeletal muscle fibers is mediated by the chemical transmitter agent acetylcholine at the motor end plate (8). Release of acetylcholine from its vesicular storage sites in the nerve terminal is triggered by arrival of the nerve impulse, forming what is in effect a physicochemical mechanism for current amplification to levels that excite muscular contraction.

3.1 Biosynthesis of Acetylcholine

The biosynthesis of acetylcholine (46.**4**) occurs in two phases, choline synthesis and choline acetylation. Choline (46.**3**), which is also required for phospholipid synthesis, is synthesized in the liver by a pathway from serine (46.**1**) via ethanolamine (46.**2**).

Because of the widespread requirement for choline it is normally present in human blood plasma at concentrations of the order of 1 μg/ml. The second and final phase of acetylcholine synthesis, however, takes place within the nerve terminals. The enzyme responsible for acetylation, choline *O*-acetyltransferase (choline acetylase) is synthesized by ribosomes of the nerve cell body, and transported to the axon terminal, where biosynthesis utilizing acetylcoenzyme A occurs in the axoplasm (9).

Since choline is cationic it is not lipid-soluble, but like a number of other low molecular weight hydrophilic organic compounds it seems able to penetrate most cell membranes, presumably by nonspecific aqueous diffusion rather than lipid diffusion. It has, however, also been clearly demonstrated (10) that cholinergic axon terminals possess a high affinity choline-specific active transport mechanism. Such a mechanism is essential to effect choline uptake at a rate sufficient to maintain acetylcholine synthesis and to ensure the maintenance of acetylcholine stores under conditions of peak demand.

3.2 Interference with Acetylcholine Synthesis

Interference with acetylcholine synthesis, thereby reducing the availability of acetylcholine, offers one approach to neuro-

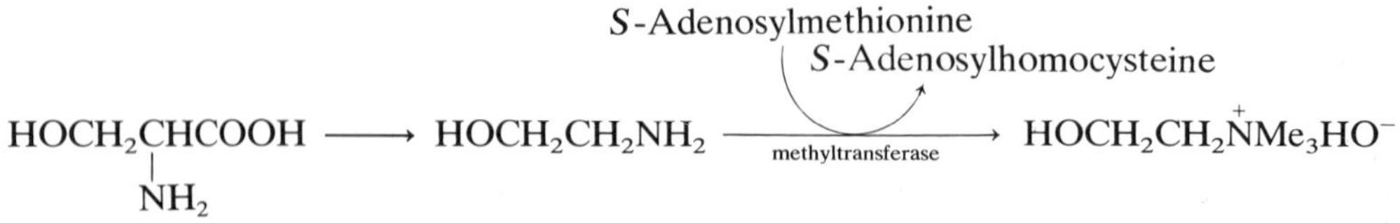

$$S\text{-Adenosylmethionine}$$
$$S\text{-Adenosylhomocysteine}$$

$$\text{HOCH}_2\text{CHCOOH} \longrightarrow \text{HOCH}_2\text{CH}_2\text{NH}_2 \xrightarrow[\text{methyltransferase}]{} \text{HOCH}_2\text{CH}_2\overset{+}{\text{N}}\text{Me}_3\text{HO}^-$$
$$\underset{\text{NH}_2}{|}$$

Serine	Ethanolamine	Choline
46.**1**	46.**2**	46.**3**

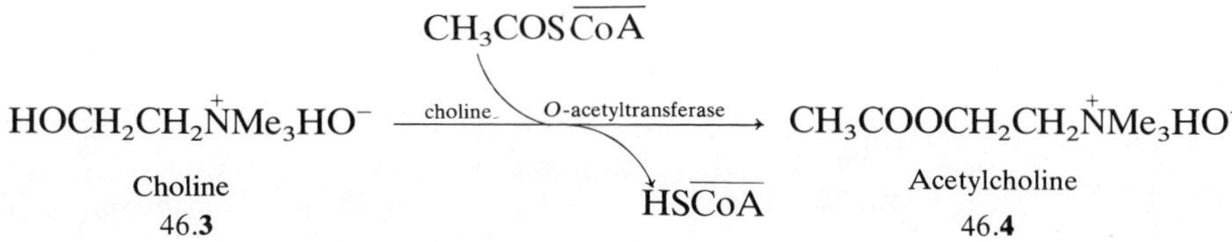

$$CH_3COS\overline{CoA}$$

$$HOCH_2CH_2\overset{+}{N}Me_3HO^- \xrightarrow[\text{choline}]{\text{O-acetyltransferase}} CH_3COOCH_2CH_2\overset{+}{N}Me_3HO^-$$

Choline
46.**3**

$$\overline{HSCoA}$$

Acetylcholine
46.**4**

muscular blockade. Substances that inhibit the choline carrier mechanism, such as hemicholinium (HC-3) (11–13), are believed to act by competing with choline for the carrier, thereby rendering the nerve terminal deficient in choline. The resulting neuromuscular blockade is consequently slow in onset and dependent on the frequency of nerve stimulation, since it becomes effective only as existing stores of acetylcholine are used up and fail to be replaced. There is some evidence, however, that HC-3 is transported by the carrier mechanism in place of choline, and that it also competes with choline at intracellular binding sites. The failure in nervous transmission induced by HC-3 is nonetheless reversed by excess choline, indicating that inhibition of the carrier mechanism is reversible. HC-3 is a bis-phenacylcholine (46.**5**) and exists in solution as the tautomeric bis-hemiketal (46.**6**), from which its name is derived.

The compound WIN 4981 (46.**7**) appears to act in the same way as HC-3 (14). Triethylcholine (46.**8**), the triethyl analog of choline, also acts similarly, competing with choline for the transport mechanism and being transported by it. It is also readily acetylated by choline O-acetyltransferase (15) to acetyltriethylcholine, which is devoid of stimulant action on acetylcholine receptors. As a result triethylcholine produces a slowly developing paralysis under rapid stimulation of the nerve. Its action also is markedly antagonized by choline, and during paralysis an injection of acetylcholine produces a normal response, indicating that the sensitivity of the motor end plate is unaltered.

A number of substances that act as *in vitro* inhibitors of choline O-acetyltransferase are known, of which one of the more potent is 4-NVP, *trans*-4-(1-naphthylvinyl)pyridine (46.**9**; 16, 17). This compound appears to be ineffective *in vivo*,

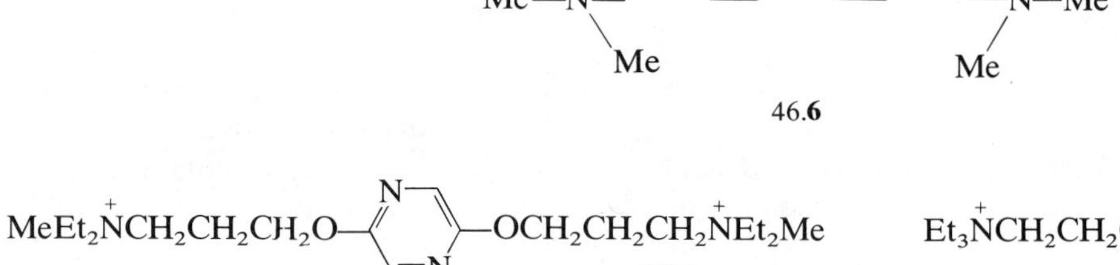

$$HOCH_2CH_2\overset{+}{N}CH_2CO \underset{Me\ \ \ Me}{\diagdown} \text{(biphenyl)} COCH_2\overset{+}{N}CH_2CH_2OH$$
$$\underset{Me\ \ \ Me}{}$$

46.**5**

46.**6**

$$MeEt_2\overset{+}{N}CH_2CH_2CH_2O- \text{(pyrazine)} -OCH_2CH_2CH_2\overset{+}{N}Et_2Me$$
$$2I^-$$

46.**7**

$$Et_3\overset{+}{N}CH_2CH_2OH\ I^-$$

46.**8**

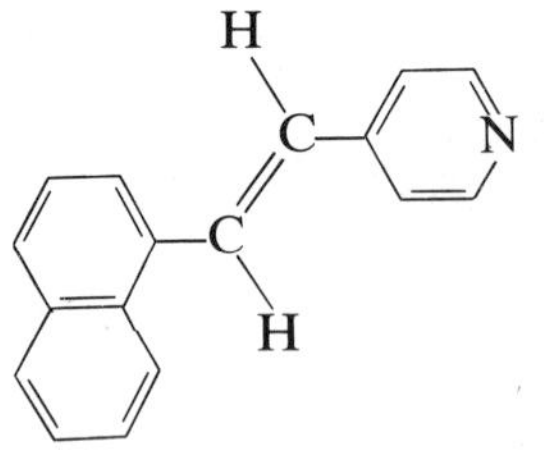

46.**9**

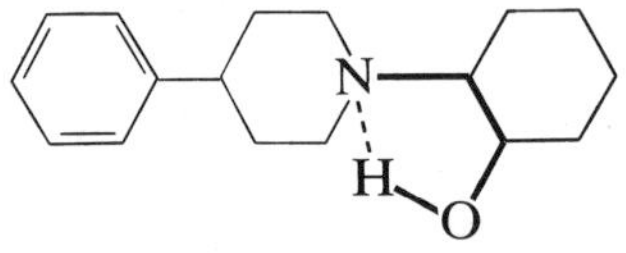

46.**10**

however, and also appears to have a direct effect on muscle contraction (18). To date, no substance that specifically inhibits the enzyme *in vivo* has emerged.

3.3　Acetylcholine Storage

The principal storage sites of acetylcholine in the nerve terminals consist of small vesicles (19–21). These are small cellular bodies with phospholipid membranes about 40–50 nm in diameter, which are visible by electron microscopy (22) in the axoplasm of the nerve terminals (Fig. 46.1). Similar vesicles have been separated from nervous tissue of the electric organ of *Torpedo* by homogenization and centrifugation, and the separated vesicles shown to contain some 80% of the acetylcholine present in the preparation (23). Experiments with rat (24) and snake (25) muscle show that each vesicle contains some 9000–10,000 molecules of acetylcholine.

The vesicles also contain ATP, prostagladin (26), and a soluble acidic protein, *vesiculin* (27), of molecular weight about 10,000, which probably serves to bind the positively charged acetylcholine in a stable form. Vesicular-bound acetylcholine, unlike that present in the axoplasm, is protected from hydrolysis by acetylcholinesterase (28).

3.4　Acetylcholine Release

Even in the absence of nerve stimulation, small amounts of acetylcholine are steadily and continuously released at the nerve terminals in discrete amounts or quanta (29), each quantum being considered to correspond to the rupture of a single storage vesicle. Acetylcholine so released produces a continuous series of miniature end plate potentials, each leading to depolarization of the postjunctional membrane. The depolarization produced by these mini potentials, however, is too small to initiate muscular contraction.

In contrast, stimulation of the motor nerve and receipt of the nerve impulse lead to the simultaneous release of some 4.2×10^6 molecules of acetylcholine (24) with the disruption and disappearance (21) of around 200–400 vesicles (23) in each axon terminal. The precise mechanism of vesicle disruption and acetylcholine release is still not fully understood. Electron microscopy, however, shows that the vesicles become concentrated in parallel bands close to the terminal membrane at *release sites* which lie opposite the folds in the muscle membrane (30–32). Arrival of the nerve impulse at the axon terminal depolarizes the terminal membrane, increasing its permeability to Ca^{2+} ions. This permits a rapid buildup of calcium ion concentration to the threshold value of $10^{-6} M$, which is essential for vesicle disruption (33). In this, Ca^{2+} is specific. Only Sr^{2+} can replace it, and it is about 100 times less effective (34, 35), whereas Mg^{2+} and a number of other ions (Be^{2+}, Mn^{2+}, and La^{2+}) competitively antagonize the action of Ca^{2+} in promoting vesicle disruption (36, 37).

Calcium ion activation promotes fusion of the vesicles with the axon terminal membrane, with concomitant release of their contents into the synaptic cleft. This is the first step in a cycle of events (Fig. 46.2). It is followed by invagination and infolding of the terminal membrane to produce new

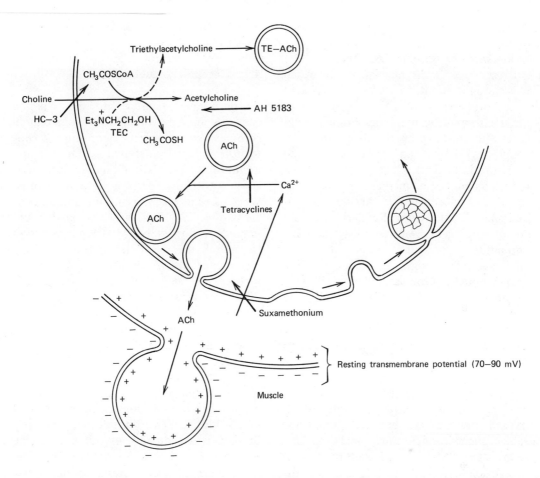

Fig. 46.2 Biosynthesis, storage and release of acetylcholine and their inhibition at the motor end plate.

vesicles which break off in clusters to migrate away from the inside of the membrane (38, 39).

It has been suggested that the role of calcium ions in stimulating fusion of the vesicles with the terminal membrane lies in a specific ability to neutralize the surface negative charge of the vesicles (40) which in the resting phase of the nerve ensures their repulsion (41, 42) from the negatively charged inner surface of the terminal membrane. There are good physico-chemical grounds for this view. Thus the distribution of gangliosides in aqueous lipid systems is influenced by Ca^{2+} ion concentrations (43) in the same way as the addition of cations promotes the aggregation of anionic detergent micelles (44). Similar effects have also been observed with negatively charged liposomes (45), the synthetic phospholipid-based cellular structures for which high body clearance rates have been ascribed to charge neutralization by Ca^{2+} ions and consequent aggregation. There is good reason to suppose, therefore, that the rise in axoplasmic Ca^{2+} ion concentration following membrane depolarization similarly promotes complexation, leading to changes in the orientation of phospholipids in the vesicle membrane which promote fusion with the terminal membrane.

Irrespective of the mechanism by which it is brought about, loss of surface charge would promote fusion of the vesicles with the depolarized terminal membrane. In accord with this hypothesis, drugs that uncouple oxidative phosphorylation, and therefore induce release of Ca^{2+} ions from mitochondria, also increase spontaneous release of acetylcholine at the neuromuscular junction (46). Similarly, calcium complexing agents, such as the tetracycline antibiotics, inhibit the release of acetylcholine, and in high doses can cause a prejunctional neuromuscular block (47).

Other substances act elsewhere in the life cycle of the vesicles blocking the process whereby they are refilled with acetylcholine from the axoplasm. The base AH 5183 (46.**10**) appears to act in this way, though part of its action is also postjunctional (48, 49). It is interesting, therefore, to note that in its most probable conformation its oxygen and nitrogen functions adopt the same gauche configuration (46.**11**) as that seen in the NMR-derived conformation of acetylcholine (46.**12**; R = H; 50) and the crystal structure of (S)-(+)-acetyl-β-methylcholine (46.**12**; R = CH$_3$; 51; 52).

4　ACTION AND FATE OF RELEASED ACETYLCHOLINE

4.1　Receptor Combination

Acetylcholine released into the synaptic cleft by nerve stimulation immediately combines with a specific lipoprotein receptor on the postjunctional surface of the motor end plate. Combination of acetylcholine with the receptors is accompanied by changes in receptor and membrane conformation (19). This causes a massive and immediate flow of Na^+ and K^+ ions across the muscle membrane through the opening of ion channels, which results in a transient increase in membrane conductance (53, 29). The inward movement of Na^+ ions and much smaller and slower outward movement of K^+ ions amount to a minimum net flow of 3000 univalent cations per acetylcholine molecule released (25). The ionic imbalance lowers the normal negative charge on the inside of the muscle membrane, thereby reducing the normal resting end plate 70–90 mV (inside negative) potential. This reduction of potential is the so-called end plate depolarization (54). The time scale of these events from acetylcholine release to depolarization is of the order of 0.5 msec.

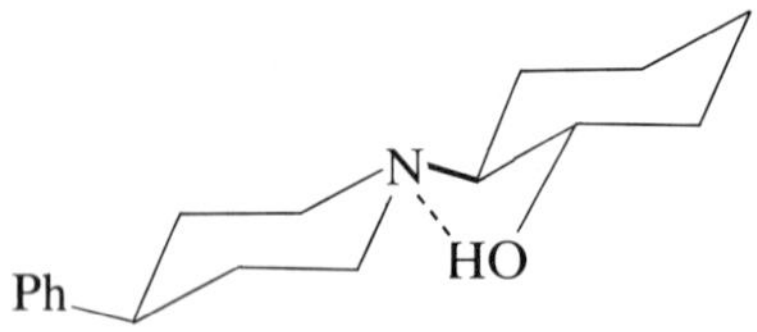

46.**10**

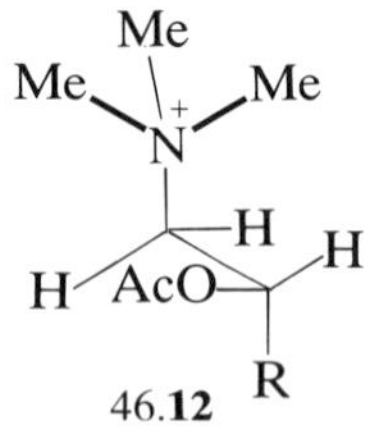

46.**12**

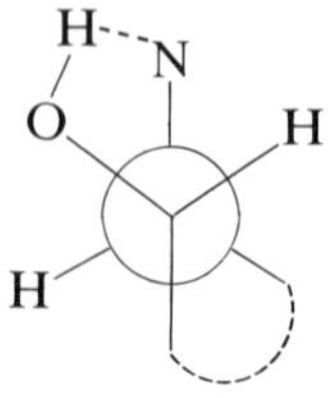

46.**11**

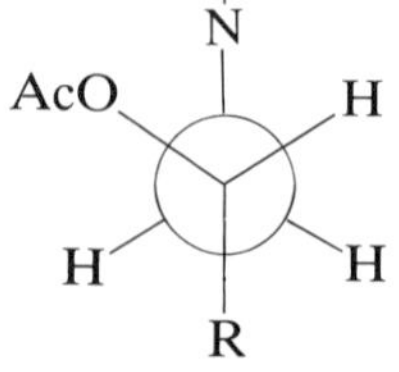

46.**12**

4.2   Muscle Contraction

Depolarization of the motor end plate region by acetylcholine creates a center at
lower electrical potential than the surrounding muscle membrane. Provided a
critical threshold level of depolarization is
achieved, current flows from the adjacent
higher potential areas toward the depolarized end plate (Fig. 46.3, A). In consequence, the effect of the initially localized end
plate depolarization is transmitted outward
over the muscle membrane, increasing permeability first to Na$^+$ and then to K$^+$ ions.
This movement of ions across the muscle
membrane is such that the potential difference between muscle and end plate is
rapidly and completely reversed (Fig. 46.3,
B) before fading to zero. The rapid passage of
this self-propagating action potential over
the muscle fiber membrane sets off the
contraction mechanism.

4.3   Nature and Isolation of
Acetylcholine Receptors

The nature of acetylcholine receptors has
been established not only by experiments
on mammalian nerve–muscle preparations,
but also on the electric tissue of the giant
South American freshwater eel, *Electrophorus electricus*, and that of the gaint electric ray, *Torpedo marmorata*. The electric
organs in these fish are developed from
embryonic tissue similar to that which gives
rise to muscle. They consist, however, almost completely of large flat cells, known
as electroplaques, which are innervated and
stimulated by acetylcholine in the same way
as skeletal muscle. These electroplaques
also respond to other cholinergic receptor
agonists, and their response is inhibited by
the same antagonists that block neuromuscular transmission in mammals. As in
skeletal muscle, receipt of a nervous im-

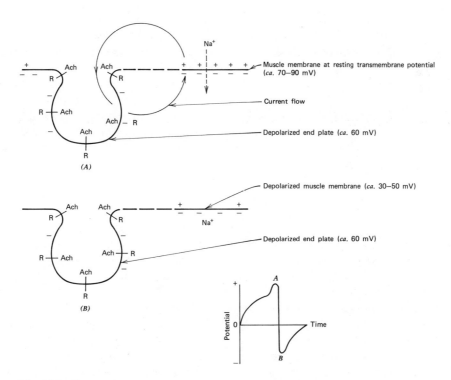

Fig. 46.3   Current flow across muscle membrane and potential difference–time curves.

pulse at the nerve–electroplaque junction stimulates the release of acetylcholine, causing a massive ion flow across the electroplaque membrane which is responsible for the generation of a net electric current flow.

In contrast to the mammalian neuromuscular junction, where despite the large number of cholinergic receptors the actual amounts of receptor tissue are very small, fish electric tissue provides an extremely rich source of receptor protein. This is especially high in *Torpedo marmorata* where the concentration of receptors is so great that all the current generated flows directly through the acetylcholine receptor channels. In *Electrophorus electricus*, however, although the proportion of electric to nonelectric tissue is much higher, the density of receptors is lower. The electroplaques, therefore, resemble muscle more in that the acetylcholine–receptor response is merely the trigger that opens the ion channels and induces current flow elsewhere in the postsynaptic membrane.

The earliest attempts to isolate and purify cholinergic receptor protein capable of reacting specifically with typical agonists and antagonists were only partially successful (55–57). The discovery that the venom of certain crotalid and elapid snakes is irreversibly bound to isolated electroplax tissue (56, 57, 2), blocking the normal acetylcholine-induced depolarization, provided a much more effective tool for receptor isolation. α-Bungarotoxin (α-BGT) from the Taiwan banded krait, *Bungaris multicinctus*, radiolabeled with ^{131}I, has been used as a marker in the isolation of lipid-soluble receptor protein fractions from *Torpedo marmorata* (58) and frog, rat, and mouse (59, 60) neuromuscular tissue. Solubilization of toxin-tagged receptor homogenates from *Torpedo* with the detergent Triton-X 100 gave a series of protein fractions separable by gel filtration (58). The labeled α-Bgt–receptor protein complex

eluted ahead of acetylcholinesterase, indicating its molecular weight to be somewhat greater than that of the enzyme (mol wt 240,000), whereas deaggregation in sodium dodecylsulfate revealed the existence of α-Bgt–receptor protein fractions of mol wt 88,000 and 180,000, respectively. Allowing for the molecular weight (7983) of α-Bgt (61), these results were interpreted as implying that the purified cholinergic receptor lipoprotein is isolable with Triton-X 100 as a tetramer of apparent mol wt 320,000, capable of dissociation in sodium dodecylsulfate to a monomer and dimer.

More highly purified receptor protein has been obtained by affinity chromatography (62) of similar fractions, from *Electrophorus electricus*, solubilized with Triton-X 100. These were absorbed on 1,3-bis(trimethylammoniumethoxy) - 4 - iodoacetamidobenzene diiodide (an analog of gallamine) linked to Sepharose 2B, and eluted with gallamine (63), to give a purified product with a specific activity of 5400 nmol of *Naja nigricollis* ^{3}H-α-toxin binding site per gram of protein, and an apparent mol wt of 230,000 by detergent extraction. Dissociation of this purified protein in the presence of sodium dodecylsulfate shows the presence on polyacrylamide electrophoresis of two subunits of mol wt 45,000 and 54,000, respectively (64). Similar subunit mol wts between 40,000 and 45,000 have also been reported for fractions isolated with the aid of ^{3}H-α-toxin (65) and specific affinity reagent (66) labels.

Cross-linking experiments with suberimidate (67) also suggest the presence of two distinct types of subunit in the native receptor protein. Semiquantitative assessment of their relative proportions is consistent with an associated (quaternary) structure composed of five subunits, three of mol wt 45,000 and two of 54,000 (64), which electron microscopy shows to be arranged in rosette-like structures. Purified receptor protein from *Torpedo californica* has likewise been shown to consist of four subunits (mol wt 39,000, 48,000, 58,000, and 64,000) in association, of which only the subunit with mol wt 39,000 exclusively binds specific receptor site affinity labels (68). It is perhaps also significant that even the purest receptor protein fractions from *Electrophorus electricus* when bound either to ^{3}H-α-toxin or ^{3}H-decamethonium are capable only of partial dissociation to units of mol wt 100,000 or 150,000 which closely combine two or more lower molecular weight subunits (63, 64, 69).

4.4   Density and Life-Span of Acetylcholine Receptors

Radiolabeled α-bungarotoxin has also been used to determine the number and distribution of receptors. In this way, rat and mouse diaphragm preparations have been shown to have about 4×10^7 and $2-3 \times 10^7$ acetylcholine binding sites (receptors) per end plate, respectively (70). These figures compare favorably with that found by autoradiography in mouse diaphragm (71) using the depolarizing neuromuscular blocking agent ^{14}C-decamethonium (7.5×10^7), but significantly are some 10 times greater than that found from similar autoradiographic experiments with the nondepolarizing blocking agents ^{14}C-curarine (4×10^6) and ^{14}C-toxiferine (4×10^6). Thus we have a situation in which each nerve stimulation leads to the release of some 4×10^6 molecules of acetylcholine (24) at each axon terminal in proximity to some 4×10^7 receptor sites.

Experiments with inhibitors of protein synthesis on denervated muscle *in vivo* (72) and in tissue culture (73) show that individual receptors have a finite life, and that whereas the turnover rate of receptors may be measured in days in adult muscle, in developing muscle the half-life may be no more than some 90 min (74).

4.5   Receptor Protein Characteristics

Similarity in the properties (75) and amino acid constituents (63) of purified acetylcholine receptor protein and acetylcholinesterase forms the basis of speculation that the anionic, cation-binding subsite for acetylcholine is similarly constituted, if not actually structurally and stereochemically identical (76, 77) in the two proteins. The relatively high proportion of glutamate and aspartate residues present in the purified cholinergic receptor protein (63) lends support to the view, widely held but experimentally unproved, that the anionic center is constituted just as it is believed to be in acetylcholinesterase (78, 79). The topography of the acetylcholine receptor site and its behavior in response to agonists and antagonists has been largely defined by the combination of two complementary methods of approach. These are founded on the one hand on the technique of specific affinity labeling developed by Karlin and his collaborators, and on the other hand on the synthesis and study of specific antagonists of defined structure and stereochemistry, which are described in the latter part of this chapter.

Del Castillo and Katz (80) noted that the cholinergic receptor is inactivated by heavy metals, a response that is often but not necessarily associated with the presence of sulfhydryl (SH) or chemically related groups. The presence in close proximity to the receptor anionic subsite of a readily reducible disulfide (—S—S—) group was established by Karlin and Bartels (81) in experiments which showed that the response of the electroplax of *Electrophorus electricus* to acetylcholine and other agonists is specifically inhibited by prior exposure to dithiothreitol (DTT; 46.**13**; 82). This inhibition, however, is completely reversed by subsequent treatment with the sulfhydryl oxidizing agent, 5,5'-dithiobis(2-nitrobenzoate) (DTNB; 46.**14**; 83), but is sus-

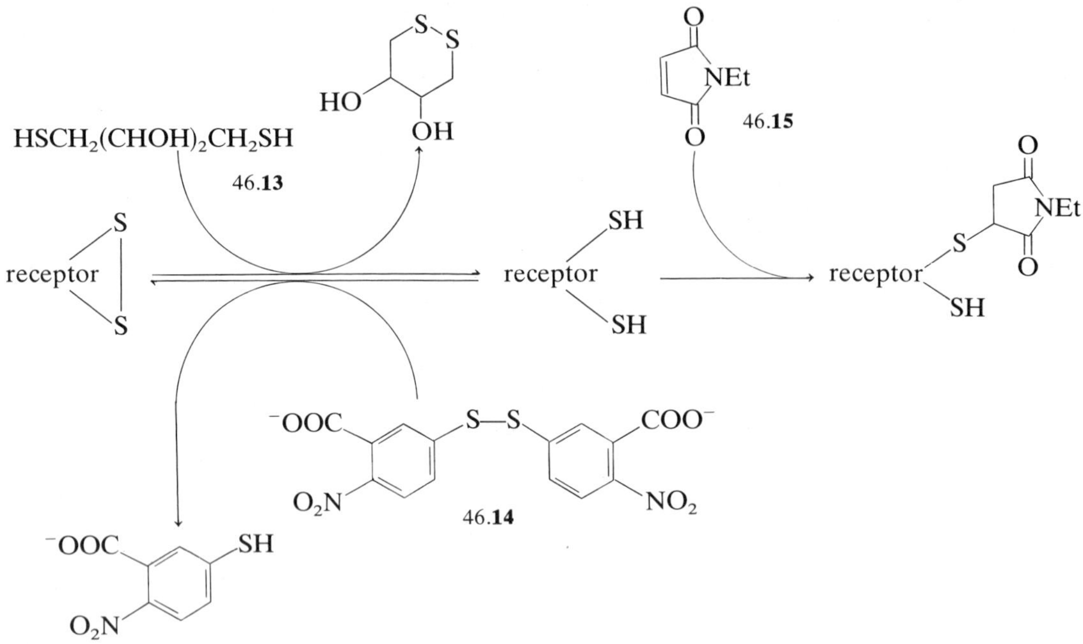

HSCH$_2$(CHOH)$_2$CH$_2$SH

46.**13**

46.**15**

receptor

receptor

receptor

46.**14**

tained by application of the sulfhydryl blocking agent N-ethylmaleimide (NEM; 46.**15**).

Maleimide derivatives which incorporate the electroplax depolarizing phenyltrimethylammonium group (84), such as 4-(N-maleimido) phenyltrimethylammonium iodide (MPTA; 46.**16**; 85), 4-(N-maleimido)benzyltrimethylammonium iodide (MBTA; 46.**17**; 86), and related compounds, have provided a sensitive method for mapping the relationship between the anionic and disulfide receptor subsites. Thus in the absence of prior SS-bond reduction with DTT, both MPTA and MBTA are merely competitive receptor inhibitors. Reaction of such compounds with the DTT-reduced receptors, however, shows that combination of a quaternary ammonium group and a sulfhydryl-reactive double bond in the same molecule leads not only to irreversible inhibition but also to a substantial enhancement in the rate of reaction with the DTT-reduced disulfide group over that of N-ethylmaleimide.

There is some evidence that changes in

receptor response following DTT reduction of the receptor subsite are brought about by changes in receptor conformation. Thus reduction and alkylation of the SS-bond receptor subsite lead not only to complete inhibition of the normal agonist response to acetylcholine, but also to a similar inhibition in response to other receptor agonists, such as carbamylcholine and, to a lesser extent, tetramethylammonium. In contrast, however, response to the depolarizing neuromuscular blocking agent decamethonium is increased after receptor reduction, but decreased by subsequent alkylation or reoxidation. Also, hexamethonium, which is a competitive inhibitor of acetylcholine at the electroplax and a weak neuromuscular blocking agent at vertebrate neuromuscular junctions, partially protects DTT-reduced receptors against alkylation by MPTA (85, 86) and MBTA (86, 87). However, since alkylation of reduced receptors by NEM is not slowed by hexamethonium, its hindrance to SH alkylation must be due solely to competition at the anionic subsite. Nonetheless, in contrast to its action as a weak competitive inhibitor of acetylcholine at native cholinergic receptors, hexamethonium acts as an agonist, causing depolarization of DTT-reduced receptors. Moreover, reoxidation of the DTT-reduced receptors or NEM alkylation restores the receptors to their native specificity in response to hexamethonium.

The conclusion that these changes in receptor response are linked to corresponding changes in receptor conformation is supported by correlation of the properties of the maleimide affinity reagents with their molecular dimensions. Thus their potency as agonists of DTT-reduced receptors, as measured by depolarization, increases (Table 46.1) as the intramolecular distance between the reactive double bond and the quaternary ammonium group decreases (86). The powerful agonistic response to bromoacetylcholine bromide (46.**18**) and *p*-nitrophenyl 4-*NN*-dimethylaminobezoate methiodide (46.**19**) in which the subsite-reactive groups are only 9.4 and 9.0 Å apart, respectively, supports the general conclusion that this latter subsite spacing is characteristic of the active agonist-sensitive conformation of reduced receptors. Hexamethonium, with a similar inter-onium group spacing is clearly capable of holding reduced receptors in the same active conformation by ionic bonding at both subsites.

The further conclusion that lack of agonistic activity in maleimide derivatives with a 12 Å separation of subsite-reactive groups is attributable to an inactive reduced receptor conformation however, is less well founded. Firstly, there is no certainty that the same sulfhydryl group is involved in all the reactions. Secondly, it fails to account rationally for the enhanced depolarizing (agonistic) activity of decamethonium in a way that is entirely consistent with the response to hexamethonium, since it is assumed that both compounds react with the same sulfhydryl group but with chain shortening and bending only in the case of decamethonium. Notwithstanding these uncertainties, affinity labeling of DTT-reduced receptors provides a useful insight into the behavior and topography of the native cholinergic receptor site.

Although the presence of an SS-bond receptor subsite in close proximity to the anionic subsite is clearly established, there is no evidence to suggest that this bond or its cleavage plays any direct part in agonist–receptor interaction at the neuromuscular junction. Karlin (86), however, suggests reasonably that noncovalently bound agonists of native receptors, such as acetylcholine, align themselves with the receptor subsites in a way that resembles the bridging of DTT-reduced receptor subsites by MBTA (46.**17**) and other agonistic affinity labels. It is further inferred that the disulfide bridge functions merely as a conformation stabilizer for an adjacent hydrophobic bonding subsite. Evidence for the involvement of such a hydrophobic subsite comes not only from the lack of depolarizing activity in choline (46.**3**), which in contrast to acetylcholine (46.**4**) would be repelled from hydrophobic sites (88), but also from the increasing potency of alkyltrimethylammonium compounds with increasing alkyl chain length (89–92).

The idea that receptor activity is associated with changes in tertiary structure (conformation) of the receptor protein is supported by fluorescence probe studies (93) with 1-anilinonaphthalene-8-sulfonic acid (ANS) on native electroplax tissue. This compound, which is reversibly bound to excitable electroplax tissue, shows an increase in fluorescence intensity during the generation of action potentials, which parallels the increase in membrane potential and reflects corresponding changes in membrane conformation. Binding experiments with purified receptor protein from *Electrophorus electricus* (94, 63) and receptor-rich fragments from *Torpedo marmorata* (95) also support the view that agonists cooperatively stabilize the receptor

Table 46.1   Relative Reaction Rates of Affinity Reagents with DTT-Reduced Receptors, Intramolecular Distances, and Agonist Activity

Compound[a]	Relative Reaction Rate	Intramolecular Distance between SH-Reactive Group and Me_3N^+ Group, Å	Agonist Activity (Depolarization, mV)
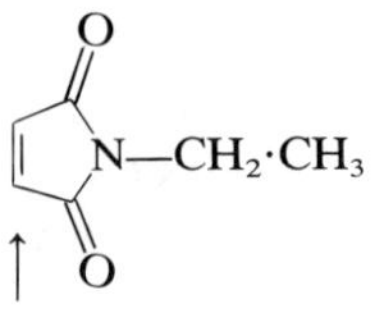 (maleimide)N—$CH_2 \cdot CH_3$ **46.15**	1	—	—
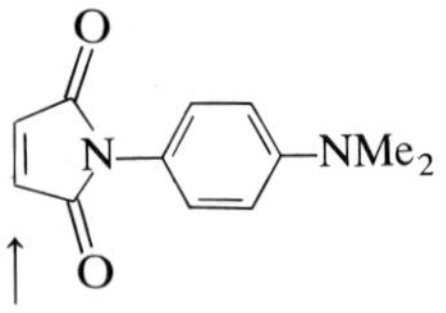 (maleimide)N—(C$_6$H$_4$)—NMe_2	0.6	—	—
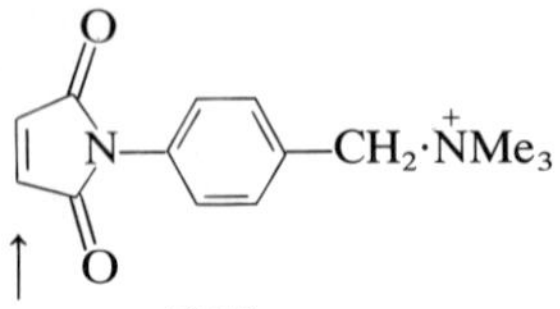 (maleimide)N—(C$_6$H$_4$)—$CH_2 \cdot \overset{+}{N}Me_3$ **46.17**	1100	12.0	0
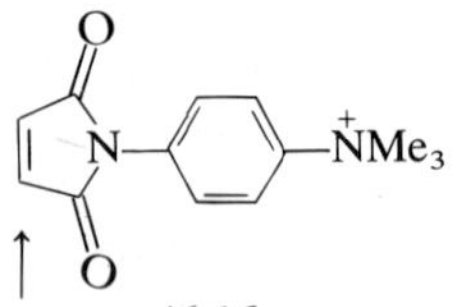 (maleimide)N—(C$_6$H$_4$)—$\overset{+}{N}Me_3$ **46.16**	460	11.3	1
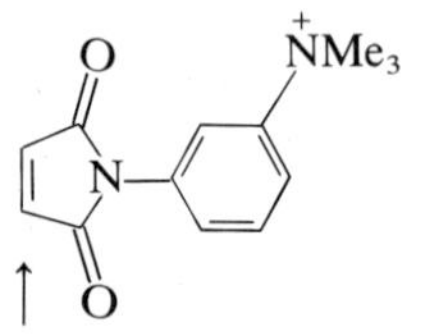 (maleimide)N—(C$_6$H$_4$)—$\overset{+}{N}Me_3$ (meta)	270	10.6	2
$BrCH_2 \cdot CO \cdot OCH_2 \cdot CH_2\overset{+}{N}Me_3Br^-$ **46.18**	b	9.4	30
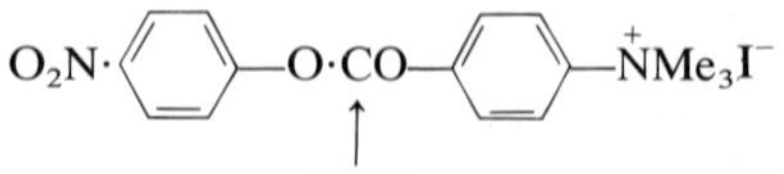 $O_2N \cdot$(C$_6$H$_4$)—$O \cdot CO$—(C$_6$H$_4$)—$\overset{+}{N}Me_3I^-$ **46.19**	b	9.0	30

[a] Arrow indicates SH-reactive group.
[b] Not measured.

444

protein in a conformation which promotes high agonist affinity. Thus pretreatment of solubilized receptor preparations with carbamylcholine progressively decreases the rate at which *Naja nigricolla* ^{3}H-α-toxin is bound, with at the same time a marked parallel increase in receptor affinity for carbamylcholine. It appears, therefore, that in the resting state the receptor protein exists in a low agonist affinity conformation, and that cholinergic agonists regulate their own affinity through stabilization of an alternative high affinity conformation.

Changes in the quaternary structure of the cholinergic receptor protein affecting its dissociation into subunits (64–66) are also implicated in the receptor mechanism for the creation of ion channels (96, 84). Even in the purest receptor protein the molecular weight per ^{3}H-α-toxin or ^{3}H-decamethonium binding site is never less than, 100,000–150,000 (64), suggesting that these compounds form molecular bridges linking receptor subunits and in this way inhibit both receptor $\rightleftharpoons$ subunit dissociation and the creation of ion channels.

The similarity in behavior of the snake venoms to that of relatively simple bis-onium compounds such as decamethonium is clarified by the elucidation of the complete amino acid sequences of α-bungarotoxin (97, 61, 98) and the cobra toxins (99–105). These proteins, which range in length from some 61 to 74 amino acids units, have a number of molecular features in common. They are characterized by the possession of multiple (four to six) disulfide bridges, which stabilize the molecule in a conformation essential for activity. Thus reduction of the disulfide bridges in native Formosan cobra toxin with β-mercaptoethanol results in a major conformational change from a right-handed α-helix to a random coil structure, which is accompanied by complete loss of lethal (neuromuscular blocking) activity (106, 107). Moreover, both conformation, as determined by ORD measurements, and lethal activity are re-

stored by reoxidation. A second and seemingly equally important common feature of all these neuromuscular blocking snake venoms is the possession of at least one and frequently two or more sets of adjacent strongly basic amino acid units as, for example, in α-bungarotoxin (^{25}Arg–^{26}Lys; ^{51}Lys–^{52}–Lys; ^{70}Lys–^{71}Arg; Refs. 97, 61, 98), the integrity of which is relevant to blocking potency (105). Each pair of adjacent basic amino acids is therefore capable of binding to and bridging across receptor subunits in exactly the same way as simple bisquaternary ammonium neuromuscular blocking agents (64) such as tubocurarine (46.**30**, R = H) and decamethonium (46.**32**; $n = 10$), thereby blocking the normal response to acetylcholine.

4.6   Termination of Acetylcholine Action

A considerable body of indirect evidence exists to suggest that enzymatic hydrolysis rather than acetylcholine–receptor dissociation is the rate-controlling step in terminating transmitter function. Thus decay of the end plate current is more rapid than diffusion of acetylcholine out of the synaptic cleft (108), whereas the action of acetylcholine is prolonged in the presence of cholinesterase inhibitors such as neostigmine (109, 110). Waser (71) has demonstrated by autoradiographic studies with the anticholinesterases ^{32}P-DFP and ^{14}C-DFP on mouse diaphragm that acetylcholinesterase is located in specific sites facing onto the junctional cleft on the surface of the postjunctional membrane. These same studies showed the presence of some 2.4×10^7 cholinesterase centres per motor end plate, i.e., in equal numbers to and in close proximity to the acetylcholine receptors. Grob and co-workers (111–114) have also described the isolation from human skeletal muscle of a ribonucleoprotein with potent anticholinesterase activity, which is also precipitable *in vitro* by tubocurarine at neuromuscular blocking concentrations and resolubilized by tubocurarine antagonists.

Equally, there is a significant body of evidence that indicates beyond doubt that anticholinesterase activity and cholinergic receptor activity reside in discrete units of the postsynaptic membrane. Thus, although α-bungarotoxin binds irreversibly (115) to the acetylcholine receptor, it does not bind to acetylcholinesterase (116). Similarly, the receptor is blocked by sulfhydryl-sensitive reagents (117, 118), but acetylcholinesterase is not (119), whereas enzymatic digest studies have shown that collagenase is capable of abolishing the cholinesterase activity of the postsynaptic junctional membrane (120) by releasing acetylcholinesterase into solution.

5 STRUCTURE–ACTIVITY RELATIONSHIPS

Although the acetylcholine receptor has been partially characterized by receptor protein studies, many aspects of the molecular events that follow agonist–receptor association are still unresolved. Detailed structural and stereochemical studies have, however, established a number of well-defined parameters, which are essential requirements of drugs capable of inducing neuromuscular blockade.

5.1 History

The effects of neuromuscular blocking agents were first recorded in 1510 by Pieter Martyr d'Anglera, who described the use of poisoned arrows by South American Indians in attacks on travelers in the Amazon region (121). These poisons were described in 1596 by one of Sir Walter Raleigh's lieutenants, Keymis, as *ourari*. This term, which is related to the modern word *curare*, is said to be derived from *eor*, meaning to kill, and *uira*, a bird, in South American

Indian tongue, and hence is descriptive of the traditional use of arrow poisons in hunting. The poisons, which are soft extracts prepared from the bark of various trees of *Strychnos* and *Chondodendron* species, were recognized as being of two distinct types distinguished by the containers in which they are packed and known as *tube*, and *calabash* curare, respectively.

It was not until the middle of the nineteenth century that the work of Claude Bernard (122, 123) established the site of action of curare as the neuromuscular junction by demonstrating that both nerve and muscle remain separately excitable after curarization. Within a few years, the realization that curare extracts contain quaternary ammonium salts prompted Crum Brown and Fraser (124, 125) to examine the effects of other similar compounds, and show that the methiodides of atropine, brucine, codeine, coniine, morphine, strychnine, and thebaine all produce similar paralytic action. The work of Hunt and Renshaw (126) and Ing and Wright (127, 89), however, established that the ability to produce neuromuscular block is not confined to quaternary ammonium salts (46.**20**), and that other strongly cationic compounds, including sulfonium (46.**21**), phosphonium (46.**22**), arsonium (46.**23**), and stibonium (46.**24**) salts exhibit similar properties.

$$R_4\overset{+}{N}X^- \qquad Me_3\overset{+}{S}X^- \qquad Me_4\overset{+}{P}X^-$$
$$46.\mathbf{20} \qquad\quad 46.\mathbf{21} \qquad\quad 46.\mathbf{22}$$

$$Me_4\overset{+}{As}X^- \qquad Me_4\overset{+}{Sb}X^-$$
$$46.\mathbf{23} \qquad\qquad 46.\mathbf{24}$$

5.2 Bonding Characteristics

Holmes et al. (128) showed that the ability of simple onium ions to block frog sartorius muscle is related to the charge density of the central onium ion, on the assumption that the charge distribution depends on electronegativity differences between the central onium atom and alkyl carbon, and the electron-repelling properties of the alkyl substituent. Thus with dipole moment as the criterion of charge distribution over the N–H($\xrightarrow{1.31}$), S–H($\xrightarrow{0.68}$), P–H($\xrightarrow{0.36}$), and As–H($\xleftarrow{0.10}$) bonds, curariform potency runs parallel to the charge density on the onium ion. Similarly, the electron-repelling power of alkyl substituents Me > Pr > Et determines the potency order of tetramethylammonium > tetra-n-propylammonium > tetraethylammonium ions. Studies of complex metal ions have also shown that in the series of ammono– and ethylenediamine–cobalt complexes,

$$[Co(NH_3)_6]^{3+}, \quad [Co(en)_3]^{3+},$$

$$[Co(NH_3)_5(NO_2)]^{2+}, \quad [Co(NH_3)_4(NO_2)_2]^+,$$

and $[Co(NH_3)_2(NO_2)_4]^-$, only the cationic complexes are active, and decreasing peripheral charge on the complex cation is associated with decreasing neuromuscular blocking potency (129).

Other factors in addition to charge density are important in determining the level of potency of simple onium compounds. These include secondary binding characteristics due to hydrophobic interactions, van der Waals bonding, charge-transfer complexing, and stereochemical factors affecting antagonist–receptor association. Thus the increasing potency of alkyltrimethylammonium compounds with increasing alkyl chain length (89–91) reflects the increasing influence of hydrophobic effects. Similarly, the greater potency of complex metal ions embodying such heteroaromatic amines as 2,2′-bipyridyl and 1,10–phenanthroline in place of aliphatic diamines or ammonia can be ascribed to the greater propensity of flat heteroaromatic molecules to engage in van der Waals bonding and charge-transfer complexing.

5.3 Stereochemistry

The influence of stereochemistry in and around the quaternary ammonium ion is evident in the potency difference shown by optical enantiomers (46.**25**) of the molecularly asymmetric complexes [Ru(1,10-phenanthroline)$_3$]$^{2+}$, [Ni(1,10-phenanthroline)$_3$]$^{2+}$, and [Os(1,10-phenanthroline)$_3$]$^{2+}$, of which the (+) isomers are some 1.5–2 times more potent than the corresponding (−) isomers in both the toad rectus abdominis and rat diaphragm preparations (129).

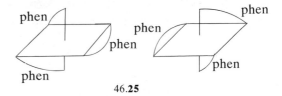

46.**25**

Similarly, the β isomers in a series of N,N-dialkyl-D-coniinium and N,N-dialkyl-L-conhydrinium ions (130), in which the N-benzyl group on the asymmetric quaternary nitrogen is equatorial (131), are all more potent than their corresponding axial α isomers. In this respect the more active isomers adopt conformations about nitrogen which parallel those of the more active isomers of N-ethyl-N-methyltetrahydropapaverinium iodides, in which the larger substituent is also equatorial.

Stereochemical requirements at the centers immediately adjacent to the quaternary nitrogen atom are still incompletely resolved. Thus, whereas (S) isomers of the monoquaternary compounds laudanosine methiodide (131, 132), laudanosine ethiodide (131), and glaucine methiodide (132) are more potent than the corresponding (R) isomers, the reverse is true in the norcoralydine methiodides (133). Somewhat surprisingly the (R,R) isomers of polymethylenebis- and related bisquaternary compounds incorporating laudanosinium (134), pavinium (135), and even simple alkyl groups (136) are more potent than their corresponding (*S,S*) isomers. Analysis of this complex situation is complicated by the flexibility of the laudanosinium and polymethylene bisquaternary compounds, but detailed interpretation (137) of agonist–receptor and antagonist–receptor interactions in the succinylbis-*α*- and *β*-methylcholines and the rigid norcoralydine methiodides, supported by conclusions based on a nonbiologic antagonist–receptor model (138), suggest that the recorded potency ratios are best accommodated by antagonist–receptor interaction at the right-hand and rear faces, where they are oriented as in 46.**12** and 46.**26**–46.**29**. Thus neuromuscular blocking potency compared to that of tubocurarine

(potency = 100) decreases in the order 46.**26** (potency = 13.6), 46.**27** (potency = 4.5), 46.**28** (potency = 3.2), 46.**29** (potency = 2.1) as steric hindrance to receptor association in the right-hand octants of these molecules (as drawn) increases.

This interpretation of antagonist–receptor stereochemistry also provides a rational explanation of the relative potencies of (+)-tubocurarine and the synthetic (+)-isotubocurarine (139), (+)-chondocurarine, and (+)- and (−)-curarines, which are discussed below.

5.4 Bisquaternary Salts

The isolation and structural studies of (+)-tubocurarine by King (140–143) provided

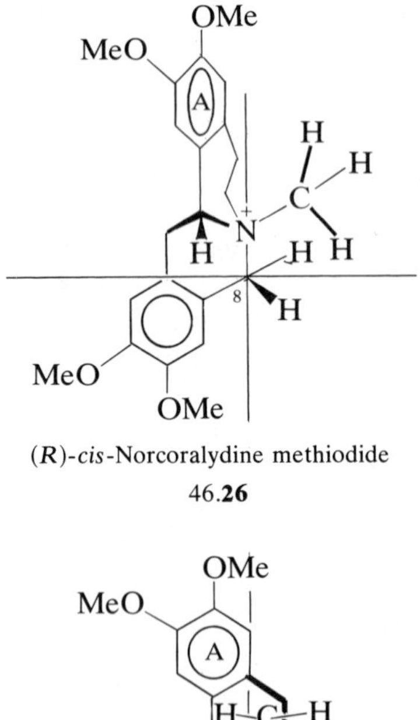

(*R*)-*cis*-Norcoralydine methiodide

46.**26**

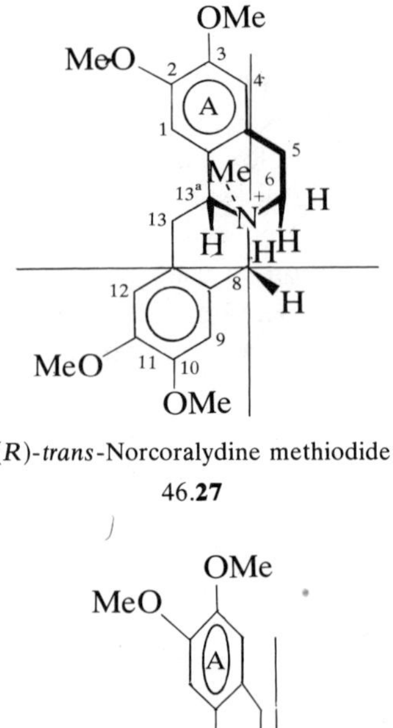

(*R*)-*trans*-Norcoralydine methiodide

46.**27**

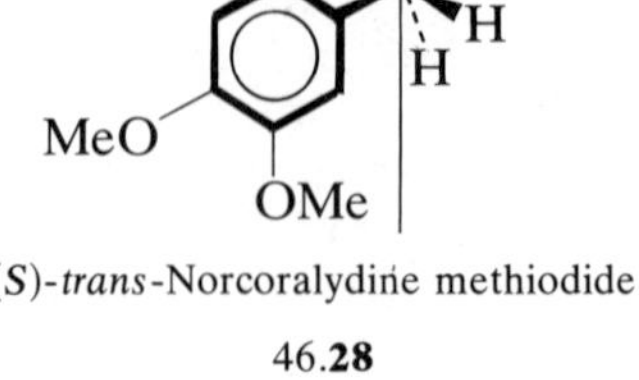

(*S*)-*trans*-Norcoralydine methiodide

46.**28**

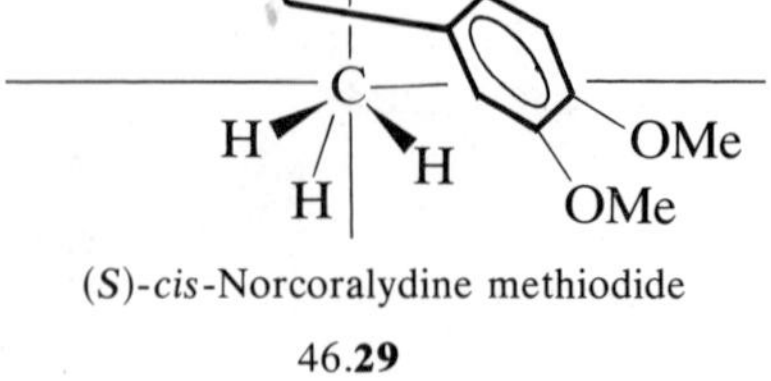

(*S*)-*cis*-Norcoralydine methiodide

46.**29**

the key to the development of clinically useful neuromuscular blocking agents. Although the structure assigned by King to (+)-tubocurarine was characterized and accepted for many years as the bisquaternary ammonium salt, 46.**30** (R = Me), the work of Everett et al. (144) has established that (+)-tubocurarine chloride is in fact the monoquaternary salt of structure 46.**30** (R = H, X = Cl), that the corresponding bisquaternary compound, 46.**30** (R = Me), is identical with the alkaloid chondocurarine, and the so-called dimethyltubocurarine is in fact O,O,N-trimethyltubocurarine, 46.**31**.

Identification of tubocurarine as a monoquaternary salt explains the deepening of neuromuscular block, which is observed when plasma pH is lowered by respiratory or metabolic acidosis (144a). Increased ionization of the tertiary amino nitrogen at lower pH increases the proportion of the drug present as the active dicationic species. Likewise, the small decrease in potency shown by tubocurarine with increased plasma pH under respiratory or metabolic alkalosis is probably a reflection of partial ionization of the free phenolic groups in the molecule. In contrast, the potency of the nonphenolic bisquaternary ammonium

compound O,O,N-trimethyltubocurarine is marginally decreased by acidosis and marginally increased by alkalosis to an extent compatible with the effect of pH on ionization of the plasma proteins, and with concomitant changes in drug–protein binding and the concentration of unbound drug.

The isolation of (+)-tubocurarine from tube curare not only established a source of pure material for use in surgery (1, 2), but also provided the stimulus and model for the synthetic variants, which were to follow. Considering the inherent difficulties in purifying and characterizing high molecular weight quaternary salts such as tubocurarine with the techniques available to King, the error in its identification as a bisquaternary salt is very understandable. In any event, this misidentification, although unfortunate for King, was indeed fortunate for pharmacology and medicine in that, although accidentally, it focused attention on the bis and polyquaternary salts which have proved so useful.

The significance of a bisquaternary ammonium structure was confirmed by the studies of Barlow and Ing (145, 146) and Paton and Zaimis (147), which demonstrated anticholinergic properties of the polymethylene bisquaternary ammonium

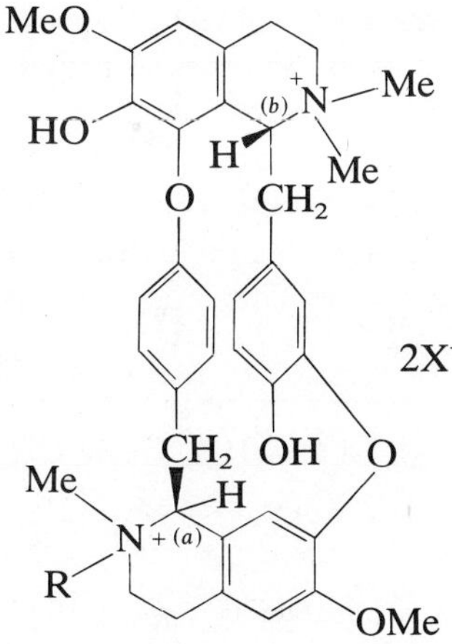

46.**30**

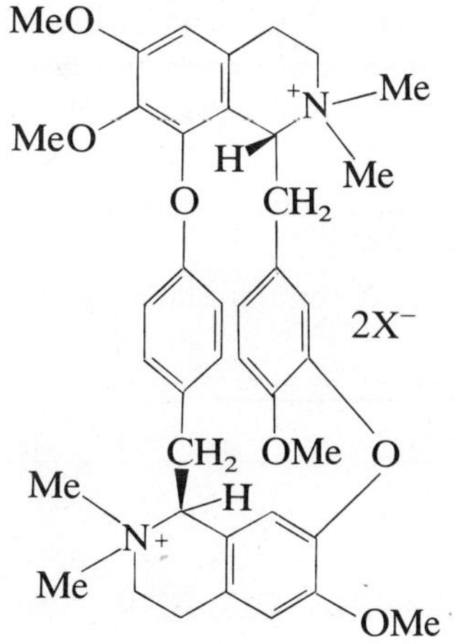

46.**31**

compounds, 46.**32**. Neuromuscular potency varies with chain length, rising from negligible levels in pentamethonium (46.**32**, $n = 5$) and hexamethonium (46.**32**, $n = 6$) to a maximum in decamethonium (46.**32**, $n = 10$), and thereafter declining again. In contrast, pentamethonium and hexamethonium are potent blockers of cholinergic transmission at sympathetic and parasympathetic ganglia (Chapter 44), a property that declines with increasing inter-onium distance to negligible levels in decamethonium.

5.5 Depolarizing Neuromuscular Blocking Agents

Despite its intrinsic resemblance to the tube curare alkaloids as a bisquaternary ammonium salt, decamethonium differs markedly from tubocurarine in the characteristics of the blockade that is produced at the neuromuscular junction. Thus block by decamethonium is accompanied by prolonged depolarization of the postjunctional membrane, which is similar to that produced when the action of acetylcholine is prolonged by the effects of cholinesterase inhibitors (148). Paralysis is preceded by muscle fasciculations and by potentiation of the maximum twitch tension (149). The action of decamethonium is prolonged, owing in part to its resistance to metabolism, and is characterized by penetration of the postsynaptic membrane (150) and nonreversibility by anticholinesterases such as neostigmine and edrophonium (149), which increase the local concentration of acetylcholine.

The distinction between depolarizing and curariform or antidepolarizing agents is complicated because in some animal species the block that is produced, although depolarizing at first, subsequently displays characteristics of antidepolarizing drugs. The two phases, described as phase I and phase II block, have been shown to be characteristic of block in the guinea pig (151), the rabbit (152), the soleus muscle of the cat (153), and in human subjects suffering from myasthenia gravis (154). Block by decamethonium in most other muscles of the cat and in healthy human subjects is purely depolarizing (phase I) and shows no phase II component (155).

The discovery of neuromuscular blocking activity in decamethonium revived interest in the isosteric suxamethonium chloride (46.**33**, $n = 2$, $m = 2$), which was first described in 1906 (156). Reexamination by Bovet and his collaborators (157) in 1949 revealed suxamethonium to be a potent, short-acting neuromuscular blocking agent. Similar properties are shown by its homologs and analogs, including the reversed esters (46.**34**) and monoesters (46.**35**), all of which show a similar distribution of potencies within the series (157, 158).

Interpolation of aromatic ester (159) and aromatic ether (160, 161) links in the center of the polymethylene chain of decamethonium also leads to compounds with depolarizing activity, but maximum potency occurs at somewhat greater inter-onium distances. The prime requirement for a depolarizing block in all these compounds is a molecule that is long and slender in shape, a characteristic that led Bovet and his collaborators (162) to describe them as *leptocurares*. This requirement is met in the

$$\overset{+}{Me_3N}(CH_2)_n \overset{+}{N}Me_3 \quad 2X^-$$

46.**32**

$$\overset{+}{Me_3N}(CH_2)_n OCO(CH_2)_m COO(CH_2)_n \overset{+}{N}Me_3 \quad 2X^-$$

46.**33**

$$\overset{+}{Me_3N}(CH_2)_n COO(CH_2)_m OCO(CH_2)_n \overset{+}{N}Me_3 \quad 2X^-$$

46.**34**

$$\overset{+}{Me_3N}(CH_2)_n COO(CH_2)_m \overset{+}{N}Me_3 \quad 2X^-$$

46.**35**

compounds 46.**32**–46.**35**, which have in common small quaternary head groups (trimethylammonium) and linking chains which are unbranched, particularly in close proximity to the onium groups. Any major departure from these requirements leads to a change in the characteristics of the block from depolarizing to antidepolarizing.

These strict structural requirements suggest that the anionic receptor is situated in some sort of pit or cleft on the receptor surface. Access to the cleft for anionic and hydrophobic bonding is essential for induction of the typical agonist response giving rise to conformational changes in the receptor protein, ion channeling, and depolarization. Chain branching and/or increase in N-alkyl group dimensions inhibit entry to the cleft. Compounds with such features are less tightly bound and hence unable to induce the conformational changes leading to depolarization. They can, however, deny access of acetylcholine to the receptors, and therefore act as competitive inhibitors.

5.6   Curariform (Antidepolarizing) Neuromuscular Blocking Agents

Block by tubocurarine differs from that induced by decamethonium and suxamethonium in that it is not accompanied by depolarization of the postsynaptic membrane. Such action is best described as *curariform*, though the term has unfortunately been carelessly misused in a wider sense by some authors to cover all neuromuscular blocking agents. Other terms that have been used to describe this particular type of block are *competitive*, *nondepolarizing*, or *antidepolarizing*. The action of such compounds is reversed by the action of anticholinesterases such as neostigmine and edrophonium which permit the buildup of sufficiently high localized concentrations of acetylcholine to displace the blocking agent (163, 164). In this sense there is competition between agonist and antagonist for the receptor site. The term *competitive*, however, has been criticized on the grounds that it could also be applied to depolarizing agents (165). Similar objections apply to the term *nondepolarizing* on the grounds that it fails to distinguish between compounds which act prejunctionally as opposed to postjunctionally (165, 166). The term *antidepolarizing* (167), although widely used, suffers also from the disadvantage that although the action of this class of drugs is not accompanied by depolarization, there is no evidence for postulating direct interference with the mechanism of depolarization at the molecular level.

The effects of different curariform agents are additive when coadministered, but they are antagonized by drugs that act by a depolarizing mechanism (168). Also, in contrast to depolarizing agents they do not penetrate the muscle membrane, and are displaced by high localized concentrations of acetylcholine when these are allowed to build up under the action of acetylcholinesterases (163). These properties are consistent with the much higher affinity of the end plate receptors for the small trimethylammonium head groups and elongated unbranched chain structures of the typical depolarizing agents compared with the characteristically large onium substituents and large inter-onium linking groups of the archetypal curariform compounds, tubocurarine and its derivatives 46.**30** and 46.**31**. Compounds with these distinctive structural features were described by Bovet and his collaborators (162) as *pachycurares*.

Modification of either the onium groups or the inter-onium chain of both decamethonium and suxamethonium in accord with these requirements leads to compounds with curariform action. Thus both decaethonium (46.**36**; 169) and suxaethonium (46.**37**; 157, 170) are less potent than the corresponding methonium compounds, and decaethonium has curariform activity (171).

$$\overset{+}{\text{Et}_3\text{N}}(\text{CH}_2)_{10}\overset{+}{\text{NEt}}_3 \quad 2\text{X}^-$$

46.**36**

$$\text{Et}_3\overset{+}{\text{N}}(\text{CH}_2)_2\text{OCO}(\text{CH}_2)_2\text{COO}(\text{CH}_2)_2\overset{+}{\text{NEt}}_3 \quad 2\text{X}^-$$

46.**37**

Similarly, replacement of one or more methyl groups at each end of decamethonium by much larger alkyl groups such as *n*-heptyl or *n*-decyl, also reduces potency and alters the mechanism of action from depolarizing to curariform (172). Suxaethonium has been used clinically (173), but is significantly less potent and of much shorter duration of action than suxamethonium owing to its more rapid hydrolysis by plasma cholinesterase (174). For this reason it has not found favor in practice, although postoperative pain has been reported to be less severe than with suxamethonium (175), an advantage that probably reflects its nondepolarizing mechanism of action.

Other ethonium and related compounds with similar properties include prodeconium bromide (46.**38**; 176–178), the linear polyethonium compounds (46.**39**; 179–186), gallamine (46.**40**; 187, 188). hexafluorenium (46.**41**; 189–191), and benzoquinonium (46.**42**; 192–194). Pro-

deconium has only about one-fifth the potency of decamethonium in man and is histamine-releasing, whereas the linear polyonium compounds were found to produce recurarization in some patients. Hexafluorenium (195) and benzoquinonium (194) are both potent anticholinesterases, and the level of this activity was too high for these compounds to be useful clinically. Of all these compounds, only gallamine has become established in clinical practice.

Incorporation of the quaternary ammonium groups into heterocyclic rings, which do not form part of the inter-onium structure, also leads to compounds with curariform activity. Numerous compounds of this type have been prepared. Heteroaromatic systems as in decamethylenebispyridinium, decamethylenebisquinolinium, and decamethylenebisisoquinolinium iodides all reduce potency markedly, but introduction of methoxyl groups in the bisquinolinium compounds restores activity

$$\text{Me}_2\overset{+}{\text{N}}(\text{CH}_2)_2\text{O}(\text{CH}_2)_{10}\text{O}(\text{CH}_2)_2\overset{+}{\text{NMe}}_2 \quad 2\text{Br}^-$$
$$| \qquad\qquad\qquad\qquad\qquad\qquad | $$
$$\text{CH}_2\text{COOPr} \qquad\qquad\qquad \text{CH}_2\text{COOPr}$$

46.**38**

$$\text{Et}_3\overset{+}{\text{N}}(\text{CH}_2)_6\overset{+}{\text{N}}(\text{CH}_2)_6\overset{+}{\text{NEt}}_3 \quad 3\text{I}^-$$
$$\text{Et} \quad \text{Et}$$

46.**39**

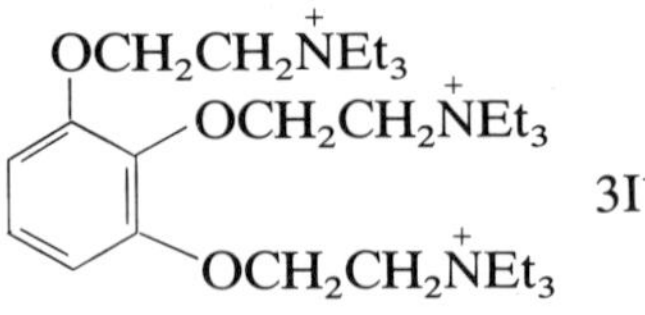

46.**40**

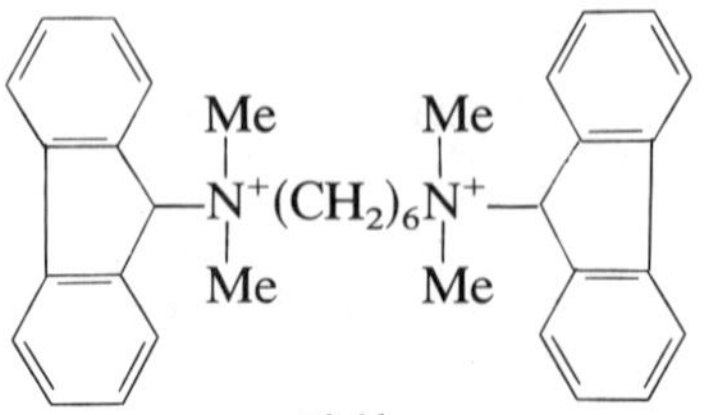

46.**41**

$$\text{Et}_3\overset{+}{\text{N}}(\text{CH}_2)_3\text{NH}\text{—}\overset{O}{\underset{O}{\bigcirc}}\text{—NH}(\text{CH}_2)_3\overset{+}{\text{NEt}}_3 \quad 2\text{X}^-$$

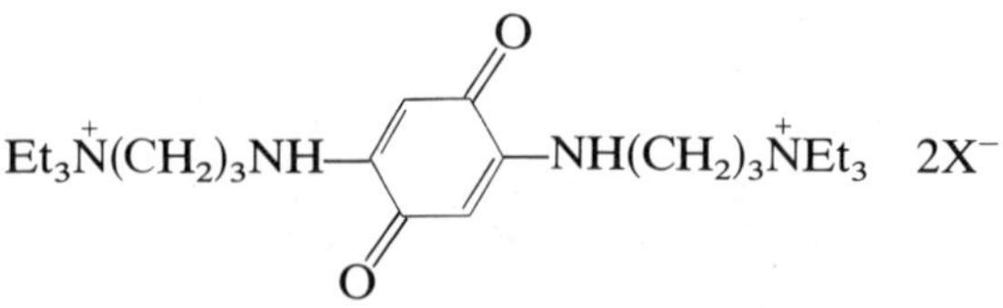

46.**42**

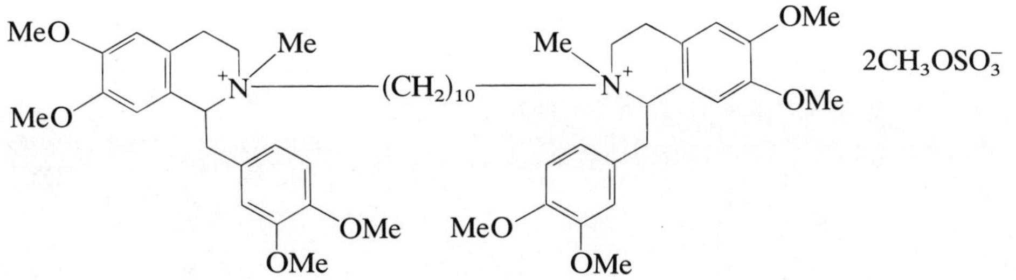

46.**43**

(196). Decamethylenebistetrahydroquino-linium and decamethylenebistetrahydroiso-quinolinium compounds showed similar patterns of activity, with potency increasing in parallel with methoxyl substitution in the aromatic rings (197). Laudexium (46.**43**), prepared in extension of these studies, combines the optimum features of these compounds in 1-benzyltetrahydroisoquino-linium moieties closely resembling those in tubocurarine (198–200). It is a typical curariform neuromuscular blocking agent, about half as potent as tubocurarine in man (201–205), but slower in onset and of longer duration of action. Histamine-releasing activity is lower than with tubo-curarine, and in keeping with its curariform activity its action is readily reversed by neostigmine. Like tubocurarine and its de-rivatives it is not readily metabolized, and may therefore give rise to recurarization in some patients.

Chain modification, particularly that in-corporating large lipophilic groups in the center of the chain of decamethonium and suxamethonium in general leads to a loss of depolarizing characteristics. Thus whereas the (S,S) and (R,R) isomers of succinylbis-α-methylcholine are depolarizing, the cor-responding (S,S) and (R,R) isomers of succinylbis-β-methylcholine have tubo-curarine-like properties (206). Similarly, succinylbis-β-phenylcholine (46.**44**) is also tubocurarine-like, though its monophenyl analog is decamethonium-like (207). The largest single group of compounds of this type, however, are steroids, which for the most part carry quaternary ammonium sub-stituents in rings A and D. The discovery of curariform neuromuscular blocking activity in the steroidal alkaloid, malouetine (46.**45**; 208, 209) stimulated interest in the steroid nucleus as a carrier moiety capable of providing fixed interquaternary spacing and orientation. Malouetine is almost as potent as tubocurarine, giving a typical curariform block that is readily reversed by neostigmine, but of considerably shorter duration than that of tubocurarine in the rabbit. Investigation of the $3\beta,20\beta$-, $3\alpha,20\alpha$-, and $3\alpha,20\beta$-stereoisomers (210, 211) of malouetine ($3\beta,20\alpha$), the related $3\alpha,17\alpha$-bisquaternary ammonium-5α-androstane (46.**46**) and its $3\alpha,17\beta$-, $3\beta,17\alpha$-, and $3\beta,17\beta$-stereoisomers (212–214), and the corresponding conessine derivatives (46.**47**; R^1, R^2 = alkyl; 215) has shown that the effect of stereochemistry at these positions is negligible. Thus the malouetine stereo-isomers all have similar potencies (211), and not only do the $3\alpha,17\alpha$- and $3\beta,17\beta$-androstane isomers have similar potencies, but those of the corresponding $3\alpha,17\beta$- and $3\beta,17\alpha$-isomers, in which the onium groups project from opposite faces of the steroid nucleus, also have activities of the same order. A number of steroid compounds have undergone extensive examination in man, but only one, pancuronium (46.**48**) has found an established place in general anesthetic practice.

Modification of both chain and onium groups by incorporation of both in large heterocyclic structures as in the calabash

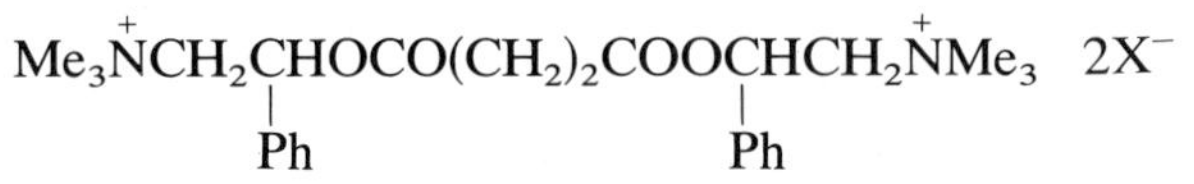

$$Me_3\overset{+}{N}CH_2CHOCO(CH_2)_2COOCHCH_2\overset{+}{N}Me_3 \quad 2X^-$$

$$\underset{Ph}{|} \qquad\qquad\qquad \underset{Ph}{|}$$

46.**44**

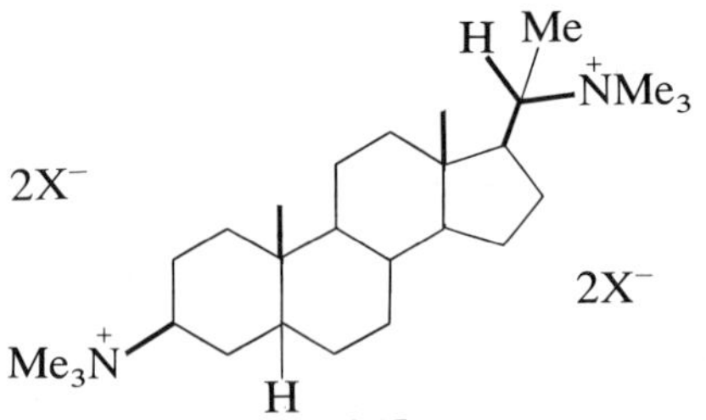

46.**45**

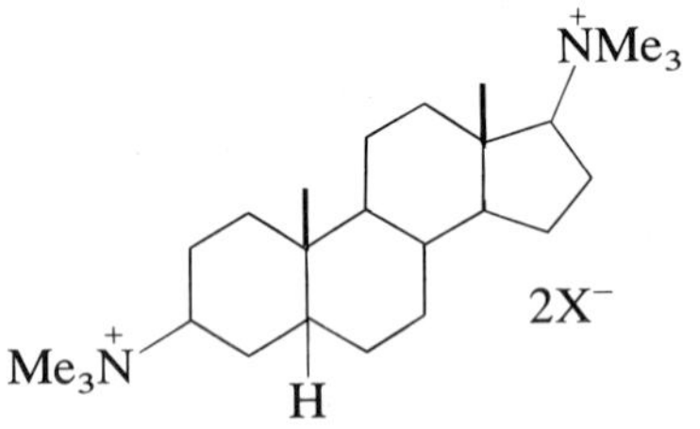

$2X^-$

46.**46**

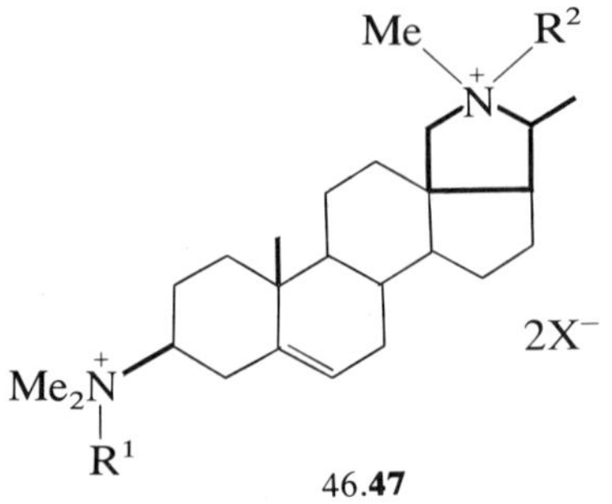

$2X^-$

46.**47**

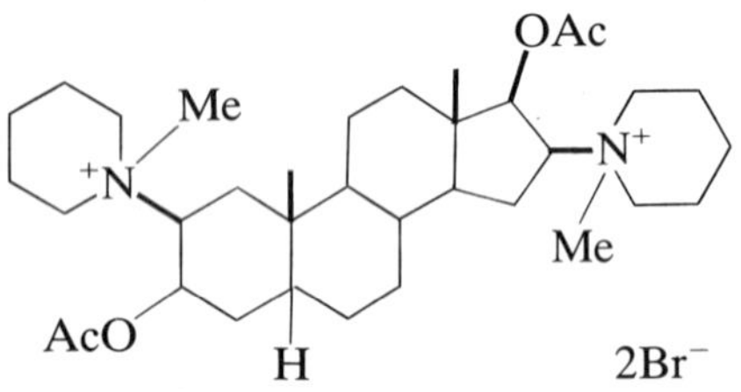

46.**48**

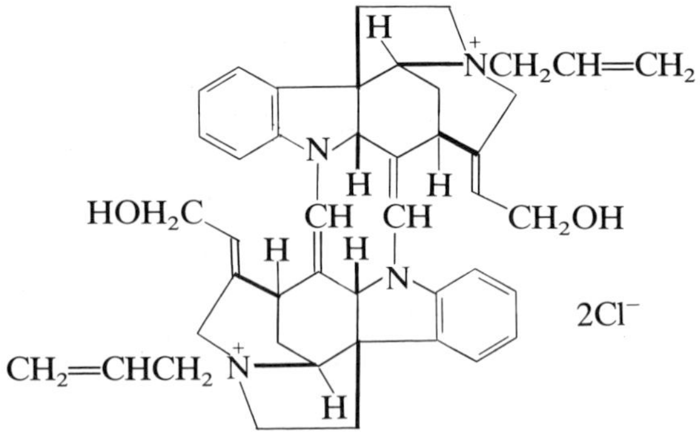

$2Br^-$

46.**49**

$2Cl^-$

curare alkaloids, the toxiferines (216–223), also leads to compounds that are tubo-curarine-like in action. The alkaloids themselves are long-acting in man (224) owing to lack of metabolism (225, 226) but chemical modification of toxiferine-I has led to a clinically useful product, N,N'-diallylbis-nortoxiferine, alcuronium chloride (46.**49**; 227).

5.7 Significance of the Second Quaternary Center

The much greater potency of bisquaternary compounds compared with their simple monoquaternary counterparts raises the question of the role of the second quaternary center. Autoradiographic studies with radiolabeled α-Bgt have shown the presence of approximately one receptor per 5000 Å^2 of the postsynaptic membrane in mouse, rat, chick, and rhesus monkey preparation (228). This puts the average distance between receptors at *ca.* 70 Å. Other estimates based on frog tissue put the average distance at *ca* 32 Å (59), but even at this minimum distance it is clear that bisquaternary compounds almost certainly do not span receptors. It is also evident that they do not span identical receptor subunits. Thus, although conformational changes in the receptor membrane follow- ing binding to one of the quaternary cen- ters might conceivably be invoked to sup- port the concept of binding to more than one receptor subunit, the exacting stereo- chemical requirements for potency seen in the norcoralydines (46.**26**–46.**29**) implies that if one quaternary center in an asym- metric molecule such as tubocurarine (46.**30**; R = H) has the optimum require- ments for fit, the second quaternary center could not meet these requirements at a second receptor subunit that is in all re- spects identical to the first. The function of the second quaternary center in bis- quaternary compounds must therefore be to promote antagonist–receptor association at a subsidiary anionic site, which nonethe- less forms an integral part of the receptor. The observation that the cholinergic recep- tor protein is capable of only partial dis- sociation in presence of snake neurotoxins and decamethonium to units of mol wt 100,000 or 150,000 suggests that the subsidiary anionic binding site brought into play in curariform block is located in those subunits that do not bind acetylcholine (64).

The concept of principal and subsidiary anionic binding sites with preferred recep- tor geometry at the principal site is sup- ported by the relative potency (=231) of isotubocurarine (46.**50**; 139) compared to that of tubocurarine (=100). Consideration of models leads to the conclusion that center (*a*) (absolute stereochemistry *S*) in tubocurarine is most likely to present itself to the receptor in a manner that approxi- mates most closely to that adopted by (*R*)- *cis*-norcoralydine (46.**26**), whereas center (*b*) (absolute stereochemistry *R*) would similarly be most likely to present itself to the receptor in a manner analogous to (*R*)- *trans*-norcoralydine (46.**27**). Since (*R*)-*cis*- norcoralysine is more potent than (*R*)- *trans*-norcoralydine, center (*a*) in the tubo- curarines should be bound preferentially to the principal anionic binding site of the receptor. This accords, therefore, with the

observation of greater potency in isotubo- curarine (46.**50**), in which the quaternary ammonium group is at center (*a*), com- pared with tubocurarine which has the quaternary ammonium group at center (*b*). It is significant, too, that the potency of iso- tubocurarine is only marginally less than that of the corresponding bisquaternary compound chondocurarine (46.**51**; 229; re- lative potency = 290), and that the bis- quaternary (+)-curarine with the doubly fa- vored (*S,S*) stereochemistry (46.**52**) has a potency relative to tubocurarine of 350, whereas (−)-curarine with the doubly unfa- vored (*R,R*) configuration (46.**53**) has a relative potency of only 130 (230).

Receptor association involving primary and secondary anionic binding sites, as op- posed to a simple one-point attachment– adumbration theory (231) in which the re- ceptor is then shielded against agonist ap- proach by the sheer bulk of the antagonist molecule, is emphasized by the properties of various monoquaternary steroids. Thus in contrast to the high potency of pancuro- nium (46.**48**) monoquaternary salts derived from 2β-amino-3-acetoxy- and 3α-amino- 2-acetoxyandrostane and pregnane (232) are all very weak neuromuscular blocking agents, despite their acetylcholine-like con- figuration and the large steroidal skeleton. At the same time the monoquaternary con- essine derivative (46.**47**, R^1 = butyl, R^2 = H; 118), which has a second nonquaternary basic group capable of acquiring a positive charge by ionization, is almost as potent as the bisquaternary *N,N'*-dimethylconessine (46.**47**, R^1 = R^2 = Me).

6 CLINICALLY USEFUL AGENTS

6.1 Clinical Requirements

Although neuromuscular blocking agents are used primarily as muscle relaxants in major surgery (1, 2), they are also used in clinical practice to produce muscle relaxa- tion for intubation (4), in orthopedics (5),

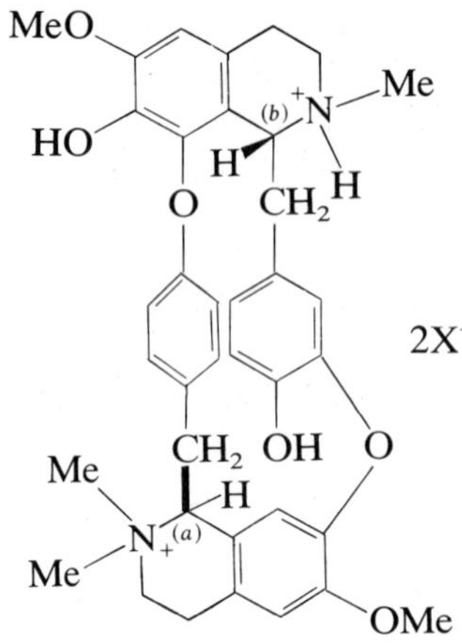

46.**50**

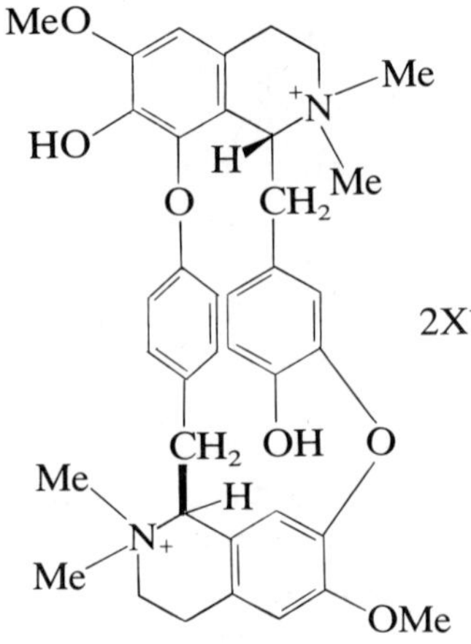

46.**51**

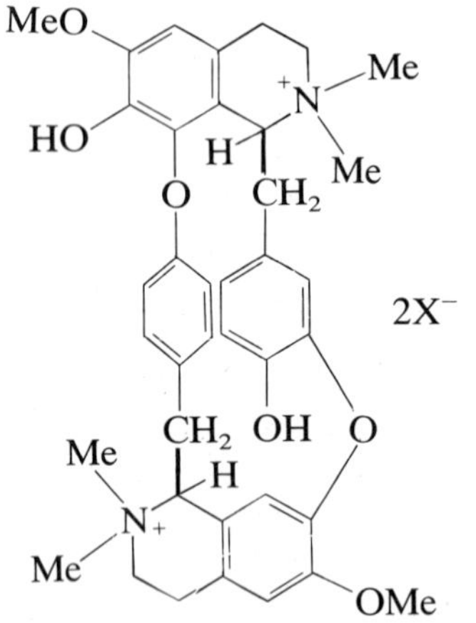

46.**52**

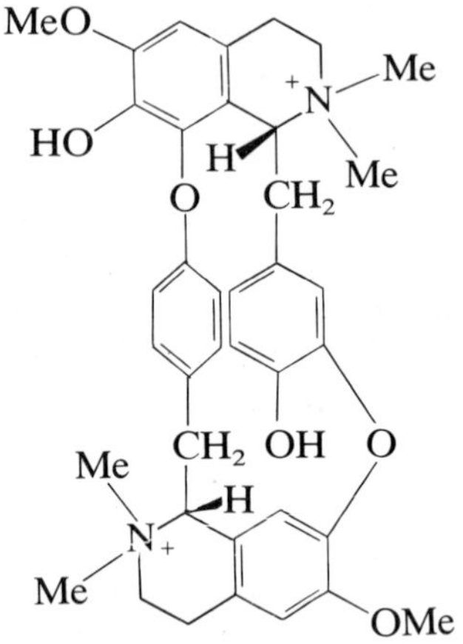

46.**53**

in electroshock therapy (7), and in the control of certain spastic conditions (6). The properties required of agents for use in these different spheres differ, but irrespective of the intended field of use, there are certain properties that are required as a prerequisite in any agent for use in clinical practice. These include the following:

1. Specificity of action and adequate potency for controlled muscle relaxation.
2. Freedom from undue toxicity and side reactions.
3. Ready reversibility by anticholinesterases or other appropriate agents.

4. Rapid onset of paralysis.
5. Optimum duration of action for the required use.
6. Rapid elimination or deactivating metabolism.
7. Freedom from undesirable interaction with other anesthetics and substances used as adjuncts to anesthesia or surgery.
8. Freedom from unpleasant side effects.

According to Savarese and Kitz (233) three types of neuromuscular blocking drugs are required to cover the needs of anesthetists. All should be curariform in their mode of action and hence capable of rapid reversal by anticholinesterases. One, for use in intubation and similar procedures, should be rapid in onset (1–2 min) giving complete paralysis for 5–10 min and complete recovery in 10–20 min. Somewhat longer duration of action is required for more general surgical work. Many operations are complete within 20–30 mins, so that a second group of compounds with a duration of some 15–20 min is required for general surgery. Such compounds should not produce cumulative effects on repetitive administration, and should preferably be rapidly metabolized, giving speedy recovery (15–20 min). This decreases the need for reversal of neuromuscular blockade by neostigmine at the end of the operation, and thus reduces the hazards of postoperational recurarization. A third group of long-acting drugs similar to those presently used but devoid of cardiovascular effects were also considered to be desirable for use in heart surgery. Of the compounds presently used, only dimethyltubocurarine, 46.**31**, meets these requirements (234). A further requirement is that placental transfer should be low, as found for tubocurarine, gallamine, suxamethonium (235), dimethyltubocurarine, and pancuronium (236, 237).

6.2 Duration, Metabolism, and Fate

None of the currently used neuromuscular blocking agents meets all the ideal criteria, but with the exception of suxamethonium,

all are curariform in action, and hence are readily reversible by neostigmine. This lack of reversibility in suxamethonium (46.**54**), however, is compensated for by its rapid metabolism in normal subjects by plasma esterases, which also accounts for its short duration of action. Hydrolysis occurs in two stages to produce products with negligible motor end plate activity (238, 239) which are readily excreted.

A small proportion of subjects with particular genetic defects are deficient in plasma esterases (240) and such patients may suffer unduly prolonged muscle paralysis and hence apnea (241). The numbers affected arc quite small; about 1 in 30 persons has a limited esterase deficiency, but completely atypical pseudocholinesterases occur with a frequency of no more than about 1 in 3000.

Metabolism is much more limited and excretion considerably slower in tubocurarine, gallamine, and pancuronium. Excretion occurs mainly in the urine, but only 36% of the dose of tubocurarine was excreted 3 hr after intravenous administration in dogs, even though 75% was accounted for after 24 hr (242). Excretion of pancuronium is more rapid, some 84% of an intravenous dose in cats being accounted for in urine, bile, and liver within 8 hr. Of this, 58% was unchanged, 14.5% as the 3-hydroxy, 7% as the 17-hydroxy, and 4.5% as the 3,17-dihydroxy derivative. The much slower rate of metabolism and excretion of these compounds is evident in their much longer duration of action (Table 46.2; 234) compared to that of suxamethonium. It is

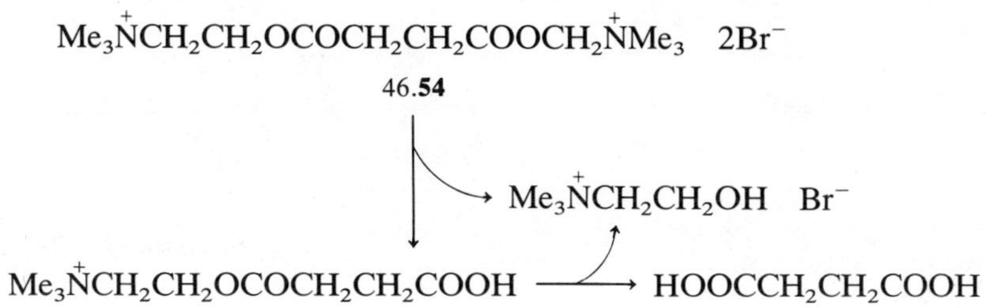

$$Me_3\overset{+}{N}CH_2CH_2OCOCH_2CH_2COOCH_2\overset{+}{N}Me_3 \quad 2Br^-$$

46.**54**

$$Me_3\overset{+}{N}CH_2CH_2OCOCH_2CH_2COOH \longrightarrow HOOCCH_2CH_2COOH$$

$$Me_3\overset{+}{N}CH_2CH_2OH \quad Br^-$$

Table 46.2   Recovery Times and Cardiovascular and Autonomic Effects at Full Paralyzing Doses of Neuromuscular Blocking Agents in the Cat (234)

Agent	Full Paralysing Dose, mg/kg i.v.	Mean Recovery Time, min	Arterial Blood Pressure (Initial = 100)	Heart Rate (Initial = 100)	Vagal Response % Inhibition	Nictitating Membrane, % Inhibition
Tubocurarine	0.40	44	54	86	80	55
Dimethyltubo-curarine	0.08	76	99	98	2	1
Gallamine	2.4	64	98	103	74	1
Alcuronium	0.16	71	79	96	39	0
Pancuronium	0.04	27	92	98	33	2
Fazadinium	2.0	20	47	88	89	8

also evident in the increased biliary secretion of tubocurarine (242) and in the increased duration of action of both tubocurarine (46.**30**, R = H) and pancuronium (46.**48**) that follows ligation of the renal arteries (243, 244). Similar metabolic information on alcuronium (46.**49**), gallamine (46.**40**), and the so-called *dimethyltubocurarine* (*O,O,N*-trimethyltubocurarine; 46.**31**) appears not to be available but their prolonged action (Table 46.2; 145) indicates that any breakdown is slow, at least by comparison with suxamethonium, and that the bulk of the drug is excreted unchanged.

In contrast fazadinium (AH8615, 46.**55**), which is also curariform in action and readily reversed by anticholinesterases, is relatively short-acting and rapidly metabolized by liver azoreductase in most laboratory animals (245, 246). It is, however, somewhat longer acting in the cat (234) and man (247, 248), although metabolized by the same pathway with cleavage of the molecule into inactive excretable fragments.

The related compound AH10407 (46.**56**; 249, 250) is reported to be ultra-short-acting in the cotton-eared marmoset. It gives a 63% block in man at 0.4 mg/kg intravenously with recovery in 1 min, but is also readily reversible by neostigmine. It is relatively stable in acid media, but very unstable in alkali, and in human blood in which some 90% was degraded within 1.5 min. It was suggested that chemical degradation, by nucleophilic attack of bicarbonate and other basic ions, yields products in which the curarizing quaternary centers are destroyed.

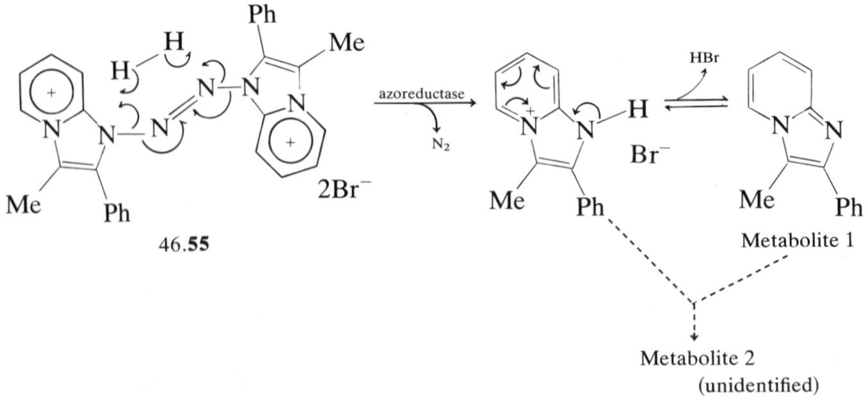

46.**55**   Metabolite 1

Metabolite 2 (unidentified)

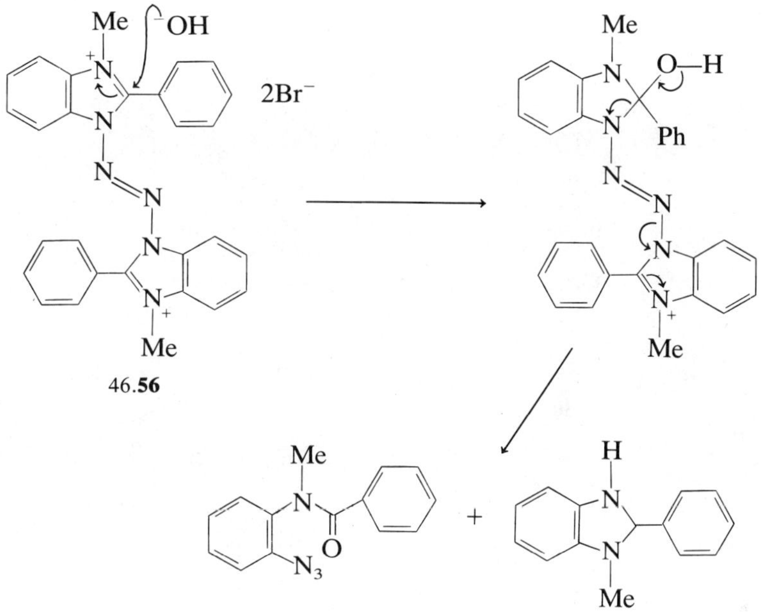

46.**56**

An alternative approach to the preparation of biodegradable neuromuscular blocking agents (250a, 250b) is based on a combination of esterase hydrolysis and base-catalyzed Hofmann elimination initiated at the natural pH of human plasma. Atracurium Besylate (46.**57**; $m = 2$; $n = 5$; $X^- = PhSO_2O^-$) based on this concept (250c, 250d) is potent, non-depolarizing, readily reversed by neostigmine, and potentiated by halothane in the cat and rhesus monkey (250e) and man (250f). Relative potency losses after incubation in standard buffer pH 7.4, and cat and human plasma show that atracurium besylate degrades by Hofmann elimination at physiological pH (route 1) as well as by ester hydrolysis (route 2). In accord with this conclusion, increase of plasma pH by hyperventilation decreases the intensity and duration of blockade, and lowering of plasma pH enhances potency.

6.3 Side Effects

Most neuromuscular blocking agents currently in use suffer from one or more side effects which for the most part are disadvantageous. Thus although suxamethonium (46.**54**) is a valuable short-acting blocking agent, it is depolarizing and the onset of paralysis is, therefore, preceded by muscle twitching which often results in severe postoperative muscle cramp (251). Its depolarizing action also raises plasma potassium, which can lead to cardiac arrest in patients with hyperkalemia (252), and repeated doses can in certain circumstances give rise to asystole due to vagal stimulation (253). Suxamethonium has also been reported to cause histamine release (174), which may give rise to bronchospasm in susceptible patients.

The major disadvantages of the curariform agents are their cardiac and autonomic effects. Gallamine (46.**40**), alcuronium (46.**49**), pancuronium (46.**48**), and fazadinium (46.**55**) all show a selective atropine-like block of muscarinic receptors in the heart, blocking the reflex slowing mechanism of the vagus (254–256, 234; Table 46.2), and leading to tachycardia and hypertension in man. Tubocurarine, on the other hand, blocks the cardiac vagus by the parasympathetic ganglion (257), but does

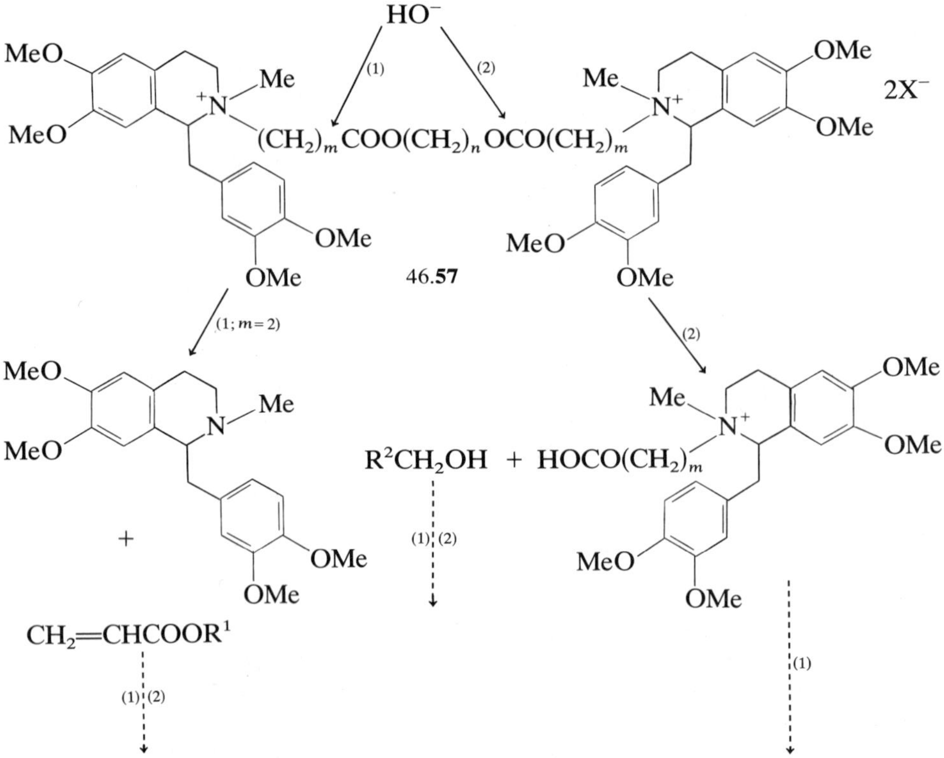

46.**57**

not cause tachycardia in man presumably because of the concomitant blockade of sympathetic ganglia (257–259). *Dimethyltubocurarine* (*O,O,N*-trimethyltubocurarine, 46.**31**), alone, is relatively free from cardiovascular effects, but is too long-acting for most purposes (Table 46.2; 234).

Other important side effects of tubocurarine (46.**30**; R = H) include histamine release (260) and ganglion block. This is probably a reflection of its monoquaternary structure, and can be sufficiently pronounced to cause a marked fall in blood pressure in most patients (261). Pancuronium (46.**48**) and alcuronium (46.**49**) have been shown to be free from histamine-releasing activity (255), but fazadinium (46.**55**) produces a substantial lowering of blood pressure in the cat (234). Pancuronium has also been shown to possess some activity against pseudocholinesterase (255), which may account for the slight miosis and fall of intraocular tension shown by most patients.

6.4 Interactions with General Anesthetics and other Medicaments

Most general anaesthetics, including ether (1, 203, 262), chloroform (263, 264), cyclopropane (263, 265, 266), halothane (263, 267), and methoxyfluorane, depress neuromuscular transmission. These effects are considered to be due to increased membrane fluidity resulting from changes in dielectric constant and viscosity (268). The effect is additive with both depolarizing and curariform neuromuscular blocking agents. Higher molecular weight ethers also show similar but diminished effects. A number of other substances, including pentobarbitone (262), chlorothiazide (269), chlorpromazine (270, 271), various sulfonamides (272), and antibiotics (47) have also been reported to interact with neuromuscular blocking agents.

REFERENCES

1. S. C. Cullen, *Surgery*, **14**, 261 (1943).

2. H. R. Griffith and G. E. Johnson, *Anesthesiology*, **3**, 418 (1942).

3. J. R. Roche, *Am. J. Ophthalmol.*, **33**, 91 (1950).

4. B. R. Simpson, T. M. Savage, E. I. Foley, L. A. Ross, L. Strunin, B. Walton, M. P. Maxwell, and D. M. Harris, *Lancet*, **1972-I**, 516.

5. F. Koch and O. Lundskog, *Nord. Med.*, **44**, 1211 (1950).

6. M. S. Burman, *J. Bone Joint Surg.*, **20**, 754 (1938).

7. A. E. Bennett, *Am. J. Psychiatr.*, **97**, 1040 (1941).

8. B. Katz, *Nerve, Muscle and Synapse*, McGraw-Hill, New York, 1966.

9. F. Fonnum, *Biochem. J.*, **103**, 262 (1967).

10. R. Birks and F. C. MacIntosh, *Can. J. Biochem. Physiol.*, **39**, 787 (1961).

11. J. P. Long and F. W. Schueler, *J. Am. Pharm. Assoc. Sci. Ed.*, **43**, 79 (1954).

12. F. W. Schueler, *J. Pharmacol. Exp. Ther.*, **115**, 127 (1955).

13. F. C. MacIntosh, R. I. Birks, and P. B. Sastry, *Nature*, **178**, 1181 (1956).

14. R. M. Gesler, A. B. Lasher, J. O. Hoppe, and E. A. Steck, *J. Pharmacol. Exp. Ther.*, **125**, 323 (1959).

15. A. S. V. Burgen, G. Burke, and M. Desbarats-Schonbaum, *Brit. J. Pharmacol. Chemother.*, **11**, 308 (1956).

16. J. C. Smith, C. J. Cavallito, and F. F. Foldes, *Biochem. Pharmacol.*, **16**, 2438 (1967).

17. H. L. White and C. J. Cavallito, *Biochem. Biophys. Acta*, **206**, 343 (1970).

18. B. A. Hemsworth and F. F. Foldes, *Eur. J. Pharmacol.*, **11**, 187 (1970).

19. J. I. Hubbard, *Physiol. Rev.*, **53**, 674 (1973).

20. M. Israel, J. Gautron, and B. Lesbats, *C. R. Acad. Sci. Paris*, **266**, 273 (1968).

21. A. W. Clark, A. Mauro, H. E. Longenecker, and W. P. Hurlburt, *Nature*, **225**, 703 (1970).

22. H. A. Lester, *Sci. Am.*, **236**, 106 (1977).

23. J. I. Hubbard and D. F. Wilson, *J. Physiol.* (London), **228**, 307 (1973).

24. L. T. Potter, *J. Physiol.* (London), **206**, 145 (1970).

25. S. W. Kuffler and D. Yoshikami, *J. Physiol.* (London), **251**, 465 (1975).

26. P. W. Ramwell, J. E. Shaw, and J. Kucharski, *Science*, **149**, 1390 (1969).

27. J. Musick and J. I. Hubbard, *Nature* **237**, 279 (1972).

28. W. Feldberg, *Physiol. Rev.*, **25**, 596 (1945).

29. P. Fatt and B. Katz, *J. Physiol.* (London), **115**, 320 (1951).

30. R. Birks, H. E. Huxley, and B. Katz, *J. Physiol.* (London), **150**, 134 (1960).

31. J. I. Hubbard and S. Kwanbunbumpen, *J. Physiol.* (London), **194**, 407 (1968).

32. V. J. McMahan, N. C. Spitzer, and K. Peper, *Proc. Roy. Soc.* (London) *Ser. B*, **181**, 421 (1972).

33. E. M. Kosower and R. Werman, *Nature New Biol.* (London), **233**, 121 (1971).

34. F. A. Dodge, R. Miledi, and R. Rahamimoff, *J. Physiol.* (London), **200**, 267 (1969).

35. U. Meiri and R. Rahamimioff, *J. Physiol.* (London), **215**, 709 (1971).

36. J. I. Hubbard, S. F. Jones, and E. M. Landau, *J. Physiol.* (London), **194**, 355 (1968).

37. *Ibid.*, **196**, 75 (1968).

38. A. W. Clark, W. P. Hurlburt, and A. Mauro, *J. Cell Biol.*, **52**, 1 (1972).

39. J. Heuser and R. Miledi, *Proc. Roy. Soc.* (London) *Ser. B*, **179**, 247 (1971).

40. R. W. Abers and G. J. Koval, *Biochim. Biophys. Acta*, **60**, 359 (1962).

41. Z. L. Blioch, I. M. Glagoleva, E. A. Liberman, and V. A. Nenashev, *J. Physiol.* (London), **199**, 11 (1968).

42. L. L. Simpson, *J. Pharm. Pharmacol.*, **20**, 889 (1968).

43. R. Quarles and J. Folch-Pi, *J. Neurochem.*, **12**, 543 (1965).

44. P. H. Elworthy, *Pharm. J.*, **18**, 566 (1976).

45. G. Gregoriadis, P. D. Leatherwood, and B. E. Ryman, *FEBS Lett.*, **14**, 95 (1971).

46. I. M. Glagoleva, E. A. Liberman, and Z. Kh-M. Khashaev, *Biofizka*, **15**, 76 (1970).

47. C. B. Pittinger and R. Adamson, *Ann. Rev. Pharmacol.*, **12**, 169 (1972).

48. R. I. Brittain, G. P. Levy, and M. B. Tyers, *Eur. J. Pharmacol.*, **8**, 93, (1969).

49. I. G. Marshall, *Brit. J. Pharmacol.*, **38,** 502 (1970).

50. C. C. J. Culvenor and N. S. Ham, *Chem. Commun.*, 537 (1966).

51. C. Clothia and P. Pauling, *Chem. Commun.*, 626 (1969).

52. C. Clothia and P. Pauling, *Nature*, **223,** 919 (1969).

53. J. C. Eccles, B. Katz, and S. W. Kuffler, *J. Neurophysiol.*, **4,** 363 (1941).

54. B. L. Ginsborg, *Pharmacol. Rev.*, **19,** 289 (1967).

55. C. Chargas, E. Penna Franca, K. Nishie, and E. J. Garcia, *Arch. Biochem. Biophys.*, **76,** 251 (1958).

56. S. Ehrenpreis, *Biochim. Biophys. Acta*, **44,** 561 (1960).

57. J. L. La Torre, G. S. Lunt, and E. De Robertis, *Proc. Natl. Acad. Sci. U.S.*, **65,** 716 (1970).

58. R. Miledi, P. Molinoff, and L. T. Potter, *Nature*, **229,** 554 (1971).

59. R. Miledi and L. T. Potter, *Nature*, **233,** 599 (1971).

60. D. K. Berg, R. B. Kelly, P. B. Sargent, P. Williamson, and Z. W. Hall, *Proc. Natl. Acad. Sci. U.S.*, **69,** 147 (1972).

61. D. Mebs, K. Narita, S. Iwanaga, Y. Samejima, and C. Y. Lee, *Z. Physiol. Chem.*, **353,** 243 (1972); (through *Chem. Abstr.*, **76,** 109380 (1972)).

62. R. W. Olsen, J. C. Meunier, and J. P. Changeux, *FEBS Lett.*, **28,** 96 (1972).

63. J. C. Meunier, R. Sealock, R. Olsen, and J. P. Changeux, *Eur. J. Biochem.*, **45,** 371 (1974).

64. F. Hucho and J. P. Changeux, *FEBS Lett.*, **38,** 11 (1973).

65. J. C. Meunier, R. W. Olsen, A. Menez, P. Fromageot, P. Boquet, and J. P. Changeux, *Biochemistry*, **11,** 1200 (1972).

66. M. J. Reiter, D. A. Cowburn, J. M. Prives, and A. Karlin, *Proc. Natl. Acad. Sci. U.S.*, **69,** 1168 (1972).

67. G. E. Davies and G. R. Stark, *Proc. Natl. Acad. Sci. U.S.*, **66,** 651 (1970).

68. C. L. Weill, M. G. McNamee, and A. Karlin, *Biochem. Biophys. Res. Commun.*, **61,** 997 (1974).

69. J. Schmidt and M. A. Raftery, *Biochemistry*, **12,** 852 (1973).

70. D. M. Fambrough and H. C. Hartzell, *Science*, **176,** 189 (1972).

71. P. G. Waser, *Ann. N. Y. Acad. Sci.*, **144,** 737 (1967).

72. W. Grampp, J. B. Harris, and S. Thesleff, *J. Physiol.* (London), **221,** 743 (1972).

73. D. M. Fambrough, *Science*, **168,** 372 (1970).

74. H. C. Hartzell and D. M. Fambrough, *Proc. Ann. Meet. Soc. Neurosci., 1st, 1971,* p. 161.

75. J. P. Changeux, T. R. Podleski, and J. C. Meunier, *J. Gen. Physiol.*, **54,** 225 (1969).

76. A. O. Župančič, *Ann. N. Y. Acad. Sci.*, **144,** 689 (1967).

77. D. Nachmansohn, *Chemical and Molecular Bases of Nerve Activity*, Academic Press, New York, 1959.

78. R. M. Krupka, *Biochemistry*, **5,** 1988 (1966).

79. *Ibid.*, **6,** 1183 (1967).

80. J. Del Castillo and B. Katz, *J. Physiol.* (London), **128,** 157 (1955).

81. A. Karlin and E. Bartels, *Biochem. Biophys. Acta*, **126,** 525 (1966).

82. W. W. Cleland, *Biochemistry*, **3,** 480 (1964).

83. G. L. Ellman, *Arch. Biochem. Biophys.*, **82,** 70 (1959).

84. T. Podleski and D. Nachmansohn, *Proc. Natl. Acad. Sci. U.S.*, **56,** 1034 (1966).

85. A. Karlin and M. Winnik, *Proc. Natl. Acad. Sci. U.S.*, **60,** 668 (1968).

86. A. Karlin, *J. Gen. Physiol.*, **54,** 245S (1969).

87. A. Karlin, *The Chemical Nature of the Acetylcholine Receptor, Drug Cholinergic Mech CNS Proc. Conf., 1970,* E. Heilbronn, Ed., Foersvarats Forskningsanst, Stockholm, p. 489; through *Chem. Abstr.*, **76,** 95507 (1972).

88. H. G. Mautner, E. Bartels, and G. D. Webb, *Biochem. Pharmacol.*, **15,** 187 (1966).

89. H. R. Ing and W. M. Wright, *Proc. Roy. Soc. Ser. B.*, **109,** 337 (1931).

90. M. J. Dallemagne and E. Phillipott, *Arch. Int. Pharmacodyn.*, **87,** 127 (1951).

91. J. Thomas and G. A. Starmer, *J. Pharm. Pharmacol.*, **13,** 752 (1961).

92. T. R. Podleski, *Biochem. Pharmacol.*, **18,** 211 (1969).

93. J. Patrick, B. Valeur, L. Monneric, and J. P. Changeux, *J. Membrane Biol.*, **5,** 102 (1971).

94. J. C. Meunier and J. P. Changeux, *FEBS Lett.*, **32,** 143 (1973).

95. M. Weber, T. David-Pfeuty, and J. P. Changeux, *Proc. Natl. Acad. Sci. U.S.*, **72,** 3443 (1975).

96. E. De Robertis, *Science*, **171,** 963 (1971).

97. K. Nanta, D. Mebs, S. Iwanaga, Y. Samejima, and C. Y. Lee, *Biochem. Biophys. Res. Commun.*, **44,** 711 (1971).

References

463

98. C. Y. Lee, S. L. Chang, S. T. Kau, and S-H. Luh, *J. Chromatogr.*, **72,** 71 (1972).

99. D. P. Botes and D. J. Strydom, *J. Biol. Chem.*, **244,** 4147 (1969).

100. H. Kyozo, N. Kenji, T. Sasaki, and T. Suzuki, *Biochem. Biophys. Res. Commun.*, **36,** 482 (1969).

101. K. Nakai, C. Nakai, T. Sasaki, K. Kakiuchi, and R. Hayashi, *Naturwissenschaften*, **57,** 387 (1970).

102. C. C. Yang, *Radiat. Sensitivity Toxins Anim. Poisons, Proc. Panel 19–22 May, 1969* IAEA, Vienna, 1970, p. 63; through *Chem. Abstr.*, **74,** 11556 (1971).

103. D. P. Botes, D. J. Strydom, C. G. Anderson, and P. A. Christensen, *J. Biol. Chem.*, **246,** 3132 (1971).

104. D. P. Botes, *J. Biol. Chem.*, **246,** 7383 (1971).

105. E. Karlson, D. Eaker, and G. Ponterius, *Biochem. Biophys. Acta*, **257,** 235 (1972).

106. C. C. Yang, *Biochem. Biophys. Acta*, **133,** 346 (1967).

107. C. C. Yang, *J. Biochem.* (Tokyo), **61,** 272 (1967); through *Chem. Abstr.*, **66,** 101872 (1967).

108. A. G. Ogston, *J. Physiol.* (London), **128,** 222 (1955).

109. J. C. Eccles and W. V. Macfarlane, *J. Neurophysiol.*, **12,** 59 (1949).

110. M. Kordas, *J. Physiol.* (London), **224,** 333 (1972).

111. D. Grob and T. Namba, *Fed. Proc. Fed. Am. Soc. Exp. Biol.*, **22,** 215 (1963).

112. D. Grob, T. Namba, M. A. Solomon, and D. S. Feldman, *J. Clin. Invest.*, **41,** 1363 (1962).

113. T. Namba and D. Grob, *Ann. N. Y. Acad. Sci.*, **144,** 772 (1967).

114. T. Namba and D. Grob, *Biochem. Pharmacol.*, **16,** 1135 (1967).

115. C. C. Chang, *J. Formosan Med. Ass.*, **59,** 416 (1960).

116. *Ibid.*, **59,** 315 (1960).

117. C. C. Chang, S. E. Lu, P. N. Wang, and S. T. Chuang, *Eur. J. Pharmacol.*, **11,** 195 (1970).

118. S. Ellis and S. B. Beckett, *J. Pharmacol. Exp. Ther.*, **112,** 202 (1954).

119. A. Karlin, *Biochem. Biophys. Acta*, **139,** 358 (1967).

120. Z. W. Hall and R. B. Kelly, *Nature New Biol.* (London), **232,** 62 (1971).

121. K. Bryn Thomas, *Curare. Its History and Usage*, Lippincott, Philadelphia, 1963.

122. C. Bernard, *C. R. Soc. Biol.*, **2,** 195 (1851).

123. C. Bernard, *C. R. Acad. Sci. Paris*, **43,** 825 (1856).

124. A. Crum Brown and T. R. Fraser, *Trans. Roy. Soc. Edinburgh*, **25,** 151–93 (1868).

125. A. Crum. Brown and T. R. Fraser, *Proc. Roy. Soc. Edinburgh*, **6,** 556 (1869).

126. R. Hunt and R. R. Renshaw, *J. Pharmacol. Exp. Ther.*, **25,** 315 (1925).

127. H. R. Ing and W. M. Wright, *Proc. Roy. Soc. Ser. B.*, **109,** 337 (1931).

128. P. E. B. Holmes, D. J. Jenden, and D. B. Taylor, *Nature*, **159,** 86 (1947).

129. F. P. Dwyer, E. C. Gyarfas, R. D. Wright, and A. Schulman, *Nature*, **179,** 425 (1957).

130. H. Hildebrandt, *Arch. Exp. Pathol. Pharmakol.*, **53,** 76 (1905).

131. J. B. Stenlake, W. D. Williams, N. C. Dhar, and I. G. Marshall, *Eur. J. Med. Chem.*, **9,** 233 (1974).

132. P. W. Erhardt and T. O. Soine, *J. Pharm. Sci.*, **64,** 53 (1975).

133. J. B. Stenlake, W. D. Williams, N. C. Dhar, R. D. Waigh, and I. G. Marshall, *Eur. J. Med. Chem.*, **9,** 248 (1974).

134. J. B. Stenlake, W. D. Williams, N. C. Dhar, and I. G. Marshall, *Eur. J. Med. Chem.*, **9,** 239 (1974).

135. A. A. Genenah, T. O. Soine, and N. A. Shaath, *J. Pharm. Sci.*, **64,** 62 (1975).

136. T. O. Soine, W. S. Hanley, N. A. Shaath, and A. A. Genenah, *J. Pharm. Sci.*, **64,** 67 (1975).

137. J. B. Stenlake, in *Progress in Medicinal Chemistry*, Vol. 16, G. P. Ellis and G. B. West, Eds., Elsevier/North Holland, Amsterdam, 1979, p. 257.

138. J. B. Stenlake and N. C. Dhar, unpublished.

139. T. O. Soine and J. Naghaway, *J. Pharm. Sci.*, **63,** 1643 (1975).

140. H. King, *J. Chem. Soc.*, **1935,** 1381.

141. H. King, *Nature*, **158,** 515 (1946).

142. H. King, *J. Chem. Soc.*, **1947,** 936.

143. H. King, *J. Chem. Soc.*, **1948,** 265.

144. A. J. Everett, L. A. Lowe, and S. Wilkinson, *Chem. Commun.*, **1970,** 1020.

144a. R. Hughes, *Brit. J. Anaesth.*, **42,** 658 (1970).

145. R. B. Barlow and H. R. Ing, *Nature*, **161,** 718 (1948).

146. R. B. Barlow and H. R. Ing, *Brit. J. Pharmacol. Chemother.*, **3,** 298 (1948).

147. W. D. M. Paton and E. J. Zaimis, *Nature*, **161,** 718 (1948).

148. Z. M. Bacq and G. L. Brown, *J. Physiol.* (London), **89,** 45 (1937).

149. W. D. M. Paton and E. J. Zaimis, *Brit. J. Pharmacol. Chemother.,* **4,** 381 (1949).

150. R. Creese and J. MacLagan, *J. Physiol.* (London), **210,** 363 (1970).

151. R. A. Hall and M. W. Parkes, *J. Physiol.* (London), **122,** 274 (1953).

152. D. J. Jenden, K. Kamijo, and D. B. Taylor, *J. Pharmacol. Exp. Ther.,* **111,** 229 (1954).

153. P. A. Jewell and E. J. Zaimis, *J. Physiol.* (London), **124,** 417 (1954).

154. H. C. Churchill-Davidson and A. T. Richardson, *Nature,* **170,** 617 (1952).

155. T. H. Cannard and E. J. Zaimis, *J. Physiol.* (London), **149,** 112 (1959).

156. R. Hunt and R. De M. Taveau, *Brit. Med. J.,* **1906-II,** 1788.

157. D. Bovet, F. Bovet-Nitti, S. Guarino, V. G. Longo, and M. Marotta, *R. C. 1st Sup. Sanit.,* **12,** 106 (1949).

158. R. Fusco, G. Palazzo, S. Chiavarelli, and D. Bovet, *Gazz. Chim. Ital.,* **79,** 836 (1949).

159. V. Rosnati, *Gazz. Chim. Ital.,* **87,** 215 (1957).

160. V. Rosnati, H. Angelini-Kothny, and D. Bovet, *Gazz. Chim. Ital.,* **88,** 1293 (1958).

161. S. Levis, S. Preat, and J. Dauby, *Arch. Int. Pharmacodyn.,* **93,** 46 (1953).

162. D. Bovet, F. Bovet-Nitti, S. Guarino, V. G. Longo, and R. Fusco, *Arch. Int. Pharmacodyn.,* **88,** 1 (1951).

163. G. Briscoe, *Lancet,* **1936-I,** 469.

164. W. T. Riker, *Pharmacol. Rev.,* **5,** 1 (1953).

165. D. B. Taylor and O. A. Nedergaard, *Physiol. Rev.,* **45,** 523 (1965).

166. W. C. Bowman, in *Progress in Medicinal Chemistry,* Vol. 2, G. P. Ellis and G. B. West, Eds., Butterworths, London, 1962, p. 88.

167. F. F. Foldes, *Brit. J. Anaesth.,* **26,** 394 (1954).

168. O. F. Hutter and J. E. Pascoe, *Brit. J. Pharmacol. Chemother.,* **6,** 691 (1951).

169. R. B. Barlow, T. D. M. Roberts, and D. A. Reid, *J. Pharm. Pharmacol.,* **5,** 35 (1953).

170. K. Kalow, *Anaesthesiology,* **20,** 505 (1959).

171. S. Thesleff and K. R. Unna, *J. Pharm. Exp. Ther.,* **111,** 99 (1954).

172. J. M. van Rossum and E. J. Anino, *Arch. Int. Pharmacodyn.,* **118,** 393 (1959).

173. P. Valdoni, *R. C. 1st sup. Sanit.,* **12,** 255 (1949).

174. W. D. M. Paton, *Anaesthesiology,* **20,** 453 (1959).

175. G. E. Hale-Enderby, *Brit. J. Anaesth.,* **31,** 530 (1959).

176. R. Frey, in *Proc. World Congr. Anaesthesiol., Scheveningen, 1955,* Burgess, Mineapolis.

177. L. Rendell-Baker, F. F. Foldes, J. H. Birch, and P. B. D'Souza, *Brit. J. Anaesth.,* **29,** 303 (1957).

178. A. R. Hunter, *Anaesthesist,* **8,** 82 (1959).

179. D. Edwards, J. J. Lewis, J. B. Stenlake, and M. S. Zoha, *J. Pharm. Pharmacol.,* **9,** 1004 (1957).

180. *Ibid.,* **10,** 106T, 122T.

181. F. C. Carey, D. Edwards, J. J. Lewis, and J. B. Stenlake, *J. Pharm. Pharmacol.,* **11,** 70T (1959).

182. D. Edwards, J. J. Lewis, J. B. Stenlake, and F. Stothers, *J. Pharm. Pharmacol.,* **11,** 87T (1959).

183. D. Edwards, J. B. Stenlake, J. J. Lewis, and F. Stothers, *J. Med. Pharm. Chem.,* **3,** 369 (1961).

184. D. Edwards, D. E. McPhail, T. C. Muir, and J. B. Stenlake, *J. Pharm. Pharmacol.,* **12,** 137T (1960).

185. J. J. Lewis, D. E. McPhail, T. C. Muir, and J. B. Stenlake, *J. Pharm. Pharmacol.,* **13,** 543 (1961).

186. F. C. Carey, J. J. Lewis, J. B. Stenlake, and W. D. Williams, *J. Pharm. Pharmacol.,* **13,** 103T (1961).

187. D. Bovet, F. Depierre, and Y. De Lestrange, *C. R. Acad. Sci., Paris,* **225,** 74 (1947).

188. D. Bovet, F. Depierre, S. Courvoisier, and Y. De Lestrange, *Arch. Int. Pharmacodyn.,* **80,** 172 (1949).

189. C. J. Cavallito, A. P. Gray, and E. C. Spinner, *J. Am. Chem. Soc.,* **76,** 1862 (1954).

190. V. F. Cordaro and J. G. Arrowood, *Curr. Res. Anaesth. Analg.,* **34,** 112 (1955).

191. J. G. Arrowood and J. S. Kaplan, *Curr. Res. Anaesth. Analg.,* **35,** 412 (1956).

192. C. J. Cavallito, E. A. Sorta, and J. O. Hoppe, *J. Am. Chem. Soc.,* **72,** 2661 (1950).

193. J. O. Hoppe, *J. Pharmacol. Exp. Ther.,* **100,** 333 (1950).

194. J. O. Hoppe, *Ann. N.Y. Acad. Sci.,* **54,** 395 (1951).

195. F. F. Foldes, R. E. Molloy, E. K. Zsigmond, and J. A. Zwartz, *J. Pharmacol. Exp. Ther.,* **129,** 400 (1960).

196. H. O. J. Collier and E. P. Taylor, *Nature,* **164,** 491 (1949).

197. E. P. Taylor, *J. Chem. Soc.,* **1951,** 1150.

198. *Ibid.,* **1952,** 142.

199. E. P. Taylor and H. O. J. Collier, *Nature,* **167,** 692 (1951).

200. H. O. J. Collier and B. Macauley, *Brit. J. Pharmacol.*, **7,** 398 (1952).

201. R. I. Bodman, H. J. V. Morton, and W. D. Wylie, *Lancet,* **1952-II,** 517.

202. R. Binning, *Anaesthesia,* **8,** 268 (1953).

203. J. W. Dundee, T. C. Gray, and J. E. Riding, *Brit. J. Anaesth.,* **26,** 13 (1954).

204. G. M. Wyant and M. S. Sadove, *Curr. Res. Anaesth. Analg.,* **33,** 178 (1954).

205. A. R. Hunter, *Brit. J. Anaesth.,* **27,** 73 (1955).

206. E. Lesser, *J. Pharm. Pharmacol.,* **1,** 703 (1961).

207. V. Rosnati and H. Angelini-Kothny, *Gazz. Chim. Ital.,* **88,** 1284 (1958).

208. M. M. Janot, F. Lainé, and R. Goutarel, *Ann. Pharm. Fr.,* **18,** 673 (1960).

209. A. Quévauviller and F. Lainé, *Ann. Pharm. Fr.,* **18,** 678 (1960).

210. R. Goutarel, *Tetrahedron,* **14,** 126 (1961).

211. F. Khuong Huu-Lainé and W. Pinto-Scognamiglio, *Arch. Int. Pharmacodyn.,* **147,** 209 (1964).

212. M. Alauddin, B. Caddy, J. J. Lewis, M. Martin-Smith, and M. F. Sugrue, *J. Pharm. Pharmacol.,* **17,** 55 (1965).

213. D. G. Bamford, D. F. Biggs, M. Davis, and E. W. Parnell, *Brit. J. Pharmacol.,* **30,** 194 (1967).

214. M. Martin-Smith, in *Drug Design,* Vol. 2, E. J. Ariens, Ed., Academic, New York-London, 1971, p. 505.

215. D. Busfield, K. J. Child, A. J. Clarke, B. Davis, and M. G. Dodds, *Brit. J. Pharmacol.,* **32,** 609 (1968).

216. W. von Philipsborn, H. Schmid, and P. Karrer, *Helv. Chim. Acta,* **39,** 913 (1956).

217. K. Bernauer, F. Berlage, W. von Philipsborn, H. Schmid, and P. Karrer, *Helv. Chim. Acta,* **41,** 2293 (1958).

218. F. Berlage, K. Bernauer, H. Schmid, and P. Karrer, *Helv. Chim. Acta,* **42,** 2650 (1959).

219. A. R. Battersby and H. F. Hodson, *Proc. Chem. Soc.,* **1958,** 287.

220. A. R. Battersby and H. F. Hodson, *J. Chem. Soc.,* **1960,** 736.

221. J. Kebrle, H. Schmid, P. G. Waser, and P. Karrer, *Helv. Chim. Acta,* **36,** 102 (1953).

222. P. G. Waser and P. Harbeck, *Anaesthesist,* **8,** 193 (1959).

223. F. F. Foldes, O. Wolfram, and M. D. Sokoll, *Anaesthesist,* **10,** 210 (1961).

224. P. G. Waser, *Helv. Physiol. Pharmacol. Acta,* **8,** 342 (1950).

225. *Ibid.,* Suppl. VIII, 1 (1953).

226. P. G. Waser, H. Schmid, and K. Schmid, *Arch. Int. Pharmacodyn.,* **96,** 386 (1954).

227. P. G. Waser and P. Harbeck, *Anaesthesist,* **11,** 33 (1962).

228. E. A. Barnard, J. Wieckowski, and T. H. Chiu, *Nature,* **234,** 207 (1971).

229. O. Wintersteiner, in *Curare and Curare-like Agents,* D. Bovet, F. Bovet-Nitti, and G. B. Marini-Bettôlo, eds., Elsevier, London, 1959, p. 160.

230. H. A. Holiday and R. F. Varney, quoted by O. Wintersteiner, Ref. 229.

231. S. Loewe and S. C. Harvey, *Arch. Exp. Pathol. Pharmakol.,* **214,** 214 (1952).

232. J. J. Lewis, M. Martin-Smith, T. C. Muir, and H. H. Ross, *J. Pharm. Pharmacol.,* **19,** 502 (1967).

233. J. J. Savarese and R. J. Kitz, *Anesthesiology,* **42,** 236 (1975).

234. R. Hughes and D. J. Chapple, *Anesthesiology,* **48,** 59 (1976).

235. C. Bérenger, M. Galluser, and P. Gauthier-Lafaye, *Anesth., Analg., Réanim.,* **28,** 2 (1971).

236. I. Spiers and A. W. Sim, *Brit. J. Anaesth.,* **44,** 370 (1972).

237. I. Kivalo and S. Saarikoski, *Brit. J. Anaesth.,* **44,** 557 (1972).

238. V. P. Witticker and S. Wijesundera, *Biochem. J.,* **52,** 475 (1952).

239. F. I. Tsuji and F. F. Foldes, *Fed. Proc. Fed. Am. Soc. Exp. Biol.,* **12,** 321, 374 (1953).

240. W. Kalow and W. Staron, *Can. J. Biochem. Physiol.,* **35,** 1305 (1957).

241. H. Lehman and E. Ryan, *Lancet,* **1956-II,** 124.

242. E. N. Cohen, W. H. Brewer, and D. Smith, *Anesthesiology,* **28,** 309 (1967).

243. R. D. Miller, W. C. Stevens, and W. L. Way, *Anesth. Analg.,* **52,** 661 (1973).

244. M. Gibaldi, G. Levy, and W. L. Hayton, *Brit. J. Anaesth.,* **44,** 163 (1972).

245. E. E. Glover and M. Yorke, *J. Chem. Soc.* **1971,** 3280.

246. L. Bolgar, R. T. Brittain, D. Jack, M. R. Jackson, L. E. Martin, J. Mills, D. Pointer, and M. B. Tyers, *Nature,* **238,** 354 (1972).

247. R. T. Brittain and M. B. Tyers, *Brit. J. Anaesth.,* **45,** 837 (1973).

248. C. E. Blogg, T. M. Savage, J. C. Simpson, L. A. Ross, and B. R. Simpson, *Proc. Roy. Soc. Med.,* **66,** 1023 (1973).

249. E. E. Glover, R. T. Rowbottom, and D. C. Bishop, *J. Chem. Soc., Perkin Trans.,* **I,** 842 (1973).

250. C. E. Blogg, R. T. Brittain, B. R. Simpson, and M. B. Tyers, *Proc. Brit. Pharmacol. Soc., Commun.*, **1975**, 35.

250a. J. B. Stenlake, J. Urwin, R. D. Waigh, and R. Hughes, *Eur. J. Med. Chem.*, **14,** 77 (1979).

250b. J. B. Stenlake, J. Urwin, R. D. Waigh, and R. Hughes, *Eur. J. Med. Chem.*, **14,** 85 (1979).

250c. J. B. Stenlake, R. D. Waigh, G. H. Dewar, J. Urwin, and N. C. Dhar, U.K. Prov. Pat. Appl. 50589/75 and 45028/76; Belg. Pat. 76355 (1977).

250d. J. B. Stenlake, in *Advances in Pharmacology and Therapeutics*, Vol. 3, J. C. Stoclet, Ed., Pergamon, Oxford–New York, 1979, p. 303.

250e. R. Hughes and D. J. Chapple, *Brit. J. Anaesth.*, **52,** 238 (1980).

250f. T. M. Hunt, R. Hughes, and J. P. Payne, *Brit. J. Anaesth.*, **52,** 238–239 (1980)

251. H. C. Churchill-Davidson, *Brit. Med. J.*, **1,** 746 (1954).

252. R. Roth and H. Wüthrick, *Brit. J. Anaesth.*, **41,** 311 (1969).

253. J. A. Mathias and C. D. G. Evans Prosser, *Progr. Anaesth.*, 1153 (1970).

254. W. F. Riker and W. C. Wesco, *Ann. N. Y. Acad. Sci.*, **54,** 373 (1951).

255. T. M. Speight and G. S. Avery, *Drugs*, **4,** 163 (1972).

256. I. G. Marshall, *J. Pharm. Pharmacol.*, **25,** 530 (1973).

257. A. C. Guyton and R. C. Reeder, *J. Pharmacol. Exp. Ther.*, **98,** 188 (1950).

258. L. O. Randall, *Ann. N. Y. Acad. Sci.*, **54,** 460 (1951).

259. R. Hughes, *Brit. J. Anaesth.*, **28,** 392 (1956).

260. W. Sniper, *Brit. J. Anaesth.*, **24,** 232 (1952).

261. F. F. Foldes, *Clin. Pharmac. Ther.*, **1,** 345 (1960).

262. E. P. Pick and G. V. Richards, *J. Pharmacol. Exp. Ther.*, **90,** 1 (1947).

263. D. C. Watland, J. P. Long, C. B. Pittinger, and S. C. Cullen, *Anesthesiology*, **18,** 883 (1957).

264. K. Naess, *Acta Physiol. Scand.*, **19,** 187 (1949).

265. F. F. Foldes, T. S. Machaj, R. D. Hunt, P. G. McNall, and P. C. Carberry, *J. Am. Med. Assoc.*, **150,** 1559 (1952).

266. D. A. Lang, K. K. Kimura, and K. R. Unna, *Arch. Int. Pharmacodyn.*, **85,** 257 (1951).

267. M. Johnstone, *Brit. J. Anaesth.*, **28,** 392 (1956).

268. P. W. Gage and O. Hamill, *Neurosci. Lett.*, **1,** 61 (1975).

269. W. Ferrari, G. L. Gessa, and S. Sangiori, *Nature*, **184,** 1235 (1959).

270. V. Dyrberg and W. Hougs, *Acta Pharmacol. Toxicol.*, **14,** 138 (1958).

271. C. Su and C. Y. Lee, *Brit. J. Pharmacol.*, **15,** 88 (1960).

272. J. Cheymol and F. Bourillet, *J. Physiol. Paris*, **51,** 483 (1959).

CHAPTER FORTY-SEVEN

Skeletal Muscle Relaxants

R. J. MOHRBACHER

McNeil Laboratories, Inc.
Camp Hill Road
Fort Washington, Pennsylvania 19034, USA

CONTENTS

1 INTRODUCTION

The drugs discussed in this chapter are used primarily to reduce localized muscle contraction and spasm following musculoskeletal trauma. To date, most drugs are of minimal therapeutic value in the treatment of the general muscle rigidity and spasticity associated with neurological disorders (e.g., cerebral palsy), cerebral injury, or transection of the spinal cord. Drugs to induce relaxation during surgical procedures (neuromuscular blocking agents) and agents to reduce the muscular tremors of parkinsonism are presented in Chapters 46 and 45, respectively. Because there is a poor correlation between animal experiments with artificially induced spasticity/spasm and clinical efficacy, attention in this chapter is directed primarily to those compounds in which at least one member of the class was tested clinically. The intensity of synthesis and testing of compounds for skeletal muscle relaxation has subsided somewhat since the 1955–1965 period of vigorous activity. This may be due to the recognition of the limited therapeutic utility of orally administered muscle relaxants and to the evolution of selected members of known CNS-depressant classes (i.e., benzodiazepines, aminoalkyltricyclic compounds) as skeletal muscle relaxants.

Several new compounds with different mechanistic spectra of activity are discussed. The biochemical events that occur following administration of some skeletal muscle relaxants are beginning to be unraveled, but the studies reported to date offer limited guidance to the medicinal chemist or pharmacologist.

2 CLINICAL ASPECTS

Skeletal muscle spasm is usually caused by trauma such as overextension or a bruising blow which results in an *acute* episode of involuntary contraction of a muscle or group of muscles. This is often attended by pain, interference with function, and occasionally, postural distortion. In some cases, tension headaches are claimed to be responsible for local, sustained muscle contractions which can be treated with muscle relaxant–analgesic combinations or muscle relaxant–antianxiety drugs.

Spasticity can be described as hyperactivity of motor reflexes caused by chronic malfunction of spinal or supraspinal neural pathways as seen in hemiplegia, paraplegia, spinal cord transection, and multiple sclerosis. A lesion to a motoneuronal pathway anywhere from the cerebral cortex to the spinal cord can be responsible for the exaggerated muscle tone of spasticity. In general, acute muscular spasms are the result of excessive spinal and brain stem polysynaptic neural activity whereas chronic spastic conditions may involve a greater proportion of supraspinal monosynaptic neurons (1, 2).

The currently available CNS muscle relaxants are likely to be more effective in treating acute spasm than in providing long-term relief to spastic conditions such as hemiplegia. Another approach to the treatment of spasticity might be direct inhibition of the contractile mechanism of skeletal muscle as exemplified by dantrolene sodium (see Section 6.17).

3 PHYSIOLOGY OF MUSCLE CONTROL

The physiology of the musculospinal reflex arc and the influence of supraspinal control centers on this arc are extremely complex and incompletely understood in most types of spasticity or spasm. Comprehensive discussions of the abnormal physiology of spasticity are presented by Burke (3), Hilson (4), and in a symposium (5). The probable pathways involved in nerve signal transmission for normal muscle reflexes are presented in simplified form in Fig. 47.1.

The resting tension and flexor–extensor activity of skeletal muscle are maintained by a group of motor nerves, Ia, II, α, and γ, which synapse in the spinal cord at alpha or gamma motoneuronal sites. The spinal cord serves as a control center for afferent signals from the muscle and higher brain centers. The alpha and gamma motoneurons, in addition to dispatching efferent signals to

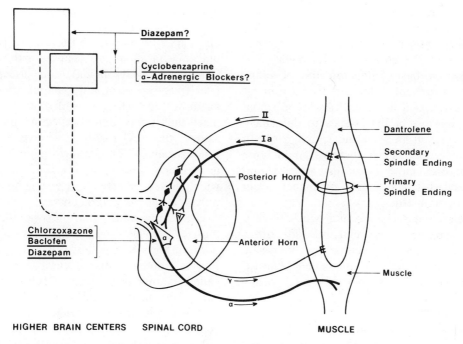

Diazepam?

Cyclobenzaprine
α-Adrenergic Blockers?

II

Ia

Dantrolene

Secondary
Spindle Ending

Primary
Spindle Ending

Posterior Horn

Chlorzoxazone
Baclofen
Diazepam

α

Anterior Horn

Muscle

γ

α

HIGHER BRAIN CENTERS   SPINAL CORD   MUSCLE

Fig. 47.1 Simplified basic reflex pathways and probable sites of drug action [after Brogden et al. (58) and Burke (3)].

the muscles, receive and modulate signals from supraspinal areas. The muscle spindle is a tension-sensitive organ within the muscle which receives gamma efferent and initiates group Ia and II afferent nerve impulses in the flexor–extensor activity of body movement.

When a muscle is stretched, specialized stretch receptors (primary and secondary) in the muscle spindle transmit signals to the spinal cord along group Ia and group II afferent fibers. The incoming afferent volley carried along group Ia fibers makes a direct (monosynaptic) connection with the alpha motoneurons of the stretched muscle, which then reflexively contracts. Afferent signals initiated at the secondary muscle-spindle endings activate polysynaptic pathways (group II fibers) involving a number of interneurons before actual stimulation of the alpha motoneurons. The sensitivity of muscle-spindle receptors is affected by the gamma motoneurons. One of the principal physiological abnormalities in spastic-

ity is an increase in gamma motoneuronal activity, lowering the threshold of the muscle spindles to stretching of the muscles (1).

The higher brain centers have both inhibitory and facilitatory actions; interruption of these pathways leads to abnormal stretch reflexes. Many forms of spasticity are due to a net excess of excitatory influences. In animals, the decerebrate rigid cat mimics this latter neural imbalance. Unfortunately, these supraspinal circuits are also involved in other CNS-mediated functions and the depressant effect of muscle-relaxant drugs on these pathways may give rise to intolerable side effects such as sedation or muscular weakness.

4 PHARMACOLOGY

The pharmacological actions of the muscle relaxants are thought to be due to their inhibition of nervous impulses within the spinal cord and at supraspinal levels, such as the reticular formation. The complexity and lack of information on the interaction of the spinal cord and higher motor control systems of the cortex, basal ganglia, and cerebellum have hampered the development of animal tests for the action of muscle-relaxant drugs on these supraspinal centers. Most of the studies to date have been concentrated on the spinal cord. In the future, medicinal chemists could hope for more selective animal tests which would be related to the effect of higher brain centers on spasticity.

Skeletal muscle relaxants which have a wide separation between relaxant doses and doses causing sedation or other side effects still elude the medicinal chemist. Intense muscle-relaxant activity can rarely be observed in humans following oral administration. These are the challenges facing the medicinal chemist today.

Thorough reviews on pharmacological methods of evaluating muscle relaxants in animals are those by Smith (6) and Domino (7). The pharmacologist must try to define the intensity and mechanistic profile of muscle relaxation observed and assess other CNS effects, particularly depressant effects, which are frequently present. The starting point is often observations in intact rodents—loss of righting reflex, reversible hind leg weakness and paraplegia, without concomitant respiratory depression and general stupor. Antagonism of the tonic extensor phase of convulsions induced by electroshock, strychnine, or pentylenetetrazole (also properties of many anticonvulsants) are exhibited by most muscle relaxants. Antagonism of spinal, polysynaptic reflex activity preferentially over monosynaptic reflexes is an identifying characteristic of many muscle relaxants leading to their classification as interneuronal blocking agents. In the cervically transected cat dosed with a polysynaptic relaxant, the knee jerk reflex (monosynaptically mediated) is unaffected but the flexor and crossed extensor reflexes

(polysynaptically mediated) are diminished or blocked. However, this difference in effect may be merely a reflection of partial blocking on all spinal synapses with multisynaptic pathways being more susceptible (8). Thus the term polysynaptic blocking agent is satisfactory provided it is recognized that it may merely reflect an additive, rather than a highly selective, effect. Mephenesin (47.**2**), methocarbamol (47.**10**) and chlorzoxazone (47.**72**), the latter two widely used clinically, are examples of polysynaptic blocking agents.

Hypertonia and hyperreflexia of skeletal muscles can be produced by a variety of decerebration techniques; it is usually done in cats. Intercollicular decerebration (also called gamma decerebrate rigidity) of the cat causes an increased activity of gamma motoneurons (fusimotor neurons) (9). Decerebrate rigidity produced by ischemia involves primarily alpha efferents directly to skeletal muscle cells (Fig. 47.1) (7). Both forms of decerebrate rigidity involve transmission over spinal interneurons, but apparently of different types. Phenothiazines, such as chlorpromazine (47.**87**), are generally more potent in gamma, relative to alpha, decerebrate rigidity, suggesting that their major site of action is supraspinal (7, 9). Compounds such as mephenesin (47.**2**) are less selective, producing depression of both alpha and gamma supraspinal efferent systems (6). Spinal cord transected cat preparations can be used to assess supraspinal versus spinal sites of action. Since more neurons in spinal and supraspinal sites are polysynaptic, there must be great differences in drug transport and/or in receptor sensitivity for those polysynaptic muscle relaxants that act predominantly at the spinal cord.

CNS-depressant drugs, such as the barbiturate-hypnotic agents, phenothiazine-tranquilizing agents, and the benzodiazepine-antianxiety agents, have pharmacological profiles that are somewhat similar to those of muscle relaxants. At present, drugs in each of the latter two classes [e.g., cyclobenzaprine (47.**90**), diazepam (47.**76**)] show both muscle-relaxant and sedative properties in clincial use. The supposed predominant sites of actions of the different types of muscle relaxants are indicated in Fig. 47.1. A more detailed discussion of the mode of action for certain drugs is presented below (Section 6).

5   HISTORICAL BACKGROUND

In 1910 Gilbert and Descomps (11) reported that antodyne (47.**1**), clinically used as an analgetic–antipyretic agent, caused reversible paralysis in animals. Goodman (12), in 1943, reported similar effects for benzimidazole (47.**67**). In 1946 Berger and Bradley (13, 17) made a study of analogs of antodyne that resulted in the clinical introduction of mephenesin (47.**2**) as a muscle relaxant. Since that time, an extremely wide variety of compounds have been reported to have muscle-relaxant properties; excellent reviews are those by Landes et al (14), Engelhardt and Stone (15), and Donahoe and Kimura (16).

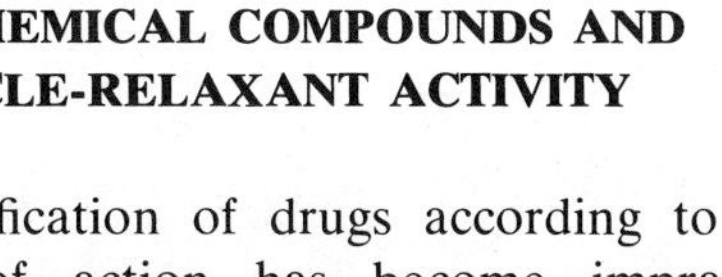

$$\text{OCH}_2\text{CHOHCH}_2\text{OH}$$
R

47.**1**   R = H
47.**2**   R = CH$_3$

6   CHEMICAL COMPOUNDS AND MUSCLE-RELAXANT ACTIVITY

Classification of drugs according to their site of action has become impractical, partly because of our incomplete knowledge of the pathophysiology of spasticity/spasm, and partly because many drugs are now known to have several sites of action. Drugs are presented in this section by chemical structural class in generally increasing complexity of structure.

6.1   Glycerol Ethers and Derivatives

Mephenesin (47.**2**) was the most potent and had the widest safety margin among 143 α-aryl ethers tested in mice by Berger and Bradley (17). These investigators found that the aryl group could be replaced by alkyl groups (47.**3**), particularly *n*-pentyl. However, maximal activity was only about one-third that of mephenesin (47.**2**). For an excellent review of analogs of mephenesin, the reader is referred to Donahoe and Kimura (16). Though Berger concluded that α,γ-diethers were inactive at sublethal doses, Hine et al. (18) reported that α,γ-diether 47.**4** was equipotent to mephenesin following intraperitoneal administration to mice.

$$\text{ROCH}_2\text{CHOHCH}_2\text{OR}'$$

47.**3**   R = CH$_3$, C$_2$H$_5$, *n*-C$_5$H$_{11}$, R' = H
47.**4**   R = C$_6$H$_5$, R' = C$_2$H$_5$

Mephenesin (47.**2**) is completely metabolized in man within 24 hr to major inactive metabolite 47.**5** and minor metabolite 47.**6** (19). In an effort to inhibit the rapid metabolic oxidation of mephenesin, Berger (20) tested ester 47.**7** and found that it had a significantly longer duration of action with one-third the potency. Other esters of glycerol ethers (18) increased the duration of paralysis in animals, but the potency varied. Another related approach to improving the potency and duration of action of

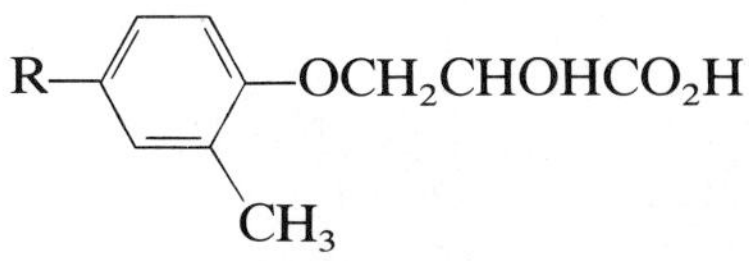

$$R\text{—}\bigcirc\text{—OCH}_2\text{CHOHCO}_2\text{H}$$
CH$_3$

47.**5**   R = H
47.**6**   R = OH

$$\bigcirc\text{—OCH}_2\text{CHOHCH}_2\text{OCO(CH}_2)_2\text{CO}_2\text{H}$$
CH$_3$

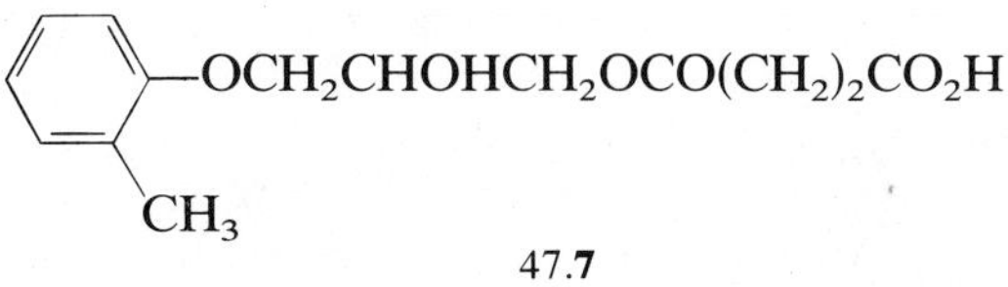

47.**7**

$$ArOCH_2CHOHCH_2OCONH_2$$

47.**8** Ar = o-CH$_3$C$_6$H$_4$
47.**9** Ar = p-ClC$_6$H$_4$
47.**10** Ar = o-CH$_3$OC$_6$H$_4$

mephenesin led to the study of γ-carbamates 47.**8**–47.**10**. Mephenesin carbamate (47.**8**) is similar in potency and duration of paralysis to mephenesin following intraperitoneal administration to mice (21), but has a longer duration of action than mephenesin following oral administration. This is due to the carbamate being more slowly absorbed from the gastrointestinal tract. At equal concentrations in the blood, mephenesin and its carbamate (47.**8**) produce equivalent degrees of muscle relaxation (22). Of the three carbamates that have been in clinical use, the p-chloro analog (47.**9**) has a significantly longer duration of action. This is probably due to the chlorine atom inhibiting hydroxylation of the phenyl ring (as seen in 47.**6**). Although chlorphenesin carbamate (47.**9**) exhibits a longer duration of pharmacological action it is rapidly excreted in the urine of rats and man, with 85% of the dose recovered as glucuronide 47.**11** 24 hr after administration to man (23). In man, methocarbamol (47.**10**) has a biologic half-life (1.2 hr) intermediate between that of mephenesin carbamate (47.**8**) and chlorphenesin carbamate (3.1 hr) (24). Methocarbamol and its metabolites are extensively conjugated before urinary excretion, with approximately equal amounts of 47.**12** and 47.**13** being isolated from human urine (25).

The mechanism of action for muscle relaxation activity of the glycerol ethers described above is thought to be due to inhibition of nerve impulse transmission in the polysynaptic (also called internuncial) pathways in the spinal cord, hence the name polysynaptic depressants. Mephenesin is one of the most widely studied drugs of this type and could be looked on as a "primary standard" of polysynaptic muscle relaxants. Unfortunately. it is only weakly active in man and has slight clinical use in the United States, western Europe, and Japan. Methocarbamol (47.**10**) is one of the three most commonly used skeletal muscle relaxants in the United States, chlorphenesin carbamate (47.**9**) being used about one-tenth as often.

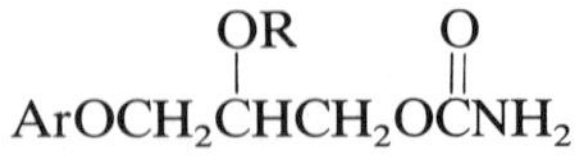

Several structures (47.**14**, 47.**15**), which can be considered to be cyclic derivatives of aryl glycerol ethers, have shown muscle-relaxant activity in animals (26, 27). Epoxy ether 47.**14** has a longer duration of action than mephenesin and was shown to be converted to mephenesin by guinea pig liver homogenase (26).

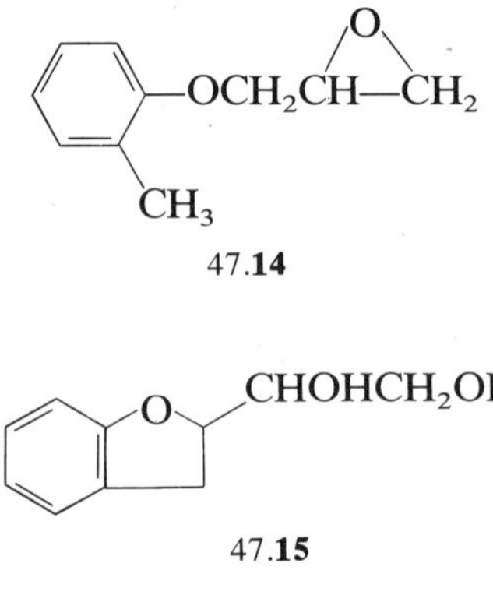

47.**14**

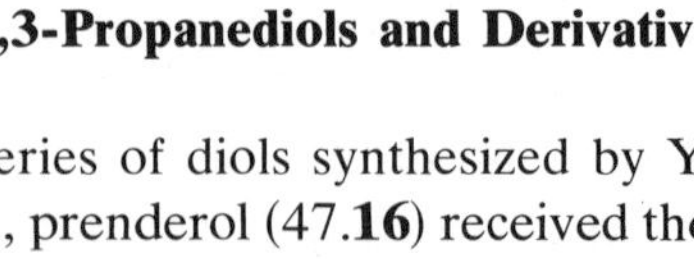

47.**15**

6.2 1,3-Propanediols and Derivatives

Of a series of diols synthesized by Yale et al. (28), prenderol (47.**16**) received the most study as a muscle relaxant. Its pharmacological profile (29, 30) resembled that of mephenesin with a higher ratio of anticonvulsant activity to muscle-relaxant activity. In an effort to obtain longer duration of activity, a variety of mono- and diesters of 47.**16** were tested with little success (16).

$$ArOCH_2\overset{\overset{\displaystyle OR}{|}}{C}HCH_2O\overset{\overset{\displaystyle O}{\|}}{C}NH_2$$

47.**11** Ar = p-ClC$_6$H$_4$, R = C$_6$H$_9$O$_6$
47.**12** Ar = p-OH, o-CH$_3$OC$_6$H$_3$; R = C$_6$H$_9$O$_6$ or SO$_3$H
47.**13** Ar = o-HOC$_6$H$_4$, R = C$_6$H$_9$O$_6$ or SO$_3$H

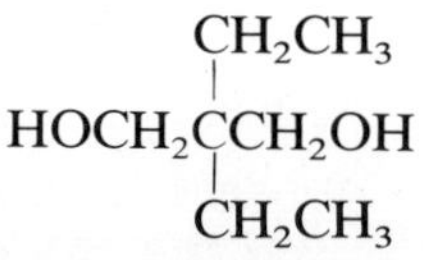

$$\underset{\textbf{47.16}}{\overset{\displaystyle CH_2CH_3}{\underset{\displaystyle CH_2CH_3}{HOCH_2CCH_2OH}}}$$

Among a series of mono- and dicarbamates, Berger (31) discovered that meprobamate 47.**17** possessed unique muscle-relaxant activity of duration approximately eight times that of mephenesin. In addition to the spinal cord polysynaptic inhibitory activity of mephenesin, meprobamate inhibits internuncial circuits in the central nervous system. Currently, meprobamate finds more use as a minor tranquilizer than as a muscle relaxant. The N-isopropyl derivative of meprobamate, carisoprodol (47.**18**), is more potent as a muscle relaxant than either mephenesin or meprobamate (6) and receives significant use in the United States and western Europe. Other monoalkyl analogs (47.**19**) have received considerable study (32, 33). The major metabolites of both meprobamate (47.**17**) and carisoprodol (47.**18**) are the penultimate carbon oxidation products 47.**20** and 47.**21**, respectively.

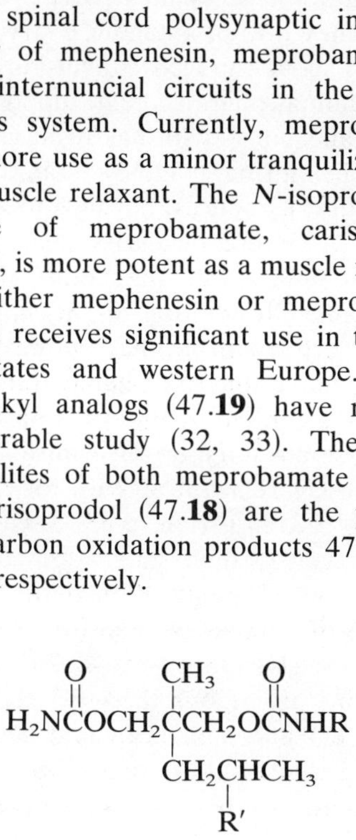

$$H_2NCOCH_2\underset{\underset{\displaystyle R'}{\overset{|}{\underset{|}{CH_2CHCH_3}}}}{\overset{\overset{\displaystyle CH_3}{|}}{\underset{}{C}}}CH_2OCNHR$$

47.**17** R, R′ = H
47.**18** R = (CH₃)₂CH, R′ = H
47.**19** R = n-C₄H₉, CH₂—CH; R′ = H
                              $\diagdown$ CH₂
47.**20** R = H, R′ = OH
47.**21** R = (CH₃)₂CH, R′ = OH

6.3 Ethylene Glycols and Derivatives

A number of arylethylene glycols are reported to possess muscle-relaxant activity (16). Styramate (47.**22**) has a pharmacolog-

ical profile similar to that of mephenesin in animals (36, 37) and receives minor clinical use in Europe. Phenaglycodol (47.**23**) has polysynaptic inhibitory activity in animals (38).

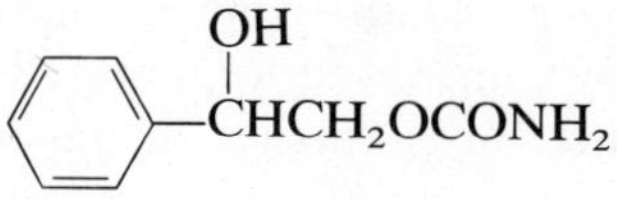

47.**22**

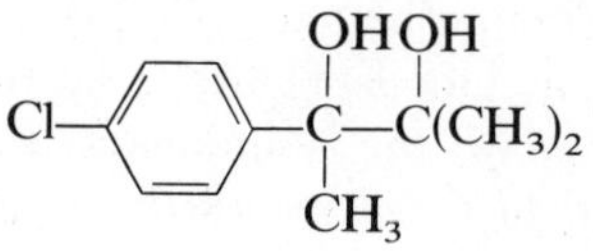

47.**23**

6.4 Cyclized Polyols

The initial observation that the glycerol ketal of cyclohexanone 47.**24** exhibited weak paralyzing activity similar to that of the monoethers of glycerol led to the synthesis and study of approximately 100 analogs (16). In most of these analogs the 4 substituent is CH₂OH (39) or its carbamate derivative (40). R and R′ are generally one- to five-carbon alkyl groups, as in glyketal (47.**25**) and promoxolane (47.**26**), both of which have fallen into obscurity after clinical trials. A 2-aryl-substituted analog (47.**27**) has been reported to show muscle-relaxant activity in animals (41).

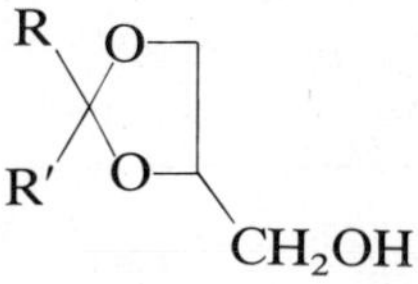

47.**24** R, R′ = -CH₂(CH₂)₃CH₂-
47.**25** R, R′ = CH₃, n-C₅H₁₁
47.**26** R, R′ = (CH₃)₂CH
47.**27** R, R′ = p-ClC₆H₄, C₂H₅

6.5 Simple Monohydric Alcohols and Carbamates

A variety of carbinols and carbamates have been reported to possess tranquilizing and muscle-relaxant activity (16). Trials of emylcamate (47.**28**) and phenprobamate (47.**29**) in humans led to minor clinical use of the latter in Germany and Japan. Phenprobamate appears to be a spinal polysynaptic depressant of the chlorzoxazone (47.**72**) range of potency in animals (6, 42). Phenprobamate (47.**29**) undergoes extensive metabolism in man so that more than 65% of the administered dose is eliminated in the urine as the glycine conjugate of benzoic acid. A minor metabolite, 3-hydroxy analog 47.**30**, is equivalent to phenprobamate in anticonvulsive and tranquilizing activity (43).

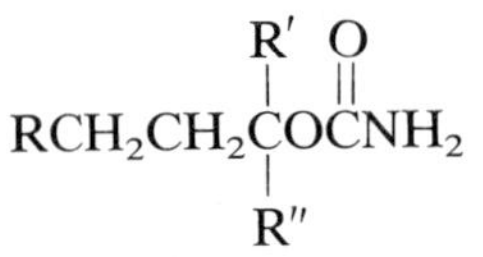

$$R'\ \ O$$
$$|\ \ \ ||$$
$$RCH_2CH_2COCNH_2$$
$$|$$
$$R''$$

47.**28** R = H, R' = CH$_3$, R'' = C$_2$H$_5$
47.**29** R = C$_6$H$_5$, R', R'' = H

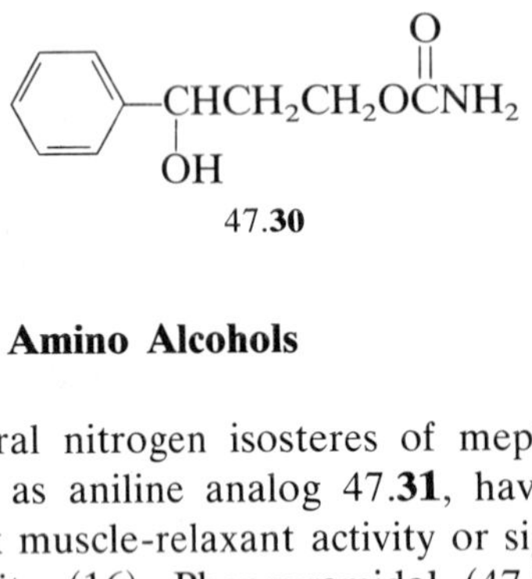

47.**30**

6.6 Amino Alcohols

Several nitrogen isosteres of mephenesin, such as aniline analog 47.**31**, have either weak muscle-relaxant activity or significant toxicity (16). Phenpyramidol (47.**32**) was originally used as a muscle relaxant (44) but now finds its principal use as an analgetic.

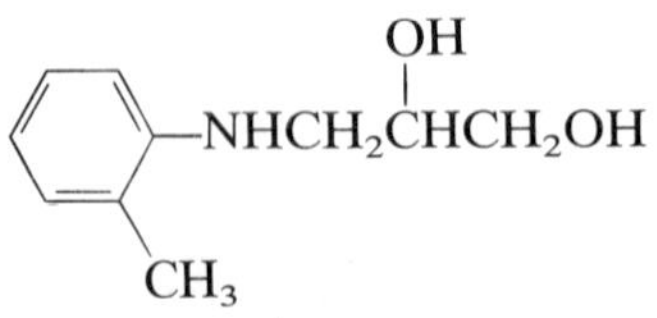

47.**31**

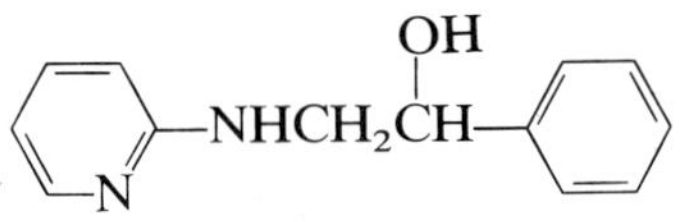

47.**32**

6.7 Amino Ethers

Few of the amino ethers that have been studied as muscle relaxants possess spinal, polysynaptic depressant activity; e.g., in animals they do not antagonize strychnine- or electroshock-induced convulsions. Only limited animal pharmacology supportive of muscle-relaxant activity has been reported for orphenadrine (47.**33**). Smith (45) showed that it reduces, but fails to abolish, rigidity in intercollicularly decerebrated cats, resembling the anticholinergic drug scopolamine. In addition to anticholinergic activity, orphenadrine has antihistaminic activity comparable to diphenhydramine (6) and finds use in the treatment of parkinsonism. A small number of clinical papers claim muscle relaxant activity for orphenadrine (47.**33**) in various types of back pain (46). However, there are no meaningful structure–muscle-relaxant activity studies available in animals or man for orphenadrine. Curiously, diazepam (47.**76**) and orphenadrine are among the most prescribed muscle relaxants and both find significant use in the treatment of other CNS diseases.

Metabolic studies of orphenadrine in man reveal at least seven products in the urine (47) with the conjugated acid (47.**37**) being the major metabolite. The other metabolites (47.**34**–47.**39**) and unchanged drug are present in only small amounts in the urine. The N-demethylated metabolite, tofenacin (47.**35**), demonstrated possible antidepressant activity in one clinical trial (48).

A number of aminoalkylbenzodioxane derivatives have both adrenergic-blocking and muscle-relaxant activity in animals and man. Quiloflex (47.**40**) and other adrenolytic CNS-sedative drugs (e.g., chlorprom-

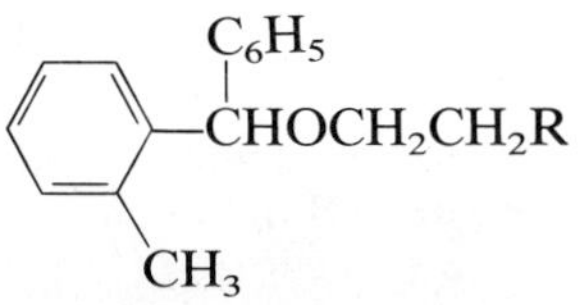

$$
\underset{\underset{\displaystyle CH_3}{|}}{C_6H_5} \\
\text{—CHOCH}_2\text{CH}_2\text{R}
$$

47.**33**   R = N(CH₃)₂
$$\overset{O}{\underset{\uparrow}{}}$$
47.**34**   R = N(CH₃)₂
47.**35**   R = NHCH₃
47.**36**   R = NH₂

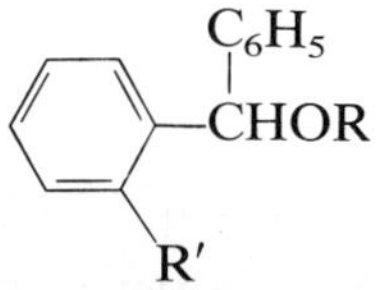

$$
\underset{\underset{\displaystyle R'}{|}}{C_6H_5} \\
\text{—CHOR}
$$

47.**37**   R = CH₂CO₂H, R′ = CH₃
47.**38**   R = H, R′ = CH₃
47.**39**   R = CH₂CH₂N(CH₃)₂
          R′ = CO₂H

azine) may induce muscle relaxation by interaction with adrenergic neurotransmitters in the central nervous system. However, the multiplicity of sites and actions of drugs possessing adrenergic blockade as a minor component of their pharmacological profile preclude any unanimous conclusion as to their mechanism of action. In cats treated with Quiloflex, decerebrate rigidity is abolished and the crossed extensor reflex is depressed, but it has no effect on convulsions induced by strychnine, pentylenetetrazole, or electroshock (6). In humans, Quiloflex has a beneficial effect on spasticity caused by spinal cord lesions but cerebral spasticity was not affected (49). Side effects of nausea, light-headedness, and sedation may limit its usefulness. Ambenoxan (47.**41**) causes skeletal muscle flaccidity without loss of the righting reflex when administered orally or parenterally to rats, rabbits, dogs, and monkeys and has been in clinical trial (50). In mice 47.**41** gave a greater separation of effect between loss of righting reflex and hypotonia (vertical ladder test) than mephenesin (47.**2**), meprobamate (47.**17**), and methocarbamol (47.**10**) (51).

Thymoxamine (47.**42**), an α-adrenergic blocker (52) with no reported muscle-

relaxant activity in animals, produced a transient reduction in spasticity in patients with lower limb spasticity. In normal volunteers it reduced the ankle jerk reflex by approximately 34% following an intravenous dose of 0.1 mg/kg with no observed sedation (53).

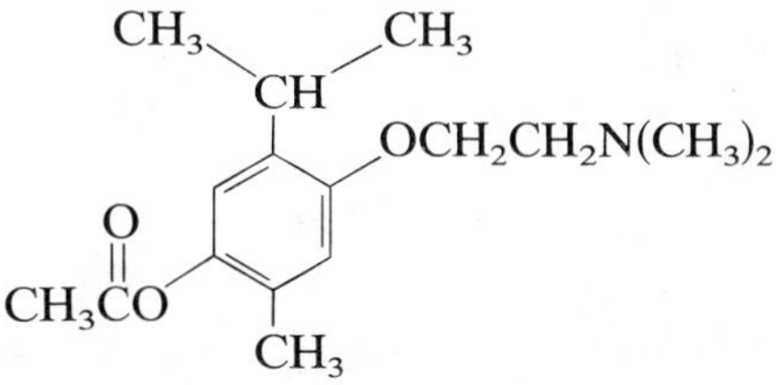

$$
\underset{\underset{CH_3CO}{\overset{O}{\uparrow}}}{}\text{...}\;\;
\begin{array}{c}
CH_3 \quad CH_3 \\
CH \\
OCH_2CH_2N(CH_3)_2 \\
CH_3
\end{array}
$$

47.**42**

6.8   Amides

A variety of relatively simple amides (15, 16) exhibit mephenesin-like, polysynaptic depressant activity in animals, but apparently have not been tested clinically as

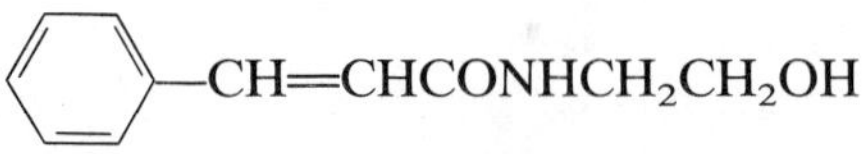

$$
\text{—CH}{=}\text{CHCONHCH}_2\text{CH}_2\text{OH}
$$

47.**43**

muscle relaxants. Idrocilamide (47.**43**) depressed spinal polysynaptic pathways in rodents and baboons (54, 55). A double-blind clinical trial in patients with spasticity of spinal or cerebral origin failed to show a significant incidence of beneficial therapeutic effects (55).

$$
\text{CH}_2\text{NHCH}_2\text{CH}_2\text{R}
$$

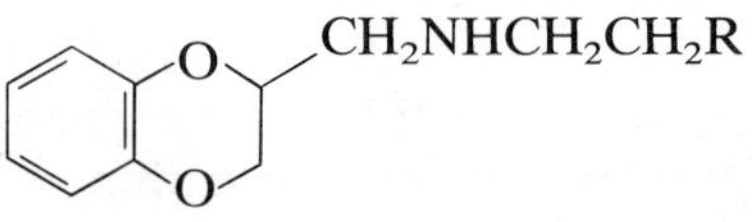

47.**40**   R = CH₂OCH₃
47.**41**   R = OCH₂CH₂OCH₃

6.9   Amino Acids

Khaunina (56) discovered the CNS-depressant effects of the α-, β-, and γ-aminobutyric acids leading to the current use in Russia of β-phenyl-γ-aminobutyric acid (Phenigan) (47.**44**) as a tranquilizing agent. Faigle and Keberle selected the *p*-chloro analog (baclofen) (47.**45**), probably because of its metabolic stability in animals and man (57), for development as a muscle relaxant.

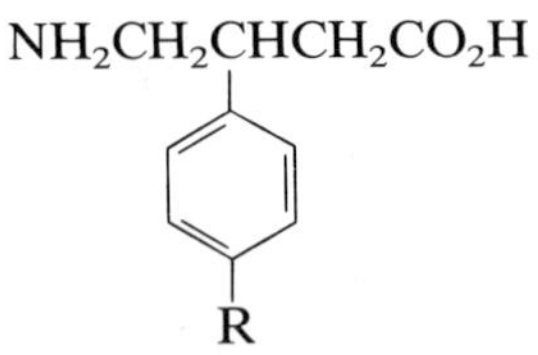

$$NH_2CH_2CHCH_2CO_2H$$

47.**44** R = H
47.**45** R = Cl

A variety of arylaminobutyric acids, such as the α- or γ-aryl analogs, and analogs (47.**46**–47.**50**) are essentially inactive except for guanidine (47.**49**), which apparently is somewhat active (57). The ethyl ester of baclofen (47.**45**) and γ-lactam (47.**51**) are also inactive as central inhibitors. Unfortunately, neither the exact chemical structure of the aryl group nor the pharmacological tests employed are described in the literature. Baclofen is rapidly and completely absorbed after oral administration to rats, dogs, and man (57).

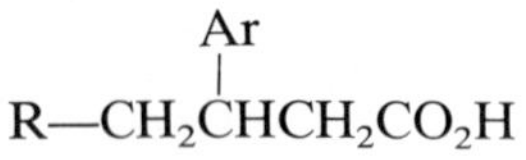

$$Ar$$
$$|$$
$$R—CH_2CHCH_2CO_2H$$

47.**46** R = NHCH$_3$
47.**47** R = N(CH$_3$)$_2$
47.**48** R = NHCOCH$_3$
                NH
                ||
47.**49** R = NH—C—NH$_2$
47.**50** R = OH

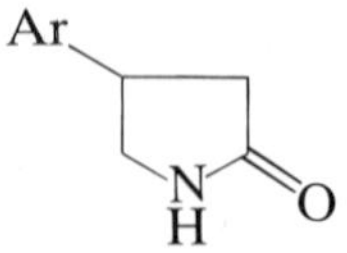

47.**51**

The plasma half-life in man is approximately 3 hr and about 85% of the oral dose is excreted unchanged. One of the major metabolites is oxidation product 47.**50**.

Baclofen (47.**45**), in placebo-controlled and open therapeutic trials, is useful in alleviating spastic symptoms such as clonus, spinal automatic movements, flexor spasms, and pain in patients with multiple sclerosis and various spinal disorders (58). It does not appear to be useful in spasticity of cerebral origin. Baclofen does not inhibit strychnine-induced convulsions, but inhibits both monosynaptic extensor and polysynaptic flexor transmission (58). In cats, it inhibits decerebrate rigidity induced by either intercollicular transection or ischemic procedures. These results suggest that baclofen influences both the alpha and gamma motoneuronal systems, predominantly at the spinal cord (Fig. 47.1).

A number of biochemical studies in animals demonstrates that baclofen has similar biochemical effects to γ-hydroxybutyric acid in causing a marked rise in the brain concentration of dopamine with little effect on the brain concentration of norepinephrine (59, 60). Baclofen, although structurally related to γ-aminobutyric acid (GABA), does not seem to interact at GABA receptors (61). Baclofen also inhibits the activation of polysynaptic receptors by substance P in the rat spinal cord (62). Unlike GABA, baclofen enters the CNS easily according to the pharmacokinetic data (57) and as indicated by its alleviation of spinal spasticity in animals and man. The relationship of the biochemical events reported following administration of baclofen and the muscle relaxation observed is unclear.

6.10   Pyrrolidines

A group of diversely substituted pyrrolidines show muscle-relaxant activity in animals. AHR-2666 (47.**52**) blocks cat spi-

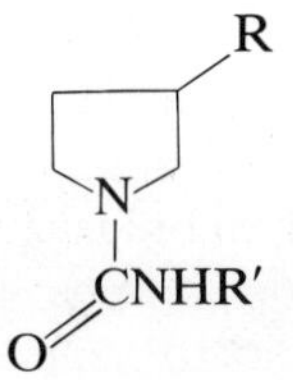

47.52   R = m-ClC$_6$H$_4$O, R' = CH$_3$
47.53   R = m-CF$_3$C$_6$H$_4$, R' = C$_2$H$_5$

nal interneurons and directly depresses skeletal muscle, indicating both central and peripheral effects. In spite of the direct effect on skeletal muscle, no impairment of respiration was observed (63). Like AHR-2666, AHR 2776 (47.53) prevented strychnine-induced convulsions and, in general, mimicked the activity of mephenesin (64). AHR-2666 is rapidly absorbed and excreted in rats, dog, and man. Major urinary metabolites in dog and man are 47.54 and 47.55 (65).

HA-966 (47.56) elevates the threshold to strychnine-induced convulsions in mice and abolishes the polysynaptic flexor reflex in cats. (66). A reversible, long-lasting CNS depression is produced following administration to cats, dogs, or monkeys. Judging from papers published to date, HA-966 appears to draw more interest' as a biochemical tool than as a skeletal muscle relaxant. Hillen and Noach (67) showed that HA-966 blocks dopamine release, causing an increase in its concentration in the rat striatum. The effect of HA-966 (47.56) on cerebral metabolism of glucose and acetate (68) and its effect on dopamine synthesis (69) are discussed with no obvious conclusion as to the relationship of these effects to muscle relaxation or sedation.

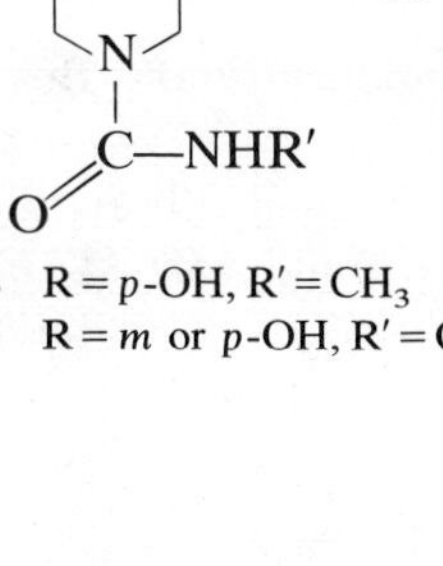

47.54   R = p-OH, R' = CH$_3$
47.55   R = m or p-OH, R' = CHO

Rasmussen et al. (70) discovered a series of pyrrolidinylideneureas with muscle-relaxant activity. Xilobam (47.57) is a potent polysynaptic muscle relaxant with minimal sedative effects in animals. This was judged by comparing the relative dose required to antagonize strychnine-induced convulsions to that necessary to elevate the

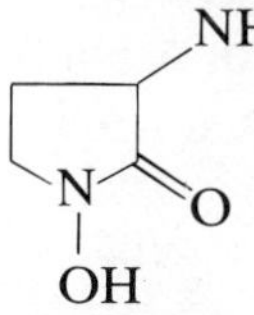

47.56

pseudo and persistent convulsive threshold induced by pentylenetetrazole (71). Antagonism of certain effects· of pentylenetetrazole is a measure of sedative activity (7). Xilobam, currently in clinical trial, is well absorbed. It is rapidly metabolized and excreted in rats, dogs, and man. Surprisingly, changing the aryl group of 47.57 to m-chlorophenyl gives minimal muscle-relaxant activity and stronger antianxiety activity.

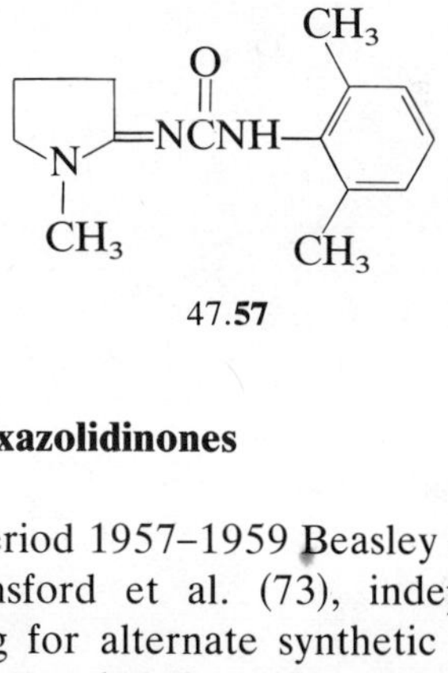

47.57

6.11   Oxazolidinones

In the period 1957–1959 Beasley et al. (72) and Lunsford et al. (73), independently searching for alternate synthetic routes to mephenesin (47.2) and methocarbamol (47.10), isolated unexpected oxazolidinone products 47.58 and 47.59. Further study of these reactions led to the synthesis of metaxalone (47.60). Mephenoxalone (47.59) shows weak muscle-relaxant activity in animals and was subsequently introduced as a minor tranquilizer. Metaxalone

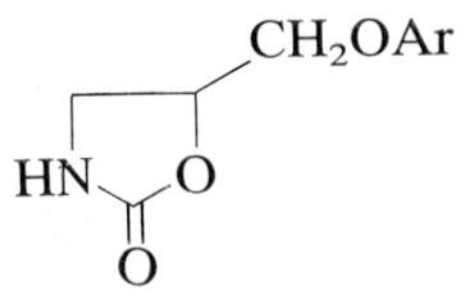

CH$_2$OAr

47.**58** Ar = o-CH$_3$C$_6$H$_4$
47.**59** Ar = o-CH$_3$OC$_6$H$_4$
47.**60** Ar = 3, 5-(CH$_3$)$_2$C$_6$H$_3$

(47.**60**) has a muscle-relaxant profile generally characteristic of a polysynaptic depressant (6) and receives only minor clinical use.

Human urinary metabolites of metaxalone (47.**60**) include carboxylic acid 47.**61** and oxazolidinone 47.**62** (74). The acid and its glucuronide are the major metabolites with minor amounts of 47.**62**. These, and similar observations in dogs, indicate that the oxazolidin-2-one ring is relatively stable to metabolism.

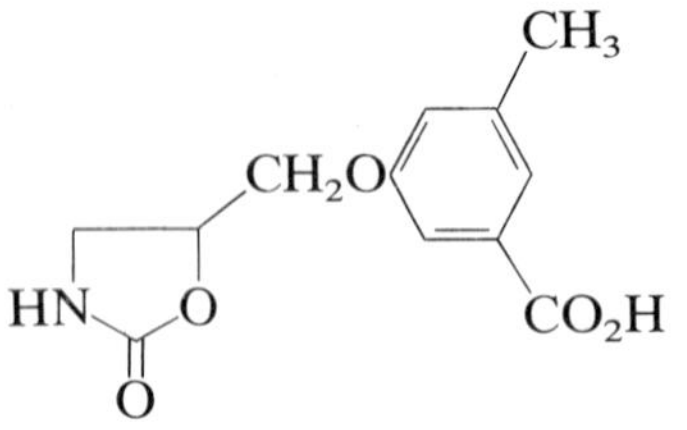

47.**61**

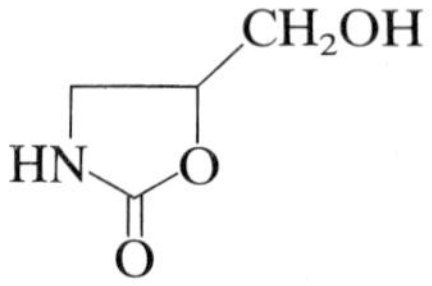

CH$_2$OH

47.**62**

6.12   Oxadiazoles

Yale and Losee (75) reported muscle-relaxant activity in a series of 5-imino-2-phenyl-1,3,4-oxadiazolines. One of the more potent analogs was compound 47.**63**.

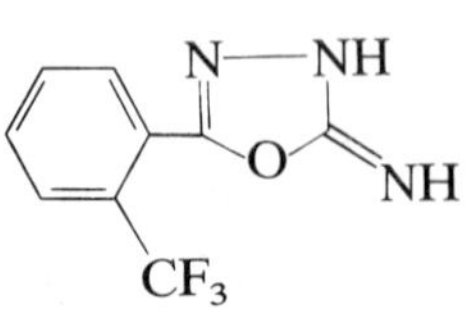

47.**63**

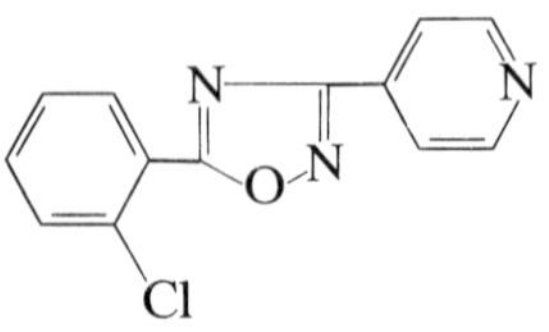

47.**64**

Pifexole (47.**64**), the most active of 35 1,2,4-oxadiazoles studied (76), has a similar profile of muscle-relaxant activity in animals to that of chlorzoxazone (77). In rats, pifexole is reported to be seven times more potent than chlorzoxazone in inhibition of strychnine-induced convulsions.

6.13   Thiazanones

Surrey et al. (78) synthesized a series of substituted 1,3-thiazanones (47.**65**); Gesler and Surrey (79) found the N-alkyl sulfones (Y = SO$_2$) to be more potent and better absorbed following oral administration than the sulfides (Y = S). The pharmacological profiles of chlormezanone (47.**66**) and meprobamate (47.**17**) in animals as both muscle relaxants and tranquilizing agents are qualitatively similar (6), with chlormezanone being more potent. It was initially introduced into the United States as a muscle relaxant but finds more use as an antianxiety agent. Chlormezanone (47.**66**) is widely used in western Europe and Japan as a muscle-relaxant/antianxiety agent. Less than 2% of the oral dose of chlormezanone administered to man is excreted intact. The major urinary metabolite is p-chlorobenzoic acid eliminated as 4-chlorohippuric acid (80).

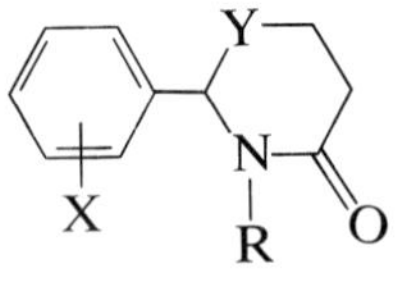

47.**65**   R = H, CH$_3$, C$_2$H$_5$
            X = H, Cl
            Y = S, SO$_2$
47.**66**   R = CH$_3$, X = p-Cl, Y = SO$_2$

6.14   Benzimidazoles and Benzoxazoles

Goodman's original observation (12) in 1943 that benzimidazole (47.**67**) produces flaccid paralysis in a variety of animal species was followed by a detailed

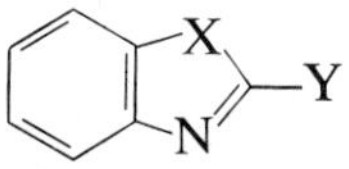

47.**67** X = NH, Y = H
47.**68** X = O, S, NH: Y = H
47.**69** X = S, Y = NH₂
47.**70** X = O, Y = NH₂

structure–activity study of a series of heterobicyclic compounds of general structure 47.**68**–47.**70** by Domino (81). Substituted 2-aminobenzthiazole 47.**69** and 2-aminobenzoxazole (47.**70**) were among the most potent compounds in producing paralysis in mice.

Marsh (82) reported the potent mephenesin-like properties of zoxazolamine (47.**71**) in 1955. It was used clinically for several years, but was withdrawn from clinical use because of the reported development of severe hepatitis in some patients (6). Chlorzoxazone (47.**72**), a minor metabolite of zoxazolamine (47.**71**), has muscle-relaxant activity of the same order as zoxazolamine (83) and has replaced it in clinical use. The major urinary metabolites of both drugs are the inactive 6-hydroxylated products 47.**73** and 47.**74**. Approximately 60% of the oral dose of zoxazolamine and 90% of the oral dose of chlorzoxazone are isolated as conjugates of their 6-hydroxy metabolites 47.**73** and 47.**74**, respectively (84). Chlorzoxazone antagonizes convulsions induced by strychnine or maximal electroshock in rodents and is a spinal polysynaptic depressant with little effect on higher CNS centers (83) (see Fig. 47.1). In man, chlorzoxazone (47.**72**) is rapidly absorbed after oral administration and is one of the three most widely used skeletal muscle relaxants in the United States.

6.15 Benzodiazepines and Benzoxazocines

Both chlordiazepoxide (47.**75**) and diazepam (47.**76**) have muscle-relaxant activity, diazepam being significantly more potent than chlordiazepoxide in animal tests. The pharmacology of benzodiazepines has been reviewed (85); substantial evidence is presented that this class of compounds shows both depressant and facilitatory effects on the CNS in animals.

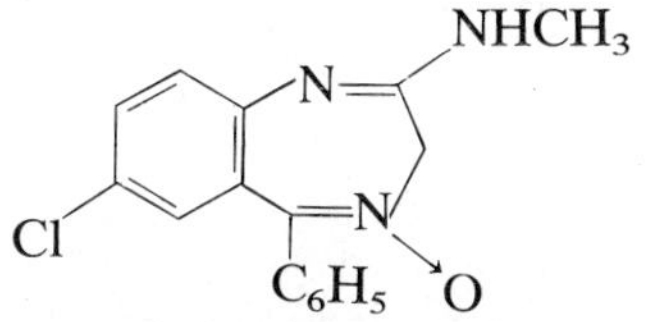

47.**75**

At the spinal level, enhancement of presynaptic inhibition and depression of polysynaptic activity have been demonstrated. At supraspinal levels, probably in the brainstem reticular formation, very small doses of benzodiazepines produce marked depressant effects most likely on the reticular facilitatory system (86, 87).

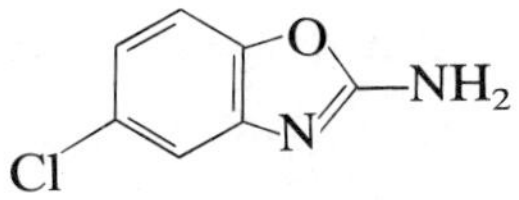

47.**71**

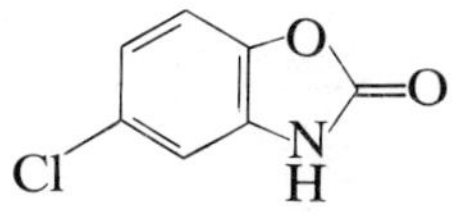

47.**73**

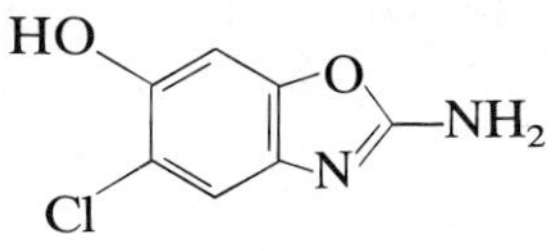

47.**72**

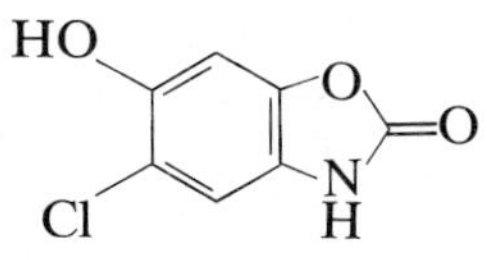

47.**74**

Significant effects on supraspinal sites differentiate the muscle-relaxant mechanism of action of the benzodiazepines from that of chlorzoxazone and methocarbamol-type compounds (see Fig. 47.1). Although there has been considerable investigation of the biochemical events following administration of diazepam to animals (85), no definitive relationship to muscle relaxation has been established.

In humans, diazepam (47.**76**) effectively suppresses activity in spinal reflex pathways and is of proved benefit in relieving painful flexor and extensor spasms and in controlling muscle tone in patients with spinal spasticity (including multiple sclerosis). However, it is of little value in patients with cerebral lesions (3). Diazepam appears to be the current agent of choice for the spastic patient. Baclofen (Section 6.9) is another promising drug for relief of spinal spasticity. A comparative clinical trial of these two drugs in spasticity has been reported (88).

In addition to being the most-prescribed antianxiety agent, diazepam (47.**76**) is one of the three most widely used muscle relaxants. The widespread acceptance of this antianxiety muscle relaxant suggests that this combination of activities is uniquely useful in relieving muscle spasms due to psychogenic or local pathological causes such as trauma or inflammation. A significant incidence of sedation is the major limiting side effect of diazepam.

A number of analogs of diazepam have

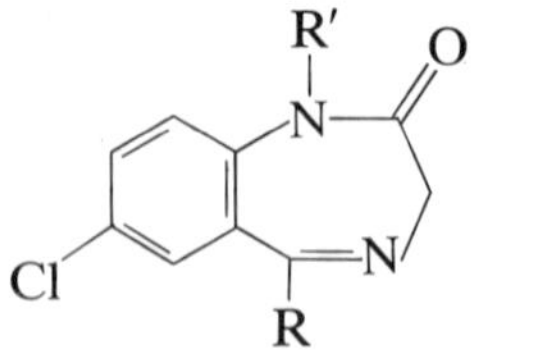

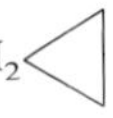

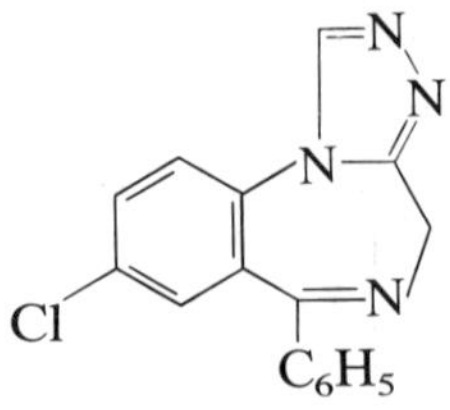

47.**79**

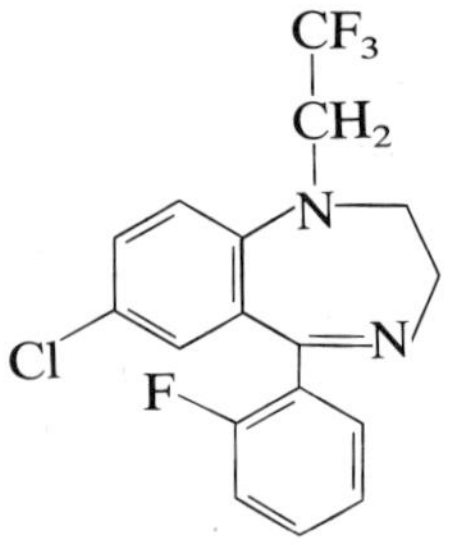

47.**80**

been studied. Tetrazepam (47.**77**) has muscle-relaxant activity in animals and man (89), where it appears to be more effective in reducing skeletal muscle hypertonia in patients with multiple sclerosis (90) than in patients with cerebral palsy (91). There are few reports in animals or man (92) to support the claim for the muscle-relaxant activity of prazepam (47.**78**). Two benzodiazepines (47.**79**, 47.**80**), structurally somewhat different from either chlordiazepoxide (47.**75**) or diazepam (47.**76**), have significant muscle-relaxant activity in animals. The activity of estazolam (47.**79**) (93) was compared to that of chlorzoxazone (47.**72**), methocarbamol (47.**10**), and chlormezanone (47.**66**) in cats (94). Like other benzodiazepines, estazolam depresses spinal and supraspinal polysynaptic reflexes, primarily by depression of the reticular facilitatory system versus direct interneuronal inhibition by chlorzoxazone and methocarbamol. In cats, fletazepam (47.**80**) appears to have a greater separation of doses between muscle-relaxant activity (antagonism of etonitazine-induced rigidity) and depressant activity (ataxia and impairment of avoidance performance) than diazepam (95, 96). All the benzodiazepines reported to date are qualitatively similar in their pharmacological profiles and it appears unlikely that any of these analogs of diazepam (47.**77**–47.**80**) will provide significant clinical advantage over diazepam.

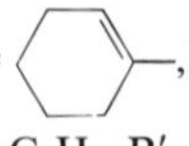

The metabolism of diazepam (47.**76**) and several other benzodiazepines is presented

47.**76**   R = C_6H_5, R' = CH_3

47.**77**   R = ⬡ , R' = CH_3

47.**78**   R = C_6H_5, R' = CH_2 ◁

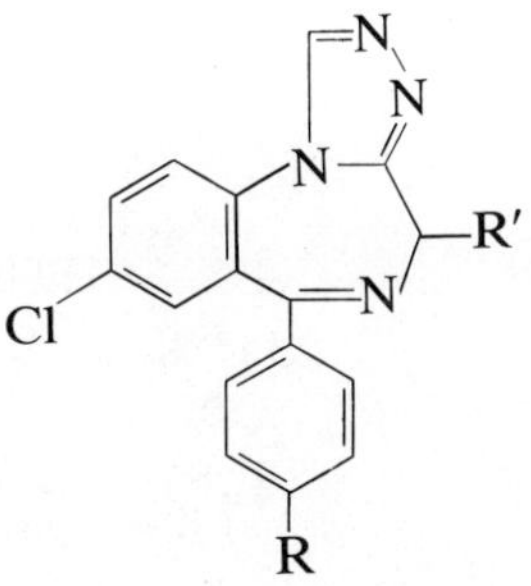

47.**81** R = OH, R′ = H
47.**82** R = H, R′ = OH

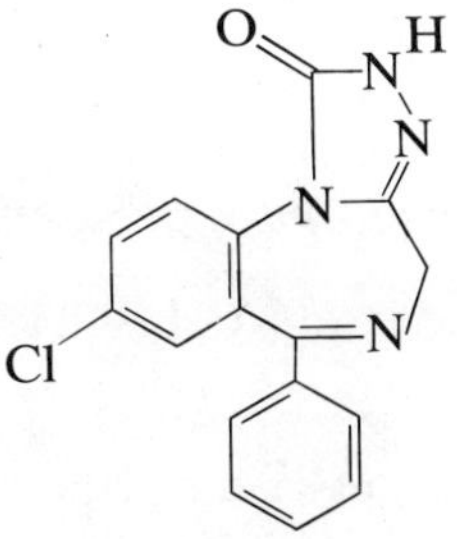

47.**83**

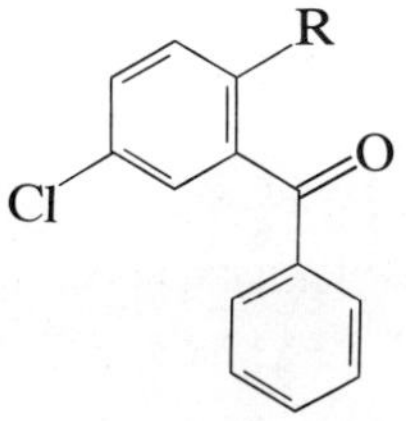

47.**84** R =

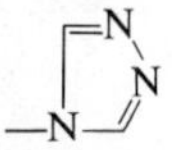

47.**85** R =

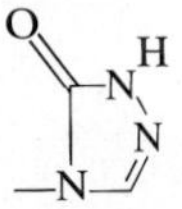

in Chapter 57. Estazolam (47.**79**) is extensively metabolized in rats, dogs, and man with similar metabolic profiles in dogs and man (97). Human urinary metabolites include hydroxylated products 47.**81** and 47.**82** and oxidation product 47.**83**, which is a much less potent muscle relaxant in rats (98). Metabolic cleavage of the diazepine ring leads to benzophenones 47.**84** and 47.**85**.

Nefopam (47.**86**), which could be considered a cyclized analog of orphenadrine (47.**33**), has significantly less antihistaminic and anticholinergic activity than orphenadrine (99). A double-blind clinical study showed beneficial effect on muscle spasm as compared to placebo (100), but the compound may be developed as an analgetic rather than as a skeletal muscle relaxant (101).

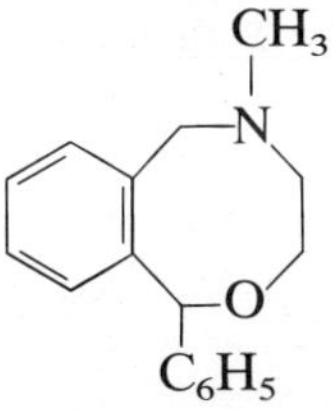

47.**86**

6.16 Aminoalkyltricyclic Compounds

The phenothiazine tranquilizers have muscle-relaxant activity among their CNS-depressant profiles. Chlorpromazine

(47.**87**) has been shown to reduce intercollicular decerebrate rigidity in cats by inhibition of the discharge of γ-motoneurons, possibly by depression of neuronal activity at some supraspinal site. Maxwell (102, 103) studied a group of phenothiazines in a search for an improved ratio of potency in reduction of decerebrate rigidity and sedative potential, which led to the clinical trial of dimethothiazine (47.**88**). In an effort to find a more potent antispastic agent with even less sedative side effects, the same group chose M & B 18,706 (47.**89**) as a compound worthy of detailed study (104). It appears to be equipotent to chlorpromazine in reducing intercollicular decerebrate rigidity in cats with 1/20 to 1/100 the potency of chlorpromazine in central depressant/sedative tests in rats.

The antidepressant aminoalkyltricyclic drugs, imipramine, desipramine, and amitriptyline (Chapter 58), have a similar

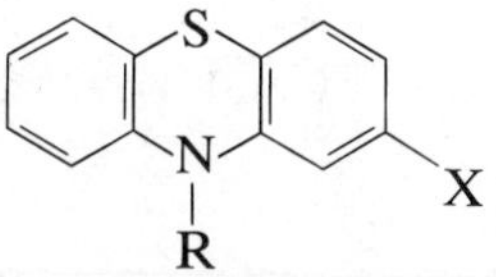

47.**87** R = $CH_2CH_2CH_2N(CH_3)_2$, X = Cl
47.**88** R = $CH_2CHN(CH_3)_2$, X = $SO_2N(CH_3)_2$
　　　　　　CH_3
47.**89** R = $CH_2CHCH_2N(CH_3)_2$, X = $CO(CH_2)_3CH_3$
　　　　　　CH_3

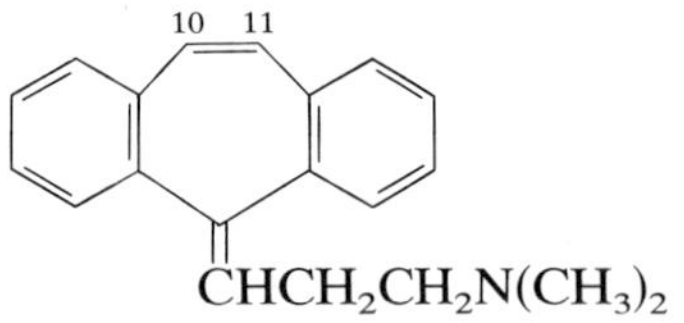

CHCH$_2$CH$_2$N(CH$_3$)$_2$

47.90

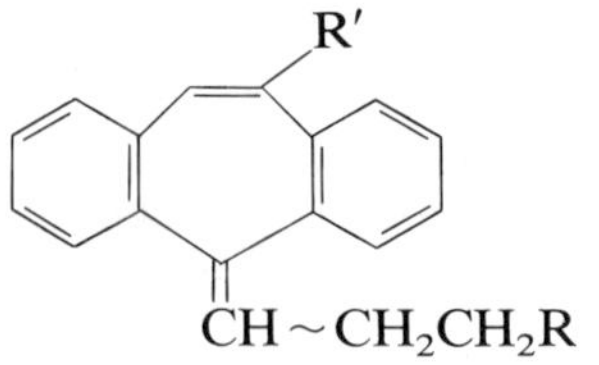

CH $\sim$ CH$_2$CH$_2$R

O
$\uparrow$

47.**91** R = N(CH$_3$)$_2$, R' = H

O
$\uparrow$

47.**92** R = N(CH$_3$)$_2$, R' = OH
47.**93** R = NHCH$_3$, R' = H
47.**94** R = NHCH$_3$, R' = OH
47.**95** R = N(CH$_3$)$_2$, R' = OH

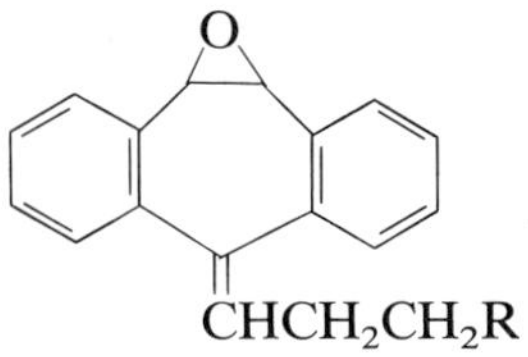

CHCH$_2$CH$_2$R

47.**96** R = N(CH$_3$)$_2$

pharmacological profile to the phenothiazines (47.**87**–47.**89**) as muscle relaxants (10, 105). Cyclobenzaprine (47.**90**), the 10,11-dehydro analog of amitriptyline, shows antidepressant and muscle-relaxant activity in animals and man (10, 106). It apparently exerts its action at a supraspinal site (see Fig. 47.1). Compared to chlorpromazine (47.**87**) and diazepam (47.**76**), cyclobenzaprine (47.**90**) appears to be more consistent in reducing tonic α-motoneuronal activity in cats and less potent in inducing ataxia (10). In humans 47.**90** may be more effective in treating local muscle spasm than spasticity (107, 108). Cyclobenzaprine was introduced onto the U.S. market in 1977.

Cyclobenzaprine (47.**90**) undergoes extensive metabolism in rats, giving rise to at least six metabolites (47.**91**–47.**96**). The stereochemistry of the substituents on the *exo* double bond in 47.**92**, 47.**94**, and 47.**95** is not known. In addition to unchanged drug, major urinary metabolites appear to be 47.**91** and 47.**92** (109).

Dantrolene (47.**98**) is clearly the most potent with some activity observed in the *m*- and *o*-nitro analogs (47.**97**, R = *o*- and *m*-NO$_2$) as well as the *p*-amino *p*-cyano, and *p*-chloro analogs (47.**97**, R = *p*-NH$_2$ *p*-CN, *p*-Cl). Replacement of the chlorine atom with bromine or fluorine decreases activity markedly. Replacement of the 4-carbonyl group of dantrolene (47.**98**) with methylene (47.**99**) reduces the activity slightly, and changing the position of the amino group (47.**100**) greatly decreases activity (111).

After further testing in animals and man the muscle-relaxant activity of dantrolene (47.**98**) is now believed to be essentially independent of the CNS (112). Apparently, it acts directly on the contractile mechanism of skeletal muscle to decrease the force of contraction with no demonstrable effect on neuromuscular transmission or polysynaptic reflexes. A review of the pharmacological and clinical properties of dantrolene sodium has been published (112). It probably interferes with the re-

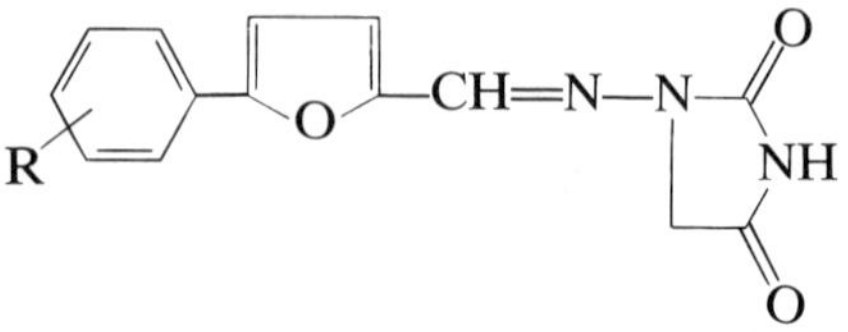

6.17 Miscellaneous Compounds

Synder et al. (110) found classical muscle-relaxant activity (inhibition of cat flexor reflex) among a series of relatively insoluble furfurylideneaminohydantoins 47.**97**.

47.**97** R = NO$_2$, NH$_2$, Cl, CN
47.**98** R = *p*-NO$_2$

lease of calcium from the sarcoplasmic reticulum of muscle fibrils, thereby uncoupling the excitation–contraction mechanism of skeletal muscle (113) (see Fig. 47.1). A number of clinical trials have demonstrated that dantrolene sodium is beneficial in treatment of spasticity caused by multiple sclerosis, spinal and cerebral lesions, and cerebral palsy (112). A high incidence of side effects of CNS, hepatic, or gastrointestinal origin and general muscular weakness would seem to limit broad clinical use of dantrolene sodium (112).

Dantrolene (47.**98**) is slowly and incompletely absorbed following oral administration to man (112). The major urinary excretion products are dantrolene, its hydroxylated derivative 47.**101** (114), and its acetamido derivative 47.**102** (115).

Thiocolchicoside (47.**103**) has muscle-relaxant activity in animals (116) and is used clinically in France and Italy (117).

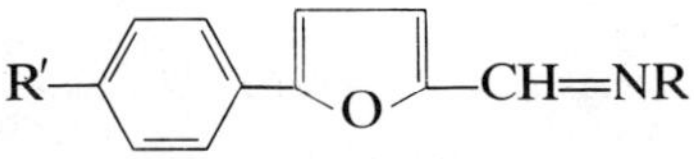

47.**103**

47.**99** R = 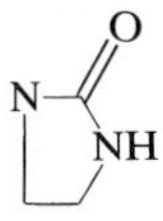 , R′ = NO₂

47.**100** R = 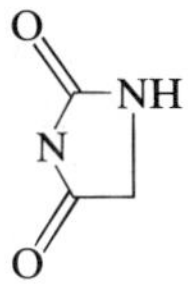 , R′ = NO₂

47.**101** R = 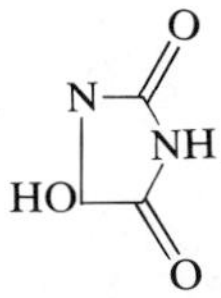 , R′ = NO₂

47.**102** R = 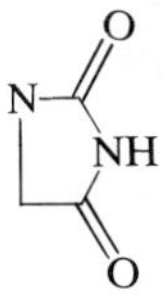 , R′ = CH₃CONH

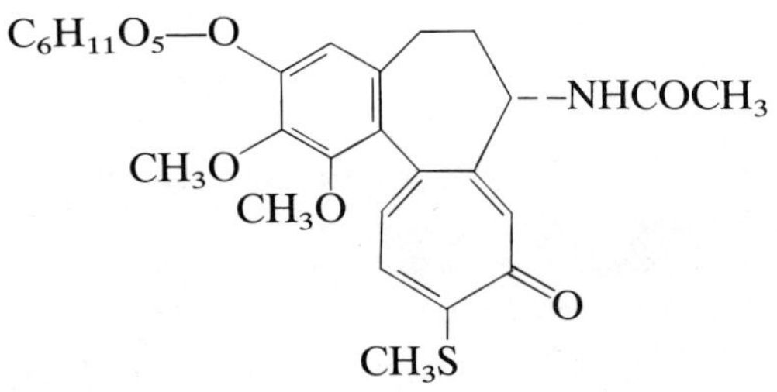

REFERENCES

1. D. L. McLellan, *J. Neurol. Neurosurg. Psychiatr.*, **36**, 555 (1973).
2. R. Herman, W. Freedman, and N. Mayer, *Arch. Phys. Med. Rehab.*, **55**, 338 (1974).
3. D. J. Burke, *Drugs*, **10**, 112 (1975).
4. A. Hilson, *Postgrad. Med. J.*, **48**, 25 (1972).
5. *Arch. Phys. Med. Rehab.*, **55**, 332–392 (1974).
6. C. M. Smith, in *Physiological Pharmacology*, Vol. II, W. S. Root and F. G. Hofmann, Eds., Academic, New York., 1965.
7. E. F. Domino, in *Evaluation of Drug Activities: Pharmacometrics*, Vol. I, D. R. Laurence and A. L. Bacharach, Eds., Academic, New York, 1964.
8. C. N. Latimer, *J. Pharmacol. Exp. Ther.*, **118**, 309 (1956).
9. R. Granit, in *Basis of Motor Control*, Academic, New York, 1970.
10. N. N. Share and C. S. McFarlane, *Neuropharmacol.*, **14**, 675 (1975).
11. A. Gilbert and R. Descomps, *C. R. Soc. Biol.*, **69**, 145 (1910).
12. L. Goodman, *Bull. N. Engl. Med. Cent.*, **5**, 97 (1943).
13. F. M. Berger, *Pharmacol. Rev.*, **1**, 243 (1949).
14. R. C. Landes, R. J. Stopkie, and V. T. Spaziano, in *Annual Reports in Medicinal Chemistry*, Vol. 8, R. V. Heinzelman, Ed., Academic, New York, 1973.
15. E. L. Engelhardt and C. A. Stone, in *Medicinal Chemistry*, Part II, 3rd ed., A. Burger, Ed., Wiley-Interscience, New York, 1970.
16. H. B. Donahoe and K. K. Kimura, in *Drugs Affecting the Central Nervous System*, A. Burger, Ed., Dekker, New York, 1968.
17. F. M. Berger and W. Bradley, *Brit. J. Pharmacol.*, **1**, 265 (1946).
18. C. H. Hine, H. E. Christensen, F. J. Murphy, and H. Davis, *J. Pharmacol. Exp. Ther.*, **97**, 414 (1949).

19. R. F. Riley, *J. Am. Chem. Soc.*, **72,** 5712 (1950).

20. F. M. Berger and R. F. Riley, *J. Pharmacol. Exp. Ther.*, **96,** 269 (1949).

21. F. M. Berger, *J. Pharmacol. Exp. Ther.*, **104,** 468 (1952).

22. L. S. Goodman and A. Gilman, Eds., *The Pharmacological Basis of Therapeutics*, 4th ed., Macmillan, New York, 1970, p. 227.

23. D. R. Buhler, *J. Pharmacol. Exp. Ther.*, **145,** 232 (1964).

24. A. A. Forist and R. W. Judy, *J. Pharm. Sci.*, **60,** 1686 (1971).

25. R. B. Bruce, L. B. Turnbull, and J. H. Newman, *J. Pharm. Sci.*, **60,** 104 (1971).

26. K. Söllner and K. Irrgang, *Arzneim.-Forsch.*, **15,** 1355 (1965).

27. H. E. Zaugg, *J. Am. Chem. Soc.*, **76,** 5818 (1954).

28. H. L. Yale, E. J. Pribyl, W. Braker, J. Bernstein, and W. A. Lott, *J. Am. Chem. Soc.*, **72,** 3716 (1950).

29. W. A. Lott, *Trans. N.Y. Acad. Sci.*, **11,** 1 (1948).

30. F. M. Berger, *Proc. Soc. Exp. Biol. Med.*, **71,** 270 (1949).

31. F. M. Berger, *J. Pharmacol. Exp. Ther.*, **112,** 413 (1954).

32. F. M. Berger, M. Kletzkin, and S. Margolin, *Med. Exp.*, **10,** 327 (1964).

33. B. W. Horrom, U.S. Pat. 3,037,045 (1962).

34. J. Edelson, A. Schlosser, and J. F. Douglas, *Biochem. Pharmacol.*, **14,** 901 (1965).

35. J. F. Douglas, B. J. Ludwig, and A. Schlosser, *J. Pharmacol. Exp. Ther.*, **138,** 21 (1962).

36. S. J. DeSalva, G. R. Clements, and N. Ercoli, *J. Pharmacol. Exp. Ther.*, **126,** 318 (1959).

37. E. Macko, G. Wilfon, L. Greene, A. D. Bender, and R. E. Tedeschi, *Arch. Int. Pharmacodyn. Ther.*, **168,** 220 (1967).

38. I. H. Slater, G. T. Jones, and W. K. Young, *Proc. Soc. Exp. Biol. Med.*, **93,** 528 (1956).

39. F. M. Berger, V. Boekelheide, and D. S. Tarbell, *Science*, **108,** 561 (1948).

40. B. W. Horrom and H. E. Zaugg, U.S. Pat. 3,121,094 (1964).

41. J. Chladt and H. Braunlich, *Acta. Biol. Med. Ger.*, **15,** 79 (1965).

42. G. Stille, *Arzneim.-Forsch.*, **12,** 340 (1962).

43. D. S. Farrier, *Arzneim.-Forsch.*, **25,** 813 (1975).

44. T. B. O'Dele, L. R. Wilson, M. D. Napoli, H. D. White, and J. H. Miraby, *J. Pharmacol. Exp. Ther.*, **128,** 65 (1960).

45. C. M. Smith, *Proc. Soc. Exp. Biol. Med.*, **116,** 75 (1964).

46. T. Tervo, L. Petaja, and P. Lepisto, *Brit. J. Clin. Pract.*, **30,** 62 (1974); K. Hingorani, *ibid.*, **25,** 227 (1971).

47. D. E. Hathway, in *Foreign Compound Metabolism in Mammals*, Vol. 2, The Chemical Society, Burlington House, London, 1972, p. 214.

48. G. Bram and N. Shanmuganathan, *Curr. Ther. Res. Clin. Exp.* **13,** 625 (1971).

49. G. Zervopoulos and G. Michailides, *Arzneim.-Forsch.*, **2,** 161 (1962).

50. M. Shapero and P. J. Southgate, *Brit. J. Pharmacol.*, **38,** 263 (1970).

51. M. A. Cymbolist and M. Shapero, *J. Pharm. Pharmacol.*, **26,** 109 (1974).

52. J. Mercier, J. Canellas, and J. Roquebert, *Therapie*, **26,** 785 (1971).

53. S. J. Phillips and A. Richens, *Electroenceph. Clin. Neurophysiol.*, **30,** 470 (1971).

54. M. Grand, J. C. Depin, L. Fontaine, and M. Bayssat, *Eur. J. Med. Chem.*, **9,** 205 (1974).

55. G. D. Perkin and M. J. Aminoff, *Brit. J. Clin. Pharmacol.*, **3,** 879 (1976).

56. R. A. Khaunina, *Farmakol. Toksikol.*, **31,** 202 (1968); through *Chem. Abstr.*, **69,** 9495 (1969).

57. J. W. Faigle and H. Keberle, *Postgrad. Med. J.*, **48,** 9 (1972).

58. R. N. Brogden, T. M. Speight, and G. S. Avery, *Drugs*, **8,** 1 (1974).

59. M. DaPrada and H. H. Keller, *Life Sciences*, **19,** 1253 (1976).

60. N. Arden and H. Wachtel, *Acta. Pharmacol. Toxicol.*, **40,** 310 (1977).

61. A. Nistri and A. Constanti, *Experientia*, **31,** 64 (1975).

62. K. Saito, S. Konishi, and M. Otsuka, *Brain Res.*, **97,** 177 (1975).

63. D. N. Johnson, W. H. Funderburk, A. E. Hakala, and J. W. Ward, *Fed. Proc.*, **31,** 535 abstr. (1972).

64. D. N. Johnson, W. H. Funderburk, and J. W. Ward, *Fed. Proc.*, **29,** 779 abstr. (1970).

65. L. B. Turnbull, L. Teng, J. Newman, R. B. Bruce, and W. R. Maynard, *Drug Metab. Disp.*, **4,** 379 (1976).

66. I. L. Bonta, C. J. DeVos, H. Grijsen, F. C. Hillen, E. L. Noach, and A. W. Sim, *Brit. J. Pharmacol.*, **43,** 514 (1971).

67. F. C. Hillen and E. L. Noach, *Eur. J. Pharmacol.*, **16,** 222 (1971).

68. H. Möhler, A. J. Patel, A. L. Johnson, A. P. Reynolds, and R. Balázs, *J. Neurochem.*, **24,** 865 (1975).

69. B. J. Van Zivieten-Boot and E. L. Noach, *Eur. J. Pharmacol.*, **33,** 247 (1975).

70. C. R. Rasmussen, J. F. Gardocki, J. N. Plampin, B. L. Twardzik, B. E. Reynolds, A. J. Molinari, N. Schwartz, W. W. Bennetts, B. E. Laky, and J. Marakowski, *J. Med. Chem.*, **21**, 1044 (1978).

71. J. F. Gardocki, *Arch. Int. Pharmacodyn. Ther.*, **233**, 326 (1978).

72. Y. M. Beasley, V. Petrow, O. Stephenson and A. S. Thompson, *J. Pharm. Pharmacol.*, **9**, 10 (1960).

73. C. D. Lunsford, R. P. Mays, J. A. Richman, and R. S. Murphey, *J. Am. Chem. Soc.*, **82**, 1166 (1960).

74. R. B. Bruce, L. Turnbull, J. Newman, and J. Pitts, *J. Med. Chem.*, **9**, 286 (1966).

75. H. L. Yale and K. Losee, *J. Med. Chem.*, **9**, 478 (1966).

76. G. P. Leszkovszky and L. Tardos, *Acta. Physiol. Hung.*, **37**, 319 (1970).

77. G. P. Leszkovszky and L. Tardos, *Arzneim.-Forsch.*, **20**, 1778 (1970).

78. A. R. Surrey, W. G. Webb, and R. M. Gesler, *J. Am. Chem. Soc.*, **80**, 3469 (1968).

79. R. M. Gesler and A. R. Surrey, *J. Pharmacol. Exp. Ther.*, **122**, 517 (1958).

80. E. W. McChesney, W. F. Banks, Jr., G. A. Portmann, and A. V. R. Crain, *Biochem. Pharmacol.*, **16**, 813 (1967).

81. E. F. Domino, K. R. Unna, and J. Kerwin, *J. Pharmacol. Exp. Ther.*, **105**, 486 (1952).

82. D. F. Marsh, *Fed. Proc.*, **14**, 366 (1955).

83. A. P. Roszkowski, *J. Pharmacol. Exp. Ther.*, **129**, 75 (1960).

84. A. H. Conney and J. J. Burns, *Ann. N.Y. Acad. Sci.*, **86**, 167 (1960).

85. W. Schallek, W. Schlosser, and L. O. Randall, in *Advances in Pharmacology and Chemotherapy*, Vol. 10, S. Garattini, A. Goldin, F. Hawking, and I. J. Kapin, Eds., Academic, New York, 1972, p. 119.

86. R. Polyin and C. D. Barnes, *Neuropharmacology*, **15**, 133 (1976).

87. A. C. Przybyla and S. C. Wang, *J. Pharmacol. Exp. Ther.*, **163**, 439 (1968).

88. N. E. F. Cartlidge, P. Hudgson, and D. Weightman, *J. Neurol. Sci.*, **23**, 17 (1974).

89. J. Schmitt, P. Comoy, M. Wuquet, J. Boitard, J. LeMeur, J. J. Basselier, M. Brunard, and J. Salle, *Chem. Ther.*, **2**, 254 (1967).

90. J. Lavagna, J. Becle, M. Gizy, and G. Darcourt, *Marseille Med.*, **108**, 73 (1971).

91. P. Grimaud and J. Chevrier, *Sem. Hop. Paris*, **47**, 953 (1971).

92. I. M. Levine, P. B. Jossmann, D. G. Friend, and V. DeAngelis, *Neurology*, **19**, 510 (1969).

93. K. Kamiya, Y. Wada, and M. Nishikaura, *Chem. Pharm. Bull.*, **21**, 1520 (1973).

94. S. Chiba and Y. Nagawa, *Jap. J. Pharmacol.*, **23**, 83 (1973).

95. M. Steinman, J. G. Topliss, R. Alekel, Y. Wong, and E. E. York, *J. Med. Chem.*, **16**, 1354 (1973).

96. A. Barnett, J. Goldstein, E. P. Fiedler, and R. I. Taber, *Arch. Int. Pharmacodyn. Therap.*, **212**, 164 (1974).

97. Y. Kanai, *Xenobiotica*, **4**, 441 (1974).

98. R. Nakajima, Y. Saji, Y. Kozato, R. Mikoda, S. Tanayama, and Y. Nagawa, *Tekeda Kenkyusho Ho*, **32**, 264 (1973) quoted in Ref. 97.

99. M. W. Klohs, M. D. Draper, F. J. Petracek, K. H. Ginzel, and O. N. Re, *Arzneim.-Forsch.*, **22**, 132 (1972).

100. W. E. Tobin and R. H. Gold, *J. Clin. Pharmacol.*, **43**, 514 (1971).

101. M. M. Gassel, E. Diamantopoulos, V. Petropoulos, A. C. R. Hughes, M. L. F. Ballesteros, and O. N. Re, *J. Clin. Pharmacol.*, **16**, 34 (1976).

102. D. R. Maxwell and M. A. Read, *Neuropharmacology*, **11**, 849 (1972).

103. E. M. Keary and D. R. Maxwell, *Brit. J. Pharmacol. Chemother.*, **29**, 400 (1967).

104. D. R. Maxwell, M. A. Read, and E. A. Sumpter, *Brit. J. Pharmacol.*, **50**, 35 (1974).

105. J. N. Sinha, B. P. Jaju, and R. C. Srimal, *Jap. J. Pharmacol.*, **16**, 250 (1966).

106. M. Protiva, *Farm. Ed. Sci.*, **21**, 76 (1966).

107. P. Ashby, D. Burke, S. Rao, and R. J. Jones, *J. Neurol. Neurosurg. Psychiatr.*, **35**, 599 (1972).

108. N. A. Bercel, *Curr. Ther. Res. Clin. Exp.*, **22**, 462 (1977).

109. G. Belvedere, C. Pantarotto, V. Rovei, and A. Frigerio, *J. Pharm. Sci.*, **65**, 815 (1976).

110. H. R. Synder, Jr., C. S. Davis, R. K. Bickerton, and R. P. Halliday, *J. Med. Chem.*, **10**, 807 (1967).

111. T. J. Schwan and K. O. Ellis, *J. Pharm. Sci.*, **64**, 1047 (1975).

112. R. M. Pinder, R. N. Brogden, T. M. Speight, and G. S. Avery, *Drugs*, **13**, 3 (1977).

113. K. O. Ellis and J. F. Carpenter, *Arch. Phys. Med. Rehab.*, **55**, 362 (1974).

114. R. L. White and T. J. Schwan, *J. Pharm. Sci.*, **65**, 135 (1976).

115. P. P. Cox, J. P. Heotis, D. Polin, and G. M. Rose, *J. Pharm. Sci.*, **58**, 987 (1969).

116. C. Plotka and R. Jequier, *Arch. Int. Pharmacodyn. Ther.*, **109**, 386 (1957).

117. R. Ceccarelli, C. Conti, G. Ballabio, *Minerva Med.*, **59**, 4669 (1968); see also *Minerva Med.*, **59**, 2570, 4665, 4678, 4682 (1968).

CHAPTER FORTY-EIGHT

Histamine H₂-Receptor Agonists and Antagonists

C. ROBIN GANELLIN

and

GRAHAM J. DURANT

The Research Institute
Smith Kline & French Laboratories Limited
Welwyn Garden City, Hertfordshire, England

CONTENTS

1   BACKGROUND

Histamine [4(5)-imidazolylethylamine] was
first reported in 1907 by Windaus and Vogt
(1), who synthesized the compound because
of its chemical resemblance to the naturally
occurring alkaloid pilocarpine and to the
amino acid histidine; these authors had no
idea of its physiological activity or of its
potential interest. Subsequently, in 1910,
histamine was shown to be produced from
histidine by bacterial decarboxylation (2),
to occur in ergot extracts (3), and to cause
pronounced pharmacological effects (4, 5).
In their classic papers Dale and Laidlaw
(5, 6) showed that histamine was a potent
stimulant of smooth muscle contraction and
that it caused pronounced vascular effects
which closely resembled the effects seen
after anaphylactic shock. The first chemically characterized isolation of histamine
from animal tissues was in 1911 (7) (from
ox intestinal mucosa) but there remained
the strong possibility that the histamine had
been generated from histidine during the
extraction procedure; thus it was some
time before the biologic significance of
naturally occurring histamine was appreciated.

These classic investigations laid the foundation for the intensive study that was to
follow. Histamine was later found to be a
constituent of many tissues (8) and came to
be regarded as a substance liberated in
response to injurious stimuli (9a). Although
histamine had been shown by Popielski
(10) to stimulate secretion of gastric acid,
attention was directed toward a pathological role for histamine rather than a
physiological function (9). It is probably no
accident, therefore, that the first antihistamine drugs arose out of the search for
substances to counteract the toxic manifestations of histamine release. The initial discovery of antihistamines by Bovet and
Staub (11) in 1937 was followed by a vigorous search for other compounds in many
laboratories, and within a few years various
potent specific antagonists had been developed (reviewed in Chapter 49 and Refs.
12 and 13). These drugs were introduced
for clinical use in allergy, e.g., in hay fever
and acute urticaria (14).

Pharmacologically, the antihistamines
were found to be effective antagonists of
the action of histamine in stimulating contractions of smooth muscle, notably from
the bronchi, gut, and uterus. They were
also shown to antagonize many of the actions of histamine on the vascular system,
in particular, the histamine-induced increase in capillary permeability and certain
vasoconstrictor actions; it was also found
that these antagonists reduced the intensity
of, but did not abolish, vasodilator actions.
Quantitative pharmacology, from studies
on blood pressure (15) or on isolated
smooth muscle (16), suggested that the
mode of antagonism was competitive and,
in 1947, Schild (17) introduced pA_x values
to characterize the antagonism. Two typical
compounds, mepyramine (48.**1**) and
diphenhydramine (48.**2**), were thereby
shown to be specific in antagonizing histamine-stimulated contractions of the isolated ileum of the guinea pig, relative to
other stimulants; they were effective at low
concentrations and the antagonism they
produced was surmountable.

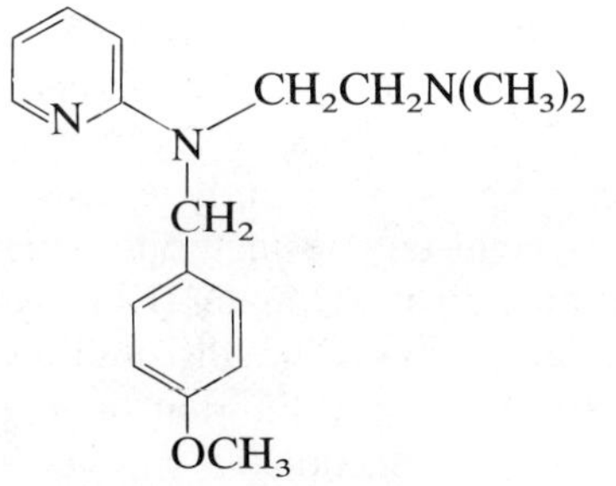

48.1 Mepyramine

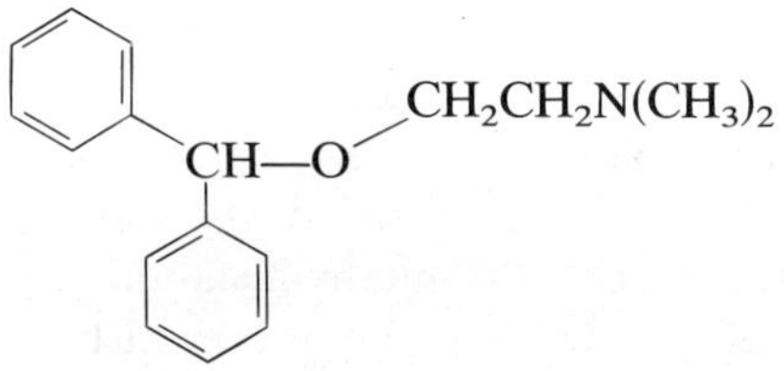

48.2 Diphenhydramine

These antagonists came to be regarded as competing with histamine for occupation of its specific receptor sites (17, 18) and they were used to establish the criteria for comparing receptors in different tissues and species (19, 20); for example, mepyramine gave similar pA_2 values when tested against histamine on the perfused lung of the guinea pig, the isolated ileum and trachea of the guinea pig, and human bronchi; the results indicated a homogeneity for the histamine receptors in these tissues. The antagonists were also used to identify different agonists which acted on the same receptors (21); thus the potencies of histamine and 2-(2-pyridyl)ethylamine (48.7 in Fig. 48.8) on the guinea pig ileum were found to vary in the ratio of approximately 1:30, but the same pA_2 values were obtained with mepyramine or diphenhydramine against either agonist (20); this is the expected result if the agonists are acting on the same receptors and the antagonism is competitive. The pharmacological receptors involved in these mepyramine- and diphenhydramine-sensitive histamine responses were subsequently defined by Ash and Schild in 1966 (22) as histamine H_1 receptors.

Several other actions of histamine had been noted which could not be specifically antagonized by mepyramine and related drugs: for example, stimulation of gastric acid secretion (see Refs. 23 and 24 for comprehensive bibliographies), stimulation of isolated atria (25), inhibition of rat uterus (26), and the vasodilator effects of large doses of histamine (27). Various workers suggested that these nonantagonizable actions of histamine might involve other histamine receptors (22, 25, 27–32), but proof was lacking.

Some pointers to the differentiation of different histamine receptors had been obtained by considering the relative activities of agonists on different tissue systems. For example, Grossman and co-workers (33) compared the histamine-like activities of some 60 compounds chemically related to histamine, and noted the apparent lack of uniform correlation between activity on gastric secretion in the dog, and activities on guinea pig intestinal strip or cat blood pressure. A more extensive list was later compiled by Jones (34a); he, too, pointed out that certain compounds were relatively selective, mimicking histamine in only some pharmacological actions. Ash and Schild (22) made quantitative estimates of the relative activities of different histamine congeners on the isolated guinea pig ileum, on the isolated rat uterus, and in vivo as stimulants of rat gastric acid secretion; they obtained a correlation in activity ratios which suggested that a common receptor mechanism might be involved in rat gastric acid secretion and rat uterus inhibition. Further indications of two receptor populations were provided from quantitative studies of methylhistamines: Black and co-workers (35) estimated activities relative to histamine on guinea pig ileum (H_1) and guinea pig atrium (non-H$_1$), i.e., two *in vitro* systems taken from the same animal species. They found that the two assays gave indistinguishable estimates of the relative activities of N^α-methylhistamine, N^α,N^α-dimethylhistamine, α-methylhistamine, and β-methylhistamine (see Fig. 48.1 for numbering). 4-Methylhistamine, however, was much more active on the atrium (43% of histamine) than on the ileum (0.23%). Conversely 2-methylhistamine was significantly less active (4.4%) on the atrium than on the ileum (16.5%). Similar results were obtained using rat tissues, viz; gastric motility *in vivo* (H$_1$), gastric acid secretion *in vivo* (non-H$_1$), and uterine muscle *in vitro* (non-H$_1$). These results, analyzed statistically, were in keeping with the notion of there being a homogeneous population of histamine receptors in these three non-H$_1$ systems. However, in order to classify these receptors, it was necessary to use a specific antagonist. Work to produce such a compound had started in 1964 at Smith Kline & French Laboratories in England, and in 1972 Black et al. (35) were able to announce the discovery of burimamide, *N*-methyl-*N'*-[4-(imidazol-4-yl)butyl]thiourea (48.**30** in Table 48.9), a specific competitive antagonist of histamine on these non-H$_1$ tissue systems, thereby defining histamine H$_2$ receptors. Studies of the action of the H$_2$-receptor antagonists in blocking histamine-stimulated secretion of gastric acid have established beyond doubt a role for histamine in normal physiological maintenance.

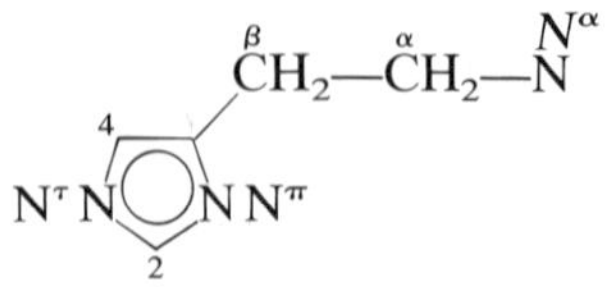

Fig. 48.1 Histamine numbering according to Black and Ganellin (36).

A considerable research effort in many laboratories using selective histamine-like agonists and the specific histamine antagonists has subsequently characterized actions of histamine in terms of H$_1$ and H$_2$ receptor types for many tissue systems and animal species. The distribution of these receptor types in different tissue systems is discussed in Section 7.

2 CHEMICAL CHARACTERIZATION OF HISTAMINE

The existence of two receptor populations for histamine raises an interesting question for the medicinal chemist, viz., whether the chemical mechanism of histamine interaction differs between the two receptor types. At present, very little is known about the structure of these receptors at the molecular level so that to attempt an answer one has to rely on studies of histamine chemistry. It is thus necessary to identify chemical properties of histamine which may differentiate its action at H$_1$ and H$_2$ receptors.

One approach is to characterize histamine chemically in great detail in the expectation that certain specialized properties will become evident. This method is unlikely to provide conclusive answers but it ought to be capable of posing some pertinent questions. A complementary approach is to identify chemical properties of histamine which may be critical for its biological activity, by investigating closely related structural analogs. The procedure requires chemical comparisons to be made between such analogs and histamine in a manner that leads to correlations between chemical properties and biological activity. Structure–activity analysis is, however, complicated by the fact that histamine in aqueous solution is a mixture of various ionic species, tautomers, and conformers; which of these species may be biologically important is not self-evident. Furthermore, the various sepcies are in equilibria; i.e., they are undergoing interconversion, and indeed, these very processes may have biological significance.

2.1   Histamine Protonation and Tautomerism

Titration of histamine in aqueous solution gives three stoichiometric pK_a values (37). Fully protonated histamine is a dication

(48.**3a**; Fig. 48.2) and the first stoichiometric ionization constant ($pK_{a_1} = 5.80$ at 37°C) corresponds to dissociation from the ring NH to give the monocation. The second ionization constant ($pK_a = 9.40$ at 37°C) corresponds to dissociation at the side chain NH_3^+ group to give the uncharged molecule. At high pH, the ring again ionizes at NH ($pK_{a_3} = 14$) to give an anion. The relative populations of the species as a function of pH are shown graphically in

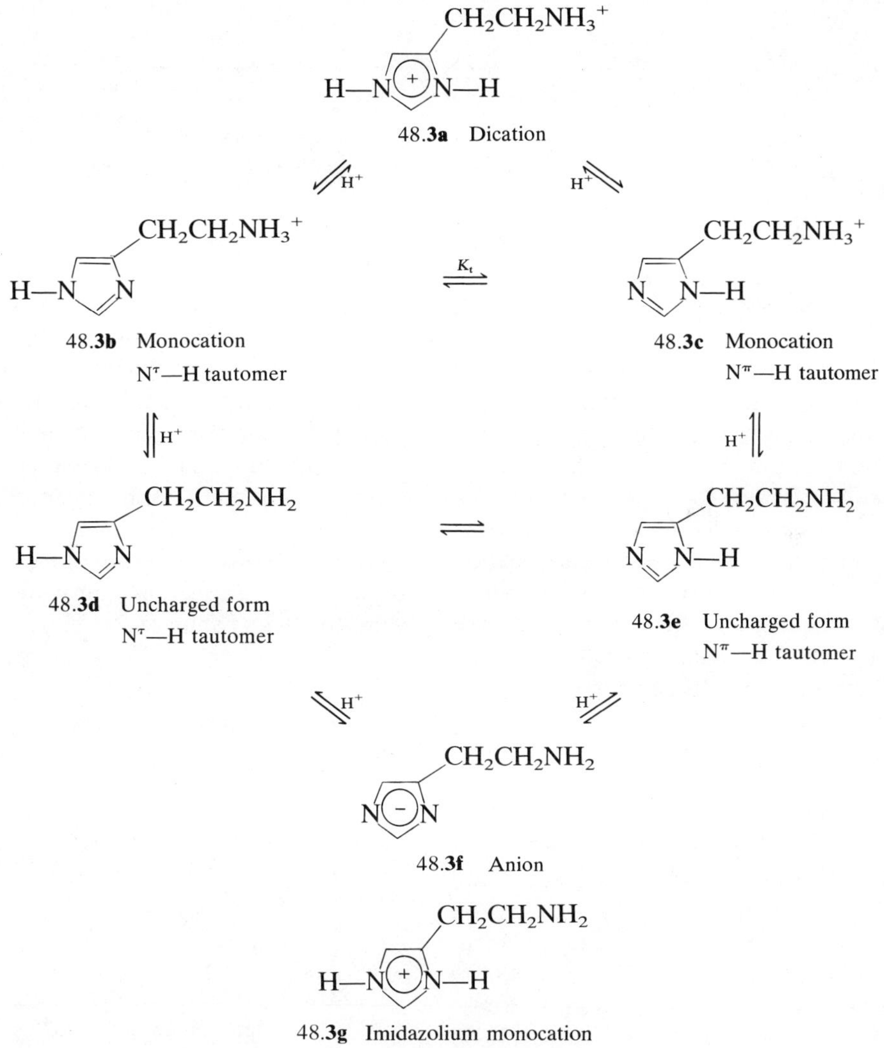

Fig. 48.2   Ionic and tautomeric equilibria between histamine species. Side chain deprotonation of dication 48.**3a** furnishes the monocation 48.**3g** and this must also be present, although the concentration of 48.**3g** is likely to be less than 1 part in 100 relative to 48.**3b** and 48.**3c**.

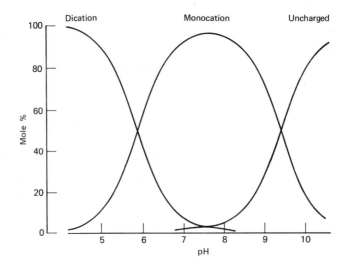

Fig. 48.3   Species composition of histamine at 37°C in water as a function of pH, using the values $pK_{a_1} = 5.80$ and $pK_{a_2} = 9.40$.

Fig. 48.3. The curve for the monocation reaches a maximum in the pH range 7–8; since this is also the physiological pH range it suggests (but does not prove) that the physiologically important species is the monocation. At pH 7.4, 96% of histamine is present as the monocation; however, it must be remembered that the pH could be considerably lower in the vicinity of some membranes, and below pH 5.8 the dication predominates. Values for the relative populations of species at pH 7.4 and 5.4 are given in Table 48.1. Because the imidazole ring possesses two nitrogen sites for proton dissociation, both monocation and uncharged forms can exist as two distinct tautomers; the full series of equilibria relating the various species is given in Fig. 48.2.

In the crystalline state the equilibrium is "frozen"; histamine monocation has been examined by X-ray crystallography as the monohydrobromide salt (38) and found to exist entirely in the N$^\tau$—H tautomer (48.**3b**) whereas the crystalline histamine base has been found (39) exclusively as the N$^\pi$—H tautomer (48.**3e**); see Fig. 48.1 for histamine numbering. In solution the various forms are in equilibrium and it is of considerable interest to measure their relative concentrations.

The relative population of tautomers has been estimated for histamine monocation in aqueous solution from pK_a data by comparing the corresponding N-methyl or N-benzyl derivatives (40). The ratio of concentrations of the two monocation tautomers, given by the tautomeric equilibrium constant K_t, was found to be 4.37 and 4.07, respectively, giving an approximate mean value of 4.2 (Table 48.2). Thus according

Table 48.1   Population of Histamine Species in Aqueous Solution[a]

Species	Mole Percentage of Species	
	At pH 7.4	At pH 5.4
Dication 48.**3a**	2.4	71.5
Monocation 48.**3b** + 48.**3c**	96.6	28.5
Uncharged 48.**3d** + 48.**3e**	1	3×10^{-3b}
Anion 48.**3f**	2.5×10^{-7b}	1×10^{-11b}

[a] Derived from pK_a values at 37°C (37): $pK_{a_1} = 5.80$; $pK_{a_2} = 9.40$; $pK_{a_3} = 14$.
[b] These values replace those originally published in Ref. 79, in which an error was made in the calculations.

Table 48.2 Ratio of Tautomer Concentrations (K_t) for Histamine Monocation in Water, by Different Procedures

A. Direct Method, by pK_a Comparisons (40)

$$\log K_t = pK_{a(N^\tau - H)} - pK_{a(N^\pi - H)}$$

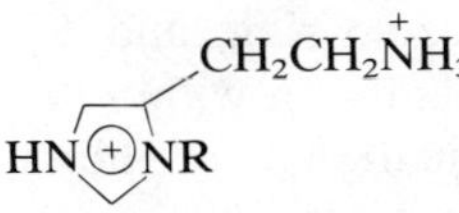

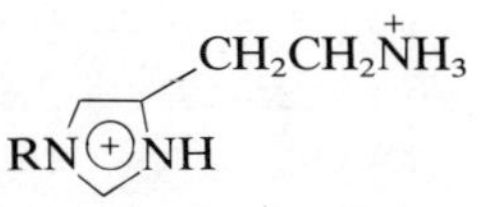

R	$pK_{a(N^\tau - H)}$	$pK_{a(N^\pi - H)}$	K_t
CH_3	6.63	5.99	4.37
$CH_2C_6H_5$	6.23	5.62	4.07

B. Indirect Method, from Hammett Equation (41)

$$\log K_t = (\rho_{N^\tau - H} - \rho_{N^\pi - H})\sigma_{CH_2CH_2NH_3^+};$$

$$\sigma_{CH_2CH_2NH_3^+} = +0.11$$

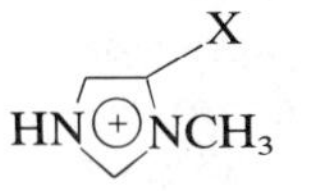

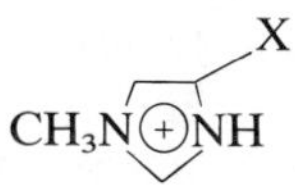

$\rho_{(N^\tau - H)}$	$\rho_{(N^\pi - H)}$	K_t
−7.0	−10.4	2.4

C. Direct Observation, by ^{13}C NMR Shift Analysis (43a)

K_t

ca. 4

to these measurements, about 80% of histamine monocation in water is in the N^τ—H tautomeric form, and 20% is in the N^π—H form. An alternative method based on the Hammett equation provided a value for K_t of 2.4 (41); this was obtained by Charton's method (107) comparing ρ values for the respective series of 1-methyl 4- or 5-substituted imidazoles in the equation:

$$\log K_t = (\rho_5 - \rho_4)\sigma_{m,x}$$

$$= (\rho_{N^\tau - H} - \rho_{N^\pi - H})\sigma_{CH_2CH_2NH_3^+}$$

where the substituent constant σ for the ammonium-ethyl side chain was taken as +0.11, this value being derived from the pK_a of isohistamine [2-(2-aminoethyl)-imidazole] and the plot of pK_a vs. σ_m for a series of 2-substituted imidazoles (41). The value given by Charton's method may be less reliable because it is obtained indirectly and requires added assumptions, but it provides a qualitative confirmation of the previous work. It also demonstrates that the tautomer preference is in accord with the generality that electron-withdrawing substituents (X) favor the N^τ—H tautomer (42). Charton's method is useful for estimating K_t for substituted histamines (see Section 3, and Table 48.8). Further confirmation that the N^τ—H tautomer (48.**3b**) of histamine monocation is preferred in aqueous solution has been obtained more recently by direct estimates using ^{13}C NMR spectroscopy (43). Observation of ^{13}C chemical shifts as a function of pH also indicates a tautomer ratio of ca. 4 : 1 in favor of the N^τ—H tautomer (43a).

A precise value for the tautomeric equilibrium constant for the uncharged histamine molecule has not yet been published but recent work based on ^{13}C chemical shift analysis (43b) indicates that the N^τ—H tautomer (48.**3d**) is preferred in aqueous solution; furthermore it appears that the uncharged molecule closely resembles the monocation in this respect, thus indicating that side chain protonation appears to have little effect on tautomer preference in solution. These results are in contrast to the crystal structure findings (*vide supra*; 38, 39).

Molecular orbital calculations have been used to predict tautomer stability (44, 45) but the absolute energies are very sensitive to the molecular geometry used as input data. The monocation is predicted to occur overwhelmingly as the N^τ—H tautomer whereas the uncharged molecule is predicted to be in the N^π—H form. These predictions agree with the crystal structure data but do not agree with the measurements made on solutions. For a very polar molecule such as histamine, tautomeric stability is likely to depend on the nature of the solvent, and this is difficult to take into account in theoretical calculations.

2.2 Histamine Conformation

Histamine is a conformationally flexible molecule. Being a 1,2-disubstituted ethane, rotation occurs about the single bonds shown in structure 48.**4** (Fig. 48.4) and the

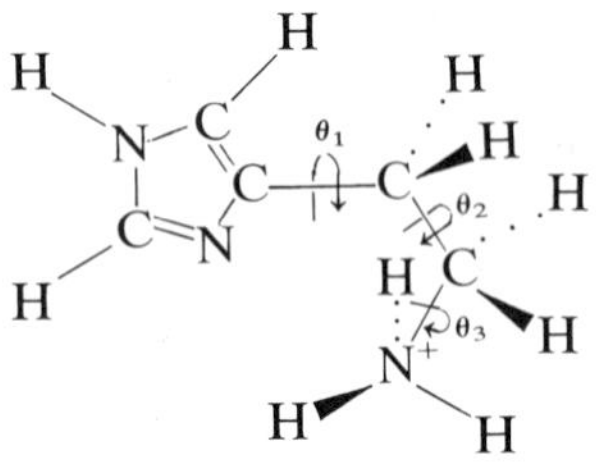

48.**4**

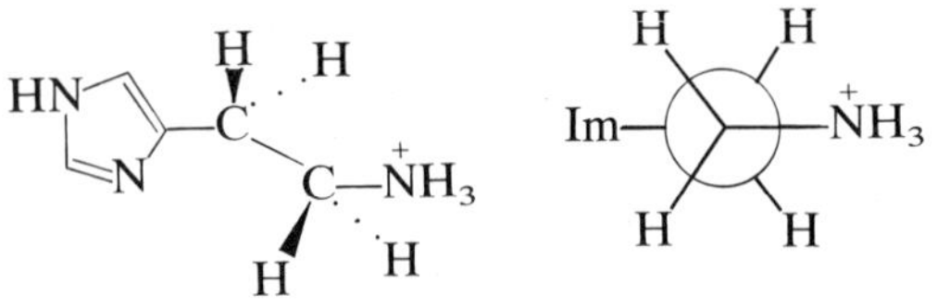

48.**5**   Trans (extended) conformation, $\theta_2 = 180°$, (antiperiplanar)

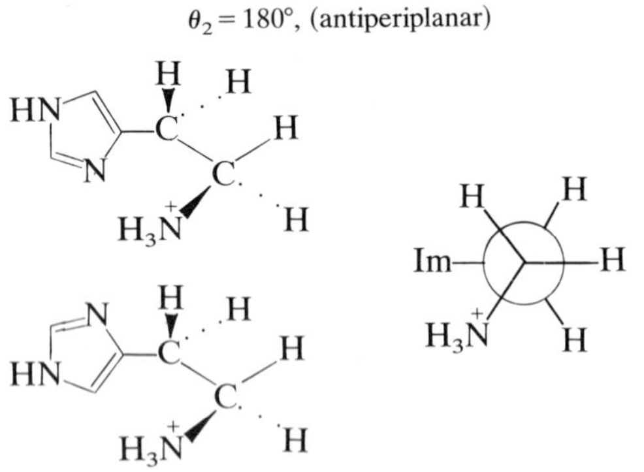

48.**6**   Gauche (folded) conformation, $\theta_2 = 60°$ or $300°$, (synclinal)

Fig. 48.4 Histamine monocation (N^τ—H tautomer) showing torsion angles (θ), and trans and gauche conformations; θ_1 measures the rotation of the imidazole ring, and θ_2 measures the rotation within the side chain. The form shown in 48.**4** corresponds to $\theta_1 = 180°$, $\theta_2 = 0°$.

conformation can be described in terms of the three torsion angles θ_1, θ_2, and θ_3. For histamine itself, θ_3 is relatively unimportant (since the NH_3^+ group is symmetrical) and the spatial characteristics of the molecule are determined by θ_1, which describes the orientation of the imidazole ring, and θ_2, which represents the orientation within the side chain. The conformational equilibria for the various ionic species have been widely studied using nuclear magnetic resonance spectroscopy (NMR) and molecular orbital calculations (see Table 48.3 for references).

As with other disubstituted ethanes, the most favored conformers are the trans (fully extended, $\theta_2 = 180°$) and gauche (folded, $\theta_2 = 60°$ or $300°$) in which the hydrogen atoms within the side chain have a staggered arrangement, structures 48.**5** and 48.**6** (Fig. 48.4). However, the different methods of calculation disagree as to the relative stabilities of the conformers. The less sophisticated EHT (see Table 48.3 for key to abbreviations) or empirical treatments predict stability for both trans and gauche conformations in histamine monocation and dication, with the trans conformer being slightly more stable by approximately 1 kcal/mol. These conclusions agree with experimental results derived from NMR studies for aqueous solution. Surprisingly, the more sophisticated PCILO method gives strikingly different results and predicts conformation to depend on the type of cation; i.e., the dication is entirely trans but the monocation is overwhelmingly gauche. Calculations using the CNDO/2 and INDO methods give results similar to the PCILO calculations, and these have also been confirmed by STO-3G calculations *ab initio* on the isolated molecule. The discrepancy between these calculations for the isolated molecule and the data from aqueous solution have been partly resolved by modifications that take account of a counterion or include molecules of water (the "supermolecule" approach of Pullman in which the hydration sites in histamine are bound by water of solvation); the results are summarized in Table 48.3. However, it is unlikely that the discrepancy is due solely to the presence or absence of water. Similar discrepancies are found for histamine base; the INDO and PCILO procedures predict a strong preference for the gauche conformer, yet both trans and gauche conformers of histamine base ap-

Table 48.3   Calculated and Observed Preferred Conformers of Histamine Species by Different Procedures[a]

Procedure	Dication	Mono-cation	Un-charged	Ref.
Calculations on the Isolated Molecule				
EHT		T+G		46
EHT	T+G	T+G		47
Empirical	T+G	T+G		48
INDO		G	G	49
PCILO		G	G	50
PCILO	T	G		51a
CNDO/2	T	G		47
STO-3G	T	G		51a
FSGO		G		51b
Calculations on the Modified Molecule				
Hydrated PCILO	T+(G)	T+G		51a
F⁻ counter ion CNDO	T+G	G		52
Measurement of Solutions				
NMR in D₂O	T+G	T+G		53
				54
				47
NMR in CDCl₃			T+G	55, 56
IR in CHCl₃			T+G	56
Measurement of Solid				
Crystal	T	T	T	see Table 48.4

[a] The abbreviations used are as follows: EHT, extended Hückel theory; INDO, intermediate neglect of differential overlap; PCILO, perturbative configuration interaction using localized orbitals; CNDO, complete neglect of differential overlap; NMR, nuclear magnetic resonance spectroscopy; IR, infrared spectroscopy; T, trans conformation, $\theta_2 = 180°$, antiperiplanar; G, gauche conformation, $\theta_2 = 60°$ or $300°$, synclinal; FSGO, floating spherical Gaussian orbital.

pear to be present in chloroform solution. Furthermore, in the anhydrous crystal, histamine monocation and base are present as the trans conformer, yet both species are predicted by the INDO and PCILO procedures to be overwhelmingly in gauche forms.

The preferred orientation θ_1 of the imidazole ring also varies according to the molecular orbital calculation procedure, but the only physical measurements are crystallographic. Crystallography cannot identify relative preference under equilibrium conditions but it does indicate stable forms under a particular set of circumstances, viz., when "frozen" in the crystal lattice. So far, for the dication, monocation, and uncharged (free base) species, only the trans conformation has been obtained but various orientations of the imidazole ring have been found, depending on the salt used for crystal determination. Values of θ_1, the dihedral angle between the two planes formed respectively by the imidazole ring and the C—C—N

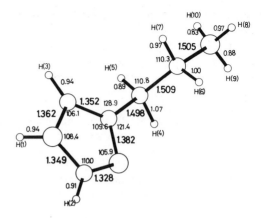

Fig. 48.5 Bond lengths and angles of N$^\tau$—H tautomer of histamine monocation (from crystal structure of histamine monohydrobromide, Ref. 38).

side chain, are given in Table 48.4 together with the counterions and literature references. The geometry found crystallographically for histamine monocation (as the hydrobromide) is given in Fig. 48.5 (38).

The molecular orbital calculations also show that there are substantial energy barriers to interconversion between trans and guache conformations but that rotation of the imidazole ring is much less restricted. These results are in keeping with the crystallographic findings, viz., a single value for θ_2 but a multiplicity of values for θ_1.

Table 48.4 Orientations, θ_1, of the Imidazole Ring in the Various Histamine Species Found by Crystallography^a

Salt	Di-cation θ_1°	Mono-cation θ_1°	Un-charged θ_1°	Ref.
Base			66.3	39
Monobromide		89.7		38
Dibromide	30			57
Dichloride	26.7			58
Diphosphate H$_2$O	82.5			59
Sulfate, H$_2$O				
I	4.4			60
II	9.2			
Tetrachloro-cobaltate	7			61

^{a} In each case the side chain has the trans conformation; θ_1 represents the dihedral angle between the two planes formed respectively by the imidazole ring and the C—C—N side chain.

2.3 Histamine as a Receptor Ligand

It is conceivable that when histamine interacts with its receptors it functions in the chemical sense as a ligand binding to a specific molecular site, so that it is pertinent to mention briefly some of the properties that may have importance for ligand–receptor interaction.

Histamine is a very polar hydrophilic molecule; the partition coefficient for histamine free base between 1-octanol and water buffer at pH 11.8 is low ($P = 0.2$) (62). Histamine has a strong capacity for hydrogen bonding, in which the ammonium

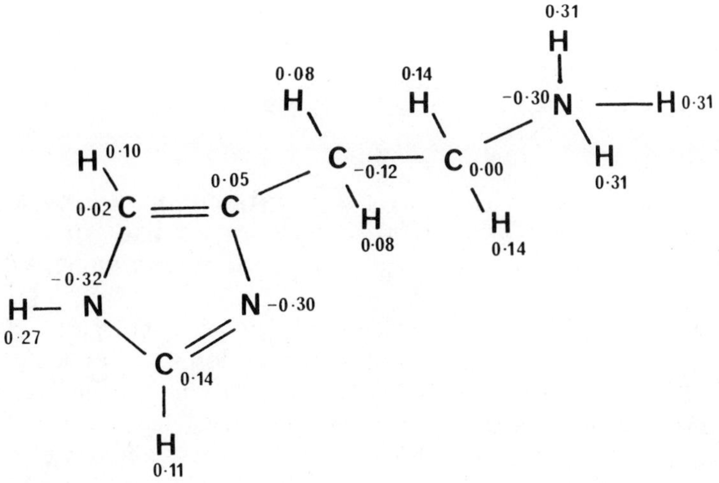

Fig. 48.6   Net electronic charges (in electron units) for trans conformer of the N^τ—H tautomer of histamine monocation, calculated *ab initio* (51a).

and imidazolium cations act as hydrogen donors and the uncharged ring (as in the monocation or free base) acts both as hydrogen donor and acceptor.

Electronic charge distributions within the histamine molecule which provide a fundamental basis for considering molecular interactions have been calculated by several research groups (for Mulliken population analyses on histamine monocation see Refs. 45, 46, 49-51). The individual calculations differ in the numerical values predicted but they appear to be consistent in indicating that all the nitrogen atoms are negatively charged, that there is little net charge on the carbon atoms, and that the positive charge is distributed widely over all the hydrogen atoms in the molecule although tending to be concentrated on the N—H hydrogens (see Fig. 48.6 for an example). A more sophisticated approach by Richards and Wallis (64) considers the electron density with respect to the covalent radii of atoms; this method gives a better indication of the electron densities for the outermost electrons and has obvious merit since it is the outermost electrons that are first "felt" in molecular interactions. The results suggest that the positive charge in the monocation is evenly dispersed over the whole molecule.

Most work on histamine as a ligand has been concerned with metal complexes, either in solution (formation constants) or in the solid state. Histamine forms stable complexes with the divalent transition metal cations Cu, Ni, Co, Zn, and Cd, and the measured stability constants (Table 48.5) show that the Irving–Williams order of stabilities Co<Ni<Cu>Zn is maintained. Crystal structure determinations have established the geometry for coordination between histamine and Cu(II) (69) or Ni(II) (70), and confirm earlier suggestions that the stability of the complexes in solution is due to chelation of histamine base between the metal cation and the side chain NH_2 and ring—N^π nitrogen atoms, forming a six-membered ring. The complex may contain more than one molecule of histamine per metal atom (e.g., structure in Fig. 48.7); in solution 1:1, 2:1, and in the case of Ni, Co, and Zn 3:1 complexes are formed. The values of the successive formation constants given in Table 48.5 indicate that chelation of the first molecule of

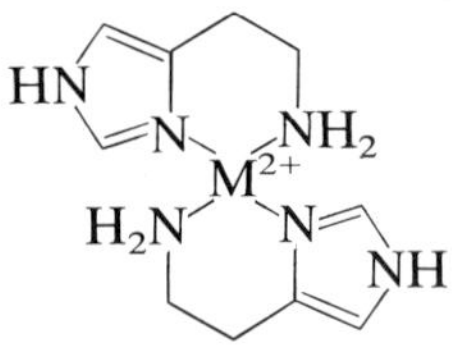

Fig. 48.7 Chelate complex between two molecules of histamine base and a divalent cation, M^{2+}, as in (histamine)$_2$Cu(ClO$_4$)$_2$ (69b).

histamine to metal cation has higher stability than chelation of the second and third molecules. In the crystal structures so far determined, the histamine : metal ratio is 2 : 1 for Cu(II), and 2 : 1 or 3 : 1 for Ni(II). Interactions of histamine, histidine, and other imidazole derivatives with transition metal ions in chemical and biological systems have been reviewed by Sundberg and Martin (72). The binding of alkaline earth divalent cations Mg, Ca, Sr, and Ba to histamine has had only limited study; values of log K_1 have been reported (71) (Table 48.5) and indicate that histamine forms weak 1 : 1 complexes.

Much past interest has centered on the binding of histamine in mast cells, and the nature of the complex presumed to form with heparin (73). The possibility of a ternary histamine–zinc–heparin complex has also been explored (74) but the role of zinc

has since been questioned (75). The state of the histamine molecule (e.g., conformation or protonation) in this complex is not yet known.

3 CHEMICAL EVIDENCE FOR THE ACTIVE FORM OF HISTAMINE AT H$_1$ AND H$_2$ RECEPTORS

The possible biological significance of the various forms of histamine must be considered. The best indications of their likely importance have come from structure–activity considerations of analogs (congeners). For a description of structure–activity studies see articles by Jones (34a) and Paton (34b).

More than 30 years ago, Niemann and Hays (76) concluded that the active form of histamine was the monocationic tautomer 48.**3b**. This conclusion followed from the original finding (77) that 2-pyridylethylamine (48.**7**) was a histamine-like stimulant of guinea pig smooth muscle contraction, whereas 4-pyridylethylamine (48.**11**) was not active (see Fig. 48.8). Niemann and Hays also noted that since 3-pyridylethylamine (48.**10**) was not active, the histamine tautomer 48.**3c** must also be devoid of histamine-like activity; they also suggested

Table 48.5 Stability Constants of Histamine Metal Complexes in Aqueous Solution at 37°C

	Cu^{2+}	Ni^{2+}	Zn^{2+}	Co^{2+}	Cd^{2+}	Ca^{2+}	Sr^{2+}	Ba^{2+}	Mg^{2+}
Ref.	65	66a	66b	66b	68	71	71	71	71
log K_1^a	9.28	6.60	5.03	4.89	4.54	3.07	2.96	2.87	2.50
log K_2	6.30	4.84	4.78	3.54	3.25				
log K_3		2.93	2.28	2.03^b					
log β_2^c	15.58	11.44	9.81	8.43	7.79				

^{a} log K_1 refers to the first formation constant, with stoichiometry histamine : metal cation = 1 : 1; log K_2 and log K_3 are the successive second and third formation constants with 2 : 1 and 3 : 1 stoichiometry, respectively.
^{b} At 25°C (67).
^{c} log $\beta_2 = $ log K_1K_2.

2-Pyridylethylamine monocation 48.**7** compared with N$^\tau$ – H tautomer 48.**3b** of histamine monocation. Formally, these have fragment 48.**8** in common and can chelate a proton between the nitrogen atoms as in structure 48.**9**, but see text:

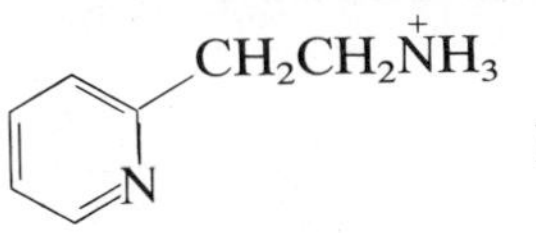

3-Pyridylethylamine 48.**10** and 4-pyridylethylamine 48.**11** monocations compared with N$^\pi$—H tautomer 48.**3c** of histamine monocation:

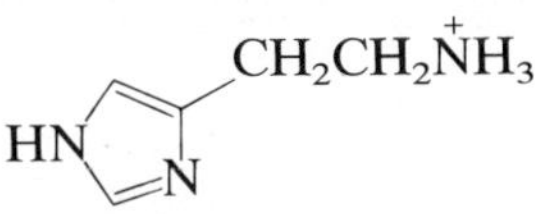

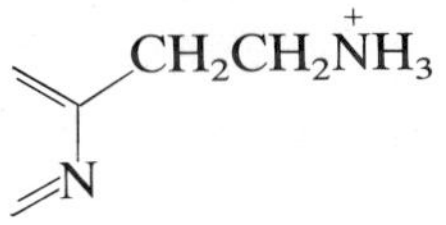

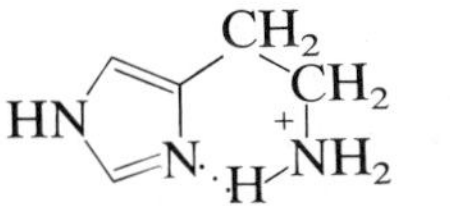

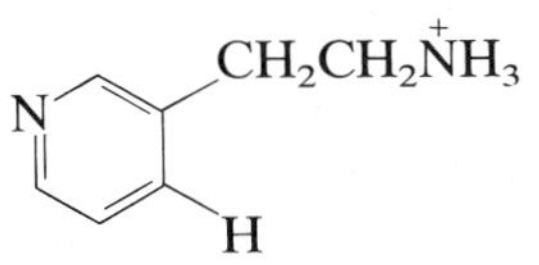

Fig. 48.8 The three isomeric pyridylethylamine structures compared with histamine tautomers.

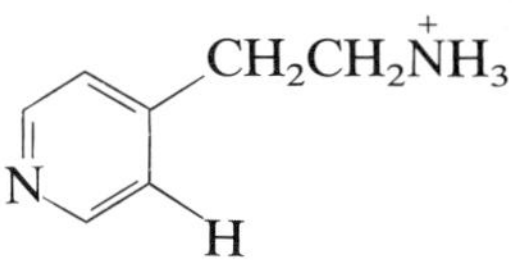

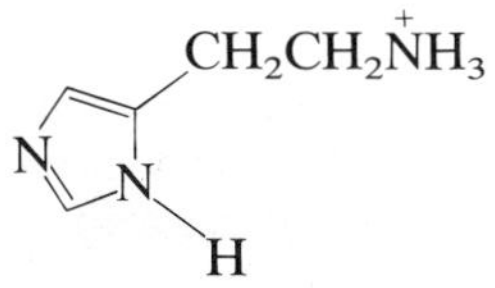

that tautomer 48.**3b** would be stabilized by intramolecular hydrogen bonding and asserted that for activity, chelation between the nitrogen atoms should occur in the cation (e.g., structure 48.**9**). Chemical evidence for such stabilization has been lacking, however, and recent work on histamine argues against such structures as having particular stability, at least in aqueous solution, e.g., the pK_a studies on the thermodynamics of proton dissociation (37) and on the relative tautomer stabilities (40), and the NMR investigations on conformer stabilities (47, 54).

Extensive examinations of other heterocyclic analogs of histamine have been carried out and comparison made with various actions of histamine, e.g., for stimulating contractions of the isolated guinea pig ileum (78), causing a depression of the blood pressure of the anesthetized cat (29, 78), stimulating mammalian gastric acid secretion (22, 29, 33), and inhibiting the isolated rat uterus (22). The finding that some compounds showed a separation in activities relative to histamine has complicated the consideration of structure–activity relationships (discussed in Refs. 32 and 34). This has become less of a problem now that the activities can be classified in terms of H$_1$- or H$_2$-receptor mediation (22, 35). Some examples of compounds showing relative selectivity as H$_1$ or H$_2$ agonists are shown in Table 48.6.

3.1 Evidence for the Monocation as an Active Form

At pH 7.4, the main form of histamine is the monocation, but at low pH (e.g., 5.4, as may occur in the vicinity of some membranes) the dication predominates (*vide supra*, Table 48.1). Thus both monocation and dication are sufficiently prevalent to be considered as active forms in histamine–receptor interactions. Indications that the dication is probably not an active form come from comparing active histamine analogs which have a heterocyclic ring with a very low pK_a so that the population of dication is extremely small. Examples such as 2-thiazolylethylamine (48.**21**), 3-(1,2,4-triazolyl)ethylamine (48.**22**), and 4-chloro-histamine (48.**23**) are shown in Table 48.7. These compounds have very low dication populations even at pH 5.4; e.g., 3-(1,2,4-triazolyl)ethylamine has only 0.01% of molecules in the dication at pH 5.4 but it has at least 10% of the potency of histamine at either H$_1$ or H$_2$ receptors; likewise, the dication is unlikely to be an active

Table 48.6 H$_1$ and H$_2$ Receptor Agonist Activities of Methylhistamines (Assayed at Smith Kline & French Laboratories Limited, Welwyn Garden City, England)

Compound Name and Structure	Agonist Activity Relative to Histamine = 100 (95% Confidence Limits)		
		H$_2$	
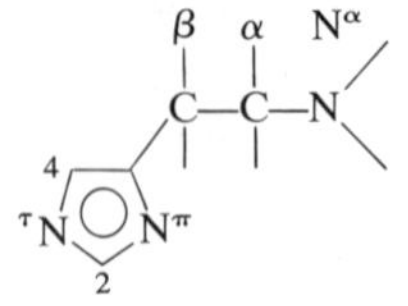	**H$_1$: Ileum**[a]	**Gastric Stimu-ation**[b]	**Atrium**[c]
48.**12** N^π-Methylhistamine	<0.01[d,e,f]	<0.2[e,g]	<0.1
48.**13a** 2-Methylhistamine	16.5(15.1–18.1)[h,i]	2.0[h]	4.4(4.1–4.8)[h]
48.**13b** 2,N^α,N^α-Trimethylhistamine	16.8(15.8–17.7)[e]	1.4[e]	
48.**14** N^τ-Methylhistamine	0.42(0.16–1.0)[j]	<0.1[k]	<0.01[k]
48.**15a** 4-Methylhistamine	0.23(0.20–0.27)[h,l]	39[h,m]	43(40–46)[h]
48.**15b** 4,N^α-Dimethylhistamine	0.16(0.1–0.2)[e,n]	8.2[e,o]	36(26–49)
48.**15c** 4,N^α,N^α-Trimethylhistamine	0.1[e]	3.0[e,p]	13.5(12.7–14.2)
48.**16a** N^α-Methylhistamine	72(62–84)[j,q]	74[e,r]	74(71–78)[j]
48.**16b** N^α,N^α-Dimethylhistamine	44(38–51)[j,s]	19[e]	51(42–61)[j]
48.**17** N^α,N^α,N^α-Trimethylhistamine	0.09[t,u]	Weak[t]	
48.**18** α-Methylhistamine	0.36(0.18–0.73)[j]	0.8[e]	0.74(0.42–1.3)[j]
48.**19** β-Methylhistamine	0.83(0.42–1.6)[j]	0.4[e]	0.89(0.79–1.1)[j]
48.**20** β,β-Dimethylhistamine	<0.001[e]	<0.1[e]	

[a] Tested for stimulating contraction of isolated guinea pig ileum in the presence of atropine (Ref. 79, unless otherwise indicated).

[b] Tested by rapid intravenous injection for stimulation of gastric acid secretion in the atropinized and vagotomized anesthetized rat (Ref. 79, unless otherwise indicated).

[c] Tested for stimulation of rate in the spontaneously beating isolated guinea pig right atrium in the presence of propranolol (previously unreported results are from R. C. Blakemore and M. E. Parsons, The Research Institute, Smith Kline & French Laboratories Ltd., Welwyn Garden City, England).

[d] Approximate value obtained by comparison of single doses required to cause equal contractile responses in a minimum of two preparations.

[e] Ref. 80.   [f] Reported inactive by Lee and Jones (78).

[g] Approximate value obtained by comparison of doses required to produce equal acid secretory responses in a minimum of two preparations.

[h] Ref. 35.

[i] Lee and Jones (78) report 30%.

[j] Ref. 91.

[k] R. C. Blakemore and M. E. Parsons.

[l] Bertaccini et al. (83a) report 1%; they name this compound 5-methylhistamine.

[m] Bertaccini et al. (83a) report 40%.

[n] Bertaccini et al. (83b) report 0.2%; they name this compound 5-methyl-N-methylhistamine.

[o] Bertaccini et al. (83b) report 25%.

[p] Also studied by Impicciatore et al. (83c) in the cat.

[q] A. Vertiainen (84) reports 100%.

[r] Ash and Schild (22) report 51%.

[s] Craver et al. (85) report 80% Lin et al. (29) report 18%.

[t] Ref. 79.   [u] Bertaccini and Vitali (83d) report 1%.

Table 48.7 Histamine Congeners with Weakly Basic Rings. Ring pK_a Values, Mole Percentages at 37°C of Dication at pH 7.4 and 5.4, and H$_1$ or H$_2$-Agonist Activities. For all Compounds Except Histamine, the Mole Percentage of Monocation is Greater than 97% at Either pH

Compound Name	Structure	Ring pK_a (37°C)	Mole percentage of Dication pH 7.4	Mole percentage of Dication pH 5.4	H$_1$: Ileum	H$_2$: Gastric Stimulation
Histamine	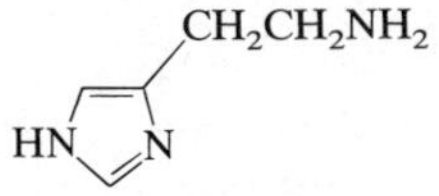	5.8	2.4	71.5	100	100
48.**21** 2-Thiazolylethyl-amine	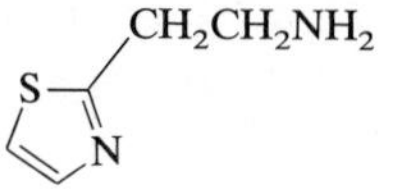	~1.5[b]	10^{-4}	10^{-2}	26	0.3
48.**22** 1,2,4-Triazol-3-ylethylamine	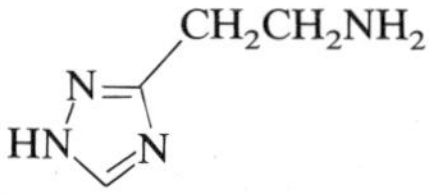	1.4[c]	10^{-4}	10^{-2}	12.7[d]	13.7[d]
48.**23** 4-Chlorohist-amine	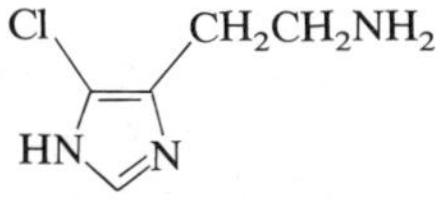	3.1[e]	5×10^{-3}	0.5	1.7[f]	12

[a] Agonist activities as indicated in Table 48.6.
[b] Holmes and Jones (87) report pK_{a_1} 1.68 and pK_{a_2} 9.53 at 25°C for the isomeric 4-thiazolylethylamine.
[c] E. S. Pepper in Ref. 79.
[d] Ref. 35.
[e] Ganellin (41) reports pK_{a_1} 3.23 and pK_{a_2} 9.34 at 25°C.
[f] R. C. Blakemore in Ref. 41; H$_1$ activity is probably an overestimate since the compound may have been contaminated with histamine.

species for 2-thiazolylethylamine at H$_1$ receptors or for 4-chlorohistamine at H$_2$ receptors.

There is less evidence as to whether the uncharged (free base) form is active. All compounds so far known to be active are strong bases, viz., amines or amidines (see Ref. 34), which exist mainly in cationic forms at physiological pH. The tertiary amine N^α,N^α-dimethylhistamine (48.**16b**) is active at H$_1$ and H$_2$ receptors but the quaternary ammonium derivative

$N^\alpha,N^\alpha,N^\alpha$-trimethylhistamine (48.**17**) is extremely weak (Fig. 48.9) (Table 48.6). Therefore, a proton on the N^α-ammonium group appears to be important for agonist activity at both H$_1$ and H$_2$ receptors (79). If the main function of the proton were hydrogen bonding then activity would appear to reside exclusively with the monocation, but if the proton were required to dissociate then the uncharged form would be generated, possibly as a transient species. The uncharged form might be required for

N^α,N^α-Dimethylhistamine (48.**16b**) is active at H$_1$ and H$_2$ receptors, but $N^\alpha,N^\alpha,N^\alpha$-trimethylhistamine (48.**17**) is extremely weak (see Table 48.6):

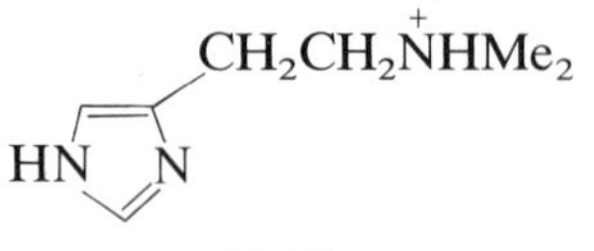

$$CH_2CH_2\overset{+}{N}HMe_2$$

48.**16b**

$$CH_2CH_2\overset{+}{N}Me_3$$

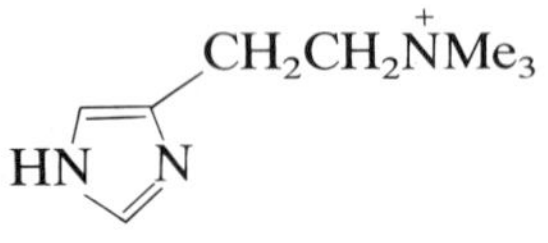

48.**17**

Thus agonist activity is associated with the presence of the side chain unit:

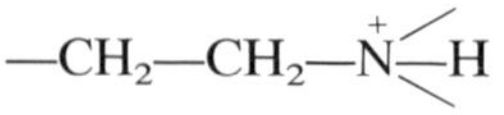

$$-CH_2-CH_2-\overset{+}{N}{\Large\langle}^{\diagup}_{H}$$

The side chain may form a hydrogen bond to a base, B:

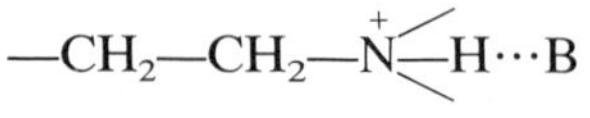

$$-CH_2-CH_2-\overset{+}{N}{\Large\langle}^{\diagup}_{H\cdots B}$$

or it may dissociate, giving up its proton to a base B$^-$ and becoming uncharged:

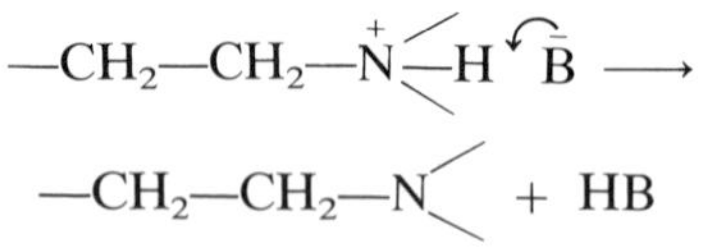

$$-CH_2-CH_2-\overset{+}{N}{\Large\langle}^{\diagup}_{H}\;\overset{\frown}{B} \longrightarrow$$

$$-CH_2-CH_2-N{\Large\langle} \;+\; HB$$

Fig. 48.9   Side chain N-methylhistamines.

access (e.g., penetration of membranes) or be involved in assisting imidazole-mediated proton transfer at the receptor site (45).

3.2 Evidence for the Involvement of Tautomerism at H$_2$ Receptors

Although histamine is tautomeric it is probable that imidazole tautomerism is not functionally involved in H$_1$-receptor stimulation. This follows from the finding that 2-pyridylethylamine (48.**7**) (77, 88) and 2-thiazolylethylamine (48.**21**) (78), which cannot tautomerize, have histamine-like activity in stimulating contractions of the guinea pig ileum (an H$_1$ receptor system). The activity of these compounds, taken together with the inactivity of their isomers [3-pyridylethylamine (48.**10**) and 5-thiazolylethylamine] also indicates that the N$^\tau$—H tautomer of histamine monocation is the active form at H$_1$ receptors (79), in agreement with the previous suggestions of Niemann and Hays (76). These non-tautomeric heterocyclic ethylamines are only weakly active at H$_2$ receptors, however, and it appears that effective H$_2$-receptor agonists are compounds that can undergo a 1,3-prototropic tautomerism (79). Further indications of the importance of tautomerism for H$_2$-receptor agonist activity come from a comparison of the activities of 4-substituted histamine derivatives (Table 48.8). 4-Methylhistamine (48.**15a**) is about half as active as histamine; replacement of methyl by electron-withdrawing substituents reduces activity. Thus 4-chloro- and 4-bromohistamine (48.**23** and 48.**24**) have about $\frac{1}{10}$ and 4-nitrohistamine (48.**25**) has less than $\frac{1}{100}$ of the activity of histamine. Electron-withdrawing substituents in the 4 position of the imidazole ring change the relative tautomer concentrations since they alter the electron densities at the nitrogen atoms and affect proton acidities; the effect is more pronounced at the nearer nitrogen atom so that the relative stabilities of the tautomers change in comparison with histamine (41). The population of the N$^\tau$—H tautomer of 4-methylhistamine is similar to that of histamine but is reduced by one order of magnitude for 4-chlorohistamine and by two orders of magnitude for 4-nitrohistamine (Table 48.8). These reductions in populations of the N$^\tau$—H tautomer approximately parallel the changes in H$_2$-receptor agonist activities. The tautomeric effect may not be the only factor affecting receptor activity; the substituent will exert other effects, e.g., steric, polarity, and lipid water distribution.

Table 48.8 Tautomer Concentration Ratios, K_t, Percentage Mole Fractions of N^τ – H Tautomer, and H_2 Receptor Agonist Activities (Relative to Histamine=100) of 4-Substituted Histamine Monocations

$$K_t = \frac{R \quad CH_2CH_2NH_3^+}{R \quad CH_2CH_2NH_3^+}$$

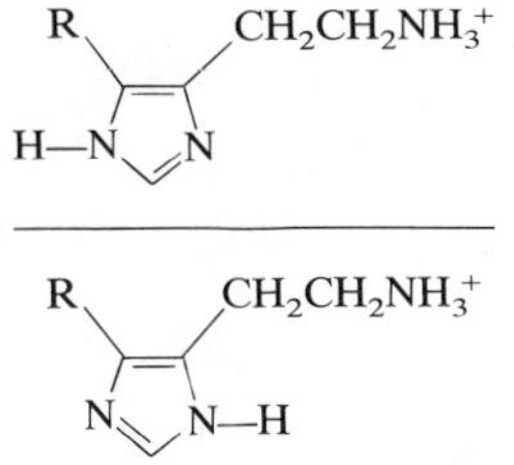

Compound Number	R	K_t^a	% Mole Fraction[b] N^τ—H	H_2-Receptor Agonist Activity[c]
Histamine	H	2.4	71	100
48.**15a**	CH$_3$	4.1	80	43[d]
48.**23**	Cl	0.13	12	11
48.**24**	Br	0.11	10	9[e]
48.**25**	NO$_2$	0.009	0.9	0.6

[a] $K_{t,R}$ = antilog [3.4 ($\sigma_{m,CH_2CH_2NH_3^+} - \sigma_{m,R}$)], with $\sigma_{m,CH_2CH_2NH_3^+}$ taken as +0.11 (41).
[b] Mole fraction of monocation, not the mole fraction of total species, which would be pH dependent.
[c] Activities determined *in vitro* on guinea pig right atrium, in the presence of propranolol, expressed relative to histamine = 100 (R. C. Blakemore in Ref. 41).
[d] 95% fiducial limits 40–46.
[e] 95% fiducial limits 7.4–10.1.

The results lead to the speculative deduction that the N^τ—H tautomer is a biologically active form of histamine at the H_2 receptor, or that the free-energy difference between the tautomers must be small for effective biological activity. If the interaction is static and it is the tautomer *per se* that is active then the *pros*-nitrogen (N^π) may function as an electron-pair donor and the N^τ—H may act as a hydrogen donor in multiple hydrogen bonding. Alternatively if the interaction is dynamic and the process of tautomerism is involved then histamine

might act as a proton transfer agent (41). Pictorially (Fig. 48.10) one can envisage the imidazole ring catalyzing the transfer of a proton from site A to site B, and perhaps a catalytic mechanism of some kind may be involved in the events leading to an effective H_2-receptor response (79). Such a proton transfer mechanism is analogous to the function of imidazole in the histidyl residues of certain enzymes, e.g., the catalytic site in chymotrypsin (89). A similar mechanism has also been proposed on theoretical grounds (45).

The highly selective H_2-receptor agonist dimaprit, 48.**26**, [S-(3-N,N-dimethylaminopropyl)isothiourea] (86, 90) (Fig. 48.11, Table 48.19) provides additional

H_1 *Receptors*

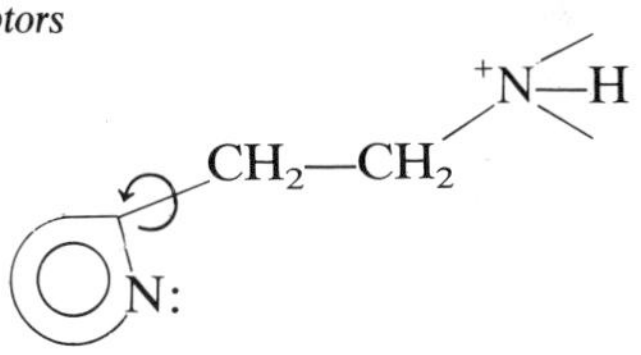

indicating (1) Side chain cation and N—H
(2) Heterocyclic ring with basic N: (with lone pair of electrons) in ortho position
(3) Ring rotation or possible "essential" conformation

H_2 *Receptors*

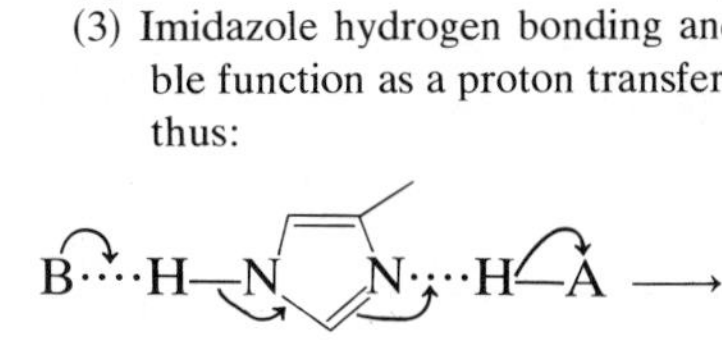

indicating (1) Side chain cation and N—H
(2) N^τ—H tautomer and amidine system
(3) Imidazole hydrogen bonding and possible function as a proton transfer agent, thus:

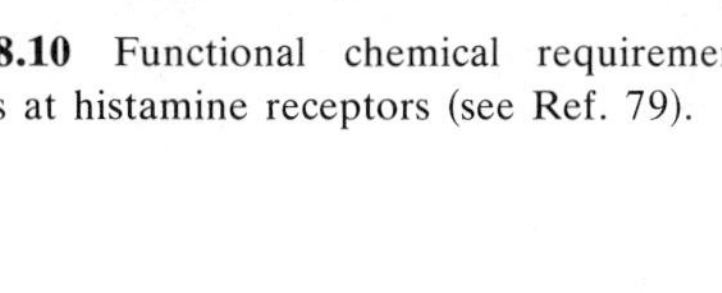

Fig. 48.10 Functional chemical requirements of agonists at histamine receptors (see Ref. 79).

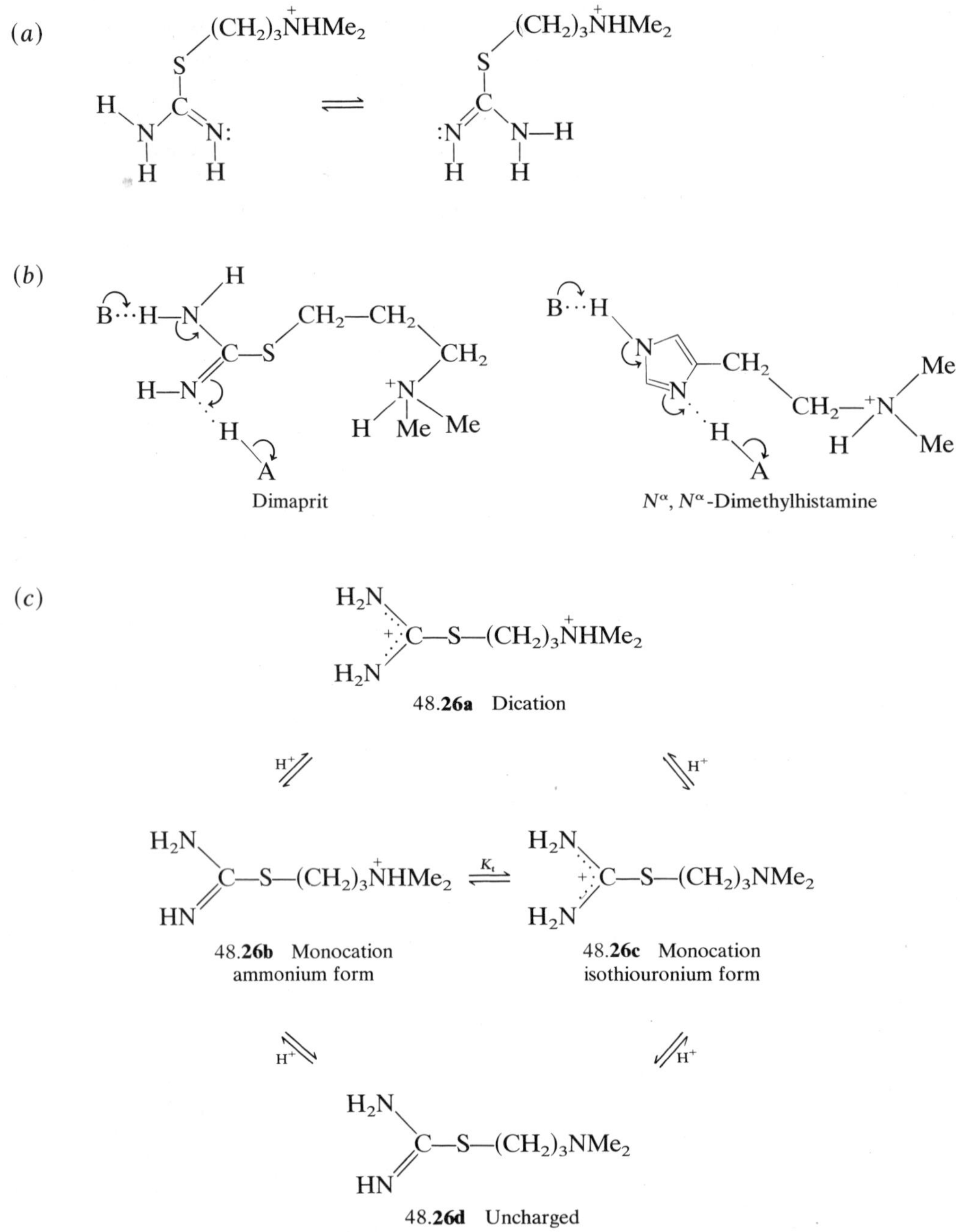

Fig. 48.11 Dimaprit formulas (48.**26**), illustrating (*a*) tautomerism of isothiourea group, (*b*) comparison with N^{α}, N^{α}-dimethylhistamine to show a possible similarity in function in hydrogen bonding and as proton transfer agents (see Ref. 90), (*c*) equilibria between different ionic species. The apparent stoichiometric pK_a values measured at 40°C in water are pK_{a_1} 8.23, pK_{a_2} 9.23. At pH 7.4 the relative concentrations of species are approximately dication (87%), monocation (13%), uncharged (0.2%). The relative concentrations of the two monocations was measured using NMR spectroscopy, and afforded $K_t = [C]/[B] \approx 1.4$; whence percentage of ammonium monocation 48.**26b** is approximately 5.4% (90).

504

evidence for the involvement of tauto-merism. Dimaprit has two basic centers and pK_a studies indicate that at pH 7.4 about 5% of the molecules are present as the monocation analogous to histamine mono-cation. Chemical comparison suggests that the $NHMe_2^+$ group corresponds to the NH_3^+ of histamine (or more correctly, to the $NHMe_2^+$ group of N^α,N^α-dimethyl-histamine) and that the isothiourea group of dimaprit may simulate the imidazole ring of histamine (90). Isothioureas resemble imidazoles in that both are planar 6π-electron systems which incorporate an amidine; the latter in the uncharged form has N—H and N (lone pair of electrons) and undergoes 1,3-prototropic tauto-merism. Tautomerism of dimaprit is de-picted in Fig. 48.11 and a comparison is made with N^α,N^α-dimethylhistamine show-ing a possible similarity in function in hyd-rogen bonding and as proton transfer ag-ents. In this comparison, isothiourea and imidazole represent a very interesting and novel example of bioisosterism. Dimaprit also poses an interesting problem for con-formational analysis since the higher and lower homologs are not active (90).

3.3   Evidence for an Active Conformation

Methyl substitution in histamine may dramatically affect agonist activity; in the imidazole ring, substituents may also im-part selectivity of action. Thus 4-methyl-histamine is a selective H_2-receptor agonist whereas 2-methylhistamine is a relatively selective H_1-receptor agonist (35). Presum-ably, such selectivity is caused by the methyl group interfering with molecular function; this may occur as a simple steric inhibition of agonist receptor fit but, since this is difficult to verify, alternative expla-nations should also be sought. Methyl-substituted histamines may provide a homogeneous series with respect to many chemical properties and form a useful set for study (Table 48.6).

A series of methyl-substituted histamines was studied with respect to conformational properties and receptor selectivities (91), and it was suggested (92) that the striking receptor selectivity of 4-methylhistamine (which has 40% of the potency of hist-amine as an H_2-receptor stimulant but only 0.2% at H_1 receptors) could be accounted for in the difference between its conforma-tional properties and those of histamine; this permitted the definition of an "H_1-essential" conformation, (see also Ref. 93), i.e., a conformation essential to drug activ-ity that has to be adopted by histamine at some stage during productive interaction at the H_1-receptor site. This is the fully ex-tended trans conformation where $\theta_1 = 0°$ and $\theta_2 = 180°$, in which the carbon and nitrogen atoms are coplanar with the ring (illustrated in Fig. 48.12), and there is a maximum separation (interatomic distance of 5.1 Å) between the charged ammonium group and the ring N^π-nitrogen atom. Furthermore, in this conformation any effect from the side chain in obscuring the lone electron pair at N^π is minimal. This would be a very satisfactory situation if the nitrogen atom were involved in donating its electron pair during productive drug–receptor interaction.

The described "H_1-essential" conforma-tion is apparently not a minimum energy form. Indeed, for histamine, the trans rotamer ($\theta_2 = 180°$) is predicted by EHT calculations to be at a minimum energy when $\theta_1 = 120°$, whereas the "H_1-essential" con-formation at $\theta_1 = 0°$ is calculated to have an energy about 3 kcal/mol above this (al-though the value may be an overestimate; see Ref. 94). That this planar conformation is capable of stable existence is demon-strated by the crystal structure of histamine sulfate (60) (see Table 48.4). These findings lead to the speculation that histamine may undergo a conformational change during H_1-receptor stimulation. A histamine

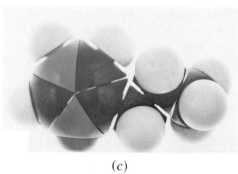

(a)

$\theta_1 = 0°;\ \theta_2 = 180°$

(b)

(c)

Fig. 48.12 (a) Steric interaction between the C$_4$-methyl and α-methylene groups in 4-methylhistamine in the coplanar $(\theta_1 = 0°)$, trans $(\theta_2 = 180°)$ conformation; intersecting arcs represent the overlap of van der Waals zones. (b) H$_1$ receptor "essential" conformation of histamine proposed by Ganellin (92). (c) CPK model of histamine monocation in the proposed H$_1$ receptor "essential" conformation. The model illustrates the close approach between the hydrogen atoms of the side chain α-CH$_2$ and the ring 4 positions.

molecule, arriving in the neighborhood of the site of action in one of its most probable (minimum energy) conformations, could either interact with the receptor and undergo a change involving the "H$_1$-essential" conformation or, under a perturbing influence of the receptor, might adopt the "H$_1$-essential" conformation prior to forming a drug–receptor complex. The described conformation may be only

one of several forms involved during receptor stimulation or, indeed, may be involved in only a transient manner while the agonist undergoes a required conformational change. Thus rotation of the imidazole ring may also be involved in the action of histamine at H$_1$ receptors.

Since 4-methylhistamine is an effective agonist at H$_2$ receptors it follows that conformations inaccessible to 4-methylhistamine, such as those where θ_1 approaches 0°, are not involved in H$_2$-receptor interactions.

3.4 Chemical Functional Requirements of Agonists at Histamine Receptors

The chemical functional requirements revealed by structure–activity analysis are summarized in Fig. 48.10. The active form of histamine for both receptors is likely to be the N$^\tau$—H tautomer of the monocation (48.**3b**), which is also the most prevalent species in water at around neutrality, and a side chain N—H appears to be needed. However, different chemical properties of histamine may be associated with interactions at the two receptor types. At the H$_1$ receptor, imidazole tautomerism is not a functional requirement, but the presence of the nitrogen atom ortho to the ammonium-ethyl group appears to have special significance. The ring may also need to be able to freely rotate or at least to achieve coplanarity with the side chain. At the H$_2$ receptor, the tautomeric property of the imidazole ring of histamine appears to be important and histamine might be involved in multiple hydrogen bonding or as a proton-transfer agent.

These suggestions for the chemical properties of histamine needed for agonist activity are obviously incomplete. Furthermore, to define the chemical constitution of other agonist molecules much remains to be done in studying their chemistry. Substituents may have pronounced effects; at some positions a methyl or ethyl group is tolerated without much loss in activity, but larger alkyl groups hinder agonist function e.g., 4-ethylhistamine is a selective H$_2$-receptor agonist (243–245) but 4-propylhistamine is only a weak partial agonist (244). Similar effects on H$_1$-receptor agonist activity have been observed with N^α- or 2-substituted analogs (246, 247). There may also be different effects depending on the polarity of substituents; e.g., a 5-amino substituent in 3-(1,2,4-triazolyl)ethylamine (48.**22**) is reported to impart selectivity towards H$_2$ receptors, whereas the 5-methyl derivative (analogous to 2-methylhistamine) appears to be a specific H$_1$-receptor agonist (248).

4   DEVELOPMENT OF H₂-RECEPTOR ANTAGONISTS

4.1   The Search for an Antagonist

The inability of the antihistaminic drugs (H$_1$-receptor antagonists) to inhibit histamine-stimulated gastric acid secretion has been known for many years (95), but there have been few published reports of concerted efforts to discover a specific antagonist to this action of histamine. Robertson and Grossman (23) screened compounds in a search for inhibitors of gastric acid secretion, and Grossman et al. (33) reported on an extensive study of compounds, chemically related to histamine, which were examined for their action on acid secretion and also tested as possible inhibitors of histamine stimulation. Lin et al. (29), Ash and Schild (22), and van den Brink (81) also examined close analogs of histamine for possible antagonism of histamine-stimulated acid secretion. However, none of these studies established a histamine antagonist.

At the Smith Kline & French Laboratories in England the approach taken by Black and his colleagues in seeking an antagonist also took histamine as the chemical starting point; however, the studies were not restricted to close structural analogs but an attempt was made to design an antagonist by modifying the structure and chemistry of histamine. Compounds were tested for ability to inhibit histamine-stimulated gastric acid secretion in anesthetized rats. Gastric acid secretion was measured by the pH of the lumen perfusate from the stomach of the anesthetized rat (96); a plateau of gastric acid secretion was established by continuous intravenous infusion of histamine at a dose high enough to produce a near maximal response and potential inhibitors were then given by rapid intravenous injection. Since other types of inhibitors of gastric secretion could also act in this test, compounds found to be active were also tested on isolated tissue systems to provide additional criteria for specific antagonism to histamine (see Section 6.1).

The working hypothesis was to seek a molecule that would compete with histamine for its receptor site. It was thought that an antagonist would have to be recognized by the receptor, then bind more strongly than histamine, but not trigger off the usual response. In attempting to design an antagonist, many different approaches were tried, including the use of analogies derived from known examples of chemical–biologic relationships between other types of receptor agonists and antagonists, or enzyme substrates and inhibitors, or antimetabolites. Taking histamine as the starting point, its structure was modified to alter deliberately some definite aspect of its chemical properties. Some examples, summarized in Fig. 48.13, have been more fully discussed elsewhere (63, 97). Modifications were made to the imidazole ring of histamine to change ionization properties (pK_a and tautomerism); e.g., electronegative substituents were introduced into the 4 position (Fig. 48.13a) and other heterocyclic analogs were examined; an analogy

(a) Electron with-drawing substituents R alter ring pK_a and tautomerism:

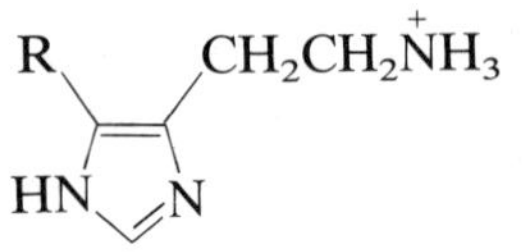

$$R \qquad CH_2CH_2\overset{+}{N}H_3$$
$$HN \diagdown N$$

(b) Ring fusion, by analogy with β-adrenergic blockers:

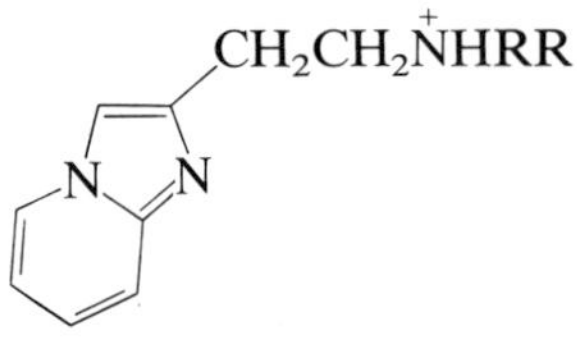

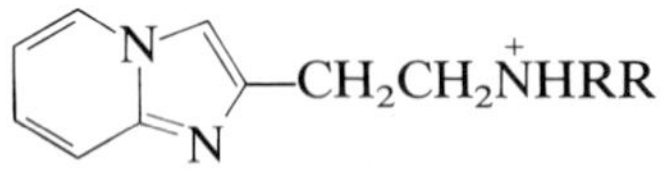

$$CH_2CH_2\overset{+}{N}HRR$$

$$-CH_2CH_2\overset{+}{N}HRR$$

(c) Nonpolar lipophilic substituents for hydrophobic bonding:

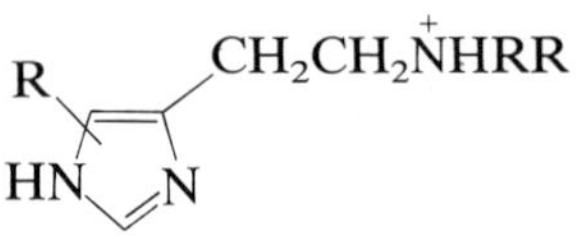

$$R \qquad CH_2CH_2\overset{+}{N}HRR \quad R = H \text{ or } -(CH_2)_n CH_3$$
$$HN \diagdown N \qquad\qquad\qquad\qquad\quad \text{or } -(CH_2)_n C_6H_5$$
$$\qquad\qquad\qquad\qquad\qquad\qquad n = 0\text{–}5$$

(d) For H$_2$-receptor *agonists*, methyl substituents can be accommodated at positions 4 and N$^\alpha$; a methyl group is accommodated less well at position 2, and poorly accommodated elsewhere (cf. Table 48.6):

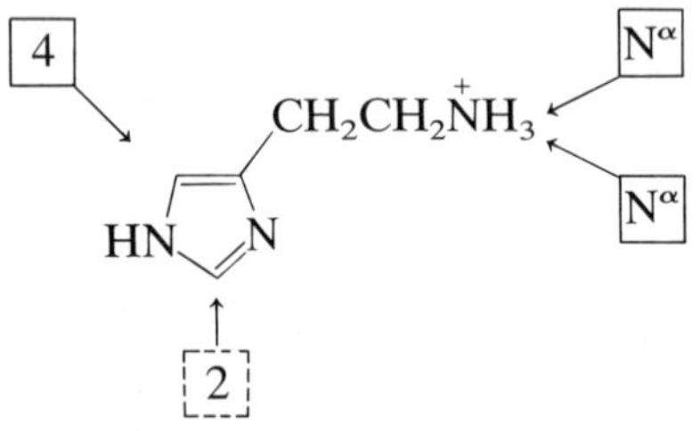

$$\boxed{4} \qquad\qquad\qquad \boxed{N^\alpha}$$
$$CH_2CH_2\overset{+}{N}H_3$$
$$HN \diagdown N \qquad\qquad \boxed{N^\alpha}$$
$$\boxed{2}$$

Fig. 48.13 Some attempts to design a histamine antagonist.

with the β-adrenergic blockers led to fusion of a benzene ring to the imidazole ring of histamine (Fig. 48.13b), as in the relationship between the β-adrenergic agonist isoproterenol and its antagonist pronethalol (98). In another approach, nonpolar lipophilic substituents were introduced at vari-

ous positions in histamine (Fig. 48.13c), since many competitive antagonist drugs contain such groups that are thought to contribute to drug–receptor association through hydrophobic interaction at nonpolar regions of the receptor at the active site or its immediate vicinity (cf. Ref. 99). A range of alkyl- and arylalkyl-substituted histamines was examined since it was not possible to know in advance which groups might match molecular requirements.

By analogy with active-site-directed enzyme inhibitors designed from substrates, where both position and nature of a lipophilic substituent can be critical (100), it was considered essential to identify sites in the histamine molecule where a substituent can be accommodated without loss of receptor binding. Methyl was selected as a suitable small nonpolar substituent on the basis that if a methyl-substituted histamine possessed a good level of histamine-like agonist activity one could deduce that receptor binding had been retained. This study established that methyl substitution markedly influences the level of H$_2$-receptor agonist activity and that the position of substitution is critical. A methyl group is tolerated well at the ring 4 position or on the side chain N$^\alpha$ atom (Fig. 48.13d); it is tolerated less well at the ring 2 position or on the side chain α- or β-carbon atoms (Table 48.6). Thus two positions, 4 and N$^\alpha$, in the histamine molecule were identified where methyl substitution does not result in appreciable loss in H$_2$-receptor binding (80).

The above approaches were concerned mainly with modifications to the imidazole ring of histamine, or with making the molecule lipophilic, but none of the compounds was found to antagonize the non-H$_1$ actions of histamine. Attention was also directed to compounds in which the imidazole ring was unaltered, and where the side chain had been modified. For example (Fig. 48.14a), the NH$_3^+$ group was replaced by SH or OH to see whether an altera-

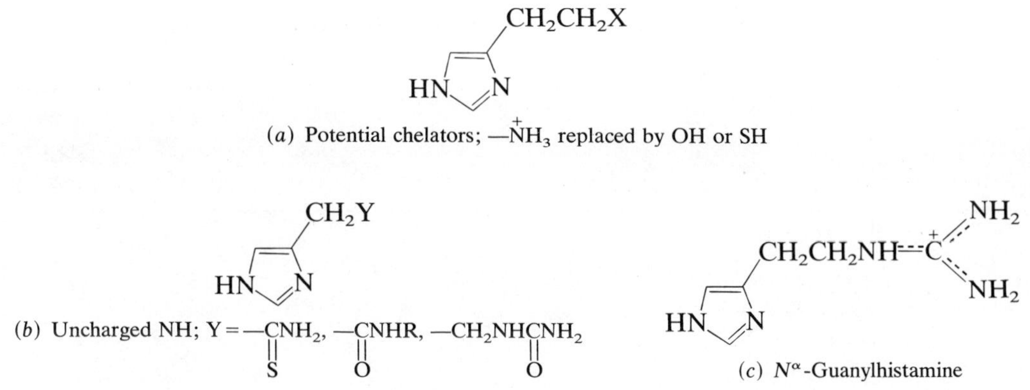

(a) Potential chelators; —$\overset{+}{N}H_3$ replaced by OH or SH

(b) Uncharged NH; Y = —$\underset{\underset{S}{\|}}{C}NH_2$, —$\underset{\underset{O}{\|}}{C}NHR$, —$CH_2NH\underset{\underset{O}{\|}}{C}NH_2$

(c) N^α-Guanylhistamine

Fig. 48.14   Further attempts to obtain potential antagonists by modifying the side chain of histamine.

tion of potential chelating properties might provide an antagonist. A number of other polar-substituted imidazoles resembling histamine were also examined; some amidic derivatives (shown in Fig. 48.14b) differ from histamine in having side chain nitrogen atoms uncharged. Ultimately, the guanidine analog of histamine, N^α-guanylhistamine (Fig. 48.14c) provided the "breakthrough." In this compound, the imidazole ring of histamine is retained, but the side chain amino group is modified, although it is still polar and charged.

N^α-Guanylhistamine (48.**27**) was found (101) to be a partial agonist [as defined by Stephenson, (102)] (see Table 48.9). Thus using the lumen perfused stomach of the anesthetized rat preparation, stimulant activity was found at doses in the range 16–128 × 10^{-6} mol/kg (given by rapid intravenous injection); the compound was a weak agonist having less than 0.5% the activity of histamine and was able to achieve only 50–60% of the maximum response of histamine. Antagonist activity was demonstrated by injecting high doses of guanylhistamine intravenously, having first established a near maximal plateau of secretion to an intravenous infusion of histamine. The approximate intravenous ID$_{50}$ (that is, the dose to produce 50% inhibition of near

maximal secretion) was 800 × 10^{-6} mol/kg. The partial agonist activity was also demonstrated on the isolated guinea pig right atrium *in vitro*.

4.2   Development of Burimamide

The antagonist activity of guanylhistamine was barely detectable but the compound provided a basis for further drug development. Guanylhistamine contains the more strongly basic guanidine group in place of the amino group of histamine and should be protonated throughout the physiological pH range, existing mainly as the guanidinium ion. Guanidinium cations differ from ammonium cations in being planar (instead of tetrahedral) and having a π-electron system extending over four sp^2-hybridized atoms; since the positive charge is delocalized, it is more diffuse on the guanidinium N atoms than on the ammonium N. This may alter the hydrogen-bonding characteristics.

Examination of other **guanidine** derivatives for histamine antagonism indicated that the ability to antagonize histamine was not a property of guanidines *per se*; thus the presence of an imidazole ring appears to be of importance, so that the imidazole and guanidine groups probably act

Table 48.9   Some Key Compounds in the Development of H_2-Receptor Antagonists

Compound	Structure	Antagonist In Vitro K_B,[a] 10^{-6} M	Activity In Vivo ID_{50},[b] μmol/kg
48.27 N^α-Guanylhistamine: the "lead"; a weakly active partial agonist	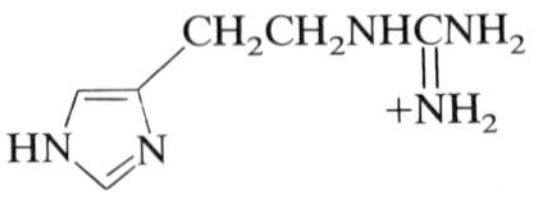 CH$_2$CH$_2$NHCNH$_2$ / +NH$_2$ / HN—N	130	800
48.28 SK&F 91486: lengthening the side chain increases activity	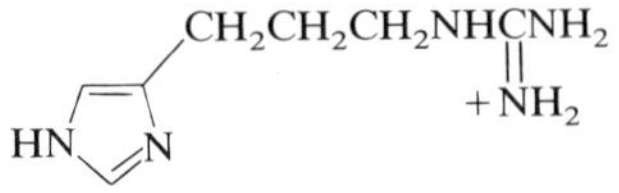 CH$_2$CH$_2$CH$_2$NHCNH$_2$ / +NH$_2$ / HN—N	22	100
48.29 SK&F 91581: thiourea analogue is much less active as an antagonist, but is not an agonist	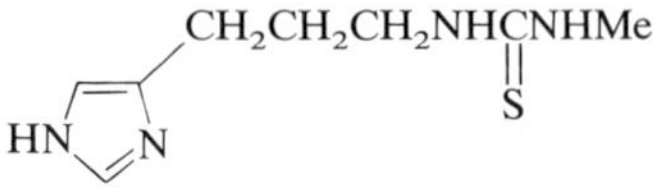 CH$_2$CH$_2$CH$_2$NHCNHMe / S / HN—N	115[c]	[d]
48.30 Burimamide: lengthening the side chain again dramatically increases antagonist activity	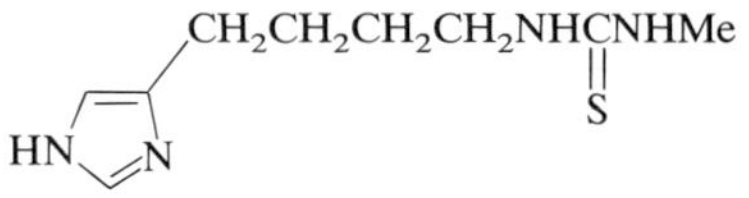 CH$_2$CH$_2$CH$_2$CH$_2$NHCNHMe / S / HN—N	7.8	6.1
48.31 Metiamide: introducing —S— in the side chain and CH$_3$ in the ring alters imidazole tautomerism and increases activity	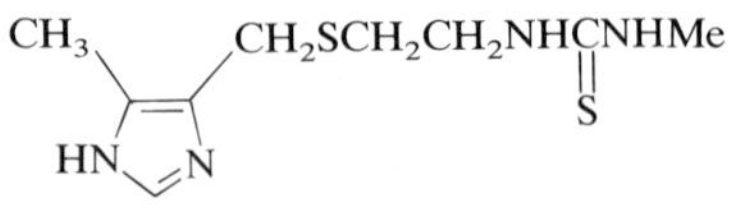 CH$_3$ / CH$_2$SCH$_2$CH$_2$NHCNHMe / S / HN—N	0.92	1.6
48.32 Guanidine isostere: replacing C=S by C=NH gives a basic side chain and reduces activity	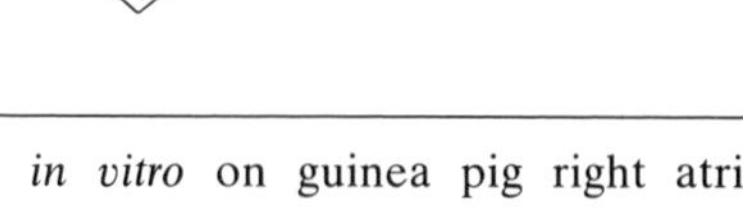 CH$_3$ / CH$_2$SCH$_2$CH$_2$NHCNHMe / +NH$_2$ / HN—N	16	12
48.33 Cimetidine: introducing a CN substituent reduces basicity and increases activity	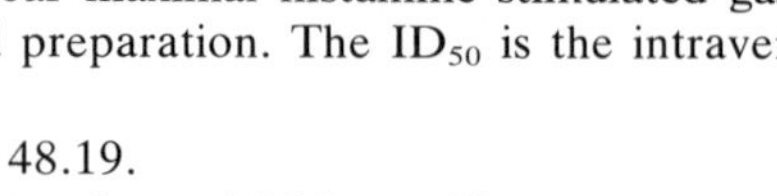 CH$_3$ / CH$_2$SCH$_2$CH$_2$NHCNHMe / N—CN / HN—N	0.79	1.4

[a] Dissociation constant, K_B, determined *in vitro* on guinea pig right atrium against histamine stimulation.
[b] Activity *in vivo* as an antagonist of near maximal histamine-stimulated gastric acid secretion in anesthetized rats using a lumen perfused preparation. The ID_{50} is the intravenous dose required to produce 50% of inhibition.
[c] Refined data. See footnote *h* in Table 48.19.
[d] No antagonism seen up to an intravenous dose of 256 μmol/kg.

cooperatively. One may note that in extended conformations, guanylhistamine has a greater intramolecular distance between the imidazole ring and side chain terminal nitrogen atoms than does histamine; a greater interatomic distance seems to be necessary, since extension of the side chain to increase the separation furnishes homologs which are considerably more active as antagonists, although they are still partial agonists. The simple homolog 3-(imidazol-4-yl)propylguanidine (48.**28**, SK & F 91486) was found (103) to be six to eight times more potent as an antagonist (see Table 48.9). Various related amidinium and isothiouronium structures (Fig. 48.15) have been found to have activity as antagonists and are described in several patents (104); many of these compounds have also been found to be partial agonists. There is a strong resemblance between these structures and histamine in that they incorporate an imidazole ring and a cationic side chain. It seems likely that these features permit receptor recognition and provide binding for a competitive antagonist, but also allow the molecule to mimic histamine as an agonist. Such thoughts prompted attempts to remove the agonist effect by replacing the guanidinium group with other nonbasic polar hydrogen-bonding groups which would not be charged, e.g., the thioureido derivative SK & F 91581 (48.**29**, Table 48.9) in which thione S replaces imino NH and makes the remaining nitrogen atoms relatively nonbasic. This compound did not act as a partial agonist but was only weakly active as an antagonist. Extending the length of the alkylene chain resulted in a marked increase in antagonist potency exemplified by the drug burimamide (48.**30**, Table 48.9). Burimamide was found to be about 100 times more potent than N^α-guanylhistamine as a histamine antagonist and did not act as a partial agonist. Burimamide was shown to be a highly specific competitive antagonist of histamine on non-H$_1$ tissue systems, thereby defining histamine H$_2$ receptors (see Section 6.1), and allowing burimamide to be defined as an H$_2$-receptor antagonist.

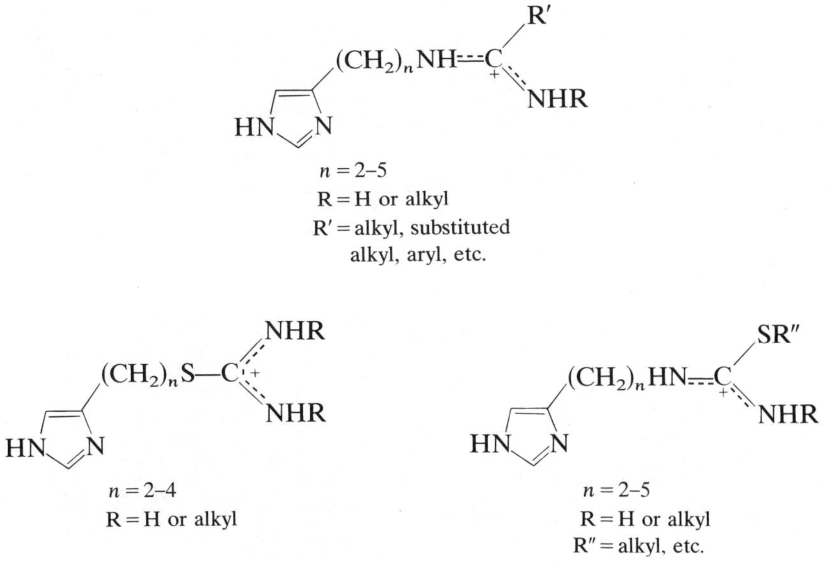

$n = 2\text{--}5$
R = H or alkyl
R' = alkyl, substituted
alkyl, aryl, etc.

$n = 2\text{--}4$
R = H or alkyl

$n = 2\text{--}5$
R = H or alkyl
R'' = alkyl, etc.

Fig. 48.15 Amidinium and isothiouronium analogs of the guanidine partial agonists.

4.3 Development of Metiamide

Although burimamide was sufficiently selective pharmacologically it lacked adequate oral activity needed for exploring its therapeutic potential, and it appeared that a more active compound was required. Of various attempts made to produce a more suitable drug, a successful approach was based on the realization that burimamide in aqueous solution is a mixture of many chemical species in equilibrium (105). At physiological pH there are three main forms of the imidazole ring, three planar configurations of the thioureido group (a fourth is theoretically possible but is disfavored by internal steric hindrance), and various trans and gauche rotamer combinations of the side chain CH$_2$—CH$_2$ bonds

(Fig. 48.16). This means that at any given instant only a small proportion of the drug molecules would be in a particular form.

The existence of a mixture of species leads one to question which may be biologically active and whether altering drug structure to favor a particular species would alter drug potency, that is, to use the technique of dynamic structure–activity analysis (DSAA) (106). There are substantial energy barriers to interconversion between the species of burimamide so that it is quite likely that a drug molecule, presenting itself to the receptor in a form unfavorable for drug–receptor interaction, might diffuse away again before having time to rearrange into a more favorable form. The relative population of favorable forms might therefore determine the

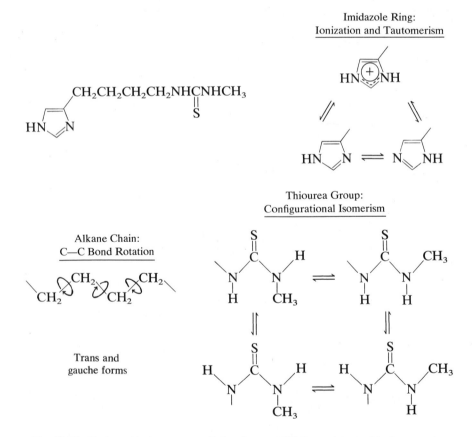

Fig. 48.16 Burimamide in aqueous solution is an equilibrium mixture of various species.

amount of drug required for a given effect. The various species do not interconvert instantaneously, but whereas the rotamers of the side chain and thioureido groups are interconverted simply by internal rotation of a C—C or C—N bond, interconversion of the ring forms probably involves a water-mediated proton transfer. If a molecule presents itself to the receptor with the ring in an unfavorable form it might not readjust, unless there were suitably oriented water molecules (or other hydrogen donor–acceptors) present. The form of the ring therefore merits special consideration.

The above arguments led to a study of the population of imidazole species in burimamide. At physiological pH the main species (Fig. 48.17) are the cation (48.**34a**) and two uncharged tautomers (48.**34b** and 48.**34c**). The populations of these species were estimated qualitatively from the electronic influence of the side chain using pK_a data, since the substituent R in the 4(5) position of imidazole alters the electron densities at the ring nitrogen atoms and affects proton acidity. The substituent effect is more marked at the nearer nitrogen atom so that if R is an electron-withdrawing group, the 1,4 tautomer 48.**34b** should predominate (107). The fraction present as cation 48.**34a** is determined by the ring pK_a

and the pH of the medium. The electronic influence of the side chain was assessed from the measured ring pK_a using the Hammett equation: $pK_{a,R} = pK_{a,H} + \rho\sigma_m$. The p$K_a$ values of relevant compounds are given in Table 48.10. For burimamide the ring pK_a is 7.25, which is greater than that of imidazole itself; it was argued that the side chain [R = (CH$_2$)$_4$NHCSNHCH$_3$] must therefore be releasing electrons and should favor tautomer 48.**34c**. Electronically, the side chain appears to resemble a methyl group since the pK_a is close to that of 4(5)-methylimidazole (48.**37**). At pH 7.4 the cation is one of the main species for burimamide (mole percentage is 40%) and tautomer 48.**34b** would be the least favored. For histamine the ammonium-ethyl side chain (R = —CH$_2$CH$_2$NH$_3^+$) lowers the pK_a of the imidazole ring; i.e., it withdraws electrons and favors tautomer 48.**34b**; there is only a small proportion of cation present at pH 7.4 (about 3%), and nearly 80% of histamine molecules are in the form 48.**34b** (see Section 2.1).

Thus although both histamine and burimamide are monosubstituted imidazoles, the structural similarity is misleading in that the predominant species of the respective imidazole rings are chemically different. If the active form of the antagonist were species 48.**34b**, the form most preferred for

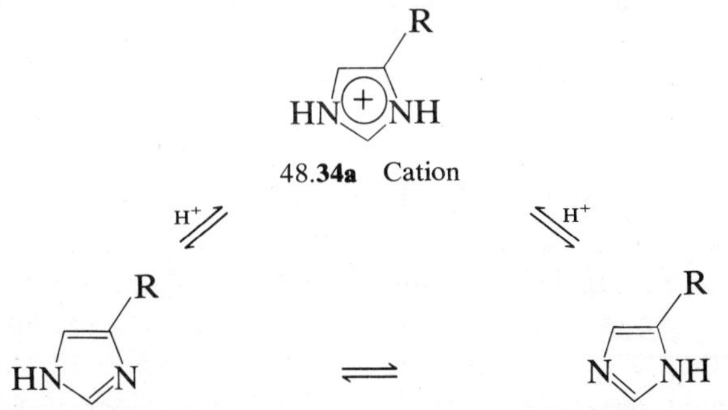

48.**34a** Cation

48.**34b** [1, 4] tautomer
Favored when R is electron-withdrawing

48.**34c** [1, 5] tautomer
Favored when R is electron-releasing

Fig. 48.17 Equilibria between imidazole species: substituents R in 4(5) position of the imidazole ring alter tautomerism (42, 107).

Table 48.10   Apparent pK_a Values^a of Substituted Imidazole Cations at 37°C and their Mole Percentages at pH 7.4 (105)

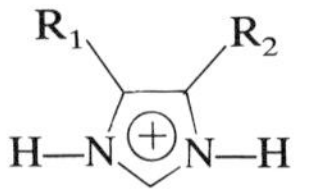

48.**35**

Compound	R$_1$	R$_2$	pK_a'	Preferred Tautomer^b	Mole % of Cation A at pH 7
48.**36** Methylburimamide	CH$_3$	—(CH$_2$)$_4$NHCSNHCH$_3$	7.80		72
48.**37** 4(5)-Methylimidazole	H	—CH$_3$	7.40	48.**34c**	50
48.**30** Burimamide	H	—(CH$_2$)$_4$NHCSNHCH$_3$	7.25	48.**34c**	40
48.**38** Imidazole	H	—H	6.80		20
48.**31** Metiamide	CH$_3$	—CH$_2$SCH$_2$CH$_2$NHCSNHCH$_3$	6.80	48.**34b**	20
48.**39** 4(5)-Methylthiomethyl imidazole	H	—CH$_2$SCH$_3$	6.35^c	48.**34b**	8
48.**40** Thiaburimamide	H	—CH$_2$SCH$_2$CH$_2$NHCSNHCH$_3$	6.25	48.**34b**	7
48.**41** 4(5)-Methoxymethyl imidazole	H	—CH$_2$OCH$_3$	6.00^c	48.**34b**	4
48.**3** Histamine	H	—CH$_2$CH$_2$NH$_3^+$	5.90	48.**34b**	3

^{a} pK_a determined potentiometrically at 25°C on 0.005 M solutions in 0.1 M KCl by titration against HCl, corrected to 37°C by subtracting 0.0225 units per degree rise for values in the range 7.5–7.0 (108), and 0.02 for the range 6.5–6.0 (37), and rounded off to the nearest 0.05 unit (105).
^{b} Structures in Fig. 48.16; R$_2$ = R.
^{c} Ref. 109.

histamine, then increasing its relative population might increase activity. Thus incorporating an electronegative atom into the antagonist side chain would convert it into an electron-withdrawing group and should favor species 48.**34b**. This would not be the only condition for activity, however; it would be necessary to minimize disturbance to other biologically important molecular properties such as stereochemistry and lipid–water partition. In this sense, the methylene group (—CH$_2$—) is isosteric with a thioether linkage (—S—), as the data in Table 48.11 show. The groups have similar van der Waals radii and give rise to similar bond angles. The C–S bond is somewhat longer than a C–C bond so that in the thioether the adjacent methylene

groups would be farther apart by 0.3–0.4 Å; this is quite a modest effect, amounting to an increase in distance between these two groups of about 15%.

Making this substitution in burimamide at the carbon atom beta to the ring afforded the compound "thiaburimamide" (Table 48.10, R$_1$ = H, R$_2$ = —CH$_2$SCH$_2$CH$_2$NHCSNHCH$_3$, 48.**40**). The effect on partition of the uncharged molecule is small. Log P (at 37°C between 1-octanol and aqueous buffer at pH 9.0) is reduced from 0.39 (burimamide) to 0.16 (thiaburimamide). The electronic influence of the modified side chain, shown by the ring pK_a, is similar in magnitude but in the opposite direction to that of a methyl group so that the main species should be tautomer

Table 48.11 Comparison of Methylene (—CH₂—), Thioether (—S—), and Ether (—O—) Linkages

	Units	RCH_2—X—CH_2R			Ref.
		X = CH₂	X = S	X = O	
C—X bond length	Å	1.54	1.81	1.43	110a,b
CXC bond angle, R = H	o	109	105	111	110c
C⋯C interatomic distances					
between centers	Å	2.51	2.87	2.37	111
van der Waals radius of X	Å	2.0	1.85	1.40	110d
Group contribution of X to					
van der Waals volume	cm³/mol	10.2	10.8	3.7	112
Molar volume increment of X	cm³/mol	16.6	10.8	6.7	113
C—X rotational energy					
barrier, R = H	kcal/mol	3.3	2.13	2.72	114, 115, 116
log P (octanol–H₂O), R = CH₃		3.39[a]	1.95	0.77	117a, 118, 119
Hydrophobic fragmental constant, f,		+0.53	−0.51	−1.54	120
of group X		+0.54	−0.79	−1.81	117a
Basicity (pK_a), R = CH₃			−6.8	−2.4	117c

[a] Previously reported value, 2.50 (117b).

48.34b. Since a further stabilization of tautomer 48.**34b** might be obtained by incorporating an electron-releasing substituent in the vacant 4(5) position of the ring, a methyl group was substituted into the ring of the antagonist; thus furnished the drug metiamide, N-methyl-N'-{2-[(5-methylimidazol-4-yl)methylthio]ethyl}-thiourea (48.**31**, Tables 48.9 and 48.10) (121). The two ring substituents are seen to have electronic effects of equal magnitude but of opposite direction. They should combine to favor tautomer 48.**34b** but have opposing effects on ring pK_a; indeed, they must exactly cancel since the pK_a's of metiamide and imidazole are identical (Table 48.10). This means that at pH 7.4 the main species of metiamide would be tautomer 48.**34b**, as for histamine, although there would still be a substantial proportion of cation present (20%). The methyl group should not interfere with receptor interaction since it has been shown that 4-methylhistamine is an effective H₂-receptor agonist (35). For metiamide, in comparison with burimamide, the ratio of tautomers is re-versed and the population of cation is decreased.

The pharamacological consequences of these manipulations are shown in Table 48.12. The results obtained in the two *in vitro* tissues are in good agreement and, taken together, show that metiamide *in vitro* is three to four times more active than thiaburimamide and eight to nine times more active than burimamide (105).

It can be seen that modifying the side chain in burimamide by isosteric replacement of —CH₂— by —S— favors tautomer 48.**34b**, reduces the ring pK_a, and gives a more active compound (thiaburimamide). Introducing a 4(5)-methyl group to give metiamide should increase further the preference for tautomer 48.**34b**, but it also decreases the combined populations of the uncharged tautomers (48.**34b** and 48.**34c**) through raising the ring pK_a. Although these are opposing effects the net result is that metiamide is more active still. By contrast, the analogous structural modification of burimamide, incorporation of a ring 4(5)-methyl group to give "methylburi-

Table 48.12 H$_2$-Receptor Antagonist Activities^a of Burimamide and Analogs, Determined *in Vitro* on Guinea Pig Atrium and Rat uterus (105)

| Compound^b | K$_B$ (95% limits), $\times 10^{-6}$ M | |
	Atrium	Uterus
Metiamide	0.92 (0.74–1.15)	0.75 (0.40–1.36)
Thiaburimamide	3.2 (2.5–4.5)	3.2 (2.5–4.5)
Burimamide	7.8 (6.4–9.6)	6.6 (4.9–8.3)
Methylburimamide	8.9 (5.6–15)	10.7 (4.5–31)
Oxaburimamide^c	28 (13–69)	6.6 (4.9–8.3)

^{a} The dissociation constant (K_B) was calculated from the equation $K_B = B/(x-1)$, where x is the respective ratio of concentrations of histamine needed to produce half-maximal responses in the presence and absence of different concentrations (B) of antagonist, and $-\log K_B = pA_2$.
^{b} Structures in Table 48.10.
^{c} Oxaburimamide is N-{2-[(imidazol-4-yl)methoxy]ethyl}-N'-methylthiourea; R$_1$ = H, R$_2$ = CH$_2$OCH$_2$CH$_2$NHCSNHCH$_3$ in structure 48.**35** of Table 48.10. Tested by R. C. Blakemore (122).

mamide" (48.**36**, Tables 48.10 and 48.12), does not increase activity. In this case the two ring substituents have nearly equal electronic effects in the same direction; the methyl group counterbalances the electronic influence of the side chain on tautomerism so that the two tautomers become equally populated, but it raises the ring pK_a to 7.80, so that at pH 7.4 the predominant species is the cation 48.**34a** (72%).

These results illustrate the problem of attempting to manipulate the biologic properties of drug molecules through altering the structure. The changes in chemical properties accompanying structural modification often impose their own inherent limitations; a structural change, biologically advantageous with respect to a given chemical property, may affect some other chemical property in a biologically disadvantageous way, and one has to discover the optimum balance of opposing influences.

Another example of the sensitivity of the system to changes in drug structure is illus-

trated by the use of an oxygen ether linkage (—O—) in place of —CH$_2$— or —S—. Comparison of the pK_a values of 4(5)-methoxymethylimidazole (48.**41** in Table 48.10) and 4(5)-methylthiomethylimidazole (48.**39** in Table 48.10) indicate that the substituents are electronically similar, which suggests that oxygen or sulfur linkages in the antagonist side chain should have comparable effects on imidazole tautomerism. Oxaburimamide is, however, less active than burimamide (Table 48.12). Although the ether linkage has a similar geometry to methylene in terms of bond lengths and angles (Table 48.11), the oxygen atom is substantially smaller, as indicated by van der Waals radii and molar volume increments. The ether oxygen atom is also more basic and hydrophilic than sulfur or methylene (Table 48.11). These differences may explain why oxygen is less successful than sulfur as an isosteric replacement for CH$_2$ in the H$_2$-receptor antagonist series. The question has been considered in greater detail elsewhere (123), particularly with regard to conformation and possible intramolecular hydrogen-bonding interactions.

4.4 Development of Cimetidine

In further studies of the structural requirements for H$_2$-receptor antagonism, the effect of replacing the thiourea group of metiamide was investigated. The importance of the investigation was emphasized by the finding of kidney damage and agranulocytosis in high dosage chronic toxicity tests with metiamide (124, 125) and the possibility that these effects were attributable to the presence of a thiourea group in the drug molecule. Isosteric replacement of the thiourea sulfur atom of metiamide by carbonyl oxygen (:O) or imino nitrogen (:NH) led to the synthesis of the urea (48.**42**) and guanidine (48.**32**). These were found to be H$_2$-receptor antagonists but were less potent than metiamide (Table 48.13). The guanidine (48.**32**) was of particular interest in being an antagonist, more potent than imidazolylalkylguanidines (48.**27** and 48.**28**), and yet not a partial agonist.

The guanidine (48.**32**) proved to be a suitable structure for molecular modification to provide compounds of increased potency. The third nitrogen atom permits the introduction of further substituents while retaining the side chain and terminal N-methyl substituent that are present

Table 48.13 Structures and H$_2$-Receptor Antagonist Activities^{a,b} of Metiamide, Cimetidine, and Isosteres (126a, 126b)

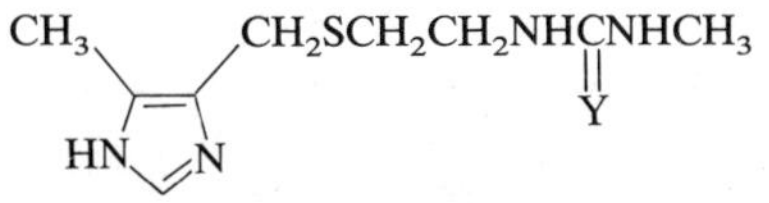

$$CH_3 \quad\quad CH_2SCH_2CH_2NHCNHCH_3$$

(with HN—N imidazole ring and Y)

Compound	Y	H$_2$-Antagonist Activity	
		in Vitro^a K_B (95% limits), $10^{-6}\,M$	in Vivo^b ID$_{50}$, μmol/kg
48.**31** Metiamide (thiourea)	S	0.92 (0.74–1.15)	1.6
48.**42** Urea isostere	O	22 (8.9–65)	27
48.**32** Guanidine isostere	NH	16 (8.1–32)	12
48.**43** Guanylurea derivative	NCONH$_2$	7.1 (4.0–14)	7.7
48.**44** Nitroguanidine isostere	NNO$_2$	1.4 (0.79–2.8)	2.1
48.**33** Cimetidine (cyanoguanidine)	NCN	0.79 (0.68–0.92)	1.4

^{a} Activities determined against histamine stimulation of guinea pig right atrium in vitro (R. C. Blakemore and M. E. Parsons, Smith Kline & French Laboratories, Welwyn Garden City, England). The dissociation constant (K_B) was calculated from the equation $K_B = B/(x-1)$, where x is the respective ratio of concentrations of histamine needed to produce half-maximal responses in the presence and absence of different concentrations (B) of antagonist, and where $-\log K_B = \mathrm{pA}_2$.

^{b} Activity as an antagonist of histamine-stimulated gastric acid secretion in anesthetized rats using a lumen perfused preparation (35). Compounds given by rapid intravenous injection during a near maximal plateau of histamine-stimulated gastric acid secretion. The ID$_{50}$ is the dose required to produce 50% inhibition, and was estimated from the linear regression of $\log[I/(100-I)]$ vs. log dose, where I = percentage inhibition (R. C. Blakemore and M. E. Parsons, Smith Kline & French Laboratories, Welwyn Garden City, England).

in metiamide. Guanidine (pK$_a$ 13.6) is strongly basic compared with thiourea, which is neutral (pK$_a$ − 1.2), and the disubstituted guanidine group of 48.**32** would exist almost exclusively in the cationic form under physiological conditions. Guanidine basicity can, however, be reduced by introducing a further substituent (Z) on the third nitrogen atom. As illustrated in Fig. 48.18, a trisubstituted guanidinium cation (48.**45a**) exists in equilibrium with three conjugate bases (48.**45b–d**) since proton dissociation can occur from each of the three nitrogen atoms. If the substituent Z is electronegative, basicity is reduced and the neutral guanidine species is stabilized.

A relationship between substituent effect and guanidine pK$_a$ was demonstrated by Charton (127) using the inductive substituent constant σ_I in the Hammett equation.

$$pK_{a,Z} = pK_{a,H} + \rho\sigma_{I,Z}$$

A plot of pK$_a$ vs. σ_I for a series of monosubstituted guanidines is shown in Fig.

48.19. The very high ρ value (−24) reflects the high sensitivity of pK$_a$ to substituent effects in guanidine; this can be attributed to the substituent being attached directly to the nitrogen atom bearing the dissociable proton. Electron-withdrawing substituents (Z) would be expected to favor the imino tautomer (48.**45b**) compared with the amino tautomers (48.**45c** and **d**) since the proton on the adjacent nitrogen atom in the cation (48.**45a**) would be more acidic than the protons on the more distant terminal nitrogen atoms (127). The groups cyano and nitro are sufficiently electron-attracting to reduce guanidinium pK$_a$ by 14 units; the ionization constants of cyanoguanidine (pK$_a$ −0.4) (128) and nitroguanidine (pK$_a$ −0.9) (129) approach that of thiourea (−1.2).

The nitroguanidine (48.**44**) and cyanoguanidine (48.**33**) analogs of metiamide were synthesized and found to be highly active H$_2$-receptor antagonists (Table 48.13). The introduction of either the nitro or the cyano group into the guanidine

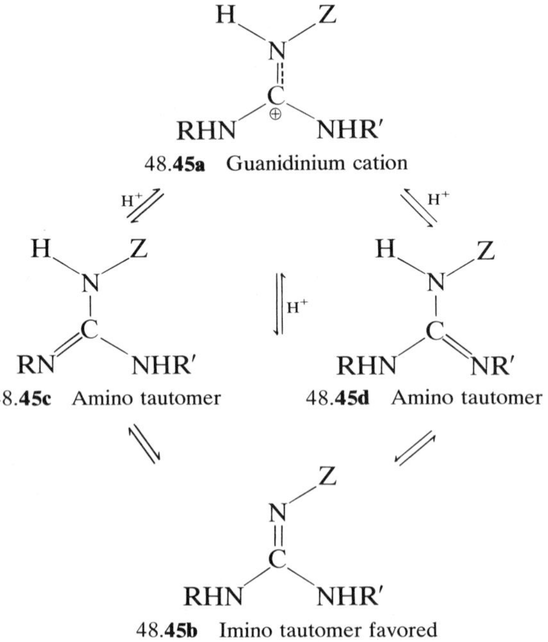

48.**45a** Guanidinium cation

48.**45c** Amino tautomer   48.**45d** Amino tautomer

48.**45b** Imino tautomer favored
when Z is strongly
electron-withdrawing

Fig. 48.18 Equilibria between guanidinium cation and the three conjugate bases.

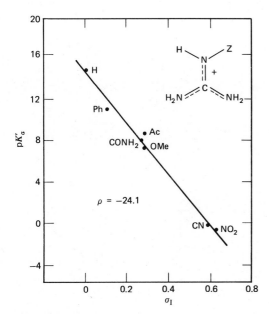

Fig. 48.19 Apparent pK_a values at 25°C of N-substituted guanidinium cations vs. σ_I substituent constants. Data from Charton (127). The line corresponds to the equation p$K'_a = 14.20 - 24.1\sigma_I$.

48.**32** thus results in a marked increase in H$_2$-receptor antagonist activity; the cyanoguanidine (48.**33**) is as active as the thiourea (48.**31**) (126a, b).

The cyanoguanidine N''-cyano-N-methyl-

N'-{2-[(5-methylimidazol-4-yl)-methylthio]-ethyl}guanidine (48.**33**) has the WHO-recommended international non-proprietary name cimetidine (126c). Many of the physicochemical properties of cimetidine and metiamide are similar and reflect the characteristics of cyanoguanidine and thiourea (Table 48.15). They are polar molecules with similar octanol–water partition coefficients. Cimetidine is slightly more water–soluble than metiamide and the solubility of both compounds is greatly increased by the addition of dilute acid to protonate the imidazole ring. The ring pK_a (6.80) is identical in the two compounds (109), which should therefore have similar species composition of the disubstituted imidazole ring. Metiamide and cimetidine possess the conformational properties expected for N,N'-disubstituted thioureas and cyanoguanidines (Fig. 48.20). NMR studies have demonstrated that, in solution, metiamide assumes three stable conformations of the thiourea group (48.**46a–c**, X = S), whereas cimetidine assumes only the two staggered configurations (48.**47a** and **b**) of the cyanoguanidine group (55). These forms are in equilibrium and interconvert

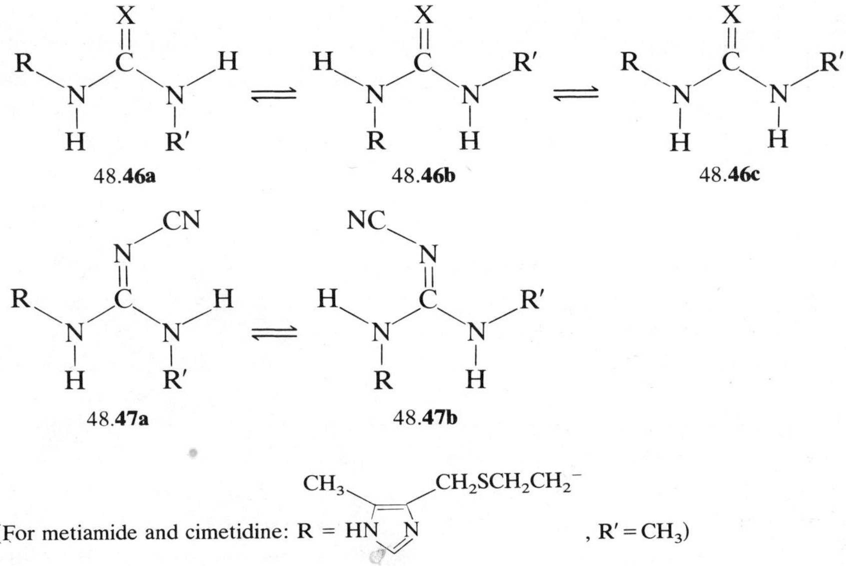

48.**46a**   48.**46b**   48.**46c**

48.**47a**   48.**47b**

(For metiamide and cimetidine: R = HN⎯N⎯CH$_3$ ... CH$_2$SCH$_2$CH$_2^-$, R' = CH$_3$)

Fig. 48.20 Planar conformations of N,N'-disubstituted thioureas and cyanoguanidines in solution.

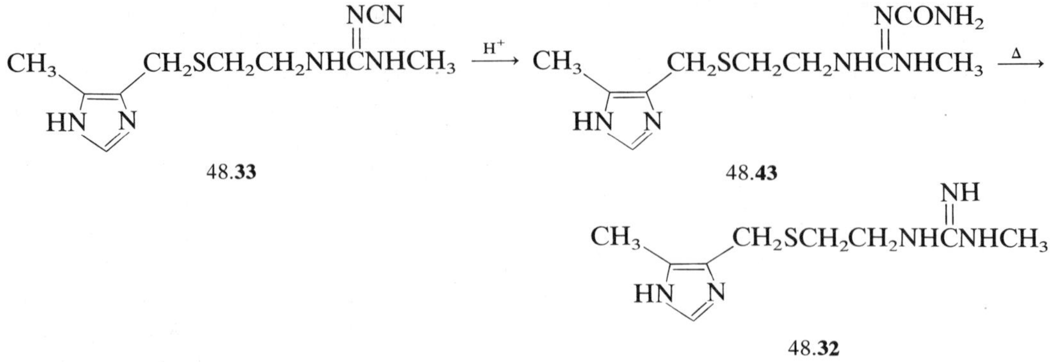

Fig. 48.21 Cimetidine (48.**33**) is converted hydrolytically into the guanylurea (48.**43**) and thence to the guanidine (48.**32**).

by C–N bond rotation. (Free energies of activation, $\Delta G\ddagger$ for the corresponding dimethyl analogs are given in Table 48.15.) Cyanoguanidines and thioureas differ sufficiently in chemical reactivity (e.g., in oxidative and hydrolytic reactions) for differences to be expected in the rates and products of biotransformation of drug molecules containing these groups. In the presence of excess dilute hydrochloric acid, cimetidine is slowly hydrolyzed to the guanylurea (48.**43**, Fig. 48.21), conversion being complete after 5 days at 20°C (126b). This guanylurea is also an H$_2$-receptor antagonist but it is less active than cimetidine and more comparable with the guanidine 48.**32** in antagonist potency (Table 48.13).

4.5 Cyanoguanidine–Thiourea Equivalence

The equieffectiveness of cyanoguanidine and thiourea groups in H$_2$-receptor antagonists, as implied by the similar antagonist potencies of cimetidine and metiamide, was also illustrated in the series of imidazole derivatives (Table 48.14) in which the thioureas (48.**30**, 48.**31**, 48.**40**, and 48.**36**) and the corresponding cyanoguanidine antagonists (48.**48**, 48.**33**, 48.**49**, and 48.**50**) were compared (126b).

The similarity in many physicochemical properties of cyanoguanidine and thiourea has been discussed (126). In Table 48.15 are listed some properties of cyanoguanidine and thiourea and also of nitroguanidine and urea. All these molecules are planar π electron systems with similar geometries, e.g., equal C–N bond distances and bond angles. They are also weakly amphoteric, that is, both weakly acidic and weakly basic with similar pK_a's. These molecules are all polar and hydrophilic with high dipole moments (μ) and low octanol–water partition coefficients (P). However, the partition coefficient of urea is even lower than that of thiourea, cyanoguanidine, or nitroguanidine. The close similarity in many physicochemical properties of thiourea and cyanoguanidine and the pharmacological equivalence of these groups in histamine H$_2$-receptor antagonists has led to the description of these groups as "true bioisosteres" (126b). Bioisosterism is not universal, however, and for other biological actions these groups may be nonequivalent (e.g., 149). Nitroguanidine may also be considered to be a bioisostere of thiourea, whereas urea may be regarded as a "partial bioisostere" of thiourea in H$_2$-receptor antagonists. Differences in polarizability and in partition of thiourea and urea groups (126) may contribute to the quantitative differences in an-

Table 48.14 *In vitro* Comparison of Thiourea and Cyanoguanidine H$_2$-Receptor Antagonists[a]

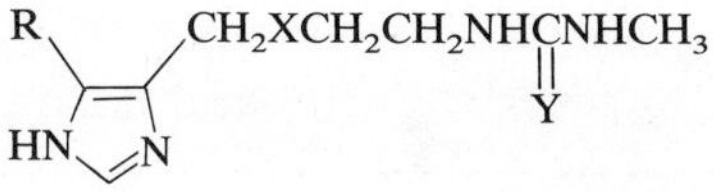

$$R\text{—}CH_2XCH_2CH_2NHCNHCH_3$$

(imidazole ring: HN, N; substituent Y on C)

Compound	R	X	Y	H$_2$-Antagonist Activity[b]: K_B (95% limits), $\times 10^{-6} M$ Atrium	Uterus
48.**30**	H	CH$_2$	S	7.8 (6.4–9.6)	6.6 (4.9–8.3)
48.**48**	H	CH$_2$	NCN	8.3 (2.0–59)	7.1 (2.9–23)
48.**31**	CH$_3$	S	S	0.92 (0.74–1.15)	0.75 (0.40–1.36)
48.**33**	CH$_3$	S	NCN	0.79 (0.68–0.92)	0.81 (0.54–1.2)
48.**40**	H	S	S	3.2 (2.5–4.5)	3.2 (2.5–4.5)
48.**49**	H	S	NCN	1.4 (0.78–2.7)	1.6 (0.83–3.2)
48.**36**	CH$_3$	CH$_2$	S	8.9 (5.6–15)	10.7 (4.5–31)
48.**50**	CH$_3$	CH$_2$	NCN	8.1 (2.3–69)	4.9 (2.4–12)

[a] Ref. 126b.

[b] Activities determined against histamine stimulation of guinea pig right atrium and rat uterus *in vitro* (R. C. Blakemore and M. E. Parsons, Smith Kline & French Laboratories, Welwyn Garden City, England). The dissociation constant (K_B) was calculated from the equation $K_B = B/(x - 1)$, where x is the respective ratio of concentrations of histamine needed to produce half-maximal responses in the presence and absence of different concentrations (B) of antagonist, and where $-\log K_B = pA_2$.

tagonist potency between metiamide and its urea analog (48.**42**). Another important factor may be the difference in conformational behavior between these groups. NMR studies indicate that the urea 48.**42** exists predominantly as the *Z,Z* conformation (Fig. 48.20, 48.**46c**, X = 0) (55), and it may be that the two conformations 48.**46a** and 48.**46b** analogous to the cyanoguanidine are more active pharmacologically but are energetically unfavorable for the urea (123).

4.6 Impromidine, a Potent H$_2$-Receptor Agonist

A fascinating result was obtained by combining the imidazolylalkyl side chains of the guanidine structures 48.**28** (a weak partial agonist) and 48.**32** (an antagonist) (Table 48.9) into a single guanidine (150). The resulting compound, impromidine (SK & F 92676, 48.**51**) (Fig. 48.22), is a very potent and selective H$_2$-receptor agonist, being nearly 50 times more potent than histamine on the guinea pig atrium preparation and achieving the same maximum response as histamine (Table 48.19). Impromidine is not as active on the rat uterus preparation (nine times more potent than histamine) and it behaves as a partial agonist, achieving only 80% of histamine's maximal response; this indicates that the increase in potency relative to histamine is due to increased affinity for H$_2$ receptors rather than to increased efficacy. The activity of impromidine has important implications in

Table 48.15   Comparison of Thiourea, Urea, Cyanoguanidine, and Nitroguanidine

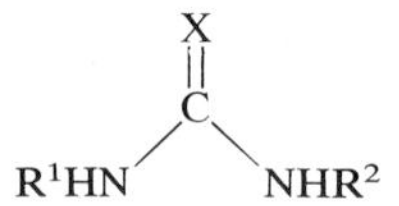

$$\underset{R^1HN \qquad NHR^2}{\overset{\overset{\textstyle X}{\|}}{C}}$$

R^1 = R^2 = H	Y = S	Y = O	Y = NCN	Y = NNO
Geometry: C—N bond length (A°)	1.34[a]	1.35[b], 1.34[c]	1.34[d], 1.32[e]	1.34[f]
N—C—N bond angle (°)	119[a]	117[b], 118[c]	124[d], 120[e]	118[f]
Basicity (pK_a); proton gained at 25°C	−1.2[g]	−0.15[h]	−0.4[i]	−0.9[j]
Acidity: proton lost at 25°C	15[k]	13.7[l]	14[m]	12.8[n]
Hydrophilicity: $P = C_{oct}/C_{H_2O}$ at 37°C	0.09[p]	0.02[p]	0.07[p]	0.13[p]
Dipole moment, μ dioxane (D)	4.89[q] (25°)	4.56[q] (25°)	8.16[r] (35°)	6.95[s] (30°)
R^1 = R^2 = CH$_3$				
Partition, P (oct–H$_2$O) 37°C	0.58[p]	~0.11[p]	0.40[p]	0.20[p]
$\Delta G^{\#}$ for interconversion between conformers (kcal/mol)	11.8[t]	~7.5[t]	12.4[u]	—

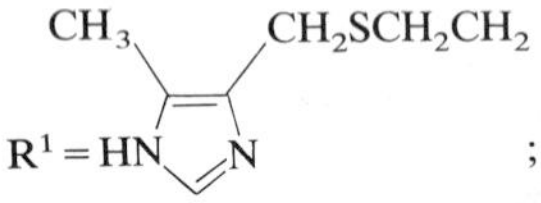

$$R^1 = HN\overset{\displaystyle CH_3 \qquad CH_2SCH_2CH_2}{\underset{N}{\diagup\diagdown}} \quad ; \ R^2 = CH_3$$

Partition, P (oct–H$_2$O) 37°C	3.2[p]	0.87[p]	2.5[p]	1.5[p]

References: [a] 130. [b] 131. [c] 132. [d] 133. [e] 134. [f] 135. [g] 136. [h] 137. [i] 128. [j] 138. [k] 139. [l] 140. [m] 141. [n] 142. [p] 143. [q] 144. [r] 145. [s] 146. [t] 147. [u] 148.

considering drug–receptor interaction, for it appears that a chemical group which contributes affinity in antagonist structures converts a weak partial agonist (48.**28**) into an agent (impromidine) which has increased efficacy as well as increased affinity. Impromidine is also a potent stimulant of gastric acid secretion, having 17–27 times the potency of histamine in rat, cat, and dog preparations, and it is suggested that impromidine may be useful as a diagnostic agent in man for the estimation of the maximal secretory capacity of the stomach (150).

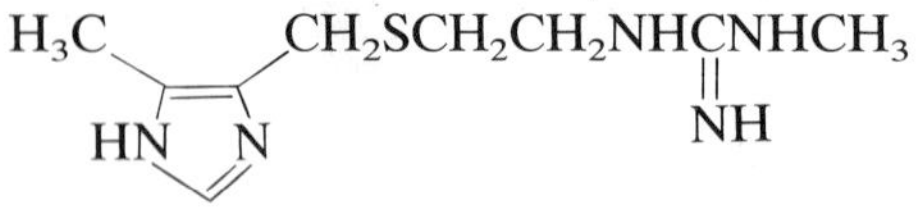

48.**32**   Antagonist 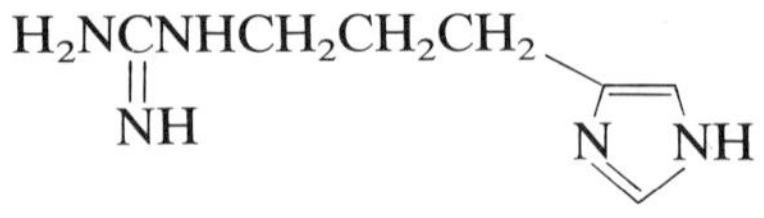   48.**28**   Weak partial agonist

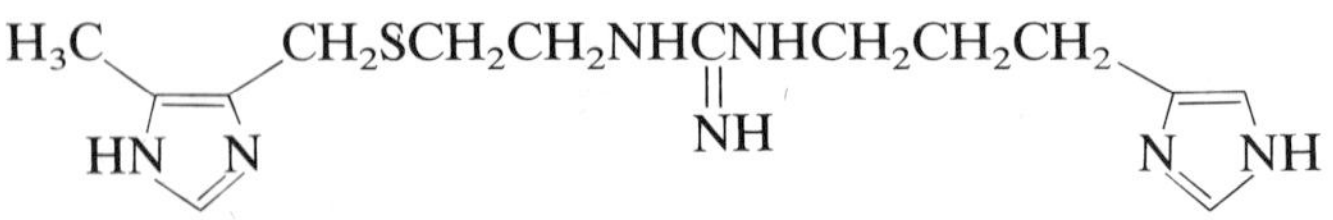

48.**51**   Impromidine, potent H$_2$ agonist

Fig. 48.22   Impromidine (48.**51**) is derived by combining partial structures from the guanidines 48.**28** and 48.**32** (150).

5   CHEMICAL MODE OF ACTION OF H$_2$-RECEPTOR ANTAGONISTS

The discovery of H$_2$-receptor antagonists is very recent and, from the limited studies made so far, it would be premature to draw far-reaching conclusions about structure–activity relationships. Furthermore, the perception of such relationships depends on the manner in which the problem has been viewed and analysed. Current notions about which structural features of these antagonists may be important in determining their activities as drugs have been conditioned by the results obtained during the development of these compounds.

Section 4 traces some of the lines of reasoning that were usefully applied to the development of improved antagonists. Special consideration was given to the chemistry of the imidazole ring, to alternative groups in place of the ammonium group of histamine, and to the length of the alkylene side chain. One should not simply use these observations to prescribe the structural requirements of antagonists, however, because it would imply that there is no other way of constituting active structures. For example, it does not follow that since these antagonists possess an imidazole ring, all active compounds must have imidazole rings; however, one should still consider the corollary that for compounds which incorporate an imidazole ring, the state of the ring and its particular chemistry may influence activity. Likewise one may consider various facets of the chemistry of the groups used in place of ammonium, and the various consequences of altering the side chain.

Pharmacologically, these compounds act as competitive antagonists; the effect is reversible and the antagonists are readily displaced from *in vitro* preparations by changing the bathing fluid; i.e., the compounds are easily washed out. Likewise, *in vivo*, the compounds appear to have a relatively short duration of action. Thus there are no grounds for suggesting that the antagonists act by irreversible binding or by forming covalent bonds. One may presume, therefore, that they form some sort of reversible association complex with the receptors. Using the simple notion of receptor-site occupancy one may seek chemical features common to agonist and its competitive antagonist to suggest chemical binding sites. Thus one may imagine that the imidazole ring of histamine engages the receptor at a specific site, and that the same site is engaged by the imidazole ring of the antagonist. Histamine substituted by a methyl group in the ring 4 position can still function well at H$_2$ receptors, and, likewise, the antagonists can accommodate a 4-methyl group in the imidazole ring without impairment of activity; methylation at other ring positions in histamine drastically reduces agonist activity and, similarly, the other ring-methyl isomers of metiamide are much less active as antagonists. However, this parallel is only partial: agonist molecules not only engage receptors, they also have to elicit a receptor response; i.e., they must possess "efficacy" or "intrinsic activity." By contrast, the antagonist merely has to "occupy" the receptors; it does not elicit a response. Thus one finds that certain heterocyclic analogs of histamine are only weakly active as H$_2$-receptor agonists (79), but such heterocyclic analogs of burimamide, metiamide, or cimetidine may be active as H$_2$-receptor antagonists (151). These observations are not contradictory to the initial suggestion that the imidazole ring of the antagonist specifically engages the receptor, but they imply that only some of the chemical properties of imidazole need be possessed by the antagonist ring.

If the antagonist ring engages the receptor at the site that would otherwise accommodate the imidazole ring of histamine, then one may envisage that the rest of the antagonist molecule contributes additional binding by interacting with some accessory region. The molecular structure of the antagonists appears to be quite critical for activity. Activity is markedly affected by altering the length of the side chain, suggesting a cooperative effect between active groups, and one may consider that the thioureido or guanidino groups make specific contributions to binding. There are various ways in which these groups may be involved but it is not yet possible to do more than speculate. For example, these groups may interact with a specific molecular site through hydrogen bonding, or by acting as electron-pair donors in metal complexation (e.g., see references cited in Refs. 152 and 153 for complexation by thiourea in solution); or, since these groups are both highly polarizable and planar, it is possible that they participate in a "stacking interaction" of the type proposed for nucleotide bases (154, 155).

Since burimamide, metiamide, and cimetidine are hydrophilic molecules, it is likely that hydrophobic binding does not make a major contribution to drug–receptor association; this contrasts with many other receptor antagonists, e.g., α- and β-adrenergic blocking agents, anticholinergics, and H₁-receptor antihistamines, which incorporate lipophilic substituents and in which hydrophobic binding

is believed to be of prime importance to drug action (cf. 99).

The importance of chain length in the antagonists raises the question of whether certain conformations may be associated with antagonist activity. The overall molecular conformation of the antagonist molecules is determined by the alkane side chain. Studies of metiamide and cimetidine in CD₃OD solution by NMR spectroscopy indicate that the ethane grouping (—CH₂CH₂—) in the side chain is probably a statistical mixture of gauche and trans-forms (cf. Figs. 48.23, 48.24); i.e., in methanolic solution about 33% of the metiamide molecules assume the trans conformation at any given instant (55). The conformation of the thiourea group was discussed in Section 4.4 (see Fig. 48.20). Infrared spectroscopic studies of solutions in bromoform indicate that mixtures of inter- and intramolecularly hydrogen-bonded species are formed (143). With the thiourea derivatives the intramolecular interaction involves a thiourea NH group and the imidazole basic nitrogen atom, hydrogen bonded in a ring. Examination of Corey-Pauling-Koltun (CPK) space-filling molecular models indicates that two

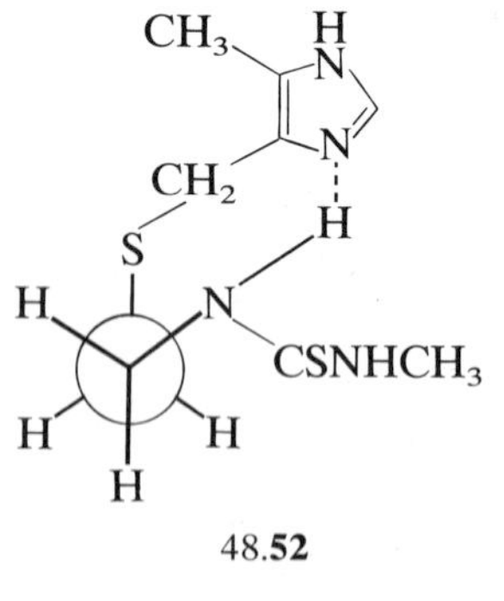

| 48.**52** | 48.**53a** | 48.**53b** |

Eight-membered ring, —CH₂CH₂— gauche, imidazole in N$^\tau$—H tautomer, thiourea group not constrained

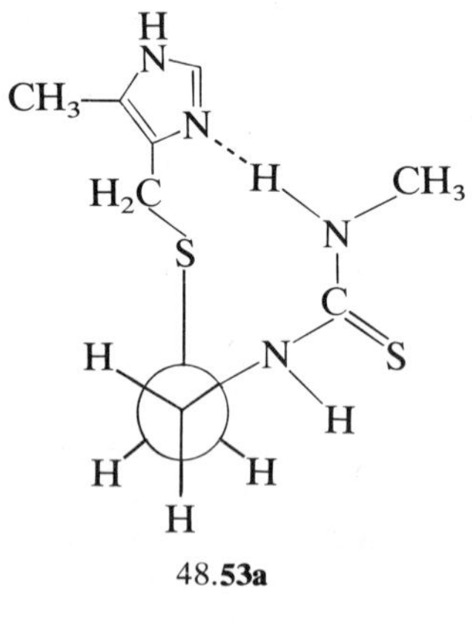

Ten-membered ring, —CH₂CH₂— gauche, imidazole in N$^\tau$—H tautomer, thiourea group in E,Z configuration

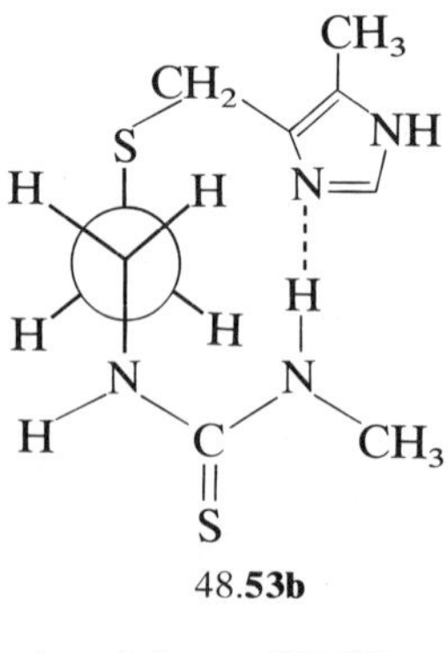

Ten-membered ring, —CH₂CH₂— trans, imidazole in N$^\tau$—H tautomer, thiourea group in E,Z configuration, as found in the crystal (158)

Fig. 48.23 Intramolecular hydrogen-bonded structures of metiamide (viewed as Newman projection formulas along CH₂CH₂ bond).

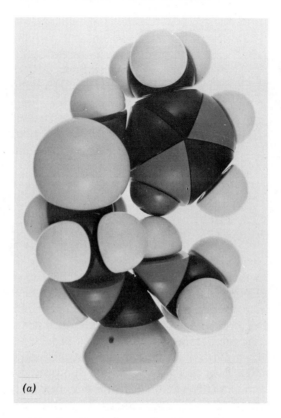

(a)

Fig. 48.24   CPK model of single molecule of metiamide as found in the crystal (158).

sizes of rings are possible, containing 8 or 10 atoms. With metiamide, the 8-membered ring (48.**52**) involves a gauche conformation about the —CH$_2$CH$_2$— bond (Fig. 48.23), but it does not restrict the thiourea configuration. The 10-membered ring, however, requires an *E,Z* configuration for the thiourea group (see Ref. 156 for definition of *E,Z*) but can accommodate either gauche (48.**53a**) or trans (48.**53b**) conformations about the —CH$_2$CH$_2$— bond. Similar considerations apply to the overall conformation of cimetidine, except that of necessity the cyanoguanidine group assumes an *E,Z* configuration.

The structure of these antagonists has been studied by crystallography. In burimamide (157), the molecules are linked together by a complex network of hydrogen bonds between the imidazole rings (NH $\cdots$ N), and between the thiourea residues (NH $\cdots$ S), but there are no thiourea–imidazole contacts. The alkyl chain is extended and approximately planar, and the thiourea group is in the staggered *E,Z* form (Figs. 48.25, 48.26). The crystal structures of metiamide and thiaburimamide (158) differ from that of burimamide; the molecules are not extended (as in burimamide) but are folded and there is an intramolecular NH $\cdots$ N hydrogen bond from a thiourea NH to the imidazole N$^\pi$ atom, forming a 10-membered ring in which the —CH$_2$CH$_2$— bond has the trans conformation (48.**53b**) in Fig. 48.23). The thiourea groups are in the staggered *E,Z* configuration, the same one as is found in crystalline burimamide, and form hydrogen-bonded pairs linked through N—H $\cdots$ S bonds.

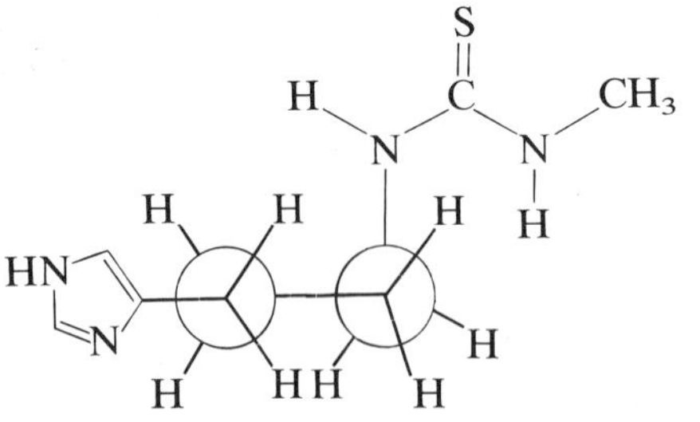

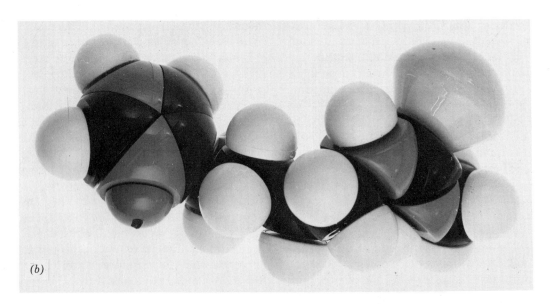

Fig. 48.25 Structure of single molecule of burimamide (157), ahowing imidazole in N$^\tau$—H tautomer; (CH$_2$)$_4$ groups in, respectively, trans, trans and half-gauche conformations; and thiourea group in *E,Z* configuration.

The molecular conformation of cimetidine is very similar to that adopted by metiamide and thiaburimamide, and a 10-membered ring is formed by an intramolecular NH $\cdots$ N hydrogen bond from a cyanoguanidine NH to the imidazole N$^\pi$ atom (159) (Figs. 48.27, 48.28). Indeed, the crystal structure is notable for its close similarity to that of metiamide. The cyanoguanidine groups are in an *E,Z* configuration and the lone electron pair on the imino nitrogen functions in the structure to form a N—H $\cdots$ N hydrogen bond between pairs of cyanoguanidine groups, thus giving rise to a 12-membered ring system. This closely resembles the 8-membered rings formed between pairs of thiourea groups in metiamide. These results provide further evidence for isosterism between the thiourea and cyanoguanidine groups.

An interesting relationship between the crystal structure and crystal stability has been demonstrated (158) for these compounds, stability being correlated with increasing melting point and reduced aqueous solubility (Table 48.16).

Replacement of CH$_2$ by S in burimamide was made initially as an "isosteric" substitution which would modify the electronic properties of the side chain; however, it was pointed out that the replacement may slightly lengthen the chain and increase conformational flexibility (105). The crystal structures provide evidence for the formation of a cyclic intramolecularly hydrogen-bonded conformation in these compounds with a thioether side chain. It is interesting that a 10-membered ring should form, and one must consider that this may contribute to the greater activity of these molecules. It is not known whether the molecule has to

Fig. 48.26 CPK model of single molecule of burimamide as found in the crystal (157).

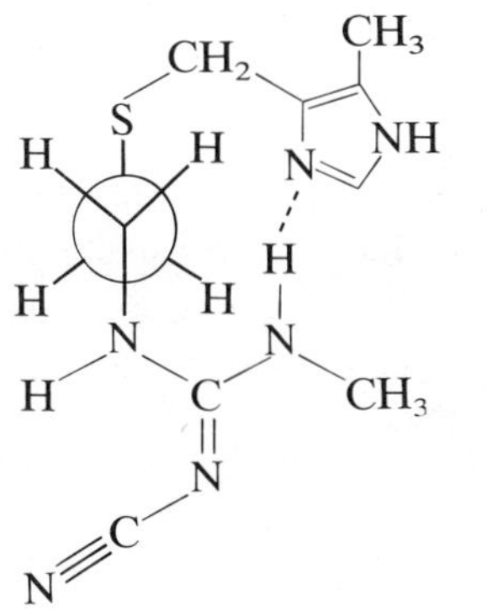

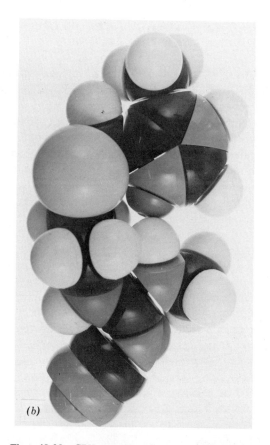

Fig. 48.27 Structure of single molecule of cimetidine (159), showing 10-membered ring, —CH_2CH_2— trans, imidazole in N^τ—H tautomer, and cyanoguanidine group in E,Z configuration.

achieve this configuration in order to be biologically active, or whether the thioether link simply functions to increase molecular flexibility in a way that is biologically advantageous. Thus, in addition to the electronic effects, it is possible that conformational effects of the thioether linkage also contribute to the activity of these compounds as histamine antagonists.

(b)

Fig. 48.28 CPK model of single molecule of cimetidine as found in the crystal (159).

Table 48.16   Physical Characteristics of Crystalline Burimamide, Metiamide, Cimetidine, and Related Compounds (158)

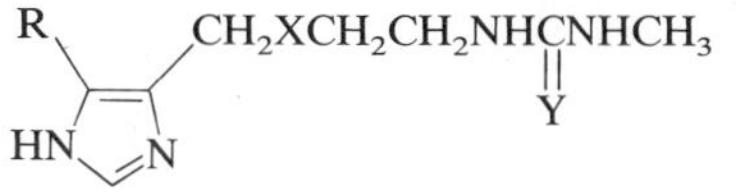

$$\underset{HN \diagdown N}{\overset{R}{\diagup}} CH_2XCH_2CH_2NHCNHCH_3 \quad \overset{||}{Y}$$

Compound	R	X	Y	M.p., °C	Intra-molecular Hydrogen Bonding	Aqueous Solubility g/1	M
Metiamide	CH_3	S	S	150–152	Yes	3.2	0.013
Cimetidine	CH_3	S	NCN	141–142	Yes	11.4	0.045
Burimamide	H	CH_2	S	129–130	No	14.7	0.069
Methylburimamide	CH_3	CH_2	S	110–112	No[a]	25.4	0.112
Thiaburimamide	H	S	S	96–98	Yes	70.4	0.306

[a] The absence of intramolecular hydrogen bonding is inferred from the solid state infrared spectrum for methylburimamide (158).

6 PHARMACOLOGICAL PROPERTIES OF H$_2$-RECEPTOR ANTAGONISTS

Pharmacological properties are reviewed in this section by first outlining the pharmacological criteria which may be used for defining an H$_2$-receptor antagonist. These criteria derive mainly from dose–response relationships on tissue preparations *in vitro*. Pharmacological studies *in vivo* are prefaced by a brief description of the pharmacokinetics and bioavailability of H$_2$-receptor antagonists. Stimulation of gastric acid secretion is the most clearly defined phenomenon of physiological importance that is known to involve histamine H$_2$ receptors, and studies in animals are reviewed, followed by a summary of clinical findings and therapeutic applications of H$_2$-receptor antagonists. The possible involvement of gastric adenyl cyclase in H$_2$-receptor-mediated stimulation of gastric acid secretion and possible relationships between H$_2$-receptor blockade and effects on histamine formation, catabolism, and uptake are reviewed briefly. Some pharmacological properties of H$_2$-receptor antagonists that are not entirely explained on the basis of H$_2$-receptor blockade are also outlined.

6.1 Pharmacological Characterization of H$_2$-Receptor Antagonists

The selective blockade of the actions of histamine in increasing atrial rate and inhibiting evoked contractions in the rat uterus *in vitro* led to the definition of burimamide as a histamine H$_2$-receptor antagonist in 1972 by Black and co-workers (35) (see Section 4.2). Burimamide produces a dose-related parallel displacement of cumulative histamine dose–response curves on atrium and uterus without affecting their slopes or maxima (Fig. 48.29), for both tissues the regression of log(histamine dose ratio −1) on log-(antagonist concentration) i.e., Schild plot (20), is linear with a slope not significantly different from unity (Fig. 48.30). These results allow the definition of burimamide as a competitive histamine H$_2$-receptor antagonist. The calculated dissociation constants (K_B) for the putative drug receptor complex (Table 48.12) are not significantly different between the two tissues, thereby also defining the homogeneity of the two receptor populations. Additional evidence for H$_2$-receptor antagonism by burimamide was obtained using 2-methyl- and 4-methylhistamines as agonists. Although

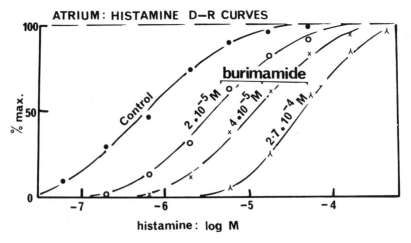

Fig. 48.29 Histamine cumulative log dose–response curves from a guinea pig atrium, without antagonist and after equilibration with increasing concentrations of burimamide (35).

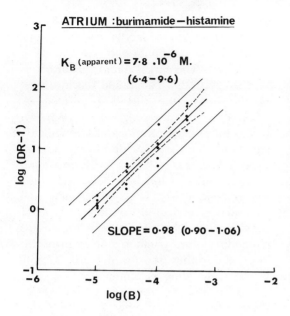

ATRIUM :burimamide—histamine

K_B (apparent) = 7·8 .10^{-6} M.

(6·4 – 9·6)

SLOPE = 0·98 (0·90 – 1·06)

Fig. 48.30 Antagonism of histamine by burimamide on guinea pig atrium. Antagonism is expressed by histamine dose ratios (DR) needed for equal responses before and after burimamide (B) equilibration. For competitive inhibition $\log(DR-1) = \log(B) - \log K_B$, where K_B = (apparent) dissociation constant for antagonist–receptor interaction (35).

of the antagonist should be independent of the equilibrium constant of the agonist that has been used (20). The specificity of the antagonism is illustrated by the weak activity of burimamide on atrium or uterus against isoproterenol (catecholamine β receptors), or against carbachol (cholinergic muscarinic receptors) and histamine (H$_1$ receptors) on guinea pig ileum (35). Subsequently, metiamide (121, 160, 161) and cimetidine (126c, 162) were also shown to meet the criteria for specific competitive antagonism of histamine H$_2$ receptors (See Sections 4.3 and 4.4). The estimated K_B values indicate that metiamide and cimetidine are nearly 10 times more active than burimamide as H$_2$-receptor antagonists (Table 48.14). The specificity of cimetidine as an H$_2$-receptor antagonist is indicated in Table 48.17.

6.2   Pharmacokinetics of H$_2$-Receptor Antagonists

An understanding of the action of a drug in a whole animal situation is assisted by knowledge of its bioavailability and pharmacokinetic behavior. Since this in turn is assisted by an appreciation of the physical properties of the drug molecule, it is worth emphasizing that each of the H$_2$-receptor antagonists, burimamide, metiamide, and cimetidine, are polar and hydrophilic molecules. They have low parti-

these histamine analogs have widely different potencies on guinea pig atrium, the estimated K_B values for burimamide were not significantly different from those obtained using histamine as agonist (35). These results are consistent with burimamide acting as a competitive antagonist since on theoretical grounds the K_B value

Table 48.17   The Antagonist Activity of Cimetidine *in Vitro* (126c, 162)

Tissue	Agonist	Apparent Dissociation Constant (K_B) $\times 10^{-7}$ M with 95% Confidence Limits	Slopes of $\log(DR-1)$ vs. $\log(B)$
Atrium	Histamine	7.9 (6.8–9.2)	0.81(0.62–1.00)
	Isoprenaline	1330 (410–6200)	1.44 (1.17–1.71)
Uterus	Histamine	8.1 (5.4–12.1)	0.96(0.82–1.10)
	Isoprenaline	2620 (121–31110)	0.61 (0.39–0.82)
Ileum	Histamine	4460 (2020–10700)	1.47 (1.34–1.60)
	Carbachol	360 (208–658)	0.79 (0.72–0.86)

tion coefficients and contain a basic imidazole ring (p$K_a \simeq 7$) that exists largely in a protonated form in an acidic environment. Both metiamide and cimetidine are well absorbed in all species studied (rat, dog, and man) when administered orally (163, 164). Griffiths et al. (164) report that the bioavailability of an oral dose of cimetidine is at least 70% that of an intravenous dose. Studies using intestinal segments of rats suggest that absorption of cimetidine is most rapid from the ileum and duodenum (164). For both metiamide and cimetidine, a substantial proportion of drug is excreted in the urine unchanged (164–166). A main metabolite for each compound is the respective thioether monosulfoxide, and the ring hydroxymethyl compound (48.**55**) has also been identified as a minor metabolite of cimetidine. The guanylurea (48.**47**) has been detected in the urine from cimetidine-treated animals but is probably formed nonenzymatically by acid hydrolysis. The structures of identified metabolites of cimetidine are shown in Fig. 48.31. The production of the sulfoxide metabolite (48.**54**) in human subjects was found to be independent of the dose or route of administration of labeled cimetidine and accounted for about 10% of the radioactivity eliminated in the urine (164). The plasma protein binding of burimamide, metiamide, and ci-

metidine, is insignificant (163, 164). A two-compartment kinetic model has been proposed for the distribution of cimetidine in man (164). The large volume of distribution suggests that cimetidine reaches most of the body, and this is confirmed by whole-body autoradiography (WBAR) (167). From considerations of lipophilicity, cimetidine and metiamide would not be expected to easily cross the blood–brain barrier, and this has also been confirmed by WBAR (167, 168). Metiamide and cimetidine are cleared from the body quite rapidly with a half-life of elimination for cimetidine of just under 2 hr in man and dogs and rather shorter (53 min) in rats (164). Cimetidine is eliminated from the blood mainly by the kidney. However, there is evidence that other routes of excretion are available and may become important in cases of renal impairment (164). Differences between cimetidine and metiamide have been observed in studies of the retention of these drugs in a variety of cells in bone marrow smears from rats which have been injected with these substances. Whereas the radioisotope from ^{3}H-metiamide, like that from ^{35}S-thiourea, was retained, particularly in the basophils, there was no uptake of radioisotope into bone marrow cells after injection of ^{3}H-cimetidine (168).

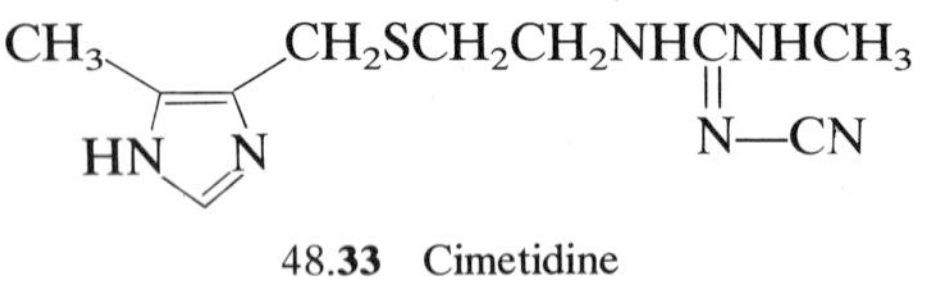

CH$_3$ CH$_2$SCH$_2$CH$_2$NHCNHCH$_3$
HN   N   N—CN

48.**33**   Cimetidine

HOCH$_2$ CH$_2$SCH$_2$CH$_2$NHCNHCH$_3$
HN   N   N—CN

48.**55**   5-Hydroxymethyl derivative of cimetidine

O
↑
CH$_3$ CH$_2$SCH$_2$CH$_2$NHCNHCH$_3$
HN   N   N—CN

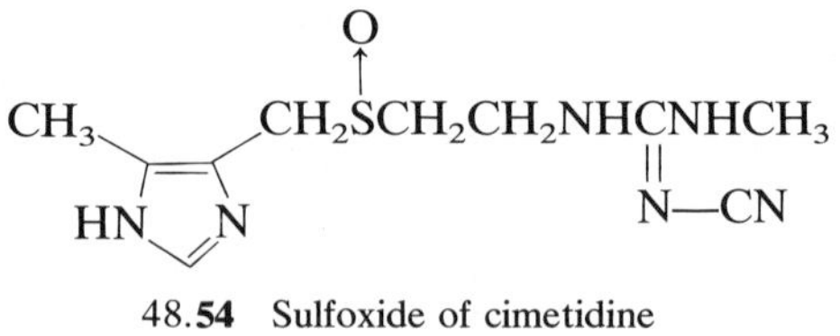

48.**54**   Sulfoxide of cimetidine

CH$_3$ CH$_2$SCH$_2$CH$_2$NHCNHCH$_3$
HN   N   NCONH$_2$

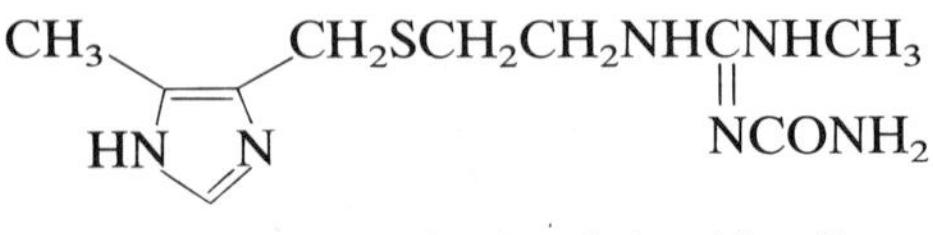

48.**47**   Guanylurea derivative of cimetidine (formed nonenzymatically)

Fig. 48.31   Cimetidine and possible metabolites (164).

6.3   H$_2$-Receptor Antagonists and Mammalian Gastric Acid Secretion

6.3.1 ACTIONS IN ANIMALS. Burimamide, metiamide, and cimetidine inhibit gastric acid secretion, stimulated by histamine, in all preparations and species studied (35, 121, 126c, 160, 161). That the inhibition of gastric acid secretion is competitive and surmountable is evident from experiments in which the antagonists given by intravenous infusion cause a parallel displacement of the dose–response curves for histamine in stimulating gastric acid secretion in the lumen perfused rat preparation and the Heidenhain pouch dog. Using labeled burimamide and metiamide regressions were calculated between log(plasma concentration of drug) and log(dose ratio -1) to provide data homologous to that obtained *in vitro* (35, 160). The slope of the regressions were not significantly different from unity and the calculated apparent dissociation constants for burimamide and metiamide were not significantly different from those estimated on isolated preparations. The dose that produces 50% reduction in stimulated gastric acid secretion (ID$_{50}$) in the anesthetized rat for burimamide, metiamide, cimetidine, and other H$_2$-receptor antagonists correlate well with *in vitro* data when expressed as a plot of atrial or uterine pA$_2$ against $-\log(ID_{50})$ for gastric secretory inhibition (35, 160, 162). Additionally, using lumen perfused rat stomachs *in vitro*, it has been shown that metiamide causes parallel displacement of dose–response curves to histamine with dose ratios not significantly different from those obtained on guinea pig atria and rat uterus (169). Thus there is a reasonable body of experimental evidence to support the view that burimamide, metiamide, and cimetidine inhibit histamine-stimulated gastric acid secretion by competitive antagonism of H$_2$ receptors in the gastric mucosa. The inhibition by cimetidine of gastric acid secretion stimulated by histamine in the rat is illustrated in Fig. 48.32.

Histamine H$_2$-receptor antagonists also inhibit the secretion of gastric acid stimulated by pentagastrin with ID$_{50}$ values similar to those for inhibition of histamine (35, 121, 126c). Significant inhibitory effects are also exerted by metiamide and cimetidine against cholinergically stimulated secretion, although higher concentrations are required than for comparable inhibition of histamine- or pentagastrin-stimulated secretion. Results with H$_2$-receptor antagonists against various other stimulants of gastric secretion and against basal secretion have been reviewed by Parsons (170). Findings with H$_2$-receptor antagonists have led to much discussion and speculation concerning the receptors involved in the physiological control of gastric acid secretion (171–173). The hypothesis, propounded by Code (174), that histamine is the final common mediator for all forms of stimulation of gastric acid secretion has been reviewed (170) in the light of evidence provided by H$_2$-receptor antagonists.

6.3.2 ACTIONS IN MAN. Burimamide was the first H$_2$-receptor antagonist to be studied in man (175). In healthy human subjects, inhibition of maximally stimulated gastric acid secretion by burimamide was far more impressive than inhibition by anticholinergic drugs, and it was estimated that an intravenous infusion of burimamide produced 50% inhibition of histamine- or pentagastrin-stimulated acid secretion at an average burimamide plasma concentration (IC$_{50}$) of 15.3 μM, in agreement with estimates made in other species (35). Subsequently, metiamide was found to be more effective than burimamide as an inhibitor of histamine- or pentagastrin-stimulated acid secretion in healthy man with an average IC$_{50}$ of 3.3 μM (176). Of particular interest was the finding of good oral absorption

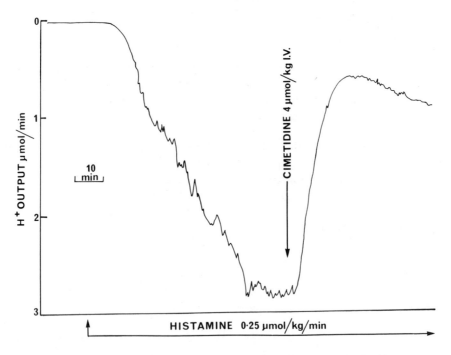

Fig. 48.32   The inhibitory effect of a single injection of cimetidine on the near maximal acid secretory response to an intravenous infusion of histamine, using the lumen perfused stomach of the anesthetized rat (162).

with metiamide and its effectiveness as an inhibitor of gastric acid secretion when given by mouth. Metiamide was subsequently investigated in the treatment of clinical conditions, known collectively as peptic ulceration, that are associated with gastric acid hypersecretion.

Peptic ulcers are often classified by their site of occurrence, i.e., gastric, duodenal, or lower esophageal, of which duodenal ulcers are the most common. Although the precise etiology of gastric and duodenal ulceration is unknown, secretion of acid and pepsin appear to play an important role in ulcer formation (177, 178). Hypersecretion is usually observed in patients with duodenal ulceration, although not in patients with gastric ulcers. The involvement of gastric acid in the formation or aggravation of gastric and duodenal ulcers is reflected in the existing drugs used in their treatment, which are intended to neutralize acid, to

reduce its rate of secretion (anticholinergic agents), or to protect the gastric mucosa from its damaging effects (178).

Metiamide was shown to inhibit both histamine- and pentagastrin-stimulated secretion of acid in patients with duodenal ulcer (179, 180). and was also shown to inhibit vagally stimulated gastric secretion (181), nocturnal acid secretion (182), and basal and meal-stimulated secretion (183, 184). Clinically, metiamide gives marked symptomatic relief to patients suffering from peptic ulcer, (185) and healing of recalcitrant multiple ulcers has been reported following treatment with metiamide (179, 186). In a multi center double-blind trial (187) in patients with endoscopically confirmed duodenal ulceration, healing of ulcers was significantly increased in patients receiving metiamide compared with those on placebo. The only side effects that were reported in trials with metiamide were five cases of readily reversible granulocytopenia (188, 189). It is noteworthy that in chronic toxicity tests at doses of metiamide at least 20 times the effective dose in the dog, some animals developed kidney damage and agranulocytosis (190). Clinical trials with metiamide were consequently limited to more seriously ill patients.

Since the induction of agranulocytosis was considered to be associated with the thiourea group in metiamide, clinical studies were pursued with the non-thiourea H$_2$-receptor antagonist cimetidine, which did not show any signs of hematopoietic toxicity in chronic tests in animals (126c, 191). Initial studies in healthy human subjects confirmed previous studies in animals that, both qualitatively and quantitatively, the pharmacological properties of cimetidine and metiamide are similar. However, cimetidine may be slightly more potent than metiamide in man (EC$_{50} \simeq 2 \mu$M) (192). Extensive clinical studies have been conducted with cimetidine, and its therapeutic effectiveness has been demonstrated in the treatment of peptic ulcer and associated gastrointestinal disorders. Thus in both open and controlled clinical trials in patients with endoscopically diagnosed duodenal ulcers, cimetidine has been shown to produce rapid ulcer healing and symptomatic relief (193, 194). Results of additional clinical studies including a double-blind multicenter trial of cimetidine in the treatment of duodenal ulcer were reported at a symposium (195–198). Cimetidine has also been investigated in the treatment of gastric ulcer (199, 200) and peptic esophagitis (201). In the treatment of a particularly severe and rare form of hypersecretory disease, Zollinger–Ellison syndrome, patients who had been constantly secreting many times their normal amount of acid were returned to normal within 24–48 hr (202). Both metiamide and cimetidine have been shown to be effective in the treatment of gastrointestinal hemor-

rhage in patients with fulminant hepatic failure, severe hepatitis, and cirrhosis (203, 204). It has been suggested that cimetidine may have an important role in the prophylaxis and treatment of bleeding in patients with liver disease (204). No cases of agranulocytosis or any other unacceptable side effects have been reported in clinical studies with cimetidine. Cimetidine was introduced into clinical practice in the United Kingdom in late 1976.

6.4 H$_2$ Receptors and Gastric Mucosal Cyclic AMP

It is now widely accepted that cyclic adenosine 3′,5′-monophosphate (cyclic AMP) serves as an intracellular "second messenger" mediating the actions of a number of hormones including histamine (205a). In recent years there has been increasing evidence for the hypothesis that histamine stimulates gastric acid secretion by increasing the intracellular cyclic AMP levels in the gastric mucosa (205b). The discovery of the specific H$_2$-receptor antagonists burimamide and metiamide has provided powerful tools for further study of the involvement of cyclic AMP in histamine-stimulated gastric acid secretion, and several groups of workers have reported that burimamide and metiamide competitively inhibit histamine-stimulated adenylate cyclase from gastric mucosa (205–208). Scholes and co-workers (209) have reported that burimamide and metiamide competitively inhibited histamine-stimulated cyclic AMP formation in cells from dog gastric mucosa with apparent K_B values very similar to values found by Black and co-workers on guinea pig atrium and rat uterus. The relative activities of 2- and 4-methylhistamines in elevating cyclic AMP in these cells is similar to their relative activities on guinea pig atrium, rat uterus, and rat gastric secretion. Furthermore, the H$_1$-receptor antagonist mepyramine does not inhibit cyclic AMP formation in this preparation. This work adds to the considerable body of evidence that the histamine receptor, the H_2 receptor, involved in the stimulation of gastric acid is linked to an adenylate cyclase system and that cyclic AMP may act as an intracellular mediator of the action of histamine on the parietal cells of gastric mucosa. There is also evidence suggesting a link between H_2 receptors and adenylate cyclase systems in the heart and various other tissues (see Section 7).

6.5 Influence of H₂-receptor Antagonists on Histamine Formation, Catabolism, and Uptake

Histamine H_2-receptor antagonists have been studied for their effects on histamine production, catabolism, and uptake since these events can be envisaged as influencing or modulating the inhibitory effects of the antagonist drug on the agonist molecule.

The main pathways of synthesis and catabolism of histamine are shown in Fig. 48.33. The conversion of L-histidine into histamine is catalyzed by a specific L-histidine decarboxylase (EC 4.1.1.22). Both burimamide and metiamide are reported to markedly increase histidine decarboxylase activity in the glandular stomach of rats (210). Other inhibitors of acid secretion are also known to increase histidine decarboxylase activity. It has been suggested by Håkanson et al. (211) that this is a general effect due to the raising of intragastric pH, which results in increased circulating levels of gastrin and a consequent stimulation of histidine decarboxylase activity. Results with burimamide and metiamide are in accord with this hypothesis (210).

Histamine catabolism was reviewed by Schayer (212) in 1959. Oxidative deamination by diamine oxidase (histaminase, EC 1.4.3.6) or methylation of the imidazole

ring by histamine N-methyltransferase (EC 2.1.1.8) are the main pathways for inactivating histamine. In the gastric mucosa the principal pathway involves histamine N-methyltransferase, the enzyme that catalyzes the transfer of the methyl group of S-adenosylmethionine (SAM) to the N^τ nitrogen atom of histamine (213). This enzyme is competitively inhibited by H_1-receptor antagonists in the presence of histamine concentrations less than $10 \, \mu M$ (214a). The H_2-receptor antagonists, burimamide and metiamide, also inhibit the enzyme (214b, 214c) but there does not appear to be a correlation between enzyme activity and receptor activity (214c). Schayer and Reilly (215) have suggested that burimamide occupies histamine binding sites in some tissues since burimamide modifies the distribution of injected histamine. However metiamide has virtually no effect on the distribution of injected histamine, indicating that this is not an inherent property of H_2-receptor antagonists.

Some H_1- and H_2-receptor antagonists appear to block histamine uptake and metabolism by guinea pig isolated atrium and mouse neoplastic mast cells. However, burimamide ($IC_{50} \, 0.47 \, \mu M$) is much more active than metiamide ($IC_{50} \, 30 \, \mu M$) and H_1-receptor antagonists in inhibiting histamine methylation in guinea pig atria and also in blocking histamine uptake by mast cells ($IC_{50} \, 1.8 \, \mu M$ for burimamide and $28 \, \mu M$ for metiamide). These effects clearly do not correlate with H_2-receptor antagonist potency, and it is suggested that they are related to inhibition of histamine-methylating enzymes or competition at binding sites for histamine uptake (216).

6.6 Catecholamine Release and α-Adrenoreceptor Blockade

Some differences have been noted between certain pharmacological effects of the H_2-receptor antagonists burimamide and meti-

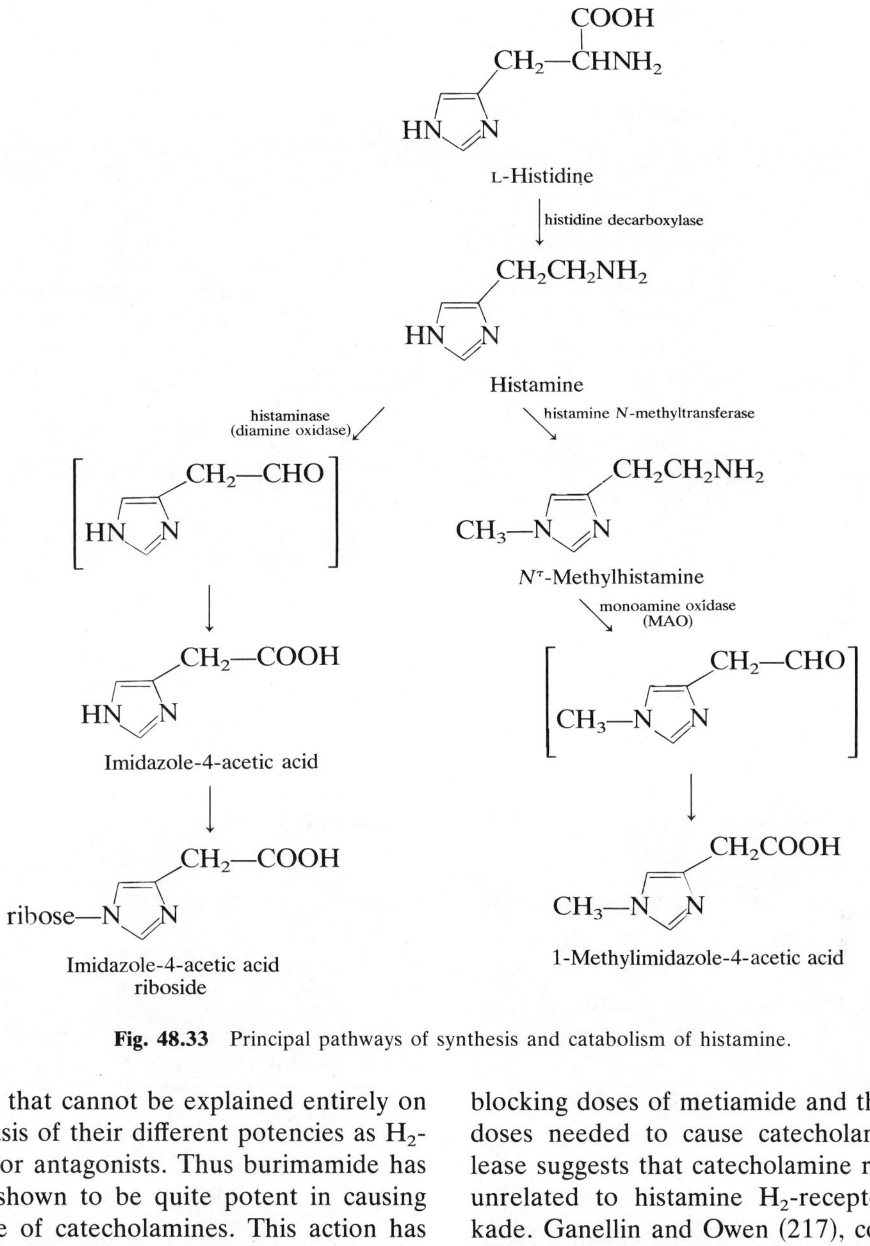

Fig. 48.33   Principal pathways of synthesis and catabolism of histamine.

amide that cannot be explained entirely on the basis of their different potencies as H$_2$-receptor antagonists. Thus burimamide has been shown to be quite potent in causing release of catecholamines. This action has been demonstrated using the chronically denervated nictitating membrane of the cat, where burimamide causes contractions that may be abolished by pretreatment with the α-adrenoreceptor blocking drug phentolamine and reduced by adrenalectomy (161). Metiamide is much less active than burimamide in causing catecholamine release in this preparation, and the separation between effective histamine H$_2$-receptor

blocking doses of metiamide and the larger doses needed to cause catecholamine release suggests that catecholamine release is unrelated to histamine H$_2$-receptor blockade. Ganellin and Owen (217), compared catecholamine release in rats caused by burimamide, metiamide, and two close chemical analogs, methylburimamide and thiaburimamide. Although differences are less marked than in the cat, the results (Table 48.18) show a clear trend in relating catecholamine release to ring pK_a; i.e., catecholamine release increases with increasing pK_a. The pK_a differences mean that 70% of methylburimamide (which is

Table 48.18   Structures, Pressor Activities, H$_2$-Receptor Antagonist Activities (pA$_2$), Ionization Constants (pK$_a$), Mole Fractions of Imidazolium Cation (n_c), and Octanol–Water Partition Coefficients (P) of Four Histamine H$_2$-Receptor Antagonists (217)

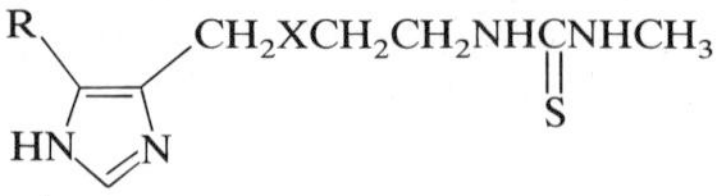

$$\underset{HN \diagdown N}{R \diagdown} \begin{array}{c} CH_2XCH_2CH_2NHCNHCH_3 \\ \| \\ S \end{array}$$

	Methylburimamide, R = CH$_3$, X = CH$_2$	Burimamide, R = H, X = CH$_2$	Metiamide, R = CH$_3$, X = S	Thiaburimamide, R = H, X = S
Pressor Responses, mm Hg ± S.E. Mean				
10 μm/kg	7.2 ± 1.5	7.4 ± 2.0	5.5 ± 1.3	3.4 ± 1.8
20 μm/kg	13.7 ± 1.6	10.0 ± 2.0	6.8 ± 1.4	3.4 ± 0.8
40 μm/kg	19.8 ± 3.6	15.8 ± 1.2	9.2 ± 1.5	4.8 ± 1.8
80 μm/kg	25.7 ± 3.8	20.7 ± 4.9	19.5 ± 4.4	7.6 ± 1.9
pA$_2$ (atrial histamine H$_2$ receptors)[a]	5.03	5.11	6.03	5.49
pK$_a$ at 37°C[a]	7.8	7.25	6.8	6.25
n_c at pH 7.4[a]	0.72	0.40	0.20	0.07
$P = \dfrac{C_{octanol}}{C_{aq.buffer}}$[b]	7.1	2.5	3.2	1.4

[a] Ref. 105.
[b] Partition at 37°C between 1-octanol and aqueous buffer at pH 9.2.

most active at releasing catecholamines) would be protonated at pH 7.4, whereas for thiaburimamide only 7% of molecules would be protonated. Burimamide (40%) and metiamide (20%) are intermediate. It seems likely, therefore, that it is the cationic forms of these histamine H$_2$-receptor antagonists that act to release catecholamines.

Another property of burimamide that is not shared by metiamide is its α-adrenoreceptor blocking activity. This can be shown in the anesthetized cat where burimamide antagonizes the pressor response to norepinephrine and *in vitro* where, using the rat seminal vesicle preparation, a pA$_2$ value for burimamide against epinephrine was measured as 4.7 (161). It was not possible to demonstrate α-blockade with metiamide.

7   HISTAMINE RECEPTOR CLASSIFICATION OF TISSUE SYSTEMS

In the original definition and characterization of histamine H$_1$ and H$_2$ receptors (22, 35; Sections 1 and 6.1), mepyramine-sensitive H$_1$ receptors were identified in the actions of histamine in stimulating contractions of smooth muscle from organs such as gut and bronchi, while mepyramine-refractory, burimamide-sensitive H$_2$ receptors were identified in histamine-stimulated tachycardia of isolated guinea pig atria, in the inhibition by histamine of evoked contractions of the isolated rat uterus, and in the action of histamine in stimulating gastric acid secretion. However, histamine exerts many additional biological actions in various tissues and the availability of selective H_1- and H_2-receptor agonists and antagonists has provided valuable tools for analyzing these actions in terms of H_1- or H_2-receptor involvement. The subject of tissue distribution of histamine receptors was reviewed in 1975 by Chand and Eyre (218).

7.1   Compounds Used for Pharmacological Characterization of Histamine Receptors

The respective classes of histamine antagonists (Table 48.19) provide valuable tools for analyzing biological actions of histamine in terms of H_1- or H_2-receptor involvement. In situations where administered histamine gives good dose–response relationships, and these are shifted in a parallel fashion in the presence of a selective antagonist, such that the Schild plot of $\log(DR-1)$ vs. $\log$(concentration of antagonist) has a linear regression of slope not significantly different from unity, the case for inferring receptor involvement is very strong.

There may be instances, however, where analysis is more complex e.g., where both H_1 and H_2 receptors are involved in mediating the response. Under these circumstances the highly selective agonists that are now available may be used to assist in the analysis (Table 48.19). The selective agonists may also be useful in providing additional evidence for the involvement of histamine receptors in cases where quantitative studies on histamine prove to be difficult. Where the antagonists act in an apparently noncompetitive manner, one must also consider whether other mechanisms are interfering; for example, the antagonist might affect histamine distribution (such as access to the receptor, uptake to other tissues, metabolism; see Section 6.5) or it may interfere with the response mechanism e.g., by affecting the transport of metal ions or by altering energy regulating systems.

In cases where histamine is not administered but the possible involvement of endogenous histamine is being investigated, the problems are much greater. Here one must be extremely cautious; if an antagonist interferes with a particular biologic response one should not simply presume that it owes its actions to an antagonism of endogeneous histamine at its receptors, but further evidence should be sought. Although the antagonists are highly selective agents, they are still chemical substances and are therefore potentially able to exert other affects.

Obviously, because a drug (whether antagonist or agonist) acts at a particular population of receptors, it does not follow that all observed effects of the drug are due to receptor interactions. In this sense it may be helpful to use chemical control substances that match many of the chemical properties of the active drugs but that lack the specific structural properties needed for effective receptor interactions. Such compounds are included in Table 48.19, viz., telemethylhistamine for use in conjunction with histamine or 2- or 4-methylhistamines; 4-pyridylethylamine for use in conjunction with the selective H_1-receptor agonist, 2-pyridylethylamine; SK & F 91487 [2-(S-dimethylaminoethyl)isothiourea], "nordimaprit," for use in conjunction with the highly selective H_2-receptor agonist, dimaprit; and SK & F 91581 [N-methyl-N'-[3-(imidazol-4-yl)propyl]thiourea], "norburimamide," for use in conjunction with the H_2-receptor antagonists burimamide or metiamide. Many other control substances may be devised, but the compounds mentioned in Table 48.19 have the merit of being available synthetically. The use of such controls should be considered whenever the analysis of histamine-mediated effects appears to be complex. If, in a particular test system, the active agent and the chemical control are found to be similarly active, one must seriously question whether the effect arises from direct interaction with histamine receptors.

Table 48.19   Compounds used for Pharmacological Characterization of Histamine Receptors

Name	Structure	Activity	H_1 Ileum (95% limits)	H_2 Gastric Stimulation	H_2 Atrium (95% limits)
			Agonist Activity Relative to Histamine = 100[a]		
Histamine	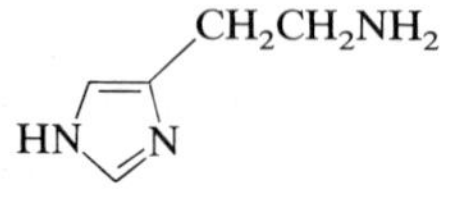	Agonist (H_1 and H_2)	100	100	100
Telemethylhistamine[b]	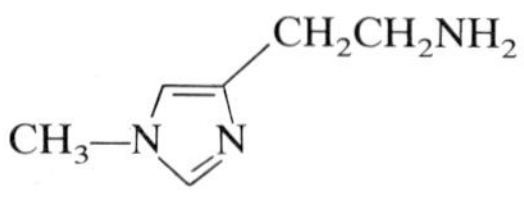	"Inactive" control	~0.5	<0.01	<0.1

H_1-Receptor Selective Agonists

Name	Structure	Activity	H_1 Ileum	H_2 Gastric	H_2 Atrium
2-Methylhistamine[b]	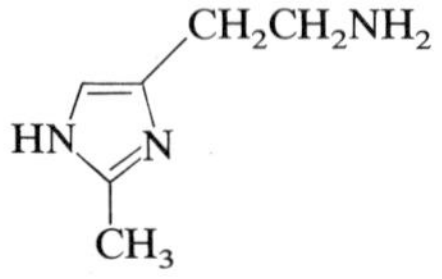	Relatively selective H_1	16.5(15.1–18.1)	2.0	4.4(4.1–4.8)
2-Pyridylethylamine[c]	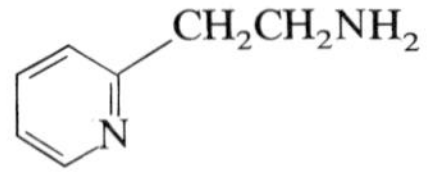	Selective H_1	5.6[d](5.0–6.3)	~0.2[e]	"2.5"[f]
N^α-Methyl-2-pyridylethylamine (Betahistine)[g]	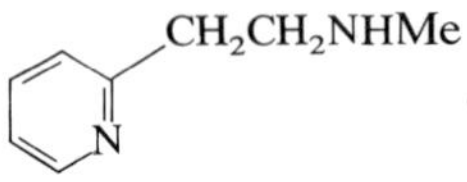	Selective H_1	8.0(7.2–8.8)	~0.2	"1.5"[h]
2-Thiazolylethylamine	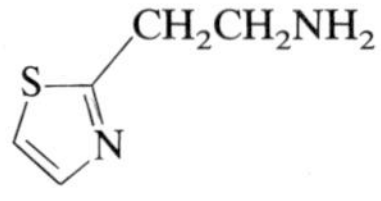	Selective H_1	26[i](20–33)	~0.3	2.2(2.0–2.5)
4-Pyridylethylamine[c]	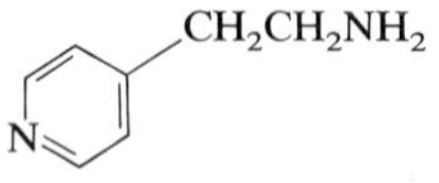	"Inactive" control	<0.001	~0.4	<0.01

H_2-Receptor Selective Agonists

Name	Structure	Activity	H_1 Ileum	H_2 Gastric	H_2 Atrium
4-Methylhistamine[b]	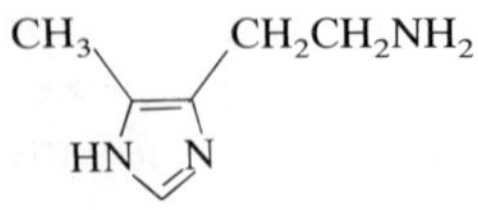	Relatively selective H_2	0.23(0.20–0.27)	39	43(40–46)

Table 48.19   (*Continued*)

Name	Structure	Activity	Agonist Activity Relative to Histamine = 100^a		
			H_1	H_2	
			Ileum (95% limits)	Gastric Stimulation	Atrium (95% limits)
3-Pyrazolylethylamine (Betazole)^j	CH$_2$CH$_2$NH$_2$ (pyrazole ring, N-N-H)	Relatively selective H_2	0.12^k (0.10–0.14)	$\sim 0.5^l$	2.1(1.4–2.8)
Dimaprit^m	HN= C—SCH$_2$CH$_2$CH$_2$N(CH$_3$)$_2$, H$_2$N	Highly selective H_2	<0.0001	19.5	71(61–81)
SK & F 91487^n (Nordimaprit)	HN= C—SCH$_2$CH$_2$N(CH$_3$)$_2$, H$_2$N	"Inactive" control	<0.01	0.1	<0.1
SK & F 92676° (Impromidine)	CH$_3$ — CH$_2$SCH$_2$CH$_2$NHCNH(CH$_2$)$_3$ (NH), HN—N , N—NH				
N-[3-(Imidazol-4-yl) propyl]-N′-{2- [(5-methylimidazol-4-yl) methylthio]ethyl} guanidine		Potent selective H_2	<0.001	1680	4810

Name	Structure	pA$_2$ (Guinea Pig Ileum)
H$_1$-Receptor Antagonists		
Mepyramine^p	CH$_3$O— (benzene)—CH$_2$—N—CH$_2$CH$_2$N(CH$_3$)$_2$ (pyridine, N)	9.4
Diphenhydramine^p	CH—O—CH$_2$CH$_2$N(CH$_3$)$_2$ (two phenyl groups)	8.0

Table 48.19 (*Continued*)

Name	Structure	pA$_2$ (Guinea Pig Ileum)
Triprolidine[p]	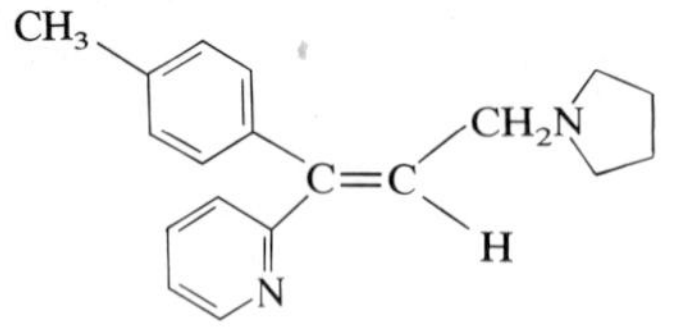	9.9
Chlorpheniramine[q]	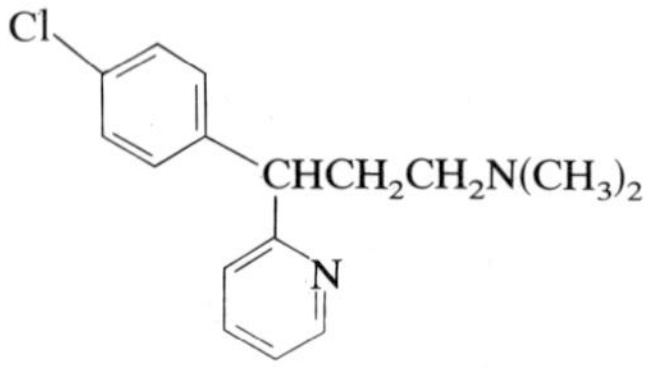	d (+) enantiomer 9.3 l (−) enantiomer 7.8

Name	Structure	pA$_2$ (Guinea Pig Atrium)

H$_2$-Receptor Antagonists[r]

Name	Structure	pA$_2$ (Guinea Pig Atrium)
Burimamide	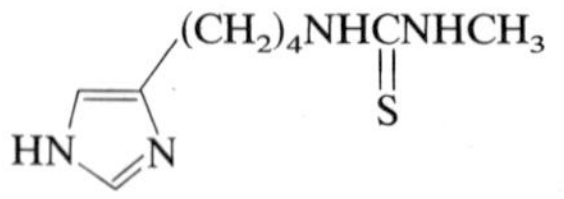	5.1
Metiamide	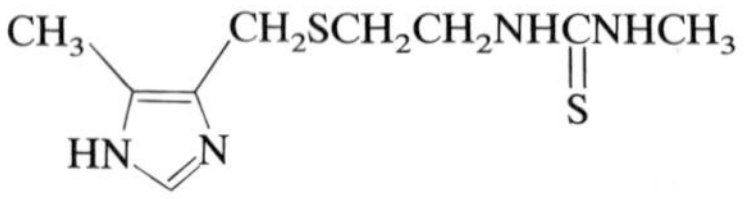	6.0
Cimetidine	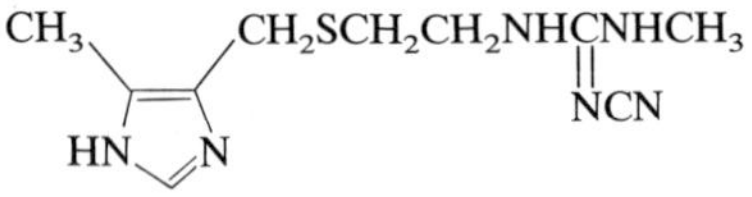	6.1
SK & F 91581 (Norburimamide)	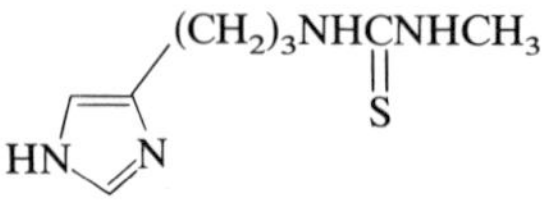	3.9[s]

[a] Assay methods and data from R. C. Blakemore and M. E. Parsons, The Research Institute, Smith Kline & French Laboratories Limited, Welwyn Garden City, England (see Table 48.6).
[b] Full data in Table 48.6.
[c] Ref. 79.
[d] Ash and Schild (22) report 0.3%; see also Arunlakshana and Schild (20).
[e] Ash and Schild (22) report 0.7%.
[f] Partial agonist; only achieved 49% (±2.5% S.E.M.; $n = 8$) of the maximal response to histamine (R. C. Blakemore and M. E. Parsons).
[g] Serc.
[h] Partial agonist; only achieved 39% (±10% S.E.M.; $n = 4$) of the maximal response to histamine (R. C. Blakemore and M. E. Parsons).
[i] Lee and Jones (78) report 30%.
[j] Histalog (from Eli Lilly and Co.).
[k] Ash and Schild (22) report 0.06%; Lin et al. (29) report 1%; van den Brink (81) reports 0.02%.
[l] Ash and Schild (22) report 4.2%. Rosiere and Grossman (82) tested this compound given subcutaneously in dogs and later reported (33) that it had approximately 1.4% of the activity of histamine.

7.2 Histamine Receptors in the Peripheral Vasculature

Histamine lowers blood pressure, by causing widespread vasodilatation, in most animal species. However, the effects of histamine have always appeared complex since responses are species-sensitive, sometimes biphasic, and only partially inhibited by classical antihistaminic drugs. Thus depressor and vasodilator responses to small doses of histamine can be abolished by treatment with mepyramine, whereas responses to larger doses of histamine are refractory even to very large doses of classical antihistamines (27). The dual receptor hypothesis and the advent of selective antagonists and agonists had shed some light on the complexities of the vascular effects of histamine. Indeed, observations in the first human pharmacological experiments with burimamide created considerable interest, since the combination of H_1- and H_2-receptor antagonists used (mepyramine and burimamide) had dramatic effects on dermal wheal and flare caused by histamine (35). In animal experiments, it was shown that burimamide, on its own, is not effective as an antagonist of histamine depressor responses in cats, whereas administration of mepyramine, followed by burimamide or metiamide, completely abolishes such responses (35, 220). Results were consistent with the involvement of both H_1 and H_2 receptors in depressor responses to histamine and were additionally consistent with the affinity for H_1 receptors being higher than for H_2 receptors (220). Additional evidence for the involvement of both H_1 and

H_1 receptors has been provided by use of selective agonists (221, 222). The distribution and classification of histamine receptors in various blood vessels from many species are included in the review by Chand and Eyre (218). A comprehensive review of histamine receptors in the vascular system has recently been published by Owen (223). There is a growing body of evidence to support the original suggestion by Folkow et al. (27), and restated by Furchgott (224), that two types of receptor are involved in the vascular effects of histamine.

7.3 Histamine Receptors in the Heart

The effect of histamine on the heart *in vivo* is complex, and as a consequence most useful studies on the cardiac effects of histamine have been made *in vitro* using a variety of preparations, usually from the guinea pig. The increase in rate of guinea pig right atrium (positive chronotropic effect) which is blocked by burimamide is one of the original H_2-receptor systems characterized by Black and co-workers (35). The receptors involved in the inotropic response (increased force of contraction) to histamine are more complex, but in isolated whole hearts the inotropic effect is suppressed by H_2-receptor antagonists (225). Histamine also causes a decrease in atrioventricular conduction (negative dromotropic effect), and this effect appears to be mediated by H_1 receptors (226). There is therefore pharmacological evidence for the presence of both H_1 and H_2 receptors in the

---

^{m} Ref. 86.
^{n} Ref. 90.
^{o} Ref. 150.
^{p} Ref. 219 (30 minute contact times).
^{q} Ref. 246.
^{r} $pA_2 = -\log K_B$, where K_B is the dissociation constant (see Tables 48.9 and 48.14).
^{s} 95% Confidence limits 3.64–4.25 ($n = 6$), slope of regression $= 0.90 \pm 0.07$ (R. C. Blakemore and M. E. Parsons); this result was obtained by computer-assisted calculation and is a more refined figure than that previously quoted in Ref. 126a and 168).

heart. The classification of cardiac histamine receptors has been reviewed
(223, 227).

Histamine is known to stimulate cardiac
adenylate cyclase in a washed membrane
preparation from guinea pig ventricle. A
quantitative *in vitro* study using selective
agonists and antagonists indicated that cardiac adenylate cyclase can be classified as
an H$_2$-receptor system and that the enzyme
is intimately involved in both the positive
inotropic and chronotropic effects of histamine on the intact heart (228).

7.4 Histamine Receptors in the Nervous System

The role of histamine in the central and
peripheral nervous system is not well understood and a detailed discussion of this
complex subject is outside the scope of this
review. However, a neurotransmitter role
for histamine in mammalian brian has been
claimed (229).

There is some evidence for the presence
of both H$_1$ and H$_2$ receptors in the brain,
based mainly on studies of adenylate cyclase activation in brain slices by selective
agonists and on the use of selective antagonists as inhibitors of histamine-induced
cyclase activation (230, 231). The situation
is complicated, however, by variation in
responses depending on the source of enzyme (tissue or animal species). Investigation of selective neuronal firing using
microiontophoretic techniques also indicates an H$_2$-receptor involvement (232).
Discussions on the possible role of histamine in the brain, including the evidence
for its function as a synaptic transmitter,
are contained in recent reviews (229, 233).

7.5 Histamine Receptors Associated with Immunologic Function

Histamine appears to have an important
modulating effect on the function of a variety of cells involved in immunity and in-

flammation. Evidence has been presented
for histamine H$_2$ receptors on mast cells
(234), basophils (235a), T-lymphocytes
(235b), and neutrophils (236). Characterization of the receptors has depended
mainly on studying the interaction between
histamine and the H$_2$-receptor antagonists
burimamide and metiamide. In some cases,
cyclic adenosine monophosphate levels
have been used as the response. For a
discussion on histamine receptors in leuco-
cytes, including their role in immuno-
pathological conditions, the review by
Chand and Eyre (218) should be consulted.

7.6 Ligand Binding Studies and Histamine Receptors

The specific binding of high affinity ligands
has been used to explore various pharmacological receptors and such studies have
been applied to examination of histamine
receptors.

^{3}H-Mepyramine, synthesized from the 5-
bromopyridyl derivative by catalytic hydrogenation with tritium gas (249), has been
studied (250) with respect to its specific
binding to homogenates of the longitudinal
muscle-myenteric plexus preparation from
guinea pig small intestine. Inhibition of ^{3}H-
mepyramine by other compounds, viz., ($\pm$)
chlorpheniramine, promethazine, tripoli-
dine, burimamide, and lachesine, gave
affinity constants in good agreement with
values for *in vitro* inhibition of the
contractile reponse to histamine on intact
segments of guinea pig ileum, suggesting
that specific binding to histamine H$_1$ receptors had been observed. Binding of ^{3}H-me-
pyramine to membrane fractions from
guinea pig or rat whole brains was later
demonstrated (251, 252), and good agreement obtained between inhibition of binding and potency as H$_1$-receptor histamine
antagonists, for a group of compounds including the two stereoisomers of chlorpheniramine, which showed a striking 240-
fold difference in affinity constants. It ap-

pears that the binding of ^{3}H-mepyramine in guinea pig and rat brain is to sites that have the character of histamine H$_1$ receptors. However, there are some indications that the binding of ^{3}H-mepyramine may not represent a simple equilibrium with a single set of binding sites (251).

Binding of ^{3}H-cimetidine to homogenates of guinea pig whole brain has been studied (253) but this probably does not represent H$_2$-receptor binding, since the measured IC$_{50}$ values for inhibition of binding by unlabeled cimetidine or metiamide are in the range $3–5 \times 10^{-8}\,M$, nearly a hundredfold lower than the affinity constants for H$_2$-receptor histamine antagonism on peripheral tissue systems.

High affinity binding of ^{3}H-histamine to homogenized regions of rat brain has been observed (254) but it would be premature to conclude that this represents binding to histamine receptors. Sites for selective localization of histamine (not apparently connected with receptor binding) have been seen previously in other tissue systems, notably in the heart (216) and aorta (255).

There have been attempts to isolate and purify the histamine H$_1$ receptor from a membrane fraction of smooth muscle of cat small intestine. Binding of ^{3}H-histamine to this fraction appears to be to H$_1$ receptors, and is consistent in comparison with the selective agonists 2- and 4-methylhistamine (256). Affinity labeling with the β-haloalkylamine Dibenamine was investigated, but it appears that this drug does not have a sufficiently high degree of specificity (257); there is clearly a need for specific affinity labels for both H$_1$ and H$_2$ receptors.

8   CHEMICAL COMPARISON OF H$_1$- AND H$_2$-RECEPTOR ANTAGONISTS

There is a marked chemical distinction between the recently discovered H$_2$-receptor antagonists and the conventional H$_1$-receptor antagonists. Ariens et al. (238)

remarked, "for many of the antihistamines used in therapy, the only resemblance in chemical structure with the histaminomimetics seems to be the amino group." Thus the H$_1$-antagonists possess aryl or heteroaryl rings (as in the general formula, 48.**56**) but these need not have a structural relationship to the imidazole ring of histamine (81, 239); the aryl groups confer considerable lipophilicity (the octanol–water partition ratio P is often greater than 1000; see Table 48.20) and probably contribute to receptor association by hydrophobic binding. Effective H$_1$-receptor antagonists resemble histamine in possessing a side chain group (usually ammonium) that is positively charged at physiological pH. In marked contrast burimamide, metiamide, and cimetidine are hydrophilic molecules, having low octanol–water partition ratios; they bear a structural relationship to histamine in having an imidazole ring but differ in the side chain which, though polar, is

Table 48.20   Partition ratios, P, of Uncharged Forms of Some Histamine Antagonists and Imidazole Derivatives, Together with Percentages (% C_{aq}) Remaining in Aqueous Layer After Equilibration

Antagonist	$P = \dfrac{C_{octanol}}{C_{aq.buffer}}$ [a]	% $C_{aq.} = \dfrac{100}{P+1}$
Histamine[b]	0.2	83
Imidazole[c]	0.5	67
4(5)-Methylimidazole[c]	1.5	40
Thiaburimamide[c]	1.4	42
Burimamide[c]	2.5	29
Cimetidine[c]	2.5	29
Metiamide[c]	3.2	24
Mepyramine[d]	700	0.14
Diphenhydramine[d]	2500	0.04
Triprolidine[d]	8300	0.012

[a] Partition between 1-octanol and aqueous buffer at 37°C (143).
[b] Measured at pH 11.8.
[c] Measured at pH 9.0.
[d] From Ref. 237.

Table 48.21   Chemical Differentiation between Histamine and its Antagonists[a]

H₂ Antagonist	Histamine (Agonist)	H₁ Antagonist
Imidazole—hydrophilic Thiourea	Imidazole—hydrophilic	Aryl Rings—lipophilic
Cyanoguanidine—uncharged	Ammonium—charged	Ammonium—charged

[a] General formula of H₁ antagonists:

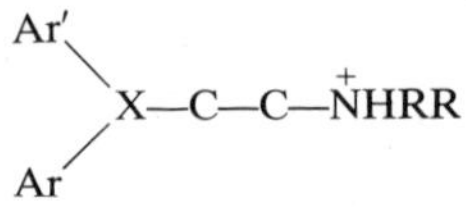

$$\begin{array}{c} Ar' \\ \diagdown \\ \diagup \\ Ar \end{array} X{-}C{-}C{-}\overset{+}{N}HRR$$

48.**56**

uncharged. These substantial chemical differences (indicated in Table 48.21) probably account for the considerable degree of selectivity shown by the respective antagonists in distinguishing the two types of receptor (63).

The chemical structural features associated with respective receptor activities of these compounds are shown schematically in Fig. 48.34. The two functional groups of histamine, viz., the imidazole ring and the ammonium group, appear to have different roles at the two receptors. Compounds acting at the H₁-receptor have ammonium (or similarly charged) groups; the compounds having H₂-receptor activity are derivatives of imidazole (or an analogous heterocycle). In the sense used by Ariens and Simonis (240) H₁-receptor recognition is determined by the ammonium group, but at H₂-receptors it is determined by the imidazole ring. Thus in the development of H₂-receptor antagonists, it was found necessary to retain the imidazole ring and

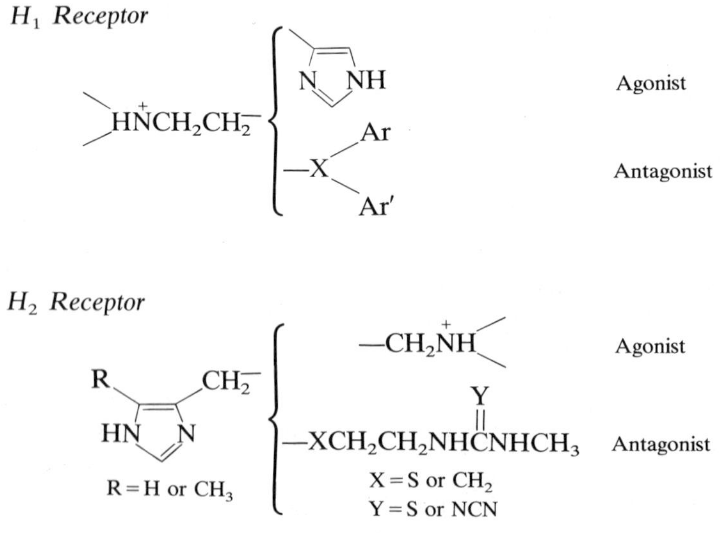

H₁ Receptor

Agonist

Antagonist

H₂ Receptor

Agonist

Antagonist

X = S or CH₂
Y = S or NCN

Fig. 48.34 Chemical features of histamine and its antagonists associated with receptor activity.

to modify the ammonium side chain. In each case the nature of the activity (i.e., agonist, antagonist, or no effect) is determined by the rest of the molecule.

It appears that certain chemical properties of imidazole, and thiourea or cyanoguanidine, determine the H_2-receptor antagonist activities of burimamide, metiamide, and cimetidine and impart biological selectivity. Being uncharged in the side chain, these compounds are unable to mimic the stimulant actions of histamine; they are not agonists. Having low lipophilicity probably limits access to the central nervous system and avoids some of the "side effects" normally associated with use of the H_1-receptor antagonists. Antihistaminic drugs often possess local anesthetic and anticholinergic properties and many exert CNS-depressant effects (13). Unlike the lipophilic H_1-receptor antagonists, burimamide, metiamide, and cimetidine do not produce overt signs of CNS action in behavioral tests and have only weak local anesthetic or anticholinergic activities (241, 242).

REFERENCES

1. A. Windaus and W. Vogt, *Chem. Ber.*, **40,** 3691 (1907).

2. D. Ackermann, *Z. Physiol. Chem.*, **65,** 504 (1910).

3. G. Barger and H. H. Dale, *Proc. Chem. Soc.*, **26,** 128 (1910); *J. Chem. Soc.*, **97,** 2592 (1910).

4. D. Ackermann and Fr. Kutscher, *Z. Biol.*, **54,** 387 (1910).

5. H. H. Dale and P. P. Laidlaw, *J. Physiol.*, **41,** 318 (1910).

6. H. H. Dale and P. P. Laidlaw, *J. Physiol.*, **43,** 182 (1911).

7. G. Barger and H. H. Dale, *J. Physiol.*, **41,** 499 (1911).

8. J. J. Abel and S. Kubota, *J. Pharm. Exp. Ther.*, **13,** 243 (1919).

9. H. H. Dale, *Lancet*, (a) 1233 (1929). (b) 1285 (1929).

10. L. Popielski, *Arch. Ges. Physiol.*, **178,** 214 (1920).

11. D. Bovet and A. M. Staub, *C. R. Soc. Biol.*, **124,** 547 (1937).

12. W. W. Douglas, in *The Pharmacological Basis of Therapeutics*, 4th ed., L. S. Goodman and A. Gilman, Eds., Macmillan, New York, 1970, pp. 621–645.

13. D. T. Witiak, in *Medicinal Chemistry* Part 2, 3rd ed., A. Burger, Ed., Wiley-Interscience, New York, 1970, pp. 1643–1668.

14. J. H. Gaddum, *Brit. Med. J.*, 867 (1948).

15. J. A. Wells, H. C. Morris, H. B. Bull, and C. A. Dragstedt, *J. Pharmacol. Exper. Ther.*, **85,** 122 (1945).

16. B. N. Halpern and G. Mauric, *C. R. Soc. Biol.*, **140,** 440 (1946).

17. H. O. Schild, *Brit. J. Pharmacol.*, **2,** 189 (1947).

18. H. O. Schild, *Brit. J. Pharmacol.*, **4,** 277 (1949).

19. D. F. Hawkins and H. O. Schild, *Brit. J. Pharmacol.*, **6,** 682 (1951).

20. O. Arunlakshana and H. O. Schild, *Brit. J. Pharmacol.*, **14,** 48 (1959).

21. H. O. Schild, *Pharmacol. Rev.*, **9,** 242 (1957).

22. A. S. F. Ash and H. O. Schild, *Brit. J. Pharm. Chemother.*, **27,** 427 (1966).

23. C. Robertson and M. I. Grossman, *Arch. Int. Pharmacodyn.*, **90,** 223 (1952).

24. A. C. Ivy and W. H. Bachrach, in *Hand. Exp. Pharm.*, XVIII/I, *Histamine and Antihistaminics*, M. Rocha e Silva, Ed., Springer-Verlag, Berlin, 1966, pp. 810–891.

25. U. Trendelenburg, *J. Pharm. Exp. Ther.*, **130,** 450 (1960).

26. P. B. Dews and J. D. P. Graham, *Brit. J. Pharmacol.*, **1,** 278 (1946).

27. B. Folkow, K. Haeger, and G. Kahlson, *Acta Physiol. Scand.*, **15,** 264 (1948).

28. H. D. Janowitz and F. Hollander, *Proc. Soc. Exp. Biol.*, **95,** 320 (1957).

29. T. M. Lin, R. S. Alphin, F. G. Henderson, D. N. Benslay, and K. K. Chen, *Ann. N. Y. Acad. Sci.*, **99,** 30 (1962).

30. A. L. Bartlet, *Brit. J. Pharmacol.*, **21,** 450 (1963).

31. E. J. Ariens, A. M. Simonis, and J. M. Van Rossum, in *Molecular Pharmacology*, Vol. 1, E. J. Ariens, Ed., Academic, New York, 1964, pp. 217, 221.

32. R. B. Barlow, *Introduction to Chemical Pharmacology*, 2nd ed., Methuen, London, 1964, pp. 344–377.

33. M. I. Grossman, C. Robertson, and C. E. Rosiere, *J. Pharm. Exp. Ther.*, **104,** 277 (1952).

34a. R. G. Jones, Ref. 24, pp. 1–43.

34b. D. M. Paton, in *Histamine and Antihistaminics*, M. Schachter, Ed., Pergamon, New York, 1973, pp. 3–24.

35. J. W. Black, W. A. M. Duncan, G. J. Durant, C. R. Ganellin, and M. E. Parsons, *Nature*, **236,** 385 (1972).

36. J. W. Black and C. R. Ganellin, *Experientia*, **30,** 111 (1974).

37. T. B. Paiva, M. Tominaga, and A. C. M. Paiva, *J. Med. Chem.*, **13,** 689 (1970).

38. K. Prout, S. R. Critchley, and C. R. Ganellin, *Acta Crystallogr.*, **B30,** 2884 (1974).

39. J. J. Bonnet and J. A. Ibers, *J. Am. Chem. Soc.*, **95,** 4829 (1973).

40. C. R. Ganellin, *J. Pharm. Pharmacol.*, **25,** 787 (1973).

41. C. R. Ganellin, in *Molecular and Quantum Pharmacology*, E. D. Bergmann and B. Pullman, Eds., D. Reidel Publishing Co., Dordrecht, Holland, 1974, pp. 43–53.

42. A. R. Katritzky and J. M. Lagowksi, in *Advances in Heterocyclic Chemistry*, Vol. 2, Academic, New York-London, 1963, p. 32.

43a. W. F. Reynolds and C. W. Tzeng, *Can. J. Biochem.*, **55,** 576 (1977).

43b. R. E. Wasylishen and G. Tomlinson, *Can. J. Biochem.*, **55,** 579 (1977).

44. S. Kang and D. Chou, *Chem. Phys. Lett.*, **34,** 537 (1975).

45. H. Weinstein, D. Chou, C. L. Johnson, S. Kang, and J. P. Green, *Mol. Pharmacol.*, **12,** 738 (1976).

46. L. B. Kier, *J. Med. Chem.*, **11,** 441 (1968).

47. C. R. Ganellin, E. S. Pepper, G. N. J. Port, and W. G. Richards *J. Med. Chem.*, **16,** 610 (1973).

48. M. Kumbar, *J. Theor. Biol.*, **53,** 333 (1975).

49. J. P. Green, S. Kang, and S. Margolis, *Mem. Soc. Endocrinol.*, **19,** 727 (1971).

50. J. L. Coubeils, P. Courrière, and B. Pullman, *C. R. Acad. Sci. Paris, Ser. D.*, **272,** 1813 (1971).

51a. B. Pullman and J. Port, *Mol. Pharmacol.*, **10,** 360 (1974).

51b. G. Simons and E. R. Talaty, *J. Am. Chem. Soc.*, **99,** 2407 (1977).

52. R. J. Abraham and D. Birch, *Mol. Pharmacol.*, **11,** 663 (1975).

53. A. F. Casy, R. R. Ison, and N. S. Ham, *Chem. Commun.*, **1970,** 1343.

54. N. S. Ham, A. F. Casy, and R. R. Ison, *J. Med. Chem.*, **16,** 470 (1973).

55. Personal communication from Dr. E. S. Pepper, The Research Institute, Smith Kline & French Laboratories, Welwyn Garden City, Hertfordshire, England.

56. S. R. Byrn, C. W. Graber, and S. L. Midland, *J. Org. Chem.*, **41,** 2283 (1976).

57. D. F. Decou, Dissertation No. 64–9987, Univ. Microfilms Inc., Ann Arbor, Mich. (1964).

58. J. J. Bonnet, Y. Jeannin, and M. Laaouini, *Bull. Soc. Fr. Mineral. Cristallogr.*, **98,** 208 (1975).

59. M. V. Veidis, G. J. Palenik, R. Schaffirin, and J. Trotter, *J. Chem. Soc. A*, 2659 (1969).

60. T. Yamane, T. Ashida, and M. Kakudo, *Acta Crystallogr.* **B29,** 2884 (1973).

61. J. J. Bonnet and Y. Jeannin, *Acta Crystallogr.*, **B28,** 1079, (1972).

62. R. C. Mitchell, in Ref. 63.

63. G. J. Durant, J. C. Emmett, and C. R. Ganellin, in *International Symposium on Histamine H₂-Receptor Antagonists*, C. J. Wood and M. A. Simkins, Eds., Smith Kline & French Laboratories, Welwyn Garden City, 1973, pp. 13–21.

64. W. G. Richards and J. Wallis, *J. Med. Chem.*, **19,** 1250 (1976).

65. D. D. Perrin, I. G. Sayce, and V. S. Sharma, *J. Chem. Soc. A*, **1967,** 1755.

66a. D. D. Perrin and V. S. Sharma, *J. Chem. Soc. A*, **1968,** 446 (log $K_3 = 2.93$).

66b. D. D. Perrin and V. S. Sharma, *J. Chem. Soc. A*, **1969,** 2060.

67. B. L. Mickel and A. C. Andrews, *J. Am. Chem. Soc.*, **77,** 5291 (1955).

68. at 40°; W. C. Nicholas and W. C. Fernelius, *J. Phys. Chem.*, **65,** 1047 (1951).

69. J. J. Bonnet and Y. Jeannin, (a) *C. R. Acad. Sci. Paris, Ser. C*, **270,** 1329 (1970). (b) *Acta Crystallogr.*, **B26,** 318 (1970).

70a. J. J. Bonnet and Y. Jeannin, *Bull. Soc. Fr. Mineral. Cristallogr.* **93,** 287 (1970).

70b. J. J. Bonnet and Y. Jeannin, *Bull. Soc. Fr. Mineral Cristallogr.*, **95,** 61 (1972).

71. P. A. Kramer, J. R. Hazlett, and D. O. Kildsig, *J. Pharm. Sci.*, **66,** 542 (1977).

72. R. J. Sundberg and R. B. Martin, *Chem. Rev.*, **74,** 471 (1974).

73. See discussion by J. P. Green (a) in U. S. von Euler, S. Rosell, and B. Uvnäs, Eds., *Mechanisms of Release of Biogenic Amines*, Pergamon, London, 1966, pp. 125–145. (b) *Fed. Proc.*, **26,** 211 (1967).

74. L. Kerp, *Int. Arch. Allergy Appl. Immunol.*, **22,** 112 (1963).

75. B. Uvnäs, C. H. Aborg, and U. Bergqvist, *Acta Physiol. Scand.*, **93,** 401 (1975).

76. C. Niemann and J. T. Hays, *J. Am. Chem. Soc.*, **64,** 2288 (1942).

77. L. A. Walter, W. H. Hunt, and R. J. Fosbinder, *J. Am. Chem. Soc.*, **63,** 2771 (1971).

78. H. M. Lee and R. G. Jones, *J. Pharmacol. Exper. Ther.*, **95,** 71 (1949).

79. G. J. Durant, C. R. Ganellin, and M. E. Parsons, *J. Med. Chem.*, **18,** 905 (1975).

80. G. J. Durant, J. C. Emmett, C. R. Ganellin, A. M. Roe, and R. A. Slater, *J. Med. Chem.*, **19,** 923 (1976).

81. F. G. van den Brink, in *Histamine and Antihistamines. Molecular Pharmacology, Structure–Activity Relations, Gastric Acid Secretion*, Drukkerij Gebr. Janssen N.V., Nijmegen, 1969, pp. 179–180.

82. C. E. Rosiere and M. I. Grossman, *Science*, **113,** 651 (1951).

83a. G. Bertaccini, M. Impicciatore, T. Vitali, and V. Plazzi, *Farm. Ed. Sci.*, **27,** 680 (1972).

83b. G. Bertaccini, M. Impicciatore, and T. Vitali, *Farm. Ed. Sci.*, **31,** 934 (1976).

83c. M. Impicciatore, F. Mossini, V. Plazzi, M. Chiavarini, and G. Bertaccini, *Atteneo Parmense, Acta Bio-Med.*, **45,** 145 (1976).

83d. G. Bertaccini and T. Vitali, *J. Pharm. Pharmacol.*, **16,** 441 (1964).

84. A. Vartiainen, *J. Pharmacol. Exp. Ther.*, **54,** 265 (1935).

85. B. N. Craver, W. Barrett, A. Cameron, and E. Herrold, *Arch. Int. Pharmacodyn. Ther.*, **87,** 33 (1951).

86. M. E. Parsons, D. A. A. Owen, C. R. Ganellin, and G. J. Durant, *Agents Actions*, **7,** 31 (1977).

87. F. Holmes and F. Jones, *J. Chem. Soc.*, 2398 (1960).

88. W. H. Hunt and R. J. Fosbinder, *J. Pharmacol. Exp. Ther.*, **75,** 299 (1942).

89. D. Blow, *Acc. Chem. Res.*, **9,** 145 (1976).

90. G. J. Durant, C. R. Ganellin, and M. E. Parsons, *Agents Actions*, **7,** 39 (1977).

91. C. R. Ganellin, G. N. J. Port, and W. G. Richards, *J. Med. Chem.*, **16,** 616 (1973).

92. C. R. Ganellin, *J. Med. Chem.*, **16,** 620 (1973).

93. L. Farnell, W. G. Richards, and C. R. Ganellin, *J. Med. Chem.*, **18,** 662 (1975).

94. W. G. Richards, J. Hammond, and D. G. Aschman, *J. Theor. Biol.*, **51,** 237 (1975).

95. E. R. Loew, *Physiol. Rev.*, **27,** 542 (1947).

96. M. E. Parsons, Ph.D. thesis, University of London, 1969.

97. C. R. Ganellin, G. J. Durant, and J. C. Emmett, *Fed. Proc.*, **35,** 1924 (1976).

98. G. J. Durant, J. M. Loynes and S. H. B. Wright, *J. Med. Chem.*, **16,** 1272 (1973).

99. E. J. Ariens and A. M. Simonis, *Arch. Int. Pharmacodyn. Ther.*, **127,** 479 (1960).

100. B. R. Baker, *J. Chem. Educ.*, **44,** 610 (1967).

101. G. J. Durant, M. E. Parsons, and J. W. Black, *J. Med. Chem.*, **18,** 830 (1975).

102. R. P. Stephenson, *Brit. J. Pharmacol.*, **11,** 379 (1956).

103. M. E. Parsons, R. C. Blakemore, G. J. Durant, C. R. Ganellin, and A. C. Rasmussen, *Agents Actions*, **5,** 464 (1975).

104. J. W. Black, G. J. Durant, J. C. Emmett, and C. R. Ganellin, Brit. Pat. 1,296,544 (1972); 1,305,546 (1973); 1,305,547 (1973); 1,305,549 (1973).

105. J. W. Black, G. J. Durant, J. C. Emmett, and C. R. Ganellin, *Nature*, **248,** 65 (1974).

106. C. R. Ganellin, in *Drug Action at the Molecular Level*, G. C. K. Roberts, Ed., Macmillan, London, 1977, pp. 1–39.

107. M. Charton, *J. Org. Chem.*, **30,** 3346 (1965).

108. S. P. Datta and A. K. Grzybowski, *J. Chem. Soc., B*, **1966,** 136.

109. Personal communication from M. J. Graham, The Research Institute, Smith Kline & French Laboratories, Welwyn Garden City, Hertfordshire, England.

110. L. Pauling, *The Nature of the Chemical Bond*, Cornell University, New York, 1960, (a) p. 224. (b) p. 229. (c) p. 112. (d) pp. 260–261.

111. By geometry.

112. A. Bondi, *J. Phys. Chem.*, **68,** 441 (1964).

113. O. Exner, *Coll. Czech. Chem. Commun.*, **32,** 1 (1967).

114. E. L. Eliel, *Stereochemistry of Carbon Compounds*, McGraw-Hill, New York, 1962, p. 319.

115. L. Pierce and M. Hayashi, *J. Chem. Phys.*, **35,** 479 (1961).

116. P. H. Kasai and R. J. Myres, *J. Chem. Phys.*, **30,** 1096 (1959).

117a. A. Leo, P. Y. C. Jow, C. Silipo, and C. Hansch, *J. Med. Chem.*, **18,** 865 (1975).

117b. C. Hansch, J. E. Quinlan, and G. L. Lawrence, *J. Org. Chem.*, **33,** 347 (1968).

117c. E. M. Arnett and G. Scorrano, in *Advances in Physical Organic Chemistry*, Vol. 13, V. Gold, Ed., Academic, London, 1976, pp. 130.

118. C. Hansch and S. M. Anderson, *J. Org. Chem.*, **32,** 2583 (1967).

119. S. Anderson and C. Hansch, result quoted in A. Leo, C. Hansch, and D. Elkins, *Chem. Rev.*, **71,** 525 (1971).

120. G. G. Nys and R. F. Rekker, *Eur. J. Med. Chem.*, **9,** 361 (1974).

121. J. W. Black, W. A. M. Duncan, J. C. Emmett, C. R. Ganellin, T. Hesselbo, M. E. Parsons, and J. H. Wyllie, *Agents Actions*, **3,** 133 (1973).

122. Personal communication from Dr. M. E. Parsons, The Research Institute, Smith Kline & French Laboratories, Welwyn Garden City, Hertfordshire, England.   •

123. G. J. Durant in *Proceedings of the Sixth International Symposium on Medicinal Chemistry*, M. A. Simkins, Ed., Cotswold Press, Oxford, 1979.

124. R. W. Brimblecombe, W. A. M. Duncan, and M. E. Parsons, *S. Afr. Med. J.*, **48,** 2253 (1974).

125. R. W. Brimblecombe, W. A. M. Duncan, and T. R. Walker, in Ref. 63, pp. 53–72.

126a. G. J. Durant, J. C. Emmett, and C. R. Ganellin, in *Cimetidine, Proceedings of the Second International Symposium on Histamine H$_2$-Receptor Antagonists*, W. L. Burland and M. A. Simkins, Eds., Excerpta Medica, Amsterdam-Oxford, 1977, pp. 1–12.

126b. G. J. Durant, J. C. Emmett, C. R. Ganellin, P. D. Miles, M. E. Parsons, H. D. Prain, and G. R. White, *J. Med. Chem.*, **20,** 901, (1977).

126c. R. W. Brimblecombe, W. A. M. Duncan, G. J. Durant, J. C. Emmett, C. R. Ganellin, and M. E. Parsons, *J. Int. Med. Res.*, **3,** 86 (1975).

127. M. Charton, *J. Org. Chem.*, **30,** 969 (1975).

128. R. C. Hirt, R. G. Schmitt, H. L. Strauss, and J. G. Koren, *J. Chem. Eng. Data*, **6,** 610 (1961).

129. J. G. Bonner, and J. C. Lockhardt, *J. Chem. Soc.*, **1958,** 3858.

130. M. Truter, *Acta Crystallogr.*, **22,** 556 (1967).

131. J. E. Worsham, H. A. Levy, and S. W. Peterson, *Acta Crystallogr.*, **10,** 319 (1957).

132. P. Vaughan and J. Donohue, *Acta Crystallogr.*, **5,** 530 (1952).

133. E. W. Hughes, *J. Am. Chem. Soc.*, **62,** 1258 (1940).

134. N. V. Rannev, R. P. Ozerov, I. D. Datt, and A. N. Kshnyskina, *Kristallografiya*, **11,** 175 (1966).

135. J. M. Bryden, L. A. Burkardt, E. W. Hughes, and J. Donohue, *Acta Crystallogr.*, **9,** 573 (1956).

136. M. J. Janssen, *Rec. Trav. Chim.*, **81,** 650 (1962).

137. D. W. Farlow and R. B. Moodie, *J. Chem. Soc B*, **1971,** 407.

138. J. G. Bonner and J. C. Lockhardt, *J. Chem. Soc.*, **1958,** 3858.

139. M. Herlem, *Bull. Soc. Chim. Fr.*, **1965,** 3329.

140. G. Charlot and B. Tremillon, in *Les Réactions Chimiques dans les Solvents et les Sels Fondus*, Gauthier-Villars, Paris, 1963, p. 90.

141. N. Kameyama, *J. Chem. Ind. (Japan)*, **24,** 1263 (1921); through *Chem. Abstr.*, **16,** 2247.

142. J. E. DeVries and E. St. Clair Gantz, *J. Am. Chem. Soc.*, **76,** 1008 (1954).

143. Personal communication from Dr. R. C. Mitchell, the Research Institute, Smith Kline & French Laboratories, Welwyn Garden City, Hertfordshire, England.

144. W. D. Kumler and G. M. Fohlen, *J. Am. Chem. Soc.*, **64,** 1944 (1942).

145. W. C. Schneider, *J. Am. Chem. Soc.*, **72,** 761 (1950).

146. W. D. Kumler and P. T. Sah, *J. Org. Chem.*, **18,** 669 (1953).

147. M. L. Filleux-Blanchard and A. Durand, *Org. Magn. Resonance*, **3,** 187 (1971).

148. C. G. McCarty and D. M. Wieland, *Tetrahedron Lett.*, 1787 (1969).

149. D. E. Beattie, R. Crossley, A. C. W. Curran, D. G. Hill, and A. E. Lawrence, *J. Med. Chem.*, **20,** 718 (1977).

150. G. J. Durant, W. A. M. Duncan, C. R. Ganellin, M. E. Parsons, R. C. Blakemore, and A. C. Rasmussen, *Nature*, **276,** 403 (1978).

151a. G. J. Durant, J. C. Emmett, C. R. Ganellin, and G. R. White, Brit. Pat. 1,307,539 (1973).

151b. G. J. Durant, J. C. Emmett, and C. R. Ganellin, Brit. Pat. 1,338,169 (1973).

152. D. Gattegno, A. M. Guiliani, M. Bossa, and G. Ramunni, *J. Chem. Soc. Dalton*, **1973,** 1399.

153. D. R. Eaton and K. Zaw, *Canad. J. Chem.*, **49,** 3315 (1971).

154. P. O. P. Ts'o, I. S. Melvin, and A. C. Olson, *J. Am. Chem. Soc.*, **85,** 1289 (1963).

155. W. Saenger and D. Suck, *Eur. J. Biochem.*, **32,** 473 (1973).

156. When two groups are on the same side of the reference plane they are assigned the descriptor Z (*zusammen*); when on opposite sides they are assigned the descriptor E (*entgegen*); see J. E. Blackwood, C. W. Gladys, K. L. Loening, A. E. Petracra, and J. E. Rush, *J. Am. Chem. Soc.*, **90,** 509 (1968).

157. B. Kamenar, K. Prout, and C. R. Ganellin, *J. Chem. Soc. Perkin Trans. II*, **1973,** 1734.

158. K. Prout, S. R. Critchley, C. R. Ganellin, and R. C. Mitchell, *J. Chem. Soc. Perkin Trans. II*, **1977,** 68.

159. E. Hädicke, F. Frickel, and A. Franke, *Chem. Ber.*, **111,** 3222 (1978).

160. M. E. Parsons, in Ref. 63, pp. 207–216.

161. R. W. Brimblecombe, W. A. M. Duncan, D. A. A. Owen, and M. E. Parsons, *Fed. Proc.*, **35,** 1931 (1976).

162. M. E. Parsons, in Ref. 126a, pp. 13–20.

163. T. Hesselbo, in Ref. 63, pp. 29–42.

164. R. Griffiths, R. M. Lee, and D. C. Taylor, in Ref. 126a, pp. 38–51.

165. D. C. Taylor, in Ref. 63, pp. 45–51.

166. D. C. Taylor and P. R. Cresswell, *Biochem. Soc. Trans.*, **3,** 884 (1975).

167. S. A. M. Cross, in *Proc. 18th Meet. Eur. Soc. Toxicol. Edinburgh, 1976*; *Excerpta Medica*, **18,** 288–290 (1970).

168. S. A. M. Cross, in Ref. 63, pp. 73–83.

169. K. T. Bunce and M. E. Parsons, *J. Physiol.* (London), **258,** 453 (1976).

170. M. E. Parsons, in *Topics in Gastroenterology*, Vol. 3, S. C. Truelove and M. J. Goodman, Eds., Blackwell Scientific Publications, Oxford, 1975, pp. 323–341.

171. J. W. Black, in Ref. 63, pp. 219–221.

172. J. W. Black, in *Proc. 6th Int. Congr. Pharmacol.*, *1975*, **1,** 3–16 (1976).

173. M. J. Grossman and S. J. Konturek, *Gastroenterology*, **3,** 323 (1975).

174. C. F. Code, *Fed. Proc.*, **24,** 1311 (1965).

175. J. H. Wyllie, T. Hesselbo, and J. W. Black, *Lancet*, **1972-II,** 1117.

176. J. H. Wyllie and T. Hesselbo, in Ref. 63, pp. 371–378.

177. P. Goadby, *Pharm. J.*, **216,** 347 (1976), and references cited therein.

178. P. Bass, in *Advances in Drug Research*, Vol. 8, Academic, New York-London, 1974, p. 205.

179. S. J. Haggie, C. G. Clark, J. W. Black, and J. H. Wyllie, *Fed. Proc.*, **35,** 1948 (1976).

180. B. Thjodleifsson and K. G. Wormsley, *Brit. Med. J.*, **2,** 304 (1974).

181. D. C. Carter, J. A. H. Forrest, M. Werner, R. C. Heading, J. Park, and D. J. C. Shearman, *Brit. Med. J.*, **3,** 554 (1974).

182. G. J. Milton-Thompson, J. G. Williams, D. J. A. Jenkins, and J. J. Misiewicz, *Lancet*, **1974-II,** 693.

183. M. Mainardi, V. Maxwell, R. A. L. Sturdevant, and J. I. Isenberg, *New Engl. J. Med.*, **291,** 373 (1974).

184. C. T. Richardson and J. S. Fordtran, *Gastroenterology*, **66,** A207/861 (1974).

185. R. E. Pounder, J. G. Williams, G. J. Milton-Thompson, and J. J. Misiewicz, *Brit. Med. J.*, **2,** 307 (1975).

186. M. H. Thompson, C. W. Venables, I. T. Miller, J. D. Reed, D. J. Sanders, E. R. Grund, and E. L. Blair, *Lancet*, **1975-I,** 35.

187. Report of multicentre trial. L. R. Celestin et al., *Lancet*, **1975-II,** 779.

188. J. A. H. Forrest, D. J. C. Shearman, R. Spence, and L. R. Celestin, *Lancet*, **1975-I,** 392.

189. W. L. Burland, P. C. Sharpe, D. G. Colin-Jones, P. R. G. Turnbull, and P. Bowskill, *Lancet*, **1975-II,** 1085 (1975).

190. R. W. Brimblecombe, W. A. M. Duncan, and T. F. Walker, in Ref. 63, pp. 53–70.

191. G. B. Leslie and T. F. Walker, in Ref. 126a, pp. 24–33.

192. W. L. Burland, W. A. M. Duncan, T. Hesselbo, J. G. Mills, P. C. Sharpe, S. J. Haggie, and J. H. Wyllie, *Brit. J. Clin. Pharm.*, **2,** 481 (1975).

193. S. J. Haggie, D. C. Fermont, and J. H. Wyllie, *Lancet*, **1976-II,** 983.

194. W. S. Blackwood, D. P. Maudgal, R. G. Pickard, D. Lawrence, and T. C. Northfield, *Lancet*, **1976-II,** 174.

195. K. D. Bardhan et al., in Ref. 126a, pp. 260–271.

196. G. Gillespie, G. R. Gray, I. S. Smith, I. Mackenzie, and G. A. Crean, Ref. 126a, pp. 240–247.

197. W. Domschke, S. Domschke, and L. Demling, in Ref. 126a, pp. 217–223.

198. G. Bodemar, B. Norlander, and A. Walan, in Ref. 126a, pp. 224–239.

199. P. J. Ciclitira, R. J. Machell, M. J. Farthing, A. P. Dick, and J. Hunter, in Ref. 126a, pp. 283–286.

200. J. P. Bader, T. Morin, J. J. Bernier, J. Bortrand, C. Bétourné, J. Gastard, R. Lambert, A. Ribet, H. Sarhes, and J. Toulet, in Ref. 126a, pp. 287–292.

201. R. A. McCluskie, K. D. Bardhan, D. M. Saul, H. L. Duthrie, M. G. Greaney, and T. P. Irvin, in Ref. 126a, pp. 297–304.

202. J. G. Stage, S. J. Rune, F. Stadil, and H. Worning, in Ref. 126a, pp. 306–310.

203. R. J. Bailey, B. R. D. MacDougall, and R. Williams, *Gut*, **17,** 389 (1976).

204. B. R. D. MacDougall, R. J. Bailey, and R. Williams, *Clin. Sci. Mol. Med.*, **51,** 1p (1976).

205a. S. C. Verma and J. H. McNeill, *Can. J. Pharm. Sci.*, **13,** 1 (1978).

205b. For a brief summary of earlier literature see T. P. Dousa and C. F. Code, in Ref. 63, pp. 319–330.

206a. H. O. Karppanen, P. J. Neuvonen, P. R. Bieck, and E. Westermann, *Naunyn-Schmiedebergs Arch. Pharm.*, **284**, 15 (1974).

206b. H. O. Karppenen and E. Westermann, *Naunyn-Schmiedebergs Arch. Pharm.*, **279**, 83 (1973).

207. J. H. McNeill and S. C. Verma, *Brit. J. Pharmacol.*, **52**, 104 (1974).

208. G. Sachs, J. G. Spenney, R. L. Shoemaker, C. P. Sung, B. D. Jenkins, and V. D. Wiebelhaus, in Ref. 63, pp. 331–340.

209. P. Scholes, A. Cooper, D. Jones, J. Major, M. Walters, and C. Wilde, *Agents Actions*, **616**, 677 (1976).

210. D. V. Maudsley, Y. Kobayashi, L. Bovaird, and M. Zeidel, *Biochem. Pharmacol.*, **23**, 2963 (1974).

211. R. Håkanson, G. Liedberg, and J. Oscarson, *Brit. J. Pharmacol.*, **47**, 498 (1973).

212. R. Schayer, *Physiol. Rev.*, **39**, 116 (1959).

213. W. Lorenz, H. Barth, and E. Werle, *Arch. Pharmacol.*, **267**, 421 (1970).

214a. K. M. Taylor and S. H. Snyder, *Mol. Pharmacol.*, **8**, 300 (1972).

214b. H. Barth, J. Niemeyer, and W. Lorenz, *Agents Actions*, **3**, 138 (1973).

214c. K. M. Taylor, *Biochem. Pharmacol.*, **22**, 2775 (1973).

215. R. W. Schayer and M. A. Reilly, in Ref. 63, pp. 87–95.

216. R. Fantozzi, F. Franconi, P. F. Mannaioni, E. Masini, and F. Moroni, *Brit. J. Pharmacol.*, **53**, 569 (1975).

217. C. R. Ganellin and D. A. A. Owen, *Agents Actions*, **7**, 93 (1977).

218. N. Chand and P. Eyre, *Agents Actions*, **5**, 277 (1975).

219. R. R. Ison, F. M. Franks, and K. S. Soh, *J. Pharm. Pharmacol.*, **25**, 887 (1973).

220. J. W. Black, D. A. A. Owen, and M. E. Parsons, *Brit. J. Pharmacol.*, **54**, 319 (1975).

221. R. W. Brimblecombe, S. B. Flynn, and D. A. A. Owen, *J. Physiol.*, **249**, 31P (1975).

222. D. A. A. Owen, *Brit. J. Pharmacol.*, **55**, 173 (1975).

223. D. A. A. Owen, *Gen. Pharmacol.*, **8**, 141 (1977).

224. R. F. Furchgott, *Pharmacol. Rev.*, **7**, 183 (1955).

225. J. H. McNeill and S. C. Verma, *J. Pharmacol. Exp. Ther.*, **188**, 180 (1974).

226. R. Levi, N. Capurro, and C. N. Lee, *Eur. J. Pharmacol.*, **30**, 328 (1975).

227. R. Levi, G. Allan, and J. H. Zavecz, *Fed. Proc.*, **35**, 1942 (1976).

228. C. L. Johnson and H. Mizoguchi, *J. Pharmacol. Exp. Ther.*, **200**, 174 (1977).

229. J. C. Schwartz, *Life Sci.*, **17**, 503 (1975); *Ann. Rev. Pharmacol. Toxicol.*, **17**, 325 (1977).

230. M. Baudry, M. P. Martres, and J. C. Schwartz, *Nature*, **253**, 362 (1975).

231a. M. Rogers, K. Dismukes, and J. W. Daly, *J. Neurochem.*, **25**, 531 (1975).

231b. K. Dismukes, M. Rogers, and J. W. Daly, *J. Neurochem.*, **26**, 785 (1976).

232. H. L. Haas and U. M. Bucher, *Nature*, **255**, 634 (1975).

233. C. R. Calcutt, *Gen. Pharmacol.* **7**, 15 (1976).

234. L. W. Chakrin, R. D. Knell, J. Mengel, D. Young, C. Zaher, and J. R. Wardell, *Agents Actions*, **4**, 297 (1974).

235a. L. M. Lichtenstein and E. Gillespie, *Nature*, **224**, 287 (1973).

235b. M. Plaut, L. M. Lichtenstein, and C. S. Henney, *J. Clin. Invest.*, **55**, 856 (1975).

236. W. W. Busse and J. Sosman, *Science*, **194**, 737 (1976).

237. A. Leo, C. Hansch, and D. Elkins, *Chem. Rev.*, **71**, 525 (1971).

238. E. J. Ariens, A. M. Simonis, and J. M. Van Rossum, in Ref. 31, p. 214.

239. F. G. Van den Brink, *Arch. Pharmacol. Exp. Pathol.*, **259**, 9 (1976).

240. E. J. Ariens and A. M. Simonis, *Arch. Int. Pharmacodyn. Ther.*, **127**, 479 (1960).

241. J. W. Black and K. E. V. Spencer, in Ref. 63, pp. 23–26.

242. R. W. Brimblecombe and W. A. M. Duncan, in Ref. 126a, pp. 54–65.

243. G. Bertaccini, G. Coruzzi, and T. Vitali, *Pharmacol. Res. Commun.*, **10**, 747 (1978).

244. M. Impicciatore, G. Morini, F. Bordi, and G. Bertaccini, *Ital. J. Gastroenterol.*, **10**, 10 (1978).

245. H. G. Lennartz, M. Hepp, and W. Schunack, *Eur. J. Pharmacol.*, **13**, 229 (1978).

246. F. G. van den Brink and E. J. Lien, *Eur. J. Pharmacol.*, **44**, 251 (1977).

247. P. Dziuron and W. Schunack, *Eur. J. Med. Chem.*, **10**, 129 (1975).

248. L. L. Grechishkin, L. K. Gavrovskaya, and V. L. Goldfarb, *Pharmacologia*, **15**, 512 (1977).

249. D. H. Marrian, S. J. Hill, J. K. M. Sanders, and J. M. Young, *J. Pharm. Pharmacol.*, **30**, 660 (1978).

250. S. J. Hill, J. M. Young, and D. H. Marrian, *Nature*, **270**, 361 (1977).

251. S. J. Hill, P. C. Emson, and J. M. Young, *J. Neurochem.*, **31,** 997 (1978).

252. R. S. L. Chang, V. T. Tran, and S. H. Synder, *Eur. J. Pharmacol.*, **50,** 449 (1978).

253. W. P. Burkard, *Eur. J. Pharmacol.*, **50,** 449 (1978).

254. J. M. Palacios, J. C. Schwartz, and M. Garbarg, *Eur. J. Pharmacol.*, **50,** 443 (1978).

255. F. R. Goodman, G. Debbas, and G. B. Weiss, *Arch. Int. Pharmacodyn. Ther.*, **218,** 212 (1975).

256. M. K. Uchida and K. Takagi, *Jap. J. Pharmacol.*, **27,** 9 (1977).

257. M. K. Uchida, *Gen. Pharmacol.*, **9,** 145 (1978).

CHAPTER FORTY-NINE

Inhibitors of
the Allergic Response

DONALD T. WITIAK

and

RICHARD C. CAVESTRI

Division of Medicinal Chemistry
College of Pharmacy
Ohio State University
Columbus, Ohio 43210, USA

CONTENTS

1 INTRODUCTION

Allergic or hypersensitivity reactions cause many chronic and acute illnesses including hay fever, pruritus, contact dermatitis, drug rashes, urticaria, atopic dermatitis, and anaphylactic shock (1, 2). The anaphylactic phenomenon may be defined as an acute and rapid physiological reaction of an animal or human having an immediate hyper-

553

sensitivity to a specific type of foreign substance, i.e., a biological response to an antigenic challenge (3). Sensitizing antigens derived from a variety of sources, such as foodstuffs, animal hair, pollen, and dust, may cause allergic manifestations in susceptible animals. The antigen or allergen, which may be a polysaccharide, protein, or simple compound covalently bound to a protein (4), combines with a specific antibody in a previously sensitized individual, thereby initiating a series of steps leading to the symptoms observed in allergy or anaphylaxis. Human allergy and anaphylaxis in most mammals involve similar physiological reactions, i.e., increased capillary permeability, edema, general fall in blood pressure, and contraction of smooth muscle. Although Dale and Laidlow (5, 6) first suggested that histamine [β-(4-imidazolyl)ethylamine] might be involved in anaphylaxis, subsequent studies by numerous investigators have revealed that histamine alone cannot account for all the symptoms of allergic manifestations.

Sensitization involves antibody production stimulated by the antigen (or immunogen). These macromolecules are serum proteins, often referred to as immunoglobulins, and are synthesized from the globulin fraction of blood. Two major types of anaphylaxis have been characterized. One type is termed "active" and results when immunogens in the animal initate production of the antibodies. A second type is termed "passive" and occurs when the animal receives preformed antibodies from an exogenous source. Passive cutaneous anaphylaxis (PCA) is considered a localized reaction, but systemic anaphylaxis also exists (3). Serum antibodies or immunoglobulins (Ig) have been divided into four chemical types and are named IgG, IgM, IgA, and IgE (3). Allergic phenomena are mainly concerned with IgE or reagin (7). IgE is directly implicated in hay fever, some forms of asthma, and some drug hypersensitivities (3, 8). The im-

mediate type of hypersensitivity is mediated by IgE antibodies (9) which are tightly bound to target cells (10). A delayed type of anaphylactic reaction, which may take up to 8 hr before onset, has been attributed to the IgG antibody (11), which is weakly bound to the target cell (10). This may explain its slow onset of action. Through studies using rat peritoneal cells, Bach et al. (10) have proposed that both IgE and IgGa antibodies occupy the same site on target cells. These proposals are in agreement with the results of Stanworth (7), who suggested that the receptor site, although unknown, may be a complex having both binding and activation sites for histamine release (10).

Target cells may be basophils, platelets, or tissue-bound mast cells. The mast cell is a granule containing structure surrounded by a continuous membrane (12, 13). The binding interaction of antigen (7, 14, 15) with the antibody, fixed on the surface membrane of mast cells, results in undefined damage to the cell. Such damage results in the release of pharmacological mediators into extracellular tissue space. Subsequent interaction of the mediators with effector structures on smooth muscle affords the pharmacological response.

The release and response of pharmacological mediators in many mammalian systems has been reviewed (16). Histamine, serotonin (5-hydroxytryptamine, 5-HT), bradykinin, prostaglandins E_2 (PGE$_2$) and $F_{2\alpha}$ (PGF$_{2\alpha}$), slow-reacting substance of anaphylaxis (SRS-A), and aorta-contracting substance (RCS) (17) are among the many important chemical mediators thus far characterized. Antagonists to these agents are considered in this chapter. Additionally, heparin (18), acetylcholine (19), catecholamines, and adenyl compounds (20) play a role in the allergic phenomenon. These substances and/or their antagonists are considered in other chapters. Since a long-term cure of allergic symptoms must by achieved by the slow and tedious process involving desensitization to usually multiple and overlapping antigens, various antagonists to the chemical mediators have been sought. Additionally, ascorbic acid and bioflavanoids have been used because of their antiallergenic activity (21). Symptomatic relief of bronchial asthma is obtained with epinephrine, isoproterenol, and by some more selective β_2-receptor stimulants. Epinephrine may contribute some α-receptor action that constricts bronchial mucosal vessels, thereby reducing congestion and edema, but the principal relief is obtained by direct muscle relaxation of the bronchioles (1). In prolonged attacks of asthma, which may or may not be due to an allergy, both adrenocorticosteroids and aminophylline are useful (1).

2 HISTAMINE RELEASE

Rat peritoneal mast cells (22) and monkey lung mast cells (23) isolated from sensitized animals release histamine by the interaction of antigen with IgE antibodies bound to the cell surface. Although the binding reaction does not seem to involve an energy requirement (24), the anaphylactic release of histamine does (25). The release of histamine in chopped sensitized lung tissue is markedly inhibited by anoxia (25). Others have also observed that anoxia, glucose deficiencies, and metabolic inhibitors (antimycin-A, oligomycin, or 2-deoxyglucose) block histamine release (26, 27) and that Ca^{2+} and intracellular ATP are required for the biochemical event (27, 28). Histamine is released from its ionic binding sites on a heparin–protein complex found in the intracellular granules within the continuous cell wall (13) or plasma membrane of mast cells (29). After membrane alteration of intact mast cells a passive exchange of histamine for cations, possibly Na^+, by the granules takes place in the extracellular fluid (29). The release of histamine is accompanied by a decrease of intracellular

ATP (27) and morphological changes on the mast cell surface after exposure to either antigen, compound 48/80, or extracellular ATP (30–33).

Application of exogenous ATP causes a dose-dependent (33, 34) release of histamine from isolated normal mast cells only in the presence of Ca^{2+}. This response is not uniform for all cells in the same medium. Morphological changes, such as granule alteration, externalized granules, and some vacuole formation are observed (33, 34). Ca^{2+} may release histamine by inducing the formation of vacuoles within the mast cell and serves to fuse the perigranular membrane with the plasma membrane thus forming cellular pores (33). Alternatively, antigen-induced anaphylactic release of histamine from sensitized mast cells, irrespective of the concentration of Ca^{2+}, is inhibited in a dose-dependent fashion by preincubating such cells with ATP (3–12 μM) (35). Apparently, inhibition by extracellular ATP occurs at a step in the release process which follows the binding of antigen or compound 48/80 to the plasma membrane of the mast cell (35, 36). Recent findings show that mast cell active agents (i.e., antigens) do not have a direct action on the granules within the cell (37). In fact, isolated granules are insensitive to horse serum antigen or compound 48/80, with or without the presence of Mg^{2+} or Ca^{2+} (37).

Histamine release from the isolated granules by the ionophore A23187 depends on the presence of Ca^{2+} or Mg^{2+} (37). Alternatively, ATP requires Mg^{2+} for the release of histamine from granules (37); the reverse is found for intact mast cells (34, 38). Ca^{2+} has been shown to exert an extracellular effect on sensitized rat mast cells. This serves to stabilize IgE in a reactive conformation on the cell surface (39). Antigen binding initiates a passing state of increased permeability of the plasma membrane. Ca^{2+} enters the cell, owing to a concentration gradient, and becomes available for energy-requiring intracellular reactions. These reactions promote the influx of Na⁺ and the concomitant release of histamine (40). Antigen, like ATP, causes an increased uptake of $^{45}Ca^{2+}$ into mast cells (28, 41, 42). Foreman and Mongar (43) have proposed that histamine release is the consequence of Ca^{2+} passing into the mast cell through gates in the cell membrane formed subsequent to the antigen-antibody reaction. If Ca^{2+} is added to the incubation mixture subsequent to antigen challenge, no release of histamine is observed. Thus Ca^{2+} must be present when the proposed gates are opened during antigen challenge. Apparently, after some time, such gates close. Owing to its transport properties, A23187 stimulates histamine release subsequent to gate closing (44).

Since cyclic AMP (cAMP) inhibits histamine release induced by antigen, but not by A23187, cAMP has been proposed to act on the Ca^{2+} channel involved in the antigen-evoked histamine release mechanism (44, 45). Presumably, the Ca^{2+} channel is closed by cAMP. A23187 is suggested to be involved in the formation of an artificial channel in parallel to the normal one initiated by antigen stimulation (44). Further work is required to define more precisely the role of antigen, Ca^{2+}, cAMP, and ATP on histamine release.

3 DEVELOPMENT OF ANTIHISTAMINES

3.1 Early Antihistamines

Research on antihistaminic drugs was initiated in 1933 in France by Fourneau and Bovet (46), who observed that 2-(N-piperidinomethyl)-1,4-benzodioxane (49.1) pro-

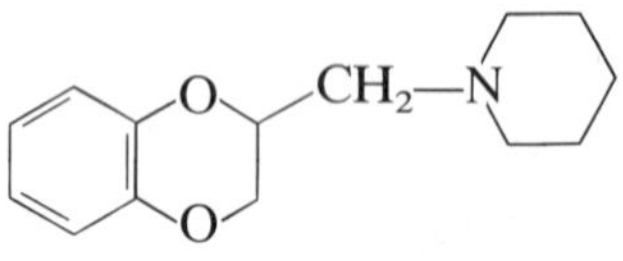

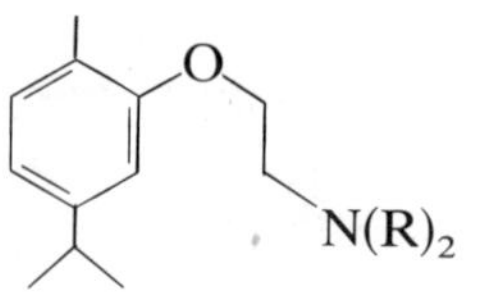

49.2a   R = C₂H₅
49.2b   R = CH₃

tected animals from bronchial spasm caused by inhaled histamine aerosol. Compound 49.**1** had been synthesized from cathachol and epichlorohydrin, followed by treatment with piperidine, and then screened for other activities, among them antispasmodic properties (47). This initiated an eventually worldwide interest in the synthesis and study of related antihistaminic compounds of the H₁ type.

Since 49.**1** may be regarded as an ether, other aryl ethers containing basic side chains were investigated. Of these, β-(5-isopropyl - 2 - methylphenoxyethyl)diethylamine (49.**2a**), a compound synthesized by Fourneau in 1933 (46) and designated 929F or thymoxyethyldiethylamine, counteracted two to three lethal doses of histamine (48). The dimethyl homolog 49.**2b** was less toxic, but neither compound is of value clinically because they are not tolerated by humans.

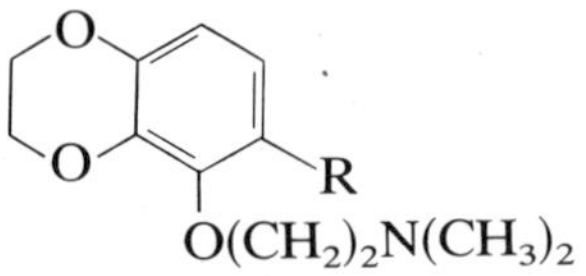

49.3a   R = H
49.3b   R = (CH₂)₄CH₃

Compound 49.**3a**, 5-[2-(dimethylamino)-ethoxy]-1,4-benzodioxane, which possesses the original ring system and is also an aryl ether containing a basic side chain, has antihistaminic properties. Substitution in the 6 position with an alkyl group increased antihistaminic potency with the C-6 pentyl derivative 49.**3b** being the most potent in this series. Compounds 49.**3a** and 49.**3b**

49.1

protected guinea pigs exposed to histamine aerosol and antagonized the contractions of the guinea pig ileum induced by histamine (49).

3.2   Derivatives of Ethylenediamine

Isosteric replacement of the ether oxygen by an amino group affords the ethylenediamine series. As early as 1937 Staub (50) of the Pasteur Institute showed that Fourneau's compound 1571F (*N*-phenyl-*N*,*N*′,*N*′-triethylethylenediamine) was superior to 49.**2a** and 49.**2b** since it counteracted two to six lethal doses of histamine. From her studies with a series of compounds, Staub reasoned that the best hope for clinically useful antihistamines lay in further variations of the structures $RR'NCH_2CH_2NR''_2$ or $ROCH_2CH_2NR''_2$, where R is phenyl or substituted phenyl, R′ is alkyl or aralkyl, and R″ is a small alkyl group.

From these and similar observations, it was concluded that substitution of the benzene ring with alkyl groups increasing in size up to four carbon atoms raised antihistamine activity and decreased antiacetylcholine potency. Variations in the relative nuclear positions of the two alkyl substituents were without effect on the activity, but usually increased toxic side reactions. The findings of the French investigators were corroborated by many others (51), and the search for superior antihistaminic agents was begun.

Not until nine years after Fourneau and Bovet's original work was a clinically useful antihistaminic drug discovered. In 1942 Halpern (52) reported a study of 24 derivatives of *N*-phenyl-*N*,*N*′,*N*′-triethylethylenediamine. Of these compounds, which were prepared by Mosnier (53), the two most potent were *N*,*N*-dimethyl-*N*′-ethyl-*N*′-phenylethylenediamine (49.**4a**), and *N*-benzyl-*N*′,*N*′-dimethyl-*N*-phenylethylenediamine (phenbenzamine, 49.**4b**). Phen-

49.**4a**   R = C_2H_5

49.**4b**   R =

benzamine, which was prepared from *N*-benzylaniline and dimethylaminoethyl chloride in the presence of potassium carbonate (53), served as a model for the compounds of this series.

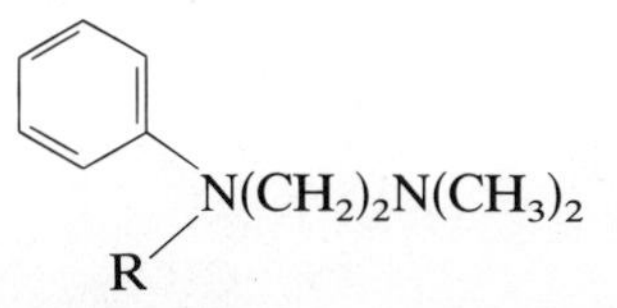

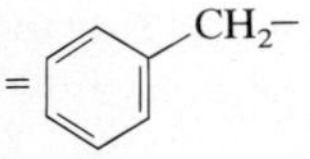

Pyrilamine [*N*,*N*-dimethyl-*N*′-(4-methoxybenzyl)-*N*′-(2-pyridyl)ethylenediamine, 49.**5**, results when the benzyl group of phenbenzamine is replaced by 4-methoxybenzyl and the phenyl group is replaced by 2-pyridyl (54–56). This compound, introduced by Bovet and his associates in 1944, produces fewer side effects such as drowsiness. This initiated a search for other heterocyclic analogs that led to some of the most effective and least toxic drugs in this group. Mepramine, potent in the prevention of bronchospasm in guinea pigs, was synthesized by a method that is typical of the preparation of many similar compounds (57, 58); condensation of 2-aminopyridine with dimethylaminoethyl chloride in the presence of sodamide or lithamide yields the desired compound after subsequent reaction with 4-methoxybenzyl chloride. Most other antihistaminic drugs in this series were developed between 1945 and 1950.

Isosteric replacement of the benzyl group of phenbenzamine (49.**4b**), by 2-thenyl

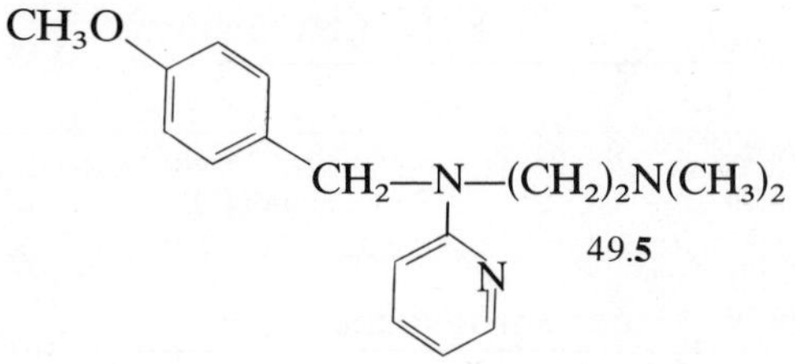

49.**5**

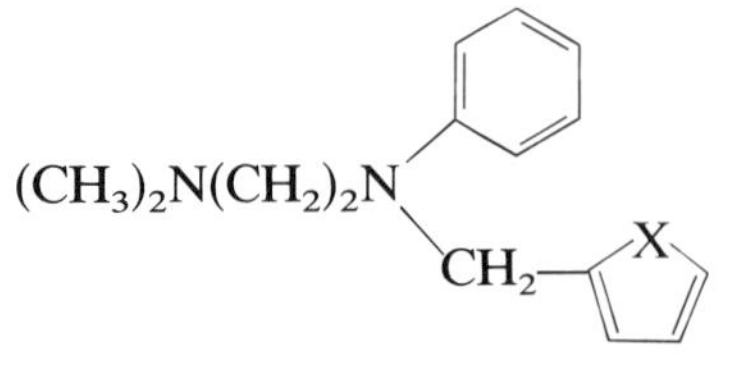

49.**6a** X = S
49.**6b** X = O

(59) affords methaphenilene [*N*,*N*-dimethyl-*N'*-phenyl-*N'*-(2-thenyl)ethylenediamine, 49.**6a**], which is less toxic, but also less active (60, 61). The 2-furfuryl compound, 49.**6b**, has similar properties. Tripelennamine (49.**7a**), the earliest substituted ethylenediamine developed independently in American laboratories, was introduced in 1946 (57). This compound, which is equal in potency to mepyramine on the guinea pig ileum, is widely prescribed for hay fever and other allergies, although it produces many minor side effects. The 4-chloro compound, chloropyramine (49.**7b**), has similar properties (62).

The pyridine homolog, 49.**7c**, of tripelennamine, having a terminal dimethylamino group, exhibited similar potency to the pyrrolidino derivative 49.**7d** (63). Compound 49.**7c** ($ED_{50} = 8 \times 10^{-8}$ M) and 49.**7d** ($ED_{50} = 2.5 \times 10^{-7}$ M) inhibited the action of histamine on the guinea pig ileum. Further, 10 mg/kg and 15 mg/kg i.p., respectively, protected guinea pigs against dosages of i.p. injection of histamine up to 2.9 mg/kg.

A study designed to produce compounds with selective anesthetic properties yield-

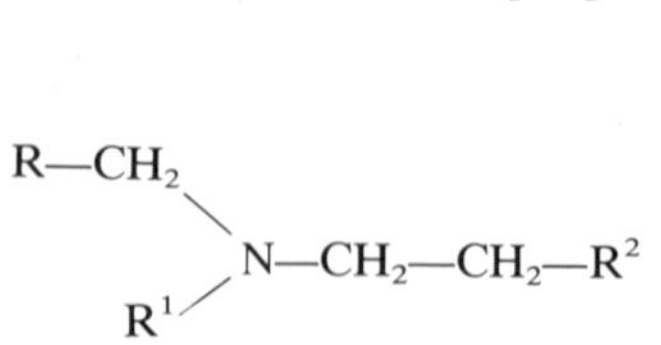

49.**7a** R = phenyl, R^1 = 2-pyridyl, R^2 = N(CH₃)₂
49.**7b** R = *p*-Cl-phenyl, R^1 = 2-pyridyl, R^2= N(CH₃)₂
49.**7c** R = 2-pyridyl, R^1 = phenyl, R^2 = N(CH₃)₂
49.**7d** R = 2-pyridyl, R^1 = phenyl, R^2 = N

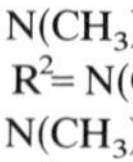

ed the potent antihistamine *N*-(3-fluoro-4-ethoxybenzyl)-*N*-(2-pyridyl)-*N'*, *N'*-dimethylethylenediamine (49.**8**) (64). Similar results were observed with compounds 49.**9a** and 49.**9b**; these compounds inhibited the action of histamine (80 and 100%, respectively, at 1×10^{-6} M) on the guinea pig ileum (65).

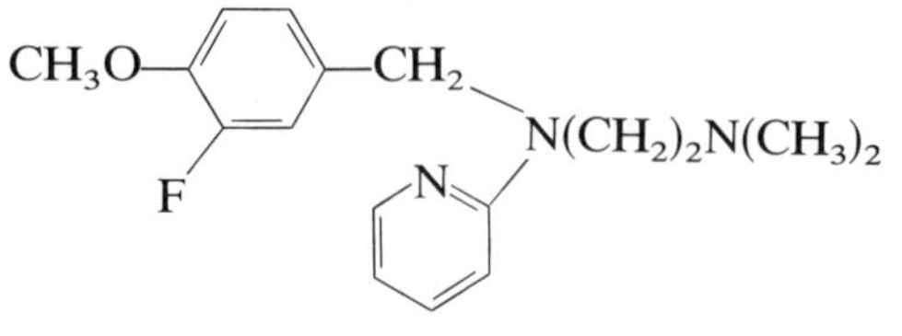

49.**8**

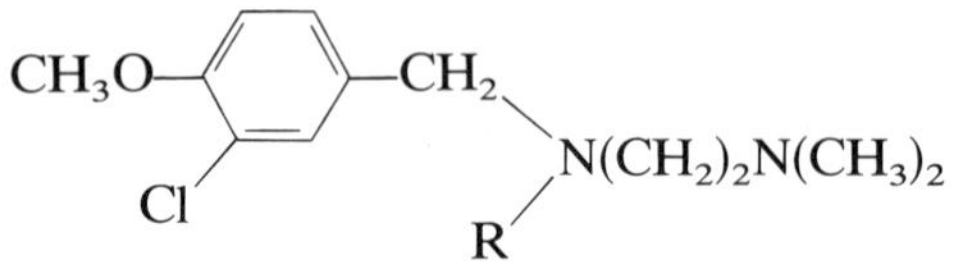

49.**9a** R = phenyl
49.**9b** R = 2-pyridyl

Subsequent to the discovery of mepyramine and tripelennamine, many ethylenediamine-type antihistamines have become available; the choice of a suitable agent often becomes one of personal preference, except where side effects are more pronounced in a particular patient. Deficiencies in potency and duration of action, failure to relieve severe allergic symptoms, and toxic side reactions (66) in existing antihistaminic drugs prompted synthesis of new ethylenediamines. Zolamine (49.**10a**), the 2-thiazole isostere of mepyramine (49.**5**), is reported to have a low incidence of side reactions. Thonzylamine (49.**10b**), a pyrimidine analog of pyrilamine, compares in activity with tripelennamine, but is reported to have lower toxicity (67–69). This compound became the active component of some cold remedies.

Methapyrilene (49.**11a**), the 2-thenyl isostere of tripelennamine (49.**7a**), is

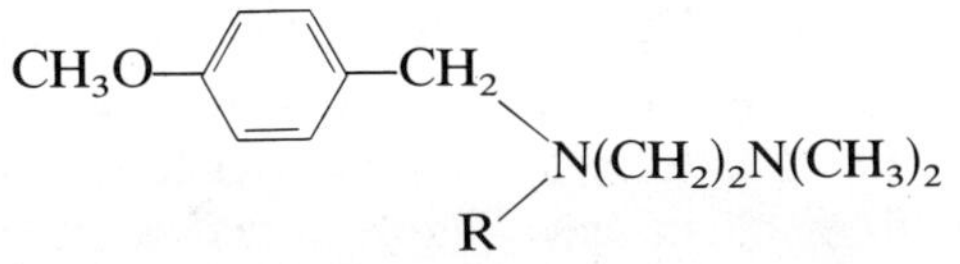

CH_3O—⟨benzene⟩—CH_2
$N(CH_2)_2N(CH_3)_2$
R

49.**10a**   R = ⟨thiazole⟩

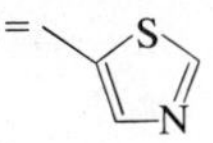

49.**10b**   R = ⟨pyrimidine⟩

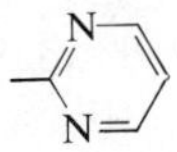

closely related to the latter in toxicity and activity (70). Chloropyrilene (49.**11b**), which results from substitution of chlorine in the thiophene ring of methapyrilene, shows a slight increase in potency and lower toxicity (71–73). In methafurylene (49.**11c**), the 2-thenyl group is replaced by 2-furfurylmethyl without significant change in antihistaminic potency (74–77). The 3-thenyl derivative, thenyldiamine (49.**12**), has about 1.5 times the potency of methapyrilene (78, 79).

An unusual isosteric replacement of the aromatic ring in tripelennamine (49.**7a**) is found in the two selenophenes 49.**13a** and 49.**13b**. Thus N,N-dimethyl-N'-(α-pyridyl) - N' - (2 - seleninyl)ethylenediamine

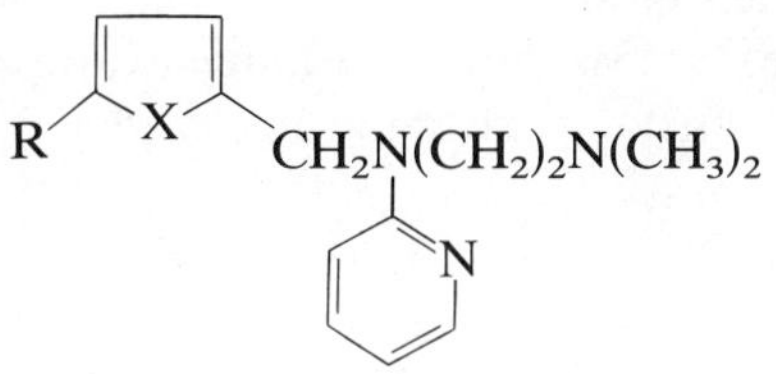

R—⟨X⟩—$CH_2N(CH_2)_2N(CH_3)_2$
⟨pyridyl, N⟩

49.**11a**   R = H; X = S
49.**11b**   R = Cl; X = S
49.**11c**   R = H; X = O

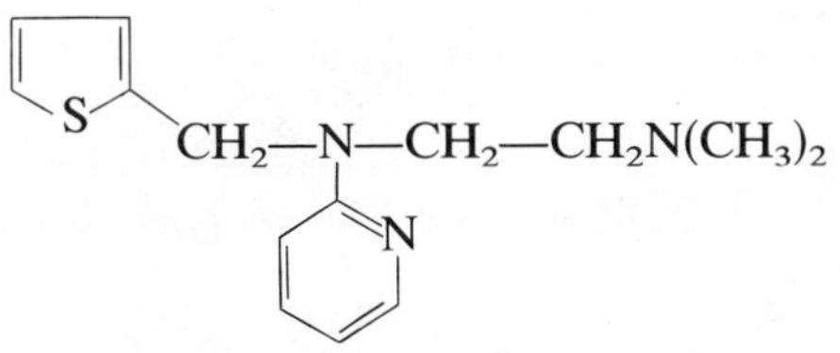

⟨thiophene, S⟩—CH_2—N—CH_2—$CH_2N(CH_3)_2$
⟨pyridyl, N⟩

49.**12**

(49.**13a**) ($LD_{50} = 90$ mg/kg for mice), at a drug concentration of 1×10^{-8} to 1×10^{-7} g/ml, inhibited the response of histamine (2×10^{-6} g/ml) on the guinea pig ileum; at 1×10^{-5} g/ml this compound abolished the effect of histamine in the same test system (80). Selene-4 (49.**13b**), (N,N-dimethyl-N'-(α-pyridyl)-N'-(2-selenyl)ethylenediamine [$LD_{50} = 90$ mg/kg (dogs)], is capable of counteracting 150 times the lethal dose of histamine in dogs (81).

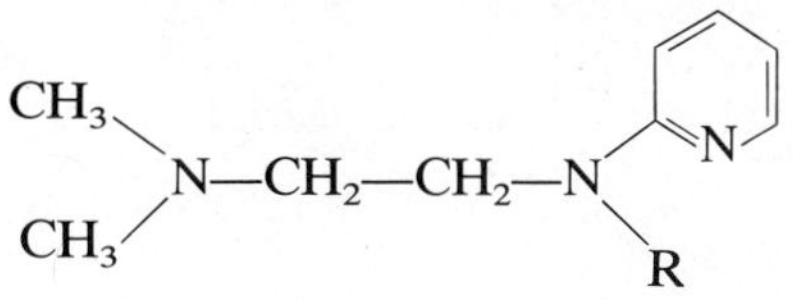

CH_3\
CH_3/ N—CH_2—CH_2—N ⟨pyridyl, N⟩
R

49.**13a**   R = —CH_2—⟨selenophene, Se⟩

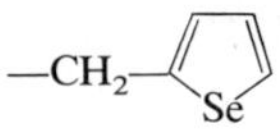

49.**13b**   R = —⟨selenophene, Se⟩

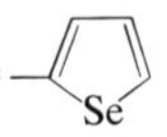

3.3   Derivatives of Aminoalkyl Ethers

Concurrent with the development of the ethylenediamines series, antihistaminic research with aminoalkyl ethers took place between 1943 and 1954. Investigations in the United States began in 1943, and some of the earliest experiments with basic ethers were performed by Rieveschl and Huber (82, 83). In 1946 they introduced diphenhydramine (49.**14a**) the first widely used drug in this series. Chemically, diphenhydramine is β-dimethylaminoethyl benzhydryl ether, a compound patterned on the structure of antispasmodics of the dialkylaminoethyl diphenylacetate type. The compound was synthesized by condensing benzhydryl bromide with dimethylaminoethanol in the presence of sodium carbonate (83, 84).

Diphenhydramine is two to four times more effective than N-phenyl-N',N'-triethylethylenediamine (compound 1571F, 49.**2a**), 16 times more effective than papaverine, and 33 times more so than

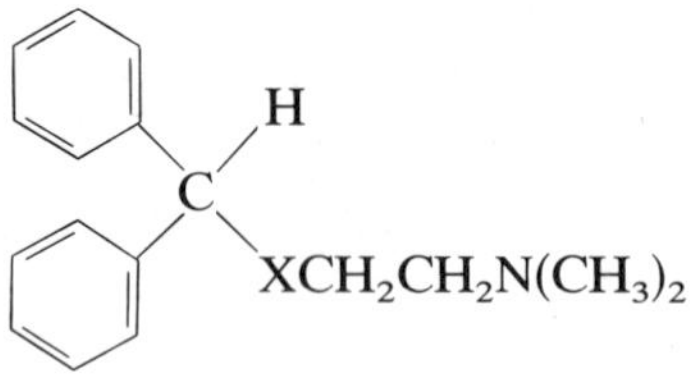

49.**14a**   X = O
49.**14b**   X = S

aminophylline in protecting guinea pigs from lethal doses of inhaled histamine. Diphenhydramine is used extensively in human hay fever, urticarial dermatoses, mild cases of wheezing, and many other allergic conditions; this drug is of little value in vasomotor rhinitis and asthma (85), which may be caused by release of substances other than histamine.

Analogs of diphenhydramine (49.**14a**) that substitute a sulfur atom in place of oxygen at the ether linkage (49.**14b**) are less effective than diphenhydramine, but have increased anticholinergic activity. Apparently, the required hydrophilic ether oxygen link provides compounds of greater potency than their sulfur analogs; presumably, thioethers have sufficient steric bulk which prevents a suitable fit at the receptor surface (86).

Diphenhydramine, dispensed as the hydrochloride, exhibits the usual side effects of drowsiness and nervousness in many individuals. In an attempt to overcome these symptoms, salts of diphenhydramine with centrally excitant purine derivatives were tested. Only 8-chlorotheophyllinate was sufficiently acidic to furnish an isolable salt. This salt, dimenhydrinate (N,N-dimethyl-2-diphenylmethoxyethylamine 8-chlorotheophyllinate, 49.**15**), achieved fame when Gay and Carliner reported it to be 100% effective against seasickness in a study carried out on the rough Atlantic Ocean (87, 88). This study was criticized for the lack of controls, but later work confirmed the compound's good anti-motion sickness activity (89).

Subsequently, diphenhydramine was tested and found to be equiactive with dimenhydrinate in air- and seasickness. This finding might have implied that antihistaminic and anti-motion sickness potency were related, but extensive studies revealed only a few antihistaminic drugs to be effective against motionsickness; the diethyl analog of diphenhydramine, some phenothiazines, diphenylpyraline (4-diphenylmethoxy-1-methylpiperidine), 2-(N-phenyl-N-benzylaminomethyl)imidazoline, and some others have this activity (89). Side effects continue to be a problem with dimenhydrinate. Sedation is the most common complaint, but anticholinergic activity and consequently the symptoms of dry mouth, dizziness, blurred vision, and fatigue are often experienced. Other compounds in the aminoalkyl ether series acosely related to diphenhydramine. Monosubstitution in one para position, as in medrylamine [4-methoxybenzhydryl β-dimethylaminoethyl ether (49.**16a**)], bromodiphenhydramine (49.**16b**), and chlorodiphenhydramine (49.**16c**) may be advantageous because fewer side effects are elicited in some cases (90–94). Utilization of a para methyl group affords the active antihistamine p-methyldiphenhydramine (49.**16d**), whereas insertion of an ortho methyl group causes a loss of antihistaminic properties and enhances atropine-like activity (95–96).

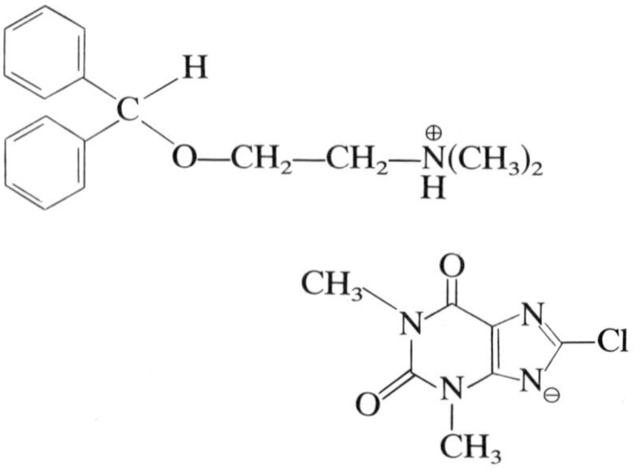

49.**15**

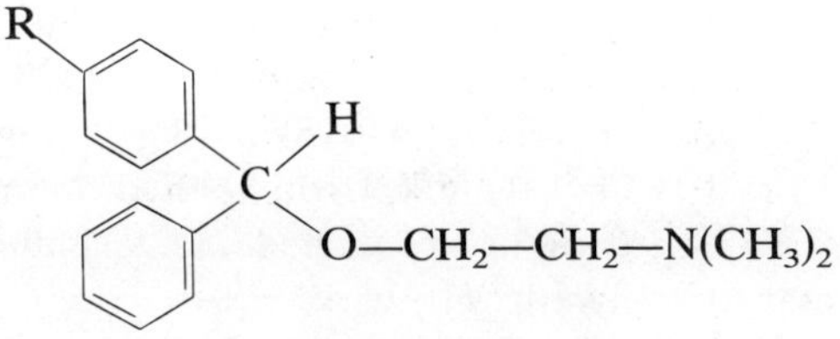

49.**16a** R = CH$_3$O
49.**16b** R = Br
49.**16c** R = Cl
49.**16d** R = CH$_3$

The 4,4′-dimethyl analog of diphenhydramine is less potent than the racemic mixture of the mono-substituted 4-methyl analog (49.**16d**). However, the dextrorotatory isomer is more potent than the levorotatory enantiomorph (97). The low potency of the levoisomer was rationalized on the basis of a possible poor fit at the receptor; the unacceptable protrusion of the 4-methyl group onto the aromatic ring of a proposed phenylalanine residue in the receptor was suggested to account for decreased potency (97).

A series of silicon analogs of known potent antihistamines has been synthesized and investigated for antihistaminic properties (98–100). The silicon analogs, *N,N*-dimethyl-2-(methyldiphenylsilyloxy)ethylamine (49.**17a**) (98), *N,N*-dimethyl-2-(methylphenyl-*p*-tolylsilyloxy)ethylamine (49.**17b**) (98), *N,N*-dimethyl-2-(*p*-chlorophenylmethylphenylsilyloxy)ethylamine (49.**17c**) (99), and *N,N*-Dimethyl-2-(*p*-bromophenylmethylphenylsilyloxy)ethyl-

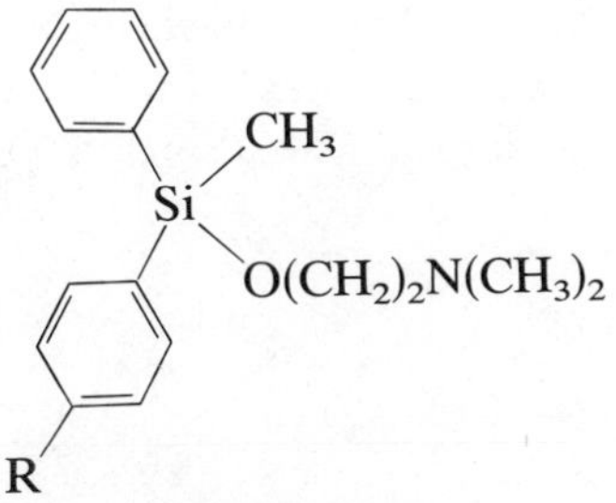

49.**17a** R = H
49.**17b** R = CH$_3$
49.**17c** R = Cl
49.**17d** R = Br

amine (49.**17d**) (100) were competitive antagonists against the spasmogenic effects of histamine on the guinea pig ileum. Generally, they were slightly less potent than the corresponding carbon compounds. The duration of action for 49.**17a** (20 min), 49.**17b** (25 min), 49.**17c** (15 min), and 49.**17d** (14 min) in Tyrode solution at 37°C paralleled the rate of hydrolysis of the silyloxy bond (98–100).

Homologs of diphenhydramine, having the terminal dimethylamino nitrogen in strained rings, also exhibit antihistaminic activity; *p*-methylaryl-substituted analogs containing small basic rings have pA$_2$ values 0.8 times greater than the unsubstituted derivative. Those derivatives having an azetidine ring have pA$_2$ values of approximately 8.7 (i.e., 49.**18a**); the *p*-methyl-substituted compound, 49.**18b**, has a pA$_2$ value of 10.0. Compound 49.**18b** was 250 times more potent than either the substituted or unsubstituted diphenhydramine.

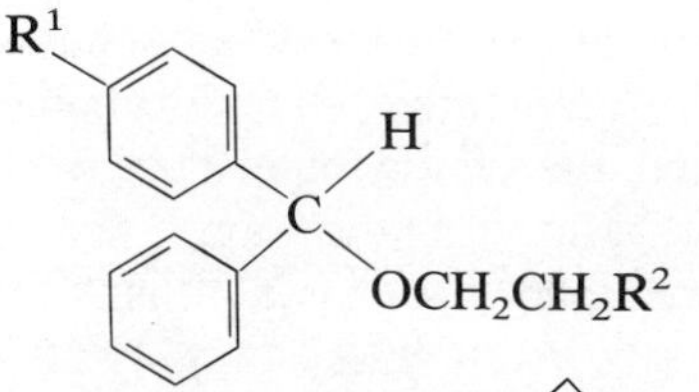

49.**18a** R^1 = H, R^2 = —N⟨⟩

49.**18b** R^1 = CH$_3$, R^2 = —N⟨⟩

49.**18c** R^1 = H, R^2 = —N◁

49.**18d** R^1 = CH$_3$, R^2 = —N◁

Use of an aziridine ring (49.**18c** and 49.**18d**) afforded compounds that were slightly less potent (pA$_2$ = 8.0 and 7.4, respectively). These compounds were classified as irreversible short-acting antagonists when tested on the guinea pig ileum (101).

The *p*-chloro analog, 1-{2-[α-(*p*-chlorophenyl)benzyloxy]ethyl}piperidine (HT-11, 49.**19**), when tested as an antitussive agent, was 0.78–1.36 times as potent as codeine in

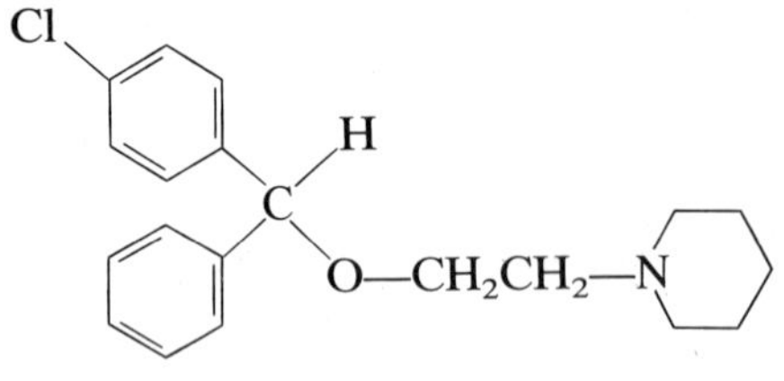

49.**19**

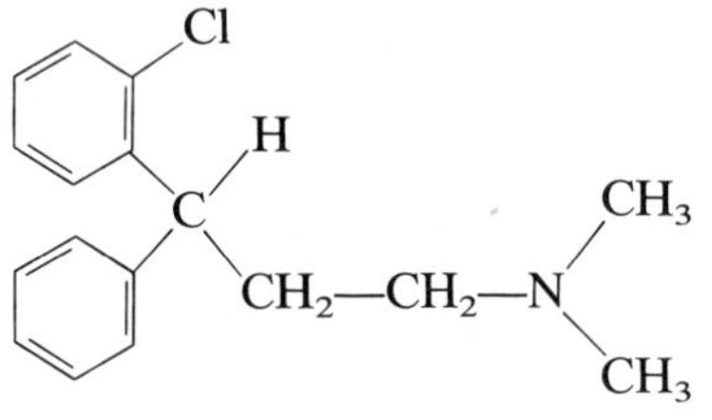

49.**20**

the dog and cat, respectively. When tested against contractions induced by histamine $(1 \times 10^{-5}\,\text{g/ml})$ on the guinea pig tracheal muscle, the potencies of 49.**19** $(5 \times 10^{-7}\,\text{g/ml}, 77\%$ inhibition) and diphenhydramine $(2 \times 10^{-7}\,\text{g/ml}, 89\%$ inhibition) are comparable (102). Chophendianol, α-(dimethylaminoethyl)-o-chlorobenzhydrol, inhibited the action of histamine by 79% $(5 \times 10^{-5}\,\text{g/ml})$ in the same test system; chophendianol also has antitussive properties (103). Both 49.**19** and 49.**20** exhibit cough suppressant and nasal decongestant activity (102, 103).

Quaternization of the amino group of diphenhydramine with methyl bromide affords Paradryl, a potent antihistamine with strong anticholinergic properties (104–107). Similar results were observed with the quaternized p-methyl diphenhydramine analog (108).

Diphenhydramines containing a tropane

ether (i.e., 49.**21**), are able to protect guinea pigs injected with histamine (10 mg/kg s.c.) for 1 hr $(\text{ED}_{50} = 0.185\,\text{mg/kg})$ up to 3 hr $(\text{ED}_{50} = 1.0\,\text{mg/kg})$; diphenhydramine $(\text{ED}_{50} = 1.0\,\text{mg/kg})$ protected the test animal for only 1 hr (109).

Doxylamine, 1-(β-dimethylaminoethoxy)-1-phenyl-1-(2-pyridyl)ethane (49.**22a**), is derived (110) by isosteric replacement of one phenyl group of diphenhydramine (49.**14a** and 2-pyridyl and by substitution of methyl on the carbon α to the ether function. The potency of (49.**22a**) is comparable in activity to diphenhydramine (49.**14a**) and tripelennamine (49.**7a**) (111). In these ether-type antihistamines, substitution of 2-thienyl for the 2-pyridyl group decreased activity. Removal of the α-methyl group and insertion of chlorine into the para position of the phenyl ring in doxylamine afforded another good antihistaminic agent, carbinoxamine (49.**22b**); the dextrorotatory isomer is the most potent enantiomer (112). Phenyltoloxamine (β-dimethylaminoethyl o-benzylphenyl ether, 49.**23**) is an isomer of diphenhydramine that belongs to a most active class of dialkylaminoalkyl ethers of o-benzylphenol and has some effect in preventing histamine induction of asthma in the guinea pig (113–115).

Thymoxamine (49.**24**), which has a dimethylaminoethoxy side chain, is a specific α-adrenergic blocker which lacks β-adrenergic and serotonin receptor activity and is less effective than diphenhydramine as an antihistamine (116). However, 49.**24** can block airway resistance in man induced by histamine aerosol with a single 400 mg dose (117).

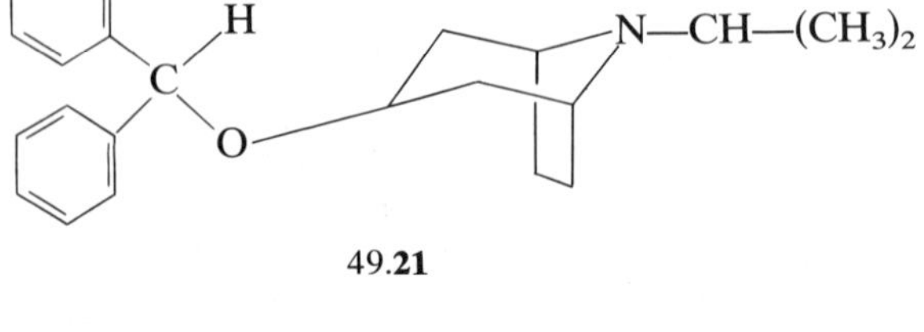

49.**21**

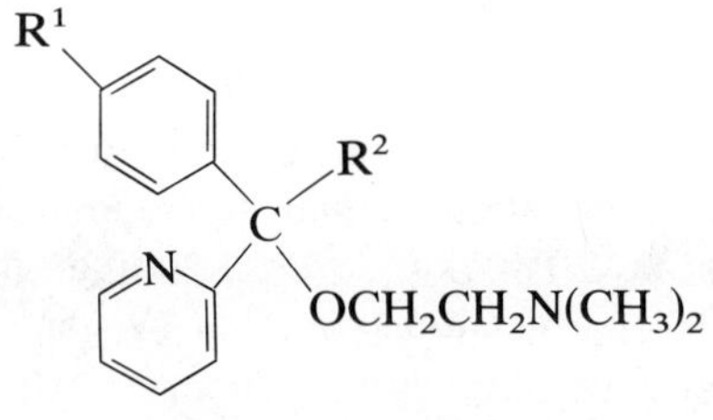

49.**22a** $R^1 = H$, $R^2 = CH_3$
49.**22b** $R^1 = Cl$, $R^2 = H$

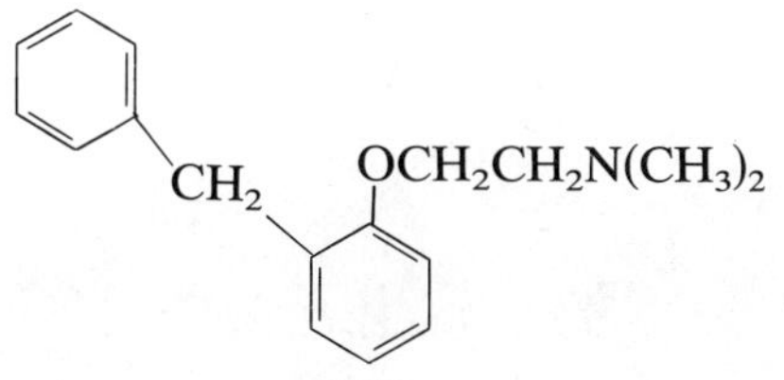

49.**12**

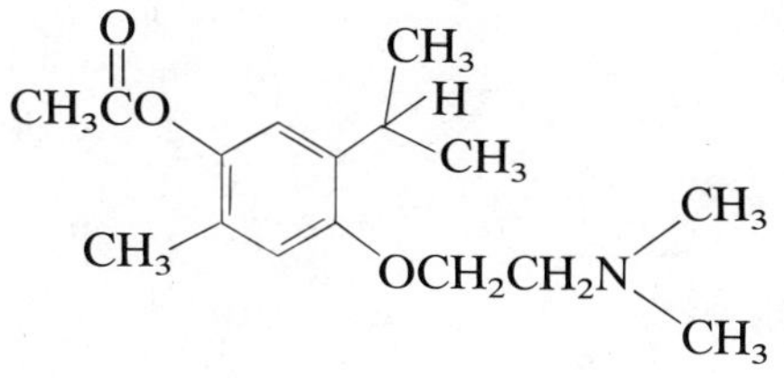

49.**24**

3.4   Derivatives of Cyclic Basic Chains

The search for new antihistaminic drugs was not limited to the proved activity of compounds containing the dimethylamino group; early investigations also included nitrogen-heterocyclic ring systems. 4-(2-Benzhydryloxyethyl)morpholine (49.**25**), having a morpholine heterocycle (83) and diphenylpyraline (4-diphenylmethoxy-1-methylpiperidine, 49.**26**), which contains a piperidine ring (118), are representatives of

49.**25**

49.**26**

simpler heterocyclic compounds found to be active.

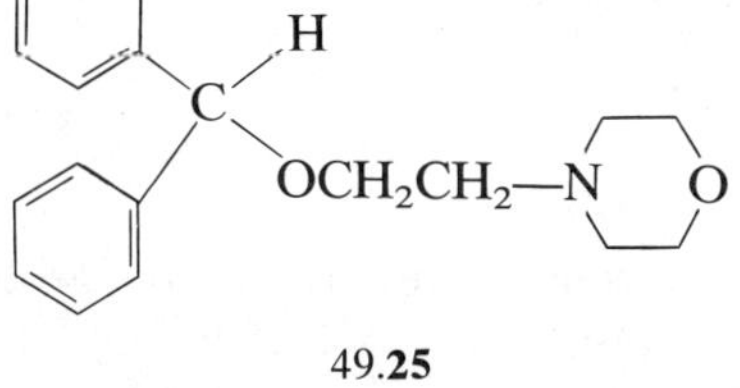

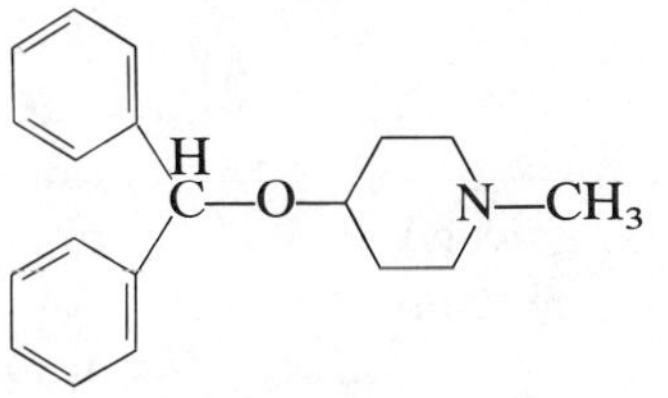

Tavist (clemastine), (+)-2-{2-[(p-chloro-α-methyl-α-phenylbenzyl)oxy]ethyl}-1-methylpyrrolidine (49.**27**), has excellent antihistaminic properties accompanied by a minimal amount of anticholinergic and CNS-depressant effects (119). At an ED_{50} of 0.026 mg/kg s.c., Tavist antagonizes endogenously produced histamine; albumin-induced edema in guinea pigs is also inhibited by this drug ($ED_{50} = 0.0013$ mg/kg s.c.). Tavist also inhibits capillary permeability ($ED_{50} = 1.4$ mg/kg s.c.) as visualized with Evans blue dye (120, 121). Chlorpheniramine (4 mg/kg orally) and Tavist (1 mg/kg) both inhibit intradermal induced wheals by histamine. However, Tavist is more potent (122) and requires at least 8 hr to obtain the maximal antihistaminic response (123). The absolute configuration of Tavist (49.**27**) has been determined by X-ray crystallography (124).

Antazoline [2-(N-phenyl-N-benzylaminomethyl)imidazoline (49.**28**)] belongs to the ethylenediamine series; this compound contains an imidazoline heterocycle and is similar in properties to phenbenzamine

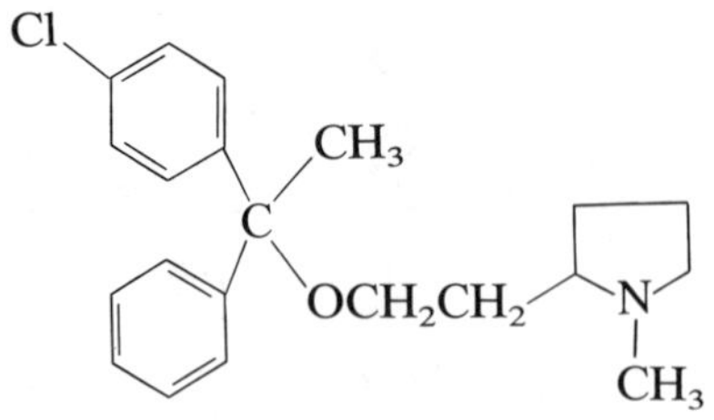

49.**27**

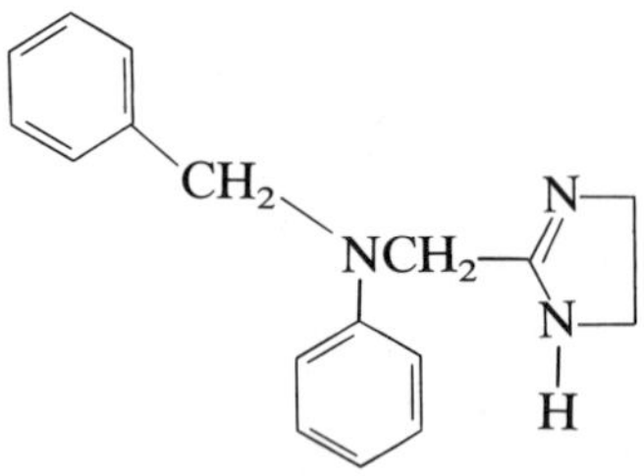

49.**28**

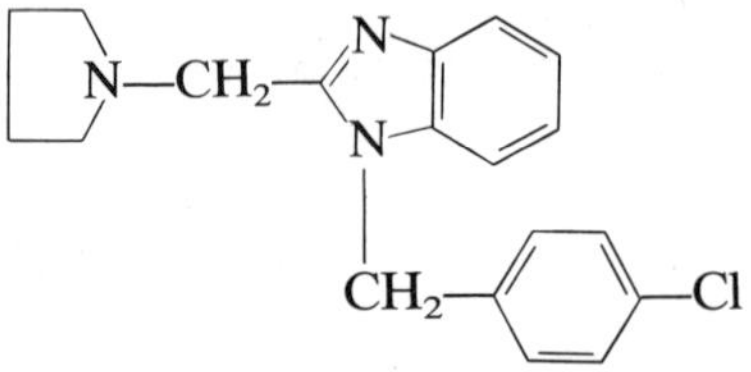

49.**29**

most promising of a series studied (132). The antihistaminic potency of 49.**30** ($ED_{50} = 0.0085$ μg/ml) on the guinea pig ileum was about equal to diphenhydramine; a 20 mg/kg dose protected guinea pigs from histamine aerosol. When compared to diphenhydramine, compound 49.**30** induced less depression, coordinated motor activity, and had anticholinergic effects.

Isosteric replacement of benzyl with 2-thenyl and replacement of the imidazolinylmethyl group of antazoline with 1-methyl-4-piperidyl affords thenalidine (49.**31**), one of many active compounds of the *N*-(2-thenyl)-*N*-substituted aniline type (133). Thenalidine tartrate, in the form of coated tablets, is claimed to be useful in acute allergy colds (134).

Cyclizine, chlorcyclizine, meclizine, and buclizine (49.**32a,b** and 49.**33a,b**, respectively) contain a piperazine ring system (136–142). These four compounds are characterized by a slow onset and prolonged duration of activity and are among the most potent antihistamines (137). Meclizine is also effective against motion sickness (127).

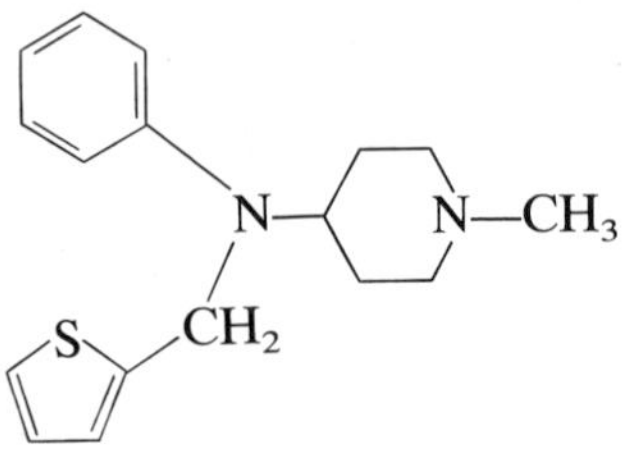

(49.**4b**). Recommended as a nonirritating agent for local application to the eye (125–128), the analog is synthesized by two methods (129, 130). The related benzimidazole, clemizole (49.**29**), similarly contains the ethylenediamine system (131) and has good antihistaminic activity.

Replacement of the imidazoline group in clemizole with a tetrahydropyridine function afforded a series of 2-[1-methyl-1,2,5,6-tetrahydro-3(and 4)-pyridyl]indoles that have histamine and 5-HT antagonist activity; the 4-pyridyl analog 49.**30** was the

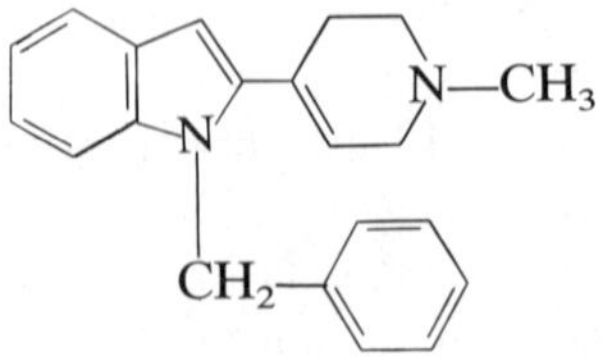

49.**31**

Substitution of the *N*-methyl group in cyclizine (49.**32a**) with a β-methyl styrene moiety affords cinnarizine (49.**34**), a potent antihistamine (143). Cinnarizine antagonizes histamine on isolated tissue ($pA_2 = 7.43–8.1$; 5–90 min incubation time, respectively) in both a competitive and noncompetitive manner (144). The mechanism of action seems to involve inhibition of Ca^{2+} transfer from outside to

49.**30**

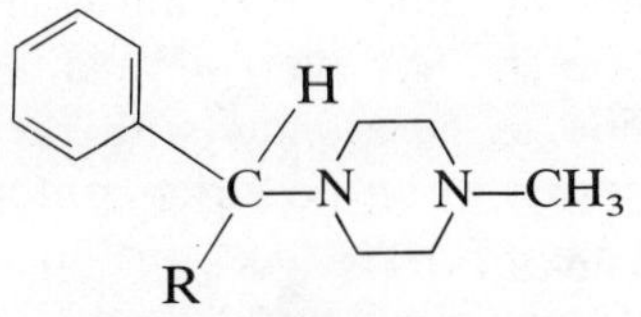

49.**32a** R = phenyl
49.**32b** R = p-chlorophenyl

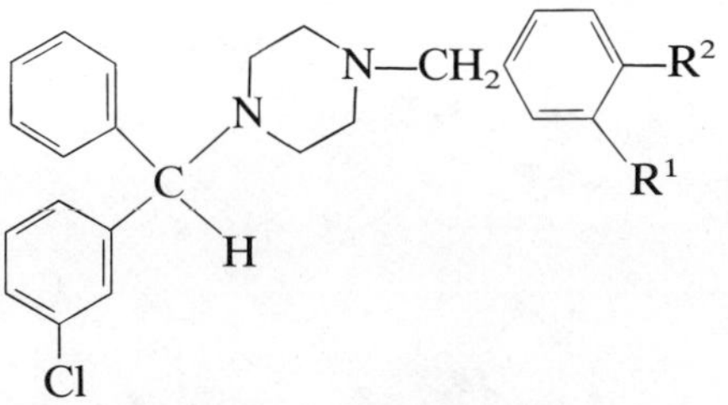

49.**33a** R¹ = CH₃, R² = H
49.**33b** R¹ = H, R² = C(CH₃)₃

inside the cell; such Ca^{2+} migration takes place during contraction of smooth muscle following stimulation with spasmogenic agents (145, 146). This effect is not observed in the resting noncontracted vascular smooth muscle (146).

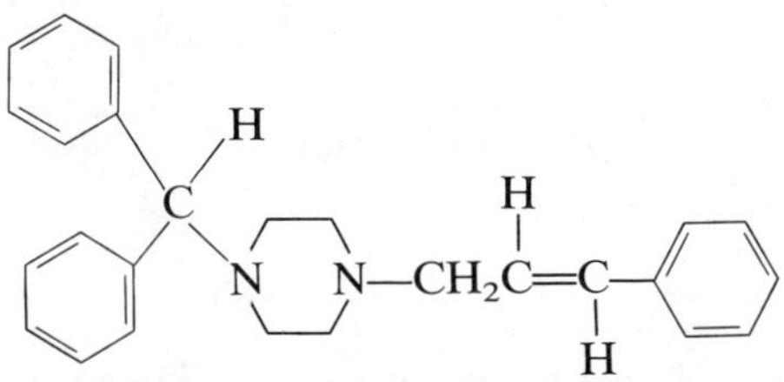

49.**34**

Owing to their lack of solubility, 2,6-dialkylpiperazine analogs of cinnarizine could not easily be assessed for their antiallergenic actions *in vitro* (147). All derivatives of the general structure 49.**35** exhibited limited antihistaminic activity *in vitro* (148). The most potent of the series, 1-(p-chlorobenzyl)-2-phenyl-4-methylpiperazine (49.**35**) ($ED_{50} = 0.19 \mu g/ml$), antagonized histamine(0.1 $\mu g/ml$)-induced contraction on the guinea pig ileum and

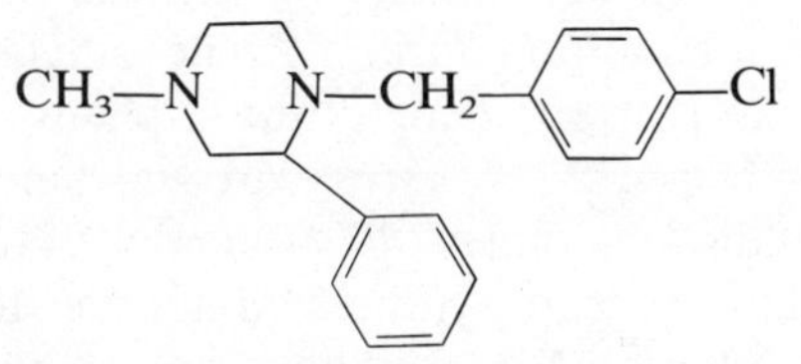

was less potent than diphenhydramine and cyclizine ($ED_{50} = 0.012 \mu g/ml$) (148).

The procainamide derivative, Sl688 (49.**36**), which contains a piperazine ring, protected guinea pigs ($ED_{50} = 7.46 mg/kg$ i.p.) from bronchospasm induced by histamine and anaphylactic shock induced by egg albumin (149, 150). Structural modification of 49.**36** always resulted in decreased potency; alteration of the p-aminophenyl group produced the major decrease in potency (150).

A number of fused ring analogs have appeared in the literature; these contain basic ethylenediamine chains and have antagonistic activity toward histamine in a

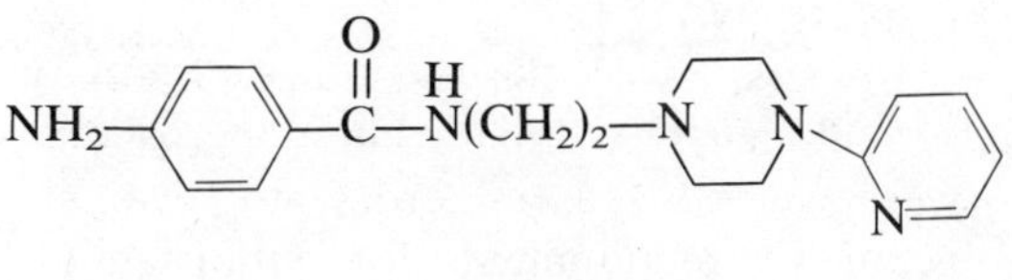

49.**36**

variety of test systems. From a series of diazabicycloalkanes, 2-benzhydryloctahydro-2H-pyrido-[1,2-a]pyrazine (49.**37**) was the most potent antihistamine ($ED_{50} = 4.2 \times 10^{-8} g/ml$ vs. diphenhydramine $ED_{50} = 2.4 \times 10^{-8} g/ml$) when tested against contractions induced by histamine ($1 \times 10^{-7} g/ml$) on the guinea pig ileum (151). In the whole animal, 49.**37** protected the guinea pig from histamine shock (5 mg/kg s.c.) and exhibited activity comparable to diphenhydramine ($ED_{50} = 2.01 mg/kg$ vs. $ED_{50} = 1.14 mg/kg$).

49.**35**

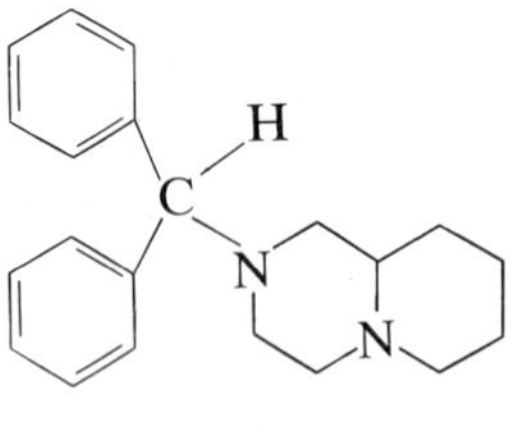

49.**37**

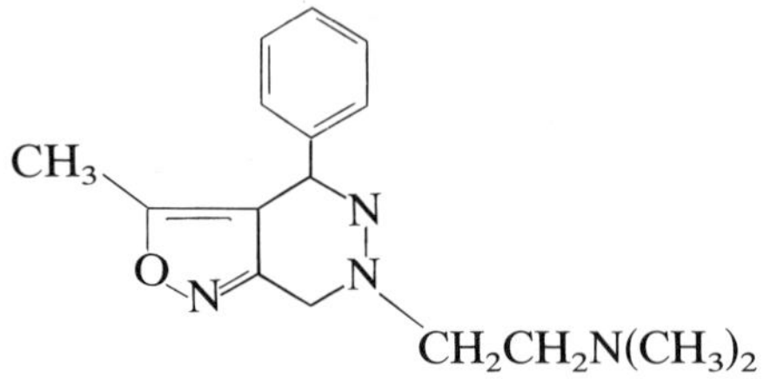

49.**38**

The isoxazolopyridazinone 49.**38** protected rabbits against 20 times the lethal dose of histamine after a single 20 mg/kg i.v. injection of the drug (152).

Carbocyclic derivatives of the hypotensive agent indoramin (49.**39a**) afforded potent histamine antagonists. Substituting the indole nucleus with an acetophenone moiety (49.**39b**) or a benzyl group (49.**39c**) produced compounds exhibiting pA_2 values on the guinea pig ileum of 9.6 and 8.6, respectively (153).

Isomers, cis-49.**40a** and trans-49.**40b**, of 1,5-diphenyl-3-dimethylaminopyrrolidine were synthesized in order to evaluate geometric requirements for antihistaminic

activity (154–156). Both isomers were potent H_1 antagonists; trans-49.**40b** was the most potent and long-acting isomer (154). Both isomers, however, were antagonists to histamine in vitro; thus with these agents there seems to be no strict conformational requirement for H_1 receptor blockade. The trans isomer is active at 2×10^{-9} M and is not easily reversed (155). In a later study (156) 49.**40b** was shown to be an inhibitor of histamine methyl transferase (HMT) while tripelennamine and 49.**40a** potentiated HMT activity. The potentiation of

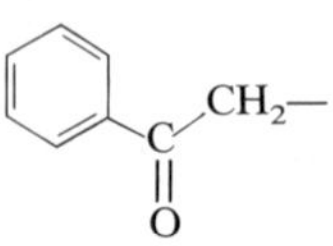

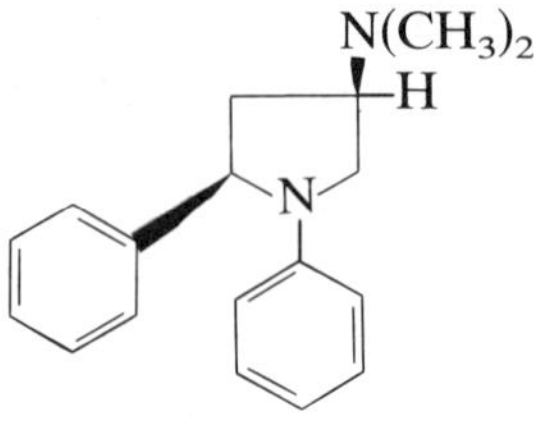

49.**40a**

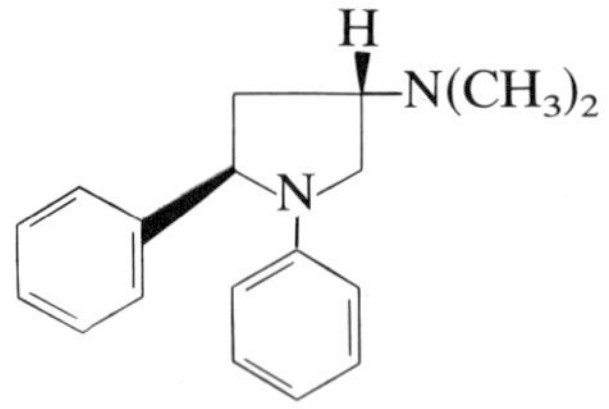

49.**40b**

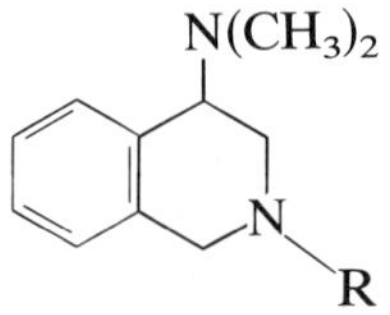

49.**41a**   R = phenyl
49.**41b**   R = benzyl

HMT was found to be due not to enzyme activation, but rather to a reversal of substrate inhibition (156). Cyclic ethylenediamine analogs, namely, the 2-phenyl- and 2-benzyl-1,2,3,4-tetrahydro-4-dimethylaminoisoquinolines (49.**41a** and 49.**41b**, respectively) were synthesized in order to obtain additional information concerning conformational requirements for H_1 receptor

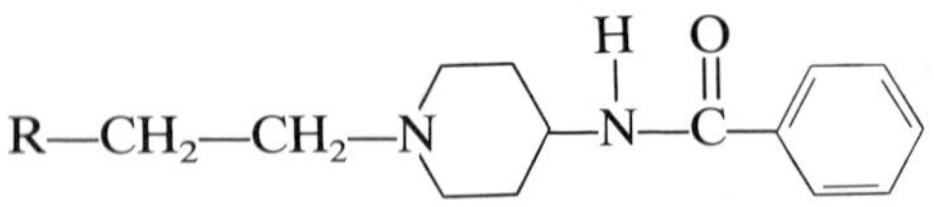

49.**39a**   R =

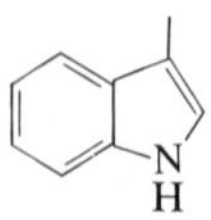

49.**39b**   R =

antagonism. Compounds 49.**41a** and 49.**41b** were found to be weak and non-specific inhibitors of acetylcholine and histamine *in vitro*. The lack of H_1 antagonist activity observed for these two analogs may be due to conformational restriction owing to ortho bonding of the molecule (157).

3.5   Derivatives of Monoaminopropyl Groups

Shortly after the introduction of early ethylenediamine and aminoalkyl ether derivatives, it was observed that appropriately substituted monoaminopropyl compounds exhibited antihistaminic activity. Pheniramine (49.**42a**) and chlorpheniramine (49.**42b**) were described in 1948–1949 (158, 159), whereas brompheniramine (49.**42c**) was introduced in 1952 (160).

Chlorpheniramine [1-dimethylamino-3-(4-chlorophenyl)-3-(2-pyridyl)propane] is a highly active, long-lasting antihistamine that exerts useful protection with a minimum of side effects at doses 50 times lower than those of other widely used agents (161–163).

These monoaminopropyl derivatives contain an asymmetric carbon atom; histamine does not. The region adjacent to the receptor for histamine seems to be asymmetric, however, since stereoselective antihistaminic activity is observed for 4-methyl diphenyhydramine (49.**17a**), Tavist (49.**27**), chlorpheniramine (49.**42b**), and brompheniramine (49.**42c**), with the dextrorotatory

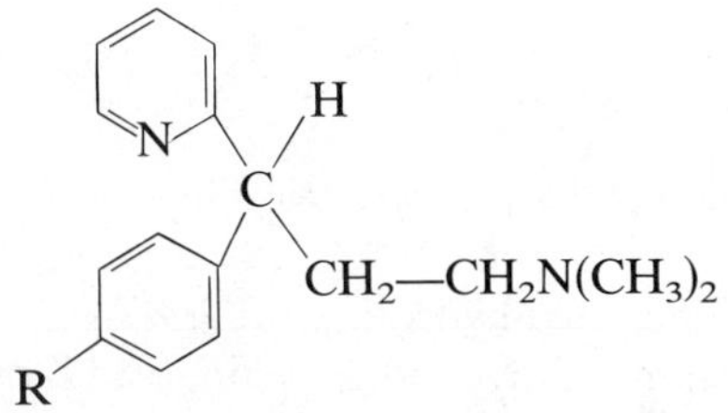

49.**42a**   R = H
49.**42b**   R = Cl
49.**42c**   R = Br

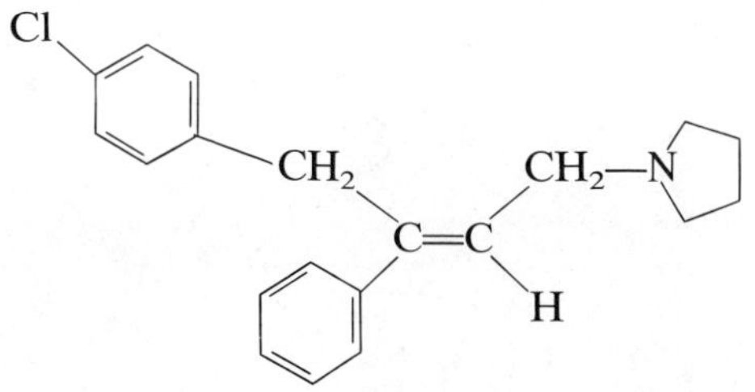

49.**43**

isomers exhibiting the greater potency (100, 124, 164).

Stereoselective activity was also observed with pyrrobutamine [1-(4-chlorophenyl)-2-phenyl-4-pyrrolidino-2-butene, 49.**43**]; the *Z* isomers shows the greatest antihistaminic activity (165). Similarly, triprolidine (49.**44**) is used as the more active *trans*-1-(4-methylphenyl)-1-(2-pyridyl)-3-pyrrolidino-1-propene isomer (166) and has a potency similar to that of chlorpheniramine.

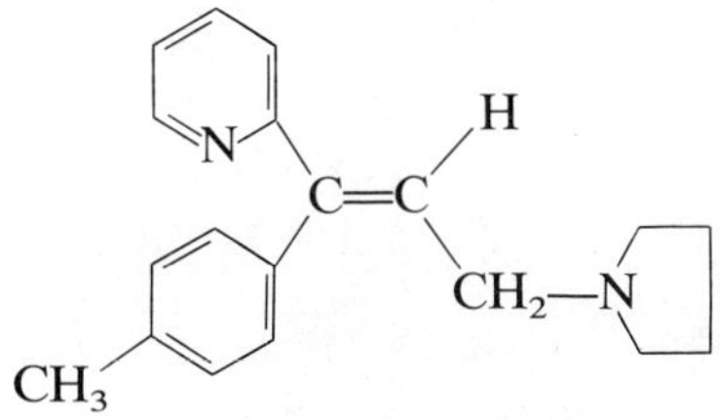

49.**44**

The influence of steric factors at the receptor is further emphasized with the *cis*-1,2-diaryl-2-butene (49.**45a**), which appears to be optimal for antihistaminic potency (167). Triprolidene has similar structural features and may interact with the same drug receptor. The *cis*-piperidino analog 49.**45b** and pyrrolidino analog 49.**45c** are equipotent at 0.01 μg/ml when tested on the guinea pig ileum (168). Related 3-amino-1-aryl-1-(2-pyridyl)propenes exhibit a sharp increase in antihistaminic potency following replacement of the dimethylamino function by a 1-pyrrolidino group (169). The potency of these compounds has been attributed to the influence of the pyrrolidino group on the orientation

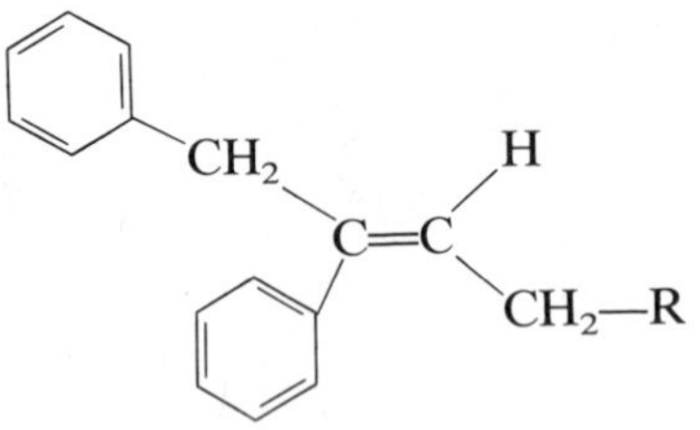

49.**45a** R = —N(CH$_3$)$_2$

49.**45b** R = —N

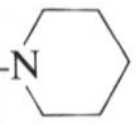

49.**45c** R = —N

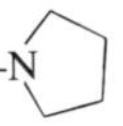

Two epimeric hexahydroindenopyridines were studied to determine the influence of a fused basic nitrogen-containing ring system on antihistaminic activity (172). Analog 49.**48**, which has the basic center coplanar with the aromatic ring, antagonizes the effects of histamine in a competitive manner (172).

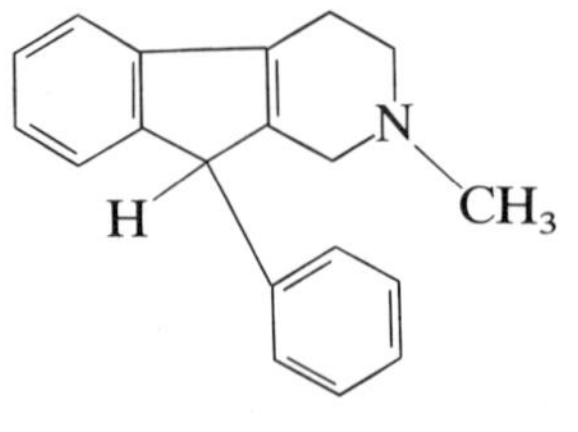

of the adjacent aromatic substituent. Any deviation from coplanarity of the aromatic ring and carbon–carbon double bond alters the biological response. Related 1,2-diaryl-4-(1-pyrrolidino)butenes are potent antihistamines, but exhibit diminished geometrical dependence on biological activity (169).

In dimethylpyrindene {1-[1-(2-pyridyl)ethyl]-2-(2-dimethylaminoethyl)indene} (49.**46**) the activity is found mainly in the levorotatory isomer, which is about four times as potent as dexchlorpheniramine (170).

In phenindamine (2-methyl-9-phenyl-1,2,3,4-tetrahydro-1-pyridindene, 49.**47**), the aminoalkyl side chain becomes part of a tetrahydropyridindene ring. The LD$_{50}$ of this drug in small animals is approximately the same as that of diphenhydramine or tripelennamine, but the substance is reportedly more potent (171). Phenindamine, synthesized in four steps beginning with a Mannich reaction on acetophenone, has found wide use in various allergies and in paralysis agitans.

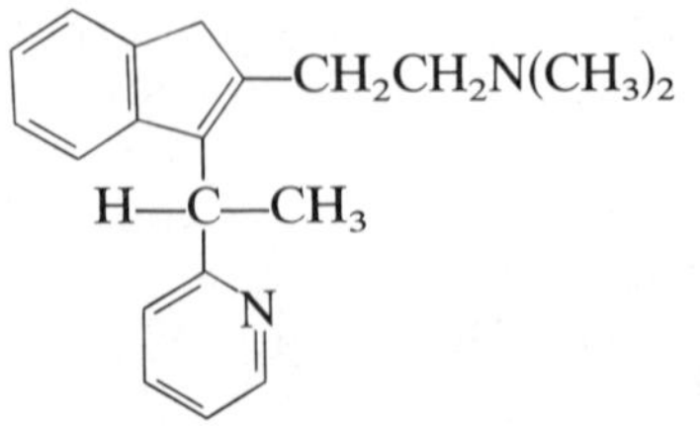

49.**47**

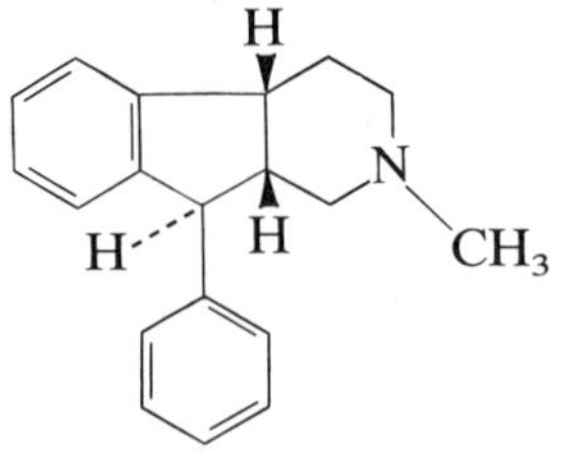

49.**48**

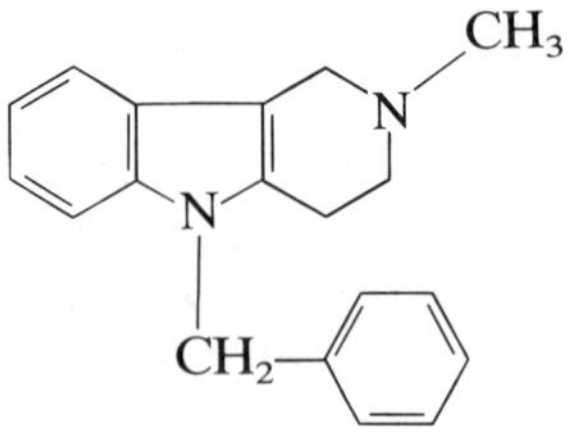

49.**49**

49.**46**

A somewhat similar tricyclic compound, 3-methyl-9-benzyl-1,2,3,4-tetrahydro-γ-carboline (mebhydroline, 49.**49**) is said to be a nonsedative, long-lasting, and orally active antihistamine. It has been used under various names, as the innocuous naphthalene-1,5-disulfonate salt (173, 174).

3.6 Derivatives of Tricyclic Systems

In the case of molecules of the general structure 49.**50** (Y = CH$_2$, a heteroatom, or CH$_2$—heteroatom) it is understandable that the same kinds of R substituents as are found in alkylamino ethers (X = CH$_2$O), ethylenediamines (X = N), and alkylamino-propyl compounds (X = C) are necessary for antihistaminic activity. The structure 49.**50** may be conceived as a molecule in

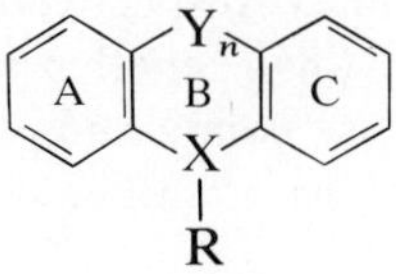

49.**50**

which the benzene rings of diphenyl—X—R, an important requirement for H$_1$ anti-histaminic activity, are ortho connected by Y. The nature of the tricyclic system and the side chain R, as well as the substituents on the A and C rings, have a profound influence on the potency and nature of activity of such molecules. A variety of tricyclic systems have been investigated for their antiallergenic, antidepressant, and antipsychotic properties.

The phenothiazines, introduced in 1945 by Halpern (175, 176), were the first class of potent tricyclic systems to be discovered. The first of the 10-amino alkyl phenothia-zine group, fenethazine (49.**51a**), was capable of counteracting 700 lethal doses of histamine in the guinea pig at a 20 mg/kg dose level (176). Branching of the side chain, as in promethazine (49.**51b**), im-proves antihistaminic potency (176). Pro-methazine, prepared from 10-(2-chloro-N-propyl)phenothiazine in the presence of copper powder (177, 178), at 10–20 mg/kg, counteracts 1500–1600 times the lethal dose of histamine in guinea pigs (176, 177). The duration of action of fenethazine and promethazine is three times that of phen-benzamine (177). Extension of the side chain by one carbon (49.**51c**) and/or exces-sive branching (49.**51d**) inactivates the phenothiazine ring system to H$_1$ histamine antagonism properties (176, 177).

Pyrathiazine (49.**51e**), prepared by N-alkylation of phenothiazine by N-pyrro-lidylethyl chloride and sodium amide (179), is three to four times as potent as tripelen-namine (49.**7a**) and has low toxicity (LD$_{50}$ = 1.5 g/kg s.c. in mice) (180). Pyra-thiazine and tripelennamine are equipotent in the Schultz–Dale anaphylactic test using sensitized animal tissue (180).

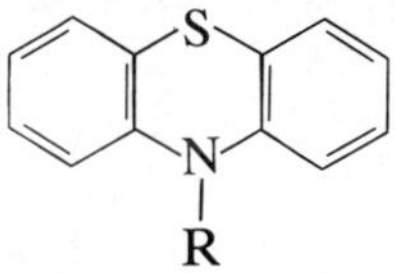

49.**51**

a   R = —CH$_2$CH$_2$N(CH$_3$)$_2$

b   R = —CH$_2$C—N(CH$_3$)$_2$ (with H above and CH$_3$ below the central C)

c   R = —CH$_2$C(CH$_3$)$_2$CH$_2$N(CH$_3$)$_2$

d   R = —CH—CHN(CH$_3$)$_2$ (with CH$_3$ and CH$_3$ substituents)

e   R = —CH$_2$CH$_2$—N (pyrrolidine ring)

f   R = —CH$_2$— (methylpyrrolidine ring with N—CH$_3$)

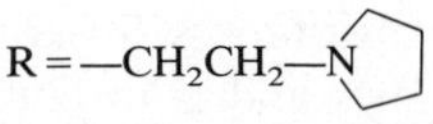

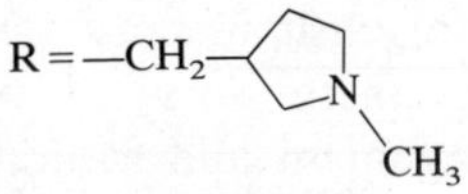

g   R = —(CH$_2$)$_3$N(CH$_3$)$_2$

Clinically, Methdilazine (49.**51f**) and chlorpheniramine (49.**42b**) were found to be equally effective in reducing the symptoms of allergy in patients sensitive to airborne pollen (181). Methdilazine has an outstanding ability to inhibit capillary permeability induced by histamine. The drug is rapidly absorbed by the gastrointestinal tract and is cleared from the body within 48 hr after a typical 12 mg oral dose (182).

Minor variation of structure and salt forms within a new class of drugs changes the activity in a series both qualitatively and quantitatively. 10-{3-[1-(4-N-Methylcarbamyl)piperidyl]propyl}-2-trifluoromethylphenothiazine (49.**52**), one of a series of 20 related analogs, was found to be 3.5 times more potent than trifluoperazine hydrochloride ($ED_{50} = 2.1 \pm 0.8$ mg/kg) or the free base ($ED_{50} = 7.2 \pm 1.15$ mg/kg) in the guinea pig test system (183). Three carbon atoms bridging the pyrrolidino nitrogen to the phenothiazine nitrogen afforded the most potent compounds. Further extension of the chain length resulted in a complete loss of activity (183).

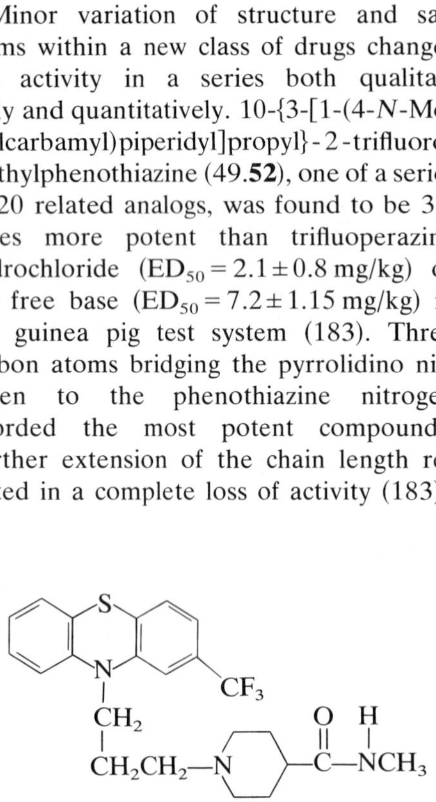

49.**52**

Modification (substituents or ring enlargement) of rings A and C in phenothiazines may either result in increased potency or lead to complete loss of activity (184, 185). Enlargement and saturation of ring C afforded analogs of the types 49.**53a** and 49.**53b**, which were 50–200 times less potent than chlorpheniramine (49.**42b**) on the guinea pig ileum (184).

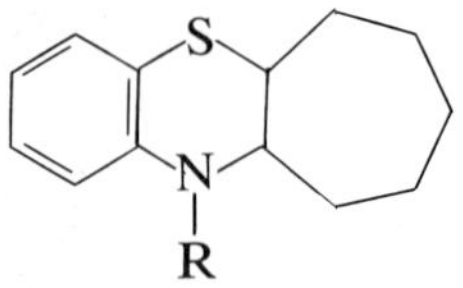

49.**53a**   R = —CH₂N(C₂H₅)₂

49.**53b**   R = —CH₂CH₂—N

Substitution with functional groups known to enhance biologic activity afforded compounds 49.**54a** and 49.**54b**, which were 8 and 600 times, respectively, less potent antihistamines than fenethazine (49.**51a**) *in vitro*. Also these compounds exhibited notable CNS activity (185).

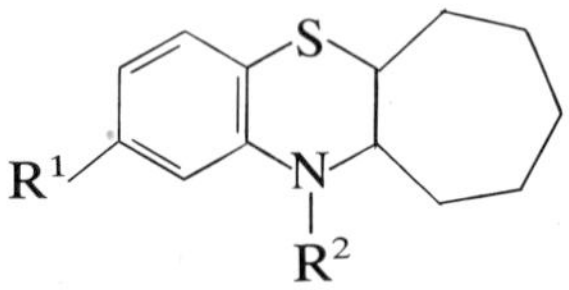

49.**54a**   R¹ = CF₃, R² = (CH₂)₂N(C₂H₅)₂
49.**54b**   R¹ = Cl, R² = (CH₂)₂N(CH₃)₂

The diazabicycloalkane-substituted phenothiazine (49.**55**) inhibited 79.8% of the effects of histamine (0.1 μg/ml) on the guinea pig ileum when 0.02 μg/ml of antagonist was added 5 min after the addition of histamine; under these conditions, diphenhydramine afforded 83.7% inhibition (186). Increasing the linking chain to three carbon atoms increased CNS effects, whereas two carbon chains afforded molecules with the best antihistamine activity (186).

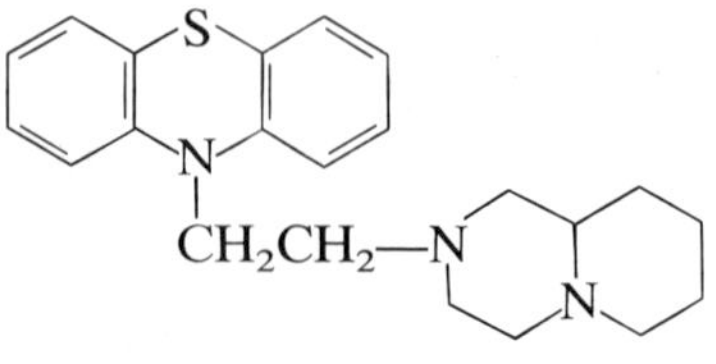

49.**55**

Potent antiallergenic agents were discovered through investigation of a number of 1-azaphenothiazine (thiophenylpyridylamine) analogs (187–189). Generally, derivatives of the 1-azaphenothiazine ring system exhibit more pronounced central and antihistaminic effects over the same derivatives in the phenothiazine series (188). Optimal antihistaminic potency was observed *in vitro* with the 10-substituted *N,N*-dimethylaminoethyl (49.**56a**), *N,N*-dimethylaminoisopropyl (49.**56b**), and *N*-ethylpyrrolidino (49.**56c**) 1-azaphenothiazine analogs (188, 189). The most potent of the series, isothipendyl (49.**56b**) was four times more potent than promethazine on the isolated guinea pig ileum (188). Clinically, this analog exhibits satisfactory activity with single 4–12 mg doses (188). Isothipendyl, in clinical studies carried out in the United States, was shown to be less effective than methdilazine and to have greater sedative properties (181).

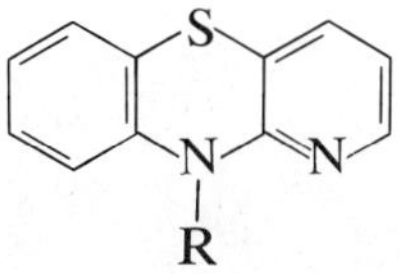

49.**56a** R = —CH$_2$CH$_2$N(CH$_3$)$_2$

49.**56b** R = —CH$_2$CH—N(CH$_3$)$_2$ (CH$_3$)

49.**56c** R = —CH$_2$CH$_2$—N

The 4-azaphenothiazine system (49.**57**) also affords active antihistamines when the *N,N*-dimethylaminoethyl side chain is employed (190). Contrary to what is observed for the phenothiazine tricyclic ring system, 2,7-diazaphenothiazine (49.**58**) was found to be active; introduction of a dimethylaminopropyl group into position 10 (49.**58b**) increases antihistaminic potency (191).

The tricyclic thioxanthene series of compounds, largely investigated for their psychotherapeutic properties (192–194), have

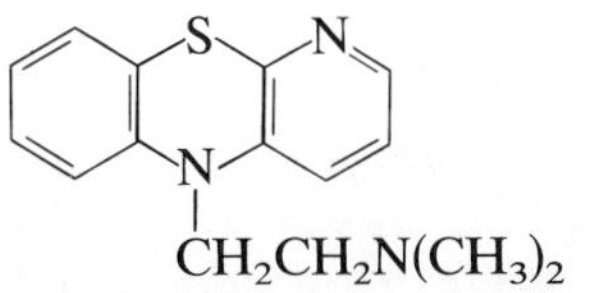

CH$_2$CH$_2$N(CH$_3$)$_2$

49.**57**

R

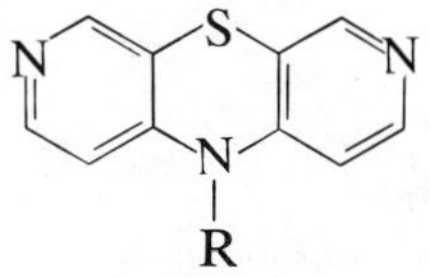

49.**58a** R = H
49.**58b** R = —(CH$_2$)$_3$N(CH$_3$)$_2$

potent H$_1$ antihistaminic activity (193). The nitrogen atom in the phenothiazine ring system may be substituted by an *sp*^{2} hybridized carbon atom without loss of biologic activity (192). One compound, chlorprothixene (49.**59**), exists in two isomeric forms (191, 193, 194). The cis isomer (195) exhibits the greater psychotherapeutic activity, whereas the trans isomer has 17 times more potent antihistaminic activity than diphenhydramine on the isolated guinea pig ileum (193). It is the trans isomer that is the clinical candidate (194).

The related 9-(*N*-methyl-4-piperidylidene)thioxanthene (Calmixen, 49.**60**) exhibits antiserotonin, antibradykinin, anticholinergic, and antihistaminic activity (196, 197); in the rat, 49.**60** is a diuretic (198). Calmixen has clinical efficacy in the relief of allergic rhinitis; 69% of the human subjects receiving 1 mg three times daily responded favorably (196). Calmixen also provides protection in the passive Arthus phenomenon, and also protects rabbits against anaphylactic shock (197). However,

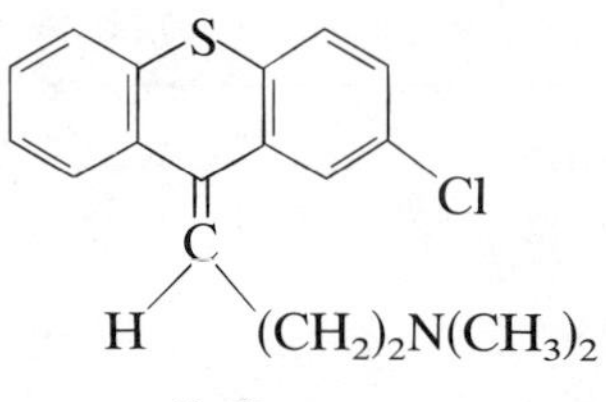

Cl

H (CH$_2$)$_2$N(CH$_3$)$_2$

49.**59**

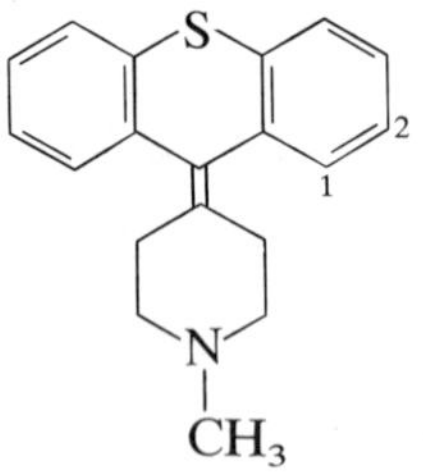

49.**60**

this compound does not reduce or alter the anaphylactic shock induced by antigen in rats sensitized to chick albumin (199). This competitive inhibition of histamine receptors is reported to reduce wheals in human skin induced by polymyxin B, at a dose of 4 mg i.v. (200). Substitution with chlorine in the 2 position of Calmixen decreases the antihistaminic potency, whereas formation of the sulfoxide produces optimal antihistaminic effects (201).

Structurally related 4-azathioxanthenes (49.**61**) and their sulfoxides (with appropriate R groups) exhibit antihistaminic and antiserotonin properties (202), but additional pharmacological data will be needed to determine their clinical usefulness as antiallergenic or antidepressant drugs.

Replacement of sulfur in 49.**61** by oxygen affords the 1-azaxanthenes. One representative of this class, namely, 1-methyl-4-piperidylene maleate (49.**62**) is a potent bronchodilator and mild antihistamine. The bronchospasms induced by egg albumin anaphylaxis are relaxed by 49.**62** in the isolated perfused lung. Analog 49.**62** also protects guinea pigs against histamine

aerosol (ED_{200} sec, 12.2 mg/kg). Compound 49.**62** has *in vitro* an ED_{50} of 0.0009 mg/l. on the guinea pig ileum (203). Interestingly, 49.**62** lowers pulmonary resistance in the anesthetized dog (0.025 mg/kg i.v.), inhibits the release of histamine from rat peritoneal mast cells, and inhibits phosphodiesterase activity by a mechanism different from the β-adrenergic pathway. Substitution of chlorine in the 7 position of 49.**62** diminishes potency.

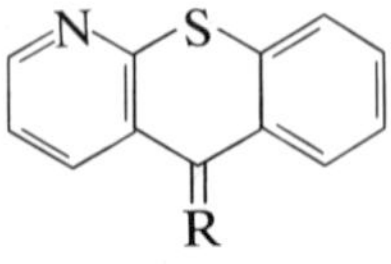

The related 4-azaxanthene, 1-methyl-4-piperidylidene-4-azaxanthene (49.**63**), as the fumarate salt, is more potent than 49.**62** when assessed for its ability to protect guinea pigs from histamine aerosol (ED_{200} sec, 0.71 mg/kg for 49.**63**). Compound 49.**63** exhibits *in vitro* an ED_{50} of 0.0003 mg/l. against histamine, but gives inconsistent results in the bronchial relaxation test (203).

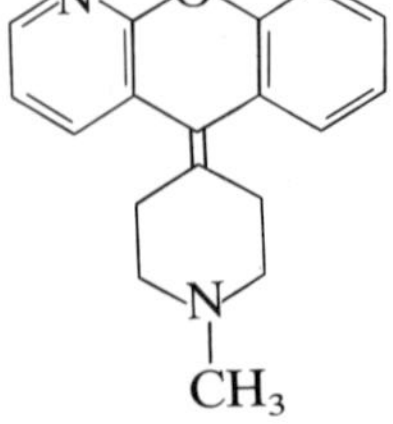

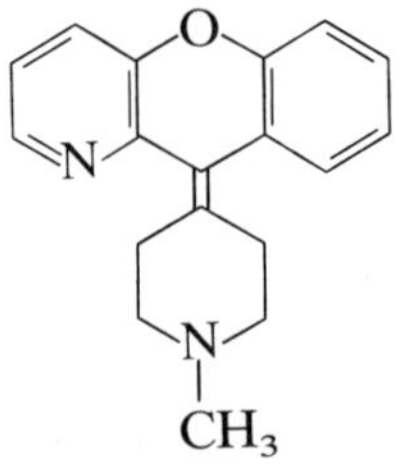

49.**63**

Bioisosteric replacement of the sulfur atom in the phenothiazine 49.**51a** with —CH_2CH_2— or —CH=CH— affords the 10,11-dihydro-5H-dibenz[b, f]azepine (49.**64**) and the 5H-dibenz[b, f]azepine (49.**65**) analogs, respectively. Greater attention has been devoted to the study of psychotherapeutic and antidepressant activity of compounds where R = dialkylaminopropyl, but agents in this series also have antiallergenic activity, especially when R = dimethylaminoethyl (204).

Dibenz [b, e] azepine (49.**66a**) represents the monoaza analog of 5H-dibenzo[a, d] cycloheptene (49.**66b**) and was studied because of its relationship to antihistamines of

49.**61**

CH$_3$

49.**62**

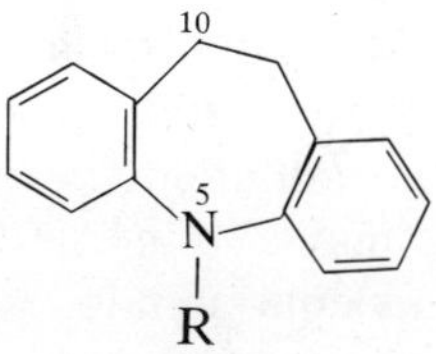

49.64

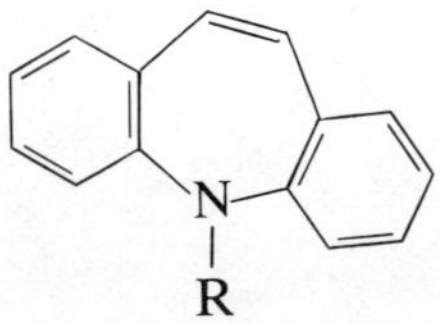

49.65

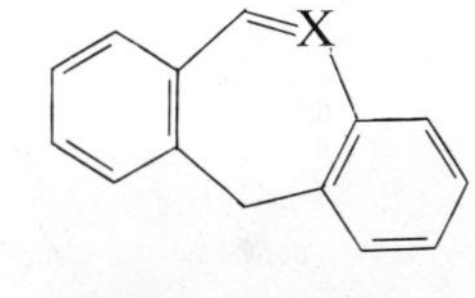

49.66a X = —N—
49.66b X = —CH$_2$—

the benzylaniline type (205, 206). The 5-(2-dimethylaminoethyl)-5,6-dihydromorphanthridine (49.**67**), a 5,6-dihydro derivative of dibenz[b, e]azepine (205, 207, 208), shows high antihistaminic potency, whereas the 5-(3-dimethylaminopropyl) analog 49.**68** is 800 times more potent than diphenhydramine on the guinea pig ileum (209). This observation is in contrast to studies with most other antihistaminic agents where the propyl analog generally exhibits a decrease in antihistaminic potency. The dimethylaminopropyl compound was originally introduced as an antihistamine, but its structural relationship to imipramine (49.**69**) (201) prompted investigation of its CNS activity. The corresponding 6-substituted 5,6-dihydro-11H-dibenz[b, e]azepines (49.**70**) (210), 6-substituted 11H-dibenz[b, e]-azepines (49.**71**), and 11-substituted 5,6-dihydrodibenz[b, e]azepines (49.**72**) are mainly of interest as antidepressants (211),

although utilization of appropriate R groups yields compounds with antihistaminic activity.

Derivatives of 6,11-dihydrodibenz[b, e]-oxepin (49.**73a**) and 6,11-dihydrodibenzo-[b, e]thiepin (49.**73b**) are interesting because of their psychotherapeutic and antiallergenic properties (212, 213). Prothiaden (49.**74a**) protects guinea pigs from histamine aerosol (PD$_{50}$ = 0.46 mg/kg) and can detoxify the guinea pig with a single 0.76 mg/kg s.c. injection 30 min after the intrajugular injection of 10 mg/kg of histamine (213). The combination of equal mounts of prothiaden and Bromadryl, termed Prothiadryl, increases the antihistaminic response in dogs (214). Prothiaden, when not in combination with other drugs, is of greater value as an antidepressant (215). In the 6,11-dihydrodibenzo[b, e]-thiepin series, methiadene (49.**74b**) also is a potent antihistamine (PD$_{50}$ = 0.3 mg/kg) *in*

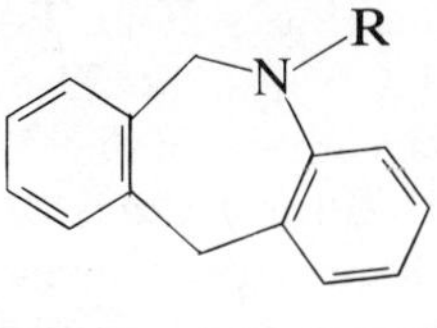

49.67 R = (CH$_2$)$_2$N(CH$_3$)$_2$
49.68 R = (CH$_2$)$_3$N(CH$_3$)$_2$

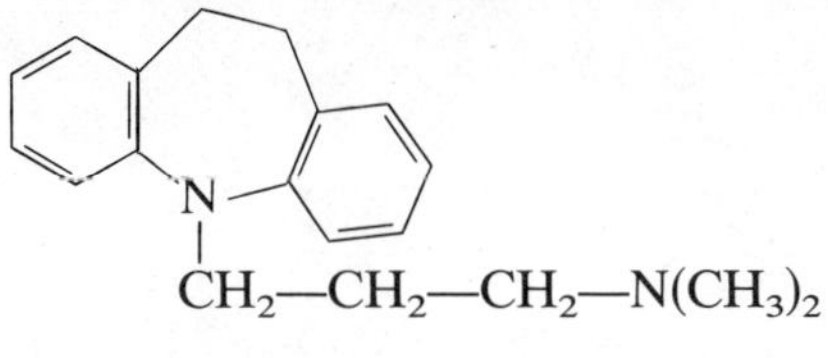

CH$_2$—CH$_2$—CH$_2$—N(CH$_3$)$_2$

49.69

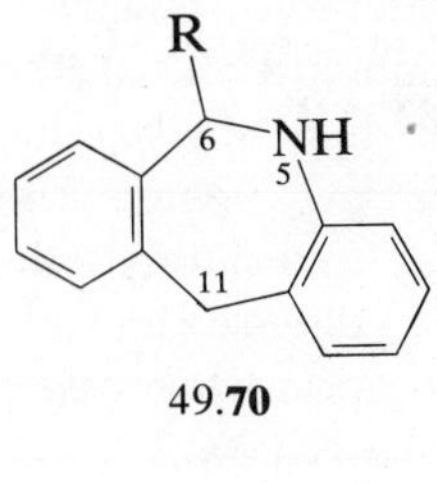

49.70

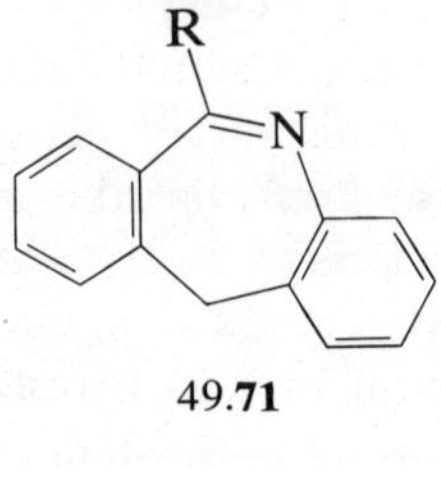

49.71

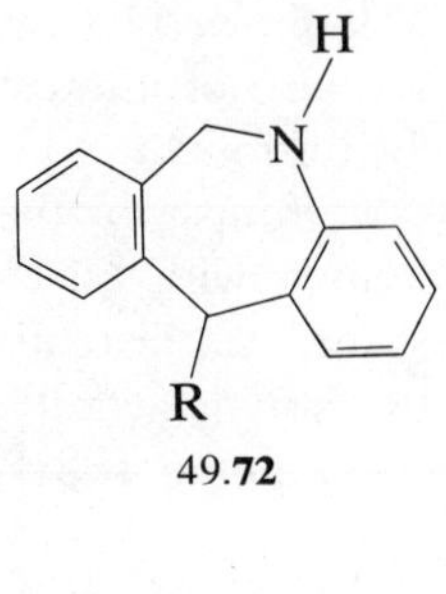

R
49.72

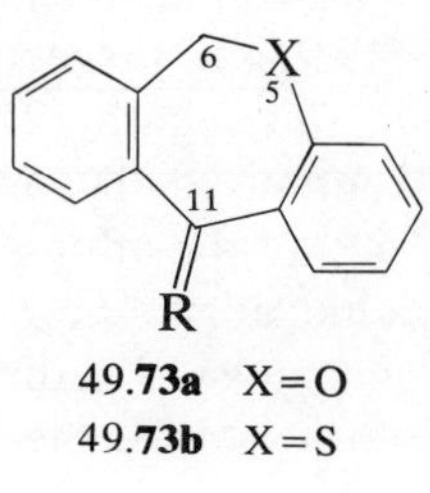

49.73a X = O
49.73b X = S

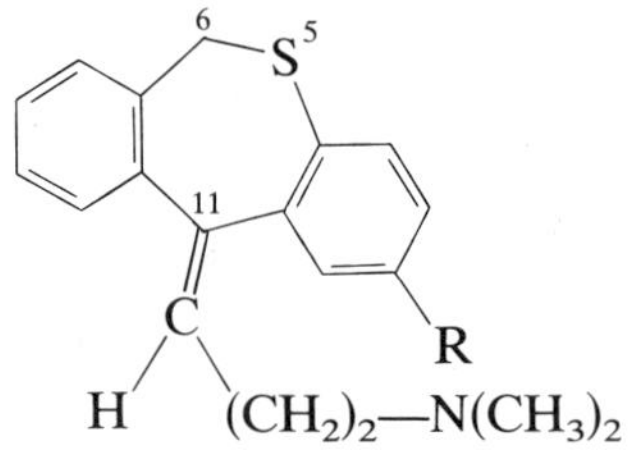

49.**74a**　R = H
49.**74b**　R = CH$_3$

vivo, and detoxifies the guinea pig with a single 0.53 mg/kg dose of drug (215). The trans isomer (PD$_{50}$ = 0.3 mg/kg) *in vivo* is more potent than the cis isomer (PD$_{50}$ = 5.0 mg/kg) or prothiaden (216). However, the cis isomer is more potent than the trans isomer when assessed for its CNS-depressant activities as determined by the rotating-rod test (216).

11 - (4 - Methylpiperazino) - 6,11 - dihydro-dibenzo[*b*, *e*]thiepin (49.**75a**) is also of interest for its anti-reserpine and CNS-depressant activity (217). Amethobenz-epine, 11-(2-dimethylaminoethoxy)-6,11-dihydrodibenzo[*b*, *e*]thiepin (49.**75b**), is a very active antihistamine with only weak antiserotonin and sedative properties. The compound is devoid of antireserpine activity (215, 218).

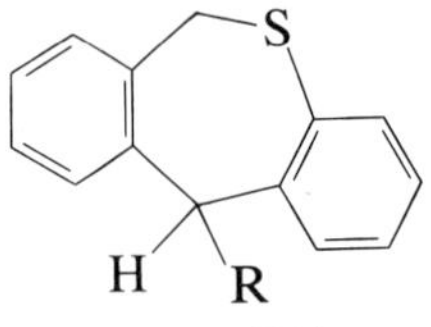

49.**75a**　R = —N⟨　⟩N—CH$_3$

49.**75b**　R = —O(CH$_2$)$_2$N(CH$_3$)$_2$

The related 10-substituted dibenz[*b*, *f*]-oxepin and dibenzo[*b*, *f*]thiepin derivatives (49.**76a,b**, respectively) are also of interest in this regard (219). Substitution by appropriate dialkylaminoalkyl groups at the site of R affords compounds with CNS-stimulating, CNS-depressant, antihistaminic, antispasmodic, and adrenolytic activity. For example; the 11-dimethylaminopropyl-

idenyl derivative of 49.**73a** (doxepin) exhibits antispasmodic and vasodilator activity as well as antihistaminic properties. This compound may also interfere with the uptake of norepinephrine into storage sites (220).

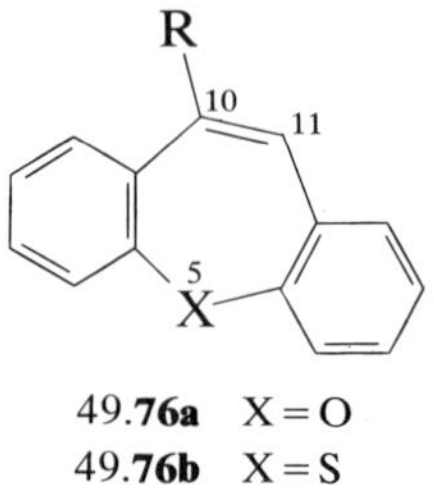

49.**76a**　X = O
49.**76b**　X = S

Using conventional methods 10,11-dihydrodibenzo[*b*, *f*]thiepin 49.**77** was converted (221) to the highly active antihistamine amethothepine (49.**78a**). This analog has strong CNS-depressant activity. The antihistaminic potency is increased by substitution of chlorine into the 7 position. The related 10-(4-methylpiperazine) compound, perathiepine (49.**78b**), also has considerable CNS-depressant, antiserotonin, anti-histaminic, and analgetic activity (205).

As early as 1949 it was observed that the dimethylaminoethyl ether derived from fluorenol (49.**79**) was 100 times less potent than the benzhydryl ether analog, diphen-hydramine (49.**14a**) (218). Protiva (205) suggested that this was the result of a planar tricyclic ring system. For high activity the A and C rings should not be coplanar (205); enlargement of the B ring to six or seven atoms affords active compounds. This observation prompted investigation of the dimethylaminoethyl ether of dibenzo-suberol (10,11-dihydro-5*H*-dibenzo[*a*, *d*]-cyclohepten-6-ol, 49.**80a**) (223, 224). The ether 49.**80a** shows considerable antiacetyl-choline activity and exhibits 10% of the antihistaminic activity of diphenhydramine (49.**14a**) on the guinea pig ileum. The related 5-[2-(1-methyl-2-pyrrolidinyl)eth-yl] - 10, 11 - dihydro - 5*H* - dibenzo[*a*, *d*]cy-cloheptene (49.**80b**) is reported to possess strong antihistaminic activity (225).

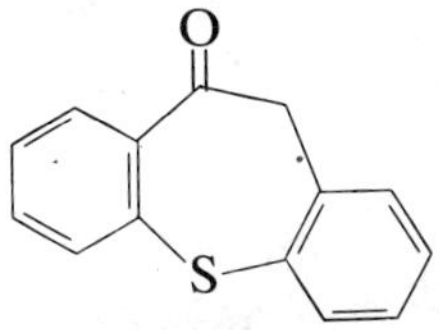

O

49.**77**

R H

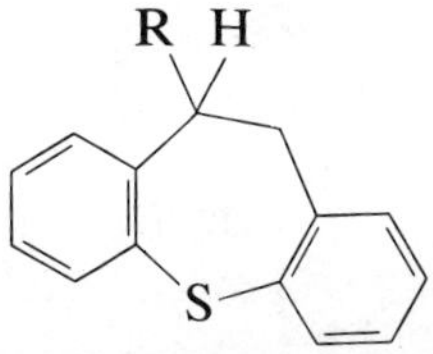

49.**78a** R = —O—(CH$_2$)$_2$N(CH$_3$)$_2$

49.**78b** R = —N⟨ ⟩N—CH$_3$

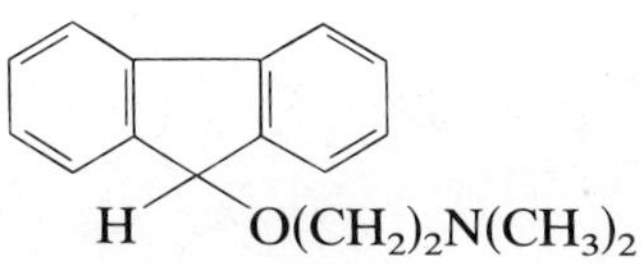

H   O(CH$_2$)$_2$N(CH$_3$)$_2$
49.**79**

Cyproheptadine, 5-(1-methylpiperidy-lidene-4)-5H-dibenzo[a, d]cycloheotene (49.**81**), has no notable CNS action, but has exceptionally high antihistamine and anti-serotonin activity (226), which prompted its use as an antipruritic drug (227). The thi-oxanthene analog (49.**60**) has similar activ-ity, illustrating bioisosterism between sulfur and vinylene in a condensed aromatic ring (227). The xanthene analog is considerably less potent. Saturating the 10,11 double bond of cyproheptadine does not affect antihistaminic activity, but lowers anti-serotonin potency slightly. Alkyl groups larger than methyl or ethyl on the piperi-dine nitrogen, or nuclear halogenation, cause a decrease in both antihistaminic and antiserotonin activity. Introduction of a 5-(1,2-dialkylpyrrolidyl) group into a 10,11-dihydro-5H-dibenzo[a, d]cyclohept-ene (49.**82**) affords a compound that is less potent than promethazine or diphenhydra-mine in antagonizing the actions of his-tamine on the guinea pig ileum (228).

Azatadine, 6,11-dihydro-11-(1-methyl-4-piperidylidenyl)-5H-benzo[5, 6]cyclohep-

ta[1, 2-b]pyridine (49.**83**) as the maleate salt, is the most potent analog in this series. This tricyclic compound protects mice from fatal anaphylaxis (PD$_{50}$ = 0.014 mg/kg) and inhibits the effects of histamine (ED$_{50}$ = 0.72 μg/l.) on the guinea pig ileum; the compound is 3.4 times as potent as chlor-

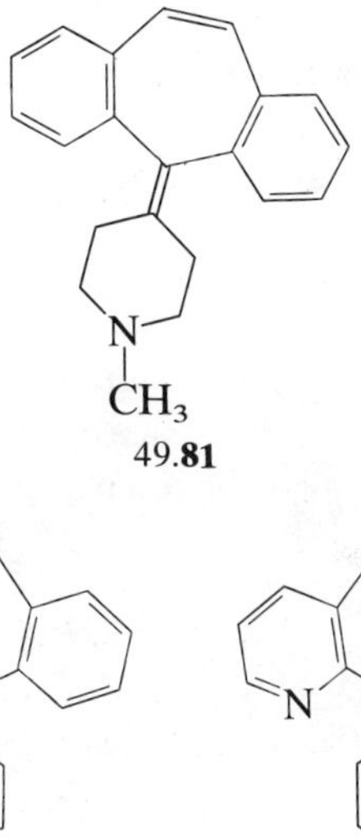

N
CH$_3$
49.**81**

R

N
R
49.**82**

N

N
CH$_3$
49.**83**

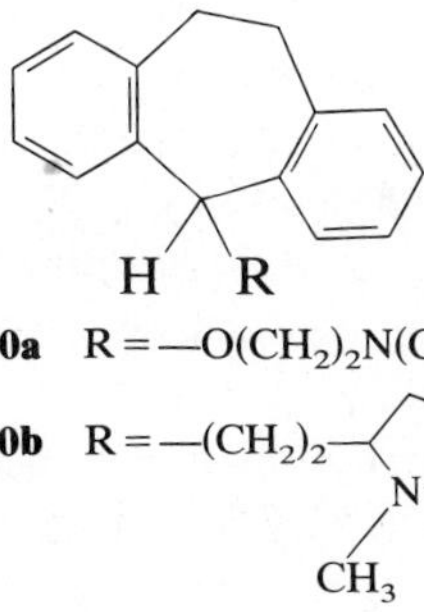

pheniramine maleate. The 10,11-un-saturated compound and the 7- or 8-chloro-substituted derivatives are less po-tent. For arylaza analogs the order of de-creasing potency is 4-aza > 2-aza > 1-aza > 3-aza, when R is 1-methyl-4-piperidy-lidene (229). Azatadine is an effective oral anaphylactic agent in guinea pigs and mice (0.24 and 0.019 mg/kg, respectively), being

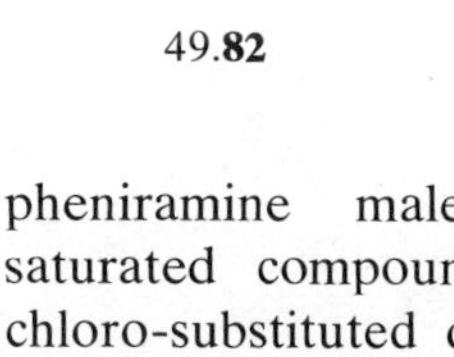

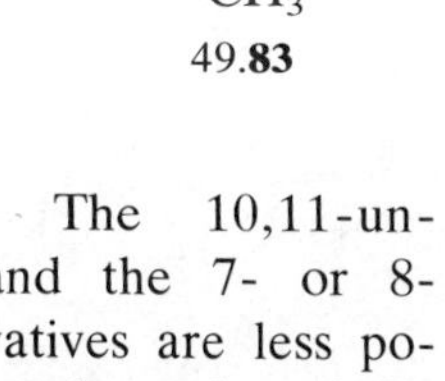

H R
49.**80a** R = —O(CH$_2$)$_2$N(CH$_3$)$_2$

49.**80b** R = —(CH$_2$)$_2$—⟨N⟩
CH$_3$

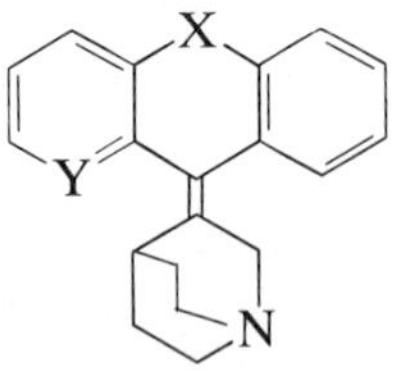

49.**84a** X = —CH₂—CH₂—, Y = —N—
49.**84b** X = —CH=CH—, Y = —CH—
49.**84c** X = —O—, Y = —N—
49.**84d** X = —S—, Y = —CH—

8.7 and 4.4 times, respectively, less toxic than cyproheptidine (230). Replacement of R with a quinuclidylidene ring affords analog 49.**84a**, which is a potent antihistamine (ED$_{200}$ sec, 620 μg/kg) which does not act through direct muscle relaxation (231).

Other tricyclic ring analogs having the quinuclidylidene base, such as 5H-dibenzo[a, d]cycloheptene (49.**84b**) (ED$_{200}$ sec, 2.1 mg/kg), 4-azaxanthene (49.**83c**) (ED$_{200}$ sec, 4.03 mg/kg), and the thioxanthene (49.**84d**) (ED$_{200}$ sec, 3.93 mg/kg), were less potent as antihistamines in guinea pigs. Generally, introduction of the quinuclidylidene base into these compounds in place of a piperidylidene group yields analogs that are more toxic (231). Saturation of the exocyclic double bond and replacement of the piperidine ring with a piperazino group as in 5-(4-methyl-1-piperazino)-10,11-dihydro-5H-dibenzo[a, d]-

49.**85a** R = —N   N—CH₃

49.**85b** R = —O   N—CH₃

49.**85c** R = —O   N—CH₂CN

cycloheptene (49.**85a**) also affords effective antiallergenic agents (232).

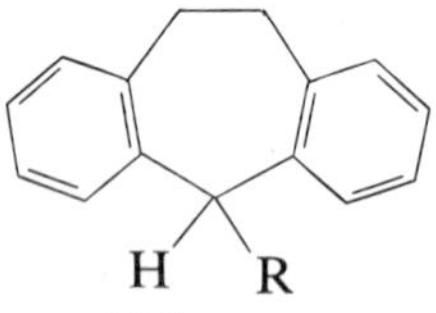

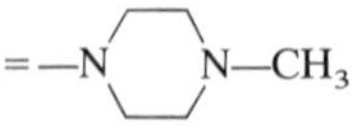

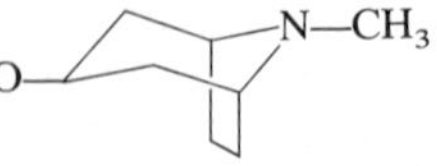

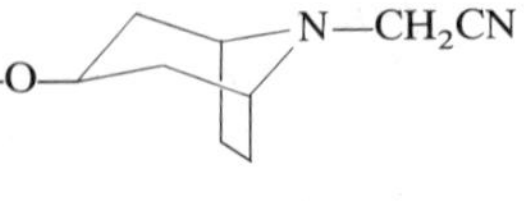

Deptropine (49.**85b**), also known as dibenzheptropine, contains a tropanyl ether group; it is one of many basic dibenzosuberyl ethers studied (233), and exhibits strong antihistaminic, antiserotonin, and anticholinergic activity. Although the compound has only 1/70 the antiserotonin activity of lysergic acid diethylamide on the rat uterus, it exhibits considerable protection against serotonin-induced asthma. Deptropine has 55–110 times the antihistaminic potency of diphenhydramine (49.**14a**) on the guinea pig ileum, but it has no effect on histamine-induced gastric secretion in the cat. Considerable protection is afforded guinea pigs during anaphylactic shock upon oral or parenteral administration of deptropine.

The methobromide salt of deptropine citrate and the maleate of 49.**86a** are reported to be as potent as the tertiary bases, but have little or no central effects; it was assumed that quaternary compounds do not pass the blood–brain barrier (234). Considerably weaker peripheral anticholinergic, but more potent antihistaminic properties are observed with the 1-aza-10,11-dihydrodibenzocycloheptene analog BS-7723 (49.**86b**) (235). BS-7723 protects guinea pigs from histamine aerosol; in bronchial asthma this analog may have the advantageous property of stimulating the cilia of the tracheal strip (235). Many related derivatives of 5H-dibenzo[a, d]cycloheptene have been prepared for evaluation as psychotherapeutic agents (236). Other substituted systems, with longer alkylaminoalkyl side chains, have only very weak antihistaminic activity. The N-substituted alkyl nitrile analog 49.**85c** is only two to four times as potent as diphenhydramine, but is reported to have significantly less anticholinergic activity (237).

Structurally related hepzidine, 4-[10,11-dihydro-5H-[a, d]cyclohepten-5-yl)oxy]-1-methylpiperidine (49.**87**), as the hydrogen

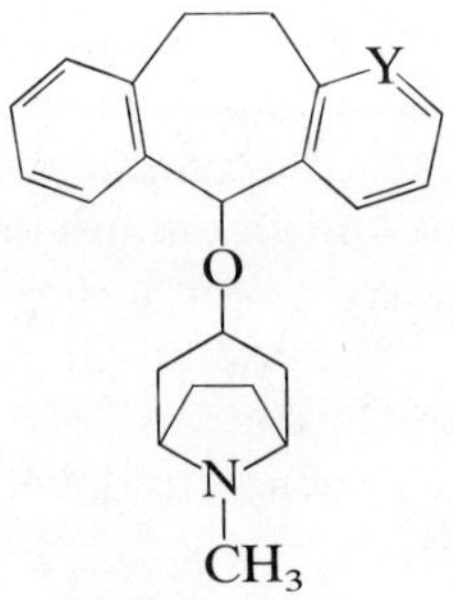

49.**86a** Y = —CH—
49.**86b** Y = —N—

maleate (238), has antidepressant properties. However, it is two to four times more
potent than diphenhydramine in antagonizing the effects of histamine in the
peripheral vasculature. Hepzidine is 10–20
times less effective in reducing histamine-
induced anaphylactic shock in guinea pigs
when compared to deptropine and cyproheptadine (239, 240). This compound also
exhibits anticholinergic and antiserotonin
properties. Tricyclic spirodioxolanes, having the general structure 49.**88**, also have
antihistaminic and antiserotonin properties
(241).

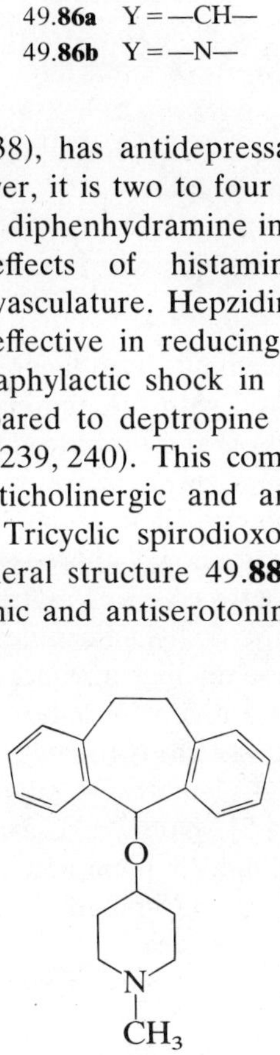

49.**87**

Compounds of the structure 49.**88**, where
R = CH$_3$, X = —OCH$_2$—, —CH$_2$CH$_2$—,
and —CH=CH—, exhibited the more pronounced antihistaminic activity; such compounds antagonize the effects of histamine
(50 μg/ml) at a concentration of 0.25–0.3
μg/ml of drug on the guinea pig ileum.
Generally, increasing the size of the
R group results in decreased anti-

histaminic potency; compounds with X =
—CH$_2$CH$_2$— were generally more potent
antiserotoninergic agents (241).

Antiallergenic compounds may also be
derived from the isomeric 10,11-dihydro-
5H-dibenzo[a, d]cyclohepten-10-one [di-
benzosuber-10-one ring system (49.**89**)]
(238, 242). The corresponding amine
49.**90a** (205) and its N-methyl and N,N-di-
methyl derivatives show CNS-depressant
and antihistaminic activity. 10-(4-Methyl-
1-piperazino)-10,11-dihydro-5H-dibenzo-
[a, d]cycloheptene (49.**90b**) (243) and ame-
thoptene (49.**90c**), a 10-(2-dimethylamino-
ethyl) ether of 10-dibenzosuberol, are reported (205) to have a high degree of antihistaminic and CNS-depressant activity.

Homophenothiazine, dihydrodibenzo-[b,
f](1,4)thiazepin (49.**91**) (205, 244), prepared in a four-step synthesis from methyl
2-thiosalicylate and 2-chloronitrobenzene,

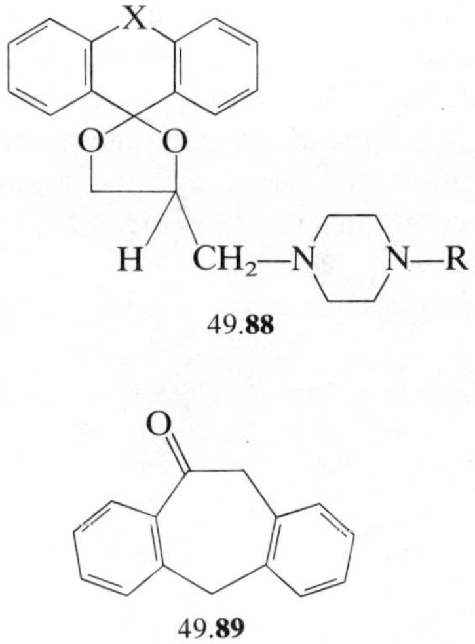

49.**88**

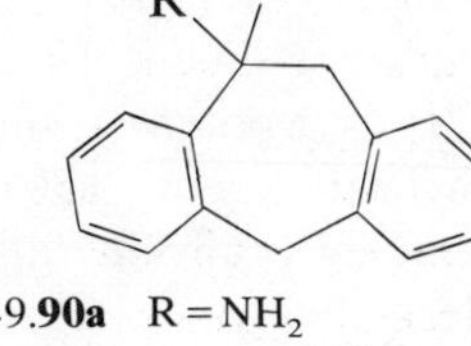

49.**89**

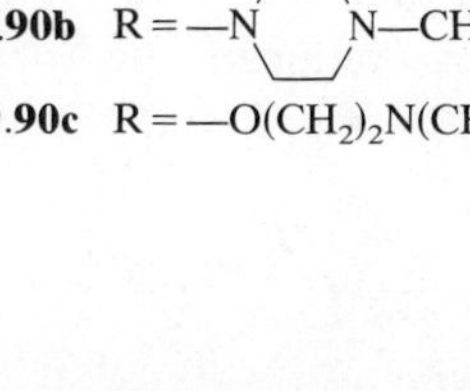

49.**90a** R = NH$_2$
49.**90b** R = —N( )N—CH$_3$
49.**90c** R = —O(CH$_2$)$_2$N(CH$_3$)$_2$

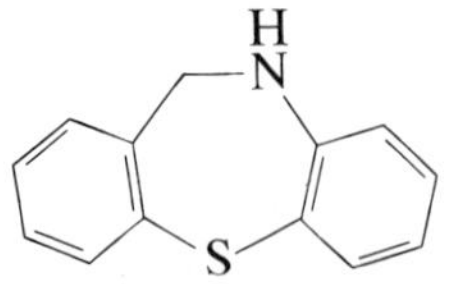

49.**91**

yields active antiallergenic and anti-depressant drugs upon appropriate sub-stitution at the site of the amino nitrogen or alicyclic carbon atom (244, 245). The re-lated dibenz[b, f](1, 4)oxazepines (49.**92a**), with suitable substitution (246), show neurotropic, antireserpine, antiserotonin, antihistaminic, and antispasmodic activities, but are not outstanding in any one area. The 5-(2-dimethylaminoethyl) derivative of the isomer 5,11-dihydrodibenz[b, e](1, 4)-oxazepine (49.**92b**) is about five times as potent as mepyramine (49.**5**) on the guinea pig ileum and 12 times as potent in inhibit-ing anaphylactoid edema induced by dex-tran in rats (247). The latter activity is potentiated by the antiserotonin agent 2'-(3-dimethylaminopropylthio)cinnamanilide (248). Compound 49.**92b** causes an in-crease in central motor activity in animals; its effect on barbiturate-induced hypnosis is questionable (249).

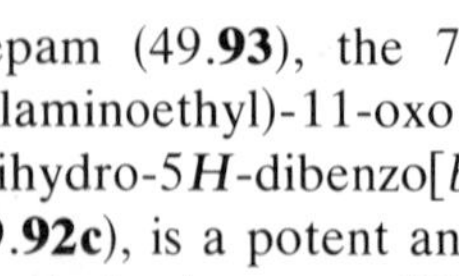

49.**92a** X = NH, Y = O
49.**92b** X = O, Y = N(CH₂)₂N(CH₃)₂
49.**92c** X = Y = NH

Clobenzepam (49.**93**), the 7-chloro-10-(β-dimethylaminoethyl)-11-oxo derivative of 10,11-dihydro-5H-dibenzo[b, e](1, 4)di-azepine (49.**92c**), is a potent antihistaminic and antianaphylactic agent (250) with an ED₅₀ of 0.13 mg/kg orally in rats. This is 2000 times less than the LD₅₀ for this compound (251).

Activity is reduced by deleting the halogen in position 7 and the carbonyl at

position 11; the corresponding 10,11-di-hydro-11-deoxy compounds are practically inactive *in vivo* although they are structur-ally related to known antihistamines of the benzylaniline type. An unsubstituted nit-rogen bridge at position 5 affords the high-est activity. Derivatives of benzanilide (49.**94**) and of phenanthridone (49.**95**) are inactive (252).

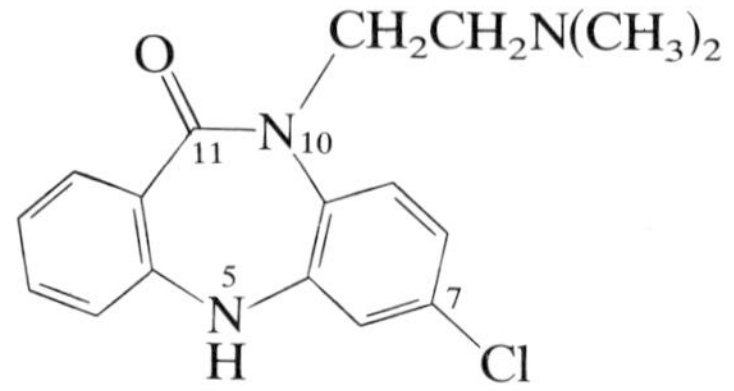

49.**93**

An enhancement of antianaphylactic po-tency appeared with the elimination of the 11-oxo function and the introduction of an aliphatic amine in position 5 of the di-benzodiazepines. Their mechanism of ac-tion remains unknown; there seems to be a correlation between α-chymotripsin inhibi-tion and antianaphylactic potency, but in addition, these analogs may act by prevent-ing antibody–antigen formation (253).

Ketotifene (49.**96**) is the hydrogen fumu-rate salt of 4-(1-methyl-4-piperidylidene)-4H-benzo[4, 5]cyclohepta[1, 2-b]thiophen-10(9H)-one and is completely absorbed through the gut (254–256). The antihist-

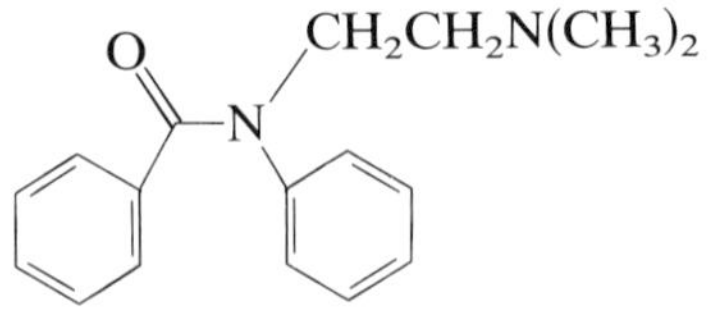

49.**94**

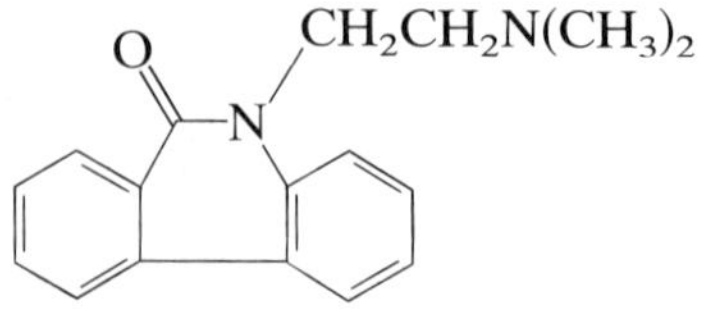

49.**95**

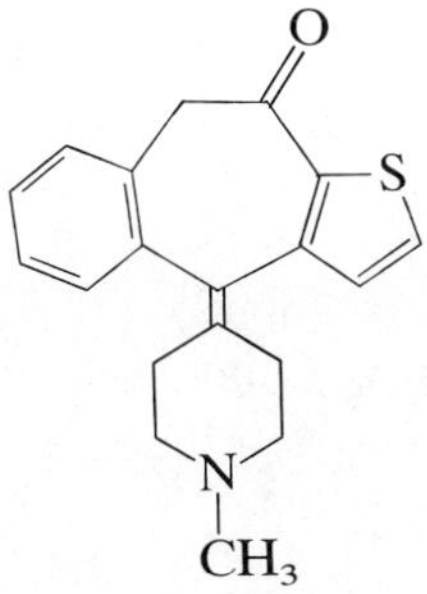

49.**96**

aminic potency of ketotifene has been confirmed in man (255). In patients, the symptoms of chronic urticaria were relieved when ketofifene was administered orally, 1 mg twice daily, over a 4 week period (255). At the same dose level and route of administration, ketotifene protected 24 asthma patients against allergenic bronchospasms induced by inhaled antigen (256). The antiallergenic effect of 49.**96** is immediate and lasts for 4–6 hr after taking 1.0 mg of the drug (256). Ketotifene may not only exert its antiallergenic activity by blocking histamine receptors, but may also act as a mastocyte-protecting agent by inhibiting the release of histamine from storage sites (257). The introduction of a 7-chloro moiety into ketotifene affords HL-22-914 (CPP 22-914; 49.**97**), which is a very potent long-acting antihistamine showing sedation only at higher doses (258).

Dithiadene, 4-(3-dimethylaminopropylidene)-4,9-dihydrothieno[2, 3-*b*]benzo[*e*]-thiepin (49.**98**), exhibits an antihistaminic effect that exceeds that of promethazine in

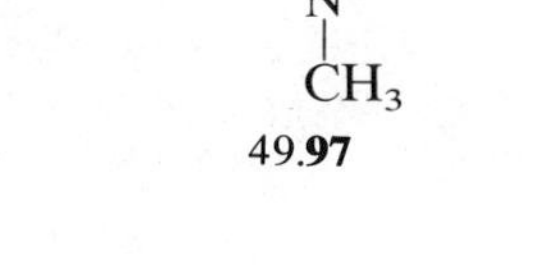

49.**97**

guinea pigs in the histamine aerosol and detoxification tests (259, 260). The cis isomer of 49.**98** ($ED_{50} = 0.04$ mg/kg i.p.) appears to be somewhat less potent than the trans isomer ($ED_{50} = 0.02$ mg/kg i.p.) in the histamine aerosol test and are by an order of magnitude more potent than the standards promethazine (49.**51b**; $ED_{50} = 0.47$ mg/kg i.p.) and cyproheptadine (49.**81**; $ED_{50} = 0.23$ mg/kg i.p.) in the same test (261). A tricyclic system containing a

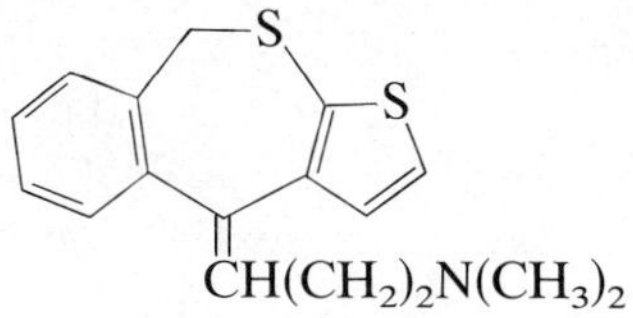

49.**98**

3-thienylsulfide, namely, 10-(3-dimethylaminopropylidene)-5, 10-dihydrothieno-[3, 2-*c*]-2-benzothiepin (49.**99**), is an effective antihistaminic (262). In the histamine aerosol test, 49.**99** ($ED_{50} = 0.209$ mg/kg i.v. in guinea pigs when administered 15 min prior to histaminic challenge) is similar in potency to cyproheptadine (49.**81**), but is an order of magnitude less potent than dithiadene (261). In the detoxification test, 49.**99** ($ED_{50} = 0.054$ mg/kg s.c. when administered 30 min prior to histamine challenge) has approximately the same potency as promethazine (49.**51b**; $ED_{50} = 0.06$ mg/kg s.c.) and cyproheptadine

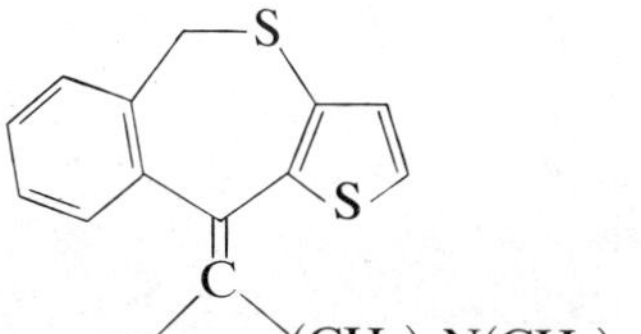

49.**99**

(49.**81**; $ED_{50} = 0.04$ mg/kg s.c.), but only 50% the potency of dithiadene (261, 262). Interestingly, analog 49.**99** has practically no antiserotonin activity and the CNS-depressant effect is low. Analog 49.**99** exhibits only a slight antianaphylactic effect against dextran-induced histamine release in rats (262).

4 NATURALLY OCCURRING AND MISCELLANEOUS ANTIHISTAMINES

Over the last decade a large number of reports have appeared describing uncharacterized natural products which have high antihistaminic potency *in vitro* or *in vivo*. Substances were obtained from hops (*Humulus lupulus*) (263), the creeper *Ipomoea pes-caprae* (L.) Roth (264), *Ruta graveolens* (265), purified Hungarian oak gall extracts (perhaps containing piperonylic acid residues) (266), musk from the deer *Moschus moschiferus* (267), crown gall-infected tomato plants (tomatine and gomatine) (268), and the skin of the frog *Rana tigrina* (269). Active compounds with known structures include fumarine (270), cannabis, and $(-)$-*trans*-Δ^9-tetrahydrocannabinol (271). The latter compound inhibits histamine, serotonin, acetylcholine, and bradykinin *in vitro* in a noncompetitive manner. Fumarine blocks histamine, serotonin, and bradykinin *in vitro*.

Benzeneboronic acid and the *p*-methyl analog are examples of synthetic materials not having the classical antihistamine structures. Benzeneboronic acid (ED$_{50}$ = 11 × 10^{-4} g/ml) and *p*-methylbenzeneboronic acid (ED$_{50}$ = 122 × 10^{-5} g/ml) inhibit the actions of histamine (2 × 10^{-4} g/ml) on the guinea pig ileum. This action is nonspecific since these compounds also exhibited anticholinergic activity and inhibited BaCl$_2$-induced spasms. Boric acid is inactive in these test systems (272).

5 METABOLISM OF ANTIHISTAMINES

A recent review is available which discusses the absorption, distribution, metabolism, and elimination of antihistamines in detail (273). Therefore, this section only gives a brief overview of antihistamine metabolism and emphasizes major metabolic pathways. On administration to small animals, antihistamines are found in the highest concentration in the lung, kidney, and spleen, although the most active tissues of metabolism of these drugs, as revealed by *in vitro* studies, are the liver, kidney, and heart. Antihistamines are not significantly metabolized in the gastrointestinal tract and can therefore be taken orally (274). When mouse hepatic function is previously damaged by injection with carbon tetrachloride, the antihistamine content of tissue is greater and longer lasting than that in untreated animals (275). Although a comparative study (276) utilizing diphenhydramine (49.**14a**), tripelennamine (49.**7a**), thonzylamine (49.**10b**), and promethazine (49.**51b**) showed that thonzylamine is removed from tissue most rapidly, more studies are needed before structural correlations with excretion rates can be drawn.

Some antihistamines are excreted in part unchanged. In rabbits 3.6–10% (diphenhydramine), 9.5–12% (tripelennamine), and 4.3–7.9% (thonzylamine) of the oral dose is found in the urine after 24 hr (276). The nature of the metabolites depends on the animal. Small animals have fairly simple excretion patterns in contrast to humans (277). Typical metabolites result from *N*-demethylation, ether cleavage, perhaps side chain degradation, and ring hydroxylation and oxidation (278).

Employing tritiated diphenhydramine labeled in the diphenylmethyl function, male and female rhesus monkeys were administered a 10 mg/kg dose either i.v. or orally. Analysis of the urine from these animals revealed the presence of diphenhydramine, the primary and secondary amine analogs of diphenhydramine, diphenhydramine *N*-oxide, diphenylmethoxyacetic acid, the glutamate conjugate of diphenylmethoxyacetic acid, and a trace of benzhydrol (279). Previous investigators (276, 278) observed benzhydrol as a metabolite of diphenhydramine from rabbits, but the benzhydrol detected (279) may arise from the subsequent acid-induced decomposition of diphenylmethoxyacetic acid or its glucuronide, both of which are acid-labile (280). A comparative study, using male guinea pigs, rats, and rabbits, confirmed previous reports (278, 281) showing that diphenhydramine, tripelennamine, and several other antihistamines are found in the highest concentration in the lungs, followed by the spleen, kidney, and liver (276). Diphenhydramine and its o-methyl analog, when incubated with rat liver microsomes, yield formaldehyde via N-demethylation (282). Male rat microsomes show a greater enzymatic activity than female rat microsomes for diphenhydramine N-demethylation (283).

Like diphenhydramine, tripelennamine (49.**7a**) rapidly leaves the blood of guinea pigs and rats and localizes in tissues, predominantly in the lung (281, 284–286). In humans, less than 1% of tripelennamine free base is recovered in the urine (281). Approximately 10% of the free base is excreted in conjugated form (286). The liver was found to be the most active organ for metabolizing tripelennamine. A study using ^{14}C-labeled tripelennamine revealed that the urine contained a compound tentatively identified as the glucuronide (287). The major metabolic modification of tripelennamine seems to be hydroxylation on one or more positions of the aromatic rings followed by conjugation with glucuronic acid (287).

The metabolic inactivation, tissue distribution, and protein binding of cyclizine (49.**32a**) and chlorcyclizine (49.**32b**), two piperazino derivatives, were studied in dogs and rats. The major route of cyclizine and chlorcyclizine metabolism in vivo and in vitro is through their corresponding N-demethylated derivatives, norcyclizine and norchlorcyclizine, both of which have little, if any, antihistaminic activity. Both drugs

exhibit a similar distribution pattern and are mainly localized in the lung, spleen, liver, and kidney (288). The formation of norchlorcyclizine probably goes through an intermediate chlorcyclizine N-oxide which is subsequently reduced to chlorcyclizine and demethylated in vivo (288, 289). In contrast to results obtained with chlorcyclizine, chronic cyclizine administration does not lead to accumulation of norcyclizine in tissue. However, there is a marked sex difference for chlorcyclizine metabolism; N-demethylation is eight times faster in male rats (288). Chronic administration of chlorcyclizine to female rats resulted in tissue accumulation of the N-demethylated analog, whereas chronic administration of cyclizine did not lead to the accumulation of norcyclizine (288). The failure of norcyclizine to accumulate in tissues was attributed to a more rapid disappearance of this compound; high tissue levels of both norchlorcyclizine and norcyclizine are found shortly after administration of the parent drugs. Norcyclizine binds less to plasma and therefore is more available to degradative liver enzymes (288). Other investigators have identified N-(p-chlorobenzhydryl)ethylenediamine as another metabolite obtained from the chronic administration of chlorcyclizine to female rats (290). The ethylenediamine metabolite disappears at a slower rate; these observations are similar to the metabolism and disappearance of piperazine ring containing neuroleptic drugs (291). A study using benzyl carbon-labeled norchlorcyclizine-^{14}C administered to male and female rats revealed no detectable radiolabeled carbon dioxide in expired air, thus eliminating the possibility of total metabolism of chlorcyclizine to the benzhydryl function (292).

Benzhydrol is a primary urine metabolite of cinnarizine (49.**34**) in adult male rats. Thirty percent of the metabolites are found in the urine, whereas 60% are found in feces. Those found in feces have been characterized as N-benzhydrylpiperazine and benzophenone. N-4 dealkylation also occurs; cinnamylpiperazine and cinnamaldehyde were identified in the urine (293).

Chlorpheniramine sulfoxide N-oxide was detected in rat urine extracts along with chlorpheniramine (13.2%) and N-demethylchlorpheniramine (5.8%) (294) as unchanged drug (294–295). Additionally, chlorpheniramine has been shown to be metabolized to two unidentified substances; the principal portion of the administered drug is excreted as polar metabolites (296). Studies in vivo revealed metabolites in urine were similar to those obtained with isolated rat liver microsomes.

Hydroxylation at positions 3 and 7, sulfoxidation, and N-demethylation are the major metabolic pathways of phenothiazine derivatives (297). Phenothiazine sulfoxide is a significant degradation product of the neuroleptic promazine (49.**51g**), which indicates that side chain cleavage may also take place (298). Studies with the structurally related psychotherapeutic dibenz[b, f]-azepine system show that they also are ring hydroxylated at position 2 and N-demethylated at the dimethylaminoalkyl group of their side chain (299). Antihistamines belonging to these tricyclic systems probably follow similar metabolic pathways.

Isolated rat liver perfusates of chlorprothixene (49.**59**) show that sulfoxidation, N-demethylation, and glucuronic acid conjugates are the main metabolites (300, 301). Metabolites isolated from dog and rat urine show that sulfoxidation and N-demethylation are the major in vivo metabolic pathways (301, 302). Aromatic ring hydroxylation was proposed as a metabolic route for chlorprothixene, but was not confirmed experimentally (302). Formation of chlorprothixene sulfoxide N-oxide was detected in rat urine extracts along with the major metabolite, chlorprothixene sulfoxide; amounts of the N-demethylated product formed were similar to the N-oxide derivative (301).

Two comprehensive surveys of cyproheptadine (49.**81**) metabolism in rats, dogs, and man have appeared (303, 304). The major metabolites isolated from dog urine include trans-10,11-dihydroxycyproheptadine (12%), cyproheptadine N-oxide (35%), 10,11-dihydro-10,11-epoxy-5H-dibenzo[a, d]cycloheptene (12%), unchanged drug (20%), and five additional uncharacterized minor substances (303, 304). Using radiolabeled drug, the principal metabolite in humans was tentatively identified as a quaternary ammonium glucuronide-like conjugate (45–55%). No evidence for metabolic alteration at the tricyclic (C-10,11) ethylene bridge was found in humans (303). Species differences were observed for tissue concentrations following cyproheptadine administration (304).

The tricyclic ether, hepzidine (49.**87**), is hydrolyzed in the stomach of male and female rats within 30 min after oral administration. The principal metabolite, 10,11-dihydro-5H[a, d]cyclohepten-5-ol is the product resulting from such hydrolysis. More than 50% of the oral dose undergoes hydrolysis in the stomach prior to absorption. The nonhydrolyzed drug is absorbed and biotransformed mainly by N-demethylation (20%). The major metabolite found in rat urine following hepzidine administration was 1-methyl-1-piperidinol, whereas bile contained unaltered drug along with various uncharacterized metabolites (305).

The tropanyl ether analog of hepzidine, namely, deptropine (49.**85b**), readily undergoes N-demethylation in the rat. Within 6 hr after i.p. administration, deptropine-N-$^{14}CH_3$ was found to be more than 22% metabolized by this route as measured by formation of radioactive carbon dioxide (305). Deptropine, on the other hand, is poorly demethylated in vitro; at concentrations greater than 3×10^{-3} M this analog inhibits the NADPH-dependent oxidase enzyme system as well as its own N-demethylation and the N-demethylation of other substances. Deptropine and related structures are found to associate and precipitate rat liver microsomes which may provide an explanation for their slow metabolism *in vitro* (305).

Many drugs, including chlorcyclizine (49.**32b**) and diphenhydramine (49.**14a**), are potent stimulants of liver microsomal enzymes (306). As a result, chronic administration of chlorocyclizine enhances the metabolism of many unrelated drugs, speeds up its own metabolism (288, 307), and leads to less toxic metabolites that are eliminated rapidly in urine and bile. This may explain why some of these drugs become less toxic during long-term toxicity studies (289, 306, 307).

Acute clinical poisoning with antihistamines is rare in adults because of the large margin of safety between the therapeutic and toxic dose; children are considerably more susceptible to the convulsant action of this class of drugs (308). This is in agreement with studies showing that the resistance of small animals to chlorpheniramine and diphenhydramine increases with age. The lack of resistance in newborn animals does not seem to be related to an inability to metabolize the drug in the liver, but rather to greater absorption (309).

6 PHARMACOLOGY AND MODE OF ACTION OF ANTIHISTAMINES

Antihistamines are evaluated *in vitro* by the Magnus procedure, i.e., by measuring the minimum amount of the drug that relaxes histamine-induced spasms in an isolated strip of the guinea pig ileum immersed in Tyrode solution (58). The Schultz–Dale reaction, an anaphylactic *in vitro* test, utilizes an isolated strip of guinea pig ileum obtained from an animal sensitized to egg albumin or to *Bordetella pertussis* vaccine (310, 311). Anaphylaxis induced by antigen or by *Bordetella* vaccine also releases other mediators of the antigen–antibody reaction. The initial inhibition of released histamine by any test antihistamine permits the continued slow contraction of the test organ

(311). To differentiate between a true antihistamine or a bronchodilating mode of action for test compounds, an *in vitro* perfused lung procedure is also employed (203). Isolated perfused lung, obtained from guinea pigs sensitized to egg albumin, when challenged with the the same antigen, undergoes severe bronchoconstriction. The antihistamines chlorpheniramine (49.**42b**), azatadine (49.**63**), and cyproheptadine (49.**81**) are inactive in this test. However, bronchodilating agents such as aminophylline, isoproterenol, and the 4-azaxanthene 49.**62** are active (203). The more common procedure *in vivo* for assessing antihistamine activity includes protection against intravenously injected or aerosolized histamine, or against anaphylactic death caused by the administration of a foreign protein to a previously sensitized animal. A test *in vivo* which closely parallels the human response to antihistamines involves relief of nasal resistance to air flow induced by histamine or allergens in rats and guinea pigs (312). In man antihistamine may be evaluated by studying the extent to which they inhibit local skin reactions to intradermally injected histamine (313). These and other test methods have been reviewed (58).

Diphenhydramine (49.**14a**), pyrilamine (49.**5**), antazoline (49.**28**), promethazine (49.**51b**), and other agents (314) caused local vasoconstriction in the mesentery of rats. However, if injected intramuscularly, these compounds produce no vascular alterations (315). In this phenomenon they differ from epinephrine, which is a strong vasoconstrictor whether applied locally or intravenously. Adrenergic or cholinergic blockers, antiserotonin compounds, and local anesthetics do not prevent the local vasoconstrictor action of antihistamines (314).

In addition to cholinergic blocking, antifibrillatory, and local-anesthetic activity (316), antihistamines of different chemical groups inhibit peristalsis in the guinea pig ileum (317) and show a depressant action on skeletal muscle (318, 319), perhaps through noncompetitive antagonism with acetylcholine at a site different from the site on the muscle membranes and contractile element (320). These compounds also potentiate the effector organ response to catecholamines (106, 321). The mechanism is similar to the one proposed for cocaine, namely, blocking the uptake of norepinephrine by the adrenergic neurons (322). The ability to potentiate norepinephrine does not depend on the antihistaminic potency of the compounds (323); some depress, whereas others potentiate the vasopressor effect of the catecholamine (324). Some antihistamines also exhibit an activating influence on carbonic anhydrase of the rat stomach, although less so than histamine (325). The pheniramines are effective inhibitors of synaptosome dopamine uptake (326) and also inhibit histamine N-methyltransferase (327). Guinea pigs treated with ethanol and chlorpheniramine (49.**42b**) tolerated higher doses of histamine aerosol (prior to shock-induced death) than did those animals not receiving the ethanol treatment (328).

Antihistamines prevent liver damage after administration of thioacetamide *in vivo* (329) and *in vitro* (330) and protect against nutritional liver injury (331), mouse virus hepatitis (332), and carbon tetrachloride necrosis (333). Like local anesthetics, which also show such protection against cell-damaging agents, antihistamines inhibit ion transport, phosphorprotein turnover, and the rate of mitochondrial swelling (334). Antihistamines seem to act as antiallergenic agents by more than one mechanism. Serotonin and bradykinin, known to be released during anaphylaxis in small animals, are also antagonized by some antihistamines.

The specific competitive antagonism of histamine on a molecular level may be studied at receptors in the guinea pig ileum (335, 336). These sites are designated H_1 receptors (335, 337) to distinguish them from other actions of histamine that are not antagonized by antihistamine compounds (51, 318, 338), such as stimulation of gastric acid secretion, inhibition of the rat uterus, and stimulation of isolated atria.

Competitive antagonism is defined by the interaction of histamine and antihistamines with a receptor rather than as an observable pharmacological response. The receptor–antihistamine (antagonist) complex, like the receptor–histamine (agonist) complex, is a reversible reaction to which the law of mass action applies (333, 337, 339).

The competitive antagonism of histamine and antihistamines on H_1 receptors is studied by use of dose ratios ($[A_2]/[A_1]$), where $[A_2]$ is the concentration of agonist needed in the presence of a given concentration of antagonist $[B]$ that is required to produce the same response as the initial concentration of agonist $[A_1]$. This dose ratio is related to $[B]$ and K_B by

$$\frac{[A_2]}{[A_1]} = 1 + [B]K_B \qquad (49.1)$$

The K_B is the association (affinity) constant of the receptor–antagonist complex for the following equation:

$$\text{receptor} + B \rightleftarrows \text{receptor–B} \qquad (49.2)$$

For agonists that have intrinsic activity, such as histamine, the negative log of the dose that causes 50% of the maximal effect ($-\log[A]_{50}$) is defined as a pD_2 value. Since antagonists, such as antihistamines, have no intrinsic activity, they cannot be defined in terms of pD_2 values. For antagonists, Schild introduced the term pA_2; here $pA_2 = -\log[B]$, where $[B]$ is the dose of antagonist that necessitates doubling the dose of agonist to compensate for the action of the antagonist (335, 336, 339, 340). In other words, when the dose ratio ($[A_2]/[A_1]$ is 2, $[B]K_B = 1$ and $K_B = 1/[B]$. Therefore, the $\log K_B = \log 1/[B] = -\log[B] = pA_2$. If a tenfold instead of a twofold increase in agonist is necessary, the designation becomes pA_{10}. Generally, then, for $[B_X]$, which produces a dose ratio of X, log $(1/B_X)$ is called pA_X.

If we know $[B]$ and the dose ratio, we can calculate K_B. If pA_2 values (or dose ratios) for two different agonists of a given antagonist are the same, the inference is that the agonists are operating on the same receptor site. This kind of analysis, using pA_2 values, can be made only if the antagonism is competitive; therefore the dose–response curves must be parallel in the presence and absence of antagonist. This is the case for the histamine–antihistamine relationship, which is competitive on H_1 receptors. On the receptors of the guinea pig ileum *in vitro*, most common antihistamines have pA_2 values between 8.5 and 10.0. Antagonists such as atropine have much lower pA_2 values. The pA_2 value obtained *in vitro* is not linearly related to the potency of the drug *in vivo*. Usually a single pA value is insufficient to characterize an antagonist fully. For accuracy, it is necessary to state both the time–action and the concentration–action relationships of the test system. Longer contact times give higher pA values and usually indicate approximate equilibrium conditions (336).

When antihistamines competitively inhibit the action of histamine at H_1 receptors, it is usually assumed that the antagonist binds to the same site as does histamine; when the antagonist binds, it has no intrinsic activity. This molecular mechanism may be a grossly simplified explanation. Indeed, to date the histamine pharmacological receptor has not been isolated. It remains to be seen whether the H_1 receptor is simply the active site on a protein or other membrane macromolecule or consists of more than one protein at proper pH and smaller molecules and ions. Furthermore, to determine what happens (on a molecular level) after histamine reacts with the receptor will require considerably more research. It is

likely, however, that histamine interacts with cell membranes, leading to an increase in membrane permeability to inorganic ions and that this causes the variety of pharmacologic actions. Facilitation of Ca^{2+} entry may explain the stimulant effect of histamine on smooth muscle contraction (1).

7   STRUCTURE–ACTIVITY RELATIONSHIPS OF ANTIHISTAMINES

According to classical receptor theory, the biologic effect of histamine and antihistamines is the result of physiocochemical interactions with the receptor molecules of an organism. Modification of the histamine–agonist structure has not generally given rise to strong H_1 antagonists but rather to less active agonists. Antihistamines differ from histamine in their structural requirements; however, both have aliphatic amino groups capable of reaction with an anionic site in the receptor. Antihistamines probably do not occupy the identical receptor area occupied by histamine but perhaps only the anionic site; the aromatic portion of the molecule seems necessary for interaction with regions adjacent to the site. Such interactions are important since they are expected to increase the affinity of the antagonist for the antihistamine receptor. This may explain why stricter structural relationships exist for histamine than for H_1-antihistamines (341). Although model systems for antihistamine–receptor binding have been proposed (97), presently available data do not preclude the possibility of multiple binding sites or the possibility that histamine and antihistamines interact with different sites through a reversible molecular perturbation (342) mechanism.

Maximum antihistaminic activity is found in structures of the type 49.**100**, where R^1 and R^2 are aromatic or heteroaromatic rings, one of which may be separated from X by a methylene group; X is CO, N, or

49.**100**

CH; R^3 is generally an ethylene group or a two-carbon fragment of a nitrogen heterocyclic system. Only in the case of tricyclic compounds, such as the piperidylalkylphenothiazines, does a three-carbon alkylene chain (R^3) elicit antihistaminic activity that is approximately 3–30 times that noted with the corresponding two-carbon analogs (343). The aromatic rings R^1 and R^2 may or may not be ortho connected by Y, where Y = CH$_2$, a heteroatom, or CH$_2$—heteroatom. R^4 and R^5 are methyl groups, but small planar cyclic groups may be employed advantageously. For data suggesting structure–activity relationships of specific groups of antihistamines, the reader is referred to various review articles (58, 344).

When two aromatic rings (R^1 and R^2) are present, maximum activity is observed if both rings are not coplanar. For example, the fluorene analog of diphenhydramine (in which both rings are coplanar) exhibits 100 times less activity than diphenhydramine (49.**14a**). In potent tricyclic systems the A and C rings do not lie in the same plane, enabling interaction with sites adjacent to the histamine (H$_1$) receptor.

Introduction of small para substituents into aralkyl groups of compounds in which the rings are not ortho-connected by Y seems to be a reliable means for maintaining or potentiating activity. Increasing the size of o-alkyl substituents causes a reduction in antihistaminic activity (345, 346). Compounds without substitution in the 2 position of the phenothiazine nucleus generally are more active (343).

A careful comparison of apparently significant physical properties, i.e., solubility, ionization constants, and surface tension, of 16 clinically useful antihistamines did not reveal any direct correlation between phys-

ical and biologic properties (343). Since the cations of histamine and the competitive antihistamines are the predominant forms of these compounds under physiological conditions, the electrostatic component of their surface forces should outweigh other factors in the attraction of the compounds to the histamine receptor. However, the ionic bond cannot be the sole factor governing this attraction because the pK_as of the drugs and their antihistaminic activity do not show a linear relationship.

It has been proposed that the extended trans conformation of histamine is the "active" conformation at H$_1$ receptors (348–350). Extended Hückel calculations indicated that the lowest energy conformation of the cation of histamine is the fully extended form. Since, by extended Hückel calculations, histamine may exist in two distinct nearly equally preferred conformations, it was suggested that one of these may be required for H$_1$ activity, whereas the other is required for H$_2$ activity (351). However, such studies cannot easily be related to "active" conformations since histamine or antihistamine interaction with a receptor may involve high energy forms wherein energy required for rotation may readily be gained and markedly exceeded through the binding process.

James and Williams (352) have proposed that a flexible histamine–antihistamine receptor protein could be responsible for the action of the agonist and antagonist. Thus the proposed receptor may be able to adopt different conformations during histamine or antihistamine binding; i.e., a reversible allosteric or molecular perturbation mechanism may be involved. Although bovine serum albumin (BSA) cannot be construed as a receptor it is of interest to note that antihistamines were shown to induce changes in BSA which prevent binding of histamine (353). In solution, histamine and various antihistamines exist as a mixture of gauche and trans forms (354–356). In solution the gauche form of antihistamines of the general type $XCH_2CH_2N(R)_2$ increases with increasing electronegativity of X (i.e., $X = O > X = N > X = C$) (357). In neutral solution, circular dichroism and PMR studies have revealed that pheniramine derivatives (49.**42a**, 49.**42b**, and 49.**42c**) exist in at least two discernible (extended and folded) conformations; by PMR the extended conformation is preferred in water (358). However, any attempt to correlate solid state (352, 359–362), solution (354–356), or calculated (348–351) conformations of drug molecules with biological activity has many pitfalls; the situation is further complicated if the binding involves allosteric or molecular perturbation mechanisms.

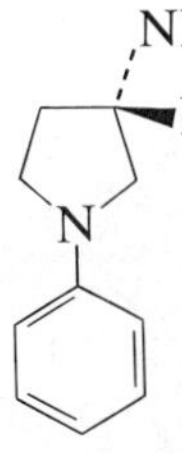

Results reported by Hanna and Ahmed (154), who employed conformationally constrained *cis*- and *trans*-1,5-diphenyl-3-dimethylaminopyrrolidine analogs (49.**40a** and 49.**40b**) of phenbenzamine (49.**4b**), do not support the suggestion (352, 359–362) that a fully extended trans conformation about the C–C bond of the dimethylamino-ethyl function is necessary for activity. In fact, both 49.**40a** and 49.**40b** are potent histamine H_1-receptor antagonists, and neither isomer is capable of attaining a fully extended trans N–C–C–N conformation (154). Geometric effects on histamine methyltransferase served to account for the differences in duration of action of the two isomers *in vitro* (156). Similarly, L(S)- and D(R)-3-ethylamino-1-phenylpyrrolidines (49.**101a** and 49.**101b** with pA_2 values of 5.92 and 4.92, respectively), which have reduced antihistaminic potency *in vitro* likely owing to the presence of only one phenyl ring, cannot achieve a fully extended trans N–C–C–N conformation (363). Utilizing a series of *cis*- and *trans*-1,2-diphenyl-4-amino-2-butenes (49.**102a** and 49.**102b**), it was observed that a *cis*-2-H,3-Ar (49.**101a**) [rather than *trans*-2-H,3-Ar (49.**102b**)] relationship provided optimal antihistaminic activity on the isolated guinea pig ileum (168). Thus Casy and Ison

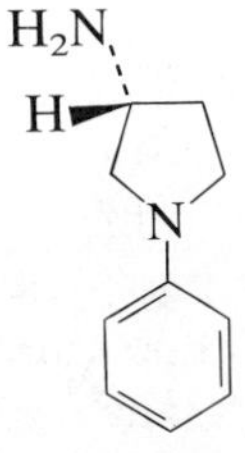

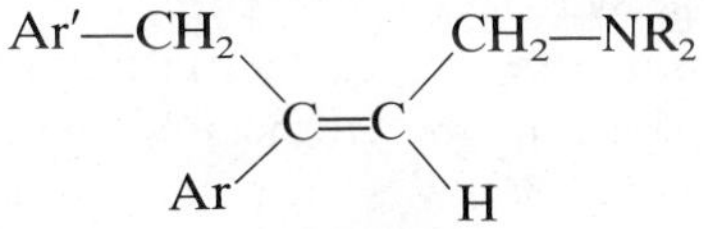

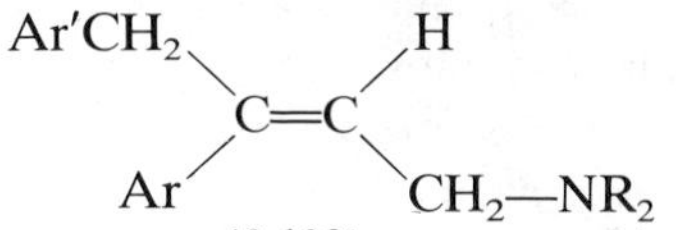

49.**101a**   49.**101b**

49.**102a**

49.**102b**

(168) proposed that conformationally less restricted drugs may adopt conformations related to the *cis*-2-H, 3-Ar configuration wherein the plane of the second aryl group (Ar′) lies at an approximate right angle to the Ar—CH=CH— plane; the Ar—CH=CHCH$_2$N function is nearly coplanar. Structural and conformational requirements emphasized by Casy and Ison (168) may represent a satisfactory approximation of receptor-bound H_1 antihistamines (154). Additionally, Hanna and Ahmed (154) have shown that there is not a strict requirement for the fully extended trans N–C–C–N conformation for H_1 receptor blockade. A range of values for the trans torsional angle may be accommodated in effective antihistamine–receptor interactions.

Stereoselective (enantiomeric) antihistaminic activity is generally observed only when the asymmetric center is located alpha to the aromatic ring functions (on carbon beta to the aliphatic N) (96, 346, 363). Stereoselective activity was observed for the dextrorotary isomer of dimethylaminoethyl 4-methylbenzhydryl ether,

which is four times as active as the levoro-
tary enantiomorph. Similarly, the D forms
of carbinoxamine (49.**22b**), pheniramine
(49.**42a**), chlorpheniramine (49.**42b**), and
brompheniramine (49.**42c**) (164, 364, 365)
are more potent their respective L enantiomorphs. The D isomers of pheniramines
49.**42a**–49.**42c** have been shown to have
the (S) configuration (366, 367). In the case
of dimethylpyrindene (49.**46**), the L isomer
possesses the greater antihistaminic potency (368). However, in the case of isothipendyl (49.**56b**), where the asymmetric
center is located beta to the aromatic rings
(alpha to the dimethylamino group), resolution affords D and L enantiomorphs that
exhibit less activity than the original DL pair
(364, 365). For promethazine (49.**51b**), in
which the asymmetric center is located
alpha to $N(CH_3)_2$, D and L isomers are
reported to have the same toxicity and activity (369). However, compounds of the
pyrrolidino type (49.**101a** and 49.**101b**), in
which the asymmetric center is located
alpha to the aliphatic amino group, do
show stereoselective activity *in vivo* (363).
Dihydrodibenzo(*b*, *f*)thiepin and related tricyclic or diaryl-substituted enantiomorphic
pyrrolidines exhibit little or no stereoselective differences in antihistaminic potency (370, 371). Stereoselective activity
observed for the structurally smaller
monoaryl analogs (49.**101a** and 49.**101b**)
may be a reflection of intra-antihistamine
receptor asymmetry (363), whereas diaryl
antihistamine stereoselective activity may
reflect asymmetry of regions further removed from the anionic binding site. Loss
of stereoselective antihistaminic activity for
the diastereoisomeric dibenzo(*b*, *f*)thiepins
(49.**103**), which have the required asymmetric center located in the aromatic tricyclic rings in addition to an asymmetric
center located alpha to the dialkylamino
function, likely is due to their nonspecific
antispasmodic activity (371).

Through use of thermodynamically derived substituent constants and hydro-

49.**103**

phobic parameters Kutter and Hansch
(372) concluded that in the diphenhydramine series steric effects from the ortho and
meta positions are so similar that they can
be treated together in one term. The selection of substituents in the study did not
allow a separation between the roles of
hydrophobic parameters (π) and steric
parameters (E_S). Although the activity does
not parallel π nearly so well as it parallels
$E_S^{o,m}$, it seems unlikely that hydrophobic
effects of substituents are unimportant.
From their mathematical analysis Kutter
and Hansch observed that substituents in
the ortho and meta positions of the more
highly substituted ring have parallel deactivating effects, and substituents in the
ortho and meta positions of the less substituted ring have little effect. Mono-para-
substitution has an activating effect up to
an optimum size and then a deactivating
effect; a second para substituent appears to
have a deactivating effect.

8 RELEASE AND ANTAGONISM OF BRADYKININ

Bradykinin (373), a nonapeptide (Arg-Pro-
Pro-Gly-Phe-Ser-Pro-Phe-Arg) (374–376),
is not only released, but is actually formed
during anaphylaxis (377–380) by a kinin-
forming enzyme, kallikrein (381–382).
Bradykinin has a $t_{1/2}$ of less than 15 sec in
the cat (383) and less than 30 sec in the
human (384). Since bradykinin has a short
$t_{1/2}$ in the circulation, kallikrein, which has
a longer $t_{1/2}$ (120 sec in the cat), may be

responsible for prolonging the physiological activity of the nonapeptide (383). Bradykinin has five basic physiological actions: (1) smooth muscle contraction, (2) vasodilation, (3) increased capillary permeability, (4) promotion of the accumulation and migration of leukocytes, and (5) production of pain (385). In man vasodilation is perphaps the most significant physiological action of bradykinin (386). This peptide, which has been synthesized (375, 376), induces bronchiolar constriction in the anesthetized guinea pig (387). On the adrenal medulla, bradykinin causes the release of catecholamines that antagonizes its action (388). Bradykinin is found in increased concentration in guinea pig lungs during anaphylactic shock (389) and the subsequent release of catacholamines, *in vivo*, relaxes the guinea pig trachea (390).

Bradykinin or some other polypeptide may be responsible for chymotrypsin-mediated release of known bronchoconstrictory histamine from mast cells (391). Little has appeared in the literature regarding the release of kinins in allergy of the human respiratory tract. During severe bronchial asthma, a tenfold increase in levels of kinins over those of normal subjects has been reported (392). Bronchoconstriction by bradykinin aerosol in normal human subjects is thought to occur by nonspecific irritation of vagal irritant receptors; these receptors are blocked by atropine (393).

Bradykinin bronchoconstriction (394–396) in the guinea pig anesthetized with urethane is antagonized (in order of decreasing potency) by indomethacin and mefenamate > aspirin > salicylate (17, 397). Bradykinin may be acting either directly on the effector organ or indirectly by liberating other active substances. Piper and Vane (17) have shown that bradykinin and SRS-A releases a recently identified (397a) rabbit-aorta contracting substance (RCS). Histamine has little effect on the release of RCS. Proteases also seem to be

involved in the release of RCS (398). Thus the chain of events during anaphylaxis involves the antigen–antibody mediated release of kinins (382) and SRS-A, which in turn stimulate the release of RCS; all these substances cause bronchoconstriction. Aspirin and other antiphlogistic acids apparently prevent the bradykinin and SRS-A-induced release of RCS from the guinea pig lung during anaphylaxis (17, 399). Aspirin blocks the release of bradykinin and arachidonic acid-induced release of RCS in the guinea pig lung (399), whereas quinacrine only antagonizes the action of bradykinin (400). Bradykinin likely activates endogenous phospholipase A or some other acylhydrolase. Quinacrine seems to antagonize the process at an earlier stage, whereas aspirin-like drugs interfere at later steps in the process. Studies utilizing phenylbutazone, soybean trypsin (401), pyrilamine (49.5), and ascorbic acid in experimentally induced anaphylaxis in rats indicate the presence of two phases; that is, an early phase in which bradykinin is the mediator and against which a mixture of pyrilamine and ascorbic acid protects and a late phase that does not involve bradykinin (401, 402). Neither pyrilamine nor ascorbic acid is effective alone, whereas phenylbutazone or soybean trypsin are individually active. An important step in the protection seems to involve reduction of the kinin-forming enzyme and not a reduction in circulating bradykinin levels (401).

Bradykinin is among the agonists available for studies of potential antagonists (403, 404). Garcia Leme and Rocha e Silva (405) studied the inhibitory potencies (pK_i) of certain dibenzocycloheptene and thiaxanthene derivatives as competitive antagonists of bradykinin on the guinea pig ileum. Cyproheptadine (49.**81**) was a noncompetitive antagonist ($pK_i = 7.00$–7.30) to bradykinin in this test. Various benzodiazepines, cycloalkindols, and dibenzazepines are also reported to be noncompetitive antagonists. Chlorpromethazine

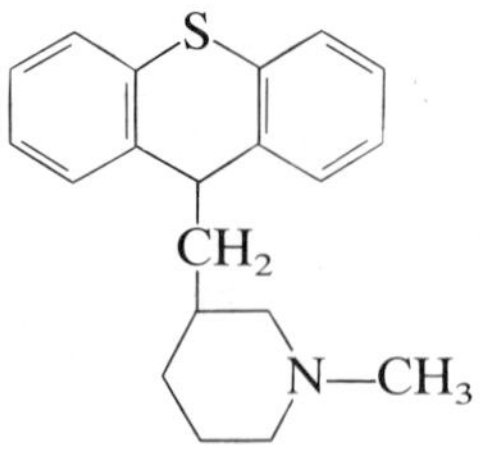

49.**104**

($pK_i = 6.50$–6.60) and promethazine (49.**51b**) ($pK_i = 5.30$) inhibit the action of bradykinin on the guinea pig ileum (405). Methixene [9-(1-methyl-3-piperidyl-methyl)thioxanthene] (49.**104**) was first regarded to be a competitive antagonist ($pK_i = 6.60$–6.80) (405). Later studies by VanRiezen (406) showed that this compound is a noncompetitive inhibitor in a cumulative dose fashion on the guinea pig ileum. Methixene also noncompetitively antagonizes histamine, acetylcholine, and serotonin on the guinea pig ileum to the same extent. Using the same test procedure, VanRiezen (407) found that N-(3-benzylthio-2,6-dichlorophenyl)anthramyl acid (ASD-30) (49.**105**) is a noncompetitive antagonist of bradykinin, which is only partially reversible in the higher dose ranges of 2×10^{-5} M/ml. A closely related phenothiazine derivative, dimethothiazine (49.**106**), abolished the effects of bradykinin in the rabbit ear vein at 100 μg/ml. On the rat colon and the duodenum, this compound was active at 10 μg/ml; on the rat uterus this compound exhibited a potency equal to cyproheptadine which is active at 100 μg/ml (408). The cycloheptathiophene analog pizotyline (49.**107**) at $6\times$

10^{-5} to 6×10^{-6} g/ml is a weak noncompetitive antagonist to bradykinin on the guinea pig ileum (409). Pizotyline did not modify the direct vascular effects of the peptide in the rat, but potentiated the action of bradykinin on the adrenal medulla. These data suggest that at least two types of bradykinin receptors are present in rats (409).

A variety of structurally diverse compounds having antihistaminic activity also antagonize bradykinin in various preparations. The antihistamine chlorpyramine (49.**7b**) at 5–10 mg/kg i.p. reduces thermic edema in the rat's paw from released endogenous bradykinin (410). At concentrations of 1×10^{-7} g/ml, this compound reduces the contraction induced by 0.5 or 1.0 ng of bradykinin on the rat uterus by 49 and 35%, respectively. At 2×10^{-7} g/ml 49.**7b** had no effect on the response induced by 5-HT, but did antagonize the action of histamine (410). Tribenoside (49.**108**), a relatively nontoxic glucofuranoside, antagonizes the action of histamine, serotonin, and bradykinin and has an antianaphylactic effect in actively sensitized guinea pigs and mice (411). In the normal rat, 49.**108** antagonizes the hypotensive affect of bradykinin by 50–80% (412); the ED_{50} of 49.**108** on bradykinin induced contractions on the guinea pig ileum *in vitro* varied between 1 and 10 μg/ml (411). Tribenoside antagonizes the smooth muscle stimulant action of norepinephrine on rat seminal vesicles ($ED_{50} = 100$ μg/ml), but is inactive against the same actions of epinephrine on the rat vas deferens (411, 413).

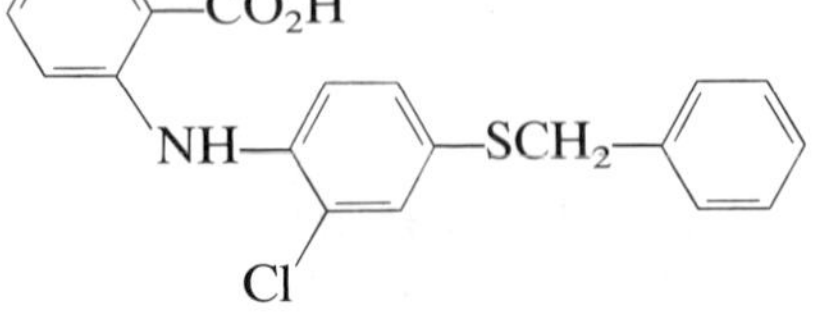

49.**105**

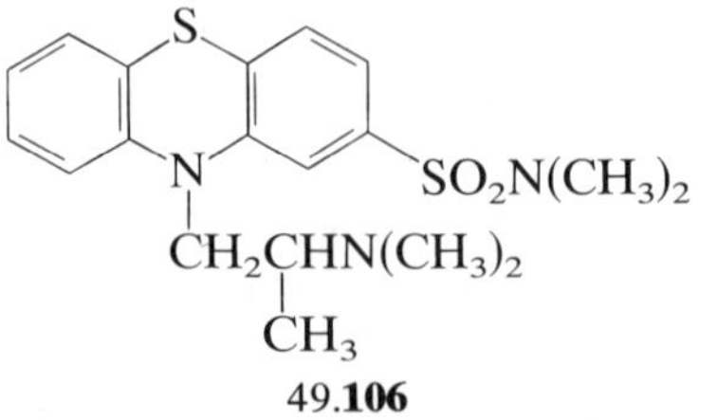

49.**106**

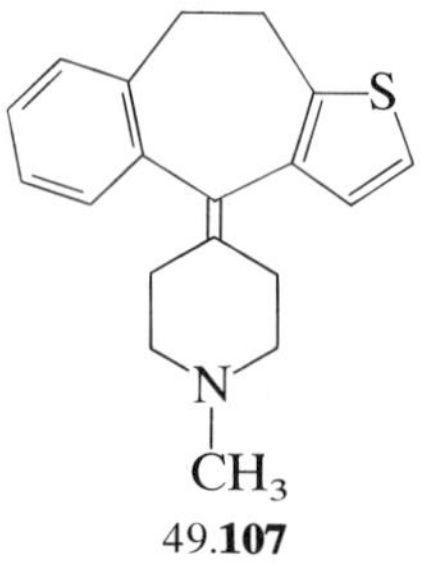

49.**107**

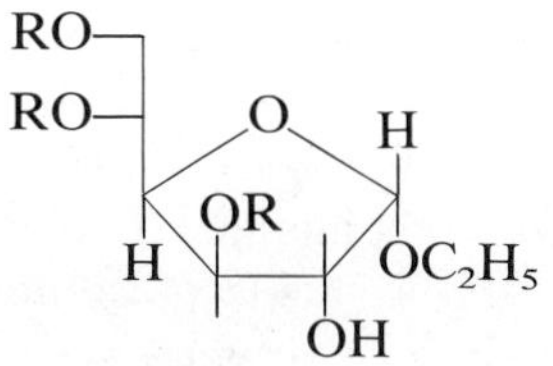

49.**108**   R = CH$_2$Ph

Two long chain esters, α-phenylglycine-N-heptyl ester (414) and N-hexyl gallate (415), have been reported to have anti-bradykinin activity. α-Phenylglycine N-heptyl ester (414) at $2-4 \times 10^{-5}$ M competitively reduced the relaxation induced by bradykinin on the rat duodenum. Esters of gallic acid also suppressed the effects of bradykinin on the guinea pig ileum. The apparent competitive antagonism increased with increasing chain length, up to six carbons. Inhibition by longer chain esters, four to six carbons, could only partially be reversed by 0.2 μg/ml of bradykinin (415).

A number of SH compounds, such as 2-mercaptoethylamine, glutathione, cysteine, 2,3-dimercaptopropanol, and 2-mercaptoethanol, are known to potentiate bradykinin-induced contraction of the guinea pig ileum (416–420). Potter and Walaszek (421, 422) concluded that cysteine potentiates the action of bradykinin on the guinea pig ileum via release of acetylcholine and that free NH$_2$ and SH groups were essential for such potentiation. To further investigate stereochemical requirements for this activity Witiak et al. (423) studied various cis- and trans-2-mercaptocyclobutylamines (49.**109a**), their aminomethyl homologs (49.**109b**), and their benzylmercapto analogs (49.**109c**). Only cis-49.**109c** was observed to be a potent

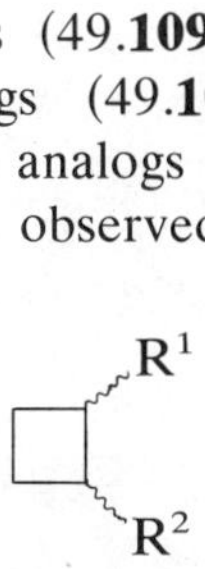

49.**109a**   R^1 = NH$_2$, R^2 = SH
49.**109b**   R^1 = CH$_2$NH$_2$, R^2 = SH
49.**109c**   R^1 = NH$_2$, R^2 = SCH$_2$Ph

potentiator of bradykinin-induced contraction of the guinea pig ileum, exerting its effect through release of acetylcholine. Large functions such as SCH(Ph)$_2$ and SC(Ph)$_3$ have been shown by Potter and Walaszek (421, 422) to afford cysteine analogs which block bradykinin-induced contractions of the guinea pig ileum, whereas smaller functions (SCH$_3$ and SCH$_2$Ph) afford analogs having 1/10 and 1/5 the potentiating activity of cysteine.

At higher concentrations (10^{-4} M) both cis- and trans-49.**109c** reduced by 21 and 31%, respectively, bradykinin-induced contractions; similarly 49.**109a** isomers were weak, but nonstereoselective antagonists. The cis-aminomethyl homolog (49.**109b**) at 10^{-4} M exhibited a small but significant reduction in bradykinin-induced contraction of the guinea pig ileum, whereas trans-49.**109b** was inactive. Since cis-49.**109b** exhibited no inhibitory effects against histamine and acetylcholine, it was proposed that this structure may provide clues for the development of more potent bradykinin antagonists (423).

9   RELEASE AND ANTAGONISM OF SEROTONIN

Serotonin (5-hydroxytryptamine; 5-HT) is implicated as a causative factor in allergic disorders (424). Anaphylactic reactions in rodents (425–427) are a result of the simultaneous release of 5-HT (428) with histamine (429–430). Both rat (431, 432) and mouse (433, 434) peritoneal mast cells were shown to contain 5-HT which is released in vitro by an anaphylactic reaction (433–435). Antigen challenge of actively sensitized guinea pig lung, aorta, and small intestine in vitro demonstrated that 5-HT and histamine are released at a constant rate (436); increased amounts of antigen caused increased release of histamine, but not of 5-HT. Mast cells found in rodents are histochemically identical to mast cells

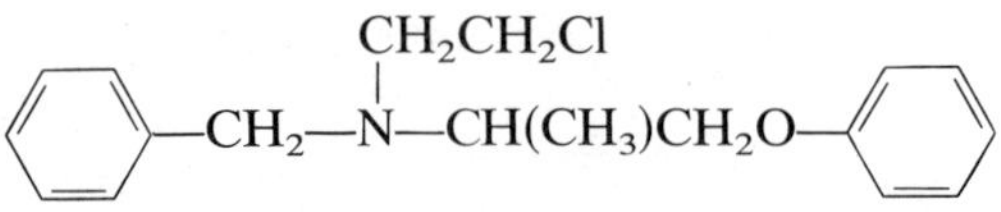

49.**110**

found in humans and have similar proteins and morphological characteristics, but human mast cells apparently lack 5-HT (437). Thus the significance of 5-HT in human anaphylaxis remains obscure (438–440).

The spasmogenic action of 5-HT on the guinea pig ileum is partially antagonized by morphine and completely eliminated by phenoxybenzamine (49.**110**) (441). Receptors blocked by morphine are termed M receptors and are located in nervous tissue, whereas those blocked by phenoxybenzamine are termed D receptors and are likely located in smooth muscle (441, 442). Reflex bradycardia is produced by the action of 5-HT and abolished by Tipindol (49.**111**) on afferent nerve endings of the cardiopulmonary reflexogenic system that are called T receptors (443, 444). Offermeier and Ariens (442) found calf tracheal muscle and rat fundus strip preparations to be more suitable for studying M and D receptors since these tissues exhibit cumulative dose responses. Both morphine and atropine antagonize 5-HT in the calf tracheal muscle preparation, whereas lysergic acid diethylamide (LSD, 49.**112a**) antagonizes the response of 5-HT only on the rat fundus strip. Morphine and atropine are inactive in the latter preparation. Additionally, acetylcholine esterase inhibitors potentiate the response of 5-HT on the calf tracheal muscle, but not on the rat fundus strip.

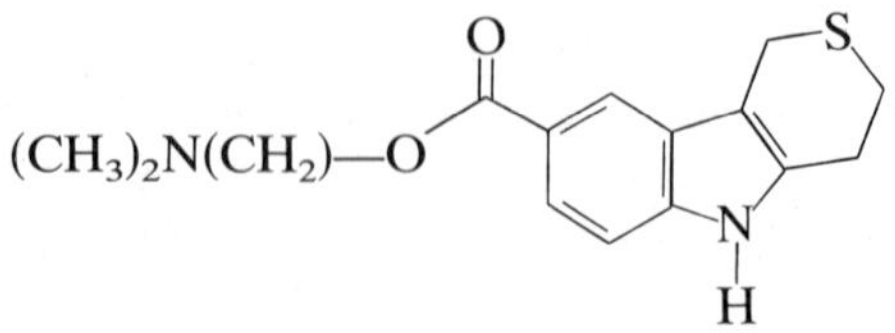

49.**111**

The protective action of some proteolytic enzyme inhibitors may partially be due to antagonism of the vascular response during shock to catecholamines and 5-HT (445). ε-Aminocaproic acid, a competitive inhibitor of the proteolytic enzymes plasmin and trypsin, and the ethyl ester of L-tyrosine, a competitive inhibitor of chymotrypsin, antagonize the vascular effects of 5-HT in the rat (445). ε-Aminocaproic acid (446) and the ethyl esters of both tyrosine and lysine (447) protect mice against anaphylactic shock.

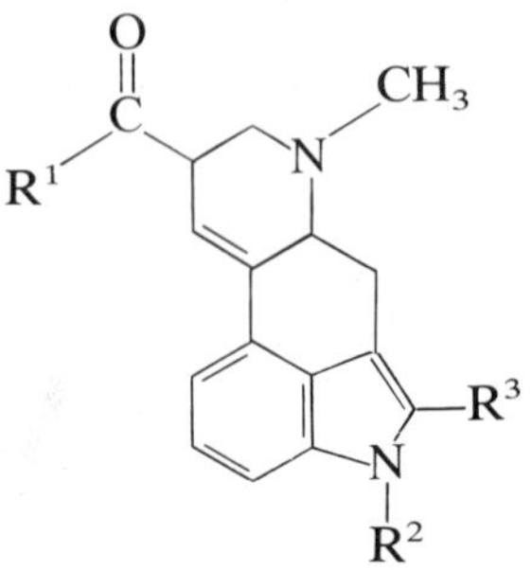

49.**112a** $R^1 = N(C_2H_5)_2$, $R^2 = R^3 = H$
49.**112b** $R^1 = NH[CH(C_2H_5)CH_2OH]$, $R^2 = CH_3$, $R^3 = H$
49.**112c** $R^1 = N(C_2H_5)_2$, $R^2 = H$, $R^3 = Br$
49.**112d** $R^1 = N(C_2H_5)_2$, $R^2 = CH_3$, $R^3 = H$

Partial protection against anaphylaxis in mice can be achieved using a variety of drugs. LSD (49.**112a**) significantly reduces anaphylactic mortality in white mice (448, 449). At the same dose methylsergide (49.**112b**) and 2-bromolysergic acid diethylamide (49.**112c**) are less effective. However, reserpine, a 5-HT releaser, has approximately the same activity (67% mortality) as 1-methyllysergic acid diethylamide (49.**112d**) (65% mortality) and is somewhat less active than 49.**112c** (55% mortality). In reducing serotonin-induced edema of the rat's paw 49.**112b** is four times as potent as 49.**112a** (450). In the same test 49.**112c** and 49.**112d** exhibit 28 and 91%, respectively, the potency of LSD. These relative differences in potency correlate with the observed protection against anaphylaxis by these compounds. At twice

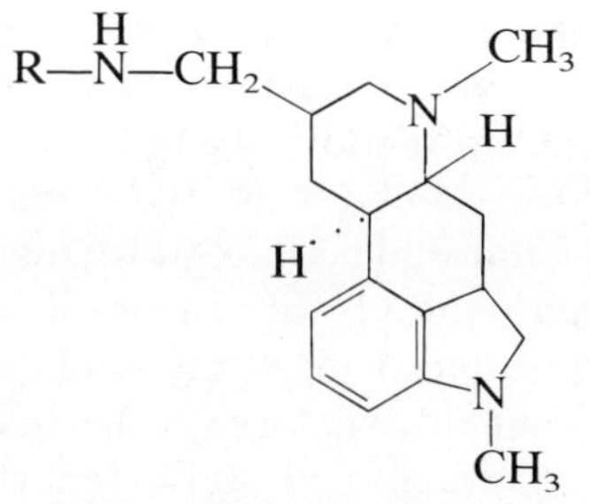

49.**113a** R = CO₂C₂H₅
49.**113b** R = CO₂(CH₂)₃CH₃

the dose of LSD, methylergide exhibits a significant increase in ability to protect against anaphylactic shock (36% mortality).

Natural ergot alkaloids and their derivatives are not specific in their biological properties. In addition to blocking 5-HT, these analogs have oxytoxic and adrenolytic actions. However, selective 5-HT antagonist activity is reported for the dihydrolysergamine derivative 49.**113a** on the isolated rat uterus (451). Minimal oxytocic and potent 5-HT antagonist activity was also reported for the butyl urethane derivative 49.**113b** (451). Also B and C ring deficient analogs methylsergide, 49.**114**, where the indole N function is replaced by a cinnamoyl group, are reported to be more potent than methylsergide in the rat uterus test (452).

Several cinnamanilides related to 49.**114** exhibit 5-HT blocking properties. Cinanserin [2′-(3-dimethylaminopropylthio)cinnamanilide, 49.**115a**] was observed to be 157 times more potent than phenoxybenzamine (49.**110**) as a 5-HT antagonist in

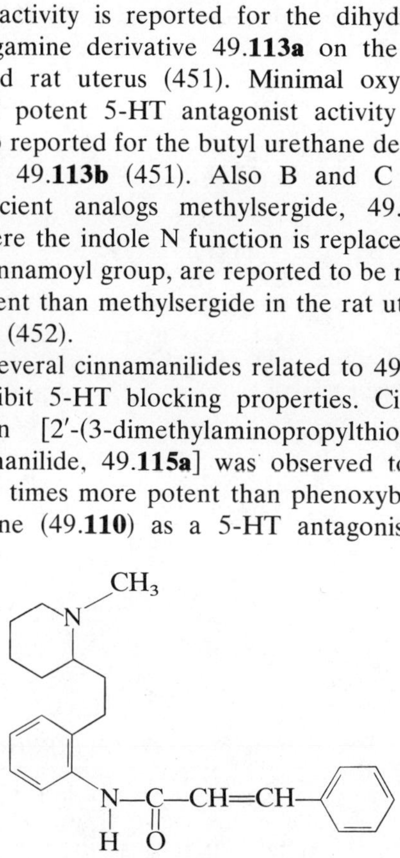

49.**114**

dogs and mice (453); carbonyl analog 49.**115b** and piperazino compound 49.**116a** exhibited three times more activity than cinanserin in the rat uterus test (454). When compared against 5-HT in the dog bronchoconstrictor assay, 49.**115a**, 49.**115b**, and 49.**116a** were equipotent. Benzyl (49.**116b**) and phenethyl (49.**116c**) substituted piperazino analogs were equipotent to cinanserin in the rat uterus assay (454). Chloro analog 49.**117a** is reported to be a weak immunosuppressive

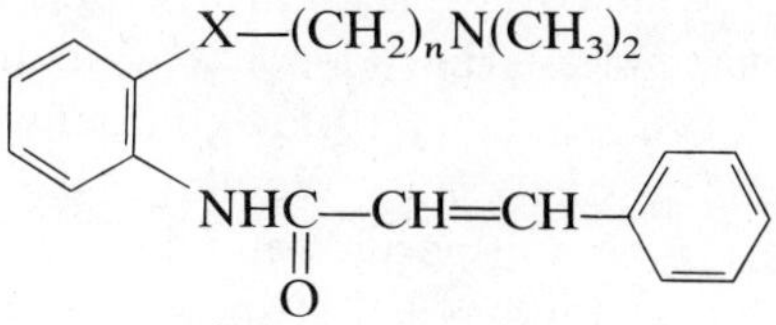

49.**115a** X = S, n = 3
49.**115b** X = CO, n = 2

agent having potent noncompetitive 5-HT antagonist activity on the rat uterus (455, 456). Toluidide 49.**117b** was characterized as a good immunosuppressive (mouse-sheep red blood cell assay) and a weak antagonist of 5-HT. Although methylsergide potentiates the action of acetylcholine on smooth muscle, 49.**117a** and 49.**117b** do not (455, 456).

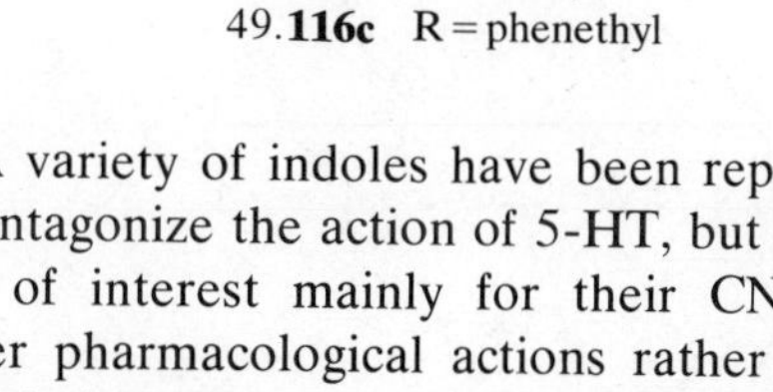

49.**116a** R = 2-pyridyl
49.**116b** R = benzyl
49.**116c** R = phenethyl

A variety of indoles have been reported to antagonize the action of 5-HT, but these are of interest mainly for their CNS or other pharmacological actions rather than for their antiallergenic properties. Tryptamine is more spasmogenic than 3-amino-

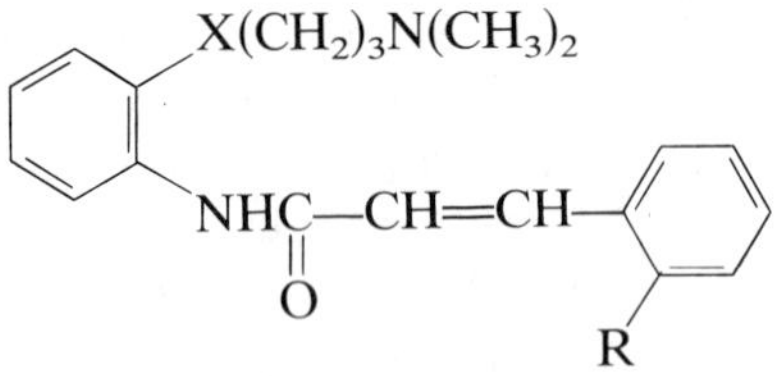

49.**117a**   X = S, R = Cl
49.**117b**   X = O, R = H

methylindole on smooth muscle (457). Increasing the number of side chain methylene groups in tryptamine increases the antiserotonergic effect and decreases the spasmogenic activity (457). An irreversible antagonist of 5-HT (1-benzyl-2-methyl-5-methoxytryptamine; 49.**118**), initially introduced by Shaw and Woolley (458, 459), seems to be nonspecific for 5-HT receptors on the rat fundus test strip (442). The related oxypertine (49.**119**) at 1 mg/kg i.v. antagonizes (37–55%) 5-HT-induced hy-

pertension in choralose anesthetized dogs treated with hexamethonium bromide (460). Dihydroindole 49.**120** is a potent competitive inhibitor of 5-HT on the rat fundus and guinea pig uterus (461). Serotonin-induced hypertension in the pithed and anesthetized rat was blocked by 49.**120**, but this analog was inactive in the rabbit. Pidevich et al. (444) reported that indole analogs 49.**121a** and 49.**121b** were potent antagonists of D receptors in the isolated rabbit atrium; the related tricyclic analog 49.**122** (K-277) was a better antagonist of M receptors, whereas the debenzylated analog, Tipindol (49.**111**), was the better T-receptor inhibitor. The quaternary derivative 49.**123a** was 38 times more potent than Tipindol in reducing reflex bradycardia. The gamma carboline derivative 49.**123b** is a 5-HT T-receptor antagonist and the ethyl ester analog 49.**123c** is

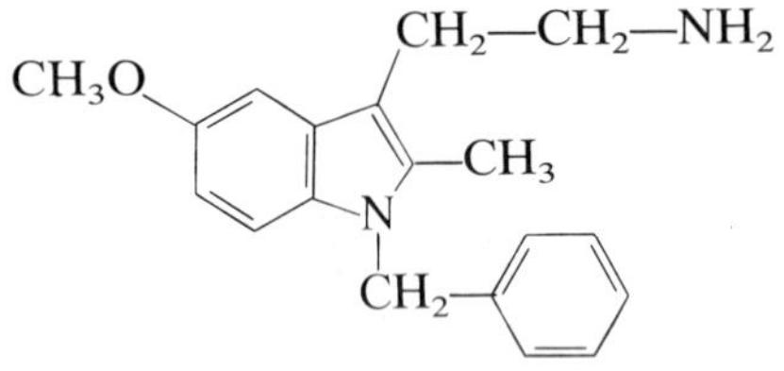

49.**118**

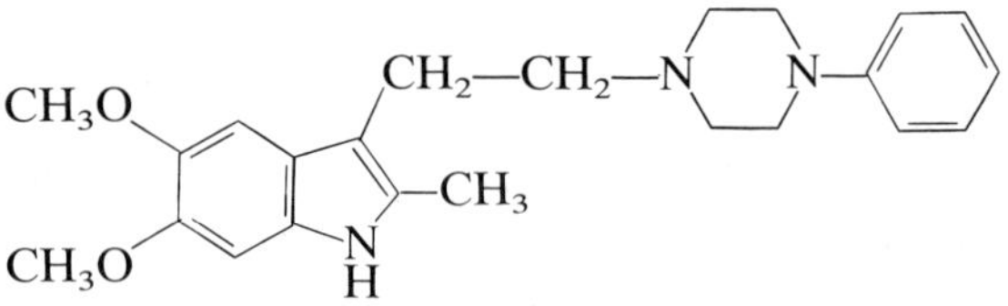

49.**119**

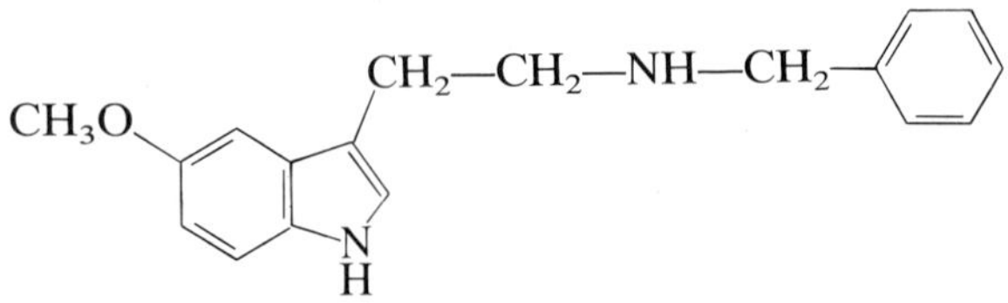

49.**120**

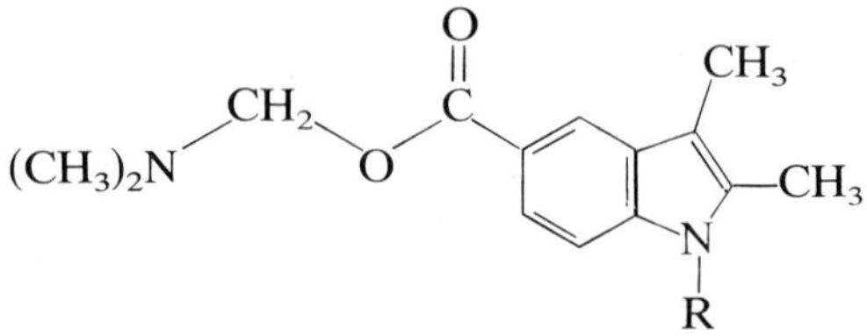

49.**121a**   R = $(CH_2)_2N(CH_3)_2$
49.**121b**   R = benzyl

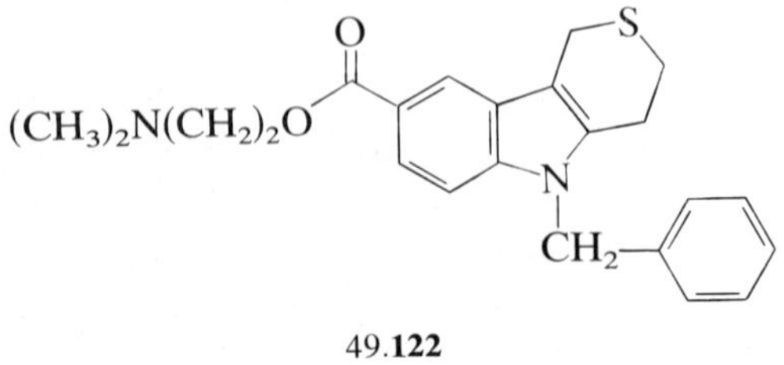

49.**122**

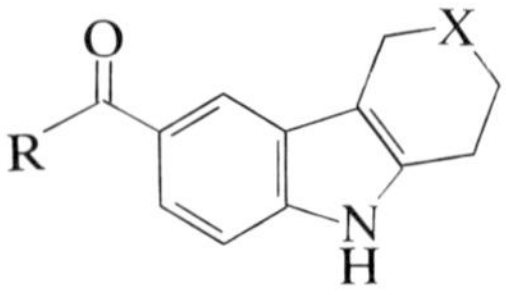

49.**123a**   R = —$O(CH_2)_2\overset{+}{N}H(CH_3)_2I^-$
         X = S
49.**123b**   R = —$O(CH_2)_2N(CH_3)_2$
         X = N
49.**123c**   R = —OCH_2CH_3
         X = N

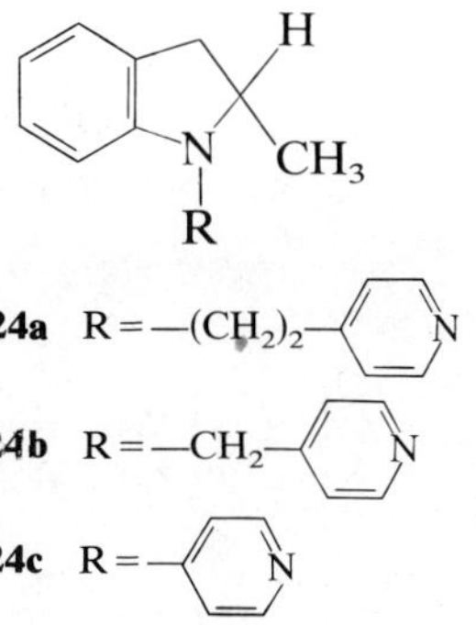

49.**124a** R = —(CH₂)₂—⟨pyridyl⟩

49 **124b** R = —CH₂—⟨pyridyl⟩

49.**124c** R = ⟨pyridyl⟩

inactive, suggesting the necessity of an amino bearing side chain (443).

A remarkable separation in receptor antagonist activity was observed with 1-[2-(4-pyridylethyl)-2-methyl]-2,3-dihydroindole (49.**124a**); this analog is an irreversible inhibitor of 5-HT on D receptors in the rat stomach muscle, whereas the 1-(4-pyridyl)-methyl analog 49.**124b** was an equally effective antagonist of 5-HT on all three receptors. The related 4-pyridyl derivative 49.**124c** was a weak 5-HT antagonist on D and M receptors, but was an agonist on T receptors (462).

Benzindoles 49.**125** and 49.**126** are respectively 5 and 32 times more potent antagonists of 5-HT than 49.**118** on the rat uterus (463). On the rat uterus, 49.**127** completely blocked the contractile effect of 5-HT; the ring-opened analog 49.**128** was found to be 25 times as potent as 49.**118** (464).

The related bromo derivative 49.**129a** at 0.1 μg/ml inhibited the contractile response of 0.01 μg/ml 5-HT on the rat uterus; 49.**126** is 24 times as potent as 49.**115** in this assay (465). The chloro analog 49.**129b** exhibited three to four times the potency of

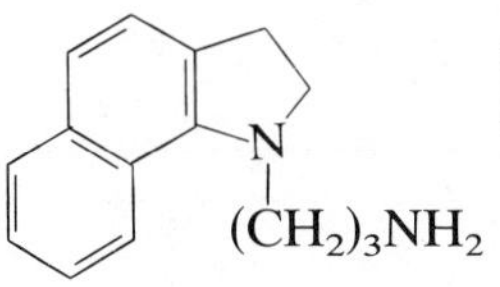

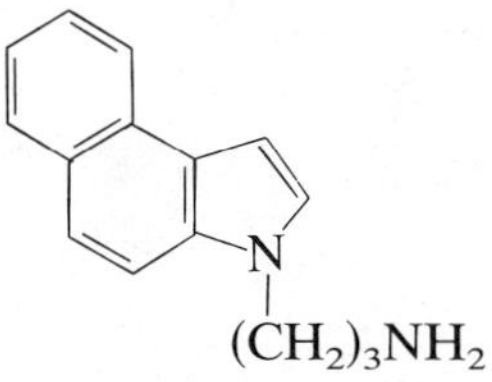

49.**118** (465). Carbazole, 49.**130a**, one of a series, was a potent competitive inhibitor of 5-HT on the rat uterus (466). Analog 49.**130a** is thought to be more potent than closely related compounds 49.**130b** and 49.**130c** owing to enhanced binding; after application of 49.**130b** and 49.**130c** the rat uterus recovered in 1 hr, but recovery required 72 hr after application of 49.**130a**. The acetamide of 5-methoxytryptamine, Melatonin (49.**131a**), competively blocked

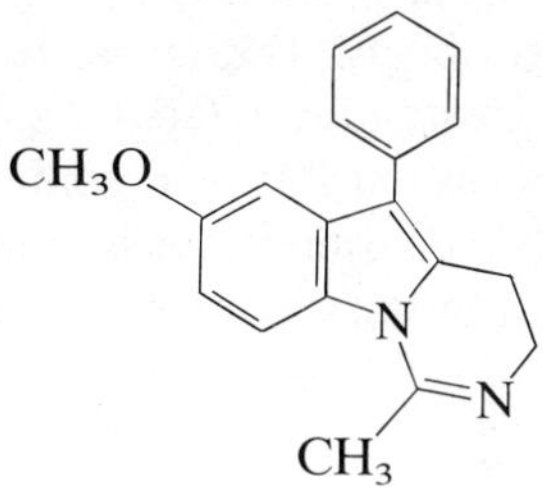

49.**127**

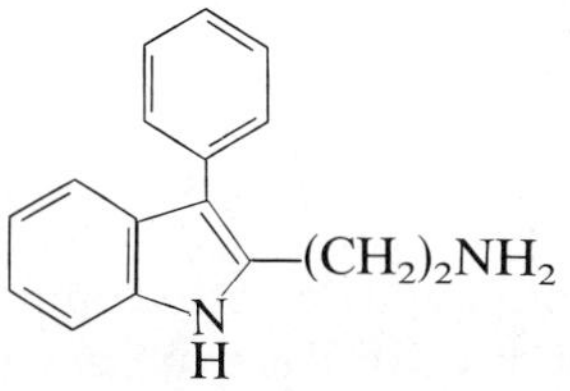

49.**128**

5-HT-induced contractions in the isolated rat stomach strip (467); the demethoxy analog 49.**131b** was less potent in the rat uterus (466). Additionally, several isosterically related indane (468), indene (469), and benzo[*b*]thiophene (470) analogs have been shown to inhibit 5-HT activity in a variety of pharmacological tests.

Numerous analogs having structures related to the classical antihistamines, antipsychotics, or antidepressants have been reported to inhibit 5-HT activity in a variety of biological tests. Since the significance of 5-HT involvement in the allergic syndrome in man is questionable, most of

49.**125**

49.**126**

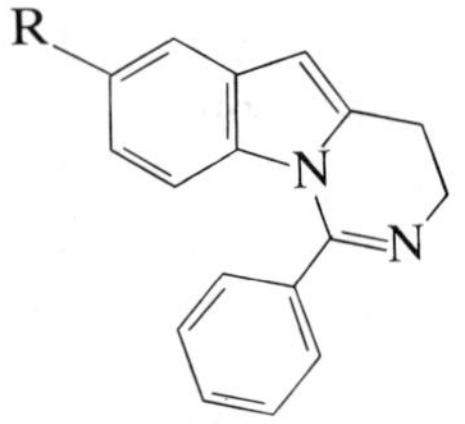

49.**129a** R = Br
49.**129b** R = Cl

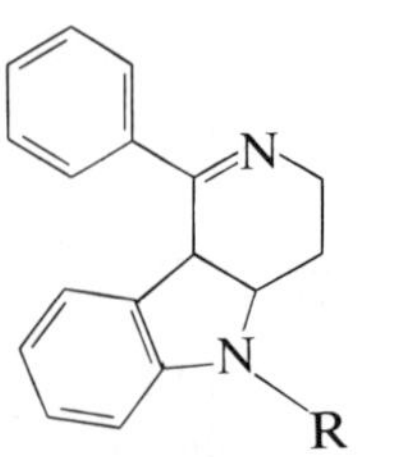

49.**130a** R = —C₂H₅
49.**130b** R = H
49.**130c** R = —CH₃

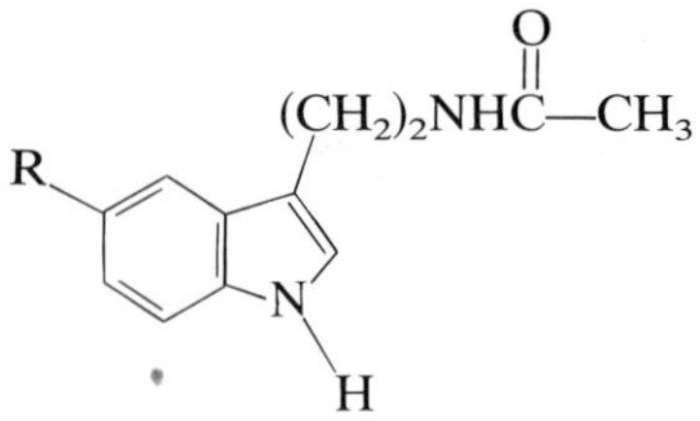

49.**131a** R = OCH₃
49.**131b** R = H

these analogs are studied for their anticipated CNS effects. Therefore, blocking 5-HT by antihistamine-related analogs may in fact be responsible for some of their undesirable pharmacological properties. For these reasons, a brief discussion of some of the analogs which modify 5-HT activity is presented in this section.

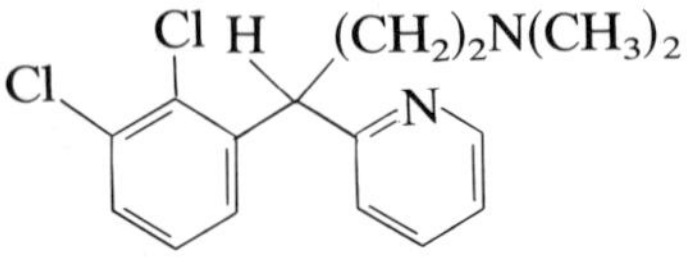

49.**132**

Many structurally diverse compounds inhibit or modify 5-HT activity *in vivo* and *in vitro*. Several investigations concerned with the effects of tricyclic analogs on 5-HT brain levels and uptake by nerve endings have been reported (471–473). The 3,4-dichloro analog 49.**132** of pheniramine is reported to be 30 times more potent than desipramine as an inhibitor of 5-HT uptake into the rat and mouse brain (474). Pheniramine analogs have been shown to inhibit 5-HT uptake by the synaptosomes of rat corpus striatum (474). The anti-5-HT activity observed for cyproheptidine (49.**81**) prompted its use as an antipruritic drug (226, 227). On an equal-dose basis, benzcyclan (49.**133**), as the maleate salt, exerts a pronounced 5-HT antagonist effect on the rat fundus strip which equals the effect produced by methylsergide (475). Pretreatment of guinea pigs with this reversible antagonist is prophylactic to 5-HT aerosol.

Mianserin (49.**134**), a novel piperazine tetracyclic ring analog, is a selective 5-HT antagonist reportedly more potent than cyproheptadine (476). A structural requirement for activity in this series appears to be related to the intersectional angle of 120° formed by the two planes of the aromatic rings (476). When the intersectional angle is changed, by construction of seven-membered B rings, activity is lost. The benzocycloheptathiophene analog, pizotyline (49.**107**), is a potent antagonist to the effects of 5-HT (477) in the burned rat skin test (478) and aids in the prevention of abortion in pregnant women (479).

Piperazine analog 49.**135** (AF-1161) has been compared to chlorpromazine by the bronchographic method (480). This compound preferentially inhibited the effects of 5-HT at a dose of 0.002–0.003 mg/kg i.v.; a dose of 0.26 μg/ml inhibited all responses

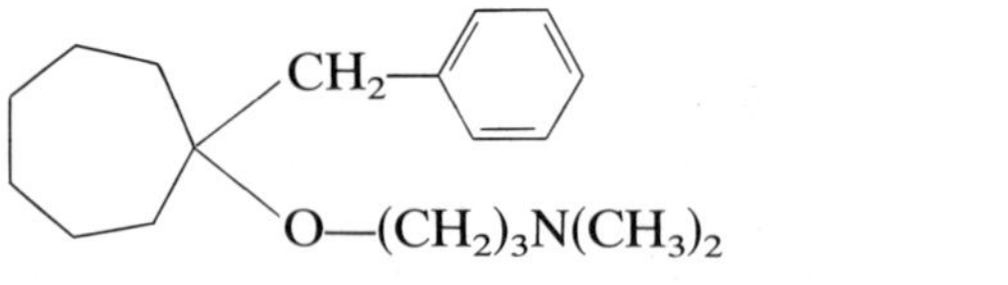

49.**133**

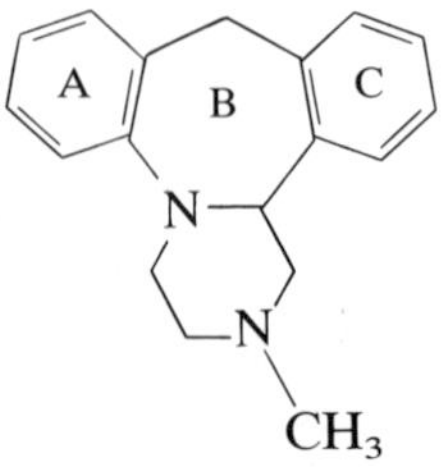

49.**134**

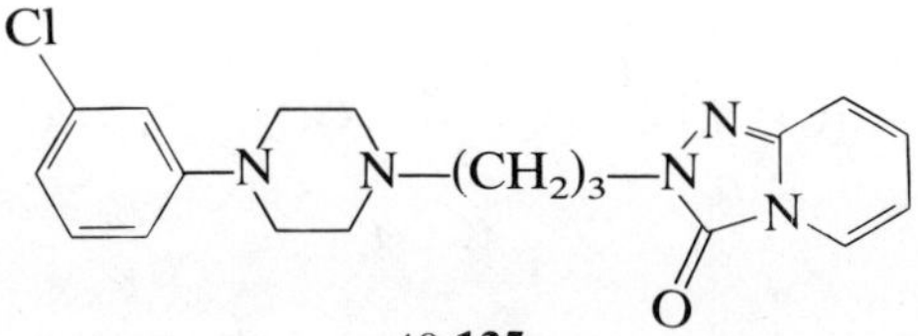

49.135

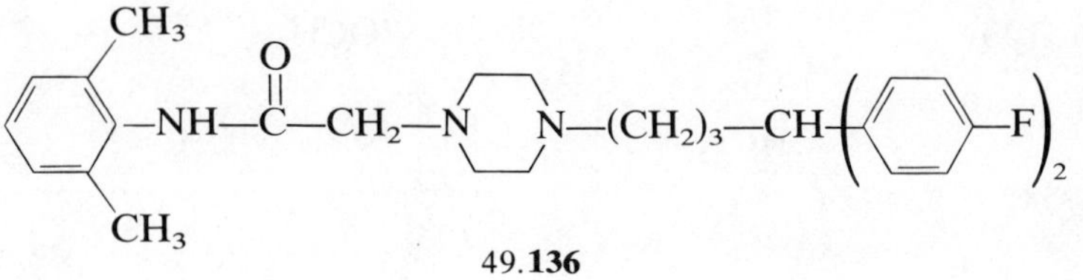

49.136

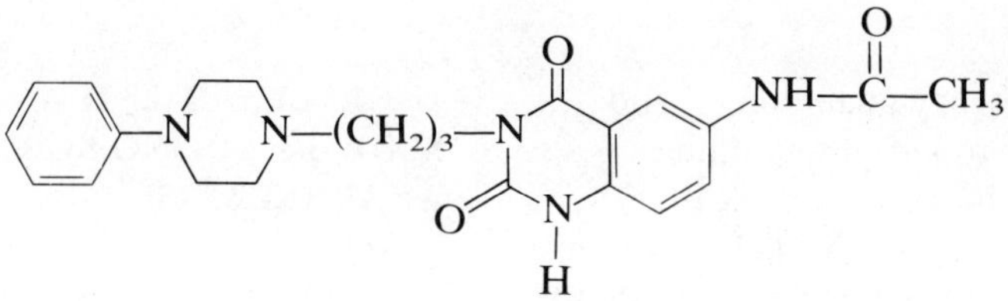

to 5-HT on the rat uterus. The drug lido-flazine (49.**136**) also exerts a selective dose-dependent competitive antagonism of 5-HT on the isolated rabbit aortic strip and the rat stomach fundus strip (481, 482). The effects of PGE_1 on the rat stomach fundus was blocked by 49.**136** (482). Concentrations of 49.**136** which blocked the effects of histamine, 5-HT, and PGE_1 did not antagonize the effects of acetylcholine, methacholine, and bradykinin; the later agonists were antagonized only at higher concentrations of drug (482). The antagonism between 49.**136**, 5-HT, and PGE_1 led the authors to propose that PGE_1 acts partially by means of serotonin receptors. Quinazolinedione analog 49.**137** is also a potent competitive antagonist when compared to methylsergide and cyproheptadine (49.**81**) in four different biological systems (483, 484). In the isolated rat uterus and in the 5-HT-induced hypertensive ganglion-blocked dog, 49.**137** was more potent than methylsergide. Antagonism of 5-HT in the guinea pig lung and rat's paw edema assays by cyproheptadine was less effective than with 49.**137** (483, 484).

The α-adrenergic blocker 49.**138** exhibits weak anti-5-HT properties at a dose level where methylsergide acts as a spasmogen (485). The structurally diverse nature of 5-HT antagonists is further illustrated by dihydroquinoline (49.**139**), which antagonizes 5-HT on the guinea pig ileum, but has no apparent activity against histamine or potassium (486). Further, the basic long chain aromatic ketone enantho-penone (49.**140**) is a 5-HT antagonist on rabbit jejunum and the rat uterine horn

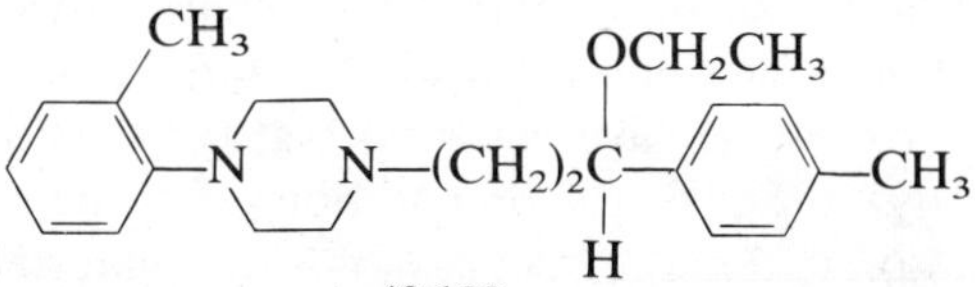

49.138

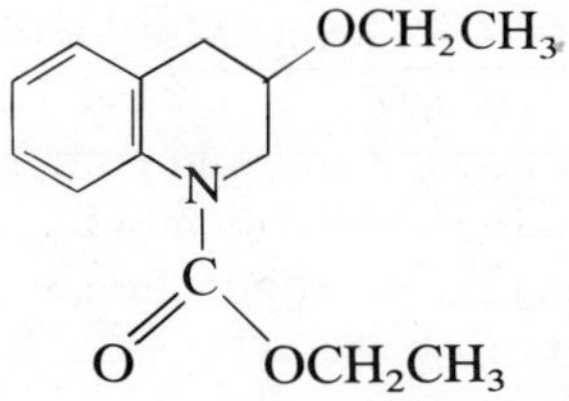

49.139

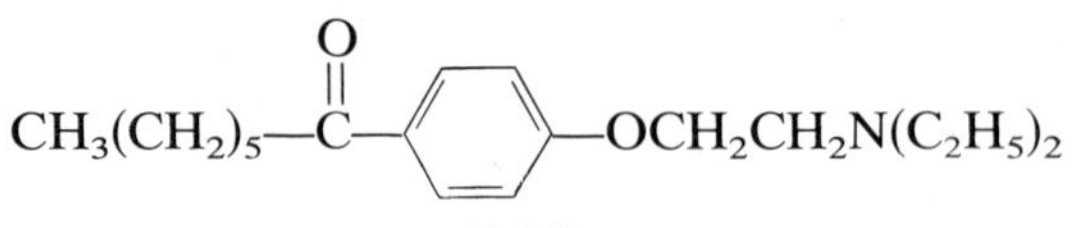

$$CH_3(CH_2)_5-\overset{\overset{\text{O}}{\|}}{C}-\langle\text{benzene}\rangle-OCH_2CH_2N(C_2H_5)_2$$

49.**140**

$$CH_3O-\langle\text{benzene}\rangle-O\overset{\overset{\text{CH}_3}{|}}{C}HCH_2NH\overset{\overset{+}{N}H_2}{\underset{\|}{C}}CH_2-\langle\text{benzene, }OCH_3\rangle \qquad CH_3-\langle\text{benzene}\rangle-SO_3^-$$

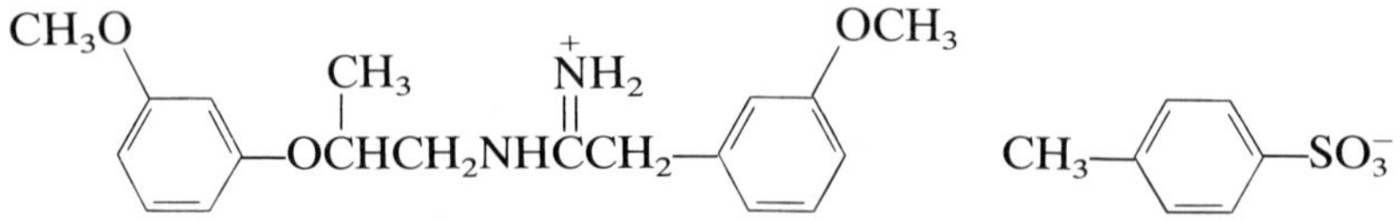

49.**141**

(487). 1,3-Dibenzylguanidine and 1-benzyl-3-(*o*-chlorobenzyl)guanidine also block 5-HT in the rat colon (488).

A new peripheral 5-HT antagonist, xylamidine tosylate (BW 545C64) (49.**141**) abolishes the pressor effect of 5 μg/kg of 5-HT in the pithed rat with a single 0.1 mg/kg i.v. injection (489). Taken orally 1 hr prior to 5-HT injection, 49.**141** is one-tenth as potent as methylsergide. Taken 5 hr before 5-HT challenge the drug is twice as potent as methylsergide. In addition to the many analogs which block 5-HT, an antibody has been produced to this amine which antagonizes its effects on the aortic strip, prevents its uptake by platelets, and sequesters free compound in solution (490).

Although the structures of gangliosides have not been completely characterized, Offermeier and Ariens (442) and Veinberg et al. (491) have observed that the sensitivity of 5-HT test preparations may be restored through the use of such materials. Serotonin-ganglioside micelles have been reported to reversibly bind to serotonin receptors (492, 493). If this is the case, this system may serve as a model for the co-operative role of serotonin and gangliosides in the postsynaptic membrane and/or the role of 5-HT in conduction of nerve impulses through the synapse.

10 RELEASE AND ANTAGONISM OF SLOW-REACTING SUBSTANCE OF ANAPHYLAXIS

The term "slow-reacting substance" (SRS) was first used by Feldberg and Kellaway (494) in 1938 to describe a substance that caused prolonged contraction of smooth muscle and that was released by perfusion of lung tissue with cobra venom. Interaction of an appropriate antigen with a perfused sensitized lung or mast cell challenged under the same conditions also released SRS (496–498). After antigen injection, SRS was found in the perfusate of the guinea pig lung and was identified by its resistance to mepyramine antagonism (499–500). Brocklehurst (501) used the term "SRS of anaphylaxis" (SRS-A) to denote the release of SRS by any antigenic challenge.

It is now known that IgE and IgGa mediated allergic reaction in the rat causes the release of both histamine and SRS-A. The release of SRS-A is influenced by intracellular levels of cAMP and antagonized in the rat by PGE_1 and PGE_2 in a dose-dependent fashion (502). The release of histamine and SRS-A from the perfused monkey lung is inhibited by chlorophenesin (49.**142**) in a dose-dependent fashion. Chlorophensin medi-

$$Cl-\langle\ \rangle-O-CH_2-\underset{\underset{H}{|}}{\overset{\overset{OH}{|}}{C}}-CH_2OH$$

49.**142**

ates this inhibition by activating adenyl-cyclase, thus causing an intracellular increase of cAMP (503). Exogenous addition of dibutyryl-cAMP resulted in inhibition of the release of SRS-A from rat peritoneal cells (504) and from human lung tissue (505) challenged with antigen. Alternatively, cholinergic stimulation or increased intracellular levels of cGMP, caused by the exogenous addition of 8-bromo-GMP to human lung tissue, enhanced the release of SRS-A (506). Thus it appears that target cells in human lung tissue are involved in the immunologic release of mediators which may interact with adrenergic and cholinergic receptor sites. When these sites are stimulated, they are capable of modulating the complex immunologic reaction through changes in the levels of the two cyclic nucleotides, cAMP and cGMP (506). Circulating levels of epinephrine may effectively modulate allergic activity by stimulating rapid formation of cAMP (507). The possible antianaphylactic effect may involve receptors other than those categorized as either β_1 or β_2 (508).

The strong contraction observed by released SRS-A on the guinea pig ileum is well maintained and used as a standard test procedure for detecting the presence of SRS-A (509). Guinea pig-produced SRS-A causes contraction in asthmatic and non-asthmatic human bronchioles (500, 510) as well as guinea pig bronchiole strips (511, 512) *in vitro*. A solution of SRS-A, administered in aerosol form, also produces bronchoconstriction in humans (513). After prolonged contact with SRS-A, smooth muscle does not return to its fully relaxed state, suggesting that SRS-A either alters the smooth muscle cell biochemistry or

binds to the cell surface, thereby preventing its own metabolism by normal body processes (509).

Characterization of those cells that are responsible for the release of SRS-A has received considerable attention (514–517). Initially, the rat neutrophil was thought to be a prerequisite for SRS-A synthesis (518), but subsequent studies demonstrated that the rat peritoneal mast cell was required for IgE-mediated release of SRS-A (519). Ishizaka et al. (23) observed that a substance released by antigen challenge from a suspension of sensitized monkey lung containing mast cells also had the pharmacological activity of SRS-A. Antigen challenge *in vitro* of human leukocytes obtained from sensitized individuals initially released histamine followed by SRS-A (520). No SRS-A was found in sonicated sensitized leukocytes. Thus SRS-A obtained from leukocytes appeared to be synthesized *de novo* after allergin challenge (520). In all studies *in vitro*, SRS-A was always released more slowly than the preformed chemical mediators, histamine, and eosinophil chemotactic factor of anaphylaxis (ECF-A). These observations further indicate that SRS-A formation takes place after antigen challenge (501, 521). Further, after antigen challenge, normal or passively sensitized human lung fragments or isolated human lung cells contain no detectable amounts of intracellular SRS-A at time zero. After 1 min, SRA-A appears; the intracellular concentration plateaus at 2 min. SRS-A continues to be released up to 15–30 min after antigen challenge (522). The polycationic compound 48/80 also induces the release of histamine and the formation and release of SRS-A from the perfused cat's paw. This is suspected to be an energy requiring process (523).

SRS-A is an acidic lipid-like material (524), previously proposed to contain an abundance of calcium and sulfur [perhaps due to sulfate ester group(s)] (525) and originally thought not to be a prostaglandin (526), protein, peptide, or carbohydrate (527). This substance is soluble in chloroform, 80% ethanol, and dilute NaOH solution (522, 528) and has a reported mol wt of 500 (525, 529), but travels as though it had a mol wt of 2000–5000 on acrylamide gel (527). SRS-A has been characterized as leukotriene C, having a C-6 substituent consisting of cysteine, glutamic acid and glycine as the tripeptide glutathione (527a, b) (See Chapter 62, diagram 16). SRS-A is inactivated by aryl sulfatases (525), phenylisocyanate, and iodine monobromide (530), is stable to heat, and is more sensitive to acid than to base (526).

As in the case of histamine, Ca^{2+} plays an important role in the release of SRS-A. Tissues that were depleted in Ca^{2+} by use of Ca^{2+}-free water or EDTA exhibited decreased ability to release histamine and SRS-A when stimulated with compound 48/80. Stanberg (530) suggested that Ca^{2+} may be needed for activation of an endogenous phospholipase A which promotes the release of anaphylactic mediators. The selective action and dissociated release of histamine and SRS-A by cytochalasins A and B from human lung fragments suggests that the immunologic stimulus causing the release of histamine and SRS-A may be identical (531). However, the subsequent biochemical events leading to the release of histamine and the formation and release of SRS-A may be very different (531). It also seems that cysteine may be acting as a cofactor for an enzyme(s) involved in SRS-A formation since cysteine enhances the formation and release of SRS-A from human peripheral leukocytes, monkey lungs, guinea pig lung fragments, and rat peritoneal cells (532).

Histamine and ECF-A are found as preformed anaphylactic mediators in sensitized rat pleural and peritoneal cavity mast cells (521). The quantities of histamine and ECF-A secreted by nasal polyps after antigen challenge are comparable to those released by human lung tissue, but the amount of SRS-A released from nasal polyps is significantly less. This may partly explain why antihistamines are efficacious in the control of allergic rhinitis (533).

The interaction of antigen with antibody attracts eosinophils to the site of injury or inflammation (534). Arylsulfatases extracted from purified human eosinophils also destroy purified human SRS-A (535). Arylsulfatases are also found in human lung tissue (536) and arylsulfatase B, isolated from eosinophils obtained from human lung tissue, similarly inactivated SRS-A (537). Human lung arylsulfatase B inactivated SRS-A obtained from either the rat peritoneal cavity or sensitized human lung in a linear time-dependent reaction. In a competitive experiment, the cleavage of p-nitrocatechol sulfate by arylsulfatase B was shown to be suppressed by the addition of SRS-A (537). Since human lung tissue contains predominantly arylsulfatase B, it would appear that this enzyme is responsible for controlling the concentration of SRS-A at or near the site of its generation in the lung (535, 537). Human lung tissue passively sensitized with ragweed antibody and challenged with specific antigen E yielded human SRS-A that was separated into four biologically active fractions (538). Contrary to the results observed with crude human SRS-A, only the first fraction was inactivated by arylsulfatase type H-1. However, all four active SRS-A fractions exhibited an inhibitory effect on arylsulfatase-catalyzed hydrolysis of nitrocatechol sulfate (538). These data are consistent with the proposal that SRS-A has a sulfate group (525, 535, 537), but now it appears that the function is a thioether (527a, b).

The anthelmintic diethylcarbamazine citrate (49.**143**), which does not antagonize the release of histamine, is reported to block the release of SRS-A in a dose-dependent fashion at a stage subsequent to the antigen-antibody interaction (519, 539, 540). A number of amide derivatives, (pi-

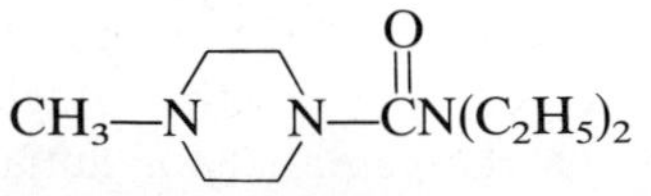

$$CH_3-N \qquad N-CN(C_2H_5)_2$$

with an O (=O) above the carbonyl carbon.

49.**143**

pecolamide, nicotinamide, isonicotinic acid hydrazide, and benzamide) afford greater than 30% inhibition of antigen-induced release of SRS-A from rat peritoneal cells (541).

Renewed interest in the search for active antiallergenic agents was initiated by the discovery and synthesis of disodium cromoglycate [1,3-bis(2-carboxychroman-5-yloxy)-2-hydroxypropane, disodium salt (DSCG), 49.**144**] by Fisons Laboratories. The bischromone 49.**144** is one of several chromone-2-carboxylic acids having anti-allergenic activity (542–544). Since DSCG is poorly absorbed orally, owing to its size and the acidic nature of the chromone carboxylic acid groups, the compound is administered in the form of a powder aerosol (543). For DSCG to be prophylactic, it must be inhaled prior to or at the time of antigen challenge. It has been proposed that DSCG acts by a nonspecific inhibition of the release of histamine and SRS-A at a stage following the reaction of antigen with IgE type reagin antibodies, but prior to the release of pharmacological mediators from mast cells (543).

Taylor et al. (545) found DSCG to have a synergistic action with theophylline, iso-prenaline, and PGE_1. Thus these investigators concluded that DSCG has a specific inhibitory effect on mast cell cAMP phosphodiesterase (546). Taylor et al. (546)

proposed that two phosphodiesterase iso-enzymes may be present in mast cells; one is more sensitive to theophylline-like drugs and is dominant in smooth muscle, whereas the other is more sensitive to DSCG. Tolerance to DSCG may also be explained in terms of the two isoenzymes. Taylor et al. (546) suggested that the rise in the intracellular cAMP level, induced by inhibition of DSCG-sensitive phosphodiesterase, might result in a compensatory activation of additional cyclic nucleotide phosphodiesterase. Alternatively, tolerance to DSCG may result from its ability to stimulate the production of an inhibitor to histamine release in the mast cell. Since the amount of formed inhibitor is limited, additional DSCG produces no effect (547, 548). A third proposal considers the possibility that interaction of DSCG with receptors is only slowly reversible and that DSCG more or less continually occupies receptors on the surface and/or inside the mast cell, thereby leading to tachyphylaxis (549). Although the phenomenon of tachyphylaxis is unclear, the maximal effect is observed when the interval between the predose and challenge dose is between 5 and 30 min. Tachyphylaxis is absent after 2 hr.

Interestingly, concentrations of DSCG necessary to obtain 50% inhibition of histamine release in rat peritoneal mast cells increased from 6 μM in buffered H_2O to 80 μM when 10% D_2O was added, and to greater than 500 μM in the presence of 25% D_2O (550). These data suggest that the interaction between DSCG and histamine release is not a simple one (550). Additionally, DSCG does not antagonize

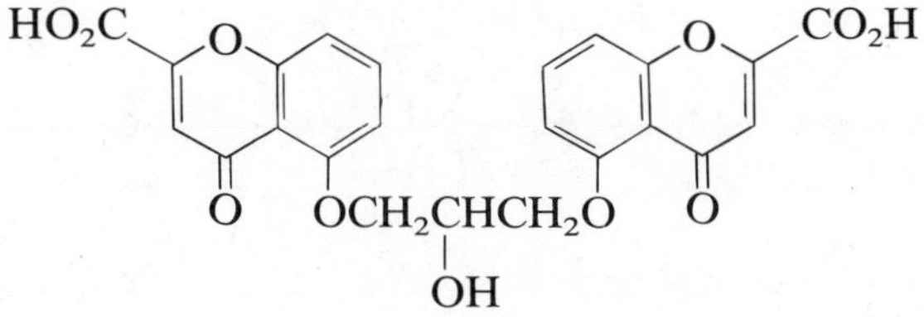

49.**144**

with HO₂C and CO₂H chromone structures connected by OCH₂CHCH₂O with OH.

the contraction of the guinea pig ileum induced by histamine, 5-HT, bradykinin, or SRS-A *in vitro* (551).

Structure–activity studies have shown that coplanarity of the two chromone rings is probably the most important requirement for biological activity (551). The fused chromone analog 49.**145** retains activity (49.**144** $ID_{50} = 0.7$ mg/kg vs. 49.**145** $ID_{50} = 0.5$ mg/kg) in the PCA test. The length and position of the linking chain in bis-chromone structures seems not to be critical for antiallergenic activity unless the chain is bonded to the 8 positions of the chromone rings. Thus 8,8′-substituted bis-chromones and 8-substituted mono-chromone-2-carboxylic acids are inactive. No antiallergenic activity is observed with bischromone structures bonded through a single methylene group or when the linking

chain $[O—(CH_2)_n—O]$ is longer than $n = 6$. The oxygen atoms in the bridging chain seem not to be essential for antiallergenic potency since the isosteric analog 49.**147** (49.**146** $ID_{50} = 0.3$ mg/kg vs. 49.**147** $ID_{50} = 0.25$ mg/kg) is active in the rat PCA test. The bischromone 49.**148**, having a carbox-amido methane linking chain, is equally as active as DSCG, but very insoluble (552).

A variety of compounds related to DSCG have been synthesized in an effort to obtain orally active and/or prophylactive drugs. Screening methods generally make use of the PCA test. Unfortunately, it does not necessarily follow that agents that fail in the rat PCA test are also inactive as antiallergenic agents of the immediate type-I allergic reaction (551). Although the rat PCA test is convenient and rapid, other species and allergic hypersensitivity reac-

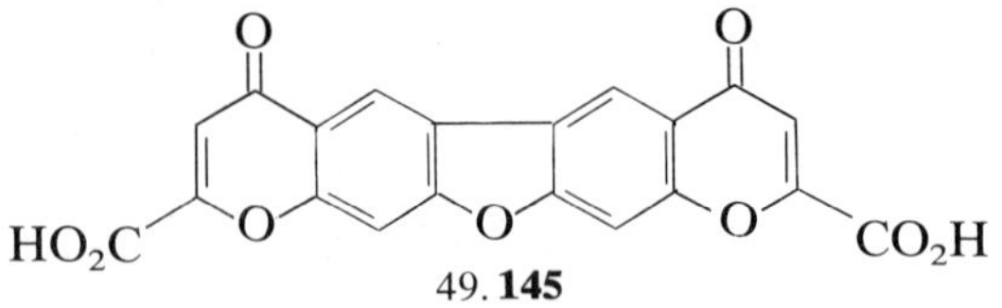

49. **145**

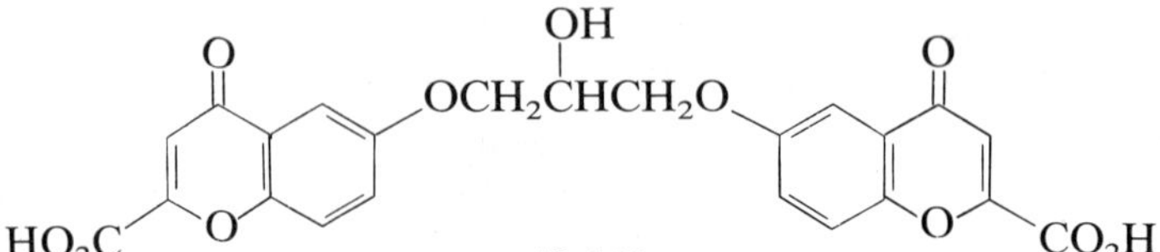

49. **146**

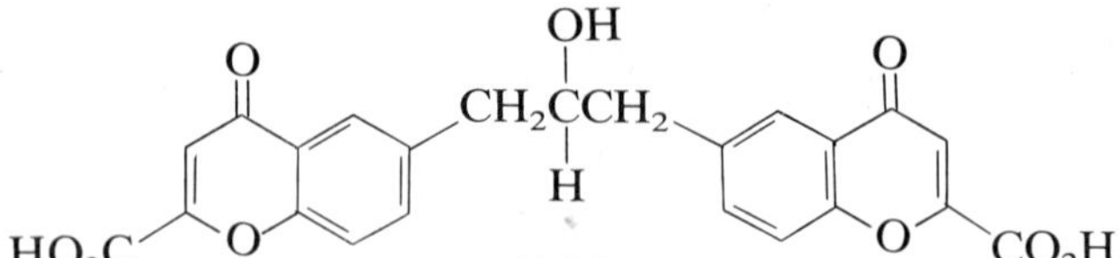

49.**147**

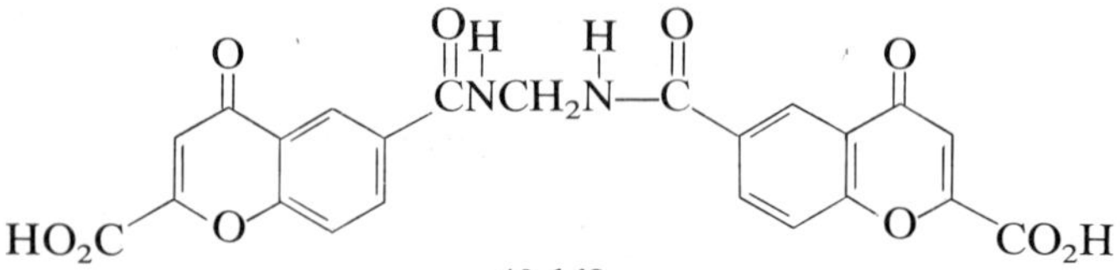

49.**148**

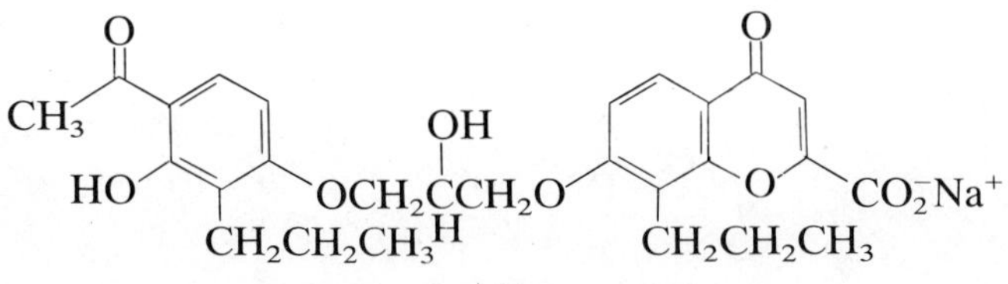

49.**149**

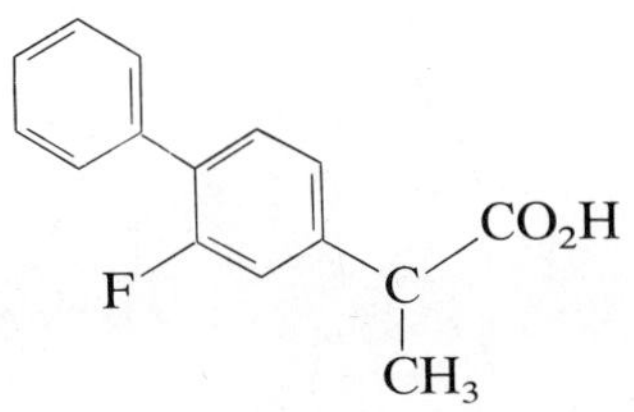

49.**150**

tion tests should be employed for assessing drug activity. Recently, anaphylactic bronchoconstriction was produced in guinea pigs with IgE antibodies; thus the guinea-pig may be a potential experimental model of human allergic asthma (553).

Unlike DSCG, the monosodium salt of 7-[3-(4-acetyl-3-hydroxy-2-propylphenoxy)-2-hydroxypropoxy]-4-oxo 8-propyl-4H-chromone-2-carboxylate (49.**149**), is a potent and selective inhibitor of SRS-A-induced contractions on the guinea pig ileum (554, 555). Compound 49.**149** also antagonizes PGE_1, $PGF_{2\alpha}$, histamine, 5-HT, acetylcholine, and bradykinin, but requires 11000–6000 times greater concentration than those needed to antagonize the effects of SRS-A on the guinea pig ileum. Unlike any other compounds, 49.**149** (0.005–0.008 μg/ml) reverses the effects of an existing response to SRS-A on the guinea pig ileum in a dose-dependent manner (554, 555). The guinea pig preformed mediator, ECF-A, is antagonized by 49.**149**, whereas DSCG and hydrocortisone exhibited no similar inhibition in this test (556). The inhibitory effect of 49.**149** on the guinea pig ECF-A-induced chemotaxis of eosinophils may be a direct action on the ECF-A molecule or be a reflection of the inability of eosinophils to recognize the chemotactic stimulus (556). Although flurbiprofen (49.**150**) differs markedly from 49.**149** in structure, its action against SRS-A at a concentration of 0.0032 μg/3 ml antagonized bradykinin (0.32 μg/3 ml) 81% in this preparation. The dextrorotatory isomer of 49.**150** is estimated to be approx-

imately eight times more potent than the racemic compound (557).

The flavanoid baicalein (49.**151**), obtained from the radius of *Scutellaria biacalensis* Georg, had been used in ancient Chinese medicine as a diuretic and antiallergenic. A derivative of 49.**151**, 5-hydroxy-7-methoxychromone-2-carboxylic acid (49.**152**), is more potent than DSCG (20 mg/kg vs. 1.25 mg/kg, respectively; 100% inhibition), whereas the saturated chromanone 49.**153** has virtually no activity in the rat PCA test (558). The inactivity of 4-oxo-4H-1-benzopyran-3-carboxylic acid (49.**154**) in the rat PCA test may be due to intramolecular hydrogen bonding of the carboxyl hydrogen to the chromone ketone. Acrylic acid 49.**155** does not allow for such hydrogen bonding and is active (4–10 mg/kg) in the same test. Introduction of an alkoxy or an alkyl group at C-6 or C-8 of 49.**155** afforded analogs having enhanced biological activity (1–3 mg/kg); the

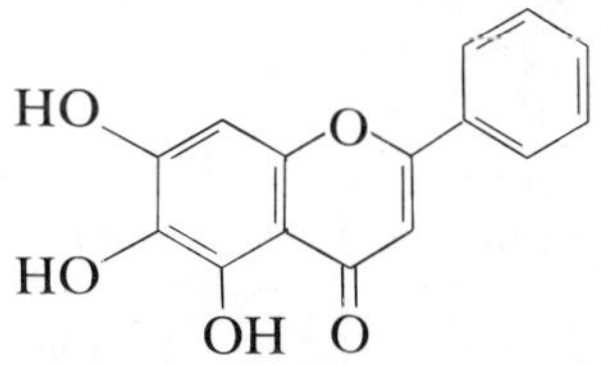

49.**151**

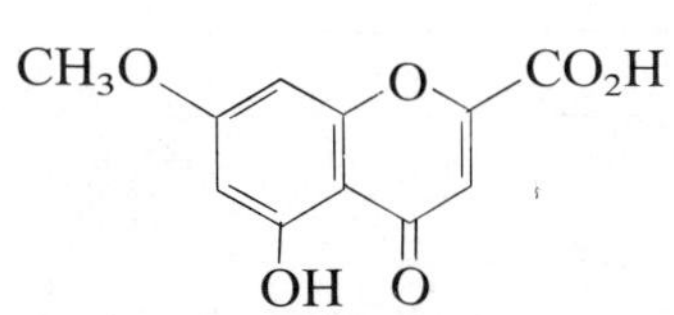

49.**152**

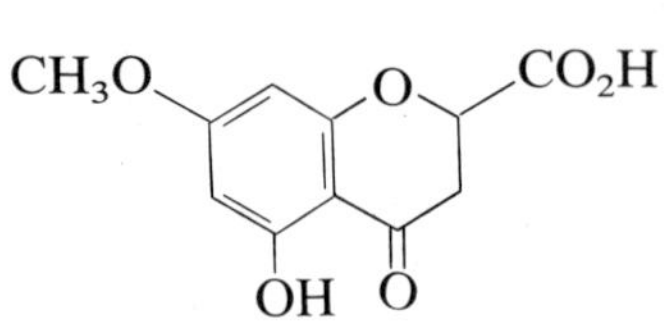

49.**153** 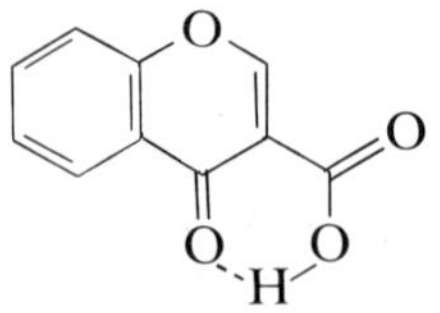   49.**154** 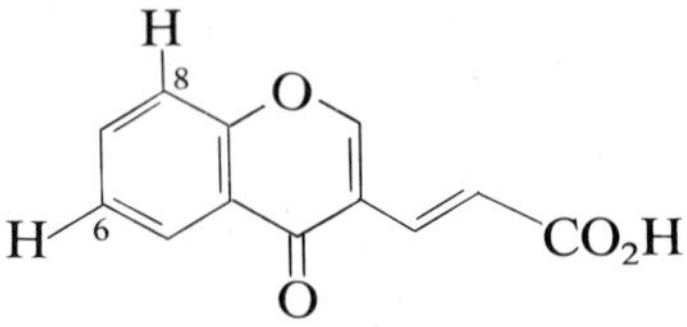   49.**155**

greatest activity was obtained with the C-6 isopropyl derivative (<1 mg/kg) after either i.v. or oral administration. The C-6 di-methylamino derivative of 49.**155** is also active (1–3 mg/kg), whereas the C-6 car-boxyl analog is inactive in the rat PCA test (559).

Replacement of a carboxyl group by a 5-tetrazolyl group has in some cases resulted in retention of, but rarely improved, bio-logic activity. Unsubstituted 2-(5-tetra-zolyl)chromone 49.**156a** and certain C-6 (49.**156b**) and C-7 (49.**156c**) methyl-sub-stituted derivatives are more potent than DSCG. For similar responses in the rat PCA test, doses required for DSCG were 5 mg/kg, and for 49.**156a** and 49.**156c**, 1 mg/kg given at the time of antigen chal-lenge. Analog 49.**156b** required 50 mg/kg when administered 15 min after challenge (560, 561). Alkyl or halogen substitution at C-3 or C-8 or replacement of the 5-oxo function by a 4-thioxo moiety resulted in loss of activity (560, 561).

Tetrazole derivatives of biologically inac-tive chromone acids exhibit an enhanced antiallergenic potency. The unsubstituted tetrazole derivative 49.**157** is active intra-venously, but not orally. The tetrazole de-

rivative of 49.**155** shows no improvement in potency (562). In fact, 49.**157** was 2.5 times as potent as tetrazole 49.**156** in the PCA test. Analogs of 49.**157** (6-ethyl; 6-chloro; 6-nitro; 6-hydroxy; 6,8-dimethyl), 49.**158** and 49.**159** are 4–10 times as po-tent as DSCG and are orally active (562).

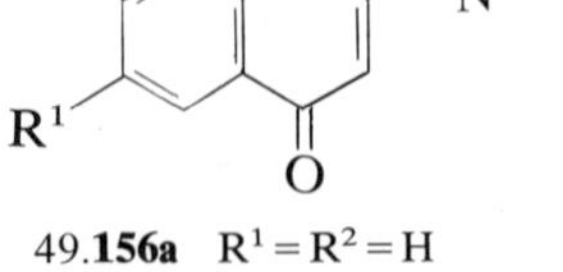

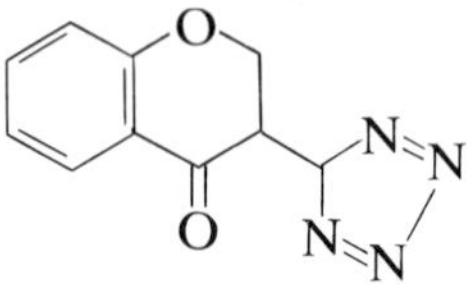

49.**157**

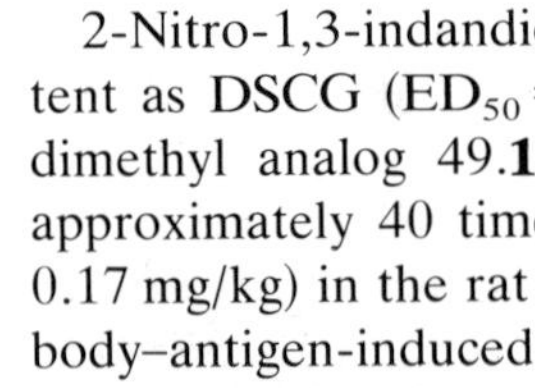

49.**158** 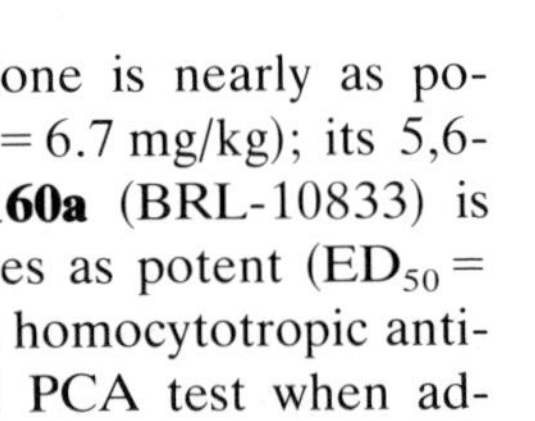   49.**159**

2-Nitro-1,3-indandione is nearly as po-tent as DSCG ($ED_{50} = 6.7$ mg/kg); its 5,6-dimethyl analog 49.**160a** (BRL-10833) is approximately 40 times as potent ($ED_{50} = 0.17$ mg/kg) in the rat homocytotropic anti-body–antigen-induced PCA test when ad-ministered 10 min prior to antigen chal-lenge. Elimination of the nitro group in 49.**160a** abolished biologic activity (563). Compound 49.**160a** is more effective than DSCG in inhibiting the extravasation of dye, induced by released histamine, in the passive peritoneal anaphylaxis test. Addi-tionally, 49.**160a** is more effective orally than i.p., whereas DSCG is only active by i.p. administration in this test (564). Partial

49.**156a** $R^1 = R^2 = H$
49.**156b** $R^1 = CH_3$; $R^2 = H$
49.**156c** $R^1 = H$; $R^2 = CH_3$

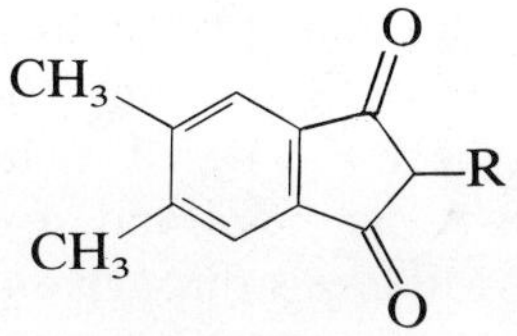

49.**160a** R = NO$_2$
49.**160b** R = —CN

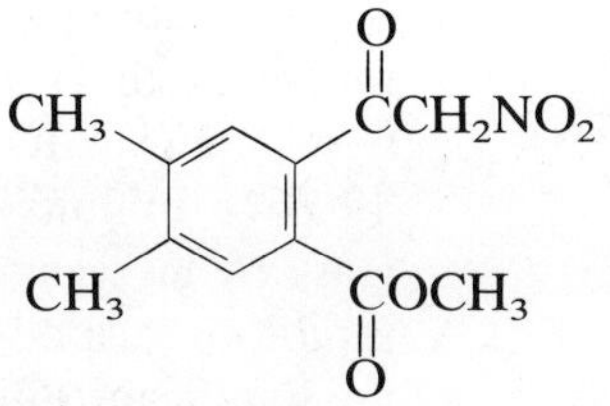

49.**161**

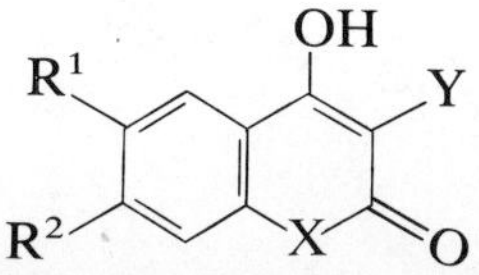

49.**162a** R^1 = R^2 = CH$_3$, X = O, Y = NO$_2$
49.**162b** R^1 = R^2 = CH$_3$, X = NH, Y = NO$_2$
49.**162c** R^1 = R^2 = H, X = NH, Y = NO$_2$
49.**162d** R^1 = R^2 = CH$_3$, X = O, Y = CN

or complete reduction of the aromatic ring in 49.**160a** afforded a decrease or complete loss of potency (565). Formation of 49.**160a** *in vivo* accounts for the activity of nitroacetophenone analog 49.**161** (566). Structurally related six-membered lactone 49.**162a** and lactam 49.**162b** analogs of the coumarin type were more potent than DSCG (ED$_{50}$ = 1.0 mg/kg for 49.**162a**; 3.8 mg/kg for 49.**162b**) in the rat PCA test (567, 568). No increase in potency was observed upon insertion of nitrogen (analog 49.**163**) into the carbocyclic ring of 49.**162c** (568). For these analogs and various carbocyclic reduced forms, the planarity of the strain-free olefinic ring function seems to be most important for biologic activity (568).

Replacement of the nitro group in 49.**160a** and 49.**162a** with a nitrile function affords analogs 49.**160b** and 49.**162d** with retention of antiallergenic activity. A substantial loss of antiallergenic activity was observed when the hydroxyl group of 49.**162a** was replaced with a hydrogen, alkyl, halogen, methoxyl, amino, or ethylamino function. These results further supported the apparent significance of the 1,3-dicarbonyl system (569).

Since the function O—C=C—C=O in the hetero ring of DSCG seemed to be particularly important for biologic activity, tricyclic xanthone analogs 49.**164a**–49.**164c**, having this same function in the central ring, were constructed and tested (570). In the PCA test 49.**164a** was approximately one-half as potent as DSCG. Linear or branched alkoxy substitution at C-5 or C-7 resulted in potency increases with the orally or i.v. active 7-isopropoxy analog 49.**146b** being eightfold more potent than DSCG. The 7-(2-hydroxyethoxy) analog 49.**164c** (AH 7725) is reportedly more potent than DSCG after i.v. (ID$_{50}$ = 50 μg/kg vs. 1.3 mg/kg for DSCG) administration to the rat (571). A single dose (200–500 mg of AH 7725 was orally active in man as a prophylactic agent against the immediate type of asthma induced by inhaled antigen (572). It has been proposed that DSCG and AH 7725 may be acting by similar mechanisms (571).

The tetrazole analog, 7-methoxy-2-(1*H*-tetrazol-5-yl)xanthen-9-one (AH 7079),

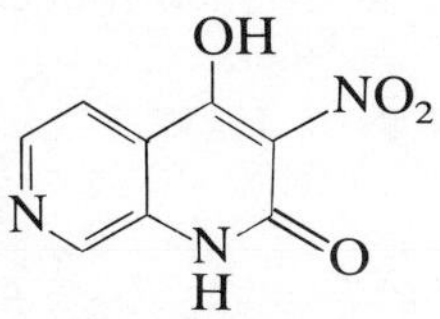

49.**163**

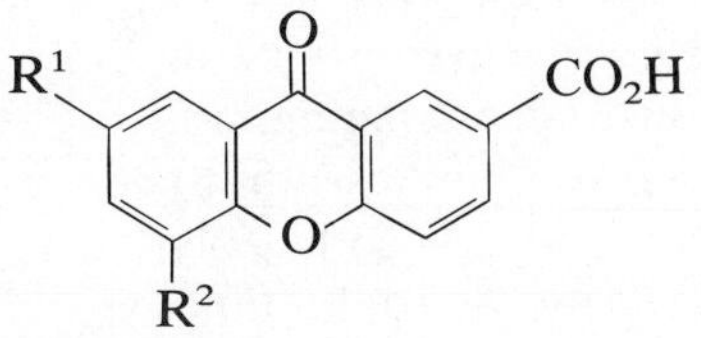

49.**164a** R^1 = R^2 = H
49.**164b** R^1 = H, R^2 = —OCHCH$_3$
49.**164c** R^1 = H, R^2 = —OCH$_2$CH$_2$OH

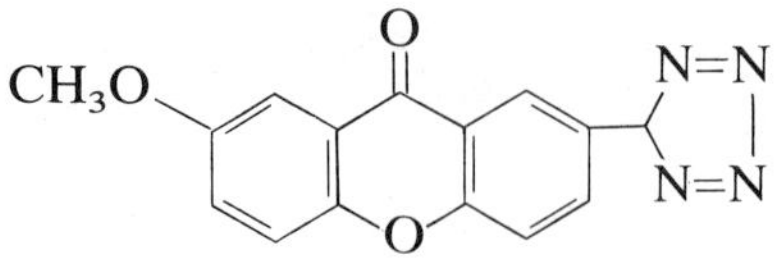

49.**165**

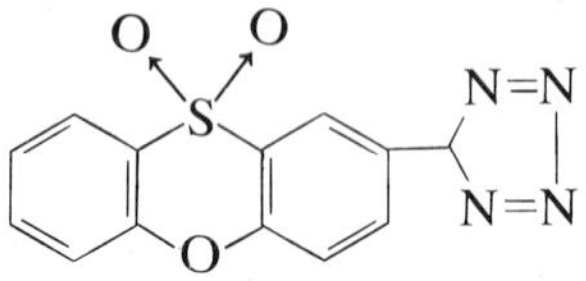

49.**166**

49.**165**, protects against allergic airway disease (573) and is 100 times more potent than DSCG in antagonizing the release of histamine in the human leukocyte preparation (575). The thioxanthone Doxantrazol (49.**166**) is active in human subjects given a single oral dose (200 mg). The compound blocks the release of histamine from passively sensitized human lung tissue (575, 576).

Methylxanthines inhibit histamine release in the rat PCA test, but are ineffective in this test when nonreaginic antigens are employed during challenge. Thus methylxanthines may have a mode of action similar to that of DSCG (577). During a study of 1- and 3-substituted 8-azaxanthines, 1-methyl-3-(p-nitrobenzyl)-8-azaxanthine was observed to be nearly as potent as DSCG in the rat PCA test (577). Activity in this series could not be interpreted on the basis of a consideration of partition coefficients. However, 2-substituted 9-azapurin-6-ones, capable of undergoing intramolecular hydrogen bonding, exhibited improved potency. Whereas 2-pyridyl analog 49.**167a** was nearly inactive, N-oxide 49.**167b**, capable of hydrogen bonding, was equipotent to DSCG in this test (578); 4-thiazolyl 49.**167c** and 3-isothiazolyl 49.**167d** were, respectively, 2 and 2.5 times more potent than DSCG (578). 2-Propoxy analog 49.**167e** (M+B 22,948) was 20–50 times more potent than DSCG in inhibiting reagin-mediated anaphylaxis in a number

of test systems (579, 580) and strongly antagonizes the release of SRS-A from calf tissue (581). It has been proposed that 49.**167e** inhibits SRS-A synthesis and release by increasing cAMP levels through an inhibition of phosphodiesterase. DSCG has no significant effect in the calf test system (581). Again, intramolecular hydrogen bonding is possible in 49.**167e**. Decreases in potency parallel presumed decreases in intramolecular hydrogen bonding capability as alkoxy substituents increase in size. Coplanarity of the phenyl substituent with the azahypoxanthine moiety seems to be a requirement for high antiallergenic potency (579).

Several tricyclic (49.**168a,b** 49.**169**, 49.**170**, 49.**171**) and tetracyclic (49.**172**) γ-pyrones, as well as their structurally related bicyclic (49.**173**) and tricyclic (49.**174**, 49.**175**, 49.**176**) quinolone acids have been tested (549, 581–590). 4-Oxo-4H-[1]-benzofuro[3, 2-b]pyran-2-carboxylic acid (49.**168a**) and its thio analog 49.**168b** were one-half as potent as DSCG in the rat PCA test. (582). Benzothieno analog 49.**168b** was 18 times more potent than DSCG in the Prausnitz–Kustner (PK) reaction test, whereas 49.**168a** was less active.

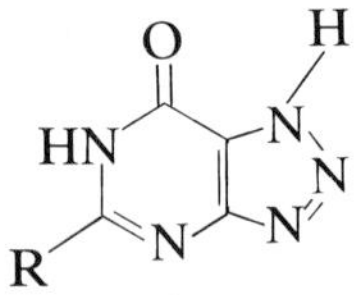

49.**167**

a   R = 2-pyridyl
b   R = 2-pyridyl N-oxide

c   R =

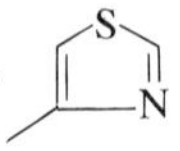

d   R =

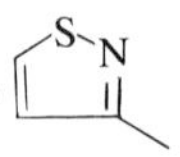

e   R =

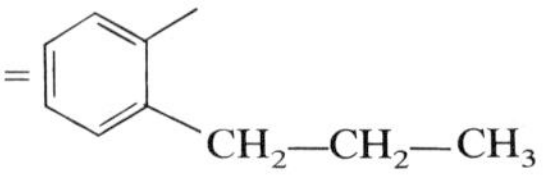

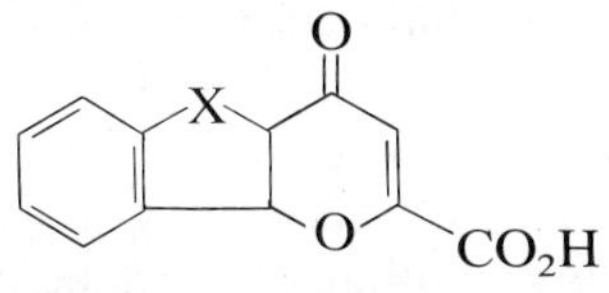

49.**168a** X = O
49.**168b** X = S

A series of planar benzodipyrans, having two strongly acidic conjugated carboxyl groups (49.**169**, 49.**170**, and 49.**171**), show antiallergenic activity as determine by the rat PCA test (583). Generally, linear benzodipyrans (49.**169** and 49.**170**) are more potent (ID_{50} = 0.18 and 0.68 mg/kg i.v., respectively) than angular isomers such as 49.**171** (ID_{50} = 7.6 mg/kg i.v.). Propyl or N-butyl substitution at R^1 in 49.**169** significantly increased antiallergenic potency (ID_{50} = 0.05 mg/kg i.v.), whereas alkoxy substitution (R^2 = OCH_3) produced no enhancement in activity. Interestingly, alkoxy groups in angular analogs such as 49.**171** (R^1 = OCH_3, OC_2H_5, and $OCH_2CH = CH_2$; ID_{50} = 0.73, 0.38, and 0.62 mg/kg i.v., respectively) show a marked increase in antiallergenic potency, whereas an ethyl function at R^2 in 49.**171** had little or no effect on potency (583). Alkyl- and alkoxy-

substituted analogs 49.**171** (R^1 = OCH_3 and R^2 = propyl) resulted in a further increase in potency (ID_{50} = 0.18 mg/kg i.v.) in the rat PCA test. Introduction of electron-withdrawing groups into either the linear 49.**169** (R^2 = NO_2) or angular 49.**171** (R^2 = Cl) benzodipyran systems resulted in less potent compounds.

The novel tetracyclic analog 5,5-dimethyl - 11 - oxo - 5H, 11H - (2) - benzopyrano-[4, 3 - g](1) - benzopyran - 9 - carboxylic acid (49.**172a**) was effective at 0.43 mg/kg i.v. in the rat PCA test (584, 585) and is reported to be a potent antagonist of SRS-A release from calf tissue (581). Significant enhancement of antiallergenic potency over 49.**172a** was observed with analog 49.**172b** (ED_{50} = 0.11 mg/kg i.v.) in the rat PCA test. Simple substitution at C-4 and C-12 in 49.**172a** caused little or no change in potency, whereas complete loss in activity was observed utilizing SO_3H functions at C-3. Loss of activity was attributed to disruption of polarity (584).

Quinaldic acid (49.**173**), 7-amino-1,4-dihydro-8-methyl-4-oxoquinaldic acid, and its tricyclic analog (49.**174**), a 7-amino-1,4-dihydro-4-oxobenz[H]quinoline-2-carboxylic acid, are both 25 times more potent than DSCG in the rat PCA test (586).

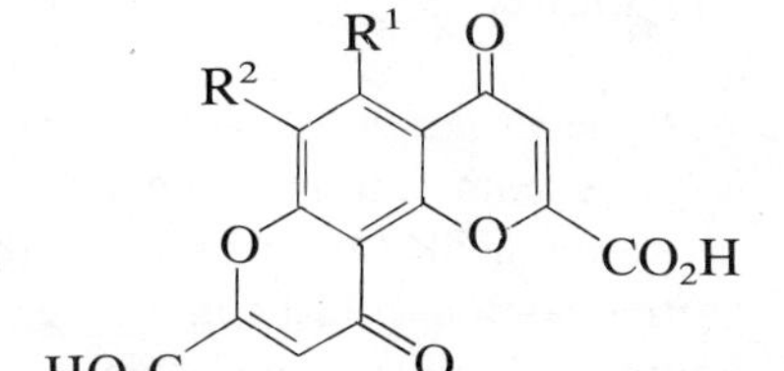

49.**169**

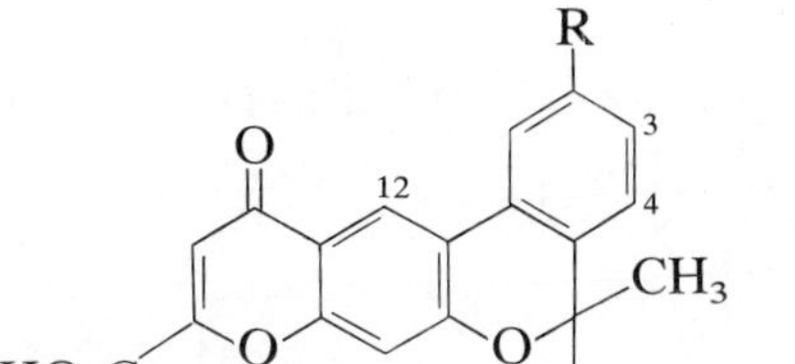

49.**170**

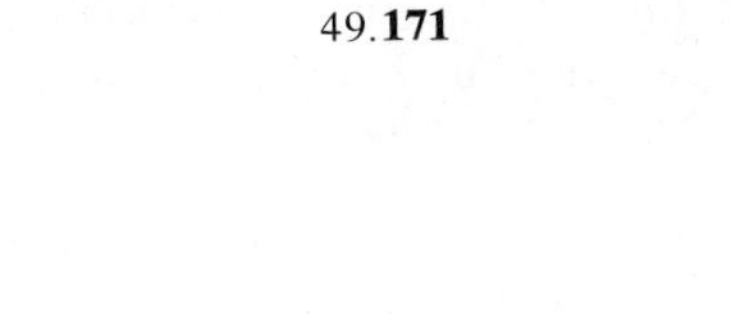

49.**171**

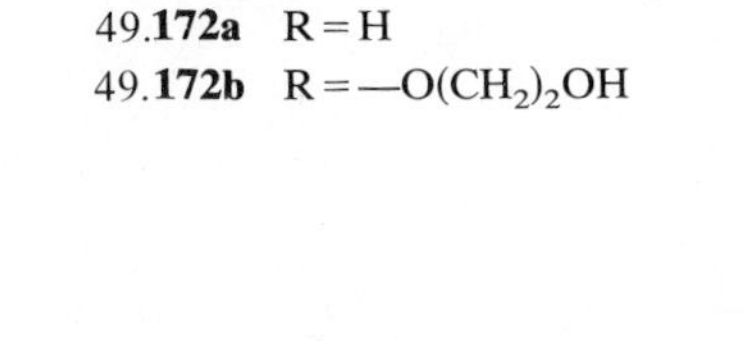

49.**172a** R = H
49.**172b** R = —$O(CH_2)_2OH$

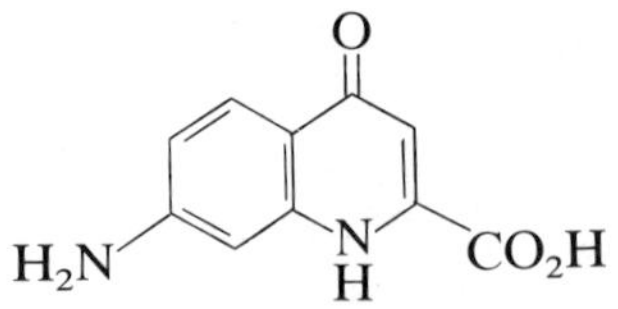

49.**173**

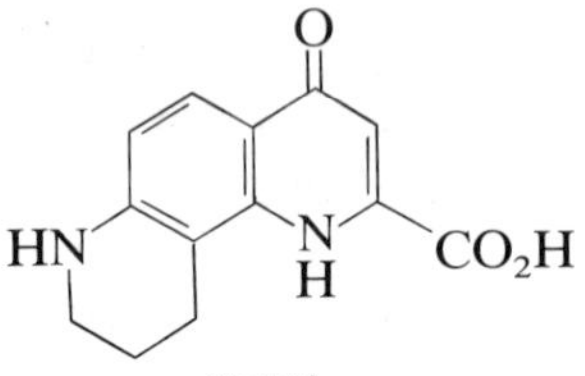

49.**174**

Tricyclic analog 49.**175**, 10-chloro-1,4,6,9-tetrahydro - 4, 6 - dioxopyrido[3, 2 - g]quinoline-2,8-dicarboxylic acid, was 50 times more potent than DSCG in the same test. At 1–10 mg/kg, 49.**175** inhibited the antigen-induced release of SRS-A in the peritoneal cavity of the rat (587). No adenyl cyclase stimulation or rat lung cAMP phosphodiesterase inhibition was observed (587). Intravenous administration of the tricyclic quinoline acid (49.**176**) (ICI 74,917), a 6-(n-butyl)-2,8-dicarboxy-4,10-dioxo-1, 4, 6, 10 - tetrahydro-1, 7-phenanthroline, is 300 times more potent than DSCG in the rat PCA test (588, 589). Like DSCG, 49.**176** does not antagonize the

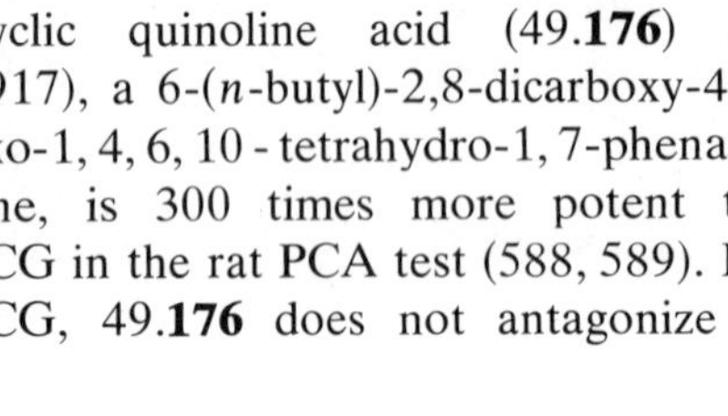

49.**175**

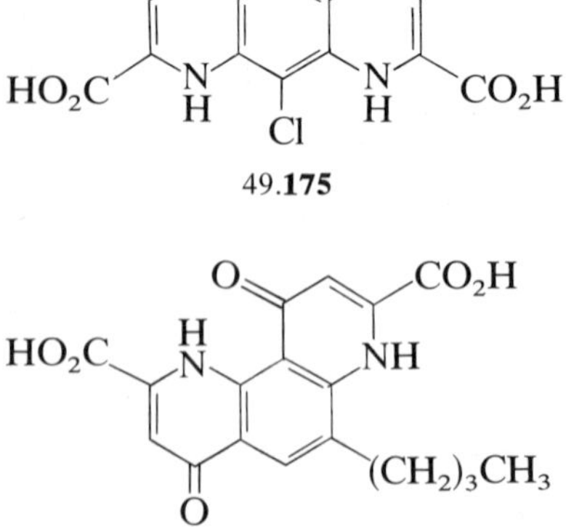

49.**176**

spasmogenic action of released histamine and 5-HT, but at 10^{-8} and 10^{-6} M does antagonize the release of histamine (590). Compound 49.**176** seems to produce tachyphylaxis by a continuous blocking of receptor sites on the surface or inside the mast cell, thereby preventing access of additional drug to these sites (549).

Evaluation of a large series of anthranilic acid analogs revealed that analog 49.**177**, originally found as a contaminant of quinazoline 49.**178**, was one of the most potent compounds in the series when assessed in the rat PCA model (591). Compound 49.**177**, unlike DSCG, was orally active (200 mg/kg p.o.), providing 91% inhibition of the PCA reaction. Intraperitoneally,

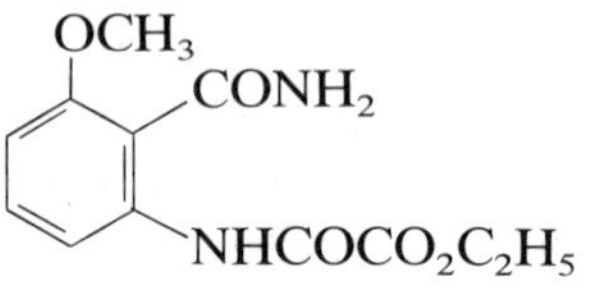

49.**177**

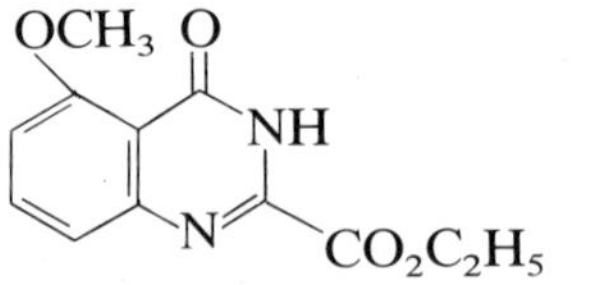

49.**178**

DSCG and 49.**177** showed 86 and 100% inhibition, respectively, at 200 mg/kg. Oxalic acids of the types 49.**177** and 49.**179** were active provided they contained a terminal group easily removable in plasma; bulky or polar (quaternary salts) esters afforded inactive derivatives. Acidic tetrazole 49.**180** was more potent than 49.**179** and showed 85% inhibition at 200 mg/kg p.o.

A new series of orally active antiallergenic compounds based on cinnoline-3-propionic acids (49.**181a**–49.**181c**) have activities comparable to known clinical compounds. Simple uncrowded alkyl substituents at C-6 are preferable to electron-releasing methoxy and benzyloxy groups.

49.**179**

49.**180**

49.**181a** $R^1 = H$, $R^2 = C_2H_5$, $R^3 = H$
49.**181b** $R^1 = H$, $R^2 = R^3 = C_2H_5$
49.**181c** $R^1 = CH_3$, $R^2 = R^3 = C_2H_5$

The activity of 49.**181a**–49.**181c** was thought to be due to β-oxidation *in vivo*, yielding the cinnolonecarboxylic acid. However, when 49.**181b** was administered to a rhesus monkey no metabolic product resulting from β-oxidation was detected. Thus cinnoline-3-propionic acids seem to have intrinsic antiallergenic activity (592).

REFERENCES

1. W. W. Douglas, in The *Pharmacological Basis of Therapeutics*, 5th ed., L. S. Goodman and A. Gilman, Eds., Macmillan, London, 1975, Chap. 29.

2. D. T. Witiak, in *Principles of Medicinal Chemistry*, W. O. Foye, Ed., Lea and Febiger, Philadelphia, 1974, Chap. 20.

3. M. K. Bach, *Ann. Rep. Med. Chem.*, **7**, 238 (1972).

4. B. B. Levine, *Ann. Rev. Med.*, **17**, 23 (1966).

5. H. H. Dale and P. P. Laidlow, *J. Physiol.* (London), **41**, 318 (1910).

6. H. H. Dale and P. P. Laidlow, *J. Physiol.* (London), **43**, 182 (1911).

7. D. R. Stanworth, *Nature*, **233**, 310 (1971).

8. J. Pepys, in *Identification of Asthma*, R. Porter and J. Bach, Eds., Churchill, Livingstone, London, 1971, p. 88.

9. K. Block, in *Mechanisms in Allergy*, L. Goodfriend, A. H. Sehon, and R. P. Orange, Eds., Marcel Dekker, Inc., New York, N.Y., 1972, p. 11.

10. M. K. Bach, K. L. Bloch, and K. F. Austen, *J. Exp. Med.*, **133**, 752 (1971).

11. J. Peyes, W. M. Turner, P. L. Dawson, and K. E. W. Hinson, in *Allergology*, B. Core, M. Richter, A. Sehon, and A. W. Frankland, Eds., Excerpta Medica, Amsterdam, 1968, p. 221.

12. J. W. Combs, *J. Cell. Biol.*, **31**, 563 (1966).

13. D. E. Smith, *Int. Rev. Cytole*, **14**, 328 (1963).

14. I. Mota, *Ann. N.Y. Acad. Sci.*, **103**, 264 (1963).

15. K. F. Austen, R. O. Orange, and D. M. Valentine, *Biochem. Acute Allerg. React. Symp.*, Italy, *1967*, Blackwell Scientific, Oxford, England, 1968, p. 283.

16. K. J. Bloch, *Progr. Allergy*, **10**, 84 (1967).

17. P. J. Piper and J. R. Vane, *Nature*, **223**, 29 (1969).

18. L. B. Jaques and W. T. Waters, *Am. J. Physiol.*, **129**, 389 (1940).

19. A. Kuntz, *Ann. Allergy.*, **3**, 91 (1945).

20. M. Rocha e Silva, in *Handbook of Experimental Pharmacology* (Hefter-Heuber), Vol. XVIII, Part 1, O. Eichler and A. Farah, Eds., Springer, Berlin, 1966, p. 431.

21. E. M. Saporiti and A. Marino, *Semana Med.*, **123**, 1267 (1963).

22. M. K. Bach and J. R. Brashler, *J. Immunol.*, **111**, 324 (1973).

23. T. Ishizaka, K. Ishizaka, and H. J. Tomioka, *J. Immunol.*, **108**, 513 (1972).

24. B. Diamant, *Acta Physiol. Scand.*, **56**, 1 (1962).

25. J. L. Parrot, *C. R. Soc. Biol.*, **136**, 361 (1942).

26. B. A. V. Perera, and J. L. Mongar, *Immunology*, **8**, 519 (1963).

27. T. Johansen and N. Chakravarty, *Int. Arch. Allergy Appl. Immunol.*, **49**, 208 (1975).

28. J. C. Foreman and J. L. Mongar, *J. Physiol.* (London), **224**, 753 (1972).

29. B. Uvnas, C. H. Aborg, and A. Bergendorff, *Acta Physiol. Scand.*, **78**: Suppl. 336, 1 (1970).

30. P. Anderson, S. A. Slorach, and B. Uvnas, *Acta. Physiol. Scand.*, **90**: Suppl. 396, 122 (1974).

31. G. D. Bloom and N. Chakravarty, *Acta Physiol. Scand.*, **78**, 410 (1970).

32. P. G. Krüger and G. D. Bloom, *Experientia*, **29**, 329 (1973).

33. P. G. Krüger, G. D. Bloom, and B. Diamant, *Int. Arch. Allergy Appl. Immunol.*, **47**, 1 (1974).

34. B. Diamant and P. G. Kruger, *Acta. Physiol. Scand.*, **71**, 291 (1967).

35. N. Grosman and B. Diamant, *Agents Actions,* **5,** 108 (1975).

36. R. Dahlquist, B. Diamant, and K. Elwin, *Acta. Physiol. Scand.,* **87,** 145 (1973).

37. N. Grosman and B. Diamant, *Agents Actions,* **6,** 394 (1976).

38. R. Dahlquist and B. Diamant, *Acta. Pharmacol. Toxicol.,* **34,** 368 (1974).

39. N. Grosman and B. Diamant, *Acta. Pharmacol. Toxicol.,* **35,** 284 (1974).

40. B. Diamant, N. Grosman, P. S. Skov, and S. Thomle, *Int. Arch. Allergy Appl. Immunol.,* **47,** 412 (1974).

41. J. C. Foreman, J. L. Mongar, and B. D. Gomperts, *Nature,* **245,** 249 (1973).

42. R. Dahlquist and B. Diamant, *Proc. 5th Int. Congr. Pharmacol., San Francisco, 1972.*

43. J. C. Foreman and J. L. Mongar, *J. Physiol.* (London) **230,** 493 (1973).

44. J. C. Foreman and B. D. Gomperts, *Int. Arch. Allergy Appl. Immunol.,* **49,** 179 (1975).

45. J. C. Foreman, J. L. Mongar, B. D. Gomperts, and L. G. Garland, *Biochem. Pharmacol.,* **24,** 538 (1975).

46. E. Fourneau and D. Bovet, *Arch. Int. Pharmacodyn.,* **46,** 178 (1933).

47. G. Ungar, J. I. Parrot, and D. Bovet, *C. R. Soc. Biol.,* **124,** 445 (1937).

48. D. Bovet and A. M. Straub, *C. R. Soc. Biol.,* **124,** 547 (1937).

49. V. Rocka and H. Polukordas, *Sin. Izuch. Fiziol. Akt. Veshchestv. Mater. Kmf.,* 87 (1971); through *Chem. Abstr.,* **79,** 87572.

50. A. M. Straub, *Ann. Inst. Pasteur,* **63,** 400, 420, 485 (1939).

51. E. R. Loew, *Phys. Rev.,* **27,** 542 (1947).

52. B. N. Halpern, *Arch. Int. Pharmacodyn.,* **68,** 339 (1942).

53. M. M. Mosnier, *Fr. Pat.,* 913, 161 (1943).

54. D. Bovet, R. Horclois, and F. Walthert, *C. R. Soc. Biol.* **138,** 99 (1944).

55. B. N. Halpern and F. Walthert, *C. R. Soc. Biol.,* **139,** 402 (1945).

56. R. J. Horclois, U.S. Pat. 2,501,151 (1950).

57. C. P. Huttrer, C. Djerassi, W. L. Beears, R. L. Mayer, and C. R. Scholz, *J. Am. Chem. Soc.,* **68,** 1999 (1946).

58. F. Leonard and C. P. Huttrer, *Histamine Antagonists,* Chemical Biological Coordination Center, National Research Council, Washington, D.C., 1950.

59. L. P. Kyrides, F. C. Meyer, and F. B. Zienty, *J. Am. Chem. Soc.,* **69,** 2239 (1947).

60. F. Leonard and U. V. Solmssen, *J. Am. Chem. Soc.,* **70,** 2064 (1948).

61. N. Ercoli, R. J. Schachter, W. C. Hueper, and M. N. Lewis, *J. Pharmacol. Exp. Ther.,* **93,** 210 (1948).

62. J. R. Vaughan, Jr., G. W. Anderson, R. C. Clapp, J. H. Clark, J. P. English, K. L. Howard, H. W. Marson, L. H. Sutherland, and J. J. Denton, *J. Org. Chem.,* **14,** 228 (1949).

63. S. Miyano, A. Abe, Y. Kase, T. Yuizono, K. Tachibana, T. Miyata, and G. Kito, *J. Med. Chem.,* **13,** 704 (1970).

64. A. Quevauviller, B. Maziere, and M. Maziere, *Anesth. Analg. Reanim.,* **25,** 53 (1968).

65. M. A. Iradyan, L. V. Shakhbazyan, S. N. Asratyan, and A. A. Aroyan, *Arm. Khim. Zh.,* **23,** 808 (1970); through *Chem. Abstr.,* **74,** 86503.

66. T. B. Bernstein and S. M. Feinberg, *J. Lab. Clin. Med.,* **34,** 1007 (1949).

67. E. Schwartz and J. Reicher, *Ann. Allergy,* **7,** 320 (1949).

68. H. L. Friedman and A. V. Tolstoouslov, U.S. Pat. 2,465,865 (1949).

69. A. R. Judd and A. R. Henderson, *Ann. Allergy,* **7,** 306 (1949).

70. A. W. Weston, *J. Am. Chem. Soc.,* **69,** 980 (1947).

71. R. C. Clapp, J. H. Clark, J. R. Vaughan, Jr., J. P. English, and G. W. Anderson, *J. Am. Chem. Soc.,* **69,** 1549 (1947).

72. J. H. Clark, R. C. Clapp, J. R. Vaughan, Jr., L. H. Sutherland, R. Winterbottom, G. W. Anderson, J. D. Forsythe, J. Blodinger, S. L. Elberlin, and J. P. English, *J. Org. Chem.,* **14,** 216 (1949).

73. L. P. Kyrides, F. C. Meyer, F. B. Zienty, J. Harvey, and L. W. Bannister, *J. Am. Chem. Soc.,* **72,** 745 (1950).

74. J. H. Biel, *J. Am. Chem. Soc.,* **71,** 1306 (1949).

75. K. Hayes, G. Gever, and J. Orcutt, *J. Am. Chem. Soc.,* **72,** 1205 (1950).

76. J. A. Orcutt and J. P. Prytherch, *J. Pharmacol. Exp. Ther.,* **99,** 479 (1950); J. A. Orcutt, S. M. Michaelson, J. P. Prytherch, and I. P. Duprey, *ibid.,* **99,** 488 (1950).

77. G. Viaud, *Produits Pharm.,* **2,** 53 (1947).

78. E. Campaigne and W. M. LeSuer, *J. Am. Chem. Soc.,* **71,** 333 (1949).

79. A. M. Lands, J. O. Hoppe, O. H. Siegmund, and F. P. Luduena, *J. Pharmacol. Exp. Ther.,* **95,** 45 (1949), J. O. Hoppe and A. M. Lands, *ibid.,* **97,** 371 (1949).

80. L. F. Chernysheva, *Tr. Nauchn. Konf. Aspirantov. Ordinatorov. 1-yi, Mosk. Med. Int.,* Moscow,

162–164 (1969); through *Chem. Abstr.*, **66**, 36513.

81. L. F. Chernysheva, A. N. Kudrin, and V. S. Gigauri, *Vop. Farmakol. Regol. Deyatel Serdtsa Mater. Simp.*, 106 (1969); through *Chem. Abstr.*, **73**, 129437.

82. G. R. Rieveschl, Jr., U.S. Pat. 2,421,714 (1947).

83. G. R. Rieveschl, Jr., and W. F. Huber, *Abstr. 109th Meet. Am. Chem. Soc.*, *1946*, p. 50K.

84. E. R. Loew, M. E. Kaiser, and V. Moore, *J. Pharmacol. Exp. Ther.*, **83**, 120 (1945).

85. S. M. Feinberg, *J. Am. Med. Assoc.*, **132**, 702 (1946).

86. H. Timmerman, R. F. Rekker, A. F. Harms, and W. Th. Nauta, *Arzneim.-Forsch.*, **20**, 1258 (1970).

87. L. N. Gay and P. E. Carliner, *Bull. Johns Hopkins Hosp.*, **84**, 470 (1949).

88. L. N. Gay and P. E. Carliner, *Science*, **109**, 359 (1949).

89. H. I. Chinn and P. K. Smith, *Pharmacol. Rev.*, **7**, 33 (1955).

90. G. Barac, *C. R. Soc. Biol.*, **143**, 550 (1949).

91. B. Folkow, K. Haeger, and G. Kahlson, *Acta Physiol. Scand.*, **15**, 264 (1948).

92. T. H. McGavack, A. H. Shearman, J. Weissberg, A. M. Fuchs, P. M. Schulman, and I. J. Drekter, *J. Allergy*, **22**, 31 (1951).

93. J. W. Thomas and F. R. Kelley, Jr., *Ann. Allergy*, **9**, 481 (1951).

94. N. Brock, D. Lorenz, and H. Veigel, *Arzneim.-Forsch.*, **4**, 262 (1954).

95. U. G. Bijlsma, A. F. Harms, A. B. H. Funcke, H. M. Tersteege, and W. T. Nauta, *Arzneim.-Forsch.*, **5**, 72 (1955).

96. M. J. Jarrousse and M. T. Regnier, *Ann. Pharm. Fr.*, **9**, 321 (1951).

97. R. F. Rekker, H. Timmerman, and A. F. Harms, *Arzneim.-Forsch.*, **21**, 688 (1971).

98. R. Tacke and U. Wannagat, *Monatsh. Chem.*, **106**, 1005 (1975).

99. R. Tacke and U. Wannagat, *Monatsh. Chem.*, **107**, 111 (1976).

100. R. Tacke and U. Wannagat, *Monatsh. Chem.*, **107**, 439 (1976).

101. W. Th. Nauta, T. Bultsma, R. F. Rekker, and H. Timmerman, *Med. Chem. Spec. Contrib. Int. Symp. 3rd.*, 125 (1972).

102. K. Takagi, T. Yuizono, and Y. Kase, *Yakugaku Zasshi*, **87**, 907 (1967).

103. T. Yuizono and Y. Kase, *Yakugaku Zasshi*, **87**, 915 (1967).

104. K. Wilken-Jensen, *Acta Allergol.*, **3**, 341 (1950).

105. E. R. Loew, M. E. Kaiser, and M. Anderson, *Fed. Proc.*, **5**, 190 (1946).

106. E. R. Loew, R. MacMillan, and M. E. Kaiser, *J. Pharmacol. Exp. Ther.*, **86**, 229 (1946).

107. C. V. Winder, M. E. Kaiser, M. M. Anderson, and E. M. Glassco, *J. Pharmacol. Exp. Ther.*, **87**, 121 (1946).

108. R. F. Rekker, H. Timmerman, A. F. Harms, and W. Th. Nauta, *Chim. Ther.*, **7**, 279 (1972).

109. A. Engelhardt and H. Wick, *Arzneim.-Forsch.*, **17**, 876 (1967).

110. C. H. Tilford, R. S. Shelton, and M. G. Van Campen, Jr., *J. Am. Chem. Soc.* **70**, 4001 (1948).

111. J. Cany and H. Huidoboro, *Therapie*, **15**, 159 (1960).

112. A. P. Roszkowski and W. M. Grovier, *Pharmacologist*, **1**, 60 (1959).

113. L. C. Cheney, R. R. Smith, and S. B. Binkley, *J. Am. Chem. Soc.*, **71**, 60 (1949).

114. J. Fakstorp and E. Ifversen, *Acta Chem. Scand.*, **4**, 1610 (1950).

115. J. B. Hoekstra, D. E. Tisch, N. Rakieten, and H. L. Dickison, *J. Am. Pharm. Assoc.*, **42**, 487 (1953).

116. J. Mercier, J. Cannellas, and J. Roquebert, *Therapie*, **26**, 785 (1971).

117. F. J. Prime, S. Bianco, J. P. Griffin, and P. L. Kamburoff, *Bull. Physiopathol. Resp.*, **8**, 99 (1972).

118. W. Kunz, *Arch. Pharm.*, **287**, 463, 468 (1954).

119. D. Roemer and H. Weidmann, *Med. Welt*, **27**, 2794 (1966).

120. H. Weidmann, J. Grauwiler, R. Griffith, D. Romer, M. Taeschler, and Z. Zehnder, *Bull. Chim. Farm.*, **106**, 467 (1967).

121. P. Wodniansky and F. X. Wohlzogen, *Wien. Klin. Wochenschr.*, **79**, 500 (1967).

122. A. Hedges, M. Hills, W. P. Mallay, A. J. Newman-Taylor, and P. Turner, *J. Clin. Pharmacol. New Drugs*, **11**, 112 (1971).

123. L. DeCaro and S. C. Rizzo, *Folia Allergol.* **16**, 234 (1969).

124. A. Ebnother and H-P. Weber, *Helv. Chim. Acta.* **7**, 2462 (1976).

125. J. B. Bourquin, *Schweiz. Med. Wochenschr.*, **76**, 296 (1946).

126. W. Brack, *Schweiz. Med. Wochenschr.*, **76**, 316 (1946).

127. R. Meier and K. Bucher, *Schweiz. Med. Wochenschr.*, **76**, 294 (1946).

128. O. Schindler, *Schweiz. Med. Wochenschr.*, **76**, 300, (1946).

129. C. Djerassi and C. R. Scholz, *J. Am. Chem. Soc.*, **69**, 1688 (1947).

130. K. Miescher and W. Klarer., U.S. Pat. 2,449,241 (1948).

131. M. Protiva, *Chemie Antihistaminovych Latek a Histaminove Skupiny*, *Ceskoslovensker Akademie ved.*, Praha, 1955.

132. R. N. Schut, F. E. Ward, O. J. Lorenzetti, and E. Hong, *J. Med. Chem.*, **13**, 394 (1970).

133. D. Jerchel, H. Fischer, and M. Kracht, *Ann. Chem.*, **575**, 162 (1952); W. Schulemann and H. Friebel, *Deut. Med. Wochenschr.*, **78**, 540 (1953).

134. M. Kerenyi and I. Szent-Gyorgy, *I Gyogyszereszet*, **16**, 255 (1972).

135. N. J. Ehrlich and M. A. Kaplan, *Ann. Allergy*, **8**, 682 (1950).

136. S. Y. P'an, J. F. Gardocki, and J. C. Reilly, *J. Am. Pharm. Assoc.*, **43**, 653 (1954).

137. E. A. Brown, L. A. Fox, J. P. Maher, C. Nobili, R. C. Norton, and T. Sannella, *Ann. Allergy*, **8**, 32 (1950).

138. B. H. Chase and A. M. Downes, *J. Chem. Soc.*, **3874** (1953).

139. R. Baltzly, S. BuBreuil, W. S. Ide, and E. Lorz, *J. Org. Chem.*, **14**, 775 (1949).

140. K. E. Hamlin, A. W. Weston, F. E. Fischer, and R. J. Michaels, Jr., *J. Am. Chem. Soc.*, **71**, 2731 (1949).

141. H. C. Murfitt and T. Dewing, Brit. Pat. 656,043 (1951).

142. H. Morren, S. Trolin, R. Denaver, E. Grivsky, and J. Maricq, *Bull. Soc. Chim. Belge*, **60**, 282 (1951).

143. B. N. Halpern, C. Stiffel, M. Liacopoulos-Briot, and L. Conovici, *Arch. Int. Pharmacodyn. Ther.*, **142**, 170 (1963).

144. J. M. Van Nueten and P. A. J. Janssen, *Arch. Int. Pharmacodyn. Ther.*, **204**, 37 (1973).

145. T. Godfraind and A. Kaba, *Brit. J. Pharmacol.*, **36**, 549 (1969).

146. T. Godfraind and A. Kaba, *Arch. Int. Pharmacodyn. Ther.*, **196**, 35 (1972).

147. G. Cignarella and E. Testa, *J. Med. Chem.*, **11**, 612 (1968).

148. Y. Ikeda, Y. Nitta, I. Hirano, K. Noda, and K. Yamada, *Yakugaku Zasshi*, **90**, 1452 (1970).

149. J. L. Duhault, F. P. Tisserand, and G. L. Regnier, *Arzneim.-Forsch.* **24**, 1970 (1974).

150. G. L. Regnier, R. J. Canevari, J. L. Dahault, and M. L. Laubie, *Arzneim.-Forsch.*, **24**, 1964 (1974).

151. I. Uesaka, S. Kubo, Y. Takamatsu, K. Yamada, T. Tanabe, and H. Yamazoe, *Yakuguka Zasshi*, **92**, 1339 (1972).

152. P. V. Dal, P. Lacrimini, and S. Pinzauti, *Bull. Chem. Farm.*, **112**, 517 (1973).

153. J. L. Archibald, P. Fairbrother, and J. L. Jackson, *J. Med. Chem.*, **17**, 739 (1974).

154. P. E. Hanna and A. E. Ahmed, *J. Med. Chem.*, **16**, 463 (1973).

155. P. E. Hanna, A. E. Ahmed, V. R. Grund, and R. L. Merriman, *J. Pharm. Sci.*, **62**, 512 (1973).

156. P. E. Hanna and R. T. Borchardt, *J. Med. Chem.*, **17**, 471 (1974).

157. P. E. Hanna, V. R. Grund, and M. W. Anders, *J. Med. Chem.*, **17**, 1020 (1974).

158. A. LaBelle and R. Tislow, *Fed. Proc.*, **7**, 236 (1948).

159. R. Tislow, A. LaBelle, A. J. Makovsky, M. A. G. Reed, M. D. Cunningham, J. F. Emele, A. Grandage, and R. J. M. Roggenhofer, *Fed. Proc.*, **8**, 338 (1949).

160. N. Sperber, D. Papa, and E. Schwenk, U.S. Pat. 2,676,964 (1954), S. Saijo, *J. Pharm. Soc. Japan*, **72**, 1529 (1952).

161. C. P. Huttrer, *Experientia*, **5**, 53 (1949).

162. N. Sperber, D. Papa, E. Schwenk, and M. Sherlock, *J. Am. Chem. Soc.*, **71**, 887 (1949).

163. D. W. Adamson and J. W. Billinghurst, *J. Chem. Soc.*, 1039 (1950).

164. F. E. Roth, *Chemotherapia*, **3**, 120 (1961).

165. D. W. Adamson, P. A. Barrett, J. W. Billinghurst, A. F. Green, and T. S. G. Jones, *Nature*, **168**, 204 (1951).

166. A. F. Green, *Brit. J. Pharmacol.*, **8**, 171 (1953).

167. A. F. Casy and A. P. Parulkar, *Can. J. Chem.*, **47**, 423 (1969).

168. A. F. Casy and R. R. Ison, *J. Pharm. Pharmacol.*, **22**, 270 (1970).

169. R. R. Ison and A. F. Casy, *J. Pharm. Pharmacol.*, **23**, 848 (1971).

170. C. F. Huebner, E. Donoghue, P. Wenk, E. Sury, and J. A. Nelson, *J. Am. Chem. Soc.*, **82**, 2077 (1960).

171. J. T. Pati and W. Wenner, U.S. Pats. 2,470,108, and 2,470,109 (1949); G. Lehmann, L. O. Randall, and E. Hagen, *Arch. Int. Pharmacodyn. Ther.*, **78**, 253 (1949).

172. J. Augstein, A. L. Ham, and P. R. Leeming, *J. Med. Chem.*, **15**, 466 (1972).

173. U. Horlein, *Chem. Ber.*, **87**, 463 (1954).

174. F. Mietzsch, *Angew. Chem.*, **66**, 363 (1954).

175. B. N. Halpern, *J. Am. Med. Assoc.*, **129**, 1219 (1945).

176. B. N. Halpern and R. Ducrot, *C. R. Soc. Biol.*, **140,** 361 (1946).

177. C. P. Huttrer, *Enzymologia*, **12,** 277 (1948).

178. A. Charpentier, *Compt. Rend.*, **225,** 306 (1947).

179. W. B. Reid, J. B. Wright, H. G. Kolloff, and J. H. Hunter, *J. Am. Chem. Soc.*, **70,** 3100 (1948).

180. M. J. VanderBrook, K. J. Olson, M. T. Richmond, and M. H. Kuizenga, *J. Pharmacol. Exp. Ther.*, **94,** 197 (1948).

181. H. W. Wahner and G. A. Peters, *Proc. Mayo. Clinic*, 35, 161 (1960).

182. J. H. Weikel and P. M. Lish, *Pharmacologist*, **1,** 64 (1959).

183. W. B. McKeon, Jr., and H. J. Bronstein, *Arch. Int. Pharacodyn. Ther.*, **168,** 55 (1967).

184. F. M. Moralli, F. Liberatore, P. Marchini, G. Liso, and M. Cardellini, *J. Med. Chem.*, **17,** 463 (1974).

185. M. Cardellini, F. Claudi, U. Gulini, F. M. Moralli, G. DeCaro, and F. Venturi, *Eur. J. Med. Chem.*, **9,** 513 (1974).

186. K. Yamada, H. Yamazoe, T. Tanabe, H. Kato, Y. Kinoshita, and T. Mouri, *Yakugaku Zasshi*, **93,** 854 (1973).

187. K. Stach and W. Poldinger, in *Fortschritte der Anzneimittel Forschung*, Vol. 9, E. Jucker, Ed., Birkhauser, Basel, 1966, pp. 146–148

188. A. Von Schlichtegroll, *Arzneim.-Forsch.*, **7,** 237 (1957).

189. P. Von Schlichtegroll, *Arzneim.-Forsch.*, **8,** 489 (1958).

190. W. A. Schuler and H. Klebe, *Ann. Chem.*, **653,** 172 (1962).

191. E. Werle, K. Kopp, and G. Leysath, *Arzneim.-Forsch.*, **12,** 443 (1962).

192. P. V. Peterson, N. Lassen, T. Holm, R. Kopf, and I. Møller Nielsen, *Arzneim.-Forsch.*, **8,** 395 (1958).

193. I. Møller Nielsen and K. Neuhold, *Acta Pharmacol. Toxicol.*, **15,** 335 (1959).

194. J. O. Jilek, M. Rajsner, J. Pomykacek, and M. Protiva, *Cesk. Farm.*, **14,** 294 (1965).

195. J. D. Dunitz, H. Eser, and P. Strickler, *Helv. Chim. Acta.*, **47,** 1897 (1964).

196. B. C. Eisenberg, *Ann. Allergy*, **20,** 523 (1962).

197. J. P. Girard, *Med. Exp.*, **9,** 400 (1963).

198. J. H. Trapold and U. Briner, *Fed. Proc.*, **21,** 430 (1962).

199. J. Lecomte, *C. R. Soc. Biol.*, **161,** 1155 (1967).

200. J. Sondergaard, T. Castellani, S. J. Henningsen, and H. Zachariae, *Acta. Allergol.*, **23,** 282 (1968).

201. D. Romer and A. Cerletti, *Arch. Exp. Pathol. Pharmakol.*, **250,** 174 (1965).

202. E. Jucker and A. Ebnother, Belg. Pat. 638,971 (1964); E. Jucker, A. Ebnother, and E. Rissi, Fr. Pat. 1,392,046 (1965); J. Renz, J. P. Bourquin, C. Brueschweiler, H. Winkler, and G. Schwarb, Fr. Pat. 1,377,694 (1964).

203. F. J. Villani, T. A. Mann, E. A. Wefer, J. Hannon, L. L. Larca, M. J. Landon, W. Spivak, D. Vashi, S. Tozzi, G. Danko, M. del Prado, and R. Lutz, *J. Med. Chem.*, **18,** 1 (1975).

204. R. Kuhn, *Wien. Med. Wochenschr.*, **110,** 245 (1960); *Schweiz. Med. Wochenschr.*, **94,** 590 (1964); *ibid.*, **87,** 1135 (1957). W. Schindler and F. Hafliger, *Helv. Chim. Acta*, **37,** 472 (1954).

205. M. Protiva, *Farm. Ed. Sci.*, **21,** 76 (1966).

206. M. Protiva, M. Borovicka, V. Hach, Z. Votava, J. Sranmkova, and Z. Horakova, *Experientia*, **13,** 291 (1957); M. Borovicka and M. Protiva, *Collect. Czech. Chem. Commun.*, **23,** 1330 (1958).

207. F. Hunziker, F. Kunzle, O. Schindler, and J. Schmutz, *Helv. Chim. Acta*, **47,** 1163 (1964).

208. G. Garonna and S. Palazzo, *Gazz. Chim. Ital.*, **83,** 533 (1953); **84,** 1135 (1954).

209. Z. Votava, J. Metysova, and Z. Horakova, *Cesk. Farm.*, **7,** 125 (1958).

210. M. Protiva and J. Jilek, Czech Pat. 113,250 (1965).

211. S. O. Winthrop, M. A. Davis, F. Herr, J. Stewart, and R. Gaudry, *J. Med. Chem.*, **5,** 1199 (1962).

212. S. O. Winthrop, M. A. Davis, F. Herr, J. Stewart, and R. Gaudry, *J. Med. Chem.*, **5,** 1207 (1962). M. Protiva, M. Rajsner, V. Seidhova, E. Adlerova, and Z. J. Vejdelek, *Experientia*, **18,** 326 (1962). M. Rajsner and M. Protiva, *Cesk. Farm.*, **41,** 404 (1962). K. Stach and H. Springler, *Angew. Chem.*, **74,** 31 (1962); *Monatsh. Chem.*, **93,** 889 (1962). K. Stach and F. Bickelhaupt, *ibid.*, **93,** 896 (1962). F. Gadient, E. Jucker, A. Lindenmann, and M. Taeschler, *Helv. Chim. Acta*, **45,** 1860 (1962).

213. J. Metysova, J. Metys, and Z. Votava, *Arzneim.-Forsch.*, **13,** 1039 (1963).

214. Z. Votova, J. Metys, and A. Dlabac, *Act. Nerv. Super.*, **14,** 120 (1972).

215. J. Metysova, J. Metys, and Z. Votova, *Arzneim.-Forsch.*, **15,** 524 (1965).

216. M. Rajsner, J. Metys, E. Svatek, and M. Protiva, *Collect. Czech. Chem. Commun.*, **34,** 1015 (1969).

217. V. Seidlova, M. Rajsner, E. Adlerova, and M. Protiva, *Monatsh. Chem.*, **96,** 650 (1965).

218. M. Protiva, M. Rajsner, E. Adlerova, V. Seid-

lova, and Z. J. Vejdelek, *Collect. Czech. Chem. Commun.*, **29,** 2161 (1964).

219. M. Protiva, E. Adlerova, and J. Metys, Belg. Pat. 646,051 (1964); C. L. Zirkle, U.S. Pat. 3,100,207 (1963); J. R. Geigy A. G., Netherlands Pat. Appl. 6,404,862 (1963). C. F. Boehringer Sohn G.m.b.H., Belg. Pat. 623,259 (1963).

220. J. W. Constantine, A. Scriabine, S. G. Smith, W. K. McShane, and K. D. Booher, *J. New Drugs,* **4,** 249 (1964).

221. J. O. Jilek, V. Seidlova, E. Svatek, M. Protiva, J. Pomykacek, and Z. Sedivy, *Monatsh. Chem.,* **96,** 182 (1965).

222. J. Jilck, J. Urban, and M. Protiva, *Chem. Listy,* **43,** 56 (1949).

223. V. Mychajlyszyn and M. Protiva, *Collect. Czech. Chem. Commun.,* **24,** 3955 (1959).

224. W. Treibs and H. Klinkhammer, *Chem. Ber.,* **83,** 367 (1950); *ibid.,* **84,** 671 (1951); A. C. Cope and S. W. Fenton, *J. Am. Chem. Soc.,* **73,** 1673 (1951); T. W. Campbell, R. Ginsig, and D. Schmid, *Helv. Chim. Acta,* **36,** 1489 (1953).

225. E. Jucker and A. Ebnother, Swiss Pat. 401,055 (1966).

226. C. A. Stone, H. C. Wenger, C. T. Ludden, J. M. Stavorskii, and C. A. Ross, *J. Pharmacol. Exp. Ther.,* **131,** 73 (1961).

227. E. I. Engelhardt, H. C. Zell, W. S. Saari, M. E. Christy, C. D. Colton, C. A. Stone, J. M. Stavorskii, H. C. Wenger, and C. T. Ludden, *J. Med. Chem.,* **8,** 829 (1965).

228. S. Umio, H. Hitomi, H. Nojima, N. Kumaoaki, I. Ueda, T. Kanaya, Y. Deguchi, *J. Med. Chem.,* **15,** 891 (1972); M. Hitomi, N. Watanabe, N, Kumadaki, and S. Kumada, *Arzneim.-Forsch.,* **22,** 961 (1972).

229. F. J. Villani, P. J. L. Daniels, C. A. Ellis, T. A. Mann, K. C. Wang, and E. A. Wefer, *J. Med. Chem.,* **15,** 750 (1972).

230. S. Tozzi, F. E. Roth, and I. I. A. Tabachnick, *Agents Actions,* **4,** 264 (1974).

231. F. J. Villani, T. A. Mann, and E. A. Wefer, *J. Med. Chem.,* **18,** 666 (1975).

232. A. F. Harms, Brit. Pat. 969,023 (1964).

233. A. B. H. Funcke, D. Mulder, M. C. DeJonge, H. M. Tersteege, A. F. Harms, and W. Th. Nauta, *Arch. Int. Pharmacodyn.,* **148,** 135 (1964); A. F. Harms and W. Th. Nauta, *J. Med. Chem.,* **2,** 57 (1960); C. Vanderstelt, A. F. Harms, and W. Th. Nauta, *ibid.,* **4,** 335 (1961).

234. H. Timmerman, U. L. Lavy, and D. Mulder, *Arch. Int. Pharmacodyn. Ther.,* **187,** 291 (1970).

235. U. I. Lavy, A. B. H. Funcke, G. VanHell, and H. Timmerman, *Arzneim.-Forsch.,* **23,** 854 (1973).

236. M. A. Davis, S. O. Winthrop, J. Stewart, F. A. Sunahara, and F. Herr, *J. Med. Chem.,* **6,** 251 (1963); M. A. Davis, F. A. Sunahara, F. Herr, and R. Gaudry, *ibid.,* **513,** (1963); M. A. Davis, S. O. Winthrop, R. A. Thomas, F. Herr, M. P. Charest, and R. Gaudry, *ibid.,* **7,** 88, 439 (1964).

237. C. Van der Stelt, P. S. Hofman, A. B. H. Funcke, and W. Th. Nauta, *Arzneim.-Forsch.,* **17,** 1446 (1967).

238. C. Van der Stelt, A. F. Harms, and W. Th. Nauta, *J. Med. Chem.,* **4,** 335 (1961).

239. D. Mulder, and C. J. Van Eeken, *Arch. Int. Pharmacodyn. Ther.,* **162,** 497 (1966).

240. A. B. H. Funcke, W. J. Louwerse, H. M. Tersteege, A. F. Harms, and W. Th. Nauta., *Arch. Int. Pharmacodyn. Ther.,* **167,** 334 (1967).

241. G. Raynaud, J. Thomas, C. Gouret, B. Pourrias, N. Dorme, G. Bregeon, C. Euvrard, and C. Pinon, *Eur. J. Med. Chem.-Chim Ther.,* **9,** 634 (1974).

242. J. Rigaudy and I. Nedelec, *C. R. Soc. Biol.,* **236,** 1287 (1953). *Bull. Soc. Chim. Fr.,* **638,** (1959); N. J. Leonard, A. J. Kresge, and M. Oki, *J. Am. Chem. Soc.,* **77,** 5078 (1955).

243. Rhone-Poulenc, Netherlands, Pat. Appls. 6,506,504 and 6,506,574 (1965).

244. V. Hach and M. Protiva, *Chem. Listy,* **51,** 1909 (1957); *Collect. Czech. Chem. Commun.,* **23,** 1941 (1958).

245. G. Seidl (to Farbwerke Hoechst, A. G.), Ger. Pat. 1,217,958 (1966).

246. J. O. Jilek, J. Pomykacek, J. Metysova, J. Metys, and M. Protiva, *Collect. Czech. Chem. Commun.,* **30,** 463 (1965).

247. H. L. Yale and F. Sowinski, *J. Med. Chem.,* **7,** 609 (1964).

248. B. Rubin, J. J. Piala, R. Millonig, and B. N. Craver, *Arch. Int. Pharmacodyn.,* **155,** 47 (1965).

249. A. R. Furgiucle, J. P. High, Z. P. Horowitz, and J. C. Burke, *Arch. Int. Pharmacodyn.,* **160,** 4 (1956).

250. A. R. Hanze, R. E. Strube, and M. E. Greig, *J. Med. Chem.,* **6,** 767 (1963). F. Hunziker, F. Kunzle, and J. Schmutz, *Helv. Chim. Acta,* **46,** 2337 (1963).

251. H. Ackermann, E. Eichenberger, F. Hunziker, H. Lauener, and J. Schmutz, *Med. Exp.,* **6,** 205 (1962).

252. F. Hunziker, H. Lauener, and J. Schmutz, *Arzneim.-Forsch.,* **13,** 324 (1963).

253. M. E. Greig, A. T. Gibbons, and G. A. Young, *J. Med. Chem.,* **14,** 153 (1971).

254. E. Waldvogel, G. Schwarb, J. M. Bastian, and J. P. Bourquin, *Helv. Chim. Acta.,* **59,** 866 (1976).

255. K. Kuokkanen, *Acta Allergol.*, **30,** 73 (1975).

256. J. P. Girard and M. Cuevas, *Allergologia et Immunopathologia*, **4,** 198 (1976).

257. U. Martin and D. Roemer, *Monographs of Allergy*, in press, 1976.

258. A. Petrin, *Int. J. Clin. Pharmacol.*, **12,** 199 (1975).

259. J. Metys and J. Metysova, *Acta Biol. Med. Ger.*, **15,** 871 (1965).

260. M. Rajsner, J. Metys, and M. Protiva, *Collect. Czech. Chem. Commun.*, **32,** 2854 (1967).

261. M. Rajsner, E. Svatek, J. Metys, and M. Protiva, *Collect. Czech. Chem. Comm.*, **39,** 1366 (1974).

262. M. Rajsner, S. Metys, B. Kakal, and M. Protiva, *Collect. Czech. Chem. Comm.*, **40,** 2905 (1975).

263. F. Coujolle, P.-H.-Chanh, P. Duch-Kan, and L. D. Bravo, *Agressologie*, **10,** 405 (1969).

264. S. Wasuwat, *Nature*, **225,** 758 (1970).

265. I. Novak, G. Buzas, E. Minker, M. Koltai, and K. Szendrei, *Acta Pharm. Hung.*, **37,** 131 (1967).

266. D. Chu and B. A. Kovacs, *Arch. Int. Pharmacodyn. Ther.*, **214,** 155 (1975); D. Chu, T. H. Chan, and B. A. Kovacs, *ibid.*, **214,** 141 (1975).

267. S. D. S. Seth, A. Mukhopadhyay, N. Bagchi, M. C. Prabhakar, and R. B. Arora, *Jap. J. Pharmacol.*, **23,** 673 (1973).

268. J. A. Wakkary, L. Goodfriend, and B. A. Kovacs, *Arch. Int. Pharmacodyn. Ther.*, **183,** 303 (1970).

269. S. Jayasunder, S. M. Periyasamy, and N. K. Bhide, *Indian J. Physiol. Pharmacol.*, **17,** 213 (1973).

270. A. H. Dil, *Therapie*, **28,** 767 (1973).

271. R. K. Turker, S. Kaymakcalan, and Z. S. Ercan, *Arch. Int. Pharmacodyn. Ther.*, **214,** 254 (1975).

272. P. H. Chanh, I. Sokan, and M. H. Quessada, *Aggressologie*, **15,** 131 (1974).

273. D. T. Witiak and N. J. Lewis, in *Handbook of Experimental Pharmacology*, Vol. XVIII, Part II, G. V. R. Born, O. Eichler, A. Farah, H. Herken and A. D. Welch, Eds., M. Rocha e Silva, Ed., Springer, Berlin, 1977, pp. 514–560.

274. P. Naranjo and E. Banda de Narranjo, *Arch. Int. Pharmacodyn.*, **94,** 383 (1953); *J. Allergy*, **24,** 442 (1953).

275. I. Iwasaki, *Yakugaku Zasshi*, **53,** 375 (1957).

276. M. Kikkawa, D. Sasaki, T. Iwasaki, and J. Vedo, *Osaka City Med. J.*, **3,** 69 (1956).

277. H. Goldenberg and V. Fishman, *Biochem. Biophys. Res. Commun.*, **14,** 404 (1964).

278. A. J. Glazko and W. A. Dill, *J. Biol. Chem.*, **179,** 417 (1949); A. J. Glazko, D. A. McGinty, W. A. Dill, M. L. Wilson, and C. S. Ward, *ibid.*, **179,** 409 (1949).

279. J. C. Drach, and J. P. Howell, *Biochem. Pharmacol.*, **17,** 2125 (1968).

280. D. Robinson, *Biochem. J.*, **68,** 584 (1958).

281. E. L. Way and R. E. Dailey, *Proc. Soc. Exp. Biol.*, **73,** 423 (1950).

282. R. C. Roozemond, *Biochem. Pharmacol.*, **14,** 699 (1965).

283. R. Kato, K-I, Onoda, and A. Takanaka, *Jap. J. Pharmacol.*, **20,** 562 (1970).

284. H. M. Jones and E. S. Brady, *J. Am. Pharm. Assoc. Sci. Ed.*, **38,** 579 (1949).

285. T. H. McGavack, J. J. Drekter, S. Schutzer, and A. Heisler, *J. Allergy*, **19,** 251 (1948).

286. E. Perlman, *J. Pharmacol. Exp. Ther.*, **95,** 465 (1949).

287. E. O. Weinman and T. A. Geissman, *J. Pharmacol. Exp. Ther.*, **125,** 1 (1959).

288. R. Kuntzman, A. Klutch, I. Isai, and J. J. Burns, *J. Pharmacol. Exp. Ther.*, **149,** 29 (1965).

289. R. Kuntzman, A. Phillips, I. Tsai, A. Klutch, and J. J. Burns, *J. Pharmacol. Exp. Ther.*, **155,** 337 (1967).

290. H. J. Gaertner, and U. Breyer, *Arzneim.-Forsch.*, **22,** 1084 (1972); H. J. Gaertner, U. Breyer, and G. Liomin, *J. Pharmacol. Exp. Ther.*, **185,** 195 (1973).

291. U. Breyer and H. J. Gaertner, *Advan. Biochem. Psychopharmacol.*, **9,** 167 (1974); U. Breyer, H. J. Gaertner, and A. Prox, *Biochem. Pharmacol.*, **23,** 313 (1974); H. J. Gaertner, U. Breyer, and G. Liomin, *Biochem. Pharmacol.*, **23,** 303 (1974).

292. J. A. Close, J. G. Gobert, and A. M. Rodriguez, *Proc. Eur. Soc. Study Drug Toxicity*, **9,** 144 (1968).

293. W. Soudin and I. van Wijangaarden, *Life Sci.*, **7,** 231 (1968).

294. P. Kabasakalian, M. Taggart, and E. Townley, *J. Pharm. Sci.*, **57,** 856 (1968).

295. A. H. Beckett and G. R. Wilkinson, *J. Pharm. Pharmacol.*, **17,** 256 (1965).

296. E. A. Peets, M. Jackson, and S. Symchowicz, *J. Pharmacol. Exp. Ther.*, **180,** 464 (1972); A. E. Peets, R. Weinstein, W. Hillard, and S. Symchowicz, *Arch. Int. Pharmacodyn. Ther.*, **199,** 171 (1972).

297. J. Christensen and A. W. Wase, *Fed. Proc.*, **15,** 410 (1956); G. H. Benham, *Canada J. Res.*, **23E** 71 (1945); H. B. Collier, D. E. Allen, and W. E. Swales, *ibid.*, **210,** 151 (1943); N. P. Salzman and B. B. Brodie, *J. Pharmacol. Exp. Ther.*, **118,** 46 (1956; F. DeEds, C. W. Eddy, and J. O. Thomas, *ibid.*, **64,** 250 (1938); J. D. Davidson,

L. L. Terry, and A. Sjoerdsma, *ibid.*, **121,** 8 (1957); S. S. Walkenstein and J. Seifter, *ibid.*, **125,** 283 (1959); I. Hoffman, O. Nieshulz, K. Popendiker, and E. Fauchert, *Arzneim.-Forsch.*, **9,** 133 (1959); H. Goldenberg., V. Fishman, A. Heaton, and R. Burnett, *Proc. Soc. Exp. Biol. Med.*, **115,** 1044 (1964).

298. V. Fishman and H. Goldenberg, *J. Pharmacol. Exp. Ther.*, **150,** 122 (1965).

299. R. Kuhn, *Psychopharmacologia*, **8,** 201 (1965).

300. A. Cordelli, M. Ferrari, and E. Savonitto, *Arch. Int. Pharmacodyn.*, **180,** 121 (1969).

301. J. Raaflaub, *Arzneim.-Forsch.*, **17,** 1393 (1967).

302. I. Huus and A. R. Khan, *Acta. Pharmacol. Toxicol.*, **25,** 397 (1967).

303. C. C. Porter, B. H. Arison, V. F. Gruber, D. C. Titus, and W. J. A. Vandeheuvel, *Drug Metab. Distrib.*, **3,** 189 (1975).

304. H. B. Hucker, A. J. Balletto, S. C. Staufer, A. G. Zallhei, and B. H. Arison, *Drug. Metab. Distrib.*, **2,** 406 (1974); K. L. Hintze, J. S. Wold, and L. J. Fischer, *ibid.*, **3** (1975).

305. W. Hespe, H. Prins, W. F. Kafoe, and W. Th. Nauta, *Biochem. Pharmacol.*, **17,** 655 (1968).

306. J. J. Burns, A. H. Conney, and R. Koster, *Ann. N.Y. Acad. Sci.*, **104,** 881 (1963).

307. A. H. Conney and A. Klutch, *Fed. Proc.*, **21,** 182 (1962); A. H. Conney, I. A. Michaelson, and J. J. Burns, *J. Pharmacol. Exp. Ther.*, **132,** 202 (1961).

308. J. B. Wyngaarden and M. H. Seeves, *J. Am. Med. Assoc.*, **145,** 277, (1951).

309. C. C. Lee, *Toxi ol. Appl. Pharmacol.*, **8,** 210 (1966).

310. M. Cirstea and G. Suhaciu, *Arch. Int. Physiol. Biochem.*, **76,** 344 (1968).

311. B. Csaba and M. Went, *Acta. Physiol.*, **39,** 369 (1971).

312. H. Salem and E. Clemente, *Arch. Otolaryngol.*, **96,** 524 (1972).

313. M. A. Green, *Ann. Allergy*, **12,** 273 (1954); E. Dundas, J. H. Toogood, and T. Wanklin, *J. Allergy*, **32,** 1 (1961); A. Reinberg and E. Sidi, *J. Invest. Derm.*, **46,** 415 (1966).

314. B. M. Altura and B. W. Zweifach, *Am. J. Physiol.*, **209,** 545, 550 (1965).

315. V. Conrad, *C. R. Soc. Biol.*, **145,** 1875 (1951); B. M. Altura and B. W. Zweifach., *Angiology*, **17,** 493 (1966).

316. J. M. Robson and C. A. Keele, *Recent Advances in Pharmacology*, 1st ed., Blakiston, Philadelphia, 1951, pp. 72–73.

317. M. I. Sharma, P. G. Dashputra, and M. V. Rajapurkar, *Ind. J. Med. Res.*, **52,** 511 (1964).

318. N. K. Dutta, *Brit. J. Pharmacol.*, **4,** 281 (1949).

319. M. V. Rajapurkar, M. I. Sharma, N. K. Joshi, and P. G. Dashputra, *Ind. J. Med. Res.*, **52,** 502 (1964).

320. H. K. Choksey and M. N. Jindal, *Arch. Int. Pharmacodyn.*, **157,** 339 (1965); E. Schubert and H. Schwartze, *Med. Pharm. Exp.*, **14,** 457 (1966).

321. F. F. Yonkman, D. Chess, D. Mathieson, and N. Hansen, *J. Pharmacol. Exp. Ther.*, **87,** 256 (1946); K. Kuriaki and T. Uchida, *ibid.*, **113,** 228 (1955); I. R. Innes, *Brit. J. Pharmacol.*, **13,** 6 (1958).

322. J. H. McNeill and T. M. Brody, *J. Pharmacol. Exp. Ther.*, **152,** 478 (1966); L. Isaac and A. Goth, *Life Sci.*, **4,** 1899 (1965); L. Isaac and A. Goth, *J. Pharmacol. Exp. Ther.*, **156,** 463 (1967).

323. G. L. Johnson and J. B. Kahn, Jr., *J. Pharmacol. Exp. Ther.*, **152,** 458 (1966).

324. J. Lecomte, A. Cession-Fossion, and G. Cession, *C. R. Soc. Biol.*, **159,** 515 (1965).

325. D. Dobreseu, *C. R. Soc. Biol.*, **160,** 717 (1966).

326. M. Kumbar and D. V. S. Sankar; *Res. Commun. Chem. Path. Pharmacol.*, **4,** 707 (1972).

327. H. Barth, I. Niemeyer, and W. Lorenz, *Agents Actions*, **3,** 138 (1973).

328. R. B. Smith, G. V Rossi, and R. F. Orzechowski, *Toxicol. Appl. Pharmacol.*, **28,** 280 (1974).

329. C. H. Gallagher, D. N. Gupta, J. D. Judah, and K. R. Rees, *J. Pathol. Bacteriol.*, **72,** 193 (1956).

330. J. D. Judah, *Nature*, **185,** 390 (1960).

331. A. E. M. McLean, *Nature*, **185,** 191, 936 (1960).

332. J. D. Judah, G. Bjotvedt, and T. Vainio, *Nature*, **187,** 507 (1960).

333. K. R. Rees, K. P. Sinha, and W. G. Spector, *J. Pathol. Bacteriol.*, **81,** 107 (1961).

334. J. D. Judah, *Biochem. Biophys, Acta*, **53,** 375 (1961); *Fed. Proc.*, **21,** 1097 (1962).

335. H. O. Schild, *Brit. J. Pharmacol.*, **4,** 277 (1949).

336. H. O. Schild, *Brit. J. Pharmacol.*, **2,** 189 (1947).

337. R. F. Furchgott, *Ann. Rev. Pharmacol.*, **4,** 21, 24 (1964).

338. C. A. Ashford, H. Heller, and G. A. Smart, *Brit. J. Pharmacol.*, **4,** 153 (1949); U. Trendelenburg, *J. Pharmacol. Exp. Ther.*, **130,** 450 (1960).

339. D. Arunlakshana and H. O. Schild, *Brit. J. Pharmacol.*, **14,** 48 (1959).

340. A. S. F. Ash and H. O. Schild, *Brit J. Pharmacol.*, **27,** 427 (1966).

341. E. J. Ariens and A. M. Simonis, *Farm. Ed. Sci.*, **21,** 581 (1966).

342. B. Belleau, *J. Med. Chem.*, **7,** 776 (1964).

343. W. B. McKeon, Jr., *Arch. Int. Pharmacodyn.*, **145**, 396 (1963).

344. R. B. Barlow, *Introduction to Chemical Pharmacology*, 2nd ed., Wiley, New York, 1964, pp. 344–377.

345. A. H. Beckett, *Proc. First Int. Pharm. Meet.*, **7**, 5 (1961).

346. A. F. Harms and W. Th. Nauta, *J. Med. Pharm. Chem.*, **2**, 57 (1960).

347. N. G. Lordi and J. E. Christian, *J. Am. Pharm. Assoc.*, **45**, 300 (1956).

348. P. E. Periti, *Pharmacol. Res. Commun.*, **2**, 309 (1970).

349. C. R. Ganellin, G. N. J. Port, and W. G. Richards, *J. Med. Chem.*, **16**, 616 (1973).

350. C. R. Ganellin, *J. Med. Chem.*, **16**, 620 (1973).

351 L. B. Kier, *J. Med. Chem.*, **11**, 441 (1968).

352. M. N. G. James and G. J. B. Williams, *Can. J. Chem.*, **52**, 1880 (1974).

353. L. B. Kier, *J. Med. Chem.*, **11**, 915 (1968).

354. M. S. Ham, *J. Pharm. Sci.*, **65**, 612 (1976).

355. M. S. Ham, *J. Pharm. Sci.*, **60**, 1764 (1971).

356. M. S. Ham, A. F. Casy, and R. R. Ison, *J. Med. Chem.*, **16**, 470 (1973).

357. B. Pullman, P. Courriere, and H. Berthod, *Mol. Pharmacol.*, **11**, 268 (1975).

358. B. Testa, in *Molecular and Quantum Pharmacology, Proceedings of the 7th Jerusalem Symposium on Quantum Chemistry and Biochemistry*, E. D. Bergmann and B. Pullman, Eds., Reidel, Dordrecht, Netherlands, 1974, pp. 241.

359. M. N. G. James and G. J. B. Williams, *J. Med. Chem.*, **14**, 670 (1971).

360. M. N. G. James and G. J. B. Williams, *Can. J. Chem.*, **52**, 1872 (1974).

361. G. R. Clark and G. L. Palenik, *J. Am. Chem. Soc.*, **92**, 1777 (1970).

362. G. R. Clark and G. L. Palenik, *J. Am. Chem. Soc.*, **94**, 4005 (1974).

363. D. T. Witiak, Z. Muhi-Eldeen, N. Mahishi, O. P. Sethi, and M. C. Gerald, *J. Med. Chem.*, **14**, 24 (1971).

364. F. E. Roth and W. M. Govier, *Am. J. Pharmacol.*, **124**, 347 (1958).

365. R. T. Brittain, P. F. D'Arcy, and J. H. Hunt, *Nature*, **183**, 734 (1959).

366. G. Hite and A. Shafièe, *J. Pharm. Sci.*, **56**, 1041 (1967).

367. A. Shafiée and G. Hite, *J. Med. Chem.*, **12**, 266 (1969).

368. W. E. Barrett, R. Rutledge, A. Dietrich, and A. J. Plummer, *Fed. Proc.*, **19**, 210 (1960).

369. I. Toldy, L. Vargha, I. Toth, and J. Borsy, *Acta. Chim. Acad. Sci. Hung.*, **19**, 273 (1959).

370. D. T. Witiak, S. Y. Hsu, J. E. Ollmann, R. K. Griffith, S. K. Seth, and M. C. Gerald, *J. Med. Chem.*, **17**, 690 (1974).

371. D. T. Witiak, B. R. Vishnuvajjala, T. K. Gupta, and M. C. Gerald, *J. Med. Chem.*, **19**, 40 (1976).

372. E. Kutter and C. Hansch, *J. Med. Chem.*, **12**, 647 (1969).

373. *Handbook Exp. Pharmacol.*, **25**, (1970).

374. D. F. Elliot, G. P. Lewis, and E. W. Horton, *Biochem. Biophys. Res. Commun.*, **3**, 87 (1960).

375. R. A. Boissonas, S. Guttmann, P. A. Jaquenoud, J. Pless, and E. Sandrin, *Ann. N.Y. Acad. Sci.*, **104**, 5 (1963).

376. S. Sakkihara, N. Nakamizo, Y. Kishida, and S. Yoshimura, *Bull. Chem. Soc. Jap.*, **41**, 1477 (1968).

377. M. Rocha e Silva, W. T. Beraldo, and G. Rosenfeld, *Am. J. Physiol.* **156**, 261 (1949).

378. D. F. Hawkins and L. Rosa, *Int. Arch. Allergy Appl. Immunol.*, **14**, 312 (1959).

379. W. Feldberg, *Arch. Klin. Exp. Dermatol.*, **213**, 343 (1961).

380. F. K. Austen and J. H. Humphrey, *Advan. Immunol.*, **3**, 1 (1963).

381. O. Jonasson and E. L. Becker, *J. Exp. Med.*, **123**, 509 (1966).

382. E. Brocklehurst and S. C. Lahiri, *J. Physiol.*, **160**, 15P (1962).

383. S. H. Ferreira, and J. R. Vane, *Nature*, **215**, 1237 (1967).

384. K. Sahmeli and T. K. A. B. Eskes, *Am. J. Physiol.*, **203**, 261 (1962).

385. G. P. Lewis, *Ann. N.Y. Acad. Sci.*, **104**, 236 (1963).

386. R. H. Fox, R. Goldsmith, D. J. Kidd, and G. P. Lewis, *J. Physiol.* (London), **157**, 589 (1961).

387. H. O. J. Collier, J. A. Holgate, M. Schachter, and P. G. Shorley, *Brit. J. Pharmacol.*, **15**, 290 (1960).

388. H. O. J. Collier, G. W. L. James, and P. J. Piper, *J. Physiol.* (London), **180**, 13P (1965).

389. V. Libro and L. Mariani, *Atti. Accad. Med. Lombarda*, **16**, 244 (1961).

390. G. W. L. James, *J. Pharm. Pharmacol.*, **21**, 379 (1969).

391. A. M. Rothschild, M. P. O. Antonio, J. J. Dias, A. Castania, and L. C. Neves, *Advan. Exp. Med. Biol.*, **21**, 317 (1972).

392. K. Abe, N. Watanabe, N. Kumagai, T. Mouri, T. Seki, and K. Yoshinaga, *Experientia*, **23**, 626 (1967).

393. B. G. Simonsson, B-E. Skoogh, N. P. Bergh, R. Andersson, and N. Svedmyr, *Respiration*, **30**, 278 (1973).

394. H. O. J. Collier and G. W. L. James, *J. Physiol.* (London), **185**, 71P (1966).

395. H. O. J. Collier, A. R. Hammond, and B. Whiteley, *Nature*, **200**, 176 (1963).

396. H. O. J. Collier and G. W. L. James, *Brit. J. Pharmacol.*, **25**, 283 (1965).

397. H. O. J. Collier, *Biochem. Pharmacol.*, **10**, 47, 1962.

398. J. Pickens, G. B. West, and C. J. Whelan, *Brit. J. Pharmacol.*, **45**, 140P (1972).

399. H. O. J. Collier, *Proc. R. Soc. Med.*, **64**, 1 (1971).

400. B. B. Vargaftig and N. Daoltai, *J. Pharm. Pharmacol.*, **24**, 159 (1972).

401. M. S. Starr and G. B. West, *Brit. J. Pharmacol.*, **37**, 178 (1969).

402. W. Dawson, M. S. Starr, and G. B. West, *Brit. J. Pharmacol.*, **27**, 249 (1966).

403. E. J. Walaszck, C. G. Huggins, and C. M. Smith, *Ann. N.Y. Acad. Sci.*, **104**, 281 (1963).

404. H. O. J. Collier, *Proc. Int. Pharmacol. Meet. 1st*, Stockholm, **9**, 47 (1961).

405. J. Garcia Leme and M. Rocha e Silva, *Brit. J. Pharmacol.*, **25**, 50 (1965).

406. H. Van Riezen, *J. Pharm. Pharmacol.*, **18**, 688 (1966).

407. H. VanRiezen and E. Bettink, *J. Pharm. Pharmacol.*, **20**, 474 (1968).

408. J. D. Horowitz and M. L. Mashford, *J. Pharm. Pharmacol.*, **21**, 51 (1969).

409. J. Damas, *Arch. Int. Pharmacodyn. Ther.*, **204**, 150 (1973).

410. A. Gecse, L. Szekeres, and G. B. West, *J. Pharm. Pharmacol.*, **21**, 544 (1969).

411. R. Jaques and B. Schar, *Schweiz Med. Wochenschr.*, **97**, 553 (1967).

412. J. Lecomte, *C. R. Soc. Biol.*, **163**, 1469 (1969).

413. R. Jaques, G. Huber, L. Neipp. A. Rossi, B. Schar, and R. Meier, *Experientia*, **23**, 149 (1967).

414. A. Gecse, E. Zsilinszky, J. Lonovics, and G. B. West, *Int. Arch. Allergy Appl. Immunol.*, **41**, 174 (1971).

415. L. P. Posati, K. K. Fox, and M. J. Pallansch, *J. Agric. Food. Chem.*, **18**, 632 (1970).

416. W. T. Sherman and R. F. Gautieri, *J. Pharm. Sci.*, **58**, 971 (1969).

417. E. G. Erdos and J. R. Wohler, *Biochem. Pharmacol.*, **12**, 1193 (1963).

418. S. H. Ferreira and M. Rocha e Silva, *Biochem. Pharmacol.*, **11**, 1123 (1962).

419. M. Cirstea, *Brit. J. Pharmacol.*, **25**, 405 (1965).

420. D. A. Tewksbury, *Arch. Int. Pharmacodyn.*, **173**, 426 (1968).

421. D. E. Potter and E. J. Walaszek, *Pharmacology*, **5**, 359 (1971).

422. D. E. Potter and E. J. Walaszek, *Fed. Proc. Fed. Am. Soc. Exp. Biol.*, **28**, 799 (1969); **27**, 662 (1968).

423. D. T. Witiak, B. K. Sinha, R. R. Ruffolo, Jr., and P. N. Patil, *J. Med. Chem.*, **16**, 232 (1973).

424. R. A. MacHaffie, L. R. Menebroker, D. J. Mahler, and A. J. Barak, *J. Allergy*, **31**, 106 (1960).

425. D. A. Rowley and E. P. Benditt, *J. Exp. Med.*, **103**, 399 (1956)

426. G. B. West in *5-Hydroxytryptamine*, G. P. Lewis, Ed., Oxford, Pergamon, England, 1958, pp. 168–171.

427. E. T. Iff and N. M. Vaz, *Int. Arch. Allergy Appl. Immunol.*, **30**, 313 (1966).

428. B. N. Halpern, T. Neveu, and S. Spector, *Brit. J. Pharmacol.*, **20**, 389 (1963).

429. M. D. Gershon and L. L. Ross, *J. Exp. Med.*, **115**, 367 (1962).

430. G. B. West in *Fortschritte der Arzneimittel-forschung*, Vol. 3, E. Jucker, Ed., Birkhauser, Basel, 1961, p. 412.

431. Ref. 430, pp. 417, 418, and 420.

432. I. Mota, *Brit. J. Pharmacol.*, **12**, 453 (1957).

433. B. K. Bhattacharya and G. P. Lewis, *Brit. J. Pharmacol.*, **11**, 202, 411 (1956).

444. J. R. Parratt and G. B. West, *J. Physiol.* (London), **137**, 169 (1957).

435. M. A. Fink, *Proc. Soc. Exp. Biol. Med.*, **92**, 673 (1956).

436. M. Kurihara and K. Shibata, *Jap. Pharmacol.*, **23**, 853 (1973).

437. L. Hodinka and G. Csaba, *Acta. Morphol. Acad. Sci. Hung.*, **22**, 11 (1974).

438. J. H. Humphrey and R. Jaques, *J. Physiol.* (London), **124**, 305 (1954).

439. G. B. West, *J. Pharm. Pharmacol.*, **11**, 513 (1959).

440. J. F. Riley and G. B. West, in *Handbook of Experimental Pharmacology* (Hefter-Heuber). Vol. XVIII, Part I, O. Eichler and A. Farah, Eds., Springer, Berlin, 1966 pp. 130–131.

441. J. H. Gaddum and Z. P. Picarelli, *Brit. J. Pharmacol.*, **12**, 323 (1957).

442. J. Offermeier and E. J. Ariens, *Arch. Int. Pharmacodyn.*, **164**, 192 (1966).

443. I. N. Pidevich and N. F. Kucherova, *Farmakol. Toksikol.*, **36,** 214 (1973).

444. I. N. Pidevich, Z. P. Senova, and I. B. Fedorova, *Farmakol. Toksikol.*, **34,** 155 (1971).

445. R. Weiner and B. W. Zweifach, *Am. J. Physiol.*, **211,** 725 (1966).

446. B. W. Zweifach, A. L. Nagler, and W. Troll, *J. Exp. Med.*, **113,** 437 (1961).

447. W. M. Meyers and K. L. Burdon, *Experientia*, **16,** 52 (1960).

448. C. L. Fox, Jr., J. M. Finbinder, and C. T. Nelson, *Am. J. Physiol.*, **192,** 241 (1958).

449. F. H. Dunne and L. E. Hollister, *Agressologie*, **7,** 487 (1966).

450. W. Doepfner and A. Cerletti, *Int. Arch. Allergy Appl. Immunol.*, **12,** 89 (1958).

451. G. B. Fregnan and A. H. Glasser, *Experientia*, **24,** 150 (1968).

452. H. C. Ferguson and K. W. Dungan, *J. Med. Chem.*, **16,** 1015 (1973).

453. J. Krapcho, B. Rubin, A. M. Drungis, E. R. Spitzmiller, C. F. Turk, J. Williams, B. N. Craver, and J. Fried, *J. Med. Chem.*, **6,** 219 (1963).

454. J. Krapcho and C. F. Turk, *J. Med. Chem.*, **9,** 809 (1966).

455. J. Krapcho, R. C. Millonig, C. F. Turk, and B. J. Amrein, *J. Med. Chem.*, **12,** 164 (1969).

456. M. Kirby, *J. Pharm. Pharmacol.*, **24,** 67 (1972).

457. T. K. Trubitsyna and M. N. Mashkovskii, *Farmakol. Toksikol.*, 33, 387 (1970).

458. E. N. Shaw and D. W. Woolley, *J. Pharmacol. Exp. Ther.*, **116,** 164 (1956).

459. E. N. Shaw, *J. Am. Chem. Soc.*, **77,** 4319 (1955).

460. J. VandenDriessche, P. Allain, and E. Eben-Moussi, *C. R. Sol. Biol.*, **162,** 238 (1968).

461. K. Takagi, I. Takayanagi, T. Irikura, K. Nishino, M. Ito, H. Ohkubo, and N. Ichinoseki, *Jap. J. Pharmacol.*, **19,** 234 (1969).

462. I. V. Komissarov, *Farmakol. Toksikol.*, **33,** 392 (1970).

463. L. D. Basanagoudar, S. Siddappa, and M. Sirsi, *J. Karnatak Univ. Sci.*, **17,** 43 (1972).

464. G. S. Gadaginamath, S. Siddappa, and S. Namjappa, *J. Karnatak Univ. Sci.*, **19,** 194 (1974).

465. G. A. Bhat, S. Siddappa, and M. Sirsi, *J. Karnatak Univ. Sci.*, **18,** 34 (1973).

466. S. P. Hiremath, M. G. Purohit, and K. G. S. Bhat, *J. Karnatak Univ. Sci.*, **19,** 202 (1974).

467. M. C. Fioretti, E. Menconi, and C. Riccardi, *Riv. Farmacol. Ter.*, **5,** 43 (1974).

468. J. B. Data, M. L. Taylor, and M. Forcione, *J. Pharm. Sci.*, **63,** 848 (1974).

469. S. J. Dykstra, J. M. Berdahl, K. N. Campbell, C. M. Combs, and D. G. Lankin, *J. Med. Chem.*, **10,** 418 (1967).

470. M. B. Chapman, K. Clarke, A. J. Humphries, and S. U-D Saraf, *J. Chem. Soc., C,* **6,** 1612 (1969).

471. K. Hole, *Eur. J. Pharmacol.*, **19,** 156 (1972).

472. H. S. Alpers and H. E. Himwich, *J. Pharmacol. Exp. Ther.*, **180,** 531 (1972).

473. P. K. Parkhomets, A. V. Palladin, and V. J. Kocherha, *Ukr. Biokhim. Zh.*, **42,** 687 (1970).

474. C. A. Korduba, J. Veals, and S. Symchowicz, *Life Sci.*, **13,** 1557 (1973).

475. B. Csaba, S. Toth, and G. Molnar, *Arzneim.-Forsch.*, **19,** 1726 (1969).

476. W. J. Van derBurg, I. L. Bonta, J. Delobelle, C. Ramon, and B. Vargaftig, *J. Med. Chem.*, **13,** 35 (1970).

477. F. Sicuteri, G. Franchi, and P. L. Del Bianco, *Int. Arch. Allergy Appl. Immunol.*, **31,** 78 (1967).

478. K. Rao and K. Krishna, *J. Indian Med. Assoc.*, **60,** 238 (1973).

479. E. Sadovsky, D. Weinstein, Y. Pfeifer, W. Z. Polishuk, and F. G. Salman, *Arch. Int. Pharmacodyn.*, **205,** 305 (1973).

480. B. Silvestrini, V. Cioli, S. Burberi, and B. Catanese, *Int. J. Neuropharmacol.*, **7,** 587 (1968).

481. R. K. Turker and S. O. Kayaalp, *Experientia*, **23,** 647 (1967).

482. R. K. Turker, S. O. Kayaalp, and A. Ozer, *Arzneim.-Forsch.*, **18,** 1209 (1968).

483. E. Hong, *Arzneim.-Forsch.*, **23,** 1726 (1973).

484. H. Fujimori and D. P. Cobb, *J. Pharmacol. Exp. Ther.*, **148,** 151 (1965).

485. M. S. K. Ghouri and T. J. Haley, *Eur. J. Pharmacol.*, **3,** 303 (1968).

486. S. Kalsner, *Brit. J. Pharmacol.*, **47,** 386 (1973).

487. P. H. Chanh, N. P. Buu-Hoi, and M. Th. Richert, *Arch. Int. Pharmacodyn. Ther.*, **180,** 450 (1969).

488. A. A. Lubas, A. Stankevicius, and A. Skadurskii, *Farmakol. Toksikol.*, **33,** 17 (1970).

489. C. F. Copp, A. F. Green, H. F. Hodson, A. W. Randall, and M. F. Sim, *Nature*, **214,** 200 (1967).

490. R. A. O'Brien, M. Boublik, and S. Spector, *J. Pharmacol. Exp. Ther.*, **194,** 145 (1975).

491. A. Ya. Veinberg, B. N. Manukhin, N. A. Reshetnikova, N. E. Chupriyanova, and G. I.

Samokhvalov, *Vopr. Med. Khim.*, **18**, 477 (1972).

492. A. Ya. Veinberg, *Khim. Zhizn.*, **7**, 50 (1975).

493. A. Ya. Veinberg, N. E. Chupriyanova, Yu. V. Rodionov, and G. I. Samokhvalov, *Biofizika*, **20**, 388 (1975); Engl. Transl. p. 391.

494. W. Feldberg and C. H. Kellaway, *J. Physiol.* (London), **94**, 187 (1938).

495. C. H. Kellaway and E. R. Trenthewie, *Quart. J. Exp. Physiol.*, **30**, 121 (1940).

496. N. Chakravarty, *Acta Physiol. Scand.*, **48**, 167 (1960).

497. N. Chakravarty and B. Uvnas, *Acta Physiol. Scand.*, **48**, 302 (1960).

498. N. Chakravarty, B. Hogberg, and B. Uvnas, *Acta Physiol. Scand.*, **45**, 255 (1959).

499. W. E. Brocklehurst, *J. Physiol.* (London), **120**, 16P, (1953).

500. W. E. Brocklehurst, in *Ciba Foundation Symposium on Histamine*, Churchill, London, 1956 p. 175.

501. W. E. Brocklehurst, *J. Physiol.* (London), **151**, 416 (1960).

502. W. J. Koopman, R. P. Orange, and K. F. Austen, *Proc. Soc. Exp. Biol. Med.*, **137**, 64 (1971).

503. A. Malley and L. Baecher, *J. Immunol.*, **107**, 586 (1971).

504. W. J. Koopman, R. P. Orange, and K. F. Austen, *J. Immunol.*, **105**, 1096 (1970).

505. R. P. Orange, W. G. Austen, and K. F. Austen, *J. Exp. Med.*, **134**, 136S (1971).

506. M. Kaliner, R. P. Orange, and K. F. Austen, *J. Exp. Med.*, **136**, 556 (1972).

507. E. S. K. Assem and H. O. Schild, *Int. Arch. Allergy Appl. Immunol.*, **40**, 576 (1971).

508. E. S. K. Assem and H. O. Schild, *Int. Arch. Allergy Immunol.*, **45**, 62 (1973).

509. W. E. Brocklehurst, *Advan. Drugs Res.* **5**, 109 (1970).

510. W. E. Brocklehurst, *J. Physiol.* (London), **128**, 1P (1955).

511. P. A. Berry, H. O. J. Collier, and J. A. Holgate, *J. Physiol.* (London), 165, 41P (1963).

512. P. A. Berry and H. O. J. Collier, *Brit. J. Pharmacol.*, **23**, 201 (1964).

513. H. Herxheimer and E. Stresemann, *J. Physiol.* (London), **165**, 78P (1963).

514. B. Uvnas and I. L. Thon, *Exp. Cell. Res.*, **18**, 512 (1959).

515. L. O. Boreus and N. Chakravarty, *Acta Physiol. Scand.*, **48**, 315 (1960).

516. K. F. Austen and J. H. Humphrey, *Advan. Immunol.*, **3**, 1 (1963).

517. W. E. Brocklehurst, *Progr. Allergy*, **6**, 539 (1962).

518. R. P. Orange, M. D. Valentine, and K. F. Austen, *Science*, **157**, 318 (1967).

519. R. P. Orange, J. D. Stechschulte, and K. F. Austen, *J. Immunol.*, **105**, 1087 (1970).

520. J. A. Grant and L. M. Lichtenstein, *J. Immunol.*, **112**, 897 (1974).

521. S. I. Wasserman, E. J. Goetzl, and K. F. Austen, *Fed. Proc.*, **32**, 819 (1973).

522. R. A. Lewis, S. I. Wasserman, E. J. Goetzl, and K. F. Austen, *J. Exp. Med.*, **140**, 1133 (1974).

523. K. Strandberg, *Acta. Physiol. Scand.*, **82**, 47 (1971).

524. K. Strandberg, *Acta. Physiol. Scand.*, **82**, 500 (1971).

525. R. P. Orange, R. C. Murphy, and K. F. Austen, *J. Immunol.*, **113**, 316 (1974).

526. K. Strandberg and B. Uvnas, *Acta. Physiol. Scand.*, **82**, 358 (1971).

527. O. H. Callaghan, *U.S. Natl. Tech. Inf. Sev.*, A.D. Rep., No. 764614/4.

527a. R. C. Murphy, S. Hammarstrom and B. Samuelsson, *Proc. Natl. Acad. Sci. USA*, **76**, 4275 (1979).

527b. S. Hammarstrom, R. C. Murphy and B. Samuelsson, *Biochem. biophys. Res. Comm.*, **91**, 1266 (1979).

528. B. O. Linn, C. H. Shunk, K. Folkers, O. Ganley, and H. J. Robinson, *Biochem. Pharmacol.*, **8**, 339 (1961).

529. R. P. Orange, R. C. Murphy, M. L. Karnousky, and K. F. Austen, *J. Immunol.*, **110**, 760 (1973).

530. K. Strandberg, *Acta. Physiol. Scand.*, **82**, 509 (1971).

531. R. P. Orange, *J. Immunol.*, **114**, 182 (1975).

532. R. P. Orange and E. G. Moore, *J. Immunol.*, **116**, 394 (1976).

533. M. Kaliner, S. I. Wasserman, and K. F. Austen, *New Engl. J. Med.*, **289**, 277 (1973).

534. M. Litt, *Ann. N.Y. Acad. Sci.*, **116**, 964 (1964).

535. S. I. Wasserman, E. J. Goetzl, and K. F. Austen, *J. Immunol.*, **114**, 645 (1975).

536. K. S. Dodgson, B. Spencer, and C. H. Wynn, *Biochem. J.*, **62**, 500 (1956).

537. S. I. Wasserman and K. F. Austen, *J. Clin. Invest.* **57**, 738 (1976).

538. H. Takahashi, M. E. Webster, and H. H. Newball, *J. Immunol.*, **117**, 1039 (1976).

539. R. P. Orange and K. F. Austen, *Cell. Humoral Mech. Anaphylaxis, Allergy Proc. Int. Symp. Can. Soc. Immunol.*, 3rd 1968, **1**, 196 (1968).

540. R. P. Orange and K. F. Austen, *Int. Arch. Allergy Appl. Immunol.*, **41**, 79 (1971).

541. R. P. Orange and K. F. Austen, *Advan. Immunol.*, **10**, 105 (1969).

542. J. S. G. Cox, *Nature* (London), **216**, 1328 (1967).

543. J. S. G. Cox, J. E. Beach, A. M. J. N. Blair, A. J. Clark, J. King, T. B. Lee, D. E. E. Loveday, G. F. Moss, T. S. C. Orr, J. T. Ritchie, and P. Sheard., *Adv. Drug Res.*, **5**, 115 (1970).

544. R. N. Brogden, T. M. Speight, and G. S. Avery, *Drugs*, **7**, 164 (1974).

545. W. A. Taylor, D. H. Francis, D. Sheldon, and I. M. Roitt, *Int. Arch. Allergy Appl. Immunol.*, **46**, 104 (1974).

546. W. A. Taylor, D. H. Francis, D. Sheldon, and I. M. Roitt, *Int. Arch. Allergy Appl. Immunol.*, **47**, 175 (1974).

547. E. J. Kusner, B. Dubnick, and D. J. Herzig, *J. Pharmacol. Exp. Ther.*, **184**, 41 (1973).

548. D. S. Thomson and D. P. Evans, *Clin. Exp. Immunol.*, **13**, 537 (1973).

549. P. W. Marshall, D. S. Thomson, and D. P. Evans, *Int. Arch. Allergy Appl. Immunol.*, **51**, 274 (1976).

550. D. J. Herzig and E. J. Kusner, *J. Pharmacol. Exp. Ther.*, **194**, 457 (1975).

551. H. Cairns, C. Fitzmaurice, D. Hunter, P. B. Johnson, J. King, T. B. Lee, G. H. Lord, R. Minshull, and J. S. G. Cox, *J. Med. Chem.*, **15**, 583 (1972).

552. G. Barker, G. P. Ellis, and D. Shaw, *J. Med. Chem.*, **16**, 87 (1973).

553. J. F. Carney, *Int. Arch. Allergy Appl. Immunol.*, **50**, 322 (1976).

554. J. Augstein, J. B. Farmer, T. B. Lee, P. Sheard, M. L. Tattersall, *Nature, New Biol.*, **245**, 215 (1973).

555. R. A. Appleton, J. R. Bantick, T. R. Chamberlain, D. N. Hardern, T. B. Lee, and A. D. Pratt, *J. Med. Chem.*, **20**, 371 (1977).

556. D. G. Jones and A. B. Kay, *J. Pharm. Pharmacol.*, **26**, 917 (1974).

557. M. E. Greig and R. L. Griffin, *J. Med. Chem.*, **18**, 112 (1975).

558. Y. Sanno, A. Nohara, H. Kuriki, and A. Koda, *Takeda Kenkyusho*, **33**, 225 (1974).

559. A. Nohara, H. Kuriki, T. Saijo, K. Ukawa, T. Murata, M. Kanno, and Y. Sanno, *J. Med. Chem.*, **18**, 34 (1975).

560. G. P. Ellis and D. Shaw, *J. Med. Chem.*, **15**, 865 (1972).

561. G. P. Ellis and D. Shaw, *J. Chem. Soc. Perkin Trans. I*, **1972**, 779.

562. A. Nohara, *Tetrahedron Lett.*, **1187**, 1974.

563. D. R., Buckle, N. J. Morgan, J. W. Ross, H. Smith, and B. A. Spicer, *J. Med. Chem.*, **16**, 1334 (1973).

564. J. W. Ross, H. Smith, and B. A. Spicer, *Int. Arch. Allergy Appl. Immunol.*, **51**, 226 (1976).

565. D. R. Buckle, N. J. Morgan, and H. Smith, *J. Med. Chem.*, **18**, 203 (1975).

566. D. R. Buckle, B. C. C. Cantello, N. J. Morgan, H. Smith, and B. A. Spicer, *J. Med. Chem.*, **18**, 733 (1975).

567. D. R. Buckle, N. J. Morgan, H. Smith, and B. A. Spicer, *J. Med. Chem.*, **18**, 391 (1975).

568. D. R. Buckle, B. C. C. Cantello, H. Smith, and B. A. Spicer, *J. Med. Chem.*, **18**, 726 (1975).

569. D. R. Buckle, B. C. C. Cantello, H. Smith, and B. A. Spicer, *J. Med. Chem.*, **20**, 265 (1977).

570. J. R. Pfister, R. W. Ferraresi, I. T. Harrison, W. H. Rooks, A. P. Roszkowski, A. VanHorn, and J. H. Fried, *J. Med. Chem.*, **15**, 1032 (1972).

571. J. Fullarton, L. E. Martin, and C. Vardey, *Int. Arch. Allergy Appl. Immunol.*, **45**, 84 (1973).

572. E. S. K. Assem, J. A. Evans, and M. K. McAllen, *Brit. Med. J.*, **2**, 93 (1974).

573. E. S. K. Assem, M. K. McAllen, *Int. Arch. Allergy Appl. Immunol.*, **45**, 697 (1973).

574. E. S. K. Assem, *Int. Arch. Allergy Appl. Immunol.*, **45**, 705 (1973).

575. J. F. Batchelor, L. G. Garland, A. F. Green, D. T. D. Hughes, M. J. Follenfant, J. H. Gorvin, H. F. Hodson, and J. E. Tateson, *Lancet*, **1975-I**, 1169.

576. S. P. Haydu, J. L. Bradley, and D. T. D. Hughes, *Brit. Med. J.*, **3**, 283 (1975).

577. C. J. Coulson, R. E. Ford, E. Lunt, J. Marshall, D. L. Pain, and I. H. Rogers, *Eur. J. Med. Chem.*, **9**, 313 (1974).

578. A. Holland, D. Jackson, P. Chaplen, E. Lunt, S. M. Marshall, D. L. Pain, and K. R. A. Wooldridge, *Eur. J. Med. Chem.*, **10**, 447 (1975).

579. B. J. Broughton, P. Chaplen, P. Knowles, E. Lunt, S. M. Marshall, D. L. Pain, and K. R. H. Wooldridge, *J. Med. Chem.*, **18**, 1117 (1975).

580. B. J. Broughton, P. Chaplen, P. Knowles, E. Lunt, D. L. Pain, K. R. H. Wooldridge, R. Fords, S. M. Marshall, J. L. Walker, and D. R. Maxwell, *Nature*, **251**, 650 (1974).

581. J. F. Burka and P. Eyre, *Int. Arch. Allergy Appl. Immunol.*, **49**, 774 (1975).

582. J. B. Wright and H. G. Johnson, *J. Med. Chem.*, **16**, 861 (1973).

583. J. R. Bantick, H. Cairns, A. Chambers, R. Hazard, J. King, T. B. Lee, and R. Minshull, *J. Med. Chem.*, **19**, 817 (1976).

584. P. B. Stewart, J. B. Devlin, and K. R. Freter,

Fed. Proc. Fed. Am. Soc. Exp. Biol., **33,** 762 (1974).

585. J. P. Devlin, K. Freter, and P. B. Stewart, *J. Med. Chem.*, **20,** 205 (1977).

586. C. M. Hall, H. G. Johnson, and J. B. Wright, *J. Med. Chem.*, **17,** 685 (1974).

587. H. G. Johnson and C. A. VanHout, *Int. Arch. Allergy Appl. Immunol.*, **50,** 446 (1976).

588. E. P. Evans and D. S. Thompson, *Brit. J. Pharmacol.*, **53,** 409 (1975).

589. E. P. Evans, P. W. Marshall, and D. S. Thompson, *Int. Arch. Allergy Appl. Immunol.*, **49,** 417 (1975).

590. D. P. Evans, D. J. Gilman, D. S. Thomson, and W. S. Waring, *Nature*, (London), **250,** 592 (1974).

591. J. H. Sellstedt, C. J. Guinosso, A. J. Begany, S. C. Bell, and M. Rosenthale, *J. Med. Chem.*, **18,** 926 (1975).

592. D. Holland, G. Jones, P. W. Marshall, and G. D. Tringham, *J. Med. Chem.*, **19,** 1225 (1976).

CHAPTER FIFTY

General Anesthetics

KEITH W. MILLER

Departments of Anesthesia and Pharmacology
Harvard Medical School and Massachusetts
General Hospital
Boston, Massachusetts, USA

CONTENTS

1 INTRODUCTION

It is now 130 years since the first public demonstration of ether anesthesia took place at the Massachusetts General Hospital in Boston. In that period, with the sole exception of the introduction of nonflammable agents, essentially no major pharmacological improvements have been made in the volatile agents available to the anesthetist. The perspective is even worse when one considers that Paracelsus wrote in the sixteenth century of diethyl ether that "... it has an agreeable taste, so that even chickens take it gladly, and thereafter fall asleep for a long time, awaking unharmed ... its use may be recommended for painful illnesses, and it will mitigate the disagreeable complications of them" (1). Whether, in fact, volatile agents more satisfactory than those employed today do await discovery is an open question. However, recent advances in the understanding of the action of anesthetics, and of their pharmacokinetics, toxicity, and metabolism, provide grounds fo believing that further improvements may yet be forthcoming.

There are a number of characteristics of general anesthetics which together distinguish them as a unique class of agent. Prime amongst these is their relative lack of structural specificity. Within the constraint that lipophilicity is required, substances as disparate as xenon and certain steroids produce general anesthesia. The conclusion that anesthetics do not interact with specific receptors is reinforced by the high concentrations required for anesthesia, and the lack of specific pharmacological antagonists. The implication that anesthetics are simple general cellular poisons is at least partially true, and the margin of safety between depressing consciousness and other vital functions, such as respiration, is small. Therapeutic ratios in the region of two to four are indeed normal. These characteristics, together with very steep dose–effect curves and the clinical need for rapid induction, place a high demand on the skill of the anesthetist. Fortunately these disadvantages are partially, and uniquely, offset by the mode of administration of the volatile agents. Thus it is possible to precisely control the concentration administered to the patient and, at least for agents with rapid pharmacokinetics, to rapidly reduce the level of anesthesia. This, of course, is not true of the intravenous agents and accounts for their lack of popularity for all but brief procedures.

One final problem associated with general anesthetics stems from the high concentrations of these agents required. At the end of a prolonged operation a patient exposed to halothane will have absorbed more than a mole of the agent! Complete elimination of the anesthetic then requires days. The potential for toxicity resulting from such agents or their metabolities cannot be ignored.

The production of improved agents thus requires consideration of factors leading to improving their specificity of action in depressing neuronal function, while providing rapid pharmacokinetics and low toxicity. These are areas where our knowledge is far from complete, but the remainder of this chapter is devoted to exploring approaches and ideas that may be helpful in attaining these objectives.

2 MECHANISMS OF ACTION

2.1 Introduction

Two points must be kept in mind when considering how anesthetics work. First, these agents are nonspecific in action, are used at high concentration, and have access to all areas of the organism. It is therefore probable that even if the primary action is produced by a single mechanism, other modes of action may occur at, or somewhat above, clinical concentrations. Second, general anesthetics form such a diverse group of agents structurally that certain agents, or groups of agents, may have structures conferring some rather specific pharmacological property in addition to that of general anesthesia.

One might thus usefully think of several types of specificity occurring with these agents. First, agants acting by a single type of mechanism on different cellular processes may exhibit specificity. Thus halothane blocks the response of the postsynaptic neuromuscular junction to agonists at about twice the clinical concentration (2), whereas axonal conduction block requires concentrations about an order of magnitude higher than clinical (3). Although this is true of many anesthetics, other agents, such as ethanol and urethane, block axonal conduction at lower doses than required for synaptic block (4). The range of selectivity covers little more than an order of magnitude, and it is probable that in all cases the underlying mechanism is similar and involves a fairly nonspecific interaction with the excitable membranes. Second, agents acting nonspecifically by a mechanism different from that involved in general anesthesia. For example, the ability of volatile anesthetics to inhibit purified brain cholinesterase is unrelated to their anesthetic potency, and in most, but not all, cases the effect is insignificant at clinical doses (5). Third, quite specific interactions may occur; thus some, but not all, barbiturates produce a bicuculline-antagonized GABA-mimetic effect in frog spinal motoneurons, whereas volatile agents have no such effect (6). This effect may be related to the displacement by some of these compounds of tritiated picrotoxinin from a specific binding site in brain (6a).

Thus in seeking to bring our rather incomplete knowledge of how anesthetics work to bear on the problem of the design of agents of superior selectivity, the challenge is, first, to achieve selectivity within the framework of a single type of general mechanism (i.e., nonspecific depression of excitable membranes), so that the higher centers of consciousness may be depressed independently of peripheral function, and, second, to avoid agents that produce relatively specific effects on other structures. It will be apparent from what follows that we are not in a strong position to predict the properties of such agents; nonetheless it is important to the ultimate goal not to fall into the opposite trap provided by the success of unitary hypotheses of anesthetic action.

2.2   The Physicochemical Approach

The objective of this approach is to find a model in which both the distribution of molecules surrounding the anesthetic molecule, and the intermolecular forces between them, resemble closely those between the anesthetic and its unknown physiological site of action. If the model fulfills these conditions, a correlation between the anesthetic potency and the affinity of the anesthetic for the model is to be expected. A limitation of the method is that the intermolecular forces between unlike molecules tend to be systematically related to those between the two like molecules (7). Because of this relationship many of the physical properties of anesthetics correlate with each other and with anesthetic potency. It is thus important to include in such correlations anesthetics whose intermolecular forces with other molecules vary anomalously. In particular, fully fluorinated compounds have much weaker interactions with hydrocarbons, for example, than would be expected. Thus although anesthetic potency has been correlated in the literature with a multitude of physical properties, few of these correlations pass the test when fluorinated anesthetics (e.g., CF_4, SF_6) are included (7). Even when successful, however, such a correlation can only be said to be consistent with the data; in no way is any model based on a correlation proved by it. Critically applied, however, this approach severely restricts the number of acceptable models (8). Furthermore, since these models are based on potency data obtained with intact animals, they are complementary to, and form a conceptual link with, detailed studies of a biophysical, biochemical, or electrophysiological nature. Indeed the correspondence between such models and recent studies of membrane–anesthetic interactions has been rewarding. No detailed account is given here of the critical testing of the many proposed correlations. Several recent reviews deal with this subject (3, 7, 9). Instead, a brief development of the ideas most pertinent to currently held views is presented.

2.3   Solubility Theories

The lipophilicity of anesthetics has long been noted and still provides one of the best predictors of anesthetic potency.

The most generalized form of the solubility theories is that given by Ferguson (10), who noted that although the equilibrium concentrations of various anesthetics producing a given level of anesthesia vary widely, the corresponding thermodynamic activities lie in a relatively narrow range. The activity of a volatile anesthetic is defined as

$$a_{50} = \frac{P_{50}}{p^0} \qquad (50.1)$$

where a_{50} is the thermodynamic activity at the anesthetic partial pressure P_{50} (or at the ED_{50}), and p^0 is the saturated vapor pressure of the pure liquid anesthetic. The thermodynamic activity a_{50} is found to be approximately equal to 0.01–0.04 for many anesthetics (10, 11; Table 50.1), so that the anesthetic partial pressure of any other agent may be predicted by Ferguson's principle. Since many empirical rules have been developed (12) for prediction of vapor pressure this is quite a useful relationship. However, from the foregoing discussion one limitation should be immediately apparent. Only the derived quantity a_{50} contains any information about the anesthetic site; p^0 is a property dependent only on the agent's own intermolecular forces. Thus the estimate is reliable only to the degree that the intermolecular forces between the unknown agent and the site of action of anesthesia are related to its own forces by the same relationship governing those anesthetics used to derive a_{50}. Thus the highest degree of accuracy is obtained when an additional member of an homologous series is considered, whereas low reliability may be expected with highly fluorinated agents.

Figure 50.1 shows that, although the fully fluorinated gases show marked deviations, most common liquid anesthetics have a potency that is well within an order of magnitude of that predicted (Table 50.1). Thus if the underlying physical shortcomings of Ferguson's approach are recognized it provides a reliable first estimate of an agent's potency.

Ferguson's approach may be classified as a solubility theory because $(1/p^0)$ is the ideal (statistical) solubility predicted by Raoult's law (7). An obvious improvement would be to substitute for ideal solubility the solubility in a solvent which closely resembles the site of action of anesthetics. Historically such an approach preceded Ferguson's; the well-known correlation of anesthetic potency with lipid (e.g., olive oil) solubility proposed by Meyer and by Overton at the turn of the century provides in fact a much more accurate method for predicting anesthetic potency even for the fluorinated gases (Fig. 50.1, Table 50.2). This correlation was recently tested against self-consistent data for 18 agents and found to have a standard deviation of only 24% over a potency range of four orders of magnitude (13)!

The model based on this correlation is that anesthesia "occurs when a certain molar concentration is attained in the lipids of the cell." For mice this concentration is 0.08 M, a rather high figure, which serves to emphasize the dangerously nonspecific nature of general anesthetics.

The Meyer–Overton hypothesis may be written

$$P_{50}x_2 = \text{constant} \qquad (50.2)$$

where x_2 is the mole fraction solubility of the anesthetic in olive oil at a partial pressure of 1 atm. Equations 50.1 and 50.2 provide useful predictive rules that are not improved on by more precise models in practice. The latter, however, do develop our concepts to the point at which molecular level considerations now intrude and thus offer the best hope for future developments. Thus Mullins (14) suggested that the

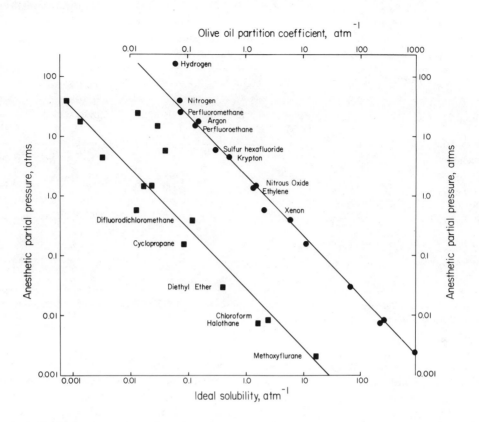

Fig. 50.1 A comparison of the correlation of anesthetic potency with ideal solubility (Ferguson's rule) (■) and with olive oil solubility (●). The lines are drawn with unit slope as required by equations 50.1 and 50.2. The ideal solubility is $(1/P^0)$. This and the Ostwald partition coefficient are given at 37°C and are taken from Ref. 7. Anesthetic data are for mice from Ref. 13.

Table 50.1 Some Commonly Used Volatile Anesthetics

Agent	Formula	Partition Coefficient (59)	
		Blood/Gas	Oil/Gas
Nitrous oxide	N_2O	0.47	1.4
Cyclopropane	$\begin{array}{c} CH_2 \\ \diagup \quad \diagdown \\ CH_2 — CH_2 \end{array}$	0.5	12
Diethyl ether	$C_2H_5OC_2H_5$	12	65
Halothane (fluothane)	$CF_3CHClBr$	2.3	224
Methoxyflurane (penthrane)	$CHCl_2CF_2OCH_3$	12	970
Fluroxene (Fluoromar)	$CF_3CH_2OCHCH_2$	1.4	48
Enflurane (Ethrane)	$CHClFCF_2OCHF_2$	1.8	98
Isoflurane (Forane)	$CF_3CHClOCHF_2$	1.4	98

Table 50.2   Comparison of Thermodynamic Activity and Concentration in Olive Oil at the Equilibrium Anesthetic Concentration for Some Common Anesthetics

Agent[a]	ED_{50} % atm (8)	Vapor Pressure at 37°C, atm	Thermodynamic activity $\times 10^2$	Olive Oil Partition Coefficient 37°C, α	$\alpha \times P_{50}$
Fluroxene	3.4	0.78	4.3	47.8	1.63
Diethyl ether	3	1.09	2.8	65	1.95
Chloroform	0.84	0.44	1.9	265	2.23
Halothane	0.77	0.62	1.3	224	1.72
Methoxyflurane	0.22	0.062	3.6	970	2.13
Mean			2.8		1.93
Standard deviation, %			44		13

[a] Fluroxene is 2,2,2-trifluroethyl vinyl ether. Halothane is 1,1,1-trifluoro-2,2-chlorobromoethane. Methoxyflurane is 1,1-difluoro-2,2-dichloroethyl methyl ether.

volume of the anesthetic might also be important: "...equal degrees of anesthesia with equal volume fraction in the membrane." This may be written as

$$P_{50}x_2\bar{V}_2 = \text{constant} \qquad (50.3)$$

where $\bar{V}_2$ is the partial molar volume of the anesthetic at its site of action. Unfortunately values of $\bar{V}_2$ vary so little from agent to agent that it is difficult to distinguish equations 50.2 and 50.3 experimentally. Mullins suggested that the anesthetic's volume was important because it might act by occluding free space in excitable membranes. Thus he also accounted for the greater than expected potency of diethyl ether by observing that ether caused unusual volume contractions when mixed with liquids such as benzene and suggested that this occurred "...because part of the volume occlusion necessary for anesthesia has been achieved by a rearrangement of the membrane molecules." Attractive as this concept, is, it leads to the erroneous prediction that elevated pressure would act synergistically with anesthetics, whereas the opposite is actually observed. Thus helium

and neon do not cause anesthesia at partial pressures as high as 250–300 atm (8); in fact high pressures of helium reduce the anesthetic potency of other agents, whereas similar pressures of neon have little effect (15). The occlusion interpretation of equation 50.3 is also rendered unattractive by subsequent developments in solution theory over the past 20 years, which show that free volume in liquids is not a useful concept (16, 17).

If two nonpolar liquids are mixed they expand (7, 17). If this expansion were the cause of anesthesia then the remarkable pressure antagonism would be explained. This is the concept that was embodied in the so-called critical volume hypothesis, which states that "anesthesia occurs when the volume of a hydrophobic region is caused to expand beyond a certain critical amount by absorption of molecules of an inert substance. If the volume of this hydrophobic region can be restored by changes of pressure then anesthesia will be removed." This may be written (18) as

$$E_{50} = \frac{P_{50}x_2\bar{V}_2}{V_m} - \beta P_T \qquad (50.4)$$

where E_{50} is the relative expansion which causes anesthesia, V_m is the molar volume of the anesthetic site (or model solvent), β is its isothermal compressibility, and P_T is the total ambient pressure. It can be seen that equation 50.4 reduces to equation 50.3 if P_T is constant, and in addition equation 50.2 is a good approximation if $\bar{V}_2$ is relatively constant.

The form of equation 50.4 has been verified by measuring the potency of a number of anesthetics as a function of pressure (18). Greater insight is provided by calculations using olive oil as a model, however. These show that anesthesia occurs when an expansion of 0.35% is achieved and that, further, the compressibility of the site of action is $3 \times 10^{-5} \, \text{atm}^{-1}$. The lack of anesthetic potency of helium is now explained without additional assumptions, for the expansion that occurs when a raised partial pressure of it dissolves is more than offset by the compression resulting from the elevated mechanical pressure, so that E (equation 50.4) takes on a net negative value. In the case of neon the two terms in equation 50.4 are nearly in balance ($E \simeq 0$). Thus elevated pressures of helium reduce the volume of the anesthetic site and so reduce the potency of other anesthetics, whereas neon causes very little change in either (15, 18).

2.4 Physical Characterization of the Anesthetic Site

If in fact general anesthetics do act at a number of different sites to produce different pharmacological effects (e.g., anticonvulsive action, synaptic blocking action, nerve fiber blocking action) by a single mechanism, then each of these actions should be accounted for by the models outlined above. However, one would expect that the physical characteristics (e.g., solubility, compressibility) might vary somewhat from site to site. There is some

indication that this is indeed so, and, although little systematic progress has yet been made, it is possible that this may lead to the development of a more rational molecular basis for specifying the selectivity of anesthetic agents.

One such characterization has been made on the basis of compressibility. It is observed that mammals compressed in oxyhelium atmospheres become hyperexcitable and suffer convulsions at pressures above about 75 atm. The convulsion threshold pressure may be raised by addition of anesthetics to the breathing mixture. If we assume that the convulsions are triggered by compression of a hydrophobic region, then the protective action of anesthetics results from their tendency to expand the convulsive site. Applying the critical volume hypothesis to the convulsive site, using olive oil as a model, yields a critical volume change for convulsions of -0.4% and a compressibility of $7 \times 10^{-5} \, \text{atm}^{-1}$ (19). The latter value is more than twice that observed for the site of anesthesia, thus providing clear evidence that the two sites are distinct even though the same type of mechanism is involved at each.

Other attempts at characterization have focused on the solvent properties of the sites of action (14, 20). Thus the "solvent power" of the site may be characterized by a solubility parameter, δ, which is defined as

$$\delta^2 = \frac{E_v}{V_m} \tag{50.5}$$

where E_v is the energy of vaporization of the solvent and V_m its molar volume (17). This parameter provides a measure of the cohesive energy density or internal pressure of a solvent. It is thus related to the energy that must be expended to make a cavity in the solvent of sufficient size to accept a solute (anesthetic) molecule. Some of this energy is recovered when the solute molecule is added to the cavity. This may be estimated from the solubility parameter of the solute. This approach essentially attempts to apply the concepts of regular solution theory to the anesthetic site. All the assumptions inherent in this theory thus apply (e.g., ideal entropy of solution, equal size of solvent and solute molecule, etc., see Ref. 17). In practice, although regular solution theory is only strictly applicable in narrowly defined circumstances, it provides a useful semiempirical predictive framework in a wider range of situations. It is, for example, widely used by the chemical engineering community for assessing solvent power. The only direct tests of its applicability to biomembranes show that it offers a self-consistent framework when applied semiempirically (21, 22).

Mullins (14) applied this approach to the action of alcohols on the perfused stellate ganglion of the cat (4) and obtained $\delta =$ 11.5 and 10 $(\text{cal/cm}^3)^{1/2}$ for nonsynaptic and for synaptic block, respectively, implying a less polar or cohesive site in the latter case. Thus ethanol with a δ of 13 selectively blocks the nonsynaptic pathway (at concentrations lower than those required to block the synaptic pathway); butanol with an intermediate δ of 11 blocks both pathways at similar concentrations, whereas octanol with a δ of 9 blocks the synaptic pathway selectively. This reflects the relation of the solubility of the agents at each site to the difference between their solubility parameter and that of the site (17, 20). At a given partial pressure the concentration of octanol is higher at the synaptic than at the nonsynaptic site and, other things being equal, this explains its selectivity. Thus in general agents with δ greater than 11.5 depress the nonsynaptic pathways selectively, whereas those with δ less than 10 are selective for synaptic pathways. Apolar compounds, such as general anesthetics, generally have δs less than nine and thus are predicted to be selective for synaptic pathways, as is found to be the case. Indeed, analysis of the general anesthetic potency data for mice suggests that the best correlations are obtained with nonpolar solvents having $\delta \simeq 10\text{--}11$ (13, 22a), consistent with the notion that general anesthesia results from synaptic block.

More recently attempts have been made to rationalize the balance of excitation and depression found with many volatile agents (20). In a series of fluorinated ethers it was found that convulsant agents all had $\delta \lesssim 7$. Although some of the inert gases break this rule, their δs do have to be estimated at low temperatures or by long extrapolation (17). The common anesthetics have $\delta > 7$ (e.g., halothane 7.7, diethyl ether 7.4, chloroform 9.2). The rule may therefore have some validity, possibly limited to homologous series. An explanation consistent with this might be that two sites are depressed by all the agents. One might be an inhibitory synapse and the other an excitatory synapse of somewhat higher δ. The agents of low δ might then selectively depress the inhibitory synapse leaving on balance an excited state. Whether such is the case remains to be demonstrated, however.

In, fact general anesthetics all seem to cause excitation at low doses and depression at high doses, so that the situation is probably more complex than suggested. Nonetheless, attempts to characterize the solubility parameters of unidentified sites of action may well go some way toward rationalizing the selectivity of these nonspecific agents. Since δ may be characterized according to an anesthetic's solubility in known solvents (17, 23), as well as by equation 50.5, it should be possible to extend this approach to nonvolatile agents. When the small perturbations in structure required to convert an anesthetic barbiturate to a convulsant are considered, however, it seems probable that the approach will not meet with universal success. In fact recent studies show that, in addition to solubility-related specificity, certain groups of anesthetics, for example, barbiturates and steroids, can selectively order or fluidize the membranes in which they dissolve (24). This emphasizes the limitations of the bulk solvent approach and suggests more detailed studies of anesthetic–membrane interactions may be required for a complete description.

2.5   Conclusions

The physicochemical approach to the mechanisms of anesthetic action thus provides a number of useful correlations that enable one to predict an agent's anesthetic potency with a fair degree of certainty. Attempts to characterize the solubility properties of various sites, both in the autonomic and central nervous system, may extend the usefulness of this approach even further. In addition to these correlations, the physicochemical approach leads to detailed models of anesthetic action. By the very nature of the approach these models are merely consistent with the available data; their support does not constitute a proof of their validity. However, the approach does rule out most of the models that have been proposed in the past, and the remaining models point to areas where more direct studies may be fruitful (7, 8).

The most successful of these models is the critical volume hypothesis. It suggests that the site of action of anesthesia behaves much like a bulk phase with a solubility parameter of about 10. Furthermore, anesthesia results from an anesthetic-induced expansion of this phase, and pressure reversal studies suggest it has a compressibility comparable to that of a hydrocarbon liquid. On the basis of these observations two general types of site have been invoked.

The first type is the hydrocarbon core of the lipid bilayer region of membranes, which provides a fluid region that is extensive in two dimensions and 30–40 Å thick. Thus even the third dimension must appear extensive to an anesthetic with a molecular diameter of some 5 Å, although for larger

molecules a divergence between the behavior in a membrane and in a bulk solvent might be expected. Thus on ascending the homologous series of normal alcohols all produce anesthesia until tridecanol and higher homologs are examined. The failure of the higher members to be anesthetics represents a failure of the simple bulk solvent models so far examined. As we will see, however, detailed studies of membranes provide an explanation for this.

The second class of sites involves protein. This protein is unlikely to be cytoplasmic or loosely bound to membranes, because the interior hydrophobic regions of such proteins are densely packed and exhibit little motion. Except for specific pockets that may accommodate a nonpolar molecule of a given size, any generalized penetration of this region leads to destabilization of the protein's structure. Some such proteins do nonetheless show marked sensitivity to anesthetics, the classical example being the luciferases of luminous bacteria and fireflies (25). However, when a wide range of agents is examined the interaction between the anesthetics and the enzyme does not correlate with oil solubility (8, 26). It cannot be ruled out, however, that at clinical doses some specific anesthetic(s) may inhibit a particular enzyme. Thus diethyl ether partially inhibits brain acetylcholine esterase at clinical doses, whereas most other clinical agents do not (5). Even a saturated solution of one of these agents produces no effect.

If cytoplasmic proteins are unlikely sites of action for clinical anesthetics, integral membrane proteins are more probable candidates. Our knowledge of these is far from complete, but with long sections of apolar amino acid residues embedded in the lipid bilayer they are likely targets. Furthermore electrophysiological studies of peripheral synapses strongly point to the involvement of receptor–ionophores in the postsynaptic membrane (2, 27). However, even if this is the mechanism by which anesthetics act,

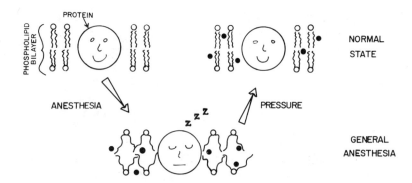

Fig. 50.2 A schematic interpretation of the critical volume hypothesis at the molecular level. Anesthetic (●) dissolves in the lipid bilayer of an excitable membrane, expanding it and increasing its fluidity. This disordering of the lipid interferes with the function of an excitable protein, whose identity is unknown, thus resulting in general anesthesia. Increasing the pressure restores the lipids to their original state, thus reversing the anesthesia even though the anesthetic is still present in the membrane.

they might do so indirectly by modifying the properties of the lipid bilayer in which these proteins function (Fig. 50.2).

We now examine how molecular level studies of model and isolated membranes generally corroborate the bulk solvent models and rectify some of their shortcomings, without at present resolving the question of the site of anesthetic action.

3 ANESTHETIC–MEMBRANE INTERACTIONS

3.1 Introduction

The lipid solubility hypothesis has long been used as evidence that anesthetics act on cell membranes, but ignorance of the cell membrane's structure held back further developments. However, in the past decade fundamental advances in concepts of cell structure have occurred which have precipitated a deeper understanding of anesthetic–membrane interactions. Nonetheless this understanding remains limited by knowledge of membrane structure and function.

Several recent texts adequately review developments in the membrane field (28, 29). The bilayer of amphiphatic lipid molecules provides the cell with a passive permeability barrier with which to maintain its integrity. Proteins attached to, or embedded in, the membrane provide for specific functions such as maintenance of cell shape and of ion gradients, access for nutrients unable to diffuse across the lipid bilayer, and exo- and endocytosis. The lipid bilayer may be readily reconstituted *in vitro* and its properties have been extensively studied. On the other hand, the functions of integral membrane proteins, which may span the bilayer and are thus probably intimately involved in electrical and chemical excitability, are often lost when they are extracted, and correspondingly little progress has been made in elucidating the relation between their structure and function. It follows that our knowledge of anesthetic–bilayer interactions is good, though surprisingly incomplete, whereas the question of anesthetic–bilayer–integral protein interactions remains largely speculative. Thus it should be clear that, although the physicochemical approach is rather fully developed, a molecular level approach upon which future advances may be based has not yet been elaborated in any detail.

3.2 The Solvent Properties of Membranes

One might hope to find that lipid bilayers have solvent properties parallel to those of bulk solvents, such as olive oil and benzene, while deviating from these solvents sufficiently to allow specificity through differential solubility in various cell membranes, or regions of membranes within a cell. Unfortunately few systematic studies have been made and we are far from resolving questions such as, how far does solubility in a cell membrane depend on its composition?

Seeman (3) has measured the partition coefficients of a number of alcohols, barbiturates, and related compounds in red blood cell ghosts. He concludes that at doses of these agents which block nerve conduction the concentration in erythrocytes is fairly constant. This suggests that the correlation with synaptic block may be less good. Unfortunately few other studies have been sufficiently systematic to allow such correlations to be made. However, a number of other studies of simple solutes in biologic and lipid membranes suggests that these membranes do have solubility properties roughly similar to those of bulk solvents (30, 31).

The dependence of solubility on lipid bilayer composition has been studied recently. The partition coefficients of hydrocarbon gases in egg phosphatidylcholine bilayers change little when cholesterol or negatively charged lipids are incorporated in the bilayer (32), whereas the partition coefficient of benzyl alcohol and pentobarbital depends markedly on lipid composition in both bilayers and biomembranes (33, 34). Thus some specificity of action might then be possible from differential partitioning of barbiturate, but not hydrocarbon, anesthetics, Apparently at odds with this concept is the fact that pentobarbital has a lower partition coefficient in bilayers with lipid compositions similar to

nerve than in those typical of organelles (e.g., the cholesterol composition of neurons is very much greater than that of mitochondria). However, since the lipid in cell membranes may be heterogeneously distributed (35), simple extrapolation from lipid bilayers and total biomembrane composition may not be warranted unless the composition in the specific membrane region of interest is known.

The available evidence suggests that the solubility parameter concept may be applicable directly to erythrocyte ghosts at least in the case of gaseous solutes, but that such an application has to proceed on a rather semiempirical basis (21). Furthermore the partition coefficient of hydrocarbon gases varies little with lipid composition (32), and if this is true of other nonpolar solutes and biomembranes, there may be little point in characterizing membranes with this parameter.

We may tentatively conclude, at least for apolar anesthetics, that the lipid regions of membranes behave in such a way that equation 50.2 may well be valid. However, much work remains to be done.

3.3 Changes in Membrane Dimensions

Measurements of this property provide a direct test of the critical volume hypothesis. Unfortunately the considerable technical difficulties have been discouraging.

The surface area of lipid monolayers may be readily measured, and is found to increase in the presence of general anesthetics (36). Significantly nitrogen, but not neon and helium, also causes an area increase (37).

Seeman and colleagues measured the surface area of erythrocytes and found that alcohols (38) and pentobarbital (39) cause expansions larger than would be predicted from their partition coefficients and molecular volume (3). This may arise from the anisotropic structure of the membrane

(8, 18), because increasing the head group area of the phospholipids decreases the anisotropy of their acyl chains, thus reducing the bilayer thickness. Indeed membrane surface area and thickness are observed to have a positive and a negative coefficient of thermal expansion respectively (40). Seeman (3), however, believes that the extra expansion involves a contribution from membrane protein. The question remains unresolved.

It is thus still unclear whether the use of bulk solvent values of the partial molar volume in equations 50.3 and 50.4 is entirely justified; however, membranes do expand qualitatively as predicted by the critical volume hypothesis, and recent unpublished measurements in the author's laboratory show that the partial molal volume of halothane in egg lecithin bilayers, at least, has a value close to that expected.

3.4 Membrane Fluidity

The phospholipids in both biological and model lipid membranes assume a bilayer structure in which their polar head groups face the aqueous regions on either side of the membrane, whereas their acyl chains, sandwiched between, form a fluid array oriented perpendicular to the plane of the membrane. The fluidity of this lipid bilayer is important to the function of membrane protein. This has been most clearly demonstrated in *E. coli* mutants auxotrophic for unsaturated fatty acids, where it is found that β-glucoside and β-galactoside transport is greater in those cells with more fluid acyl chains (29, 41). Moreover, as the temperature is lowered transport slows abruptly at a temperature that is characteristic of the acyl chains incorporated into the membrane and that is perhaps also related to the transition from liquid crystal to gel observed in lipid bilayers. This relation between lipid fluidity and protein function is more difficult to demonstrate in mam-

malian systems, but provides the underlying rationale for models of anesthetic action based on anesthetic-induced increases in lipid fluidity (Fig. 50.2).

The evidence that a change in membrane fluidity may be the primary perturbation leading to general anesthesia rests on two points. First, the critical volume hypothesis may be modified by the assumption that membrane expansion results in a less anisotropic distribution of lipid acyl chains, thus linking conceptually the *in vivo* data and the membrane model (42). This is supported by the observation that pressure reverses the effects of anesthetics on simple lipid bilayers (42–44). Second, a close qualitative correlation is observed between a hydrophobic compound's ability to fluidize membranes and its potency as an anesthetic.

The ability of radiolabeled monovalent cations to cross lipid bilayers is readily monitored. Addition of various ionophores, such as the carrier valinomycin, to the bilayer suspension increases the ion permeability and provides a model of lipid–protein interactions. General anesthetics increase this permeability. In one study, five general anesthetics were added to lipid bilayer suspensions and the increase in valinomycin-mediated K^+ permeability was measured (43). Bilayers that contained a high proportion of cholesterol (as do nerves) had their permeability increased equally by all the anesthetics when they were applied at their respective physiological nerve-blocking doses. This increase in permeability was opposed by pressure. For example, ether (25 mM) increases the permeability by 23% over the control value, and a pressure of 84 atm exactly cancels the increase in permeability caused by ether. If reasonable assumptions are made about ether's bilayer/buffer partition coefficient, it is possible to calculate that it expands the membrane about 0.3%. Since 84 atm counters this expansion, the compressibility of the bilayer is $3.7 \times 10^{-5}\,\text{atm}^{-1}$ (43). This value is strikingly close to that calculated for the site of general anesthesia in mice by the critical volume hypothesis (19). Thus this model correlates closely with *in vivo* behavior, although the analogy is not exact since the potency correlation is with nerve rather than synapse block.

Spectroscopic studies provide a more direct and molecular measure of membrane fluidity, but their sensitivity to small changes is less than that of the permeability measurements discussed above. Most studies have utilized paramagnetic probes covalently attached in the acyl region of lipid bilayers. This spin-label technique has proved quite powerful and a number of important points have been established. Halothane and methoxyflurane both decrease the anisotropy of the acyl chains (measured by an order parameter, S) in cholesterol containing phospholipid bilayers, and this disordering or fluidizing effect is opposed by elevated pressures (44). Anesthetics of widely differing struc-

tures have all been shown to fluidize these bilayers (Fig. 50.3), whereas a number of lipid-soluble nonanesthetics, such as the higher alkanols, do not fluidize them (45–47). Compounds such as Δ^9-tetrahydrocannabinol and chlorpromazine are partial anesthetics, being unable to produce anesthesia alone but reducing the concentration of an anesthetic required to cause anesthesia (48). They are only capable of partially fluidizing lipid bilayers (50) (Fig. 50.3). Elevated pressures of helium increase the order parameter (49).

Thus taken as a whole the lipid bilayer model is quite a good predictor of anesthetic potency. However, a number of problems remain. The sensitivity of the spectroscopic techniques is such that the changes observed are barely detectable at anesthetic concentrations. Even when a more sensitive technique is employed the changes are not large—around a 25% increase in valinomycin-mediated K^+ permeability, for example (43). This makes it

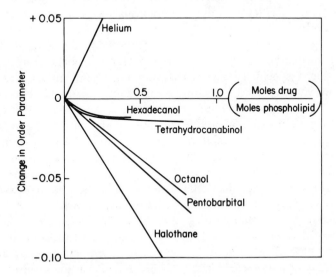

Fig. 50.3   Relation between the change in order parameter (ΔS), measured using spin-labeled fatty acids or phospolipids, and the concentration of various perturbants in phosphatidylcholine:cholesterol (2:1) lipid bilayers. Data for helium from Ref. 49, for hexadecanol and tetrahydrocanabinol from Ref. 46, and the remainder from Ref. 24.

difficult to define a correlation with anesthetic potency, and nothing as quantitative as the olive oil solubility correlation has been presented. It also raises the question of whether such changes are large enough to result in general anesthesia (47). In fact, however, the anesthetic-induced changes observed in the kinetics of post-synaptic conductance at the neuromuscular junction are not very large, even though they are sufficient to block conduction (27). Recently a modified bilayer model of anesthetic action has been proposed which may overcome this objection. This assumes that anesthetics increase the proportion of fluid lipid in a region of a membrane that requires the coexistence of solid- and liquid-like lipid for the protein to function (51, 52). If sufficient anesthetic is added to "melt" the solid phase by a process analogous to depression of the freezing point anesthesia might result. Since this effect would be proportional to the concentration of anesthetic in the membrane, and since pressure would favor the more dense phase, thus opposing the action of the anesthetic, this model is also qualitatively consistent with the critical volume hypothesis. It has been questioned recently, however (52a).

Another problem of the lipid fluidity model is the question of specificity to which we have alluded previously, for if anesthetics fluidize membranes indiscriminately then the model fails to provide a unique mechanism for their selective depression of neuronal function. Any such selectivity would then depend only on solubility or on special structural features of the functional units involved. Recently, however, a number of studies have shown that fluidization may be achieved selectively (24, 53, 54), and the concept of fluidizing efficacy has been introduced (24). All the early work was carried out in phospholipid bilayers containing at least 33 mol % cholesterol. It now appears that bilayers with lower cholesterol content may actually be ordered

by some anesthetics, particularly intravenous agents with rigid ring structures. Thus pentobarbital ordered bilayers with less than, and fluidized those with more than, 10% cholesterol (24). It thus exhibited negative and positive fluidizing efficacy, respectively. Since changes in either direction of bilayer fluidity could lead to pharmacological effects (55), these differences in fluidizing efficacy might underlie such phenomena as the delicate balance between anesthetic and convulsant activities seen in many barbiturates (24).

4 PHARMACODYNAMICS OF VOLATILE ANESTHETICS

The ability to control continuously the partial pressure of anesthetic in the brain is unique to the inhalation anesthetics. It is this advantage above all others that renders them acceptable clinically. One only has to compare the restricted use of intravenous anesthetics, such as barbiturates, to recognize the dangers of using agents with such low therapeutic ratios in the absence of pharmacological antagonists. The ability to pharmacodynamically reverse anesthesia in a controlled manner is thus of paramount importance. Fortunately a good understanding of the uptake and distribution of inhalation agents has been obtained in recent decades (56–59). It is clear that agents differ significantly in their pharmacodynamics, but in a rational way that may be exploited by the medicinal chemist. It is thus worth presenting the principles underlying the pharmacodynamics of inhalation anesthetics.

The anesthetist has under his control only the partial pressure of anesthetic delivered by the anesthesia machine. Between this and the brain a series of partial pressure drops occur until, eventually, equilibrium is attained and the partial pressure is the same throughout the system. Thus the delivered partial pressure is initially higher

than that required for steady-state anesthesia; for most anesthetics this may remain
true throughout a surgical procedure and
the possibility exists for changes in
physiological parameters to modulate the
brain partial pressure even though the inspired partial pressure is constant. However, it is simpler to first consider the physical properties that determine the rate of
uptake under constant physiological conditions.

Early studies showed that neither in the
lung nor in the tissues was diffusion a limiting factor in anesthetic uptake (56). Since
the prime purpose of the circulatory system
is the rapid delivery of oxygen to all tissues
this finding is not surprising, for diffusion
would be a relatively slow process. Distribution from the lung to tissues is thus perfusion controlled. Those tissues with highest blood flow and lowest capacity to dissolve anesthetic saturate most rapidly, and
vice versa. Although multitissue compartment mathematical models can readily be

written, the available data are adequately
represented by grouping the tissues into
three compartments perfused in parallel
(58) (Fig. 50.4). These are (1) a very highly
perfused, low capacity group, e.g. brain,
kidney, and heart; (2) a moderately well
perfused group of high capacity, e.g., muscle and skin; and (3) a poorly perfused,
very high capacity group—the fatty tissues.
The relative capacities of these groups of
course depend on the partition coefficients
of the agents involved. In the diagram the
distributions of halothane and nitrous oxide
are contrasted (Fig. 50.4).

Thus arterial blood leaving the lung contains anesthetic dissolved at the alveolar
partial pressure. On reaching a tissue the
anesthetic diffuses rapidly down the partial
pressure gradient, so that the venous partial
pressure is always at equilibrium with that
in the tissue. The magnitude of this partial
pressure depends inversely on the capacity
of the tissue to dissolve anesthetic (and thus
is lowest for the fatty tissues) and on the

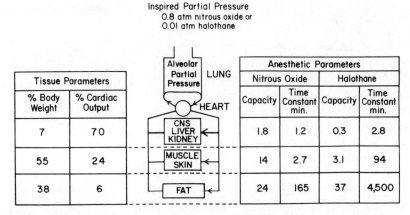

Fig. 50.4   A schematic representation of the three tissue compartment perfusion limited model for the uptake of
volatile anesthetics given by equations 50.6 and 50.7. Physiological parameters are for a person weighing 70 kg.
Anesthetic partition coefficients used were taken from Ref. 59. The capacity of the tissue for anesthetic is given as
milliliters of gas (37°C, 1 atm partial pressure) dissolved in 1 ml tissue, and is for the tissue equilibrated with the
inspired partial pressure of anesthetic. The time constant is the time to reach 63% of equilibrium, and three to
four time constants are equivalent to 95–98% equilibration (59). The time constants given are those for
equilibration between a constant alveolar partial pressure and the tissue. Equilibration with the inspired partial
pressure takes a little longer for nitrous oxide and much longer for halothane (see following figures). The time
constant is given by $\lambda_{tissue/blood} \times$ tissue volume/perfusion rate, where the cardiac output is taken as 6 l/min.

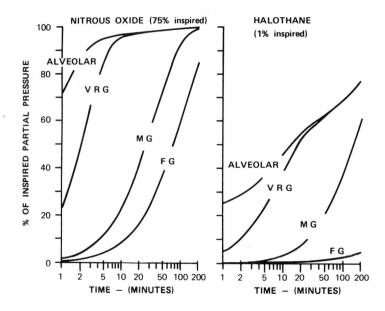

Fig. 50.5 The change of dissolved partial pressure in various tissues with time calculated for the perfusion limited model. VRG is vessel rich group (brain, liver, etc.), MG is muscle group (muscle, skin), and FG is fat group. Tissues with highest perfusion and lowest solubility tend to equilibrate most rapidly. Partition coefficients for nitrous oxide and halothane, respectively, are brain/blood 1.06 and 2.9; muscle/blood 2.3 and 3.5; fat/blood 2.3 and 60. Reproduced with permission from Ref. 59.

current difference between alveolar and tissue partial pressures. This difference declines on every circuit of the blood and equilibrium is approached in an exponential manner. Calculation shows that the brain actually equilibrates very rapidly with the alveolar partial pressure (Figs. 50.4, 50.5), so that to a first approximation we may assume that the rate of change of alveolar partial pressure is equivalent to that in the brain. With this in mind we now consider the rate processes in ventilation, which usually turn out to provide the rate-determining steps in overall equilibration between the anesthesia machine and the brain.

The inspired partial pressure of a completely insoluble gas would equilibrate with the alveolar partial pressure in about 2 min (Fig. 50.6). (This assumes a functional residual capacity of 3 l and a minute volume of 6 l/min.) In practice, however, anesthetic is being removed from the alveoli at a rate proportional to the cardiac output and the

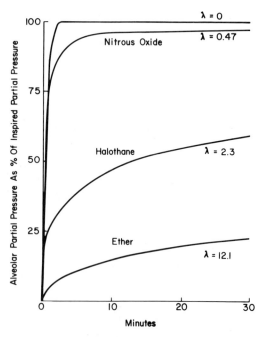

Fig. 50.6 The rate of rise of alveolar partial pressure toward a constant inspired partial pressure is inversely related to the anesthetic's blood/gas partition coefficient, λ. Adapted from Ref. 59.

blood/gas partition coefficient. Thus the achieved alveolar partial pressure is given by the balance of two rate processes. In Fig. 50.6 the ratio of alveolar partial pressure to inspired partial pressure is represented schematically for four different situations to illustrate this point. Thus the single most important physical variable in determining the rate of equilibration of an anesthetic with the brain is its blood/gas partition coefficient. The smaller this coefficient, the more rapid equilibration, and the higher the degree of control that a skilled anesthetist may exercise over anesthetic level.

These qualitative arguments may be stated quantitatively so that the role of physical and physiological parameters may be fully appreciated (58, 59). Assume that perfusion is limiting and that instantaneous equilibrium is achieved between blood and tissues. Then for a system of i tissues the rate of change of alveolar partial pressure is given by

$$\frac{dP_A}{dt} = \frac{M}{V}(P_I - P_A) - \lambda_{b/g}\frac{Q}{V}(P_A - P_V)$$

$$(50.6)$$

and for the ith tissue

$$\frac{dP_i}{dt} = \frac{q_i}{\lambda_i V_i}(P_A - P_i) \qquad (50.7)$$

where P_I = Inspired anesthetic partial pressure
P_A = Alveolar partial pressure
P_V = Mixed venous partial pressure
P_i = Partial pressure in ith tissue
M = Minute volume
V = Lung volume
V_i = Volume of ith tissue
Q = Cardiac output
q = Blood flow to ith tissue
$\lambda_{b/g}$ = Blood/gas partition coefficient
λ_i = ith tissue/gas partition coefficient

These four simultaneous first-order differential equations may be readily solved by numerical integration on a computer.

For our purposes the rate of rise of alveolar partial pressure toward a constant inspired partial pressure provides a useful index of the changing partial pressure in the brain. In Fig. 50.5 the solutions of all four equations are presented graphically for rapid (nitrous oxide) and intermediately fast (halothane) anesthetics. Note that with nitrous oxide the alveolar partial pressure is two-thirds of that inspired in less than 1 min, whereas for halothane the corresponding time is more than 1 h. It follows that the anesthetics with high blood/gas partition coefficients would require enormously long times for induction of anesthesia unless the inspired partial pressure is raised initially, in order to speed induction, and then reduced as an adequate level is achieved in the brain. Since the clinical indicators of anesthetic level are somewhat subjective and may vary from agent to agent, it is important to be able to predict for a new or unfamiliar agent how long such an induction period might be. Thus when halothane first replaced the more slowly saturating diethyl ether in the United States overdosage resulting from a too prolonged induction period was not uncommon.

A further factor to be considered is the available vapor pressure of the agent. Thus with methoxyflurane the partial pressure that can be delivered by a vaporizer is only some four times that finally required to maintain anesthesia. Induction is then very lengthy (the blood/gas partition coefficient is 12), perhaps as much as 20 min unless given with adjuvants (60).

The role of physiological parmeters may be readily appreciated from the uptake model. Some examples are illustrated in Fig. 50.7. Increasing minute volume or decreasing cardiac output enables the alveolar partial pressure to rise more rapidly. These changes are in practice most important for the less rapidly saturating anesthetics, for in these at any given time the alveolar to inspired partial pressure difference is greatest. With these agents the combination of

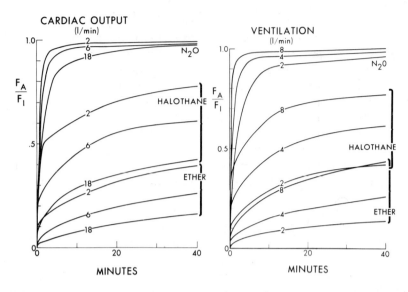

Fig. 50.7 The rate of rise of alveolar partial pressure toward a constant inspired partial pressure also depends on the physiological variables. Increased ventilation and decreased cardiac output both increase this rate, but the effects are least important with nitrous oxide because after 10–20 min equilibrium is very nearly achieved. From Ref. 59 with permission.

prolonged induction together with the anesthetic-induced depression of cardiac output and ventilation lead to a situation in which alveolar partial pressure rises continuously at constant inspired partial pressure. This rise may itself further depress respiration and cardiac output, resulting in an additional elevation of alveolar partial pressure, and so on. The need for constantly modulating the inspired partial pressure is clear. Similar arguments apply to occasions such as the commencement of controlled respiration and onset of hemorrhagic shock. (See Ref. 59 for a complete discussion.)

Large changes in the alveolar partial pressure are most likely with the most slowly saturating agents (Fig. 50.7). Thus anesthetic levels in an agent with rapid kinetics, such as nitrous oxide, tend to vary less during undetected or unexpected changes of physiological parameters, and, moreover, more rapid responses to such changes in anesthetic levels are possible. Nitrous oxide is, therefore, often to be pre-

ferred for low risk patients although its limited potency requires the use of an adjuvant such as a barbiturate or opiate. On the other hand, with the most slowly saturating agents trouble tends to develop more slowly, and they may therefore be preferred for inexperienced operators. Diethyl ether is a classic instance of this and illustrates a further advantage for agents with high blood/gas partition coefficients. That is, when the alveolar partial pressure is allowed to rise sufficiently for respiratory arrest to occur, perfusion may be adequate to reduce the alveolar partial pressure sufficiently rapidly for respiration to recommence spontaneously (59). In essence the anesthetic redistributes toward the fatty and muscle tissues. This safety factor probably contributed to ether's long popularity for use under relatively uncontrolled circumstances.

The rate of recovery from anesthesia is a mirror image of uptake, being most rapid for agents of low blood/gas partition coefficient. The rate also depends on how

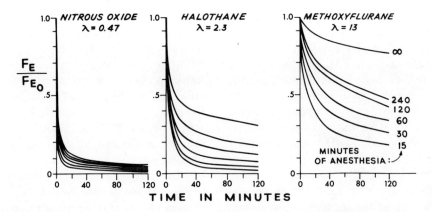

Fig. 50.8   The rate of fall of alveolar partial pressure, P_A, from a value, P_{A_0}, attained just before the inspired partial pressure is reduced to zero, increases with both the duration of anesthesia and the anesthetic's blood/gas partition coefficient. Reproduced with permission from *Anesthesiology*, **30**, 290 (1969).

saturated the tissues have become during exposure to anesthetic. With the soluble agents prolonged recovery times may result (Fig. 50.8). More important than time to recovery of consciousness are the sequelae of prolonged exposure to low levels of anesthetics. With an agent such as methoxyflurane this may provide a degree of postoperative analgesia. More significant, however, is the increased opportunity for metabolic degradation that low levels of anesthetic remaining in the body for days may provide. There is now good evidence that such prolonged low level exposures have deleterious effects on the health of operating room personnel (61). (In this sense the operating room may be a microcosm of our polluted society!) The modes of metabolism are discussed below. It is clear, however that given an equal rate of metabolism, use of an agent with fast kinetics results in a lower exposure to metabolites. If induction of the metabolism occurs fast kinetics assumes even greater importance.

5   METABOLISM AND TOXICOLOGY OF ANESTHETICS

The demonstration that all the commonly used volatile anesthetics are appreciably metabolized in rats (62) has been followed by much work aimed both at elucidating the metabolic pathways involved and at characterizing the possible toxic consequences of such metabolism. How far metabolism is related to those rare adverse reactions to anesthetics exhibited by patients, to hepatotoxicity, and so on, is hard to assess (61) in the absence of a suitable experimental model, although attempts to produce such a model are progressing (63). However, anesthesiologists provide for the epidemiologist a group who are constantly exposed to low levels of anesthetic vapors. Several studies have demonstrated that anesthesia personnel may exhibit a somewhat elevated incidence of cancer, as well as of miscarriages of pregnancy and of congenital abnormalities in offspring (64, 65).

Thus, in addition to the gross toxic effects associated with a number of anesthetics, such as chloroform and trichlorethylene, whose use is now discontinued, carcinogenicity of a new anesthetic, its metabolites, and its contaminants must be considered. As suggested in the preceding section, the use of anesthetics with rapid kinetics may minimize this problem, but it is clearly important to obtain a deeper understanding of the mechanisms involved. Currently the biotransformation of a number of anesthetics has been investigated (reviewed in Ref. 66), but much remains to be learned (67), and the possible mechanisms of toxic injury remain largely conjectural (66). Our ability to predict the probability of a compound being metabolized and of its metabolites having toxic consequences is thus not complete. An example of the sort of systematic approach that is generally lacking is a study of the dechlorination of 15 chloroethanes *in vitro* (68), and a subsequent quantum mechanical analysis of this data (69), which emphasized the importance of the extent of electron deficiency in the most electron-deficient carbon valence atomic orbital of these compounds. Studies such as those on the structure–activity relationships of the carcinogenicity of compounds such as haloethers (70) may also prove useful.

Detailed studies of individual anesthetics illustrate the metabolic routes that may be involved. Dechlorination and debromination of methoxyflurane and halothane have been demonstrated, may be induced by phenobarbital or by methoxyflurane, and

may be brought about *in vitro* by rat liver microsomes, presumably via an oxidative pathway (62, 71). Defluorination of halothane also occurs under hypoxic conditions and is associated with a selective increase of covalent binding to microsomal lipid over that to protein (67). In man as much as 10–20% of halothane absorbed may be accounted for by urinary metabolites, which can be detected over a period of many days (72). A recent thorough study of the urinary metabolites of ^{14}C-halothane in man (73) confirmed and extended earlier observations (66). The three major metabolic products were trifluoroacetic acid, *N*-trifluoroacetylethanolamide, and *N*-acetyl-*S*-(2-bromo-2-chloro-1,1-difluoroethyl)- cysteine. The authors proposed the scheme shown in Fig. 50.9 for the production of these metabolites. Of these, bromochlorodifluoroethylene, and perhaps an intermediate bromochlorotrifluoroethane anion, are also likely intermediates in the covalent binding of radioactivity to other cellular organelles. This would be consistent with the known ability of glutathione to inhibit such binding

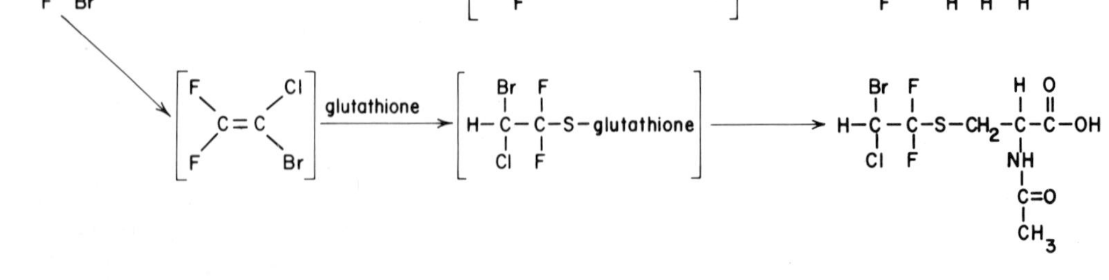

Fig. 50.9 Proposed scheme for the formation of three identified urinary metabolites of halothane in man. Reproduced from Ref. 73 with permission.

during exposure to chloroform and halothane (74). Further studies of the products of such reactions in the liver may be important in defining the mechanism of toxicity.

ACKNOWLEDGEMENT

This chapter was written during the tenure of a U.S. Public Health Service Research Career Development Award from the National Institute of General Medical Sciences.

REFERENCES

1. Paracelus (von Hohenheim), *Opera Medico-Chemica sive Paradox*, 1605; through M. H. Armstrong Davis, "History of Anaesthesia," in *General Anaesthesia*, Vol. 1, 3rd ed., T. C. Grey and J. F. Nunn, Eds., Appleton-Century-Crofts, New York, 1971, p. 711.

2. B. E. Waud and D. R. Waud, *Anesthesiology*, **43,** 540 (1975).

3. P. Seeman, *Pharmacol. Rev.*, **24,** 583 (1972).

4. M. G. Larrabee and J. M. Posternak, *J. Neurophysiol.*, **15,** 19 (1952).

5. L. Braswell and R. J. Kitz, *J. Neurochem.*, **29,** 665 (1977).

6. R. A. Nicoll, *Proc. Natl. Acad. Sci. U.S.*, **72,** 1400 (1975).

6a. M. K. Ticku, M. Ban, and R. W. Olsen, *Mol. Pharmacol.*, **14,** 391 (1978).

7. K. W. Miller and E. B. Smith, "Intermolecular Forces and the Pharmacology of Simple Molecules," in *A Guide to Molecular Pharmacology-Toxicology*, Part II, R. M. Featherstone, Ed., Dekker, New York, 1973, p. 427.

8. J. C. Miller and K. W. Miller, "Approach to the Mechanisms of Action of General Anaesthetics", in *International Review of Science, Biochemistry Series I*, Vol. 12, H. Blaschko, Ed., University Park Press, Baltimore, Md., 1975, p. 33.

9. R. D. Kaufman, *Anesthesiol.*, **46,** 49 (1977).

10. J. Ferguson, *Proc. Roy. Soc.*, (London), **127B,** 387 (1939).

11. A. Cammarata, *J. Pharm. Sci.*, **64,** 2025 (1975).

12. R. C. Reid and T. K. Sherwood, *The properties of Liquids and Gases, Their Estimation and Correlation*, 2nd. ed., McGraw-Hill, New York, 1966, p. 114.

13. K. W. Miller, W. D. M. Paton, E. B. Smith, and R. A. Smith, *Anesthesiology*, **36,** 339 (1972).

14. L. J. Mullins, *Chem. Rev.*, **54,** 289 (1954).

15. M. J. Halsey, E. I. Eger, D. W. Kent, and P. J. Warne, *Progr. Anesthesiol.*, **1,** 353 (1974).

16. J. A. Pryde, *The Liquid State*, Hutchinson, London, 1966. pp. 98–110.

17. J. H. Hildebrand, J. M. Prausnitz, and R. L. Scott, *Regular and Related solutions*, Van Nostrand-Reinhold, New York, 1970.

18. K. W. Miller, W. D. M. Paton, R. A. Smith, and E. B. Smith, *Mol. Pharmacol.*, **9,** 131 (1973).

19. K. W. Miller, *Science*, **185,** 867 (1974).

20. S. Cohen, A. Goldschmid, G. Sctacher, S. Srebrenik, and S. Gitter, *Mol. Pharmacol.*, **11,** 379 (1975).

21. L. J. Bennett and K. W. Miller, *J. Med. Chem.*, **17,** 1124 (1974).

22. L. S. Koehler, W. Curley, and K. A. Koehler, *Mol. Pharmacol.*, **13,** 113 (1977).

22a. K. W. Miller, M. W. Wilson, and R. A. Smith, *Mol. Pharmacol.*, **14,** 950 (1978).

23. S. Srebrenik and S. Cohen, *J. Phys. Chem.*, **80,** 996 (1976).

24. K. W. Miller and K-Y. Y. Pang, *Nature*, **253** (1976).

25. F. H. Johnson, D. E. Brown, and D. Marsland, *J. Cell. Comp. Physiol.*, **20,** 269 (1942).

26. D. C. White and C. R. Dundas, *Nature*, **226,** 456 (1970).

27. P. W. Gage and O. P. Hamill, *Brit. J. Pharmacol.*, **57,** 263 (1976).

28. G. Weissmann and R. Claiborne, Eds., *Cell Membranes, Biochemistry, Cell Biology and Pathology*, H. P. Publishing, New York, 1975.

29. C. F. Fox and A. Keith, Eds., *Membrane Molecular Biology*, Sinauer, Stamford, Conn., 1972.

30. G. G. Power and H. Stegall, *J. Appl. Physiol.*, **29,** 145 (1970).

31. Y. Katz and J. M. Diamond, *J. Membrane Biol.*, **17,** 101 (1974).

32. K. W. Miller, L. Hammond, and E. G. Porter, *Chem. Phys. Lipids*, **20,** 229 (1977).

33. C. M. Colley and J. C. Metcalfe, *FEBS Lett.*, **24,** 241 (1972).

34. K. W. Miller and S-C. T. Yu, *Brit. J. Pharmacol.*, **61,** 57 (1977).

35. S. E. Gordesky and C. V. Marinetti, *Biochem. Biophys. Res. Commun.*, **50,** 1027 (1973).

36. J. A. Clements and K. W. Wilson, *Proc. Natl. Acad. Sci. U.S.*, **48,** 1009 (1962).

37. P. B. Bennett, D. Paphadjopoulos, and A. D. Bangham, *Life Sci.*, **6**, 2527 (1967).

38. P. Seeman, W. O. Kwant, T. Sauks, and W. Argent, *Biochim. Biophys. Acta*, **183**, 490 (1969).

39. S. Roth and P. Seeman, *Biochim. Biophys. Acta*, **255**, 190 (1972).

40. V. Luzzatti, "X-ray Diffraction Studies of Lipid–Water Systems," in *Biological Membranes*, D. Chapman, Ed., Academic London New York, 1968, p. 119.

41. G. Wilson and C. F. Fox, *J. Mol. Biol.*, **55**, 49 (1971).

42. S. M. Johnson and K. W. Miller, *Nature*, **228**, 75 (1970).

43. S. M. Johnson, K. W. Miller, and A. D. Bangham, *Biochim. Biophys. Acta*, **307**, 42 (1973).

44. J. R. Trudell, W. L. Hubbell, and E. N. Cohen, *Biochim. Biophys. Acta*, **291**, 328 (1973).

45. J. C. Metcalfe, P. Seeman, and A. S. V. Burgen, *Mol. Pharmacol.*, **4**, 87 (1968).

46. D. K. Lawrence and E. W. Gill, *Mol. Pharmacol.*, **11**, 280 (1975).

47. J. M. Boggs, T. Yoong, and J. C. Hsia, *Mol. Pharmacol.*, **12**, 127 (1976).

48. T. S. Vitez, W. L. Way, R. D. Miller, and E. I. Eger, *Anesthesiol.*, **38**, 525 (1973).

49. J. H. Chin, J. R. Trudell, and E. N. Cohen, *Life Sci.*, **18**, 489 (1976).

50. D. K. Lawrence and E. W. Gill, *Mol. Pharmacol.*, **11**, 595 (1975).

51. J. R. Trudell, D. G. Payan, J. H. Chin, and E. N. Cohen, *Proc. Natl. Acad. Sci. U.S.* **72**, 210 (1974).

52. J. R. Trudell, *Anesthesiol.*, **46**, 5 (1977).

52a. M. J. Pringle and K. W. Miller, *Biochem. Biophys. Res. Commun.*, **85**, 1192 (1978).

53. P. H. Rosenberg, H. Eible, and A. Stier, *Mol. Pharmacol.*, **11**, 879 (1975).

54. M. J. Neal, K. W. Butler, C. F. Polnaszek, and I. C. P. Smith, *Mol. Pharmacol.*, **12**, 144 (1976).

55. J. C. Metcalfe, J. R. S. Hoult, and C. M. Colley, "The Molecular Implications of a Unitary Hypothesis of Anaesthetic Action," in M. J. Halsey, R. A. Millar, and R. A. Sutton, Eds., *Molecular Mechanisms of General Anaesthesia*, Churchill Livingston, Edinburgh, 1974, p. 145.

56. S. S. Kety, *Pharmacol. Rev.*, **3**, 1 (1951).

57. E. M. Papper and R. J. Kitz, *Uptake and Distribution of Anesthetic Agents*, McGraw-Hill, New York, 1963.

58. W. W. Mapleson, *J. Appl. Physiol.*, **18**, 197 (1963).

59. E. I. Eger, *Anesthetic Uptake and Action*, Williams and Wilkins, Baltimore, Md., 1974, pp. 77–159.

60. H. Wollman and T. C. Smith, "Uptake, Distribution, Elimination and Administration of Inhalation Anesthetics," in *The Pharmacological Basis of Therapeutics*, 5th ed., L. S. Goodman and A. Gilman, Eds., Macmillan, New York, 1975, pp. 71–80.

61. M. H. M. Dykes, J. P. Gilbert, P. H. Schur, and E. N. Cohen, *Can. J. Surg.*, **15**, 1 (1972).

62. R. A. VanDyke, M. B. Chenoweth, and A. VanPoznak, *Biochem. Pharmacol.*, **13**, 1239 (1964).

63. I. G. Sipes and B. R. Brown, *Anesthesiology*, **45**, 622 (1976).

64. E. N. Cohen, *Anesthesiology*, **41**, 321 (1974).

65. T. H. Corbett, R. G. Cornell, K. Lieding, and J. L. Endres, *Anesthesiology*, **38**, 260 (1973).

66. E. W. VanStee, *Ann. Rev. Pharmacol.*, **16**, 67 (1976).

67. L. A. Widger, A. J. Gandolfi, and R. A. VanDyke, *Anesthesiol.*, **44**, 197 (1976).

68. R. A. VanDyke and C. G. Wineman, *Biochem. Pharmacol.*, **20**, 463 (1971).

69. G. Loew, J. R. Trudell, and H. Motulsky, *Mol. Pharmacol.*, **9**, 152 (1973).

70. B. L. Van Duuren, C. Katz, B. M. Goldschmidt, K. Frenkel, and A. Sivak, *J. Natl. Cancer Inst.*, **48**, 1431 (1972).

71. R. A. VanDyke, *J. Pharm. Exp. Ther.*, **154**, 364 (1966).

72. H. F. Cascorbi, D. A. Blake, and M. Helrich, *Anesthesiol.*, **32**, 119 (1970).

73. E. N. Cohen, J. R. Trudell, H. N. Edmunds, and E. Watson, *Anesthesiol.*, **43**, 392 (1975).

74. B. R. Brown, I. G. Sipes, and A. M. Sagalyn, *Anesthesiol.*, **41**, 554 (1974).

CHAPTER FIFTY-ONE

Local Anesthetics

BERTIL H. TAKMAN

and

H. JACK ADAMS

Chemistry and Pharmacology Sections,
Astra Pharmaceutical Products, Inc.
Framingham, Massachusetts 01701, USA

Poor human nature, so richly endowed with nerves of anguish, so splendidly organized for pain and sorrow, is so slenderly equipped for joy.—George DuMaurier, *Peter Ibbetson* (1893)

CONTENTS

1 INTRODUCTION

Local anesthetic agents belong to that special class of pharmacological agents that is purposely administered as close to the site of action as possible. A local effect is, in fact, specifically desired, and absorption into the general circulation and subsequent redistribution in the body can lead to undesirable systemic effects and toxicity. The desired local effect is a selective analgesia or anesthesia of some part of the body, ranging from a small skin wheal to the entire abdomen and lower limbs. The phrase "regional anesthesia" informs us that specific regions of the body may be selectively anesthetized. This is done by administering the local anesthetic solution around nerve trunks or plexuses that innervate the region to be anesthetized.

As with many pharmacological agents, the usefulness of local anesthetic agents depends on the reversibility of their effects. Although irreversible block of nerve fibers may be desirable in some conditions, such as the chronic pain of cancer, these agents are most commonly used in situations in which pain is obtunded and motor activity blocked for a few minutes or several hours. It is required of such agents that they not exhibit neurotoxic effects at the concentrations normally used. However, all known local anesthetics possess the potential of causing damage to neural tissue if applied in sufficiently high concentrations. Much time, money, and effort have been spent in the synthesis and testing of compounds that possess good local anesthetic activity accompanied by low local and systemic toxicity. Recently, there has been a resurgence of interest in long-acting and ultra-long-acting agents. In addition to keeping patients free of pain during prolonged operative procedures, such products reduce the need for narcotic analgesics in the postoperative period. Furthermore, long-acting agents can reduce the number of injections of local anesthetic required to keep a patient free of pain for long periods, and this in turn reduces the demands on the time of professional personnel.

As for the future, several intriguing challenges await the enterprising and ingenious chemist and pharmacologist: ultra-long-acting compounds that produce reversible blocks that last days rather than hours; drugs that selectively block sensory fibers while producing a minimal block of motor fibers; and agents to reverse local anesthetic blocks quickly and completely. To the skeptical let us say that there is evidence, some of which is presented in this chapter, for the feasibility of obtaining each of these goals. What remains is the discovery of the agents that can pass the rigorous tests of efficacy and safety that must be applied in order to establish the clinical usefulness of any pharmacological agent.

2 ANATOMY AND PHYSIOLOGY OF THE NERVE MEMBRANE

Our concepts of the anatomy of the nerve membrane have changed continually over the past 50 years as new techniques and instrumentation have enabled the scientist to probe ever deeper into its mysteries. These changing concepts have been reviewed and summarized by Strichartz (1) and Meymaris (2), among others, and the collaboration of art and science has provided superb artwork to help us visualize the molecular structure of this incredible membrane (3). Without this membrane and its ability to transmit impulses, many of the life-forms on this planet—including that apotheosis of the animal kingdom, man—would not exist. It is this membrane that transmits messages of pleasure and pain that affect us so profoundly, and it is toward alleviation of the latter that local anesthetic agents are employed. In order to discuss local anesthetic agents meaningfully, we must learn something about this membrane that transmits impulses and with which local anesthetic agents interact.

The lipid properties of the membrane have been recognized for many years (4) and have been invoked to explain the penetration of the membrane by lipid-soluble substances. Most clinically useful local anesthetic agents of the amine type have pK_a's between 7 and 9. At the pH of body fluids a sufficient proportion of the molecules is in the lipid-soluble uncharged form, emphasizing the importance of this physico-chemical property for penetration through lipid-containing barriers. The importance of proteins in the membrane was also recognized early, and, in fact, proteins equal or exceed the quantity of lipids in nearly all membranes (3), but only recently have investigators begun to elucidate the functions of proteins in the membrane.

Ionic conditions and events when the membrane is in the "resting" state and during transmission of an impulse have been described. The interested reader should see, for example, Aidley (5), Covino and Vassallo (6), or de Jong (7). Those who want a more detailed discussion of the subject should see Hille (8) or Ulbricht (9). For the purposes of this discussion, we are concerned primarily with that implosive rush of sodium ions that occurs following depolarization of the membrane by a natural or artificial stimulus. To explain this phenomenon and to understand the current theories of the modes of action of agents that prevent this influx of sodium ions and thereby block the propagated impulse, we invoke such concepts as channels, selectivity filters, and gates. The description presented here is generally accepted; other investigators have proposed different concepts and hypotheses, however, and some of these are discussed below.

We first describe briefly the anatomy of the nerve trunk. Enveloping a nerve trunk, which may comprise a number of groups of axons, is the external sheath known as the epineurium. Each bundle of axons within the epineurium is surrounded by a connective tissue sheath called the perineurium, and each axon in such a bundle is, in turn, surrounded by a nucleated cell known as the Schwann cell. An *unmyelinated* axon is surrounded only by the Schwann cell. If, on the other hand, the Schwann cell has deposited layers of a lipoprotein known as myelin around the axon, then the axon is *myelinated*. For a discussion of the role of the myelin sheath in impulse propagation, the interested reader should see, for example, de Jong (7).

The anatomic relationships of these several barriers are shown in Fig. 51.1. Although it is obvious that local anesthetic agents must penetrate all these barriers in order to effect local anesthesia, we are concerned in this discussion only with the axonal membrane itself. The membrane of the axon, like the membranes of all living cells, is the interface between the internal milieu of the cell and the external milieu in which it exists. It is not impermeable to ions and molecules, although some pass through it with more difficulty than others. One of the most important features of the nerve membrane is the "sodium channel," the nature of which has been the subject of intense investigation in recent years. Evidence strongly suggests it is a protein, possibly a lipoprotein, that is embedded in the

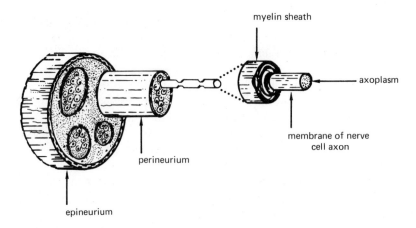

myelin sheath

axoplasm

membrane of nerve
cell axon

perineurium

epineurium

Fig. 51.1 Diagram of a peripheral nerve showing the various barriers that local anesthetic agents must penetrate
in order to arrive at the membrane of a nerve fiber.

matrix of the axonal membrane and that
has an aqueous pore traversing it from ex-
terior to interior. Figure 51.2 shows an
artist's conception of the membrane and a
sodium channel. The nerve membrane in
the resting, polarized state appears to
exhibit a selective impermeability to
sodium ions. Sodium ions can indeed
diffuse across the membrane, but most of
them are actively extruded from the interior by the so-called sodium pump. This
active extrusion of sodium ions results in a
lower concentration of sodium inside the
membrane than outside it. Potassium,
which can also diffuse across the membrane, is not actively extruded, and the
extrusion of sodium results in an ionic imbalance compensated for by a retention of
potassium ions within the cell. The net result is a situation in which the concentration of sodium ions is higher outside than
inside and the concentration of potassium
ions is higher inside than outside. Although
the concentration gradient favors outward
diffusion of potassium ions, this tendency is
counterbalanced by the presence in the
axoplasm of negative charges that are associated with nondiffusible substances such
as protein. The membrane is thus
polarized, its inside being negative relative

to the outside. The result is a set of conditions across the membrane that allow it to
conduct a propagated impulse. One further
item is required: a mechanism for the influx
of cations. Permeability to the cations must
rise and fall sharply, something like a flood-
gate that is suddenly opened fully and then
almost as suddenly closed, since the inward
rush of cations must be of sufficient magnitude and duration to depolarize the
membrane but must be terminated
promptly as soon as this has been accomplished. This, as far as we know, is precisely
what the sodium channel does. The most
obvious way to control the movement of
sodium would be by the opening and closing
of the aqueous pore of the sodium channel
by means of a constriction at some site
along the pore. Results obtained in, for
example, voltage clamp studies indicate
there are, rather, two sites, one more external in the pore than the other, that control
sodium influx. These are referred to as
gates and have been identified with the m
and h processes in Hodgkin–Huxley ter-
minology. They are known as m and h
gates, and a schematic representation of the
events thought to take place during sodium
activation and inactivation is shown in Fig.
51.3. At the normal resting potential the m

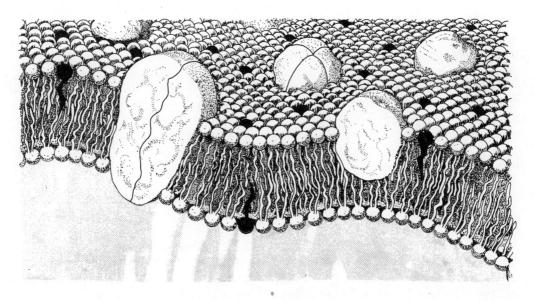

Fig. 51.2 Current membrane model according to Singer. The drawing shows the protein molecules embedded in the bilayer of lipids and cholesterol. Some of the proteins have access to both the inside and outside of the membrane, and some of these may contain pores for the transport of ions, for example. Reprinted with permission from S. J. Singer, "Architecture and Topography of Biologic Membranes," *Hospital Practice*, **8**° 5, and from *Cell Membranes: Biochemistry, Cell Biology & Pathology*, G. Weissmann and R. Claiborne, Eds., Copyright © 1975 by HP Publishing Co., Inc., New York.

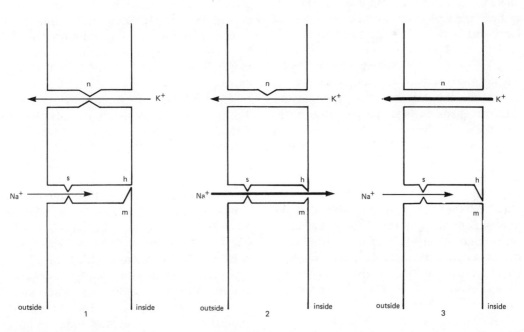

Fig. 51.3 Schematic representation of membrane showing sodium and potassium channels, selectivity filters, and the h, m, and n gates.

gate is closed and the h gate is open. As the internal potential becomes less negative, the m gate starts to open rapidly and the h gate starts to close slowly. The m gate allows an inward rush of sodium ions through the channel before the h gate closes it and before the n gate, which controls potassium efflux, opens sufficiently to allow a significant flow of potassium ions. Finally, an efflux of potassium ions through the n gate reestablishes the resting membrane potential. The m gate is closed and the h gate is open as at the start of this cycle.

Studies with blocking agents such as tetrodotoxin and saxitoxin and with specific tertiary amines and quaternary ammonium compounds have helped investigators define the sodium channel, although they do not all visualize it in the same way (10–14). Since the sodium channel is the sole route for the influx of sodium ions during membrane excitation, the simplest way to prevent depolarization of the membrane and block the propagated impulse would be to close this channel. This is, in fact, what blocking agents and classical local anesthetic agents do. Not all of them do it in the same way, however, and Takman has proposed a classification of blocking agents based on their sites of action, e.g., at the external end of the pore, at the internal (axoplasmic) end of the pore, within the membrane, or a combination of the latter two (15). Hille has shown that it is possible to interpret the effects of the various types of blocking agents on the electrophysiological parameters of a myelinated nerve fiber in such a way that all these agents may be regarded as acting at the sodium channel (12). If this is true, then it is not necessary to postulate an indirect effect on the channel from events occurring some distance from it. There is convincing evidence that saxitoxin and tetrodotoxin block by fitting into the external opening of the pore and need not get into or across the membrane to produce block. Classical local anesthetic agents, on the other hand, must

get into and across the membrane. A further restriction is placed on those agents that block by fitting a cationic receptor site in the channel: they can gain access to the receptor site only when the h gate is open. A schematic diagram of the sodium channel showing the routes of entry and sites of action of the several kinds of blocking agents is shown in Fig. 51.4.

3 CHEMICAL STRUCTURE OF AGENTS THAT BLOCK PROPAGATED IMPULSES

3.1 Introduction

Compounds that block the conduction of impulses when applied to a nerve fiber can be separated into two main groups: those that cause a persistent depolarization of the membrane, thus precluding the maintenance of transmembrane potentials and consequently preventing the impulse-conducting function of the fiber; and those that block the conduction without concomitant depolarization, the block being caused by an inhibition of the influx of sodium ions through the sodium channels. Only the latter group contains compounds that have found use as local anesthetic agents.

Based on their different sites of action, the nondepolarizing agents can also be divided into two groups: those that block the sodium channel at the selectivity filter, the constriction located close to the outer surface of the axonal membrane (16); and those that block the influx of sodium ions at a site other than the selectivity filter. For at least some compounds this site has been shown to be within the channel and closer to its axoplasmic opening (12, 13, 17, 18).

We cannot state with complete assurance whether all agents of this type exert their blocking effect directly at sites inside the channel or indirectly at sites some distance removed from the channel. As a consequence of this, we must use somewhat more arbitrary principles to classify further the

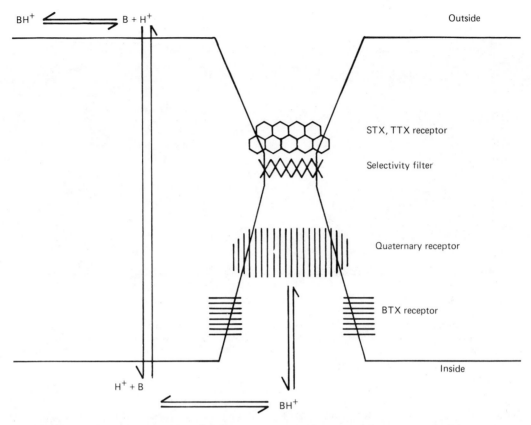

Fig. 51.4   Schematic representation of sodium channel showing selectivity filter and postulated receptor sites

agents belonging to the second group and for the sake of convenience and clarity have selected a structural phenomenological approach to this classification:

1. Quaternary ammonium compounds. These usually act well only when applied from the axoplasmic side of the membrane. Quaternary blocking agents show frequency dependence (*vide infra*).

2. Amines that are sufficiently strong bases to exist in both the charged and uncharged forms within the range of physiological pH. Most of these can produce block regardless of whether they are applied outside or inside the membrane. As a group, they possess various degrees of frequency dependence.

3. Compounds that are either very weak bases, such as certain aromatic amines,

or lack an amine or similar base function. This group comprises agents that are essentially uncharged molecular species at pH 7.4. They do not show frequency dependence.

There are exceptions to these classifications: a quaternary ammonium compound exists as a charged species at all pH values, but at pH 7.4 an amine with a pK_a of 10.5 also is present almost exclusively as the charged species; in a series of compounds with pK_a values ranging from 10.5 to 4.5, this ratio of charged to uncharged species ranges from 10^3 to 10^{-3}, and the weaker a base is, the more it resembles an electrically neutral species (Fig. 51.5).

Furthermore, classifying compounds according to the ease with which they penetrate the membrane can lead to inconsisten-

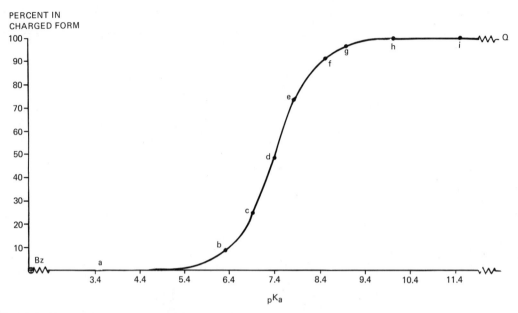

Fig. 51.5 The relationship between the pK_a value of a base and the percent charged form in a dilute aqueous solution at pH 7.4 ($f = 1$). (*a*) 2,6-Xylidine; (*b*) 2-[*N*-[2-methoxyethyl)methylamino]-2′,6′-acetoxylidide; (*c*) 2-(2-methoxyethylamino)-2′,6′-acetoxylidide (*d*) 2-dimethylamino-2′,6′-acetoxylidide; (*e*) lidocaine; (*f*) tetracaine; (*g*) piperocaine; (*g*) 9-aminoacridine; (*i*) tetrodotoxin.

cies. For example, a quaternary compound can be made increasingly lipophilic and its ability to penetrate the membrane can be thereby enhanced. Amines and uncharged molecules can also be made more or less lipophilic, and thus it is possible, by having compounds with both good and poor penetration characteristics in each group, to obliterate any well-defined boundaries among these three classes of agents.

As mentioned above, information available to date indicates that quaternaries and uncharged molecules are frequency dependent and frequency independent, respectively. The intermediate group, however, contains compounds whose frequency dependence ranges from very low to quite pronounced (12).

3.2 Depolarizing Agents

There is a group of compounds that interferes with the normal mechanism of sodium

permeability by obliterating the inactivation process. The resulting increase in resting sodium permeability eventually leads to a state in which the electrical potential differences across the membrane become too small to allow the conduction of impulses along the nerve membrane: the conduction is blocked by increased rather than by decreased sodium permeability.

No compounds of this group have found use as local anesthetic agents. They constitute an important group, however, because their interference with specific parts of normal function renders them useful as tools in the study of the mechanisms of action and the topology of the sodium channel (19). The batrachotoxins, grayanotoxins, and veratrum alkaloids are discussed as examples of the agents that block conduction by depolarization.

Batrachotoxin, 51.**1**, (20, 21) selectively increases the resting sodium permeability of the squid axon and causes a depolarization of the membrane in a concentration of

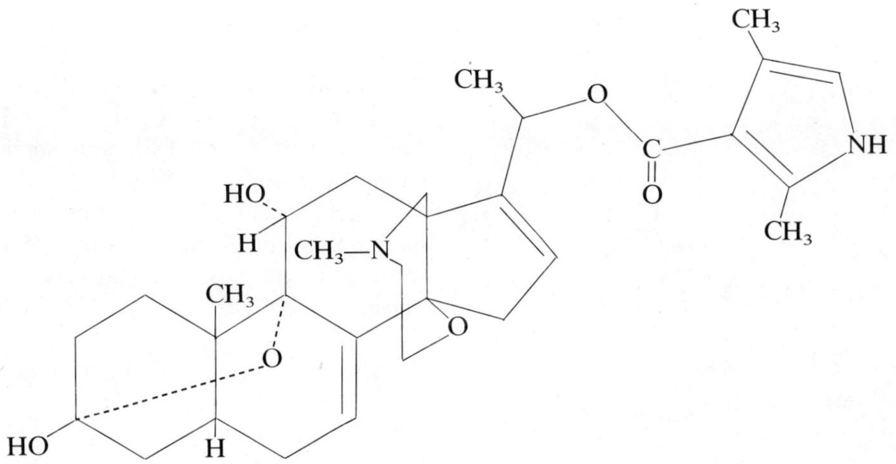

51.1

about 10^{-7} M (22). This process is relatively slow unless the batrachotoxin (BTX) is applied inside the membrane rather than outside (23). The *in vitro* studies indicate that the binding of BTX is, if not actually irreversible, extremely strong. *In vivo* studies of spinal anesthesia in sheep have shown that regional anesthesia can be produced by means of a depolarizing agent such as BTX and that both the sensory and motor components of the block are reversible (24) (Table 51.1).

A sodium channel held in the "open" condition by BTX can be blocked by agents such as tetrodotoxin (22) and procaine (22, 25). Although a concentration of 5×10^{-4} M procaine is sufficient to block an untreated node of the isolated nerve fiber of the frog, a tenfold increase in concentration is required for total block of the BTX-treated node (25). On the other hand, a channel blocked by tetrodotoxin (TTX) or procaine cannot be "unblocked" by the application of BTX. Depolarization occurs during washout after a membrane has been exposed to BTX and TTX simultaneously; however, it does not occur, under the same conditions, if procaine is substituted for TTX (22).

The grayanotoxins I–III are tetracyclic diterpenoids (51.**2a–c**) found in plants of several genera of the family Ericaceae, e.g.,

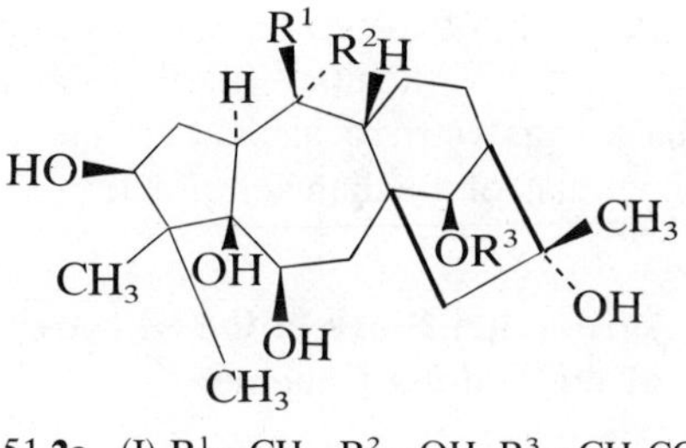

Table 51.1 Spinal Anesthesia in Sheep[a] with Batrachotoxin (24)

Animal Number	Concn.,[b] μg/ml	Total dose, μg	Duration of Analgesia in Perianal Region, hr
1	1	2	12–22
2	1	2	22
3	1	2	25
4	1	2	23
5	2	4	27
6	2	4	36–47

[a] For technique, see Lebeaux (36).
[b] All solutions contained 5% glucose, pH 4.

51.**2a** (I) $R^1 = CH_3$, $R^2 = OH$, $R^3 = CH_3CO$
51.**2b** (II) R^1, $R^2 = CH_3$, $R^3 = H$
51.**2c** (III) $R^1 = CH_3$, $R^2 = OH$, $R^3 = H$

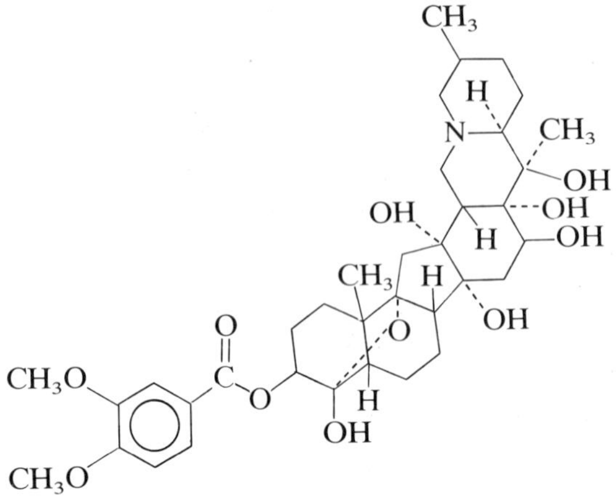

51.**3**

Rhododendron and Kalmia. Their chemistry has been described (26–30) and, although they are chemically unrelated to BTX, they possess a blocking action on the nerve membrane that is identical to that of BTX. Studies on the isolated squid axon indicate that binding of the grayanotoxins to the membrane is much more reversible than the binding of BTX (31).

The third group, the depolarizing veratrum alkaloids, is exemplified by veratridine, 51.**3**, (32); its action is similar to that of BTX and the grayanotoxins (19, 33). Only a few of the alkaloids of Veratrum and related genera are known to possess depolarizing properties; the other alkaloids either have little effect on the action potential or, if they do block it, do so without causing depolarization. For structure–activity relationships on the nerve, see, for example, Ohta et al. (34) and Honerjäger (35). A note of caution: veratrine is a mixture of veratrum alkaloids, and Narahashi has warned against its use as a tool in studies of mechanism of action (19).

3.3 Agents that Block at the Selectivity Filter of the Sodium Channel

There are presently only two compounds, tetrodotoxin (TTX) (51.**4**, Fig. 51.6), and saxitoxin (STX), 51.**5**, that have been

shown unambiguously to block the sodium channel at the narrow part situated close to the outside of the membrane: the selectivity filter of the channel (16). In addition, some derivatives of TTX and some close chemical relatives of TTX and STX probably interact with this site; however, these have not yet been subjected to such intense scrutiny in the laboratory as have the two marine toxins proper.

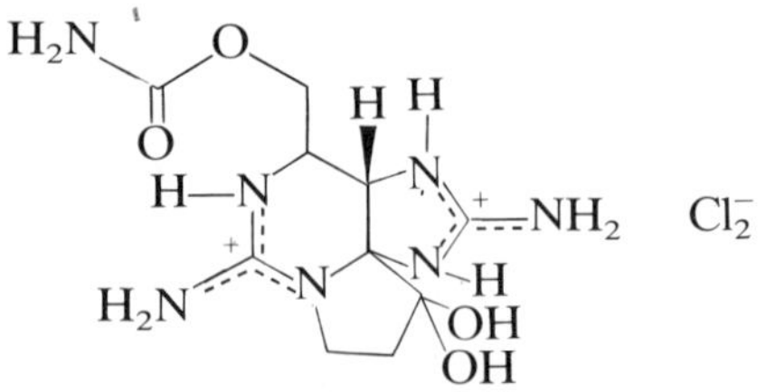

51.**5**

Both compounds are the causative agents in forms of food poisoning that have been known for centuries. TTX is the toxic constituent of several species of pufferfish of the suborder Gymnodontes which cause serious poisoning if not properly prepared before ingestion (e.g., fugu poisoning in Japan); see Kao (37) for details and further references.

More recently, TTX has been identified as the toxic principle of a species of goby, *Gobius criniger*, which is taxonomically unrelated to the Gymnodontes (38). TTX has also been found in Californian newts, e.g., *Taricha torosa* (39), as well as in Central American frogs of the genus *Atelopus* (40). The maculotoxin from the venom of the Australian octopus, *Hapalochlaena maculosa*, has recently been found to be identical to TTX (41). The wide distribution taxonomically and ecologically of this remarkable chemical structure is intriguing.

The structure of TTX was elucidated conclusively by Woodward (42, 43) and was confirmed synthetically by Kishi et al. (44–47). The other specific sodium blocker, STX, is produced by certain dinoflagellates, e.g., *Gonyaulax catenella*, which are responsible for the phenomenon referred to

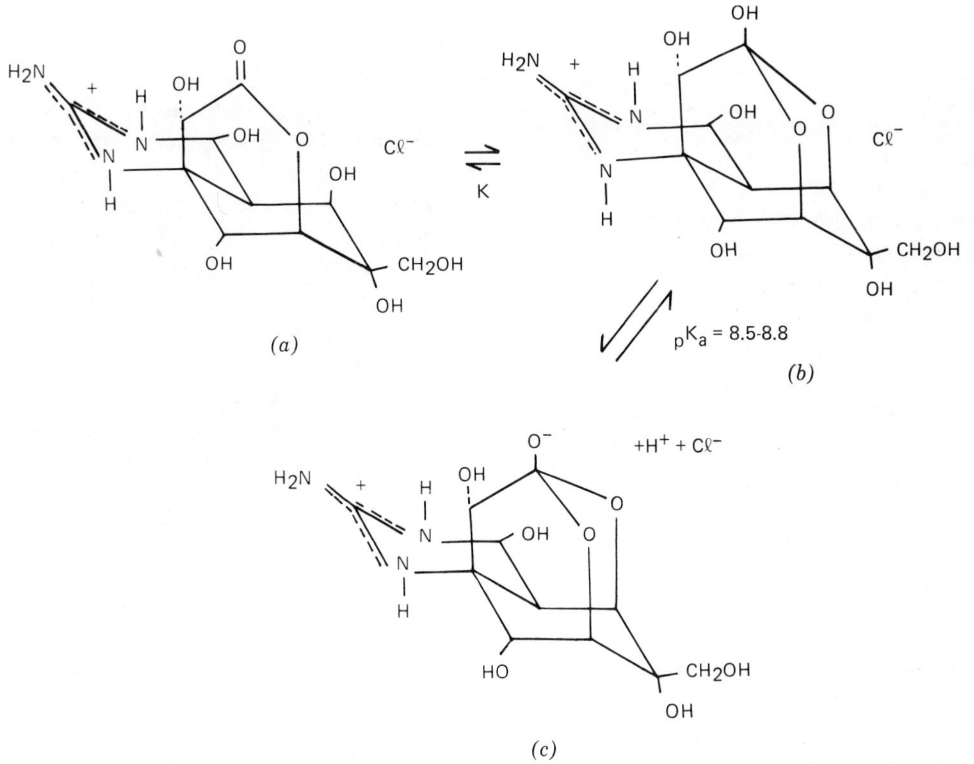

Fig. 51.6 Tetrodotoxin (51.4). (*a*) Cationic lactone form; (*b*) cationic hemilactal form; (*c*) zwitterionic hemilactal form. The numerical value of K (the equilibrium constant between the cationic forms) is not known. The pK_a for the acid function at C-10 = 8.5–8.8.

as "red tide." They can become concentrated in the siphons of several species of shellfish (e.g., *Saxidomus giganteus*, hence saxitoxin). Contaminated clams can, when eaten, cause toxic manifestations and death (shellfish poisoning); see Evans (48) for an extensive review of various aspects of STX.

The structure of STX has been determined by X-ray crystallography by Schantz et al. (49), and a successful total synthesis was recently reported by Tanino et al. (50).

Although pharmacologically very similar, the two toxins are structurally quite different. However, when inspected sterically some common features emerge, and the identity of these structural elements and arrangements have been of signal importance in adding information to our understanding of the outer parts of the sodium

channel and its function (16). Except for the structural features alluded to, these two compounds have in common pronounced hydrophilic properties and at physiological pH almost permanently positively charged regions residing in their guanidino moieties (pK_a 11.5, 12) (51a, b). Their actions at the membrane are almost identical; both block sodium permeability exclusively without any effect on the slow potassium permeation (52). This effect is observed only when they are applied to the membrane from the outside; application inside the axonal membrane of the squid or frog has no effect (53, 54).

Their potency is high, liminal blocking concentrations being of the order of 10^{-10}–10^{-9} M on single nerve fibers of small dimension. The dissociation constant, $K =$

k_2/k_1, for the reaction

$$\text{toxin} + \text{receptor} \underset{k_2}{\overset{k_1}{\rightleftharpoons}} \text{toxin-receptor}$$

on the desheathed rabbit vagus nerve was found to be $(3.0 \pm 0.4)10^{-9}$ M for TTX and $(6.7 \pm 0.3)10^{-9}$ M for STX (55, 56). Values of similar magnitude were found for TTX in the isolated frog nerve (57).

Adams et al. have studied the local anesthetic activity of STX and TTX administered to experimental animals topically, subdurally, epidurally, and around peripheral nerve trunks. In general, local anesthesia was effected with low concentrations on those areas of application in which there were no major barriers to the diffusion of these highly hydrophilic agents; epidurally and around peripheral nerve trunks, i.e., in the presence of barriers such as the peripheral nerve sheath or the *dura mater*, the toxins required higher concentrations in order to effect anesthesia. As is the case with conventional local anesthetic agents, latency, frequency of block, and duration were improved in the presence of these barriers by the addition of a vasoconstrictor such as epinephrine to the solutions. Of special interest is the synergism between these toxins and conventional local anesthetic agents demonstrated in the studies of peripheral nerve block in the rat and epidural anesthesia in the cat and dog (64, 65). As would be expected, local anesthesia produced by mixtures of a local anesthetic agent and STX or TTX reflect the short latency and high frequency of block of the former and the extremely long duration of block of the latter. All this is effected by lower concentrations—and, therefore, lower total doses—of toxin than are required when the toxins are administered by themselves.

3.4 Quaternary Ammonium Compounds

It was often stated in older literature that the formation of a quaternary ammonium compound from a local anesthetic molecule resulted in loss of anesthetic activity. About 25 years ago, it became clear that this observation was erroneous when it was demonstrated that alkylation of benzoyltropines (Table 51.2) (58) as well as of procaine, tetracaine, and dibucaine (59) yielded quaternary compounds with a surprising amount of blocking activity. However, the onset times were found to be very long, which is possibly why quaternaries had earlier been assumed to be without blocking properties. Later, experiments by Hach and Horáková (60, 61) confirmed the possibilities of obtaining nerve block with quaternaries and also demonstrated *in vivo* prolongation of duration of anesthesia when quaternaries and basic amine local anesthetics were given in combination.

Frazier and co-workers (62) showed that the monoquaternaries QX 314, 51.**6**, QX 572, 51.**7**, as well as the bisquaternary hemicholinium-3, 51.**8**, block much more effectively if they are applied from the axoplasmic side of the membrane than from

Table 51.2 Benzoyl-ψ-tropine and Quaternary Derivatives. Duration of Infiltration and Conduction Block (Procaine = 1) (58)

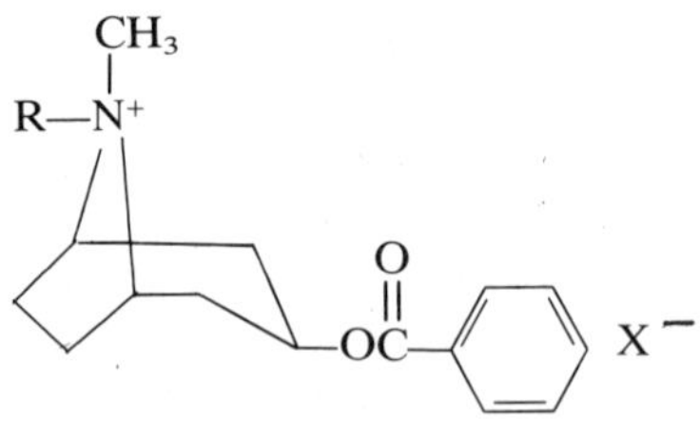

R	X	Infiltration[a]	Conduction[b]
H	Cl	2.2	2.6
CH_3	I	0.25	0.4
C_2H_5	Br	0.58	2.8
C_3H_7	Br	0.80	3.0
i-C_5H_{11}	I	1.55	4.3
Benzyl	Br	2.2	2.0

[a] Rat abdomen.
[b] Frog plexus.

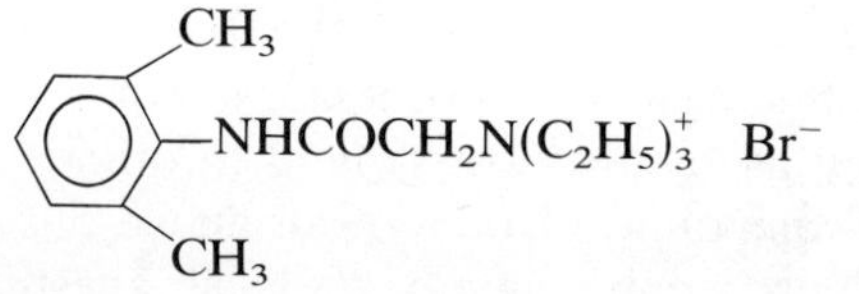

$$\text{51.6}$$

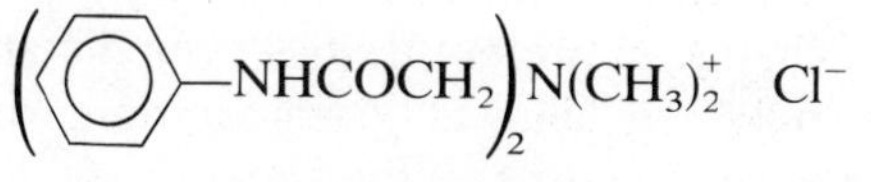

$$\text{51.7}$$

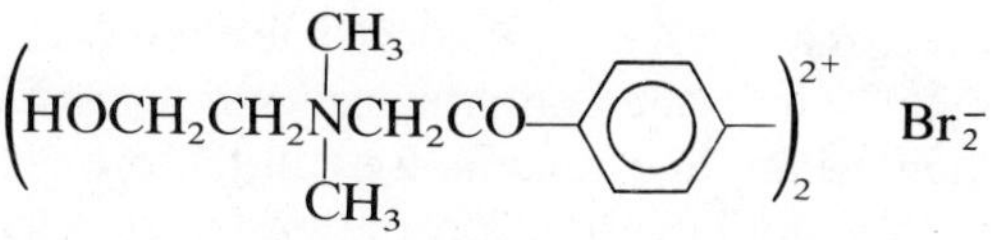

$$\text{51.8}$$

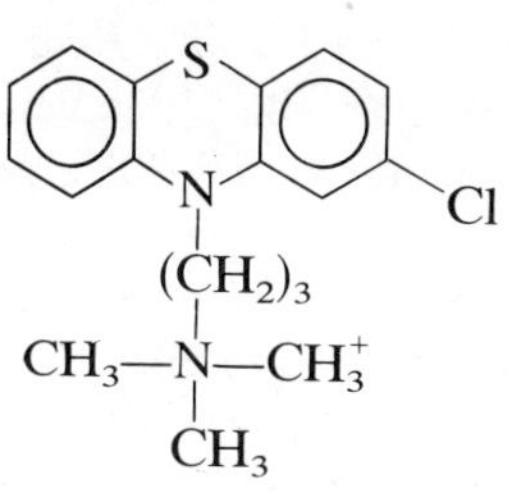

$$\text{51.9}$$

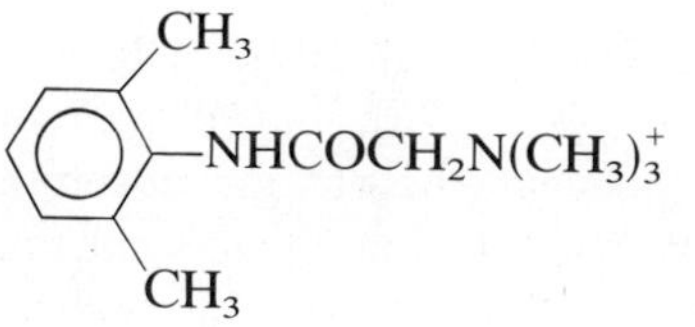

$$\text{51.10}$$

the outside. If applied externally, the structure and physiochemical properties of the agent determine whether they block quickly, slowly, or not at all. In general, the more lipophilic the quaternary, the more easily it will penetrate. Thus N-methylated chlorpromazine, 51.9, was found to block both fast and effectively when applied outside the nerve (63), whereas QX 222, 51.10, the trimethyl homolog of QX 314, does not block at all when administered outside the nerve.

The quaternary blocking agents have so far not contributed to practical anesthesiology but have been significant tools in the unraveling of the structure and function of the axoplasmic part of the sodium channel

and, particularly, in the elucidation of the mechanism of action of the classical local anesthetic agents (Section 4). It should be noted by the investigator that quaternized blocking agents must be carefully checked for absence of the corresponding basic amines before experiments are undertaken.

3.5 Amines of Intermediate Basic Strength

The compounds treated in this section are those amines that are present to a significant degree as uncharged (base) form as well as charged (acid or ionic) form in the physiological pH range. They can be defined, somewhat loosely, as amines with pK_a values in the range 5.5–9.5, i.e., with base/acid ratios in the range 1–99% at pH 7.3–7.5. The pK_a values for the agents used as injectable local anesthetics are, however, to be found almost exclusively in the upper half of this range, that is, between 7.5 and 9.5. This is dictated by the solubility properties of the agents. If the pK_a is low, an amine will exist to a great extent in the base form and this usually has only a limited water solubility. Thus increasing the pK_a increases the total aqueous solubility of the agent.

The ratio of the two forms of any base in aqueous solution is defined by the Henderson–Hasselbalch equation, written here in the form:

$$\log \frac{[B]}{[BH^+]} = pK_a - pH \qquad (51.1)$$

where [B] is the concentration (mol/l) of the base form, $[BH^+]$ is the activity of the ionic form (i.e., the product of the concentration and the activity coefficient), pK_a refers to the thermodynamic ionization constant, and pH has the meaning applied to it when describing aqueous solutions.

At pH 7.4, equation 51.1 becomes

$$\log \frac{[B]}{[BH^+]} = pK_a - 7.4 \qquad (51.2)$$

which expresses the ratio between the two forms at normal physiological pH. If the total concentration, C, of the agent is known, the concentrations of ionized and un-ionized forms of any agent with known pK_a can be calculated at pH 7.4 from equations 51.2 and 51.3.

$$C = [B] + \frac{[BH^+]}{f} \qquad (51.3)$$

Equation 51.3 demands that the activity coefficient, f, be either known or calculable. Often, it is arbitrarily set equal to 1, although this is true only in solutions that are very dilute with respect to ionic species. The investigator should be cautioned to consider carefully the implications of equating concentration and activity. If necessary, the error involved should be estimated in order to minimize the risk of arriving at misleading conclusions. For a short but more detailed discussion, including practical considerations, see Albert and Serjeant (66).

In 1884 local anesthesia and local anesthetic agents became firmly established as clinical concepts through the introduction of cocaine in ophthalmologic practice by Carl Köller in Vienna (67). In the same year interest was awakened in moderately strong amines as local anesthetic agents.

Attempts had been made prior to 1884 to use local application of various agents as a means of alleviating pain, for the benefit of both the patient and surgeon, but they had not met with the necessary success and approval to gain general acceptance. The reader interested in the historical development is referred to Liljestrand's treatise (68), which gives an especially clear analysis of the complex story surrounding the introduction of cocaine.

The blocking agents discussed in this section are subdivided into groups according to structural features.

3.5.1 ESTERS OF AMINO ALCOHOLS. It is mainly a concession to historical tradition to start with a presentation of the amino alcohol esters. Although they held a do-

minant position through the first two-thirds of the history of local anesthetic agents, they have since lost ground to other types of compounds. Today, well above 50% of all procedures involving local anesthesia are performed with agents of other types. This change in preference has been dictated not only by clinical considerations but perhaps even more by the superior stability shown by the more modern agents. However, many ester-type local anesthetics remain in the pharmaceutical armamentarium, and several are still the preferred agents in certain procedures.

3.5.1.1 *Cocaine and Related Agents.* Even though the medicinal acceptance of cocaine as a local anesthetic took place without much resistance, the configurational assignment of the molecule offered some formidable problems. Preceded by some earlier attempts (69–71), the isolation of cocaine from *Erythroxylon coca* Lam. took place in 1860 (72). Its structure was determined by Willstätter and Müller in 1898 (73), but it took almost another 60 years before the absolute configuration was elucidated and cocaine was shown to be 2(*R*)-carbomethoxy-3(*S*)-(−)-benzoxy-1(*R*)-tropane (51.**11a**); for a review of the chemical aspects of the cocaines see Ref. 74.

The curiosity and interest aroused by the various pharmacological properties of cocaine led to manipulations of the molecule even before its structure had been ascertained. Thus the identification of ester functions in the largely unknown cocaine structure prompted the use of alcohols other than methanol and acids other than benzoic acid in the preparation of analogs and homologs from the hydrolysis products of cocaine (75–81).

The fact that (−)-cocaine was not the only alkaloid with anesthetic properties present in *Erythroxylon* species was also observed early. The truxillines, e.g., α-truxilline, (51.**12**) (78–80), cinnamoyl cocaine (80–83), tropacocaine (benzoyl-ψ-tropeine,

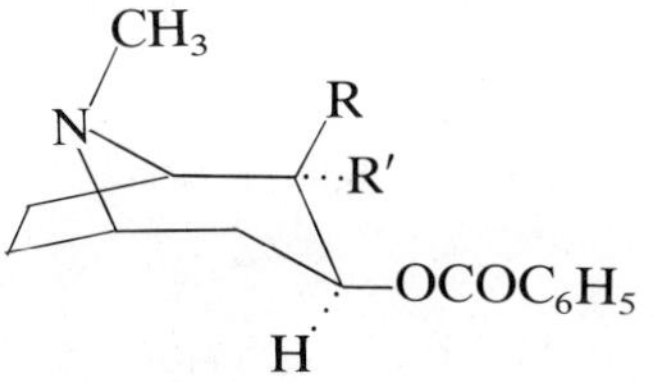

51.**11a**   R = CO$_2$CH$_3$, R′ = H
51.**11b**   R = H, R′ = CO$_2$CH$_3$

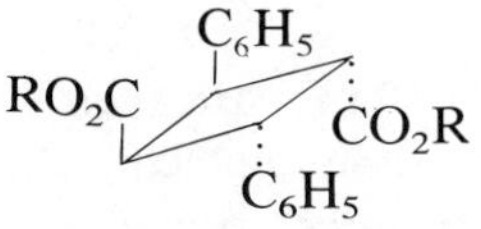

51.**12**   R = methylecgonine residue

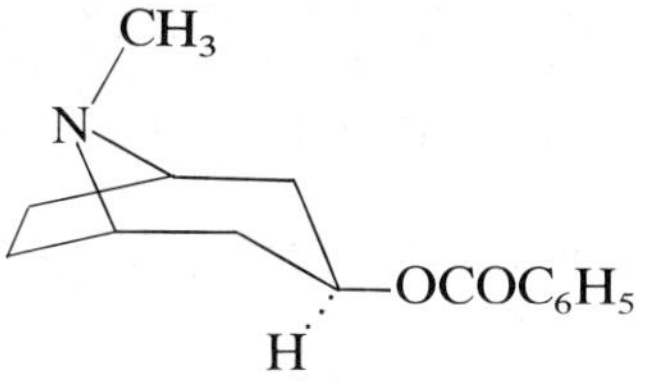

51.**13**

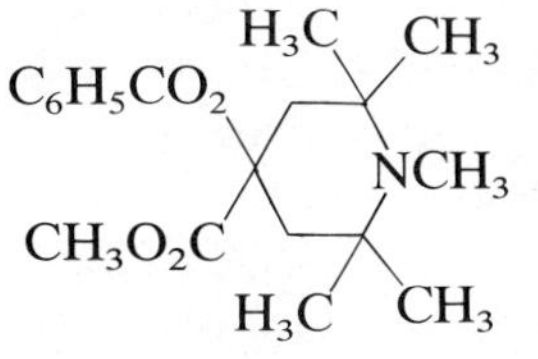

51.**14**

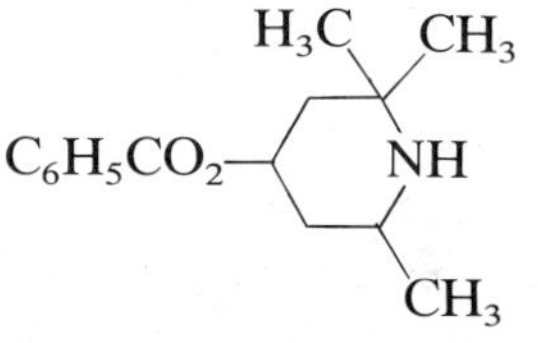

51.**15**

(51.**13**) (84, 85), and (+)-pseudococaine (51.**11b**) (86, 87), were isolated and characterized around 1890. Whereas tropacocaine found early use, (+)-ψ-cocaine did not find its way into the clinic until 1924, under the name of psicaine (88, 89).

The main direction of local anesthetic research depended on the slow elucidation of the structure of cocaine; the development in 1895 of eucaine A, or α-eucaine (51.**14**), by Merling (90, 91) was an attempt to simplify the structure of the alkaloid and yet to retain its desirable properties. This was the first useful compound obtained by this approach, which later would give us almost all the clinically accepted local anesthetics. α-Eucaine possesses sufficient potency (92) but suffers from pronounced tissue-irritating properties; therefore the related and better tolerated β-eucaine (51.**15**) (93) was tested and soon replaced it.

3.5.1.2   *Aminoalkyl Benzoates and Related Esters.*   A further step in varying the structures was the substitution of simple alkylamino alcohols for the ecgonine part of cocaine first represented by Fourneau's stovaine [1-dimethylaminomethyl-1-methylpropyl benzoate, (51.**16a** (94). This compound, the first recorded aminoalkyl benzoate, turned out to be irritating and less potent than cocaine; it was superior to cocaine only as a spinal anesthetic (95). Another related ester, amydricaine [1,1-bis(dimethylaminomethyl)propyl benzoate, 51.**16b** (96)], is more potent than cocaine, especially on addition of epinephrine, but it too suffers from a pronounced liability to cause irritation.

A definitive step toward providing the practitioner with a synthetic agent superior to cocaine was taken by Einhorn when he prepared procaine, 2-diethylaminoethyl 4-aminobenzoate (51.**17**) (95, 97). The toxicity of this compound is low, and it is unusually well tolerated by tissue. Its stability in

$$\underset{\substack{\displaystyle | \\ C_2H_5}}{C_6H_5CO_2\overset{\displaystyle R \atop \displaystyle |}{C}CH_2N(CH_3)_2}$$

51.**16a**   R = CH$_3$
51.**16b**   R = CH$_2$N(CH$_3$)$_2$

p-NH$_2$C$_6$H$_5$CO$_2$CH$_2$CH$_2$N(C$_2$H$_5$)$_2$

51.**17**

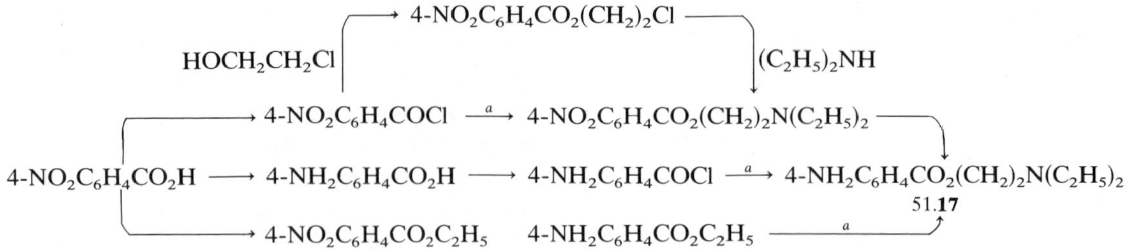

$$4\text{-NO}_2\text{C}_6\text{H}_4\text{CO}_2(\text{CH}_2)_2\text{Cl}$$

$$\text{HOCH}_2\text{CH}_2\text{Cl} \quad\quad\quad\quad\quad (\text{C}_2\text{H}_5)_2\text{NH}$$

$$4\text{-NO}_2\text{C}_6\text{H}_4\text{COCl} \xrightarrow{a} 4\text{-NO}_2\text{C}_6\text{H}_4\text{CO}_2(\text{CH}_2)_2\text{N}(\text{C}_2\text{H}_5)_2$$

$$4\text{-NO}_2\text{C}_6\text{H}_4\text{CO}_2\text{H} \longrightarrow 4\text{-NH}_2\text{C}_6\text{H}_4\text{CO}_2\text{H} \longrightarrow 4\text{-NH}_2\text{C}_6\text{H}_4\text{COCl} \xrightarrow{a} 4\text{-NH}_2\text{C}_6\text{H}_4\text{CO}_2(\text{CH}_2)_2\text{N}(\text{C}_2\text{H}_5)_2$$

51.17

$$4\text{-NO}_2\text{C}_6\text{H}_4\text{CO}_2\text{C}_2\text{H}_5 \quad\quad 4\text{-NH}_2\text{C}_6\text{H}_4\text{CO}_2\text{C}_2\text{H}_5 \xrightarrow{a}$$

Fig. 51.7 Synthetic routes to procaine (51.**17**) $[a = \text{HO}(\text{CH}_2)_2\text{N}(\text{C}_2\text{H}_5)_2]$.

solution, although not ideal, was sufficient to satisfy the practitioner, and this compound soon became the leading local anesthetic in almost all procedures except topical anesthesia, a position it held for almost 50 years.

Even if the toxic properties of procaine, both general and local, are very satisfactory, it is not a particularly potent agent in itself, and had its conception not come at a time when Braun (98, 99) was extending the duration of local anesthesia by the addition of epinephrine to the anesthetic solution, procaine might not have been recognized as a valuable agent so soon. The most common synthetic routes leading to procaine or procaine analogs are shown in Fig. 51.7.

The success of procaine led to an enormous effort to find an even better compound. Hundreds of amino alcohol esters were prepared (for reviews see Refs. 100, 101), and some were found that offered improvements over procaine in certain respects such as potency, longer duration of anesthesia, or better surface-anesthetic properties, but none were found that could compete on an overall basis.

The efforts were now directed mostly toward further improvements of the existing drugs of the amino alcohol ester type, essentially with procaine (51.**17**) and stovaine (51.**16a**) as starting points. Occasionally cocaine and its congeners or the other early local anesthetics were studied for ideas in the design of new compounds. Early in this post-procaine period there were attempts to prepare agents that would contain in the same molecule the necessary structural attributes to make them vasoconstrictors as well as local anesthetics (see end of this section).

It was observed relatively early that the duration of anesthesia and often the topical-anesthetic properties of the procaine-like compounds are favored by an increase of the aminoalkyl group and the intermediate alkylene chain. Thus the diisopropyl homolog of procaine, isocaine-Schmitz (51.**18a**) (102, 103), is about as effective as cocaine on the rabbit cornea. In 3-dibutylaminopropyl 4-aminobenzoate (butacaine, 51.**18b**) (104, 105), both chain length and N-alkyl groups are enlarged. Butacaine was also found to be about as active topically as cocaine (103, 106).

3-Dimethylamino-1,2-dimethylpropyl 4-aminobenzoate (tutocaine, 51.**19**) (107), is another example of a molecule with changes in both the chain and N-alkyls; in this case the end groups were decreased and the chain was increased in length and bulk. The structural changes were accompanied by an increase in duration of anesthesia in the rabbit cornea (108). Similar manipulations led to the clinical introduction of 3-diethylamino-2,2-dimethylpropyl 4-aminobenzoate (dimethocaine, 51.**20**) (109, 110), 2-isobutylaminoethyl 4-amino-

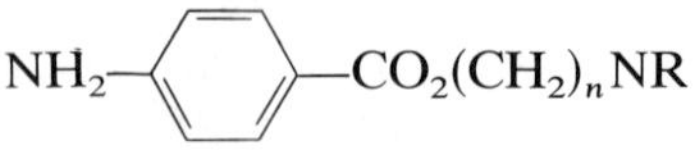

$$\text{NH}_2\text{—}\langle\text{—}\rangle\text{—CO}_2(\text{CH}_2)_n\text{NR}$$

51.**18a** $n = 2$, R = $[\text{CH}(\text{CH}_3)_2]_2$
51.**18b** $n = 3$, R = $(\text{C}_4\text{H}_9)_2$

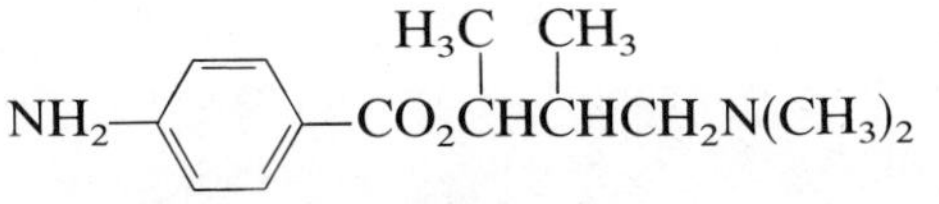

$$NH_2 - \langle \rangle - CO_2CHCHCH_2N(CH_3)_2$$
$$\overset{H_3C}{|} \quad \overset{CH_3}{|}$$

51.**19**

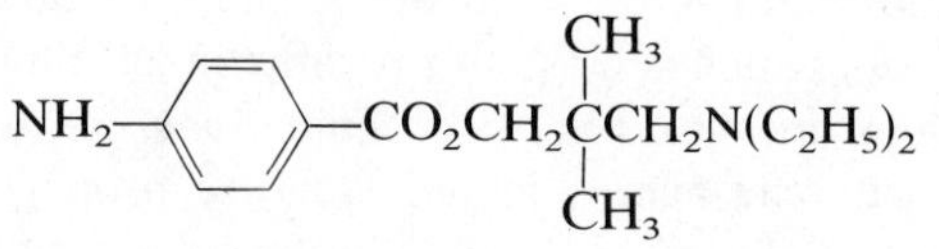

$$NH_2 - \langle \rangle - CO_2CH_2CCH_2N(C_2H_5)_2$$
$$\overset{CH_3}{\underset{CH_3}{|}}$$

51.**20**

$$NH_2 - \langle \rangle - CO_2CH_2CH_2NHR$$

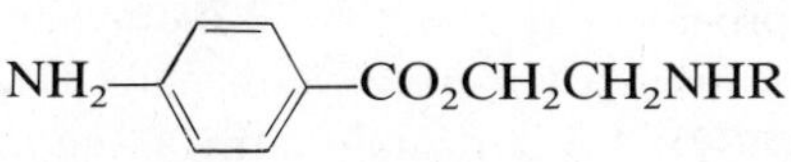

51.**21a**   R = CH$_2$CH(CH$_3$)$_2$
51.**21b**   R = C$_5$H$_{11}$

benzoate (butethamine, 51.**21a**) (111–113), and 2-*n*-pentylaminoethyl 4-amino-benzoate (naepaine, 51.**21b**) (111–113). The latter two differ from the previously mentioned agents in that they are secondary amines.

Besides butacaine (51.**18b**) two other heavily substituted compounds, 2-diethyl-amino-4-methylpentyl 4-aminobenzoate (panthesin, 51.**22**) (114–116) and 2-(2-octylamino)-2-methylpropyl 4-aminobenzoate (octacaine, 51.**23**) (117, 118), are the extreme cases among local anesthetics of this group that have been accepted or at least seriously considered for practical use.

Introduction of alkyl groups into the 4-amino group of the procaine-type compounds has provided local anesthetics with prolonged duration, among which 2-dimethylaminoethyl 4-butylaminobenzoate

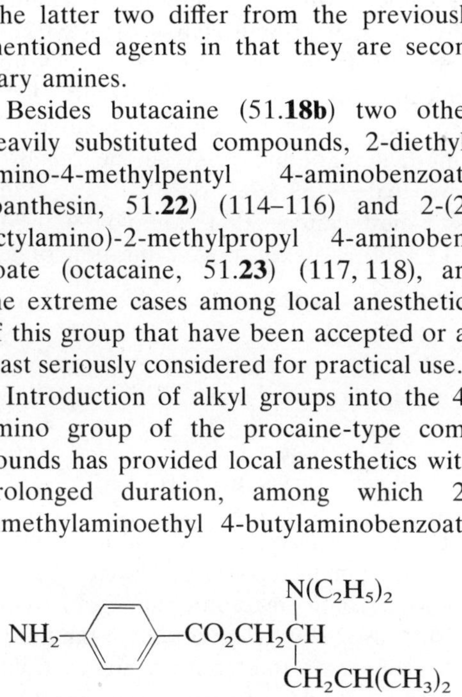

$$NH_2 - \langle \rangle - CO_2CH_2CH$$
$$\overset{N(C_2H_5)_2}{\underset{CH_2CH(CH_3)_2}{|}}$$

51.**22**

$$H_2N - \langle \rangle - CO_2CH_2CNHCHC_6H_{13}$$
$$\overset{CH_3 \ CH_3}{\underset{CH_3}{|}}$$

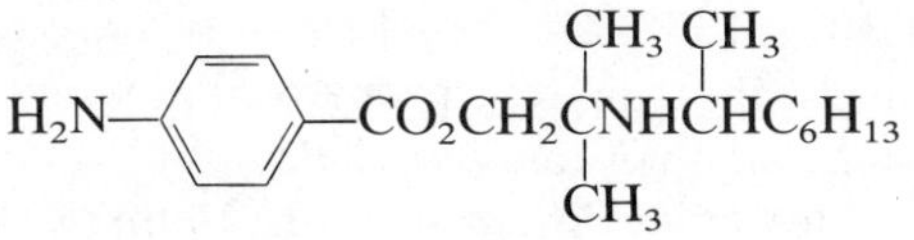

51.**23**

(tetracaine, 51.**24**) (119, 120) seems to possess optimal properties for clinical use. It is a rather toxic long-acting agent, but it has shown itself to be quite safe when used in low concentrations and at the prescribed doses. Tetracaine is currently the most widely used agent for spinal anesthesia.

The increases in potency that characterize some of these variations of the procaine theme were to be gained at the price of increased toxicity, a phenomenon that has been a most persistently negative factor in almost all efforts to increase the potency of local anesthetics.

The structural evolution from cocaine (51.**11a**) via α-eucaine (51.**14**) and β-eucaine (51.**15**) to stovaine (51.**16a**) was explored further during the same period and resulted in a number of local anesthetics that are of clinial use.

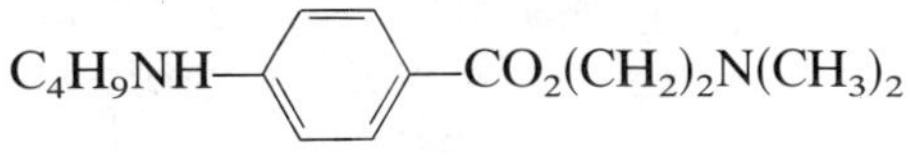

$$C_4H_9NH - \langle \rangle - CO_2(CH_2)_2N(CH_3)_2$$

51.**24**

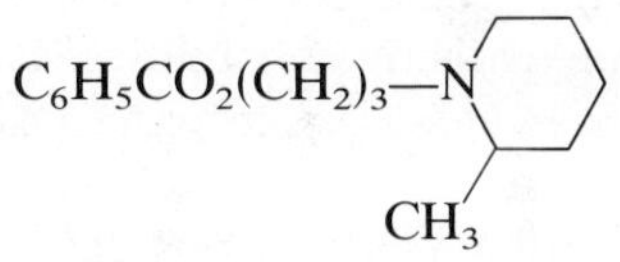

$$C_6H_5CO_2(CH_2)_3 - N \langle \rangle$$
$$\overset{}{\underset{CH_3}{}}$$

51.**25**

$$C_6H_5CO_2CHCH_2NH - \langle \rangle$$
$$\overset{}{\underset{CH_3}{|}}$$

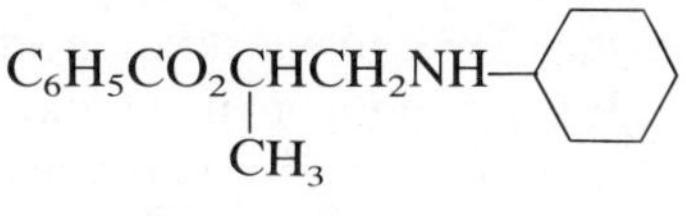

51.**26**

Piperocaine [3-(2-methylpiperidino)-propyl benzoate, 51.**25** (121)], which is somewhat more potent and toxic than procaine (122), and hexylcaine (2-cyclohexylamino-1-methylethyl benzoate, 51.**26**) (123), which is even more potent (122), have found use topically and in infiltration anesthesia, and also as spinal and epidural anesthetics.

Meprylcaine (2-methyl-2-propylamino-propyl benzoate, 51.**27a**) (124, 125), and

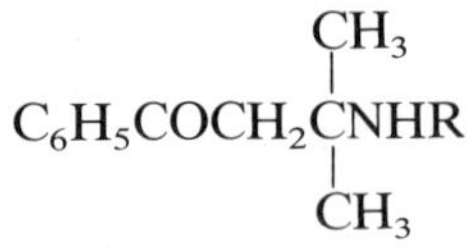

$$CH_3$$
$$C_6H_5COCH_2CNHR$$
$$CH_3$$

51.27a R = C_3H_7
51.27b R = CH_2CH(CH_3)_2

the closely related isobucaine (2-isobutylamino-2-methylpropyl benzoate, 51.**27b** (126, 127) are two other members of this class whose local anesthetic and toxic characteristics place them between the two preceding compounds and procaine.

Because there were already early examples of local anesthetics with other substituents on the benzene ring (e.g., phenacaine, 51.**67**, and the Orthoforms, 51.**75a, b**, the introduction of groups other than 4-amino in the benzoic acid moiety did not add anything new in principle to local anesthetic drug design. Nor is it particularly surprising that we encounter the largest number of structures that have found their way to the clinic in this category; the number of synthetic possibilities clearly becomes tremendously increased by this added feature.

Of the compounds in this category that have been seriously considered for clinical use, the majority still contain an amino group in the ring and most often in the 4 position. Introduction of an alkoxy group into the benzene nucleus was the most successful procedure for obtaining clinically acceptable drugs of this type. By the same manipulations shown in preceding examples, it was possible to prolong duration

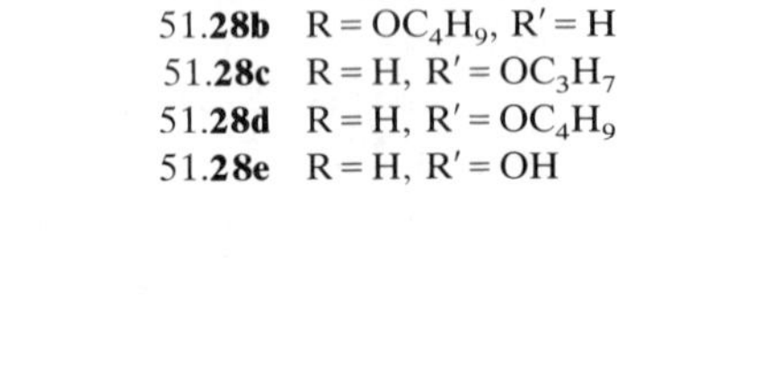

R   R'
$$NH_2 - \text{[benzene ring]} - CO_2CH_2CH_2N(C_2H_5)_2$$

51.28a R = H, R' = Cl
51.28b R = OC_4H_9, R' = H
51.28c R = H, R' = OC_3H_7
51.28d R = H, R' = OC_4H_9
51.28e R = H, R' = OH

and to enhance both potency and topical anesthetic properties over those of procaine.

A compound that adds other variation in qualities is 2-diethylaminoethyl 4-amino-2-chlorobenzoate (chloroprocaine, 51.**28a**) (128), which is close to procaine in anesthetic properties but is probably one of the least toxic agents in use (129), a property that is due to its rapid biotransformation (130). However, it is less stable in solution than procaine. Benoxinate (2-diethylaminoethyl 4-amino-3-*n*-butoxybenzoate, 51.**28b**) (131, 132), 2-diethylaminoethyl 4-amino-2-propoxybenzoate (propoxycaine, 51.**28c**) (133–135), and 2-diethylaminoethyl 4-amino-2-*n*-butoxybenzoate (ambucaine, 51.**28d**) (133, 134) are three closely related compounds that have found applications in the clinic. Hydroxyprocaine (diethylaminoethyl 4-amino-2-hydroxybenzoate, 51.**28e**) (136, 137) is an agent that has been tested clinically and is of moderate activity (138), whereas its two tetracaine-like relatives, 2-dimethylaminoethyl 4-butylamino-2-hydroxybenzoate (51.**29a**) (137, 139), and its 2-diethylaminoethyl homolog (51.**29b**) (137, 139), possess longer duration of action.

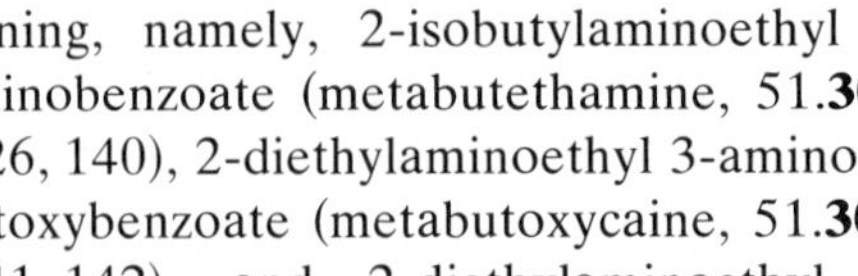

OH
$$C_4H_9NH - \text{[benzene ring]} - CO_2CH_2CH_2NR$$

51.29a R = (CH_3)_2
51.29b R = (C_2H_5)_2

Three 3-aminobenzoic esters merit mentioning, namely, 2-isobutylaminoethyl 3-aminobenzoate (metabutethamine, 51.**30a**) (126, 140), 2-diethylaminoethyl 3-amino-2-butoxybenzoate (metabutoxycaine, 51.**30b**) (141, 142), and 2-diethylaminoethyl 3-amino-4-propoxybenzoate (proparacaine, 51.**30c**) (133, 143). The former two are relatively short acting; proparacaine is more potent than cocaine but is also of considerable toxicity. Piridocaine [2-(2-piperidyl)-ethyl 2-aminobenzoate, 51.**31**] (144) seems

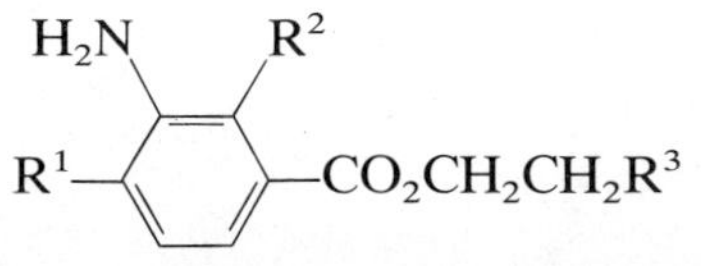

51.**30a** $R^1 = H$, $R^2 = H$, $R^3 = NHCH_2CH(CH_3)_2$
51.**30b** $R^1 = H$, $R^2 = OC_4H_9$, $R^3 = N(C_2H_5)_2$
51.**30c** $R^1 = OC_3H_7$, $R^2 = H$, $R^3 = N(C_2H_5)_2$

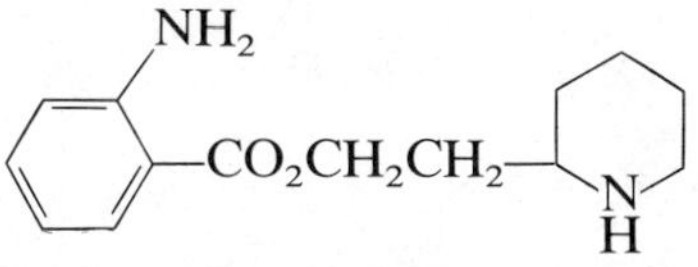

51.**31**

to be the only 2-aminobenzoic acid derivative that has passed preliminary pharmacological testing into the clinic (145).

The absence of an aromatic amino group
and the presence of a 4-substituted ether
moiety are the common features among the
following examples: parethoxycaine [2-
diethylaminoethyl 4-ethoxybenzoate, 4-
$C_2H_5OC_6H_4CO_2(CH_2)_2N(C_2H_5)_2$] (146–
148) and cyclomethycaine [3-(2-methyl-
piperidino)propyl 4-cyclohexyloxybenzo-
ate, 51.**32**] (149). Cyclomethycaine possess
the longest anesthetic effect of them and
enjoys a certain use as a topical agent (150).
The piperonylic acid derivative 2-diethyl-
aminoethyl 3,4-methylenedioxybenzoate
(51.**33**) (151, 152) was among the earlier
representatives of the whole group; however, it never found any particular practical
application.

The same is true of another example of
ring substitution, 2-diethylaminoethyl 4-

51.**32**

51.**33**

isopropylbenzoate [4-$(CH_3)_2CHC_6H_4CO_2$-
$(CH_2)_2N(C_2H_5)$] (153, 154), which failed
because of its irritating properties. The biphenyl derivative 2-diethylaminoethyl 2-
hydroxy-3-phenylbenzoate (biphenamine,
51.**34**) (155, 156) has found some use for
topical application.

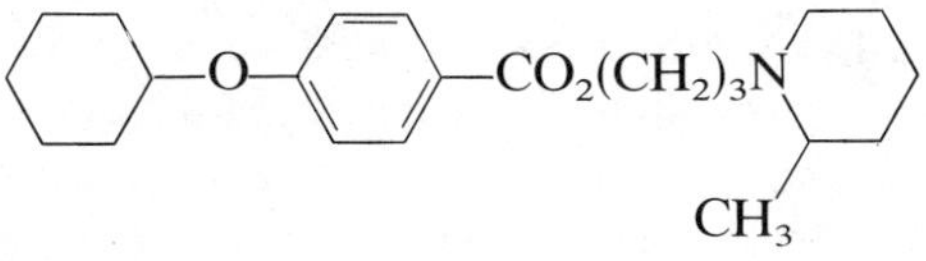

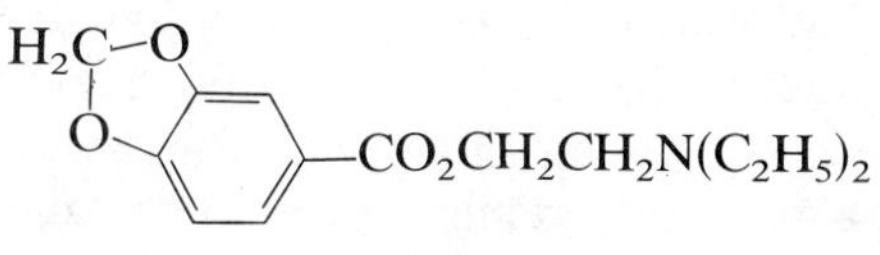

Of the compounds that are derived from
acids other than the benzoic acids, few have
achieved clinical use, although many have
been prepared and tested. The first American synthetic product, 3-diethylaminopro-
pyl cinnamate [$C_6H_5CH{=}CHCO_2(CH_2)_3$-
$N(C_2H_5)_2$] (157, 158), belongs to this
group; it achieved a certain use during
World War I (159) but soon fell by the
wayside for other, better tolerated drugs
(160, 161). Two naphthoic acid esters, 2-di-
ethylaminoethyl   4-amino-1-naphthoate

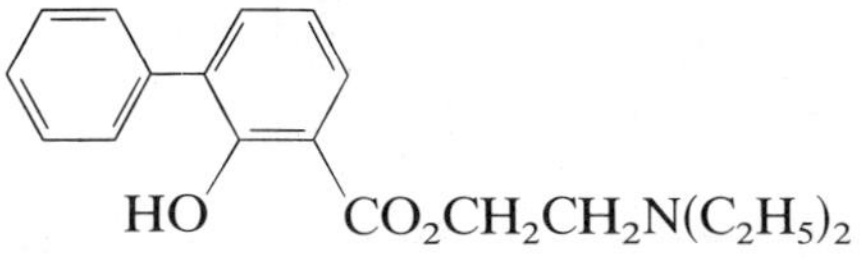

51.**34**

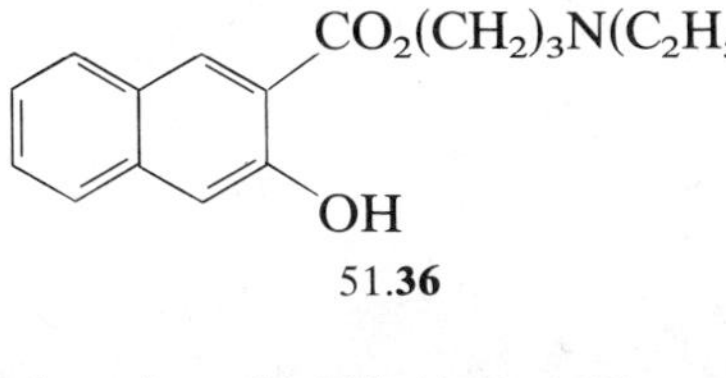

51.**35**

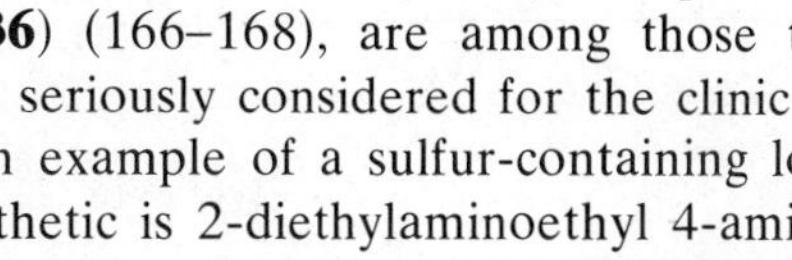

51.**36**

(naphthocaine, 51.**35**) (162–165) and 3-di-
ethylaminopropyl 3-hydroxy-2-naphthoate
(51.**36**) (166–168), are among those that
were seriously considered for the clinic.

An example of a sulfur-containing local
anesthetic is 2-diethylaminoethyl 4-amino-
thiobenzoate [thiocaine, 4-$NH_2C_6H_4COS$-
$(CH_2)_2N(C_2H_5)_2$] (169–171). Its claim to
acceptance, based on superior anesthetic

parameters, was denied because of a pronounced liability to cause irritation.

Introduction of various functional groups in the amino alcohol part seems to have met with little success. As a prospect for clinical recognition we may mention 3-diethylamino-2-hydroxypropyl 4-propyl-aminobenzoate [cornecaine, 4-$C_3H_7NHC_6$-$H_4CO_2CH_2CH(OH)CH_2N(C_2H_5)_2$] (172, 173).

The propensity for hydrolysis of many esters in aqueous solution causes a practical stability problem in the storage of their parenteral preparations, but successful attempts to overcome this stability problem have been made. Rabjohn et al. prepared esters of benzoic acids with 2,6 substitution, e.g., 51.**37** (174) and Honkanen synthesized, among others, the 2,6-dimethyl analog of procaine, 51.**38** (175). The durations were often improved by these substitutions, but for other reasons, e.g., local irritation, none of their compounds were acceptable as local anesthetics.

Fairly soon after the introduction of epinephrine as an adjunct to prolong the action of local anesthetic solutions (98, 99), the first attempt was made to combine the effects of the two agents into the same molecule. 2-Diethylamino-1-phenylpropyl benzoate (Allocaine-S, 51.**39**), (176, 177)

$$CH_3$$
$$C_6H_5CO_2CHCHN(C_2H_5)_2$$
$$C_6H_5$$
51.**39**

51.**40**

$$C_6H_5CO_2CHCH_2N(CH_3)_2$$
$$C_6H_5$$
51.**41**

was reported to possess both properties. Because of side effects, however, it did not offer any improvement over procaine solutions containing epinephrine and was soon dropped from consideration. It shared this fate with later compounds that were designed with the same goal in mind—for instance, epicaine [2-diethylaminoethyl 4-(3,4-dihydroxyphenacylamino)benzoate, (51.**40**)] (178, 179) and a close relative of 51.**39**, 2-dimethylamino-1-phenethyl benzoate (locaine, 51.**41**) (180–182).

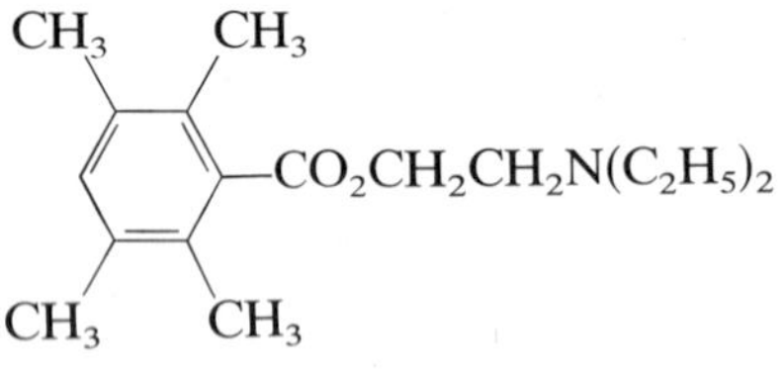

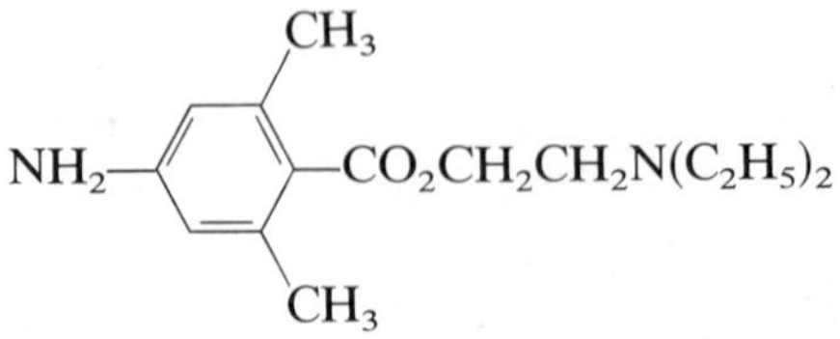

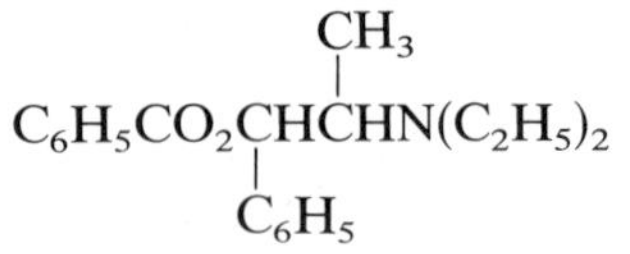

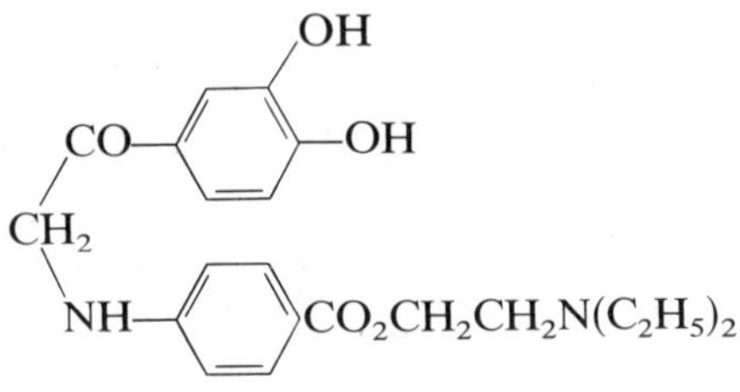

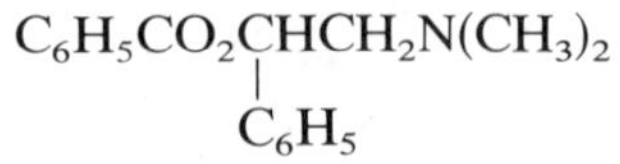

3.5.2 AMINOACYLANILIDES. Einhorn and Oppenheimer reported the synthesis of the first acylanilide possessing local anesthetic properties in 1900. The compound, 2-diethylamino-4'-hydroxy-3'-methoxycarbonylacetanilide (nirvanine, 51.**42**) (183), was too irritating to become a substitute for cocaine and this line of synthesis was not pursued further by these researchers.

The renewed interest in acylanilides in the 1930s was not based on nirvanine but had its beginning in a chemical study of the structure of gramine [3-(dimethylaminomethyl)indole, 51.**43**] (184) to determine

51.**37**

51.**38**

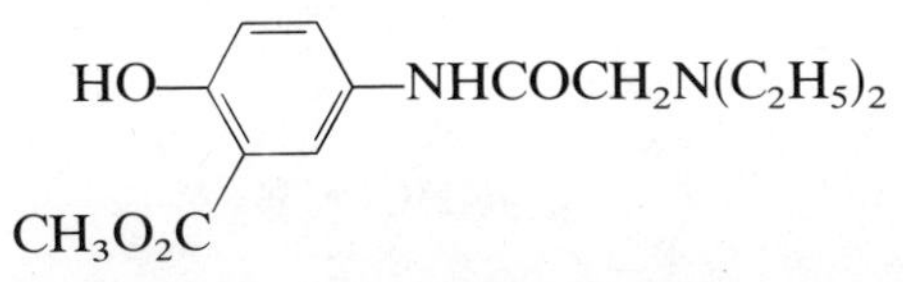

HO—⟨benzene ring⟩—NHCOCH$_2$N(C$_2$H$_5$)$_2$

CH$_3$O$_2$C

51.**42**

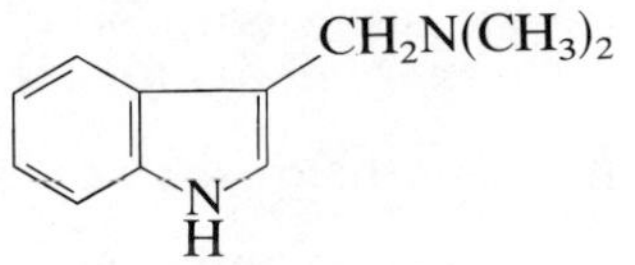

⟨indole ring⟩—CH$_2$N(CH$_3$)$_2$

N
H

51.**43**

CH$_3$

⟨benzene ring⟩—NHCOCH$_2$N(CH$_3$)$_2$

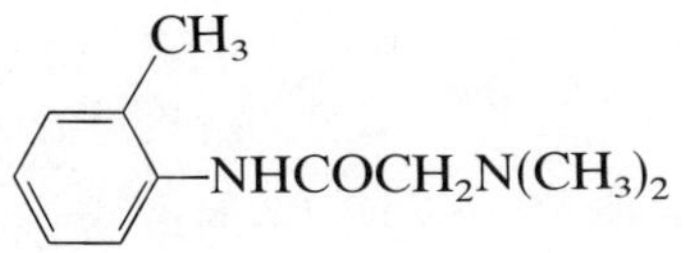

51.**44**

the position of the side chain. The 2-dimethylaminomethyl derivative as well as the intermediate in its synthesis, 2-dimethylamino-2′-acetotoluidide (51.**44**), turned out to produce the typical local anesthetic response when tested on the tongue.

A series of related compounds was prepared by Erdtman and Löfgren (185). Intrigued by the results, Löfgren continued his studies of this class of compounds and arrived after further syntheses of 30 compounds at lidocaine (2-diethylamino-2′,6′-acetoxylidide (Fig. 51.8, 51.**45**) (186, 187).

With the synthesis of lidocaine, two objectives on the road to a better all-around local anesthetic were reached. The new drug is far more stable in solution, a particular advantage for heat sterilization, and it is also more potent and faster in onset (188).

The stability of lidocaine to hydrolysis is striking in comparison with several of the ester compounds. Thus a lidocaine solution can be heated with 50% sulfuric acid or with 20% ethanolic potassium hydroxide for 5 hr without causing more than 3 and 0.5% decomposition, respectively (189). This property is explained by the presence of two methyl groups ortho to the amide group that stabilize the amide bond, perhaps by steric as well as electronic effects. An illustration of the influence of the two ortho methyl groups in this respect is obtained by comparing the pseudo rate constants for the hydrolysis of lidocaine with those of its o-toluidine and aniline analogs (190). They are in the ratio 1:36:112, which shows that one o-methyl group gives some added stability to the amide bond, whereas the introduction of the second o-methyl group adds remarkable protection to the bond against hydrolysis.

Even if lidocaine's toxicity is somewhat higher than that of procaine, the drug is

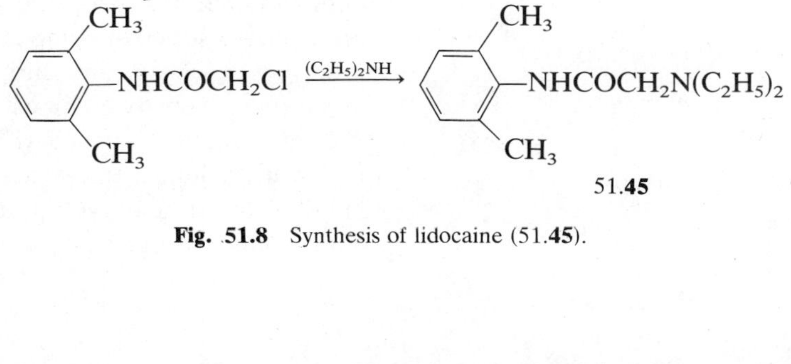

CH$_3$

⟨benzene ring⟩—NH$_2$ + ClCOCH$_2$Cl

CH$_3$

CH$_3$

⟨benzene ring⟩—NHCOCH$_2$Cl $\xrightarrow{(C_2H_5)_2NH}$ ⟨benzene ring⟩—NHCOCH$_2$N(C$_2$H$_5$)$_2$

CH$_3$ CH$_3$ CH$_3$

51.**45**

Fig. 51.8 Synthesis of lidocaine (51.**45**).

nonetheless relatively nontoxic in comparison with most other local anesthetics. Furthermore, it is well tolerated by the tissues. The favorable properties of lidocaine had as a consequence the increased use of local anesthetics in surgery, and many procedures are now performed with certain forms of local, rather than general, anesthesia (191). Examples are the currently widespread use of epidural (peridural) and other major nerve-block procedures (192, 193).

The simplest route to lidocaine and its derivatives is presented in Fig. 51.8.

The success of lidocaine started a surge of investigations of anilide derivatives. At the same time Löfgren prepared the analog trimecaine (2-diethylaminoacetomesidide, 51.**46**) (186, 194), which has become one of the more commonly used agents in eastern Europe (101), and somewhat later prilocaine (2-propylamino-2'-propionotoluidide, 51.**47a**) (195, 196).

Examples of other members of this class that have found clinical application are 2-diethylamino-2'-ethyl-6'-methylacetanilide (51.**48a**) (197, 198); 2-butylamino-6'-chloro-2'-acetotoluidide (butanilicaine, 51.**48b**) (199, 200); 2-(1-pyrrolidino)-2',6'-acetoxylidide (pyrrocaine, 51.**48c**) (201–203); 2-diethylamino-2'-methoxycarbonyl-6-methylacetanilide (tolycaine, 51.**48d**)

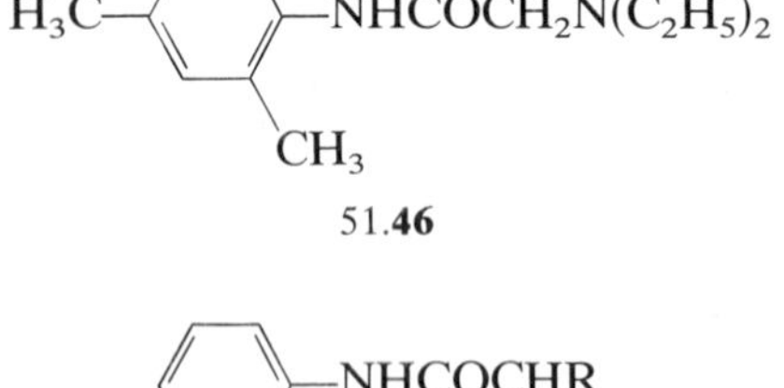

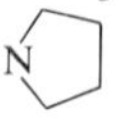

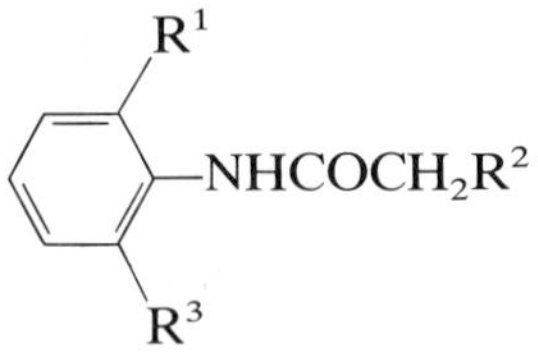

51.**48a** $R^1 = CH_3$, $R^2 = N(C_2H_5)_2$, $R^3 = C_2H_5$
51.**48b** $R^1 = Cl$, $R^2 = NHC_4H_9$, $R^3 = CH_3$
51.**48c** $R^1 = R^3 = CH_3$, $R^2 = N$
51.**48d** $R^1 = CH_3$, $R^2 = N(C_2H_5)_2$, $R^3 = CO_2CH_3$

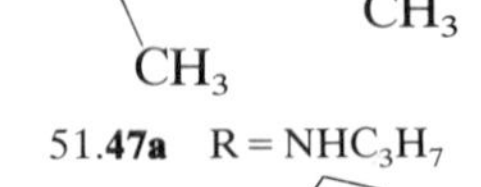

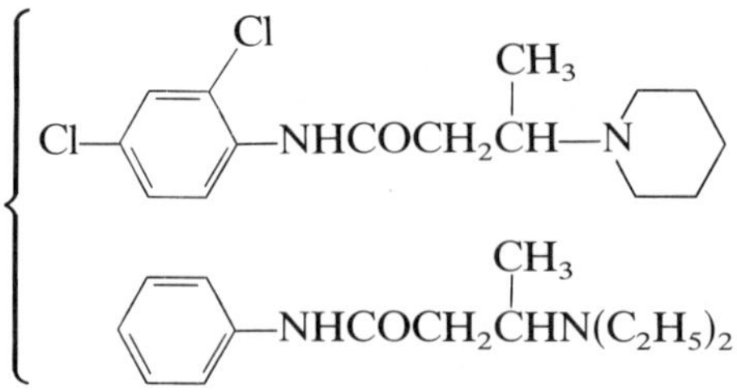

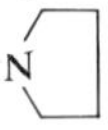

51.**49**

(204, 205); and a mixture of 3-diethylaminobutyranilide and 3-piperidino-2',4'-dichlorobutyranilide (51.**49**) (206, 207).

Two modifications of prilocaine (51.**47a**) that are said not to cause methemoglobinemia are 2-methyl-2-propylamino-2'-propionotoluidide (quatacaine, 51.**50**) (208) and 2-(1-pyrrolidino)-2'-propionotoluidide (aptocaine, 51.**47b**) (209).

The need for longer durations of anesthesia prompted the exploration of acylanilides of increased molecular weight. One of the lidocaine homologs from these efforts, 2-(N-ethylpropylamino)-2',6'-butyroxylidide, (etidocaine, 51.**51**) (210) has recently been introduced.

By making the amine function part of a ring system—that is, by joining one of the aminoalkyl groups with the intermediate acyl chain—a series of compounds was prepared by af Ekenstam and co-workers; among these were two clinically acceptable local anesthetics, 1-methyl-2',6'-hexahydropicolinylxylidide (mepivacaine, 51.**52a**) (211–213) and 1-butyl-2',6'-hexahydropicolinylxylidide (bupivacaine, 51.**52b**) (211,

51.**46**

51.**47a** $R = NHC_3H_7$
51.**47b** $R = N$

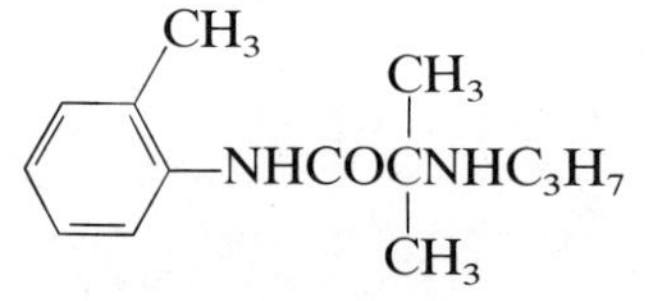

CH$_3$

NHCOCNHC$_3$H$_7$

CH$_3$ / CH$_3$

51.**50**

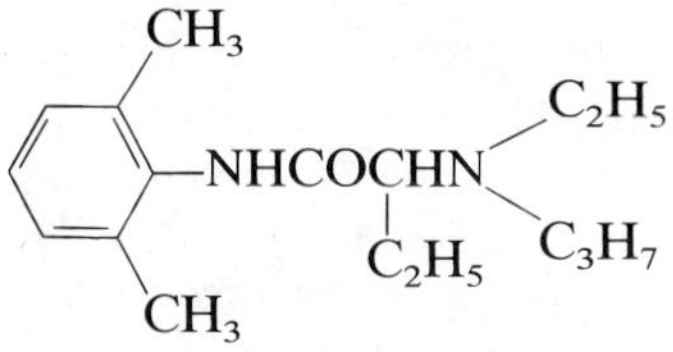

CH$_3$

NHCOCHN—C$_2$H$_5$ / C$_2$H$_5$ / C$_3$H$_7$

CH$_3$

51.**51**

CH$_3$

R / N

NHCO—

CH$_3$

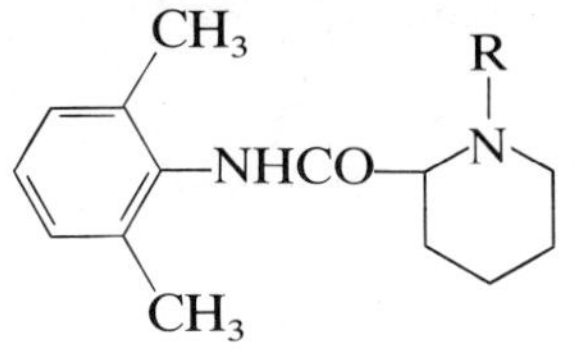

51.**52a**   R = CH$_3$
51.**52b**   R = C$_4$H$_9$

214). Mepivacaine possesses clinical properties of the lidocaine type, whereas bupivacaine is characterized by longer duration but also higher general toxicity and liability to cause irritation. Bupivacaine has been proved a valuable addition to the clinically useful agents when long anesthesia is desired, particularly in major nerve blocks. Curiously, mepivacaine seems to be much less active than lidocaine as a surface anesthetic.

A recent addition to the agents of this type, of even higher molecular weight than bupivacaine, is *trans*-2'-chloro-6'-methyl-3-(octahydro-1*H*-1-pyrindino) propionanilide (rodocaine, 51.**53**) (215). It is a more

Cl

CH$_2$CH$_2$CONH—

H / N

CH$_3$

H

51.**53**

potent agent than lidocaine (51.**45**) in the rat, and produces longer blocks, but is in addition more toxic.

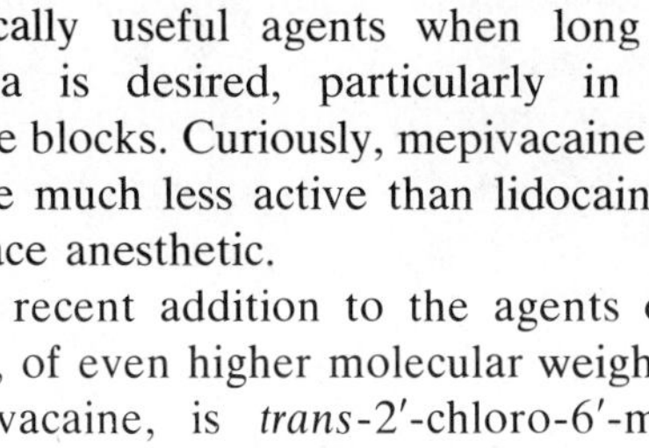

N—OC$_4$H$_9$

CONHCH$_2$CH$_2$N(C$_2$H$_5$)$_2$

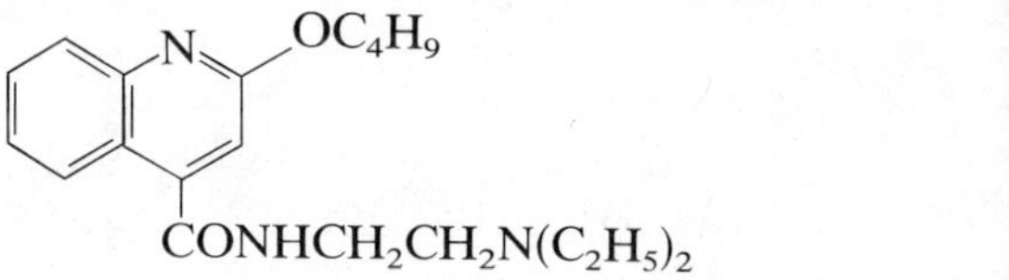

51.**54**

3.5.3 NON-ANILIDE AMIDES. An unexpected effect in a series of compounds prepared for one purpose may lead to a product in a different area. This is illustrated by the development of the earliest member of this type of compound—the very potent local anesthetic 2-butoxy-*N*-(2-diethylaminoethyl)cinchoninamide (dibucaine, 51.**54**) was prepared by Miescher (216) in a synthetic program directed toward antipyretics. The toxicity of dibucaine is considerable, yet it is used because of its extraordinary potency, which permits use at low concentrations (217). The type of amide arrangement that is present in dibucaine can be characterized as the opposite of the anilide type; both types of amide bond obviously can be useful in local anesthetic structures. Reversing this bond in dibucaine as well as in lidocaine, however, results in compounds whose pharmacological properties are inferior to those of their useful structural isomers.

The most potent local anesthetic that has found clinical use is 2,2'-(2-hydroxyethylamino)-bis[*N*-(1,1-dimethyl-2-phenethyl)-*N*-methylacetamide] (oxethazaine, 51.**55**) (218). The type of compound to which it belongs was found among by-products in reactions designed to obtain the monomeric amines. For some time it was thought that these were the active anesthetics, until it was realized eventually that the bis compounds in the mixture carried the observed potent local anesthetic effect. Oxethazaine is approximately 2000 times more potent than lidocaine on the rabbit cornea but it

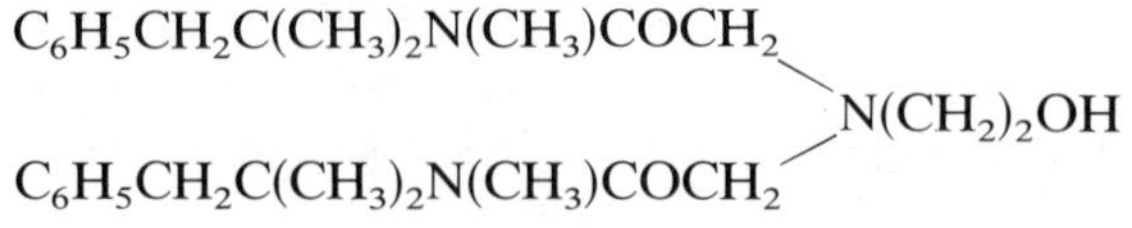

$$C_6H_5CH_2C(CH_3)_2N(CH_3)COCH_2$$
$$N(CH_2)_2OH$$
$$C_6H_5CH_2C(CH_3)_2N(CH_3)COCH_2$$

51.**55**

has a high systemic toxicity and a long onset time (219, 220); it has been used in certain gastrointestinal conditions.

3.5.4 AMINOCARBAMATES. At the time of the synthesis of dibucaine (51.**54**) incorporation of the carbamate group into a molecule was achieved, yielding a clinically acceptable local anesthetic. It was already known that, for example, phenylurethane ($C_6H_5NHCO_2C_2H_5$) exerts effects on isolated systems similar to those observed with local anesthetics (221). A useful dicarbamate, 3-piperidinopropylene dicarbanilate, diperodon (51.**56**), was now realized (222–224). Shortly thereafter a second carbamate, 9-(2-diethylaminoethoxycarbonyl)-carbazole (51.**57**) (225, 226), was found to possess satisfying properties; it was not clinically accepted, however. A more complex molecule that shared the same fate was 1,3-bis[4-(2-diethylamino-ethoxy-carbonyl)phenylcarbamoyloxy]propane (tridiurecaine, 51.**58**) (227, 228), which contains two procaine molecules joined at the 4-amino nitrogens via carbamate groups to a propyl chain.

In general, the carbamates share the stability problems of the esters. Stability can be improved by introducing protecting groups in the vicinity of the carbamate group as in 1-butyl-3-piperidyl 2′-chloro-6′-methylcarbanilate, 51.**59** (229), a compound that is similar to bupivacaine, 51.**52b**, although its action is somewhat shorter in duration.

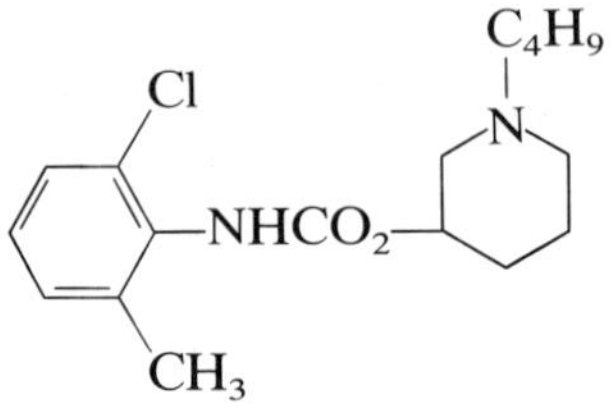

51.**59**

3.5.5 AMINOETHERS. Two compounds that have been introduced contain an ether link instead of the ester or amide groups of previously described agents: 3-butyl-1-(2-dimethylaminoethoxy)isoquinoline, dimethisoquin, 51.**60**) (230) and 4-[3-(4-butoxyphenoxy)propyl]-morpholine(pramoxine, 51.**61**) (231, 232). In a general way their

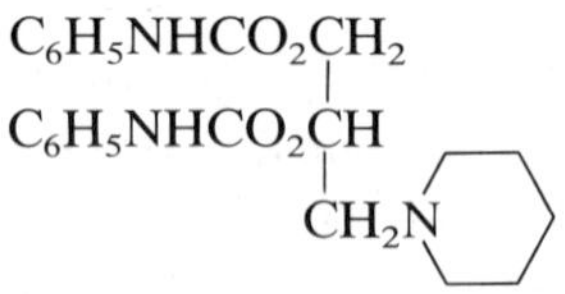

$$C_6H_5NHCO_2CH_2$$
$$C_6H_5NHCO_2CH$$
$$CH_2N$$

51.**56**

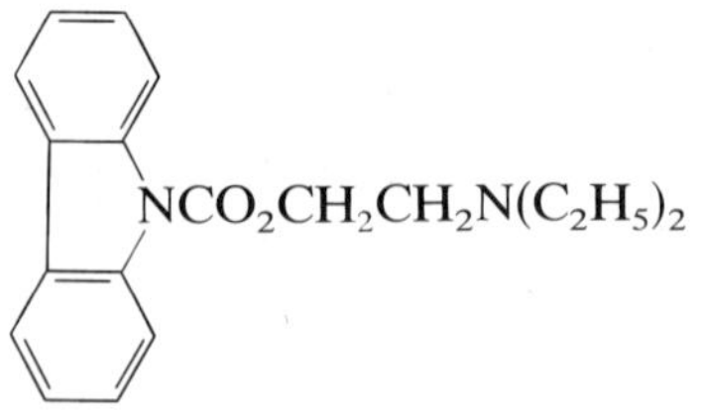

$$NCO_2CH_2CH_2N(C_2H_5)_2$$

51.**57**

$$CH_2O_2CNH\!-\!\langle\ \rangle\!-\!CO_2(CH_2)_2N(C_2H_5)_2$$
$$CH_2$$
$$CH_2O_2CNH\!-\!\langle\ \rangle\!-\!CO_2(CH_2)_2N(C_2H_5)_2$$

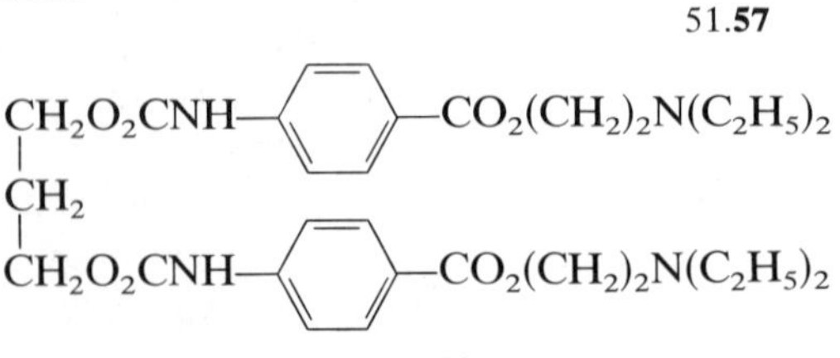

51.**58**

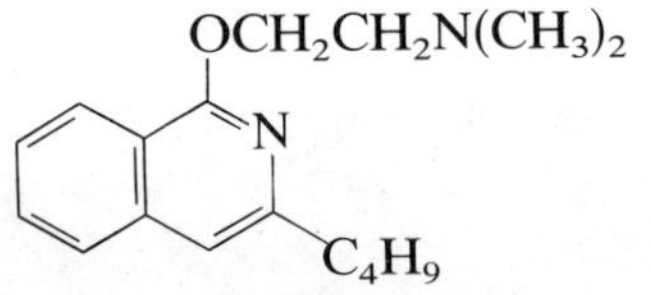

51.**60**

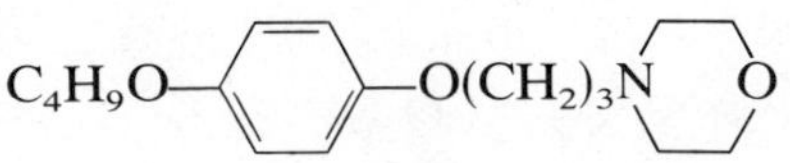

51.**61**

structures resemble dibucaine (51.**54**) and the procaine- or lidocaine-type agents, respectively. Dimethisoquin produces local anesthesia of considerable duration both in surface (corneal) and infiltration test methods in animals; this is accompanied by increased toxicity (233). From animal experiments it seems to be more potent and somewhat less generally toxic than dibucaine. Both dimethisoquin and pramoxine are recommended only for topical use.

Another compound, {4-[3-(4-morpholino)propyl]benzyloxy}benzene (fomocaine, 51.**62**) (234), bears some structural likeness to pramoxine. It produces topical anesthesia of the cornea similar to tetracaine (51.**24**) and is reported to be rather nontoxic, systemically as well as locally.

An aminoether of different and more complex structure is 1-(2-anilinoethyl)-4-[2-(diethylamino)ethoxy]- 4 -phenylpiperidine (diamocaine, 51.**63**) (235). This agent appears to be equipotent to tetracaine in conduction anesthesia in the rat but is less toxic.

Another agent belonging to this class is o-[2-(diisopropylamino)ethoxy]butyrophenone (ketocaine, 51.**64**) (236), a potent topical anesthetic that can be used on intact skin effectively if incorporated into a suitable vehicle (237–239) (see also Section 5.2.3). Also of more recent date is 1-(2-methylphenoxy) -3-(2,2,5,5-tetramethyl- 1 -pyrrolidino)-2-propanol (lotucaine, tolcaine, 51.**65**) (240, 241). It is more potent than lidocaine as an infiltration and topical agent.

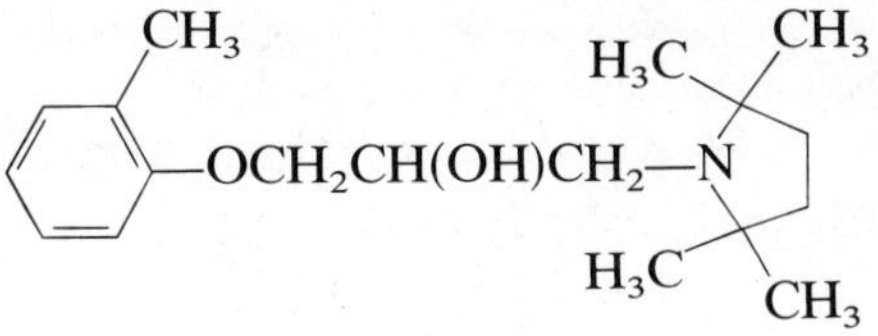

51.**65**

3.5.6 AMINOKETONES. Falicain (3-piperidino-4'-propoxypropiophenone, 51.**66a**) (242–244) and dyclonine (3-piperidino-4'-butoxypropiophenone, 51.**66b**) (243–245), are the two representatives of this type that

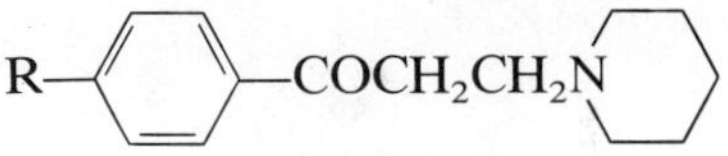

51.**66a**   R = OC_3H_7
51.**66b**   R = OC_4H_9

have found some clinical use. Because of tissue irritation dyclonine is used topically only. The same irritation liability is characteristic of falicain; nonetheless this agent has been used as a parenteral drug in eastern and central Europe.

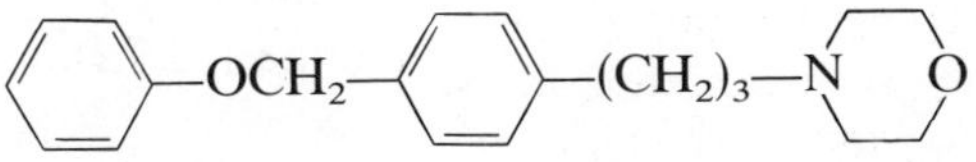

51.**62**

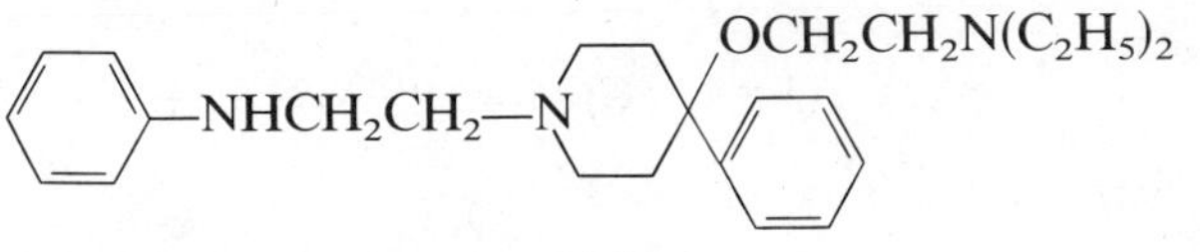

51.**63**

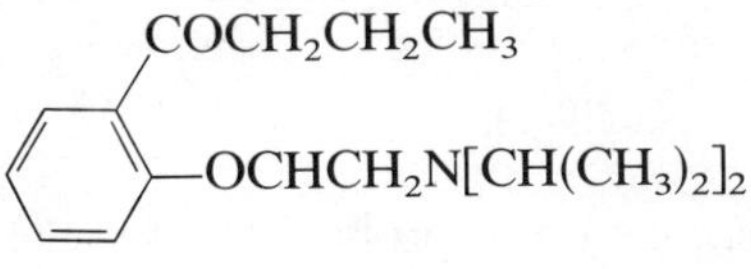

51.**64**

3.5.7 AMIDINES AND GUANIDINES. A departure from cocaine as a guide in search of new synthetic local anesthetics took place when Täuber (246) and Gutmann (247) described the anesthetic properties of N,N'-bis(4-ethoxyphenyl)acetamidine (phenacaine, 51.**67**), an agent still in use in ophthalmology. This structure led later to similar guanidine derivatives, one of which, N^1,N^3-bis(4-methoxyphenyl)-N^2-(4-ethoxyphenyl)guanidine (acoin-C, 51.**68**) (248, 249), found some limited use about the turn of the century.

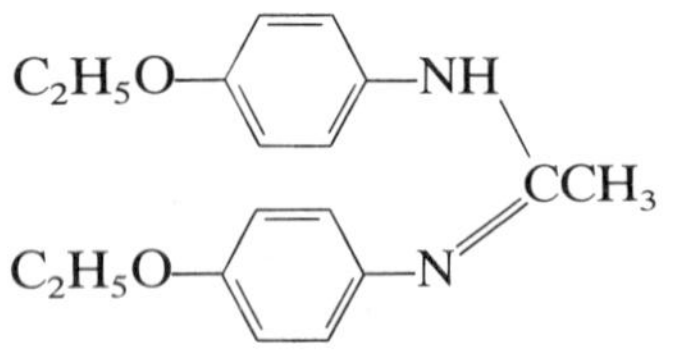

51.**67**

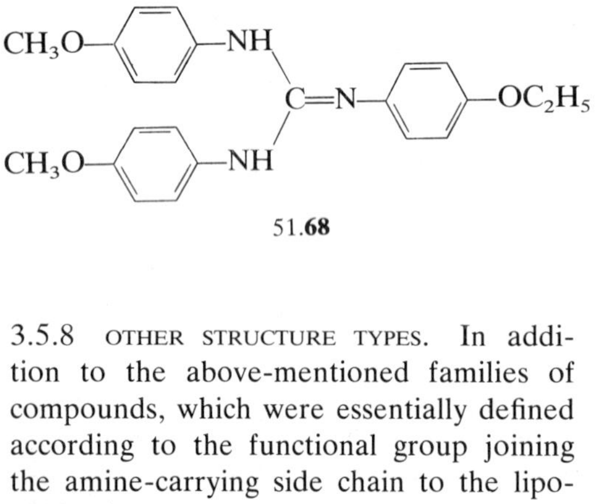

51.**68**

3.5.8 OTHER STRUCTURE TYPES. In addition to the above-mentioned families of compounds, which were essentially defined according to the functional group joining the amine-carrying side chain to the lipophilic (most often aromatic part of the molecule), there are many other types of amines that possess blocking properties.

Monofunctional amines are perhaps the most fundamental type, as exemplified by 6-methyl-2-heptylamine, $(CH_3)_2(CH_2)_4$-$CH(CH_3)NH_2$ (octodrine, 51.**69**) (249a), a fairly strong base [$pK_a = 10.3$ (249b)], that differs from agents discussed previously in being a primary aliphatic amine. It produces topical anesthesia on the rabbit cornea but is probably better classified as a

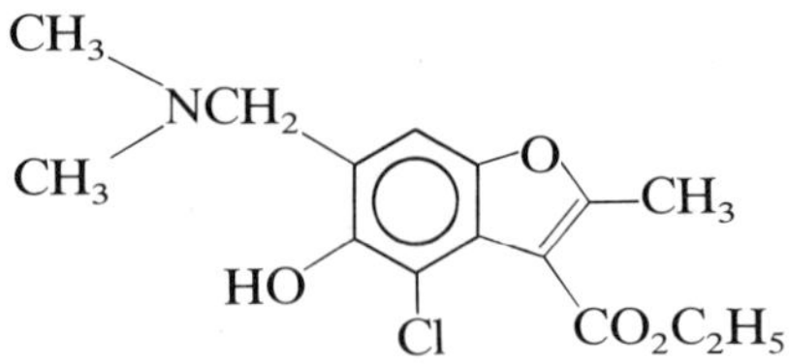

51.**70**

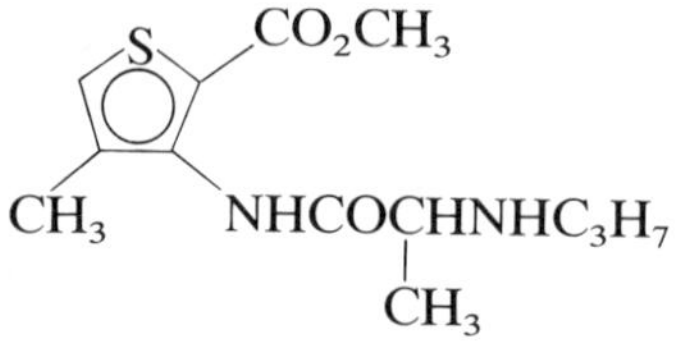

51.**71**

sympathomimetic drug than as a local anesthetic.

The benzofuran derivative furocaine (51.**70**) has been proposed as a local anesthetic agent (249c), as has also the amide-type agent 2-methoxycarbonyl-4-methyl-3-(2-propylaminopropionylamino)thiophene (carticaine, 51.**71**) (249d), which possesses lidocaine-like properties in isolated nerve preparations.

As is the case with octodrine (51.**69**), local anesthetic properties are often found in agents that demonstrate their characteristic and clinically useful properties in other pharmacological fields; this includes sympatholytics, spasmolytics, sympathomimetics, antiarrhythmics, and analgetics (101). In some cases, the local anesthetic component in the pharmacodynamic spectrum of a drug can be rather pronounced—for instance, in chlorpromazine and in antihistaminics such as diphenhydramine or zolamine (51.**72**).

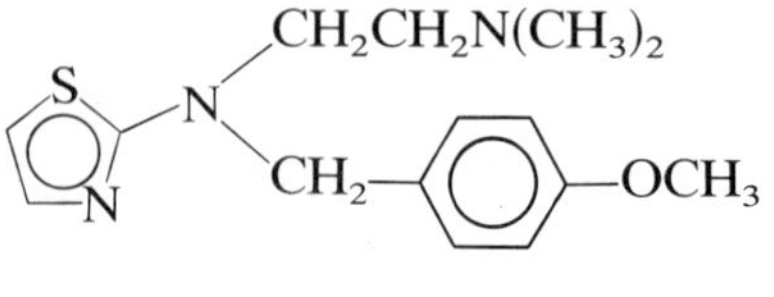

51.**72**

3.6 "Neutral" Agents

Blocking agents that are essentially un-charged (un-ionized) at physiological pH (See Section 3.1) are often labeled *neutral* in the local anesthetic literature. This group includes certain weakly basic amines, some weak acids, and a number of alcohols, ethers, and carbamates, that do not possess an amine function. Because of the poor aqueous solubility of many of these compounds they cannot, with few exceptions, be used effectively except in topical preparations.

However, in basic research on nerve function as well as in studies of mechanisms of action of local anesthetics, many of these agents have been and are important pharmacological tools. This is made possible by the low concentration levels that are effective in work on isolated and especially desheathed nerve preparations.

3.6.1 WEAKLY BASIC AMINES. Reasoning from the anesthetic properties of some aromatic compounds and the requirement that benzoyloxy and carbomethoxy groups be present to give local anesthetic effects to the tropane portion of cocaine, Einhorn and Heinz (249e) prepared the ester 51.**73**, which, however, was only slightly effective on the cornea. They expected to find a complete disappearance of the anesthetic properties when they tested the unbenzoylated parent compound, analogous to the lack of activity of methylecgonine (51.**74**), the debenzoylated cocaine. They were surprised to find that their debenzoylated compound was more potent than the more complex derivative 51.**73**. As a result of this observation two surface anesthetics, namely, the methyl ester of 4-amino-3-hydroxybenzoic acid (Orthoform Old, 51.**75a**) and orthocaine (Orthoform New, methyl-3 amino-4-hydroxybenzoate, 51.**75b**) were introduced (249f, 249g).

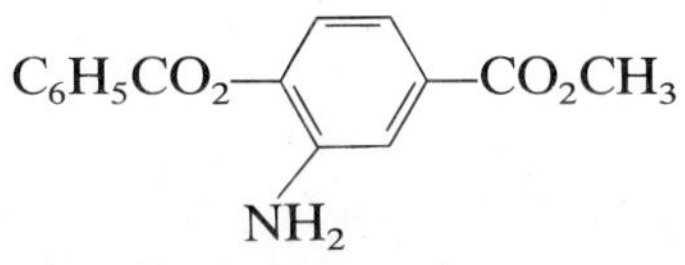

A sequence of events similar to the development of 51.**75a**, **b**, although directed

51.**73**

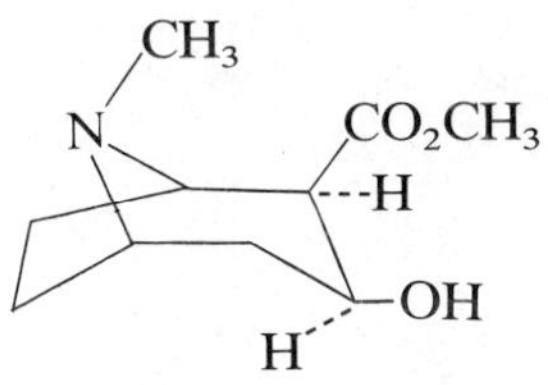

51.**74**

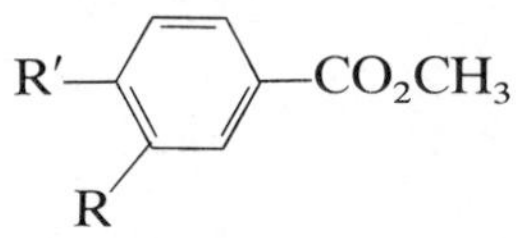

51.**75a**   R = OH, R' = NH₂
51.**75b**   R = NH₂, R' = OH

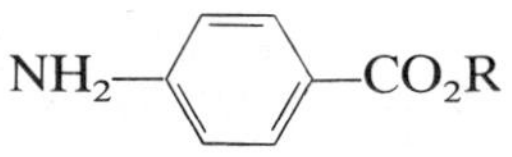

51.**76a**   R = C₂H₅
51.**76b**   R = C₄H₉

toward goals in another field, led Ritsert in 1890 to the identification of ethyl 4-amino-benzoate (benzocaine, 51.**76a**) (249h, 249i), a sparingly water-soluble local anesthetic. However, at the time the hope was to find an improvement over cocaine usable by the same techniques of administration. Therefore, this compound was put aside for more than 10 years before it reached the clinic (249j, 250); a synthesis of benzocaine in the meantime (251) was not accompanied by recognition of its medicinal effects.

Like 51.**75a**, **b**, benzocaine is not suitable as an injectable local anesthetic because of its very weakly basic properties. Efforts to provide a suitable salt that would make it more soluble at pH values tolerated by tissue understandably failed. But it is indeed a useful surface anesthetic, still widely used, and the parent compound of several

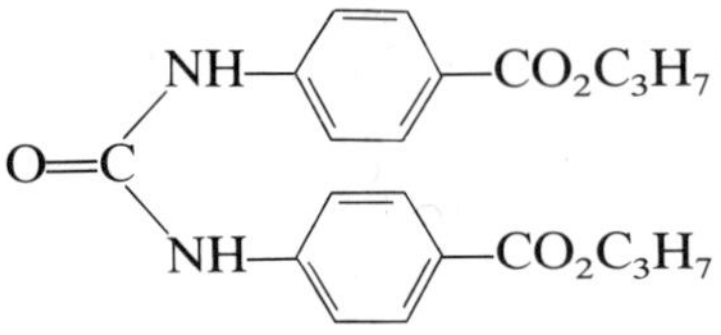

51.**77**

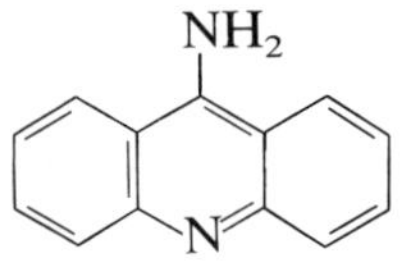

51.**78**

other higher alkyl 4-aminobenzoates that have found similar use (e.g., 51.**75b**) (252).

An attempt to improve on this type of structure by joining two molecules to each other with a bridge via their 4-amino groups resulted in dipropäsin (51.**77**), formally a urea derivative (253). It is very insoluble and was introduced for anesthesia of the intestinal tract; however, it met with only limited recognition.

Certain simpler weak amines possess nerve blocking activity although they are not clinically useful; this group includes many aromatic amines, e.g., 2,6-xylidine [2,6-$(CH_3)_2C_6H_3NH_2$]. The pronounced blocking effects of strong aromatic amines such as 4-aminopyridine [$pK_a^{25°} = 9.11$ (254)], which blocks potassium channels exclusively (255), or 9-aminoacridine (51.**78**) [$pK_a^{20°} = 9.99$ (256)], a blocker of sodium as well as potassium (257), indicate that weakness of the aromatic base is not a criterion for interaction with the ionic-conducting channels of the membrane (also octodrine, 51.**69**, Section 3.5.8).

3.6.2 NON-AMINE AGENTS. Fairly successful clinical attempts to produce local anesthesia were the topical application of phenol in olive oil to burns and wounds (258) and the use of 80–85% phenol solution on the intact skin over an area of intended incision (259, 260). Related to phenol was the early use of guaiacol (261) and eugenol in dentistry. The observation

that 1,1-dimethyl-2,2,2-trichloroethanol [chlorobutanol, $Cl_3CC(CH_3)_2OH$] could be used in the same manner was also made during the last century (262). About 1920 the local anesthetic properties of benzyl alcohol ($C_6H_5CH_2OH$) and its relatives were established (263–265). Of more recent date is the introduction of certain polyglycol ethers [e.g., thesit, $C_{12}H_{25}(OCH_2CH_2)_9OH$], which have found limited use in Europe in topical preparations (266). Characteristic of all these agents is a fairly high degree of tissue irritation.

Some kavakava constituents, such as pyrones (e.g., dihydrokavain, 51.**79**) (267, 268), have been identified as compounds with some intradermal local anesthetic effect.

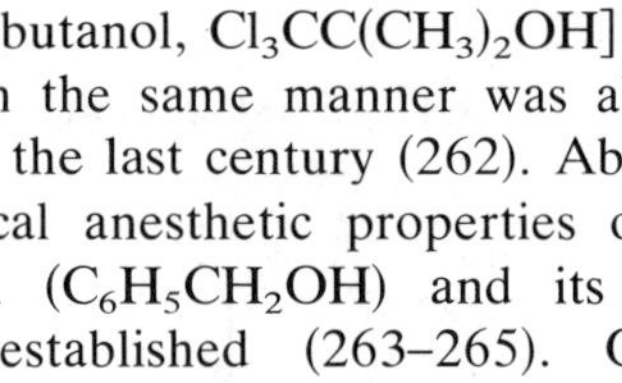

51.**79**

Many other compounds of this type have been used to produce conduction block, especially in basic neurophysiological and neuropharmacological research. Lower aliphatic alcohols, e.g,, ethanol and butanol, barbituric acids, ethylurethane, and many simple aromatic amides, such as N,N-diethyl-2-methylbenzamide, interfere with normal sodium channel function. It should also be noted that high concentrations of ethanol and phenol are used clinically to cause irreversible blocks of nerves (nerve destruction) in certain cases of intractable pain; in sufficiently low concentrations, however, both these agents produce fully reversible blocks.

4 MECHANISMS OF ACTION AT THE MEMBRANE LEVEL

In spite of great advances that have been made in recent years, our understanding of how blocking agents act is far from complete. This seems to be particularly true for the chemical structure types among which the clinically useful local anesthetics are found.

4.1   Depolarizing Agents

Blockers of nerve conduction are divided into three groups in Section 3.1. The first contains the agents that cause depolarization of the nerve membrane and thereby block the propagation of impulses along the nerve. The most potent agents acting in this manner are rather large and bulky molecules (51.**1**–51.**3**). It is therefore unlikely that the effect is caused by their presence inside the sodium channel where they would interfere with the fast passage of ions. Since they must interfere with the closing of the gates of the channel, near the axoplasmic surface of the membrane, it is likely that they find their important reaction sites close to this interior surface. That they act faster when applied from the inside of the membrane than from the outside supports this conclusion (23). Therefore, they apparently act on the channel protein from within the membrane rather than from within the sodium channel and at such a part of the protein that the conformational changes necessary for a closing of the "gate" under electric field changes across the membrane are effectively inhibited; i.e., they act relatively close to the inner membrane surface.

4.2   Tetrodotoxin and Saxitoxin

There has now accumulated much solid evidence for the identification of the site of action for the second group, e.g., the two marine toxins tetrodotoxin (TTX) (51.**4**) and saxitoxin (STX) (51.**5**), which block sodium ion flux. The work of Hille (16, 269) and others leaves no doubt that TTX and STX act at the same site (55, 270): fairly close to the outer surface of the membrane, possibly at a constricted portion (the selectivity filter) of the sodium channel, and certainly not deeper inside the membrane than that. It has also been made quite clear that a strong negative charge at or close to this constriction, probably a carboxylate group, is involved in the binding of the toxins (269, 56). In addition, it is most likely that the spatial organization of other binding centers of the channel protein are so organized in the vicinity of the constriction that they allow binding to the 4-hydroxyl group of TTX and the hydrated carbonyl groups of the STX molecule.

The entrance portion of the channel is probably so organized that it facilitates transfer of entering sodium ions down the channel by accomplishing smooth loss of several water molecules of the fully hydrated sodium ion and facile substitution of the sodium–water bonds of the hydrated ion for similar bonds to suitably situated polar groups on the protein structure of the inside channel wall (cf. Refs. 271, 272). Therefore, essentially lipophilic compounds cannot easily reach the biotoxin receptor by passage through the channel, whereas TTX and STX, with the assistance of their hydrophilic groups, can move down the channel toward the selectivity filter. A true receptor for the biotoxins thus exists at this end of the channel, which can be seen as a critical receptor for partially dehydrated sodium ions also. Pharmacologically, the biotoxins can, in a sense, be looked upon as antagonists to a partly dehydrated sodium ion, possibly $[Na(H_2O)]^+$ or $[Na(H_2O)_2]^+$. The steps leading to the understanding of the concepts outlined above are presented in several articles (16, 56, 269–274), and additional experimental evidence can also be obtained from other critical studies (275, 276).

4.3   Quaternary Ammonium Compounds

Absolutely convincing evidence for the mechanism of action for the remaining types of blocking agents is available only for the quaternary derivatives of local anesthetics and some other quaternary ammonium compounds.

It can be stated that the quaternary blocking agents, which in general penetrate the membrane with great difficulty must, in order to exert their effect, first reach the axoplasm and then move into the sodium channel through its interior opening (277, 17). Furthermore, the channel must be in the open state for them to block. When the channel is inactivated or closed, these agents cannot pass into the interior regions of the channel. Conversely, the quaternary ions cannot easily escape from the channel unless it is in the open state.

The significant observation that the channels have to be in the open state for block to occur was made by Strichartz (17) while studying the blocking properties of the quaternary ammonium derivatives of lidocaine (51.**6**, 51.**10**) under voltage clamp conditions. Applying the agent from the axoplasmic side of the membrane, he found that the block obtained after one depolarizing pulse was significantly enhanced as more pulses were applied, eventually reaching an equilibration when a sufficient number of pulses had been given. Since these pulses normally open the channels, one can infer that the use of the channels enhances the block. The phenomenon that has been called use dependence or frequency dependence is not unique to the quaternaries but has been observed for a variety of tertiary and secondary amine anesthetics (see below). It is, however, not a property of TTX and STX, which is in agreement with their quite different site and mechanism of action (18, 278).

It may be necessary to point out that not all quaternary ammonium compounds block the sodium channel. It is well-known that certain tetraalkylammonium ions, e.g., tetraethylammonium (TEA), do not block the sodium channels of nerve membranes but do block the potassium channels selectively, a property that has been utilized in order to facilitate the study of the electric phenomena of the membrane; by adding TEA to the test solutions applied to the nerve, the investigator can separate the sodium currents and study them independently. Armstrong (10) found that, among the tetraalkylammonium ions, the maximal blocking effect on potassium channels was obtained with the nonyltriethyl ammonium ion. Quaternized local anesthetic molecules, as well as the corresponding tertiary and secondary amines, do block both channels, but there is a variability in the ratio of preference to the two channel types.

4.4 Local Anesthetics Proper—Amines and "Neutral" Agents

For the remainder of the blocking agents and thus for all clinically used local anesthetics, there does not yet exist a theory that has been universally accepted. Presently, the mode of action of local anesthetics has been interpreted in terms of at least three hypotheses, supported by varying types of experimental evidence. For reviews see, e.g., Refs. 13, 279, and 280.

4.4.1 BLOCK THROUGH EXPANSION OR PHASE TRANSITIONS. The first hypothesis proposes changes in the membrane organization induced by the local anesthetic agents. It thus goes back to the Meyer–Overton explanation for general anesthesia, that is, direct correlation between the lipophilicity of an agent and its anesthetic effect. The modern and more sophisticated developments obviously can take into consideration the accumulated knowledge of membrane structure and physicochemical properties of the major membrane constituents as well as of the anesthetic agents.

This hypothesis suggests that the primary event takes place by hydrophobic bonding between the agent and certain membrane constituents, either lipids or proteins or both. During the time interval in which agent–constituent bonding is increasing, a concomitant change in volume, an expansion, takes place (see also Chapter 50). Shanes presented the effects as resulting from agent–lipid interactions (281), and Seeman considered the possibility that proteins and/or lipids may be actively involved in the events (282, 283). As a result of the disordering of the normal membrane organization, dysfunciton of sodium flux is eventually obtained and thus block of conduction.

A somewhat different explanation inside the same paradigm suggests that phase transitions in the membrane may play a significant role when anesthetic concentration (and volume) increase (284). The facts that both natural and artificial membranes become more fluid and disordered under anesthetic attack (283, 285), that erythrocyte and synaptosome membranes expand about 50 times more than pure lipid membranes under comparable conditions (286), and that increase of pressure can counteract the anesthetic effects of several agents *excluding* TTX and STX (287, 288) lend credence to some of the above hypotheses. Even though it would be pleasing to have a unifying theory for general and local anesthesia at the membrane level (cf. Refs. 287–289), there is *still* no compelling evidence available to let us single out a mechanism of this kind as fully satisfactory for explaining all the observed features of local anesthesia at the membrane level.

4.4.2 BLOCK THROUGH CHANGE IN MEMBRANE SURFACE CHARGE. Another and completey different approach to explaining local anesthesia has been proposed in different forms by, for instance, Feinstein (290) and McLaughlin (291) and is based on the influence of changes of the membrane surface charge following administration of local anesthetic agents. This hypothesis suggests that when the

molecules reach the membrane they interact with the lipid bilayer so that their polar portions point outward (in proximity to the negative charges of the phospholipids of the bilayer) and the lipid portions dip down into the lipid core of the membrane. Some of the polar ends of the anesthetic carry positive charges and thus increase the total surface charge. This could happen either at the inside or the outside surface of the membrane. Clearly a noncharged molecule like benzocaine or benzyl alcohol could not change the surface charge in this manner and this is also an argument used against this hypothesis as a general explanation for the action of all local anesthetics. However, for such agents that possess charged portions, it could obviously present an explanation for their blocking ability. See further Ref. 13.

Although it does not postulate a change in surface charges, the hypothesis that the cationic local anesthetic molecules would compete with calcium for sites at the phospholipid anionic groups (290, 292, 293) suggests a certain similarity in site of action and molecular orientation. An arrangement similar to that described above, with the lipid portions of the anesthetic inserted into the membrane core, would result. This antagonism to structural calcium would lead to secondary events (e.g., expansion) and finally to block.

4.4.3 BLOCK THROUGH ANESTHETIC RECEPTORS: ACTIVE FORM OF AMINE ANESTHETICS. The third principal current hypothesis postulates specific receptors at or in the sodium channels. The action is thus direct and antagonistic to sodium and not mediated through an event or a series of events or changes in the organization or physical chemical properties of the membrane outside of the sodium channel.

The concept that receptors for local anesthetic molecules exist somewhere in the nerve membrane is not new. The foundation for this proposition has not been the same through the years, however. The early suggestion that nerve block is caused by a competition between the local anesthetic agent and acetylcholine (294) was based on the identity of certain portions of procaine and acetylcholine, structures 51.**17** and 51.**80** (both are alkylamino ethanol esters), and on certain anticholinergic responses of procaine and other local anesthetic drugs (cf. Ref. 295). However, there are a number of distinct difficulties involved with the application of this idea to axonal nerve block; for discussions, see e.g., Refs. 280 and 296.

$$CH_3CO_2CH_2CH_2\overset{\overset{\displaystyle CH_3}{|+}}{\underset{\underset{\displaystyle CH_3}{|}}{N}}\!-\!CH_3$$

51.**80** (Cation)

Before continuing with the later developments of the receptor hypothesis, it is necessary to present the essentials of the arguments concerning the identity of the active form of the local anesthetic molecule.

The question of which form of a tertiary and secondary local anesthetic amine is the active one has been debated for more than 50 years. Is it the ion, the base, or both? The first systematic study of the problem was published in 1910 by Gros (297), who compared the effect of various local anesthetic hydrochloride solutions with and without the addition of sodium hydroxide. Much faster blocks were obtained on the frog sciatic nerve preparation when sodium hydroxide was added. Since the simple equilibrium $BH^+ + OH^- \rightleftharpoons B + H_2O$ tells us that the base form B increases in a hydrochloride solution when OH^- ions are added to it, the conclusion was drawn that the base form is the more active one.

Trevan and Boock (298), in studies on the rabbit cornea, observed changes in the minimal-effective blocking concentrations of local anesthetic solutions as the pH of the solutions was varied. They found that the minimal effective concentration decreased with increasing pH and arrived at the conclusion that the uncharged base must be the active form. Their conclusion, they felt, was substantiated by benzyl alcohol, a nonionic agent at physiological pH, showing the same anesthetic activity at all pH values. Skou (299) used a desheathed frog sciatic nerve–muscle preparation and applied local anesthetic solutions of varying concentrations and pH to the isolated nerve portion. The minimal effective concentration values obtained were in agreement with those of Trevan and Boock (298). There remained, however, in both investigations the increase in the minimum blocking concentration of base (B) with increasing pH and with decreasing minimal blocking concentration of the total amount of local anesthetic $(B + BH^+)$. If the base form were the active form, one would expect the minimum effective concentration of this form to stay constant over the pH range studied. Skou (299) therefore abstained from designating the base form as being solely involved in blocking the nerve.

A suggestion that the ionic form might be the active one came from Krahl et al. (300), who studied the influence of local anesthetic amines on eggs and larvae of the sea urchin species *Arbacia punctata* with variation of pH. To equate these test objects with nerve might be questionable, but the same conclusion was arrived at by Ritchie and Greengard (301).

They found that dibucaine (51.**54**) was a stronger anesthetic at lower than at higher pH values when studying its effect on the C fibers of the desheathed rabbit vagus. Ritchie et al. (302) noticed the effect of pH on the rate of block of dibucaine and lidocaine (51.**45**) was faster at pH 7.2 than at pH 9.2 in the desheathed preparations and the opposite in nerves whose sheaths were intact. However, the experimental results for procaine were the opposite (303), pointing out that a simple relationship did

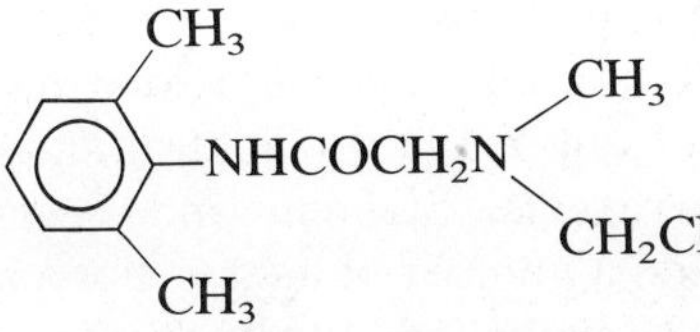

CH$_3$

—NHCOCH$_2$N

CH$_3$

CH$_3$

CH$_2$CH$_2$OCH$_3$

51.**81**   (W 6211)

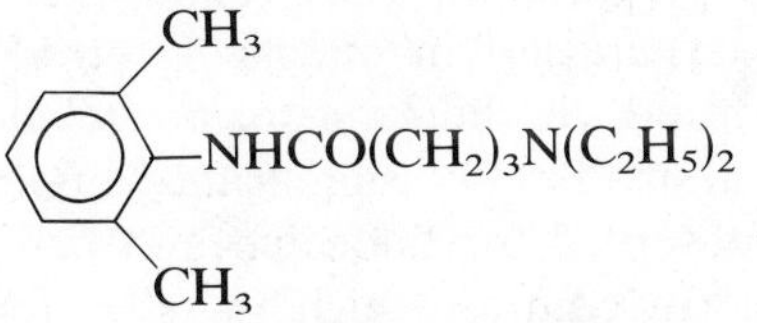

CH$_3$

—NHCO(CH$_2$)$_3$N(C$_2$H$_5$)$_2$

CH$_3$

51.**82**   (W 6603)

not exist for the variables studied for all agents. See further Ref. 296.

Ariëns and Simonis (304) arrived at the conclusion that the ion is the active form: they showed that if certain reasonable assumptions are made, Skou's data (299) favor the ion as being the active form.

Finally, Narahashi et al. (305) showed on the squid axon preparation, a single unmyelinated nerve fiber, that an increase of the pH value of a solution of amine-type local anesthetics applied *inside* the membranes lowered the blocking potency. When two chemically related local anesthetic agents with pK_a values 6.3 (51.**81**) and 9.8 (51.**82**), respectively, were studied in carefully designed experiments with application of the agents outside and inside the axonal membrane at different concentrations and pH values, the data allowed the conclusion that it is the cationic form that is the more potent species, and that this ion (like its quaternary congeners) acts on or from the inside (axoplasmic) surface of the membrane (cf. Ref. 62).

Thus as improvements in technique, models, and data analysis have added new information to the growing body of knowledge about normal nerve function, the weight of evidence currently seems to favor the ionic form as the more likely bearer of the anesthetic potency.

However, the base form must possess some blocking properties (306, 15), and we cannot exclude the possibility that for some molecular structures the base form may possess considerable activity compared to its corresponding ion. In addition to pK_a, ability to penetrate to the site of action is an important characteristic of a molecular species, and it is the neutral species, the base, that most easily penetrates not only the external barrier but, in all probability, the nerve membrane itself. That the question of "the active molecular species" by no means is completely settled yet is evident from recent studies on the pH dependence of rate of action on the nodal membrane of single fibers of sciatic nerve (11); see Section 4.4.4.

The hypothesis that relatively strong local anesthetic amines interfere directly with the transmembrane inward flux of sodium ions by occupying sites inside the channel structure followed from investigations by Courtney (18, 278) of several such compounds on voltage clamped single nerve fiber, with particular attention directed to their propensity for use dependence (frequency dependence) (cf. Section 4.3). It turned out that the agents studied showed the type of use dependence found by Strichartz for the quaternary lidocaine derivatives (17). The glycylglycylxylidide derivative GEA 968 (51.**83**) showed this property especially clearly. Courtney concluded that GEA 968 in its ionic form, like the quaternaries, can enter the sodium channel only when the channel is in its open state and reacts, possibly, at the same site as the quaternaries. The same kind of voltage dependence applied to the tertiary amines and the quaternaries, which

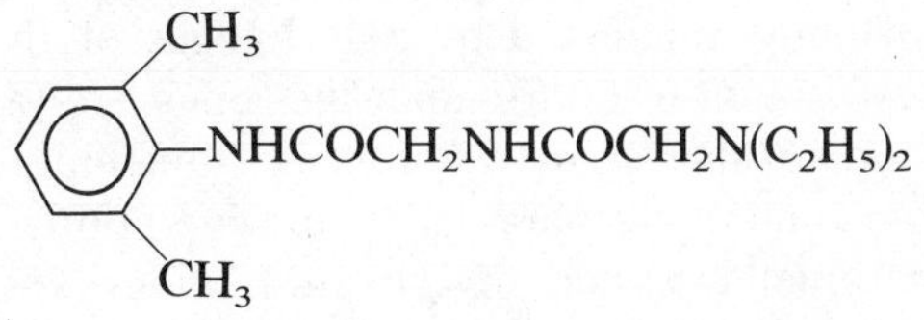

CH$_3$

—NHCOCH$_2$NHCOCH$_2$N(C$_2$H$_5$)$_2$

CH$_3$

51.**83**

51.**84**

suggested to Courtney that the ionic species was the blocking agent. This was further supported by the demonstration that the two optical antipodes RAC-109I, RAC-109II, a tertiary amine, 51.**84** (307), had the same potency ratio of 2:1 as the optical antipodes of the corresponding *N*-ethylated quaternary derivatives at the node of the single myelinated nerve fiber of the frog (308).

4.4.4 AGENTS ESSENTIALLY UNCHARGED AT pH 7.4 ("NEUTRAL" AGENTS).   It has been inferred from the available evidence that electrically neutral agents, i.e., those that do not carry a positive charge to a significant degree at physiologic pH values, probably act in a more nonspecific way outside the sodium channel and therefore exert their blocking effect through a disordering of the general normal membrane structure, for instance, through expansion or phase transitions (Section 4.4.1) (see e.g., Ref. 15).

In this group we find such agents of clinical use as benzocaine, 51.**76a**, and benzyl alcohol. The potency of a "neutral" anesthetic like benzocaine is about the same as that of procaine, 51.**17**, when compared on desheathed nerve in concentrations allowed by the limited aqueous solubility of the former (296). The blocking properties of neutral agents *in vitro* are virtually unaffected by pH changes of the test solution (296), and the ones so far studied also show differences from amine type and quaternary agents in several other parameters when investigated under vol-

tage clamp conditions (12).

There is pharmacological evidence for different sites of action for neutral and for amine-type agents. Staiman and Seeman (309) studied a number of agents alone and paired in formally (additively) equipotent mixtures on the desheathed frog sciatic nerve preparation. They found a potentiation (synergism) in effects if tetrodotoxin was mixed with lidocaine or benzyl alcohol; also a smaller but significant potentiation was observed for lidocaine and benzyl alcohol. In contrast, such pairs as tetrodotoxin–saxitoxin, benzyl alcohol–urethane, benzyl alcohol–phenol, and lidocaine ($pK_a = 7.9$)–RAC-109II (51.**84**) (pK_a 9.4) showed only additive effects. Additional contributions of similar experimental data show that lidocaine and benzocaine act synergistically but that neither lidocaine in combination with bupivacaine nor benzocaine–benzyl alcohol do (310). These results agree with the assignment of different sites of action for the two toxins and for conventional local anesthetics; among the latter, they would agree with differences in sites for the tertiary amines of $pK_a > 7.4$ and for the neutral agents.

In aqueous media, the amine agents exist as equilibrium mixtures of an ion and a neutral base form of which the latter has a greater propensity for partitioning into lipid environments. The two factors that decide the distribution of an agent are its pK_a and its partition coefficient. Strictly speaking, this is true only under equilibrium conditions, and dynamic factors (diffusion, partition, and penetration rates) may be of significant importance in a biosystem.

For the amines, however, we must consider that its two forms may exert blocking effects at different sites and through different mechanisms. For an individual drug this means that its total effect could depend on its reactivities at the different sites, and thus be at least partly determined by its pK_a and partitioning. A strongly basic hydrophilic agent would be more like the quaternary ammonium compounds in its general distribution and choice of pathways in the membrane environment, whereas a weaker base of lipophilic character should be more like the "neutral" blocking agents in these respects. If, indeed, different sites exist for charged and uncharged species, it should be possible to show synergistic behavior for suitably chosen pairs of amine agents such as a lipophilic weaker base and a hydrophilic stronger base. For agents that possess properties that allow them to exert a significant effect at both sites, we might expect that their total effect would be greater than the sum of the contributions of each of the two forms: they would possess an autosynergistic property (cf. Ref. 311).

Hille suggested that amine-type and neutral local anesthetics *as well as* quaternary blocking agents act at the same site at the sodium channel (12). This unifying hypothesis (the modulated receptor model) explains the differences observed between these three structural classes of agents in terms of access to the receptor structure by means of differing pathways: the pathway an agent takes is determined by its hydrophilicity and also by the conformational changes of the *channel* and receptor induced by drug interactions and by variations in the electric field (voltage). This very important interpretation of available experimental data should prove provocative and stimulating for future research in the local anesthetic field.

An interesting aspect of this hypothesis is that the hydrophobic interactions between receptor and agent are more important than charge–charge interactions. Implicit in this is a new answer to the question of the active species of the amine type anesthetics: both forms may be active, and the important parameter for the ultimate interaction may in some cases be only remotely related to the ion–base duality.

5 PHARMACOLOGICAL PROPERTIES IN MAN AND OTHER ANIMALS

5.1 Local Anesthetic Activity

Although distribution and metabolism of classical local anesthetic agents may and do differ from one species to another, the physicochemical processes that take place when a local anesthetic agent is injected around a nerve trunk, for example, are remarkably similar for many species. Different doses may be required to produce local anesthetic block and, because of differences in distribution and metabolism, systemic toxic effects may differ qualitatively and quantitatively; nevertheless, we can with reasonable assurance predict that an agent that blocks the sciatic nerve in *Rana pipiens* will block the sciatic nerve— or the ulnar nerve or brachial plexus—in *Homo sapiens.*

Having made this generalization, we now examine the similarities and differences between man and other species of animals when local anesthetic agents are administered by various routes.

5.2 Specific Applications

5.2.1 PERIPHERAL NERVE BLOCKS. Sciatic nerve blocks in rats and guinea pigs are a rapid and simple means of evaluating potentially useful local anesthetic agents and comparing them with known compounds (210, 312). The local anesthetic agent can be tested with and without vasoconstrictor agents and the method provides data on frequency, onset, and duration of block. If a series of increasing concentrations is tested, dose–duration curves may be obtained. Furthermore, systemic toxic signs may be manifested at one or more of the concentrations, and acute toxicity relative to other agents can be assessed. One of the disadvantages of the rat sciatic nerve block is that with many compounds a sharp break occurs in the dose–duration curve at the higher concentrations: recovery times become inordinately long, sometimes requiring days or weeks for complete recovery of normal motor function in the limb (313). This can make comparison of agents difficult. We have not established the cause of this phenomenon, but it has not been observed when the local anesthetic solutions are injected into the hip rather than the mid-thigh region. We infer from this that the long recovery times may be due to the effects of local anesthetic agents on skeletal muscle (314) rather than on the nerve fibers. Another disadvantage of using a small animal such as the rat or guinea pig is that dose–duration data may be misleading when comparisons between compounds are extrapolated to man. For example, we found that dose–duration curves of etidocaine and bupivacaine obtained with rat sciatic nerve blocks were quite similar, implying that at equal doses the durations of these two agents should be equivalent to each other in the clinical situation (210). However, clinical studies have shown that in ulnar nerve and brachial plexus blocks up to twice the dose of etidocaine may be required to produce the same duration of block as a selected dose of bupivacaine (315, 316). Although the reason for this disparity between results obtained in small and large animals is not known for certain, it has been suggested that the difference in the relative masses of neural tissue involved may be a critical factor.

5.2.2 CENTRAL NEURAL BLOCKS

5.2.2.1 *Epidural Anesthesia.*

Epidural anesthesia in the rat, guinea pig, cat, dog, and sheep has been used to test and compare local anesthetic agents. Of these, the sheep is, for a number of reasons, the best animal model. Because of the structure of the vertebrae in the lumbosacral region of the cat and dog, for example, insertion of a needle into the epidural space is difficult

and surgical implantation of a catheter is often done when these animals are to be used for studying local anesthetic agents or epidural block (317, 318). The sheep, in addition to being relatively docile, possesses a lumbosacral interspace that is easily palpated and allows epidural injections to be made easily and reproducibly (36). Furthermore, the sheep's spinal cord and roots are comparable in size to man's, sensory analgesia and motor block can be assessed independently with a reasonable degree of certainty, the spread and regression of anesthesia can be followed on the cutaneous dermatomes of the dorsum as is done in man in clinical studies, and blood samples can be drawn repeatedly from the jugular veins when it is desirable to follow concentrations of local anesthetic agents in the systemic circulation. Full evaluation of this animal model must await publication of results obtained with standard agents such as procaine, lidocaine, and bupivacaine and comparison of these with results obtained in clinical studies. It is worth noting that pregnant ewes have been used to study the effects of epidural anesthesia on uterine blood flow and fetal acid–base balance (319).

5.2.2.2 *Spinal Anesthesia.*

Subarachnoid injections have been given to a variety of species, from the rat to the sheep, for testing and comparison of local anesthetic agents, and many of the comments made in the previous section on epidural anesthesia in animal models apply here. The same behavioral and anatomic characteristics that make the sheep a good model for epidural anesthesia also make it a good model for spinal anesthesia. Subarachnoid injections can be made easily and reproducibly without surgical intervention (36). We must, however, keep in mind that there is a major difference between man and sheep in the anatomy of the spinal cord and its relation to the vertebral canal: in man the cord terminates at L1–L2, but in sheep it terminates at about S2. Consequently, when subarachnoid injections are made at the L6–S1 interspace, the local anesthetic solution is, in the sheep, deposited around the cord rather than around the caudal roots as in man. Nevertheless, several studies have shown this to be an extremely useful animal model. As with epidural anesthesia in the sheep, analgesia and motor block in the hind limbs can be assessed independently with an acceptable degree of certainty (320). Furthermore, although similarities between data obtained in man and in other animals may often be merely fortuitous, there are several examples of correspondence between data obtained with bupivacaine and tetracaine in sheep by Adams and Doherty (321) and data obtained with these two agents in man (322).

5.2.3   TOPICAL ANESTHESIA.   Topical anesthesia, as Covino and Vassallo remind us, refers to a diversity of sites of application that includes, for example, the skin, the cornea, the tracheobronchial tree, and the gastrointestinal tract (6). Because of differences in the anatomy, biochemistry, and physiology of the barriers to penetration at these various sites of application, one would assume *a priori* that a single agent would not be the drug of choice at all sites. Clinical experience has shown this to be the case. Depending on the characteristics of the site of application, specific agents and even specifically formulated vehicles may be required in order to effect local anesthesia of acceptable intensity and duration.

These differences in the characteristics of the several sites of application must be kept in mind when testing local anesthetic agents by topical applications to animals. One of the easiest and most widely used is corneal anesthesia in the intact animal. Rabbits are, in general, used in this procedure, but smaller animals such as the guinea pig (323) and even the mouse (324) can be used. Local anesthetic agents have been applied to the nasal mucosa of the rabbit to evaluate effectiveness and relative systemic toxicity (325). In order to test local anesthetic agents on skin, Campbell et al. developed a method using application of test substances to abraded and burned areas of skin in the intact guinea pig (326). Åkerman has reported a method for testing local anesthetic agents on the tracheobronchial tree of the guinea pig (327); the method also permits determination of concentrations of the drugs in the blood. The diversity of animal models for testing topically applied local anesthetic agents allows the investigator to evaluate a new compound or formulation on the site of application, be it cornea or skin or mucosa, on which it is to be used in man or to ascertain, by testing on different sites, that one on which the agent or formulation is most effective in animals and may therefore be the area in which it will be most useful clinically.

For the purposes of this discussion, we limit ourselves to topical anesthesia of the tracheobronchial tree and the skin, the former because it represents one of the most common uses of topical anesthetic agents and the latter because it poses special problems and challenges to the synthetic and pharmaceutical chemists.

Topical anesthesia of the tracheobronchial tree in relatively easy, and a number of agents, including lidocaine, prilocaine, and tetracaine, have been used for this purpose. However, absorption of local anesthetic agents from the tracheobronchial tree is quite rapid, owing in part to the large surface area that may be exposed to the substance, and the curves of blood level vs. time may simulate those obtained following a moderately rapid intravenous infusion. Toxic levels can be reached quite rapidly, and a number of fatalities occurred when tetracaine, one of the most potent and toxic agents, was used for producing topical anesthesia of this region (328). Less potent agents such as lidocaine and prilocaine have subsequently come into wide-spread use, and clinical experience with these agents has borne out Åström and Persson's observations that they are effective but less toxic than tetracaine when applied to the nasal and tracheobronchial mucosa of the rabbit (325). Awareness of the rapid absorption of these substances from the tracheobronchial tree and the attendant potential danger has led to a more cautious approach to the use of even those agents known to be inherently less toxic (329). Studies conducted by Åkerman on the cornea and nasal mucosa of the rabbit and on the tracheobronchial tree of the guinea pig show that the new long-acting agent etidocaine may be of value for certain types of applications: when applied to the mucosal surfaces of the respiratory tract, for example, etidocaine exhibited a greater margin of safety than bupivacaine and tetracaine (327).

Intact skin presents a more formidable barrier to the passage of many substances, including local anesthetic agents (330). The permeability of the skin has been the subject of intensive research, and a number of excellent review articles are available (331–333). Penetration and permeation of the skin can be facilitated by the use of sorption promoters (334, 335) and by disruption of the principal barrier, the horny layer (333). Campbell et al. (326) studied diperodon (51.**6**), benzocaine, and lidocaine on the guinea pig after abrasion or thermal injury of the skin and found that diperodon was the most effective of the three on abraded skin, all three were about equieffective on one type of experimentally induced burn, and benzocaine was the most effective in two other types of burn. Dalili and Adriani evaluated the efficacy of a number of local anesthetic agents and commercial preparations on volunteers in which localized burns were produced by ultraviolet light or in which itching and burning sensations were elicited by means of electrical stimuli (336). In general, they found

that formulations and preparations containing salts of local anesthetic agents were ineffective but that concentrated solutions of bases were effective in obtunding the itching and burning sensations. It has been recognized for a long time that the solubilized bases of local anesthetic agents penetrate and permeate skin better than solutions of their salts, and the reason for this is that the buffering capacity of the stratum corneum is considerably less than that of other tissues to which solutions of local anesthetic agents are presented.

Topical anesthesia of the intact skin, in contrast to abraded or burned, poses special problems. As Adriani and Dalili have shown, many formulations containing low concentrations of the salt forms of local anesthetic agents in various vehicles simply are not efficacious when applied topically (336). In order to produce adequate anesthesia, one must use a combination of a high concentration of the base form of the "right" local anesthetic agent in the "right" vehicle; even then, occlusive dressings and long exposure times may be required to produce anesthesia of clinically acceptable depth and duration. Åkerman et al., using the guinea pig as the model, addressed this problem and recommended for clinical trials a formulation containing ketocaine base in a special vehicle (237). Clinical studies to date indicate this formulation may be sufficiently superior to other formulations currently available to warrant a place for it in certain types of surgical procedures (238, 239).

5.3 Toxicity

The toxicity of local anesthetic agents is understood to include local and systemic toxicity. When a solution of a local anesthetic agent is injected around the nerve trunk, for example, the surrounding skeletal muscles, blood vessels, and connective tissue are also exposed to the solution, and the effects of the local anesthetic agent on these tissues must be taken into consideration. Furthermore, the local anesthetic agents are absorbed into the general circulation, and there is the potential of systemic toxic effects resulting from the agent itself or from its metabolites. It is often convenient to think of local toxic effects as depending on the concentration of drug to which the tissue is exposed and of systemic toxicity as depending on the total dose administered, although the severity of both local and systemic toxic effects are dose dependent.

The cytotoxic effects of local anesthetic agents on neural tissue have been extensively studied. Co Tui and co-workers demonstrated many years ago that the severity and reversibility of the adverse effects induced in neural tissue by these agents is dose dependent: morphological changes are absent at low concentrations, mild and reversible at higher concentrations, and severe and irreversible at still higher concentrations (337). Since all local anesthetic agents do not possess the same intrinsic potency and cytotoxic potential, it is necessary to establish for each compound the range of concentrations that produces these graded responses. Adams and co-workers used methods similar to those described by Co Tui et al. to evaluate and compare the neurotoxic proclivities of etidocaine and tetracaine on the spinal cord of the rabbit (338). Although studies of this kind establish the neurotoxicity of an agent relative to other agents, it must be kept in mind that the results may apply only to the species used and the conditions of that study: in a different species or under different conditions, the dose–response curve may shift to the left or right. The whole issue of neurotoxicity of local anesthetic agents is of paramount importance, but, as in most areas of pharmacology and toxicology, the investigator must rely on tests conducted in several species and hope that the results predict what will happen when the agent is administered to man.

Intradermal wheals on the back of the rabbit or guinea pig are often used routinely to determine the relative tissue irritating properties of local anesthetic agents (339–341). Such studies are useful in screening procedures in which extremely irritating compounds are to be eliminated from further study, but they are probably of limited value in predicting neurotoxic potential. Initial clinical studies may also involve the use of intradermal wheals in man as a means of evaluating both duration of action and tissue irritation (342–344).

Although the phenomenon has been known for some time (345), recent studies have redirected attention to the degeneration of skeletal muscle fibers exposed to local anesthetic agents (346, 347). Benoit and Belt showed that mepivacaine, bupivacaine, lidocaine, prilocaine, and cocaine cause destruction of skeletal muscle fibers and that degenerative changes can be detected by light microscopy as early as 15 min after an injection of the agent (314, 348). The concentrations they injected, which are those used clinically, exhibited highly selective effects: destruction of skeletal muscle fibers occurred, but the structural integrity of the peripheral nerves and smooth muscle of the arterioles at the injection site were unaffected. They concluded that, although indirect effects could not be unequivocally excluded, direct effects of the agents seem to be the important factors in the destruction of the skeletal muscle fibers.

Although in small doses most local anesthetic agents exhibit anticonvulsant activity, sufficiently high doses cause generalized clonic–tonic convulsions. The CNS effects of local anesthetic agents have been the subject of numerous studies, and it is now generally accepted that three phases can be demonstrated: the initial phase, which occurs at a certain range of concentrations in the CNS, is sedation; higher concentrations produce frank convulsive activity; and still higher concentrations produce profound CNS depression (6, 349). The convulsive activity is apparently due to the selective blocking of inhibitory systems in the CNS; this leaves excitatory systems unopposed, and intense CNS stimulation, manifested as convulsive episodes, can occur (350, 351). Differential block of fibers in a mixed nerve trunk by local anesthetic agents has been recognized for a long time (352, 353), and the phenomena of "differential rate of blocking" and "absolute differential block" as defined by Nathan and Sears (354) may explain both the triphasic sequence of sedation, excitement, and depression, on the one hand, and the anticonvulsant activity on the other.

The CNS toxicity of local anesthetic agents has been studied in numerous species, including primates. Electroencephalographic recordings in the rhesus monkey, for example, have apparently revealed differences in the patterns of changes that occur with various kinds of local anesthetic agents: some, such as lidocaine and procaine, are reported to produce characteristic preconvulsive patterns in the EEG, but others, such as etidocaine and bupivacaine, do not (355–357).

Whether or not these differences are real probably has not been unequivocally established. Scott reports that electroencephalography was found to be of little value as a means of predicting impending CNS toxicity in man during infusions of lidocaine, etidocaine, and bupivacaine (358). In the unpremedicated volunteer, in contrast to the premedicated patient being prepared for surgery, for example, there are certain signs and symptoms that may be interpreted as early indications of CNS effects and serve as warnings of impending ictal episodes. These adumbrative signs and symptoms include feelings of light-headedness and dizziness, disorientation, slurred speech, and localized muscle twitches and tremors (358).

Recent studies in man and in the rhesus monkey reemphasize the effect the rate of infusion may have on the acute toxicity of an agent. Because of differences in pharmacokinetic behavior, two agents may be affected unequally by changes in rates of infusion. This has been shown to be true of etidocaine and bupivacaine; for example, at high rates of infusion they are about equitoxic but at slower rates etidocaine is less toxic than bupivacaine (358, 359).

Kortilla and co-workers have examined the effects of lidocaine, etidocaine, and bupivacaine on psychomotor performance in volunteers. Intramuscular lidocaine, 200 mg in subjects weighing an average of about 70 kg, impaired reactive skills for 30–90 min after the injection (360), and intramuscular etidocaine, 2.6 mg/kg, or bupivacaine, 1.3 mg/kg, impaired performance for at least 2 hr (361). The investigators conclude that the possibility of adverse effects of local anesthetic agents on the psychomotor skills related, for example, to driving an automobile should not be ignored.

The CNS-stimulant effects of local anesthetic agents can be antagonized by means of CNS depressants. Diazepam and short-acting barbiturates such as thiopental are specifically indicated to control the CNS effects of overdosage, including convulsions (6, 362, 363). Inherent in the routine use of barbiturates and tranquilizers in the premedication of patients scheduled for regional anesthesia is the possibility that the doses used may be sufficient to mask the early signs of CNS toxicity due to inadvertent overdosage with a local anesthetic agent without preventing the convulsions that may ensue.

5.4 Distribution, Biotransformation, and Excretion

5.4.1 DISTRIBUTION. Solutions of local anesthetic agents are deposited in circumscribed sites in the body in order to effect analgesia or anesthesia in specific regions. Immediately after injection there is a competition for the agent: some of it diffuses into the nerve trunk or trunks in that area and some of it diffuses into non-nervous tissues and is taken into the circulation and carried away. If the local anesthetic solution is deposited too far away from the nerve trunk, then it may never reach the nerves in sufficient concentration to produce adequate anesthesia. Chances of producing the desired anesthetic block are increased, therefore, by depositing the solution as close as possible to the nerve trunk and by using a vasoconstrictor in the solution to reduce blood flow through the area and maintain a high concentration of local anesthetic agent locally for a longer time.

Once the local anesthetic agent is absorbed into the circulation, it is distributed through the body just as is any other drug. The concentration of drug within an organ system or body compartment at any time after its administration depends on such factors as the physicochemical properties of the local anesthetic agent; the physical and chemical properties of the tissue, organ system, or body compartment; and the relative blood flow through the tissue, organ system, or body compartment.

A generalized scheme for absorption of a local anesthetic agent from the site of deposition and subsequent distribution to various organs and tissues is shown in Fig. 51.9. If we were to substitute the term "site of action" for "nerve trunk" in this figure, we would have a scheme applicable to drugs in general. Both intact drug and its metabolites are distributed and redistributed to the various tissues and organs. In some cases, undesirable systemic effects may be due to one or more of the metabolites.

Unequal distribution of a drug in the body is due primarily to (1) binding to plasma proteins, (2) cellular binding, (3) sequestration by fatty tissues, and (4) the blood–brain barrier. Since local anesthetic agents vary considerably in structure and

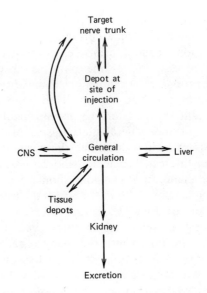

Fig. 51.9 Absorption, distribution and excretion of a local anesthetic.

therefore possess physical and chemical properties different from one another, the pattern of distribution of each local anesthetic agent is unique. Furthermore, all the metabolites of a drug may have distributions that are different from one another and from the parent compound. Those readers who are interested in the profiles of absorption and distribution of specific compounds should see the more detailed discussions and references to the literature by Covino and Vassallo (6) and de Jong (7). Examples of recent studies of hepatic clearance of local anesthetics in man and blood concentration curves after regional block are the publications of Tucker et al. (364) and Wildsmith et al. (365), respectively.

5.4.2 BIOTRANSFORMATION. The pathways for and overall patterns of biotransformation of local anesthetic agents are numerous and depend on, among other things, the chemical structures of the agents and the species in which they are studied. When discussing biotransformation of local anesthetic agents, one has the choice of either describing specific pathways for each of a number of different agents or setting forth some general principles. Since even a brief description of the patterns of bio-transformation of the major chemical types of local anesthetic agents is beyond the scope of this chapter, we instead highlight some of the general mechanisms of bio-transformation of local anesthetic agents in man. Interested readers who would like more elaborate discussions should see, for example, Boyes (366), Covino and Vassallo (6), and de Jong (7).

Local anesthetic agents may, like other drugs introduced into the living organism, undergo oxidative, reductive, hydrolytic, and synthetic reactions. Precisely what reactions occur, in what order, and to what extent depends, as we stated previously, on the chemical structure of the agent, the route of administration, and the species. Nearly all clinically useful local anesthetic agents have the general structure:

Aromatic moiety–ester
or amide linkage–amino group

The obvious points of attack, therefore, are as follows:

1. *Dealkylation of the amino group.* Oxidative deethylation of the amino nitrogen to a secondary amine is one of the first steps in the degradation of lidocaine; prilocaine, which is a secondary amine, does not require dealkylation before metabolic attack on the amide linkage occurs. *O*-Dealkylation, or ether cleavage, may occur during the bio-transformation of dibucaine, benoxinate, phenacaine, proparacaine, and promaxine, since these agents have alkoxy substitutions on the aromatic rings.
2. *Hydrolysis of the ester or amide linkage.* The pseudocholinesterases in plasma are responsible for splitting the ester linkage in chloroprocaine, procaine, and tetracaine. The ester linkages in cocaine un-

dergo hydrolytic cleavage but not by plasma pseudocholinesterases. The aminoacyl amide linkage of lidocaine is hydrolyzed by enzymes present in the endoplasmic reticulum of the liver. Perhaps because of steric hindrance, the cleavage of the amide linkage is not a major route of metabolism for mepivacaine and bupivacaine. Hydrolysis of the aminoalkyl amide linkage in dibucaine apparently can and does occur, but the biotransformation of this agent has not been well studied (7).

3. *Hydroxylation of the aromatic ring moiety.* This occurs during the bio-transformation of lidocaine, prilocaine, mepivacaine, and presumably, bupivacaine.
4. *Conjugation.* Some of the metabolites of local anesthetic agents may appear in the urine as conjugation products, chiefly glucuronides.

5.4.3 EXCRETION. The kidneys are the principal route of excretion of both intact local anesthetic agent and its metabolic breakdown products.

5.5   Other Pharmacological Properties

As we stated in the introduction to this chapter, local anesthetic agents belong to that special class of pharmacological agents that is administered as close as possible to the desired site of action, be it a nerve trunk or plexus. Although local anesthetic agents possess a variety of pharmacological actions, most of these actions, such as anti-cholinergic, antihistaminic, and anti-bacterial, are of little importance at the concentrations and doses most commonly used in clinical practice. Even though it has been shown that ganglionic blockade—specifically, block of the dorsal root ganglia—may occur following subarachnoid administration of a local anesthetic agent

(367), the significance of this action during spinal anesthesia has not been fully evaluated.

The cardiovascular effects of local anesthetic agents are manifold and complex and in spinal and epidural blocks are a combination of direct effects on various parts of the cardiovascular system and indirect effects due to block of autonomic fibers. The presence of vasoconstrictor agents such as epinephrine further complicates the picture, and sophisticated studies have been conducted to sort out and identify the effects of the vasoconstrictor and the direct and indirect effects of the local anesthetic agent (368–370).

The antiarrhythmic activity of local anesthetic agents has been recognized for some time and has served as a source of inspiration and endeavor for chemists and biologists for decades. Second only to its use as a local anesthetic agent, for example, is lidocaine's use as an antiarrhythmic agent (371, 372) (Chapter 38). Lidocaine is extremely effective against certain types of arrhythmias when administered parenterally. Oral administration is unsatisfactory: large doses are required to produce effective blood levels, and the incidence of side effects, due to circulating metabolites of lidocaine, is high. This is explained by the observation that a large percentage of an orally administered dose of lidocaine is metabolized or biotransformed on its first passage through the liver, the so-called "first-pass effect" in the argot of pharmacokineticists (373, 374).

Because of lidocaine's success in the treatment of certain kinds of cardiac arrhythmias, it has served as a starting point for a variety of chemical modifications and subsequent biological investigations. Two agents that have received attention are the quaternary compound "methyllidocaine" QX372 (51.**85**) (375) and tocainide (51.**86**). The latter, which is 2-amino-2′,6′-propionoxylidide, is effective after oral administration, and its half-life is sufficiently

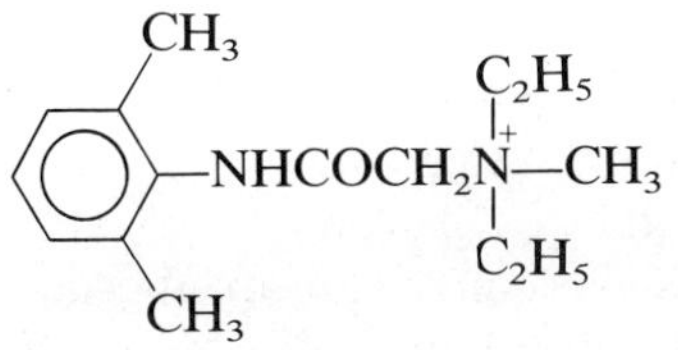

51.**85**   (Cation)

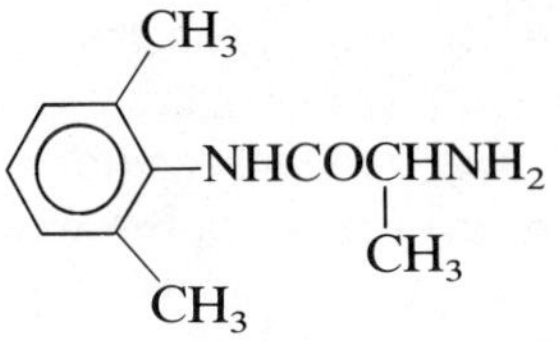

51.**86**

long so that dosing at frequent intervals is not required (376–378).

The CNS effects of local anesthetic agents have been discussed in Section 5.3. Not all the CNS effects of these agents are undesirable, and their CNS depressant and anticonvulsant activities have been studied in laboratory animals and man. Procaine and lidocaine have been employed prophylactically and therapeutically in epileptic and electrically induced seizures in man (379, 380). The mild sedation and analgesia that may occur following parenteral administration of lidocaine have led to its use as an adjunct in general anesthetic procedures (381). Himes et al. have examined this phenomenon quantitatively in patients and in experimental animals and have shown that plasma concentrations of 3–6 μg/ml decreased the anesthetic requirements of nitrous oxide and of halothane approximately 10–30% (382).

6   FUTURE DEVELOPMENTS

One can properly infer from the preceding sections that chemists, pharmacologists, and clinicians are still searching for the "ideal" local anesthetic agent. This does not necessarily mean that they are looking for a single compound that will satisfy the requirements of all the areas in which local anesthetic agents are used. It should be obvious that a single agent probably cannot be all things: it cannot be ultra-short-acting, as required for diagnostic blocks, and also ultra-long-acting, as required for relief of chronic pain; it is also highly unlikely that a single agent would have the physical and chemical properties requisite for producing topical anesthesia of the skin and at the same time have those physical and chemical properties appropriate to an agent used for peripheral nerve blocks or spinal anesthesia. Therefore, the anesthesiologists' armamentarium must include a variety of local anesthetic agents, each of which may be the agent of choice for a specific use.

We have not dwelt on pharmaceutical manipulations, i.e., formulation, as a means, for example, of shortening latency, decreasing toxicity, or increasing the duration of action of local anesthetic agents. It is well-known that certain attempts at modifying the behaviour of a local anesthetic agent by means of the vehicle produced some tragic consequences (383, 384), and it may be for this reason that, except for a flurry of activity stimulated by the properties of dimethyl sulfoxide (385), this area has received so little attention. Nevertheless, it remains an approach that might be extremely fruitful in certain areas of anesthesiology, for example as we have discussed in Section 5.2.3, topical anesthesia.

The effects of carbon dioxide on solutions of local anesthetic agents have been known for some time (386), and carbonated solutions of several of these agents have been studied *in vitro* (387, 388) and in the clinic (389–393). There seems little doubt that a potentiating effect can be demonstrated *in vitro*; shorter latency and improved blocks have been claimed for carbonated solutions used in the clinic for peripheral and central neural blocks. Carbonated solutions of lidocaine and bupivacaine are commercially available,

and the place of carbonated solutions of local anesthetic agents in anesthesiology may be established within the next few years.

Although the use of mixtures of local anesthetic agents is sound, if properly formulated, the practice has never been widespread, and for a number of reasons, mixtures of local anesthetic agents are not commerically available. Anesthesiologists who wish to administer simultanesously an agent that has a rapid onset and a short duration and another that has a slow onset and a long duration must either have such mixtures prepared for them or must prepare the mixtures themselves (394). If one keeps in mind that the onset of block is that of the agent with the shorter latency, the duration is that of the agent with the longer duration, and the toxicities are additive, the use of such mixtures is rational and will almost certainly continue to find proponents while the search for improved agents continues.

The remarkable substances STX and TTX offer a new approach to the chemistry of agents capable of producing reversible block of nerve conduction. Adams et al. have demonstrated that mixtures of either of these blocking agents with a conventional local anesthetic agent can produce reversible blocks of rapid onset and extremely long duration (64, 65). Certainly, even if these two substances never become clinically acceptable, their structures may provide synthetic chemists with a whole new approach to the synthesis of clinically useful agents for nerve block.

There is no question that in the past 10 years there have been tremendous advances in the elucidation of the mechanisms of action of agents that block propagated impulses, our understanding of the structure of the nerve membrane, and the delineation of the topography of the sodium channel. In fact, the strides made in these areas far outstrip the advances made in the introduction of new and better local anesthetic agents. However, the knowledge gained in this interval may well serve as the foundation for a whole new era of synthetic chemistry in the field of local anesthetic agents.

REFERENCES

1. G. R. Strichartz, "The Composition and Structure of Excitable Nerve Membrane," in *Mammalian Cell Membranes*, Vol. 3, G. A. Jamieson and O. H. Robinson, Eds., Butterworth, Woburn, Mass., 1977.

2. E. Meymaris, *Brit. J. Anaesth.*, **47**, 164 (1975).

3. G. Weissmann and R. Claiborne, Eds., *Cell Membranes: Biochemistry, Cell Biology and Pathology*, HP Publishing Co., New York, 1975.

4. H. H. Meyer, "The Theory of Narcosis," *Harvey Lect.*, *1905–1906, pp.* 11–17.

5. D. J. Aidley, *The Physiology of Excitable Cells*, University Press, Cambridge, 1971.

6. B. G. Covino and H. G. Vassallo, *Local Anesthetics: Mechanisms of Action and Clinical Use*, Grune and Stratton, New York, 1976.

7. R. H. de Jong, *Local Anesthetics*, 2nd ed., Charles C Thomas, Springfield, Ill., 1977.

8. B. Hille, "Ionic Basis of Resting and Action Potentials," in *Handbook of Physiology—The Nervous System*, Vol. 1, American Physiology Society, Bethesda, Md., 1977, p. 99.

9. W. Ulbricht, *Biophys. Struct. Mech.*, **1,** 1 (1974).

10. C. M. Armstrong, *Quart. Rev. Biophys.*, **7,** 179 (1975).

11. B. Hille, *J. Gen. Physiol.*, **69,** 475 (1977).

12. B. Hille, *J. Gen. Physiol.*, **69,** 497 (1977).

13. G. Strichartz, *Anesthesiology*, **45,** 421 (1976).

14. J. R. Smythies, F. Benington, R. J. Bradley, W. F. Bridgers, and R. D. Morin, *J. Theor. Biol.*, **43,** 29 (1974).

15. B. H. Takman, *Brit. J. Anaesth.*, **47,** 183 (1975).

16. B. Hille, *Biophys. J.*, **15,** 615 (1975).

17. G. Strichartz, *J. Gen. Physiol.*, **62,** 37 (1973).

18. K. R. Courtney, *J. Pharmacol. Exp. Ther.*, **195,** 225 (1975).

19. T. Narahashi, *Physiol. Rev.*, **54,** 813 (1974).

20. T. Tokuyama, J. Daly, and B. Witkop, *J. Am. Chem. Soc.*, **91,** 3931 (1969).

21. R. Imhof, E. Gössinger, W. Graf, L. Berner-Fenz, H. Berner, R. Schaufelberger, and H. Werli, *Helv. Chim. Acta*, **56,** 139 (1973).

22. E. X. Albuquerque, I. Seyama, and T. Narahashi, *J. Pharmacol. Exp. Ther.*, **184,** 308 (1973).

23. T. Narahashi, E. X. Albuquerque, and T. Deguchi, *J. Gen. Physiol.*, **58,** 54 (1971).

24. H. J. Adams, A. R. Mastri, D. Doherty, Jr. and D. Charron, *Pharmacol. Res. Commun.*, **10,** 719 (1978).

25. B. I. Khodorov, E. M. Peganov, S. V. Revenko, and L. D. Shishkova, *Brain Res.*, **84,** 541 (1975).

26. H. Kakisawa, T. Kozima, M. Yanai, and K. Nakanishi, *Tetrahedron*, **21,** 3091 (1965).

27. Z. Kumazawa and R. Iriye, *Tetrahedron Lett.*, **1970,** 927.

28. D. Narayanan, M. Röhrl, K. Zechmeister, and W. Hoppe, *Tetrahedron Lett.*, **1970,** 3943.

29. N. Hamanaka and T. Matsumoto, *Tetrahedron Lett.*, **1972,** 3087.

30. S. Gasa, N. Hamanaka, S. Matsunaga, T. Okuno, N. Takeda, and T. Matsumoto, *Tetrahedron Lett.*, **1976,** 553.

31. I. Seyama and T. Narahashi, *J. Pharmacol. Exp. Ther.*, **184,** 299 (1973).

32. S. M. Kupchan and A. W. By, "Steroid Alkaloids: The Veratrum Group," in R. H. F. Manske, Ed., *The Alkaloids, Chemistry and Physiology*, Vol. **10,** Academic, New York, 1968, p. 193.

33. W. Ulbricht, *Ergeb. Physiol. Biol. Chem. Exp. Pharmakol.*, **61,** 18 (1969).

34. M. Ohta, T. Narahashi, and R. F. Keeler, *J. Pharmacol. Exp. Ther.*, **184,** 143 (1973).

35. P. Honerjäger, *Naunyn-Schmiedeberg's Arch. Pharmacol.*, **280,** 391 (1973).

36. M. Lebeaux, *Lab. Animal Sci.*, **25,** 629 (1975).

37. C. Y. Kao, *Pharmacol. Rev.*, **18,** 997 (1966).

38. T. Noguchi and Y. Hashimoto, *Toxicon*, **11,** 305 (1973).

39. H. S. Mosher, F. A. Fuhrman, H. D. Buchwald, and H. G. Fischer, *Science*, **144,** 1100 (1964).

40. Y. H. Kim, G. B. Brown, H. S. Mosher, and F. A. Fuhrman, *Science*, **189,** 151 (1975).

41. D. D. Sheumack, M. E. H. Howden, I. Spence, and R. J. Quinn, *Science*, **199,** 188 (1978).

42. R. B. Woodward, *Pure Appl. Chem.*, **9,** 49 (1964).

43. R. B. Woodward and J. Z. Gougoutas, *J. Am. Chem. Soc.*, **86,** 5030 (1964).

44. Y. Kishi, F. Nakatsubo, M. Aratani, T. Goto, S.

Inoue, H. Kakoi, and S. Sugiura, *Tetrahedron Lett.*, **1970**, 5127.

45. Y. Kishi, F. Nakatsubo, M. Aratani, S. Inoue, and H. Kakoi, *Tetrahedron Lett.* **1970**, 5129.

46. Y. Kishi, M. Aratani, T. Fukuyama, F. Nakatsubo, T. Goto, S. Inoue, H. Tanino, S. Sigiura, and H. Kakoi, *J. Am. Chem. Soc.*, **94**, 9217 (1972).

47. Y. Kishi, T. Fukuyama, M. Aratani, F. Nakatsubo, T. Goto, S. Inoue, H. Tanino, S. Sugiura, and H. Kakoi, *J. Am. Chem. Soc.*, **94**, 9219 (1972).

48. M. H. Evans, *Int. Rev. Neurobiol.*, **15**, 83 (1972).

49. E. J. Schantz, V. E. Ghazarossian, H. K. Schnoes, F. M. Strong, J. P. Springer, J. O. Pezzanite, and J. Clardy; *J. Am. Chem. Soc.*, **97**, 1238 (1975).

50. H. Tanino, T. Nakata, T. Kaneko, and Y. Kishi, *J. Am. Chem. Soc.*, **99**, 2818 (1977).

51. (a) T. Goto, Y. Kishi, S. Takahashi, and Y. Hirata, *Tetrahedron*, 21, 2059 (1965). (b) J. Bordner, W. E. Thiessen, H. A. Bates, and H. Rapoport, *J. Am. Chem. Soc.*, **97**, 6008 (1975).

52. T. Narahashi, *Fed. Proc.*, **31**, 1124 (1972).

53. T. Narahashi, N. C. Anderson, and J. W. Moore, *Science*, **153**, 765 (1966).

54. E. Koppenhöffer and W. Vogel, *Eur. J. Physiol.*, **313**, 361 (1969).

55. D. Colquhoun, R. Henderson, and J. M. Ritchie, *J. Physiol.* (London), **227**, 95 (1972).

56. J. M. Ritchie, *Phil. Trans. R. Soc. London. Ser. B*, **270**, 319 (1975).

57. J. R. Schwartz, W. Ulbricht, and H. H. Wagner, *J. Physiol.* (London), **233**, 167 (1973).

58. L. Gyermek, *Nature*, **171**, 788 (1953).

59. K. Nador, F. Herr, G. Pataky, and J. Borsy, *Nature*, **171**, 788 (1953).

60. V. Hach and Z. Horáková, *Experientia*, **12**, 112 (1956).

61. Z. Horáková and V. Hach, *Česk. Farm.*, **6**, 36 (1957).

62. D. T. Frazier, T. Narahashi, and M. Yamada, *J. Pharmacol. Exp. Ther.*, **171**, 45 (1970).

63. W. E. Kirkpatrick and P. Lomax, *Res. Commun. Chem. Pathol. Pharmacol.*, **1**, 149 (1970).

64. H. J. Adams, M. R. Blair, Jr., and B. H. Takman, *Anesth. Analg.*, **55**, 568 (1976).

65. H. J. Adams, M. R. Blair, Jr., and B. H. Takman, *Arch. Int. Pharmacodyn. Ther.*, **224**, 275 (1976).

66. A. Albert and E. P. Serjeant, *The Determination of Ionization Constants*, 2nd ed., Chapman and Hall, London, 1971.

67. C. Köller, Lancet, **1884-II**, 990; *Wien. Med. Bl.*, **7**, 1224, 1352 (1884).

68. G. Liljestrand, "The Historical Development of Local Anesthesia", in *Int. Encycl. Pharmacol. Ther.*, Sect. 8, *Local Anesthetics*, Vol. I, P. Lechat, Ed., Pergamon, Oxford, 1971, p. 1

69. Johnston, *Chem. Gaz.*, **11**, 438 (1853).

70. H. Wackenroder, *Arch. Pharm.*, **125**, 23 (1853).

71. F. Gaedcke, *Arch. Pharm.*, **132**, 141 (1855).

72. A. Niemann, *Vierteljahresschr. Prakt. Pharm.*, **9**, 489 (1860); *Arch. Pharm.*, **153**, 129, 291 (1860).

73. R. Willstätter and W. Müller, *Chem. Ber.*, **31**, 2655 (1898).

74. G. Fodor, in *The Alkaloids*, Vol. VI, R. H. F. Manske, Ed., Academic, New York, 1960, p. 145.

75. W. Merck, *Chem. Ber.*, **18**, 2952 (1885).

76. A. Einhorn, *Chem. Ber.*, **21**, 3029, 3441 (1888).

77. A. Einhorn and O. Klein, *Chem. Ber.*, **21**, 3335 (1888).

78. C. Liebermann, *Chem. Ber.*, **22**, 130 (1889).

79. C. Liebermann, *Chem. Ber.*, **21**, 2342 (1888).

80. C. Liebermann, *Chem. Ber.*, **22**, 2240 (1889).

81. C. Liebermann, *Chem. Ber.*, **21**, 3372 (1888).

82. C. Liebermann, *Chem. Ber.*, **22**, 2661 (1889).

83. B. H. Paul and A. J. Cownley, *Pharm. J.*, [3], **20**, 166 (1889–1890).

84. C. Liebermann, *Chem. Ber.*, **24**, 2336 (1891).

85. A. P. Chadbourne, *Brit. Med. J.*, **11**, 402 (1892).

86. A. Einhorn and A. Marquardt, *Chem. Ber.*, **23**, 468, 979 (1890).

87. C. Liebermann and F. Giesel, *Chem. Ber.*, **23**, 508 (1890).

88. R. Willstättter, *Münch. Med. Wochenschr.*, **71**, 849 (1924).

89. R. Gottlieb, *Münch. Med. Wochenschr.*, **71**, 850 (1924).

90. Chem. Fabrik Schering, Ger. Pat. 90,245 (1895); *Chem. Zentralbl.*, **68-I**, 1111 (1897).

91. G. Merling, *Ber. Deut. Pharm. Ges.*, **6**, 173 (1896).

92. G. Vinci, *Berl. Klin. Wochenschr.*, **33**, 605 (1896); *Arch. Pathol. Anat. Physiol.*, **145**, 78 (1896).

93. G. Vinci, *Arch. Pathol. Anat. Physiol.*, **149**, 217 (1897).

94. E. Fourneau, *Compt. Rend.*, **138**, 766 (1904).

95. H. Braun, *Deut. Med. Wochenschr.*, **31**, 1667 (1905).

96. E. Impens, *Arch. Gesamte Physiol. Menschen Tiere*, **110,** 21 (1905).

97. A. Einhorn and E. Uhlfelder, *Ann. Chem.*, **371,** 131 (1909).

98. H. Braun, *Arch. Klin. Chir.*, **69,** 541 (1903).

99. H. Braun, *Muench. Med. Wochenschr.*, **50,** 352 (1903).

100. T. P. Carney, "Benzoates and Substituted Benzoates as Local Anesthetics," in *Medicinal Chemistry*, Vol. I, C. M. Suter, Ed., Wiley, New York, 1951, p. 280.

101. S. Wiedling and C. Tegnér, *Progr. Med. Chem.*, **3,** 332 (1963).

102. A. Einhorn, K. Fiedler, C. Ladisch, and E. Uhlfelder, *Ann. Chem.*, **371,** 142 (1909).

103. H. L. Schmitz and A. S. Loevenhart, *J. Pharmacol. Exp. Ther.*, **24,** 159, 167 (1924–1925).

104. O. Kamm, R. Adams, and E. H. Volwiler, U.S. Pat. 1,358,751 (1920); through *Chem. Abstr.*, **15,** 412 (1921).

105. W. B. Burnett, R. L. Jenkins, C. H. Peet, E. E. Dreger, and R. Adams, *J. Am. Chem. Soc.*, **59,** 2248 (1937).

106 M. L. Bonar and T. Sollmann, *J. Pharmacol. Exp. Ther.*, **18,** 467 (1921).

107. W. Schulemann, L. Schütz, and K. Meisenburg, U.S. Pat. 1,474,567 (1923); through *Chem. Abstr.*, **18,** 569 (1924).

108. W. Schulemann, *Klin. Wochenschr.*, **3,** 676 (1924).

109. C. Mannich, B. Lesser, and F. Silten, *Chem. Ber.*, **65,** 378 (1932).

110. K. Fromherz, *Naunyn-Schmiedebergs Arch. Exp. Pathol. Pharmakol.*, **158,** 368 (1930).

111. S. D. Goldberg and W. F. Whitmore, *J. Am. Chem. Soc.*, **59,** 2280 (1937).

112. D. I. Abramson and S. D. Goldberg, *J. Pharmacol. Exp. Ther.*, **62,** 69 (1938).

113. S. Kuna and A. O. Seeler, *J. Pharmacol. Exp. Ther.*, **90,** 181 (1947).

114. P. Karrer, E. Horlacher, F. Locher, and M. Giesler, *Helv. Chim. Acta*, **6,** 905 (1923).

115. O. Winterstein, *Muench. Med. Wochenschr.*, **74,** 1746 (1927).

116. E. Rothlin, *Naunyn-Schmiedebergs Arch. Exp. Pathol. Pharmakol.*, **144,** 197 (1929).

117. W. F. Ringk and E. Epstein, *J. Am. Chem. Soc.*, **65,** 1222 (1943).

118. F. W. Co Tui, A. Preiss, M. I. Nevin, and I. Barcham, *Curr. Res. Anesth. Analg.*, **22,** 301 (1943).

119. I. G. Farbenindustrie A.-G., Ger. Pat. 582,715 (1933); through *Chem. Abstr.*, **28,** 778 (1934).

120. R. Fussgänger and O. Schaumann, *Naunyn-Schmiedebergs Arch. Exp. Pathol. Pharmakol.*, **160,** 53 (1931).

121. S. M. McElvain, *J. Am. Chem. Soc.*, **49,** 2835 (1927).

122. K. H. Beyer, A. R. Latven, W. A. Freyburger, and M. P. Parker, *J. Pharmacol. Exp. Ther.*, **93,** 388 (1948).

123. E. M. Hancock and A. C. Cope, *J. Am. Chem. Soc.*, **66,** 1738 (1944).

124. J. R. Reasenberg, U.S. Pat. 2,767,207 (1956); through *Chem. Abstr.*, **51,** 5831 (1957).

125. A. P. Truant, *Arch. Int. Pharmacodyn.*, **115,** 483 (1958).

126. J. R. Reasenberg and S. D. Goldberg, *J. Am. Chem. Soc.*, **67,** 933 (1945).

127. J. Adriani, R. Zepernick, J. Arens, and E. Authement, *Clin. Pharmacol. Ther.*, **5,** 49 (1964).

128. H. C. Marks and M. I. Rubin, U.S. Pat. 2,460,139 (1949); through *Chem. Abstr.*, **44,** 5390 (1950).

129. F. F. Foldes and P. G. McNall, *Anesthesiology*, **13,** 287 (1952).

130. F. F. Foldes, D. S. Davis, S. Shanor, and G. Van Hees, *J. Am. Chem. Soc.*, **77,** 5149 (1955).

131. A. Wander A.-G., Swiss Pat. 265,343 (1950); through *Chem. Abstr.*, **44,** 9480 (1950).

132. H. E. Schlegel and K. C. Swan, *Arch. Ophthalmol.* (Chicago), **51,** 663 (1954).

133. R. O. Clinton, U. J. Salvador, S. C. Laskowski, and M. Wilson, *J. Am. Chem. Soc.*, **74,** 592 (1952).

134. F. P. Luduena, *Anesthesiology*, **16,** 751 (1955).

135. O. B. Crawford, *Anesthesiology*, **14,** 278 (1953).

136. A. Wander A.-G., Swiss Pat. 270,986 (1950); through *Chem. Abstr.*, **46,** 2578 (1952).

137. W. Grimme and H. Schmitz, *Chem. Ber.*, **84,** 734 (1951).

138. W. Keil and E. Rademacher, *Arzneim.-Forsch.*, **1,** 154 (1951); W. Keil and H. H. Bräutigam, *ibid.*, **1,** 270 (1951).

139. W. Keil and E. Rademacher, *Arzneim.-Forsch.*, **1,** 218 (1951).

140. D. H. MacDonald, *Dent., Items Interest*, **73,** 1074 (1951).

141. E. Epstein and M. Meyer, *J. Am. Chem. Soc.*, **77,** 4059 (1955).

142. W. S. Kramer, *J. Am. Dent. Assoc.*, **56,** 820 (1958).

143. A. R. McIntyre and R. F. Sievers, *J. Pharmacol. Exp. Ther.*, **63,** 369 (1938).

144. L. A. Walter and R. J. Fosbinder, *J. Am. Chem. Soc.*, **61**, 1713 (1939).

145. W. H. Hunt and R. J. Fosbinder, *Anesthesiology*, **1**, 305 (1940).

146. C. Rohmann and B. Scheurle, *Arch. Pharm. Ber. Deut. Pharm. Ges.*, **274**, 110 (1936).

147. A. R. McIntyre and R. F. Sievers, *J. Pharmacol. Exp. Ther.*, **61**, 107 (1937).

148. R. S. Sappenfield and E. A. Rovenstine, *Anesth. Analg., Curr. Res.* **19**, 48 (1940).

149. S. M. McElvain and T. P. Carney, *J. Am. Chem. Soc.*, **68**, 2592 (1946).

150. C. L. Rose, T. P. Carney, K. K. Chen, and S. M. McElvain, *Anesthesiology*, **9**, 373 (1948).

151. K. Kuwahata, A. Ochiai, and Y. Nukita, *Folia Pharmacol.* Japon., **7**, 408 (1928); through *Chem. Abstr.*, **23**, 5236 (1929).

152. R. P. Perry, D. C. Jones, and C. Pratt, *J. Am. Chem. Soc.*, **78**, 3403 (1956).

153. J. T. Bryan and P. A. Foote, *J. Am. Pharm. Assoc., Sci. Ed.*, **39**, 644 (1950).

154. M. B. Moore, *J. Am. Pharm. Assoc., Sci. Ed.*, **40**, 388 (1951).

155. W. G. Christiansen and A. W. Harvey, U.S. Pat. 1,976,922 (1934); through *Chem. Abstr.*, **28**, 7429 (1934).

156. M. Sahyun, U.S. Pat. 2,594,350 (1952); through *Chem. Abstr.*, **47**, 1190 (1953).

157. E. A. Wildman and L. Thorp, U.S. Pat. 1,193,649 (1916); through *Chem. Abstr.*, **10**, 2387 (1916).

158. H. C. Brill and C. F. Cook, *J. Am. Chem. Soc.*, **55**, 2062 (1933).

159. A. D. Bevan, *Surg. Clin.* (Chicago), **1**, 21 (1917).

160. T. Sollmann, *J. Pharmacol. Exp. Ther.*, **11**, 69 (1918).

161. W. R. Meeker and E. B. Frazer, *J. Pharmacol. Exp. Ther.*, **22**, 375 (1924).

162. S. I. Sergievskaya and V. V. Nesvad'ba, *Zh. Obsh. Khim.*, **8**, 924 (1938); through *Chem. Abstr.*, **33**, 1307 (1939).

163. F. F. Blicke and H. C. Parke, *J. Am. Chem. Soc.*, **61**, 1200 (1939).

164. L. W. Rowe, *J. Am. Pharm. Assoc., Sci. Ed.*, **29**, 241 (1940).

165. V. G. Haury, C. M. Gruber, and M. E. Drake, *J. Pharmacol. Exp. Ther.*, **70**, 315 (1940).

166. G. M. Sieger, W. M. Ziegler, D. X. Klein, and H. Sokol, *J. Am. Pharm. Assoc., Sci. Ed.*, **47**, 734 (1958).

167. M. E Fisk and F. P. Underhill, *J. Pharmacol. Exp. Ther.*, **49**, 329 (1933).

168. D. J. Graubard, L. Breidenbach, A. Alpin, and H. Soroff, *N.Y. State J. Med.*, **52**, 1909 (1952).

169. H. L. Hansen and L. S. Fosdick, *J. Am. Chem. Soc.*, **55**, 2872 (1933).

170. N. F. Albertson and R. O. Clinton, *J. Am. Chem. Soc.*, **67**, 1222 (1945).

171. L. S. Fosdick and H. L. Hansen, *J. Pharmacol. Exp. Ther.*, **50**, 323 (1934).

172. Farbwerke Hoechst A.-G., Brit. Pat. 717,516 (1954); through *Chem. Abstr.*, **49**, 13291 (1955).

173. H. J. Küchle, *Muench. Med. Wochenschr.*, **96**, 689 (1954).

174. N. Rabjohn, J. W. Fronaberger, and W. W. Lindstromberg, *J. Org. Chem.*, **20**, 271 (1955).

175. E. Honkanen, *Ann. Acad. Sci. Fenn. Ser.* A2, **99**, 1 (1960).

176. W. N. Nagai, U.S. Pat. 1,399,312 (1921); through *Chem. Abstr.*, **16**, 990 (1922).

177. S. Kubota, *J. Pharmacol. Exp. Ther.*, **12**, 361 (1918–1919).

178. R. Hill and G. Powell, *J. Am. Chem. Soc.*, **66**, 742 (1944).

179. R. L. Osborne, *Science*, **85**, 105 (1937).

180. S. L. Shapiro, H. Soloway, E. Chodos, and L. Freedman, *J. Am. Chem. Soc.*, **81**, 203 (1959).

181. G. A. Alles and P. K. Knoefel, *Arch. Int. Pharmacodyn.*, **47**, 96 (1934).

182. E. W. Ferber, *J. Am. Dent. Assoc.*, **23**, 788 (1936).

183. A. Einhorn and M. Oppenheimer, *Ann. Chem.*, **311**, 154 (1900).

184. *H. von Euler and H. Erdtman, Ann. Chem.*, **520**, 1 (1935).

185. H. Erdtman and N. Löfgren, *Sven. Kem. Tidskr.*, **49**, 163 (1937).

186. N. Löfgren, *Ark. Kemi Mineral. Geol.*, **22A**:18 (1946).

187. N. Löfgren, *Studies on Local Anesthetics. Xylocaine, a New Synthetic Drug*, Haeggströms, Stockholm, 1948.

188. S. Wiedling, *Xylocaine: The Pharmacological Basis of Its Clinical Use*, 2nd ed., Almqvist and Wiksell, Stockholm, 1964.

189. K. Bullock and J. Grundy, *J. Pharm. Pharmacol.*, **7**, 755 (1955).

190. A. Sekera, J. Sova, and Č. Vrba, *Experientia*, **11**, 275 (1955).

191. G. Haglund and W. A. Conroy, *Ill. Med. J.*, **99**, 132 (1951).

192. J. E. Davis, J. C. Frudenfeld, K. Frudenfeld, J. H. Frudenfeld, and A. N. Webb, *Am. J. Obstet. Gynecol.*, **89**, 366 (1964).

193. P. F. Kandel, W. E. Spoerel, and R. A. H. Kinch, *Can. Med. Assoc. J.*, **95,** 947 (1966).

194. L. Goldberg, *Acta Physiol. Scand.*, **18,** 1 (1949).

195. N. Löfgren and C. Tegnér, *Acta Chem. Scand.*, **14,** 486 (1960).

196. S. Wiedling, Ed., *Citanest*®, *Acta Anaesthesiol. Scand. Suppl.*, **16** (1965).

197. Farbenfabriken Bayer A.-G., Ger. Pat. 1,010,526 (1957); through *Chem. Abstr.*, **54,** 410 (1960).

198. Anon., *Dent. Echo Berlin*, **23,** 33 (1957); cited in Ref. 101.

199. Cilag Ltd., Brit. Pat. 726,080 (1955); through *Chem. Abstr.*, **50,** 4210 (1956).

200. L. Ther, *Naunyn–Schmiedebergs Arch. Exp. Pathol. Pharmakol.*, **220,** 300 (1953).

201. N. Löfgren, C. Tegnér, and B. Takman, *Acta Chem. Scand.*, **11,** 1724 (1957).

202. A. Schlesinger and S. Gordon, U.S. Pat. 2,813,861 (1957); through *Chem. Abstr.*, **52,** 10222 (1958).

203. P. P. Koelzer and K. H. Wehr, *Arzneim.-Forsch.*, **8,** 270 (1958).

204. R. Hiltmann, F. Mietzsch, and W. Wirth, U.S. Pat. 2,921,077 (1960); through *Chem. Abstr.*, **54,** 17326 (1960).

205. G. Björlin, *Odontol. Revy*, **14,** 32 (1963); through *Chem. Abstr.*, **59,** 15830 (1963).

206. E. Hofstetter, *Nature*, **170,** 980 (1952).

207. A. E. Wilder Smith and E. Hofstetter, *Helv. Chim. Acta*, **38,** 1085 (1955).

208. T. Takada, M. Tada, and A. Kiyomoto, *Nippon Yakurigaku Zasshi*, **62,** 64 (1966); through *Chem. Abstr.*, **67,** 72325 (1967).

209. F. Reynolds, T. H. L. Bryson, and A. D. G. Nicholas, *Brit. J. Anaesth.*, **48,** 347 (1976).

210. H. J. Adams, G. H. Kronberg, and B. H. Takman, *J. Pharm. Sci.*, **61,** 1829 (1972).

211. B. af Ekenstam, B. Egnér, and G. Pettersson, *Acta Chem. Scand.*, **11,** 1183 (1957).

212. H. R. Ulfendahl, *Acta Anaesthesiol. Scand.*, **1,** 81 (1957).

213. M. Sadove and G. D. Wessinger, *J. Int. Coll. Surg.*, **34,** 573 (1960).

214. F. Henn and R. Brattsand, *Acta Anaesthesiol. Scand. Suppl.*, **21,** 9 (1966).

215. W. F. M. van Bever, A. G. Knaeps, J. J. M. Willems, B. K. F. Hermans, and P. A. J. Janssen, *J. Med. Chem.*, **16,** 394 (1973).

216. K. Miescher, *Helv. Chim. Acta*, **15,** 163 (1932).

217. W. Lipschitz and W. Laubender, *Klin. Wochenschr.*, **8,** 1438 (1929).

218. M. E. Freed, W. F. Bruce, R. S. Hanslick, and A. Mascitti, *J. Org. Chem.*, **26,** 2378 (1961).

219. D. H. Beader, J. M. Glassman, G. M. Hudyma, and J. Seifter, *Proc. Soc. Exp. Biol. Med.*, **89,** 645 (1955).

220. J. M. Glassman, G. M. Hudyma, and J. Seifter, *J. Pharmacol. Exp. Ther.*, **119,** 150 (1957).

221. O. Gros. *Arch. Exp. Pathol. Pharmakol.*, **62,** 380 (1909–1910).

222. T. H. Rider, *J. Am. Chem. Soc.*, **52,** 2115 (1930).

223. T. H. Rider, *J. Pharmacol. Exp. Ther.*, **47,** 255 (1933).

224. G. F. McKim, P. G. Smith, T. W. Rush, and T. H. Rider, *J. Urol.*, **29,** 277 (1933).

225. A. W. Weston, R. W. DeNet, and R. J. Michaels, Jr., *J. Am. Chem. Soc.*, **75,** 4006 (1953).

226. P. K. Knoefel, *J. Pharmacol. Exp. Ther.*, **47,** 69 (1933).

227. N. Rabjohn, T. R. Hopkins, and R. C. Nagler, *J. Am. Chem. Soc.*, **74,** 3215 (1952).

228. G. C. Rau and B. A. Westfall, *J. Pharmacol. Exp. Ther.*, **99,** 421, (1950).

229. J. L. G. Nilsson, H. Sievertsson, R. Dahlbom, and B. Åkerman, *J. Med. Chem.*, **14,** 710 (1971).

230. J. W. Wilson, III, N. D. Dawson, W. Brooks, and G. E. Ullyot, *J. Am. Chem. Soc.*, **71,** 937 (1949).

231. H. B. Wright and M. B. Moore, *J. Am. Chem. Soc.*, **76,** 4396 (1954).

232. J. L. Schmidt, L. E. Blockus, and R. K. Richards, *Anesth. Analg., Curr. Res.*, **32,** 418 (1953).

233. E. J. Fellows and E. Macko, *J. Pharmacol. Exp. Ther.*, **103,** 306 (1951).

234. H. Oelschläger, O. Nieschulz, F. Meyer, and K. H. Schulz, *Arzneim. Forsch.*, **18,** 729 (1968).

235. B. Hermans, H. Verhoeven, and P. Janssen, *J. Med. Chem.*, **13,** 835 (1970).

236. P. Da Re and I. Setnikar, *Experientia*, **20,** 607 (1964).

237. B. Åkerman, *Acta Anaesth. Scand., Suppl. 70*, **90,** 1978.

238. L.-O. Pettersson, *Läkartidningen*, **72,** 2822 (1975).

239. B. Pontén and L. Ohlsén, *Brit. J. Plast. Surg.*, **30,** 251 (1977).

240. E. Ferrero, A. Giudice, V. Guzon, *Boll. Chim. Farm.*, **110,** 330 (1971); through *Chem. Abstr.*, **76,** 30561 (1972).

241. E. Ferrero, L. Manzoni, L. Dall'Asta, and A. Pedrazolli, *Arzneim.-Forsch.*, **23**, 1596 (1973).

242. E. Profft, *Chem. Tech.* (Berlin), **3**, 210 (1951).

243. E. Profft, *Chem. Tech.* (Berlin), **4**, 241 (1952).

244. B. E. Abreu, A. B. Richards, L. C. Weaver, G. R. Burch, C. A. Burch, C. A. Bunde, E. R. Bockstahler, and D. L. Wright, *J. Pharmacol. Exp. Ther.*, **115**, 419 (1955).

245. R. B. Arora and V. N. Sharma, *J. Pharmacol. Exp. Ther.*, **115**, 413 (1955).

246. E. Täuber, Ger. Pat. 79,868 (1894); *Chem. Zentralbl.*, **66-I**, 1048, (1895).

247. G. Gutmann, *Deut. Med. Wochenschr.*, **23**, 165 (1897).

248. Chem. Fabrik v. Heyden, Ger. Pat. 104,361 (1899); *Chem. Zentralbl.* **70-II**, 950 (1899).

249. P. Trolldenier, *Ther. Monatsh.*, **13**, 36 (1899); *Z. Thiermed.*, **5**, 81 (1901).

249a. E. J. Fellows, *J. Pharmacol. Exp. Ther.*, **90**, 351 (1947).

249b. E. B. Leffler, H. M. Spencer, and A. Burger, *J. Am. Chem. Soc.*, **73**, 2611 (1951).

249c. A. N. Grinev, A. A. Stolyarchuk, P. A. Galenko-Yaroshevskii, V. S. Tansyura, and N. V. Archangel'skaya., Ger. Pat., 2,417,638 (1974); through *Chem. Abstr.*, **83**, 28088 (1975).

249d. A. Den Hertog, *Eur. J. Pharmacol.*, **26**, 175 (1974).

249e. A. Einhorn and R. Heinz., *Muench. Med. Wochenschr.*, **44**, 931 (1897).

249f. A. Einhorn, *Ann. Chem.*, **311**, 26 (1900).

249g. A. Einhorn and B. Pfyl, *Ann. Chem.*, **311**, 34 (1900).

249h. E. Ritsert, *Pharm. Ztg.*, **70**, 1006 (1925).

249i. Anon., *Pharm. Ztg.* **37**, 427 (1892); **47**, 356 (1902).

249j. E. Ritsert, Ger. Pat. 147,790 (1903); *Chem. Zentralbl.*, **71-I**, 131 (1904).

250. C. von Noorden, *Berl. Klin. Wochenschr.*, **39**, 373 (1902).

251. H. Salkowski, *Chem. Ber.*, **28**, 1917 (1895).

252. H. Surmont and J. Tipres, *Schweiz, Apoth. Ztg.*, **62**, 376 (1924).

253. Anon., *Pharm. Ztg.*, **53**, 817 (1908).

254. Z. Rappoport, Ed., *Handbook of Organic Compound Identification*, 3rd ed., Chemical Rubber Co., Cleveland, 1967, p. 438.

255. J. Z. Yeh and T. Narahashi, *Fed. Proc.*, **35**, 846 (1976).

256. R. M. Acheson, "Acridines," in *The Chemistry of Heterocyclic Compounds*, A. Weissberger, Ed., Interscience, New York, 1956, p. 84.

257. M. Cahalan, *Biophys. J.*, **23**, 285 (1978).

258. W. Pirrie, *Lancet*, **1867-II**, 575.

259. J. H. Bill, *Am. J. Med. Sci.*, **60**, 573 (1870).

260. A. H. Smith, *Med. Rec.*, **7**, 231 (1872).

261. J. Lucas-Championniere, *Bull. Acad. Med.* (Paris), [3] **34**, 146 (1895).

262. Z. von Vamossy, *Deut. Med. Wochenschr.*, **23**, *Ther. Beil.*, 58 (1897).

263. D. I. Macht, *J. Pharmacol. Exp. Ther.*, **11**, 263 (1918).

264. A. M. Hjort and J. T. Eagan, *J. Pharmacol. Exp. Ther.*, **14**, 211 (1919–1920).

265. A. D. Hirschfelder, A. Lundholm, and H. Norrgard, *J. Pharmacol. Exp. Ther.*, **15**, 261 (1920).

266. K. Soehring, *Naunyn-Schmiedebergs Arch. Exp. Pathol. Pharmakol.*, **212**, 129 (1950–1951).

267. H. J. Meyer and H. U. May, *Klin. Wochenschr.*, **42**, 407 (1964).

268. H. U. May and H. J. Meyer, *Naunyn-Schmiedebergs Arch. Exp. Pathol. Pharmakol.*, **250**, 273 (1965).

269. B. Hille, *Fed. Proc.*, **34**, 1318 (1975).

270. R. Henderson, J. M. Ritchie, and G. Strichartz, *J. Physiol.* (London), **235**, 783 (1973); *Proc. Natl. Acad. Sci. U.S.*, **71**, 3936 (1974).

271. B. Hille, *Proc. Natl. Acad. Sci. US.*, **68**, 280 (1971).

272. B. Hille, "Ionic Selectivity of Na and K Channels of Nerve Membranes," in *Membranes—a Series of Advances, Artificial and Biological Membranes*, Vol. 3, G. Eisenman, Ed., Dekker, New York, 1975, p. 225.

273. W. Ulbricht and H.-H. Wagner, *J. Physiol.* (London), **252**, 159 (1975).

274. *Ibid.*, 185 (1975).

275. P. F. Baker and K. A. Rubinson, *Nature*, **257**, 412 (1975).

276. J. S. D'Arrigo, *J. Membrane Biol.*, **29**, 231 (1976).

277. T. Narahashi, M. Yamada, and D. T. Frazier, *Nature*, **233**, 748 (1969).

278. K. R. Courtney, Ph.D. Thesis, University of Washington, Seattle, Wash; University Microfilms, Ann Arbor, Mich., No. 74–29 (1974).

279. J. E. Scurlock, *Reg. Anesth.* **2**, 4 (1977).

280. J. M. Ritchie, *Symp. Anesth. Loc. Anesth. Reanim., Paris, 1973*, p. 53.

281. A. M. Shanes, *Pharmacol. Rev.*, **10**, 165 (1958).

282. P. Seeman, *Progr. Anesthesiol.*, **1**, 243 (1975).

283. P. Seeman, *Pharmacol. Rev.*, **24**, 583 (1972).

284. J. R. Trudell and E. N. Cohen, *Progr. Anesthesiol.*, **1**, 315 (1975).

285. J. R. Trudell, W. L. Hubbell, and E. N. Cohen, *Biochim. Biophys. Acta*, **291**, 328 (1973).

286. P. Seeman, *Experientia*, **30**, 759 (1974).

287. J. J. Kendig and E. N. Cohen, *Anesthesiology*, **47**, 6 (1977).

288. P. Seeman, *Anesthesiology*, **47**, 1 (1977).

289. J. R. Trudell, *Anesthesiology*, **46**, 5 (1977).

290. M. B. Feinstein, *J. Gen. Physiol.*, **48**, 357 (1964).

291. S. McLaughlin, *Progr. Anesthesiol.*, **1**, 193 (1975).

292. D. E. Goldman and M. P. Blaustein, *Ann. N.Y. Acad. Sci.*, **137**, 967 (1966).

293. M. P. Blaustein and D. E. Goldman, *J. Gen. Physiol.*, **49**, 1043 (1966).

294. K. V. Thimann, *Arch. Biochem. Biophys.*, **2**, 87 (1943).

295. E. Bartels and D. Nachmansohn, *Biochem, Z.* **342**, 359 (1965).

296. J. M. Ritchie, "The Mechanism of Action of Local Anesthetic Agents," in *Int. Encycl. Pharmacol., Ther., Local Anesthetics*, Vol. 1, P. Lechat, Ed., Oxford, England, 1971, p. 131.

297. O. Gros, *Arch. Exp. Pathol. Pharmakol.*, **63**, 80 (1910).

298. J. W. Trevan and E. Boock, *Brit. J. Exp. Pathol.*, **8**, 307 (1927).

299. J. C. Skou, *Acta Pharmacol. Toxicol.*, **10**, 281 (1954).

300. M. E. Krahl, A. K. Keltch, and G. H. A. Clowes, *J. Pharmacol. Exp. Ther.*, **68**, 330 (1940).

301. J. M. Ritchie and P. Greengard, *J. Pharmacol., Exp. Ther.*, **133**, 241 (1961).

302. J. M. Ritchie, B. Ritchie, and P. Greengard, *J. Pharmacol. Exp. Ther.*, **150**, 152, 160 (1965).

303. J. M. Ritchie and B. R. Ritchie, *Science*, **162**, 1394 (1968).

304. E. Y. Ariëns and A. M. Simonis, *Arch. Int. Pharmacodyn.*, **141**, 309 (1963).

305. T. Narahashi, D. T. Frazier, and M. Yamada, *J. Pharmacol. Exp. Ther.*, **171**, 32 (1970).

306. T. Narahashi and D. T. Frazier, *Neurosci. Res.*, **4**, 65 (1971).

307. S. B. A. Åkerman, G. Camougis, and R. V. Sandberg, *Eur. J. Pharmacol.*, **8**, 337 (1969).

308. B. Hille, K. Courtney, and R. Dum, "Rate and Site of Action of Local Anesthetics," in B. R. Fink, Ed., *Molecular Mechanisms of Anesthesia*, New York, 1975.

309. A. L. Staiman and P. Seeman, *Can. J. Pharmacol.*, **53**, 513 (1975).

310. H. E. Mrose and J. M. Ritchie, *J. Gen. Physiol.*, **71**, 223 (1978).

311. S. M. Waraszkiewicz, W. O. Foye, H. J. Adams, and B. H. Takman, *J. Med. Chem.*, **19**, 541 (1976).

312. B. Åkerman, *Acta Pharmacol. Toxicol.*, **32**, 97 (1973).

313. H. J. Adams and B. H. Takman, unpublished observations.

314. P. W. Benoit and W. D. Belt, *Exp. Neurol.*, **34**, 264 (1972).

315. H. Radtke, H. Nolte, H. Fruhstorfer, and M. Zenz, *Acta Anaesth. Scand. Suppl.*, **60**, 17 (1975).

316. K. H. Wencker, H. Nolte, and H. Fruhstorfer, *Brit. J. Anaesth.*, **47**, 301 (1975).

317. B. R. Duce, K. Zelechowski, G. Camougis, and E. R. Smith, *Brit. J. Anaesth.*, **41**, 579 (1969).

318. M. I. Lebeaux, *Brit. J. Anaesth.*, **45**, 549 (1973).

319. K. L. Wallis, S. M. Schnider, J. S. Hicks, and H. T. Spivey, *Anesthesiology*, **44**, 481 (1976).

320. H. J. Adams, *Pharmacol. Res. Commun.* **7**, 551 (1975).

321. H. J. Adams and D. D. Doherty, Jr., *Acta Anaesth. Scand.*, **21**, 445 (1977).

322. A. E. Pflug, G. M. Aasheim, and H. A. Beck, *Anesth. Analg. Curr. Res.*, **55**, 489 (1976).

323. M. R. A. Chance and H. Lobstein, *J. Pharmacol. Exp. Ther.*, **82**, 203 (1944).

324. W. R. Jones and L. C. Weaver, *J. Pharm. Sci.*, **52**, 500 (1963).

325. A. Åström and N. H. Persson, *J. Pharmacol. Exp. Ther.*, **132**, 87 (1961).

326. A. H. Campbell, J. A. Stasse, G. H. Lord, and J. E. Willson, *J. Pharm. Sci.*, **57**, 2045 (1968).

327. S. B. A. Åkerman, *Brit. J. Anaesth.*, **47**, 923 (1975).

328. J. Adriani and D. Campbell, *J. Am. Med. Assoc.*, **162**, 1527 (1956).

329. S. S. Chu, K. H. Rah, M. D. Brannan, and J. L. Cohen, *Anesth. Analg. Curr. Res.*, **54**, 438 (1975).

330. J. Adriani and H. Dalili, *Anesth. Analg. Curr. Res.*, **50**, 834 (1971).

331. R. J. Scheuplein and I. H. Blank, *Physiol. Rev.*, **51**, 702 (1971).

332. B. J. Poulsen, "Design of Topical Drug Products: Biopharmaceutics," *Drug Design*, Vol. IV, E. J. Ariëns, Ed., Academic, New York and London, 1973, p. 149.

333. B. Idson, *J. Pharm. Sci.*, **64,** 901 (1975).

334. W. A. Ritschel., *Angew. Chem. Int. Ed.*, **8,** 699 (1969).

335. G. Åberg and G. Adler, *Arzneim.-Forsch.*, **26,** 78 (1976).

336. H. Dalili and J. Adriani, *Clin. Pharmacol. Ther.*, **12,** 913 (1971).

337. F. W. Co Tui, A. L. Preiss, I. Barcham, and M. I. Nevin, *J. Pharmacol. Exp. Ther.*, **81,** 209 (1944).

338. H. J. Adams, A. R. Mastri, A. W. Eicholzer, and G. Kilpatrick, *Anesth. Analg. Curr. Res.*, **53,** 904 (1974).

339. M. R. Boots and S. G. Boots, *J. Pharm. Sci.*, **58,** 553 (1969).

340. M. J. Kornet, and P. A. Thio, *J. Pharm. Sci.*, **58,** 724 (1969).

341. H. J. Adams, G. H. Kronberg, and B. H. Takman, *J. Pharm. Sci.*, **62,** 1677 (1973).

342. M. Morgan and W. J. Russell, *Brit. J. Anaesth.*, **47,** 586 (1975).

343. F. Reynolds, T. H. L. Bryson, and A. D. G. Nichols, *Brit. J. Anaesth.*, **48,** 347 (1976).

344. W. Swerdlow and R. Jones, *Brit. J. Anaesth.*, **42,** 335 (1970).

345. A. Brun, *Acta Anaesth. Scand.*, **3,** 59 (1959).

346. M. D. Sokoll, B. Sonesson, and S. Thesleff, *Eur. J. Pharmacol.*, **4,** 179 (1968).

347. R. Libelius, B. Sonesson, B. A. Stamenovic, and S. Thesleff, *J. Anat.*, **106,** 297 (1970).

348. P. W. Benoit and W. D. Belt, *J. Anat.*, **107,** 547 (1970).

349. J. M. Ritchie and P. J. Cohen, in *The Pharmacological Basis of Therapeutics*, Goodman and Gilman, Eds., Macmillan, 1975, pp. 379.

350. I. H. Wagman, R. H. deJong, and D. A. Prince, *Anesthesiology*, **28,** 155 (1967).

351. R. H. deJong, R. Robles, and R. W. Corbin, *Anesthesiology*, **30,** 19 (1969).

352. W. E. Dixon, *J. Physiol.*, **32,** 87 (1905).

353. H. S. Gasser and J. Erlanger, *Am. J. Physiol.*, **88,** 581 (1929).

354. P. W. Nathan and T. A. Sears, *J. Physiol.*, **157,** 565 (1961).

355. E. S. Munson, M. J. Gutnick, and I. H. Wagman, *Anesth. Analg. Curr. Res.*, **49,** 986 (1970).

356. E. S. Munson, R. W. Martucci, and I. H. Wagman, *Brit. J. Anaesth.*, **44,** 1025 (1972).

357. E. S. Munson, W. K. Tucker, B. Ausinsch, and M. H. Malagodi, *Anesthesiol.*, **42,** 471 (1975).

358. D. B. Scott, *Brit. J. Anaesth.*, **47,** 56 (1975).

359. M. H. Malagodi, E. S. Munson, and W. J. Embro, *Brit. J. Anaesth.*, **49,** 121, (1977).

360. K. Kortilla, *Acta Anaesth. Scand.*, **18,** 290 (1974).

361. K. Kortilla, S. Häkkinen, and M. Linnoila, *Acta Anaesth. Scand.*, **19,** 384 (1975).

362. J. A. Aldrete and W. Daniel, *Anesth. Analg. Curr. Res.*, **50,** 127 (1971).

363. R. H. deJong and J. E. Heavner, *Anesthesiology*, **34,** 523 (1971).

364. G. T. Tucker, L. Wiklund, A. Berlin-Wahlén, and L. E. Mather, *J. Pharmacokinet. Biopharm.*, **5,** 111 (1977).

365. J. A. W. Wildsmith, G. T. Tucker, S. Cooper, D. B. Scott, and B. G. Covino, *Brit. J. Anaesth.*, **49,** 461 (1977).

366. R. N. Boyes, *Brit. J. Anaesth.*, **47,** 225 (1975).

367. M. J. Frumin, H. Schwartz, J. J. Burns, B. B. Brodie, and E. M. Papper, *Anesthesiology*, **14,** 576 (1953).

368. J. J. Bonica, P. U. Berges, and K. Morikawa, *Anesthesiology*, **33,** 619 (1970).

369. M. Stanton-Hicks, P. U. Berges, and J. J. Bonica, *Anesthesiol.*, **39,** 308 (1970).

370. M. Stanton-Hicks, T. M. Murphy, J. J. Bonica, L. E. Mather, and G. T. Tucker, *Brit. J. Anaesth.*, **48,** 575 (1976).

371. D. B. Scott and D. G. Julian, *Lidocaine in the Treatment of Ventricular Arrhythmias—Proc. Sym. Edinburgh, September, 1970*, E. & S. Livingstone, Edinburgh–London, 1971.

372. A. J. Moss and R. D. Patton, *Antiarrhythmic Agents*, Charles C. Thomas, Springfield, Ill., 1973.

373. R. N. Boyes, D. B. Scott, P. J. Jebson, J. J. Godman, and D. J. Julian, *Clin. Pharmacol. Ther.*, **12,** 105 (1971).

374. R. N. Boyes, H. J. Adams, and B. R. Duce, *J. Pharmacol. Exp. Ther.*, **174,** 1 (1970).

375. R. A. Gillis, F. H. Levine, H. Thibodeaux, A. Raines, and F. G. Standaert, *Circulation*, **47,** 697 (1973).

376. D. J. Coltart, T. B. Berndt, R. Kernoff, and D. C. Harrison, *Am. J. Cardiol.*, **34,** 35 (1974).

377. D. G. McDevitt, A. S. Nies, G. R. Wilkinson, R. F. Smith, R. L. Woosley, and J. A. Oates., *Clin. Pharmacol. Ther.*, **19,** 396 (1976).

378. R. A. Winkle, P. J. Meffin, J. W. Fitzgerald, and D. C. Harrison, *Circulation*, **54,** 884 (1976).

379. J. A. Wikinski, J. E. Usubiaga, R. L. Morales, A. Torrieri, and L. E. Usubiaga, *Anesth. Analg. Curr. Res.*, **49,** 504 (1970).

380. C. G. Bernard, E. Bohm, and T. Wiesel, *Surv. Anesthesiol.*, **1**, 304 (1957).

381. O. C. Phillips, W. B. Lyons, L. C. Harris, A. T. Nelson, T. G. Graff, and T. M. Frazier, *Anesth. Analg. Curr. Res.*, **39**, 317 (1960).

382. R. S. Himes, C. A. DiFazio, and R. G. Burney, *Anesthesiology*, **47**, 437 (1977).

383. A. L. Angerer, H. H. Su, and J. R. Head, *J. Am. Med. Assoc.*, **153**, 550 (1953).

384. E. Clarke, R. Morrison, and H. Roberts, *Lancet*, **1955-I**, 896.

385. V. L. Brechner, D. D. Cohen, and I. Pretsky, *Ann. N.Y. Acad. Sci.*, **141**, 524 (1967).

386. G. Nordstrom and A. P. Truant, "Aqueous Solution of Local Anesthetic Maintained under Pressure," U.S. Pat. 3,136,691 (1964).

387. G. A. Condouris and A. Shakalis, *Nature*, **204**, 57 (1964).

388. R. F. H. Catchlove, *J. Pharmacol. Exp. Ther.*, **181**, 298 (1972).

389. P. R. Bromage, *Acta Anaesth. Scand.*, **16**, 55 (1965).

390. P. R. Bromage, M. F. Burfoot, D. E. Crowell, and A. P. Truant, *Brit. J. Anaesth.*, **39**, 197 (1967).

391. P. R. Bromage and M. Gertel, *Can. Anaes. Soc. J.*, **17**, 557 (1970).

392. G. L. Houle, G. S. Fox, and I. M. G. Torkington, *Brit. J. Anaesth.*, **43**, 1145 (1971).

393. T. N. Appleyard, A. Witt, R. E. Atkinson, and A. D. G. Nicholas, *Brit. J. Anaesth.*, **46**, 530 (1974).

394. N. L. Cunningham and J. A. Kaplan, *Anesthesiology*, **41**, 509 (1974).

CHAPTER FIFTY-TWO

Analgetics

M. ROSS JOHNSON

and

GEORGE M. MILNE

Central Research
Pfizer Inc.
Groton, Connecticut 06340, USA

CONTENTS

699

1 INTRODUCTION

By the early 1970s the area of analgetics had apparently become one of diminishing returns for the medicinal chemist seeking a therapeutic breakthrough. The isolation and structure elucidation of morphine, coupled with the rise of synthetic organic chemistry, had led to an intensive effort directed at compounds that dissociated the pain-relieving and addictive properties of the opioids. So pervasive was this effort that the terms "opioid research" and "analgetic research" became and remain largely synonymous. Between 1925 and 1970 literally thousands of compounds were synthesized, many containing only remote fragments of the morphine nucleus. The narcotic antagonists and the mixed agonist/antagonists were discovered and clinical methodology was developed for the evaluation of analgetic efficacy and opioid dependence liability. Despite this impressive accumulation of knowledge, only incremental progress had been made toward the ultimate objective of a nonaddictive analgetic.

In 1973 the accumulated knowledge of opioid structure–activity relationships (SAR) and newly developed hormone receptor technology led to the discovery of the opiate receptor and, subsequently, the endogenous ligands for these receptors— the endorphins and enkephalins. These ad-vances are currently providing new landmarks and directions for analgetic research, the medicinal implications of which remain to be realized.

Before examining analgetic history and these newer developments in greater detail, it is important first to review the components of human pain perception, how analgesia is evaluated in animals, and the nature of physical dependence testing, in short, the operational steps in the search for a potent analgetic lacking physical dependence liability.

2 THE EXPERIMENTAL ASSESSMENT OF ANALGESIA AND DEPENDENCE

2.1 Pain and Pain Relief—Definitions

Given the pervasiveness of injury and disease, the ability to produce a state of analgesia has always been a significant target of medical therapy. Analgesia, as distinguished from anesthesia, is defined as the reduction of awareness of pain and suffering without loss of consciousness. The term "analgetic" is properly used to describe the agents or actions required to produce a state of analgesia (1).

The multidimensional character of human pain presents significant challenges to the analgetic researcher. Pain, as each of us experiences it, is not strictly a sensory event or a protective mechanism for alerting us to tissue damage; rather it is a highly individualized perception of stimuli as modified by a wide variety of personal, attitudinal and emotional factors.

The studies of Beecher (2, 3) provide eloquent testimony to the magnitude of these higher level interpretative contributions. He found that severely wounded soldiers seldom require analgetics, quite in contrast to individuals who have received similar injuries while engaged in some more benign pursuit. One interpretation of these findings is that the soldier feels relief to be alive at all, whereas the civilian sees only the ruin of a good figure, day, or life. Such subjective, psychological factors are an important and fascinating feature of pain research. A useful review of the subjective aspects of pain perception is provided by Melzack's book *The Puzzle of Pain* (4).

Hill and co-workers (5) demonstrated an important role for anxiety not only in the perception of pain but also in the pain-relieving actions of morphine. Current understanding of the neurophysiological pathways involved in pain perception supports the clinical observation that morphine-like analgetics provide excellent relief of dull pain and the affective components of suffering, but are poorly effective against sharp, acute pain.

At the level of the nervous system, pain sensations are first generated by specific nociceptive nerve endings in the skin and viscera. These nerve terminals, when activated by mechanical, thermal, or chemical stimuli, generate an impulse that travels along small diameter afferents (Aδ, C) to the dorsal horn of the spinal column. Such nociceptive impulses do not finally produce perceived pain until they reach and are processed by higher cortical centers. The view of pain as an affective experience is reinforced by the involvement of limbic structures.

Early researchers were inclined to view the dorsal horn and other brain stem structures as little more than synaptic way stations. More recently, with the discovery of nocisponsive interneurons and descending modulatory pathways, the dorsal horn has been accorded a much larger role in pain modulation. Based at first on theoretical considerations and later on experimental evidence, Melzack and Wall (6) proposed a significant role for the dorsal horn in pain perception and response. The Gate hypothesis, so-called because of its inhibitory modulation of incoming pain impulses

at the spinal level, has recently been reviewed by Wall (7). The involvement of such dorsal horn structures as the substantia gelatonisa will become important later as we examine pathways modulated by the endogenous opioids, the enkephalins.

Ascending along the spinal thalamic tract, the pain impulses appear to diverge into two pathways. Sharp, discretely localized pain is transmitted along the neospinothalamic pathway to the lateral nuclei of the thalamus and thence to various motor centers in the sensory cortex (Fig. 52.1). This phylogenetically recent tract (hence *neo*) appears to modulate acute, sharp pain—pain that is poorly relieved by the opioid analgetics. By contrast, the older paleospinothalamic system transmits a dull, less acute pain. This system ascends through the central gray region of the brainstem to the medial thalamus and to limbic structures which are important to emotional behavior. As is seen below, the localization of this system (Fig. 52.1) coincides closely with experimentally determined opiate receptor concentrations and with reports that potent morphine-like analgesia can be produced by electrical stimulation of the central gray. The neurophysiology of pain perception has been extensively reviewed (8–10).

Given the existence of such complex peripheral and central sensory pain systems, as well as significant emotional components of pain, it is not surprising that numerous classes of pharmacological agents produce analgesia. In addition to the opiates these include certain tranquilizers, aspirin and related nonsteroidal anti-inflammatories, amphetamine-like compounds, antihistamines, and cannabinoids. Lim and co-workers (11) proposed a tripartite classification scheme which divides analgetics into (1) peripherally acting, non-narcotic (e.g., aspirin); (2) centrally acting nonnarcotic (e.g., nefopam); and (3) centrally acting narcotic (e.g., morphine). Lim includes the narcotic antagonists and weak

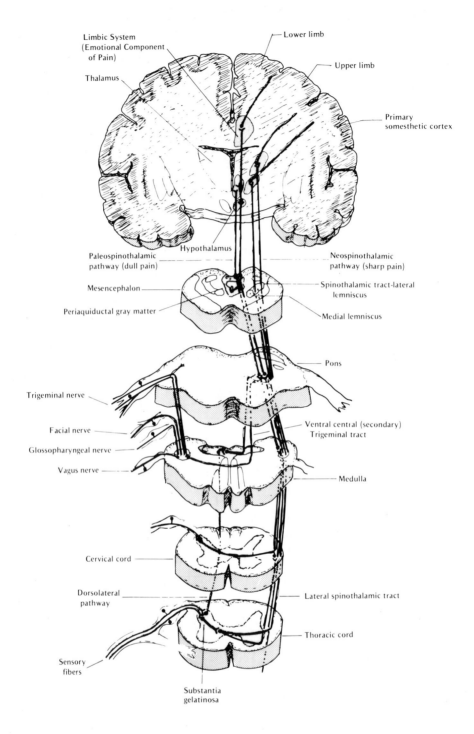

Fig. 52.1 Afferent pain systems.

The labels in the figure read:

Limbic System (Emotional Component of Pain)

Thalamus

Lower limb

Upper limb

Primary somesthetic cortex

Hypothalamus

Paleospinothalamic pathway (dull pain)

Neospinothalamic pathway (sharp pain)

Mesencephalon

Periaquiductal gray matter

Spinothalamic tract-lateral lemniscus

Medial lemniscus

Pons

Trigeminal nerve

Facial nerve

Ventral central (secondary) Trigeminal tract

Glossopharyngeal nerve

Vagus nerve

Medulla

Cervical cord

Dorsolateral pathway

Lateral spinothalamic tract

Thoracic cord

Sensory fibers

Substantia gelatinosa

agonists such as propoxyphene in category 2. We propose to include them in category 1 based on a more recent understanding of their common interaction with morphine at the opiate receptor. We confine ourselves here to the centrally active analgetics; nonsteroidal antiinflammatory analgetics are covered in Chapter 62. Several book-length reviews of the analgetic area have been published (12–14).

2.2 Analgetic Testing in Animals

The problems facing the experimenter attempting to design an animal model of human pain should be obvious. Although the overt behavior of both animals and man can reflect the intensity of the basic sensory experience, only man adequately experiences and verbalizes the wide range of affective and cognitive factors that are so important to the clinical pain experience. Although some attempts have been made to develop chronic animal models reflective of suffering, in most analgetic testing the nociceptive stimulus is acute. Common animal end points, presumably reflecting pain perception, are attempted escape and vocalization. There are four general classes of nociceptive stimuli: electrical, heat (or cold), pressure, and chemical. Extensive reviews have been published which describe the relative merits of these various procedures for the detection of centrally active analgetics (see Ref. 15 and references cited therein).

Two of the best-known rodent procedures are the D'Amour-Smith tail flick test (16) and the Woolfe-Macdonald hot plate test (17), as modified by Eddy and Leimbach (18). Both tests involve a thermal stimulus and provide good correlations with human clinical experience for the opiate agonists. In fact, the correlation between opiate agonist and hot plate/tail flick activity is so good that these tests have been considered as much predictive of physical dependence liability as of analgesia (19). The activity in man and in the hot plate test of selected clinical standards is compared in Table 52.1.

The antagonist analgetics provide an important lesson concerning overreliance on tests validated with a single class of agents. Because the narcotic antagonists (Section 3.1.3) are inactive in the classical hot plate and tail flick tests, the discovery by Lasagna and Beecher (20) that nalorphine has human clinical activity equivalent to morphine came as a surprise. As a consequence of this discovery, the phenylquinone abdominal stretching test (21) has become an important additional element of analgesic screening batteries. This test is sensitive and reasonably predictive of clinical activity not only for agonists and antagonists (22, 23), but also for a variety of peripherally acting analgetics and mechanistically distinct compounds that demonstrate some clinical evidence of analgetic effects—amphetamine, the antihistamines, and certain neuroleptics (24).

In comparing analgetic ED_{50}'s (the dose in milligrams per kilogram of body weight that produces a significant analgetic response in 50% of the animals) from various studies there are several practical caveats the medicinal chemist should heed: (1) differences in stimulus intensity that might alter sensitivity [e.g., it has been shown (25) that lowered temperatures in the hot plate test allow detection of opiate antagonists]; (2) between-study differences in the definition of "significant analgetic response" that alter the duration, and thus indirectly the intensity, of the stimulus; and (3) the spectrum of analgetic activity not in a single procedure, but across multiple tests (Mayer and Liebeskind (26) have shown that stimulation of selected brain areas may lead to evidence of analgesia in one test or at one site, but only stimulation of the central gray produces analgesia to a full spectrum of nociceptive challenges).

Recently, *in vitro* tests have assumed in-

Table 52.1   Comparative Activity of Analgetics in Mice and Man

Substance	Structure Number	Mouse ED_{50}, mg/kg[a]	Man Equivalence to 10 mg of Morphine, mg[b]
Morphine sulfate	52.1	1.0 (0.7–1.4)	10
Codeine phosphate	52.2	6.8 (4.5–10.2)	60–120
Diacetylmorphine hydrochloride	52.3	0.5 (0.4–0.6)	3–5
Dihydromorphinone hydrochloride	52.4	0.13 (.11–.16)	2–5
Dihydrocodeinone tartrate	52.5	1.6 (1.4–1.8)[c]	15
Dihydrohydroxymorphinone hydrochloride	52.6	0.09 (0.08–1.0)[e]	1.5
Dihydrohydroxycodeinone hydrochloride	52.7	0.7 (0.6–0.8)[c]	15
Levorphanol tartrate	52.19	0.2 (0.1–0.3)	2–3
Meperidine hydrochloride	52.9	4.6 (3.3–6.4)	50–100
Ketobemidone hydrochloride	52.12	0.8 (0.7–0.9)	5–15
Anileridine hydrochloride	52.10	1.5 (1.4–1.7)	25–30
(±)-Methadone hydrochloride	52.15	0.8 (0.6–1.1)	10
Phenazocine hydrobromide	52.20	0.15 (0.13–1.8)	2–3
Pentazocine	52.31	9.0 (6.5–12.4)[e]	20–30
Butorphanol tartrate	52.26	0.8 (0.6–1.0)[d,e]	2–4
Nalbuphine hydrochloride	52.29	13.0 (9.9–17.1)[d,e]	2–4
Buprenorphine hydrochloride	52.32	0.04 (0.03–0.05)[d,e]	0.3–0.6
Tilidine hydrochloride	52.96	9.2 (6.9–12.1)[d,e]	30–60
d-Propoxyphene hydrochloride	52.16	4.4 (3.4–5.1)[c]	240 (p.o.)

[a] Subcutaneous administration.
[b] Parenteral administration.
[c] A. E. Jacobson and E. L. May, *J. Med. Chem.*, **8**, 563 (1965) and Ref. 9 cited therein.
[d] Personal communication from Dr. A. E. Jacobson.
[e] As narcotic antagonist analgetics these would normally be cited as inactive in the hot plate test and, in fact, pentazocine was reported inactive by Jacobson and May in the third edition of this chapter. A change in procedure and mouse strain (see footnote c) has resulted in the above reported activity.

creasing importance in monitoring opioid SAR. Of particular importance is the opiate binding procedure that relies on stereospecific displacement of a radiolabeled opioid ligand from brain or other nervous tissue, and the guinea pig ileum and mouse vas deferens procedures that involve inhibition of smooth muscle contractions. These tests are of particular value to the medicinal chemist since they measure directly the effects of structural modification on activity without the intervening influences of distribution, absorption, and metabolism. Their particular contributions will be noted in later sections. A number of general reviews of *in vitro* methods have been published (27, 28).

2.3   Testing for Dependence Liability and Other Side Effects

In animals and man, chronic administration of opiates leads to rapid tolerance to all their effects except decreased gastric motility. Cessation of dosing or administration of a narcotic antagonist produces signs of abstinence, i.e., evidence of physical dependence. In man, symptoms begin 8–12 hr after the last dose and are similar to those produced by an influenzal attack—runny nose, sweating, and insomnia. After 24–48 hr, nausea, vomiting, gastrointestinal cramps, diarrhea, and fever can occur but these symptoms begin to diminish within 72 hr and are largely gone by 1 week. Although clearly unpleasant, withdrawal is seldom fatal and, if life threatening, can be abruptly terminated by the administration of another opiate. Even after physical dependence ends, psychological dependence remains as an important stimulus leading to readdiction.

Multiple methods have been developed for the assessment of opioid-like dependence liability which are applicable to both experimental animals and to man (29). The current status of biochemical and behavioral research into dependence mechanisms has also been reviewed (30).

Initial laboratory assessments are most often conducted in rodents. The test compound is evaluated for the reversal of its analgetic effects by a narcotic antagonist such as naloxone, as well as its ability to produce tolerance, opioid cross-tolerance, and withdrawal following chronic dosing. Recently developed opiate receptor binding techniques provide a simple yet powerful *in vitro* tool for determining the likelihood that a compound is opioid-like (see Section 3.6).

In the rhesus monkey the standard procedure for assessing dependence liability is one developed by Seevers and Deneau (32), in which a drug is examined for its ability to suppress abstinence in morphine-dependent animals. This is commonly referred to as the "single-dose suppression" test. If warranted, the drug is then administered for 30 days to naïve monkeys and the severity of nalorphine-precipitated abstinence is judged on days 14 and 28. The animals are observed for 7 days after the last dose on day 31 for evidence of non-precipitated withdrawal. Large numbers of compounds have been assessed in this way and much of this work has recently been reviewed (33).

In the past, human studies to assess addiction liability in the United States were carried out at the Addiction Research Center in Lexington, Kentucky. United States federal regulations have effectively halted this work and a suitable alternative

is not yet available. Nonetheless, large numbers of compounds have been studied in man using protocols developed by Himmelsbach, and co-workers (34) and represent an important reference base (35). As in monkeys, these studies involve substitution and direct addiction, but also add protocols designed to test for subjective liking. In this latter procedure, the experienced drug user was asked to identify the subjective effects of a test drug as opioid-like, barbiturate-like, etc. It is interesting to note that the subjective effects of morphine vary depending on whether the subject is in pain, an addict, or normal. For the patient who is experiencing pain, morphine seems to relieve both the pain and any coexistent anxiety. Similarly, in postaddicts morphine produces euphoria and some evidence of improved thought processes, whereas in naïve normals morphine is most likely to produce dysphoria and anxiety (36). A possible rodent analog of subjective drug discrimination has recently been developed (37) and could prove to be an important addition to the battery of animal tests already available to predict physical and psychological dependence liability.

In addition to analgesia and dependence liability, most potent opiate analgetics share a number of other pharmacological properties—respiratory depression, sedation, nausea, vomiting, constipation, and the suppression of the cough reflex (Chapter 53). Of these, respiratory depression is the most serious, restricting opioid use particularly where fetal exposure is possible. Fortunately the respiratory depressant effects of the opiates can be reliably assayed in dogs. The spinalized dog model developed by Martin et al. (38) has proved to be a useful tool for the comparative study of opioid effects. Sedation, constipation, and cough suppression can be either an advantage or a disadvantage, depending on the therapeutic focus. An assessment of this constellation of effects is an important feature of the comparative pharmacology of any new analgetic, but is nonetheless subservient to judgments concerning relative dependence and abuse liability.

As will be demonstrated several times in the following historical review of opioid research, it is clinical experience rather than animal pharmacology that is the final and most important arbiter of efficacy and side effect judgments.

3 HISTORICAL OVERVIEW OF OPIOID SAR AND NEWER DEVELOPMENTS IN ANALGETIC RESEARCH

3.1 Opioid SAR Development

3.1.1 EARLY HISTORY. Although the use of opium for the treatment of a variety of mental disorders and aches and pains can be traced to the beginnings of recorded medical history, attempts to treat pain with discrete medicinals began less than 200 years ago. Early workers sought to identify the active principle of opium. In 1805 Sertürner (39), a young German pharmacist, was the first to achieve the definitive

isolation of morphine (52.**1**, Fig. 52.2), which he named after Morpheus, the Greek god of sleep and dreams. His discovery was quickly followed in 1832 by the isolation of codeine (52.**2**, Fig. 52.2) from the opium poppy, *Papaver somniferum* (40).

Although the addictiveness and toxicity of morphine were recognized early, the invention of the hypodermic syringe by Wood in 1853 and the widespread use and abuse of parenteral morphine during the Civil War identified opiate addiction as a significant social problem. These and related events were responsible for initiating the search for a nonaddictive opioid, a search that still continues.

Well before the correct structure of morphine was known, attempts were made to dissect its pharmacological properties through chemical manipulations. One of the earliest products of morphine chemical transformation was its diacetyl derivative, heroin (52.**3**, Fig. 52.2), which was found to be a potent analgetic, although of shorter duration of action than morphine. Its rapid introduction into clinical use, which occur-

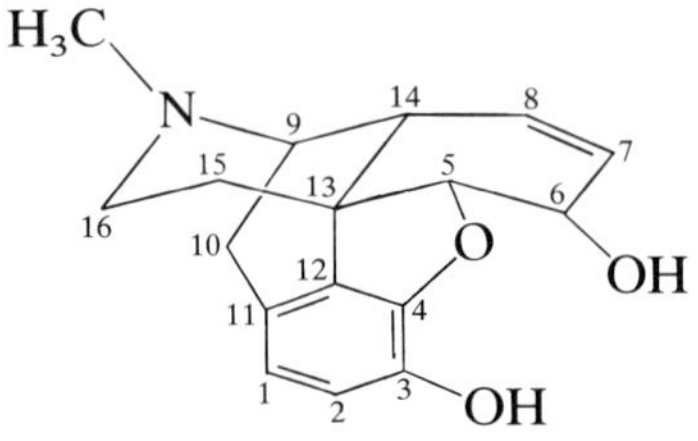

52.**1**   Morphine

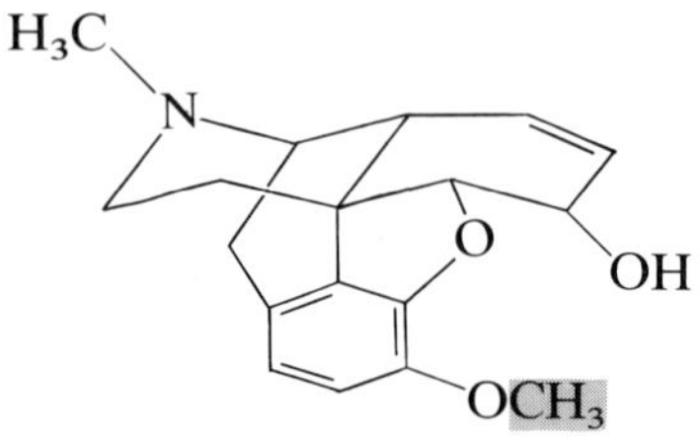

52.**2**   Codeine

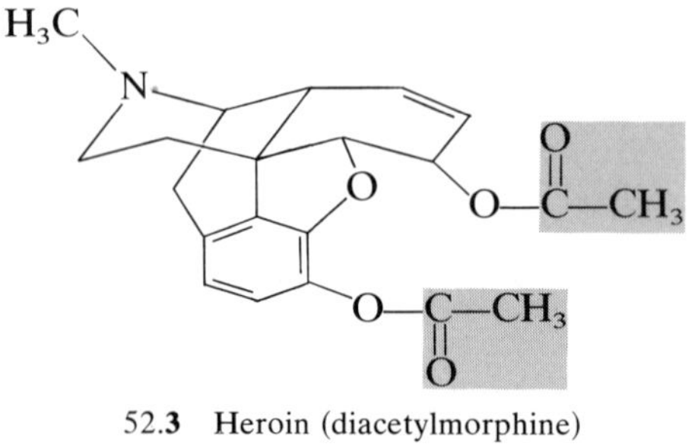

52.**3**   Heroin (diacetylmorphine)

Fig. 52.2   Structures of morphine, codeine, and heroin. Numbering system for morphine nucleus. Shaded areas indicates points of modification versus morphine.

red in 1898 (41), was based largely on claims of decreased respiratory depression in animals and reduced dependence liability based on the observation that it could be substituted for morphine in addicts without withdrawal. With time, clinical experience invalidated both these claims.

In the subsequent 25 years a number of other morphine derivatives were introduced into clinical practice. Although none are demonstrably superior to morphine, at least two, hydromorphone (52.**4**) and hydrocodone (52.**5**), remain in clinical use in a variety of proprietary analgetic and antitussive preparations.

3.1.2 SYSTEMATIC NUCLEAR MODIFICATIONS. The first systematic studies of opioid SAR, initiated in 1929, were carried out under the direction of the Committee on Drug Addiction of the National Research Council; some 150 derivatives of morphine and more than 300 synthetic products resulted (for a review, see Ref. 42). This early work

by Eddy, Mosetig, Burger, and others (42, 43) formed the basis for later systematic exploration of opioid SAR which eventually led to such early analgetics as metopon (52.**8**), and less directly to oxycodone (52.**7**) and oxymorphone (52.**6**).

The next major advance came not through thoughtful manipulation of the morphine nucleus, but through the empirical discovery of meperidine, (Demerol®, 52.**9**, Fig. 52.4) in 1939 by Eisleb and Schaumann (44). The significance of meperidine to the medicinal chemist was pointed out retrospectively by Schaumann (45), who recognized that meperidine preserves the piperidine ring and phenethylamine moieties of morphine (Fig. 52.4).

The analgetic potency of meperidine in man is approximately one-eighth that of morphine (46). Like heroin, it was initially introduced as a nonaddictive analgetic. Its dependence liability, which had been previously recognized in Germany, was confirmed in animals and man by Himmels-

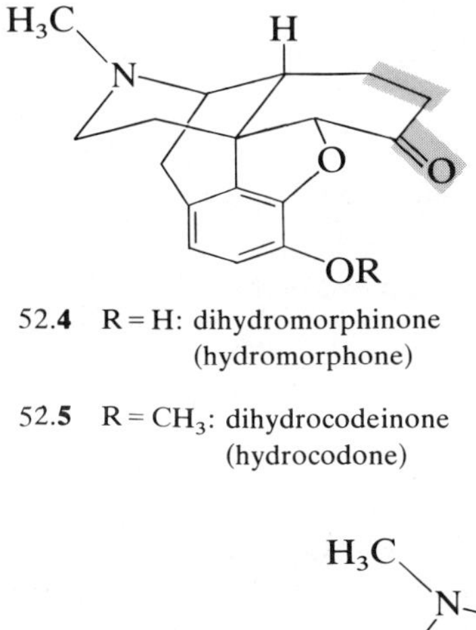

52.**4**   R = H: dihydromorphinone
           (hydromorphone)

52.**5**   R = CH$_3$: dihydrocodeinone
           (hydrocodone)

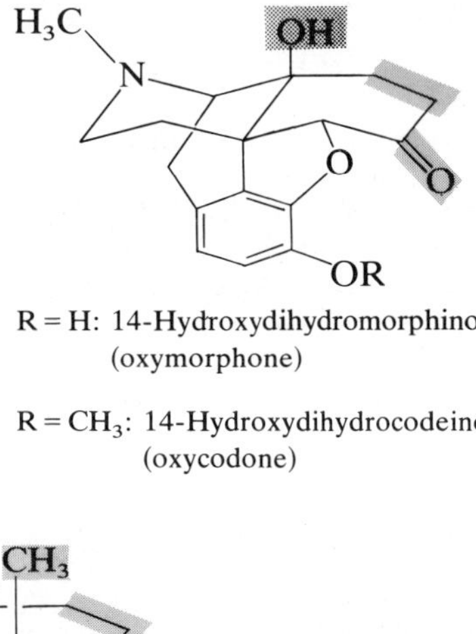

52.**6**   R = H: 14-Hydroxydihydromorphinone
           (oxymorphone)

52.**7**   R = CH$_3$: 14-Hydroxydihydrocodeinone
           (oxycodone)

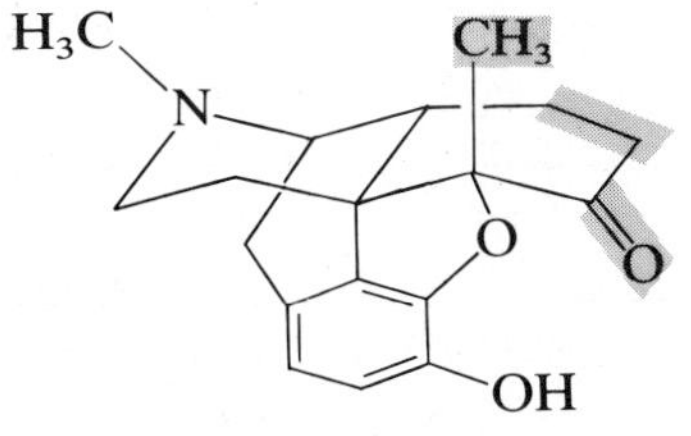

52.**8**   5-Methyldihydromorphinone
           (metopon)

Fig. 52.3 Simple transformation products of morphine. Chemical and nonproprietary names.

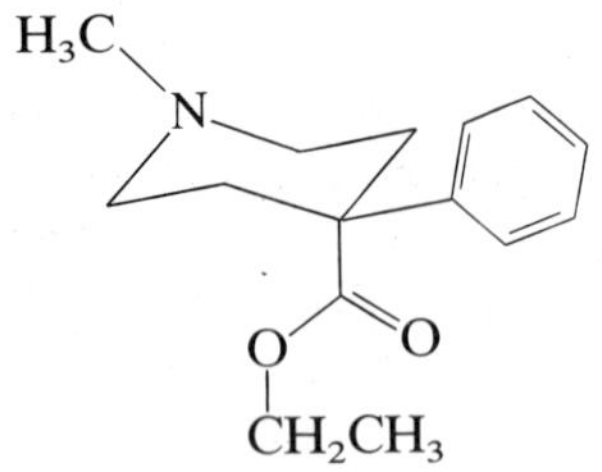

52.9
4-Carbethoxy-1-methyl-4-phenyl-
piperidine (meperidine)

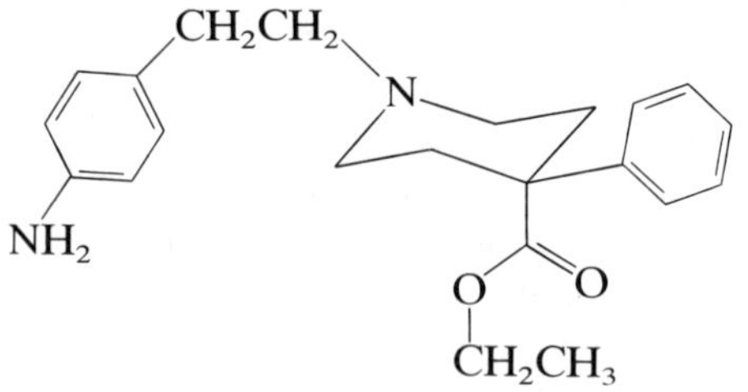

52.10
1-(*p*-Aminophenethyl)-4-carbethoxy-4-
phenylpiperidine (anileridine)

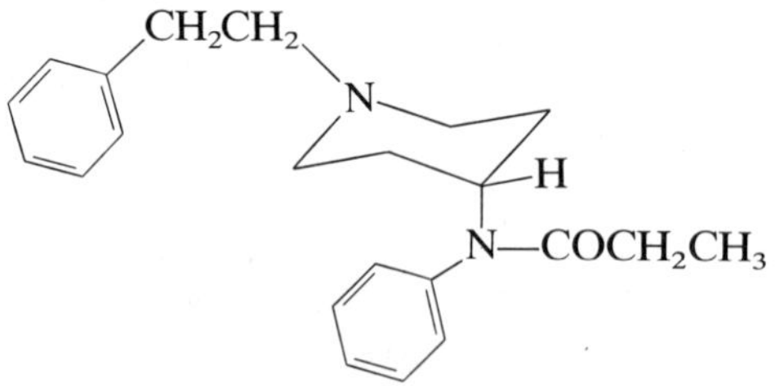

52.11
N-(1-Phenethyl-4-piperidinyl)
propiononilide (fentanyl)

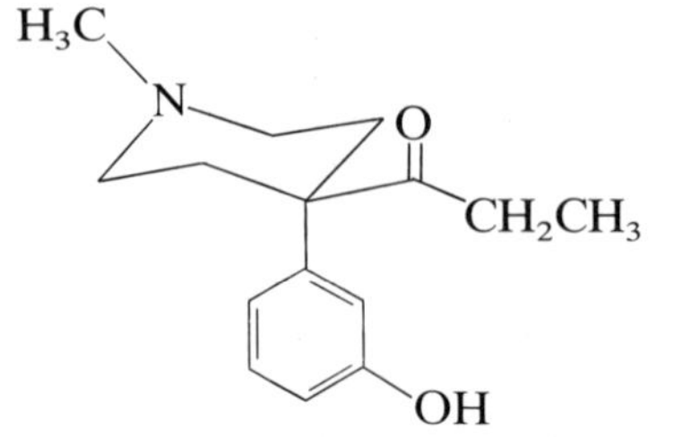

52.12
4-(*m*-Hydroxyphenyl)-1-methyl-4-propionyl-
piperidine (ketobemidone)

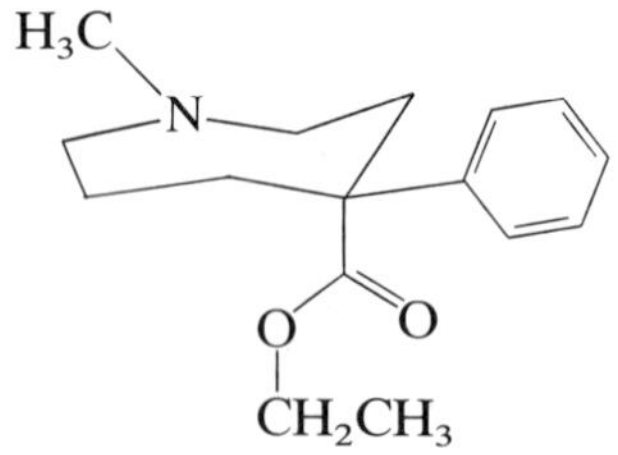

52.13
4-Carbethoxy-1-methyl-4-phenyl-
hexamethylenimine (ethoheptazine)

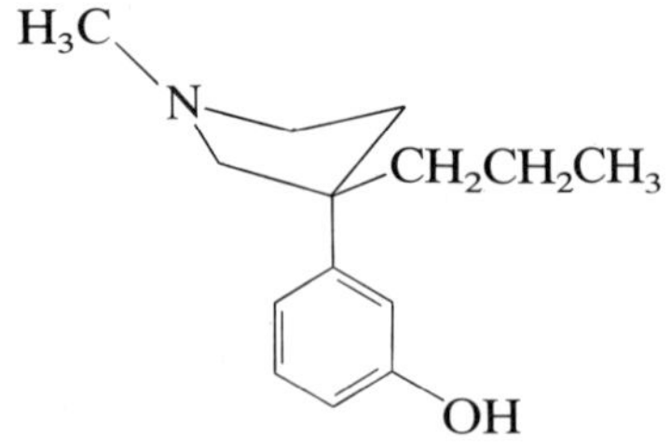

52.14
m-(1-Methyl-3-propyl-3-pyrrolidinyl)
phenol (profadol)

Fig. 52.4 Representative structures from the piperidine class of analgetics.

bach (47). Nonetheless, meperidine (De-merol) remains one of the leading substi-tutes for morphine in the parenteral treat-ment of moderate to severe pain.

Literally thousands of phenylpiperidines have been synthesized since the discovery of meperidine. Although many have de-monstrated substantially increased potency (e.g., fentanyl, 52.**11**), and some have seen clinical use (Fig. 52.4), none has achieved a significant separation of analgetic and dependence-producing effects (48).

The ultimate simplification of the mor-phine ring structure was achieved in the late 1940s with the synthesis of methadone [52.**15**, Fig. 52.5 (49)], a totally acyclic structure. Methadone differs significantly from morphine in having excellent and long-acting oral activity but otherwise very nearly duplicates morphine's total pharmacological profile, including potency and dependence liability (50, 51). Its oral activity and duration of action have contributed to its use in the outpatient treatment of individuals suffering from opioid physical dependence.

Significant numbers of methadone derivatives have been prepared. Two of the best known are dextropropoxyphene [Darvon®, 52.**16** (52)] and dextromoramide (52.**17**). Dextromoramide, like methadone, is an effective analgetic, by both the oral and parenteral routes, and is subject to substantial abuse liability (48). Although dextropropoxyphene initially was held to be a nonnarcotic analgetic, clinical experience has demonstrated that this compound also produces some degree of physical dependence (53).

Structures derived from the benzomorphan and morphinan ring systems awaited the development of the necessary synthetic chemical technology. Early attempts [see Grewe (54)] were able to produce only the basic carbocyclic skeleton of morphine. Schnider and Grüssner (55), in a pursuit of Grewe's synthetic efforts, discovered that potent analgetic activity could be retained in structures lacking the furan ring of morphine. One of these, the morphinan levorphanol (52.**19**, Fig. 52.6), proved to be an effective analgetic, three to four times more potent than morphine, but unfortunately with a concomitant degree of dependence liability.

Simplification of the morphine nucleus was extended in 1955 with the removal of an additional ring by May and Murphy (56), producing the benzomorphans. This series, for the first time, gave some evidence of separation of analgetic from dependence producing effects. Phenazocine

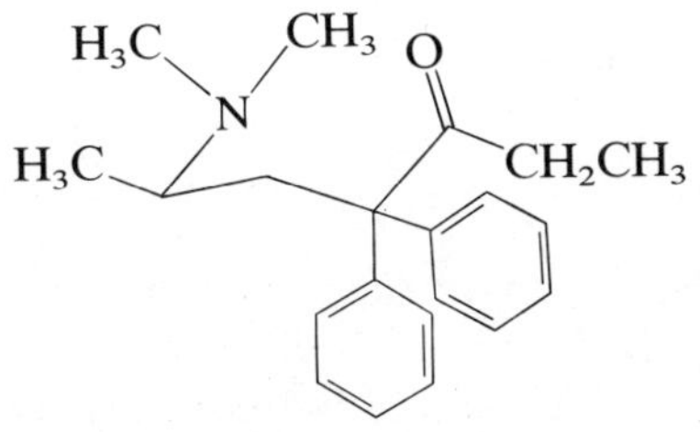

52.**15**
6-Dimethylamino-4, 4-diphenyl-
3-heptanone (methadone)

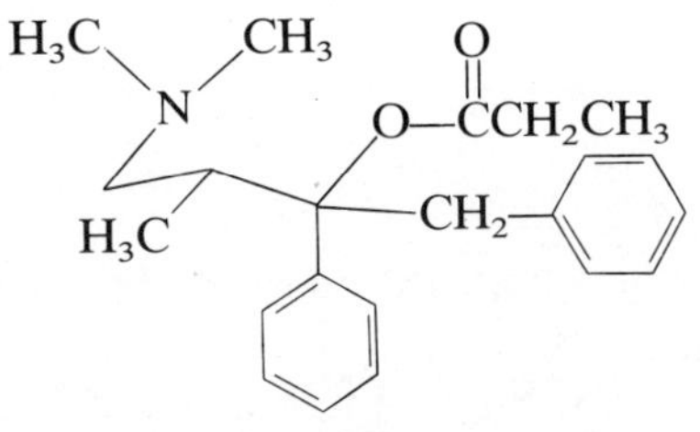

52.**16**
α-(+)-4-Dimethylamino-1, 2-diphenyl-3-
methyl-2-propionoxybutane (d-propoxyphene)

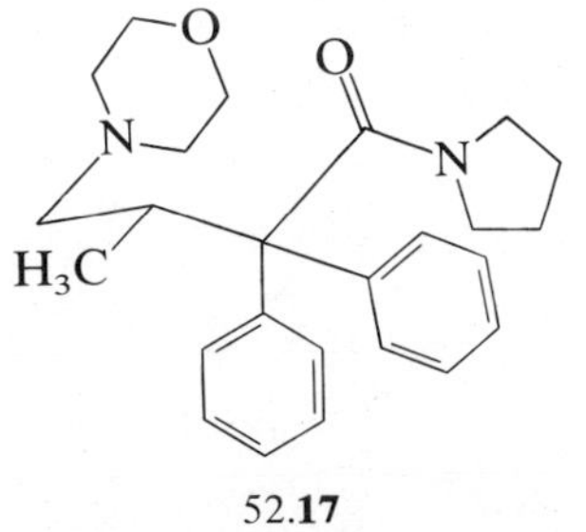

52.**17**
(+)-N-(2,2-Diphenyl-3-methyl-4-
morpholinobutryl)pyrrolidone
(dextromoramide)

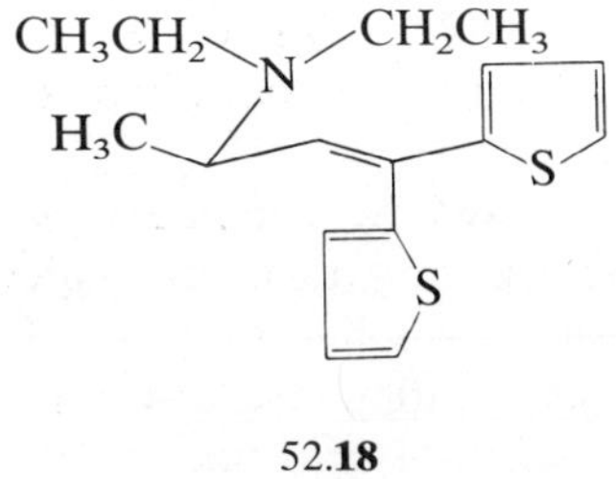

52.**18**
N,N-Diethyl-1-methyl-3,3-di-2-
thienylallylamine
(thiambutene)

Fig. 52.5 Methadone and related analgetics.

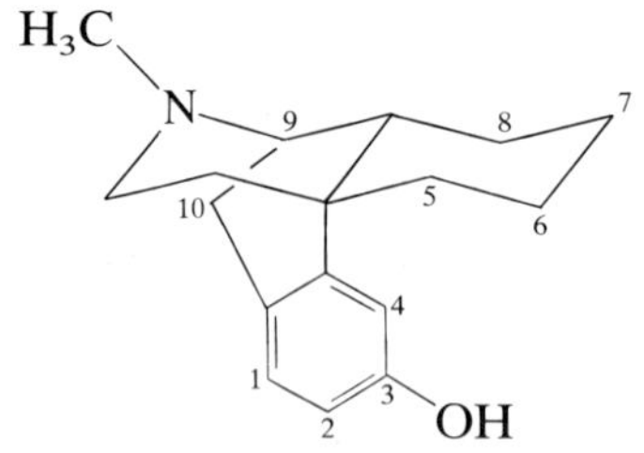

52.**19**
(−)-3-Hydroxy-*N*-methylmorphinan
(levorphanol)

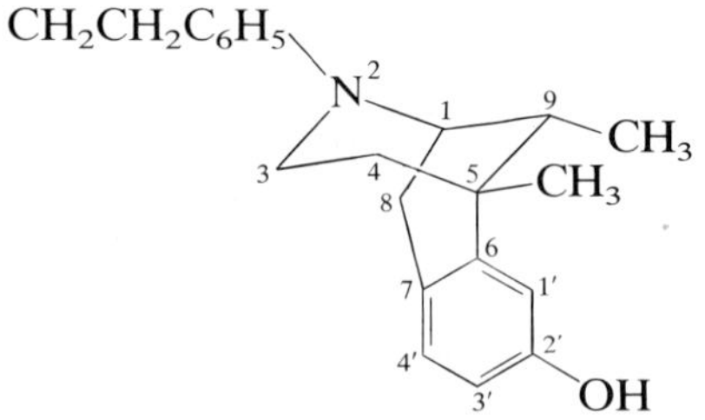

52.**20**
α-(±)-5,9-Dimethyl-2′-hydroxy-2-phenethyl-
6,7-benzomorphan (phenazocine)

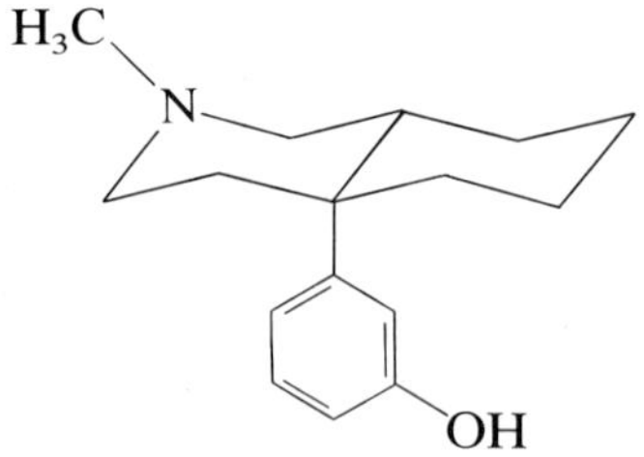

52.**21**
5-(*m*-Hydroxyphenyl)-2-methylmorphan

Fig. 52.6 Morphinans, benzomorphans, and phenylmorphans.

(52.**20**, Fig. 52.**6**), the first of the benzomorphans to be studied extensively, is orally active, is three to four times more potent than morphine parenterally, and has reduced dependence liability in monkeys (57, 58). The interest generated by the discovery of phenazocine largely obscured the discovery that an even simpler nuclear modification, 5-(*m*-hydroxyphenyl)-2-methylmorphan (52.**21**, Fig. 52.**6**), had analgetic activity equivalent to morphine in animals (56).

Although the greatest emphasis was being placed on achieving pharmacological selectivity through simplification of the morphine nucleus, Bentley and co-workers (59) were in pursuit of the concept that greater, not less, ridigity and complexity were the means for achieving selectivity. This approach led via thebaine to the oripavines, a class of compounds with excep-

tional potency. One of these, etorphine (52.**22**), is at least 2000 times more potent than morphine and is frequently used as a large animal tranquilizer (60). Although the potency of etorphine has not translated to selectivity, a related compound, buprenorphine (52.**32**), demonstrates a very low level of dependence liability and respiratory depressant side effects, as discussed in the following section.

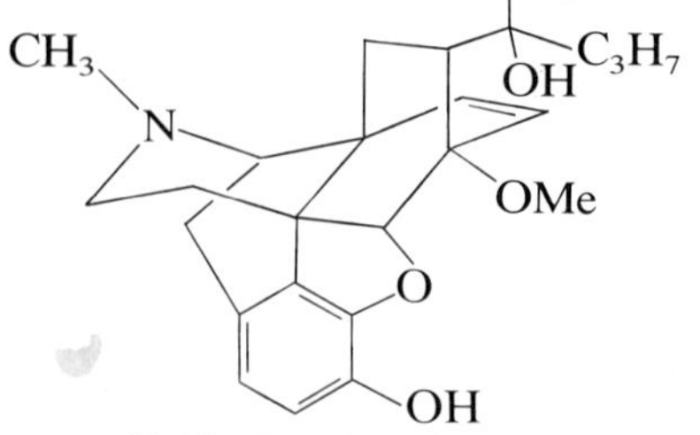

52.**22**   Etorphine (M-99)

3.1.3 NARCOTIC ANTAGONISTS. In 1915 Pohl (61) had observed that replacement of methyl by allyl in codeine produced a compound that was able to block morphine's respiratory depressant activity. However, it was not until the early 1940s (62) that a similar demonstration of specific antagonist activity was made for *N*-allylnormorphine (nalorphine, 52.**23**, Table 52.2). A second key event was the discovery in 1954 by Lasagna and Beecher (63) that nalorphine not only effectively blocked all morphine's

Table 52.2   Structural Relationships between Important Narcotic Agonist and Agonist/Antagonist Analgetics

Structure	Agonist	Antagonist
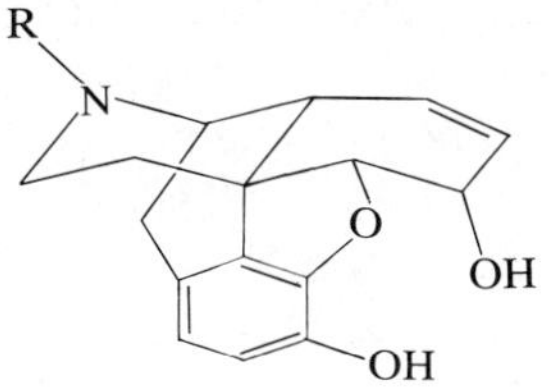	52.**2** R = CH$_3$ (morphine)	52.**23** R = CH$_2$CH=CH$_2$ (nalorphine)
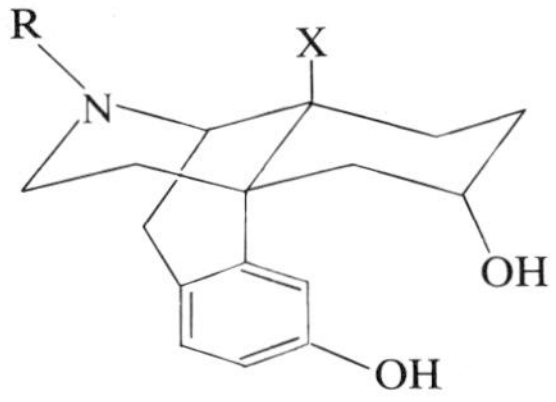	52.**19** R = CH$_3$, X = H (levorphanol)	52.**24** R = CH$_2$CH=CH$_2$, X = H (levallorphan) 52.**25** R = CH$_2$–◁, X = H (cyclorphan) 52.**26** R = CH$_2$–◇ , X = OH (butorphanol)
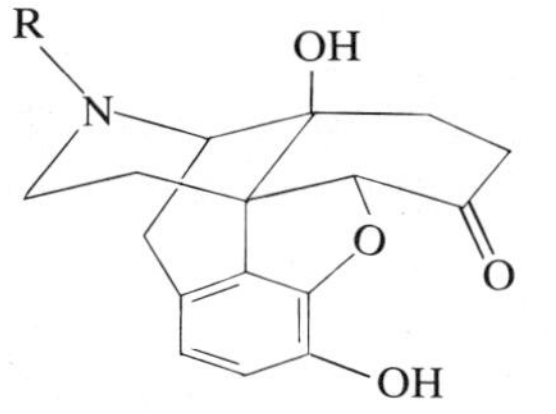	52.**6** R = CH$_3$ (oxymorphone)	52.**27** R = CH$_2$CH = CH$_2$ (naloxone) 52.**28** R = CH$_2$–◁ (naltrexone) 52.**29** R = CH$_2$–◇ (=O = —OH) (nalbuphine)
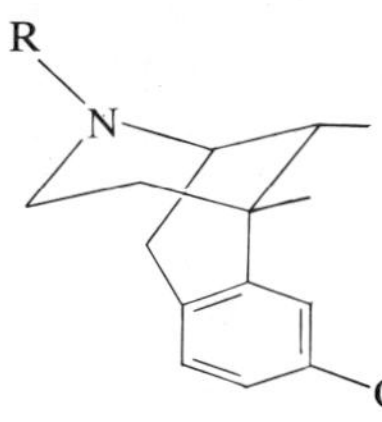	52.**20** R = CH$_2$CH$_2$Ø (phenazocine)	52.**30**, R = CH$_2$–◁ (cyclazocine) 52.**31** R = CH$_2$CH=C(CH$_3$)$_2$ (pentazocine)
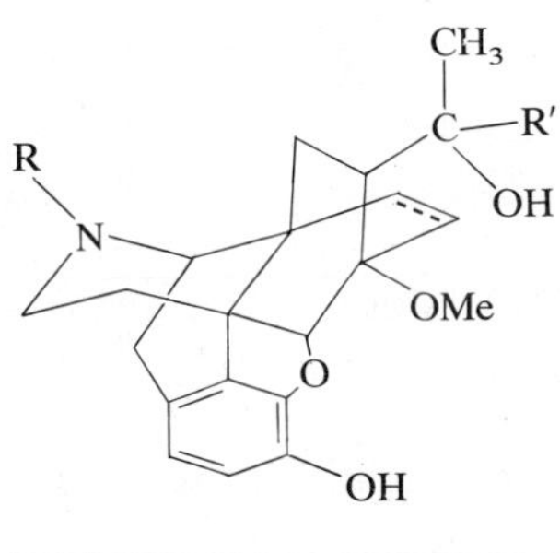	52.**22** R = CH$_3$, R' = C$_3$H$_7$ (etorphine)	52.**32** R = CH$_2$ ◁ , R' = *t*-Bu (buprenorphine) (double bond reduced)

actions in man, but was itself an analgetic of considerable potency. As was pointed out in Section 2.2, this was surprising because nalorphine like other narcotic antagonists was inactive in classical analgetic tests in animals (e.g., hot plate and tail flick) and so was assumed to be inactive in man. Also of substantial clinical importance was the demonstration that nalorphine appeared to have limited potential to produce drug dependence based on both animal and human studies (33).

Unfortunately, nalorphine's clinical utility was limited by the presence of often severe psychotomimetic side effects at analgetic doses. The historical significance of nalorphine was that it focused attention on a renewed opportunity to achieve pharmacological selectivity in compounds possessing both agonist and antagonist properties.

The respiratory depressant effects of the narcotic antagonist analgetics are modest in comparison with pure agonists such as morphine. Though they retain some ability to produce physical dependence and drug seeking behavior, their overall dependence liability is also markedly reduced. Pentazocine (52.**31**), the first narcotic antagonist analgesic to achieve broad clinical usage (64), has only recently been followed by buprenorphine (52.**32**) (65), nalbuphine (52.**29**), (66), and butorphanol (52.**26**) (67). Fewer psychotomimetic side effects are seen after these newer compounds than after nalorphine (52.**23**) and cyclazocine (52.**30**). Buprenorphine has exceptional parenteral potency (30–50 times that of morphine) and a low level of dependence liability, respiratory, and psychotomimetic side effects (65). Several comparative reviews of the clinical credentials of the narcotic agonist and antagonist analgetics have been published (68–70).

A second product of this research was the discovery of the pure narcotic antagonists—compounds able to block the effects of morphine but inactive in producing analgesia. The two most notable of these, naloxone (52.**27**) and naltrexone (52.**28**), are shown in Table 52.2. Naltrexone is more potent, orally active, and longer acting than naloxone. These compounds have proved to be extremely important to the experimental study of opioid pharmacology and in the clinical treatment of opiate overdose.

In general, opioid antagonists differ structurally from agonists only by the replacement of the N-methyl group commonly present in agonists by N-allyl, N-cyclopropyl, or related groups, although examples of antagonists with N-methyl substitution have been reported recently (71, 72). Specific SAR, predictive of the degree of mixed agonist/antagonist properties, have also been proposed (73, 74). The most important members of the narcotic antagonist family are listed in Table 52.2.

3.2 The Opiate Receptor

3.2.1 MEDICINAL CONCEPTUALIZATION. The growing body of opioid analgetic SAR, evidence of stereospecificity of action, and reversal by the narcotic antagonists first led Beckett and Casy (75) and later Portoghese (76) to speculate on the nature of receptor-based structural requirements for analgesia. In each case, a receptor surface was formulated which possessed a flat lipophilic surface binding the aromatic ring, a cavity to accommodate the hydrocarbon portion of the piperidine ring, and an anionic, amine binding site. Subsequently, more refined models have been proposed which contain an additional lipophilic binding site designed to rationalize the superior potency of the oripavines and fentanyl related analgetics (77, 73, 78). A recent modification has been the addition of different loci for amine binding to accommodate agonist and antagonist receptor states (73, 74). Such a model is shown graphically in Fig. 52.7. None of these models explains all the

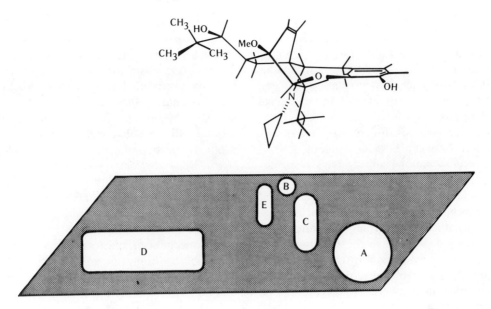

Fig. 52.7 Conceptual model of the opiate receptor. A, flat surface for aromatic ring; B, anionic site; C, cavity for C-15 and C-16; D, lipophilic site; and E, antagonist site.

anomalies (78), but this is perhaps neither damning nor surprising, given the growing recognition that there are multiple and distinct opioid receptors in analogy to the α-, β_1, and β_2-receptors of the noradrenergic system.

Although these models were primarily presented as medicinal tools capable of rationalizing opioid analgetic SAR, they also led to speculation concerning the actual existence of an opiate receptor *in vivo*. The existence of such a receptor was also suggested by the fact that the opiates have no direct pharmacological interaction with known neurotransmitter systems, although certain of the monoamine neurotransmitters, particularly serotonin, are required for the complete elaboration of morphine analgesia. Nonetheless, the idea of an opioid receptor remained largely hypothetical until 1973.

3.2.2 BIOCHEMICAL ELUCIDATION. In 1973 the presence of stereospecific opiate binding in rat brain was independently identified in three separate laboratories, headed

respectively by E. J. Simon, S. H. Snyder, and L. Terenius (79–81). These demonstrations relied on opioid stereospecificity (e.g., levorphanol and its inactive enantiomer, dextrorphan, differ by four orders of magnitude in their ability to displace ^{3}H-ligand) and on the use of ligands with high specific radioactivity (10–40 Ci/mmol). Pioneering attempts to demonstrate specificity, first by Ingolia and Dole (82) and later by Goldstein and his associates (83), had met with only marginal success, largely because these researchers were limited to high ligand concentrations resulting from the low specific activity of opioid ligands available at that time.

Stereospecific opiate binding is found in the central nervous systems of all vertebrates including man (84, 85) and in the nervous tissue of certain peripheral smooth muscle systems (80), e.g., guinea pig ileum and mouse vas deferens, but not in invertebrates (84). The pharmacological relevance of this binding is supported by its stereospecificity, reversibility, saturability in a pharmacological concentration range, and by the ability of binding studies to predict accurately pharmacological potency as measured in other more standard *in vitro* and *in vivo* tests. Thus Creese and Snyder (86) found an excellent correlation between the binding affinities and pharmacological activities of a series of opiates, both agonists and antagonists (Fig. 52.8). Similar correlations between *in vivo* analgetic activity and *in vitro* binding affinity have been demonstrated for homologous series of ketobemidones (87), benzazocines (88), and benzomorphans (89). Some important exceptions include etorphine, meperidine, and codeine (90, 91), in the first two cases due to unusually efficient distribution to the brain. A group of false positives in the opiate binding assay are the butyrophenone neuroleptics, such as haloperidol and droperidol (92). However, this may be explained by their structural similarity to the opioids, especially fentanyl (Fig. 52.9).

Since binding studies measure directly the interaction of a drug at the receptor without intervening contributions from metabolism, distribution, or absorption, they have provided an important addition to medicinal studies of opioid structure–activity relationships. For example, the low binding affinity of codeine (Table 52.3) supports the hypothesis that its *in vivo* activity depends on *O*-demethylation to morphine. Likewise, the potent binding affinity *in vitro* and the apparent absence of CNS effects for loperamide, a potent opiate-related antidiarrheal, confirms its opioid mechanism and its poor penetration of the blood–brain barrier (93).

A further, predictive feature of opiate binding came from studies of the effects of sodium ion (81, 94, 95). In a manner not duplicated by other cations, Na$^+$ increases antagonist and decreases agonist binding where added to the medium, sometimes by

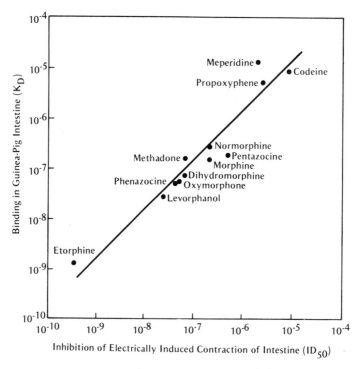

Fig. 52.8 Correlation between the pharmacological potency of opiate agonists in the guinea pig intestine and their affinity for the opiate receptor in the same tissue. [From S. H. Snyder, "Opiate Receptors and Internal Opiates," *Sci. Am.*, **236**, 44 (1977) with permission of the publisher.]

Table 52.3   Relative Potencies of Drugs in Reducing Stereospecific
^{3}H-Naloxone Binding to Rat Brain Homogenate[a]

Drug	ED_{50}, nM
(−)-Etorphine	0.3
(−)-Etonitazene	0.5
Levallorphan	1
Levorphanol	2
(−)-Nalorphine	3
(−)-Morphine	7
(−)-Cyclazocine	10
(−)-Naloxone	10
(−)-Hydromorphone	20
(−)-Methadone	30
(+)-Pentazocine	50
(+)-Methacone	300
Meperidine	1,000
(±)-Propoxyphene	1,000
(+)-3-Hydroxy-*N*-allylmorphinan	7,000
Dextrorphan	8,000
(−)-Codeine	20,000
(−)-Oxycodone	30,000
Drugs without binding effect at 0.1 m*M*	
Phenobarbital	
Norepinephrine	
Atropine	
Pilocarpine	
Arecoline	
Colchicine	
γ-Aminobutyric acid	
Bicuculline	
Serotonin	
Carbamylcholine	
Neostigmine	
Hemicholinium	
Histamine	
Glycine	
Glutamic acid	
Δ9-Tetrahydrocannabinol	
Acetylsalicyclic acid	
Caffeine	

[a] Values represent means from three log-probit determinations each using five concentrations of drug. ED_{50} is the molar concentration of drug that causes 50% reduction of ^{3}H naloxone binding. [From S. H. Snyder and C. B. Pert, *Ann. Intern. Med.* **81,** 534 (1974) with permission of the publisher.]

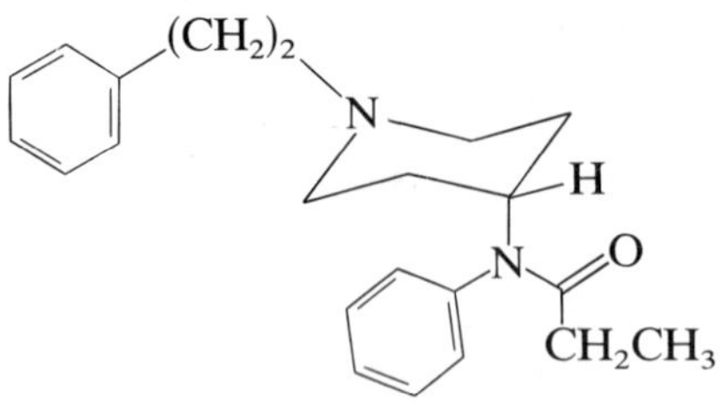

52.**11** Fentanyl 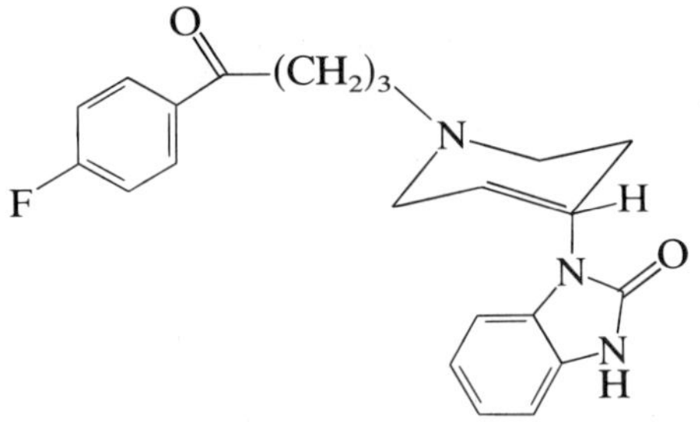   52.**33** Droperidol

Fig. 52.9   Structural similarities between the butyrophenone neuroleptics and the piperidine analgetics.

as much as fifty-fold (Fig. 52.10). This shift, which reflects the *in vivo* presence of sodium, brings relative *in vitro* agonist and antagonist potencies more closely in line with the *in vivo* superiority of most antagonists. The ratios for the mixed agonist/antagonists are variable, but generally fall at an intermediate value (~2–10). Use of this sodium effect allows the *in vitro* prediction of relative agonist and antagonist properties.

This work, coupled with related studies on the selective destruction of binding by proteolytic and thiol alkylating reagents,

has led Snyder and Simon to propose a receptor model with interconverting agonist and antagonist forms (107–109). Figure 52.11 outlines the Simon model, which is portrayed as dimeric to account for kinetic evidence of cooperation. Although this model rationalizes the relative affinities and competitive interactions of most agonists and antagonists, it does not explain the limited Na^+ sensitivity of ketocyclazocine (52.**37**, Fig. 52.16), a compound for which no antagonist properties are known; nor does it fully explain differences in the pharmacological profiles of mixed versus pure

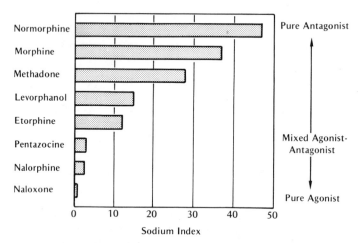

Fig. 52.10   Presence of sodium ions dramatically decreases the affinity of the opiate receptor for agonists without changing its affinity for antagonists. Bars show the ratio of the concentration of a drug required to inhibit by 50% the binding of radiolabeled naloxone to the receptor in the presence of sodium to the concentration of the drug required in the absence of sodium. Lower values indicate a lesser reduction of potency in the presence of sodium: "pure" antagonists have a sodium index of 1 or less, whereas "pure" agonists have high values. The sodium index of a new opiate drug is thus a good indicator of its agonist or antagonist properties. [From S. H. Snyder, "Opiate Receptors and Internal Opiates," *Sci. Am.*, **236**, 44 (1977) with permission of the publisher.]

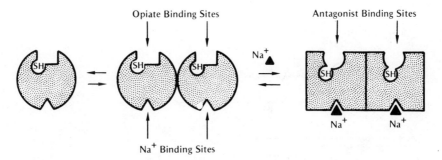

Fig. 52.11 Allosteric model for the interconversion of agonist and antagonist binding conformations of the opioid receptor. [Reproduced, with permission, from the *Annual Review of Pharmacology & Toxicology*, E. J. Simon and J. M. Miller, **18,** 371 (1978). © 1978 by Annual Reviews Inc.]

agonists and antagonists. This leaves open the possibility that there are independent populations of agonist and antagonist binding sites. The existence of just such distinct populations has recently been postulated for the noradrenergic and dopamine systems.

Overall, the localization of opiate receptors and their functional relationships to primary sensory afferents agree closely with sites and mechanisms of action derived from physiological studies (Fig. 52.1). The highest densities of opiate receptors in the brain are located in the limbic system, an area concerned with the integration of sensory input and the modulation of emotional response, and in those sensory and motor areas most directly linked to the limbic system (97, 98). It is important to note that this same brain region has been functionally linked to the actions of the opiates by electrical stimulation and lesioning experiments (e.g., Ref. 26). Interestingly, the hippocampus is one area of the limbic system with low levels of binding and with no demonstrated role in morphine pain modulation.

Dense localization of binding is also seen in the substantia gelatinosa of the spinal cord (99, 100)—an area that receives major sensory input from small caliber dorsal root afferents which convey the sensations of pain, temperature, and touch. Deafferentation of two such nerves, the accessory optic

nerve and the vagus, produces a marked decrease in autoradiographically identified receptors (101), supportive of a strategic, presynaptic role for opiate receptors in modulating the input of noxious stimuli (as proposed in the Melzack/Wall gating hypothesis). In contrast, lesions of norepineprhine, dopamine, serotonin, and acetylcholine pathways have no effect on opiate receptor binding, suggesting that the opiate receptor is not contained on or within the nerve terminals of these systems. To date, no changes in opiate binding sites or affinity have been observed in morphine-dependent animals (102–104).

Attempts to isolate the opiate receptor have met with only limited success. Based on experiments with sulfhydryl reagents and proteolytic enzymes, it is generally accepted that the receptor is composed of protein associated with membrane lipids. The evidence for a lipid component is reinforced by the ability of cerebroside sulfate and phosphatidyl serine to stereospecifically bind opiates. Cerebroside sulfate, in particular, produces a good correlation between opiate binding and *in vivo* potency (105), a finding that has led Loh et al. (106) to propose that cerebroside sulfate can fulfill many of the binding requirements dictated by the medicinal model of the opiate receptor (Fig. 52.12). This hypothesis is supported by the demonstration that mice genetically deficient in brain

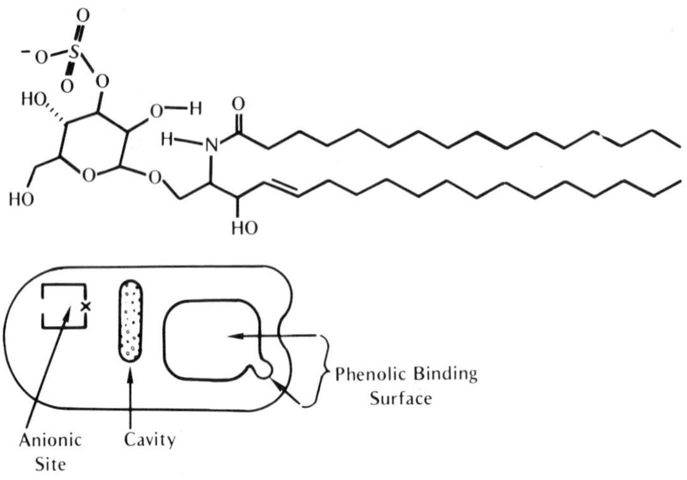

Fig. 52.12 Cerebroside as a model for the opiate receptor (106).

sulfatides and cerebrosides are markedly less sensitive to the analgetic effects of morphine (106).

The opiate receptor area has been, and continues to be, extensively reviewed (96, 110). Readers should consult such reviews for more detailed and up-to-date discussions of opiate binding and related issues.

3.3 Biochemical Transduction of Opiate Binding

No firm evidence is yet available regarding the factor(s) that transduces opiate binding into biologic activity. However, the morphine-sensitive adenylate cyclase system first described by Collier and Roy (111) provides an attractive biochemical model, not only of opiate action, but also of the phenomena of dependence and withdrawal.

In work first carried out in rat brain homogenates, but more reproducibly demonstrated by Klee, Nirenberg, Hamprecht, and co-workers (112, 113) in a neuroblastoma×glioma cell line, it was shown that opiates inhibit the prostaglandin

E_1- or E_2-stimulated production of cAMP. This effect of the opiates is stereospecific and naloxone reversible. Of relevance to the phenomenon of tolerance development, continued morphine exposure of the neuroblastoma×glioma hybrid cells produces an adaptive increase in adenylate cyclase activity and a return to nearly normal levels of cAMP (114). In analogy to *in vivo* abstinence, it was found that withdrawal of morphine or addition of the narcotic antagonist, naloxone, produced a marked increase in cAMP production to well above normal levels. A conceptualization of this process is shown in Fig. 52.13 and is suggestive of a significant role for cAMP in modulating the actions of the opiates, including tolerance development and withdrawal. This hypothetical model finds support from *in vivo* studies, wherein phosphodiesterase inhibitors (which elevate cAMP levels) can be shown in rats to produce behavioral effects mimicking withdrawal (115), whereas administration of cAMP can be shown to antagonize morphine analgesia and speed tolerance development (116).

However speculative, these and related biochemical studies do illustrate the grow-

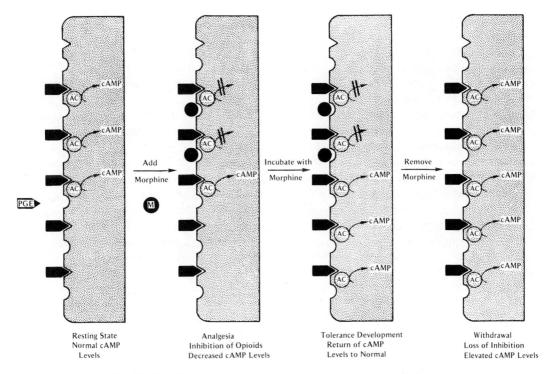

Fig. 52.13   Biochemical model of analgesia, tolerance, and withdrawal.

ing body of basic scientific information which is becoming available to provide the medicinal chemist with new and more biochemically oriented approaches to analgetic discovery.

3.4   Discovery of the Enkephalins and Endorphins

The presence of opiate receptors in all vertebrates and the obvious absence of a phylogenetic relationship between vertebrates and the poppy suggested an important physiological role for the opiate receptor. It also suggested the presence of an as yet unidentified endogenous ligand. The existence of such a ligand received considerable support from Liebeskind and his associates, who were able to demonstrate in the early 1970s that electrical stimulation of specific brain sites in the rat produces profound

analgesia (26, 117), which is naloxone reversible (118), and is subject to tolerance development and to cross-tolerance to morphine (119). These results are most readily explained by the electrically induced release of an endogenous substance with morphine-like properties. Further support for the existence of an endogenous opioid was the close correlation found between those brain areas most sensitive to stimulation-produced analgesia and regions containing a high density of opiate receptors.

Early in 1975 evidence began to emerge from three laboratories that these endogenous opioids were peptides rather than simple morphine-like molecules (120–122). The first direct evidence for the existence of such a morphine-like substance in extracts from pig brain was provided late in 1975 by John Hughes, Hans Kosterlitz, and their co-workers at Aberdeen, who reported that the endogenous ligand was not just one peptide, but two peptides (123), each with five amino acids and differing only in the carboxyl terminal amino acid (Fig. 52.14). They christened them methionine (Met) and leucine (Leu) enkephalin, the term enkephalin being coined from the Greek word meaning "in the head." Shortly thereafter Snyder's group confirmed these findings, but with one major difference. Whereas Hughes and Kosterlitz had found four times more Met- than Leu-enkephalin in porcine brain, Simantov and Snyder found that the ratio was reversed in calf brain (124). The common presence of a tyrosine residue in both the enkephalins and in morphine quickly underscored the relevance of these findings to opioid SAR.

At the same time this work was going on, Goldstein and his group were reporting the presence of pituitary opioid peptides of apparently greater molecular weight (125, 126). This was fortuitous since Hughes and co-workers in their original paper on the enkephalins had observed that the sequence of Met-enkephalin is identical to that of residues 61–65 contained in the pituitary C-fragment (residues 61–91) hormone β-lipotropin (β-LPH), first isolated by C. H. Li in 1964 (127). Subsequent studies have shown that indeed the C-fragment itself possesses potent opioid activity (128, 129). It was renamed β-endorphin. The term endorphin, following a proposal by Eric Simon, is now commonly employed as a general descriptor of opioid peptides, with the enkephalins as a specific pentapeptide subset.

The remarkable structural homology between β-LPH, β-endorphin, and Met-enkephalin suggested that Met-enkephalin might be formed by the proteolytic cleavage of β-endorphin and/or or β-LPH. Although attractive for its parsimony, this view is not supported by the recent findings of Bloom et al. (130), which point to a marked anatomic dissociation of neurons containing the enkephalins and β-endorphin—differences that suggest distinct

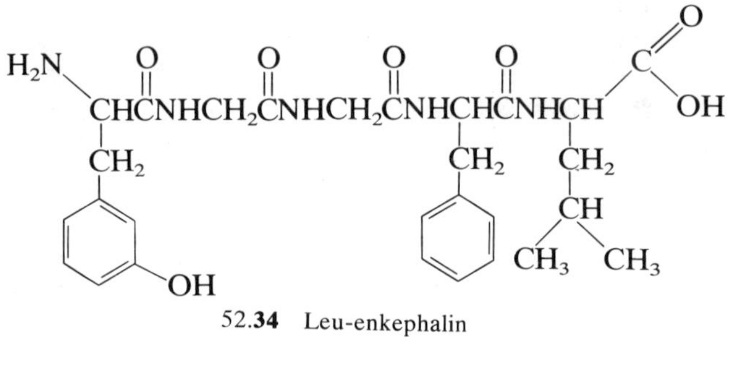

52.**34** Leu-enkephalin

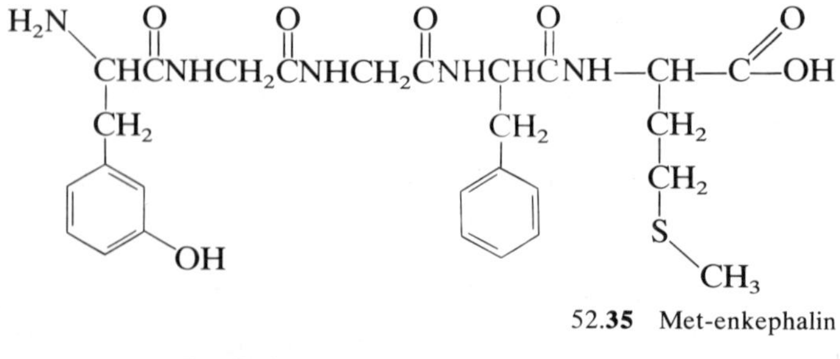

52.**35** Met-enkephalin

Fig. 52.14 Methione and leucine enkephalin.

roles for these two systems. The enkephalins appear to be the predominant opioid peptide in the CNS and gastrointestinal tract (140), while β-endorphin constitutes the major endogenous opioid in the posterior pituitary (141, 142). Furthermore, brain levels of β-endorphin and the enkephalins are unaltered up to 11 months after hypophysectomy (131), providing clear evidence that pituitary β-endorphin is not the source of either the endorphins or enkephalins found in the CNS. Taken together these results suggest the presence of at least three distinct opioid systems, the CNS β-endorphin and enkephalins as specific neurotransmitters and pituitary β-endorphin as a hormonal modulator. Differences in Met- and Leu-enkephalin distribution and pharmacology suggest yet a further subdivision. Enkephalin terminals in particular are located in many of the areas in the CNS and brainstem believed to be key to pain perception and analgesia.

In addition to β-endorphin, a number of other C-terminal β-lipotropin fragments have been identified which have opiate activity (e.g., α- and γ-endorphin (132), Table 52.4). Several other distinct non β-lipotropin-derived biologic extracts with opiate-like activity have also been described (133), including one that is apparently a nonpeptide (134). Precise structures and roles for these latter compounds are unknown.

Attempts to understand the physiological roles of these respective systems extend well beyond their ability to alter pain perception and hence the scope of this chapter. They may, however, someday provide a better understanding of the many actions of the opiates as well as providing new therapeutic directions for opioid-like drugs. This area continues to be extensively reviewed (110, 135–139).

3.5 Endorphin Biologic Function

There is growing evidence that the enkephalins function at the neuronal level as presynaptic inhibitory neurotransmitters. They are concentrated in nerve terminals and are released by depolarizing stimuli (143). The recent demonstration of a specific enkephalinase enzyme lends further credence to their role as neurotransmitters (144). Certainly in the periphery the enkephalins, like morphine, act to inhibit acetylcholine release in the guinea pig ileum and norepinephrine output in the mouse vas deferens. A similar inhibitory effect (see Fig. 52.15) on norepinephrine (157) and substance P release has also been demonstrated in CNS tissue (145). The discovery of the enkephalins in the GI tract is hardly surprising since similar distributions are observed for somatostatin, substance P, and other CNS peptides (146). Circulating

Table 52.4 Structure of Porcine Enforphins[a]

Peptide	Structure
Leu-enkephalin	H-TyrGlyGlyPheLeu-OH
Met-enkephalin	H-TyrGlyGlyPheMet OH
α-Endorphin	H-TyrGlyGlyPheMet ThrSerGluLysSerGlnThrProLeuValThr-OH
γ-Endorphin	H-TyrGlyGlyPheMet ThrSerGluLysSerGlnThrProLeuValThrLeu-OH
β-Endorphin	H-TyrGlyGlyPheMet ThrSerGluLysSerGlnThrProLeuValThrLeuPheLys- AsnAlaIleValLysAsnAlaHisLysLysGlyGln-OH

[a] All peptides except leu-enkephalin have a common sequence (61–65 of β-lipotropin). β-Endorphin corresponds to the C-terminal sequence (61–91) of β-lipotropin.

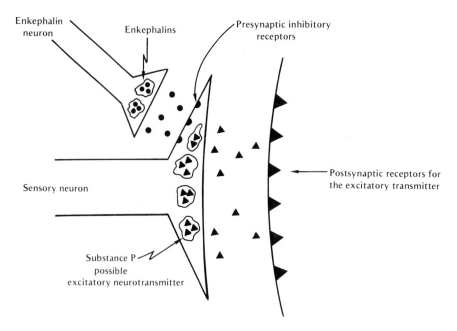

Fig. 52.15 Model of enkephalin modulation of primary sensory afferents at the point of entry into the dorsal horn of the spinal column.

levels of β-endorphin arise from the pituitary where they are released along with ACTH from a common, large molecular weight (31K) precursor (147, 148).

β-Endorphin is a potent and long-lasting (2–3 hr) analgetic in rats and cats both intracerebrally and intravenously (149, 150). Intravenous analgesia has also been reported in man (151). In contrast, the enkephalins are, at best, weakly analgetic in animals (152) and then only when injected directly into the brain. This extreme potency difference is almost certainly due to the relative metabolic lability of the enkephalins, as evidenced by the fact that their half-life is only 2–3 min in the presence of synaptic membranes as compared to 2–3 hr for β-endorphin (153).

With this evidence of morphine-like analgesia for the endorphins, the question of an endogenous role for these agents quite naturally focuses on pain modulation. Experimental evidence for such a role relies on a lowering of the pain threshold by naloxone. Using the mouse hot plate Jacob et al. (154) was the first to provide evidence

of shortened response latencies after naloxone. However, such demonstrations have proved to be very sensitive to experimental variables including diurnal variations reflective of fluctuations in endorphin release (155). The concept that the endorphins make up an endogenous pain control mechanism finds further support in reports that naloxone reverses the analgesia produced by acupuncture (156) and electrical stimulation (113) but, interestingly, not hypnosis (158). Surgical stress apparently also produces its own analgesia based on Lasagna's 1965 notation (159) of a "curious hyperalgesic effect" of naloxone in patients following surgery, an observation that has recently been confirmed in patients following dental surgery (160). In a more controversial report (161) it has been postulated that among normals, only placebo responders are naloxone sensitive. This suggests an interesting and still to be confirmed physiological rather than psychological explanation for the analgesic placebo response.

The confirmation of analgetic activity for

the endorphins created a renewed but short-lived hope that these or related peptides might lead at last to an analgesic devoid of dependence liability. Both Met-enkephalin and β-endorphin produce symptoms of physical dependence (162, 163) and evidence of tolerance and morphine cross-tolerance in animals and *in vitro* (164). Furthermore, self-administration experiments in rats indicate the development of dependence on both enkephalins (165). Drug generalization experiments indicate that Met-enkephalin is perceived by rats as subjectively comparable to fentanyl (166). In support of these findings, β-endorphin is also reported to support morphine abstinence in man (167). Rapid metabolic inactivation may partially explain why man is not addicted to his enodgenous endorphins, but part of the explanation must also be that their role is to provide tonic rather than constant neuronal modulation.

Nociception is almost certainly not the only role of the endorphins. The lack of overt naloxone activity in normals suggests that similar experiments should be designed to focus on pathological states. An interesting example of this approach is the discovery that naloxone reduces food consumption in a genetically obese strain of mice (168).

Although endorphin research has not resulted in an absolute separation of dependence liability and analgesia, it has reinforced the concept of morphologically distinct, multiple opiate receptors, an idea that becomes particularly attractive when faced with evidence that Met-enkephalin, Leu-enkephalin, and β-endorphin each subserve distinct neuronal systems.

3.6 Multiple Opiate Receptors and Selectivity

As early as 1967 Martin (169), in reviewing the pharmacological profiles of the mixed agonist antagonists, postulated that receptor dualism was required to explain compound to compound differences in analgesia, respiratory depression, and psychotomimetic effects. Using the chronic spinal dog preparation, Martin continued to accumulate data on the pharmacological fingerprints of a wide variety of opioids and in 1976 (170) expanded his hypothesis to include the presence of three discrete opiate receptors which he designated as the μ, κ, and σ receptors. The prototype agonists for these receptors are morphine (μ), ketocyclazocine (κ), and N-allylnorcyclazocine [SKF-10,047 (σ)] (Fig. 52.16). Naloxone is a prototype μ antagonist, and the novel benzomorphan antagonist recently described by Michne et al. (171) (52.**38**) shows selectivity as a κ antagonist. No selective σ antagonist is known to date.

The characteristic behavioral effects produced by each class are shown in Table 52.5. The mixed agonist/antagonists compete with morphine at the μ receptor, but do not themselves have agonist actions at this receptor. Instead their agonist activity is expressed through the other two receptors—the κ receptor mediating their analgetic actions and nalorphine-like dependence, and the σ receptor mediating their psychotomimetic effects. By this categorization, buprenorphine appears to be a partial agonist at the μ receptor, whereas nalorphine and pentazocine with their psychotomimetic side effects are μ antagonists with strong components of agonist action at the κ and σ receptors.

At the same time that evidence of discrete receptors was being accumulated by classical behavioral techniques, *in vitro* studies using receptor binding assays and the guinea pig ileum and mouse vas deferens preparations independently pointed to a similar conclusion. Hutchinson et al. (172) studied a series of benzomorphans using these assays and found that an enhanced guinea pig ileum/mouse vas deferens potency ratio coupled with poor reversal of activity by naloxone is predictive of interactions at the κ receptor, and hence of

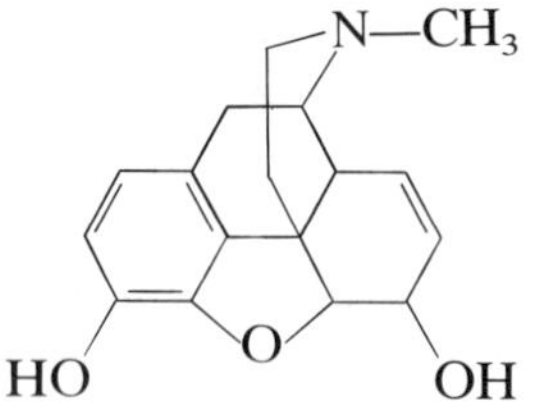

52.**1** μ-Receptor agonist
(morphine)

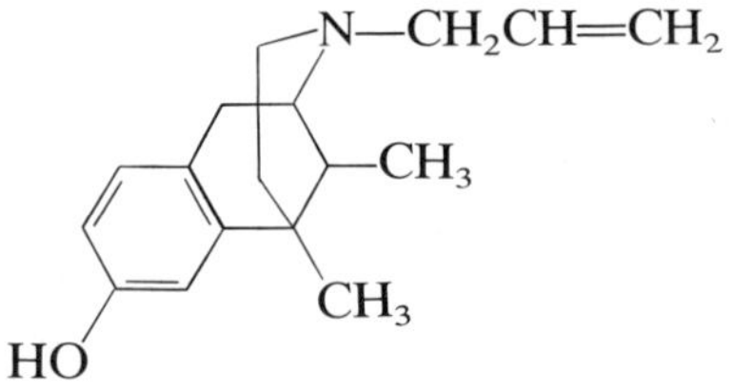

52.**36** α-Receptor agonist
(SKF 10047)

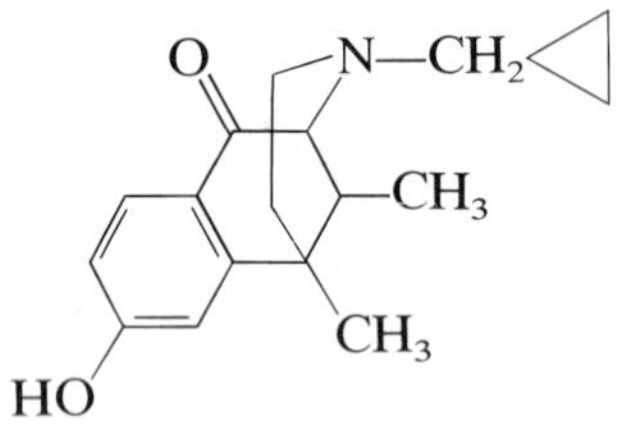

52.**37**   k-Receptor agonist
(ketocyclazocine)

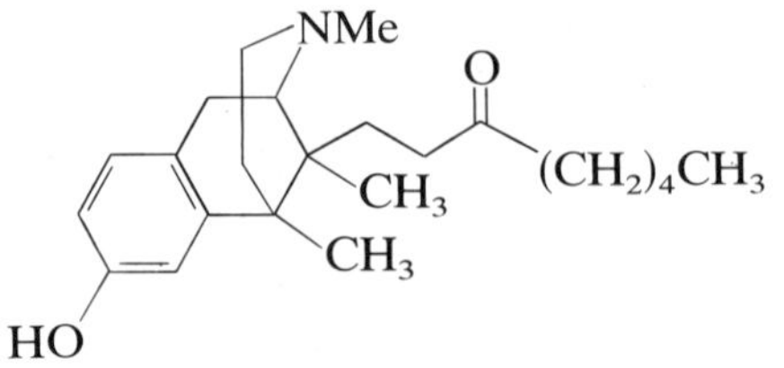

52.**38**   k-Receptor antagonist
(WIN-42,156)

Fig. 52.16   Structures of μ, k, and σ agonists and a selective k antagonist.

low morphine-like dependence liability. This conclusion is consistent with that predicted by Martin's *in vivo* work. Relatively little has been done to provide comparable *in vitro* endpoints for the σ agonists.

Initial studies of ^{3}H-enkephalin binding to opiate receptors revealed a different order of relative potencies for certain opiates than that previously seen under the ^{3}H-opiates. In addition the enkephalins were far less sensitive to the effects of sodium ion on binding affinity. Lord and Kosterlitz also found that Met- and Leu-enkephalin, but not β-endorphin, demonstrate an enhancement of mouse vas deferens activity over guinea pig ileum activity (173). This led them to suggest that, whereas β-endorphin has a large morphine-like (μ) component of action, the enkephalins interact heavily at a new group of distinct receptors which they termed the δ receptors. The suggestion is that these receptors are distinct from those outlined by Martin, although a full behavioral characterization remains to be done.

With the concepts of receptor multiplicity and the current status of analgetic research in mind, it is appropriate to turn to a detailed consideration of opioid structure–activity relationships, for it is this knowledge base and its anomalies that continue to provide the foundations for new advances in opioid analgetic research.

4   STRUCTURE–ACTIVITY RELATIONSHIPS OF THE OPIOID ANALGETICS

4.1   Naturally Occurring Opium Alkaloids

Some 27 alkaloids, including morphine and codeine, have been isolated from the dried juice of the poppy plant, *Papaver somniferum* (see Table 52.6, 174). The more important of these, in terms of their therapeutic or synthetic uses, can be classified structurally as (1) those containing the partially reduced phenanthrene skeleton (Fig. 52.17) and (2) those containing

Table 52.5 Characteristic Pharmacological Actions of μ, k, and σ Agonists

Action	μ (Morphine)	k (Keterocyclazocine)	σ (SKF-10,047)
Spinalized dog			
Pulse rate	Decrease	No change	Increase
Pupil size	Decrease	Decrease	Increase
Respiratory rate	Decrease	No change (?)	Increase
Temperature	Decrease	No change	Increase
Flexor reflex	Large decrease	large decrease	Decrease
Skin twitch reflex	Large decrease	decrease	No change
Suppression of morphine abs.	Yes	No	No
Suppression of cyclazocine abs.	Yes	Yes	No
General symptomatology	Indifference	Sedation	Delirium
In vitro			
Guinea pig ileum	Good activity	Good activity	
Mouse vas deferens	Equal or slightly less active than in ileum	4–5× less potent than in ileum using normorphine as standard	
Reversal of ileum inhibition by naloxone	Effective	3–7× more required (i.e. less sensitive)	
Reversal by Mr-1353 (a k antagonist)	Poor	Effective	
Sodium effect (^{3}H-naloxone binding)	≥50 fold	6–10 fold	

Table 52.6   Alkaloids from Opium

Morphine, 10%	Codamine
Codeine, 0.5%	Gnoscopine
Papaverine, 1%	Oxynarcotine
Noscapine, 6%	Porphyroxine
Hydrocotarine	
Thebaine 0.3%	Hydrocotarnine
Narceine, 0.2%	Lanthopine
Pseudopapaverine	Protopine
Protopapaverine	Cryptopine
Papaveramine	Neopine
Laudanine	Triptopine
Laudanidine	Pseudomorphine rheoadine
Laudanosine	Oripavine, from *Papaver orientale*
Meconidine	Isothebaine, from *Papaver orientale*

the benzylisoquinoline nucleus (Fig. 52.18). The most important phenanthrene alkaloids are morphine (52.**1**), codeine (52.**2**), and thebaine (52.**39**) (Fig. 52.17). Papaverine (52.**40**), narceine (52.**41**), and narcotine (noscapine, 52.**42**) represent the important members of the benzylisoquinolines (Fig. 52.18). Table 52.6 shows the average percentages of these alkaloids in opium (175).

In view of their structural differences, it is not surprising that the phenanthrene and benzylisoquinoline alkaloids also differ in their therapeutic indications. Narceine and narcotine are primarily employed as antitussives, whereas papaverine is a smooth muscle relaxant with little or no CNS activity. Codeine, though analgetically weaker than morphine, is distinguished by its oral activity and as such is used widely in combination with aspirin-like drugs for the treatment of mild to moderate pain and as an antitussive. Thebaine, though inactive as an analgetic, nonetheless serves as a key

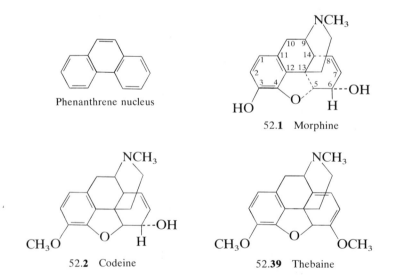

Fig. 52.17   Opium alkaloids derived from the phenanthrene nucleus.

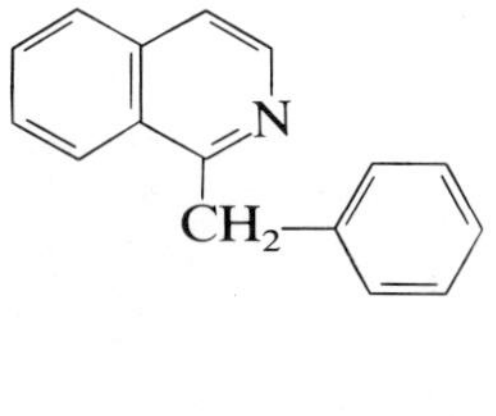

Benzylisoquinoline nucleus

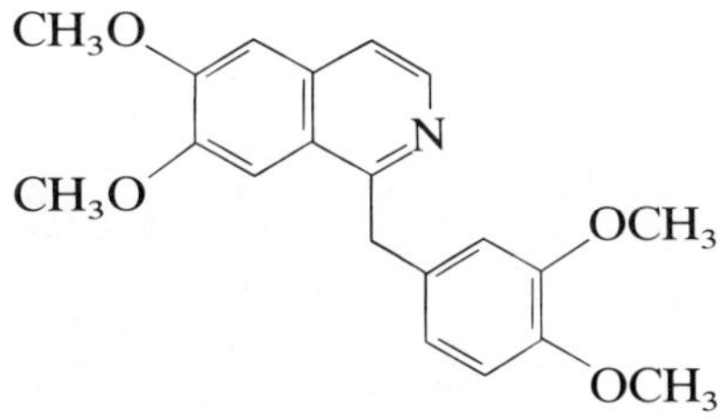

52.**40**   Papaverine

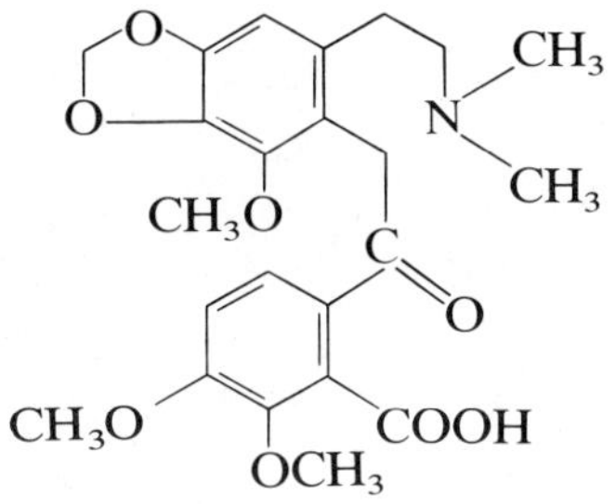

52.**41**   Narceine

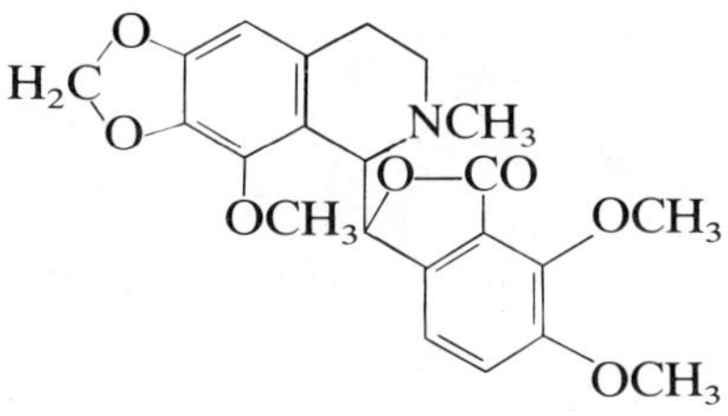

52.**42**   Noscapine

Fig. 52.18   Opium alkaloids derived from the benzylisoquinoline nucleus.

synthetic intermediate in the preparation of potent, opiate analgetics.

Historically morphine is the most important of the opium alkaloids because of its potent analgetic properties. Owing to its complex structure, more than a century elapsed following its isolation by Sertürner before Gulland and Robinson (176) proposed the correct structure of morphine in 1925. It took an additional 27 years before the accuracy of this structure was confirmed by total synthesis by Gates and Tschudi in 1952 (177, 178). The stereochemistry and absolute configuration of morphine were subsequently elucidated (179–182) and are depicted in Fig. 52.17.

Although exceptions exist, examination of the main subclasses of opiate analgetics indicates that they all have common structural features as illustrated in Fig. 52.19. Specifically, these include (1) an aromatic ring, (2) a quaternary carbon to which the aromatic ring is attached, and (3) a nitrogen atom separated from the quaternary carbon

by a two-carbon chain. The skeletal relationships of the semisynthetic and totally synthetic opiate analgetics provide the basis for the systematic treatment of the SAR contained in the following sections.

4.2   Derivatives of Codeine and Morphine

The synthesis of diacetylmorphine (heroin, 52.**3**) from morphine in the late ninteenth century (183) marked the beginning of the chemical manipulation of the natural opiates. These efforts were intensified in 1929 when a 10-year synthesis and testing program was initiated by the National Research Council of the United States. Much of this early work sought to improve the analgetic profile of morphine relative to addiction liability through modifications of the C ring. Table 52.7 summarizes some of the animal pharmacology of the C-ring modified morphine and codeine derivatives.

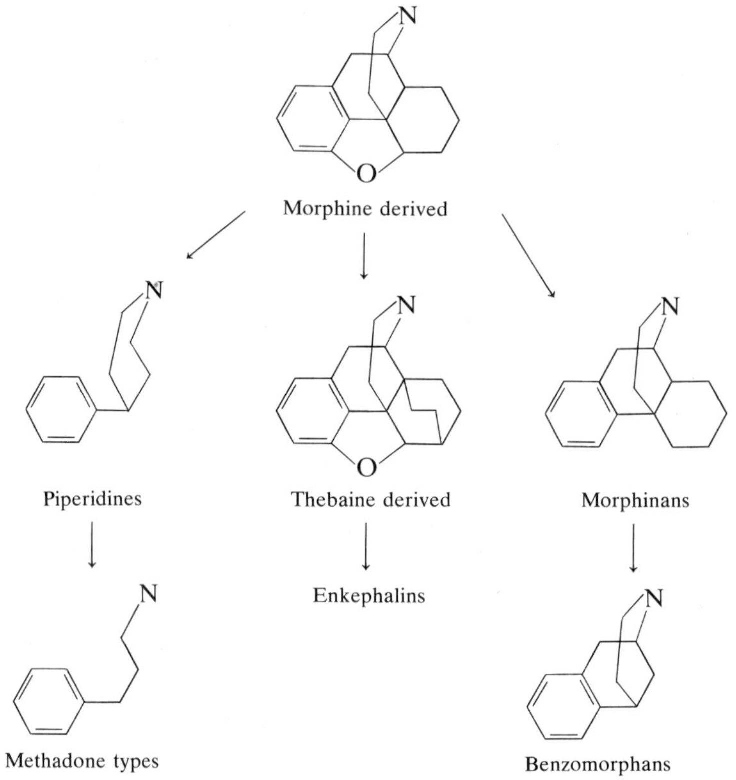

Fig. 52.19 Structural relationships of the semisynthetic and synthetic opiates.

Though some of these initial derivatives are still used clinically today, they show no real therapeutic advantage over their morphine or codeine counterparts.

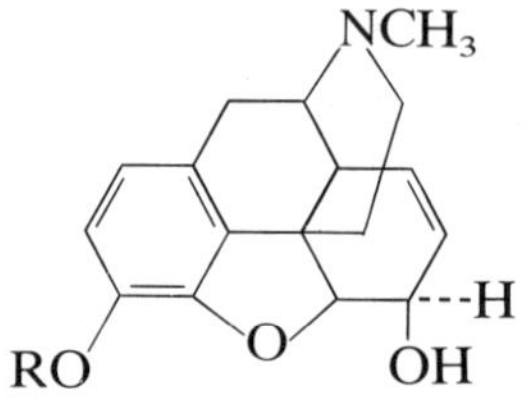

4.2.1 C-RING STRUCTURE-ACTIVITY RELATIONSHIPS. It was thus shown quite early that although the C-6 α-hydroxy group could be methylated, oxidized, or replaced by halogen (chloromorphide) to give more active analgetics, these derivatives also exhibited enhanced toxicity relative to morphine (42). Interestingly, although inversion of the 6-hydroxy group to α-isomorphine (52.**43a**) and isocodeine (52.**43b**) gave similar results, shifting of the hydroxyl to C-8 (52.**44a** and 52.**44b**) decreased analgetic activity. Since a double bond (52.**45**) and hydrogen

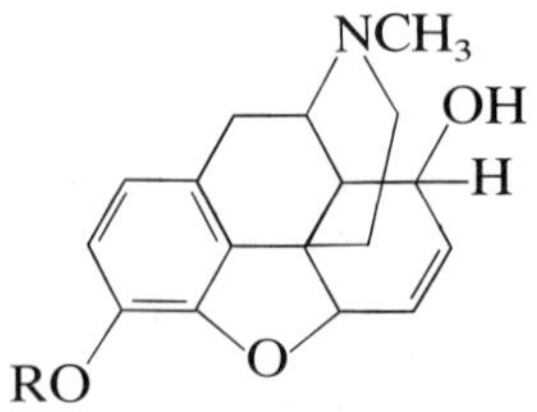

52.**43a** R = H
52.**43b** R = CH₃

52.**44a** R = CH₃
52.**44b** R = H

Table 52.7 Pharmacological Effects of Some Morphine Derivatives

Formula No.	Alkaloidal Base	LD_{50},[a] mg/kg	Median Effective Dose (ED_{50}), mg/kg					
			Analgesia[b]	Exciting Effect[c]	Emetic Action[d]	General Depression[e]	Respiratory Effects[f]	Convulsant Action[g]
52.1	Morphine	531	0.75	0.57	0.22	6.75	0.15	531
52.2	Codeine	241	8.04	8.04	16.0+	36.1	1.3	161
52.44a	Pseudocodeine	1780	17.8	22.2	4.45	89.1	48.0	
52.44b	γ-Isomorphine	2000+	7.09	7.09	1.77	133+	2.36	
52.43a	α-Isomorphine	890	0.80	0.89	0.13	22.2	0.15	
52.43b	Isocodeine	589	13.0	13.0		58.9		589
52.103	6-Acetylmorphine	293	0.18	0.18	0.18+	0.9		180
52.4	Dihydromorphinone	84	0.17	0.17	0.08	0.88	0.011	67
52.5	Dihydrocodeinone	86	1.28	0.86	2.56+	4.20	0.08	47
52.7	Dihydrohydroxycodeinone	426	1.34	0.89	0.89+	1.34	0.10	426
52.46a	Dihydrodesoxymorphine-D	104	0.08	0.16	Low	0.32	0.012	104
52.8	Metopon	25	0.07	0.10	0.07	3.00	0.012	25

[a] Subcutaneously in mice.
[b] Minimal dose administered intramuscularly that caused Eddy-pressure-test response in at least 80% of cats.
[c] Minimal dose in cats causing excitement in at least two of five animals.
[d] Minimal dose causing nausea, licking, or vomiting in cats.
[d] Smallest dose preventing immediate righting of at least 15 of 20 rats 30 min after intraperitoneal administration.
[d] As defined by Wright and Barbour (184).
[e] Minimal dose causing convulsions in mice.

(52.46) both increase morphine-like activity, it must be concluded that introduction of this C-8 functionality is directly responsible for the decreased activity. Further support of this conclusion comes from the observation that the C-8 β-halo derivatives (52.47) are more potent analgetics than morphine (185).

Catalytic rearrangement of codeine and morphine produce the potent analgetics dihydromorphinone (hydromorphone, Dilaudid, 52.4) and dihydrocodeinone (hydrocodone, Dicodid, 52.5). Clinically, hydromorphone is 10 times more potent than morphine as an analgetic, with a similar profile of side effects (186).

Introduction of a 14-hydroxy group yields the still more potent 14-hydroxydihydrocodeinone (oxycodone, Eucodal, 52.7) (187) and 14-hydroxydihydromorphonone (oxymorphone, Numorphan, 52.6) (188). Though all four of these compounds are used clinically, they offer no

real advantage over morphine because increased abuse liability parallels the increase in analgetic potency.

Introduction of a new substituent in the C ring of morphine generally produces only

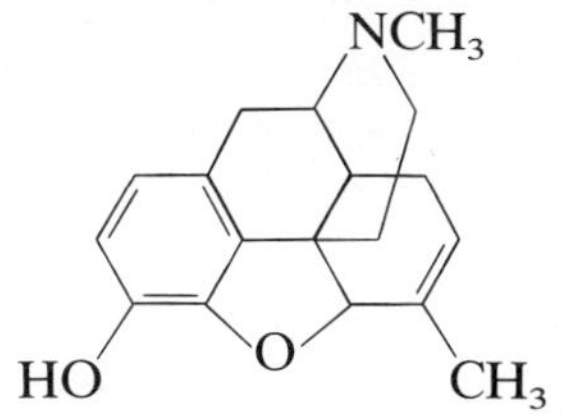

52.45

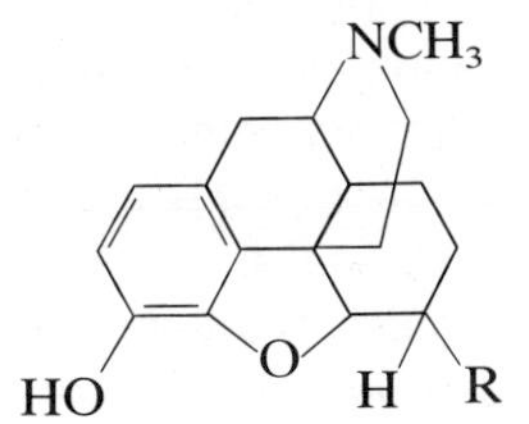

52.46a R = H
52.46b R = CH₃

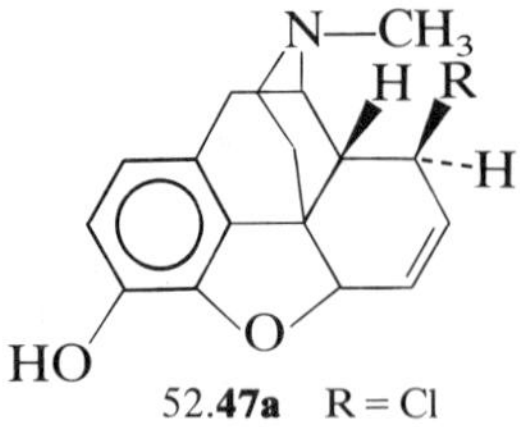

52.**47a** R = Cl
52.**47b** R = Br
52.**47c** R = I

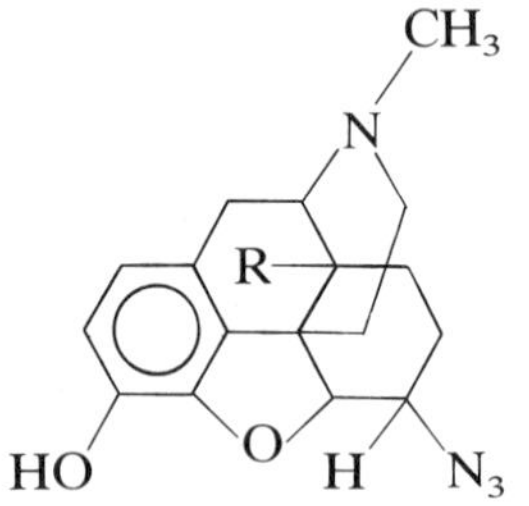

52.**48a** R = H
52.**48b** R = OH

Table 52.8 N-Substituted Normorphines

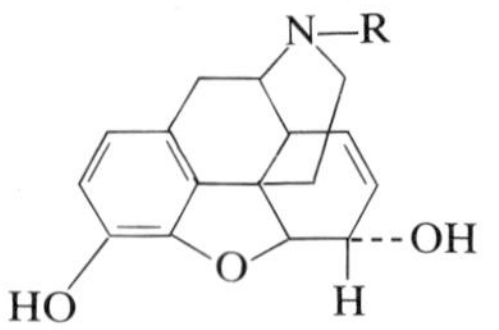

Agonist, R	Antagonist, R
CH_3	$CH_2CH{=}CH_2$
C_5H_{11}	C_3H_7
C_6H_{13}	$CH_2\text{-}c\text{-}C_3H_5$
$(CH_2)_2\text{-}c\text{-}C_6H_{11}$	$CH_2\text{-}c\text{-}C_4H_7$
$(CH_2)_2C_6H_5$	

quantitative changes in activity. Two possible exceptions to this rule are 5-methyldihydromorphine (189, 190) (metopon, 52.**8**) and azidomorphine (52.**48a**). Metopon is more efficacious than morphine orally and reputedly has fewer side effects including abuse potential (191). The difficult synthesis of metopon from thebaine has prevented widespread clinical use. Azidomorphine is 40–50 times more potent than morphine in man (192) and possesses less abuse potential at equianalgetic doses, as judged by experiments in animals (193, 194). As is the case for the parent opiates, introduction of a 14-hydroxy group (52.**48b**) produces a further improvement in therapeutic ratio (195).

4.2.2 SAR OF NITROGEN SUBSTITUTION. The replacement of the N-methyl group of morphine brings about quantitative and, more significantly, qualitative changes in SAR, yielding compounds that are potent agonists, antagonists, and mixed agonists/antagonists. Although substitution at nitrogen in the opiates is hardly new, the importance of this early work (61, 196–198) was not recognized until it was found

that N-allylmorphine (Nalorphine, 52.**23**) was a morphine antagonist (62, 199). These findings spurred the systematic SAR study of substitution at nitrogen (200, 201). Table 52.8 summarizes these and more recent findings.

The most potent agonist, N-phenethyl-normorphine (52.**49**), is six times more potent than morphine. The N-phenethyl moiety imparts similar enhanced activity to desmorphine, codeine, and heterocodeine (202–204). Likewise, use of the n-allyl group imparts antagonist activity to other family members. Substitution of potent oxymorphone series with N-allyl yields the very potent, pure narcotic antagonist naloxone (52.**27**) (205). Naltrexone (52.**28**) and nalbuphine (52.**29**) are recent examples that utilize the cycloalkylmethyl functions to produce narcotic antagonist activity. Naltrexone is a more potent and orally more effective narcotic antagonist than naloxone and it has a longer duration of action (206). Nalbuphine is an

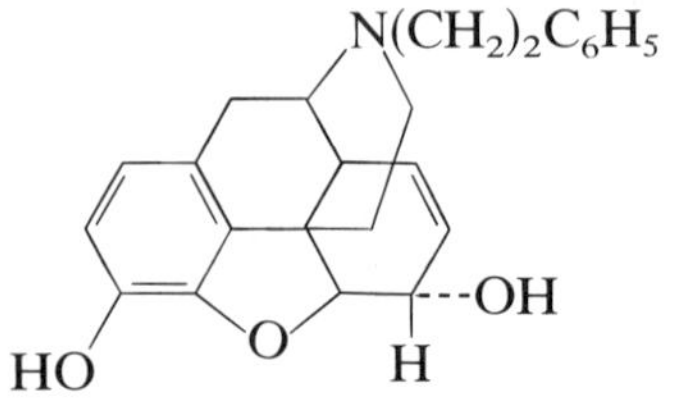

52.**49**

agonist/antagonist analgesic that is as potent as morphine, but has fewer side effects (207).

4.2.3   A-RING MODIFICATIONS. An intact A-ring is, in general, essential for analgetic activity. Masking of the phenolic hydroxyl causes a decrease in morphine's analgetic activity; heroin being a notable exception. Likewise, substitution in the phenyl ring

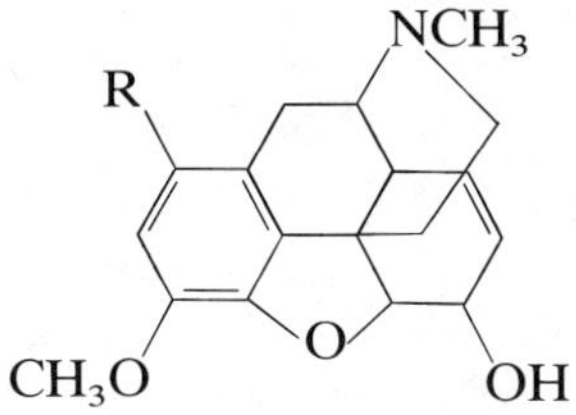

52.**50a**   R = Cl
52.**50b**   R = Br
52.**50c**   R = CH$_3$CO
52.**50d**   R = F

generally diminishes activity. Thus 1-chloro- (52.**50a**), 1-bromo- (52.**50b**), and 1-acetocodeine (52.**50c**) all have diminished potency relative to codeine (208). It is important for SAR considerations to note that 1-fluoro-codeine (52.**50d**) is as potent as codeine, allowing the conclusion that steric bulk, not electronic factors, is responsible for the decreased activity (209).

4.3   Derivatives of Thebaine and Oripavine

Since the desirable separation of analgetic effects from side effects had not been achieved with simple structures (cf. Sections 4.4–4.6), Bentley and Hardy proposed that a more rigid molecule might interact more specifically with a single, pain-relieving receptor and not with other side effect-producing centers (210). This working hypothesis led them to synthesize hundreds of substituted 6,14-*endo*-ethenotetrahydrooripavines and the corresponding O-methylated thebaines. Many of these compounds possess very high intrinsic ac-

tivity and have contributed significantly to our understanding of structural requirements for binding to the opiate receptor (211, 212).

Formally, 6,14-*endo*-ethenotetrahydrothebaine (52.**51a**) and 6,14-*endo*-ethenotetrahydrooripavine (52.**51b**) can be viewed as derivatives of thebaine (52.**52a**) and oripavine (52.**52b**), respectively. Hence members of this latter group are often designated oripavines. Like the morphine series, this series possesses the full spectrum of agonist/antagonist activity. The SAR of the oripavines parallels that of the opiates, except that they are uniformly more potent (211). This is exemplified by etorphine (52.**22**), buprenorphine (52.**32**), and diprenorphine (52.**53**). Etorphine is a pure agonist, some 1000 times more potent

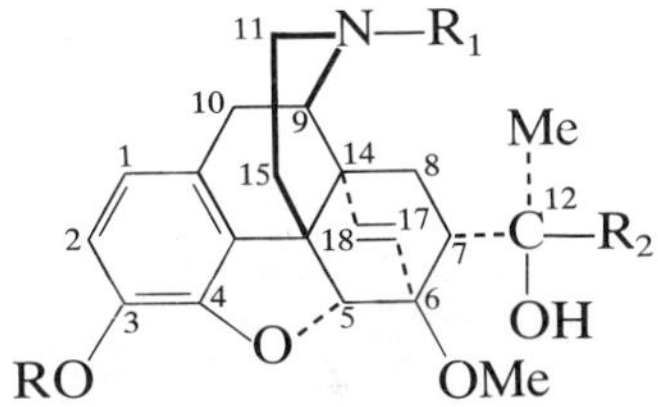

52.**51a**   R = CH$_3$
52.**51b**   R = H

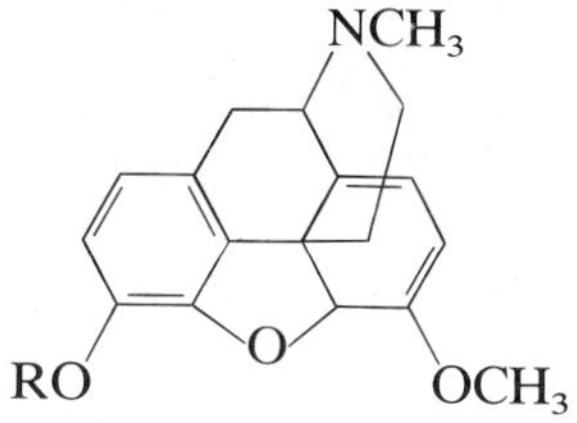

52.**52a**   R = CH$_3$
52.**52b**   R = H

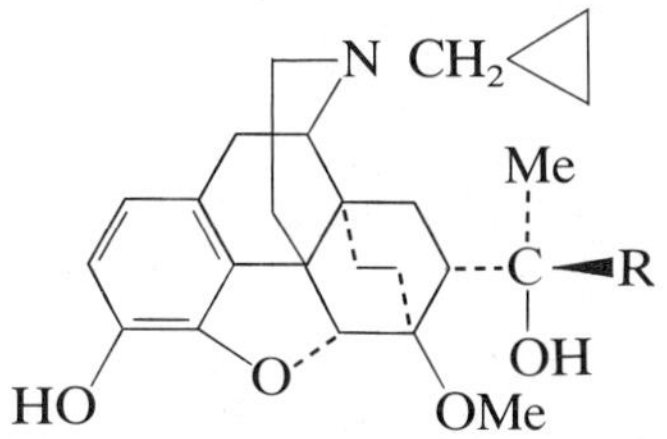

52.**32**   R = t-C$_4$H$_9$
52.**53**   R = CH$_3$

than morphine. Although it is an effective analgetic in man (214), etorphine is primarily used in veterinary medicine to immobilize large animals because of its extreme potency (214–217). At the other extreme, diprenorphine is a potent narcotic antagonist, 100 times more potent than nalorphine (218). Buprenorphine exemplifies a potent narcotic antagonist analgetic from this series, being some 10–20 times more potent than morphine in man and without psychotomimetic side effects (65).

The particular significance of this series is that it provides evidence for an additional lipophilic binding region at the opiate receptor, as witnessed by the fact that analgetic potency increases in the series 52.**54** going from R = methyl through pentyl, reaching a maximum at propyl and butyl (211). The regiospecificity of this binding is

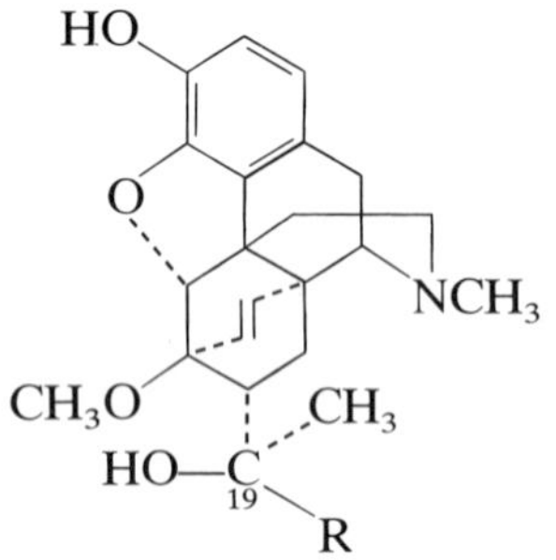

52.**56**

52.**54a** R = CH$_3$
52.**54b** R = C$_2$H$_5$
52.**54c** R = C$_3$H$_7$
52.**54d** R = C$_4$H$_9$
52.**54e** R = C$_5$H$_{11}$

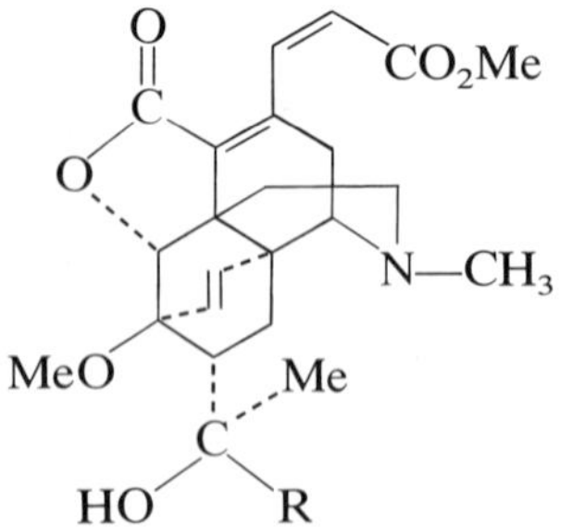

52.**55a** R = C$_3$H$_7$
52.**55b** R = C$_4$H$_9$
52.**55c** R = C$_5$H$_{11}$

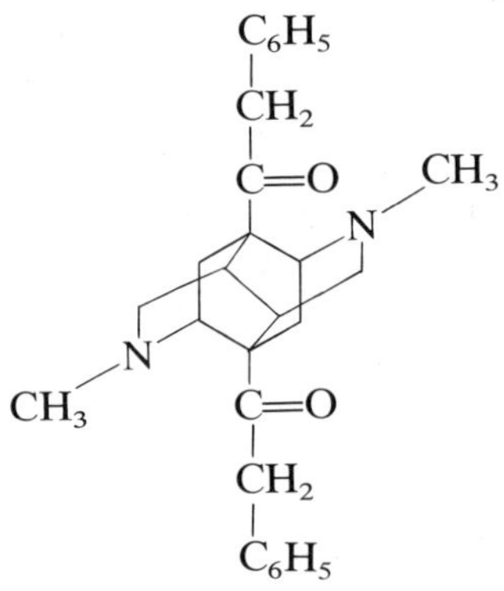

demonstrated by the observation that 52.**54c** is 50 times more potent than its diastereoisomer. The importance of the lipophilic binding region (see also Sect. 52.3.2.1) is underscored in the related alkyl series 52.**55**, which exhibits analgetic activity comparable to morphine despite the fact that the "essential" A ring is no longer present in the molecule (219)!

Similar logic may also explain the potent, narcotic analgetic activity of a recently discovered diazaditwistane 5,11-dimethyl-2,9-bis(phenacetyl)-5,11-diazatetracyclo-[6.2.2.0^{2,7}.0^{4,9}]dodecane (52.**56**) which otherwise appears to violate classic opiate SAR (220).

4.4 Piperidine Synthetics

The discovery of analgetic properties in meperidine (52.**9**) (44) represented a significant milestone and serendipitous discovery in the analgetic field since it pointed the direction to structural simplification of morphine into relatively small, uncomplicated fragments (Fig. 52.20). Modifications of the piperidine analgetics can be classified into four major families: the meperidines, the bemidones, the prodines (reversed meperidine esters), and the fentanyl group.

Many N-substituted derivatives of meperidine have been prepared with varying degrees of analgetic potency and side effect

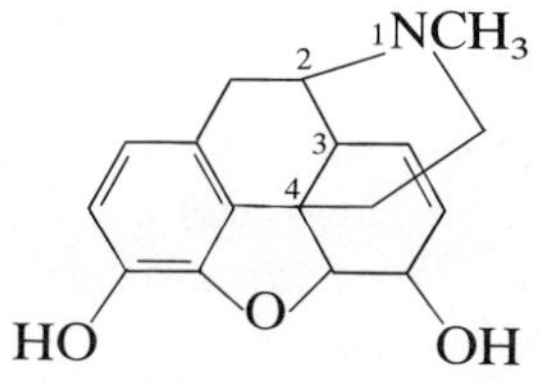

Fig. 52.20   Structural relationship of morphine and meperidine.

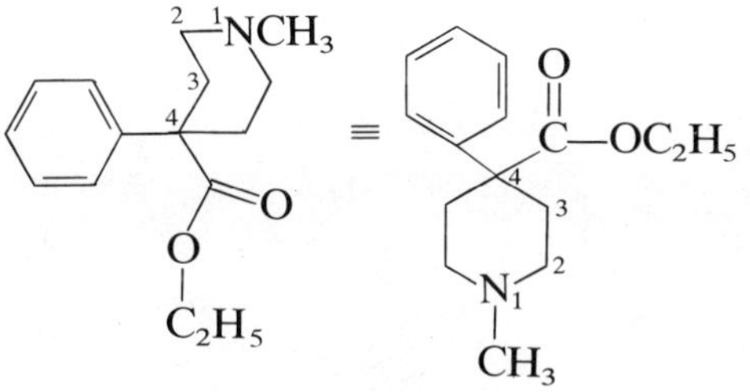

profiles (221). One of these, the *N*-*p*-aminophenethyl derivative of merperidine (anileridine, 52.**10**) is in general clinical use. Anileridine has good oral activity, two to three times more potent than meperidine, with relatively mild side effects (222). Unlike naloxone, the *N*-allyl derivative of meperidine does not possess narcotic antagonist activity. This is presumably in part due to the lack of a phenolic hydroxyl group since the closely related bemidone (52.**57**) series, which contains the hydroxyl group, has members with both strong agonist and antagonist activity depending on the nature of the *N*-substituent (223). The presence of a *m*-hydroxy group is not the only structural feature contributing to unusual antagonist SAR of the phenylpiperidines,

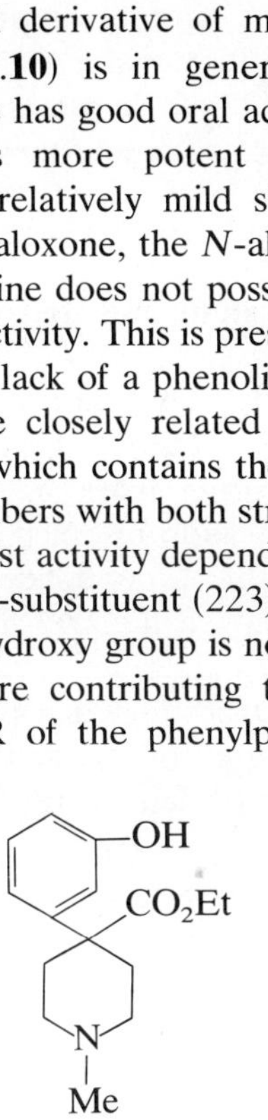

52.**57**

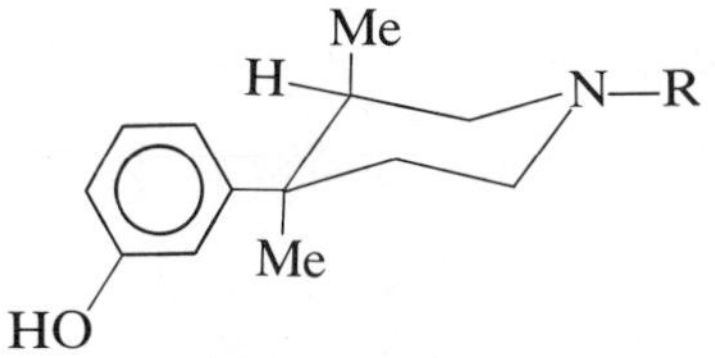

52.**58a**   R = CH$_3$
52.**58b**   R = CH$_2$CH$_2$C$_6$H$_5$

since the (+)-*N*-methyl derivative 52.**58a** possesses antagonist activity comparable to naloxone (72, 224)! The *N*-phenethyl derivative, 52.**58b**, is an even more potent antagonist. The stereochemical placement of the 3-methyl substituent is key to the antagonist properties of this unique series.

Replacement of the ester function by a ketone moiety in the bemidone series yields ketobemidone (52.**12**), which is twice as potent and more subject to abuse than is meperidine (225, 226). Similarly, replacement of the ester group of meperidine by the propionoxy function (the reversed ester of meperidine) yields compounds with greatly increased potency (221). Introduction of a methyl group into the 3 position of the reversed ester of meperidine yields the potent, diastereomeric analgetics α- and β-prodine (227, 228). Although β-prodine (52.**59**) is more potent, α-prodine (52.**60**) is used clinically in obstetrics because of its rapid onset and short duration of action (229). The *N*-substituted ester (52.**61**) is the most potent analgetic (3200 × meperidine) among the reversed esters (230). The dimethyl analog of meperidine, α-trimeperidine (52.**62**), is used clinically in the Soviet Union (221). Surprisingly, the (+) and (−) isomers of 52.**62** are equipotent (231).

Introduction of larger substituents on the piperidine ring greatly complicates stereo-structure–activity relationships relative to the rigid opiates. Thus introduction of an axial propyl group (52.**63**) substantially re-

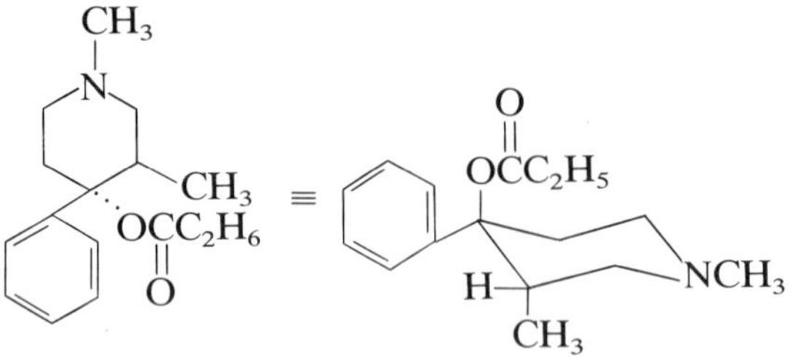

52.**59**

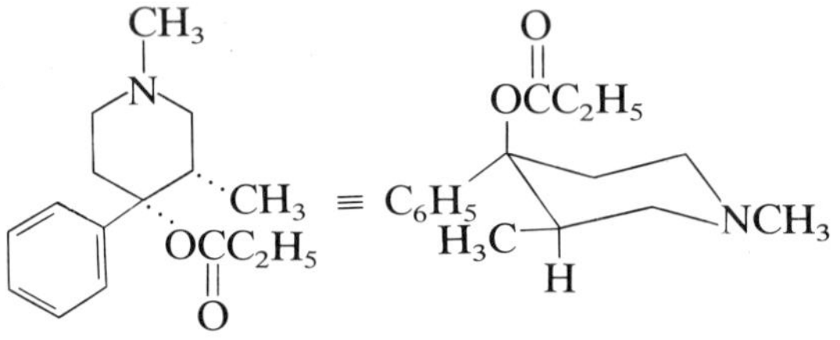

52.**60**

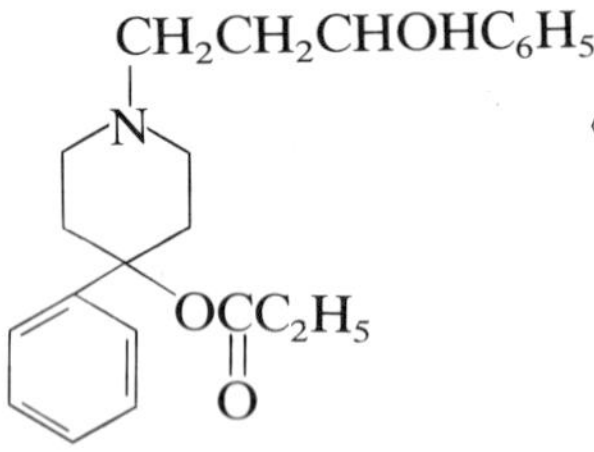

52.**61**

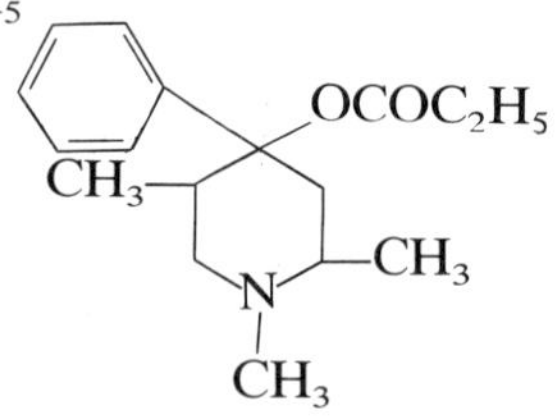

52.**62**

duces the activity in the prodine homologs, whereas the equatorial isomer (52.**64**) is as potent as morphine (232).

Ring expansion or contraction of meperidine and its reversed esters generally

results in decreased analgetic potency (233, 234). Although less potent the seven-membered ring meperidine homolog (etho-heptazine, 52.**13**) is useful in mild to moderate pain (234, 235) and has reduced addiction potential (236). The ring-contracted reversed ester, prodilidine (52.**65**), is slightly less active than codeine (237, 238).

Insertion of a nitrogen in the ketobemi-done series yields the highly potent *N*-phenylpropanamides. The parent of this series, fentanyl (52.**11**), is some 300 times more potent than morphine with a rapid onset and shorter duration of action (239, 240). Recent interest has focused on sufentanil (52.**66**) as a potential morphino-mimetic for use in anesthesia (241).

4.5 Methadone and Related Derivatives

The remarkably simple structure of methadone (52.**15**) (49, 242) is consistent with the earlier work on the meperidine analgetics, and in fact Beckett (243) suggested that a nonbonded interaction of the type shown in 52.**67** might fix methadone in a meperidine-like conformation. Gero (244) postulated a pseudopiperidine ring structure for methadone and recent conformational studies (245) of methadone

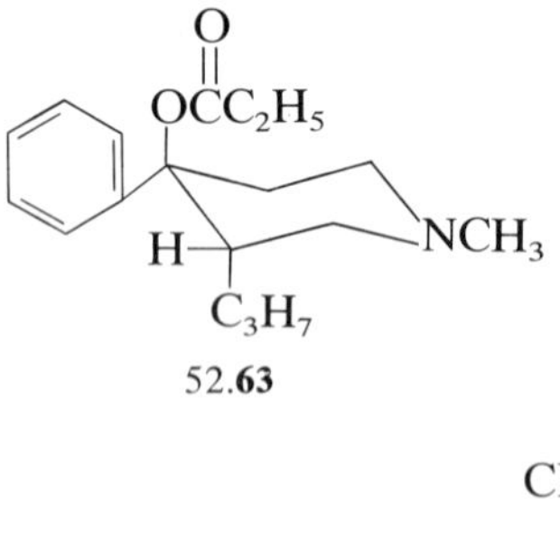

52.**63**

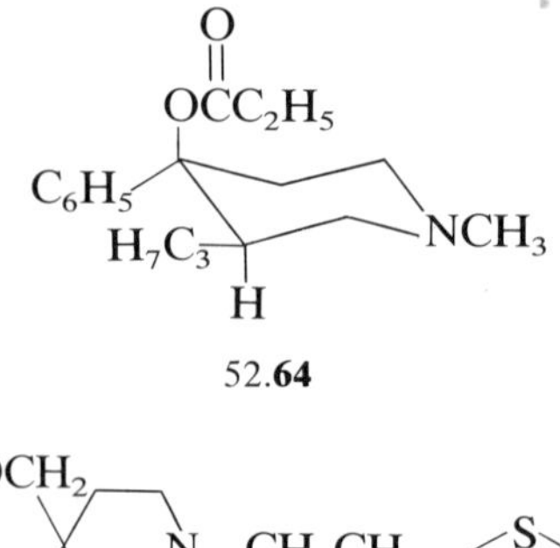

52.**64**

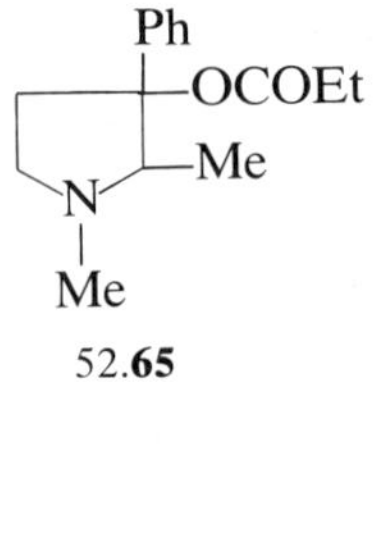

52.**65**

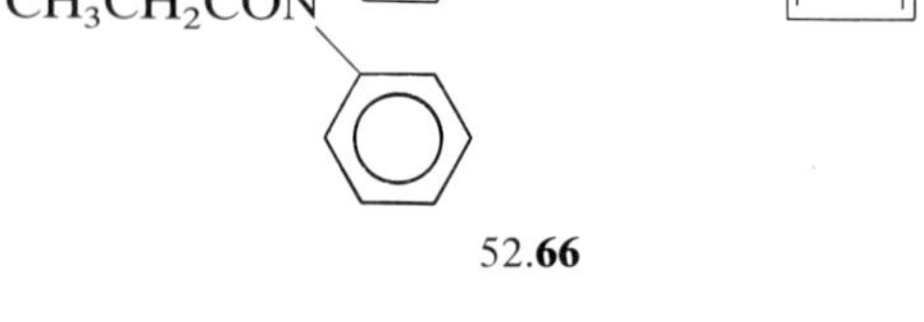

52.**66**

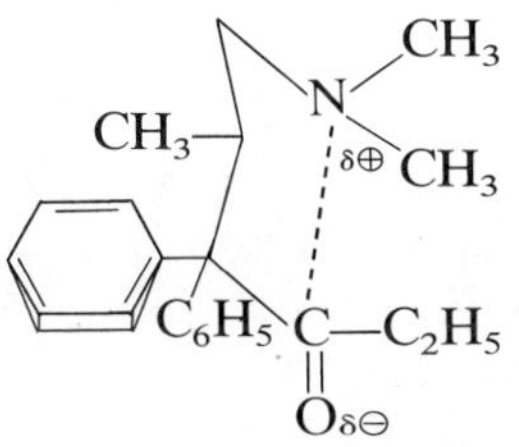

52.**67**

are consistent with such an internally stabilized structure (52.**68**). The magnitude of this stabilization is considerably weaker than was generally ascribed (245).

Clinically, methadone is equivalent to morphine as an analgetic, causes respiratory depression at equianalgetic doses, and is highly addictive (242). Today, the most important use of methadone is in the long-term treatment and rehabilitation of individuals dependent on morphine and heroin. Methadone's use in treating narcotic addicts was advocated (191) based on the fact that it is orally more effective and longer acting than morphine, and the symptoms produced on abrupt withdrawal are less severe than for morphine.

Although structural analogs of methadone generally show reduced activity or are inactive (246), (−)-isomethadone (52.**69**) is almost as potent as (−)-methadone (247, 248, 249) and generally produces fewer side effects (191). Neither 52.**69** nor any other ketone analog has gained the clinical acceptance accorded methadone. However, based on conformational studies that indicate substantially different preferred conformations for 52.**15** and 52.**69**, it has recently been proposed that isomethadone be investigated as an alternative to methadone maintenance therapy since its

greater conformational homogeneity could afford a greater selectivity of action (245).

Phenoxadone (52.**70**) and dipipanone (52.**71**), the morpholino and piperidino analogs of the dimethylamino portion of methadone, are employed clinically to a limited extent. Phenoxadone is an effective analgetic, comparable to morphine in chronic pain (250–252), but with reduced addiction liability (191, 253). Dipipanone

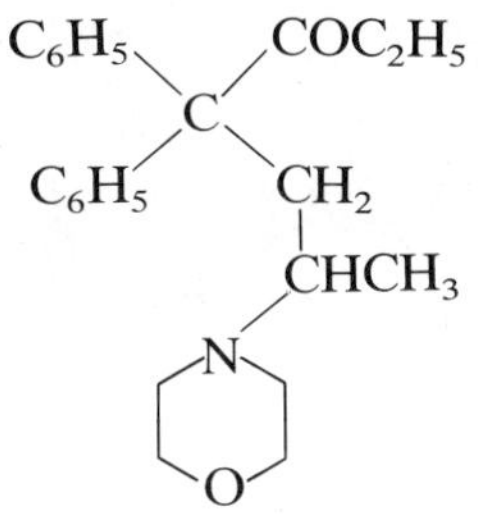

52.**70**

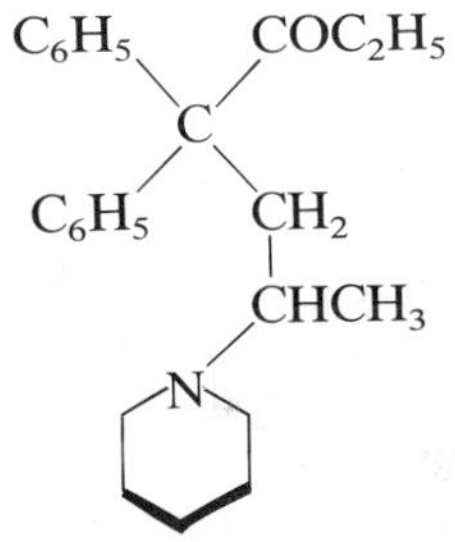

52.**71**

shares all of morphine's properties, including addiction liability (191, 254), and has been used as an adjunct to anesthesia in obstetrics and surgery (255). Methadone analogs with a tertiary amide moiety in place of the alkylketone group are potent, morphine-like analgetics (191, 256, 257). Thus (+)-N-(2,2-diphenyl-3-4-morphol-

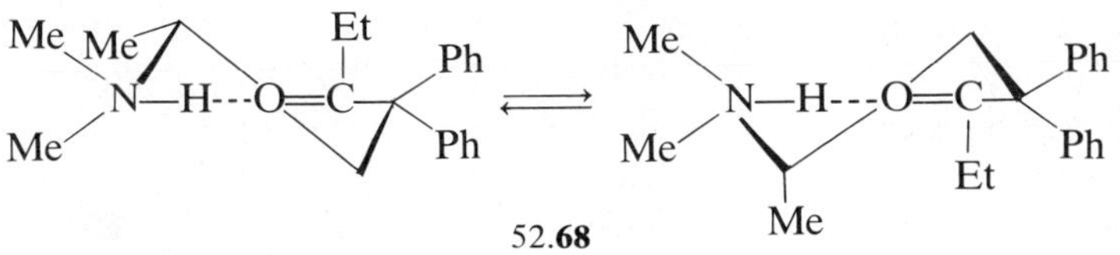

52.**68**

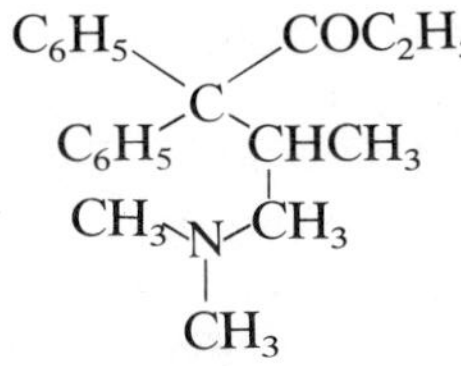

52.**69**

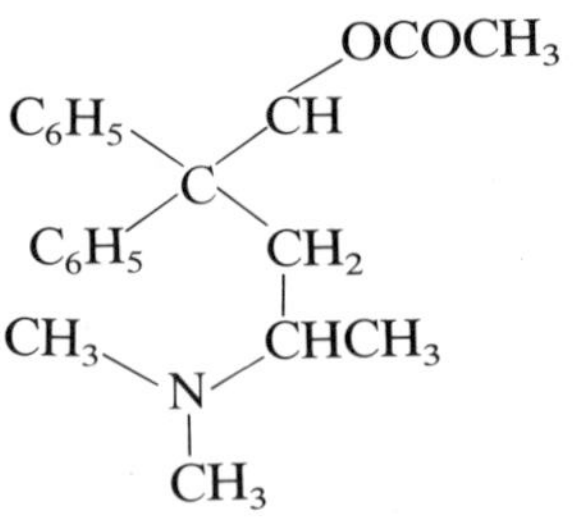

OCOCH$_3$

C$_6$H$_5$ CH

C

C$_6$H$_5$ CH$_2$

CH$_3$ CHCH$_3$

N

CH$_3$

52.**73**

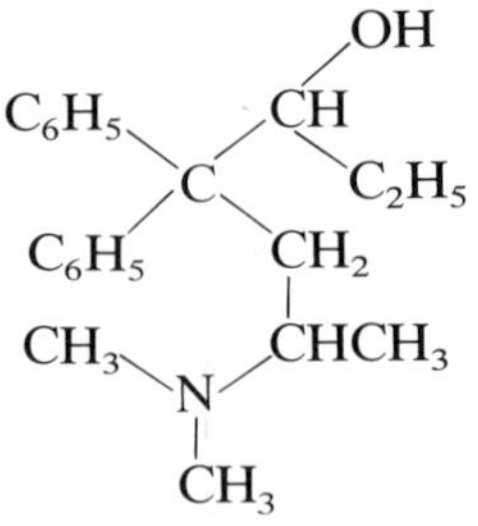

OH

C$_6$H$_5$ CH

C C$_2$H$_5$

C$_6$H$_5$ CH$_2$

CH$_3$ CHCH$_3$

N

CH$_3$

52.**72**

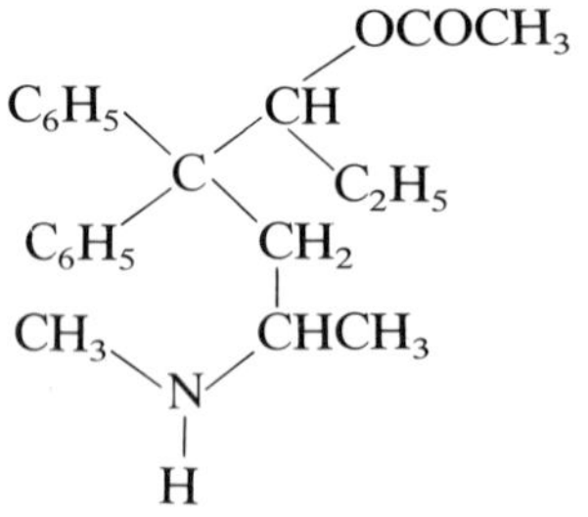

OCOCH$_3$

C$_6$H$_5$ CH

C C$_2$H$_5$

C$_6$H$_5$ CH$_2$

CH$_3$ CHCH$_3$

N

H

52.**75**

OH

C$_6$H$_5$ CH

C C$_2$H$_5$

C$_6$H$_5$ CH$_2$

CH$_3$ CHCH$_3$

N

H

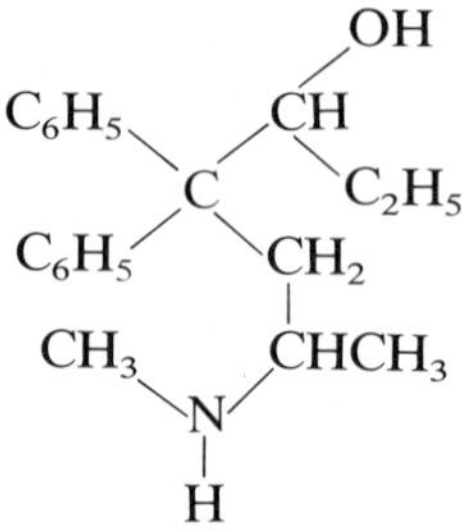

52.**74**

inobutyryl)pyrrolidine (dextromoramide) (52.**17**), the amide derivative of phenoxadone, is slightly more potent than morphine in man and is effective orally. A variant of the isomethadone structure, 4-dimethylamino-1,2-diphenyl-3-methyl-2-propionoxybutane (propoxyphene, 52.**16**) (258) is the most widely used analgetic in the United States.

The most potent analgetic of the reduced methadone isomers (259, 260) is α-(−)-methadol (52.**72**), which is obtained from the practically inert (+)-methadone. Acylation greatly enhances activity and yields the most potent isomer in the series, α-(+)-acetylmethadol (52.**73**). In man, racemic acetylmethadol is a potent, orally effective analgetic with reduced respiratory depression (261, 262). The demethylated derivatives 52.**74** and 52.**75** are metabolites in man and have been found to retain potent analgetic activity (263–266).

4.6 Morphinans and Benzomorphans

Intermediate in the structural simplification between the highly rigid opiates like morphine and the totally nonrigid methadone structures are the morphinans and benzomorphans that lack the morphine oxygen bridge.

4.6.1 MORPHINANS. N-methylmorphinan was first synthesized in 1946 by Grewe and found to be about one-fifth as potent as morphine (54, 267). The levo isomer (levorphanol, 52.**19**) was found to be four times as potent as morphine (268) and is in general clinical use today.

Although considerable potency enhancement is possible with N-substituted morphinan derivatives, especially the phenethyl type (269), interest in the series has focused on potential selectivity advantages based on antagonist substitution patterns. The N-

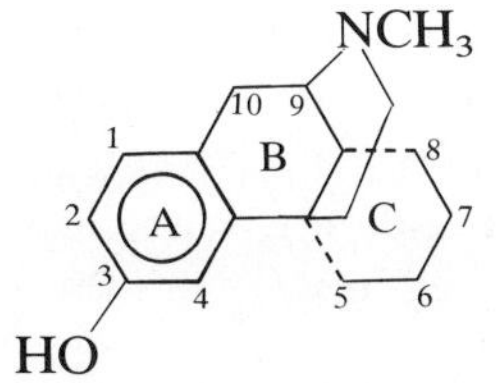

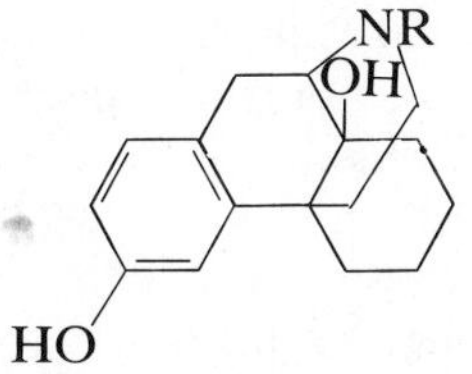

52.**76** R = CH$_2$-c-C$_3$H$_7$
52.**26** R = CH$_2$-c-C$_4$H$_9$

allyl derivative, levallorphan (52.**24**), is a potent narcotic antagonist without addiction liability (270). The cyclopropylmethyl derivative, cyclorphan (52.**25a**), is a potent analgetic and antagonist with little or no addiction liability (271).

More recently, 14-hydroxylation has yielded potent derivatives with both antagonist and agonist properties (272–274). Oxilorphan (52.**76**) and butorphanol (52.**26**) represent two of the more interesting compounds to emerge from these studies. The former is a strong antagonist with only weak analgetic activity whereas butorphanol has potent analgetic activity coupled with moderate antagonist activity (272). In man, butorphanol is 20 times more potent than pentazocine as an analgetic (275) and 4–10 times as potent as morphine. Like many of the other mixed agonist/antagonists it produces some degree of dysphoric and psychotomimetic side effects (276).

4.6.2 BENZOMORPHANS. Further structural simplification of the opiates, by deleting the C ring in the morphinans, yields the benzomorphans (52.**77**) (Table 52.9). Benzomorphan itself (52.**77**, R = R$_1$ = H) was prepared in 1947 by Barltrop (277); however, it was the synthesis of 2′-hydroxy-

2,5-dimethylbenzomorphan (52.**77**, R = R$_1$ = CH$_3$), by May and Murphy (56) that began the extensive investigation into the synthesis and pharmacology of this family which continues unabated to this day (278).

Most of the detailed SAR work in the benzomorphans has focused on the 2′,2,5, and 9 positions. At the 2′ position the following SAR is observed: OH ⩾ H > NH$_2$, NO$_2$, F, and Cl (279). 9-Hydroxylation, which is equivalent to 14-hydroxylation in the morphine series, decreases analgetic activity in 52.**78** relative to the parent 52.**79** (280). However, it has been found that 9β-hydroxylation increases relative antagonist activity. Thus whereas 52.**80** has antagonist activity that is 100 times that of cyclazocine, its analgetic activity is only 1/400 that of cyclazocine (281).

It is in the benzomorphan class that one sees a dramatic separation of analgetic activity and addiction liability in enantiomers. Thus although the levo isomers of the 5,9-dialkylbenzomorphans have the same absolute configuration as morphine (282), *l*-52.**81** possesses analgetic activity comparable to morphine without significant physical dependence capacity (PDC). Strikingly, the dextro isomer of 52.**81** has only $\frac{1}{10}$ the analgetic activity of morphine and is characterized by a high PDC (283).

A further stereotopic deviation is observed with the synthetically minor trans (β) isomers, e.g., 52.**82**, which are more potent than the cis (α) isomers (284). Similarly, the 9β-alkyl derivatives 52.**83**–52.**85** are three to five times more potent than their 9α-alkyl epimers (285). Two additional and interesting members of the β

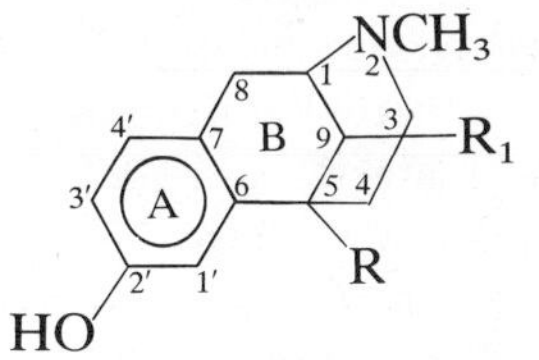

52.**77**

Table 52.9 Modified Benzomorphans

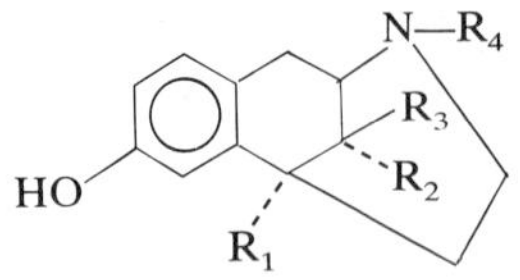

Structure Number	R₁	R₂	R₃	R₄
52.**81**	C_3H_7	CH_3	H	CH_3
52.**82**	C_2H_5	H	CH_3	CH_3
52.**83**	CH_3	H	CH_3	CH_3
52.**84**	CH_3	H	C_2H_5	CH_3
52.**85**	CH_3	H	C_3H_7	CH_3
52.**87**	H	H	CH_3	CH_3
52.**86**	C_6H_5	H	CH_3	CH_3
52.**78**	CH_3	CH_3	OH	CH_3
52.**79**	CH_3	CH_3	H	CH_3
52.**80**	CH_3	CH_3	OH	—CH₂—◁
52.**88**	CH_3	CH_3	H	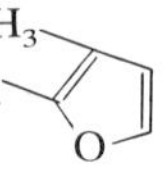 —CH₂— (furan with CH₃)
52.**89**	CH_3	CH_3	H	—CH₂— (furan)
52.**90**	CH_3	CH_3	H	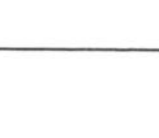 —CH₂— (furan with CH₃)
52.**91**	CH_3	CH_3	H	—CH₂— (tetrahydrofuran)
52.**92**	CH_3	H	CH_3	—CH₂— (tetrahydrofuran)

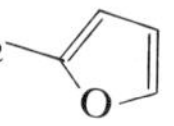

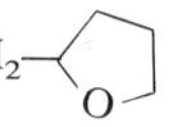

Introduction of the *N*-furfuryl group into the benzomorphans has provided a new series of potent agonists and antagonists that are currently undergoing clinical evaluation (288). Pure morphine-like agonist activity is found in 52.**88** whereas 52.**89** is a pure antagonist. 52.**90** is a pentazocine-like, mixed agonist/antagonist. Further pursuit of this series has yielded the even more potent *N*-substituted tetrahydrofurfuryl benzomorphans (289). The most active of these, 52.**91** (absolute configuration 1*R*,5*R*,9*R*,2″*R*), is 50 times more potent than morphine, does not produce Straub tail, has a high therapeutic ratio ($LD_{50}/ED_{100} = 9400$), does not suppress abstinence signs in withdrawn, morphine-dependent monkeys, and exhibits no agonist properties. The diastereoisomers with the (2″*R*) configuration, 52.**91** and 52.**92**, possess significantly greater analgetic activity than their corresponding (2″*S*) isomers. It is of interest to note that 52.**91** may share some of the unique pharmacological properties of the endogenous opiate, enkephalin (290).

Several of the early benzomorphans have been studied in humans. The *N*-phenethyl derivative, phenazocine (52.**20**), is a potent agonist, effective both orally and parenterally, with possibly less abuse liability than morphine (57, 58). *N*-Allylnormetazocine [52.**93**] is similar to levallorphan in antagonist activity (291). Pentazocine (52.**31**) and cyclazocine (52.**30**) contain classic antagonist substituents (292). The former, al-

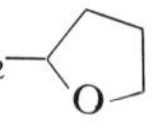

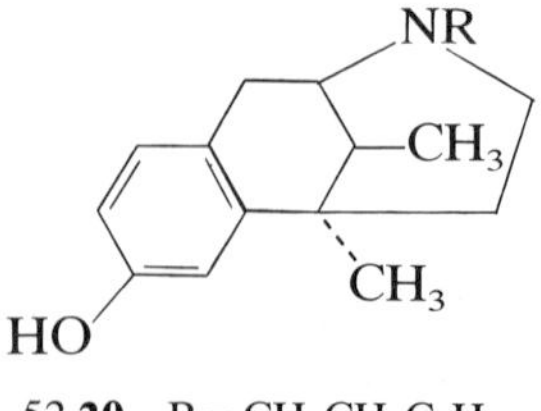

series are the 5-phenyl derivative 52.**86**, which is a potent analgetic in man, both orally and parenterally (286), and 2′-hydroxy-9β-methylbenzomorphan (52.**87**), which has analgetic activity equal to morphine in mice and does not support morphine dependence in monkeys (52.**87** actually precipitates withdrawal suggestive of antagonist properties) (287).

52.**20** R = $CH_2CH_2C_6H_5$
52.**93** R = $CH_2CH=CH_2$
52.**30** R = $CH_2\text{-}c\text{-}C_3H_5$
52.**31** R = $CH_2CH=CMe_2$

though a weak narcotic antagonist (293), was the first narcotic antagonist analgetic to be extensively studied in man and is now sold in many parts of the world. The latter, a potent narcotic antagonist and analgetic, possesses some 40 times the analgetic activity of morphine in man (294), but has a high incidence of psychotomimetic side effects.

4.7 Miscellaneous

In addition to the anomalies already cited in the preceding sections, this section provides additional examples of interesting structure types which do not fit clearly the patterns of Fig. 52.21 but, with the exception of nefopam, are opiates pharmacologically. New examples can be conveniently located by the reader on a yearly basis in *Annual Reports in Medicinal Chemistry*.

4.7.1   TETRAHYDROISOQUINOLINES. Research based on the isoquinoline nucleus, rather than the phenanthrene nucleus of the opium alkaloids, yielded the 1,2,3,4-tetrahydroisoquinoline analgetics, the most active members of which are the *N*-phenethyl-*N*-methyl derivatives (295). Although the more potent members of this class possess dependence liability, methopholine (*d,l*-1-*p*-chlorophenethyl-2-methyl-6,7-dimethoxy-1,2,3,4-tetrahydroisoquinoline, 52.**94**) has codeine-like analgetic activity with little dependence liability and is used somewhat in general clinical practice.

4.7.2   THIAMBUTENES. The thiambutene family is another example of a chemical class that at first inspection bears no re-

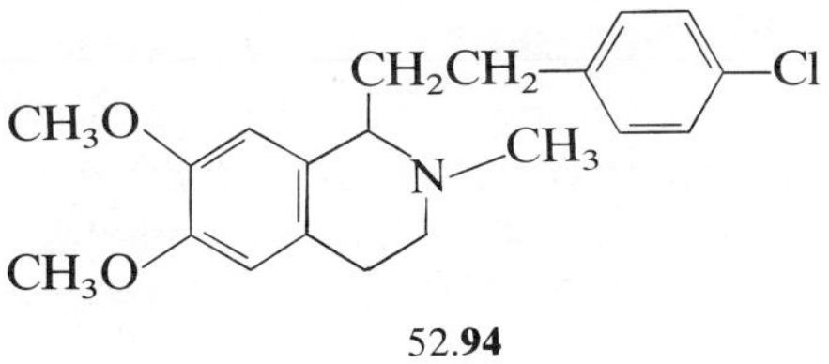

semblance to the classic opiates. In 1950, Adamson and Green developed a series of potent, morphine-like analgetics of which 3-dimethylamino-1, 1-bis(2-thienyl)-1-butene (52.**18**) is representative (296, 297). Although this series is roughly comparable to morphine in animals, it is less effective in man than predicted and its abuse liability approximates that of morphine (191). Beckett has proposed piperidine-like conformation 52.**95** to rationalize the analgetic properties of this series in terms of opioid SAR (298).

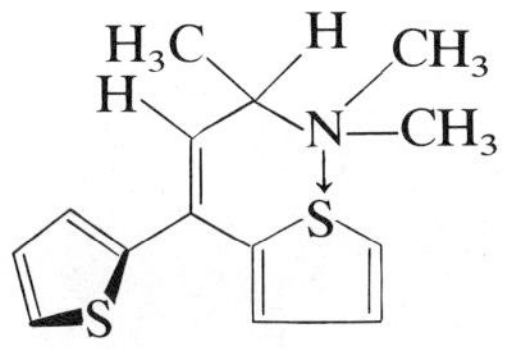

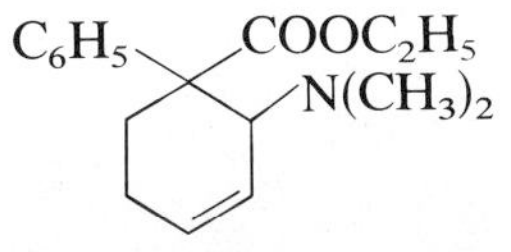

4.7.3   TILIDINE. Ethyl *trans*-2-(dimethylamino)-1-phenyl-3-cyclohexene-1-carboxylate (52.**96**, tilidine), a substituted cyclohexenylamine synthesized by Satzinger (299), is approximately twice as potent as meperidine orally in man (300). This unique analgetic lacks the three-carbon chain between the basic center and the aromatic ring, a feature that is found in classic opiate structures. Also unlike meperidine the basic center is not incorporated into a ring system. Tilidine is used on a wide scale in Germany as an analgetic.

4.7.4   VIMINOL. Viminol (*d,l*-1-[α(*N-o*-chlorobenzyl)pyrryl]-2-di-*sec*-butylaminoethanol, 52.**97**) is a mixture of three racemates, and represents both a new class of analgetics and an interesting study in stereochemistry. Although viminol possesses good, codeine-like oral analgetic activity in man (301–303) it lacks the chemical features usually associated with strong analgetics. In fact, viminol is probably more closely related structurally to the potent, high abuse potential benzimidazoles (e.g., etonitazene, 52.**98**) (304) than it is to any of the opiate types discussed in Section 4. Of

52.**95**

52.**96**

52.**94**

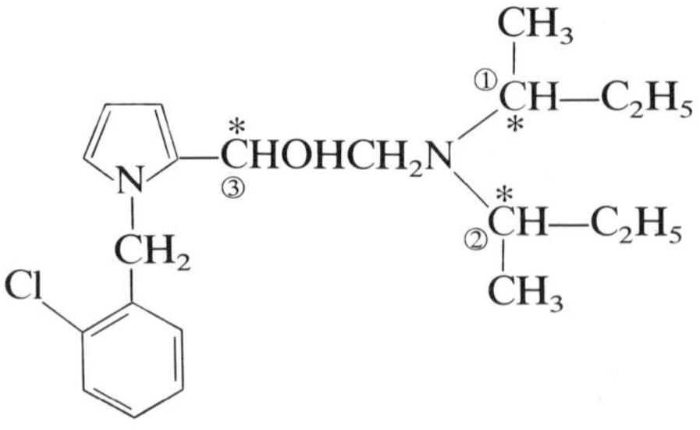

52.**97**

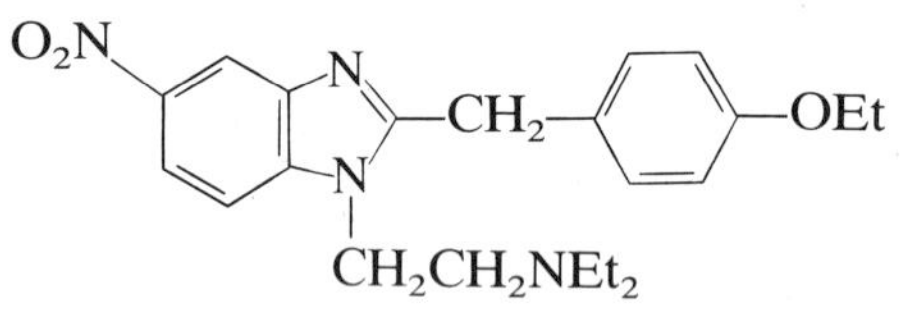

52.**98**

the six possible isomers of viminol (305), only the $(-)$-R_2 isomer [absolute configuration at starred carbons 1 and 2 in 52.**97** is (R)] exhibits potent, morphine-like analgetic activity. More significantly, $(-)$-R_2-52.**97** lacks physical dependence liability in monkeys and has only 1/100 the binding capacity of morphine to the opiate receptor (306). The analgetically inactive $(+)$-S_2 isomer [absolute configuration at 1 and 2 is (S) in 52.**97**] does not bind to the opiate receptor either, but does exacerbate abstinence in withdrawn monkeys, thus accounting for the much lower activity of the mixture of isomers (viminol) than is expected based on the potent $(-)$-R_2 component.

4.7.5 BENZYLAMINES. Two recent examples of opiate analgesia have appeared in this unique structural class. In rats $(-)$-52.**99** [$(-)$-*cis*-2-(α-dimethylamino-*m*-hydroxybenzyl)cyclohexanol] is twice as potent as morphine as an agonist and about equal to nalorphine as an antagonist (307). $(-)$-52.**99** is under active clinical evaluation in man. The $(+)$ isomer of the dioxane 52.**100** possesses naloxone reversible codeine-like analgetic activity (308).

4.7.6 NEFOPAM. Nefopam (5-methyl-1-phenyl-3, 4, 5, 6-tetrahydro-1H-2, 5-benzoxazocine hydrochloride, 52.**101**) (309) is a structurally and pharmacologically unique analgetic which exhibits potent [$\frac{1}{2}$ that of morphine (310), twice that of meperidine (311)] parenteral analgesia in man. Structurally, nefopam can be viewed as a cyclic derivative of diphenylhydramine (52.**102**). Pharmacologically the analgetic activity of nefopam is atypical. Essentially inactive in classic animal tests for potent analgetics of the morphine and meperidine group, nefopam was advanced to clinical trials based on the observation by Gassel (312) that nefopam and meperidine have similar electrophysiological profiles. Significant respiratory depression (313) and evidence of habituation or abuse (314) in man have not been observed for nefopam, placing it in a truly distinct class for a potent analgetic.

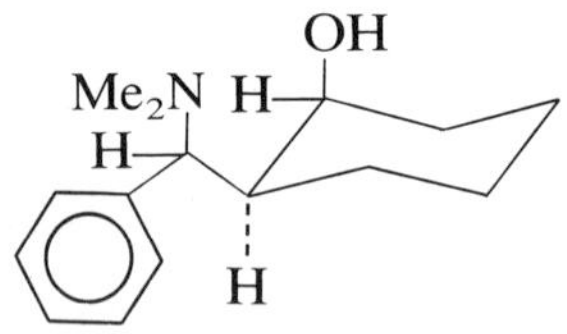

52.**99**

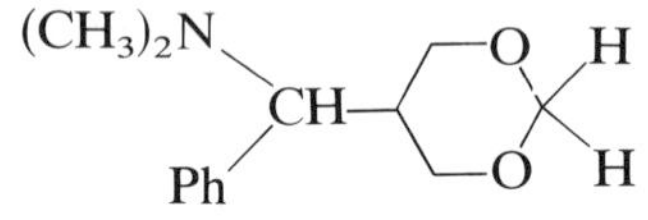

52.**100**

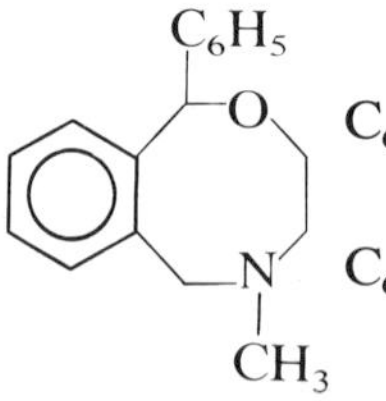

52.**101**

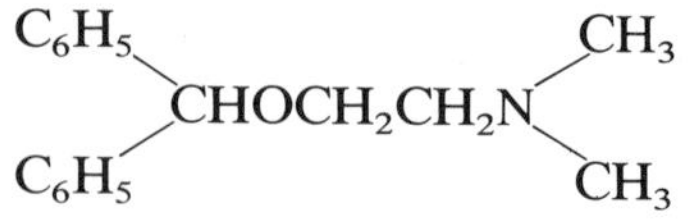

52.**102**

5   METABOLISM OF THE OPIATES

Biotransformation is a key determinate of onset, duration of action, and potency observed for the opiate analgetics. A great

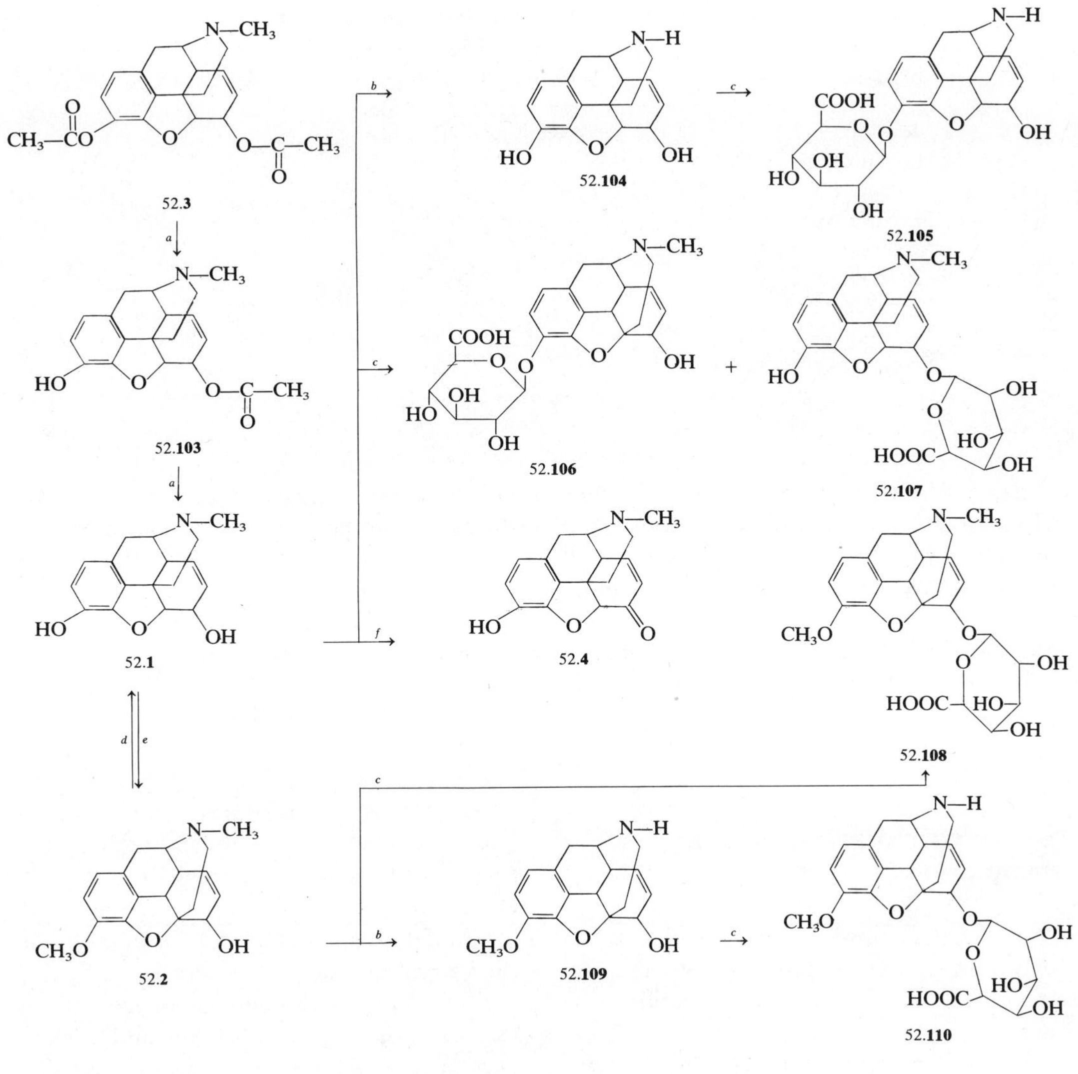

Fig. 52.21 Major metabolic pathways of heroin, morphine, and codeine. (*a*) Hydrolysis. (*b*) *N*-Dealkylation. (*c*) Conjugation. (*d*) *O*-Dealkylation. (*e*) *O*-Alkylation. (*f*) Oxidation.

deal is known about the metabolism of morphine in both animals and man and many fine reviews have been written on this subject (315, 316). This section deals primarily with morphine, heroin, and codeine. Figure 52.21 summarizes the major transformations of these derivatives resulting primarily from *N*-dealkylation, *O*-dealkylation, and hydrolysis followed by conjugation prior to excretion.

Normorphine (52.**104**) is a minor metabolite after morphine administration in man (317). Although normorphine is less analgetic and more toxic than morphine in mice (318), its contribution to the overall profile of morphine in man is probably small. *N*-Demethylation has been observed for a number of other opiate analgetics, as can be seen in Table 52.10. Opiates containing an *O*-methyl group like codeine

Table 52.10   Common Metabolic Pathways for Opiate Analgetics (315, 316)

Compound	N-Dealkylation	O-Dealkylation	Hydrolysis
Morphine (52.**1**)	+		
Heroin (52.**3**)	+		+
Codeine (52.**2**)	+	+	
Meperieine (52.**9**)	+		+
Methadone (52.**15**)	+		
Anileridine (52.**10**)	+		+
Cyclazocine (52.**30**)	+		
Nalorphine (52.**23**)	+		
Propoxyphene (52.**16**)	+		+

undergo O-dealkylation. Esterified opiates like heroin and meperidine undergo rapid hydrolysis *in vivo*. Thus heroin is excreted in the urine as free and conjugated morphine. Metabolic elimination of morphine and other opiates occurs primarily through conjugation. Approximately 65% of morphine can be accounted for as the morphine glucuronide in human urine (317).

6 SAR OF ENKEPHALINS AND ENDORPHINS

The common presence of a tyrosine β-(4-hydroxyphenyl)ethylamine moiety in both the alkaloid and peptide opioids was quickly noted (319–322), as was the presence of a lipophilic binding region for Phe^4 comparable to that postulated for the oripavine, "PET" [Fig. 52.22 (73, 319, 324, 325)]. It is important to note that several of these early structural comparisons employed incorrect absolute stereochemical assignments (323, 325). In the correct assignment the tyrosine–glycine amide linkage of enkephalin assumes the stereochemical position of the hydrogen at C-9 of morphine (noted in Fig. 52.22, 326).

Many spectroscopic (327–329) and theoretical (330–332) attempts have been made to determine the optimal conformation of the enkephalins in solution but have produced widely varied results owing to their substantial conformational mobility. Attempts have been made to refine these calculations by forcing them to account for the SAR of key enkephalin analogs. One of these (330) led to the proposal of an inverse γ-turn for Leu-enkephalin, whereas an X-ray study has indicated that Met-enkephalin adopts a β-bend conformation (324). Recent NMR studies have also favored the β_1 turn conformation with a hydrogen bond between the methionine nitrogren and the Gly^2-carbonyl (Fig. 52.22) rather than the Tyr^1-Phe^4 hydrogen bond as initially proposed by Bradbury on theoretical grounds.

While not discriminating between these two β_1 turn proposals Schiller and coworkers using fluoresence energy transfer measurements for the active analog, Trp^4 Met^5 enkephalin, have determined a 10.0 ± 1.1 Å Trp^4-Tyr^1 aromatic ring distance (325)—a value which agrees well with the 10.5 Å phenyl-phenol distance in the oripazine shown in Fig. 52.22. Maintainence of this distance between the phenol (Try) and a lipophilic center may well prove to be an important feature in the design of potent enkephalin hybrids.

Well over 1000 analogs of Met and Leu-enkephalin have been synthesized. These include specifically substituted analogs with substanially increased metabolic stability

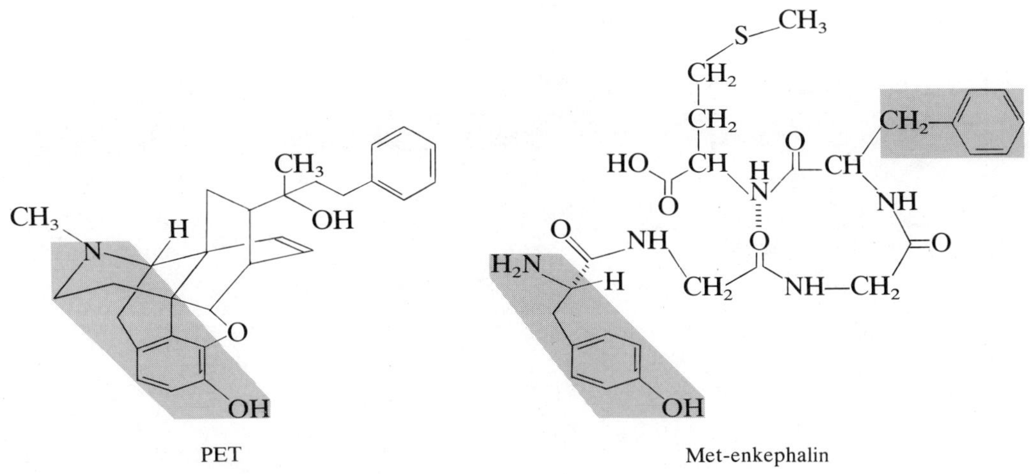

Fig. 52.22   Structural comparison of an alkaloid and peptide opioid.

and potency, several of which are active orally as well as systemically. With several notable exceptions an intact pentapeptide chain appears to be the minimum requirement for potent functional activity. The tetrapeptide Tyr-Gly-Gly-Phe, although it retains binding activity, has less than 1% of the pharmacological activity of the parent pentapeptides (333). The des-Phe tripeptide is without activity (334). Removal of the N-terminal tyrosine residue also results in total loss of activity (333, 335–337), supporting a structural homology with morphine and suggesting that cleavage of this residue may be an important *in vivo* mechanism for enkephalin inactivation. This view was supported by the early finding of greatly enhanced metabolic stability of enkephalins substituted at the 2 position by D-amino acids. More recent work has emphasized an important role for di and tricarboxypeptidases in enkephaline inactivation (see Sect 8.2). Enzymatic stability is also enhanced by conversion of the terminal carboxyl group to an amide (342, 343). With a few exceptions, increasing the size of the pentapeptide by the addition of amino acids to either terminus results in reduced activity.

Allowed substitution patterns for various portions of the pentapeptide are outlined in Table 52.11 and are discussed briefly below.

As would be anticipated from the analogy to morphine, the tyrosine group itself is very sensitive to substitution. Removal of the basic nitrogen or hydroxyl results in inactivity (333–338), as does methylation of the phenol. However, activity is retained if the basic amino acid arginine is coupled to nitrogen. A potency increase also results from monomethylation of the amine. N-Allyl-Leu-, but not Met-enkephalin, has been reported to have antagonist activity in the guinea pig ileum (348).

In contrast, the adjacent Gly^2 position is relatively amenable to modification. Substitution of D-amino acids, notably D-alanine, produces compounds with not only enhanced metabolic stability and hence potent, long-lasting analgesic activity, but also with greater intrinsic potency. With the exception of replacement of the glycyl CH by N, the Gly^3 position is extremely sensitive to substitution.

The phenyl ring of Phe^4 also seems central to activity. Although Trp has been substituted with some success and methylation

Table 52.11   Allowed Substitutions of the Enkephalins

H–Tyr		Gly	Gly	Phe	Met-OH	
NHMe	(346)	D-Ala (343)	N for CH (345)	N-CH$_3$ (346)	D-Leu	(330)
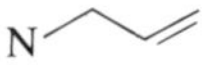 N‿ (structure)	(348)	D-Thr (341)		Trp (325)	Thz	(341)
NHArg	(349)	D-Nle (326)			CONH$_2$	(346)
NHLys	(350)	D-Met (344)			CH$_2$OH	(346)
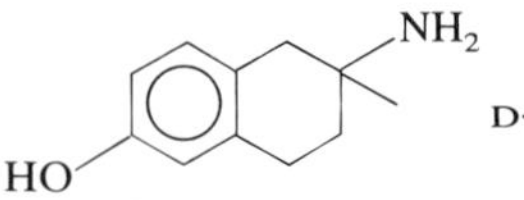 (bicyclic structure with NH$_2$, HO–)		D-Ser (344)			CO$_2$R	(344)
					S→O	(346)
		(CH$_3$)$_2$C (405)			Pro-NHEt	(344)
					Pro-NH$_2$	(344)
NHGly	(402)				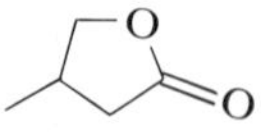 (lactone structure)	(344)
NHTyr	(402)				N-allyl	(404)

of the Phe nitrogen enhances activity, Tyr is not an allowed replacement. The inactivity of Tyr^4 and of analogs that shorten the distance between Phe^4 and Tyr^1 supports the presence of an important lipophilic binding region as proposed in Fig. 52.22.

Methionine and leucine can be modified and replaced by a number of functions. Unlike the N-terminal amine, the terminal carboxyl is not essential for activity and can be extensively modified. Conversion of the acid to the corresponding primary amide results in increased potency, presumably due to increased metabolic stability.

Notable exceptions to the early findings that the full pentapeptide is required for activity include the observation that replacement of Gly^2 by D-Ala^2 confers potent activity on the tetrapeptide H-Tyr-D-Ala-Gly-Phe-NH$_2$ and even the dipeptide H-Try-D-Ala-NH$_2$ (339). Takagi and co-workers (340) have recently reported *in vivo* analgetic activity for the dipeptide H-Tyr-D-Arg. The unique contribution of a D-amino acid at the 2 position suggests not only a role in enhanced metabolic stability but also in improved conformation to the opiate receptor.

Based on this accumulated SAR, several compounds have been prepared which have oral or i.v. activity (Fig. 52.23). Notable among these is FK-33,824 (Fig. 52.5), synthesized by Pless and co-workers. This compound is a potent analgetic in animals both subcutaneously and orally, and, like the other opioids, exhibits cross-tolerance to morphine (351). An early clinical study (352) failed to produce evidence of analgesia for FK-33,824 at low doses, but produced instead a series of atypical symptoms that were not reversed by naloxone. These results suggest that at the doses tested FK-33,824 was not exerting its effects through the classical opiate receptor.

An important feature of enkephalin SAR is the effect of structure modification on selectivity for the various opiate receptors. Kosterlitz and co-workers have shown that methylation of the N-terminal amine and amidation of the carboxyl of Met-enkephalin produces a compound with markedly enhanced μ versus δ receptor activity (353). Similar differences in the guinea pig ileum/mouse vas deferens ratios have been noted for a series of endorphin analogs.

Maximal activity and enhanced metabolic

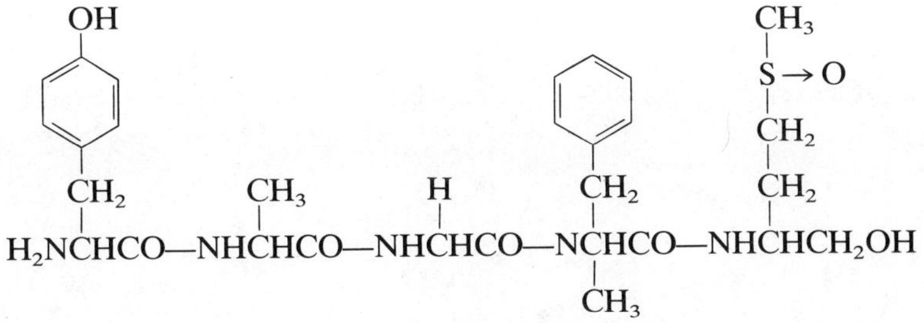

FK-33-824

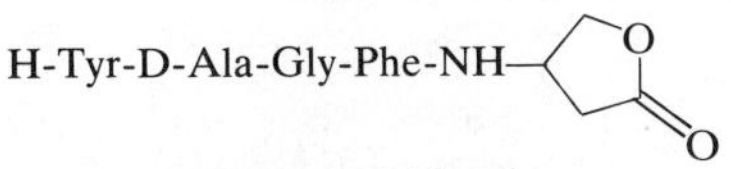

H-Tyr-D-Ala-Gly-Phe-NH—[lactone structure]

ICI-121,444 (344)

H-Tyr-D-Ala-Gly-Phe-D-Leu-OH

BW-180c (347)

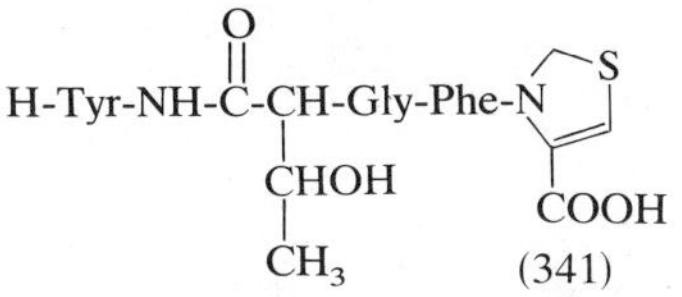

H-Tyr-NH-C-CH-Gly-Phe-N [thiazole ring with S]
          ‖ |
          O CHOH   COOH
              |
              CH₃   (341)

Fig. 52.23 Systematically active enkephalin analogs.

stability for the endorphins appear to rest with the full 31 amino acid sequence. Although the shorter α- and γ-endorphins retain analgetic activity, it has been suggested that they may arise primarily by proteolysis during extraction (354). The Leu^5-analog of β-endorphin, although not yet definitively identified *in vivo*, has been synthesized and found to possess potent opioid-like activity (355). A 15-residue peptide containing the Leu-enkephalin sequence has recently been identified, however, in extracts from pig hypothalamus (356). The remainder of its sequence is unlike that of β-LPH, further supporting the concept of a separate precursor to the enkephalins. For a more extensive discussion of β-endorphin SAR see Chapter 27.

7 CANNABINOID ANALGETICS

Various preparations from the plant *Cannabis satavia*, including marihuana and hashish, have been used for nearly 5000 years for its various social and medical properties including pain relief (357, 358). Until quite recently, reports of the analgetic activity of the natural cannabinoids in animals and man could best be described as equivocal (359, 360, 363–365). The availability of pure Δ^9-tetrahydrocannabinol (Δ^9-THC, 52.**111**; see Fig. 52.24) (361) and Δ^8-tetrahydrocannabinol (52.**112**) (362), the proposed active constituents in *Cannabis sativa*, has made possible more definitive studies. Initial results indicate that oral Δ^9-THC (10 and 20 mg) provides pain reduction equivalent to codeine (60 and 120 mg), with marked sedation being the primary side effect at the higher doses of Δ^9-THC (366–368). Although these results are preliminary, recent discoveries of cannabinoids having analgetic activity in animals and man have added impetus to the exploration of these families.

It is fitting that one of the most revealing structural probes into the analgetic activity of the cannabinoid molecules was carried

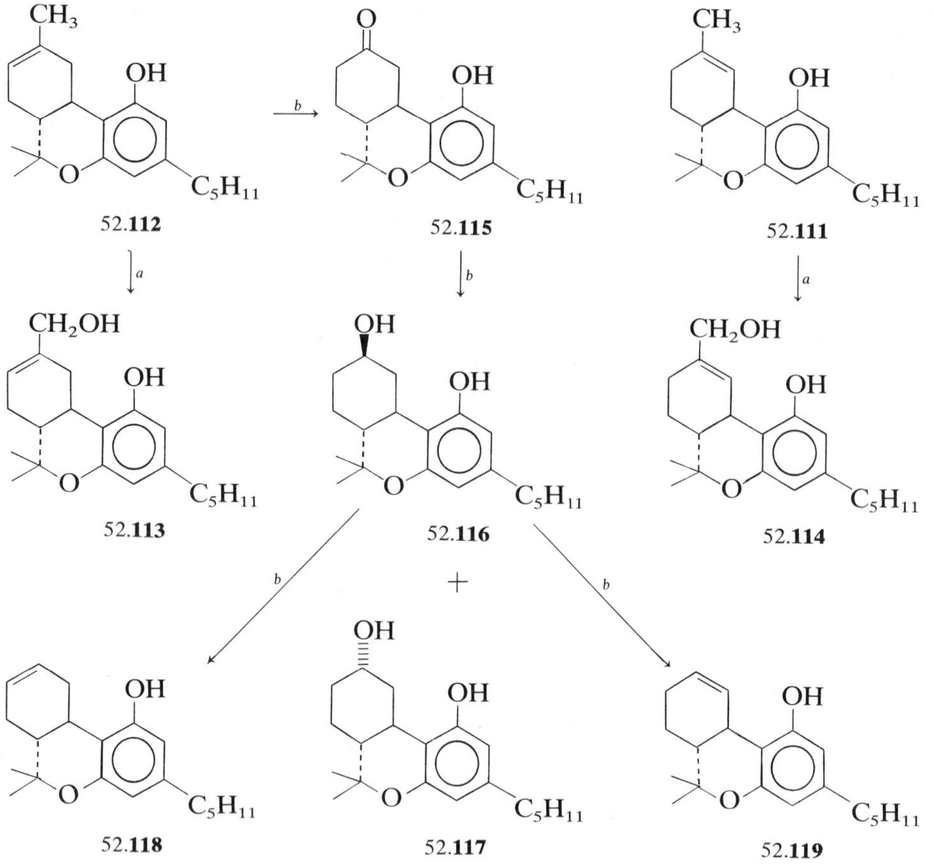

Fig. 52.24   Metabolically (a) and synthetically (b) related cannabinoid derivatives.

out in the laboratories of Everette May, an acknowledged leader in the field of opiate analgetics. In 1974, Wilson and May (369) postulated that the analgetic activity of Δ^8- and Δ^9-THC was due to their 11-hydroxy metabolites (52.**113** and 52.**114**, Fig. 52.24). This conclusion is supported by the observation that the 9-normethyl derivatives, 52.**118** and 52.**119** (370), which cannot be transformed into the 11-hydroxy metabolites, lack significant analgetic activity but elicit in the dog static ataxia and cardiovascular profiles nearly identical to those of Δ^8- and Δ^9-THC. During these studies, ($-$)-9-nor-9-β-hydroxyhexahydrocannabinol (52.**116**) was prepared and found to be an analgetic with activity in the

mouse hot plate test nearly equal to that of morphine. These findings point out that there are precise structural requirements for analgetic activity which are divergent from those features eliciting other CNS and cardiovascular effects, and further that a highly stereospecific mechanism of action is involved in cannabinoid analgesia, as is the case with the potent opiate analgetics.

Table 52.12 illustrates the regio- and stereospecificity demonstrated for this series of compounds. Key SAR points to note are as follows: (1) analgetic activity is increased by introducing the 11-hydroxyl group (compare 52.**111** and 52.**114**); (2) the nonhydroxylated derivatives 52.**115**, 52.**118**, and 52.**119** lack analgetic activity;

Table 52.12 Analgetic Activity of Some Cannabinoid Derivatives (369–372)

Compound	Analgetic ED$_{50}$, mg/kg^a
l-52.**111**	9.6
l-52.**112**	8.8
d-52.**112**	>50^b
l-52.**113**	1.9
l-52.**114**	1.9
l-52.**115**	>20^b
d,l-52.**116**	2.9
l-52.**116**	1.6
l-52.**117**	>50^b
d,l-52.**118**	>20^b
l-52.**119**	>20^b

^{a} Mouse hot plate.
^{b} Inactive at this dose.

and (3) the 9β orientation for the hydroxy group of 52.**116** is necessary for analgetic activity (the 9α derivative, 52.**117**, is inactive). It has also been shown that the phenolic hydroxyl and trans-6a,10a geometry are necessary for analgetic activity in the cannabinoids (373).

As yet, the analgetic mechanism of action for 52.**116** appears to be unresolved. Though it was originally reported (369) that naloxone (1 mg/kg) completely antagonized the analgetic effect of 52.**116**, suggesting an opiate mechanism with concomitant dependence liability, subsequent attempts have been unable to completely reverse the analgetic activity of 52.**116** with naloxone (360). In addition, unlike classical narcotic agonists, 52.**116** fails to suppress withdrawal symptoms in morphine-addicted monkeys, does not exhibit cross-tolerance with morphine (360, 374), and, most telling, does not act at the opiate receptor *in vitro*. These findings suggest that 52.**116** is a mechanistically novel analgetic in animals. No clinical studies with 52.**116** have been conducted to date. A

related compound, 52.**120** (nabilone), has analgetic activity in animals (375) and is currently undergoing evaluation as an anti-anxiety agent (376–378).

A large number of totally synthetic cannabinoids have been prepared and examined broadly for their CNS and cardiovascular effects (379, 380). However, very few systematic studies of analgetic activity have appeared. Following the synthesis of the first pharmacologically active nitrogen cannabinoid (52.**121**) (381), Pars and Razdan (382) noted some structural similarities between the azacannabinoids and other CNS agents such as LSD and morphine. A systematic SAR study (383–385) of the effect of heteroatoms in the C ring and of side chain substituents at the 1 and 3 positions ensued and culminated in the synthesis of the potent analgetic nabitan (52.**122**, SP-106, Abbott 40,656) (386). Preclinical pharmacological evaluation (387) of the propargyl derivatives 52.**122** and 52.**123** has revealed that they possess potent oral activity in classical analgetic tests equal to or exceeding anileridine and, significantly, that 52.**122** does not possess the capacity to reinforce self-administration in monkeys previously conditioned to self-inject morphine. Preliminary clinical trials in patients with postoperative and chronic pain are equivocal at doses up to 4 mg orally (388–390). A structurally distinct nitrogen-containing cannabinoid prototype, nantradol (CP-44,001, 52.**124**), was recently reported to be a potent (2-10X morphine), nonopiate analgetic in animals (391).

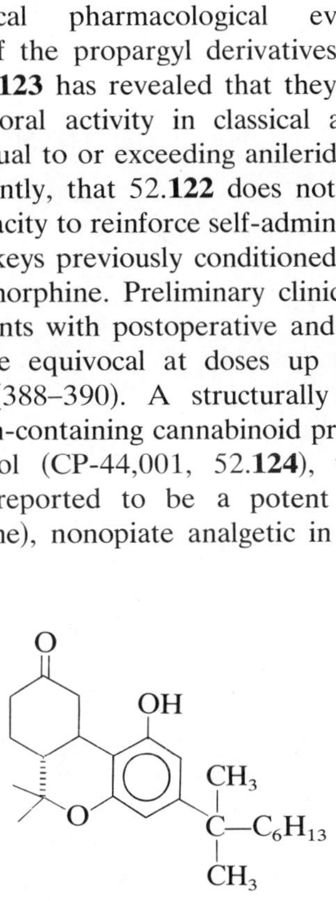

52.**120**

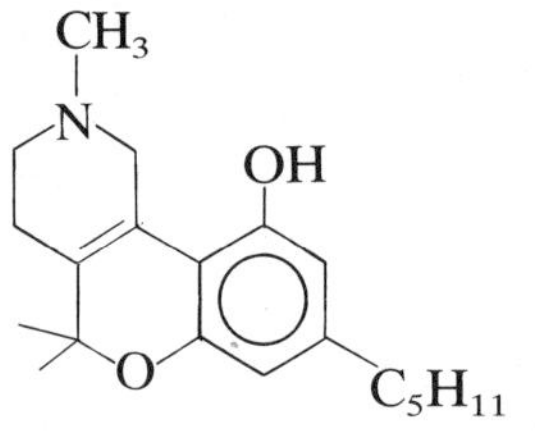

52.**121**

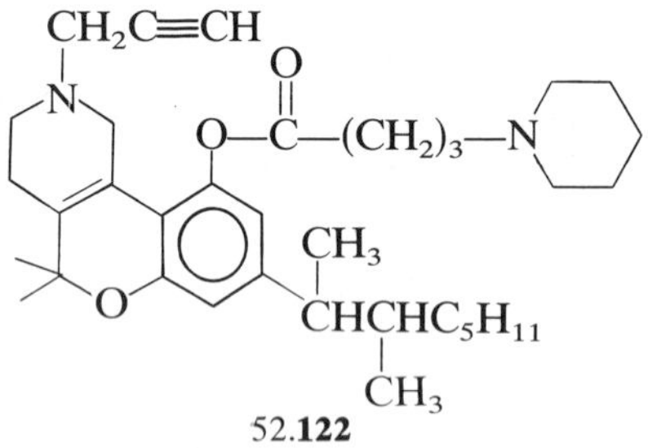

52.**122**

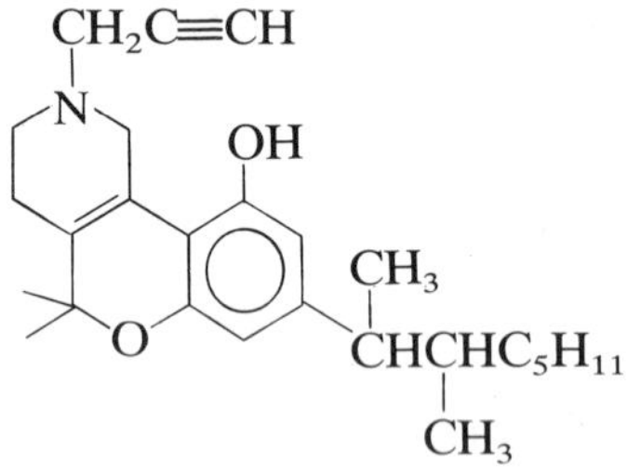

52.**123**

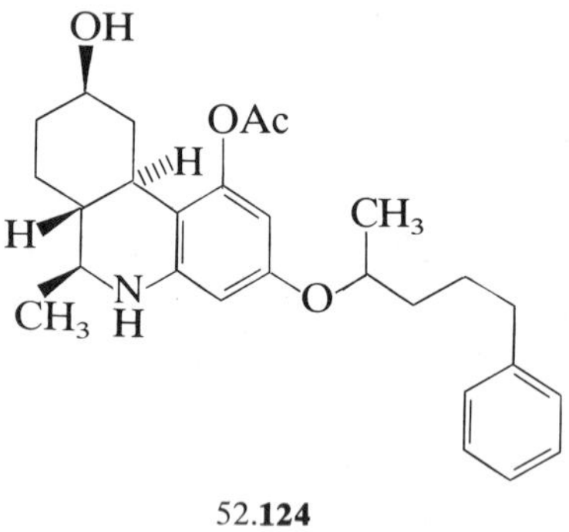

52.**124**

Confirmation of cannabinoid analgesia in man, coupled with information regarding tolerance development, side effects, and abuse potential, would provide a new avenue of exploration in the analgetic field.

8 SOME NEW DIRECTIONS IN ANALGETIC RESEARCH

In addition to the cannabinoids, recent research has identified a number of new and potentially promising approaches to potent analgetics. Some of these attempt to modulate pain by altering levels of the endogenous opioids, others seek points of neuronal intervention in systems modulated by the opioids, and still others such as the cannabinoids have no apparent connection to the opioids beyond their ability to produce broad spectrum analgesia. This section examines some of these other options, with the suggestion that they exemplify the growing possibilities for analgetic discovery.

8.1 Endorphin Release Modulation

Nitrous oxide (392), stimulation of the central gray matter (Section 3.4), and acupuncture (393) are all postulated to produce analgesia by releasing an endogenous opioid-like substance. Chronic, but not acute, haloperidol is also reported to elevate enkephalin levels in the rat (394). These data suggest that there are a number of pharmacological and physiological points of intervention that might produce analgesia by the endogenous release of endorphins, and in fact the analgetic dipeptide, Tyr-Arg has recently been proposed as an enkephalin releaser (406).

8.2 Inhibition of Endorphin Metabolism

This approach to elevating endogenous opioid levels is made particularly attractive by the recent demonstration that the structural requirements for inhibiting degradation differ from those for receptor binding (395). Specifically, L-Ala[2]-met-enkephalin, which is inactive as an opioid mimetic, is very potent as an enkephalin degradation inhibitor *in vitro*.

While early studies focused on enkephalin aminopeptidase (cleavage of Tyr) activity due to the metabolic stability provided by substitution of D-amino acids at the 2-position, recent attention has centered on the presence of di- and tricarboxypeptidases capable of degrading met and leu-enkephalin (395, 407). While the similarity of the enkephalin dicarboxypeptidase to angiotensin converting enzyme may provide some guidance in the designs of inhibitors, the actual enzymes have been demonstrated to draw different specificities.

Pursuing this conceptual approach, Ehrenphreis et al. have shown that D-phenylalanine, an inhibitor of carboxypeptidase-A, produces naloxone reversible analgesia in mice, but with no apparent tolerance development (396). Initial reports of clinical efficacy for D-phenylalanine have been reported at 250 mg four times daily. Whether or not D-phenylalanine is truly an inhibitor of enkephalin degradation and/or a clinically useful analgetic remains to be fully demonstrated. However, by analogy to cholinesterase inhibitors, the approach is medicinally attractive.

8.3 Transduction of the Opioid Response

The actions of morphine are potentiated by lowered levels of Ca^{2+}. Harris and co-workers have shown that the Ca^{2+} antagonist La^{3+} produces morphine-like analgesia, cross-tolerance, and support of abstinence in animals (397). These studies as well as earlier ones argue that morphine analgesia is expressed through alterations in Ca^{2+} levels. In this regard, it is interesting to note the involvement of Ca^{2+} in adenylate cyclase activity coupled with morphine's ability to reduce cAMP levels in some neuronal systems (see Section 3.3). This same line of

reasoning suggests (à la Collier) that a centrally active prostaglandin antagonist might be an effective analgetic, a proposition that awaits the discovery of an effective and selective antagonist.

8.4 Substance P Modulation

Substance P (SP) appears to be the major transmitter released by primary afferents at the level of the dorsal horn. This release is selectively blocked by the opiates including enkephalin (398; see Fig. 52.14). Further evidence suggestive of SP involvement in pain perception and opioid analgesia is the close correlation found between SP and enkephalin neurons in the spinal cord and SP selective excitation of cells responsive to noxious stimuli. These data would suggest that a substance P antagonist should produce analgesia at the level of the primary sensory afferents.

8.5 Noradrenergic Mechanisms

The opiates are also known to modulate noradrenergic pathways in the CNS. In support of overlapping points of mechanistic intervention for the opiate and noradrenergic systems, it has been found that the presynaptic α-agonist clonidine produces analgesia (399, 400), is subject to one-way cross-tolerance in morphine-tolerant animals, and blocks some opiate withdrawal symptoms including those in man (401). However, unlike the opiates, clonidine analgesia is not subject to naloxone reversal. One can speculate that clonidine, like enkephalin, inhibits noradrenaline release presynaptically. However, since clonidine has been reported to have central postsynaptic actions as well, the validation of this approach awaits its extension to other α-agonists.

9 CONCLUSION

In the 50 years following the structural assignment of morphine, the opioid area produced a rich record of discovery. The introduction of the new technology of receptor binding and the discovery of the endogenous opioids, the enkephalins and endorphins, has already initiated a new burst of discovery which promises to grow in vitality and scope in the coming years.

Of particular importance and promise for analgetic research is the discovery of multiple and architecturally distinct opiate receptors, pursuit of which should lead to the more accurate disection of opioid pharmacology and SAR, leading ultimately to analgetics with enhanced selectivity of action. Likewise, the recent development of technology for assaying the localization and levels of opiate receptors and endorphins should lead to the discovery of novel neurochemical means of modulating nociceptive and opioid pain pathways. The confirmation of analgetic activity in man for such mechanistic nonopioids as the cannabinoids holds out the promise of finding distinct, new directions in the search for a nonopioid analgetic. In the navigation of these as yet poorly charted waters the history of medicinal accomplishment in opioid research will continue to provide an important reference point.

REFERENCES

1. A. Burger, in *Analgetics*, Vol. 5, G. de Stevens, Ed., Academic, New York-London, 1965, pp. 1–2.

2. H. K. Beecher, *Measurement of Subjective Responses*, Oxford University Press, Oxford, 1959.

3. H. K. Beecher, *Am. J. Physiol.*, **187,** 163 (1956).

4. R. Melzack, *The puzzle of Pain*, Basic Books, New York, 1973.

5. H. E. Hill, C. H. Kornetsky, H. G. Flanary, and A. Wikler, *J. Clin. Invest.*, **31,** 473 (1952); *Arch. Neurol. Psychiatr.*, **67,** 612 (1952).

6. R. Melzack and P. D. Wall, *Science*, **150,** 971 (1965).

7. P. D. Wall, *Brain*, **101,** 1 (1978).

8. S. G. Denis and R. Melzack, *Pain*, **4,** 97 (1977).

9. R. W. Dykes, *Brain Res.*, **99,** 229 (1975).

10. M. Zimmerman, in *International Review of Physiology*, Vol. 10, R. Porter, Ed., University Park Press, Baltimore, Md., 1976, p. 179.

11. R. K. S. Lim, F. Rogers, D. W. Goto, K. Brown, G. D. Dickerson, and R. J. Engle, *Arch. Int. Pharmacodyn.*, **152,** 25 (1964).

12. G. de Stevens, Ed. *Analgetics*, Vol. 5, Academic, New York-London, 1965.

13. M. C. Brande, L. S. Harris, E. L. Way, J. P. Smith, and J. E. Villarreal, Eds., *Narcotic Antagonists*; *Advances in Biochemical Psychopharmacology*, Vol. 8, Raven press, New York, 1974.

14. H. W. Kosterlitz, H. O. J. Collier, and J. E. Villarreal, Eds., *Agonist and Antagonist Actions of Narcotic Analgenic Drugs*, University Park Press, Baltimore-London-Tokyo, 1973.

15. R. I. Taber, in Ref. 13, p. 191.

16. F. E. D'Amour and D. L. Smith, *J. Pharmacol. Exp. Ther.*, **72,** 74 (1941).

17. G. Woolfe and A. D. Macdonald, *J. Pharmacol. Exp. Ther.*, **80,** 309 (1944).

18. N. B. Eddy and D. Leimbach, *J. Pharmacol. Exp. ther.*, **107,** 385 (1953).

19. S. Archer, L. S. Harris, N. F. Albertson, B. F. Tullar, and A. K. Pieeson, 'Narcotic Antagonists as Analgesics—Laboratory Aspects, Vol. 45, *Advances in Chemistry Series*, 1964, p. 162.

20. L. Lasagna and H. K. Beecher, *J. Pharmacol. Exp. Ther.*, **112,** 306 (1954).

21. E. Siegmund, R. Cadmus, and G. Lu, *Proc. Soc. Exp. Biol. Med.*, **95,** 729 (1957).

22. R. I. Taber, D. D. Greenhouse, J. K. Rendell, and S. Irwin, *Nature*, **204,** 189 (1964).

23. H. Blumberg, P. S. Wolf, and H. B. Dayton, *Proc. Soc. Exp. Biol. Med.*, **118,** 763 (1965).

24. L. C. Hendershot and J. Forsaitti, *J. Pharmacol. Exp. Ther.*, **125,** 237 (1959).

25. F. R. Granat and J. K. Sailens, *Arch. Int. Pharmacodyn.*, **205,** 52 (1973).

26. D. J. Mayer and J. C. Liebeskind, *Brain Res.*, **68,** 73 (1974).

27. H. W. Kosterlitz and A. A. Waterfield, *Ann. Rev. Pharmacol.*, **15,** 29 (1975).

28. A. Herz, Ed., *Developments in Opiate Research*, Dekker, New York-Basel, 1978.

29. W. R. Martin, Ed., *Drug Addiction I*, Springer-Verlag, Berlin-Heidelberg-New York, 1977.

30. D. H. Clovet and K. Iwatsubo, *Ann. Rev. Pharmacol.*, **15**, 49 (1975).

31. A. E. Takemori, *Biochem. Pharmacol.*, **24**, 2121 (1975).

32. M. H. Seevers and G. Deneau, *Bull. Drug Addict Narcotics, Addendum* 1, 1 (1963).

33. W. R. Martin and D. R. Jasinski, in Ref. 29, Chap. 2.

34. C. K. Himmelsbach, *J. Am. Med. Assoc.*, **103**, 1420 (1934).

35. D. R. Jasinski, in Ref. 29, Chap. 3.

36. L. Lasagna, J. M. von Felsinger, and H. K. Beecher, *J. Am. Med. Assoc.*, **157**, 1006 (1955).

37. H. Lal, G. Giumutsos, and S. Miksic, in *Discriminative Stimulus Properties of Drugs*, H. Lal, Ed., Plenum, New York, 1977, p. 23.

38. W. R. Martin, C. B. Eudes, J. A. Thompson, R. E. Huppler, and P. E. Gilbert, *J. Pharmacol. Exp. Ther.*, **197**, 517 (1967).

39. W. A. Sertürner, *J. Pharm.*, **13**, 234 (1805).

40. P.-J. Robiquet, *Ann. Chem. Phys.*, **51**, 225 (1832).

41. H. Dreser, *Deut. Med. Wochenschr.*, **24**, 185 (1898).

42. L. F. Small, N. B. Eddy, E. Moseltig, and C. K. Himmelsbach, *Studies on Drug Addiction, Pub. Health Rep. Suppl. No.* 138, U.S. Government Printing Office, Washington, D.C., 1938.

43. E. Moseltig and A. Burger, *J. Am. Chem. Soc.*, **57**, 2189 (1935).

44. O. Eisleb and O. Schaumann, *Deut. Med. Wochenschr.*, **65**, 967 (1939).

45. O. Schaumann, *Naunyn-Schmiedebergs, Arch. Pharmacol. Exp. Pathol.*, **196**, 109 (1940); *Pharmazie*, **4**, 364 (1949).

46. L. Lasagna and H. K. Beecher, *J. Pharmacol. Exp. Ther.*, **112**, 306 (1954).

47. C. K. Himmelsbach, *J. Pharmacol. Exp. Ther.*, **75**, 64 (1942).

48. R. A. Hardy, Jr., and M. G. Howell, in Ref. 12, Chap. 5, see also Ref. 29.

49. E. C. Klerderer, J. B. Rice, V. Conquest, and J. H. Williams, *U.S. Dep. Commes. OFF. Publ. Board. Rep.*, **PP-981**, (1945).

50. H. Isbell, A. Wikler, N. B. Eddy, J. A. Wilson, and C. F. Moran, *J. Am. Med. Assoc.*, **135**, 888 (1947).

51. H. Isbell and H. F. Fraser, *Pharmacol. Rev.*, **2**, 355 (1950).

52. A. Pohland and H. R. Sullivan, *J. Am. Chem. Soc.*, **75**, 4458 (1953).

53. H. F. Fraser and H. Isbell, *Bull. Narcotics*, **12**, 9 (1960).

54. R. Grewe, *Naturwissenschaften*, **33**, 333 (1946).

55. O. Schnider and A. Grüssner, *Helv. Chim. Acta*, **32**, 821 (1949).

56. E. L. May and J. G. Murphy, *J. Org. Chem.*, **20**, 257 (1955).

57. H. F. Fraser and H. Isbell, *Bull. Narcotics*, **12**, 15 (1960).

58. N. B. Eddy and E. L. May, in *Synthetic Analgesics*, Part II, J. Rolfe, Ed., Pergamon, London, 1965.

59. K. W. Bentley, D. G. Hardy, and B. Meek, *J. Am. Chem. Soc.*, **89**, 3267, 3273 (1967); K. W. Bentley and J. W. Lewis, Ref. 14, p. 12.

60. G. F. Blane and D. S. Robbie, in *Agonist and Antagonist Actions of Narcotic Analgesic Drugs*, H. W. Kosterlitz, H. O. J. Collier, and J E. Villarreal, Eds., University Park, Baltimore, Md., 1973, p. 120.

61. J. Pohl, *Z. Exp. Pathol. Ther.*, **17**, 370 (1915).

62. J. Weijlard and A. E. Erickson, *J. Am. Chem. Soc.*, **64**, 869 (1942); K. Unna, *J. Pharmacol. Exp. Ther.*, **19**, 27 (1943); E. L. McCawley, E. R. Hart, and D. Marsh, *J. Am. Chem. Soc.*, **63**, 314 (1941).

63. L. Lasagna and H. K. Beecher, *J. Pharmacol. Exp. Ther.*, **112**, 356 (1954).

64. W. L. Dewey, *Int. Anesthesiol. Clin.*, **11**, 139 (1973); R. N. Brogden, T. M. Speight, and G. S. Avery, *Drugs*, **5**, 6 (1973) and references therein.

65. A. Cowan, J. C. Doxey, and E. J. R. Harry, *Brit. J. Pharmacol.*, **60**, 547 (1977); A. Cowan, J. W. Lewis, and I. R. Maefarlane, *Brit. J. Pharmacol.*, **60**, 537 (1977) and references therein.

66. D. R. Jasinski and P. A. Mansky, *Clin. Pharmacol. Ther.*, **13**, 78 (1972) and references therein.

67. R. C. Heel, R. N. Brogden, T. M. Speight, and G. S. Avery, *Drugs*, **16**, 473 (1978) and references therein.

68. L. Lasagna, *Pharmacol. Rev.*, **16**, 47 (1964).

69. L. M. Halpern, *Arch. Surg.*, **112**, 861 (1977).

70. R. W. Houde, in *Oncology 1970 Vol. III: Diagnosis and Management of Cancer*, R. L. Clark, R. W. Cumley, J. E. McCoy, and M. Copeland, Eds., Chicago, Year Book Medical Publishers, 1971, p. 489.

71. W. F. Michne, A. K. Pierson, T. R. Lewis, and S. J. Michalee, paper presented at the International Narcotics Research Conference, Noordwijkerhout, The Netherlands, 1978.

72. D. M. Zimmerman and R. Nicklander, "Reported to the Committee on Problems of Drug Dependence," Cambridge Mass., 1977. cited by

D. S. Fries, *Annual Reports in Medicinal Chemistry*, Vol. 13, Frank H. Clark, Ed., Academic, New York, 1978, Chap. 5.

73. A. P. Feinberg, I. Creese, and S. H. Snyder, *Proc. Natl. Acad. Sci. U.S.*, **73**, 4215 (1976).

74. S. Shiotani, T. Kometani, Y. Iitaka, and A. Itai, *J. Med. Chem.*, **21**, 153 (1978).

75. A. H. Beckett and A. F. Casy, *J. Pharm. Pharmacol.*, **6**, 986 (1954); A. H. Beckett, *ibid.*, **8**, 848 (1956).

76. P. S. Portoghese, *J. Pharm. Sic.*, **52**, 865 (1966) and references therein.

77. K. W. Bentley and J. W. Lewis, in Ref. 14, p. 12, and K. W. Bentley, A. Cowan, and J. W. Lewis, *Ann. Rev. Pharmacol.*, **11**, 241 (1971).

78. R. H. B. Galt, *J. Pharm. Pharmacol.*, **29**, 711 (1977).

79. L. Terenius, *Acta Pharmacol. Toxicol.*, **32**, 317 (1973).

80. C. B. Pert and S. H. Snyder, *Science*, **179**, 1011 (1973).

81. E. J. Simon, J. M. Hiller, and I. Edelman, *Proc. Natl. Acad. Sci., U.S.*, **70**, 1947 (1973).

82. N. A. Ingoglia and V. P. Dole, *J. Pharmacol. Exp. Ther.*, **175**, 84 (1970).

83. A. Goldstein, L. I. Lowney, and B. K. Pal, *Proc. Natl. Acad. Sci. U.S.*, **68**, 1742 (1971).

84. C. B. Pert, D. Aposhiari, and S. H. Snyder, *Brain Res.*, **75**, 356 (1974).

85. J. M. Hiller, J. Pearson, and E. J. Simon, *Res. Commun. Chem. Pathol. Pharmacol.*, **6**, 1052 (1973).

86. I. Creese and S. H. Snyder, *J. Pharmacol. Exp. Ther.*, **194**, 205 (1975).

87. R. Wilson, M. Rogers, C. B. Pert, and S. H. Snyder, *J. Med. Chem.*, **18**, 240 (1975).

88. M. E. Rogers, H. H. Ong, E. L. May, and W. A. Klee, *J. Med. Chem.*, **18**, 1036 (1975).

89. C. B. Pert, S. H. Snyder, and E. May, *J. Pharmacol. Exp. Ther.*, **196**, 316 (1976).

90. C. B. Pert and S. H. Snyder, *Proc. Natl. Acad. Sci. U.S.*, **70**, 2242 (1973).

91. C. B. Pert, S. H. Snyder, and P. S. Portoghese, *J. Med. Chem.*, **19**, 1247 (1976).

92. C. A. Clay and L. R. Brougharn, *Biochem. Pharmacol.*, **24**, 1363 (1975).

93. K. D. Stahl, W. van Bever, D. Janssen, and E. J. Simon, *Eur. J. Pharmacol.*, **46**, 199 (1977).

94. C. B. Pert and S. H. Snyder, *Mol. Pharmacol.*, **10**, 868 (1974).

95. E. J. Simon, J. M. Hiller, J. Grotti, and I. Edelman, *J. Pharmcol. Exp. Ther.*, **192**, 531 (1975).

96. E. J. Simon and J. M. Hiller, *Ann. Rev. Pharmacol. Toxicol.*, **18**, 371 (1978).

97. E. J. Simon, *Neurosci. Res. Program. Bull.*, **13**, 43 (1975).

98. M. J. Kuhar, C. B. Pert, and S. H. Snyder, *Nature*, **245**, 447 (1973).

99. S. F. Atweh and M. J. Kuhar, *Brain Res.*, **124**, 153 and **129**, 1 (1975).

100. C. B. Pert, M. J. Kuhar, and S. H. Snyder, *Life Sci.*, **16**, 1849 (1975).

101. S. F. Atweh, L. C. Murrin, and M. J. Kuhar, *Neuropharmacol.*, **17**, 65 (1978).

102. R. J. Hitzeman, B. A. Hitzeman, and H. H. Loh, *Life Sci.*, **14**, 2393 (1974).

103. W. A. Klee and R. A. Streaty, *Nature*, **248**, 61 (1974).

104. K. A. Bonnet, J. M. Hiller, and E. J. Simon, in *Opiates and Endogenous Opioid Peptides, Proc. Int. Narcotic Res. Club Meet., Aberdeen, UK*, North-Holland, Amsterdam, pp. 335–343.

105. H. H. Loh, T. M. Cho, Y. C. Wu, and E. L. Way, *Life Sci.*, **14**, 2231 (1974).

106. H. H. Loh, T. M. Cho, Y. C. Wu, R. A. Harris, and E. L. Way, *Life Sci.*, **16**, 1811 (1975).

107. S. H. Snyder, *Biochem. Pharmacol.*, **24**, 1371 (1975).

108. E. J. Simon and J. Groth, *Proc. Natl. Acad. Sci., U.S.*, **72**, 2404 (1975).

109. W. A. Klee, S. K. Sharma, and N. Nirenberg, *Life Sci.*, **16**, 1869 (1975).

110. A. Herz, Ed., *Developments in Opiate Research*, Vol. 14, *Modern Pharmacology–Toxicology*, Dekker, New York, 1978.

111. H. O. J. Collier and A. C. Roy, *Prostaglandins*, **7**, 361 (1974); *Nature*, **248**, 24 (1974).

112. S. K. Sharma, M. Nirenberg, and W. A. Klee, *Proc. Natl. Acad. Sci., U.S.*, **72**, 590 (1974).

113. J. Traber, K. Fischer, S. Latziri, and B. Hamprecht, *FEBS Lett.*, **49**, 260 (1974).

114. S. K. Sharma, W. A. Klee, and M. Nirenberg, *Proc. Natl. Acad. Sci., U.S.*, **73**, 3165 (1976).

115. D. L. Frances, A. C. Roy, and H. O. J. Collier, *Life Sci.*, **16**, 1901 (1975).

116. I. K. Ho, H. H. Loh, and E. L. Way, *J. Pharmacol. Exp. Ther.*, **185**, 336 and 347 (1973).

117. J. C. Liebeskind, D. J. Mayer, and H. Akil, *Advan. Neurol.*, **4**, 261 (1974).

118. H. Akil, D. J. Mayer, and J. C. Liebeskind, *Science*, **191**, 961 (1976).

119. D. J. Mayer and R. Hayes, *Science*, **188**, 941 (1975).

120. J. Hughes, *Brain Res.*, **88**, 295 (1975).

121. L. Terenius and W. Wahlström, *Acta. Physiol. Scand.*, **94**, 74 (1975).

122. J. Hughes, T. W. Smith, H. W. Kosterlitz, L. A. Fothergill, B. A. Morgan, and H. R. Morris, *Nature*, **258**, 577 (1975).

123. G. W. Pasternak, R. Goodman, and S. H. Snyder, *Life Sci.*, **16**, 1765 (1975).

124. R. Simantov and S. H. Snyder, *Proc. Natl. Acad. Sci. U.S.*, **73**, 2515 (1976).

125. B. M. Cox, K. E. Opheim, H. Teschemacher, and A. Goldstein, *Life Sci.*, **16**, 1777 (1975).

126. H. Teschemacher, K. E. Opheim, B. M. Cox, and A. Goldstein, *Life Sci.*, **16**, 1771 (1975).

127. C. H. Li, *Nature*, **201**, 924 (1964).

128. B. M. Cox, A. Goldstein, and C. H. Li, *Proc. Natl. Acad. Sci. U.S.*, **73**, 1821 (1976).

129. A. F. Bradbury, D. G. Smyth, C. R. Snell, N. J. M. Birdsall, and E. C. Hulme, *Nature*, **260**, 793 (1976).

130. F. Bloom, E. Battenberg, J. Rossier, N. Ling, and R. Guillemin, *Proc. Natl. Acad. Sci. U.S.*, **75**, 1591 (1978) and references therein.

131. J. Rossier, T. Vargo, S. Minnick. N. Ling, F. E. Bloom, and R. Guillemin, *Proc. Natl. Acad. Sci. U.S.*, **74**, 5162 (1977).

132. N. Ling, R. Burgus, and R. Guillemin, *Proc. Natl. Acad. Sci. U.S.*, **73**, 3942 (1976).

133. R. Schulz, M. Wuster, and A. Herz, *Life Sci.*, **21**, 105 (1977).

134. A. R. Gintzler, A. Levy, and S. Spector, *Life Sci.*, **73**, 2132 (1976).

135. L. Terenius, *Ann. Rev. Pharmacol. Toxicol.*, **18**, 189 (1978).

136. J. Hughes and H. W. Kosterlitz, *Brit. Med. Bull.*, **33**, 157 (1977).

137. R. C. A. Fredrickson, *Life Sci.*, **21**, 23 (1977).

138. S. H. Snyder and R. Simantor, *J. Neurochem.*, **28**, 13 (1977).

139. R. Guillemin, *N. Engl. J. Med.*, **296**, 226 (1977).

140. J. M. Polak, S. N. Sullivan, S. R. Bloom, P. Facer, and A. G. E. Pearse, *Lancet*, **1977-I**, 972.

141. F. Bloom, E. Battenberg, J. Rossier, N. Ling, J. Leppalvoto, T. M. Vargo, and R. Guillemin, *Life Sci.*, **20**, 43 (1977).

142. M. Ross, R. Dingledine, B. M. Cox, and A. Goldstein, *Brain Res.*, **124**, 513 (1977).

143. T. W. Smith, J. Hughes, H. W. Kosterlitz, and R. P. Sosa, in *Opiates and Endogenous Opioid Peptides*, H. W. Kosterlitz, Ed., North-Holland, Amsterdam, 1976, p. 57.

144. B. Malfroy, J. P. Swerts, A. Grayon, B. P. Roques, and J. C. Schwartz, *Nature*, **276**, 523 (1978).

145. T. M. Jessell and L. L. Iversen, *Nature*, **268**, 549 (1977).

146. A. G. E. Pearse and J. Polak, *Histochemistry*, **41**, 373 (1975).

147. R. Guillemin, T. Vargo, J. Rossier, S. Minick, N. Ling, C. Rivier, W. Vale, and F. Bloom, *Science*, **197**, 1367 (1977).

148. R. E. Mains, B. A. Eipper, and N. Ling, *Proc. Natl. Acad. Sci. U.S.*, **74**, 3014 (1977).

149. L.-F. Tseng, H. H. Loh, and C. H. Li, *Nature*, **263**, 239 (1976).

150. W. Feldberg and D. G. Smyth, *J. Physiol.*, **260**, 30P (1976).

151. Y. Hosobuchi and C. H. Li, *Commun. Psychopharmacol.*, **2**, 33 (1978).

152. L. Terenius, *Ann. Rev. Pharmacol.*, **18**, 189 (1978) and references cited therein.

153. M. Knight and W. A. Klee, *J. Biol. Chem.*, **253**, 3842 (1978).

154. J. J. Jacob, E. C. Tremblay and M. C. Colombel, *Psychopharmacologia*, **37**, 217 (1974).

155. R. C. A. Fredrickson, V. Burgis, and J. D. Edwards, *Fed. Proc.*, **36**, 965 (1977).

156. B. Pomeranz and D. Chiu, *Life Sci.*, **19**, 1757 (1976) and D. J. Mayer, *Neurosci. Res. Progr.*, **13**, 98 (1975).

157. H. D. Taube, E. Borowski, T. Endo, and K. Starlee, *Eur. J. Pharmacol.*, **38**, 377 (1976).

158. A. Goldstein and E. R. Hilgard, *Proc. Natl. Acad. Sci. U.S.*, **72**, 2041 (1975).

159. L. Lasagna, *Proc. R. Soc. Med.*, **58**, 978 (1965).

160. J. D. Levine, N. C. Gordon, R. T. Jones, and H. L. Fields, *Nature*, **272**, 826 (1978).

161. J. D. Levine, N. C. Gordon, and H. L. Fields, *Lancet*, 1978, 654.

162. E. Wei and H. Loh, *Science*, **193**, 1262 (1976).

163. J. Bläsig and A. Hertz, *Naunyn-Schmiedebergs Arch. Pharmakol.*, **294**, 297 (1976).

164. A. A. Waterfield, J. Hughes, and H. W. Kosterlitz, *Nature*, **260**, 624 (1976).

165. J. D. Belluzzi and L. Stein, *Nature*, **266**, 556 (1977).

166. F. C. Colpaert, C. J. E. Niemegeers, P. A. J. Janssen, and J. M. vanRee, *Eur. J. Pharmacol.*, **47**, 115 (1978).

167. D. H. Catlere, K. K. Hi, H. H. Loh, and C. H. Li in *Advances in Biochemical Pharmacology*, Vol. 18., E. Costa and M. Trabucchi, Eds., Raven Press, New York, 1978.

168. D. L. Margules, B. Morsset, M. J. Lewis, H. Shibuya, and C. B. Pert, *Science*, **202**, 908 (1978).

169. W. R. Martin, *Pharmacol. Rev.*, **19**, 463 (1967).

170. W. R. Martin, C. G. Eades, J. A. Thompson, R.

E. Huppler, and P. E. Gilbert, *J. Pharmacol. Exp. Ther.*, **197,** 517 (1976).

171. W. F. Michne, T. R. Lewis, S. J. Michalec, A. K. Pierson, M. G. C. Gillan, S. J. Patterson, L. E. Robson, and H. W. Kosterlitz, in *Characteristics and Functions of Opiods*, J. M. vanRee and L. Teremus, Eds., Elsevier/North Holland, 1978, p. 197.

172. M. Hutchinson, H. W. Kosterlitz, F. M. Leslie, and A. A. Waterfield, *Brit. J. Pharm.*, **55,** 541 (1975).

173. J. A. H. Lord, A. A. Waterfield, J. Hughes, and H. W. Kosterlitz, *Nature*, **267,** 495 (1977).

174. A. Osal, Ed., *Remington's Pharmaceutical Sciences*, Mack Publishing Company, Easton, Pa., 1975, p. 434.

175. A. K. Reynolds and L. O. Randall, *Morphine and Allied Drugs*, University of Toronto Press, Canada, 1957, p. 3.

176. J. M. Gulland and R. Robinson, *Mem. Proc. Manchester Lit. Phil. Soc.*, **69,** 79 (1925).

177. M. Gates and G. Tschudi, *J. Am. Chem. Soc.*, **74,** 1109 (1952).

178. *Ibid.*, **78,** 1380 (1956).

179. H. Rapoport and J. B. Lavigne, *J. Am. Chem. Soc.*, **75,** 5329 (1953).

180. K. W. Bentley and H. M. E. Cardwell, *J. Chem. Soc.*, **1955,** 3252.

181. G. Stork and F. H. Clarke, Jr., *J. Am. Chem. Soc.*, **78,** 4619 (1956).

182. J. Kalvoda, P. Buchscahcher, and O. Jeger, *Helv. Chim. Acta*, **38,** 1847 (1955).

183. C. R. A. Wright, *J. Chem. Soc.* (London), **27,** 1031 (1874).

184. C. I. Wright and F. A. Barbour, *J. Pharmacol. Exp. Ther.*, **51,** 422 (1937).

185. H. J. C. Yeh, R. S. Wilson, W. A. Klee, and A. E. Jacobson, *J. Pharm. Sci.*, **65,** 903 (1976).

186. D. L. Mahler and W. H. Forrest, *Anesthesiology*, **42,** 602 (1975).

187. M. Freund and E. Speyer, *J. Pratk. Chem.*, **94,** 135 (1916).

188. U. Weiss, *J. Am. Chem. Soc.*, **77,** 5091 (1955).

189. L. F. Small, H. M. Fitch, and W. E. Smith, *J. Am. Chem. Soc.*, **58,** 1457 (1936).

190. G. Stork, *J. Am. Chem. Soc.*, **75,** 4373 (1953).

191. N. B. Eddy, H. Halbach, and O. J. Braenden, *Bull. World Health Organ.*, **17,** 569 (1957).

192. G. Rataśági and E. Schwartzmann, *Orvostudomány*, **24,** 359 (1973).

193. J. Knoll, S. Fürst, and K. Kilemen, *J. Pharm. Pharmacol.*, **25,** 929 (1973).

194. J. Knoll, *Pharmacol. Res. Commun.*, **5,** 175 (1973).

195. J. Knoll, S. Fürst, and S. Marleit, *J. Pharm. Pharmacol.*, **27,** 99 (1975).

196. J. von Braun, *Chem. Ber.*, **49,** 971 (1916).

197. *Ibid.*, **49,** 2655 (1916).

198. J. von Braun, M. Kuhn, and S. Siddigui, *Chem. Ber.*, **59,** 1081 (1926).

199. K. Unna, *J. Pharmacol. Exp. Ther.*, **79,** 27 (1943).

200. R. L. Clark, A. A. Pessolano, J. Weijlard, and K. Pfister, *J. Am. Chem. Soc.*, **75,** 4964 (1953).

201. C. A. Winter, P. D. Orahovats, and E. G. Lehman, *Arch. Int. Pharmacodyn.*, **110,** 186 (1957).

202. R. L. Clark, A. A. Pessolano, J. Weijlard, and K. Pfister, III, *J. Am. Chem. Soc.*, **75,** 4963 (1953).

203. N. B. Eddy, L. F. Small, J. H. Ager, and E. L. May, *J. Org. Chem.*, **23,** 1387 (1958).

204. J. Weijlard, P. D. Orahovats, A. P. Sullivan, G. Purdue, F. K. Heath, and K. Pfister, III, *J. Am. Chem. Soc.*, **78,** 2342 (1956).

205. M. J. Lewenstein and J. Fishman, U.S. Pat 3,524,088 (1966).

206. R. B. Resnick, J. Volavka, A. M. Freedman, and M. Thomas, *Am. J. Physchiatr.*, **131,** 646 (1974).

207. W. T. Beaver, *Mod. Med.*, **44,** 21 (1976).

208. O. J. Braendon, N. B. Eddy, and H. Halbach, *Bull. World Health Organ.*, **13,** 937 (1955).

209. R. J. J. Ch. Lousberg and U. Weiss, *Experientia*, **30,** 1440 (1974).

210. K. W. Bently and D. G. Hardy, *J. Am. Chem. Soc.*, **89,** 3269 (1967).

211. J. W. Lewis, K. W. Bently, and A. Cowan, *Ann. Rev. Pharmacol.*, **11,** 241 (1971).

212. A. F. Bradbury, D. G. Smyth, and C. R. Snell, *Nature*, **260,** 165 (1976).

213. G. F. Blane and D. S. Robbie, *Brit. J. Pharmacol. Chemother.*, **20,** 252 (1970).

214. A. M. Harthoorn, *J. Am. Vet. Med. Assoc.*, **149,** 875 (1966).

215. J. M. King and B. Carter, II., *B. Afr. Wildlife J.*, **3,** 19 (1965).

216. J. D. Wallach, *J. Am. Vet. Med. Assoc.*, **149,** 871 (1966).

217. J. D. Wallach, *Vet. Med.*, **64,** 53 (1961).

218. G. F. Blane, *J. Pharmacol.*, **19,** 367 (1967).

219. K. W. Bently, D. G. Hardy, and P. A. Major, *J. Chem. Soc.*, **1969,** 2385.

220. M. H. Fisher, E. J. J. Grabowski, A. A. Patchett,

J. ten Broeke, L. M. Flatuker, V. J. Lotti, and F. M. Robinson, *J. Med. Chem.*, **20,** 63 (1977).

221. J. Weiglard, P. D. Orahovats, A. P. Sullivan, G. Purdue, F. K. Heath, and K. Pfister, III., *J. Am. Chem. Soc.*, **78,** 2342 (1956).

222. A. Langein, H. Merz, K. Stockhaus, and H. Wick, in *Narcotic Antagonists*, M. C. Braude, L. S. Harris, E. L. May, J. P. Smith, and J. E. Villarreal, Eds., Raven Press, New York, 1974, pp. 157–165.

224. D. M. Zimmerman, R. Nickander, J. S. Horng, and D. T. Wong, *Nature*, **275,** 332 (1978).

225. W. D. Avison and A. L. Morrison, *J. Chem. Soc.*, **1950,** 1469.

226. H. Kägi and K. Miescher, *Helv. Chim. Acta*, **32,** 2489 (1949).

227. A. Ziering and J. Lee, *J. Org. Chem.*, **12,** 911 (1947).

228. L. O. Randall and G. Lehman, *J. Pharmacol. Exp. Ther.*, **93,** 314 (1948).

229. A. C. King, *Am. J. Obstet. Gynecol.*, **71,** 1001 (1956).

230. P. A. J. Janssen and N. B. Eddy, *J. Med. Pharm. Chem.*, **2,** 31 (1960).

231. D. Fries and P. S. Portoghese, *J. Med. Chem.*, **17,** 990 (1974).

232. K. H. Bell and P. S. Portoghese, *J. Med. Chem.*, **17,** 129 (1974).

233. J. Diamond, W. F. Bruce, and F. T. Tyson, *J. Org. Chem.*, **22,** 399 (1957).

234. J. Diamond, W. F. Bruce, C. Gochman and F. T. Tyson, *J. Org. Chem.*, **25,** 65 (1960).

235. A. J. Grossman, M. Golbey, W. C. Gittinger, and R. C. Batterman, *J. Am. Geriatr. Soc.*, **4,** 187 (1956).

236. L. J. Cass, W. S. Frederik, and A. F. Bartholomay, *J. Am. Med. Assoc.*, **166,** 1829 (1958).

237. H. F. Fraser, *Fed. Proc.*, **15,** 423 (1956).

238. J. F. Cavalla, J. Davoll, M. J. Dean, C. S. Franklin, D. M. Temple, J. Wax and C. V. Winder, *J. Med. Pharm. Chem.*, **4,** 1 (1961).

239. J. Cass and W. S. Frederik, *Curr. Ther. Res.*, **3,** 97 (1961).

240. W. F. M. van Bever, C. J. E. Niemegeers, and P. A. Janssen, *J. Med. Chem.*, **17,** 1047 (1974).

241. W. F. M. van Bever, C. J. E. Niemegeers, K. H. L. Schellekens and P. A. Janssen, *Arzneim.-Forsch.*, **26,** 1548 (1976).

242. N. B. Eddy, *The National Research Council Involvement in the Opiate Problem*, National Academy of Sciences, Washington, D.C., 1973.

243. A. H. Beckett, *J. Pharm. Pharmacol.*, **8,** 848 (1956).

244. A. Gero, *Science*, **119,** 112 (1954).

245. J. G. Henkel, K. H. Bell, and P. S. Portoghese, *J. Med. Chem.*, **17,** 124 (1974).

246. P. A. J. Janssen, in *Synthetic Analgesics*, Part I, Pergamon, New York, 1960.

247. M. Bochmühl and G. Ehrhart, Ger. Pat. 711,069; through *Chem. Abstr.*, **37,** 4075 (1943).

248. A. A. Larsen, B. F. Tullar, B. Elpern, and J. S. Buck, *J. Am. Chem. Soc.*, **70,** 4194 (1948).

249. R. H. Thorp, E. Walton, and P. Ofner, *Nature*, **160,** 605 (1947).

250. A. S. Keats and H. K. Beecher, *J. Pharmacol.*, **105,** 109 (1952).

251. P. W. Nathan, *Brit. Med. J.*, **1952-II,** 903.

252. E. L. May, *J. Org. Chem.*, **21,** 899 (1956).

253. H. Isbell and H. F. Fraser, *Pharmacol. Rev.*, **2,** 355 (1950).

254. N. B. Eddy, H. Halbach, and O. J. Braenden, *Bull. World Health Organ.*, **14,** 353 (1956).

255. D. J. Coleman, J. Levin, and P. O. Jones, *Brit. Med. J.*, **1957-I,** 1092.

256. P. A. J. Janssen, *J. Am. Chem. Soc.*, **78,** 3862 (1956).

257. P. A. J. Janssen and A. H. Jageneau, *J. Pharm. Pharmacol.*, **9,** 381 (1957).

258. A. Pohland and H. R. Sullivan, *J. Am. Chem. Soc.*, **75,** 4458 (1953).

259. N. B. Eddy, E. L. May, and E. Mosettig, *J. Org. Chem.*, **17,** 321 (1952).

260. D. Leimbach and N. B. Eddy, *J. Pharmacol.*, **110,** 135 (1954).

261. N. B. Eddy, *Chem. Ind.*, **1959,** 1462.

262. N. A. David, H. J. Semler, and P. R. Burgner, *J. Am. Med. Assoc.*, **161,** 599 (1956).

263. R. E. McMahon, H. W. Culp, and F. S. Marshall, *J. Pharmacol. Exp. Ther.*, **149,** 439 (1965).

264. R. E. Billings, R. N. Booher, S. Smits, A. Pohland, and R. E. McMahon, *J. Med. Chem.*, **16,** 305 (1973).

265. R. E. Billings, R. E. McMahon, and D. A. Blake, *Life Sci.*, **14,** 1437 (1974).

266. R. N. Booher and A. Pohland, *J. Med. Chem.*, **18,** 266 (1975).

267. R. Grewe and A. Mondon, *Chem. Ber.*, **81,** 279 (1948).

268. W. M. Benson, P. L. Stefko, and L. O. Randall, *J. Pharmacol. Exp. Ther.*, **109,** 189 (1953).

269. N. B. Eddy, H. Besendorf, and B. Pellmont, *Bull. Narcotics*, **10,** 23 (1958).

270. J. Hellerbach, O. Schnider, H. Besendorf, and B.

Pellmont, *Synthetic Analgesics Part IIA. Morphinans*, Pergamon, Oxford, 1966.

271. E. L. May, in *Psychopharmacological Agents*, M. Gordon, Ed., Academic, New York, 1976, p. 47.

272. I. Monkovic, H. Wong, A. W. Pircio, Y. G. Perron, I. J. Pachter, and B. Belleau, *Can. J. Chem.*, **17**, 3094 (1975).

273. A. W. Pircio and J. A. Gylys, *J. Pharmacol. Exp. Ther.*, **193**, 23 (1975).

274. I. Monkovic, H. Wong, B. Belleau, I. J. Pachter, and Y. G. Perron, *Can. J. Chem.*, **17**, 2515 (1975).

275. A. B. Dobkin, S. Eamkaow, and F. S. Caruso, *Clin. Pharmacol. Ther.*, **68**, 547 (1975).

276. R. W. Houde, S. L. Wallenstein, and A. Rogers, in *Advances in Pain Research and Therapy*, J. J. Bonica and D. Albe-Fessard., Eds., Vol. 1, Raven Press, New York, 1976, pp. 647–651.

277. J. A. Barltrop, *J. Chem. Soc.*, **1947**, 399.

278. D. C. Palmer and M. J. Strauss, *Chem. Rev.*, **77**, 1 (1977).

279. A. E. Jacobson and E. L. May, *J. Med. Chem.*, **8**, 563 (1965).

280. E. L. May and H. Kugita, *J. Org. Chem.*, **26**, 188 (1961).

281. N. F. Albertson, *J. Med. Chem.*, **18**, 619 (1975).

282. Y. K. Sawa and J. Irisawa, *Tetrahedron*, **21**, 1129 (1965).

283. J. H. Ager, A. E. Jacobson, and E. L. May, *J. Med. Chem.*, **12**, 288 (1969).

284. N. B. Eddy and E. L. May, *Synthetic Analgesics. Part IIB, 6,7-Benzomorphans, Int. Ser. Morogr. Org. Chem.*, Vol. 8, Pergamon, Oxford, 1966.

285. K. C. Rice, A. E. Jacobson, and E. L. May, *J. Med. Chem.*, **18**, 854 (1975).

286. F. H. Clarke, R. T. Hill, J. K. Saelens, and H. Yokoyama, in Ref. 222, pp. 81–89.

287. H. Inoue, T. Oh-ishi, and E. L. May, *J. Med. Chem.*, **18**, 787 (1975).

288. H. Merz, A. Lanjbein, K. Stockhaus, G. Walther, and H. Wick, in Ref. 222, pp. 91–107.

289. H. Merz, K. Stockhaus, and H. Wick, *J. Med. Chem.*, **18**, 996 (1975).

290. G. Milne and M. R. Johnson, in *Ann. Rep. Med. Chem.*, **11**, 24 (1976).

291. M. Gordon, J. J. Lafferty, D. H. Tedeschi, N. B. Eddy, and E. L. May, *Nature*, **192**, 1089 (1961).

292. S. Archer, N. F. Albertson, L. S. Harris, A. K. Pierson, and J. G. Bird, *J. Med. Chem.*, **7**, 123 (1964).

293. L. S. Harris and A. K. Pierson, *J. Pharmacol. Exp. Ther.*, **143**, 141 (1964).

294. L. Lasagna, T. J. Dekornfeld, and J. W. Pearson, *J. Pharmacol. Exp. Ther.*, **144**, 12 (1964).

295. A. Brossi, H. Bessendorf, L. A. Pirk, and A. Rheiner, Jr., in Ref. 304, Chap. VI.

296. D. W. Adamson and A. F. Green, *Nature*, **165**, 122 (1950).

297. D. W. Adamson, *J. Chem. Soc.*, **1950**, 885.

298. A. H. Beckett, A. F. Casy, N. J. Harper, and P. M. Philips, *J. Pharm. Pharmacol.*, **8**, 860 (1956).

299. G. Satzinger, *Ann. Chem.*, **728**, 64 (1969).

300. A. I. Mauro and M. Shapiro, *Curr. Ther. Res.*, **16**, 725 (1974).

301. G. Buzzelli, M. Grazzini, and V. Monafo, *Curr. Ther. Res.*, **12**, 561 (1970).

302. L. Martinetti, E. Lodola, V. Monafo, and V. Farrari, *J. Clin. Pharmacol.*, **10**, 390 (1970).

303. F. Nobili and G. C. Bernardi, *Eur. J. Clin. Pharmacol.*, **3**, 119 (1971).

304. G. deStevens, Ed., *Analgetics*, Academic, New York, 1965, Chap. VIII.

305. D. Della Bella, V. Ferrari, V. Frigeni, and P. Lualdi, *Nature New Biol.*, **241**, 282 (1973).

306. E. L. May, *Pharmacol. Res. Commun.* **9**, 197 (1977).

307. J. P. Yardley, H. Fletcher, III, and P. B. Russell, *Experientia*, **34**, 1124 (1978).

308. R. N. Booker, S. E. Snitts, W. W. Turner, Jr., and A. Pohland, *J. Med. Chem.*, **20**, 885 (1971).

309. M. W. Klohs, M. D. Draper, F. J. Petracek, K. H. Ginzel, and O. N. Ré, *Arzneim.-Forsch.*, **22**, 132 (1972).

310. A. Sunshine and E. Laska, in *Advances in Pain Research and Therapy*, J. J. Bonica and D. Albe-Fessard, Ed., Raven Press, New York, 1976, pp. 543–551.

311. M. M. Gassel, E. Diamantopoulous, V. Petropoulos, A. C. R. Hughes, M. L. F. Ballestios, and O. N. Ré, *J. Clin. Pharmacol.*, **16**, 34 (1976).

312. M. M, Gassel, *Electromyogr. Clin. Neurophysiol.*, **3**, 342 (1973).

313. J. C. Gasser and J. W. Bellville, *Clin. Pharmacol. Ther.*, **18**, 175 (1975).

314. A. L. Klotz, *Curr. Ther. Res.*, **16**, 602 (1974).

315. L. Lemberger and A. Rubin, *Physiological Disposition of Drugs of Abuse*, Spectrum Publications, New York, 1976, Chap. 5.

316. J. T. Scrapfani and D. H. Clouet, in *Narcotic Drugs*, D. H. Clouet, Ed., Plenum Press, New York, 1971, Chap. 6.

317. S. Y. Yeh, *J. Pharmacol. Exp. Ther.*, **192**, 201 (1975).

318. J. W. Miller and H. H. Anderson, *J. Pharmacol. Exp. Ther.*, **112**, 191 (1954).

319. A. F. Bradbury, D. G. Smyth, and C. R. Snell, *Nature*, **260**, 165 (1976).

320. A. S. Horn and J. R. Rodgers, *J. Pharm. Pharmacol.*, **29,** 257 (1977).

321. B. P. Roques, C. Garbay-Jaureguiberry, R. Oberlin, M. Anteunis, and A. K. Lala, *Nature,* **262,** 778 (1976).

322. C. R. Jones, W. A. Gibbons, and V. Garsky, *Nature,* **262,** 779 (1976).

323. B. E. Maryanoff and M. J. Zelesko, *J. Pharm. Sci.,* **67,** 591 (1978).

324. G. D. Smith and J. F. Griffen, *Science,* **199,** 1214 (1978).

325. P. W. Schiller, C. F. Yam, and M. Lis, *Biochemistry,* **16,** 1831 (1977).

326. S. Bajusz, A. Z. Ronai, J. I. Szekely, Z. Dunai-Kovacs, I. Berzetei, and L. Graf, *Acta. Biochem. Biophys. Acad. Sci. Hung.,* **11,** 305 (1976).

327. M. A. Khaled, M. M. Long, W. D. Thompson, R. J. Bradley, G. B. Brown, and D. W. Lerry, *Biochem. Biophys. Res. Commun.,* **76,** 224 (1977).

328. C. Garbay-Jaureguiberry, B. P. Roques, and R. Oberlin, *Biochem. Biophys. Res. Commun.,* **71,** 558 (1976).

329. C. R. Jones, V. Garsky, and W. A. Gibbons, *Biochem. Biophys. Res. Commun.,* **76,** 619 (1977).

330. C. R. Beddell, R. B. Clark, L. A. Lowe, S. Wilkerson, K.-J. Chang, P. Cuatrecasas, and R. Miller, *Brit. J. Pharm.,* **61,** 351 (1977).

331. F. A. Momany, *Biochem. Biophys. Res. Commun.,* **75,** 1098 (1977).

332. G. H. Loew and S. K. Burt, *Proc. Natl. Acad. Sci. U.S.,* **75,** 7 (1978).

333. B. A. Morgan, C. F. C. Smith, A. A. Waterfield, J. Hughes, and H. W. Kosterlitz, *J. Pharm. Pharmacol.,* **28,** 660 (1976).

334. H. H. Büscher, R. C. Hill, D. Römer, F. Cardinaux, A. Closse, D. Hawser, and J. Pless, *Nature,* **261,** 423 (1976).

335. R. C., A. Frederickson, R. Nickander, E. L. Smithwick, R. Shuman and F. H. Norris, in *Opiates and Endogenons Opioid Peptides,* H. Kosterlitz, Ed., Elsevier/North Holland, Amsterdam, 1976, p. 239.

336. J. M. Hambrook, B. A. Morgan, M. J. Rance, and C. F. C. Smith, *Nature,* **262,** 782 (1976).

337. L. Terenius, A. Wahlström, G. Lindeberg, S. Karlsson, and V. Ragnarsson, *Biochem. Biophys. Res. Commun.,* **71,** 175 (1976).

338. J. K. Chang, B. T. W. Fong, A. Pert, and C. B. Pert, *Life Sci.,* **18,** 1473 (1976).

339. W. H. McGregor, L. Stein, and J. D. Belluzzi, *Life Sci.,* **23,** 1371 (1978).

340. H. Takagi, H. Shiomi, H. Veda, and H. Amano, *Eur. J. Pharamcol.,* **55,** 109 (1979).

341. L-Fu Tseng, H. H. Loh, and C. H. Li, *Life Sci.,* **23,** 2053 (1978).

342. L. M. Lazarus, N. Ling, and R. Grillemin, *Proc. Natl. Acad. Sci., U.S.,* **73,** 2156 (1976).

343. C. B. Pert, A. Pert, J-K Chang, and B. T. Fong, *Science,* **194,** 330 (1976).

344. A. S. Dutta, J. J. Gormley, C. F. Hayward, J. S. Morley, J. S. Shaw, G. J. Stacey, and M. J. Turnbull, *Brit. J. Pharmacol.,* **61,** 481P (1977); J. S. Shaw and M. J. Turnbull, *Eur. J. Pharmacol.,* **49,** 313 (1978).

345. J. S. Morley, lecture given at the *EMBO Workshop on Hormone Fragments and Diseases,* Leiden, The Netherlands, 1977.

346. J. Pless, W. Bauer, F. Cardinaux, A. Vlosse, D. Hauser, R. Huguenin, D. Romer, H. H. Buscher, and R. C. Hill, in *Proc. Endocrinology,* I. MacIntyre and A. G. E. Pearse, Eds., Elsevier, Amsterdam, 1978.

347. M. G. Baxter, D. Goff, A. A. Miller, and I. A. Saunders, *Brit. J. Pharmacol.,* **59,** 455P (1977).

348. E. F. Hahn, J. Fishman, Y. Shiwaku, F. F. Foldes, H. Nagashima, and D. Duncalf, *Res. Commun. Chem. Path. Pharmacol.,* **18,** 1 (1977).

349. P. Y. Law, E. T. Wei, L. F. Tseng, H. H. Loh, and E. L. Way, *Life Sci.,* **20,** 251 (1977).

350. A. S. Dutta, J. J. Gormley, C. F. Hayward, J. S. Morley, J. S. Shaw, G. J. Stacey, and M. T. Turnbull, *Life Sci.,* **21,** 559 (1977).

351. D. Roemer, H. H. Buescher, R. C. Hill, J. Pless, W. Bauer, F. Cardinaux, A. Closse, D. Hauser, and R. Hugenin, *Nature,* **268,** 547 (1977).

352. B. von Graffenried, E. del Pozo, J. Roubicek, E. Krebs, W. Poldinger, P. Burmeister, and L. Kerp, *Nature,* **272,** 729 (1978).

353. J. A. H. Lord, A. A. Waterfield, J. Hughes, and H. W. Kosterlitz, *Nature,* **267,** 495 (1977).

354. J. Rossier, A. Bayon, T. M. Vargo, N. Ling, R. Guillemin and F. Bloom, *Life Sci.,* **21,** 847 (1977).

355. R. Guillemin, N. Ling, L. Lazarus, R. Burgus, S. Minick, F. Bloom, R. Nicoll, G. Siggins, and D. Segal, *Ann. N.Y. Acad Sci.,* **297,** 131 (1977).

356. Kangawa et al., *Biochem. Biophys. Res. Commun.,* **86,** 153 (1978).

357. H. C. Li, *J. Econ. Bot.,* **28,** 437 (1974).

358. G. V. Rossi, *Am. J. Pharm.,* **142,** 161 (1970).

359. T. H. Mikuriya, *New Physician,* **18,** 902 (1961).

360. L. S. Harris, in *The Therapeutic Potential of Marihuana,* S. Cohen and R. C. Stillman, Eds., Plenum Medical Book Company, New York, 1976, pp. 299–312.

361. V. Gaoni and R. Mechoulam, *J. Am. Chem. Soc.,* **86,** 1646 (1964).

362. R. L. Hively, W. A. Mosher, and F. Hoffman, *J.*

Am. Chem. Soc., **88**, 1832 (1966).

363. R. Mechoulam, Ed., *Marijuana*, Academic, New York, 1973, pp. 220, 253, 274, 294 and references cited therein.

364. S. Y. Hill, R. Schwin, D. W. Goodwin, and B. J. Powell, *J. Pharmacol. Exp. Ther.*, **188**, 415 (1974).

365. S. L. Milstein, K. MacCannell, G. Karr, and S. Clark, *Int Pharmacopsychiat.*, **10**, 177 (1975).

366. S. F. Brunk, R. Noyes, Jr., D. H. Avery, and A. Canter, *J. Clin. Pharmacol.*, **15**, 544 (1975).

367. R. Noyes, Jr., S. F. Brunk, D. H. Avery, and A. Canter, *Clin. Pharmacol. Ther.*, **18**, 84 (1975).

368. R. Noyes, Jr., S. F. Brunk, D. A. Baram, and A. Canter, *The Pharmacology of Marihuana*, in M. C. Braude and S. Szara, Eds., Raven Press, New York, 1976, pp. 833–836.

369. R. S. Wilson and E. L. May, *Abstr. Pap. Amer. Chem. Soc.*, **168**, Meet Medi 11 (1974).

370. R. S. Wilson and E. L. May, *J. Med. Chem.*, **17**, 475 (1974).

371. R. S. Wilson and E. L. May, *J. Med. Chem.*, **18**, 700 (1975).

372. R. S. Wilson, E. L. May, B. R. Martin, and W. L. Dewey, *J. Med. Chem.*, **19**, 1165 (1976).

373. D. B. Uliss, H. C. Dalzell, G. R. Handrick, J. F. Howes, and R. K. Razdan, *J. Med. Chem.*, **18**, 213 (1975).

374. *Chemical Week*, Jan. 22, 1975, p. 39.

375. P. Stark and R. A. Archer, *Pharmacologist*, **17**, 210 (1975).

376. L. Lemberger and H. Rowe, *Clin. Pharmacol. Ther.* **18**, 720 (1975).

377. L. Lomberger, in Ref. 360, pp. 405–418.

378. L. F. Fabre, D. M. McLendon, and P. Stark, *Curr. Ther. Res.*, **24**, 161 (1978).

379. R. Mechoulam and H. Edery, in Ref. 147, pp. 101–136.

380. R. Mechoulam, M. K. McCallum, and S. Burstein, *Chem. Rev.*, **76**, 75 (1976).

381. H. G. Pars, F. E. Granchelli, J. K. Keller, and R. K. Razdan, *J. Am. Chem. Soc.*, **88**, 3664 (1966).

382. H. G. Pars and R. K. Razdan, *Ann N.Y. Acad. Sci.*, **191**, 15 (1971).

383. H. G. Pars, F. E. Granchelli, R. K. Razdan, J. K. Keller, D. G. Terger, F. J. Rosenberg, and L. S. Harris, *J. Med. Chem.*, **19**, 445 (1976).

384. R. K. Razdan, B. Z. Terris, and H. G. Pars, *J. Med. Chem.*, **19**, 454 (1976).

385. M. Winn, D. Arendsen, P. Dodge, A. Drenn, D. Dunnigan, R. Hallas, K. Hawg, J. Kyncl, Y.-H. Lee, N. Plottnkoff, P. Young, H. Zaugg, H.

Dalzell, and R. K. Razdan, *J. Med. Chem.*, **19**, 461 (1976).

386. H. G. Pars, in Ref. 360, pp. 419–437.

387. A. T. Dren, in Ref. 360, pp. 439–453.

388. R. W. Houde, S. L. Wallenstein, A. Rogers, and R. F. Kaiko, *Proc. 38th Ann. Mtg. Comm. Problems Drug Dependence*, 164 (1976).

389. M. Staquet, C. Gantt, and D. Machin, *Clin. Pharmacol. Ther.*, **23**, 397 (1978).

390. P. R. Jochimsen, R. L. Lawton, K. Versteeg, and R. Noyes, Jr., *Clin. Pharmacol. Ther.*, **24**, 223 (1978).

391. G. M. Milne, A. Weissman, B. K. Koe, and M. R. Johnson, *Pharmacologist*, **20**, 243 (1978).

392. B. A. Berkowitz, S. H. Ngai, and A. D. Finck, *Science*, **194**, 967 (1976).

393. D. J. Mayer, D. R. Price, and A. Rafii, *Brain Res.*, **121**, 368 (1977).

394. J. S. Hong, H-Y. T. Yang, J. C. Gillen, A. M. DiGiulio, W. Fralta, and E. Costa, *Brain Res.*, **160**, 192 (1979).

395. B. Malfroy, J. P. Swerts, A. Guyon, B. P. Roques, and J. C. Schwartz, *Nature*, **276**, 523 (1978).

396. S. Ehrenpreis, J. Comaty, and S. Myles, *Pharmacologist*, **22**, 168 (1978).

397. R. A. Harris, H. H. Loh, and E. L. Way, *J. Pharmacol. Exp. Ther.*, **196**, 288 (1976).

398. A. W. Mudge, S. E. Leeman, G. D. Fischbach, *Proc. Natl. Acad. Sci. U.S.*, **76**, 526 (1979), and references therein.

399. G. Paalzow and L. Paalzow, *Naunyn-Schmiedeberg's Arch. Pharmacol.*, **292**, 119 (1976).

400. S. Fielding, J. Wilker, M. Hynes, M. Szewczak, W. J. Novick, Jr., and H. Lal, *J. Pharmacol. Exp. Ther.*, **207**, 899 (1978).

401. M. S. Gold, D. E. Redmond, Jr., and H. D. Keeber, *Am. J. Psychiatr.*, **136**, 100 (1979).

402. G. Gacel, M-C. Fournie–Zaluski, E. Fellion, B. P. Roques, B. Senault, J-M. Lecomte, B. Malfroy, J-P. Swerts, and J-C. Schwartz, *Life Sci.*, **24**, 725 (1979).

403. M. L. English and C. H. Stammer, *Biochem. Biophys Res Commun.*, **85**, 780 (1978).

404. K. B. Mathur, B. J. Dhotre, R. Raghubir, G. K. Patnaik, and B. N. Dhawan, *Life Sci.*, **25**, 2023 (1979).

405. R. Nagaraj and P. Balaram, *FEBS Letters*, **96**, 273 (1978).

406. H. Takagi, H. Shiomi, H. Veda, and H. Amano, *Nature*, **282**, 410 (1979).

407. C. Gorenstein and S. H. Snyder, *Life Sci.*, **25**, 2065 (1979).

CHAPTER FIFTY THREE

Antitussives

DAVID MILLER

Research Division
Beecham Pharmaceuticals
The Pinnacles, Harlow
Essex CM19 5AD, England

CONTENTS

1 INTRODUCTION

Antitussives are drugs used in the treatment of cough and as such are used extensively often as an adjunct to other therapy, for a wide variety of respiratory diseases in which cough is a problem. These vary from mild throat infections often treated with over-the-counter preparations, to more serious complaints such as bronchitis, pneumonia, and asthma. Cough is a normal physiological response to an irritation in the laryngeal–tracheal–bronchial system, whether caused by an infecting organism or by mechanical or chemical stimulation, and serves a vital function in expelling mucus secreted in response to these stimuli. It is therefore important to distinguish between this normal or productive cough which is of benefit to the patient and needs no treatment, and nonproductive cough, which can be both painful and fatiguing and requires suppression by antitussive drugs. However, these are extreme positions and much in

759

cough therapy is devoted to converting nonproductive cough to productive cough by the use of *mucolytics*, which aid in the liquefaction of the viscid mucus frequently encountered in chronic bronchitics or asthmatics; *expectorants*, which facilitate removal of mucus from the respiratory tract; and *inhalants*, such as menthol in steam or water vapor, which soften mucus, particularly in the upper respiratory tract and aid expectoration. There is some rationale for the use of *bronchodilators* and certain *local anesthetics* in the control of cough, and *antihistamines* are often included in cough remedies. Many antitussives also have beneficial *analgetic* properties. A glance at any list of available products shows immediately that the treatment of cough is the area of polypharmacy *par excellence*, and the practice has received adverse comment (1).

The detailed discussion of antitussive compounds in this chapter is limited to those compounds falling within the definition of Gold (2), who proposed that the term antitussive be "confined to a drug which acts to raise the threshold of the cough center in the central nervous system, acts peripherally in the respiratory tract to reduce impulses which pass to this center, or a mixture which combines both these actions." However, because of the importance of nonantitussive remedies in cough treatment, a section is devoted to a brief discussion of these agents.

In order to understand how antitussive drugs may act, we must briefly consider the cough reflex arc (3) and the mechanism of cough production. This is shown schematically in Fig. 53.1. A mechanical or chemical stimulus at mucosal receptors in the pharynx, larynx, trachea, or bronchi causes an impulse to travel by the appropriate afferent nerve, which is the vagus nerve or one of its branches, to the cough center in the brain. From here, tussal impulses travel by efferent nerves to the diaphragm, inter-

costal muscles, and abdominal wall muscles. It is the contraction of these muscular systems following an initial deep inspiration of air and closure of the glottis that builds up the intrathoracic pressure. Opening of the glottis then produces a rapid expulsion of air—the cough (4).

Experiments have shown the presence of two types of receptors in the respiratory tract (5), *mechanoreceptors* responsive to mechanical stimulation and *chemoreceptors* responsive to chemical stimulation. The former are mainly located in the larynx and trachea whereas the latter appear to be distributed throughout the tracheobronchial tree. It has been postulated by Salem and Aviado (6) that irritation of the mucosa does not lead directly to stimulation of the cough receptors, but to initial bronchoconstriction, which is the primary stimulus in triggering the cough reflex.

One further group of sensory receptors should be mentioned, inhibition of which provides a possible mechanism of antitussive action. These are the *pulmonary stretch receptors* located in the alveolar walls of the lung. The impulses arising from these receptors in the act of inspiration of air are transmitted by the vagus nerve to the respiratory center and promote the following expiration, a respiratory regulation mechanism known as the Herring–Breuer reflex. It was shown in cats (7) that the extent of expiration and the intensity of coughing correlated with the amplitude of the preceding inspiration.

Mention must be made of the "cough center" in the central nervous system, since this has been the main target of attack for antitussive drugs. Early work (8) indicated that stimulation of the dorsolateral region of the medulla of the cat produced spasmodic coughing and sneezing. Very recent careful work (9) has shown that within this general area, the cough center is restricted to an area dorsomedial to the spinal trigeminal tract and nucleus. Furthermore,

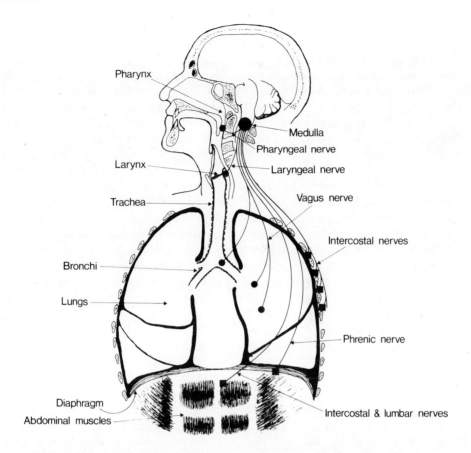

Fig. 53.1   The cough reflex arc showing afferent (●) and efferent (■) pathways.

there appears to be virtually no overlap between the cough and respiratory centers, a finding that confirms earlier work.

It is now appropriate to discuss briefly the evaluation of antitussive drugs in animals and man. Many species of animal have been used for antitussive testing, either conscious or unconscious, the most common being guinea pig, cat, and dog. The process of evaluation can be considered to be in three parts: (1) stimulation of the cough response, (2) measurement of the response, and (3) effect of the test drug on the response.

Stimulation of cough has been achieved by mechanical irritation of the tracheal mucosa (10, 11); chemical irritation by means

of, for example, ammonia vapor (12) or sulfur dioxide vapor (13) among many others; and electrical stimulation of either the trachea (14) or, much more commonly, the isolated superior laryngeal nerve of the anesthetized cat (15).

Of the various methods of stimulation used, electrical stimulation has no physiological equivalent, but it has the important advantage that an exact measurement of stimulus strength and quality can be achieved. Of great importance for site of action studies is the fact that compounds active against isolated nerve stimulated cough must be working, at least in part, via a *central* mechanism of action. Compounds acting solely by a *peripheral* mechanism at respiratory receptors would be inactive in this test. Chemical or mechanical stimulation of course have physiological counterparts; the former in particular is simple and accurately controlled and permits the use of large numbers of animals for statistical evaluation of results. It is also the method of stimulation generally used in man. Mechanical stimulation is not as reproducible.

Measurement of the cough response as described in most published work can be encompassed within three general procedures: (1) counting the number of coughs produced over a given period of time (generally recorded electronically); (2) recording of respiratory events; and (3) measurement of internal tracheal pressure. The last two procedures are particularly important in that they permit a measure of the intensity as well as the number of coughs.

Similarly, the measurement of a compound's antitussive action can be made in several ways: (1) keeping the minimal stimulus constant, the presence or absence of a response following drug dosing is noted; (2) again keeping the minimal stimulus constant, the time taken to return to the original response following dosing is measured; (3) before and after drug administration, the stimulus required to produce a given response is measured; and (4) the number of coughs on exposure to an irritant gas over a given period of time is measured before and after drug treatment.

It is apparent from the multiplicity of experimental procedures that no simple universal test for antitussive activity exists. The activity of a commonly used drug such as codeine phosphate varies widely in different animal tests, which is not really surprising when one considers the variation in parameters such as species, and route of drug administration, with all the differences in drug distribution and metabolism that this implies. A range of effective doses for codeine obtained by different investigators is shown in Table 53.1 (16), although it should be pointed out that in structure–activity studies with new series of compounds in comparison with codeine, the procedures used and the analysis of results are generally consistent and therefore the results are meaningful.

A further complication in making predictions of antitussive activity in man from

Table 53.1   Antitussive Action of Codeine in Man and Conscious Animals[a]

Cough Stimulant	Route of Administration	Effective Dose, ED_{50}, mg/kg	Species
Sulfur dioxide	s.c.	10.0	Rat
Sulfur dioxide	s.c.	19.0	Guinea pig
Ammonia	s.c.	0.3	Guinea pig
Ammonia	s.c.	2.0	Dog
Mechanical stimulation of trachea	s.c.	3.3	Dog
Mechanical stimulation of trachea	p.o.	100.0	Rabbit
Mechanical stimulation of trachea	i.v.	13.5	Rabbit
Ammonia	p.o.	10–40[b]	Man
10% Citric acid aerosol	p.o.	30[b]	Man

[a] Compiled from data in Eddy et al., Ref. 16, Table 27.
[b] Total dose. Also effective at these doses clinically.

animal data is that drugs have normally been given to animals by the intravenous or subcutaneous routes, whereas to man they are given orally almost exclusively. For the evaluation of antitussives in man, chemical stimulation of cough is the most widely used method, e.g., using ammonia diluted with air (17) or 5–10% aqueous citric acid aerosol (18). However, trials in patients are the only real test of a drug's effectiveness, and the need for carefully controlled clinical trials has been stressed (19).

2 ANTITUSSIVE DRUGS

The discussion of drugs used in the treatment of cough falls naturally into three distinct areas:

1. Centrally acting antitussives that affect the cough center in the medulla.
2. Peripherally acting antitussives that work at the receptor level in the respiratory tract.
3. Agents achieving an effect by actions other than on the cough reflex arc.

The compounds of class 3 include such types as expectorants and mucolytics, which are not antitussives within the definition of Gold (2), although they have a beneficial effect on cough. It should be pointed out that classes 1, 2, and indeed, 3 are not mutually exclusive and a compound that is mainly central in action may also have peripheral antitussive effects and vice versa. Other pharmacological actions which may contribute to an overall antitussive effect may also be present, for example, the analgetic action of codeine. In many cases, the mode of action of a compound appears to have been inferred from that of related compounds rather than established experimentally, and it is doubtful if the mode of action of very many antitussives has been worked out completely.

2.1 Antitussives Acting Mainly Centrally

This is by far the largest category of antitussive drugs. It ranges from the opium alkaloids, used for centuries in the treatment of cough, through the purified opium alkaloids, particularly codeine (53.**1b**) and noscapine (53.**8**), to the modified natural alkaloids and synthetic morphine analogs. Finally it embraces compounds totally unrelated chemically to the above categories. All this work has been carried out in the search for selective antitussive agents free from the side effects of addiction potential, respiratory depression, and constipation associated with the use of opium alkaloids.

Although morphine (53.**1a**) and codeine have been used as antitussives in man for a long time, Ernst (20, 21) was one of the first workers to show that they possessed antitussive activity in animals when they inhibited the cough reflex in cats at 0.5 and 3.0 mg/kg subcutaneously, respectively. Numerous workers, including Silvestrini and Maffii (22), have since found morphine to be a potent antitussive agent in a number of animal tests. However, because of its serious side effects in man, it is now little used in the control of cough.

(−)-Morphine occurs naturally in opium (from *Papaver somniferum*) to the extent of about 9% by weight of dried material. It is a pentacyclic tertiary base whose skeleton can be considered as being derived by internal cyclization of a benzyl isoquinoline (53.**2**). Its absolute configuration (23), and conformation are as shown in 53.**1a**. It is interesting that (+)-morphine, although devoid of analgetic activity, is also active as an antitussive (24), although less active than the (−) isomer. This would appear to indicate that the steric requirements for antitussive activity are not as rigid as those for analgetic activity, a fact that is borne out later.

All useful antitussives containing the morphine skeleton have been derived by chemical modification of (−)-morphine.

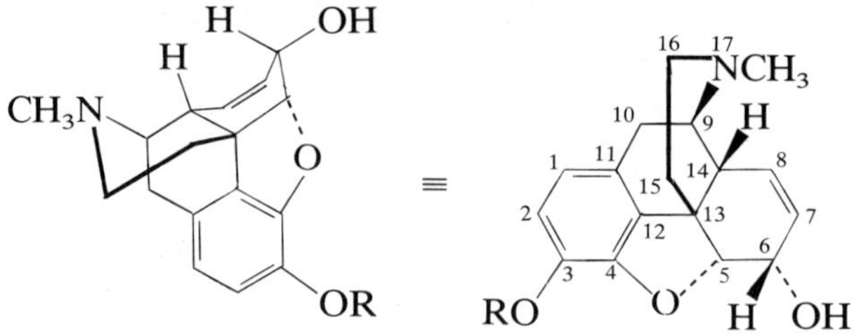

Configuration of (−) series (5*R*,6*S*,9*R*,13*S*,14*R*)

53.**1a**   R = H
53.**1b**   R = CH$_3$
53.**1c**   R = C$_2$H$_5$

53.**1d**   R = CH$_2$CH$_2$N(morpholine)

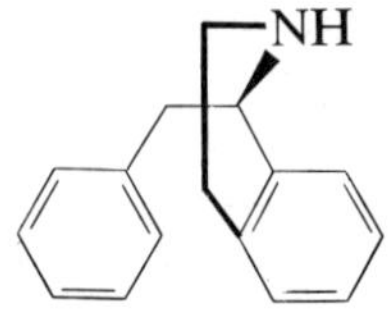

53.**2**

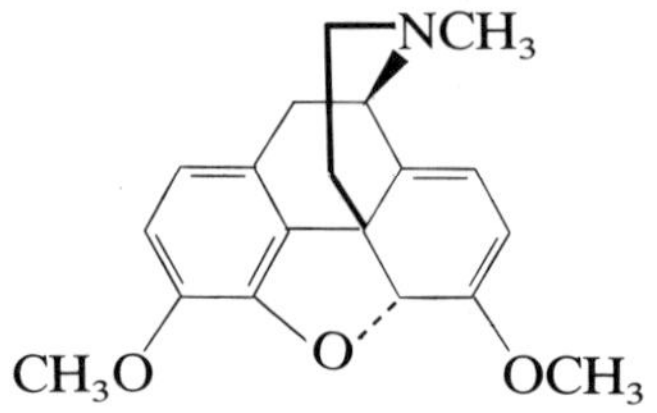

53.**3**

Chief among these is codeine (53.**1b**), the 3-methyl ether of morphine, which was first isolated in 1832 and used as early as 1838. It has a much lower addiction potential and respiratory depressant effect than morphine and is very widely used today in many cough preparations, generally as the phosphate salt. Reference has already been made to its antitussive activity in animals and man (Table 53.1), and its analgetic and calming effects probably contribute to its overall efficacy. Although occurring naturally in opium to the extent of about 0.3%, codeine is prepared commercially by methylation of morphine. Recently, an efficient conversion of thebaine (53.**3**) to codeine via codeinone has been reported (25). Thebaine, although occurring only to a very small extent in opium, is the major alkaloid constituent of *Papaver bracteatum* and hence a new potential source of codeine is available. Other morphine ethers that have found use as antitussives are ethyl morphine (53.**1c**), which is slightly less active than codeine in guinea pigs (26), and

3-morpholinoethylmorphine (pholcodine, 53.**1d**). The latter was selected from a group of basic ethers prepared and evaluated by Chabrier et al. (27) and has been shown in animals (28) and man (29) to be a useful antitussive with minimal side effects and no addiction liability.

Chemical modification of the morphine nucleus itself has been carried out extensively in an effort to prepare potent analgetics free from morphinomimetic side effects (30). At the same time, this has led to the development of some useful antitussives containing a modified C ring of morphine or codeine. 7,8-Dihydrocodeine (53.**4**) prepared by reduction of codeine has been known as an effective antitussive since 1913, and laboratory and clinical studies have supported this (31). Two other drugs worth noting are 7,8-dihydromorphinone and 7,8-dihydrocodeinone (53.**5a** and 53.**5b**). Both possess greater antitussive and analgetic activity than codeine but, unfortunately, they are also potentially addictive. In spite of this, dihydrocodeinone particu-

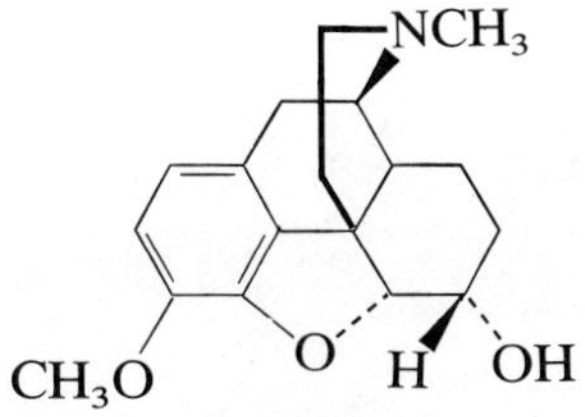

53.4

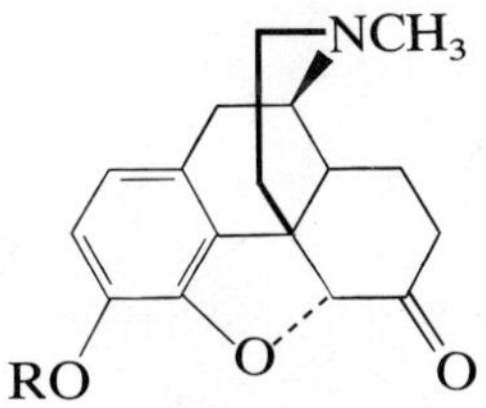

53.5a R = H
53.5b R = CH₃

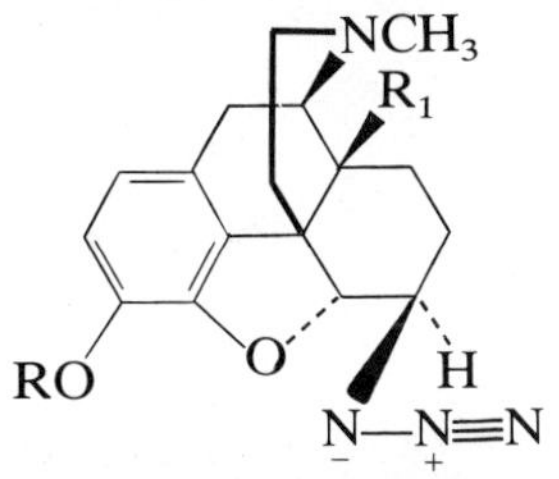

53.6a R = R₁ = H
53.6b R = H, R₁ = OH
53.6c R = C₂H₅, R₁ = H

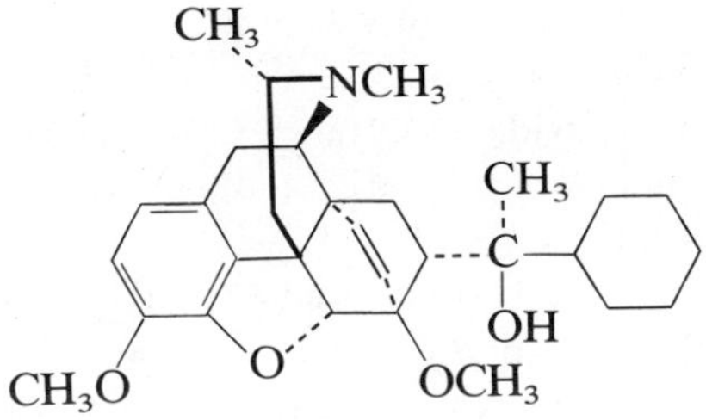

53.7

larly is quite widely used for cough suppression (32).

Recently, some interesting results on 6-azido analogs of morphine and related compounds have been reported (33, 34). When injected subcutaneously in the rat, 6-deoxy-6-azidodihydroisomorphine (azidomorphine, 53.**6a**) and its 14-hydroxy analog (53.**6b**) are, respectively, 558 and

904 times more active than codeine as antitussives. Both compounds are equipotent as analgetics but the 14-hydroxy compound is very much less toxic. Orally, azidoethylmorphine (53.**6c**) is the best compound, being 60 times more active than codeine, and its pharmacology (34a) and chemistry (34b) have been described in some detail. In contrast to morphine and codeine, the azido compounds have no effect on respiration in the cat at antitussive doses.

Commencing from thebaine (53.**3**), powerful morphine-like analgetics have been found in derivatives of 7-substituted 6, 14-*endo*-ethenotetrahydrothebaines. This work led to the finding (35) that substitution in the 16 position with an alkyl group results in the preparation of powerful antitussive agents with less prominent analgetic and morphine-like actions. The 16-methyl derivative (53.**7**) is the most active compound, being 11.6 times more active than codeine orally in the guinea pig, but some respiratory depression was noted at higher dose levels. The chemistry of the compounds has also been described (36).

It remains to be seen whether any of the new analogs described above become clinically useful.

The *N*-oxides of morphine and some of its derivatives have been reported to possess antitussive activity without analgetic activity (37, 38). Compared with the parent compounds, morphine *N*-oxide and codeine *N*-oxide are more active, whereas for dihydromorphine and dihydrocodeine *N*-oxides, the reverse is the case (38). These results are difficult to explain since in all cases, *N*-oxide formation might be expected to reduce penetration of the central nervous system and therefore reduce activity if the compounds were acting purely centrally.

Before leaving the opium alkaloids and their derivatives, mention must be made of (−)-α-narcotine (noscapine, 53.**8**) the second most common alkaloid present in opium to the extent of about 6%. First

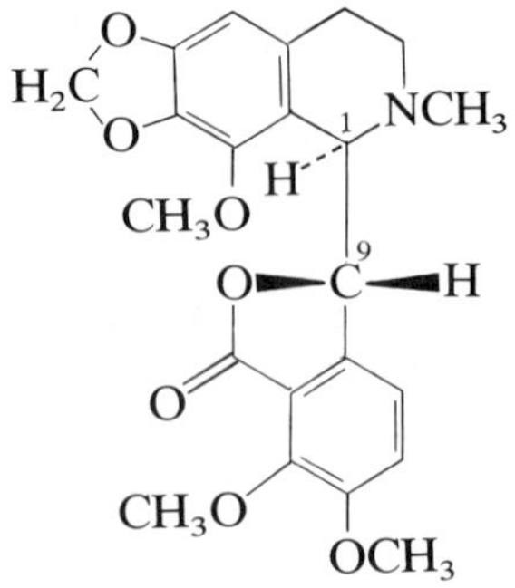

53.**8** (1R,9S)

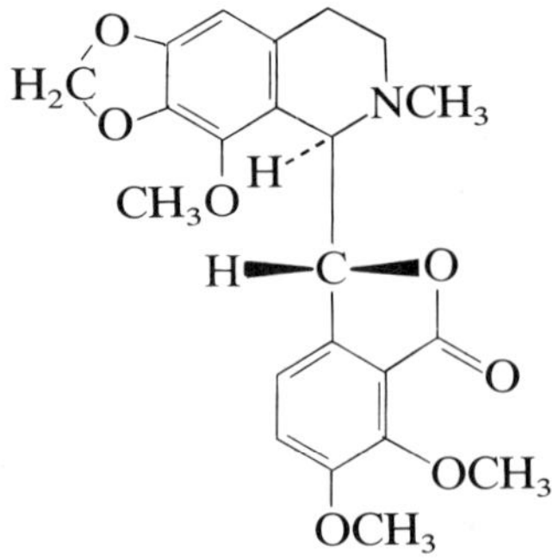

53.**9** (1R,9R)

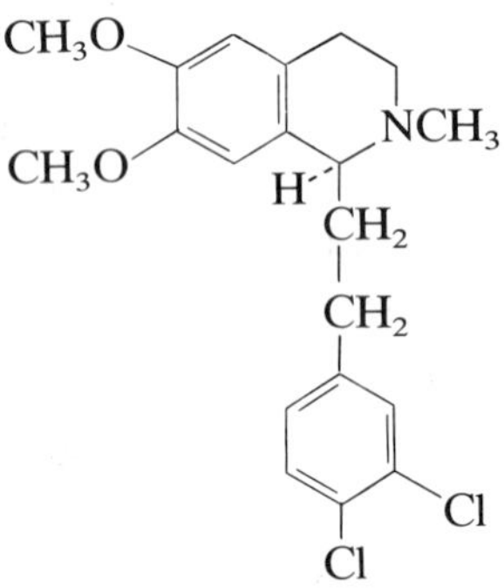

53.**10**

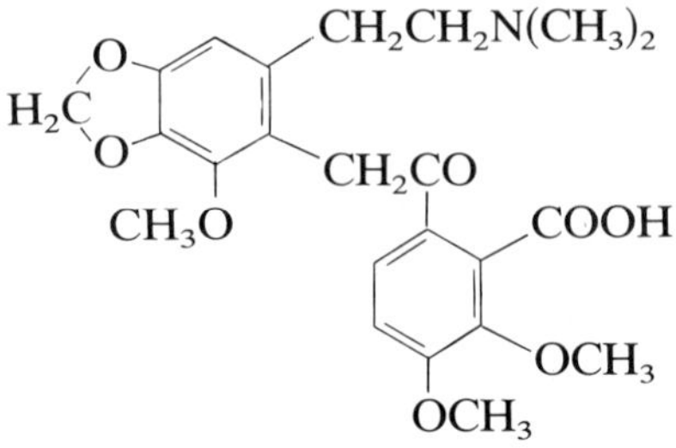

53.**11**

isolated in 1817 by Robiquet, its structure was established by Marshall et al. (39). Since the molecule contains two asymmetric centers there are two possible diastereoisomeric forms, α and β, each of which has two optically active forms. The absolute configuration of $(-)$-α-narcotine (53.**8**) along with those of its isomers has been determined by Ohta et al. (40).

Noscapine has been shown to be an effective antitussive in animals, being somewhat more active than codeine (41). It is also a bronchodilator in contrast to codeine, which causes bronchospasm, and this may contribute to its antitussive action. An important difference from the morphine congeners discussed so far is its lack of analgetic properties, addiction potential, and other morphine-like side effects, all properties that have been present to a greater or lesser extent in the morphine deriva-

tives. This demonstrates that antitussive selectivity is feasible. In man, noscapine is approximately equipotent with codeine and has found wide acceptance in the treatment of cough, particularly that of asthmatic origin (42).

It is interesting that $(-)$-β-narcotine (53.**9**) with the configuration at C-9 reversed possesses good antitussive activity (43), whereas in the synthetic analog (53.**10**) with only the C-1 asymmetric center, all the activity resides in the $(-)$ isomer (44). These results would indicate that in noscapine analogs, sterochemistry at C-1 is all important for antitussive activity. However, narceine (53.**11**), a ring-opened compound prepared by decomposition of noscapine methochloride with alkali (45), possesses antitussive activity similar to that of codeine (46). N-Methylhomopiperonylamine (53.**12**), which can be regarded as a

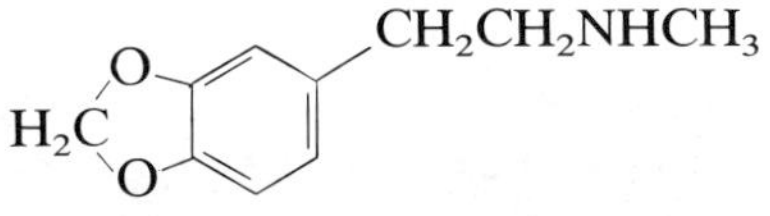

53.**12**

simplified noscapine analog related to the sympathomimetic amines, is also antitussive in humans (47).

At this point, we may turn to synthetic morphine substitutes. Early work was of course directed toward the synthesis of strong analgetics without the side effects of morphine and its congeners but from this, potent antitussive compounds were discovered of which the outstanding example is dextromethorphan, the (+) isomer of 3-methoxy-N-methylmorphinan (53.**13b**). Using the earlier Grewe synthesis of morphinans, Schnider and Grüssner (48) prepared and resolved 3-hydroxy- and 3-methoxy-N-methylmorphinans (53.**13a** and 53.**13b**). These molecules possess the basic skeleton of the morphine nucleus but lack the oxygen bridge, the 7,8 double bond, and the C-6 functionalization (morphine numbering). The absolute configuration of the (−) isomers has been shown (49, 50) to correspond with that of morphine, and not surprisingly, analgetic activity is found to reside solely in these isomers. More interestingly, antitussive activity is present in both (+) and (−) isomers, illustrating once again the lack of stereoselectivity with regard to this kind of activity.

From this work, dextromethorphan emerged as a clinically useful antitussive with much lower side effects than codeine, and no addictive properties. Pharmacological studies (51) showed it to possess a good antitussive effect similar to that of codeine in animals, and Isbell and Fraser (52) showed it to be free from addiction liability in contrast to its (−) isomer, which was very addictive. Other studies (53) showed it to be virtually free from analgetic, sedative, or other morphine-like effects. More recently, Murakami et al. (54) reported that the (+)-dimorphinan (53.**14**), the carbonate ester of (+)-3-hydroxy-N-methylmorphinan, possesses almost the same antitussive activity as dextromethorphan but is less toxic.

Since the discovery of dextromethorphan, much work has been carried out on morphinan derivatives, mainly in Japanese laboratories. Whereas for good analgetic activity a 3-oxygen function appears to be necessary, it has recently been shown (55) that compounds possessing a 3-alkyl group possess excellent antitussive activity. The preferred compound was (+)-3-methyl-N-methylmorphinan (AT 17, dimemorphan, 53.**13c**), which is 1.5 times as active as dextromethorphan with somewhat reduced toxicity. More detailed examination (56, 57) has confirmed that it is a potent centrally acting antitussive agent with minimal side effects, although, unlike dextromethorphan, it possesses some analgetic activity. An interesting chemical point to

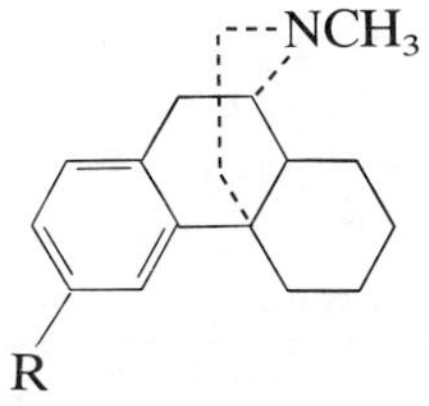

(+) Isomers
53.**13a** R = OH
53.**13b** R = OCH$_3$
53.**13c** R = CH$_3$

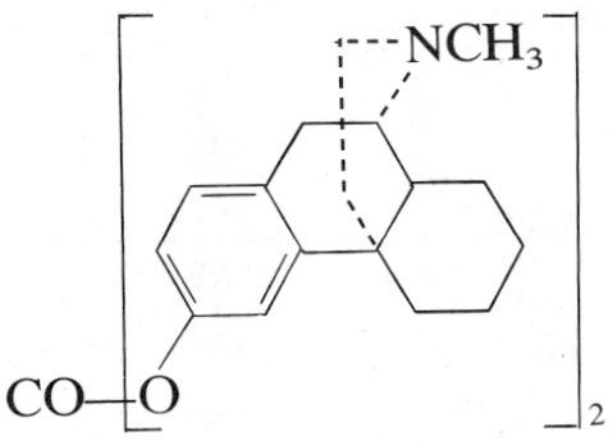

53.**14**

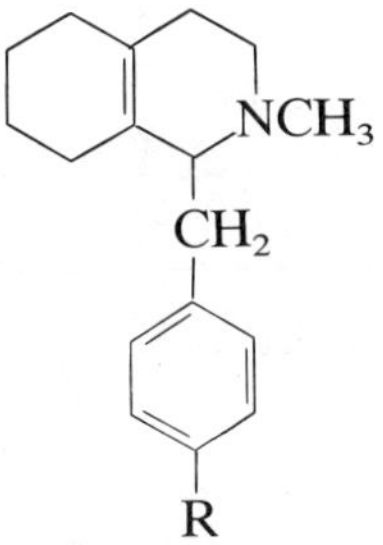

53.**15a** R = CH$_3$
53.**15b** R = OCH$_3$

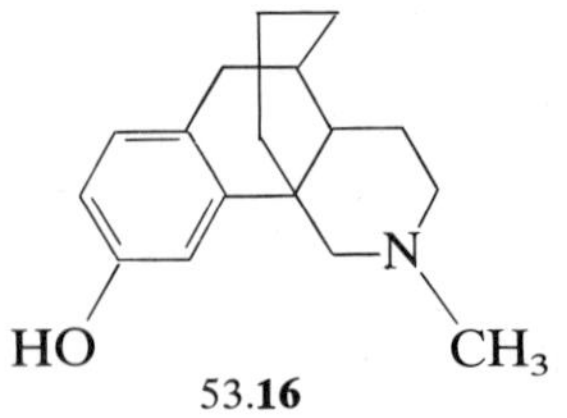

53.**16**

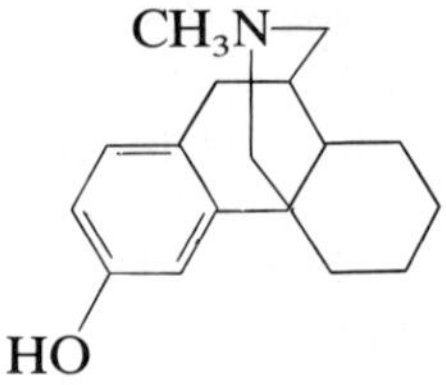

53.**17**

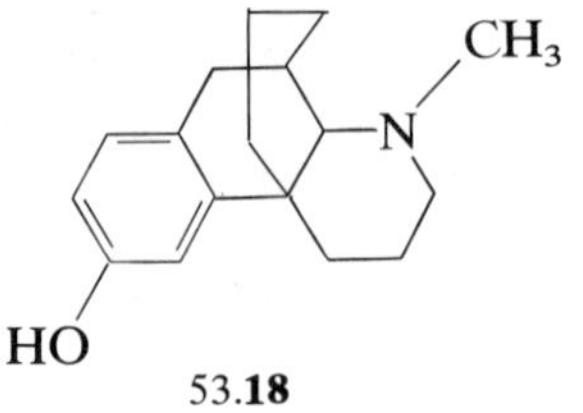

53.**18**

arise out of this work is that cyclization of the intermediate (+)-octahydroisoquinoline (53.**15a**) with hot 85% phosphoric acid solution gives the (+)-morphinan (53.**13c**), whereas the (−)-octahydroisoquinoline (53.**15b**) cyclizes to the (+)-morphinan (53.**13a**), which is remethylated to dextromethorphan (53.**13b**).

While discussing the structure–activity relationships in the morphinan series, it is worth noting that antitussive activity is not restricted to the 17-aza compounds which are the strict analogs of morphine. Thus Sugimoto and Ohshiro (58–60) claimed the 6-aza (53.**16**), 16-aza (53.**17**), and 8-aza (53.**18**) analogs to be antitussives.

It has been known for some time (e.g., 61) that introduction of a 14-hydroxyl function into the morphinan skeleton gen-

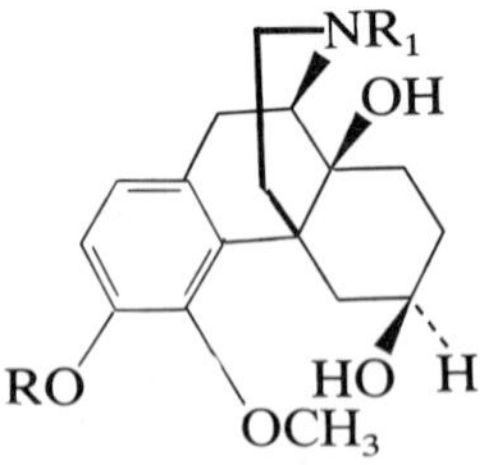

53.**19a**   R = R$_1$ = CH$_3$
53.**19b**   R = H, R$_1$ = CH$_3$
53.**19c**   R = CH$_3$, R$_1$ = H
53.**19d**   R = R$_1$ = H

erally increases antitussive activity while diminishing side effects. Two compounds of this type have been particularly commented upon in recent years. These are the 4-methyl ether of 14-hydroxydihydro-6β-thebainol (oxymethebanol, 53.**19a**) and (−)-N-cyclobutylmethyl-3,14-dihydroxy morphinan (butorphanol, 53.**20**). Oxymethebanol (62) has been shown to be an extremely potent antitussive in the guinea pig, also possessing analgetic activity and very low toxicity (63). Its metabolic fate was investigated in rodents where small amounts of the 3-O-demethylated (53.**19b**), N-demethylated (53.**19c**), and 3-O,N-demethylated (53.**19d**) compounds were detected (64). Chemical synthesis and

53.**20**

pharmacological evaluation of these metabolites (65) showed the mono-demethylated compounds to retain some antitussive activity. This study also showed that for a series of 4-ethers of 14-hydroxydihydro-6-thebainols, the 6-β epimers were consistently more active than the 6-α compounds. Butorphanol is of considerable interest in that it was synthesized as, and shown to be, a narcotic antagonist and potent analgetic (66). It also possesses powerful antitussive action and detailed pharmacological work has shown it to be much more active than codeine or dextromethorphan, both subcutaneously and orally in the guinea pig (67). It was concluded that butorphanol is a potent centrally acting antitussive with a longer duration of action than codeine, and with little abuse potential.

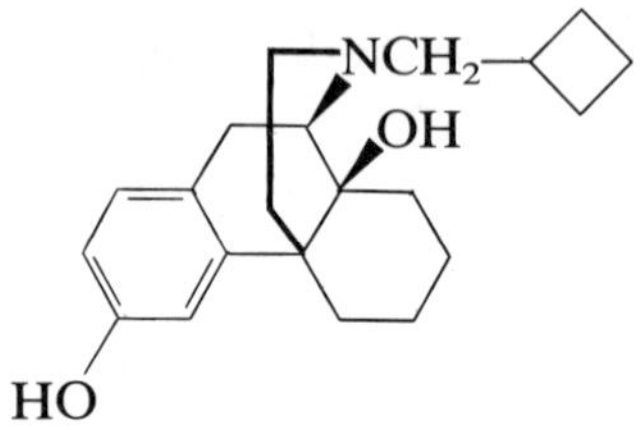

We can now examine other series of compounds derived from considerations of

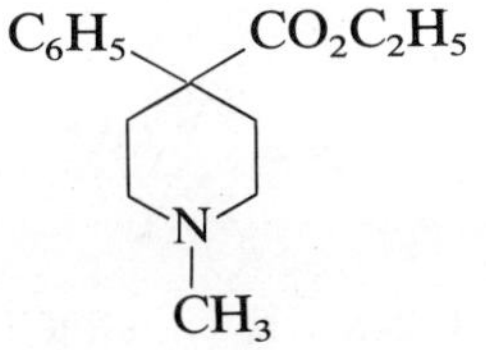

C$_6$H$_5$ CO$_2$C$_2$H$_5$

53.**21**

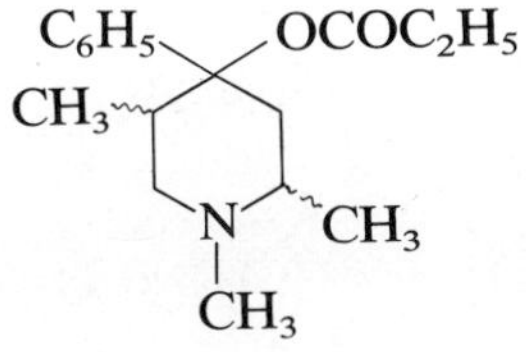

C$_6$H$_5$ OCOC$_2$H$_5$
CH$_3$ CH$_3$

53.**22**

HC≡CCH$_2$ OCOC$_2$H$_5$

CH$_2$CH$_2$C$_6$H$_5$

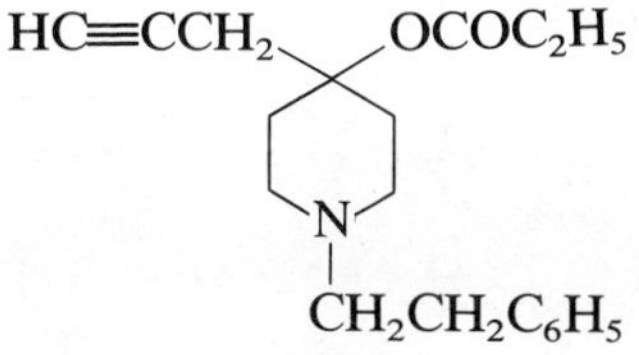

53.**23**

the morphine nucleus but which are less closely related than the morphinans. Some of these have been developed over the years to yield useful strong analgetics and it is not surprising that several have been considered as antitussives. Unfortunately, they generally possess too many morphine-like side effects for routine use in the treatment of cough.

Meperidine (53.**21**), first synthesized in 1939 (68), is both a strong analgetic and an antitussive (69) but has found little use as a cough suppressant clinically. The reversed ester trimeperidine (53.**22**) was found to be more active than codeine as a cough suppressant in the dog but, unfortunately, it also depresses respiration (70). Replacement of the 4-phenyl group by a propargyl function has been investigated and 1-phenylethyl-4-(2-propynyl)-4-propionoxy-piperidine (propinetidine, 52.**23**) was found to be much more potent than codeine as an antitussive, with little analgetic activity or narcotic side effects at effective doses (71). Recently esters of 4-propargylperhydro-azepin-4-ols (53.**24**) were also described as having antitussive activity equal to codeine, those with R = H being inactive as analgetics (72).

Methadone (53.**25a**) and isomethadone (53.**25b**) are two very important analgetics,

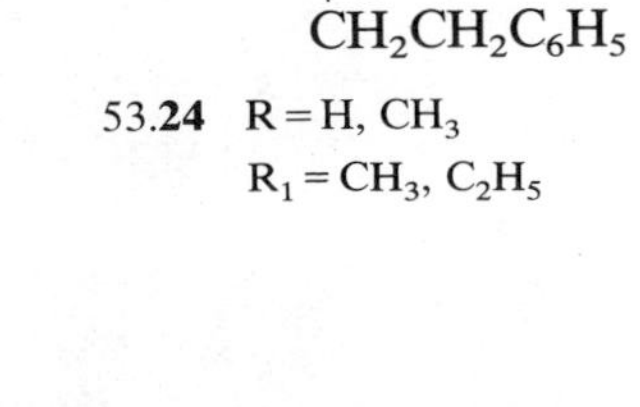

the former in its (±) form being much used clinically. Methadone has been studied extensively as an antitussive both as the racemate and in the form of its (+) and (−) optical enantiomers. Winter and Flataker (73) compared the enantiomers of methadone and isomethadone and found that the (+) isomers are extremely potent antitussives orally in the dog with very little analgetic activity, whereas the (−) isomers possess both potent antitussive and analgetic actions. Again the lack of stereospecificity for antitussive action is demonstrated. Replacement of the carbonyl function of methadone by a sulfone group (53.**26**) gives a long-lasting antitussive compound with only slight analgetic activity (74).

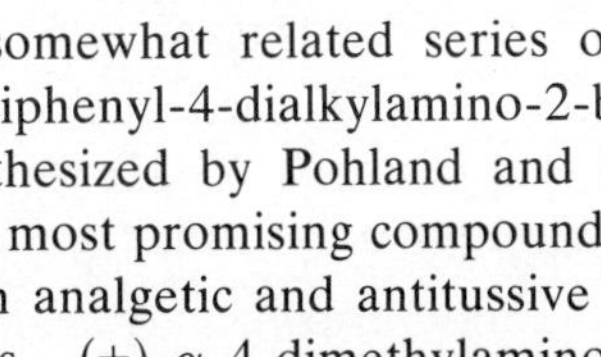

C$_6$H$_5$ COC$_2$H$_5$
C
C$_6$H$_5$ CHCHN(CH$_3$)$_2$
R R$_1$

53.**25a** R = H, R$_1$ = CH$_3$
53.**25b** R = CH$_3$, R$_1$ = H

In a somewhat related series of esters of 1,2-diphenyl-4-dialkylamino-2-butanols first synthesized by Pohland and Sullivan (75), the most promising compound possessing both analgetic and antitussive properties was (±)-α-4-dimethylamino-1,2-diphenyl-3-methyl-2-propionoxybutane (propoxyphene, 53.**27**). Pharmacological evaluation of the enantiomers of this compound (76) showed that the (−)-α isomer (levopropoxyphene) possesses useful antitussive activity, whereas analgetic activity is present mainly in the (+)-α isomer (dextropropoxyphene). It is worth noting, although

HC≡CCH$_2$ OCOR$_1$
R

CH$_2$CH$_2$C$_6$H$_5$

53.**24** R = H, CH$_3$
R$_1$ = CH$_3$, C$_2$H$_5$

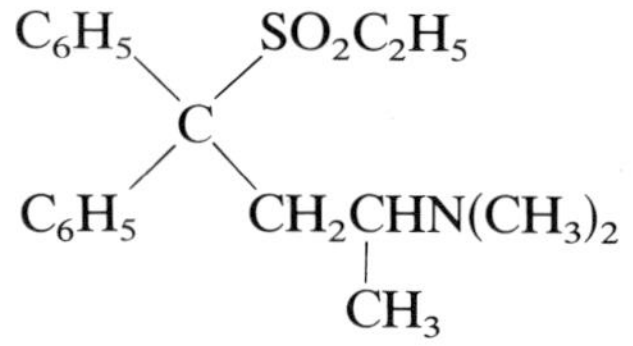

$$C_6H_5 \quad SO_2C_2H_5$$
$$\underset{|}{C}$$
$$C_6H_5 \quad CH_2CHN(CH_3)_2$$
$$CH_3$$
53.**26**

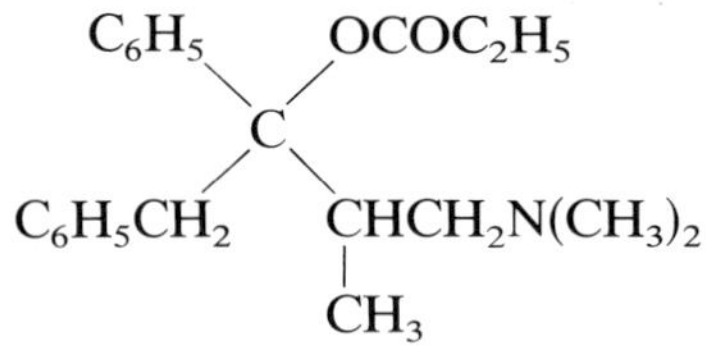

$$C_6H_5 \quad OCOC_2H_5$$
$$\underset{|}{C}$$
$$C_6H_5CH_2 \quad CHCH_2N(CH_3)_2$$
$$CH_3$$
53.**27**

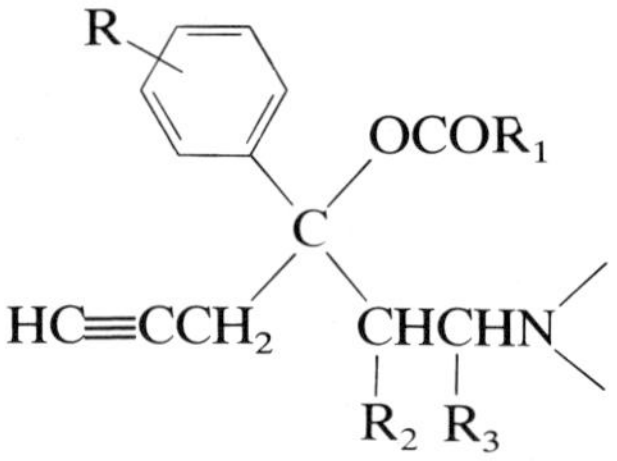

$$R$$
$$OCOR_1$$
$$\underset{|}{C}$$
$$HC{\equiv}CCH_2 \quad CHCHN$$
$$R_2 \; R_3$$
53.**28**

mainly in connection with the analgetic actions, that (+)-α-propoxyphene has the same (S) configuration at C-3 as (−)-isomethadone (77). Replacement of phenyl by ethynyl in a large series of propoxyphene analogs (53.**28**) synthesized by Prost et al. (78) gave compounds that were either inactive or only weakly active as antitussives.

Thiophene alkenylamines (53.**29**) were synthesized by Adamson (79) and many were found to be potent morphine-like analgetics (80). The most important of these, 3-diethylamino-1,1-di(2-thienyl)but-1-ene (thiambutene, 53.**29a**), was also shown to possess antitussive activity (81). Analogous compounds also possess antitussive activity and the best of these, the 3-piperidino analog (53.**29b**), particularly its (+) isomer, was stated to be a potent antitussive drug (82). Unfortunately, the compounds possess addiction liability to a varying extent.

Other related piperidino compounds claimed to have antitussive activity without analgetic effects are 53.**30**, the isomer of 53.**29b** (83), and in particular, the internally cyclized molecule 53.**31**, which is approximately equipotent with codeine in ani-

mal tests and less toxic (84). Kaśe and Yuizono (83) carried out an extensive structure–activity study with various classes of compounds possessing analgetic/antitussive activity. Almost without exception, they found that compounds containing piperidine groups possess antitussive activity associated with little or no analgetic activity.

With the discovery that antitussive activity can be separated from the analgetic and also the undesirable side effects of morphine, it is not surprising that the search for useful compounds has extended far beyond the starting point of the opium alkaloids and related molecules. Structural modification of compounds originally synthesized as, for example, antihistamines, sedatives, or parasympatholytics (anticholinergics, spasmolytics, etc.) has led to useful antitussive agents, many of them with minimal side effects. Although many of the compounds to be described have been marketed, to date none of them have had sufficient virtue to supplant codeine and its related compounds in the clinical management of cough.

Structurally, the groups of compounds displaying antitussive activity are diverse,

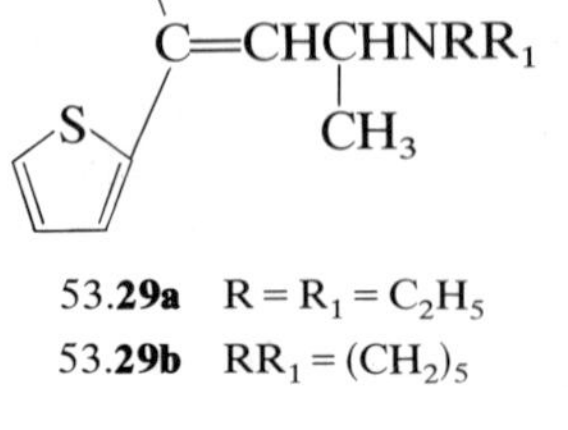

$$C{=}CHCHNRR_1$$
$$CH_3$$
53.**29a** $R = R_1 = C_2H_5$
53.**29b** $RR_1 = (CH_2)_5$

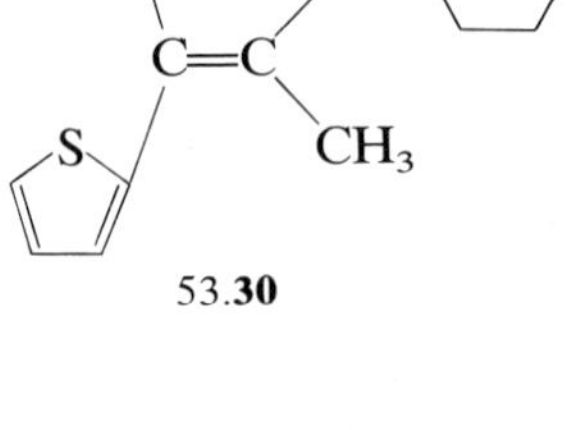

$$CH_2N$$
$$C{=}C$$
$$CH_3$$
53.**30**

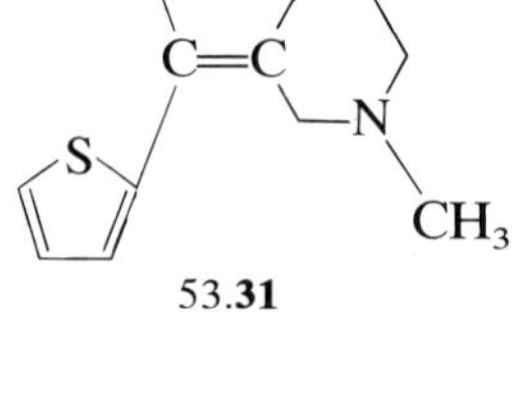

$$C{=}C$$
$$N$$
$$CH_3$$
53.**31**

but many of them, including some of the compounds already described, can be fitted into the general framework of a molecule A–B–C. In this molecule we can define the parts as follows:

1. Part A consists of a number of bulky groups such as aryl, aralkyl, cycloalkyl, or alkyl generally attached to a quaternary carbon or tertiary nitrogen atom. A quaternary carbon atom may have a polar group such as hydroxyl or nitrile as one of its substituents.
2. Part B is a chain of carbon atoms or carbon plus heteroatoms, generally two to seven units long, which may or may not be branched. Typical examples might be an alkyloxycarbonyl chain, $COOCH_2CH_2$, or simply an alkyl or alkyloxyalkyl chain.
3. Part C is a basic group which is tertiary almost without exception and is generally dimethylamino, diethylamino, or piperidino.

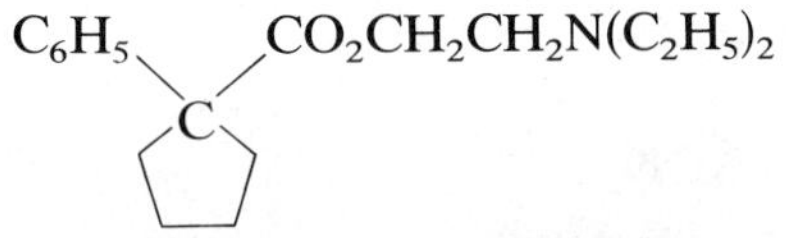

A particularly interesting group of compounds is the series of basic esters of which the prototype is 2-diethylaminoethyl 1-phenylcyclopentane-1-carboxylate (caramiphen, 53.**32**), originally developed as a spasmolytic agent. This compound as the ethanedisulfonic acid salt (85) was found to be antitussive, being somewhat less active than codeine but with a longer duration of action (86). It had little effect on respiration. Clinically, caramiphen appears to be effective in reducing cough, and there have been no reports of tolerance of dependence.

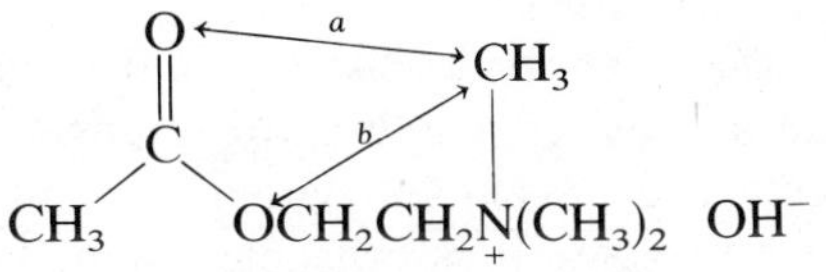

It is known (87) that for maximum parasympatholytic activity in basic esters, the distances between the carbonyl and ether oxygens of the ester function and a methyl group attached to nitrogen should be the same as those in acetylcholine (53.**33**, distances a and b), the natural transmitter in the parasympathetic nervous system. Any increase in this distance gener-

$$C_6H_5 \quad CO_2CH_2CH_2N(C_2H_5)_2$$

53.**32**

53.**33**

$$C_6H_5 \quad CO_2CH_2CH_2OCH_2CH_2N(C_2H_5)_2$$

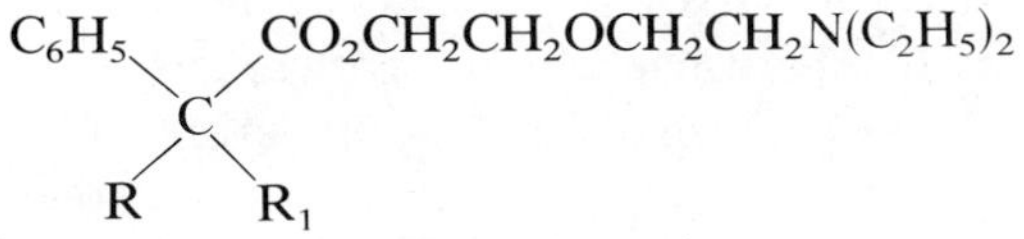

53.**34a** $RR_1 = (CH_2)_4$
53.**34b** $R = R_1 = C_2H_5$

ally leads to less active parasympatholytics. Of course other types of activity need not be affected and may in fact increase. Lengthening of the caramiphen side chain by one or two ethoxy groups (88) led to a series of compounds with antitussive activity (89) from which 2-(2-diethylaminoethyloxy)ethyl 1-phenylcyclopentane-1-carboxylate (carbetapentane, 53.**34a**) was the compound of choice, being rather more active than codeine and of low toxicity. In relation to caramiphen, it is a more active antitussive and, as expected, a less active anticholinergic. In this type of compound, maintenance of the cyclopentane ring is not necessary for good activity. The ring-opened compound oxeladin (53.**34b**) was synthesized by Petrow et al. (90) and tested by David et al. (91), who reported its activity to be similar to that of carbetapentane. As with caramiphen, this compound has found clinical application in controlling cough.

Antitussive activity has been found in basic esters of phenothiazine-10-carboxylic acid and related compounds where the phenothiazine nucleus functions as the bulky group A. Here again, use of the longer substituted aminoethyloxyethyl ester

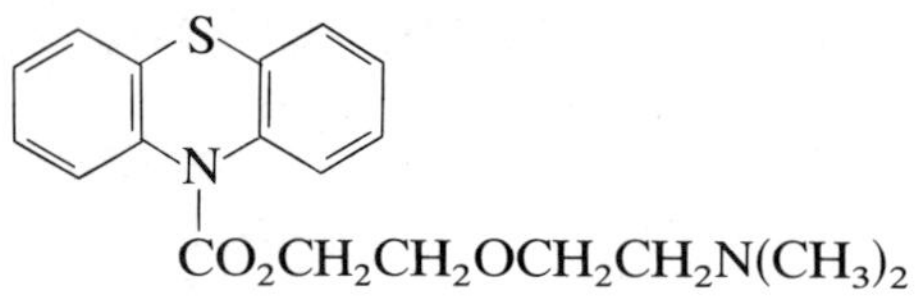

$CO_2CH_2CH_2OCH_2CH_2N(CH_3)_2$

53.**35**

side chain has been instrumental in giving good antitussive activity with reduced side effects. 2-(2-Dimethylaminoethoxy)ethyl phenothiazine-10-carboxylate (dimethoxanate, 53.**35**) was the best compound from a series synthesized by von Seemann (92) and tested by Chappel and co-workers (93). Although compounds with larger alkyl groups on nitrogen were more active, they were also more toxic. Dimethoxanate itself is slightly less active than codeine and possesses no parasympatholytic or antihistaminic activity at antitussive doses.

In a related series of compounds derived from 1-azaphenothiazine-10-carboxylic acid, the preferred compound was the 2-(2-piperidinoethyloxy)ethyl ester (pipazethate, 53.**36**). It has proved to be a clinically useful drug and has been shown to act predominantly by a central mechanism of action (94). As with dimethoxanate, pipazethate possesses no antihistaminic activity, indicating clearly that this activity is unrelated to the antitussive activity of phenothiazines in those cases where both activities are present in the same molecule.

Following a claim by Klosa (95) that basic esters of α-alkoxydiphenylacetic acids are strongly analgetic, Doyle et al. (96) prepared a series of esters of alkoxydiphenylacetic acids with 1-alkylpyrrolidyl and piperidyl alcohols. Many of these, together with some dialkylaminoalkyl esters, possess antitussive activity of the same order as codeine (97), but unfortunately, intense

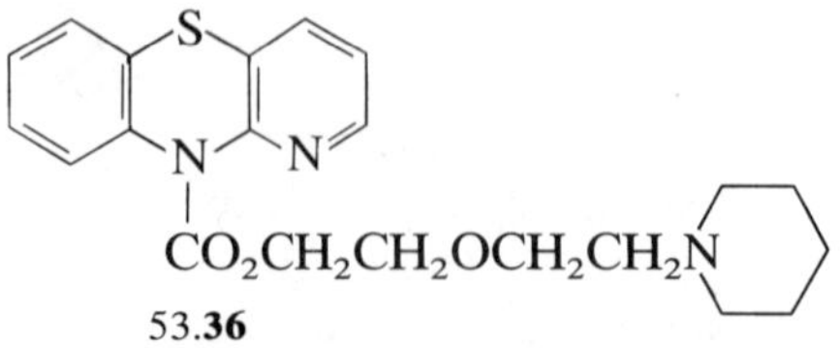

$CO_2CH_2CH_2OCH_2CH_2N$

53.**36**

salivation in cats and dogs is a limiting side effect in many cases. The best compounds exhibiting relative freedom from side effects were 3-(α-methoxy-α,α-diphenylacetoxymethyl)-1-methylpyrrolidine (53.**37a**) and its 1-ethyl homolog (53.**37b**), and 3-(α-ethoxy-α,α-diphenylacetoxy)-1-ethylpiperidine (53.**38**). In those cases where optical resolution was carried out, the optical isomers showed no improvement in activity over the racemic compounds. One further ester of note is the 2-morpholinoethyl ester of phenoxyisobutyric acid (morphethylbutyne, 53.**39**).

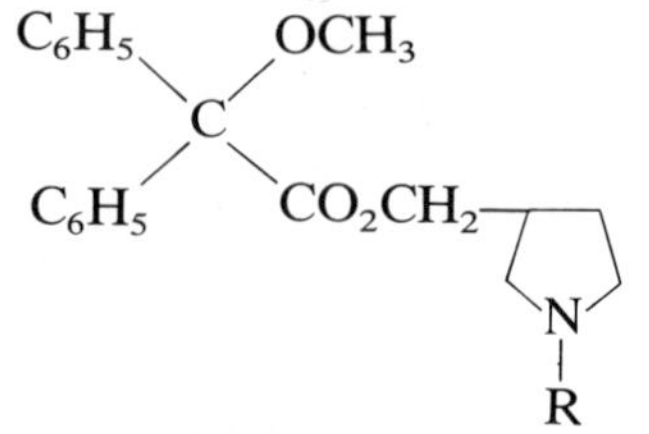

53.**37a** R = CH_3
53.**37b** R = C_2H_5

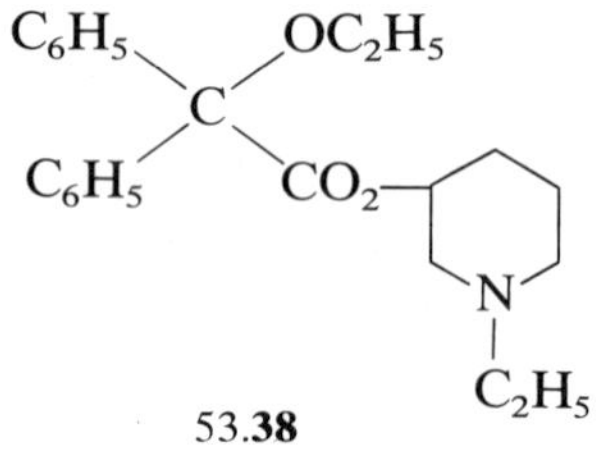

53.**38**

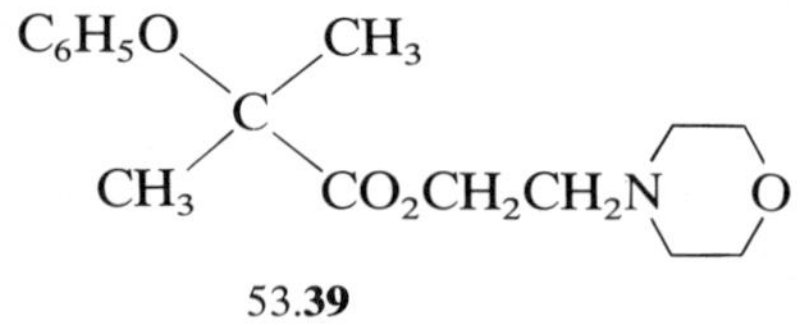

53.**39**

Pharmacologically it has been shown to have good antitussive activity in animals without serious side effects (98), and has also been claimed to have good effects in the clinic (99).

Several compounds with a simple alkyl chain between the two ends of the molecule possess important antitussive activity. The first of these is the clinically useful 4-di-

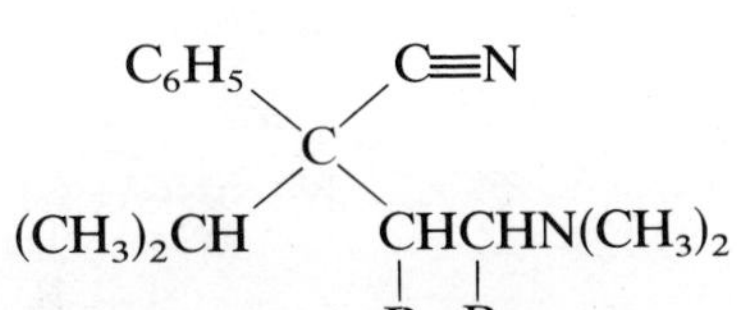

$$C_6H_5 \quad C{\equiv}N$$
$$(CH_3)_2CH \quad CHCHN(CH_3)_2$$
$$R \quad R_1$$

53.**40a**   R = H, R$_1$ = CH$_3$
53.**40b**   R = CH$_3$, R$_1$ = H

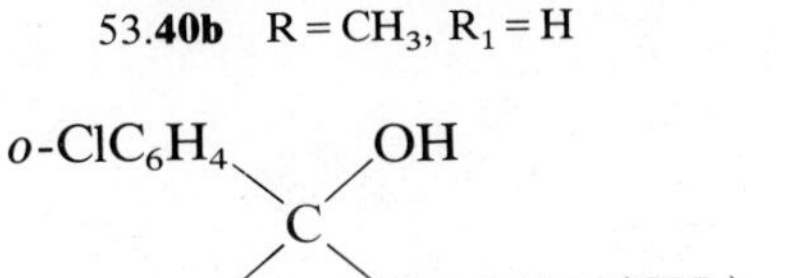

o-ClC$_6$H$_4$ \quad OH
C
C$_6$H$_5$ \quad CH$_2$CH$_2$N(CH$_3$)$_2$

53.**41**

methylamino-2-isopropyl-2-phenylvalero-nitrile (isoaminile, 53.**40a**), containing two separated centers of asymmetry, which was first described in 1957 (100). Pharmacologically, it is as active as codeine in the guinea pig and appears to possess little analgetic action (101), in contrast to its isomer with adjacent asymmetric centers (53.**40b**), which is a potent analgetic. Another compound of importance is 1-o-chlorophenyl-3-dimethylamino-1-phenyl-1-propanol (clophedianol, 53.**41**) which was the best antitussive from a series investigated by Gösswald (102). In structure–activity relationships, the position of halogenation was found to be important, the p-chloro analog having 20% of the activity of clophedianol, whereas the meta analog was inactive. Clinically, clophedianol has proved to be a useful antitussive. Another halogenated antitussive is 1-p-chlorophenyl-2,3-dimethyl-4-dimethylamino-2-butanol (53.**42**) (103) which was selected from some 300 substituted aryl butanols and pentanols. Engelhorn (104) showed it to be a centrally acting antitussive of similar potency to codeine. Recent work on the metabolism of the compound in several species including man has shown that the major metabolic pathway proceeds via successive N-demethylation to the corresponding secondary and primary amines, followed by further degradation (105).

Several recent compounds have been described with good antitussive activity containing two carbon atoms between a bulky group and basic nitrogen. Two of these are 2-(2-diethylaminoethyl)-3-phenylphthalamidine (53.**43**), with activity equal to codeine and no analgetic activity (106), and 5,7,12,13-tetrahydro-6-(2-pyrrolidinoethyl)dibenz[cg]azonine (53.**44**). The latter was the best of a series of 20 compounds synthesized by Casadio et al. (107) in terms of its therapeutic ratio. It is substantially more active in the guinea pig than isoaminile which was used as a standard. A third compound is N-(2-picolyl)-N-phenyl-N-(2-piperidinoethyl)amine (TAT-3, 53.**45**), selected from a group of 10 compounds for its antitussive activity in the dog (108). Further pharmacological

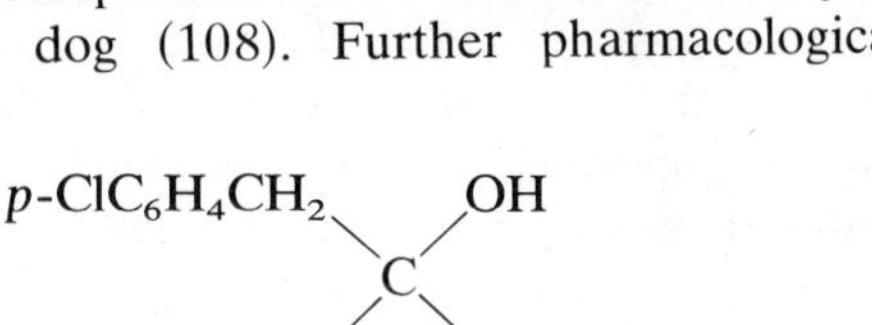

p-ClC$_6$H$_4$CH$_2$ \quad OH
C
CH$_3$ \quad CHCH$_2$N(CH$_3$)$_2$
CH$_3$

53.**42**

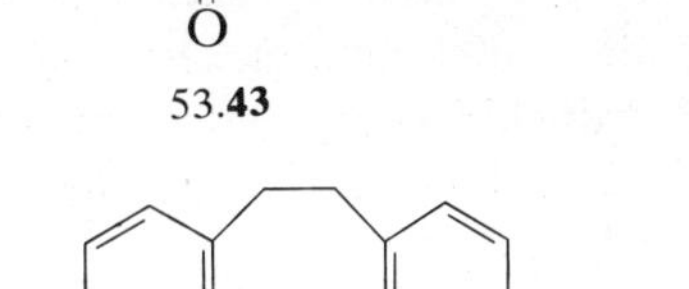

C$_6$H$_5$
NCH$_2$CH$_2$N(C$_2$H$_5$)$_2$
O

53.**43**

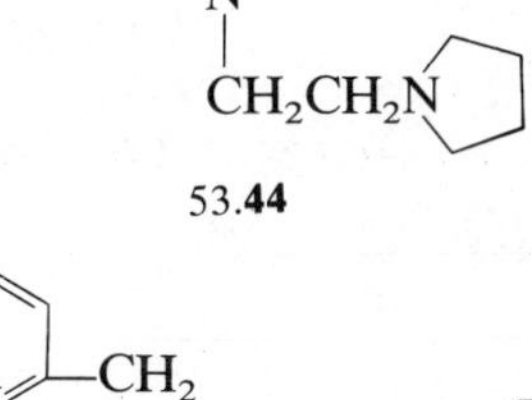

N
CH$_2$CH$_2$N

53.**44**

N \quad CH$_2$
NCH$_2$CH$_2$N
C$_6$H$_5$

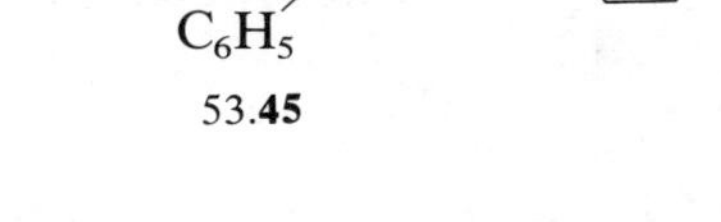

53.**45**

work (109, 110) has shown it to be slightly less active than codeine, working via a predominantly central mode of action, although a spasmolytic action on the bronchial musculature could contribute to the overall effect.

A slightly different type of compound, diphenhydramine (53.**46**), a potent antihistaminic agent, has also been shown to possess substantial antitussive action (111) and attempts have been made to increase the antitussive selectivity. Extending the side chain by one ethoxy group, as in the previously described basic ester series, achieved this aim, giving a series of antitussive compounds (112) of which *N,N*-dimethyl-2-[2-(di-2,6-xylylmethoxy)ethoxy]ethylamine (xyloxemine, 53.**47**) was selected for further evaluation (113). It proved to be a good cough suppressant free from antihistaminic properties. It is of interest that the methyl quaternary derivative of diphenhydramine, which would not be expected to pass very easily into the central nervous system, nevertheless possesses useful antitussive properties, claimed to be due to a central action at the cough center (114).

A number of piperazine derivatives have proved to be of some interest in recent years as cough suppressants. As well as central antitussive activity, these generally possess, to a greater or lesser extent, antihistaminic, anticholinergic, local anesthetic, and bronchospasmolytic actions which no doubt contribute to the overall activity observed. Some of the earliest derivatives were synthesized by Morren (115), and of

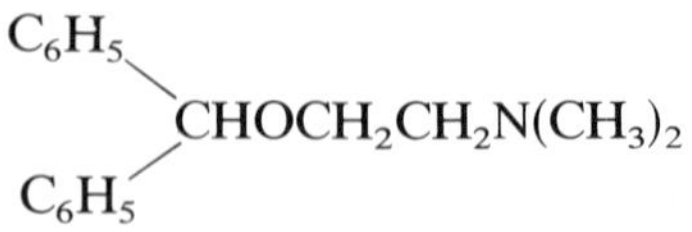

$$C_6H_5-\!\!\!\begin{array}{c} \\ \diagdown \end{array}\!\!\!CHOCH_2CH_2N(CH_3)_2$$
$$C_6H_5-\!\!\!\begin{array}{c} \diagup \\ \end{array}$$

53.**46**

$$2,6(CH_3)_2C_6H_3-\!\!\!\begin{array}{c} \\ \diagdown \end{array}$$
$$\qquad\qquad CHOCH_2CH_2OCH_2CH_2N(CH_3)_2$$
$$2,6(CH_3)_2C_6H_3-\!\!\!\begin{array}{c} \diagup \\ \end{array}$$

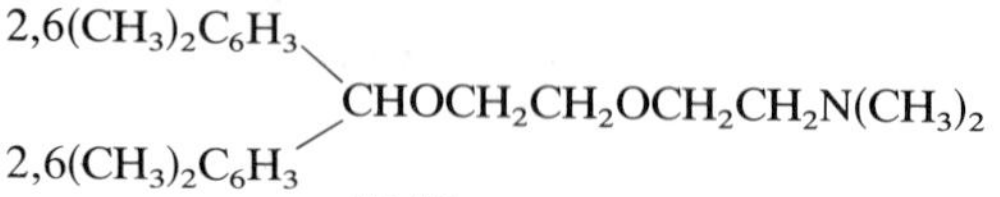

53.**47**

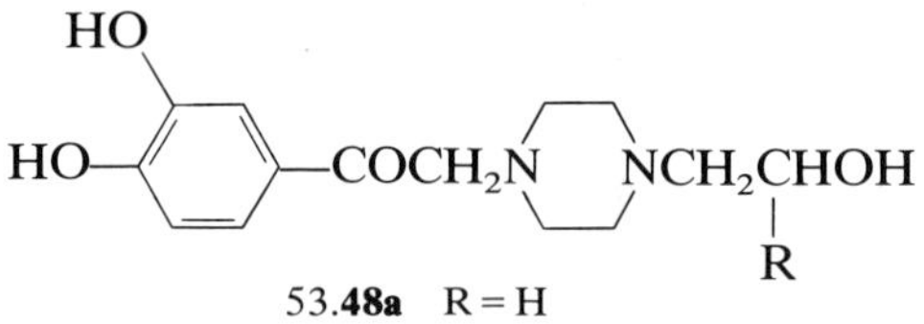

53.**48a** R = H
53.**48b** R = CH$_3$

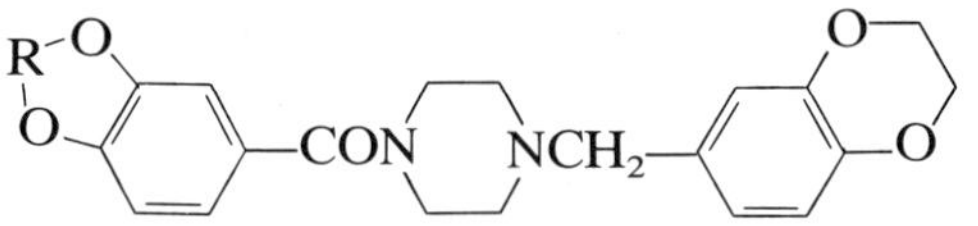

53.**49a** R = CH$_2$
53.**49b** R = (CH$_2$)$_2$

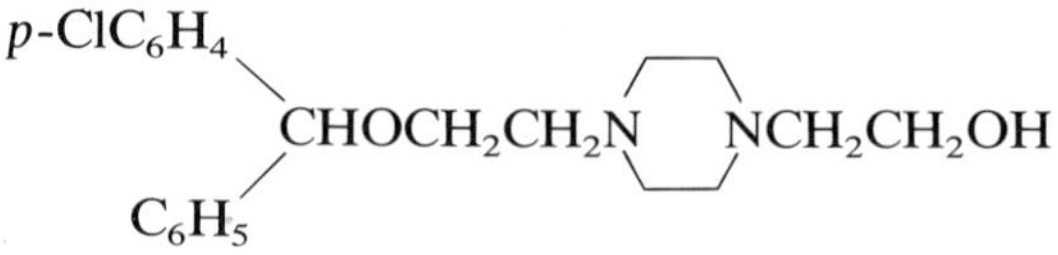

53.**50**

these 1-(3,4-dihydroxyphenacyl)-4-(2-hydroxyethyl)piperazine (53.**48a**) was one of the best compounds, being one and a half times as effective as codeine. The corresponding 2-hydroxypropyl analog (53.**48b**), however, was very much less active (116). Le Douarec et al. (117) from a series of compounds selected the two closely related piperazines 53.**49a** and 53.**49b** as being equiactive with codeine. Similarly Takagi et al. (118) claimed the halogenated benzhydryl ether of 1,4-hydroxyethylpiperazine (53.**50**), a relative of diphenhydramine, to be a good cough supressant.

Even more recently, the piperazine derivatives eprazinone [1-(2-ethoxy-2-phenylethyl)-4-(2-benzoylpropyl)piperazine, 53.**51**] (119) and zipeprol [1-(2-methoxy-2-phenylethyl)-4-(2-hydroxy-3-methoxy-3-phenylpropyl)piperazine, 53.**52**] (120) have been, mentioned as antitussives. The latter compound in particular has demonstrated a mucolytic action *in vitro* in addition to its central antitussive action *in vivo*. The metabolism of zipeprol in man, dog, and rat has been described by Constantin and Pognat (120a) and urinary metabolites from man and rat seem comparable. Although

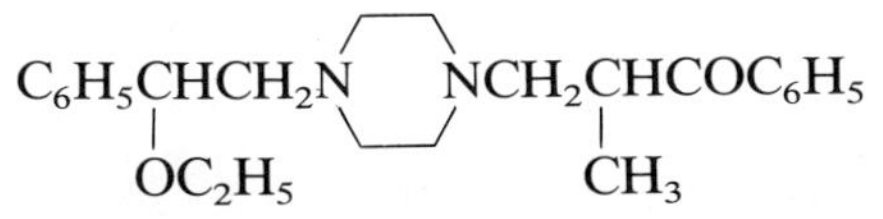

$$\underset{\underset{\text{OC}_2\text{H}_5}{|}}{\text{C}_6\text{H}_5\text{CHCH}_2\text{N}} \underset{\underset{\text{CH}_3}{|}}{\text{NCH}_2\text{CHCOC}_6\text{H}_5}$$

53.**51**

$$\underset{\underset{\text{CH}_3\text{O}}{|}\ \underset{\text{OH}}{|}}{\text{C}_6\text{H}_5\text{CH}-\text{CHCH}_2\text{N}} \underset{\underset{\text{OCH}_3}{|}}{\text{NCH}_2\text{CHC}_6\text{H}_5}$$

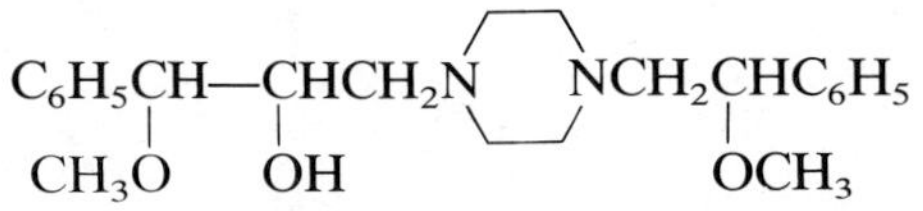

53.**52**

some material is eliminated unchanged, it is mainly metabolized by *N*-dealkylation at either piperazine nitrogen; oxidation, hydroxylation, and methylation also occur. The metabolic fate of eprazinone has been described by Takanashi et al. (121). In the rat, rabbit, and man, the major metabolic pathway appears to involve loss of the 4-(2-benzoylpropyl) group, a reaction corresponding to the *N*-dealkylation mentioned for other antitussives. This is followed by loss of the ethyl group from the ether function.

We must now look at some nonbasic naphthalene sulfonic acid derivatives, unrelated to any compounds described so far, for which important claims have been made. The first of these is sodium dibunate, a mixture of the sodium salts of 2,6 and 2,7-di-*tert*-butylnaphthalene-4-sulfonic acids (53.**53a**) (122, 123). The antitussive activity was first demonstrated by De Vleeschouwer (124), who claimed it to be peripherally acting. However, it was later demonstrated conclusively to have a predominantly central mode of action (125).

The related ethyl ester of 2,7-di-*tert*-butylnaphthalene-4-sulfonic acid (ethyl dibunate, 53.**53b**) (123) has been studied by Shemano et al. (126). Although it is not as active as codeine in animal tests, it is extremely nontoxic with a high therapeutic ratio of doses producing central nervous system side effects, including respiratory depression, to the antitussive dose. Like sodium dibunate, it appears to act mainly centrally, although lacking any of the other

pharmacological properties of the narcotic antitussives. Clinically, it has been claimed to be a very safe and effective antitussive.

A new antitussive agent of interest because of its structural relationship to the important expectorant drug bromhexine (53.**66**, Section 2.3) is 3-chloro-2-[*N*-methyl-*N*-(morpholinocarbonylmethyl)amino-methyl]benzanilide (fominoben, 53.**54**). This was selected from a large series of compounds prepared by Krüger et al. (127) as an antitussive agent equal in potency to codeine but with respiratory stimulant rather than respiratory depressant effects. The substance has no analgetic, broncholytic, or secretolytic activity (128). Clinically, fominoben appears to be a useful antitussive (128a) which recent studies have shown to be rapidly and extensively metabolized in man to a large number of metabolites (128b).

Finally in this section, mention must be made of the recently described compound 8,9b-dimethyl-4-[3-(4-methylpiper-

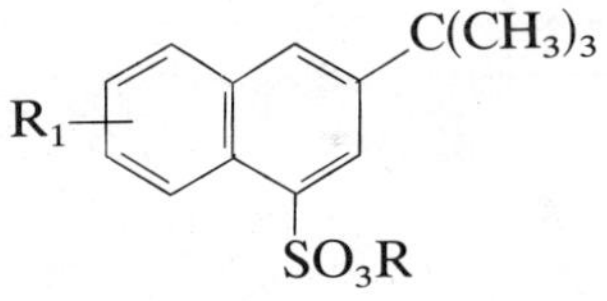

53.**53a**   R = Na, R₁ = 6-, 7-C(CH₃)₃
53.**53b**   R = C₂H₅, R₁ = 7-C(CH₃)₃

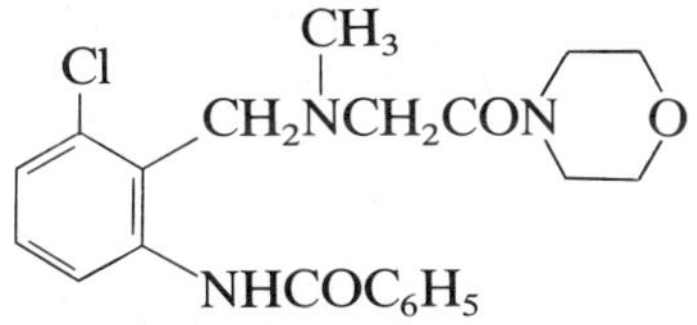

53.**54**

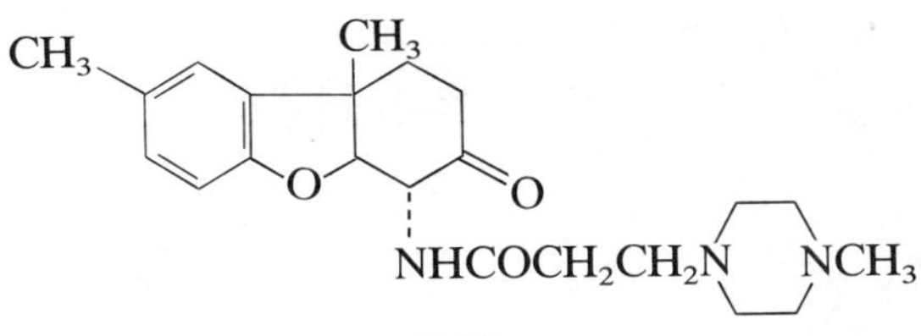

53.**54a**

azin-1-yl)propionamido]-1,2,3,4,4a,9b hexa-
hydrodibenzofuran-3-one   (azipranone,
53.**54a**), which was selected from a group
of related compounds on the basis of oral
antitussive activity in the guinea pig equal
to that of codeine, but without the side
effects of the latter (128c).

2.2   Antitussives Acting Mainly Peripherally

There are several drugs that have been
claimed to possess a predominantly
peripheral mode of action, having their
principal effects on the cough reflex arc
outside the central nervous system.
Theoretically, this could be achieved by a
selective anesthetic action on either the
cough receptors or the pulmonary stretch
receptors described earlier.

Benzonatate (nonaethylene glycol monomethyl ether *p-n*-butylaminobenzoate,
53.**55**), with a selective action on the pulmonary stretch receptors in suitable test
systems, was discovered (129) as a result of
structure–activity studies wherein a local
anesthetic molecule, *p-n*-butylamino-
benzoic acid, was combined with suitable
lipid-soluble molecules. The antitussive activity of benzonatate in animals, and its
action on stretch receptors, was confirmed
by Bucher (130). However, it is now
thought that the compound also possesses a
central component of action (131). Clinically benzonatate has been claimed to be a
nontoxic antitussive equal in effectiveness
to codeine.

Activity has also been found in 1,2,4-oxa-
diazoles. Oxolamine [5-(2-diethylaminoeth-
yl)-3-phenyl-1,2,4-oxadiazole, 53.**56**] was
the best of a series of compounds evaluated
(132) in a search for peripherally acting

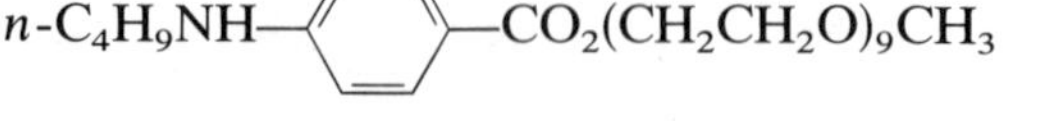

53.**56**

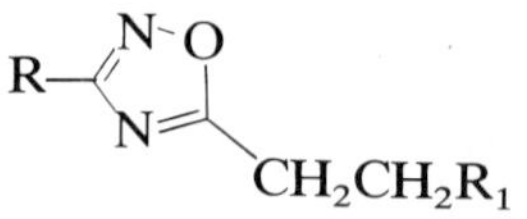

53.**57a**   R = C_6H_5CH, $R_1 = N(C_2H_5)_2$
                            |
                          C_2H_5

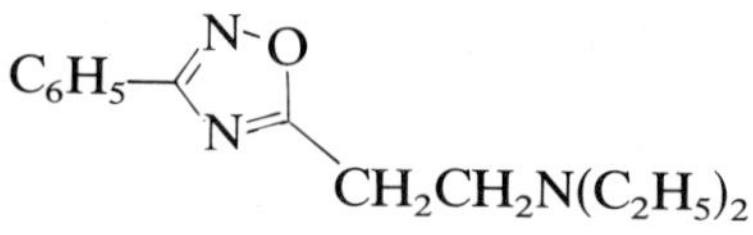

53.**57b**   R = $(C_6H_5)_2CHCH_2$, $R_1 = N$⟨ ⟩

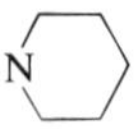

antitussives. Further pharmacological
evaluation (133) showed that the compound is more effective against acrolein-
induced cough in the guinea pig than
against cough induced by electrical stimulation of the laryngeal nerve of the cat, indicating a predominantly peripheral mechanism of action with a smaller central component. It was also suggested that the anti-
inflammatory and analgetic actions of the
compound might contribute to its overall
effect. Clinically, oxolamine has proved to
be less active than codeine but relatively
nontoxic.

It appears that in the oxadiazoles, the
group at the 3 position can be varied quite
a lot while still retaining antitussive activity.
For example, the direct analog of oxolamine with α-phenylpropyl in place of
phenyl at the 3 position (53.**57a**) is more
potent than oxolamine (134), and 3-(2,2-
diphenylethyl)-5-(2-piperidinoethyl)-1,2,4-
oxadiazole (libexin, 53.**57b**) is also a useful
cough suppressant almost equal in potency
to codeine (135).

2.3   Agents Other than Antitussives in the Control of Cough

At the beginning of this chapter, it was
stated that the treatment of cough is the
area of polypharmacy *par excellence*. The

n-C_4H_9NH—⟨ ⟩—$CO_2(CH_2CH_2O)_9CH_3$

53.**55**

majority of cough preparations on sale or prescribed today may contain a representative of several classes of drugs in addition to an antitussive. These classes of drugs include antihistamines, bronchodilators, local anesthetics, and analgetics, generally formulated in a soothing demulcent syrup. The total cough preparation is produced for the purpose of treating most of the symptoms of acute upper respiratory infection and it should be said that there is no evidence of synergism between the various ingredients in such preparations; there is of course an increased hazard of adverse interactions (1). It is clear from preceding discussions that, in any event, many antitussive compounds do in fact possess other properties that might usefully reinforce their antitussive effects, e.g., the analgetic properties of codeine or the anti-inflammatory and spasmolytic properties of oxolamine. Many antitussives also possess some bronchodilator activity and vice versa.

Antihistamines are major components of many cough preparations. As well as having a drying effect on secretions, they might be thought useful in treating cough of allergic origin. Based on experiments in animals, some antitussive activity has been attributed to many of them, e.g., diphenhydramine (111), although from studies on mepyramine (53.**58**), Boissier

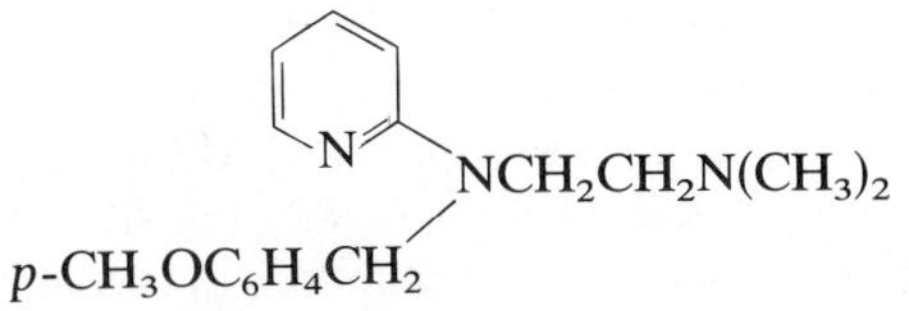

$$C_6H_5CH\!\!-\!\!CHNHR$$
$$\quad\; | \qquad\quad |$$
$$\quad\; OH \quad\; CH_3$$

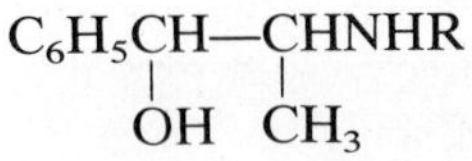

53.**60a** R = CH₃
53.**60b** R = H

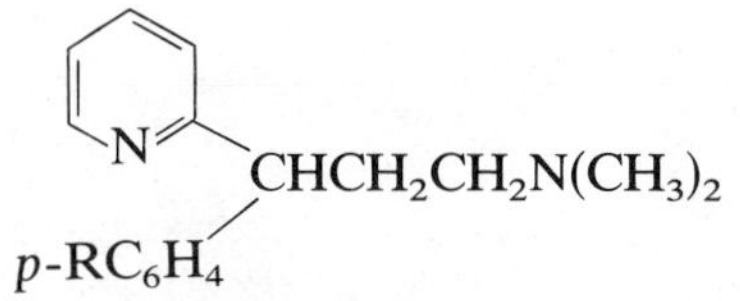

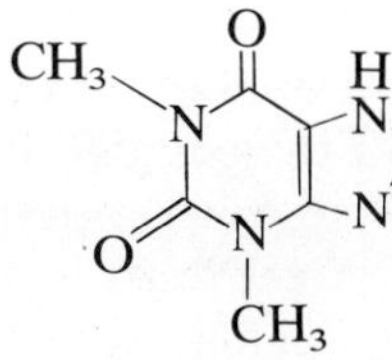

53.**61**

and Pagny (136) concluded that antihistamines are not antitussive *per se*. Two of the most commonly used antihistamines in cough preparations are brompheniramine and chlorpheniramine (53.**59a** and 53.**59b**).

Bronchodilators are also widely used in cough preparations and there is a rationale in their use as antitussives *per se* if bronchoconstriction is the initiating event in the cough reflex arc (6). Popular constituents of cough preparations are ephedrine (53.**60a**), phenylpropanolamine (53.**60b**), and theophylline (53.**61**); antitussive activity for the first two substances has been demonstrated in animals. However, as is also the case with antihistamines, clinical studies to support their widespread use are lacking.

An important way of treating cough is by converting nonproductive cough to productive cough. This can be achieved by the use of mucolytics which reduce the viscosity of bronchial mucus, or by expectorants which increase the output of respiratory tract fluid. In either case, facilitating removal of the mucus brings relief. These two classes of compounds are now examined in more detail.

Mucolytics (137) are useful mainly in dealing with the very viscous sputum characteristic of chronic bronchitics or asthmatics. Tracheobronchial secretions are formed by mucous glands and goblet cells in man and are normally composed of water (95%), mucoproteins, and mucopolysaccharides. During infection, there is a marked increase in output of mucus, and fibers of deoxyribonucleic acid (DNA) are also present owing to cellular and tissue breakdown.

$$p\text{-}CH_3OC_6H_4CH_2$$

NCH₂CH₂N(CH₃)₂

53.**58**

$$p\text{-}RC_6H_4$$

CHCH₂CH₂N(CH₃)₂

53.**59a** R = Br
53.**59b** R = Cl

The presence of DNA markedly increases the viscosity of the sputum.

Enzymes that break down protein complexes such as trypsin or chymotrypsin are very active *in vitro* in reducing the viscosity of sputum, and deoxyribonuclease (dornase) is equally effective in the case of purulent sputum containing DNA. These materials, generally administered in aerosol form, have been used clinically with some success but the incidence of side effects is high.

Derivatives of L-cysteine are currently among the most popular mucolytic agents and are thought to act by breaking disulfide bonds important in maintaining the structure of mucus. The activity apparently resides in the free sulfhydryl group since compounds with this function blocked are inactive in reducing the viscosity of mucoprotein solutions, whereas simple compounds like 2-mercaptoethanol are active. The most important derivative is *N*-acetyl-L-cysteine (53.**62**) (138), which has been found to be an effective mucolytic *in vitro*

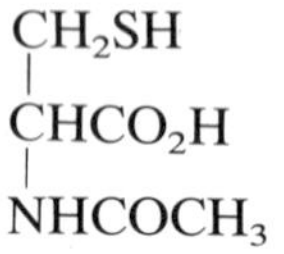

53.**62**

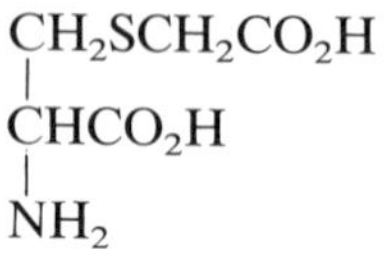

53.**63**

(139), and also in patients when administered by aerosol. *S*-Carboxymethylcysteine (53.**63**) has also been reported to be a good mucolytic in the rat (140). Recently, the clinical effects of the sodium salt of 2-mercaptoethanesulfonic acid ($HSCH_2CH_2SO_2$-Na, mistabron) have received favorable comment (141).

Expectorants are substances that increase sputum volume and promote the expulsion of secretions or exudates from the respiratory passages (142). Many of them are gastric irritants such as ammonium chloride, antimony potassium tartrate, potassium iodide, or ipecac (ipecacuanha), which at subemetic doses produce sufficient gastric or duodenal irritation to bring about a reflex increase in respiratory secretions.

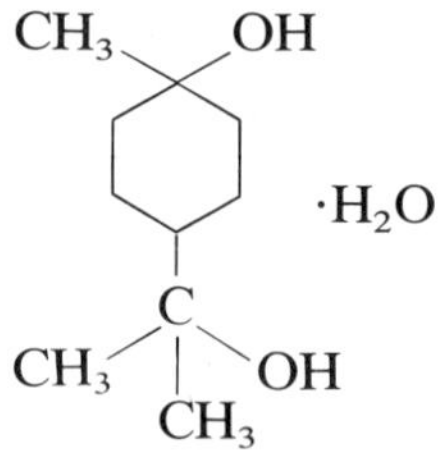

53.**64**

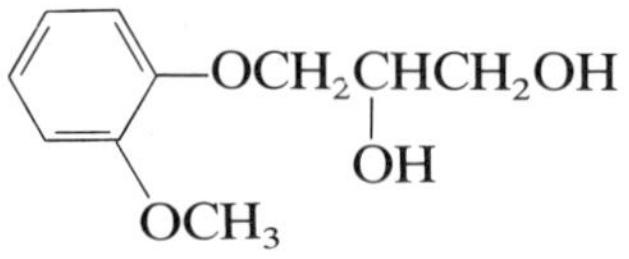

53.**65**

Other types of compounds appear to exert a direct action on the secretory cells of the respiratory tract. The essential volatile oils of eucalyptus, pine, anise, lemon, turpentine, and the drug terpin hydrate (53.**64**) all increase respiratory tract fluid in the guinea pig (143). Derivatives of phenol have been used for their expectorant properties and the glyceryl derivative of 2-methoxyphenol (glyceryl guaiacolate, 53.**65**) has attained some importance clinically. The pharmacological basis of its expectorant action was reported by Boyd et al. (144), who showed it to be active in increasing respiratory tract fluid in animals.

In recent years, the halogenated benzylamine derivative (*N*-cyclohexyl-*N*-methyl)-2-amino-3,5-dibromobenzylamine (bromhexine, 53.**66**) has been reported extensively as an expectorant drug. It was one of a group of compounds synthesized as analogs of the alkaloid vasicin (53.**67**), the active principle of the Indian indigenous

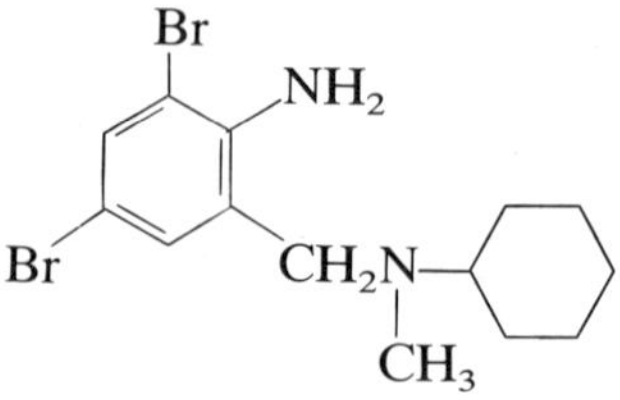

53.**66**

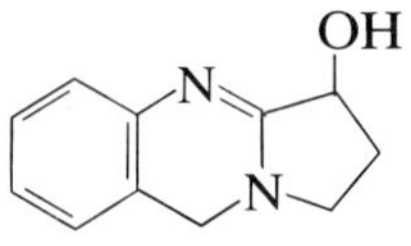

53.**67**

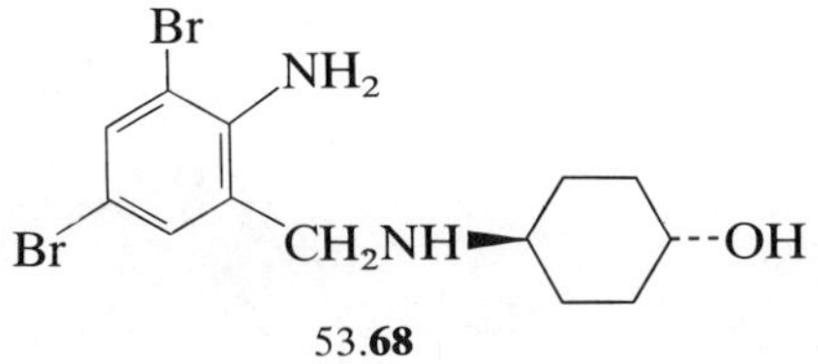

53.**68**

plant *Adhatoda vasica*, claimed to have expectorant, antitussive, and bronchodilator properties. Bromhexine was first shown to be an expectorant as well as an antitussive drug in animals by Engelhorn and Püschmann (145) and the former action has been confirmed in man in many clinical situations since. An interesting extension of this work is found in the metabolism studies. Bromhexine is extensively metabolized *in vivo* in both animals and man. In the urine of rabbits dosed with the compound, at least 10 metabolites were noted and identified (146), many of them corresponding with metabolites found in man (147). One of these metabolites, *N*-(*trans*-4-hydroxycyclohexyl)-2-amino-3,5-dibromobenzylamine (metabolite VIII, ambroxol, 53.**68**), is proving to be a potent expectorant and secretolytic agent in its own right (148, 148a).

3 CONCLUSION

The discussion of antitussive drugs and related compounds in this chapter has of course been representative rather than exhaustive. A vast number of structures have been claimed as cough suppressants, particularly in the patent literature, generally on the basis of being at least as active as codeine with fewer side effects. A few more structural types are shown in Table 53.2, along with appropriate references, but more detailed discussion of these would be out of place here since nothing would be added to our understanding of the subject. A list of the clinically more important antitussives in current use is shown in Table 53.3.

For most indications, codeine is still the most frequently prescribed antitussive probably because of its combination of antitussive, analgetic, and calming effects coupled with a low incidence of serious side effects. The dependence risk is acknowledged to be small, but where this is thought to be a problem, there are alternatives now available with no propensity for addiction. As summarized by Eddy et al. (149):

On theoretical grounds several of the codeine alternates have those properties desired in a perfect cough depressant:

(1) they possess significant cough-depressing potency;

(2) they depress cough of different pathological origins;

(3) their frequency of side-effects is no greater, perhaps less, than for codeine; and

(4) they are devoid, or practically devoid, of abuse liability.

For none of them, however, is our quantitative and practical knowledge complete enough to establish therapeutic priority.

It remains to be seen whether any of the newer drugs mentioned in this chapter will establish therapeutic priority over codeine, but what of the future? Research activity in the antitussive and mucolytic/expectorant fields is not very great compared with that in many other areas, but there is no doubt that new compounds will continue to be examined from time to time if they appear to offer significant advantages over established drugs. An interesting finding (149a, 149b) which will no doubt be followed up is the potentiation of the antitussive effect of codeine by *erythro*-1-(2′,5′-dimethoxyphenyl)-3-dimethylamino-1-butanol (53.**69**), itself possessing antitussive activity of the same order as codeine. In the guinea pig, a dose of one-seventh the effective dose of

Table 53.2   Other Compounds with Antitussive Activity

Compound	Structure	Ref.
Benzyl 2-(2-hexamethyleniminoethyl)-cyclohexanone-2-carboxylate	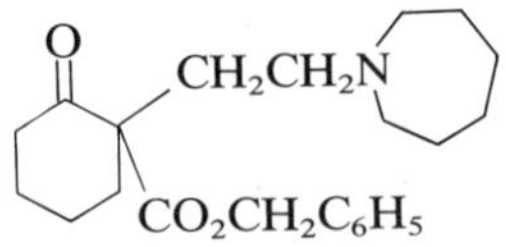	155
2-(1-Cyclopentenyl)-2-(2-morpholinoethyl)-1-cyclopentanone	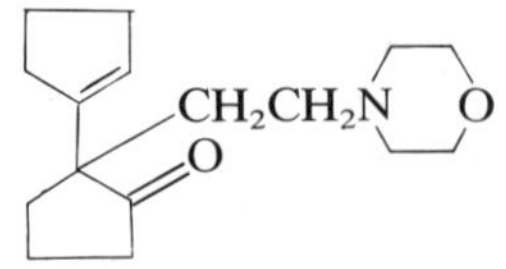	156
2-Dimethylaminomethyl-2-phenylbutyl benzoate (benzobutamine)	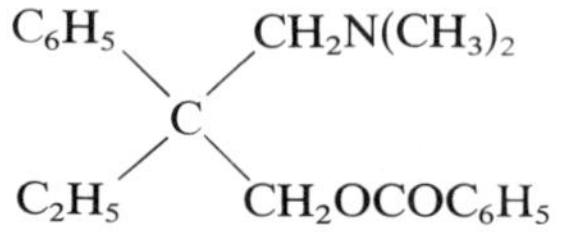	157
1-Phenylethyl-4-salicylamidomethyl-4-piperidinol (S 1592)	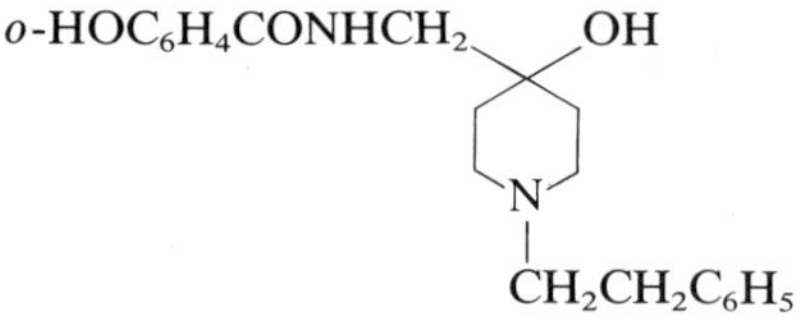	158
1-(o-Benzylphenoxy)-2-(N-piperidino) propane (benproperine)	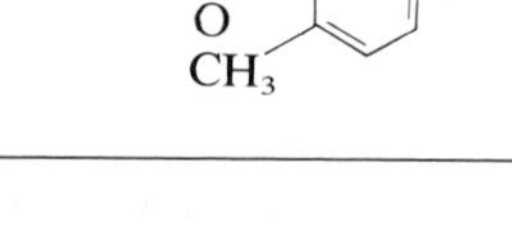	159
2-Methyl-3-o-tolyl-4-quinazolone (methaqualone)	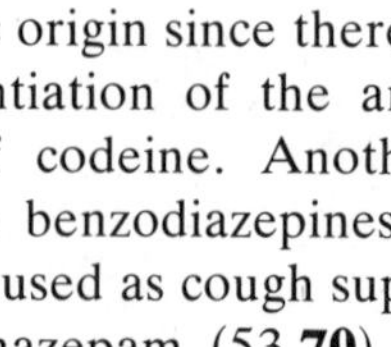	160

this compound reduced the effective dose of codeine to less than one-fifth, both drugs being given intraperitoneally. At present, the mechanism of this potentiation is unknown, although it does not appear to be of

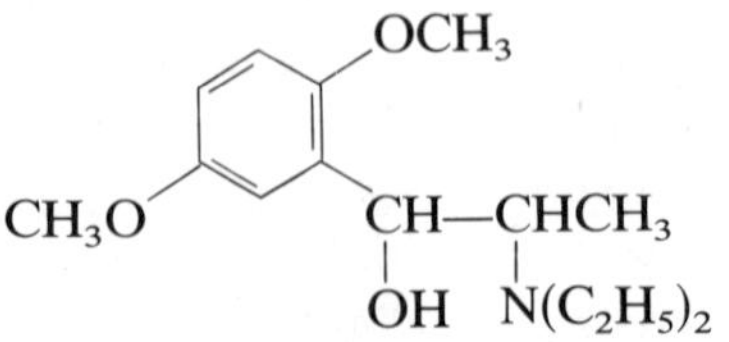

53.69

metabolic origin since there is no concomitant potentiation of the analgetic or toxic effects of codeine. Another finding concerns the benzodiazepines, which are not generally used as cough suppressants. However, clonazepam (53.**70**), a close relative of nitrazepam, has been shown to be 35 times more potent than codeine as an antitussive when tested intravenously in the cat, using electrical stimulation of the lower brain stem to elicit cough (9, 149c). This effect of clonazepam is not correlated with

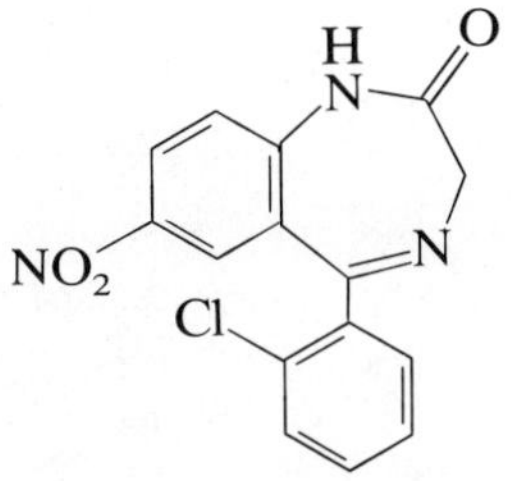

53.**70**

its muscle relaxant activity and hence it appears to be a highly selective cough suppressant in this test system.

Over the past few years, great interest in the analgetic field has centered on the demonstration of specific opiate receptor binding sites in a variety of mammalian tissues. In addition, peptide molecules such as the enkephalins (Met^5-enkephalin, H-Tyr-Gly-Gly-Phe-Met-OH and Leu^5-enkephalin, H-Tyr-Gly-Gly-Phe-Leu-OH) and β-endorphin (identical with the 61–91 amino acid fragment of β-lipotropin) have been shown to bind at opiate receptors *in vitro* and are morphine-like analgetics in animals (see Chapter 52, Section 6, and references therein). To date, no report has appeared on the testing of the above free peptides for antitussive activity, although the methyl esters of the enkephalins have

Table 53.3   Major Antitussive Drugs in Current Use

Formula No.	Chemical Name	Nonproprietary Name	Proprietary[a] Name (Country)
53.**1b**	3-Methylmorphine	Codeine	Codipront (Germany) Orthoxicol (UK)
53.**1d**	3-(2-Morpholinoethyl)morphine	Pholcodine	Copholco (UK)
53.**5**	7,8-Dihydrocodeinone	Hydrocodone	Hycomine (USA)
53.**8**	(−)-α-Narcotine	Noscapine	Conar (USA) Extil (UK)
53.**13b**	(+)-3-Methoxy-*N*-methylmorphinan	Dextromethorphan	Romilar (USA) Cosylan (UK)
53.**27**	(−)-α-4-Dimethylamino-1,2-diphenyl-3-methyl-2-propionoxybutane	Levopropoxyphene	Novrad (USA)
53.**34a**	2-(2-diethylaminoethoxy)ethyl 1-phenylcyclopentane-1-carboxylate	Carbetapentane	Toclase (Japan)
53.**36**	2-(2-Piperidinoethoxy)ethyl 1-azaphenothiazine-10-carboxylate	Pipazethate	Selvigon (USA)
53.**40a**	4-Dimethylamino-2-isopropyl-2-phenylvaleronitrile	Isoaminile	Dimyril (UK)
53.**41**	1-*o*-Chlorophenyl-3-dimethylamino-1-phenyl-1-propanol	Chlophedianol	Ulo (USA)
53.**55**	Nonaethyleneglycol monomethyl ether *p-n*-butylaminobenzoate	Benzonatate	Tessalon (USA)
Newer Drugs			
53.**13c**	(+)-3-Methyl-*N*-methylmorphinan	Dimemorphan	Astomin (Japan)
53.**52**	1-(2-Methoxy-2-phenylethyl)-4-(2-hydroxy-3-methoxy-3-phenylpropyl)-piperazine	Zipeprol	Respilene (France)

[a] A representative proprietary product containing the antitussive drug.

been shown to be inactive when administered intravenously to the cat. However, they are also inactive as analgetics when given intraventricularly to rodents (150).

With the growing realization of the importance of peptidergic transmission in the central nervous system (151) it should not be long before further studies are reported to clarify the situation and elucidate whether or not peptides are involved in the mediation of the antitussive response.

For further information on the topics discussed in this chapter, the reader is referred to the exhaustive treatise on antitussive agents edited by Salem and Aviado (Ref. 6, vols. 1–3) and the reviews of codeine and its alternates by Eddy et al. (16, 149, 152). Shorter reviews of interest are those by Doyle and Mehta (153) and Chappel and von Seemann (154).

REFERENCES

1. H. A. Bickerman, in *Drugs of Choice 1974–1975*, W. Modell, Ed., C. V. Mosby Co., St. Louis, Mo., 1974, p. 411.
2. C. Gold, *Cornell Conf. Ther.* **5,** 1 (1952).
3. K. Bucher, *Pharmacol. Rev.,* **10,** 43 (1958).
4. B. B. Ross, R. Gramiak, and H. Rahn, *J. Appl. Physiol.,* **8,** 264 (1955).
5. J. G. Widdicombe, *J. Physiol.* (London), **123,** 71 (1954).
6. H. Salem and D. M. Aviado, Eds., *Antitussive Agents, International Encyclopaedia of Pharmacology and Therapeutics*, Section 27, Vol. 1, Pergamon, New York, 1970, p. 236.
7. P. Kroepfli, *Helv. Physiol. Pharmacol. Acta,* **8,** 33 (1950).
8. H. L. Borison, *Am. J. Physiol.,* **154,** 55 (1948).
9. D. T. Chou and S. C. Wang, *J. Pharmacol. Exp. Ther.,* **194,** 499 (1975).
10. Y. Kasé, *Jap. J. Pharmacol.,* **4,** 130 (1955); through *Chem. Abstr.,* **50,** 5069 (1956).
11. R. E. Tedeschi, D. H. Tedeschi, J. T. Hitchens, L. Cook, P. A. Mattis, and E. J. Fellows, *J. Pharmacol. Exp. Ther.,* **126,** 338 (1959).
12. C. A. Winter and L. Flataker, *J. Pharmacol. Exp. Ther.,* **112,** 99 (1954).

13. H. Friebel and H. F. Kuhn, *Naunyn-Schmiedebergs Arch. Pharmakol. Exp. Pathol.,* **246,** 527 (1964).
14. P. L. Stefko and W. M. Benson, *J. Pharmacol. Exp. Ther.,* **108,** 217 (1953).
15. R. Domenjoz, *Naunyn-Schmiedebergs Arch. Pharmakol. Exp. Pathol.,* **215,** 19 (1952).
16. N. B. Eddy, H. Friebel, K. J. Hahn, and H. Halbach, *Bull. World Health Organ.,* **40,** 425 (1969).
17. U. Trendelenburg, *Acta Physiol. Scand.,* **21,** 174 (1950).
18. H. A. Bickerman and A. L. Barach, *Am. J. Med. Sci.,* **228,** 156 (1954).
19. F. B. Nicolis and G. Pasquariello, *J. Pharmacol. Exp. Ther.,* **136,** 183 (1962).
20. A. M. Ernst, *Arch. Int. Pharmacodyn. Ther.,* **58,** 363 (1938).
21. A. M. Ernst, *Arch. Int. Pharmacodyn. Ther.,* **61,** 73 (1939).
22. B. Silvestrini and G. Maffii, *Farm. Ed. Sci.,* **14,** 440 (1959).
23. J. Kalvoda, P. Buchschacher, and O. Jeger, *Helv. Chim. Acta,* **38,** 1847 (1955).
24. K. Takagi, H. Fukuda, M. Watanabe, and M. Sato, *Yakugaku Zasshi,* **80,** 1506 (1960); through *Chem. Abstr.,* **55,** 8648 (1961).
25. R. B. Barber and H. Rapoport, *J. Med. Chem.,* **19,** 1175 (1976).
26. H. Friebel, C. Reichle, and A. von Graevenitz, *Naunyn-Schmiedebergs Arch. Pharmakol. Exp. Pathol.,* **224,** 384 (1955).
27. P. Chabrier, R. Guidicelli, and J. Thuillier, *Ann. Pharm. Fr.,* **8,** 261 (1950).
28. A. J. May and J. G. Widdicombe, *Brit. J. Pharmacol. Chemother.,* **9,** 335 (1954).
29. C. E. Heffron, *J. New Drugs,* **1,** 217 (1961).
30. P. A. J. Janssen and C. A. M. Van Der Eycken, "The Chemical Anatomy of Potent Morphine Like Analgesics," in *Drugs Affecting the Central Nervous System*, Vol. 2, A. Burger, Ed., Arnold, London, 1968.
31. B. Weiss, *Am. J. Pharm.,* **131,** 286, (1959).
32. S. Hyman and S. H. Rosenblum, *Ill. Med. J.,* **104,** 257 (1953).
33. J. Knoll, S. Makleit, T. Friedmann, L. G. Hársing, Jr., and P. Hadházy, *Arch. Int. Pharmacodyn. Ther.,* **210,** 241 (1974).
34. J. Knoll, S. Fürst, and S. Makleit, *J. Pharm. Pharmacol.,* **27,** 99 (1975).
34a. J. Knoll, L. G. Hársing, Jr., and T. Friedmann, *Acta Physiol. Acad. Sci. Hung.,* **50,** 341 (1977).
34b. S. Makleit, J. Knoll, R. Bognar, S. Berenyi, G.

Somogyi, and G. Kiss, *Acta Chim. Acad. Sci. Hung.*, **93**, 169 (1977).

35. A. L. A. Boura, D. I. Haddlesey, E. J. R. Harry, J. W. Lewis, and P. A. Mayor, *J. Pharm. Pharmacol.*, **20**, 961 (1968).

36. J. W. Lewis, P. A. Mayor, and D. I. Haddlesey, *J. Med. Chem.*, **16**, 12 (1973).

37. B. Kelentey, E. Stenszky, F. Czollner, L. Szlávik, and Z. Mészáros, *Arzneim.-Forsch.*, **7**, 594 (1957).

38. K. Takagi and H. Fukuda, *Yakugaku Zasshi*, **80**, 1501 (1960); through *Chem. Abstr.*, **55**, 8648 (1961).

39. M. A. Marshall, F. L. Pyman, and R. Robinson, *J. Chem. Soc.*, **1934**, 1315.

40. M. Ohta, H. Tani, S. Moruzumi, and S. Kodaira, *Chem. Pharm. Bull.* (Tokyo), **12**, 1080 (1964).

41. J. La Barre and H. Plisnier, *Arch. Int. Pharmacodyn. Ther.*, **119**, 205 (1959).

42. M. S. Segal, *J. Am. Med. Assoc.*, **169**, 1063 (1959).

43. Y. Ota, N. Endo, and M. Hirasawa, *Chem. Pharm. Bull.* (Tokyo), **12**, 569 (1964).

44. A. Rheiner and A. Brossi, *Experientia*, **20**, 488 (1964).

45. C. R. Addinall and R. T. Major, *J. Am. Chem. Soc.*, **55**, 1202 (1933).

46. B. Kelentey, B. Stenszky, and F. Czollner, *Naunyn-Schmiedebergs Arch. Pharmakol. Exp. Pathol.*, **233**, 550 (1958).

47. H. A. Bickerman, E. German, B. M. Cohen, and S. E. Itkin, *Am. J. Med. Sci.*, **234**, 191 (1957).

48. O. Schnider and A. Grüssner, *Helv. Chim. Acta*, **34**, 2211 (1951).

49. H. Corrodi, J. Hellerbach, A. Züst, E. Hardegger, and O. Schnider, *Helv. Chim. Acta*, **42**, 212 (1959).

50. A. F. Casy and M. M. A. Hassan, *J. Pharm. Pharmacol.*, **19**, 132 (1967).

51. B. Pellmont and H. Bächtold, *Schweiz. Med. Wochenschr.*, **84**, 1368 (1954).

52. H. Isbell and H. F. Fraser, *J. Pharmacol. Exp. Ther.*, **107**, 524 (1953).

53. W. M. Benson, P. L. Stefko, and L. O. Randall, *J. Pharmacol. Exp. Ther.*, **109**, 189 (1953).

54. M. Murakami, N. Inukai, and N. Nagano, *Chem. Pharm. Bull.* (Tokyo), **20**, 1699 (1972).

55. M. Murakami, S. Kawahara, N. Inukai, N. Nagano, H. Iwamoto, and H. Ida, *Chem. Pharm. Bull.* (Tokyo), **20**, 1706 (1972).

56. Y. Kaśe, G. Kito, T. Miyata, T. Uno, K. Takahama, and H. Ida, *Arzneim.-Forsch.*, **26**, 353 (1976).

57. Y. Kasé, G. Kito, T. Miyata, K. Takahama, T. Uno, and H. Ida, *Arzneim.-Forsch.*, **26**, 361 (1976).

58. N. Sugimoto and S. Ohshiro, Jap. Pat. 3,871 (1961); through *Chem. Abstr.*, **58**, 10178 (1963).

59. N. Sugimoto and S. Ohshiro, Jap. Pat. 8,522 (1958); through *Chem. Abstr.*, **54**, 4633 (1960).

60. N. Sugimoto and S. Ohshiro, Jap. Pat. 4,084 (1963); through *Chem. Abstr.*, **59**, 11452 (1963).

61. I. Iwai, I. Seki, A. Minakami, H. Takagi, and S. Kobayashi, Jap. Pat. 24,621 (1965); through *Chem. Abstr.*, **64**, 5053 (1966).

62. I. Seki, *Yakugaku Zasshi*, **83**, 389 (1963); through *Chem. Abstr.*, **59**, 6454 (1963).

63. S. Kobayashi, K. Hasegawa, M. Mori, and H. Takagi, *Arzneim.-Forsch.*, **20**, 43 (1970).

64. H. Shindo, T. Komai, E. Nakajima, H. Murata, A. Yasumura, and I. Seki, Yakugaku Zasshi, **90**, 36 (1970); through *Chem. Abstr.*, **72**, 88520 (1970).

65. I. Seki and H. Takagi, *Chem. Pharm. Bull.* (Tokyo), **19**, 1 (1971).

66. I. Monković, H. Wong, A. W. Pircio, Y. G. Perron, I. J. Pachter and B. Belleau, *Can. J. Chem.*, **53**, 3094 (1975).

67. R. L. Cavanagh, J. A. Gylys, and M. E. Bierwagen, *Arch. Int. Pharmacodyn. Ther.*, **220**, 258 (1976).

68. O. Eisleb and O. Schaumann, *Deut. Med. Wochenschr.*, **65**, 967 (1939).

69. C. Reichle and H. Friebel, *Naunyn-Schmiedebergs Arch. Pharmakol. Exp. Pathol.*, **226**, 558 (1955).

70. E. N. Guseva, *Farmakol. Toksikol.*, **19**, 17 (1956); through *Chem. Abstr.*, **51**, 6881 (1957).

71. R. Charlier, M. Prost, F. Binon, and G. Deltour, *Arch. Int. Pharmacodyn. Ther.*, **134**, 306 (1961).

72. M. Prost, M. Urbain, and R. Charlier, *Helv. Chim. Acta*, **52**, 1134 (1969).

73. C. A. Winter and L. Flataker, *Proc. Soc. Exp. Biol. Med.*, **81**, 463 (1952).

74. Y. Kasé, T. Yuizono, H. Serikawa, S. Yamomoto, T. Yamasaki, T. Fushimitzu, N. Katayama, T. Moriza, and T. Nozuhara, *Chem. Pharm., Bull.* (Tokyo), **6**, 109 (1958).

75. A. Pohland and H. R. Sullivan, *J. Am. Chem. Soc.*, **75**, 4458 (1953).

76. E. B. Robbins and J. A. Miller, *Pharmacologist*, **2**, 98 (1960).

77. A. F. Casy and J. L. Myers, *J. Pharm. Pharmacol.*, **16,** 455 (1964).

78. M. Prost, M. Urbain, and R. Charlier, *Eur. J. Med. Chem.*, **9,** 318 (1974).

79. D. W. Adamson, *J. Chem. Soc.*, **1950,** 885.

80. D. W. Adamson and A. F. Green, *Nature*, **165,** 122 (1950).

81. A. F. Green and N. B. Ward, *Brit. J. Pharmacol. Chemother.*, **10,** 418 (1955).

82. R. Kimura and T. Yabuuchi, *Chem. Pharm. Bull.* (Tokyo), **7,** 171 (1959).

83. Y. Kasé and T. Yuizono, *Chem. Pharm. Bull.* (Tokyo), **7,** 378 (1959).

84. Y. Kasé, T. Yuizono, T. Yamasaki, T. Yamada, S. Io, M. Tamiya, and I. Kondo, *Chem. Pharm. Bull.* (Tokyo), **7,** 372 (1959).

85. J. R. Geigy A. G., Swiss Pat., 272,708 (1951); through *Chem. Abstr.*, **46,** 4563 (1952).

86. J. J. Toner and E. Macko, *J. Pharmacol. Exp. Ther.*, **106,** 246 (1952).

87. C. C. Pfeiffer, *Science*, **107,** 94 (1948).

88. H. G. Morren, Bel. Pat. 520,988 (1953); through *Chem. Abstr.*, **53,** 8174 (1959); Brit. Pat., 753,779 (1956); through *Chem. Abstr.*, **51,** 7443 (1957).

89: S. Levis, S. Preat, and F. Moyersoons, *Arch. Int. Pharmacodyn. Ther.*, **103,** 200 (1955).

90. V. Petrow, O. Stephenson, and A. M. Wild, *J. Pharm. Pharmacol.*, **10,** 40 (1958).

91. A. David, F. Leith-Ross, and D. K. Vallance, *J. Pharm. Pharmacol.*, **9,** 446 (1957).

92. C. von Seemann, U.S. Pat. 2,778,824 (1957); through *Chem. Abstr.*, **51,** 10591 (1957).

93. C. I. Chappel, M. G. P. Stegen, and G. A. Grant, *Can. J. Biochem. Physiol.*, **36,** 475 (1958).

94. K. J. Hahn and H. Friebel, *Med. Pharmacol. Exp.*, **14,** 87 (1966).

95. J. Klosa, *Arch. Pharm.*, **287,** 321 (1954).

96. F. P. Doyle, M. D. Mehta, G. S. Sach, R. Ward and P. S. Sherman, *J. Chem. Soc.*, **1964,** 578.

97. F. P. Doyle, M. D. Mehta, R. Ward, J. Bainbridge, and D. M. Brown, *J. Med. Chem.*, **8,** 571 (1965).

98. E. Marchetti, F. Samueli, and F. Stucchi, *Arch. Int. Pharmacodyn. Ther.*, **178,** 400 (1969).

99. M. Serembe and M. Barbetti, *Farm. Ed. Prat.*, **24,** 700 (1969).

100. W. Stühmer, U. Brose, and S. Funke, Ger. Pat., 964,500 (1957); through *Chem. Abstr.*, **53,** 17060 (1959).

101. D. Krause, *Arzneim.-Forsch.*, **8,** 553 (1958).

102. R. Gösswald, *Arzneim.-Forsch.*, **8,** 550 (1958).

103. A. Berg, Bel. Pat., 588,825 (1960).

104. R. Engelhorn, *Arzneim.-Forsch.*, **10,** 785 (1960).

105. K. Tatsumi, M. Nakano, S. Kitamura, and H. Yoshimura, *Yakugaku Zasshi*, **95,** 690 (1975); through *Chem. Abstr.*, **83,** 126027 (1975).

106. C. Hauna, *Arch. Int. Pharmacodyn. Ther.*, **185,** 47 (1970).

107. S. Casadio, G. Pala, A. Mantegani, E. Marazzi-Uberti, G. Coppi, and C. Turba, *J. Med. Chem.*, **13,** 1092 (1970).

108. S. Miyano, A. Abe, Y. Kasé, T. Yuizono, K. Tachibana, T. Miyata, and G. Kito, *J. Med. Chem.*, **13,** 704 (1970).

109. Y. Kasé, T. Yuizono, K. Tachibana, T. Miyata, G. Kito, and S. Miyano, *Arzneim.-Forsch.*, **19,** 1916 (1969).

110. Y. Kasé, Y. Wakita, T. Yuizono, G. Kito, and K. Kikuchi, *Arzneim.-Forsch.*, **20,** 37 (1970).

111. J. Wax, C. V. Winder, and G. Peters, *Proc. Soc. Exp. Biol. Med.*, **110,** 600 (1962).

112. C. van der Stelt, H. M. Tersteege, and W. Th. Nauta, *Arzneim.-Forsch.*, **14,** 1053 (1964).

113. H. M. Tersteege, A. B. H. Funcke, W. J. Louwerse, and W. Th. Nauta, *Arch. Int. Pharmacodyn. Ther.*, **161,** 314 (1966).

114. I. Källquist and B. Melander, *Arzneim.-Forsch.*, **7,** 301 (1957).

115. H. Morren, Bel. Pat., 556,239 (1957); through *Chem. Abstr.*, **53,** 22027 (1959).

116. Y. Kasé, T. Yuizono, M. Masuda, M. Muto, S. Miyamoto, and Y. Tagawa, *Yakugaku Zasshi*, **82,** 1298 (1962); through *Chem. Abstr.*, **58,** 11875 (1963).

117. J. C. Le Douarec, G. Régnier, and R. Canévari, *Arzneim.-Forsch.*, **15,** 1330 (1965).

118. K. Takagi, H. Fukuda, K. Fujise, K. Matsui, and M. Sato, *Yakugaku Zasshi*, **81,** 261 (1961); through *Chem. Abstr.*, **55,** 13771 (1961).

119. B . R. Anzlowar, Ed., *Unlisted Drugs*, **22,** 177 (1970).

120. G. Rispat, H. Burgi, D. Cosnier, P. Duchêne-Marullaz, and G. Streichenberger, *Arzneim.-Forsch.*, **26,** 523 (1976).

120a. M. Constantin and J. F. Pognat, *Arzneim.-Forsch.*, **28**:**I,** 64 (1978).

121. S. Takanashi, Y. Tohira, H. Suzuki, S. Ogiya, A. Sakuma, and K. Kimura, *Yakugaku Zasshi*, **95,** 897 (1975); through *Chem. Abstr.*, **84,** 25703 (1976).

122. F. W. Horner Ltd., S. A. Pat. R61/217 (1961).

123. M. Menard, L. Mitchell, J. Komlóssy, A. M. Wrigley, and F. L. Chubb, *Can. J. Chem.*, **39,** 729 (1961).

124. G. R. De Vleeschouwer, *Arch. Int. Pharmacodyn. Ther.*, **97,** 34 (1954).

125. N. K. Chakravarty, A. Matallana, R. Jensen, and H. L. Borison, *J. Pharmacol. Exp. Ther.*, **117,** 127 (1956).

126. I. Shemano, J. M. Beiler, and J. T. Hitchens, *Arch. Int. Pharmacodyn. Ther.*, **165,** 410 (1967).

127. G. Krüger, J. Keck, O. Zipp, H. Machleidt, and G. Ohnacker, *Arzneim.-Forsch.*, **23,** 290 (1973).

128. S. Püschmann and R. Engelhorn, *Arzneim.-Forsch.*, **23,** 296 (1973).

128a. C. F. Marchioni, G. Monzali, and P. Braga, *Clin. Ter.*, **79,** 443 (1976).

128b. A. Zimmer, G. Krüger, and A. Prox, *Arzneim.-Forsch.*, **28:I,** 688 (1978).

128c. S. S. Matharu, D. A. Rowlands, J. B. Taylor, and R. Westwood, *J. Med. Chem.*, **20,** 197 (1977).

129. M. Matter, U.S. Pats., 2,714,608–2,714,610 (1955); through *Chem. Abstr.*, **50,** 7137 (1956).

130. K. Bucher, *Schweiz. Med. Wochenschr.*, **86,** 94 (1956).

131. R. Sell, E. Lindner, and H. Jahn, *Naunyn-Schmiedebergs Arch. Pharmakol. Exp. Pathol.*, **234,** 164 (1958).

132. B. Silvestrini and C. Pozzatti, *Arch. Int. Pharmacodyn. Ther.*, **129,** 249 (1960).

133. B. Silvestrini and C. Pozzatti, *Brit. J. Pharmacol. Chemother.*, **16,** 209 (1961).

134. B. Silvestrini and C. Pozzatti, *Arzneim.-Forsch.*, **13,** 798 (1963).

135. K. Harsanyi, L. Tardos, I. Fehér, and G. Nagy, *Boll. Chim. Farm.*, **112,** 691 (1973).

136. J. R. Boissier and J. Pagny, *Thérapie*, **15,** 93 and 97 (1960).

137. J. Lieberman, *Am. J. Med.*, **49,** 1 (1970).

138. A. L. Sheffner, U.S. Pat., 3,091,569 (1960).

139. A. L. Sheffner, *Ann. N.Y. Acad. Sci.*, **106,** 298 (1963).

140. V. N. Huyen, S. Garcet, and L. Lakah, *C. R. Soc. Biol.*, **160,** 1849 (1966).

141. S. N. Steen, I. Ziment, D. Freeman, and J. S. Thomas, *Clin. Pharmacol. Ther.*, **16,** 58 (1974).

142. E. M. Boyd, *Pharmacol. Rev.*, **6,** 521 (1954).

143. E. M. Boyd and G. L. Pearson, *Am. J. Med. Sci.*, **211,** 602 (1946).

144. E. M. Boyd, E. P. Sheppard, and C. E. Boyd, *Appl. Ther.*, **9,** 55 (1967).

145. R. Engelhorn and S. Püschmann, *Arzneim.-Forsch.*, **13,** 474 (1963).

146. E. Schraven, F. W. Koss, J. Keck, G. Beisenherz, A. Buecheler, and W. Lindner, *Eur. J. Pharmacol.*, **1,** 445 (1967).

147. Z. Kopitar, R. Jauch, R. Hankwitz, H. Pelzer, D. Maass, and K. D. Willim, *Eur. J. Pharmacol.*, **21,** 6 (1973).

148. H. D. Renovanz, *Arzneim.-Forsch.*, **25,** 646 (1975).

148a. "Ambroxol (NA 872)," *Arzneim.-Forsch.*, **28:I,** 887–936 (1978).

149. N. B. Eddy, H. Friebel, K. J. Hahn, and H. Halbach, *Bull. World Health Organ.*, **40,** 721 (1969).

149a. Y. Kasuya, M. Watanabe, K. Miyasaka, and Y. Ishii, *Arzneim.-Forsch.*, **27:II,** 1450 (1977).

149b. H. Hamano and S. Okuda, *Chem. Pharm. Bull.* (Tokyo), **26,** 833 (1978).

149c. S. C. Wang, D. T. Chou, and M. C. Wallenstein, *Agents & Actions*, **7,** 337 (1977).

150. J. Knoll, *Eur. J. Pharmacol.*, **39,** 403 (1976).

151. J. Hughes, *Nature*, **267,** 106 (1977).

152. N. B. Eddy, H. Friebel, K. J. Hahn, and H. Halbach, *Bull. World Health Organ.*, **40,** 639 (1969).

153. F. P. Doyle and M. D. Mehta, "Antitussives," in *Advances in Drug Research*, Vol. 1, N. J. Harper and A. B. Simmonds, Eds., Academic, London-New York, 1964.

154. C. I. Chappel and C. von Seemann, "Antitussive Drugs," in *Progress in Medicinal Chemistry*, Vol. 3, G. P. Ellis and G. B. West, Eds., Butterworths, London, 1963.

155. A. E. Kaushaar, R. W. Schunk, and H. F. Thym, *Arzneim.-Forsch.*, **14,** 986 (1964).

156. M. Groszman, I. O. Berker, and F. Casimir, *Appl. Ther.*, **3,** 95 (1961).

157. G. Maffii, B. Silvestrini, and S. Banfi, *Nature*, **199,** 916 (1963).

158. J. Duhault, F. Tisserand, and G. Régnier, *Arzneim.-Forsch.*, **26,** 516 (1976).

159. B. R. Anzlowar, Ed., *Unlisted Drugs*, **27,** 173 (1975); Pharmacia A. S., Brit. Pat. 914,008 (1962); through *Chem. Abstr.*, **58,** 12523 (1963).

160. J. R. Boissier and J. Pagny, *Med. Exp.*, **1,** 368 (1959).

CHAPTER FIFTY-FOUR

Sedative–Hypnotics

JULIUS A. VIDA

Bristol-Myers Company
International Division
345 Park Avenue
New York, New York 10022, USA

CONTENTS

1   INTRODUCTION

An analysis of sedative–hypnotic drugs must first consider the state that these drugs are designed to induce, i.e., the state of sleep. Polygraphic studies have revealed that sleep consists of two different states.

787

As a rule, slow wave sleep always precedes paradoxical sleep. Alternation of the two sleep states produces a sleep pattern that is characteristic of naturally occurring sleep. Ideally, a sedative–hypnotic drug should induce sleep that is similar to naturally occurring sleep. In practice, after prolonged administration, all sedative–hypnotic drugs suppress paradoxical sleep to a degree or alter the sleep pattern that is characteristic of naturally occurring sleep. Furthermore, after prolonged administration tolerance and physical dependence to the drug may develop. In addition, many hypnotics produce a hangover effect. The benefits derived from prolonged use of sedative–hypnotics must be considered in view of these facts.

2 PHYSIOLOGY OF SLEEP

Electrophysiological recordings during sleep have demonstrated that sleep is an active process (1, 2). Furthermore, electroencephalographic (EEG) studies have revealed that the activity of the brain is not constant during sleep (3). Electrooculographic (EOG) and electromyographic (EMG) data have lent additional support to the finding that there are two opposing states of sleep (4). Based on brain function and activity in the central nervous system the following three physiological states exist:

1. Alert wakefulness.
2. Rapid eye movement (REM) sleep (also called D sleep).
3. Nonrapid eye movement (NREM sleep) (also called S sleep).

In wakefulness the EEG shows a high level of low voltage, mixed frequency activity recorded from the cortex. The EMG shows a high level of muscular activity recorded from the neck, and the EOG shows frequent eye movements.

REM sleep is characterized by tonic and phasic activities (5). Tonic phenomena include a fast, low voltage cortical activity in the electroencephalogram similar to that found in waking and a regular theta rhythm in the hippocampus. The high level of electroencephalographic activity is contrasted by the total absence of electromyographic activity, indicating no evidence of muscular activity from muscles under the chin. Because of this contrast, REM sleep is also known as paradoxical sleep (PS). Tonic phenomena persist for several minutes. The accompanying phasic phenomena include rapid eye movements displayed in the electrooculogram in a stereotyped manner. The pattern of rapid eye movement is different from that of waking and in animals is associated with jerking movements of the ears, whiskers, and paws. Phasic bursts of muscular twitches are also observed in spite of a generally relaxed muscular tonus. The phasic activity is also seen in electroencephalographic recordings from the reticular formation of the pons, from the lateral geniculate, and from the occipital cortex, giving rise to the term pontine-geniculate-occipital (PGO) spikes (6). These PGO spikes consist of high voltage waves that always precede REM sleep by some 30–45 sec. The PGO spikes occur at a fairly constant rate, probably regulated by a biochemical mechanism. Subjects awakened from REM sleep are likely to report vivid dreams. Cerebral blood flow in REM sleep is greater than that during wakefulness. It has also been suggested that REM sleep has a special role in the maintenance, restoration, and metabolism of catecholamine mechanisms (7–9).

REM sleep usually makes up 20–25% of the total amount of sleep (10, 11).

NREM sleep is devoid of rapid eye movements (12). In drowsiness and light sleep during the NREM cycle slow eye movements have been observed. Cardiovascular and respiratory activity is calm, with a slower heart rate and respiration rate than that during wakefulness. Muscle tonus is slightly decreased. The activity in the EMG is decreased compared to that in wakefulness (13).

NREM sleep is subdivided into four stages. The drowsy state (stage 1) that precedes the onset of definite sleep lasts only for a few minutes. Stage 1 is characterized by relatively low voltage, mixed frequency EEG (alpha waves). Stage 2 lasts for a somewhat longer period and is characterized by spindles in the EEG. Stage 3 is characterized by a moderate amount of high amplitude, slow wave sleep (SWS), or delta wave sleep, and in stage 4 a large amount of high amplitude, slow wave sleep is present (4–17).

It has been suggested that anabolic processes including the synthesis of neurotransmitters, biogenic amines, and other endogenous substances take place during NREM sleep (9). The fact that maximal human growth hormone secretion takes place during stage 3 and 4 sleep (18, 19) has been interpreted as support for hypothesis that NREM sleep has an anabolic restorative function (20). Although not associated with any EEG period, other hormones are also secreted in large amounts during sleep. These include prolactin (21) and, in early puberty only, luteinizing hormone and testosterone (22, 23).

3 SLEEP CYCLE

When a normal healthy person prepares for a night's rest drowsiness sets in. The alpha waves appear in the EEG, muscular tone becomes relaxed in the EMG, and slow eyeball oscillation is observed in the EOG. The state of drowsiness (NREM stage 1 sleep) quickly changes to definite sleep (NREM stage 2 sleep). A gradual change into NREM stage 3 and stage 4 state is observed within a 30–60 min period. The changes are observed in the EEG, EMG,

and EOG. A gradual decrease in heart rate, respiration, and muscular tone accompanies the sleep changes. The threshold of arousal gradually increases and reaches a maximum in stage 4. After about a 90 min period in NREM sleep a sudden burst of activities begin. The slow wave pattern in the EEG changes to a mixed frequency pattern. Simultaneously rapid eye movements are recorded in the EOG. A speedup is seen in the heart rate and respiration. Occasionally skeletal muscle jerks take place. At the same time the muscle tone below the chin is abolished. After about 10–15 min the REM sleep changes to NREM sleep. Afterward three to five 15–20 min REM periods occur during the night in 80–100 min cycles, alternating with NREM sleep. Aging and drugs have an effect on the relative proportions of REM and NREM sleep (24).

Sleep deprivation studies (25) have demonstrated the need for both NREM and REM sleep. Subjects deprived of sleep tend to spend more than a normal amount of time in NREM sleep when allowed to sleep. Similarly, if the subjects are awakened every time that REM sleep begins they become selectively deprived of REM sleep, because every time they fall asleep again, the sleep cycle begins with NREM sleep. As a result, REM sleep occurs after shorter and shorter times. Furthermore, subjects deprived of REM sleep spend more than a normal amount of time in REM sleep when allowed to follow a normal pattern. This rebound effect is also observed after REM sleep suppressing drugs are withdrawn (26).

4 NEUROTRANSMITTERS AND NREM SLEEP

Based on very elegant studies performed in cats Jouvet postulated that there is a direct relationship between 5-hydroxytryptamine (5-HT, serotonin) and NREM sleep

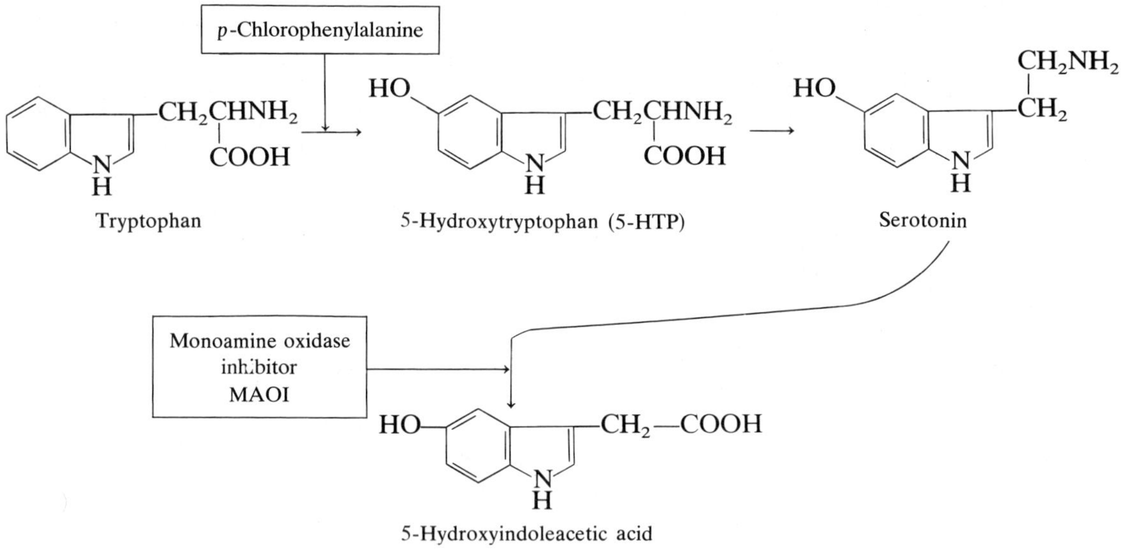

Fig. 54.1 Biogenesis and catabolism of 5-hydroxytryptamine. Inhibitors of synthesis or catabolism are set in boxes.

(27, 28). The biogenesis and catabolism of 5-hydroxytryptamine (serotonin, 5-HT) are shown in Fig. 54.1.

Although it is known that reserpine produces a tranquilizing, calming effect, it also disturbs sleep. In the cat, reserpine suppresses NREM sleep for 12 hr and REM sleep for 24 hr. The EEG recordings, however, display continuous discharges of PGO spikes, which usually precede REM sleep after NREM sleep. Reserpine is known to deplete nonspecifically the concentration of monoamines (both serotonin and catecholamines) in the brain. The hypothesis was advanced, therefore, that depletion of 5-HT levels in the brain is responsible for suppression of NREM sleep. This hypothesis is supported by the immediate reappearance of NREM in the cat if administration of reserpine is followed by injection of 5-HT, a precursor of 5-HT, which restores 5-HT levels to normal (29). On the other hand, if administration of reserpine is followed by injection of 30–50 mg/kg dihydroxyphenylalanine (dopa), which restores brain catecholamine concentration to normal, REM sleep is immediately induced

(30). This led to the theory that 5-HT is responsible for inducing NREM sleep and catecholamines are responsible for inducing REM sleep. It should be mentioned, however, that if the same dose of dopa is given to cats previously not receiving reserpine (31) a state of wakefulness is induced which lasts for 5–6 hr. Administration of *p*-chlorophenylalanine (PCPA), a known inhibitor of tryptophan hydroxylase in animals, selectively decreases brain 5-hydroxytryptophan (5-HT) and in turn 5-hydroxytryptamine (serotonin, 5-HT) levels (32). The decrease in 5-HT brain level completely prevents onset of NREM sleep (33). If PCPA administration is followed by 5-HT injection, the insomnia is reversed and NREM sleep sets in quickly (34). The animal data, however, were not confirmed in humans. On the contrary, reserpine produced an increase in REM sleep (35–38). Unlike in animals, administration of PCPA to humans had no effect on NREM sleep (39–42). Concomitant administration of PCPA and 5-HTP had no effect on the NREM sleep in humans (43).

Furthermore, in rats a high dose of the

twice-removed 5-HT precursor, tryptophan, increases the 5-HT brain levels yet induces a small decrease in total sleep duration accompanied by an increase in the frequency of REM sleep (the net result is a decrease in NREM time). On the other hand, in humans tryptophan had a marked hypnotic effect in insomniacs and increased NREM sleep in normal subjects (44).

To determine whether the hypnotic effect of L-tryptophan was due to its conversion to serotonin or to some other factor, L-tryptophan was administered to subjects whose serotonin synthesis was partially blocked by 3 weeks' administration of PCPA (45). In each case NREM sleep increased, indicating that the effect of L-tryptophan is not due to its conversion to serotonin.

NREM sleep is decreased in humans by the administration of 5-hydroxytryptophan (5-HTP) with (43) or without (46, 47) the simultaneous administration of the peripheral decarboxylase inhibitor MK-486, which blocks the conversion of 5-HTP to serotonin.

The hypothesis that 5-HT is responsible for triggering and maintaining NREM sleep is not adequately supported by human sleep studies (48).

5 NEUROTRANSMITTERS AND REM SLEEP

REM sleep is also influenced by the neurotransmitter 5-HT. Inhibition of 5-HT synthesis in animals and man with PCPA decreases not only NREM sleep but REM sleep as well (5). There is, however, a paradoxical correlation between REM sleep and 5-HT levels. It appears that a certain minimal threshold value of 5-HT is necessary to *prime* REM sleep (32). This is supported by the return of REM sleep to normal levels if PCPA administration to the cat is followed by small doses of 5-HTP. However, if PCPA administration is followed by a large dose of 5-HTP, which in turn produces large amounts of 5-HT, REM sleep is suppressed. As a result of these experiments, it appears that over a threshold value in animals thre is an indirect relationship between 5-HT levels and REM sleep (28).

In man, administration of 5-HTP increases REM sleep (49, 50, 46) unless it is coadministered with MK-486, a peripheral decarboxylase inhibitor that blocks conversion of 5-HTP to serotonin (51). In this case, no change in sleep was observed.

Similarly, L-tryptophan, the twice-removed precursor of 5-HT, in man in small doses does not significantly affect REM sleep (44). High doses of L-tryptophan, however, significantly increase REM sleep in man.

These findings suggest that the onset of REM sleep depends on a 5-HT priming mechanism, whereas the maintenance of REM sleep manifested by the duration of REM sleep depends on other mechanisms.

Further support for this hypothesis is obtained by the fact that MAO inhibitors also suppress REM sleep in the cat (52). MAO inhibitors also suppress the turnover of 5-HT. As expected, the resulting increased 5-HT levels markedly decrease REM sleep. The REM sleep suppressant effect of MAO inhibitors in animals and in man must be interpreted with some caution. MAO inhibitors increase not only 5-HT levels but other monoamine (norepinephrine, dopamine, etc.) levels as well, which also have an influence on REM sleep. Further, since MAO inhibitors interfere with the metabolism of 5-HT, it is possible that deaminated metabolites of 5-HT may be responsible for inducing REM sleep, since the absence of these metabolites (caused by the presence of MAO inhibitors) suppresses the transition from NREM to REM sleep (5, 28).

The adrenergic neurotransmitters (norepinephrine, dopamine) may also play a role in REM sleep. The effect of reserpine

α-Dopa   α-Methylnorepinephrine

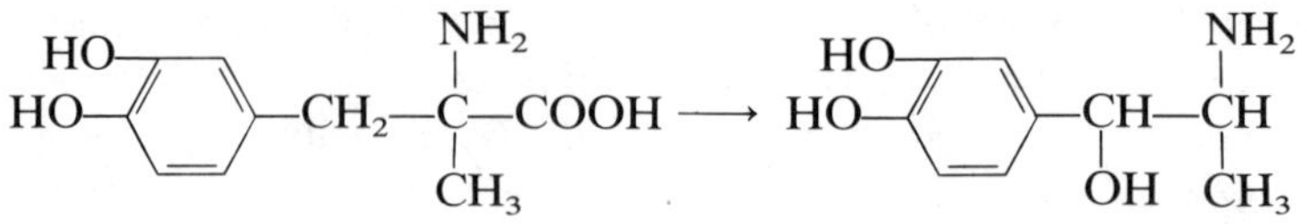

on REM sleep has been previously discussed. It was also found that a 200 mg/kg dose of α-methyldopa, which results in the synthesis of the false transmitter α-methylnorepinephrine and selectively displaces norepinephrine from the stores, increases REM sleep in the cat for 16 hr (53). Further evidence for the involvement of the adrenergic mechanism in the maintenance of REM sleep is provided by the action of disulfiram on REM sleep. Disulfiram, which blocks norepinephrine synthesis, increases REM sleep in the cat (54). The biogenesis of norepinephrine is shown in Fig. 54.2. The REM sleep-increasing effect of the drugs α-methyldopa and disulfiram is attributed to their depletion of brain norepinephrine stores.

It appears, therefore, that a minimum catecholamine threshold concentration is necessary for the onset of REM sleep. On the other hand, there is also evidence that above a minimum threshold value, which is necessary to induce REM sleep, there is an indirect relationship between the concentration of catecholamines and the amount of REM sleep. Like serotonin, the catecholamines also produce a paradoxical effect on REM sleep. This hypothesis is supported by the finding that administration of α-methyl-p-tyrosine (AMPT), an inhibitor of catecholamine synthesis, increases REM sleep in the rat and cat (55, 28) as well as in humans (56).

Further support for the indirect relationship between the concentration of catecholamines and REM sleep is obtained from the effect of 6-hydroxydopamine (6-OHDA) on REM sleep. 6-OHDA decreases catecholamine brain levels in the cat by either inhibiting catecholamine synthesis (57) or destroying catecholamine terminals (58). In any event, administration of 6-OHDA for 6 days increases REM sleep as well as the PGO period (59). It was also found that the dopamine β-hydroxylase inhibitor fusaric acid produced an increase in REM sleep in the rat 8–24 hr

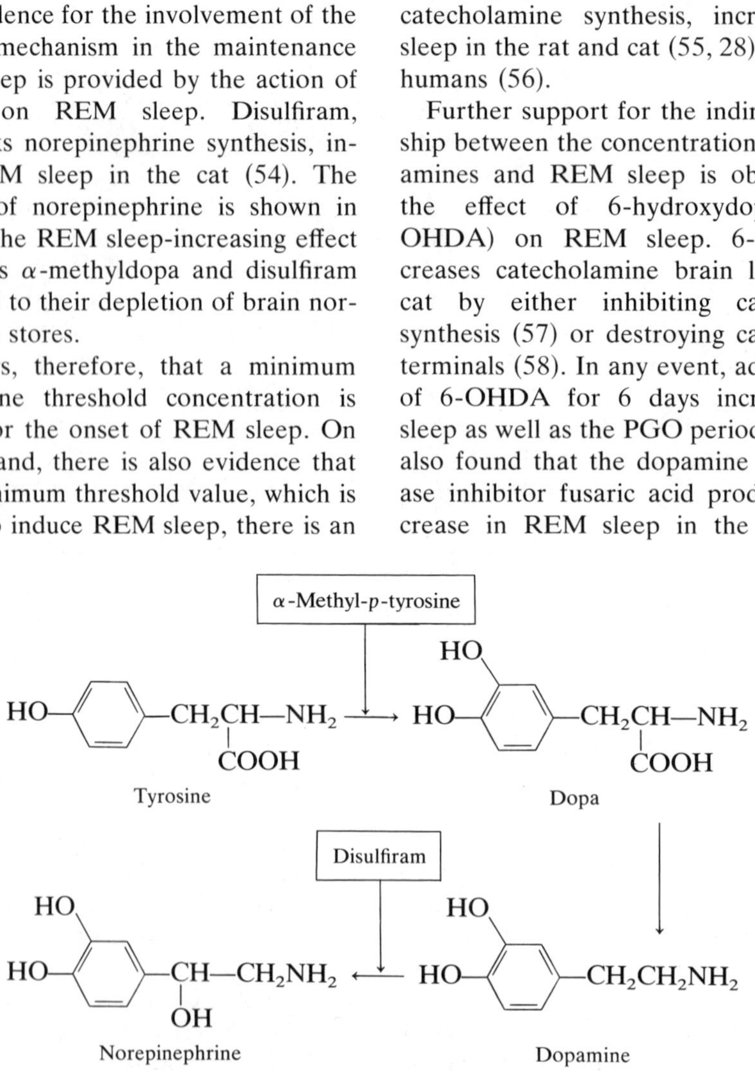

Fig. 54.2 Biogenesis of norepinephrine.

after administration (60). The selective decrease of norepinephrine levels by fusaric acid demonstrates that norepinephrine, not dopamine, is responsible for the inverse relationship.

The importance of catecholamine metabolites in determining REM sleep time is shown by the effects of MAO inhibitors. We have previously discussed the REM sleep suppressant effect of MAO inhibitors in connection with their depleting effect on the deaminated metabolites of 5-HT (61). It has also been suggested that MAO inhibitors suppress REM sleep in the cat by depleting the deaminated metabolites of norepinephrine (5). It is also possible, however, that MAO inhibitors suppress REM sleep by increasing norepinephrine levels. This would indicate again that the same type of inverse relationship exists between norepinephrine brain levels and REM sleep as does between serotonin brain levels and REM sleep. The antidepressant drugs imipramine and desipramine reduce REM sleep due to the increased norepinephrine levels at postsynaptic receptors caused by reduced reuptake of norepinephrine (62). Amphetamine, a CNS stimulant, reduces REM sleep in man by increasing norepinephrine concentration at the synapse caused by greater release from norepinephrine stores (63).

Yet another finding points out the importance of norepinephrine concentration on REM sleep. The α-adrenergic blocking agent, thymoxamine, reduces norepinephrine concentration in the brain, and in turn increases the duration of REM sleep in man (64). An increase in stage 3 and stage 4 sleep was also observed later in the night. However, the β-adrenergic receptor blocker, propranolol, had no effect on the duration of wakefulness, REM sleep, or NREM sleep, indicating that only norepinephrine acting at α-adrenergic receptors and not at β-adrenergic receptors may be involved in the maintenance of sleep (65). The theory that a cholinergic mechanism

is also involved in this maintenance but not primary mechanism of REM sleep is suggested by the finding that anticholinergic drugs, e.g., atropine (66) or hemicholinium-3 (67, 68) selectively suppress REM sleep time in the cat. It was postulated that the cholinergic system is involved in the tonic components, i.e., either the decrease of muscle tone or cortical activation of REM sleep (69–71).

6 EVALUATION OF SEDATIVE–HYPNOTICS

The methods usually employed in the evaluation of sedative–hypnotic drug candidates in small rodents (mouse or rat) involve measurements of the levels of CNS depression. These involve measurements of sleeping time (72), loss of righting reflex (73), performance on the rotarod (74), behavior in the activity cage (75–77), and finally, potentiation of other CNS depressants (78).

Recently more emphasis has been placed on the evaluation of drug candidates in the rat, cat, and monkey by measuring drug-induced changes in the sleep–wakefulness cycle. These studies have recently been reviewed (19).

The ultimate answer for the usefulness of a drug candidate is found in humans. Sleep laboratory studies in man have been increasingly used recently in the evaluation of the effectiveness of hypnotic drugs. These studies have also been reviewed (80–82).

7 CLASSIFICATION AND MECHANISM OF ACTION OF SEDATIVE–HYPNOTICS

Ideally a sedative–hypnotic drug should induce sleep that is similar in sleep pattern to natural sleep. Unfortunately almost all hypnotics distort the normal sleep pattern after repeated (one or more weeks) use. Most sedative–hypnotic drugs are general depressants of the central nervous system. Historically a drug was called a sedative if it produced calmness in anxious and disturbed patients. With the discovery of antianxiety agents (e.g., benzodiazepines) the drugs previously used as sedative–hypnotics have become less important in their role as daytime sedatives. The principal role of the sedative–hypnotics remains to induce sleep, a stronger form of depression. By virtue of their general CNS depressant properties, depending on the dose and route of administration, most sedative–hypnotic drugs can produce any degree of depression from daytime sedation to general anesthesia, and even death caused by respiratory collapse. As a result the most important common danger of sedative–hypnotics is that they are frequently used in suicide attempts. Yet another problem common to sedative–hypnotic drugs is the danger of developing physical dependence, resulting from their repeated use.

It appears that sedative–hypnotic drugs do not exert their effects by attachment to specific receptors for the following reasons. First, there is no specific antagonist that would reverse the action of hypnotics. Second, there is a lack of structural specificity since a wide variety of chemical compounds exert sedative–hypnotic properties. Third, the sedative–hypnotics lack stereospecificity; i.e., the stereoisomers display approximately the same activities (83, 84). This last point is currently under intensive investigation, however.

Soon after the discovery of the reticular activating system (85) it was postulated that the states of wakefulness and sleep are correlated with levels of activation of the reticular formation even though the direct pathways connecting the sensory organs with the cortex which travel through thalamic relays are unaffected. A decrease in the reticular activity which characterizes wakefulness brings about sleep. Supporting evidence for this theory was presented by awakening sleeping animals through stimulation of electrodes implanted in their reticular activating system (86).

On the other hand, evidence has also been presented for the existence of sleep-producing centers by inducing sleep through stimulation of electrodes implanted in the thalamus (87).

In principle, a sedative–hypnotic agent can induce sleep by either one of the following two mechanisms: by damping the activity of the reticular activating system or by stimulating the thalamic area. It appears that most sedative–hypnotics exert their action by deactivating the reticular activating system. An important exception is the class of benzodiazepines, which are known to exert an action in three distinct anatomic areas, the reticular activating system, the spinal center, and the limbic system.

Arbitrarily, the sedative–hypnotics may be classified as follows:

1. Barbiturates
2. Benzodiazepine hypnotics
3. Other cyclic nitrogen-containing hypnotics
4. Acyclic hypnotics containing nitrogen
5. Alcohols and aldehydes
6. Miscellaneous sedative–hypnotics
   a. Bromides
   b. Acids and esters
   c. Antihistamines and anticholinergics
   d. Heterocyclics
   e. Sulfones
   f. Plant extracts
   g. Endogenous sleep factors

8 BARBITURATES

8.1 History

In 1903 Fischer and von Mehring (88) decided to synthesize 5,5-diethylbarbituric acid as a hypnotic candidate based on the rationale that other compounds containing a quaternary carbon, e.g., sulfonal and amylene hydrate, displayed hypnotic properties.

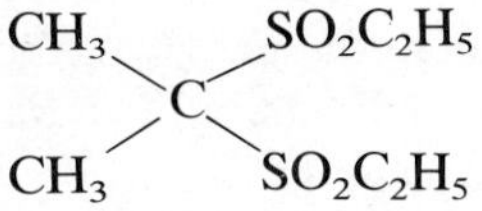

CH₃ ... SO₂C₂H₅ CH₃CH₂ ... OH
\ /   \ /
 C   C
/ \   / \
CH₃   SO₂C₂H₅   CH₃   CH₃

Sulfonal 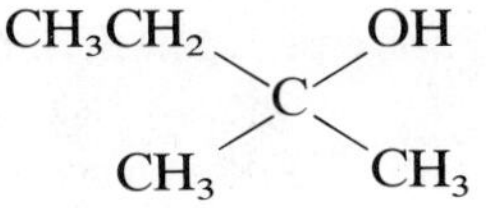   Amylene hydrate

Since 5,5-diethylbarbituric acid turned out to be a powerful hypnotic drug, Fischer and von Mehring provided one of the first examples of rational drug design. This drug is still in use. Since 1903 hundreds of barbiturates have been synthesized (89) but only a few turned out to be useful. It was not until Sandberg's publication (90) that the activity or inactivity of the barbiturates has been rationalized on the basis of two criteria, acidity and liqid/water partition coefficient.

8.2 Acidity

According to Sandberg (90) the acidity of the barbiturate must be within certain limits in order to possess hypnotic activity. On the basis of acidity values, barbiturates comprise two classes, hypnotics and inactive compounds.

Hypnotic class

  5,5-Disubstituted barbituric acids
  5,5-Disubstituted thiobarbituric acids
  1,5,5-Trisubstituted barbituric acids

Inactive class

  1-Substituted barbituric acids
  5-Substituted barbituric acids
  1,3-Disubstituted barbituric acids
  1,5-Disubstituted barbituric acids
  1,3,5,5-Tetrasubstituted barbituric acids

It should be noted, however, that although members of the 1,3,5,5-tetrasubstituted

barbituric acid series *per se* are inactive compounds, their metabolites belonging to the 1,5,5-trisubstituted barbituric acid class are hypnotics. If metabolic conversion of a 1,3,5,5-tetrasubstituted barbituric acid to a 1,5,5-trisubstituted one takes place rapidly, administration of the former may still produce a hypnotic effect.

The acidity of the various types of barbituric acids has been attributed to lactam–lactim and keto–enol tautomerism:

O   OH
‖ |
—C—NH— ⇌ —C=N—

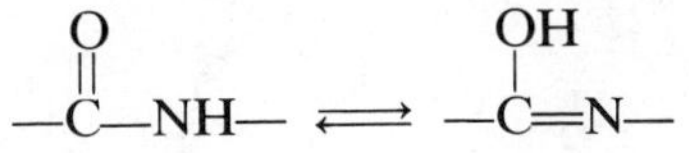

Lactam   Lactim

O   OH
‖ |
—C—CH₂— ⇌ —C=CH—

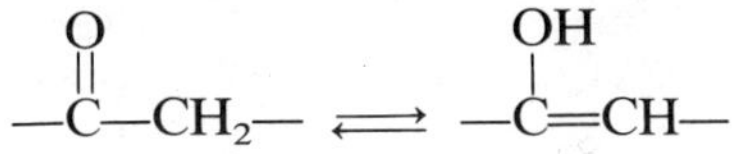

Keto   Enol

In the unsubstituted barbituric acid, all four hydrogens can be exchanged for deuterium, since all four hydrogen atoms may be involved in tautomerism:

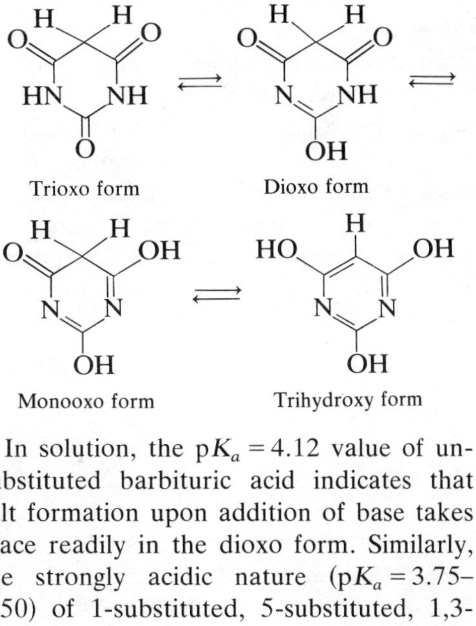

Trioxo form   Dioxo form

Monooxo form   Trihydroxy form

In solution, the $pK_a = 4.12$ value of unsubstituted barbituric acid indicates that salt formation upon addition of base takes place readily in the dioxo form. Similarly, the strongly acidic nature ($pK_a = 3.75$–5.50) of 1-substituted, 5-substituted, 1,3-disubstituted, and 1,5-disubstituted barbituric acids indicate that in solution salt formation takes place readily in the dioxo form.

The dissociation constants of 5,5-disub-stituted barbituric acids and 1,5,5-trisub-stituted barbituric acids (pK_a 7.1–8.1) reveal a mildly acidic nature for these types of compounds. The reduced acidity of these compounds can be ascribed to the fact that they exist predominantly in the trioxo form. Nevertheless, addition of a strong base converts these compounds into the salt of the dioxo tautomer:

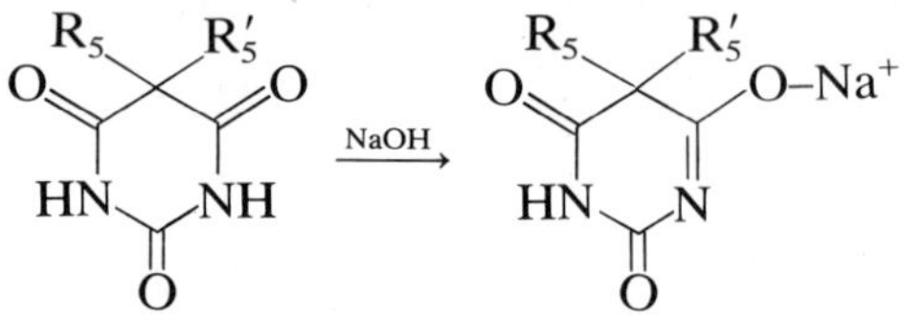

Trioxo tautomer of 5,5-disubstituted barbituric acid

Sodium salt of 5,5-disubstituted barbituric acid

The presence of the trioxo tautomer in the crystalline state can be determined by X-ray diffraction measurements (91, 92), and evidence for the existence of the dioxo tautomeric forms at various pH values can be obtained from the inspection of ultraviolet spectra.

It is interesting to note that the 5,5-disubstituted barbituric acids can undergo a second ionization (93) with a pK value of 11.7–12.7 (94). In order to convert a 5,5-disubstituted barbituric acid into a dialkali metal salt a strong base in anhydrous medium is required, as recently reported (95). The dialkali metal salt formation takes place in the monooxo form:

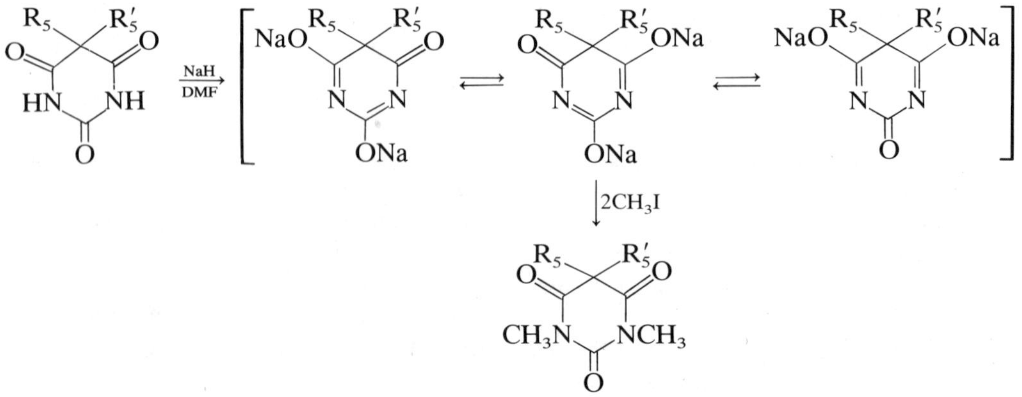

The methylation at the nitrogen rather than at the oxygen can be established with the help of ultraviolet spectroscopy. If in the last case dimethylation took place at the oxygen giving rise to enol (lactim) ethers, then the ultraviolet spectrum of the product should resemble that of the monooxo tautomeric form:

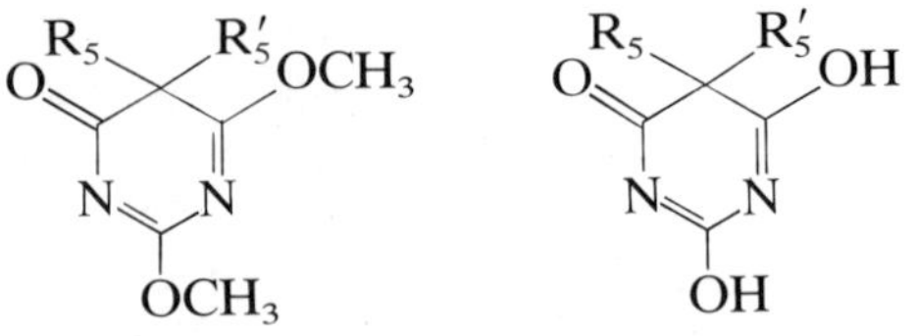

Dioxygen methylated form

Monooxo tautomeric form

On the other hand, if dimethylation took place at the two nitrogens, the ultraviolet spectrum of the product should resemble that of the trioxo tautomeric form:

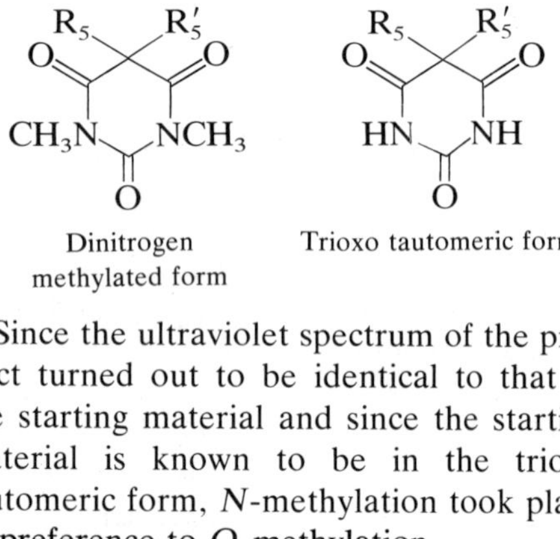

Dinitrogen methylated form

Trioxo tautomeric form

Since the ultraviolet spectrum of the product turned out to be identical to that of the starting material and since the starting material is known to be in the trioxo tautomeric form, N-methylation took place in preference to O-methylation.

Alkylation at the nitrogen, which takes place in preference to oxygen alkylation in other classes of barbituric acids as well, leads to weaker acids. If the pK_a of a representative 5,5-disubstituted barbituric acid is 7.3, the pK_a of the N-alkylated derivative is approximately 8.3.

It is possible to calculate the amount of barbituric acid in the undissociated form at various pH values from the equation

$$\log \frac{[A^-]}{[HA]} = pH - pK_a$$

where $[A^-]$ = Concentration of the anion

$[HA]$ = Concentration of the undissociated acid

The values of several examples are given in Table 54.1.

Among the given examples only 5-ethyl-5-phenylbarbituric acid and 1-methyl-5-ethyl-5-phenylbarbituric acid have a proper ratio of dissociated and undissociated forms present at physiological pH to enable them to cross the blood–brain barrier and exert an effect in the central nervous system.

Table 54.1 Percentage of Various Barbituric Acids in Undissociated Form at Physiological pH (7.4)

Compound	pK_a	Percentage of Undissociated Form
Barbituric acid	4.12	0.05
5-Phenylbarbituric Acid	3.75	0.02
5-ethyl-5-phenyl barbituric acid	7.29	43.00
1-Methyl-5-ethyl-5-phenylbarbituric acid	7.80	61.50
1,3-Diethyl-5-ethyl-5-phenylbarbituric acid	0	100

8.3 Lipid–Water Solubility

If the first criterion based on the acidity value is satisfied, a candidate barbituric acid derivative belonging to one of the active classes (e.g., 5,5-disubstituted barbituric acid, 5,5-disubstituted 2-thiobarbituric acid, or 1,5,5-trisubstituted barbituric acid) must still satisfy the second criterion concerning its lipid/water partition coefficient. In fact the partition coefficients of the most active sedative–hypnotics fall within certain values (96).

It has been found that the following structural features are required for hypnotic activity:

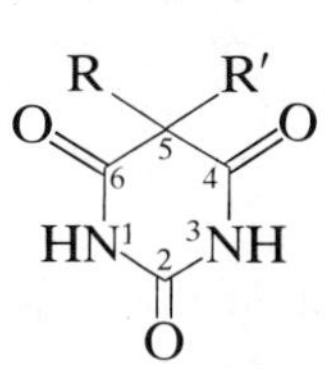

1. Hypnotic activity increases with lipid solubility until the total number of carbon atoms of both substituents at C-5 is between 6 and 10. Further increase in the sum of the carbon atoms decreases hypnotic activity in spite of further increase in lipid solubility, indicating that lipid solubility must remain within certain limits.

2. Within the same series the branched chain isomer has greater lipid solubility and hypnotic activity and shorter duration of action than the straight chain isomer. The greater the branching, the greater the activity (pentobarbital is a more potent hypnotic than amobarbital). The steroisomers, however, have approximately the same potencies.

3. Within the same series the unsaturated allyl, alkenyl, and cycloalkenyl derivatives are more hypnotic than the corresponding saturated analogs with the same number of carbon atoms. Alicyclic or aromatic substituents are more potent

than the aliphatic substituents with the same number of carbon atoms.

4. Conversion of a 5,5-disubstituted barbituric acid by methylation to a 1,5,5-trisubstituted barbituric acid does not change hypnotic activity in a significant manner.

5. Introduction of a polar substituent (OH, NH_2, COOH, CO, RNH, SO_3H) into the aromatic group at C-5 decreases lipid solubility and potency.

6. Replacement of the oxygen at C-2 by a sulfur atom increases lipid solubility and produces quick onset and short duration of action but replacement of more than one carbonyl oxygen by sulfur decreases hypnotic activity, again indicating that lipid solubility can not be increased beyond limits.

These results show that in spite of some major structural changes in the barbiturate molecule hypnotic activity can be preserved. This again points out the fact that barbiturates exert hypnotic activity in a nonspecific and nonstereospecific manner.

8.4 Metabolism

The principal site of metabolic inactivation is in the liver. In the metabolism the lipophilic character of the barbiturates decreases, which in turn decreases the ability of the barbiturates to penetrate into the central nervous system. There are four primary metabolic processes that may take place.

1. Oxidation of substituents attached to C-5 is the most important pathway of metabolism for the barbiturates. The oxidative processes may yield alcohols, ketones, and carboxylic acids. For example, thiopental is oxidized to a hydroxy compound and carboxylic acid (97) as shown (see below).

   The oxidative process may also yield phenols. If the barbiturate has a phenyl group attached to C-5, by far the most important metabolic product is the *p*-hydroxyphenyl derivative, which has been shown to be formed through the intermediate epoxide (98). For example,

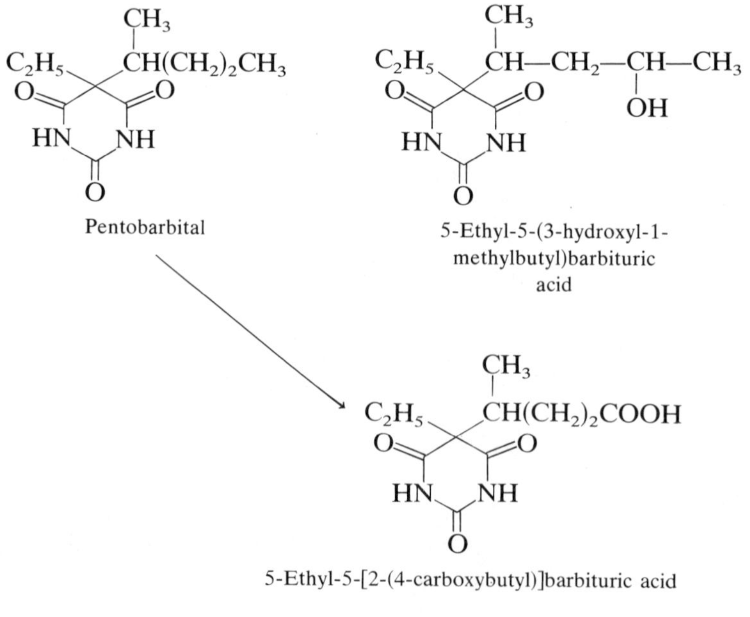

Pentobarbital

5-Ethyl-5-(3-hydroxyl-1-methylbutyl)barbituric acid

5-Ethyl-5-[2-(4-carboxybutyl)]barbituric acid

phenobarbital is metabolized to *p*-hydroxyphenobarbital.

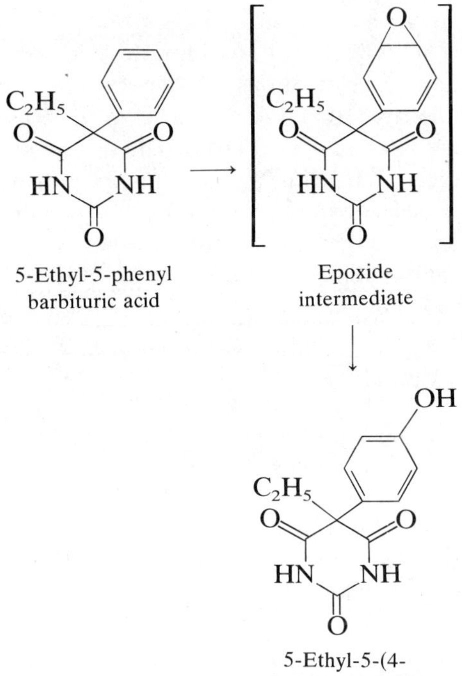

5-Ethyl-5-phenyl barbituric acid → Epoxide intermediate

5-Ethyl-5-(4-hydroxyphenyl)-barbituric acid

The oxygenated metabolites (alcohols, phenols, ketones, carboxylic acids) may be excreted in the urine in the free form or conjugated with glucuronic or sulfuric acid.

2. *N*-Dealkylation (*N*-demethylation) is an important metabolic pathway for *N*-substituted barbiturates (99):

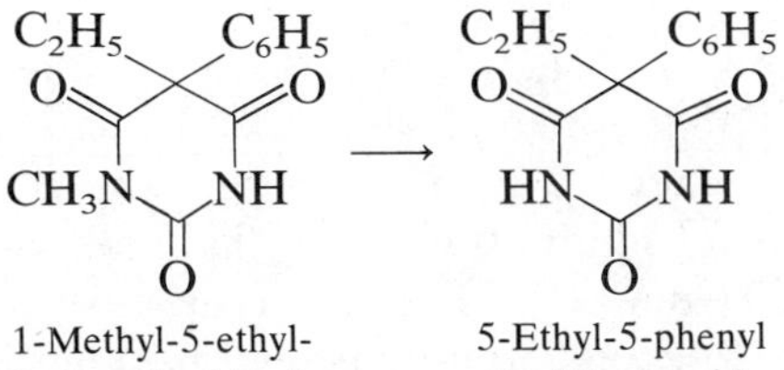

1-Methyl-5-ethyl-5-phenylbarbituric acid → 5-Ethyl-5-phenyl barbituric acid

Mephobarbital (1 methyl-5-ethyl-5-phenylbarbituric acid) is metabolized to phenobarbital (5-ethyl-5-phenylbarbituric acid), which is subject to further metabolic processes.

3. Desulfurization of 2-thiobarbiturates is a common metabolic process. For example, pentobarbital (5-ethyl-5-(1-methylbutyl)barbituric acid) is one of the metabolic products of thiopental (5-ethyl-5-(1-methylbutyl)-2-thiobarbituric acid).

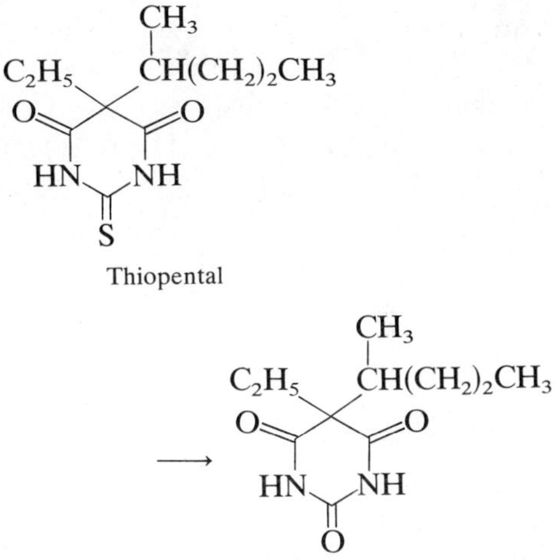

Thiopental

Pentobarbital

4. Ring scission of the barbituric ring leads to the formation of acetamides or acetylurea derivatives.

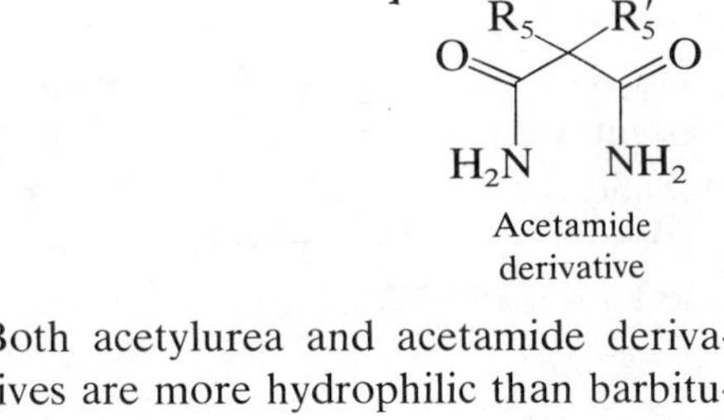

Acetylurea derivative

Acetamide derivative

Both acetylurea and acetamide derivatives are more hydrophilic than barbiturates.

The biotransformations of barbiturates have been recently reviewed (100, 101).

8.5   Mechanism of Action

Barbituric acid derivatives exert a multiplicity of effects in various anatomic formations. Most important is the effect of barbiturates in the central nervous system. In sufficient concentrations barbiturates depress the excitatory component of synaptic transmission in the reticular activating system. The general CNS-depressant properties of barbiturates are evident from the fact that increasing doses of barbiturates impart increasing degrees of CNS depression (from sedation to anesthesia). Depression has been attributed to the stabilization of the postsynaptic membrane (102) or, alternatively, to a decrease in the amount of transmitters released presynaptically (103). Adrenergic (104), serotonergic (105), and cholinergic (106) transmitters have been implicated.

Barbiturates prolong the inhibitory action of γ-aminobutyric acid (GABA). It has been suggested that the effects of barbiturates on synaptic transmission are caused by an alteration in the postsynaptic sensitivity of the neurons to excitatory and inhibitory transmitters. In high concentrations barbiturates activate GABA receptors, thereby enhancing pre- and postsynaptic inhibition (107).

It should also be noted that very small doses of barbiturates may also produce a paradoxical effect and cause hyperexcitation. This effect can be ascribed to the fact that although the concentration of the barbiturates in the reticular activating system is too small to inhibit the excitatory component of synaptic transmission, the concentration of the barbiturates is large enough to impede the inhibitory processes in the direct pathways which connect the sensory organs to the cortex through thalamic relays. The net result is exacerbation of the excitatory processes. This last phenomenon underlies the importance of the equilibrium of the neural functions of the brain between excitatory and inhibitory processes in the normal state. The role of CNS-depressant drugs is to bring about a general depressant effect of an overexcited state.

The effects of barbiturates in other anatomic formations (limbic system, thalamic, hypothalamic, cortical systems, etc.) have been reviewed (105). The biochemical effects of barbiturates are manifested by a decrease in both energy-yielding reactions (oxidative metabolic processes) and functional activities in the brain. Another very important biochemical effect of barbiturates is the induction of liver microsomal enzymes (108, 109). This effect has been correlated with the well-known rapid development of tolerance to barbiturates (110). The biochemical activities of barbiturates have been reviewed (111, 112).

The effects of barbiturates on sleep pattern is very pronounced. Administration of a barbiturate for the first time reduces the time required to fall asleep and the number of awakenings during the night and prolongs sleeping time. Initially the REM sleep is reduced but only to a small extent. On the other hand, chronic administration of barbiturates produces a severe decrease in REM sleep which lasts as long as the drug is taken (113). Upon withdrawal of the barbiturate a rebound REM sleep is observed in man that often is characterized by nightmares (114). In addition, frequent awakenings take place, with longer and longer time needed to fall asleep again. The insomnia produced by drug withdrawal can be controlled by continuing barbiturate administration, but the sleep pattern is different from that of natural sleep and the patient is not better off than he or she was before chronic administration of the barbiturate had begun (115). In order to improve sleep the dose of barbiturate may be gradually increased, which may eventually produce chronic intoxication (116). It may take several weeks after drug withdrawal for the effects of intoxication to disappear (114, 117).

Table 54.2 Sedative–Hypnotic Barbiturates in Clinical Use in the United States and Europe

Barbituric Acid	Generic Name	Trade Name	R_5	R_5'	Other Modifications	Duration of Action, hr	Onset of Action, hr	Average Adult Hypnotic Dose, g
5-Ethyl-5-isopentyl	Amobarbital	Amytal	C_2H_5	$(CH_3)_2CHCH_2CH_2$		2–8	0.25–0.5	0.1–0.3
5-Allyl-5-isopropyl	Aprobarbital	Alurate	$CH_2=CHCH_2$	$(CH_3)_2CH$		2–8	0.25–0.5	0.065–0.13
5,5-Diethyl	Barbital	Nevronidia	C_2H_5	C_2H_5		4–12	0.5–1	0.3–0.5
5-(1-Cyclohexen-1-yl)-1,5-dimethyl	Hexobarbital	Sombulex	CH_3	$(CH_2)_4CH=C—$	1-CH_3	1–4	0.25	0.25–0.4
5-Ethyl-1-methyl-5-phenyl	Mephobarbital	Mebaral	C_5H_5	C_6H_5	1-CH_3	1–4	0.25	
5-Allyl-5-(1-methyl-2-pentynyl)	Methohexital	Brevital	$CH_2=CHCH_2$	$CH_3CH_2C\equiv CCH(CH_3)$	1-CH_3			
5-Ethyl-5-(1-methyl-butyl)	Pentobarbital	Nembutal	C_2H_5	$CH_3(CH_2)_2CH(CH_3)$		2–4	0.5	0.1–0.2
5-Ethyl-5-phenyl	Phenobarbital	Luminal	C_2H_5	C_6H_5		4–12	0.5–1	0.1–0.2
5-Isopropyl-5-ethyl	Probarbital	Ipral	C_2H_5	$(CH_3)_2CH$		4–12	0.5–1	0.12–0.25
5-Allyl-5-(1-methyl-butyl)	Secobarbital	Seconal	$CH_2=CHCH_2$	$CH_3(CH_2)_2CH(CH_3)$		1–4	0.25	0.1–0.2
5-Allyl-5-sec-butyl	Talbutal	Lotusate	$CH_2=CHCH_2$	$CH_3CH_2CH(CH_3)$		2–4	0.5	0.12
5-Allyl-5-(1-methyl-butyl)-2-thio	Thiamylal	Surital	$CH_2=CHCH_2$	$CH_3(CH_2)_2CH(CH_3)$	2-S			
5-Ethyl-5-(1-methyl-butyl)-2-thio	Thiopental	Pentothal	C_2H_5	$CH_3(CH_2)_2CH(CH_3)$	2-S			

Table 54.3 Sedative–Hypnotic Barbiturates in Clinical Use Outside the United States

Barbituric Acid	Generic Name	Trade Name	R_5	R_5'	Other Modifications	Duration of Action, hr	Onset of Action, hr	Average Adult Hypnotic Dose, g
5,5-Diallyl	Allobarbital	Dial, Curral	$CH_2=CHCH_2$	$CH_2=CHCH_2$		2–8	0.25–0.05	0.1–0.3
5-(2-Bromoallyl-5-allyl	Brallo Barbital	Vespo erone	$CH_2=\overset{\mid}{C}-CH_2$ Br	$CH_2CH=CH_2$		2–4		0.15
5-sec-Butyl-5-ethyl	Butabarbital	Butisol	C_2H_5	$CH_3CH_2CH(CH_3)$		2–4	0.5	0.1
5-Allyl-5-iso-butyl	Butalbital	Sandoptal	$CH_2=CHCH_2$	$(CH_3)_2CHCH_2$		2–4	0.5	0.2–0.4
5-(2-Bromoallyl)-5-sec-butyl	Butallylonal	Pernoston	$CH_2=CBrCH_2$	$CH_3CH_2CH(CH_3)$		2–4	0.5	0.2
5-Butyl-5-ethyl	Butethal	Neonal	C_2H_5	$n\text{-}C_4H_9$		4–12	0.5–1	0.05–0.1
5-Crotyl-5-ethyl	Crotyl barbital	Melidorm	C_2H_5	$CH_2-CH=CHCH_3$		2–4		0.25
5-(1-Cyclohexen-1-yl)-5-ethyl	Cyclobarbital	Phanodorm	C_2H_5	$(CH_2)_4CH=C-$		2–8	0.25–0.5	0.1–0.2
5-Allyl-5-(2-cyclo-penten-1-yl)	Cyclopentenyl-allylbarbituric acid	Cyclopal	$CH_2=CHCH_2$	$(CH_2)_2CH=CHCH$		2–4	0.5	0.12–0.25
5-(1-Cyclohepten-1-yl)-5-ethyl	Heptabarbital	Medomin	C_2H_5	$(CH_2)_5CH=C-$		2–4	0.5	0.1–0.4
5,5-Diethyl-1-methyl	Metharbital		C_2H_5	C_2H_5	1-CH_3			
5-(1-Methylbutyl)-5-[2-(methylthio)-ethyl]-2-thio	Methitural	Neraval	$CH_3SCH_2CH_2$	$CH_3(CH_2)_2CH(CH_3)$	2-S			
1-Methyl-5-(2-bromoallyl)-5-isopropyl	Narcobarbital		$CH_2C=CH_2$ Br	$\underset{CH_3}{\overset{\mid}{CHCH_3}}$	1-CH_3	2–4		0.1–0.3
5-(2-Bromoallyl)-5-isopropyl	Propallylonal	Noctal	$CH_2-\overset{\mid}{C}=CH_2$ Br	$\underset{CH_3}{\overset{\mid}{CHCH_3}}$		2–4		0.1–0.3
5-Ethyl-5-(1-methyl-1-butenyl)	Vinbarbital	Delvinal	C_2H_5	$CH_3CH_2CH=C(CH_3)$		2–4	0.5	0.1–0.2
5-(1-Methyl-butyl)-5-vinyl	Vinylbital	Speda	$CH=CH_2$	$\underset{CH_3}{\overset{\mid}{CHC_3H_7}}$		2–8	0.5	0.15

8.6 Barbiturates Available on the Market

Table 54.2 provides a list of barbiturates available currently in the United States and in Europe; Table 54.3 lists the barbiturates available outside the United States.

9 BENZODIAZEPINE HYPNOTICS

Since benzodiazepines that are used primarily to relieve anxiety are described elsewhere in the book (Chapter 57) only those benzodiazepines are described here that are used primarily as sedative–hypnotics. The structures of these compounds are given in Table 54.4.

Since the mechanism of action of benzodiazepines is also described in Chapter 57, only the effects of benzodiazepines on the sleep pattern are discussed in this chapter. The contention that benzodiazepines have solved the problems usually associated with the use of barbiturates (117a) has been contradicted. It has been pointed out (118, 119) that in man benzodiazepines produce a considerable reduction in REM sleep and, in addition, an appreciable reduction of stage 3 and stage 4 sleep (118).

Table 54.4 Sedative–Hypnotic Benzodiazepines

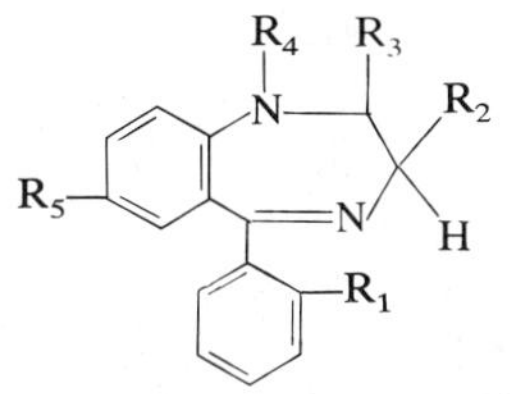

Benzodiazepine	R_1	R_2	R_3	R_4	R_5
Chlordesmethyl-diazepam	Cl	H	$=O$	H	Cl
Estazolam	H	H		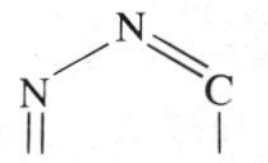 (triazole ring, N–$N=C$)	Cl
Flunitrazepam	F	H	$=O$	CH_3	NO_2
Flurazepam	F	H	$=O$	$(CH_2)_2N(C_2H_5)_2$	Cl
Fosazepam	H	H	$=O$	$(CH_2)P(CH_3)_2$ with $\downarrow O$	Cl
Lorazepam	Cl	OH	$=O$	H	Cl
Nimetazepam	H	H	$=O$	CH_3	NO_2
Nitrazepam	H	H	$=O$	H	NO_2
Nordiazepam	H	H	$=O$	H	Cl
Potassium clorazepate	H	COOK	OH OK	H	Cl
Quazepam	F	H	$=S$	CH_2CF_3	Cl
SAS 643	F	OH	$=O$	$(CH_2)_2OH$	Cl
Temazepam	H	OH	$=O$	CH_3	Cl
Triazolam	Cl	H		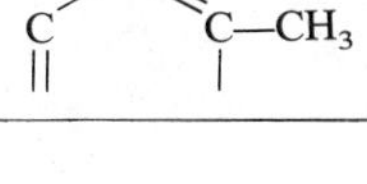 (triazole ring, $C=N$–N, C–CH_3)	Cl

Furthermore, it has also been reported that a distinction between barbiturates and benzodiazepines on the basis of withdrawal effects on the sleep pattern as documented by EEG measurements appears unwarranted (119a). On the other hand, it should also be noted that although in man larger doses of the benzodiazepines suppress REM sleep (114, 120, 121), the extent of REM sleep suppression is usually smaller with benzodiazepines than with any other type of hypnotic with the exception of chloral hydrate.

Benzodiazepine drugs are often taken in suicidal attempts but have rarely been fatal following even large overdosage. In this respect benzodiazepines possess a tremendous advantage over barbiturates and other classes of hypnotic drugs (122).

The validity of promoting a benzodiazepine as a hypnotic rather than an antianxiety agent has been questioned (123) in view of the pharmacological properties of benzodiazepines which fail to reveal any differences. On the basis of pharmacological data no prediction can be made as to which benzodiazepine in preference to others should be promoted specifically as a hypnotic. The only plausible explanation for promoting a benzodiazepine specifically as a hypnotic has been advanced on the basis of pharmacokinetic data. Namely, it has been suggested that only those benzodiazepines are suited as hypnotics that are rapidly detoxified and excreted (123).

Flurazepam, a benzodiazepine specifically promoted as a sleep inducer, is rapidly metabolized. However, the metabolites are pharmacologically more active than the parent compounds. It has been found that chronic administration of flurazepam leads to the accumulation of 1-desalkyl flurazepam for 7–10 days (124). This kinetic pattern is similar to that found with benzodiazepines used specifically as anxiolytics (125).

Benzodiazepines differ from the barbiturates in the site of their action. It is be-lieved, based on animal experiments, that barbiturates damp the cortical response to stimulation by an elevation of the arousal threshold in the reticular activating system (126). Benzodiazepines, on the other hand, have little effect on the arousal threshold; instead they exert a depressing effect on the hippocampus and other parts of the limbic system, thereby reducing alertness and vigilance and giving way to sleep (127–129).

Ideally, a hypnotic drug should not produce unwanted drowsiness or heavy-headedness upon awakening. Several studies in man have indicated that benzodiazepines produce morning aftereffects visible in EEG recordings. Nitrazepam (5–10 mg) and flurazepam (15–30 mg), for example, produce a shift to low voltage, high frequency activity in the EEG (130, 131) which is still present 12–18 hr after a single dose of the drug. There is disagreement whether benzodiazepine administration also produces an impairment of performance of intellectual and motor function. Several investigators observed impaired performance (130–133), whereas others have not confirmed these findings (134, 135). It is generally agreed, however, that even though the symptoms of hangover may not be recognized, benzodiazepines, like all other sedative–hypnotics, do produce psychomotor and EEG changes in many subjects on the morning after drug administration (123). Subjects given benzodiazepines should be warned of this fact.

The comparative evaluation of *chlordesmethyldiazepam* and *nordiazepam* in mice revealed that although only the former displays antistrychinine and spontaneous motor activity, both compounds possess narcosis potentiating muscle relaxant activity (136). Chlordesmethyldiazepam in man in 2 mg doses in a controlled trial produced a hangover effect and behavioral impairment, but no such effects were observed after a 1 mg dose of chlordesmethyldiazepam or a 100 mg dose of amylobarbital (137). The plasma levels of chlordesmethyldiazepam correlated well with sleep-inducing effects. In a single-blind study chlordesmethyldiazepam in 2 mg dose proved to be a highly effective hypnotic agent in 33 patients who suffered from long-lasting severe insomnia (138).

In a double-blind study involving 1139 patients *estazolam* in a 2 mg dose appeared to be equivalent to a 10 mg dose nitrazepam in efficacy. A higher dose of estazolam (4 mg) was more effective but also caused more incidence of side effects than a 10 mg dose of nitrazepam (139). The incidence of unsteadiness caused by 2 mg of estazolam was the same as that caused by 5 mg of nitrazepam (139).

In a double-blind crossover study estazolam (2 and 4 mg) was compared to nitrazepam (5 and 10 mg). Administration of 2 mg of estazolam prolonged total sleep time and decreased stage 1 and stage 2 sleep, whereas 4 mg of estazolam reduced stage 2 sleep and REM sleep. Nitrazepam (5 mg) produced prolongation of total sleep and a decrease in frequency of awakenings, whereas 10 mg of nitrazepam prolonged stage 2 sleep and reduced the total wakefulness during the night (140).

Flunitrazepam has been employed in 2 mg doses as a hypnotic drug before inhalation anesthesia (141), and the effects were compared to those produced by 250 mg of narcobarbital. Although a slower pulse rate and blood pressure was observed after flunitrazepam and a lower respiratory rate after narcobarbital, only minor differences (quicker onset of sleep with narcobarbital) were noted in the quality of the agents in the induction of anesthesia.

Orally administered flunitrazepam in man in 2 mg doses decreased REM sleeping time at the expense of a smaller number of REM periods and shifted it to the last two-thirds of the night (142). Flunitrazepam increased total sleep time and EEG fast activity and decreased REM sleep latency, sleep latency, total waking, and NREM sleep (142). Following withdrawal of flunitrazepam REM sleep rebound was observed only during the first one-third of the night (143). Essentially the same results were obtained in a single-blind, crossover design study, using 2 and 4 mg flunitrazepam nightly (144). Initially a reduction in REM sleep was observed. After 3 weeks of drug use, however, an internal compensation for REM sleep suppression took place; namely, in the second 3 hr of sleep an excess REM sleep was observed, whereas in the first 3 hr of sleep, REM sleep suppression persisted. On withdrawal of flunitrazepam there is a rebound excess of REM sleep. Flunitrazepam also decreases stage 3 and 4 sleep, an effect that persists during drug therapy. There is no rebound excess of NREM sleep (144). Administration of 1 mg of flunitrazepam in three consecutive nights decreased the total wake time and nightly awakenings. The REM sleep was not decreased but stage 3 and 4 sleep were moderately decreased (145). Following drug withdrawal, there was no rebound excess of NREM sleep. These authors have also examined the effects of 2 mg of flunitrazepam (233). They noted a marked decrease in time required to fall asleep, a marked decrease in the number of awakenings, no change in REM sleep time, and a marked decrease in stage 4 sleep. No REM or NREM rebound was observed after drug withdrawal (145). Flunitrazepam intravenously in 1, 2, and 4 mg doses was found to be an effective sleep-inducing agent (146). In a total of 290 patients in 2 mg doses flunitrazepam proved to be an effective hypnotic (147).

Flunitrazepam, 1 mg, was ineffective as a hypnotic (148). In 2 mg doses, flunitrazepam significantly improved both sleep induction and maintenance on short-term drug administration. Both REM and NREM sleep were significantly decreased, with the latter returning to base-line values following withdrawal of the drug and REM sleep showing a slight rebound effect (148).

On the other hand, flunitrazepam in both

1 and 2 mg doses was found to be superior to lorazepam (2.5 and 5 mg) and fosazepam (40, 60, and 80 mg) in a double-blind study consisting of 160 patients, including a placebo group. There were no objective parameters used in the evaluation of this study, however (149).

Intravenously administered flunitrazepam in 1–2 mg doses had an amnesia-producing action, indicating its usefulness as a preanesthetic agent (150).

Polygraphic sleep recordings indicated that 2 mg flunitrazepam reduced sleep latency and nocturnal awakenings, while prolonging latency time to the first REM phase. Deep sleep stages were prolonged and the duration of the REM phases were reduced slightly (151).

The efficacy of *flurazepam* in man has been demonstrated in a number of controlled studies. Flurazepam (15–30 mg) was found to be equipotent to 100 mg of secobarbital (152), 100 mg of pentobarbital (153), 50 mg of amobarbital (154), 500 mg of glutethimide (155, 156), 0.5–1.0 g of chloral hydrate (155–157), and 150–300 mg of methaqualone (157). But whereas chloral hydrate, glutethimide, methaqualone, and secobarbital were no longer effective after 4 weeks of nightly administration, flurazepam was effective during the entire 4 weeks of study.

On the one hand, it has been reported that low doses of flurazepam (10–15 mg) have little effect in man on either REM or NREM sleep (158, 159). On the other hand, Dement et al. (160) have reported a significant reduction in REM sleep duration as a result of either 15 or 30 mg of flurazepam administration. In agreement with Dement et al., Kales and Scharf reported that 30 mg of flurazepam, which is the normal adult dose, produced a moderate decrease in REM sleep and a marked decrease in eye movement density after short or intermediate term of drug use (161). At the same time stage 3 and stage 4 sleep was markedly reduced. With long-term use the reduction in REM sleep and eye movement density caused by flurazepam diminished but stage 3–stage 4 sleep remained markedly depressed (161). The efficacy of flurazepam in long-term use persisted. When flurazepam therapy was stopped, no rebound effect was noted in REM or NREM sleep duration or eye movement density (162). These facts reduce the likelihood of drug dependence to be associated with flurazepam.

In a comprehensive study extended over a 6 year period, the safety of flurazepam was evaluated in 2542 patients (163). The clinical efficacy of flurazepam as a hypnotic appeared to be substantially greater at doses of 30 mg than at doses of 15 mg. None of the adverse reactions were serious, but toxicity increased with age, especially in the higher dose (163).

Fosazepam administration improved subjective sleep quality but the feeling of morning vitality was impaired (164). Fosazepam increased the duration of sleep and decreased the number of awakenings but decreased the duration of REM and stage 3 and 4 sleep (164). Upon withdrawal of fosazepam, anxiety, impaired concentration, and a decreased morning vitality was observed. In another study both fosazepam (60–80 mg) and diazepam (5–10 mg) increased sleeping time and decreased the time required to fall asleep. The number of awakenings was also decreased, causing an improved feeling of well-being on the following day. On the following night the patients treated with fosazepam had a decreased duration of stage 1 and stage 4 and an increased duration of stage 2 sleep. It was suggested that fosazepam may be especially useful in inducing sleep in subjects with disorders of sleep secondary to psychopathology (165).

Fosazepam in a dose of 100 mg is very similar to 10 mg of nitrazepam in hypnotic effects, except that morning drowsiness and hangover effects are less pronounced after fosazepam (166). REM sleep and stage 3 and 4 sleep were decreased during fosazepam treatment (166).

Lorazepam is a potent and satisfactory preanesthetic sedative with amnesic properties, well tolerated by patients. The sedative effect of 4 mg lorazepam in man was equivalent to that produced by 100 mg of pentobarbital (167). In a controlled study lorazepam in 2 and 4 mg doses was comparable in efficacy to a 30 mg dose of flurazepam with regard to onset of sleep, depth of sleep, and number of awakenings (168). A clearly hypnotic effect was also observed in patients with acute anxiety crises after intravenous injection of 3 mg lorazepam (169). Lorazepam in doses of 1–6 mg day produced improvement of anxiety in proportionately more patients than 10–30 mg day doses of diazepam. Both compounds were well tolerated (170).

Electroencephalographic and behavioral analysis of *nimetazepam* in the cat revealed that changes induced by nimetazepam were very similar to those induced by nitrazepam (171).

Nitrazepam was the first benzodiazepine promoted specifically as a sedative–hypnotic (172–174). Nitrazepam in doses as low as 5–10 mg produces a hypnotic effect in man comparable to a 100–200 mg dose of amobarbital (175–177), 50–200 mg dose of butarbital (133, 178, 179), 100–200 mg dose of secobarbital (180), and 250–500 mg dose of glutethimide (181). Nitrazepam suppressed REM sleep (182) in man but the extent of suppression decreased with time (183). Sleep is longer lasting and less broken while using nitrazepam and no tolerance was obvious after 2 months of nitrazepam use (184). After stopping nitrazepam there is a rebound of REM sleep, which reaches a maximum in 1–2 weeks (185). Complete recovery after nitrazepam use takes 3–6 weeks (183). Nitrazepam also produces hangover effects with impairment of psychomotor performance and difficulty in falling asleep that may be longer lasting than those produced by sodium amobarbital (132). It was also found that although nitrazepam also reduced stage 3 and 4 sleep, the secretion of growth hormone during stage 3 and 4 sleep was not adversely affected (184).

The effects of *nordiazepam* and a precursor, *potassium clorazepate*, on sleep were evaluated in man (186). A dose of 5 or 10 mg nordiazepam or 15 mg of potassium clorazepate increased total sleep time and the number of awakenings, whereas the time required to fall asleep was decreased. A dose of 5 mg of nordiazepam had no effect on the duration of sleep stages. Nordiazepam (10 mg) and potassium clorazepate (15 mg) decreased the duration of stage 1 sleep and increased the duration of stage 2 sleep. During the recovery night stage 1 sleep was reduced and stage 2 sleep was increased. No effects on stage 3 sleep were observed but stage 4 sleep appeared to be suppressed. No effects were observed on REM sleep (186).

Nordiazepam in 45 patients in 10 and 20 mg doses as well as amobarbital in 200 mg dose showed significant hypnotic effects with only 20 mg nordiazepam and 200 mg amobarbital producing hangover effects (187).

Clorazepate in 22.5 mg daily doses administered for 8 days decreased REM sleep, stage 4 sleep, sleep latency, and total waking (188), whereas total sleep time was increased. During recovery, REM sleep and sleep latency were increased (188).

Quazepam (SCH 16134) is a benzodiazepine-2-thione specifically positioned as a sedative–hypnotic (189, 190). Since one of the primary processes of metabolism of benzodiazepines involves N-dealkylation and further oxidation to yield a mixture of compounds possessing various activities, the trifluoroethyl group was incorporated into the structure with the hope of obtaining a compound more resistant to N-dealkylation (191).

In a double-blind, crossover study against placebo 10 subjects received 10, 25, or 50 mg quazepam (190). All dosages reduced sleep latency and REM sleep. Stage 3 and 4 sleep remained unaffected (190).

In a controlled study in man the drug SAS 643 (5 mg) was equivalent to a 15 mg dose of flurazepam in terms of sleep induction time, sleeping time, and quality of sleep. Moreover, SAS 643 caused significantly less hangover effect compared to that caused by flurazepam (192).

Short-term administration of *temazepam* in 10 and 20 mg doses in six subjects reduced the duration of stage 1 and 2 sleep but not that of stage 3 and 4 and REM sleep. The subjects reported an improved quality of sleep (193). Temazepam has the advantage of having a short half-life (194). It is metabolized, among others, to oxazepam. In a controlled study temazepam in a mean dose of 13.2 mg/night compared favorably with a mean dose of 5.2 mg of nitrazepam in terms of quality, depth, and duration of sleep, number of awakenings, and patient satisfaction (195). In another study a 20 mg dose of temazepam was found to be equivalent to a 200 mg dose of amylobarbital in terms of onset quality and duration of sleep, but temazepam produced significantly less daytime dozing and morning hangover (196). Temazepam (20 mg dose) in man was equivalent to 5 mg of nitrazepam and 100 mg of amylobarbital but did not impair early morning behavior following nighttime medication (197).

Short-, intermediate-, and long-term administration of 30 mg temazepam was found to be ineffective in sleep induction and sleep maintenance therapy (198). On the other hand, temazepam in 10–30 mg daily doses was found to be effective, well accepted, well tolerated, and safe for general use in adults (199). This finding was confirmed in a multicenter trial in general practice (200).

Triazolam (0.5 mg) was compared with flurazepam (30 mg) and placebo in a double-blind study in 48 patients and was found to be better than the placebo in duration of sleep, onset of sleep, nocturnal awakenings, and quality of sleep (201). Flurazepam was better than the placebo in only two parameters, nocturnal awakenings and quality of sleep. Triazolam was superior to flurazepam in sleep onset and duration of sleep (201). In another study triazolam (0.5 mg) produced a significantly faster onset and longer duration of sleep than 300 mg of methyprylon (202). In three separate double-blind studies involving 104 insomniac patients, triazolam in 0.5 mg doses was preferred by physician and patient evaluation over placebo, 30 mg of flurazepam, or 500 mg of chloral hydrate (203). In another study involving 35 patients, triazolam in 0.25 mg doses was preferred over a 15 mg dose of flurazepam (203). When compared to 30 mg flurazepam, triazolam in 0.5 mg doses was better in duration of sleep, onset of sleep, and restfulness in the morning parameters (204). Evaluation in a sleep laboratory in man revealed that both sleep induction and sleep maintenance improved with short-term use of 0.5 mg triazolam. At the end of 2 weeks of drug use, all the sleep efficacy parameters were close to base-line values, indicating that triazolam loses most of its effectiveness with intermediate-term use. During both short and intermediate drug administration REM, stage 3 and 4 sleep were significantly decreased, but following drug withdrawal there was no excess REM and NREM sleep rebound. Following drug withdrawal, however, sleep difficulty increased significantly above base-line levels, indicating that triazolam withdrawal is followed by a significant worsening of sleep (205). On the other hand, in the majority of studies, in 0.25–1 mg doses triazolam proved to be an effective hypnotic, usually causing small alterations in the sleep parameters (increase in REM sleep latency and total sleep time; decrease in REM sleep, sleep latency, and stage 3–4 time) (206–214).

10 OTHER CYCLIC NITROGEN-CONTAINING HYPNOTICS

These compounds were synthesized in the hope of finding more effective, less toxic, and less dependence-producing sedative–hypnotic drugs than barbiturates. These drugs are shown in Table 54.5.

The 2,4-dioxopiperidines are similar to but less active and better tolerated sedative hypnotics than the barbiturates.

Pyrithyldione is somewhat faster acting but shorter lasting than *dihyprylone* (215). It has been suggested that dihyprylone is metabolically converted to pyrithyldione (216). Since pyrithyldione may cause blood dyscrasia, these drugs have been displaced by *methyprylone*, which does not cause blood dyscrasia (217). Methyprylone is reported to be converted metabolically to *ethypicone*, a hypnotic in its own right, in a similar manner as dihyprylone is converted to pyrithyldione (218, 219). Methylprylone, in a 300 mg dose in man exerts a hypnotic effect similar to that of secobarbital (242). In therapeutic doses methyprylone suppresses REM sleep and upon withdrawal precipitates a REM sleep rebound (220). The side effects and toxicity of methyprylone are similar to those of the barbiturates (242). Methyprylone also produces dependence (221). The piperazinedione derivative *iminophenimide* is used as a hypnotic drug in nordic countries. *Glutethimide* in man in a 500 mg dose is as potent as 100 mg of pentobarbital (222). Initial reports that glutethimide possesses fewer side effects than barbiturates are no longer held valid. In the therapeutic dose of 500 mg, glutethimide significantly suppresses REM sleep (220). Withdrawal of glutethimide produces a rebound increase of REM sleep (223, 224). Like the barbiturates, glutethimide produces dependence. Glutethimide is now regarded as a general CNS depressant with no advantages over barbiturates. Recently a warning has been issued that severe glutethimide poisoning is an even greater danger to life than comparable barbiturate overdosage (225), with glutethimide having the highest mortality of all drug-induced comas (226). A derivative of glutethimide, 3-ethyl-3-methylglutarimide (bemegride), is claimed to be a barbiturate antidote (227). Bemegride, a CNS stimulant, is reported to reverse the hypnotic effect of glutethimide, methylprylone, and pyrithyldione (228).

Many compounds with a succinimide structure are useful anticonvulsant drugs (see Chapter 55). One succinimide, *fenimide*, was found in animals to be a potent hypnotic in preference to anticonvulsant properties (229).

Ethinazone and *mecloqualone*, two methaqualone-like quinazoline-type hypnotics (230, 231), exert a potent analgesic and antitussive activity (232) as well as a hypnotic activity in man which is similar to that of barbiturates.

Methaqualone in a 150 mg dose in man is as potent as 200 mg of cyclobarbital (233). Initially promoted as a nonbarbiturate and nonaddicting sedative–hypnotic which produces only insignificant suppression of REM sleep, methaqualone in fact is widely abused (234). Later it was also shown to reduce REM sleep (120). In addition methaqualone is known to produce delusions, hallucinations, disorientation with confusion (235), and even convulsions (234).

Clomethiazole [5-(2-chloroethyl)-4-methylthiazole] is a sedative–hypnotic with anticonvulsant effect. It has been used in the treatment of agitated states, alcoholic withdrawal symptoms, and delirium tremens (236, 237). Prolonged use of clomethiazole may lead to barbiturate type dependence (238). Clomethiazole administration may produce toxic effects, e.g., digestive disturbances, dizziness, nausea, and vomiting.

It has also been reported, however, that long-term therapy in geriatrics produced favorable effects in sleep latency, usually

Table 54.5   Nonbarbiturate and Nonbenzodiazepine Cyclic Nitrogen-Containing Sedative–Hypnotics

2,4-Dioxopiperidines Structure	Chemical Name	Generic Name
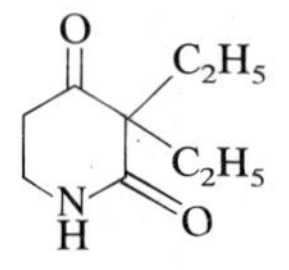	3,3-Diethyl-2,4-piperidinedione	Dihyprylone
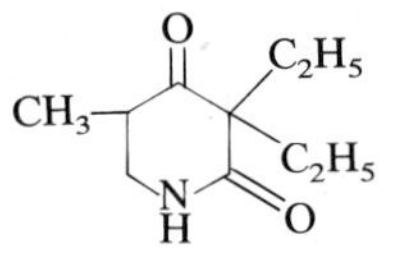	3,3-Diethyl-5-methyl-2,4-piperidinedione	Methyprylone
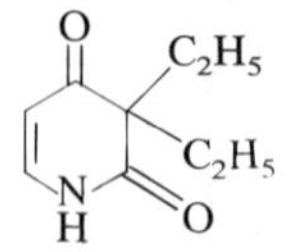	3,3-Diethyl-1,2,3,4-tetrahydropyridine-2,4-dione	Pyrithyldione
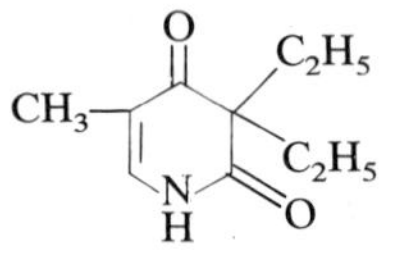	3,3-Diethyl-5-methyl-1,2,3,4-tetrahydropyridine-2,4-dione	Ethypicone
2,6-Dioxopiperazines		
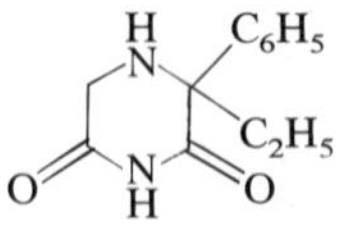	3-Ethyl-3-phenyl-2,6-piperazinedione	Iminophenimide
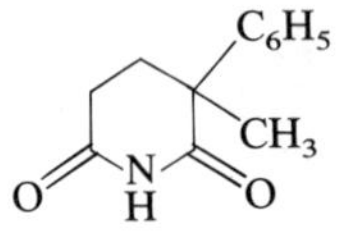	2-Ethyl-2-phenyl glutarimide	Glutethimide
Succinimides		
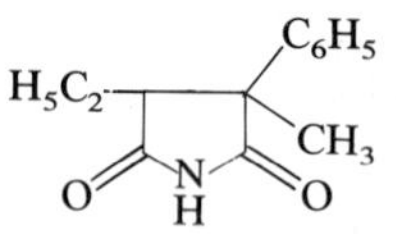	3-Ethyl-2-methyl-2-phenylsuccinimide	Fenimide
4-Oxoquinazolines		
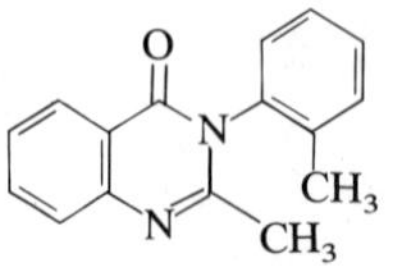	2-Methyl-3-o-tolyl-4(3H)-quinazolinone	Methaqualone

810

Table 54.5 (*Continued*)

2,4-Dioxopiperidines Structure	Chemical Name	Generic Name
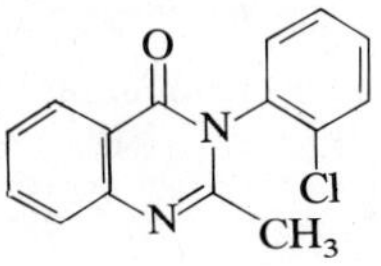	2-Methyl-*o*-chloro-phenyl-4(3*H*)-quina-zolinone	Mecloqualone
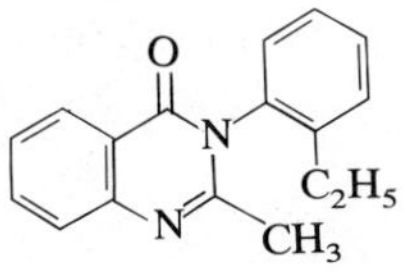	2-Methyl-*o*-ethyl phenyl-4(3*H*)-quina zolinone	Ethinazone

Thiazoles

| 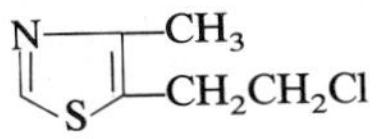 | 5-(2-Chloroethyl) 4-methylthiazole | Clomethiazole |

Oxadiazoles

| 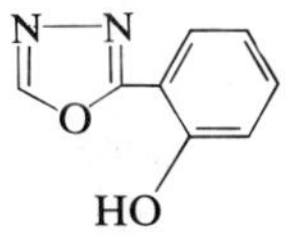 | 2-(*o*-Hydroxyphenyl)-1,3,4-oxadiazole | Fenadiazole |

after long-term, regular therapy. Hangover symptoms were not observed (239).

Fenadiazole (2-(*o*-hydroxyphenyl)-1,3,4-oxadiazole) is used primarily as a hypnotic agent in the treatment of nervous tension and frequent awakenings (240). It is used in 350 and 700 mg doses; it is well absorbed and rapidly metabolized. The effects of fenadiazole in 350 mg and 700 doses on the sleep pattern of man were investigated extensively (241). A 350 mg dose of fenadiazole produced a slight increase in sleep latency (time required to fall asleep), time awake after sleep onset, and movement time, and a decrease in percent sleep time. There were only very slight changes in the sleep pattern, with no effect on the duration of stage 3 and 4 sleep. The REM sleep was slightly suppressed, and the latency to

REM sleep was increased. A 700 mg dose of fenadiazole produced an increase in sleep latency and wakening time after sleep onset and a decrease in number of awakenings and movement time, but the percentage of sleep time was unaffected. At the same time the duration of stage 3 and 4 sleep was not affected. Unlike 350 mg of fenadiazole, which suppressed REM sleep, 700 mg of fenadiazole increased REM sleep and decreased latency to REM sleep, but the effects were very slight.

11 ACYCLIC HYPNOTICS CONTAINING NITROGEN

The importance of these types of sedative–hypnotics has diminished with time, since

Table 54.6   Acyclic Hypnotics Containing Nitrogens

Structure	Chemical Name	Generic Name
	Urethanes	
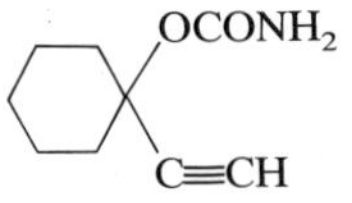 (cyclohexane with OCONH$_2$ and C≡CH)	1-Ethynyl-1-cyclo hexyl carbamate	Ethinamate
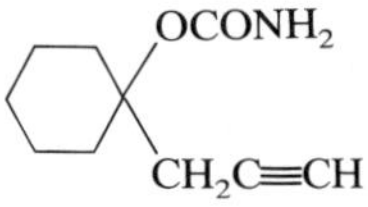 (cyclohexane with OCONH$_2$ and CH$_2$C≡CH)	1-(2-Propynyl)-1-cyclo hexyl carbamate	Hexapropymate
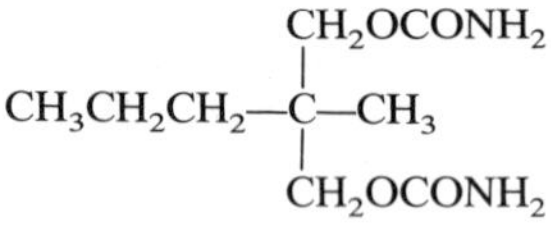 CH$_3$CH$_2$CH$_2$—C(—CH$_3$)(CH$_2$OCONH$_2$)(CH$_2$OCONH$_2$)	2-Methyl-2-n-propyl-1,3-propanediol carba mate	Meprobamate
	Amides	
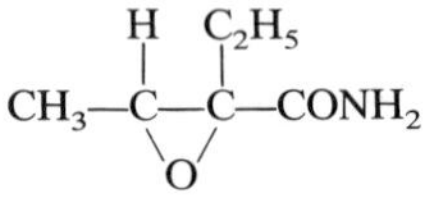 CH$_3$—C(H)—C(C$_2$H$_5$)—CONH$_2$ (epoxide O)	2,3-Epoxy-2-ethyl hexanamide	Oxanamide
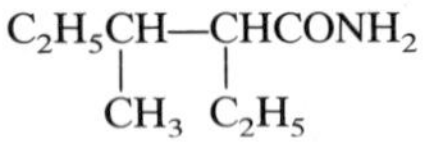 C$_2$H$_5$CH(CH$_3$)—CH(C$_2$H$_5$)CONH$_2$	2-Ethyl-3-methyl valeramide	Valnoctamide
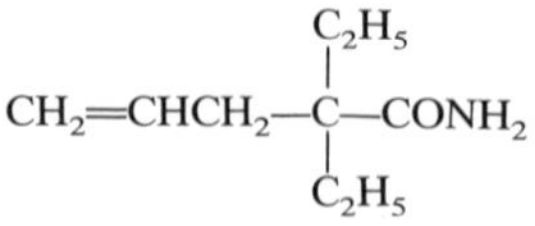 CH$_2$=CHCH$_2$—C(C$_2$H$_5$)(C$_2$H$_5$)—CONH$_2$	2,2-Diethyl-4-pentenamide	Diethylallyl-acetamide
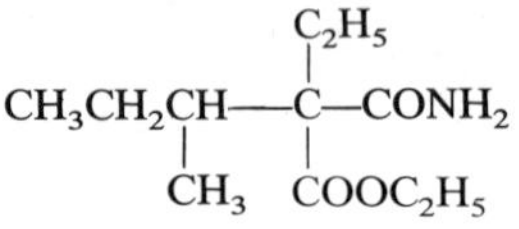 CH$_3$CH$_2$CH(CH$_3$)—C(C$_2$H$_5$)(COOC$_2$H$_5$)—CONH$_2$	2-Ethoxycarbonyl-2-ethyl-3-valeramide	Butesamide
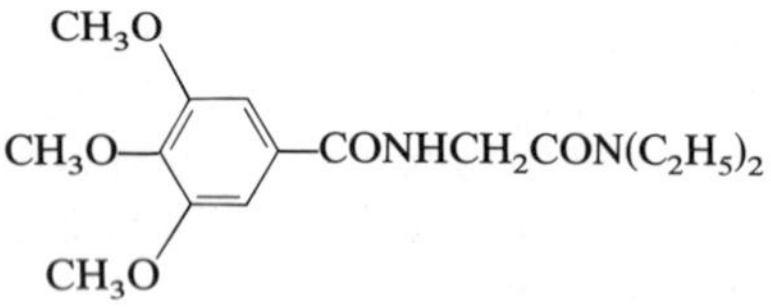 (3,4,5-trimethoxyphenyl)—CONHCH$_2$CON(C$_2$H$_5$)$_2$	α-[(3,4,5-Trimethoxy benzoyl)amino]-N,N-diethyl acetamide	Trimethobenz-glycine
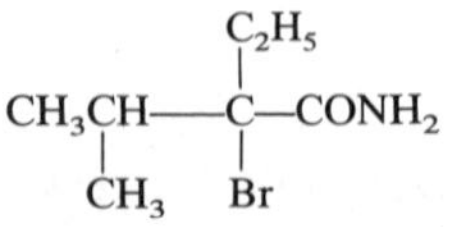 CH$_3$CH(CH$_3$)—C(C$_2$H$_5$)(Br)—CONH$_2$	2-Bromo-2-isopropyl butyramide	Ibrotamide
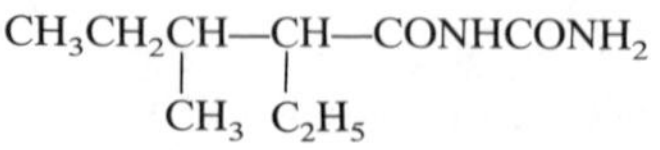 CH$_3$CH$_2$CH(CH$_3$)—CH(C$_2$H$_5$)—CONHCONH$_2$	(2-Ethyl-3-methylva leryl)urea	Capuride

Table 54.6 *(Continued)*

Structure	Chemical Name	Generic Name
$CH_3CH{=}\underset{\underset{C_2H_5}{\mid}}{C}{-}CONHCONH_2$	(2-Ethyl-*cis*-crotonyl) urea	Ectylurea
$CH_2{=}CH{-}CH_2{-}\underset{\underset{CH(CH_3)_2}{\mid}}{CH}{-}CHCONHCONH_2$	(2-Isopropyl-4-pen tenoyl)urea	Apronalide
$(CH_3)_2CH{-}\underset{\underset{Br}{\mid}}{CH}{-}CONHCONH_2$	(2-Bromo-3-methyl butyryl)urea	Bromvalurea
$(C_2H_5)_2{-}\underset{\underset{Br}{\mid}}{C}{-}CONHCONH_2$	(2-Bromo-2-ethyl butyryl)urea	Carbromal
$(C_2H_5)_2{-}\underset{\underset{Br}{\mid}}{C}{-}CONH\underset{\underset{COCH_3}{\mid}}{CONH}$	(1-Acetyl-3(2-bromo 2-ethylbutyryl)urea	Acetylcarbromal

none of these agents offers advantages over other types of hypnotics. At the same time some of these drugs have definite shortcomings in terms of therapeutic efficacy and safety. The acyclic hypnotics containing nitrogen are shown in Table 54.6.

Ethinamate (1-ethynyl-1-cyclohexyl carbamate) has a rapid onset and short duration of action. In controlled studies a 500 mg dose of ethinamate was only little better than placebo (242). It may be useful, but in doses up to 1 g, for the prompt induction of simple insomnia. Prolonged use of ethinamate may lead to dependence of the barbiturate type (243, 244).

Hexapropymate, a homolog of ethinamate, has been used to calm psychoneurotics and as a hypnotic in mild cases of insomnia (245).

Administration of 400 mg hexapropymate for three consecutive nights decreased REM sleep, nocturnal wakefulness, and sleep latency and increased REM sleep latency (246).

Meprobamate (2-methyl-2-*n*-propyl-1,3-propanediol carbamate) is used primarily as a muscle relaxant. It is used sometimes in 800 mg doses as a hypnotic. The change produced by meprobamate in EEG recordings are similar to those of barbiturates (247). The addictive properties of meprobamate are similar to those of barbiturates (248).

In a double-blind study meprobamate (1200 mg) decreased drowsiness and REM sleep, while increasing stage 2 sleep (249), whereas in another study in 400 and 800 mg doses, meprobamate produced an insignificant decrease in REM sleep (250).

Oxanamide (2,3-epoxy-2-ethylhexanamide) and *valnoctamide* (2-ethyl-3-methylvaleramide) are used principally as muscle relaxants. However, in man the two drugs in doses that produce muscle relaxation also produce sedation (251).

Diethylallylacetamide displays higher hypnotic activity than the corresponding saturated analog. The higher hypnotic activity has been ascribed to the electron density of the unsaturated group. Similarly, *butesamide*, which is characterized by the presence of an electronegative carbethoxy group, may owe its hypnotic activity to the electron density of this group. In addition to the primary amides, disubstitution on the nitrogen led to a tertiary amide, *trimetho-benzglycine*, a potent hypnotic (252). The presence of bromine atom may be responsible for the hypnotic activity of *ibrotamide*. At the same time, the presence of bromine atom is also a liability, since bromide, which possesses toxic properties, may be liberated from ibrotamide. A completely saturated ureide, *capuride*, displays hypnotic activity. The unsaturated derivative *ectylurea* is a mild sedative, and the higher homolog *apronalide* produces sleep in man but is also quite toxic. This drug may inhibit the enzyme system responsible for conjugation (253).

Bromvalurea and *carbromal* have been used in man for many years and are considered to be safe, short-acting mild hypnotics. Their prolonged use is not recommended, however, since both can release bromide, which may lead to acute intoxication (254). *Acetylcarbromal* is also a short-acting sedative-hypnotic that is similar to carbromal in every respect.

12 ALCOHOLS AND ALDEHYDES

The clinically useful alcohols are all tertiary alcohols. With the exception of amylene hydrate they all contain either a halogen atom or an acetylenic group. The presence of an electron-negative group or unsaturation characterized by electron density near the alcohol group seems to potentiate sedative-hypnotic properties.

The alcohols and aldehydes displaying sedative-hypnotic properties are shown in Table 54.7. The derivatives of chloral hydrate are shown in Table 54.8.

Amylene hydrate, which was introduced by von Mering in 1887, is one of the oldest sedative-hypnotics. The drug, a colorless liquid, has a rapid onset of action and good absorption but short duration of action. Because of its unpleasant taste and odor, it

is very seldom used. *Chlorobutanol* (*chloretone*) has sedative-hypnotic analgestic and anesthetic properties. It is most often employed in hospitals as a preanesthetic agent. It produces no gastric irritation. *Methylpentynol* (*methylparafinol*) is a powerful sedative and mild hypnotic which is employed in anxiety and tension as a psychosedative. It is metabolized quickly. Even higher doses of the drug don't produce anesthesia; the sleep induced by methylpentynol can be interrupted readily by external stimulus. Side effects caused by this liquid drug include gastric irritation (255), slurred speech (256), and after prolonged use even psychosis (257). Introduction of a bromine atom into methylpentynol yields *brommethylpentynol*, which has a more potent and longer lasting sedative-hypnotic activity than methylpentynol. Increasing the chain length and simultaneously introducing both a halogen atom and unsaturation into the methylpentynol structure leads to *ethchlorvynol*, which is equipotent to glutethimide (258). It has a rapid onset of action. It is employed as a daytime sedative and is also recommended for treating insomnia and reducing awakenings (259). Like barbiturates, glutethimide, and meprobamate, ethchlorvynol also produces changes in the electroencephalogram (260). Ethchlorvynol does not have any advantage over barbiturates as far as physical dependence capacity is concerned (261). Furthermore, etchlorvynol, like barbiturates, may also produce serious intoxication (262). *Methylphenylbutyndiol* was introduced as a hypnotic in 1964. It induces sleep in 15–30 min, with the sleep lasting at least 6 h. In 250 mg doses the compound is one-third as active as pentobarbital (263). The compound is used as a sleep inducer and sleep improver. It is also employed as an adjunct in order to reduce the amounts of neuroleptics and barbiturates administered to the patient. No side effects of the drugs have been reported (264).

Table 54.7 Alcohols and Aldehydes Employed as Sedative Hypnotics

Structure	Chemical Name	Generic Name
Alcohols		
$CH_3-\underset{\underset{OH}{|}}{\overset{\overset{CH_3}{|}}{C}}-C_2H_5$	2-Methyl-2-butanol	Amylene hydrate
$Cl_3C-\underset{\underset{OH}{|}}{\overset{\overset{CH_3}{|}}{C}}-CH_3$	2-Methyl-1,1,1-tri chloro-2-propanol	Chlorobutanol Chloretone
$H_5C_2-\underset{\underset{OH}{|}}{\overset{\overset{CH_3}{|}}{C}}-C{\equiv}CH$	3-Methyl-1-pentyn -3-ol	Methylpentynol
$C_2H_5-\underset{\underset{OH}{|}}{\overset{\overset{CH_3}{|}}{C}}-C{\equiv}CBr$	3-Methyl-1-bromo-1 -pentyn-3-ol	Brommethylpentynol
$C_2H_5-\underset{\underset{OH}{|}}{\overset{\overset{CH{=}CHCl}{|}}{C}}-C{\equiv}CH$	1-Chloro-3-ethyl-1- penten-4-yn-3-ol	Ethchlorvynol
phenyl$-\underset{\underset{OH}{|}}{CH}-\underset{\underset{OH}{|}}{\overset{\overset{CH_3}{|}}{C}}-C{\equiv}CH$	2-Methyl-1-phenyl-3- butyn-1,2-diol	Methylphenylbutyndiol
Aldehydes		
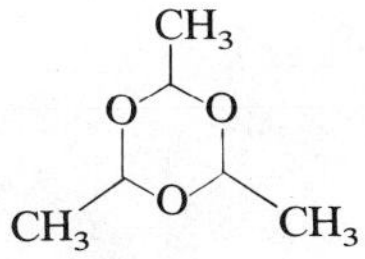 (paraldehyde ring structure)	Para-acetaldehyde	Paraldehyde
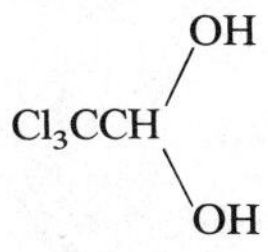 $Cl_3CCH\overset{\overset{OH}{\diagup}}{\underset{\underset{OH}{\diagdown}}{}}$	Chloral hydrate	Chloral hydrate

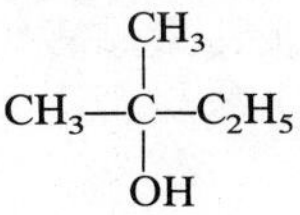

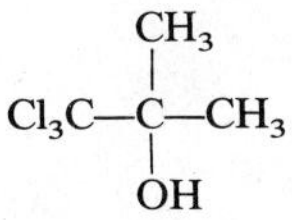

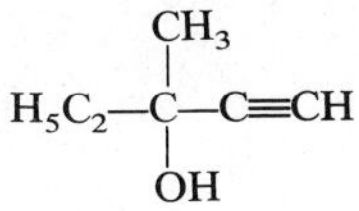

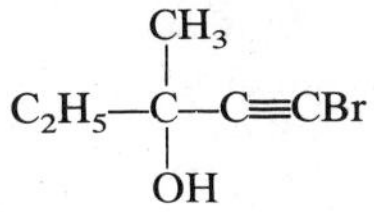

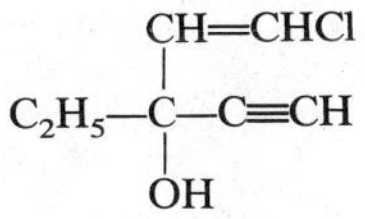

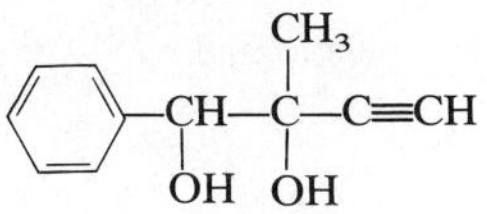

Table 54.8 Chloral hydrate Derivatives

Structure	Chemical Name	Generic Name
$Cl_3CCH(OH)_2 \cdot$ $(CH_3)_3\overset{+}{N}CH_2CO_2^-$	Chloral hydrate, compound with betaine	Chloralbetain
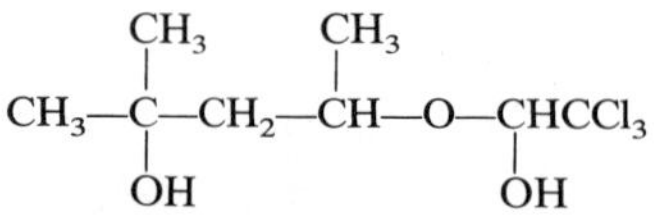 2-Methyl-2(2,2,2-trichloro-1-hydroxy ethoxy)-2-pentanol structure	2-Methyl-2(2,2,2-trichloro-1-hydroxy ethoxy)-2-pentanol	Chloralodol or chlorhexadol
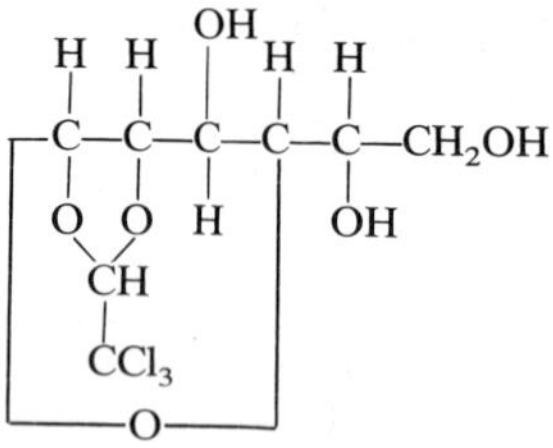 α-Mono-(trichlorethylidene)-D-glucose structure	α-Mono-(trichlorethylidene)-D-glucose	Chloralose
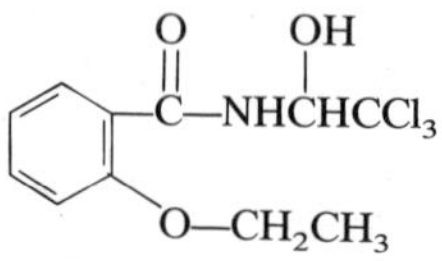 O-Ethyl-N-(2,2,2-trichloro-1-hydroxyethyl)salicylamide structure	O-Ethyl-N-(2,2,2-trichloro-1-hydroxy ethyl)salicylamide	Chloralsalicyl amide
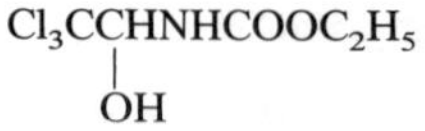 $Cl_3CCHNHCOOC_2H_5$ $\overset{\vert}{OH}$	Ethyl N-(2,2,2-tri chloro-1-hydroxyethyl carbamate	Carbochloral
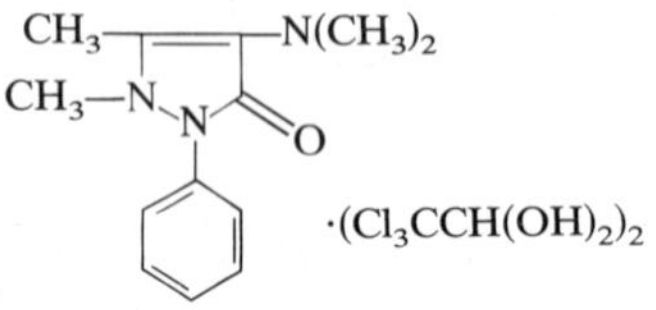 Dichloralphenazone structure $\cdot(Cl_3CCH(OH)_2)_2$	4-Dimethylamino-2,3-dimethyl-1-phenyl-3-pyrazolin-5-one compound with chloral hydrate	Dichloralphenazone
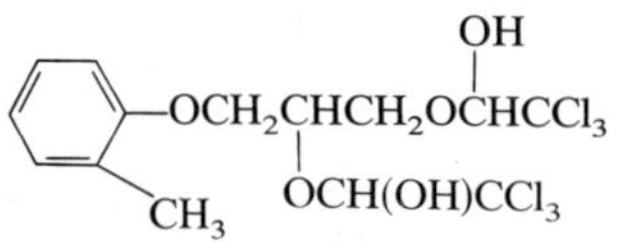 Toloxychlorinol structure	1-(o-tolyloxy)-2,3-bis(2,2,2-trichloro-1-hydroxyethoxy)propane	Toloxychlorinol
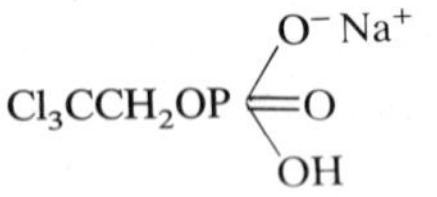 Triclofos structure Cl_3CCH_2OP	2,2,2-Trichloro ethanol, di-H-phosphate, sodium salt	Triclofos
$C(CH_2OCH(OH)CCl_3)_4$	Pentaerythritol hemiacetal with chloral	Petrichloral

Paraldehyde, the cyclic acetal of acetaldehyde, one of the oldest and safest hypnotic drugs, has been used since 1882. It quickly induces deep sleep. The side effects are minimal. It is partially excreted unchanged, but most of the drug is extensively metabolized. Its unpleasant taste, pungent odor, and mucous membrane irritating properties prevented its widespread use. Paraldehyde is still used in hospitals in emergencies, since it is safer, quicker acting, and more potent than the barbiturates. In hypnotic doses it depresses neuronal activity in the rostral segment of the reticular activating system.

Chloral hydrate, a chemically stable but volatile substance, is a potent hypnotic. In man, it has a rapid onset of action, suggesting that chloral itself exerts a hypnotic action (265). However, no chloral blood levels are found in man, since the metabolic conversion of chloral to trichloroethanol is very fast.

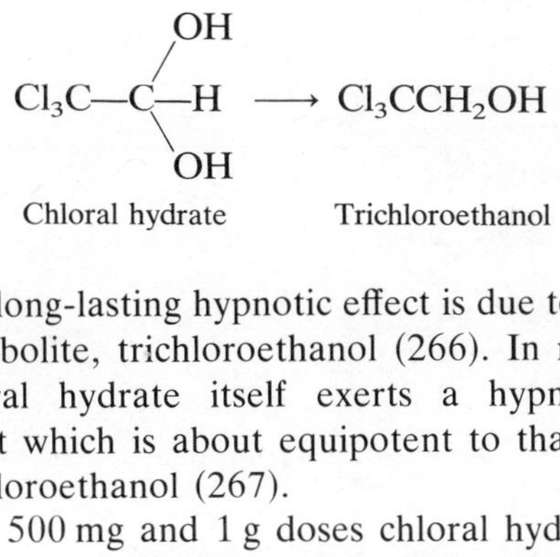

$$Cl_3C-\overset{\displaystyle OH}{\underset{\displaystyle OH}{C}}-H \longrightarrow Cl_3CCH_2OH$$

Chloral hydrate   Trichloroethanol

The long-lasting hypnotic effect is due to its metabolite, trichloroethanol (266). In rats, chloral hydrate itself exerts a hypnotic effect which is about equipotent to that of trichloroethanol (267).

In 500 mg and 1 g doses chloral hydrate did not suppress REM sleep (268, 269). A similar report claimed that chloral hydrate affected the stages of sleep less than any other hypnotics and upon withdrawal no rebound REM sleep occurred (270). On the other hand, it was reported that 800 mg of chloral hydrate initially suppressed REM sleep for up to 3 nights (271). Even these authors admitted, however, that no rebound excess REM sleep was observed when the drug was withdrawn (271).

Chloral hydrate is quite irritating to the mucous membrane and skin, and it may cause gastrointestinal distress. Chloral hydrate also has an unpleasant taste and can produce a state of physical dependence.

To overcome the unpleasant physical properties of taste and odor of chloral hydrate, a number of derivatives were prepared, which do not product gastric irritation. These derivatives, shown in Table 54.8, did not gain popularity.

13 MISCELLANEOUS SEDATIVE–HYPNOTICS

13.1 Bromides

Bromides were very popular in the middle of the nineteenth century when they were used as anticonvulsants and sedatives. Bromides have an unsatisfactory margin of safety because, in doses that are required to induce sedation; they also produce excessive drowsiness, even intoxication. Furthermore bromide ion tends to accumulate, and its excretion is extremely slow (it has a half-life of 12 days). Bromide displaces chloride ion in the CNS and causes an imbalance in the total halogen content of the body. Owing to its untoward effects, bromides are no longer used extensively.

13.2 Acids and Esters

L-*Tryptophan*, a naturally occurring substance and a precursor of serotonin, significantly reduced onset of sleep in man (44). This investigational drug is currently under extensive clinical trials as a hypnotic (272).

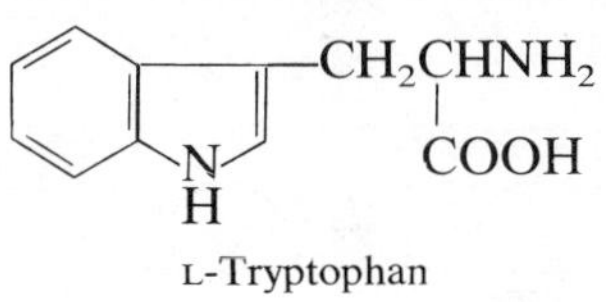

L-Tryptophan

Etomidate [(R)-(+)-ethyl 1-(1-phenyl-ethyl)-1H-imidazole-5-carboxylate]

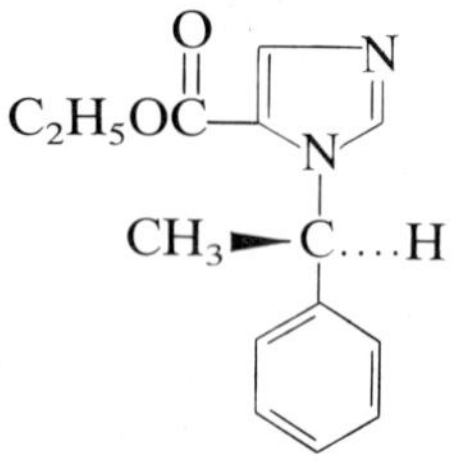

is a short-acting hypnotic drug devoid of toxic side effects (273, 274). Intravenous administration of etomidate in man in 0.15–0.30 mg/kg doses produced a fast onset of sleep, a distinct EEG pattern which is similar to that produced by other injectable hypnotics, and an extended over-all sleeping time. Disturbing effects on respiration and circulation were not observed. After etomidate treatment, assisted ventilation due to hypoxia was not necessary.

Intravenously administered etomidate quickly induces deep sleep to allow administration of normal anesthesia (275, 276).

13.3 Antihistamines and Anticholinergics

A number of antihistamines display sedative activity. Some of these drugs have been employed as sedative–hypnotics. These include the following:

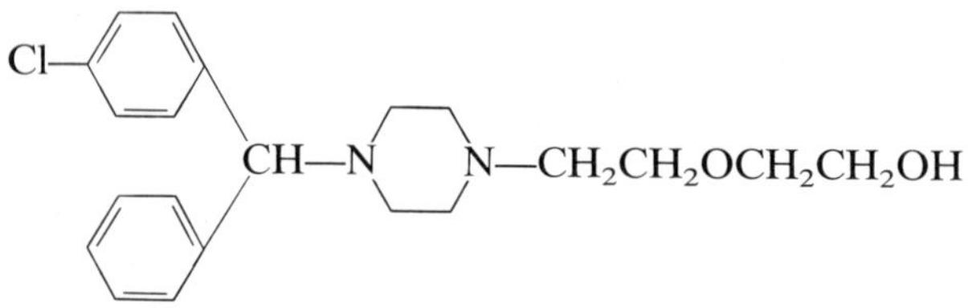

Hydroxyzine

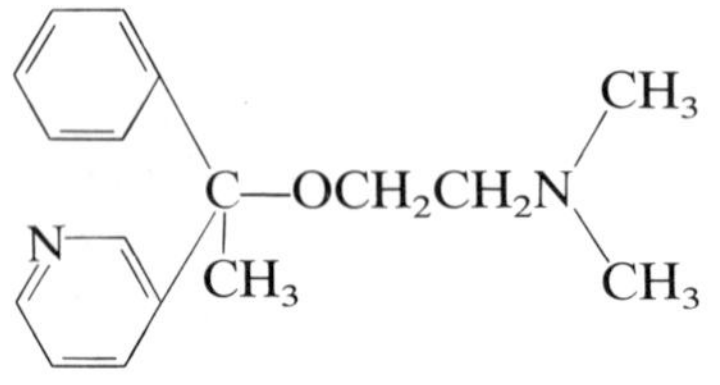

Doxylamine

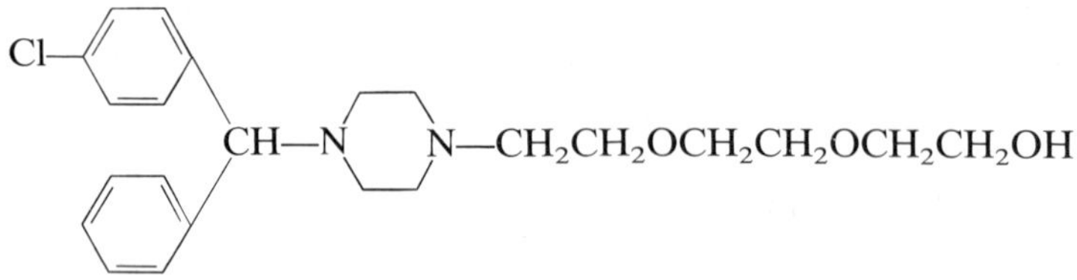

Etodroxizine

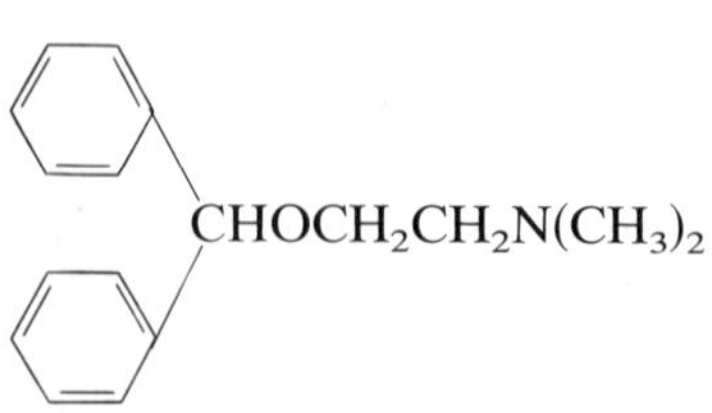

Diphenhydramine

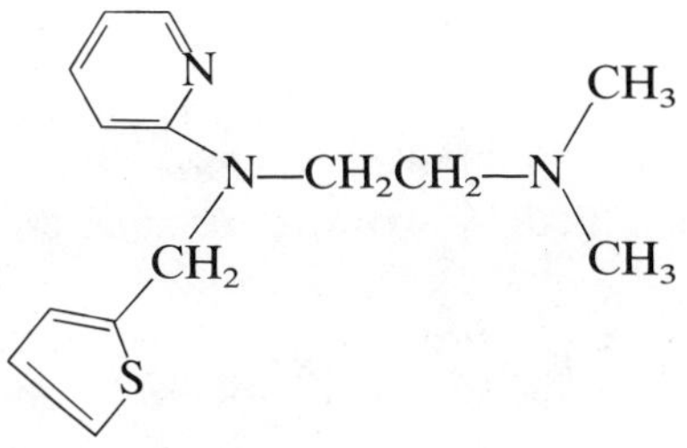

Methapyriline

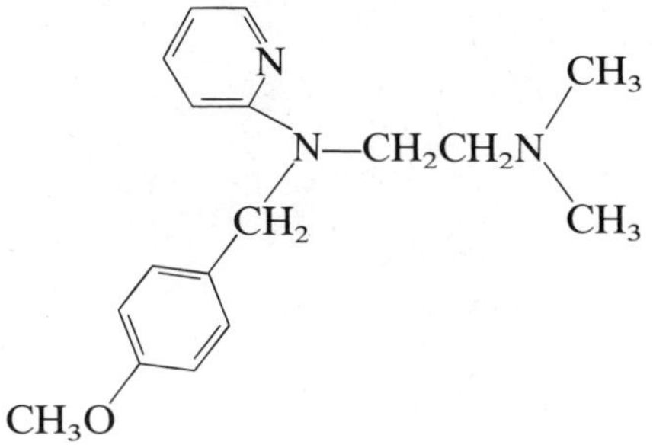

Pyrilamine

Many of the hypnotics formerly available without prescription contained *methalpyrilene* (25 mg), occasionally combined with scopolamine. A National Cancer Institute study produced tumors in rats exposed for a prolonged period to methapyrilene. As a result methapyrilene has been withdrawn from the market in the USA, Canada, UK and possibly other countries (276a). A combination of methapyrilene hydrochloride (25 g) and *hyoscine* (scopolamine) hydrobromide (0.125 mg), an anticholinergic drug was equipotent to 100 g of phenobarbital in elderly insomniacs (277). This combination can also produce intoxication (278, 279). *Etodroxizine* in man in a 12.5 mg dose had no significant effect on the sleep pattern. In larger doses (25 and 50 mg) it caused significant decreases in REM sleep during the first night (280), but the suppression of REM sleep disappeared during the following two nights of treatment. Upon drug withdrawal no rebound effects were seen. Methaqualone (250 mg) produced exactly the same effects. The combination of etodroxine (20 mg) and methaqualone (250 mg) produced a greater suppression of REM sleep (280).

Pyrilamine maleate, like methapyrilene, is often used in over-the-counter sedative formulations. *Doxylamine*, in 25 and 50 mg doses, was found to be more effective in man than 100 mg of secobarbital (281). This study provides reliable information on the hypnotic property of one of the antihistamines widely sold without prescription. On the other hand, there is no reliable information available on the hypnotic effects of other antihistamines. *Diphenhydramine* was judged to be more effective than placebo in a double-blind study in children (282).

The antihistamines employed as sedatives all contain a tertiary alkylamine group and possess mixed excitatory and inhibitory CNS effects. The CNS-depressant effects appear at low concentrations whereas the excitatory effects are observed at high concentrations. This fact explains why the hypnotic action usually cannot be intensified by simply administering larger doses of the drugs. If larger doses are administered, the excitatory effects may take over and the drug produces a paradoxical effect including restlessness and agitation.

In addition to the antihistaminic and sedative properties, these drugs also display anticholinergic and local anesthetic effects. However, the antihistaminic, spasmolytic, or local anesthetic doses are different from the sedative doses of these drugs (283). The theory has been proposed that the sedative properties of these drugs are due to their anticholinergic activities (284). This has not been proved, however. Tolerance to the sedative action of antihistamines develops rapidly; therefore, the prolonged use of these drugs is not recommended.

13.4 Sulfones

Compounds of this class show toxic effects at therapeutic doses and are no longer used as sedative–hypnotic drugs.

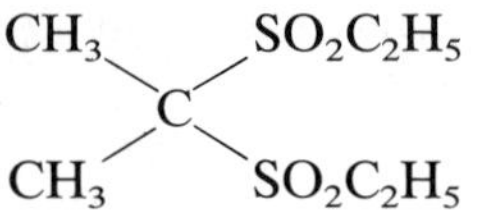

Sulfonal

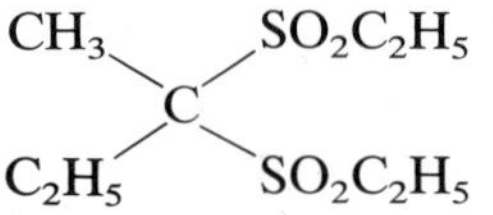

Trional

13.5 Plant Extracts

A number of plant extracts, e.g., *Radix valerianae, Glandulae lupuli, Rauwolfia serpentina, Passiflora incarnata,* and *Avana*

sativa, display sedative–hypnotic properties. It is not known which constituents are responsible for the sedative–hypnotic actions of these extracts. A number of components have been identified and found to possess pharmacological activities. These include the component of *Radix valerianae,* α-methylpyrryl ketone, valerenic acid, valepotriate, acetoxyvalepotriate, and 5,6-dihydrovalepotriate (285).

From the plant *Glandulae lupuli,* the following components were isolated and found to possess sedative hypnotic properties:

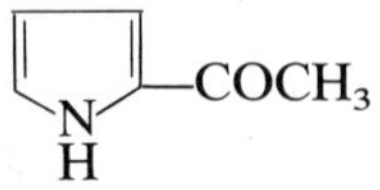

α-Methyl pyrryl ketone

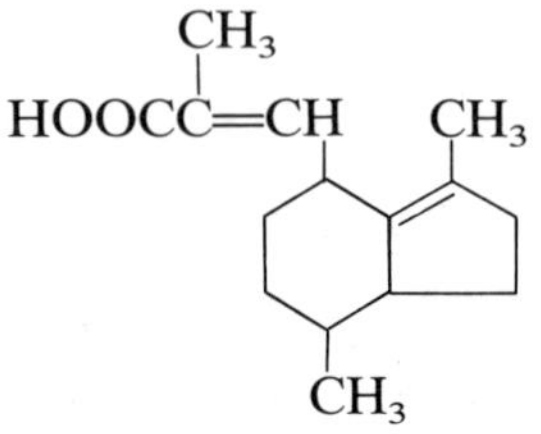

Valerenic acid

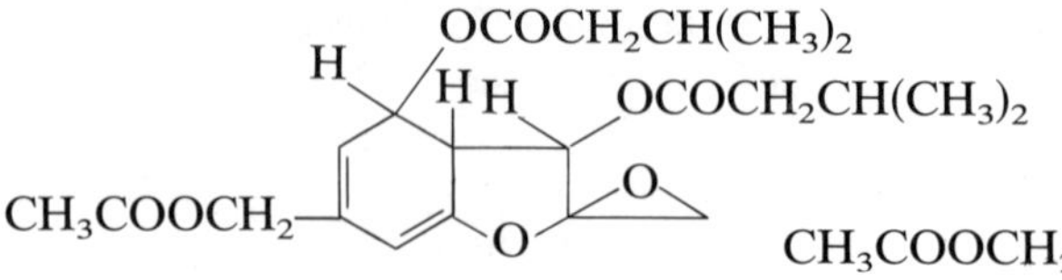

Valepotriate

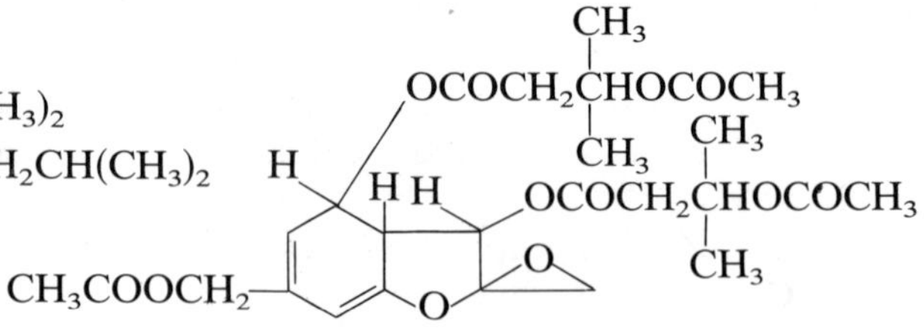

Component of *Glandulae lupuli*

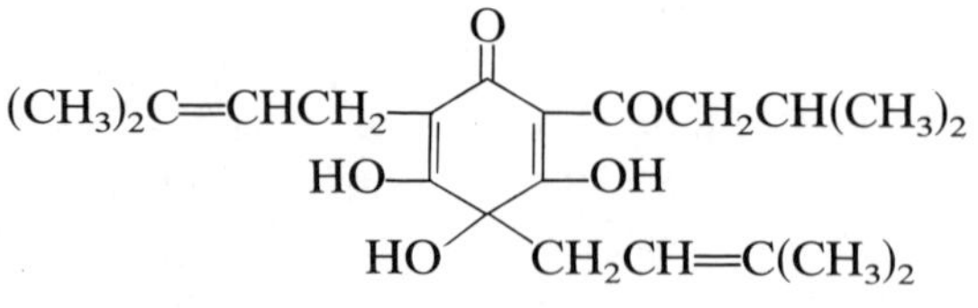

Humulon
(α-lupulinic acid)

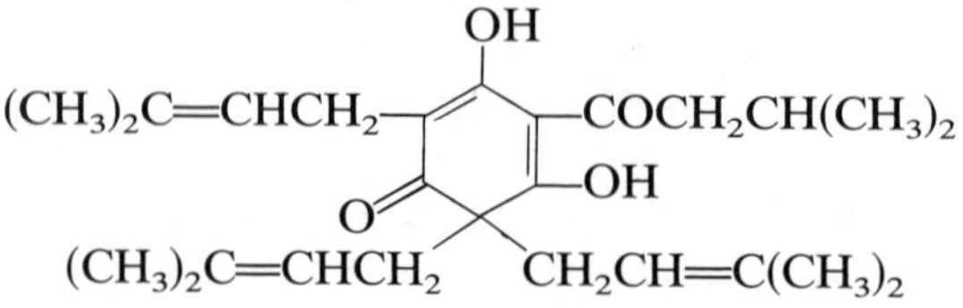

Lupulon
(β-lupulinic acid)

Various plant extracts are sold worldwide either as a single entity preparation or in combination with other sedative–hypnotics, e.g., bromides and barbiturates.

13.6 Endogenous Sleep Factors

Evidence for the synthesis or release of endogenous sleep factors was obtained as early as 1913 when Pieron and his colleagues (286, 287) transfused cerebrospinal fluid from sleep-deprived dogs to the cerebrospinal system of normal dogs, thereby inducing 6–8 h sleep in the normal dogs. At the same time dogs receiving cerebrospinal fluid from normal dogs remained alert. The validity of these experiments was confirmed in 1939 (288). More recently Pappenheimer et al. (289) repeated the Pieron phenomenon and induced sleep lasting up to 18 hr by injecting perfusate from the ventricular system of sleep-derived goat into the ventricular system of cats and rats.

Although the characterization of the sleep factor has not yet been completed, the fraction obtained from the cerebrospinal fluids of several goats with a range in mol wt of 350–500 increased sleep by about 50% in rats and rabbits following intraventricular infusion (290, 291). Indications are that the sleep factor has a peptide-like structure.

Monnier and his colleagues also confirmed the existence of sleep-inducing factors, first by a cross blood circulation technique (292–295) and later by injecting a dialysate obtained from the cerebral blood of rabbits kept asleep by electrical stimulation of the thalamus into normal rabbits (296, 297). The factor responsible for inducing sleep, called "sleep peptide delta," was later identified to be a nonapeptide (298–302).

The amino acid sequence Trp-Ala-Gly-Gly-Asp-Ala-Ser-Gly-Glu was established for the nonapeptide isolated from extra-corporal dialysates of electrically stimulated rabbits. The peptide that induces slow-wave (delta) and spindle activity enhancement in the electroencephalogram of rabbits by intraventricular infusion is called delta-sleep-inducing peptide (DSIP) (303). Subsequently, Schoenenberger and Monnier synthesized the delta-sleep-inducing peptide and compared the synthetic nonapeptide with natural DSIP. It was found that both nonapeptides showed significant and specific enhancement or induction of delta and spindle electroencephalogram patterns, whereas five possible metabolic products (fragments of the nonapeptide) were without effects. DSIP differs in its molecular weight from factor S of Pappenheimer et al. (304) extracted from goat cerebrospinal fluid or sheep brain and from the sleep-promoting material extracted from rat brain by Nagasaki et al. (305).

Further progress in the identification and characterization of endogenous sleep-producing factors may soon be expected.

REFERENCES

1. E. Aserinsky and N. Kleitman, *Science*, **118,** 273 (1953).
2. E. Aserinsky and N. Kleitman, *J. Appl. Physiol.* **8,** 1 (1955).
3. W. C. Dement and N. Kleitman, *Electroencephalogr. Clin. Neurophysiol.*, **9,** 673 (1957).
4. M. W. Johns, *Drugs*, **9,** 448 (1975).
5. M. Jouvet, *Science*, **163,** 32 (1969).
6. M. Jeanerod, J. Mouret, and M. Jouvet, *J. Physiol.* (Paris), **57,** 255 (1965).
7. L. J. West, M. Kramer, Ed., in *Dream Psychology and the New Biology of Dreaming*, Charles C Thomas, Springfield, Ill., 1969, p. XVI.
8. I. Oswald, *Postgrad. Med. J.*, **52,** 1 (1976).
9. J. C. Gillin, W. B. Mendelson, N. Sitaram, and R. J. Wyatt, *Ann. Rev. Pharmacol. Toxicol.* **18,** 563 (1978).
10. R. L. Williams, H. W. Agnew, and W. B. Webb, *Electroencephalogr. Clin. Neurophysiol.*, **17,** 376 (1964).
11. R. L. Williams, H. W. Agnew, and W. B. Webb, *Electroencephalogr. Clin. Neurophysiol.* **20,** 264 (1966).

12. I. Oswald, *Ann. Rev. Pharmacol.*, **13**, 243 (1973).

13. J. G. Salamy, in *Pharmacology of Sleep*, R. L. Williams and I. Karacan, Eds., Wiley, New York, 1976, pp. 53–82.

14. H. W. Agnew and W. B. Webb, *Psychophysiology*, **5**, 228 (1968).

15. A. Kales, G. Henser, A. Jacobsen, J. D. Kales, J. Hanley, J. R. Zweizig, and M. J. Paulson, *J. Clin. Endocrinol. Metab.*, **27**, 1593 (1967).

16. A. Kales, A. Jacobson, J. D. Kales, T. Kun, and R. Weissbuch, *Psychon. Sci.*, **7**, 67 (1967).

17. A. Kales, T. Wilson, J. D. Kales, A. Jacobson. M. J. Paulson, E. Kollar, and R. D. Walter, *J. Am. Geriatrics Soc.*, **15**, 405 (1967).

18. Y. Takahashi, D. M. Kipnis, and W. H. Daughaday, *J. Clin. Invest.*, **47**, 2079 (1968).

19. D. C. Parker, J. F. Sassin, J. W. Mace, R. W. Gotlin, and L. G. Rossman, *J. Clin. Endocrinol. Metab.*, **29**, 871 (1969).

20. I. Oswald, D. L. F. Dunleavy, S. Allen, and S. A. Lewis, in *The Nature of Sleep*, U. J. Jovanovich, Ed., Fischer, Stuttgart, p. 280.

21. J. F. Sassin, A. G. Frantz, S. Kapen, and E. D. Weitzman, *J. Clin. Endocrinol. Metab.*, **37**, 436 (1973).

22. R. M. Boyar, J. Finkelstein, H. Roffwarg, S. Kapen, E. D. Weitzman, and L. Hellman, *New Engl. J. Med.*, **287**, 582 (1972).

23. R. M. Boyar, R. S. Rosenfeld, S. Kapen, J. W. Finkelstein, H. P. Roffwarg, E. D. Weitzman, and L. Hellman, *J. Clin. Invest.*, **54**, 609 (1974).

24. W. C. Dement, *Some Must Watch while Some Must Sleep*, Freeman, San Francisco, 1972 and 1974.

25. W. Dement, *Science*, **131**, 1705 (1960).

26. E. L. Hartmann, *The Functions of Sleep*, Yale University Press, New Haven, Conn., 1973.

27. M. Jouvet, in *Psychopharmacology, A Review of Progress*, 1957–1967, D. H. Efron, Ed., U.S. Government Printing Office, Washington, D. C. 1968, pp. 523–540.

28. M. Jouvet, *Ergeb. Physiol.*, **64**, 166–307 (1972).

29. H. Corrodi, K. Fuxe, and T. Hökfelt, *J. Pharm. Pharmacol.*, **19**, 433 (1967).

30. J. Matsumoto and M. Jouvet, *C. R. Soc. Biol.* (Paris), **158**, 2137 (1964).

31. B. Jones, Ph. D. thesis, University of Delaware, 1970.

32. J. R. Mouret, P. Bobillier, and M. Jouvet, *Eur. J. Pharmacol.*, **5**, 17 (1968).

33. W. P. Koella, A. Feldstein, and J. S. Czicman, *Electroencephalogr. Clin. Neurophysiol.*, **25**, 481 (1968).

34. J. Hoyland, E. Shillito, and M. Vogt, *Brit. J. Pharmacol.*, **40**, 659 (1970).

35. J. D. Coulter, B. K. Lester, and H. L. Williams, *Psychopharmacologia*, **19**, 134 (1971).

36. E. Hartmann and J. Cravens, *Psychopharmacologia*, **33**, 169 (1973).

37. J. S. Hoffman and E. F. Domino, *J. Pharmacol. Exp. Ther.*, **170**, 190 (1969).

38. A. Carlsson, in *Psychopharmacology, A Generation of Progress*, M. A. Lipton, A. Dimascio, and K. F. Killam, Eds., Raven Press, New York, 1978, pp. 1057–1070.

39. G. W. Fenton, *Postgraduate Med. J.*, **52**, 5 (1976).

40. R. J. Wyatt, *Biol. Psychiatr.*, **5**, 33 (1972).

41. A. Sjoerdsma, W. Lovenberg, K. Engelman, W. T. Carpenter, R. J. Wyatt, and G. L. Gessa, *Ann. Intern. Med.*, **73**, 607 (1970).

42. R. J. Wyatt, K. Engelman, D. J. Kupfer, J. Scott, A. Sjoerdsma, and F. Snyder, *Electroencephalogr. Clin. Neurophysiol.*, **27**, 529 (1969).

43. R. J. Wyatt and J. C. Gillin, in R. L. Williams and I. Karacan, Eds., *Pharmacology of Sleep*, New York, Wiley, 1976, pp. 239–274.

44. E. Hartmann, J. Cravens, and S. List, *Arch. Gen. Psychiatry.*, **31**, 394 (1974).

45. R. J. Wyatt, D. Fram, D. J. Kupfer, and F. Snyder, *Lancet*, **1970–II**, 842.

46. R. J. Wyatt, V. Zarcone, K. Engelman, W. C. Dement, F. Snyder and A. Sjoerdsma, *Electroencephalogr. Clin. Neurophysiol.*, **30**, 505 (1971).

47. C. Guilleminault, J. P. Cathala, and P. Costaigne, *Electroencephalogr. Clin. Neurophysiol.*, **34**, 177 (1973).

48. R. J. Wyatt, *Biological Psychiatr.*, **5**, 33 (1972).

49. M. P. Mandell, A. J. Mandell, and A. Jacobson, in *Recent Advances in Biological Psychiatry*, J. Wortis, Ed., New York, Plenum, 1964, Vol. 7, pp. 115–122.

50. V. Zarcone, A. Kales, M. Scharf, T. L. Tan, J. Q. Simmons, and W. C. Dement, *Arch. Gen. Psychiatr.*, **28**, 843, (1973).

51. J. C. Gillin, R. Post, R. J. Wyatt, F. Snyder, F. Goodwin, and W. E. Bunney, *Sleep Res*; **1**, 45 (1972).

52. J. R. Mouret, A. Vilppula, N. Frachon, and M. Jouvet, *C. R. Soc. Biol.* (Paris), **162**, 914 (1968).

53. D. Dusan-Peyrethon, J. Peyrethon, and M. Jouvet, *C. R. Soc. Biol.* (Paris), **162**, 116 (1968).

54. D. Dusan-Peyrethon and J. L. Froment, *C. R. Soc. Biol.* (Paris), **162**, 2141 (1968).

55. D. King and R. E. Jewett, *J. Pharmacol. Exp. Ther.*, **177,** 188 (1971).

56. T. Vaughan, R. J. Wyatt, and R. Green, *Psychophysiology*, **9,** 96 (1972).

57. U. Ungerstedt, *Eur. J. Pharmacol.*, **5,** 107 (1969).

58. U. Ungerstedt and G. W. Arbuthnott, *Brain Res.*, **21,** 485 (1970).

59. E. Hartman, R. Chung, P. R. Draskoczy, and J. J. Schildkraut, *Nature*, **233,** 425 (1971).

60. E. Hartmann, V. Pochay, and G. Zwilling, *Sleep Res.*, **4,** 97 (1975).

61. M. Jouvet, in *Serotonin and Behaviour*, J. Barchas and M. Usdin, Eds., Academic, New York, 1973, p. 395.

62. D. L. F. Dunleavy, V. Brezinova, I. Oswald, A. W. MacLean, and M. Tinker, *Brit. J. Psychiatr.*, **120,** 663 (1972).

63. I. Oswald, in *Amphetamines and Related Compounds*, E. Costa and S. Garattini, Eds., Raven, New York, pp. 865–871.

64. I. Oswald, V. R. Thacore, K. Adam, V. Brezinova, and R. Burack, *Brit. J. Clin. Pharm.*, **2,** 107 (1975).

65. E. Hartmann and G. Zwilling, *Pharm. Biochem. Behav.*, **5,** 135 (1976).

66. M. Jouvet, *Arch. Ital. Biol.*, **100,** 125 (1962).

67. J. Hazra, *Eur. J. Pharmacol.*, **11,** 395 (1970).

68. E. F. Domino and M. Stawiski, *Psychophysiology*, **7,** 315 (1971).

69. B. L. Baxter, *Exp. Neurol.*, **21,** 1 (1968).

70. B. L. Baxter, *Exp. Neurol.*, **23,** 220 (1969).

71. A. G. Karczmar, V. G. Longo, and A. Scotti de Carolis, *Physiol. Behav.*, **5,** 175 (1970).

72. H. C. Carrington and J. K. Raventos, *Brit. J. Pharmacol.*, **1,** 215 (1946).

73. R. K. S. Lim, M. H. Pindell, H. G. Glass, and K. Rink, *ANN. N.Y. Acad. Sci.*, **64,** 667 (1956).

74. W. J. Kinnard and C. J. Carr, *J. Pharmacol. Exp. Ther.*, **121,** 354 (1957).

75. F. N. Fastier, R. N. Speden, and H. Waal, *Brit. J. Pharmacol.*, **12,** 251 (1957).

76. A. W. Lessin and M. W. Parkes, *Brit. J. Pharmacol.*, **12,** 245 (1957).

77. S. D. Feurt and J. P. La Rocca, *J. Am. Pharm. Assoc. Sci. Ed.*, **45,** 487 (1956).

78. J. F. Reinhard and J. V. Scudi, *Proc. Soc. Exp. Biol. Med.*, **100,** 381 (1959).

79. R. N. Straw, in *Hypnotics*, F. Kagan, T. Harwood, K. Rickels, A. D. Rudzik, and H. Sorer, Eds., Spectrum Publications, New York, 1975, pp. 65–85.

80. A. Kales and J. D. Kales, *New Engl. J. Med.*, **293,** 826 (1975).

81. A. Kales, E. O. Bixler, M. Scharf, and J. D. Kales, *Clin. Pharmacol. Ther.*, **19,** 576 (1976).

82. A. Kales, J. D. Kales, E. O. Bixler, and M. B. Scharf, in *Hypnotics*, F. Kagan, T. Harwood, K. Rickels, A. D. Rudzik, and H. Sorer, Eds., Spectrum Publications, New York, 1975, pp. 109–121.

83. E. C. Kleiderer and H. A. Shonle, *J. Am. Chem. Soc.*, **56,** 1772 (1934).

84. H. G. Mautner and H. C. Clemson, in *Medicinal Chemistry*, A. Burger, Ed., 3rd ed., Wiley, New York, 1970, pp. 1365–1385.

85. G. Moruzzi and H. W. Magoun, *Electroencephalogr. Clin. Neurophysiol.*, **1,** 455 (1949).

86. D. B. Lindsley, L. H. Schreiber, W. B. Knowles, and H. W. Magoun, *Electronencephalogr. Clin. Neurophysiol.*, **2,** 483 (1950).

87. K. Akert, W. P. Koella, and R. Hess, *Am. J. Physiol.*, **168,** 260 (1952).

88. E. Fischer and J. von Mehring, *Ther. d. Gegeuw.* **44,** 97 (1903).

89. W. J. Doran, in *Medicinal Chemistry*, F. F. Blicke and R. H. Cox, Eds., Wiley, New York, 1959.

90. F. Sandberg, *Acta Physiol. Scand.*, **24,** 7 (1951).

91. G. A. Jeffrey, S. Ghose, and J. O. Warwicker, *Acta Crystallogr.*, **14,** 881 (1961).

92. W. Bolton, *Acta Crystallogr.*, **16,** 166 (1963).

93. T. C. Butler, J. M. Ruth, and G. F. Tucker, *J. Am. Chem. Soc.*, **77,** 1488 (1955).

94. P. Zuman, J. A. Vida, A. Kardos, and M. Romer, *Anal. Lett.*, **9,** 849 (1976).

95. C. M. Samour, J. F. Reinhard, and J. A. Vida, *J. Med. Chem.*, **14,** 187 (1971).

96. J. A. Vida and E. H. Gerry, in *Anticonvulsants*, J. A. Vida, Ed., Academic, New York, 1977, pp. 151–291.

97. E. W. Maynert and J. M. Dawson, *J. Biol. Chem.*, **195,** 389 (1952).

98. D. M. Jerina, J. W. Daly, and B. Witkop, in J. H. Biel and L. G. Abood, Eds., *Biogenic Amines and Physiological Membranes in Drug Therapy*, Dekker, 1971, pp. 451–463.

99. T. C. Butler, *J. Pharmacol. Exp. Ther.*, **106,** 235 (1952).

100. W. N. Aldridge, *Enzymes Drug Action*, Ciba Found. Symp., 1962, p. 155.

101. P. Singh and J. Huot, in *Anticonvulsant Drugs*, Vol. 2, C. Raduoco-Thomas, Ed., Pergamon, Oxford, pp. 427–504.

102. S. Thesleff, *Acta Physiol. Scand.*, **37,** 335 (1956).

103. J. N. Weakly, *J. Physiol.* (London), **204,** 63 (1969).

104. N. S. Chu and F. Bloom, *Science*, **179,** 908 (1973).

105. M. Sato, G. M. Austin, and H. Yai, *Nature*, **215,** 1506 (1967).

106. E. S. Johnson, M. H. T. Roberts, and D. W. Straughn, *J. Physiol.* (London), **203,** 261 (1969).

107. R. Nicoll, in *Psychopharmacology, A Generation of Progress*, M. A. Lipton, A. Dimascio, and K. F. Killam, Eds., Raven Press, New York, 1978, pp. 1337–1348.

108. S. Orrenius, *J. Cell. Biol.*, **26,** 713 (1965).

109. S. Orrenius, *J. Cell. Biol.*, **26,** 725 (1965).

110. H. Remmer, in *Scientific Basis of Drug Dependence*, Steinberg, Ed., Churchill, London, 1969, p. 111.

111. L. Decsi, *Progr. Drug Res.*, **8,** 53 (1965).

112. D. Menard, A. Berteloot, and J. S. Hugon, *Histochemistry*, **38,** 241 (1974).

113. I. Oswald and V. R. Thacore, *Brit. Med. J.*, **2,** 427 (1963).

114. I. Oswald and R. G. Priest, *Brit. Med. J.*, **2,** 1093 (1965).

115. A. Kales, E. O. Bixler, T. L. Tan, M. B. Scharf, and J. D. Kales, *J. Am. Med. Assoc.*, **227,** 513 (1974).

116. F. A. Whitlock, *Med. J. Aust.* **2,** 391 (1970).

117. D. R. Wesson and D. E. Smith, *Barbiturates, Their Use, Misuse and Abuse*, Human Sciences Press, New York, 1977.

117a. J. Koch-Weser and D. J. Greenblatt, *New Engl. Med.*, **291,** 790 (1974).

118. E. Hartmann, *New Engl. J. Med.*, **292,** 217 (1975).

119. I. Oswald, *Brit. J. Psychiatr. Spec. Publ. No.* **9,** 272 (1975).

119a. I. Feinberg, S. Hibi, C. Cauness, and J. March, *Science*, **185,** 534 (1974).

120. A. Kales, J. D. Kales, M. B. Scharf, and T. L. Tan, *Arch. Gen. Psychiatr.*, **23,** 219 (1970).

121. E. Hartmann and J. Cravens, *Psychopharmacologia*, **33,** 233 (1973).

122. D. J. Greenblatt, M. D. Allen, B. J. Noel, and R. I. Shader, *Clin. Pharmacol. Ther.*, **21,** 497 (1977).

123. D. J. Greenblatt and R. I. Schader, *Benzodiazepines in Clinical Practice*, Raven Press, NY, 1974, pp. 183–196.

124. L. O. Randall and B. Kappell, in *The Benzodiazepines*, S. Garrattini, E. Mussini, and L. O. Randall, Eds., Raven Press, New York, 1973, pp. 27–51.

125. D. D. Beimer, *Clin. Pharmacokinet.*, **2,** 93 (1977).

126. A. Soulairac, J. Cohn, C. Gottesman, and J. Alano, *Progr. Brain Res.*, **18,** 194 (1965).

127. C. P. Gore and J. G. McComisky, in *Proc. Fourth World Congr. Psychiatry*, J. J. L. Ibor, Ed., Excerpta Medica, Amsterdam, 1968, pp. 2181–2183.

128. W. E. Haefely, in *Agents and Actions*, Vol. 7/3, Birkhauser, Basel, 1977, pp. 353–359.

129. F. E. Bloom, *Am. J. Psychiatr.*, **134,** 669 (1977).

130. A. J. Bond and M. H. Lader, *Psychopharmacologia*, **25,** 117 (1972).

131. A. J. Bond and M. H. Lader, *Brit. J. Pharmacol.*, **44,** 343P (1972).

132. A. Malpas, A. J. Rowan, C. R. B. Joyce, and D. F. Scott, *Brit. Med. J.*, **2,** 762 (1970).

133. A. J. Walters and M. H. Lader, *Nature*, **229,** 637 (1971).

134. E. O. Bixler, A. Kales, T. L. Tan, and J. D. Kales, *Curr. Ther. Res.*, **15,** 13 (1973).

135. G. Harrer, *Progr. Brain Res.*, **18,** 228 (1965).

136. L. De Angelis, V. Traversa, and R. Vertua, *Curr. Ther. Res.*, **16,** 324 (1974).

137. C. Zimmermann-Tansella, M. Tansella, and M. Lader, *J. Clin. Pharmacol., J. Clin. Pharmacol.*, **16,** 481 (1976).

138. G. Cesco, S. Giannico, I. Fabbrucci, L. Scaggiante, and N. Montanaro, *Arzneim.-Forsch.*, **27,** 146 (1977).

139. T. Momose, S. Ishii, and T. Kuge, *Curr. Ther. Res.*, **19,** 277 (1976).

140. H. Isozaki, M. Tanaka, and K. Inanaga, *Curr. Ther. Res.*, **20,** 493 (1976).

141. I. Freuchen, J. Ostergaard, and B. Ohrt Mikkelsen, *Curr. Ther. Res.*, **20,** 36 (1976).

142. J. M. Monti, H. M. Trenchi, F. Morales, and L. Monti, *Psychopharmacologia*, **35,** 371 (1974).

143. J. M. Monti and H. Altier, *Psychopharmacologia*, **32,** 343 (1973).

144. I. Oswald, S. A. Lewis, J. Tagney, H. Firth, and I. Haider, in *The Benzodiazepines*, S. Garattini, E. Mussini and L. O. Randall, Eds., Raven Press, New York, 1973, pp. 613–625.

145. A. Kales and M. B. Scharf, in *The Benzodiazepines*, S. Garattini, E. Mussini, and L. O. Randall, Eds., Raven Press, New York, 1973, pp. 577–598.

146. H. H. Chiu, *Anesthes. Intensive Care*, **4**, 355 (1976).

147. V. Samec, *Wien. Med. Wochenschr.*, **126**, 23 (1976).

148. E. O. Bixler, A. Kales, C. R. Soldatos, and J. D. Kales, *J. Clin. Pharm.*, **17**, 569 (1977).

149. J. W. Dundee, H. M. L. Johnston, J. K. Lilburn, S. G. Nair, and M. G. Scott, *Brit. J. Clin. Pharm.*, **4**, 706 (1977).

150. K. A. George and J. W. Dundee, *Brit. J. Clin. Pharm.*, **4**, 45 (1977).

151. U. J. Jovanovic, *J. Int. Med. Res.*, **5**, 77 (1977).

152. H. Jick, D. Slone, B. Dinan, and H. Muench, *New Eng. J. Med.*, **275**, 1399 (1972).

153. E. Hartmann, *Psychopharmacologia*, **12**, 346 (1968).

154. S. Fisher and P. Gal, *J. Am. Geriatr. Soc.*, **17**, 397 (1967).

155. H. Jick, *Curr. Ther. Res.*, **9**, 355 (1967).

156. A. Kales, C. Allen, M. B. Scharf, and J. D. Kales, *Arch. Gen. Psychiatr.*, **23**, 226 (1970).

157. A. Kales, J. D. Kales, M. B. Scharf, and T. L. Tan, *Arch. Gen. Psychiatr.*, **23**, 219 (1970).

158. H. Gastaut, H. Lob, and J. J. Papy, *Electroencephalogr. Clin. Neurophysiol.*, **23**, 288 (1967).

159. M. W. Johns and J. P. Masterton, *Pharmacology*, **11**, 358 (1974).

160. W. C. Dement, V. P. Zarcone, E. Hoddes, H. Smythe, and M. Carskadon, in *The Benzodiazepines*, S. Garattini, E. Mussini, and L. O. Randall, Eds., Raven Press, New York, 1973, pp. 599–611.

161. A. Kales, J. D. Kales, E. O. Bixler, and M. B. Scharf, *Clin. Pharm. Ther.*, **18**, 356 (1975).

162. D. J. Greenblatt, R. J. Shader, and J. Koch-Weser, *Ann. Intern. Med.*, **83**, 237 (1975).

163. D. J. Greenblatt, M. D. Allen, and R. I. Shader, *Clin. Pharm. Ther.*, **21**, 355 (1977).

164. S. Allen and I. Oswald, *Brit. J. Clin. Pharm.*, **3**, 165 (1976).

165. A. N. Nicholson, B. M. Stone, and C. H. Clarke, *Brit. J. Clin. Pharm.*, **3**, 533 (1976).

166. A. M. Risberg, S. Henricsson, and D. H. Ingvar, *Eur. J. Clin. Pharmacol.*, **12**, 105 (1977).

167. C. D. Blitt, W. C. Petty, W. A. Wright, and B. Wright, *Anesthesia and Analgesia*, **55**, 522 (1976).

168. R. I. H. Wang, S. L. Stockdale, and E. Hieb, *Clin. Pharmacol. Ther.*, **19**, 191 (1976).

169. P. Gomez-Lozano, *Curr. Ther. Res.*, **19**, 469 (1976).

170. I. Siassi, M. Thomas, and S. Vanov, *Curr. Ther. Res.*, **18**, 163 (1975).

171. M. Otsuka, T. Tsuchiya, and S. Kitagawa, *Arzneim.-Forsch.*, **23**, 645 (1973).

172. L. H. Sternbach, R. I. Fryer, O. Keller, W. Metlesich, G. Sach, and N. Steiger, *J. Med. Chem.*, **6**, 261 (1963).

173. L. O. Randàll, W. Schallek, C. Scheckel, R. E. Bagdon, and J. Rieder, *Schweiz. Med. Wochenschr.*, **95**, 333 (1975).

174. S. Wyss and A. Mäder, *Schweiz. Med. Wochenschr.*, **95**, 338 (1965).

175. I. Haider, *Brit. J. Phychiatr.*, **114**, 337 (1968).

176. H. Matthew, A. T. Proudfoot, R. C. B. Aitken, J. A. Raeburn, and N. Wright, *Brit. Med. J.*, **3**, 23 (1969).

177. C. Davies and S. Levine, *Brit. J. Psychiatr.*, **113**, 1005 (1967).

178. M. H. Lader and A. J. Walters, *Brit. J. Pharmacol.*, **41**, 412P (1971).

179. A. W. Peck, R. Adams, C. Bye, and R. T. Wilkinson, *Psychopharmacology*, **47**, 213 (1976).

180. W. H. Leriche, A. Csima, and M. Dobson, *Can. Med. Assoc. J.*, **95**, 300 (1966).

181. J. M. Bordeleau, G. Chovinard, and L. Tetrault, *Union Med. Can.*, **95**, 45 (1966).

182. H. E. Lehmann and T. A. Ban, *Int. Z. Klini. Pharmakol. Ther. Toxikol.*, **1**, 424 (1968).

183. I. Haider and I. Oswald, *Brit. J. Psychiatr.*, **118**, 519 (1971).

184. K. Adam, L. Adamson, V. Brezinova, W. M. Hunter, and I. Oswald, *Brit. Med. J.*, **1**, 1558 (1976).

185. I. Oswald, in *Prog. Drug Research*, E. Juckert, Ed., Birkhauser, Basel, **22**, 1978, pp. 355–372.

186. A. N. Nicholson, B. M. Stone, C. H. Clarke, and H. M. Ferres, *Brit. J. Pharm.*, **3**, 429 (1976).

187. M. Tansella, O. Siciliani, L. Burti, M. Schiavon, Ch. Zimmermann, Tansella, M. Gerna, G. Tognoni, and P. L. Morselli, *Psychopharmacologia*, **41**, 81 (1975).

188. I. Karacan, G. S. O'Brien, R. L. Williams, P. J. Salis, and J. I. Thornby, in *Sleep, Physiology, Biochemistry, Psychology, Pharmacology, Clinical Implications*, Proceedings of the First European Congress on Sleep Research, Karger, Basel, 1973, pp. 463–476.

189. M. Steinman, U.S. Pat. 3,845,039 (Oct. 29, 1964).

190. F. R. Freemon, M. S. H. Al-Marashi, and J. C. M. Lee, *J. Clin. Pharmacol.*, **17**, 398 (1977).

191. M. Steinman, J. G. Topliss, R. Alekel, Y. S. Wong, and E. E. York, *J. Med. Chem.*, **16,** 1354 (1973).

192. M. Babbini, M. V. Torrielli, E. Strumia, M. Gaiardi, M. Bartoletti, and F. de Marchi, *Arzneim. Forsch.*, **25,** 1294 (1975).

193. A. N. Nicholson and B. M. Stone, *Brit. J. Clin. Pharm.*, **3,** 543 (1976).

194. L. M. Fuccella, G. Tosolini, E. Moro, and V. Tamassia, *Int. J. Clin. Pharm.*, **6,** 303 (1972).

195. R. G. Priest and A. Z. Rizvi, *J. Int. Med. Res.*, **4,** 145 (1976).

196. A. Pines, A. R. Nandi, M. Rahman, H. Raafat, and J. F. F. Rooney, *J. Int. Med. Res.*, **4,** 132 (1976).

197. I. Hindmarch, *Arzneim.-Forsch.*, **25,** 1836 (1975).

198. E. O. Bixler, A. Kales, C. R. Soldatos, M. B. Scharf, and J. D. Kales, *Clin. Pharmacol.*, **4,** 110 (1978).

199. L. K. Fowler, *J. Int. Med. Res.*, **5,** 295 (1977).

200. L. K. Fowler, *J. Int. Med. Res.*, **5,** 297 (1977).

201. B. Matta, A. E. Franco, L. A. Lezotte, A. D. Rudzik, and W. Veldkamp, *Curr. Ther. Res.*, **16,** 958 (1974).

202. P. Lomen and O. I. Linet, *J. Int. Med. Res.*, **4,** 55 (1976).

203. L. F. Fabre, D. M. McLendon, and R. T. Harris, *J. Int. Med. Res.*, **4,** 247 (1976).

204. L. F. Fabre, L. Gross, V. Pasigajen, and C. Metzler, *J. Clin. Pharm.*, **17,** 402 (1977).

205. A. Kales, J. D. Kales, E. O. Bixler, M. B. Scharf, and E. Russek, *J. Clin. Pharmacol.*, **16,** 399 (1976).

206. T. Roth, M. Kramer, and J. L. Schwarz, *Curr. Ther. Res.*, **16,** 117 (1974).

207. T. Roth, M. Kramer, and T. Lutz, *Int. Med. Res.*, **4,** 59 (1976).

208. M. Weintraub, P. Sundaresan, W. Wardell, and L. Lasagna, *Clin. Pharm. Ther.*, **19,** 118 (1976).

209. W. B. Mendelson, D. W. Goodwin, S. Y. Hill, and J. D. Reichman, *Curr. Ther. Res.*, **19,** 155 (1976).

210. G. W. Vogel, K. Barker, P. Gibbons, and A. Thurmond, *Psychopharmacology,* **47,** 81 (1976).

211. R. B. Knapp, E. L. Boyd, G. Linsenmeyer, and O. L. Linet, *Curr. Ther. Res.*, **23,** 230 (1978).

212. K. K. Okawa, *Curr. Ther. Res.*, **23,** 381 (1978).

213. N. P. V. Nair and G. Schwartz, *Curr. Ther. Res.*, **23,** 388 (1978).

214. W. Veldkamp, R. N. Straw, C. M. Metzler, and H. V. Demissianos, *J. Clin. Pharm.*, **14,** 102 (1974).

215. T. Koppanyi, R. P. Herwick, C. R. Linegar, and R. H. K. Foster, *Arch. Int. Pharmacodyn.*, **64,** 123 (1940).

216. A. Krautwald, G. Kuschinsky, and H. Riedel, *Arch. Exp. Pathol. Pharmakol.*, **193,** 219 (1939).

217. O. Brandman, J. Coniaris, and H. E. Keller, *J. Med. Soc. N.J.*, **52,** 246 (1955).

218. L. O. Randall, V. Iliev, and O. Brandman, *Arch. Int. Pharmacodyn.*, **106,** 388 (1956).

219. O. Pribilla, *Arzneim.-Forsch.*, **6,** 756 (1956).

220. A. Kales, T. A. Preston, T. L. Tan, and C. Allen, *Arch. Gen. Psychiatr.*, **23,** 211 (1970).

221. H. Berger, *J. Am. Med. Assoc.*, **177,** 63 (1961).

222. B. Isaacs and M. B. Glass, *Lancet,* **1957–I,** 558 (1957).

223. C. Allen, A. Kales, and R. J. Berger, *Psychonomic Sci.*, **12,** 329 (1968).

224. L. Goldstein, J. Graedon, D. Willard, F. Goldstein, and R. R. Smith, *J. Clin. Pharm.*, **110,** 258 (1970).

225. J. Holland, M. J. Massie, T. C. Grant, and M. M. Plumb, *N.Y. State J. Med.*, **75,** 2343 (1975).

226. A. I. Arieff and E. A. Friedman, *Am. J. Med. Sci.*, **266,** 405 (1973).

227. K. N. V. Palmer, *Brit. Med. J.*, **1,** 1219 (1956).

228. A. Schulman and G. M. Laycock, *Aust. J. Exp. Biol. Med. Sci.*, **36,** 347 (1958).

229. G. Chen and P. Bass, *Arch. Int. Pharmacodyn.*, **152,** 115 (1964).

230. B. Dubnick and C. A. Towne, in *The Present Status of Psychotropic Drugs,* A. Cerletti and F. J. Bove, Eds., Excerpta Medica, Amsterdam, 1969, pp. 77–83.

231. J. R. Boissier, C. Dumont, and R. Ratouis, *Therapie,* **22,** 129 (1967).

232. J. R. Boissier and J. Pagny, *Med. Exp.*, **1,** 368 (1958).

233. T. W. Parsons and T. J. Thompson, *Brit. Med. J.*, **1,** 171 (1961).

234. D. S. Inaba, G. R. Gay, J. A. Newmeyer, and C. Whitehead, *J. Am. Med. Assoc.*, **224,** 1505 (1973).

235. R. H. S. Mindham, in *Meyler's Side Effects of Drugs,* Vol. VIII, M. N. G. Dukes, Ed., Excerpta Medica, Amsterdam, 1976, p. 74.

236. J. Wilson, G. W. Stephen, and D. B. Scott, *Brit. J. Anaesth.*, **41,** 840 (1969).

237. M. M. Glatt, H. R. George, and E. P. Frisch, *Brit. Med. J.*, **2,** 401 (1965).

238. M. M. Glatt, *Prescriber's J.*, **5,** 90 (1966).

239. F. Roeth, S. Lehrl, and J. Benos, *Therapiewoche,* **27,** 1462 (1977).

240. P. Berndt, *Pharmazie*, **23**, 241 (1968).

241. J. Mendels and D. A. Chernik, *Curr. Ther. Res.*, **14**, 454 (1972).

242. K. Rickels and H. Bass, *Am. J. Med. Sci.*, **245**, 142 (1963).

243. R. P. Davis, W. B. Blythe, M. Newton, and·L. G. Welt, *Yale J. Biol. Med.*, **32**, 192 (1959).

244. E. H. Ellinwood, J. A. Ewing, and P. C. S. Hoaken, *New Engl. J. Med.*, **266**, 185 (1962).

245. P. Bensoussan, *Presse Med.*, **69**, 2551 (1961).

246. A. M. Risberg, J. Risberg, and D. H. Ingvar, *J. Clin. Pharm.*, **4**, 241 (1972).

247. C. E. Henry and W. D. Obrist, *J. Nerv. Ment. Dis.*, **126**, 268 (1958).

248. C. F. Essing, *Clin. Pharm. Ther.*, **5**, 334 (1964).

249. F. R. Freemon, A. W. Agnew, Jr., and R. L. Williams, *Clin. Pharmacol. Ther.*, **6**, 172 (1965).

250. R. L. Williams and H. W. Agnew, Jr., *Exp. Med. Surg.*, **27**, 53 (1969).

251. A. P. Roszkowski and W. M. Govier, *Int. J. Neuropharmacol.*, **1**, 423 (1962).

252. J. D. Sharma and P. C. Dandiya, *Arch. Int. Pharmacodyn.*, **137**, 218 (1962).

253. O. C. De Barreiro, *Biochem. Pharmacol.*, **14**, 1694 (1961).

254. R. H. S. Myndham, in *Meyler's Side Effects of Drugs*, Vol. VIII, M. N. G. Dukes, Ed., Excerpta Medica, Amsterdam, 1976, p. 78.

255. L. Lasagna, *J. Pharmacol. Exp. Ther.*, **111**, 9 (1954).

256. E. Marley and A. A. Bartholomew, *J. Neurol. Neurosurg. Psychiatr.*, **21**, 219 (1958).

257. H. Urban, *Deut. Med. Wochenschr.*, **90**, 392 (1965).

258. K. J. R. Cuthbert, *Practitioner*, **190**, 509 (1963).

259. F. P. Johnson, L. L. Bollman, W. M. Swenson, and I. C. Nessler, *J. Am. Med. Assoc.*, **189**, 414 (1964).

260. J. E. P. Toman and E. K. Christensen, *Fed. Proc.*, **15**, 492 (1956).

261. H. S. Hudson and H. I. Walker, *Am. J. Psychiatr.*, **118**, 361 (1961).

262. C. H. Cahn, *Can. Med. Assoc. J.*, **81**, 733 (1959).

263. F. J. Kuhn and H. Wick, *Arzneim. Forsch.*, **13**, 728 (1963).

264. S. G. F. Matts, *Psychopharmacologia*, **9**, 73 (1966).

265. F. J. Mackay and J. R. Cooper, *J. Pharmacol. Exp. Ther.*, **135**, 271 (1962).

266. T. C. Butler, *J. Pharmacol. Exp. Ther.*, **95**, 360 (1949).

267. J. Grüner, J. Kriegelstein, and H. Rieger, *Arch. Exp. Pharm.*, **277**, 333 (1973).

268. A. Kales, J. Kales, M. B. Scharf, and T. Tjiauw-Ling, *Arch. Gen. Psychiatr.*, **23**, 219 (1970).

269. I. Oswald, *Brit. J. Psychiatr. Spec. Publ.*, **9**, 272 (1975).

270. E. Hartman and J. Cravens, *Psychopharmacologia* (Berlin), **33**, 219 (1973).

271. J. I. Evans and O. Ogunremi, *Brit. Med. J.*, **3**, 310 (1970).

272. E. Hartmann, *Am. J. Psychiatr.*, **134**, 366 (1977).

273. A. Doenicke, E. Wagner, and K. H. Beetz, *Anaesthesist*, **22**, 353 (1973).

274. A. Doenicke, J. Kugler, G. Peuzel, M. Lamb, L. Kalmar, I. Killan, and H. Bezecny, *Anaesthesist*, **22**, 357 (1973).

275. C. E. Famewo and C. O. Odugbesan, *Can. Anaesth. Soc. J.*, **24**, 35 (1977).

276. V. Schuermans, et al., *Anaesthesist*, **27**, 52 (1978).

276a. F.D.C. Reports **41**, (24), 15 (1979).

277. H. M. Feinblatt, *J. Gerontol.*, **13**, 48 (1958).

278. T. Sagales, S. Erill, and E. F. Domino, *Clin. Pharmacol. Ther.*, **10**, 522 (1969).

279. M. K. Thakkar and R. P. Lasser, *N.Y. State J. Med.*, **12**, 725 (1972).

280. A. M. Risberg, J. Risberg, D. Elmquist, and D. H. Ing, *Eur. J. Clin. Pharmacol.*, **8**, 227 (1975).

281. F. Sjöquist and L. Lasagna, *Clin. Pharm. Ther.*, **8**, 48 (1967).

282. R. M. Russo, V. J. Gururaj, and J. E. Allen, *J. Clin. Pharmacol.*, **16**, 284 (1976).

283. H. Weidemann and P. V. Petersen, *J. Pharm. Exp. Ther.*, **108**, 201 (1953).

284. R. P. White and L. D. Boyajy, *Arch. Int. Pharmacodyn. Ther.*, **128**, 260 (1960).

285. P. W. Thies and S. Funke, *Tetrahedron Lett.*, **11**, 1155 (1966).

286. H. Pieron, *Le Probleme Physiologique du Sommeil*, Masson, Paris, 1913, 520 pp.

287. R. Legendre and H. Pieron, *Z. Allg. Physiol.*, **14**, 235 (1913).

288. J. F. Schnedorf and A. C. Ivy, *Am. J. Physiol.*, **125**, 491 (1939).

289. J. R. Pappenheimer, T. B. Miller, and C. A. Goodrich, *Proc. Nat. Acad. Sci. U.S.*, **58**, 513 (1967).

290. J. R. Pappenheimer, *Sci. Am.*, **235**, 24 (1976).

291. V. Fencl, G. Koki, and J. R. Pappenheimer, *J. Physiol.* (London), **261**, 565 (1971).

292. M. Monnier, T. Koller, and S. Graber, *Exp. Neurol.*, **8**, 264 (1963).

293. M. Monnier, *Actual. Neurophysiol.*, **5**, 203 (1964).

294. M. Monnier and M. Fallert, *Schweiz. Med. Wechenschr.*, **79**, 509 (1967).

295. L. Hösli and M. Monnier, *Pflügers Arch. Gesamte Physiol.*, **283**, 17 (1965).

296. M. Monnier and L. Hösli, *Science*, **146**, 796 (1964).

297. M. Monnier and L. Hösli, *Progr. Brain Res.*, **18**, 118 (1965).

298. M. Monnier and A. M. Hatt, Arch. *Gesamte Physiol.*, **329**, 231 (1971).

299. M. Monnier, A. M. Hatt, L. B. Cueni, and G. A. Schoenenberger, *Arch. Gesamte Physiol.*, **331**, 257 (1972).

300. M. Monnier, L. Dudler, R. Gachter, and G. A. Schoenenberg, *Pflügers Arch. Eur. J. Physiol.*, **360**, 225 (1975).

301. G. A. Schoenenberger, *Schweiz. Rundschau Med. Praxis*, **64**, 609 (1975).

302. M. Monnier, G. A. Schoenenberger, A. Glatt, L. Dudler, and R. Gächter, *Exp. Brain Res.*, **23**, 144 (1975).

303. G. A. Schoenenberger and M. Monnier, *Proc. Natl. Acad. Sci. U.S.*, **74**, 1282 (1977).

304. J. R. Pappenheimer, G. Koski, V. Fencl, M. L. Karnovsky, and J. Kruger, *J. Neurophys.*, **38**, 1299 (1975).

305. H. Nagasaki, M. Iriki, S. Inoue, and K. Uchizono, *Proc. Jap. Acad.*, **50**, 241 (1974).

CHAPTER FIFTY-FIVE

Anticonvulsants

EUGENE I. ISAACSON

College of Pharmacy
Idaho State University
Pocatello, Idaho 83201, USA

and

JAIME N. DELGADO

College of Pharmacy
The University of Texas at Austin
Austin, Texas 78712, USA

CONTENTS

Anticonvulsants may be defined as agents that prevent, or diminish the severity of, convulsive seizures. The principal therapeutic application of anticonvulsants is in the treatment of the different varieties of epilepsy. Accordingly, a summary of the general nature of epilepsy will serve as an introduction to the anticonvulsant agents.

1 EPILEPSY

1.1 Historical Note

Epilepsy was recognized very early in the history of mankind. The disease is mentioned in the Babylonian civil code of Hammurabi (2080 BC) and in early Hebrew scripts, and full clinical descriptions were given in the Hippocratic monograph *On the Sacred Disease* (*ca.* 400 BC) (1). The English physician Sir Charles Locock made the discovery that led to the introduction of inorganic bromides as antiepileptic agents in the middle of the nineteenth century.

John Hughlings Jackson (1834–1911) is credited with the founding of the modern concepts and interpretations of epilepsy (2). Jackson's proposal that seizures are caused by "occasional, sudden, excessive, rapid, and local electrical discharges of gray matter" has been substantiated by the electroencephalogram (EEG). The introduction of the EEG demonstrated that epileptic convulsions are characterized by an excessive discharge of electricity, apparently from the dendrites of pyramidal cells of cerebral cortex neurons.

1.2 Physiological Description

In 1969, Jasper et al. (3) edited the classic monograph, *Basic Mechanisms of the Epilepsies*, which covers many important aspects of the field, including neuronal mechanisms underlying the EEG. It has been emphasized in this work that the ad-

vent of electroencephalography marked the beginning of modern studies on the characterization of the epilepsies. Thus the definition of epilepsy as a sudden paroxysmal, excessive neuronal discharge was modified to indicate not only excessive firing of individual cells, but also massive discharge of many neurons in unison, abolishing the finely organized temperospatial patterning characteristic of the integrative activity of the brain. Several investigators have developed classifications of the epilepsies. Discussion of the epilepsies and the therapeutic significance of anticonvulsants should be based on some understanding of clinical phenomena of the different types of epileptic seizures.

Gastaut and Broughton (4) reviewed the clinical aspects of epilepsy emphasizing pathophysiological mechanisms, including a description of many individual epileptic seizure types and their pathophysiological characteristics. Gastaut (1964) also is responsible for an earlier International Classification of Epileptic Seizures. The following summary, although not as comprehensive as Gastaut's, should serve as a brief introduction to this chapter. The major types of epileptic seizures include generalized seizures (without local onset); unilateral seizures (those affecting one entire side of the body); partial seizures (seizures beginning locally); erratic seizures of the newborn; and unclassified seizures. Generalized seizures have been further characterized as either convulsive or nonconvulsive. Convulsive generalized seizures include tonic–clonic seizures (grand mal seizures), tonic seizures, clonic seizures, and epileptic myoclonus. Nonconvulsive generalized seizures are represented by the classical petit mal absence, atypical absences (petit mal variant absences), and absence status. The attack of tonic–clonic seizures is frequently preceded by a succession of bilateral muscular jerks; the seizure consists of loss of consciousness and a sequence of motor and autonomic events lasting a total of 1–2 min; the ictal EEG consists of a bilateral synchronous and symmetrical epileptic discharge; it includes bursts of multiple strokes during the initial myoclonic period which are followed by transient flattening and then by a hypersynchronous discharge during the tonic phase, and multiple spike and wave discharges during the clonic phase. Classical petit mal epilepsy is characterized by impairment or loss of consciousness and of memory, of sudden onset lasting 5–15 sec; the ictal EEG contains a well-known generalized rhythmic spike and wave or multiple spike and wave discharge.

Epilepsy is a CNS malfunction that leads either to generalized hyperactivity involving essentially all parts of the brain or to hyperactivity of only a portion of the brain (5). When generalized epilepsy is manifested as seizures accompanied by general convulsions, chewing motions, and loss of consciousness, it is termed grand mal epilepsy. Grand mal epilepsy is characterized by abnormally fast brain waves, by extreme neuronal discharges originating in the mesencephalic portion of the reticular activating system; these discharges then spread throughout the central nervous system—including the cortex, the lower portions of the brain, and the spinal cord—causing tonic convulsions followed by clonic convulsions.

Another type of epilepsy in which there is generalized hyperactivity involving essentially all parts of the brain is petit mal epilepsy. It occurs in two forms, the myoclonic form and the absence form. In the former a burst of neuronal discharges lasting a fraction of a second occurs throughout the nervous system; these are similar to those that occur at the beginning of grand mal seizure; however, the entire process stops immediately and is usually over before consciousness is lost. The absence form of petit mal epilepsy is manifested by 5–20 sec of unconsciousness and some symmetrical clonic motor activity. The petit mal EEG exhibits alternately slow and fast waves.

Partial (focal) epilepsy in the form of localized convulsions that may occur without the loss of consciousness has been called cortical epilepsy or Jacksonian seizures. In many cases this disorder is a consequence of localized, organic brain lesions that can promote extremely rapid discharges in local neurons. When the discharge rate increases above ca. 1000/sec, synchronous waves spread over the adjacent cortical regions. When this phenomenon spreads to the motor cortex, it causes progressive muscular contractions. Another variety of partial epilepsy is called psychomotor seizure. It may be characterized by a short period of amnesia, an attack of abnormal rage, sudden anxiety, and a moment of incoherent speech. A typical EEG during psychomotor attack shows a low frequency between 2 and 4/sec, with superimposed 14/sec waves (5).

1.3 Therapeutic Management

Antiepileptic agents are used to reduce the number and severity of epileptic seizures. Although the specific molecular mechanism of their action is not known, a number of drugs are effective in preventing or reducing the frequency of seizures in approximately 80% of epileptic patients. The ideal antiepileptic agent should exert effective anticonvulsant action with minimal sedative–hypnotic effect. In high doses practically all hypnotics relieve convulsive attacks. However, phenobarbital, mephobarbital, and metharbital are effective anticonvulsants, even in nonhypnotic doses. Phenobarbital may be useful in the management of most types of seizures. The hydantoins (e.g., diphenylhydantoin and ethotoin) are used primarily in severe motor and psychomotor seizures. The oxazolidine-2,4-diones (trimethadione and

paramethadione), methsuximide, phensuximide, and ethosuximide are primarily useful in the treatment of absence seizures,
formerly called petit mal; ethosuximide is
considered to be the drug of choice in this
capacity. The initial drug for the treatment
of generalized tonic–clonic seizures (formerly called grand mal epilepsy) or focal
epilepsy is usually phenytoin or phenobarbital; in most cases the anticonvulsant of
choice herein is phenytoin (6, 7).

2 ETIOLOGY EPILEPSY

The nature of the biochemical reactions
leading to the CNS electrical discharges
and epileptic convulsions remains unknown. Various hypotheses have been
proposed to account for the epileptic discharge, but there is a lack of certainty
about the chemical events underlying the
convulsive reactivity of the brain. The
biochemical aspects of convulsive disorders
have been investigated by various workers
(8–10).

The neurochemistry of epilepsy and
mechanisms of action of anticonvulsants
were reviewed by Singh and Huot in 1973
(11). This review concentrates on the various neurochemical modifications that are
known to occur before, during, and after an
epileptic seizure. Hypoglycemia, pyrodox-
ine deficiency, and calcium ion and magnesium ion serum concentrations are discussed as pre-ictal changes. Intra-ictal
neurochemical modifications are the result
of increased cerebral metabolism, muscular
convulsions, and apnea. These intra-ictal
neurochemical modifications include
changes associated with the metabolism of
neurotransmitters, e.g., acetylcholine, catecholamines and serotonin, γ-amino-butyric
acid (GABA), and glycine (11).

High frequency firing in the seizure focus
of a typical epileptic patient might be due
to congenital defects, head trauma, or
neoplasm. Central nervous system vascular

malfunctions also have been implicated in
the etiology of epilepsy (3).

In 1954 Penfield and Jasper (12) provided documentation of the concept that
seizures can arise in a focus and then propagate to involve additional circuits of the
brain. Advances in neurosurgery have permitted the removal of the epileptogenic
focus, with resulting cessation of seizures
(13). Electroencephalography has proved
to be very useful in the characterization of
neurological diseases. The appearance
of rapid cortical spikes in the EEG is one of
the most specific signs of focal discharge in
epileptic patients (12). The EEG is considered to represent a summation of potentials generated largely by graded response
of the membrane of the cortex. The dendrites of the neuron generate graded responses in contrast to the all-or-none spike
responses of the axon or cell body (13).

Considering the close association of the
spike activity in the EEG with epilepsy,
Ward (13) comprehensively studied the
question as to whether or not the fundamental physiological malfunction in
epilepsy resides in the dendrites of the
neurons in epileptogenic focus. He
analyzed the data supporting the hypothesis
that the basic malfunction in epilepsy may
be at the dendritic level. According to this
hypothesis the autonomous activity that
characterizes the epileptic neuron is due to
relatively enduring dendritic depolarization, which might be the consequence of
mechanical deformation of dendritic
membrane. Another important consideration is how dendritic activity in one neuron
affects neighboring dendritic membranes.
Local field effects can induce excitability
alterations in adjacent neurons. Epileptic
neuronal dendrites are considered to be
electrically excitable since they are relatively devoid of enveloping structures (13).

Other mechanisms have been proposed
as the basis for epileptogenesis. Since spontaneous fluctuations of membrane potential
and excitability may occur under certain

conditions, pathological disturbance of the phenomena responsible for such spontaneous activity might contribute to the generation of the autonomous hyperactivity characteristic of the epileptic neuron. Epileptogenic mechanisms might involve alterations of the local circuitry of the cortex. Denervation hypersensitivity to acetylcholine has also been mentioned as a possible mechanism (13).

From a review of the neurochemistry of epilepsy (8) one can conclude that the epileptogenic cortex is characterized by an impairment of acetylcholine binding, a metabolic loss of glutamic acid, and a failure to maintain tissue K^+ concentrations.

Mechanisms that implicate excessive acetylcholine (due to overproduction or impaired binding) have been proposed as contributing factors in the etiology of seizures. However, although excessive amounts of acetylcholine may cause neuronal hyperactivity, tremors, and seizures, it seems unlikely that altered acetylcholine metabolism is a cause of human epilepsy (1). The CNS actions of acetylcholine antagonists are consistent with an important role of acetylcholine at some sites, but selective blockade solely of cholinergic transmission seems insufficient to produce complete anticonvulsant action, unless the convulsions are initiated by specific activation of cholinergic neurons (e.g., by cholinesterase inhibitors or nicotine).

A vast array of experimentation has led to much speculation regarding GABA and epilepsy, but no definite conclusions have emerged. Nevertheless, most of the experimental studies point to a possibly important role for GABA in the etiology and arrest of convulsions (11).

GABA has been regarded as a central inhibitory neurohormonal modulator (14). It appears that the GABA action is nonspecific regulation of CNS excitation. Curtis and Watkins (15, 16) applied GABA iontophoretically to the external surface membrane of spinal motoneurons, inter-

neurons, and Renshaw cells; intracellular recordings from motoneurons showed no change in resting membrane potential, but excitatory and inhibitory postsynaptic potentials were depressed or blocked. Activation of Ranshaw cells by synaptic excitation or by ionophoretic application of acetylcholine was also blocked. These results are characteristic of a nonspecific depression of neuronal activity and not of a specific inhibitory transmitter (1).

Vitamin B_6 (pyridoxine) deficiency, treatment with certain hydrazine derivatives (e.g., isoniazid), or the administration of pyridoxine antimetabolites can lead to convulsive manifestations and a decrease in GABA concentration. These convulsive disorders can be rectified by the administration of GABA or pyridoxine. Since vitamin B_6 is the precursor in the formation of pyridoxal 5-phosphate, which is the codecarboxylase responsible for the decarboxylation of glutamic acid to form GABA, and since hydrazine derivatives can inactivate pyridoxal 5-phosphate via hydrazone formation, it is possible that the convulsive disorders are due to a decrease in the availability of GABA (17, 18).

The CNS stimulant picrotoxin exerts presynaptic inhibition, and this action is blocked by GABA; hence it has been presumed that GABA plays the role of neurohormonal transmitter or modulator in presynaptic inhibition in mammals (19). The adrenal cortical steroids affect CNS excitability. Spontaneous seizures in man have been attributed to treatment with high doses of cortisone or ACTH. It is noteworthy that hydrocortisone in high doses decreases brain GABA, with an increase in brain excitability (20).

The effect of hydroxylamine or aminooxyacetic acid, which leads to an increase in GABA concentration in the brain, has also been attributed to an inhibition of the GABA–ketoglutaric transaminase system (21, 22). The CNS stimulants caffeine and centedrin also increase the GABA content of the brain (21). From studies (22) of the effect of aminooxyacetic acid on GABA transamination and GABA concentration it appears that GABA transamination is the rate-limiting step of GABA catabolism via succinate and entry into the Krebs TCA cycle. Hydroxylamine and aminooxyacetic acid have been characterized as active anticonvulsants; however, glutamic acid γ-hydrazide, another inhibitor of GABA transamination, induces an increase in brain GABA concentration and fails to protect mice against the convulsant effects of insulin or pentylenetetrazole (23).

Experimental epilepsy has been of interest to investigators in neurophysiology and neurology. The study of experimental epilepsy could achieve a model of the epileptic seizure, which might provide a better understanding of some of the pathophysiological mechanisms of the human epileptic fit. Experimental (animal) epileptogenic foci can be induced by certain drugs or by freezing (24). Local freezing of the cerebral cortex produces local discharges that may become generalized and leads to a status epilepticus and death of the animal. "Alumina" cream also has been used for producing an epileptogenic lesion; application of this cream, which is composed of ammonium hydroxide and ammonium aluminate, to the motor cortex produces, after 4–9 weeks, focal epileptic seizures that may persist for months. The focal seizure often becomes generalized, and the electrocorticographic aspect of the focal seizure resembles that of focal epileptogenic seizures in man (24). Ward (13) has described a method wherein commercial aluminum hydroxide gel is injected intracortically; the effect of this preparation most closely approximates human epilepsy. Other chemicals that have demonstrated epileptogenic properties include strychnine, penicillin, mescaline, and acetylcholine; these agents are generally applied locally to the cortex.

Experimental seizure activity useful in anticonvulsant-drug testing can also be induced by electrical stimulation (electrically induced after discharge) of a particular brain structure. The cortical epileptogenic focus generally is influenced to a minimal extent by the common anticonvulsants. The epileptogenic focus produced by minimal cortical stimulation is not affected by intracarotid phenobarbital administration (10 mg/kg). The local action of anticonvulsants has been tested in the unanesthetized rabbit on seizures elicited by electrical stimulation of the cortex, diencephalon, and rhinenencephalon. Diphenylhydantoin via the carotid artery produced some slowing in the frequency of spike discharge; administered orally, it increased the threshold only of the seizures elicited by diencephalic stimulation (25).

The triggering of epileptic seizures by sensitive or sensory stimuli has been the subject of various clinical investigations. For a review, see Ref. 26.

3 PHARMACOLOGICAL EVALUATION OF ANTICONVULSANTS

Various laboratory tests on mice and/or rats have been developed for the preliminary screening of compounds for anticonvulsant activity (1, 2, 27). The practical methods involve treatment with the potential anticonvulsant, followed by the administration of a convulsant agent, usually pentylenetetrazole, or the electrical induction of convulsions. The common electrical methods are based on the measurement of the threshold current that is necessary to induce minimal seizure, identified by the occurrence of detectable clonus of facial muscles and rhythmic twitches of whiskers and ears. This method is called the minimal electroshock test (MET). Another electroshock method measures the threshold current that delivers a supramaximal stimulus to elicit the maximal seizure (MES). Antipentylenetetrazole bioassays usually consist of the administration of pentylenetetrazole in doses ranging from convulsant to fatal, to experimental animals pretreated with the potential anticonvulsant compound; the amount of convulsant necessary to provoke seizures is determined.

Some correlations of laboratory and clinical evaluations of anticonvulsant drugs have been made by Millichap (27). Suppression of electroencephalographic seizure discharges has been correlated with control of the commonly associated clinical seizure patterns; anticonvulsants that control grand mal tonic seizures are effective against maximal electroshock tonic seizures in mice and rats, but activity against pentylenetetrazole is not essential nor constantly predictive of anti-petit mal efficacy (27).

4   GROSS EFFECTS OF ANTICONVULSANTS

Woodbury and Fingl (7) note that most antiepileptic agents modify the ability of the brain to respond to various seizure-evoking stimuli and that neurophysiological effects include reduction of posttetanic potentiation (PTP), elevation of excitatory synaptic threshold, potentiation of presynaptic or postsynaptic inhibition, and prolongation of refractory period. Accordingly, these agents affect normal functions of the brain leading to undesirable side effects.

Many anticonvulsants have sedative effects, and some cause mental disturbances. Phenacemide is reported to cause serious personality changes in some cases, including psychoses and suicidal depression (6).

Some anticonvulsants cause gastrointestinal side effects in some patients. Ataxia is a common adverse reaction due to the administration of hydantoins. Many anticonvulsants exert skin eruptions as a hypersensitivity reaction. Phenytoin often causes gingival hyperplasia in children. Hydan-

toins also have been implicated as factors leading to lymphadenopathies. Some megaloblastic anemias have been attributed to anticonvulsant hydantoins, barbiturates, and primidone. Severe blood dyscarasias have been attributed to phenacemide and mephenytoin. Hepatotoxicity has been associated with phenacemide, and nephropathies have occasionally developed during treatment with trimethadione and paramethadione (6).

Considering the foregoing, the search continues for more ideal antiepileptic agents, that is, compounds with highly selective anticonvulsant action, a broad spectrum of antiepileptic efficacy, and minimal side effects. Accordingly, the medicinal chemist endeavors to study molecular modifications and structure–activity relationships of the classic types of anticonvulsants, as well as of newer structural types of potential anticonvulsants. Moreover, as advances in neurochemistry and in the understanding of the mechanisms of the epilepsies continue to be made (3), the medicinal chemist proceeds to base drug design on more rational biochemical grounds.

5   MECHANISMS OF ANTICONVULSANT ACTION

Many mechanisms have been proposed to account for the anticonvulsant properties of the various types of antiepileptics, but none has been confirmed at the molecular level. Some of the more interesting theories implicate certain neurohormones. Carbonic anhydrase inhibition correlates with the anticonvulsant activity of certain carbonic anhydrase inhibitors. Since most anticonvulsants depress brain respiration at high concentrations, it has been conjectured that these drugs exert their actions via mechanisms involving a decrease of cerebral respiration (2).

Acetazolamide, a potent carbonic anhydrase inhibitor and diuretic, possesses anticonvulsant and antiepileptic properties. Its anticonvulsant action is due to inhibition of brain carbonic anhydrase (28) and might be due to an increased concentration of carbon dioxide resulting from inhibition of this enzyme in brain cells (29). Carbonic anhydrase conceivably plays a role in promoting the elimination of excess carbon dioxide from the brain; excess carbon dioxide decreases nerve conduction. Previously the anticonvulsant action of acetazolamide was thought to be due to acidosis since its diuretic action is associated with base loss and metabolic acidosis; acidosis was recognized as beneficial in epilepsy. We should take into consideration that the anticonvulsant action of these carbonic anhydrase inhibitors depends on catecholamine concentration in the brain (30).

The levels of serotonin in the brain are increased by various anticonvulsants: phenobarbital, diphenylhydantoin, phenacemide, paramethadione, and others. This is attributed to nonspecific depression of CNS function, resulting in decreased release of neurohormones. Since certain monoamine oxidase inhibitors possess anticonvulsant activity and resperpine is proconvulsant, the effects of these drugs on brain amine levels have led to the thought that some convulsive seizures might be due to an alteration of amine concentration, and some anticonvulsants rectify this malfunction (1).

As noted above, it has been hypothesized that excessive acetylcholine in the brain might contribute to epileptogenesis. However, it is inconceivable that specific antiacetylcholine action can be fundamental to anticonvulsant action. Acetylcholine probably performs neurohormonal functions at some specialized sites; an antiacetylcholine effect in the brain might produce anticonvulsant action only if the seizures were initiated by the excitation of the cholinergic neurons (1). Nevertheless, atropine and scopolamine, two anticholinergic alkaloids, possess some anticonvulsant properties.

Although atropine is active against convulsions induced by tetraethyl pyrophosphate, it is not considered to be an effective antiepileptic agent (1).

Johnson and Eyring's Studies (31, 32) on the mode of action of lipid-soluble depressants (e.g., alcohols, ethers, ketones, and barbiturates) should also be taken into consideration. This work indicates that anticonvulsants related to the barbiturates might exert their action(s) via conformational rearrangements of oxidative enzymes essential to brain respiration. These conformational changes appear to be functions of hydrophobic and hydrogen-bonding interactions between the depressant and the protein (see Section 8).

Finally, as has been noted, GABA has important inhibitory CNS properties and evidence indicates that many anticonvulsants may operate via GABAergic mechanisms.

6 ABSORPTION AND METABOLISM

A multiplicity of biochemical parameters must be assessed in the study of structure–activity relationships, including absorption, distribution, metabolism, and excretion phenomena. Reviews of general principles concerning these biochemical phenomena are included in the classic monograph, *Antiepileptic Drugs*, edited by Woodbury, Penry, and Schmidt (33). Animal metabolic studies are discussed by Glasson and Benakis (34), and Svensmark (35) reviewed absorption, distribution, metabolism, and excretion studies in man. A brief summary of the highlights of absorption, distribution, metabolism, and excretion is included herein. (Refer also to Chapters 2 and 3.)

Phenobarbital (55.**1**) is well absorbed from the gastrointestinal tract, and it is uniformly distributed to most mammalian tissues, including the brain. It is metabolized primarily via oxidative hydroxylation to form *p*-hydroxyphenobarbital

(55.**2**) and its glucuronide and sulfate conjugates. Phenobarbital is excreted by the
kidney in the intact form (25%) and also as
the *p*-hydroxy metabolite (75%) and its
conjugates. *p*-Hydroxyphenobarbital appears in human urine partly free and partly
conjugated, not as a glucuronide but as a
sulfate, whereas in dog urine it is detected
as the glucuronide (36). Mephobarbital
(55.**3**) is absorbed from the gastrointestinal
tract to the extent of about 50%, whereas
phenobarbital is estimated to be 70–90%
absorbed. Since *N*-demethylation is the
major route of mephobarbital metabolism,
it is conceivable that the therapeutic and
some toxic properties are due, at least in
part, to phenobarbital formed *in vivo* (36).
Metharbital (55.**4**) is also metabolized by
N-demethylation (55.**5**) in the dog and in
man (37).

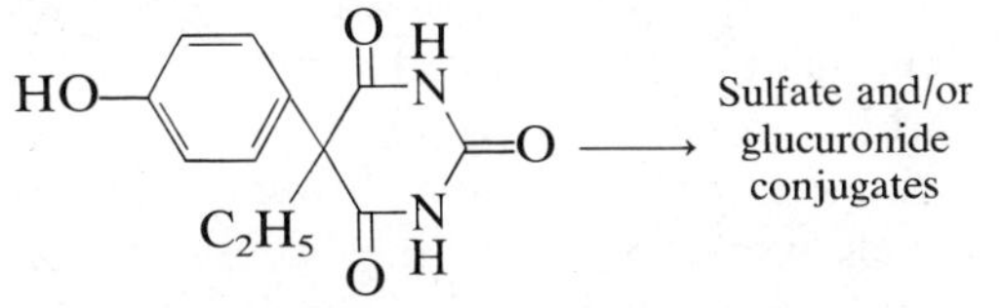

Another important metabolite of primidone is phenylethylmalondiamide (55.**7**);
50–70% of administered primidone is
excreted by the human kidney in the
form of this metabolic product. Phenylethylmalondiamide possesses only one-
fortieth of the anticonvulsant potency of
primidone (1). Alvin et al. (38) studied the
(rat) hepatic metabolism of primidone by
improved radiotracer methodology that
permits nearly quantitative accounting of
the dose as drug and identified metabolites.
^{14}C-Primidone and its metabolites were
separated by thin-layer chromatotraphy
and quantitated by liquid scintillation
counting; primidone metabolism was quantitated thus: phenobarbital formation,
15%; phenylethylmalondiamide, 80%.

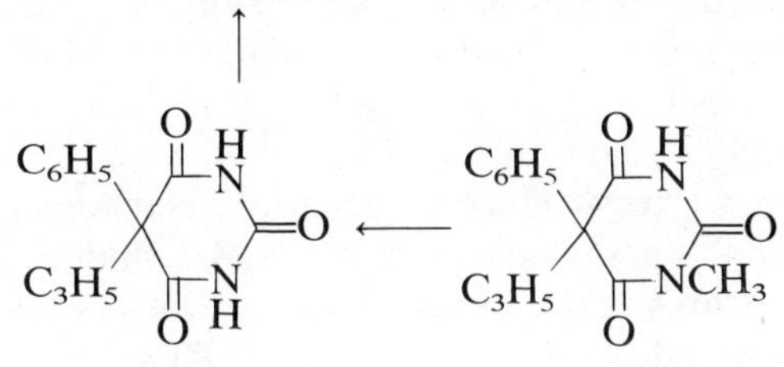

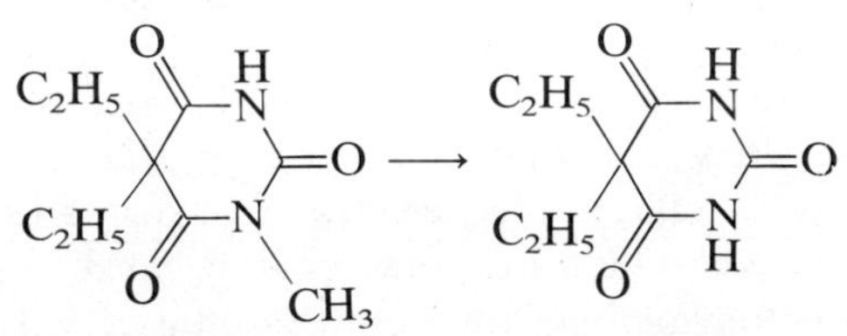

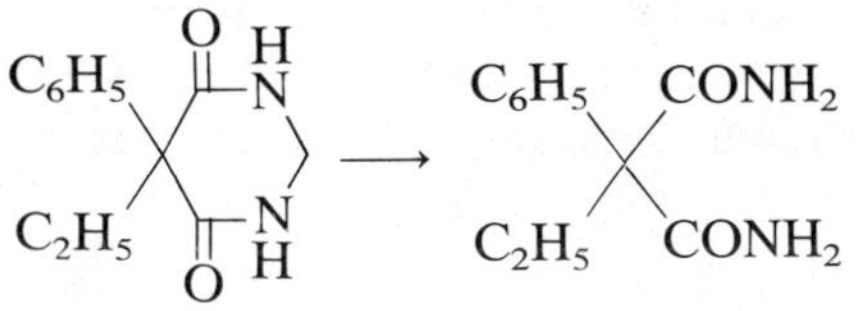

55.**6**   55.**7**

55.**2**

Diphenylhydantoin (5,5-diphenyl-2,4-
imidazolidinedione, 55.**8**) is also well absorbed when administered **orally**. The
biologic half-life in human plasma is about
24 hr. As in the case of phenobarbital, the
principal pathway of diphenylhydantoin
metabolism is via oxidative hydroxylation.
Not more than 5% of the administered
dose is excreted in the intact form, whereas
about 50% is excreted in the form of
conjugated 5-(*p*-hydroxyphenyl)-5-phenyl-
hydantoin (55.**9**) by man. The main route
of conjugation is probably via glucuronide
formation (1).

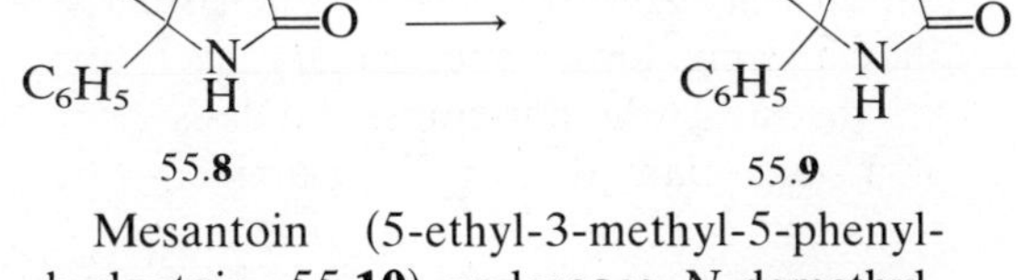

55.**1**   55.**3**

55.**4**   55.**5**

55.**8**   55.**9**

Primidone (2-desoxyphenobarbital) (55.**6**)
is absorbed well in man upon oral
administration. It is metabolized to
phenobarbital (55.**1**) and *p*-hydroxypheno-
barbital, resulting in blood concentrations
of 55.**1** in the therapeutic range (1, 36).

Mesantoin (5-ethyl-3-methyl-5-phenyl-
hydantoin, 55.**10**) undergoes *N*-demethyl-
ation to form 5-ethyl-5-phenylhydantoin

(Nirvanol, 55.**11**); then Nirvanol is *p*-hydroxylated (55.**12**).

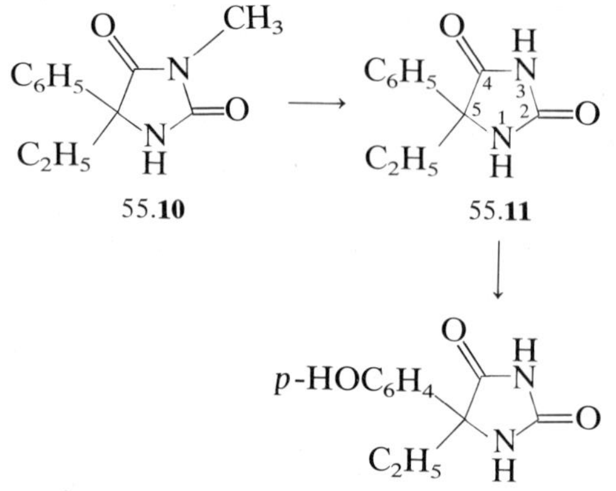

55.**10** → 55.**11**

↓

55.**12**

The metabolism of ethotoin (peganone), 3-ethyl-5-phenylhydantoin, has been studied in comparison with its *N*-methyl analog and 5-phenylhydantoin. Significant *N*-dealkylation takes place as an initial reaction in the dog. *p*-Phenyl hydroxylation also affects the two *N*-alkyl analogs but does not affect 5-phenylhydantoin. The *p*-hydroxy derivatives were detected in urine as glucuronides. Phenylhydantoic acid is reported to be a major metabolic product of these three hydantoins (39).

The therapeutic oxazolidine-2,4-diones (Section 7.4) also are metabolized by *N*-demethylation, and the *N*-demethylated products have been suggested as contribution to the anticonvulsant properties (1, 2).

Goulet et al. (40) studied the human metabolism of ethosuximide and they reported the urinary excretion of the stereoisomeric 2-(1-hydroxyethyl)-2-methylsuccinimides. These workers also noted that the plasma levels of ethosuximide among subjects receiving single daily (therapeutic) doses did not drop to the subtherapeutic range at 24 hr and that steady-state plasma levels and urinary excretion are the same whether ethosuximide is given as a single daily dose or on a divided-dose regimen.

7 STRUCTURE–ACTIVITY RELATIONSHIPS

7.1 Barbiturates

The anticonvulsant barbiturates include phenobarbital (55.**1**) and metharbital (55.**4**). Various structure–activity studies of the barbiturates have been conducted (41) and are discussed in Chapter 54. Considering that both phenobarbital and mephobarbital are phenyl-substituted at the 5 position, it is tempting to associate this structural feature with selectivity for motor cortex activity since diphenylhydantoin also possesses this type of substitution. It has been deduced that grand mal epilepsy is controlled by a variety of compounds, and the most effective possess phenyl substitution. Metharbital possesses some anti-grand mal activity, but its tropism is less strict than that of its phenylated relatives, phenobarbital and mephobarbital (2).

Samour et al. (42) found, in a series of 1,3-bis(alkoxymethyl)-5,5-disubstituted barbituric acids, tested in mice, that 1,3-bis(alkoxymethyl)phenobarbitals, including 1,3-bis(dimethoxymethyl)phenobarbital, DMMP (named eterobarb by the *USAN and the USP Dictionary of Drug Names*, 1978), were very effective against electroshock and pentylenetetrazole (PTZ)-induced seizures. The analogous derivatives of barbital were active against PTZ. Both series of compounds were inactive as hypnotics.

Additionally, it was found that 1,3-bis-(acyloxymethyl)phenobarbital derivatives were active against electroshock and PTZ and were not hypnotic in mice. 1,3-bis-(acetoxymethyl)-5,5-diethylbarbituric acid was effective against electroshock and was not hypnotic. 1,3-bis(halomethyl)phenobarbital derivatives were active against PTZ and had no hypnotic activity (43).

In a further exploration of the effect

of *N*-substituent variations, it was found that 1-methyl-3-methoxymethylphenobarbital was more effective against PTZ than 1,3-bis(dimethoxymethyl)phenobarbital or mephobarbital, but was less active against electroshock than 1,3-bis(methoxymethyl)-phenobarbital or mephobarbital. The compound was devoid of hypnotic activity. Other compounds reported in this study were 1-morpholinomethyl)phenobarbital and 1-(piperidinomethyl)phenobarbital. These compounds were active against maximal seizure (MES) and PTZ and were weaker hypnotics than phenobarbital (44).

The metabolites of DMMP appear to be important. For example, in man, phenobarbital, 1-methylphenobarbital, and 1-methoxymethylphenobarbital are major metabolites. 1,3-Dimethylphenobarbital and 1-methyl-3-methoxymethylphenobarbital also have been identified. This observation led to an investigation of 1-alkyl, 1-alkoxymethyl, 1,3-dialkyl, and 1-alkyl-3-alkoxymethyl derivatives of barbital and phenobarbital. 1,3-Dimethylphenobarbital was as potent as mephobarbital against MES and PTZ and was about as hypnotic as mephobarbital. 1,3-Diethylphenobarbital was not anticonvulsant; 1,3-dibenzyl-phenobarbital and 1-benzylphenobarbital were very weakly anticonvulsant. None of these compounds were hypnotic except at lethal doses. 1-Methyl-3-methoxymethyl-barbital possessed good activity against MES and PTZ seizures and, unlike methar-bital, was not hypnotic (45).

The effects of 5,5-diphenylbarbituric acid were examined in mice. The compound was far more active by i.p. administration than by gavage. It appeared that a limited water solubility was associated with poor gastro-intestinal absorption. The compound parenterally or by gavage was less potent than phenobarbital against MES and PTZ and less potent than diphenylhydantoin against MES (46).

7.2   Hydantoins

5-Ethyl-5-phenylhydantoin (55.**11**) nirvanol), which is analogous to phenobarbital, was one of the pioneer compounds of this class of anticonvulsants. Although it is an effective anticonvulsant, the compound is too toxic to be considered safe therapeutically (47).

In 1908 Blitz (48) prepared 5,5-diphenylhydantoin (55.**8**), phenytoin. Later in 1938, Merritt and Putnam (49) evaluated phenytoin with respect to anticonvulsant activity and found it to be effective in protecting against convulsive seizures induced by electrical stimulation in the cat. Now, after almost three decades of clinical application, phenytoin remains one of the most effective antiepileptic medicinals with minimal sedative–hypnotic side effects (50).

5-Ethyl-3-methyl-5-phenylhydantoin (55.**10**) (mesantoin), which is the *N*-3-methyl congener of nirvanol, is less toxic than nirvanol; it appears that *N*-methylation leads to a decrease in toxicity, but mesantoin is *N*-demethylated *in vivo* to form nirvanol. The 1- and 3-methyl derivatives of phenytoin (55.**13**, R′ or R″ = CH$_3$) have also been assessed but ranked as less active than phenytoin (1).

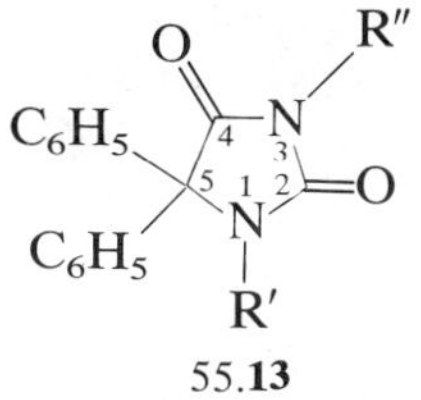

55.**13**

The 5,5-dithienyl and 5,5-dipyridyl analogs of phenytoin were studied and categorized as comparable to diphenylhydantoin as anticonvulsants (47).

Some spirohydantoins and spirothiohydantoins have interesting anticonvulsant properties. Generally, these compounds differ from the corresponding aryl-substituted hydantoins in that they are primarily effective as antipentylenetetrazole agents. However, 5,5-heptamethylenehydantoin is active against pentylenetetrazole- and electroshock-induced convulsions (1).

In a series of cycloalkanespiro-5-hydantoins, some cycloheptanespiro-5-hydantoins were active as anticonvulsants, generally most effective against pentylenetetrazole (51). Cyclopentanespiro-5-hydantoins exhibited little activity, except at near toxic doses when sedation was observed, and the cyclooctanespiro-5-hydantoins showed anticonvuslant and sedative activity reminiscent of the barbiturates.

The spirohydantoin (55.**14**) (spirodon) from 2-tetralone is active against electroshock and pentylenetetrazole seizures. This compound is effective against grand mal epilepsy and is particularly useful against psychomotor and focal attacks; however, toxic reactions have occurred in high proportion (1).

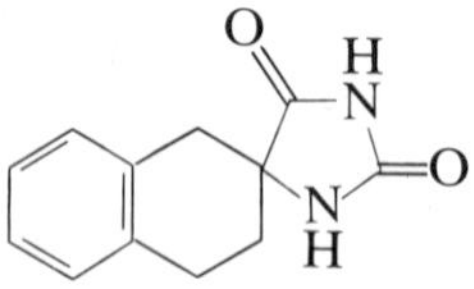

55.**14**

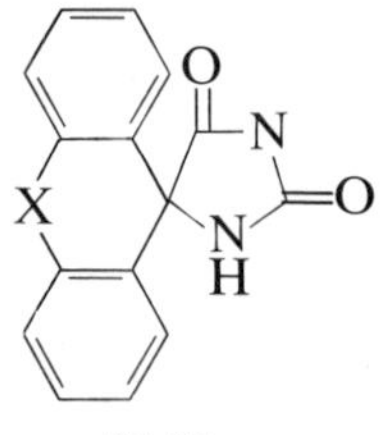

55.**15**

In a series of spirohydantoins (55.**15**) derived from tricyclic ketones, the biologic properties of the spiro analogs of diphenylhydantoin depend on the nature of the bridge X between the two aryl cycles (52). Earlier the spirohydantoin derived from fluorenone had been characterized as an anticonvulsant in humans. However,

the compounds possessing different X bridges, —CH_2CH_2—, —CH=CH—, and —$(CH_2)_3$—, are practically devoid of anticonvulsant properties. Indeed, the compound with X = —$(CH_2)_3$— proved to be a potent convulsant.

Among thiohydantoins and dithiohydantoins, 5,5-dimethyldithiohydantoin is active against pentylenetetrazole seizures but of doubtful effectiveness against electroshock (2). 5,5-Heptamethylene-2,4-dithiohydantoin is active against the same agent, and the 2-thiohydantoin has sedative–hypnotic activity (1). The 2-thio congener of diphenylhydantoin is less active than diphenylhydantoin. Albutoin is said to be active against all seizure types, especially grand mal (53).

Among 3-phenyl- and 3-tolyl-5-benzylidine-2-thiohydantoins, compounds in which the benzylidine phenyl are chloro-substituted on the 3 position have some activity against PTZ in mice (54).

The structural resemblance between thiohydantoins and the thyrotoxic thiouracils has been a matter of concern, but this side effect varies with the nature of the 5-substitution and in some cases is minimal (1).

The 3-methoxymethyl derivative of diphenylhydantoin proved to be equiactive with diphenylhydantoin in mice in the MES test and also had weak anti-PTZ activity. The 3-benzyloxymethyl and 3-butoxymethyl derivatives were active against both MES and PTZ (55).

The 3-acetoxymethyl derivative has a spectrum of activity analogous to the parent rather than to the 3-methoxymethyl derivative. It antagonized MES seizures and was inactive against PTZ (56).

In a further study, 3-acetoxymethyl and 1,3-di(acetoxymethyl) derivatives of 5-ethyl-5-phenylhydantoin and 1,3-di-(alkoxymethyl) and mixed alkyl, alkoxymethyl derivatives of 5,5-diphenylhydantoin and 5-ethyl-5-phenylhydantoin were prepared and tested in mice. Promising compounds included 1,3-di(methoxymethyl)-5,5-diphenylhydantoin and 3-acetoxymethyl-5-ethyl-5-phenylhydantoin, effective against MES, and 3-methoxymethyl-5-ethyl-5-phenylhydantoin, effective against both MES and PTZ. None of the compounds, given orally, were more active than the parent compounds against MES (57).

Young et al. (58) determined the structures of products formed when certain hydantoins (diphenylhydantoin and mephenytoin) and succinimides (ethosuximide and phensuximide) were treated with p-nitrobenzyl bromide in sodium carbonate solutions. The 3-p-nitrobenzyl derivative of diphenylhydantoin and the N-p-nitrobenzyl derivative of ethosuximide were tested against PTZ in mice and were inactive orally (58).

Derivatives of diphenylhydantoin represented by the structure 55.13) where R' = OEt, OH, NH_2, NHEt, and $NHNH_2$ were prepared and reported to have anticonvulsant activity (anticonvulsant data not given) (59).

Stella et al. (60) used the prodrug approach to circumvent the biologic problems associated with the poor water solubility of diphenylhydantoin. The prodrug reacted under physiological conditions to form diphenylhydantoin.

A report (61) states that pretreatment with lithium carbonate for 9 days significantly promoted diphenylhydantoin's decrease of the duration of MES in mice. Lithium carbonate alone had no effect on the duration of MES.

7.3 Acyl-, Aralkyl-, and Alkylureas

Phenylacetylurea (55.**16a**) (phenacemide) can be considered an open chain analog of the hydantoins. It possesses high anticonvulsant activity both against electroshock and pentylenetetrazole seizures. A derivative, α-chlorophenylacetylurea

(55.**16b**), has also been characterized as an effective anticonvulsant (1).

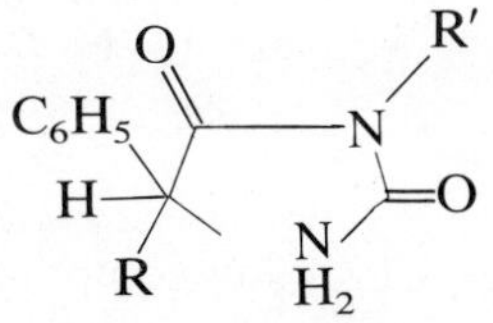

55.**16a**   R = R′ = H
55.**16b**   R = Cl, R′ = H
55.**16c**   R = C_6H_5, R′ = H

Phenylethylacetylurea (pheneturide) has properties similar to phenacemide. Since both compounds possess potential for severe toxicity, use is limited to temporal lobe epilepsy refractory to other agents (62).

The classic work of Spielman et al. (63) led to the advent of phenacemide as a medicinal agent. This study revealed that among aliphatic ureides the highest anticonvulsant activity is found in those derived from secondary and tertiary acids of about seven carbon atoms; with an increase in molecular weight the activity decreases, and the compounds tend to become hypnotic. Among aromatic ureides, phenacemide proved to be the most active, whereas the thienyl analog was practically inactive. Activity decreased with aromatic substitution of phenacemide. Also, diphenylacetylurea (55.**16c**), the acyclic analog of diphenylhydantoin, is inactive as an anticonvulsant. N-Methylation of phenacemide does not increase the anticonvulsant activity (1).

Among a series of acylurea derivatives of the type 55.**16d**, where R = iso-C_5H_{11}, $CHMe_2$, CHMePh, $CHMeCH_2Ph$, or CHPrPh, and R′ = Me, Et, Pr, Me_2CH, Bu, Me_2CHCH_2, Ph, or $PhCH_2$, the compounds where R = CHMePh, $CHMeCH_2Ph$, and R′ = n-alkyl showed the highest activity against electroshock and PTZ, reportedly because they hydrolyzed more rapidly than the other compounds to the substituted ureas (64).

A study of tert-butylurea in mice and rats revealed that it possessed pronounced ac-

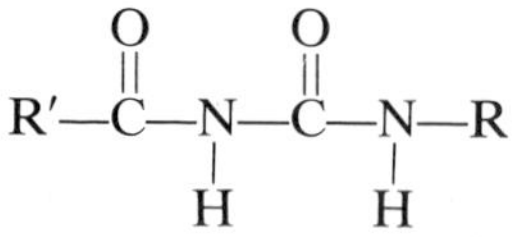

55.**16d**

tivity against PTZ. The compound did not
appear to be a potent hypnotic agent (65).

7.4 Oxazolidine-2,4-diones

The oxazolidine-2,4-dione system (55.**17**) is
a close structural congener of the hydantoin
system, differing only in that an oxygen
atom replaces the NH group at position
1. The chemical properties of the oxazoli-
dine-2,4-diones have been reviewed (66). As
in the case of the hydantoins, substitution
at the 5 position is associated with anticonvulsant activity.

The first oxazolidine-2,4-dione found to
be useful was 2,5,5-trimethyloxazolidine-
2,4-dione (trimethadione) (55.**17a**), an
effective anti-petit mal agent; it had been
synthesized as a potential analgetic agent
(67). Also important as an anti-petit mal
agent is 2,5-dimethyl-5-ethyloxazolidine-
2,4-dione (paramethadione) (55.**17b**),
somewhat less potent than trimethadione
but also less apt to induce side effects.

In Europe, two other oxazolidine-2,4-
diones have been used clinically against
petit mal: 3-ethyl-5,5-dimethyloxazolidine-
2,4-dione (dimidione) (55.**17c**) and 3-allyl-
5-methyloxazolidine-2,4-dione (malidione)
(55.**17d**) (1).

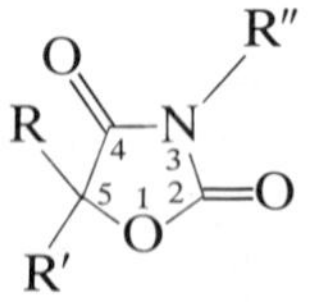

55.**17a**   R, R′, R″ = CH_3
55.**17b**   R = R″ = CH_3, R′ = C_2H_5
55.**17c**   R = R′ = CH_3, R″ = C_2H_5
55.**17d**   R = H, R′ = CH_3, R″ = allyl
55.**17e**   R = R′ = C_6H_5, R″ = H

Because several oxazolidine-2,4-diones
are effective anti-petit mal agents and are
ineffective against grand mal it might be
inferred that the oxazolidine-2,4-dione system automatically confers upon a compound anti-petit mal characteristics. However, 5,5-diphenyloxazolidine-2,4-dione
(55.**17e**) is an anti-grand mal agent and is
ineffective in petit mal (1). Thus the nature
of the substituents on C-5 is important;
lower alkyl substituents tend toward anti-
petit mal activity and aryl substituents toward anti-grand mal activity (1, 2).

It has been stated that among anti-petit
mal agents imido alkylation is mandatory
(2). Because of the characteristically small
alkyl substituents on the 5 position the
anti-petit mal oxazolidine-2,4-diones are
relatively polar molecules. The imido alkylation could serve two functions: increase
the partition coefficient and prevent the
dissociation of the imido hydrogen, in both
cases favoring more effective distribution to
the central nervous system. The N-alkyl
substituent does not appear to be necessary
at the site of action. Trimethadione, paramethadione, and dimidione are extensively
N-dealkylated and these early studies
suggested that the N-dealkylated metabolites are important for bioactivity (68–
73).

More recently, the N-demethylated
metabolite of trimethadione, dimethadione
(DMO), has been studied. It proved to be
effective against electroshock and PTZ in
mice and rats. Additional evidence that
DMO is involved in the activity of trimethadione came from studies on the electroshock seizure threshold (EST). The EST
increased rapidly after trimethadione administration, decreased somewhat after
3 hr, and then increased to above normal
levels 4–6 hr after administration. Hepatec-
tomy abolished the late rise and did not
effect the initial rise in EST (74).

The effect of chronically administered
trimadione on the PTZ seizure threshold in
mice was studied by Frey and Kretschmer

(75). They concluded that the anticonvulsant effect of trimethadione is due mainly to dimethadione.

7.5 Amides

5-Ethyl-5-phenylhexahydropyrimidine-4,6-dione (primidone) (55.**21**), the 2-methylene congener of phenobarbital, possesses interesting anticonvulsant properties. This compound was synthesized by Bogue and Carrington (76) and compared with phenobarbital, diphenylhydantoin, mesantoin, trimethadione, and phenurone. The anticonvulsant potency of primidone compares favorably with that of the other compounds (76). In another study, the molecular modification from phenobarbital to primidone did not alter the spectrum of anticonvulsant activity, but reduced this activity. Primidone is less neurotoxic than phenobarbital in mice and rats. These conclusions were reached on the basis of results from a variety of electroshock and chemoshock (pentylenetetrazole) tests in mice, rats, cats, and rabbits. Primidone also was tested in psychiatric patients for its ability to modify therapeutic electroshock seizures (77).

Certain dialkylmalondiamides have proved to possess anticonvulsant activity with no discernible sedative–hypnotic effects (78). Furthermore, the disubstituted cyanoacetamide intermediates used in the preparation of the malondiamides were more active as anticonvulsants and were also devoid of sedative–hypnotic properties. 2-Ethyl-2-propyl- (55.**18a**) and 2,2-diethylcyanoacetamide (55.**18b**) showed

significant activity against both electroshock and pentylenetetrazole; hence a series of *N*-alkylated and *N*-cyclic derivatives of the aforementioned cyanoacetamides was prepared (79). The acyclic members of this series possess interesting anticonvulsant properties, whereas the cyclic compounds are convulsants (80).

Dibenzo[*a,d*]cycloheptadiene-5-carboxamide (55.**19**) possesses a high order of anticonvulsant activity and is more potent orally than diphenylacetamide, the open ring analog. The cycloheptatriene congener and the 3-chlorocycloheptatriene compound also demonstrate promising anticonvulsant properties (in mice) with low toxicity. In general the doses required to protect against pentylenetetrazole were smaller than those required for anti-electroshock effect (81).

The importance of geometric isomerism to activity was demonstrated among *N*-alkyl-α,β-dimethylcinnamide derivatives. Members of the *E* series in mice were CNS depressant in Irwin's test and, in some instances, anticonvulsant as measured against PTZ. On the other hand, the *Z* isomers caused marked CNS stimulation, producing tremors and convulsions (82).

In a further study, the effect on activity in mice of substitution of the phenyl among selected compounds of the *E* series (*N*-cyclopropyl, *N*-allyl, and *N*-propargyl) and the *Z* series (*N*-cyclopropyl and *N*-allyl) was examined (83). In the *E* series 4-substitution with halogen increased anticonvulsant activity (PTZ). Substitution with electron-donating groups (4-methyl, 4-methoxy, and 3,4,5-trimethoxy) reduced or abolished anticonvulsant activity. In the *Z* series 4-substitution with halogen decreased CNS stimulation. *Z*-*N*-Cyclopropyl derivatives 4-substituted with chlorine or bromine became anticonvulsant. Substitution with 4-methyl decreased stimulatory activity only in the *N*-cyclopropyl compound; 4-methoxy substitution did not generally alter stimulatory properties.

C_2H_5 \qquad $CONH_2$

C

R \qquad CN

55.**18a** $R = C_3H_7$
55.**18b** $R = C_2H_5$

$CONH_2$
55.**19**

7.6 Imides

Miller and Long (84) synthesized a series of succinimides for anticonvulsant evaluation, many of which demonstrated significant activity against pentylenetetrazole and/or electrically induced convulsions. α,α-Diphenylsuccinimide (55.**20a**), which resembles diphenylhydantoin in structure, was active only against electroshock. N-Alkyl derivatives were studied, and as in the case of phenytoin, N-methylation of α,α-diphenylsuccinimide also decreased activity against electroshock. Some N-substituted phenylsuccinamic acids were compared with the corresponding imides, and the amides proved to be devoid of anticonvulsant properties. N-Methyl-α-phenylsuccinimide (phensuximide) (55.**20b**) has been compared clinically with oxazolidinediones.

Phensuximide has use in the treatment of petit mal epilepsy but is less effective than trimethadione and paramethadione (6). Another α-phenyl compound, methsuximide (N,α-dimethyl-α-phenylsuccinimide) (55.**20**, R = R' = CH$_3$), is more active than phensuximide in the treatment of petit mal and psychomotor seizures; however, it also is more toxic. [Both compounds appear to be extensively metabolized by N-demethylation and the respective N-demethylmetabolites are thought to make significant contributions to activity and toxicity (85).] The α,α-dialkyl compound, ethosuximide (α-ethyl-α-methylsuccinimide), is considered the agent of choice in the treatment of petit mal (6). It is more active than the phenyl compounds against PTZ and less active than the phenyl compounds against

electroshock. It is substantially safer than trimethadione and paramethadione.

Further studies on the activities of substituted succinimides against PTZ and electroshock have been conducted. In a series of p-alkylphenyl-N-methylsuccinimides it was found that iso-alkyl substitution tended to promote activity against PTZ. The compounds were most active against electroshock (86).

α-Methylalkoxyphenylsuccinimides and alkoxybenzylsuccinimides were active against electroshock and PTZ (87). The length of the alkoxy group influenced activity but not in a consistent pattern. In general, α-methylalkoxyphenylsuccinimides were most active against PTZ and alkoxybenzylsuccinimides were most active against electroshock.

Davis et al. (52) noted that spiro {dibenzo[a,d]cycloheptadiene-5,2'-succinimide} (55.**21**) afforded protection in mice in doses as low as 5% of its LD$_{50}$ (both against pentylenetetrazole and electroshock).

α-Methyl-α-phenylglutarimide (55.**22a**) possesses anticonvulsant activity, primarily against pentylenetetrazole. α-Ethyl-α-phenylglutarimide (glutethimide) (52.**22b**) is a useful sedative–hypnotic, whereas α-(p-aminophenyl)-α-ethylglutarimide (aminoglutethimide) (55.**22c**) is devoid of

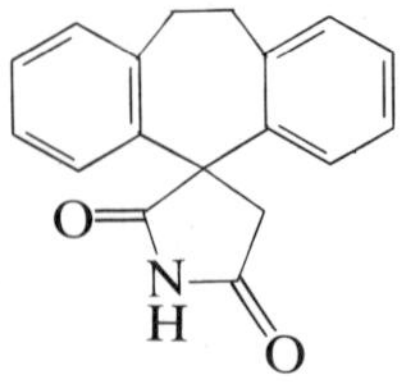

55.**21**

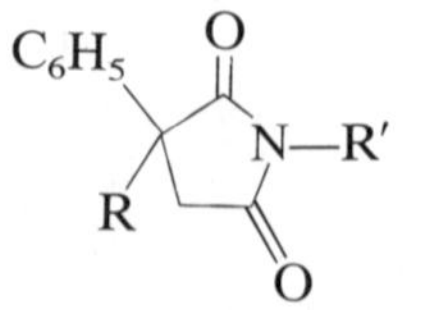

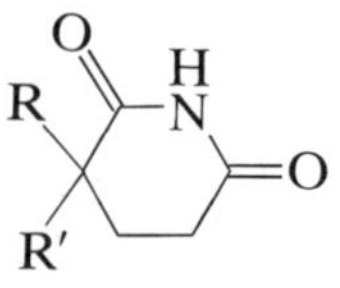

55.**20a**   R = C$_6$H$_5$, R' = H
55.**20b**   R = H, R' = CH$_3$

55.**22a**   R = CH$_3$, R' = C$_6$H$_5$
55.**22b**   R = C$_2$H$_5$, R' = C$_6$H$_5$
55.**22c**   R = C$_2$H$_5$, R' = sp-aminophenyl

sedative effects but is effective as an anti-convulsant in grand mal and to some extent in petit mal cases. Some β-substituted glutarimides possess analeptic properties. β-Ethyl-β-methylglutarimide (bemegride) has been used in medicine for its CNS-stimulatory properties.

Aminoglutethimide has been compared with diphenylhydantoin against grand mal seizures. With respect to efficacy it is equal to diphenylhydantoin in the mild and easily controlled cases, but not in the treatment of the more severe seizures. Aminoglute thimide therapy gives rise to a relatively high incidence of side effects, which approaches 50%.

The synthesis of 4-hydroxy-2-ethyl-2-phenylglutarimide, a glutethimide metabolite, and other glutethimide analogs has been reported. The 4-hydroxy compound was a potent sedative–hypnotic with anticonvulsive (MES) properties. Its 4-amino analog showed enhancement of anticonvulsive properties relative to sedative–hypnotic properties, as did 4-hydroxy-2-ethyl-2-phenylglutaconamide (88).

Wittiak and co-workers (89) synthesized acetyl[D(R)- and L(S)-N-(p-substituted phenyl) succinimides and -glutarimides and evaluated their anticonvulsive potencies against MES and PTZ in mice.

In the succinimide series, the D(R)-unsubstituted and chloro compounds had anticonvulsive activity (MES ans scMet). Several of the L(S)- isomers showed CNS-stimulatory properties. The L(S)- and D(R) methoxy-substituted isomers were neither anticonvulsant nor stimulatory. Because of their physical characteristics, the two nitro-substituted isomers were not biologically evaluated.

In the glutarimide series, the D(R) isomers were more anticonvulsive against MES than the L(S) isomers. In the scMet test stereoselectivity was observed for the nitro-phenylglutarimide compound. The results indicate that it is important to consider steric factors as well as hydrophobic and electronic factors when relating structure to activity among anticonvulsant drugs (89).

In an extension of the above work, additional N-(p-substituted phenyl)glutarimides were prepared (X = COCH$_3$, I, CN, CH$_2$CH$_3$, (CH$_2$)$_3$CH$_3$). In general, the (R) isomers had a more rapid onset of action, were more potent than their (S) isomers in eliciting minimal neurotoxicity, and were more active in protecting mice against electroshock and PTZ (90).

7.7 Sulfonamides

The carbonic anhydrase inhibitors acetazolamide (55.**23**), ethoxzolamide (55.**24**), sulthiame (55.**25**), and disamide (55.**26**) were shown to have anticonvulsant properties (29, 91). Acetazolamide and disamide are primarily effective against petit mal, ethoxzolamide against grand mal, and sulthiame against psychomotor seizures (84). In the United States and Europe acetazolamide is used in petit mal. Sulthiame is used in Europe in the treatment of psychomotor epilepsy.

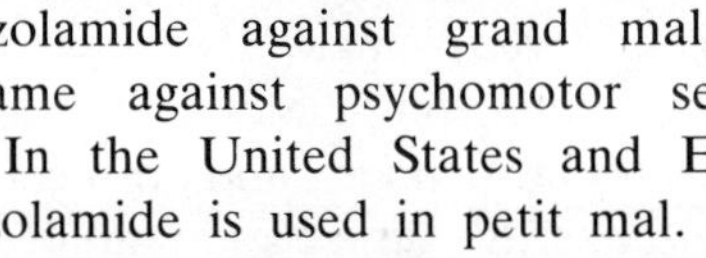

CH$_3$CONH— (thiadiazole) —SO$_2$NH$_2$

55.**23**

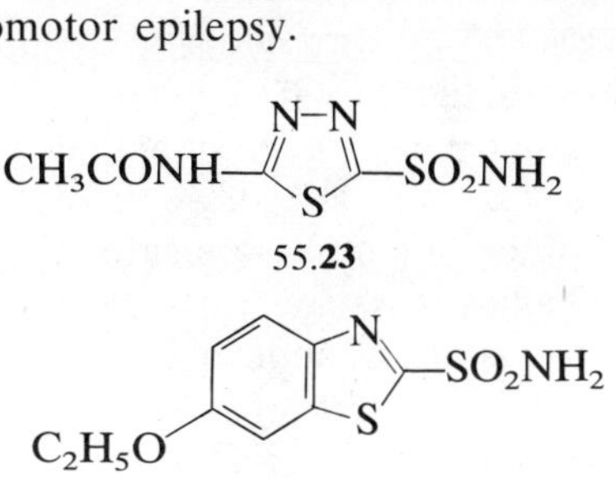

C$_2$H$_5$O— (benzothiazole) —SO$_2$NH$_2$

55.**24**

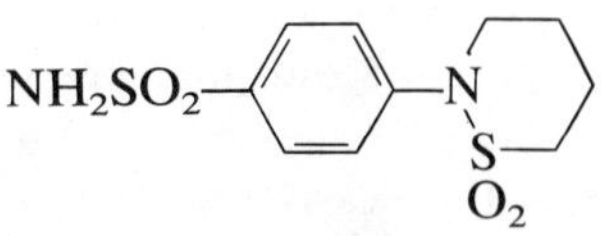

NH$_2$SO$_2$— (phenyl) —N (with S O$_2$ ring)

55.**25**

CH$_3$— (benzene ring with Cl) —SO$_2$NH$_2$, SO$_2$NH$_2$

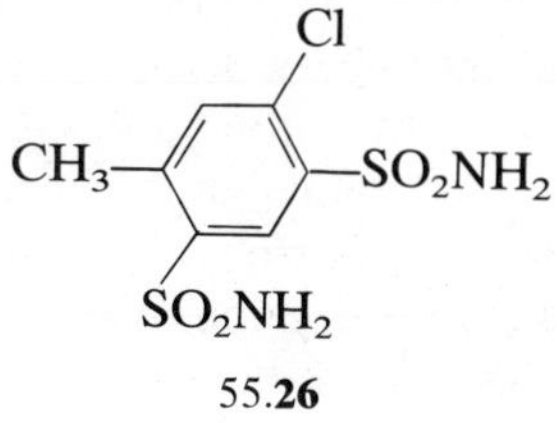

55.**26**

As noted in Section 5 the anticonvulsant effect of acetazolamide was shown to be a consequence of direct inhibition of brain carbonic anhydrase and not related to diuresis or general acidosis (30, 91, 92). Another investigation centered on the question of why the aforementioned carbonic anhydrase inhibitors are anticonvulsants whereas carbonic anhydrase inhibitors of the thiazide type, e.g. benzthiazide, are not (29). The thiazides in rats inhibited erythrocyte carbonic anhydrase but not brain carbonic anhydrase, whereas the anticonvulsant carbonic anhydrase inhibitors inhibited both erythrocyte and brain carbonic anhydrase. The thiazides did exhibit anticonvulsant effects when administered directly into the brain. Another interesting observation was made: the brain distribution patterns differed greatly for the four anticonvulsant carbonic anhydrase inhibitors. Ethoxzolamide (anti-grand mal) localized in one area, the two anti-petit mal agents, acetazolamide and disamide, in another, and the **anti-psychomotor** agent sulthiame in still another. The distribution patterns did not correlate with the probable focuses of the various epilepsies. The results support the conclusion that anticonvulsant carbonic anhydrase inhibitors act through inhibition of brain carbonic anhydrase. Failure of some carbonic anhydrase inhibitors to act as anticonvulsants could be a function of a lack of distribution to the central nervous system. Distribution patterns within the CNS could account for different antiepileptic actions. Because the distribution patterns did not correlate with the possible seizure foci it was tentatively hypothesized that carbonic anhydrase inhibitors act by inhibiting propagation of nerve impulse, i.e., act to prevent spreading of the seizure discharges.

Inasmuch as reserpine promotes depletion of catecholamines and concomitantly antagonizes the anticonvulsant action of carbonic anhydrase inhibitors, it was assumed that the catecholamines are involved in the action of the carbonic anhydrase inhibitors (30). In addition, α- or β-adrenergic blocking agents antagonize the anticonvulsant effect of carbonic anhydrase inhibitors (93).

The failure of dichloroisoproterenol to antagonize acetazolamide effectively appeared to be due to a stimulatory phase preceding blockade (94). Norepinephrine appears to be the amine required in brain for carbonic anhydrase inhibitors to have anticonvulsant effect (95), but the precise relationship between central carbonic anhydrase inhibition, levels of brain catecholamines, especially norepinephrine, and the anticonvulsant action of the carbonic anhydrase inhibitors remains to be elucidated.

Alkyl esters of 2-sulfamoylbenzoic acid and 4-amino-2-sulfamoylbenzoic acid possess interesting anticonvulsant properties (antistrychnine and anti-electroshock). Among these esters Hamor and Reavlin (96) have sought to relate the effect of substituents on the benzene ring to the rate of hydrolysis of the ester function and this to anticonvulsant activity, based on the concept that among these compounds the more resistant the ester to hydrolysis, the higher the anticonvulsant activity. Isopropyl 6-chloro-2-sulfamoylbenzoate (55.**27a**) has anti-electroshock activity, whereas isopropyl 4-bromo-2-sulfamoylbenzoate (55.**27b**) lacks this activity; the latter compound does not possess the interactions between the halogen and ester moiety that appear to be necessary for steric protection from ester hydrolysis (96).

NH$_2$SO$_2$ —— COOCH(CH$_2$)$_2$ R′

R

55.**27a** R = H, R′ = Cl
55.**27b** R = Br, R′ = H

7.8 Quinazolinones (Quinazolones)

The sedative–hypnotic agent metha-qualone, 2-methyl-2-(*o*-tolyl)-3*H*-4-quina-zolone (52.**28a**), has considerable anti-electroshock and antipentylenetetrazole properties in mice (1). According to one report, methaqualone in mice is about as active as phenobarbital against pentylene-tetrazole and approximately one-half as ac-tive as phenobarbital against electroshock (97). From studies on rat brain homoge-nates it was concluded that methaqualone acts on the respiratory chain prior to the point of the transfer of an electron from NADH to cytochrome B (98). Boltze and co-workers synthesized a large number of structural variants of methaqualone which were tested in mice to determine the rela-tionship between structure and hypnotic and anticonvulsant activities (99). Both the hypnotic and anticonvulsant actions of methaqualone are quite sensitive to struc-tural alterations: only a limited number of molecular modifications could be made with good retention of activity. Preparation of positional isomers (phthalazinones, pyrimidinones), hydrogenation of the heterocyclic ring, replacement of the ox-ygen atom with sulfur, substitution on the benzene ring of the quinazolinone nucleus, and replacement of the 3-aryl group by other groups, for example, methyl, resulted in a marked reduction or complete loss of activity. In short, only a few substitutions on the 3-phenyl function, e.g., *o*-chloro-mecloqualone (55.**28b**), replacing *o*-methyl as well as a limited number of alterations of the 2-methyl function, yielded highly active compounds. The replacement of the 2-methyl function with certain larger moieties such as the styryl or β-pyridylethenyl groups was interesting, for this led to a decrease in hypnotic activity with a con-comitant increase in the anticonvulsive activity. The compound 2-(β-pyridyl-2-ethenyl)-3*H*-(*o*-tolyl)-4-quinazolinone (55.**29**) possessed marked anticonvulsant

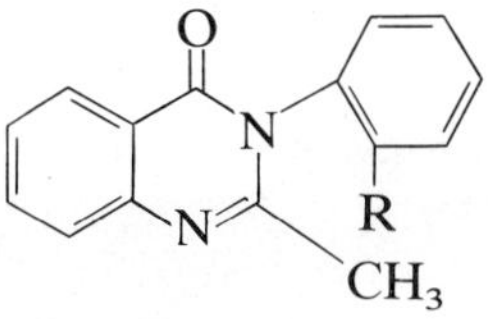

55.**28a** R = CH₃
55.**28b** R = Cl

55.**29**

activity, had a low order of toxicity, and was almost without hypnotic properties.

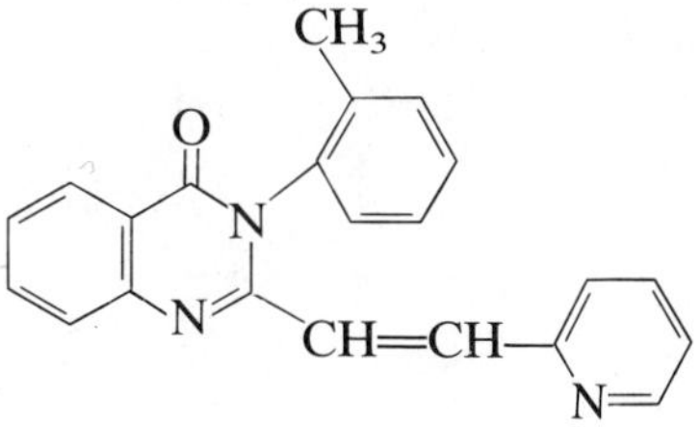

Mecloqualone is more active against electroshock in mice than its *m*-chloro or *p*-chloro isomers. Of the three isomers, it is also the least toxic and the most active as a hypnotic. Additional substitution on the phenyl function of a methyl or a second chlorine greatly decreased anticonvulsant activity or increased toxicity (100).

Some members of a series of peperazino-ethylquinazolones have anticonvulsant ac-tivity (101).

7.9 Benzodiazepines

In recent years, the area of benzodiaze-pines and related compounds has been the chemical area most explored for anti-convulsive agents.

Some general bioactivity trends among benzodiazepines are discernible. As a group they are very effective [nitrazepam (55.**30a**) and clonazepam (55.**30b**) espe-cially so] against PTZ and should be the most effective agents in controlling absence attacks. More clinical data are required. Activity against MES is varied. Most com-pounds have intermediate effectiveness.

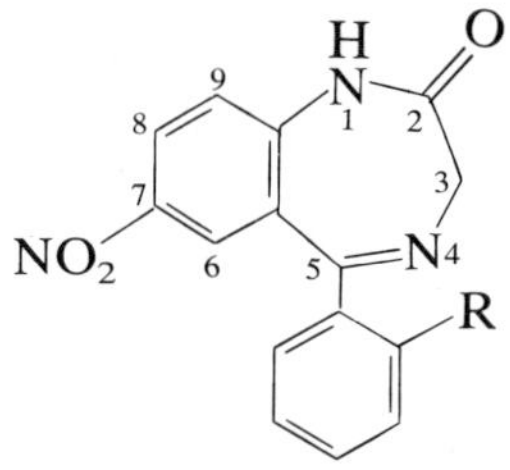

55.**30a**   R = H
55.**30b**   R = Cl

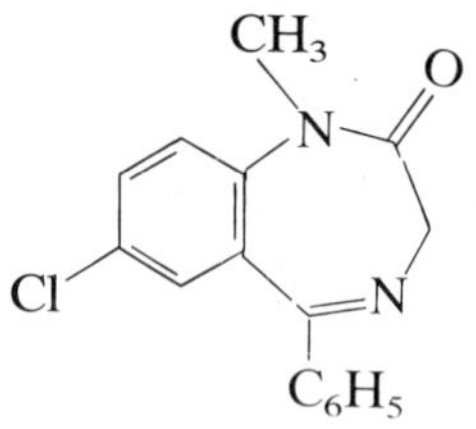

55.**31**

Exceptions are oxazepam (Chapter 57) (highly effective) and nitrazepam (ineffective). Results in the clinic against grand mal have been varied. Experimental maximal and minimal electroshock data indicate effectiveness for partial seizures. Clinical data are conflicting (102).

Two benzodiazepines appear to have attained definite clinical status. Nitrazepam is considered by some to be the drug of first choice in infantile spasms. Diazepam (55.**31**) is considered by many authorities to be the agent of choice in most cases of status epilepticus (103).

Anitconvulsant (against PTZ and MES) SAR for the benzodiazepines (55.**30**) have been tabulated by Sternback (104) and may be summarized as follows:

1. The 7 position should be substituted with an electron-withdrawing atom or group. Electron-donating substituents decrease activity.
2. Electron-withdrawing substituents at 8 or 9 decrease activity.
3. A phenyl substituent at 5 is optimal.
4. Substitution of the 5-phenyl with electron-withdrawing groups ortho or diortho increases activity. Any substitution meta or para decreases activity.
5. Methyl substitution at 1 is associated with high activity.

Additionally, it has been observed that many potently anticonvulsive benzodiazepines contain a protected or potential glycine moiety (104). It is interesting that a compound with a C—H group replacing the N at position 4 is not active as an anticonvulsant (105). Also, it has been observed that the conformation of the two aromatic rings of the benzodiazepines is similar to the conformation of the two phenyl substituents of diphenylhydantoin (106).

7.10 Alcohols

Aliphatic alcohols frequently have been evaluated as anticonvulsants and many are active in this regard. For example, experimental activities have been tabulated for more than 300 agents, ranging from simple alcohols through more complex compounds containing a number of other functional and hydrophobic groups in addition to the hydrophilic aliphatic hydroxyl function (2, 31, 32).

Among monohydric alcohols, the tertiary acetylenic carbinol ethchlorvynol (55.**32**) has been used in mixed grand and petit mal epilepsy. The closely related compound methylpentynol (55.**33**) has been used in grand and petit mal epilepsies. Both these agents possess significant sedative–hypnotic properties (1). Among polyhydric alcohols, the diol mephenesin (55.**34**) has been used in myoclonic epilepsy (107). The diol 2,2-diethyl-1,3-propanediol (Prenderol) (55.**35**) has been used in the control of petit mal (108). Phenaglycodol (55.**36**) is effective, especially against epilepsy associated with brain damage (1, 2, 109). Polyhydric alcohols tend to be more effective than the monohydric alcohols, although the dose required is quite high (2). Additionally, the

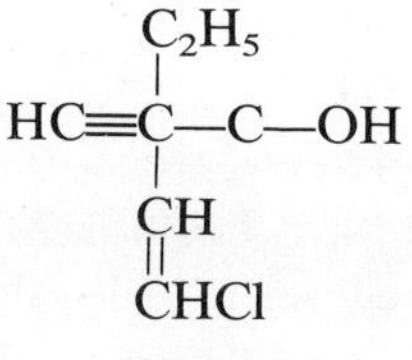

$$HC\equiv C - \underset{\underset{CHCl}{\overset{CH}{|}}}{\overset{C_2H_5}{\underset{|}{C}}} - OH$$

55.**32**

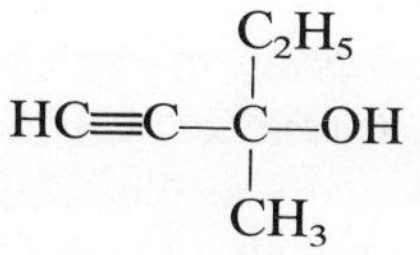

$$HC\equiv C - \underset{\underset{CH_3}{|}}{\overset{C_2H_5}{\underset{|}{C}}} - OH$$

55.**33**

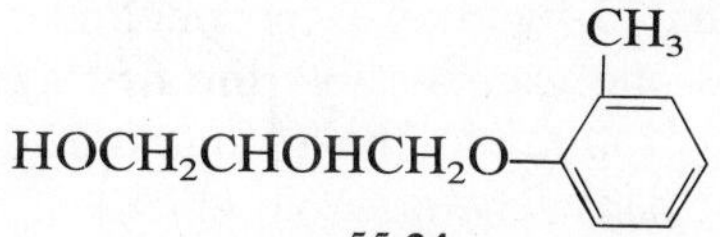

$$HOCH_2CHOHCH_2O -\!\!\!\!\!\langle\ \rangle\!\!-\!CH_3$$

55.**34**

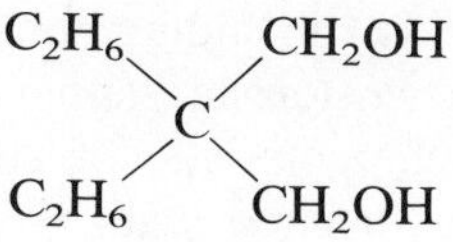

$$\underset{C_2H_6}{\overset{C_2H_6}{>}}C\underset{CH_2OH}{\overset{CH_2OH}{<}}$$

55.**35**

$$Cl -\!\!\!\!\!\langle\ \rangle\!\!-\!\underset{\underset{OH}{|}}{\overset{CH_3}{\underset{|}{C}}}\underset{\underset{OH}{|}}{\overset{CH_3}{\underset{|}{C}}} - CH_3$$

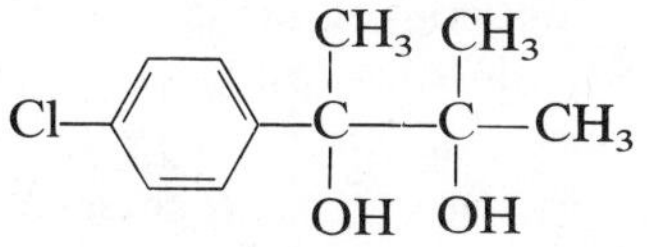

55.**36**

diols mephenesin and Prenderol are of relatively short duration of action for they are readily oxidatively degraded *in vivo* (1).

More recently, anticonvulsant activity (nicotine antagonism test, mice) has been reported in a series of 2,3-disubstituted 3-indols-3-ols, for example, compound 55.**37** (110). 2-Cyclohexylamino-1-phenylethanol (55.**38**) proved to be effective against PTZ. Cyclic ether derivatives, for example, 55.**39**, were found to be less active (111).

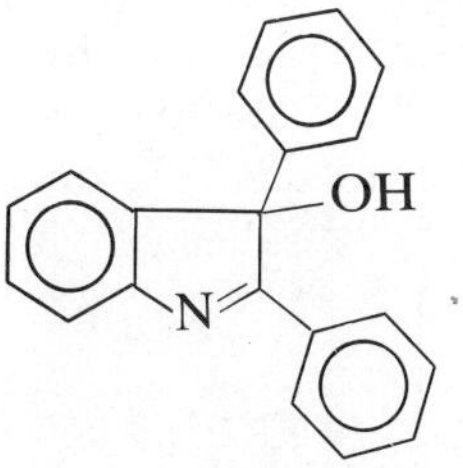

55.**37**

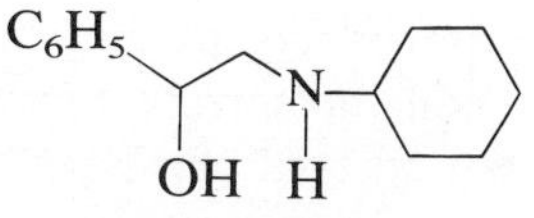

55.**38**

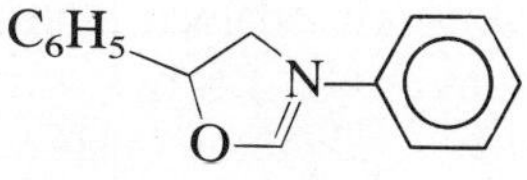

55.**39**

7.11 Carbamates

A considerable number of carbamates are active in the laboratory (2). In a general way, the structures of the anticonvulsant carbamates conform to the basic structural features common to many anticonvulsants as these have been formulated by Close and Spielman (2) and summarized for the alcohols. Of the many carbamates evaluated, meprobamate gained clinical acceptance. It has been used in the treatment of petit mal epilepsy.

A series of 1-propargyl-2-carbamoylglycerol ethers (55.**41**) has anticonvulsant properties in mice. The most effective anticonvulsants are where R = aralkyls, C_{5-6} alkyls, and trifluoromethyl- or halogen-substituted aromatic substituents (112). Among several carbamates, e.g., *tert*-butyl, benzyl, and *p*-chlorobenzyl, the *p*-chlorobenzyl compounds had higher anticonvulsant activity than meprobamate. Of the *p*-chlorobenzyl carbamates, the *N*-methylcarbamate (55.**41**) had the highest anticonvulsant activity (113). In a series of *tert*-butylphenylcarbamates of structure 55.**42**, anticonvulsant activity, in addition to other biological properties, was observed (114).

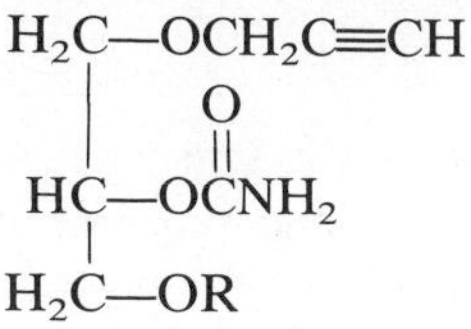

$$\underset{H_2C-OR}{\overset{\overset{\displaystyle H_2C-OCH_2C\equiv CH}{|}}{\underset{|}{HC-OCNH_2}}}$$

55.**40**

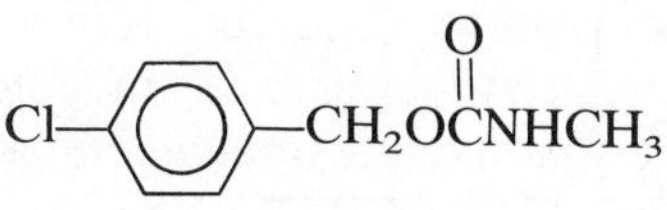

$$Cl -\!\!\!\!\!\langle\ \rangle\!\!-\!CH_2O\overset{O}{\overset{\|}{C}}NHCH_3$$

55.**41**

$$t\text{-Bu} -\!\!\!\!\!\langle\ \rangle\!\!-\!O\overset{O}{\overset{\|}{C}}NH_2$$

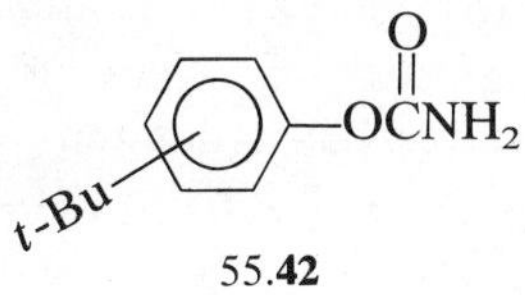

55.**42**

7.12 Miscellaneous Types

7.12.1 AMPHETAMINE AND RELATED COMPOUNDS. The psychomotor stimulants dextroamphetamine, methamphetamine, and methylphenidate are most frequently used as adjuvants with other anticonvulsants, especially the barbiturates, which tend to produce sedation. Thus their most common therapeutic role is the minimization of the sedative side effects of other agents. However, the compounds have anticonvulsant action *per se*. Dextroamphetamine and methylphenidate have a quieting effect in some children with hyperkinesia and brain damage. Dextroamphetamine and related compounds are sometimes beneficial in the treatment of petit mal. The central sympathomimetic agent phencyclidine has also been reported ro possess anticonvulsant properties (115). Agents that effect adrenergic stimulation also enhance the anticonvulsant action of carbonic anhydrase stimulation also enhance the anticonvulsant action of carbonic anhydrase inhibitors (94, 95). Conversely, adrenergic blocking agents reverse this anticonvulsant action (93). The anticonvulsant action of dextroamphetamine and related compounds probably is related to their interaction with brain catecholamines (see Chapter 41).

7.12.2 ACTH AND STEROIDS. Corticotropin (ACTH), administered intramuscularly, is considered to be the agent of choice in infants with myoclonic spasms and hypsarrythmia. The antiepileptic effects of ACTH may be due to increased levels of 3β-hydroxy-5-ene steroids. In an infant with infantile spasm and hypsarrhythmia treated with large doses of ACTH the urinary and fecal excretion of steroids increased from 0.1 mg/24 hr to 12 mg/24 hr. Metabolites of the following steroids were identified: $3\beta,16\alpha$ - dihydroxy - 5 - androsten - 17 - one, 3β-17β-dihydroxy-5-androsten-16-one, 5-pregnene-$3\beta,20\alpha$-diol, $3\beta,16\alpha$-dihydroxy-

5-pregnen-20-one, and 5-pregnene-$3\beta,17\alpha$, 20α-triol. 5-Pregnene-$3\beta,20\alpha$-diol was anticonvulsant in newborn mice (116).

Adrenocortical and sex hormones influence the electroshock seizure threshold in animals (117, 118). An investigation of several amino steroids led to the observation that 3-hydroxy-2-morpholino-5-pregnan-20-one was possibly the first synthetic steroid found to have marked activity against pentylenetetrazole (119).

The anticonvulsant activities of a number of steroids, including progesterone and deoxycorticosterone, appear to be not a general characteristic of steroids and not closely associated with progestational or other hormonal effects (120). In an evaluation of the anticonvulsant activities of a series of 3β-aminoalkyl esters of pregnenolone, the most active was 3β-(3-N-pyrrolidinylpropionyloxy)-5-pregnan-20-one, which did not possess hormonal action. It was effective in a clinical trial but had only a very low order of activity.

A study was made of the effect of substitution on 4-pregnane-3,20-dione and 5β-pregnane-3-20-dione. In both series substitutions made on rings A, B, or C produced an activity decrease. A hydroxyl group at 21 in both series increased activity. Two 5α-pregnane derivatives were not active (121).

Zinc chloride (s.c.) markedly decreased the electrical seizure threshold in mice. A number of changes were observed in the adrenal cortex. No decrease in the threshold occurred in adrenalectomized animals. Apparently the effects of zinc upon the seizure threshold is indicated via the adrenal cortex (122).

7.12.3 LOCAL ANESTHETICS. Lidocaine administered intravenously is clinically effective in the treatment of status epilepticus (1, 2). Some related local anesthetics share its anticonvulsive properties. When administered subcutaneously in mice, lidocaine and butamin have approximately the same potency as phenobarbital and diphenylhydantoin against electroshock. However, the duration of action of the local anesthetics is 1 hr, as contrasted to 8 hr for phenobarbital and diphenyl-hydantoin. Orally, lidocaine and butamin are much less potent (122). Procaine has anticonvulsant action against maximal electroshock. This activity can be enhanced by appropriate methyl substitution on the benzene ring (124).

7.12.4 ANTIMALARIALS. The most used antimalarial as an anticonvulsant is quina-crine (Chapter 20). It is of value in the treatment of petit mal resistant to other therapy. The potential for producing seri-ous side effects limits its use severely.

7.12.5 3-ACYLINDOLES. The anticonvul-sant activity (in mice and rats) of 3-acylindole compounds (55.**43**) has been compared with that of phenobarbital. Three carbons appear to be optimum in the unbranched α-carbonyl side chain (at the 3 position); however, if the chain is branched an additional carbon increases activity. The optimum compound tested was 3-iso-butyryl-1-methylindole, which was assessed as 0.36 as active as phenobarbital in rats and 0.28 as active in mice (125).

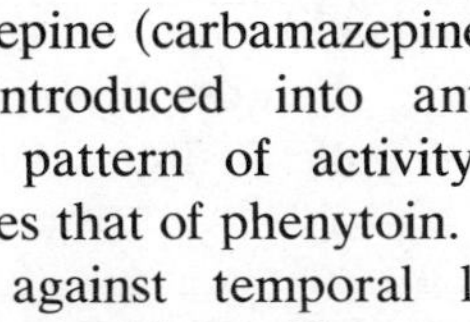

55.**43**

7.12.6 CARBAMAZEPINE. 5-Carbamyl-5H-di-benzo[b, f]azepine (carbamazepine) (55.**44**) has been introduced into antiepileptic therapy. Its pattern of activity in ani-mals resembles that of phenytoin. In man it is effective against temporal lobe and generalized convulsions. However, its use should be restricted to cases refractory to other agents until its capacity to produce serious side effects is more clearly defined (126).

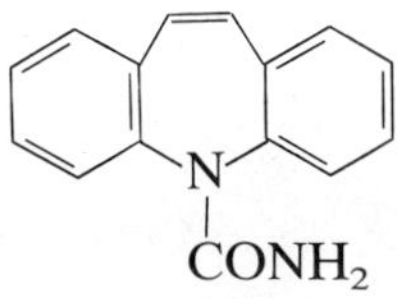

55.**45**

The analogous dibenzoxazepine is about as active as carbamazepine against electro-shock and is inactive against PTZ (127).

7.12.7 Δ^9-THC AND ANALOGS. Δ^9-Tetra-hydrocannabinol (Δ^9-THC) KMC and Δ^8-THC were active against electroshock in rodents (128–130). The isomers were equipotent in this regard. Δ^9-THC gave slight, if any, protection against PTZ. To-lerance to its anticonvulsive action is re-ported with chronic Δ^9-THC administration (128, 131, 132). Δ^9-THC and Δ^8-THC have dose-dependent properties and are equipo-tent against audiogeneic seizures in rats (130, 133). Cannabidiol (CBD), 6-oxo-CBD-diacetate, 6-hydroxy-CBD-triacetate, and 9-hydroxy-CBD-triacetate protected mice against electroshock (134). Δ^9-THC abolished spontaneous seizures in gerbils. Cannibidiol and cannabinol had no effect at doses reported to protect mice from elec-troshock (135).

In cats Δ^9-THC reduced the clinical and electrographic seizure activity produced by stimulation of subcortical brain structures. It appeared that Δ^9-THC was more active against seizures induced by hypothalamic stimulation than seizures induced by stimu-lation of the dorsomedial nucleus of the thalamus (136).

An attempt was made to correlate levels of brain Δ^9-THC and its hydroxylated metabolites (11-hydroxy- and 8α,11-di-hydroxy-Δ^9-THC) and the time course of anticonvulsant activity (MES in frogs), but a quantitative correlation was not attained (137).

Among synthetic compounds related to cannabinoids reported to have anticonvul-sant activity are dimethylheptylpyran and its isomers (128), a series of benzopyrans of

55.**45a** R = H

55.**45b** R = —CCH$_2$CH$_2$CH$_2$—N

which 55.**45a** was the most active in the audiogeneic seizure test (138), and a series of basic ester cannabinoid analogs in which 55.**45b** was very active against audiogeneic seizures (139).

7.12.8 PROSTAGLANDINS. PGE$_1$ and PGE$_2$, but not PGF$_{1\alpha}$ or PGF$_{2\alpha}$, pretreatment abolished the hind limb tonic extensor component in maximal electroshock in rabbits (140) 15(S)-15-Methyl-PGE$_2$ methyl ester and PGF$_{2\alpha}$ in nontoxic doses decreased epileptic activity in the experimental model of generalized penicillin epilepsy. The antiepileptic activity of the two compounds may be due to a direct or indirect excitatory action on brainstem neurons of the mesencephalic reticular formation and Purkinje cells (141).

Members of a series of 3-alkyl-2-(ω-carboxyalkyl)cyclopentanone derivatives were reported (142) in the patent literature to possess anticonvulsant properties.

7.12.9 DIPROPYLACETIC ACID AND CONGENERS. Dipropylacetic acid (DPA), whose anticonvulsant activity was discovered fortuitously, has been used in Europe in petit mal epilepsy for several years, and is now marketed in the United States under the name of Valproic Acid.

The animal pharmacology of dipropylacetic acid has been extensively investigated. Weichert (143) found very good anticonvulsant activity in mice against intracisternal glutamate and against audiogenic convulsions. Frey and Loescher (144) reported DPA to be weakly active in the MES test but comparable to trimethadione

and ethosuximide in the PTZ seizure threshold test. The duration of action was short and signs of neurotoxicity appeared below the ED$_{50}$ for PTZ. DPA was very active against picrotoxin, suggesting that the mode of action of DPA may involve elevation of brain GABA. Ishitobi et al. (145) noted that DPA's activity against MES, PTZ, and bemegride was so weak that effective doses were neurotoxic. However, low doses of DPA markedly potentiated the effects of DPH (phenytion(diphenylhydantoin)), nitrazepam, diazepam, and procaine, especially in the MES test. The effects of DPA on the EEG changes induced in rabbits by stimulation of the hippocampus indicated that DPA has principally an inhibiting effect on the descending reticular and limbic systems (146).

Among relatives of DPA, 3,3,4-trimethylpentanoic acid was as active, diethylacetic 2,2-dimethylbutyric, and 2,2-dimethylpropionic acids each had 80% of the activity, and dimethylacetic acid had 20% of the activity of DPA. Dibutylacetic, isovaleric, vinylacetic, isocrotonic, and tiglic acids were nonprotective, as were EtCOCO$_2$H, PrCOCO$_2$H, and BuCOCO$_2$H (147). In a series of DPA congeners (dialkylalkanoic acids <14 C atoms) and some of their alcohol precursors and amide derivatives, anticonvulsant activity (intensity and duration) increased with increased chain length (148). Introduction of a double bond decreased activity; introduction of a secondary or tertiary alcohol group or replacement of the carboxyl by hydroxyl had no effect. Among amide derivatives, dipropylacrylamide was more active than DPA amide. Dipropylpropionic was the most active anticonvulsant among dialkylpropionic acids.

From (1) a study of the competitive inhibition of GABA transaminase with respect to GABA by DPA and tripropylacetic acid (TPA) compared with the inhibition by butyric acid, valeric acid, and caproic acid, and (2) observing the anticonvulsant activity of GABA analogs and X-ray diffraction analyses of DPA, TPA, and congeners, a structural relationship between active compounds of the DPA and TPA series and GABA was made. The compounds appeared to have a structural similarity to the two preferred GABA conformations. Calculations indicated that the analogy may extend to the molecules in solution (149).

7.12.10 GABA ANALOGS. Cetyl γ-aminobutyrate applied to rabbit cortex synchronized the electroencephalogram similarly to γ-aminobutyric acid. It antagonized the effects of the GABA receptor blocking agent bicuculline. It may act by mimicking GABA (150).

A series of α-, β-, and γ-phenyl-substituted γ-aminobutyric acids and the corresponding lactams were evaluated as anticonvulsants against PTZ, electroshock, bemegride, and strychnine. The acids were all ineffective as anticonvulsants and, in some instances, potentiated convulsions. The lactams were all effective as anticonvulsants (151).

In drug(PTZ, strychnine, insulin)-induced convulsions in the mouse, γ-amino-β-hydroxybutyric acid usually reduced the duration of convulsive seizures without affecting incidence, latency, or intensity. It promoted the effectiveness of diphenylhydantoin–phenobarbital combinations (152).

α-(Butoxycarbonylamino)-γ-butyrolactone inhibited strychnine or electroshock-induced convulsions in mice (153). In a further study, the anticonvulsive and sedative effects of α-(butoxycarbonylamino)-γ-butyrolactone were compared in mice, rats, and guinea pigs and the results indicated that the compound may be useful in epilepsy (154). The compound's actions resembled those of GABA rather than γ-butyrolactone.

7.12.11 TAURINE. Taurine, by repeated i.p. or s.c. injections (3×75–200 mg/kg every 30 min), decreased experimental epileptic seizures produced in mice and cats by the application of cobalt powder to the cerebral cortex. Taurine normalized a number of the changes in the brain amino acid content caused by the cobalt treatment. The results indicated taurine could be useful in the treatment of chronic focal epilepsy in man (155).

In another study of its effect on cortical acute epileptic foci, taurine (100–150 mg/kg i.v.) decreased or abolished the spike frequency in cats with experimentally induced acute epileptic foci immediately after injection and abolished the epilepsy approximately 60–70 min after injection (156).

Van Gelder et al. (157) observed the effect of taurine on amino acids in epileptic patients. Epileptics had plasma levels of taurine and glutamic acid much higher than normal and urinary glutamic acid levels were somewhat elevated. Orally administered taurine normalized plasma glutamic acid and decreased this urinary excretion of glutamic acid. Amino acid concentrations were within normal levels and were not effected by taurine (157).

8 SUMMARY

Many of the anticonvulsant compounds possess an imido group or other polar group together with a lipophilic moiety. It is tempting to associate these features with anticonvulsant activity. It might be speculated that these features operate together to alter the structure of macromolecules associated with maintenance of CNS activity or hyperactivity. These molecular characteristics have been cited as being typical of, and fundamental to, the action of a number of CNS depressants, including anticonvulsants alcohols, carbamates, and barbiturates (32, 33). It is conceivable that many anticonvulsant barbiturates, oxazolidine-2,4-diones, hydantoins, amides, imides, carbamates, and alcohols, as well as related compounds that have been described in this chapter, might act in similar ways at the molecular level.

Among those anticonvulsants characterized by such common characteristics, highest therapeutic activity is generally seen among agents with a relatively complex hydrophobic moiety. For example, a highly branched carbon atom tends to characterize the more significant alcohols, carbamates, hydantoins, oxazolidine-2,4-diones, amides, and imides. Also, increasing the sophistication of the hydrophilic moiety seems to yield more useful agents. Thus the relatively simple hydroxyl or carbamate functions do not yield as many useful agents as do the more complex hydrophilic functions of the oxazolidine-2,4-diones, hydantoins, or barbiturates. It might be more than coincidental that within the framework of relatively simple common characteristics, increases in molecular complexity appear to parallel the increases in anticonvulsant usefulness. Thus, among molecules that possess common structural characteristics and that could possibly act by similar mechanisms, increasing the structural differentiations of both the hydrophobic and hydrophilic groups might confer increasing biologic differentiation. The simpler molecules might interact relatively indiscriminately with bioactive macromolecules, and this could be reflected in many types of action. More complex molecules might preferentially interact with one macromolecule as against another, resulting in differences in qualitative action. They could, for example, be primarily anti-grand mal or anti-petit mal. Johnson and Eyring, as well as Hansch, have emphasized that the fundamental molecular mechanism of action of several CNS depressants can be identical, even though the qualitative actions differ, and have emphasized that qualitative differences in action are a function of the agents' ability to interact with different macromolecules differently (32, 36).

Although the concept of physiocochemical differences conferring different distribution patterns and thus different qualitative actions on agents acting via similar mechanisms of action is perhaps invoked too often, still this factor cannot be overlooked and could play a role. For example, the physicochemical nature of the anti-grand mal agents tends to differ from that of anti-petit mal agents. Thus it would not be unreasonable to believe that one group of agents could localize more extensively in one area and other agents more extensively in another area, with the result that each would have different qualitative actions although both are operating via similar mechanisms at the molecular level.

Of course, there are certain types of compounds that exert anticonvulsant action through other proved mechanisms: e.g., carbonic anhydrase inhibition, norepinephrine agonism, increasing GABA levels or mimicking GABA, increasing taurine levels, and so on.

The interested reader should refer to the original literature (i.e., the following list of references) for additional information concerning the many compounds that have been investigated as anticonvulsants. The recent treatise by Vida (158) on anticonvulsants should also be consulted for more details concerning advances in anticonvulsant drug development, neuropharmacology and treatment of epilepsy, experimental evaluation of anticonvulsants, physiological disposition, and the classification and tabulation of compounds that have been tested as anticonvulsants.

REFERENCES

1. A. Spinks and W. S. Waring, in *Progress in Medicinal Chemistry* Vol. III, G. P. Ellis and G. B. West, Eds., Butterworths, Washington, D. C., 1963, p. 261.
2. W. J. Close and M. A. Spielman, in *Medicinal Chemistry*, Vol. V, W. H. Hartung, Ed., Wiley, New York, 1961, p. 1.

References

855

3. H. H. Jasper, A. A. Ward, and A. Pope, Eds., *Basic Mechanisms of the Epilepsies*, Little, Brown, Boston, 1969.

4. H. Gastaut and R. Broughton, in *Anticonvulsant Drugs*, Vol. I, *International Encyclopedia of Pharmacology and Therapeutics*, Pergamon, New York, 1973.

5. A. C. Guyton, *Textbook of Medical Physiology*, 5th ed., Saunders, Philadelphia, 1976, pp. 736–738.

6. A. M. A. Department of Drugs, American Medical Association, *A. M. A. Drug Evaluations*, 3rd ed., Publishing Sciences Group, Inc., Littleton, Mass., 1977, pp. 452–472.

7. D. M. Woodbury and E. Fingl, "Drugs Effective in the Therapy of the Epilepsies" in *The Pharmacological Basis of Therapeutics*, 5th ed., L. S. Goodman and A. Gilman, Eds., Macmillan, 1975, pp. 201–226.

8. D. B. Tower, *Neurochemistry of Epilepsy*, Charter C Thomas, Springfield, Ill., 1960.

9. A. Lajtha, in *International Review of Neurobiology*, Vol. VI, C. C. Pfeifer and J. R. Symthies, Eds., Academic, New York, 1964, p. 1.

10. A. Kreindler, in *Progress in Brain Research*, Vol. XIX, Elsevier, New York, 1965, p. 168.

11. P. Singh and J. Huot, "Neurochemistry of Epilepsy and Mechanism of Action of Antiepileptics," in *Anticonvulsant Drugs*, Vol. 2, I.E.P.T., Pergamon, New York, 1973, pp. 427–504.

12. W. Penfield and H. H. Jasper, *Epilepsy and the Functional Anatomy of the Human Brain*, Little, Brown, Boston, 1954.

13. A. A. Ward, Jr., in *International Review of Neurobiology*, Vol. III, C. C. Pfeifer and J. R. Symthies, Eds., Academic, New York, 1961, p. 137.

14. G. B. Koelle, in *The Pharmacological Basis of Therapeutics*, 3rd ed., L. S. Goodman and A. Gilman, Eds. Macmillan, New York, 1965, p. 428.

15. D. R. Curtis and J. C. Watkins, in *Inhibition in the Nervous System and γ-Aminobutyric Acid*, E. Roberts, Ed., Pergamon, Oxford, 1960, p. 424.

16. D. R. Curtis, *Pharmacol Rev.*, **15,** 333 (1963).

17. H. A. Harper, *Review of Physiological Chemistry*, Lange, Los Altos, Calif., 1973, p. 102.

18. A. White, P. Handler, and E. L. Smith, *Principles of Biochemistry*, 6th ed., McGraw-Hill, New York, 1978, pp. 1344–1345.

19. D. W. Esplin and B. Zablocka, in *The Pharmacological Basis of Therapeutics*, 3rd ed., L. S. Goodman and A. Gilman, Eds., Macmillan, New York, 1965, p. 349.

20. R. H. Travis and G. Sayers, in *The Pharmacological Basis of Therapeutics*, 3rd ed., L. S. Goodman and A. Gilman, Eds., Macmillan, New York, 1965, p. 1627.

21. A. Sytinskii and T. N. Priyatkina, *Biochem. Pharmacol.*, **15,** 49 (1966).

22. N. M. van Gelder, *Biochem. Pharmacol.*, **15,** 533 (1966).

23. R. Tapia, H. Pasantes, M. Perez de la Mora, B. G. Ortega, and G. H. Massieu, *Biochem. Pharmacol.*, **16,** 483 (1967).

24. See Ref. 10, p. 29.

25. See Ref. 10, p. 53.

26. J. R. Daube, *J. Nerv. Ment. Dis.*, **141,** 524 (1965).

27. J. G. Millichap, "Correlations of Laboratory and Clinical Evaluations of Anticonvulsant Drugs," in *Anticonvulsant Drugs*, Vol. 1, I.E.P.T., Pergamon, New York, 1973, pp. 189–202.

28. J. G. Millichap, D. M. Woodbury, and L. S. Goodman, *J. Pharmacol. Exp. Ther.*, **115,** 251 (1955).

29. H. Tanimukai, M. Inui, S. Hariguchi, and Z. Kaneko, *Biochem. Pharmacol.*, **14,** 961 (1965).

30. W. D. Gray, C. E. Rauh, and R. W. Shanahan, *J. Pharmacol. Exp. Ther.*, **139,** 359 (1963).

31. F. H. Johnson, H. Eyring, and M. J. Polissar, *The Kinetic Basis of Molecular Biology*, Wiley, New York, 1954, and references cited therein.

32. H. Eyring and E. M. Eyring, *Modern Chemical Kinetics*, Reinhold, New York, 1963, p. 73.

33. D. M. Woodbury, J. K. Penry, and R. P. Schmidt, Eds., *Antiepileptic Drugs*, Raven Press, New York, 1973.

34. B. Glasson and A. Benakis, "Absorption, Distribution, Excretion, and Metabolism of Anticonvulsant Drugs in Animals," in *Anticonvulsant Drugs*, Vol. I, I.E.P.T., Pergamon, New York, 1973, pp. 241–292.

35. O. Svensmark, "Absorption, Distribution, Metabolism and Excretion of Antiepileptic Drugs in Man," in *Anticonvulsant Drugs*, Vol. I, I.E.P.T., Pergamon, New York, 1973, pp. 293–368.

36. L. C. Mark, *Clin. Pharmacol. Ther.*, **4,** 504 (1963).

37. T. C. Daniels and E. C. Jorgensen, in *Textbook of Organic Medicinal and Pharmaceutical Chemistry*, 7th ed., C. O. Wilson, O. Gisvold, and R. F. Doerge, Eds., Lippincott, Philadelphia, 1977, pp. 105–109.

38. J. Alvin, E. Goh, and M. T. Bush, *J. Pharmacol. Exp. Ther.*, **194,** 117, (1975).

39. K. H. Dudley, D. L. Bius, and T. C. Butler, *J. Pharmacol. Exp. Ther.*, **175,** 27 (1970).

40. J. R. Goulet, A. W. Kinkel, and T. C. Smith, *Clin. Pharmacol. Ther.*, **20,** 213 (1976).

41. C. Hansch and S. M. Anderson, *J. Med. Chem.*, **10,** 745 (1967).

42. C. M. Samour, J. F. Reinhard, and J. A. Vida, *J. Med. Chem.*, **14,** 187 (1971).

43. J. A. Vida, W. R. Wilber, and J. F. Reinhard, *J. Med. Chem.*, **14,** 191 (1971).

44. J. A. Vida, M. L. Hooker, and J. F. Reinhard, *J. Med. Chem.*, **16,** 602 (1973).

45. J. A. Vida, M. L. Hooker, and C. M. Samour, *J. Med. Chem.*, **16,** 1378 (1973).

46. A. Raines, J. M. Niner, and D. J. Pace, *Pharmacol. Exp. Ther.*, **186,** 315 (1973).

47. E. Campaigne and H. L. Thomas, *J. Am. Chem. Soc.*, **77,** 5365 (1955); J. Klosa, *Arch. Pharm.*, **289,** 223 (1956).

48. H. Blitz, *Chem. Ber.*, **41,** 1379 (p. 1391) (1908).

49. H. H. Merritt and T. J. Putnam, *Arch. Neurol. Psychiatr.*, **39,** 1003 (1938); *Epilepsia*, **3,** 51 (1945); T. J. Putnam and H. H. Merritt, *Science*, **85,** 525 (1937).

50. J. C. Krantz and C. J. Carr, *Pharmacologic Principles of Medical Practice*, 6th ed., Williams and Wilkins, Baltimore, 1965, p. 412.

51. W. Oldfield and C. H. Cashin, *J. Med. Chem.*, **8,** 239 (1965).

52. M. A. Davis, S. O. Winthrop, R. A. Thomas, F. Herr, M. P. Charest, and Roger Gaudry, *J. Med. Chem.*, **7,** 439 (1964).

53. C. H. Carter, *Clin. Med.*, **78,** 33 (1971).

54. L. Musial, M. J. Korohoda, A. Szadowski, and H. Szmigielska, *Acta Pol. Pharm.*, **29,** 573 (1972); through *Chem. Abstr.*, **78,** 124503w (1973).

55. C. M. Samour, J. F. Reinhard, and J. A. Vida, *J. Med. Chem.*, **14,** 187 (1971).

56. J. A. Vida, W. R. Wilber, and J. F. Reinhard, *J. Med. Chem.*, **14,** 190 (1971).

57. J. A. Vida, M. H. O'Dea, C. M. Samour, and J. F. Reinhard, *J. Med. Chem.*, **18,** 383 (1975).

58. D. K. Yung, T. P. Forrest, M. L. Gilroy, and M. M. Vohra, *J. Pharm. Sci.*, **62,** 1764 (1973).

59. A. Blade Font, J. N. Torres Estaban, Span. Pat. 389,999 (Cl. C07D, A61K) (April 16, 1975); through *Chem. Abstr.*, **83,** 179062k (1975).

60. V. Stella, T. Higuchi, A. Hussain, and J. Truelove, *ACS Symp. Ser.*, **14** (*Prodrugs, Novel Drug Delivery Syst., Symp.*), 154–183 (1975).

61. B. Umberkoman and T. Joseph, *Indian J. Physiol. Pharmacol.*, **18,** 29 (1974).

62. D. M. Woodbury and E. Fingl, "Drugs Effective in the Therapy of the Epilepsies" in *The Pharmacological Basis of Therapeutics*, 5th ed., L. S. Goodman and A. Gilman, Eds., Macmillan, New York, 1975, p. 201.

63. M. A. Spielman, A. O. Gieszler, and W. J. Close, *J. Am. Chem. Soc.*, **70,** 4189 (1948).

64. A. G. Pechenkin, L. G. Thgnibidina, A. Pl Gilev, V. K. Gorshkova, and V. M. Kurilenko, *Khim.-Farm. Zh.*, **7,** 16 (1973); through *Chem. Abstr.*, **78,** 110819s (1973).

65. M. S. Dar, *Arch. Int. Pharmacodyn. Ther.*, **219,** 103 (1976).

66. J. W. Clark-Lewis, *Chem. Rev.*, **58,** 63 (1958).

67. M. A. Speilman, *J. Am. Chem. Soc.*, **66,** 1244 (1944).

68. T. C. Butler, *J. Am. Pharm. Assoc. Sci. Ed.*, **44,** 367 (1955).

69. T. C. Butler, *J. Pharmacol. Exp. Ther.*, **104,** 299 (1952).

70. T. C. Butler, *J. Pharmacol. Exp. Ther.*, **108,** 11 (1953).

71. T. C. Butler, *J. Pharmacol. Exp. Ther.*, **108,** 474 (1953).

72. T. C. Butler, *J. Pharmacol. Exp. Ther.*, **109,** 340 (1953).

73. T. C. Butler, *J. Pharmacol. Exp. Ther.*, **113,** 178 (1955).

74. C. D. Withrow, R. J. Stout, L. J. Barton, W. S. Beacham, and D. M. Woodbury, *J. Pharmacol. Exp. Ther.*, **161,** 335 (1968).

75. H. H. Frey and B. H. Kretschmer, *Arch. int. Pharmacodyn. Ther.*, **193,** 181 (1971).

76. J. Y. Bogue and H. C. Carrington, *Brit. J. Pharmacol.*, **8,** 230 (1953).

77. L. Goodman, E. Swinyard, W. C. Brown, D. O. Schiffman, M. S. Grewal, and E. L. Bliss, *J. Pharmacol. Exp. Ther.*, **108,** 428 (1953).

78. H. F. Schwartz and R. F. Doerge, *J. Am. Pharm. Assoc., Sci. Ed.*, **44,** 80 (1955).

79. H. F. Schwartz, L. F. Worrell, and J. N. Delgado, *J. Pharm. Sci.*, **56,** 80 (1967).

80. H. F. Schwartz, E. I. Isaacson, R. G. Brown, and J. N. Delgado, *J. Pharm. Sci.*, **57,** 1530 (1968).

81. M. A. Davis, S. O. Winthrop, R. A. Thomas, F. Herr, M.-R. Charest, and R. Gaudry, *J. Med. Chem.*, **7,** 88 (1964).

82. A. Balsamo, P. L. Barili, P. Crotti, B. Macchia, F. Macchia, A. Pecchia, A. Cuttica, and N. Passerini, *J. Med. Chem.*, **18,** 842 (1975).

83. A. Balsamo, P. L. Barili, P. Crotti, B. Macchia, F. Macchia, A. Cuttica, and N. Passerini, *J. Med. Chem.*, **20,** 48 (1977).

84. C. A. Miller and L. M. Long, *J. Am. Chem. Soc.*, **73,** 4895 (1951).

85. For example, P. J. Nicholls and T. C. Orton, *Brit. J. Pharmacol.*, **45,** 48 (1972).

86. N. E. Akopyan and D. A. Gerasimyan, *Biol. Zh. Arm.*, **24:1** (1971); through *Chem. Abstr.*, **76,** 107836y (1972).

87. N. E. Akopyan, D. A. Gerasimyan, and Dzh. A. Melkonyan, *Biol. Zh. Arm.*, **27,** 52 (1974); through *Chem. Abstr.*, **82,** 11028j (1975).

88. H. Y. Aboul-Enein, C. W. Schauber, A. R. Hansen, and L. J. Fisher, *J. Med. Chem.*, **18,** 736 (1975).

89. D. T. Witiak, S. K. Seth, E. R. Baizman, S. L. Weibel, and H. H. Wolf, *J. Med. Chem.*, **15,** 1117 (1972).

90. D. T. Wittiak, W. L. Cook, T. K. Gupta, and M. C. Gerald, *J. Med. Chem.*, **19,** 1419 (1976).

91. W. D. Gray, T. H. Maren, B. M. Sisson, and F. H. Smith, *J. Pharmacol. Exp. Ther.*, **121,** 160 (1957).

92. H. Tanimukai, T. Nishimura, and I. Sano, *Klin. Wochenschr.*, **42,** 918 (1964).

93. A. D. Rudzik and J. H. Mennear, *Proc. Soc. Exp. Biol. Med.*, **122,** 278 (1966).

94. J. H. Mennear and A. D. Rudzik, *J. Pharm. Pharmacol.*, **18,** 833 (1966).

95. W. D. Gray and C. E. Rauh, *J. Pharmacol. Exp. Ther.*, **155,** 127 (1967).

96. G. H. Hamor and B. L. Reavlin, *J. Pharm. Sci.*, **56,** 134 (1967), and references cited therein.

97. L. G. Zil'bermints, *Izv. Estestv-Nauchn. Inst. Permsk. Univ.*, **14,** 141 (1964); through *Chem. Abstr.*, **64,** 1220c (1966).

98. P. K. Seth and S. S. Parmar, *Can. J. Physiol. Pharmacol.*, **43,** 1019 (1965).

99. K. H. Boltze, H.-D. Dell, H. Lehwald, D. Lorentz, and M. Ruberg-Schwer, *Arzneim. Forsch.*, **13,** 688 (1963).

100. J. R. Boissier, Cl. Dumont, and R. Ratouis, *Therapie*, **22,** 129 (1967); through *Chem. Abstr.*, **66,** 74526 (1967).

101. K. C. Joshi, V. K. Singh, D. S. Mehta, R. C. Sharma, and L. Gupta, *J. Pharm. Sci.*, **64,** 1428 (1975).

102. T. R. Browne and J. K. Penry, *Epilepsia*, **14,** 277 (1973) and references cited therein.

103. D. J. Greenblatt and R. I. Shader, *Benzodiazepines in Clinical Practice*, Raven Press, New York, 1974, p. 121.

104. L. H. Sternback, in *The Benzoidiazepines*, S. Garattini, E. Mussini, and L. O. Randall, Eds., Raven Press, New York, 1973, p. 1.

105. B. Loev, M. M. Goodman, C. Zirkle, and E. Macko, *Arzneim.-Forsch.*, **20,** 974 (1970).

106. A. Camerman and N. Camerman, *Science*, **168,** 1457 (1970).

107. R. E. Kelly and D. R. Laurence, *Brit. Med. J.*, **1,** 456 (1955).

108. M. A. Perlstein, *Neurology*, **3,** 744 (1953).

109. C. M. Gruber and J. M. Mosier, *Proc. Soc. Exp. Biol. Med.*, **94,** 384 (1957).

110. D. Lednicher, U.S. Pat. 634,455; through *Chem. Abstr.*, **76,** P113064n (1972).

111. W. J. Irwin, D. L. Wheeler, and N. J. Harper, *J. Med. Chem.*, **15,** 445 (1972).

112. G. Huguet, C. Gouret, and G. Raynaud, *Chem. Ther.*, **4,** 474 (1969); through *Chem. Abstr.*, **73,** 54184p (1970).

113. T. Szirtes, E. Palosi, E. Ezer, L. Szporny, and L. Kisfaludi, *Acta. Pharm. Hung.*, **43,** 224 (1973); through *Chem. Abstr.*, **80,** 103936r (1974).

114. J. Peyroux, C. Derruppe, C. Tilloy, and R. Rips, *Chim. Ther.*, **8,** 387 (1973); through *Chem. Abstr.*, **81,** 114398p (1974).

115. W. D. Gray and C. E. Rauh, *J. Pharmacol. Exp. Ther.*, **155,** 127 (1967).

116. P. Eneroth, J. A. Gustafsson, H. Ferngren, and B. Hellstrom, *J. Steroid Biochem.*, **3,** 877 (1972).

117. D. E. Wooley and P. S. Timiras, *Endocrinology*, **70,** 196 (1962).

118. D. M. Woodbury, *Pharmacol. Rev.*, **10,** 275 (1958).

119. C. L. Hewett, M. S. Sugrue, and J. J. Lewis, *J. Pharm. Pharamcol.*, **16,** 765 (1964).

120. C. R. Craig, *J. Pharmacol. Exp. Ther.*, **153,** 337 (1966).

121. C. R. Crain and J. R. Deason, *Arch. Int. Pharm. Ther.*, **172,** 366 (1968).

122. Y. Santoki, *Bull. Yamaguchi Med. Sch.* **22,** 253 (1975); through *Chem. Abstr.*, **84,** 174568r (1976).

123. H. H. Frey, *Acta Pharmacol. Toxicol.*, **19,** 205 (1962).

124. K. Kapila and R. B. Arora, *J. Pharm. Pharmacol.*, **14,** 253 (1962).

125. H. H. Keasling, R. E. Wilette, and J. Szmuszkovicz, *J. Med. Chem.*, **7,** 94 (1964).

126. D. M. Woodbury and E. Fingl, "Drugs Effective in the Therapy of the Epilepsies," in *The Pharmacological Bases of Therapeutics*, 5th ed., L. S. Goodman and A. Gilman, Eds., Macmillan, New York, 1975, p. 201.

127. R. G. Babington and Z. P. Horovitz, *Arch. Int. Pharmacodyn. Ther.*, 202, 106 (1973).

128. R. Karler, W. Cely, and S. A. Turkanis, *Life Sci.*, **15**, 931 (1974).

129. J. A. McCaughran, Jr., M. E. Cocoran, and J. A. Wade, *Pharmacol. Biochem. Behav.*, **2**, 227 (1974).

130. P. F. Consroe and D. P. Man, *Life Sci.*, **13**, 429 (1973).

131. P. A. Fried and D. C. McIntyre, *Psychopharamacologia*, **31**, 215 (1973).

132. D. P. Man and P. F. Consroe, *IRCS Libr. Compend.*, **1**, 7.10.1 (1974).

133. P. F. Consroe, D. P. Man, L. Chin, and A. L. Picchioni, *J. Pharm. Pharmacol.*, **25**, 764 (1973).

134. E. A. Carlini, R. Mechoulam, and N. Lander, *Res. Commun. Chem. Pathol. Pharmacol.*, **12**, 1 (1975).

135. B. Cox, M. Ten Ham, W. J. Loskota, and P. Lomax, *Proc. West. Pharmacol. Soc.*, **18**, 154 (1975).

136. J. A. Wada, M. Sato, and M. E. Corcoran, *Exp. Neurol.*, **39**, 157 (1973).

137. R. Karler, W. Cely, and S. A. Turkanis, *Res. Commun. Chem. Pathol. Pharmacol.*, **9**, 441 (1974).

138. R. J. Razdan, G. R. Handrick, H. C. Dalsell, J. F. Howes, M. Winn, N. P. Plotnikoff, P. W. Dodge, and A. T. Dren, *J. Med. Chem.*, **19**, 552 (1976).

139. R. J. Razdan, T. Zitko, H. G. Pars, N. P. Plotnikoff, P. W. Dodge, A. T. Dren, J. Kyncl, and P. Somani, *J. Med. Chem.*, **19**, 454 (1976).

140. B. R. Madan, R. S. Gupta, and V. Madan, *Indian J. Med. Res.*, **62**, 1647 (1974).

141. L. F. Quesney, P. Gloor, L. S. Wolfe, and S. Jozsef, *Adv. Prostaglandin Thromboxane Res.*, **1**, 387 (1976).

142. R. E. Schaub, K. F. Bernady, and M. J. Weiss, Ger. Pat. 2,316,374; through *Chem. Abstr.*, **80**, 59568w (1974).

143. P. Weichert, *Zentralbl. Pharm., Pharmakother.*

144. H. H. Frey and W. Loescher, *Arzneim.-Forsch.*, **26**, 299 (1976).

145. T. Ishtiboti, Y. Kuwahara, and K. Tanaka, *Fukuoka-Igaku-Zasshi*, **60**, 806 (1969); through *Chem. Abstr.*, **72**, 109564z (1970).

146. K. Kimishima, K. Tanabe, T. Sakamoto, and A. Nishimoto, *Yango Igaku Zasshi*, **20**, 317 (1969), through *Chem. Abstr.*, **74**, 21828w (1971).

147. G. Carraz, *Agressoligie*, **8**, 13 (1967); through *Chem. Abstr.*, **67**, 9921s (1967).

148. G. Taillandier, J. L. Benoit-Guyod, A. Boucherle, M. Broll, and P. Eymard, *Eur. J. Med. Chem.—Chim. Ther.*, **10**, 453 (1975); through *Chem. Abstr.*, **84**, 159508c (1976).

149. B. Ferrandes, C. Cohen-Added, J. L. Benoit-Guyod, and P. Eymard, *Biochem. Pharmacol.*, **23**, 3363 (1974).

150. R. U. Ostrovskaya and J. Schmidt, *J. Farmakol. Toksikol* (Moscow), **36**, 179 (1973); through *Chem. Abstr.*, **78**, 154825v (1973).

151. E. Chojnacka-Wojcik, J. Hano, K. Sieroslawska, and M. Sypniewska, *Arch. Immunol. Ther. Exp.*, **23**, 747 (1975).

152. M. Maccari and M. T. Gatti, *Biochim. Biol. Sper.*, **5**, 534 (1966).

153. W. Ferrarri and M. Sandrini, *Riv. Farmacol. Ter.*, **4**, 97a (1973); through *Chem. Abstr.*, **81**, 2116e (1974).

154. M. Sandrini and W. Ferrarri, *Riv. Farmacol. Ter.*, **4**, 319 (1973); through *Chem. Abstr.*, **81**, 582246y (1974).

155. N. M. Van Gelder, *Brain Res.*, **47**, 157 (1972).

156. R. Mutani, L. Bergamini, R. Fariello, and M. Delsidime, *Brain Res.*, **70**, 170 (1974).

157. N. M. Van Gelder, A. L. Sherwin, C. Socks, and F. Anderman, *Brain Res.*, **94**, 297 (1975).

158. J. A. Vida, Ed., *Anticonvulsants*, Academic, New York, 1977.

Laboratiumsdiagn., **111**, 899 (1972); through *Chem. Abstr.*, **78**, 24095w (1973).

CHAPTER FIFTY-SIX

Antipsychotic Agents

CARL KAISER

and

PAULETTE E. SETLER

Research and Development Division
Smith Kline & French Laboratories
1500 Spring Garden Street
Philadelphia, Pennsylvania 19101, USA

CONTENTS

859

1 INTRODUCTION

Prior to the introduction of somatic therapy in the 1930s, treatment of psychotic patients was largely restricted to psychotherapy and/or custodial hospitalization. In the 1930s the introduction of insulin coma therapy and electroconvulsive shock therapy (ECT) provided a definite advance in the treatment of psychosis. Soon, however, it became obvious that ECT was less effective in schizophrenia than in affective disorders and that insulin coma was a dangerous and difficult form of therapy.

The first truly effective means of controlling the symptoms of schizophrenia became available with the discovery of the first antipsychotic agents, reserpine (56.**1**) and chlorpromazine (56.**2a**). The alkaloid reserpine is the active constituent of *Rauwolfia serpentina*, an Indian shrub. Extracts of rauwolfia have been used in Hindu medicine for centuries. In 1931 it was claimed that rauwolfia extracts were effective in calming severely disturbed patients (1). This report was confirmed by a number of investigators. In 1952 Mueller and coworkers (2) succeeded in isolating reserpine from rauwolfia and in 1954 established its structure (see Section 4.5.1) (3). At this time, Bein showed that reserpine possessed both tranquilizing and hypotensive properties (4). In 1954 Kline reported that reserpine was useful in the treatment of psychotic patients (5). Although an effective treatment for psychosis, reserpine is rarely used today.

The story of phenothiazine antipsychotics began with the synthesis of phenothiazine in 1883. Phenothiazines were introduced into human pharmacology in the 1940s as possible anthelminthic agents and as antihistamines. It was observed that promethazine (56.**2b**), a phenothiazine with potent antihistaminic activity, produced sedation and prolonged the effects of barbiturates (6). In an attempt to enhance the

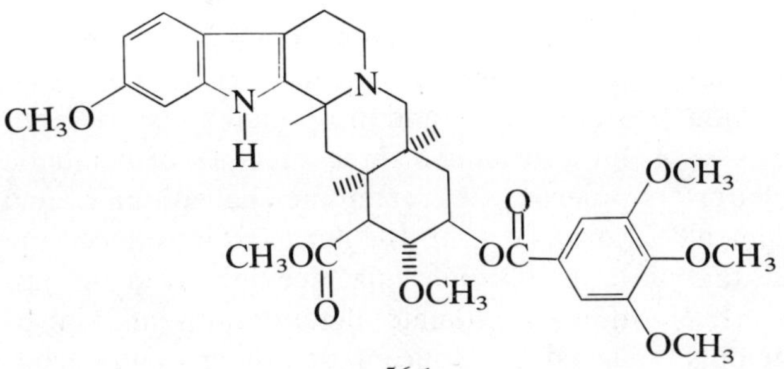

56.1

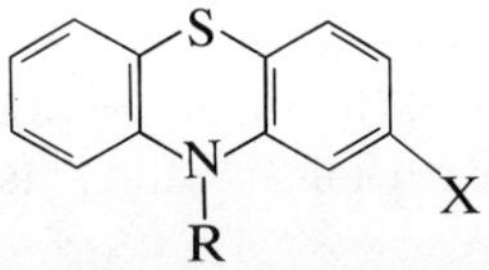

56.2a X = Cl, R(CH₂)₃N(CH₃)₂

56.2a X = Cl, R = $(CH_2)_3N(CH_3)_2$

56.2b X = H, R = $CH_2CH(CH_3)N(CH_3)_2$

56.2c X = SCH_3, R = $(CH_2)_2$—

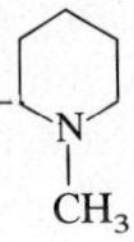

central activity of phenothiazines chlor-promazine was synthesized in 1950.

Chlorpromazine produced pronounced CNS-depressant effects in animals (7). The significance of this discovery was recognized when Delay and his colleagues (8) observed that chlorpromazine was effective in the treatment of various psychiatric disorders. In the Western Hemisphere, Lehmann and Hanrahan (9) confirmed these findings and in 1954 reported the use of chlorpromazine in the treatment of psychomotor excitement and manic states. In the same year the drug was marketed in the United States as an antiemetic agent and was quickly recognized as a very effective drug for treating nausea and vomiting. Further clinical studies soon revealed, however, that chlorpromazine's greatest usefulness was in the treatment of psychotic states.

In the nearly 30 years since the discovery of the antipsychotic drugs reserpine and chlorpromazine, a great number of derivatives of both types have been synthesized and tested, and many have found their way into clinical use. The first effective antipsychotic whose structure differed markedly from that of the prototypes was haloperidol (56.3a), a butyrophenone, whose clinical activity was essentially similar to that of the earlier antipsychotics.

The first butyrophenone of interest, i.e., the butyrophenone derivative (56.3b) of normeperidine, was discovered in 1957 in an attempt to find a novel narcotic analgetic. In addition to causing morphine-like

effects, 56.3b also produced some chlorpromazine-like effects in animals. Hundreds of related compounds were synthesized in order to increase neuroleptic activity and reduce narcotic activity. The result was haloperidol (56.3a), whose clinical antipsychotic activity was first tested in 1958 (10). A host of related compounds has been prepared and tested and a number of nontricyclic antipsychotic agents are now in use (see Section 2.2).

The first antipsychotic to show a remarkably different clinical profile was the dibenzodiazepine clozapine (56.4), which was uniquely devoid of the extrapyramidal side effects characteristic of neuroleptic drugs

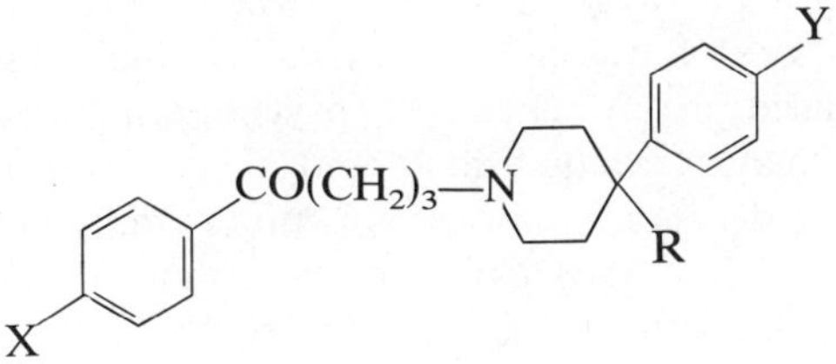

56.3a X = F, Y = Cl, R = OH

56.3b X = Y = H, R = $CO_2C_2H_5$

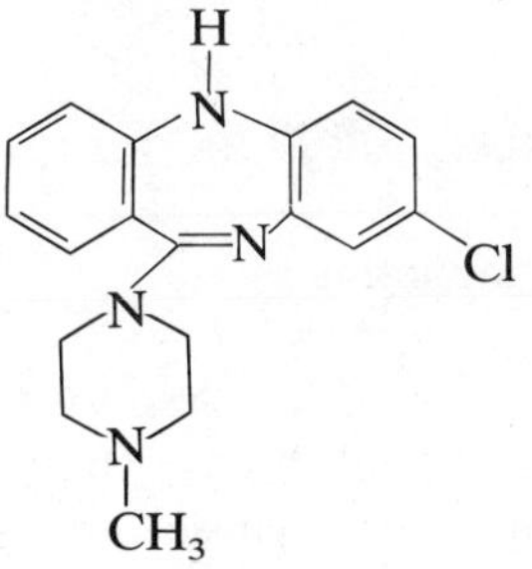

56.4

(11). Unfortunately, the production of agranulocytosis in a number of patients has impaired its clinical utility (see Section 4.3.4).

Another recent innovation in the pharmacotherapy of psychosis is the development of long-acting injectable antipsychotics that are administered every 1–2 weeks.

New terms have been coined in attempts to convey precisely the qualities of these drugs that act on the CNS and to distinguish them from other drugs that affect behavior. The general term "psychopharmacological agents" was adopted to connote drugs that influence the mind by affecting its physiological substrate, the brain. "Psychotropic" and "phrenotropic" have been used as alternative terms. Originally the antipsychotic drugs were called tranquilizers, to indicate a sedative or calming effect without sleep; ataraxics, which denotes peace of mind; neuroleptics, to denote reduction of nerve function; psycholeptics; and psychosedatives. The term "tranquilizers" was commonly used. Unfortunately, it was also applied to meprobamate and the pharmacologically related drugs that are also referred to as antianxiety agents. An attempt to distinguish between these two types of tranquilizers by calling the drugs used in treatment of psychotic patients "major tranquilizers" and those used in milder mental disorders, "minor tranquilizers" has only added to the confusion. At present the terms "neuroleptic" and "antipsychotic" are most commonly used to designate drugs for the treatment of psychosis.

2 CLINICAL ASPECTS

2.1 Schizophrenia

In 1898 Kraepelin described dementia praecox, a mental disease characterized by the lack of external causes, which occurs in young and previously healthy individuals and which is followed by eventual deterio-

ration. The phenomenology of dementia praecox includes hallucinations, delusions, stereotypies, and disordered affect. Kraepelin also named three subtypes of dementia praecox, i.e., catatonic, hebephrenic, and paranoid (12). Bleuler, who introduced the term schizophrenia, deemphasized the notion of ultimate deterioration and introduced the concept of primary and secondary symptoms. Primary symptoms include thought disorder, blunted affect, withdrawal, autistic behavior, and mannerisms, whereas hallucinations, delusions, and hostility are secondary symptoms (13, 14). Bleuler also introduced the subtype of simple schizophrenia.

Later modifications of the classification and description of schizophrenia have led to the concept of schizophrenia as a complex of diseases that include the four basic types named by Kraepelin and Bleuler. The first major subclass, catatonic schizophrenia, includes two versions: (1) *stuporous*, in which the patient may be in a stupor or at least demonstrate a marked reduction in spontaneous activity—the patient may be cataleptic or exhibit waxy flexibility of the limbs—and (2) *excited*, in which the patient demonstrates extreme psychomotor agitation—the patient speaks rapidly and incoherently and may be destructive and violent. The second major type of schizophrenia is hebephrenic, in which there is pronounced thought disorder with regression to primitive, disinhibited, unorganized behavior. Hebephrenic patients often suffer delusions and hallucinations. Paranoid schizophrenics are characterized by delusions of persecution or grandeur; they may be hostile and aggressive. The final major subtype, simple schizophrenia, is characterized by a gradual insidious loss of drive, ambition, and initiative. There is personality deterioration, withdrawal, and blunting of affect. Delusions and hallucinations are less common in this type of schizophrenia, but somatic complaints are more frequent (12). To these basic, generally accepted subtypes, some classifications add childhood schizophrenia, schizophrenia–chronic undifferentiated type, and schizo-affective disorder. Yet, despite years of attempts at description and classification of schizophrenia, "... the diagnosis of schizophrenia remains idiosyncratic, dependent on training, experience, theoretical beliefs and other biases of individual mental health clinicians" (15).

Similarly, many years of study have failed to elucidate the etiology of schizophrenia. There is little doubt that genetic factors confer a predisposition to schizophrenia. The pathophysiology which is the basis of the inherited vulnerability to schizophrenia is unknown, although several hypotheses have been advanced. Many of these hypotheses derived from concentration on hallucinations as a cardinal symptom of schizophrenia, although hallucinations occur in other disease states as well and were not considered primary symptoms by Bleuler. One group of hypotheses was based on the suggestion that symptoms of schizophrenia are caused by a toxic hallucinogenic substance produced in the body by an abnormal metabolic process. According to the adrenochrome hypothesis, epinephrine and norepinephrine could be oxidized to adrenochrome and noradrenochrome, which were claimed to have hallucinogenic properties (16, 17). The transmethylation hypothesis proposed that abnormal methylation of transmitter amines might result in the formation of endogenous hallucinogens (18). This possibility was supported by the demonstration of the *N*-methylation of tryptamine to the hallucinogenic dimethyltryptamine in brain (19). There is, however, no convincing evidence that such a process is related to schizophrenia.

The dopamine hypothesis of schizophrenia is based on the effects of drugs known to act on dopaminergic mechanisms in the brain rather than on any demonstrable abnormality of dopaminergic function in schizophrenics. Amphetamine, which causes release of catecholamines from pre-

synaptic sites, induces at high doses an acute toxic psychosis that resembles schizophrenia in some respects. L-Dopa, the precursor of dopamine, when given at high doses to nonschizophrenic subjects, occasionally induces psychotic manifestations. Both amphetamine and L-dopa, at relatively low doses, exacerbate psychotic symptomatology in schizophrenic subjects (20–22).

Although studies of unmedicated schizophrenics failed to find evidence of increased activity in dopaminergic neurons, recent controversial evidence suggests that increased dopamine receptor sensitivity may be characteristic of schizophrenic patients. Neuroleptic binding to membrane fractions, which may be one index of dopamine receptor sensitivity, is significantly elevated in some postmortem brains of schizophrenic subjects. Although this observation is confounded by the increases in dopamine receptor sensitivity on long-term administration of neuroleptics, the concomitant increase in binding observed in schizophrenic brains may reflect a characteristic of the disease process (23, 24).

2.2 Treatment of Psychosis

The principal types of therapy available to schizophrenic patients include milieu therapy, psychotherapy, and pharmacotherapy. When all three are compared, by far the greatest improvement is obtained with drug therapy (13, 25), although a combination of milieu therapy or psychotherapy with pharmacotherapy may be helpful after acute symptoms have abated and resocialization is begun. "For the therapeutic management of the vast majority of schizophrenic patients anywhere in the world today, pharmacotherapy offers higher reliability, better effectiveness, easier accessibility, greater simplicity and fewer hazards than any other treatment known today" (13). Thus neuroleptic drugs have been established as the treatment of choice for acute and chronic schizophrenia. They alleviate the primary symptoms of schizophrenia as well as some accessory symptoms (26, 27). Neuroleptic therapy may be expected to achieve cognitive restoration with normalization of psychomotor behavior in withdrawn as well as hyperactive patients (25), to shorten hospitalization, and to prevent future readmissions.

A number of antipsychotic agents are currently in clinical use in the United States. These include the aminoalkylated phenothiazines (Section 4.2.1) promethazine, chlorpromazine, triflupromazine, piperacetazine, thioridazine, and mesoridazine, as well as related piperazinyl derivatives prochlorperazine, trifluoperazine, perphenazine, fluphenazine, and acetophenazine. The esters fluphenazine enanthate and decanoate are used in antipsychotic maintenance therapy. Two thioxanthene derivatives (Section 4.2.6), chlorprothixene and thiothixene, also find clinical application as does the dibenzoxazepine (Section 4.3.2) loxapine. Nontricyclic antipsychotics that are used clinically in the United States are the butyrophenone (Section 4.4) haloperidol and the indolic β-aminoketone (Section 4.8) molindone. Many other agents described in Section 4 are employed clinically in other countries.

Antipsychotics are given to calm patients in phases of acute excitement, to control other acute psychotic manifestations, to chronically suppress psychotic symptoms, and to provide maintenance therapy for patients in remission. For these purposes many clinicians consider all the accepted antipsychotic agents to be equally effective (13, 25). The selection of antipsychotic drug is usually dictated by side effects; the drug of choice is the one best tolerated by the patient (28). When treated with the available neuroleptics, individual patients tend to respond differently to a fixed dose; therefore, the dosage must be individualized for each patient, depending on the severity of the psychoses, previous his-

tory of drug response, and sensitivity to side effects. Fairly low doses are usually administered at the onset of drug treatment, except in cases of extreme agitation, and gradually raised until the desired therapeutic effect is achieved. It is then often possible and advisable to reduce the dose once the patient is under control. Some clinicians favor the use of massive doses of antipsychotics in order to produce more rapid reduction of symptoms. It is possible to administer "mega" doses because most antipsychotics may be used safely, although not without side effects, over a wide range of doses. There is, however, little evidence for more rapid effects following administration of massive doses. Three studies of the relative rates of responding to normal and high doses of the neuroleptics, fluphenazine (29), trifluoperazine (30) (see Section 4.2.1), and haloperidol (56.**3a**) (31) revealed similar response rates in normal dose and high dose-treated patients. Other investigators using fluphenazine (32) or chlorpromazine (33) found the high dose regimen more effective in drug-resistant chronic schizophrenic patients.

A recent development in the therapy of schizophrenia is a group of long-acting neuroleptic fatty acid esters which need be given only at weekly or longer intervals. The prototype of these long-acting drugs is fluphenazine enanthate (see Section 4.2.1.2). In addition, two long-acting drugs, fluspirilene and penfluridol (see Section 4.4), which are not esters but are intrinsically long-lasting, are available outside of the United States. Penfluridol is the only one of the longer-acting neuroleptics which is active when given orally. The major advantages of long-acting injectable antipsychotic agents are (1) the assurance that the patient, especially the outpatient, is adequately medicated, because patient compliance is a major problem in the effective administration of antipsychotic drugs (13, 34) and a small number of patients fail to absorb orally administered medication, and (2) the reduction of staff time required for medication of hospitalized patients (35). The drawbacks of the depot injectable antipsychotics include a high incidence of extrapyramidal effects (36) and the requirement that outpatients visit a clinic or be treated by visiting nurses at frequent intervals in order to obtain medication.

Antipsychotic drugs are also given for maintenance therapy once the acute symptoms of schizophrenia have subsided. Proper maintenance medication is frequently the critical factor in preventing relapse. Studies of schizophrenic patients in remission show that relapse rates are much higher in patients maintained on placebo than in patients receiving maintenance doses of antipsychotic drugs (37, 38).

2.3 Therapeutically Undesirable Effects

The concept of neuroleptic activity, as originally defined (39), included the production of sedation, extrapyramidal motor disturbances, and autonomic dysfunction, together with the relief of psychotic symptoms. Inclusion of these side effects in the definition of the drug class underscores their prevalence at therapeutic doses. Extrapyramidal symptoms (EPS) occur in approximately 30–50% of patients (13, 40) and the incidence can be as high as 88%(41), depending on the antipsychotic agent, the definition of EPS used, and the diligence of observation. The drugs causing the greatest incidence of EPS are usually those of the greatest potency.

Extrapyramidal symptoms are of three types: (1) parkinsonian effects including hypokinesia, rigidity, tremor, masklike facial expression, shuffling gait, and excessive salivation; (2) akathesia, motor restlessness characterized by inability to sit still or restless limbs; and (3) dyskinesias and dystonias, uncoordinated or coordinated involuntary movements, especially of the face

and tongue. EPS are dose related. They are reversible and may be treated by concomitant administration of anticholinergic antiparkinsonism agents such as benztropine or trihexyphenidyl. It was, until recently, common practice to prophylactically administer antiparkinsonism agents concomitantly with antipsychotic drugs from the onset of antipsychotic treatment (42), but it is now considered more appropriate to use antiparkinsonism agents only when EPS appear and to withdraw the anticholinergics once the side effects are under control (13, 42, 43).

Another type of extrapyramidal syndrome, tardive dyskinesia, is produced in a smaller percentage of patients taking neuroleptic drugs. The exact incidence and the mechanism of induction of tardive dyskinesia are controversial topics, as is the question of the duration of drug treatment and dosing regimen required to produce this syndrome (44–48). It seems generally accepted that all neuroleptic drugs now commercially available have the ability to cause tardive dyskinesia. The syndrome is characterized by involuntary movements of the mouth and tongue, occasionally accompanied by choreiform movements of limbs and trunk. Tardive dyskinesia occurs most frequently in elderly patients and those who have had a long history of neuroleptic therapy. The adjective tardive is used to describe the delayed appearance of the syndrome. The most disturbing features of the syndrome are that it frequently continues after medication has been withdrawn and is only slowly reversible. Although many therapeutic approaches, including the use of reserpine (49), dopaminergic agonists (50), cholinergic agonists or precursors (49, 51, 52), benzodiazepines (53), and lithium (54) are of some benefit, no consistently effective treatment is known. In the short term, the most effective means of alleviating the symptoms is to increase the dose of neuroleptic. This is of no long-term benefit to the patient, however.

Oversedation is frequently observed in the first weeks of neuroleptic therapy, especially with tricyclic agents (13), but tolerance gradually develops and drowsiness is not usually a long-lasting problem when moderate doses are used. Very high doses of phenothiazines may occasionally cause seizures, especially in patients with organic brain damage and/or previous history of seizures. Treatment requires the use of anticonvulsant medication (55).

The autonomic effects of antipsychotics include anticholinergic effects such as dry mouth, blurred vision, constipation, and tachycardia. These effects are most commonly caused by phenothiazines except for piperazine derivatives. They are rarely caused by butyrophenones. The same is true of other autonomic effects such as orthostatic hypotension and impotence (13, 25, 55). Electrocardiographic changes are sometimes observed in patients given phenothiazines, especially thioridazine (56.2c), which causes abnormal T waves and increases the Q–R interval (13).

Metabolic and endocrine effects include weight gain, galactorrhea, amenorrhea, hyperprolactinemia, and gynecomastia in males. The most dangerous side effects are the hypersensitivity reactions. These may take the form of jaundice, agranulocytosis, cataracts, allergic skin reactions, and photosensitivity. Pigmentary retinopathy is induced by large doses of thioridazine (13). Butyrophenones rarely cause hypersensitivity reactions.

In general, the toxicity of neuroleptics is very low and there is a wide margin of safety, although uncomfortable and distressing, but not dangerous, side effects are common.

2.4   Other Uses of Antipsychotic Agents

Antipsychotic agents are the preferred treatment for schizo-affective disorders (56). They may be used in conjunction with lithium in the treatment of this condition. Antipsychotics are effective as the initial therapy for mania, with lithium gradually being substituted for them once the patient is under control. Frequently, antipsychotic agents are used in the treatment of depression. Many studies have shown that most antipsychotics are effective therapy in mixed groups of depressed patients, but they are not the drugs of choice. These agents are also generally effective in treatment of senile psychoses, but care must be used in the selection of doses for the elderly. Neuroleptics, especially haloperidol, are the only effective means of treating Gilles de Tourette syndrome, a rare neurological disorder. These drugs are also potent antiemetics. Phenothiazine neuroleptics are commonly used to control nausea and vomiting.

3   BIOLOGICAL ASPECTS

3.1   Pharmacological and Biochemical Effects

Antipsychotic agents cause a wide spectrum of behavioral, autonomic, and biochemical effects in animals (57–62). They reduce spontaneous motor activity and exploratory behavior. After high doses of antipsychotic drugs, the animals become nearly immobile and assume a hunchbacked posture with splayed hind limbs and marked palpebral ptosis. At these doses, the animals are cataleptic; that is, they maintain an induced abnormal posture for long periods of time. Still higher doses produce prostration. Clozapine, in contrast to most antipsychotics, produces only mild palpebral ptosis and little catalepsy. Marked hypotonia of skeletal muscle may mask catalepsy in the case of clozapine. Cats and monkeys may show restlessness and tremors after high doses of neuroleptics.

All neuroleptics selectively inhibit operant avoidance at doses below those required to produce overt effects (63), block the effects of injected amphetamine and apomorphine, reduce responding for electrical brain stimulation, and reduce spontaneous and provoked aggression (59, 62). They are also potent antiemetics due, presumably, to blockade of dopamine receptors in the area postrema, the chemoreceptor trigger zone. Paradoxically, these agents can themselves cause emesis in dogs when given at high doses. Neuroleptic drugs also potentiate the depressant effects of alcohol and barbiturates. The behavioral effects of antipsychotic agents are seen after acute administration. On chronic administration, tolerance develops to some of these effects. After withdrawal of an antipsychotic drug following chronic dosing, supersensitivity to the effects of dopamine agonists is observed. Although block of neuronal receptors for norepinephrine, acetylcholine, or serotonin may contribute to some of the behavioral effects of neuroleptics, especially phenothiazines and thioxanthenes, most of the low dose behavioral effects characteristic of agents with antipsychotic activity are thought to be mediated by inhibition of dopamine receptors in the brain. The same is true of the elevation of serum prolactin induced by neuroleptic drugs (64).

Antipsychotic agents produce biochemical changes in brain *in vivo* and *in vitro* that are thought to be the result of inhibition of dopaminergic neurotransmission. Except for reserpine and similar drugs which deplete brain catecholamines, neuroleptics have little effect on the level of dopamine in brain but cause consistent increases in the turnover of dopamine (65, 66). Neuroleptic drugs are believed to cause elevation of dopamine turnover (release) as the result of activation of a multineuronal feedback loop secondary to inhibition of postsynaptic dopamine receptors and/or activation of presynaptic dopamine receptors. The increase in the firing rate of dopaminergic neurons induced by neuroleptics (67) is consistent with an increase in transmitter re-

lease, as is kinetic activation of tyrosine hydroxylase by neuroleptic drugs (68).

Most neuroleptics are fairly potent inhibitors of the activation by dopamine of adenylate cyclase in brain homogenates (69). These agents displace labeled dopamine agonists and antagonists from high affinity binding sites in membrane fractions of brain. Antipsychotics also increase the turnover of norepinephrine and inhibit the noradrenergic activation of adenylate cyclase in brain slices (70). The binding of agonists and antagonists not related to dopaminergic receptors is also influenced by antipsychotic drugs which displace, for example, [^{3}H]-WB4101-[2-(2′,6′-dimethoxyphenoxy)ethylaminomethylbenzodioxan], which binds to noradrenergic binding sites (71), [^{3}H]-*N*-propylbenzilylcholine mustard (72), which binds to muscarinic binding sites, and [^{3}H]-naloxone, which binds to opiate sites (73).

Consistent with their ability to interact with a variety of neuronal systems in the brain, neuroleptics produce a number of effects mediated by actions on the autonomic nervous system. Many neuroleptics, especially among the phenothiazine and thioxanthene groups, have adrenergic and cholinergic blocking effects, and also have antihistamine and antiserotonin effects. In addition, most antipsychotics are local anesthetics.

3.1.1 MECHANISM OF ACTION. Just as the underlying biological deficit responsible for schizophrenia is unknown, so the mechanism of action of antipsychotic drugs is uncertain. Of the many biologic and biochemical actions of the known antipsychotic drugs, that which correlates best with clinical activity is blockade of dopamine receptors is the brain (74–76). The locus in the brain of the critical receptor sites is not known with any certainty, nor is it known what type or class of dopamine receptors is critical to the antischizophrenic action of neuroleptic drugs. Even more importantly, the mechanism whereby antagonism of the neurotransmitter dopamine at specific brain sites is translated to normalization of thought processes and alleviation of the other major symptoms of schizophrenia is completely unknown. It is generally accepted, however, that EPS caused by neuroleptic drugs result from blockade of dopamine receptors in the striatum.

3.2 Pharmacokinetics and Metabolism

Most neuroleptics are very fat-soluble and surface-active agents. They are rapidly absorbed following common routes of administration. Highest plasma concentrations of orally administered chlorpromazine, whose pharmacokinetics and metabolism have been the most extensively studied, depend on the dosage form (77). Also, markedly lower plasma levels result after oral versus intramuscular or intravenous administration of the drug (78). This difference is attributable to biologic conversion of chlorpromazine to inactive metabolites in the mucosal wall (79).

After absorption, the phenothiazine antipsychotics are rapidly distributed in all body tissues. Particularly high concentrations are found in the brain as well as in the lungs and liver. Few studies have compared the ability of various phenothiazines to accumulate in the brain as a whole or in discrete anatomical parts. In rats, the concentration of chlorpromazine is only slightly higher in the caudate nucleus than in the whole brain (80). An autoradiographic study of the distribution of chlorpromazine in mouse brain indicates highest concentrations in the cerebral and cerebellar cortex, but a high level is also observed in some thalamic nuclei and the hippocampus, where it remains for several days (81). A similar distribution pattern is seen in the cat brain, where significant levels of radioactivity also accumulate in the neostriatum and amygdaloid nuclei. This regional brain

accumulation of chlorpromazine does not seem related to regional blood flow (82). *In vitro*, the affinity of chlorpromazine is similar for tissue from various regions of cat brain. Thus observed differences in regional uptake *in vivo* may reflect different permeability properties of the blood–brain barrier to the sites (83).

Few studies have compared accumulation of different phenothiazines in the brain under identical conditions. The four chloro-substituted isomers of promazine, which differ markedly in their biological actions (see Section 4.2.1.3), are accumulated in the brains of mice to roughly the same extent (84). In contrast with this observation, the molar concentrations in brain of four butyrophenones were about the same after administration of ED_{50} doses for antagonism of apomorphine- and amphetamine-induced stereotyped behavior (85). In dogs, the potent antipsychotic agents chlorpromazine and prochlorperazine have similar brain distribution patterns. Highest levels of the drugs are in the medulla, hypothalamus, basal ganglia, thalamus, hippocampus, pons, amygdala, and midbrain, whereas other parts of the brain, including the cerebellum, have only low levels. In contrast, thiethylperazine, 2-ethylthio-10-[3-(4-methyl-1-piperazinyl)-propyl]phenothiazine, a potent antiemetic with relatively weak antipsychotic activity, is highly concentrated in the cerebellum (86).

After the initial distribution phase, plasma levels of neuroleptic phenothiazines fall quickly. Plasma disappearance rates of phenothiazines show a biphasic curve characteristic of highly lipophilic drugs, i.e., an initial rapid phase with a plasma half-life value as short as 2 hr, followed by a slow disappearance phase with a plasma half-life value of 16 hr (87). In the plasma, most of the phenothiazine is bound to protein; e.g., 91–99% of chlorpromazine in plasma is in the bound form (88, 89). Interestingly, the binding sites of red blood cells and rat brain synaptosomes both involve an SH group of membrane proteins (90).

Exact plasma levels of a phenothiazine antipsychotic agent are variable. A range of plasma levels, spanning almost a hundred-fold difference (about 5–500 μg/ml), is observed in patients receiving comparable clinical doses of chlorpromazine (78, 91, 92). Plasma levels in the range of 150–300 μg/ml of chlorpromazine usually correlate with clinical improvement (93). Such variations are the consequence of many factors including the time between drug administration and sampling. Further, when chlorpromazine is given orally in divided doses diurnal variations of five- to tenfold may occur even in an individual (94). Also, it is frequently observed that after initiation of a course of chlorpromazine administration plasma levels rise for about 2 weeks, reach a peak, and then decline somewhat. The decline probably reflects the induction of metabolizing enzymes by chlorpromazine (95).

Correlations between plasma levels of antipsychotic agents and therapeutic efficacy, although complicated by many methodological problems, are the object of considerable research (96). Plasma levels reflect drug availability following absorption, metabolism, and partial excretion; under ideal conditions the concentration of drug at the receptor site may be directly proportional to plasma levels (96). Evidence for such a correlation exists for phenothiazine derivatives. Plasma levels of chlorpromazine correlate with cerebrospinal fluid concentrations of the drug (97). Nevertheless, correlation of plasma levels of parent drug with therapeutic efficacy may be misleading. If metabolism is involved in tissue distribution or activity of a compound, plasma levels of a family of metabolites which may include the unchanged drug may be more relevant (98). Additionally, it is possible that plasma concentrations of unbound drug, rather than total levels, may correlate better with av-

ailability at the receptor site because only unbound drug is free to enter tissue and then cross the blood–brain barrier (99). Therapeutic concentrations of chlorpromazine, thioridazine, and haloperidol in serum water under various conditions and dosages are between 0.1 and 50 nM (75). Thus sites in the brain that are important in neuroleptic activity should be responsive to such nanomolar concentrations. Using this criterion, postsynaptic sites for haloperidol and dopamine which are stereoselectively blocked by such concentrations of (+)-butaclamol (see Section 4.3.5) are suggested as being important for neuroleptic activity (75).

The metabolic fate of phenothiazine antipsychotic agents, particularly that of chlorpromazine, has been studied more extensively than that of other drugs of this class. From 60 to 70% of the dose of phenothiazines is rapidly removed from portal circulation by the liver. A considerable amount of the drug and its metabolites, particularly in the case of piperazinylalkyl-substituted phenothiazines, is excreted via the bile into the intestine where it is partially reabsorbed. Thus fecal excretion of these piperazine derivatives is significantly greater than in the case of related phenothiazines having a dimethylaminopropyl side chain (100–102).

Like other phenothiazines, chlorpromazine is a very susceptible substrate for liver microsomal enzymes. Many of the 168 metabolites postulated for chlorpromazine have been identified and some have been tested for biologic activity (103). A large number of metabolites, and only small amounts of unchanged drug, are excreted in the urine and feces. Metabolites in the urine of psychiatric patients treated with chlorpromazine result from sulfoxidation and hydroxylation of the phenothiazine nucleus. Hydroxylation occurs mainly at position 7, and to a lesser extent at position 3, giving products excreted in the urine as conjugates of glucuronic acid. In the presence of rabbit liver microsomes further hydroxylation of hydroxychlorpromazines gives ortho-dihydroxylated derivatives which may be mono-*O*-methylated (104). The side chain of chlorpromazine undergoes further degradation to give 3-(2-chloro-10-phenothiazinyl)propionic acid, 2-chlorophenothiazine, and its sulfoxide. Some metabolites are the combination of various metabolic pathways (100–102, 105).

Despite the numerous metabolites, and perhaps artifactual products of chemical decomposition, of chlorpromazine and its metabolites that have been identified, the fate of large proportions of administered doses is not known. Some of the missing dose may be a new kind of metabolite. About 10% of the dose of chlorpromazine remains in red blood cells for a long period as a mixture of almost equal parts of "free" *N*-hydroxynorchlorpromazine and its sulfoxide. Additional concentrations of conjugated forms, sometimes equal to those of the "free" hydroxylamines, are also detected (106).

In general, other phenothiazine antipsychotic agents seem to undergo biotransformations similar to those of chlorpromazine (107, 108). In rats, thioridazine (56.**2c**) undergoes oxidative *N*-demethylation, oxidation of both sulfur atoms to sulfoxide and sulfone, and formation of glucuronides of ring-hydroxylated derivatives (109). A few studies of neuroleptic phenothiazines with a piperazinylalkyl side chain indicate degradation of the piperazine ring to give ethylenediamine derivatives (110). Several studies indicate that piperazinylalkyl and dimethylaminopropyl phenothiazines having the same nuclear substitution are degraded to identical metabolites in humans, rats, and dogs (110–114).

The question of whether or not the pharmacological actions of chlorpromazine are attributable entirely or in part to its metabolites remains unanswered. In general the metabolites are less effective in various tests for neuroleptic activity (101); however, it is possible that these more polar compounds do not readily enter the brain following systemic administration. In mice, methotrimeprazine [2-methoxy-10 - (3-dimethylamino-2-methyl-1-propyl)-phenothiazine] causes a loss of motor coordination proportionate to its presence in the brain, suggesting that it, not a metabolite, is mainly responsible for the pharmacological response (115). That a variety of other tricyclic compounds, which probably vary considerably in their metabolic patterns, are potent antipsychotics suggests that at least a considerable portion of the activity is caused by the parent drug. The activity of thioridazine (56.**2c**) may be caused in part by its 2-sulfoxide, mesoridazine, which is slightly more potent than the parent in man. 7-Hydroxychlorpromazine may be an active clinical metabolite of chlorpromazine (116, 117). Although less potent than chlorpromazine the 7-hydroxylated derivative might have useful potential as an antipsychotic agent because it causes less EPS than the parent (118). The ratio of 7-hydroxychlorpromazine to chlorpromazine sulfoxide is greater in responding than in nonresponding schizophrenic patients (119). 7-Hydroxychlorpromazine or a transformation product could be responsible for the purple pigmentation observed in some patients receiving high doses of chlorpromazine for prolonged periods (104, 115, 120). 7,8-Dihydroxychlorpromazine rapidly forms purple pigments upon incubation with microsomes, suggesting the possibility it could be a deleterious metabolite (104).

Only limited data are available concerning the metabolism of nonphenothiazine antipsychotic agents. Two thioxanthenes, i.e., chlorprothixene and thiothixene (see Section 4.2.6), afford patterns of distribution and metabolism that are similar to those of related phenothiazines (121, 122). In dogs, chlorprothixene appears to undergo ring hydroxylation, sulfoxidation, and *N*-demethylation (121).

In rats the major metabolic reaction of haloperidol is oxidative *N*-dealkylation to afford 3-(4-fluorobenzoyl)propionic acid, which is rapidly biodegraded via several steps to give 4-fluorophenylacetic acid and its glycine conjugate, 4-fluorophenaceturic acid (123, 124).

Although initial studies did not reveal reserpine (56.**1**) in the brain at the height of its antipsychotic activity, later studies with tritiated drug detected low concentrations that remained in the brain for more than 48 hr after administration. The major metabolites of reserpine are methyl reserpate and methyl trimethoxybenzoate, as well as lesser amounts of syringic acid and syringoyl methyl reserpate (125).

Tetrabenazine (see Section 4.6.1) has a relatively short biologic half-life in plasma and organs. In man, tetrabenazine cannot be detected in the blood 10 hr after administration (126). The metabolism of tetrabenazine is similar in humans, dogs, and rabbits; nine metabolites are established. These result from reduction of the carbonyl group, hydroxylation of the tertiary carbon atom in the side chain, and *O*-methylation followed by conjugation of the resulting phenol with glucuronic acid (127).

Benzquinamide (see Section 4.6.2) has a plasma half-life of only 30–40 min in dogs. It is rapidly metabolized in the liver. The major metabolite in the urinary excretion of humans and dogs is *N*-deethylbenzquinamide. Ten other metabolites, products of *N*-dealkylation, *O*-demethylation, and *O*-deacetylation, are known (128, 129).

In summary, it is clear that the various pharmacokinetic and metabolic factors, e.g., plasma levels, the form of the drug or its metabolites in the plasma, selective distribution, and metabolism, that influence the availability of an antipsychotic agent or its active metabolite at the receptor site are extremely important. So far these factors have received only relatively limited study. Investigations of this kind seem imperative before the structural requirements for antipsychotic activity can be understood. The reader is referred to Chapters 2, 3, and 4 in Part I for a fuller discussion.

4 EFFECT OF CHEMICAL STRUCTURE ON ANTIPSYCHOTIC ACTIVITY

Since the introduction of reserpine and chlorpromazine for the treatment of psychotic diseases in the early 1950s an enormous amount of structure–activity data has been accumulated. These data relate not only to structures of the reserpine and chlorpromazine type but to many different kinds of chemicals that share similar biologic actions with the pioneer antipsychotic agents. Indeed, it may be unfortunate that the modern antipsychotics were first discovered in the clinic. Subsequent pharmacological studies uncovered numerous effects elicited by these agents. These effects, in turn, have been employed to develop a variety of pharmacological screening procedures. Methods developed in this fashion, however, enable determination of only pharmacologically similar compounds with altered chemical structures, whereas they are of limited value in finding compounds with unique biologic profiles. More recently, fundamental studies of neurotransmitters, their functions, and neuroanatomic brain pathways have provided a basis for optimism that rational means for finding superior antipsychotic drugs may soon be available (130).

As a result of the enormous amounts of structure–activity data in various chemical classes that have originated from many laboratories using, e.g., different protocols, animal species, or routes of administration, comparison and correlation of this information are often difficult, if not impossible.

There is even doubt as to what constitutes a meaningful test for antipsychotic activity in animals.

4.1 Biologic Test Methods

Perhaps the most widely employed test is some form of the conditioned avoidance response test, such as the pole climb or shuttle box. This procedure distinguishes the antipsychotics from other kinds of CNS depressants and usually ranks them in the order of their clinical potencies. To some extent these tests have been replaced by anti-amphetamine and anti-apomorphine tests which do not require trained animals and seem even more selective for antipsychotics (131). Other methods that measure blockade of apomorphine-induced emesis in dogs or ptosis or catalepsy production in rodents are also used to evaluate potential antipsychotic activity. Tests that measure blockade of fighting behavior and decrease of motor activity in mice are less selective for antipsychotic agents; however, relative potencies of substances in these procedures and in man correlate reasonably well. Conversely, hypothermia production and potentiation of barbiturate-induced sleeping time, which have been used to examine compounds in some structure–activity studies, do not correlate with antipsychotic activity.

The antipsychotics also produce various biochemical responses, suggesting that they cause an increased turnover of dopamine in the brain. It is widely accepted that the neuroleptics block dopamine-sensitive postsynaptic receptors in the brain (69, 132–134), an action hypothesized to be associated with their clinical effects (21, 135). An increased turnover of dopamine results as a consequence of a compensatory increase in release of the transmitter from presynaptic neurons via a feedback mechanism (65). Various biochemical measurements of changes in dopamine metabolism have been used to evaluate antipsychotic potency, e.g., (1) enhanced accumulation of 3-methoxytyramine, the major metabolite of dopamine, after MAO inhibition (65); (2) elevated levels of homovanillic acid (HVA) and dihydroxyphenylacetic acid (DOPAC), the acid metabolites of dopamine (136–139); (3) enhanced rate of depletion of dopamine after inhibition of tyrosine hydroxylase (140–142); and (4) increased formation of [^{14}C]-dopamine from [^{14}C]-tyrosine and enhanced disappearance of amines labeled by previous injection of [^{14}C]-dopa or [^{14}C]-tyrosine (143, 144). These effects are produced by all antipsychotics that have been examined. Their ability to increase dopamine turnover seems to best distinguish neuroleptics from other kinds of drugs. In studies comparing numerous antipsychotics a good correlation is noted between potential to increase dopamine turnover and clinical efficacy; however, the data do not permit a precise rank ordering of the agents (138, 145).

Clinical potencies of tricyclic neuroleptics generally correlate with their ability to inhibit dopamine-sensitive adenylate cyclase, which is thought to be associated with the dopamine receptor (133, 146). In contrast, the relatively weak inhibitory action of the butyrophenones, which may block dopamine release (147), perhaps by facilitation of inhibitory GABA neurons (131) that synapse with central dopamine neurons (148), correlates only partially with clinical potency (149). Blockade of dopamine, an inhibitor of prolactin cells in the pituitary gland, is very likely the primary mechanism by which antipsychotics induce prolactin release, i.e., via disinhibition. This has been established by studies *in vitro* (149), *in vivo* (150, 151), and in man (135). A study of a variety of widely used antipsychotic drugs shows excellent correlation between their potency to release prolactin in man and their potency as antischizophrenic agents (152); however, some exceptions have been noted (153). Only one antischizophrenic, antidopaminergic drug—clozapine—has weak prolactin-releasing activity.

Recently, dopamine receptor binding has been demonstrated in brain membranes by labeling the receptor with the agonist [3H]-dopamine and an antagonist [3H]-haloperidol (154, 155). The relative affinities of a series of antipsychotics of various chemical classes in competing with [3H]-haloperidol binding to the dopamine receptor predict the pharmacological activities of these drugs in animal behavioral tests and their clinical potencies in schizophrenic patients (156). These binding methods provide a simple *in vitro* means for evaluating new substances as potential antipsychotic agents.

Another theory that rationalizes the actions and side effects of antipsychotic drugs is a coupling-blockade hypothesis. According to this hypothesis, fat-soluble, surface-active neuroleptics accumulate in cell membranes (157) causing membrane expansion (158), blocking nerve membrane impulses (159), displacing membrane-associated Ca^{2+} (160), and thereby enhancing the spontaneous release of neurotransmitter, e.g., dopamine (161), or modulating the coupling between impulses and neurosecretion (162). In agreement with this hypothesis, antipsychotic agents inhibit electrically stimulated release of [3H]-dopamine from rat striatal slices. Among a larger series of structurally diverse antipsychotic drugs an excellent correlation is observed for concentrations causing 50% inhibition and average daily therapeutic doses (147).

A method of prediction of clinical usefulness and estimation of the effective dosage range after single oral administration of a new compound has been developed. This method has been termed "quantitative pharmacoelectroencephalography" (163).

Despite the multitude of pharmacological and biochemical tests available as predictors of potential antipsychotic activity, in-

hibition of a conditioned avoidance response (CAR) has generally been the most widely used screening method. For this reason, in this section CAR data are given preference in comparing compounds. Where possible the potency of potential antipsychotics is compared to that of chlorpromazine as a chlorpromazine index (CI), i.e., the ED or EC value for chlorpromazine divided by the corresponding value derived for the test compound using identical experimental conditions. To illustrate the dependence of antipsychotic potency on the biologic test system, the CI's for some phenothiazines are presented in Table 56.1 (164).

4.2 Tricyclic Antipsychotic Agents; Tricyclics Having a Six-Membered Central Ring (6–6–6 Compounds)

In the general classification of tricyclic antipsychotic agents are included those substances chemically constituted by a lipophilic linearly fused tricyclic system (the tricyclic nucleus) that has a hydrophilic aminoalkyl substituent (the basic side chain) attached to its central ring. Most of these compounds have either a six-membered central ring (6–6–6 compounds), which are discussed in this section, or a seven-membered central ring (6–7–6 compounds). Substances with a larger central ring are usually devoid of significant antipsychotic activity (165–167). Although several dibenzoxazocine 56.**5a** and dibenzothiazocine 56.**5b** derivatives did show

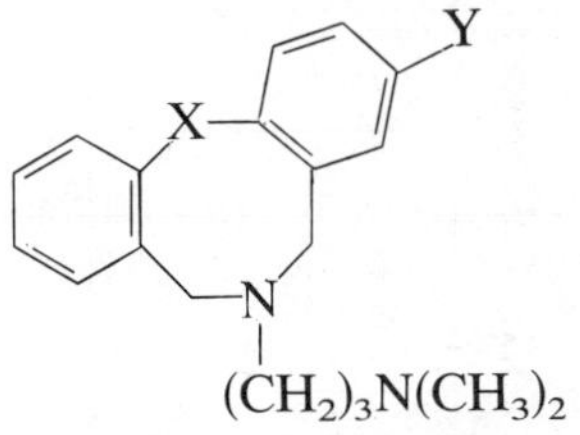

56.**5a** X = O, Y = Cl
56.**5b** X = S, Y = H

Table 56.1 Chlorpromazine Indexes (CI's)[a] of Phenothiazine Neuroleptics in Various Pharmacological Test Systems[b]

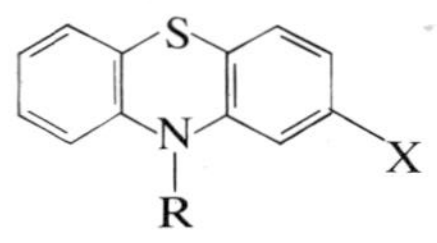

Name	X	R	Amphetamine Antagonism	Ptosis Production	Catalepsy Production	Jumping-Box Test	Apomorphine Antagonism	Open Field Test, Ambulation	Tryptamine Antagonism	Epinephrine Antagonism
Promazine	H	c	0.034	0.33	0.19	0.09	<0.08	0.09	0.065	0.95
Chlorpromazine	Cl	c	1.0	1.0	1.0	1.0	1.0	1.0	1.0	1.0
			(1.1)[d]	(10.0)[e]	(7.5)[e]	(0.93)[d]	(6.5)[d]	(4.5)[d]	(1.3)[d]	(1.6)[d]
Methopromazine	OCH_3	c	0.18	2.5	1.2	1.0	0.14	0.85	0.15	2.5
Acetylpromazine	$COCH_3$	c	5.0	8.3	0.94	1.3	0.46	1.3	0.22	16.0
Triflupromazine	CF_3	c	3.8	3.3	4.2	3.6	3.6	3.5	1.5	2.1
Trimeprazine	H	f	0.038	0.5	0.3	0.23	<0.08	0.25	0.29	0.062
Levomepromazine	OCH_3	f	0.5	2.0	1.5	1.16	0.27	0.56	0.26	1.23
Prochlorperazine	Cl	g	2.3	1.0	1.9	1.16	3.2	2.8	0.57	0.094
Trifluoperazine	CF_3	g	4.4	2.0	18.8	7.8	11.9	11.5	0.16	0.08
Thioproperazine	$SO_2N(CH_3)_2$	g	8.5	1.25	5.8	5.5	13.8	12.1	0.065	0.32
Butaperazine	$CO(CH_2)_2CH_3$	g	2.82	3.1	3.8	1.37	26.0	3.0	0.045	0.73
Perphenazine	Cl	h	6.9	5.55	24.2	9.3	20.3	20.4	1.2	1.0
Fluphenazine	CF_3	h	11.0	8.3	46.8	37.2	50.0	45.0	0.52	0.70
Acetophenazine	$COCH_3$	h	0.52	7.2	5.0	3.0	29.5	3.0	0.05	2.26
Dixyrazine	H	i	1.33	0.67	1.07	0.47	1.55	0.64	0.18	0.061
Thiopropazate	Cl	j	12.5	5.88	20.8	8.5	43.3	20.4	1.2	0.36
Pipamazine	Cl	k	1.0	8.32	4.7	1.43	0.65	2.82	1.47	1.78
Thioridazine	SCH_3	l	0.15	2.0	0.58	0.047	<0.04	0.37	0.081	1.0

[a] CI's were obtained by dividing ED (mg/kg, s.c., in rats) value for chlorpromazine by the comparable value for the test compound.

[b] Ref. 164.

[c] $R = (CH_2)_3N(CH_3)_2$.

[d] ED_{50} (mg/kg, s.c., in rats) for chlorpromazine in the indicated test.

[e] Ptosis score (ED_4) for chlorpromazine (164); catalepsy score (ED_3) for chlorpromazine (164).

[f] $R = CH_2CH(CH_3)CH_2N(CH_3)_2$.

[g] $R = (CH_2)_3N$⟨ring⟩NCH_3.

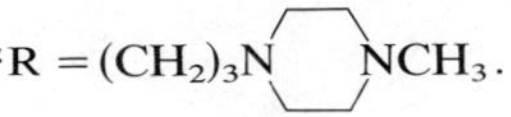

[h] $R = (CH_2)_3N$⟨ring⟩$N(CH_2)_2OH$.

[i] $R = CH_2CH(CH_3)CH_2N$⟨ring⟩$N(CH_2)_2O(CH_2)_2OH$.

[j] $R = (CH_2)_3N$⟨ring⟩$N(CH_2)_2OCOCH_3$.

[k] $R = (CH_2)_3N$⟨ring⟩$CONH_2$.

[l] $R = (CH_2)_2$⟨piperidine, H_3C–N⟩

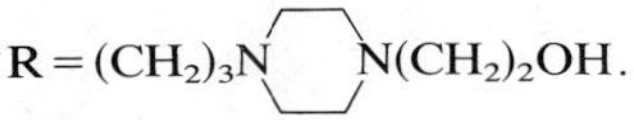

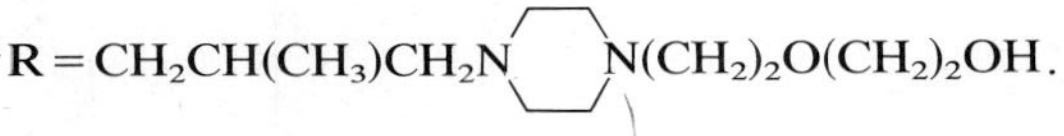

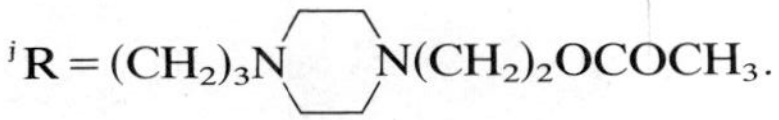

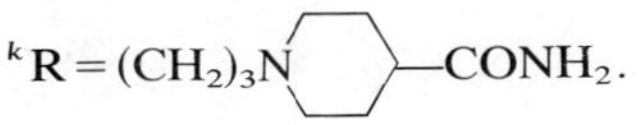

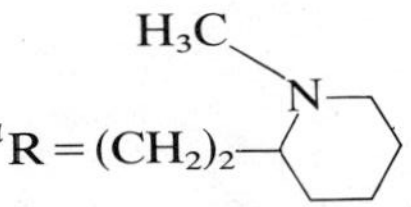

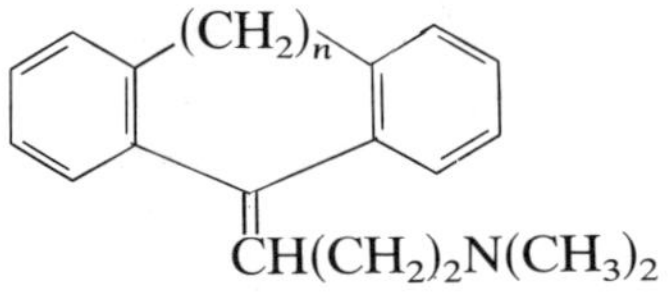

56.**6a** $n = 3$
56.**6b** $n = 0$

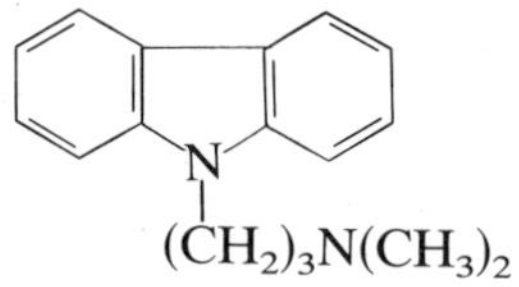

(CH$_2$)$_3$N(CH$_3$)$_2$
56.**7**

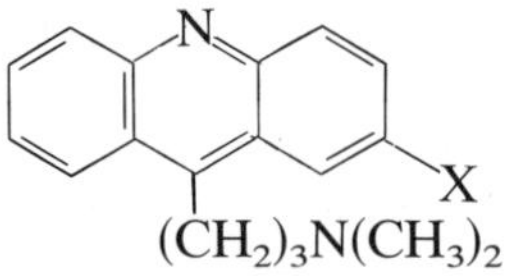

(CH$_2$)$_3$N(CH$_3$)$_2$
56.**8**   X = H, Cl, CF$_3$

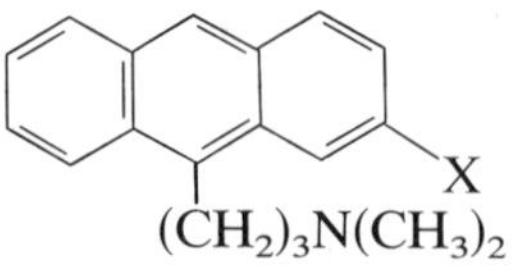

(CH$_2$)$_3$N(CH$_3$)$_2$
56.**9**   X = H, Cl, CF$_3$

weak chlorpromazine-like CNS-depressant activity in rats and mice (168), compounds such as the dibenzocyclooctane 56.**6a** lack neuroleptic properties but instead cause weak antidepressant effects (165, 166). Compounds with a five-membered central ring, e.g., the aminoalkyl derivatives of fluorene 56.**6b** (169) and carbazole 56.**7** (170), also produce only antidepressant effects. Other planar compounds, e.g., aminoalkyl derivatives of acridines 56.**8** or anthracenes 56.**9**, do not have neuroleptic properties.

Analogs of tricyclic compounds that lack a central ring, e.g., aminoalkylsubstituted diphenylamines (171, 172) and diphenylmethanes (173–175), are generally devoid of antipsychotic activity; however, some exceptions are observed. For example, several diphenylmethane derivatives of which pimozide (56.**10**) (176, 177) is the prototype are extremely potent neuroleptics. These compounds, however, appear more

closely related to butyrophenone, rather than tricyclic neuroleptics. Some other diphenylmethane derivatives, e.g., 56.**11**, have moderate CNS-depressant activity in mice (178). Another diphenylmethane derivative, 56.**12**, has a neuropharmacological profile similar to that of the tricyclic neuroleptics in animals (179).

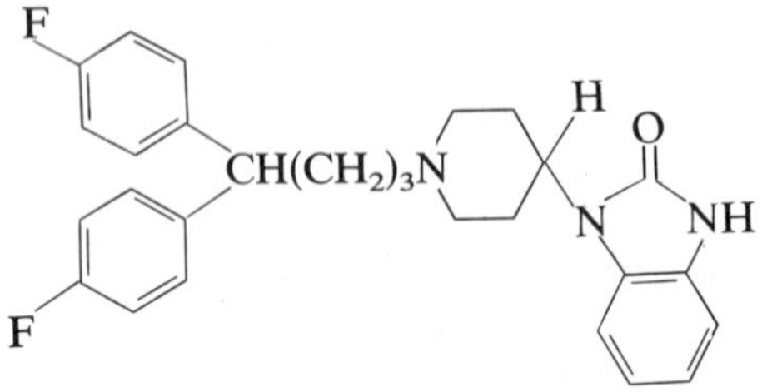

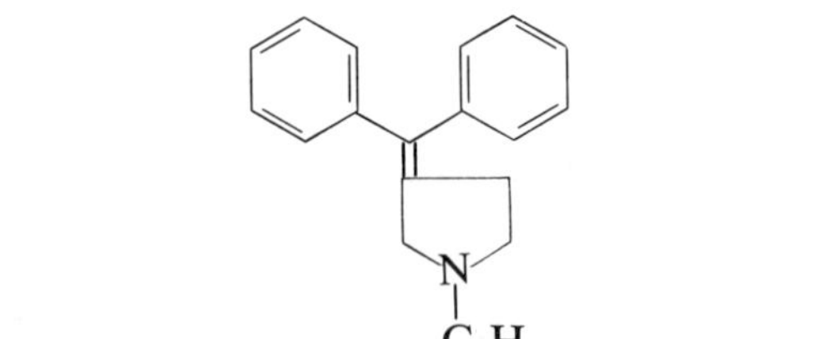

56.**11**

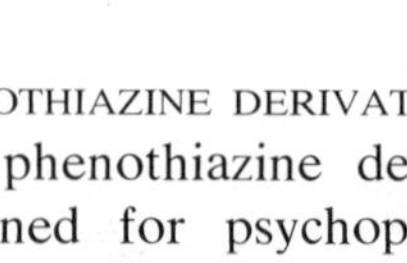

56.**12**

4.2.1   PHENOTHIAZINE DERIVATIVES. A large number of phenothiazine derivatives has been examined for psychopharmacological activity and the relationship between their structure and activity has been the subject of many reviews (101, 102, 180–189). Difficulties are encountered in any attempt to correlate these extensive

56.**10**

structure–activity data in a quantitative fashion because most studies involve a relatively small number of compounds, often tested by different methods or paradigms, and because the neuroleptic phenothiazine derivatives provide a complex pharmacological profile, affecting many different sites in the body (190).

The neuroleptic activity of phenothiazines may be affected both qualitatively and quantitatively by the nature of the chain in position 10, the amino group, and substitution of the aromatic nucleus. Consequences of some structural variations of the alkylene chain in the 10 position, the amino group, and the 2 substituent of some phenothiazines on potency in a CAR test in rats (181, 191) are presented in Table 56.2.

4.2.1.1 *Modification of the Alkyl Side Chain.* Maximum potency is observed for antipsychotic phenothiazine derivatives when there is a three-carbon spacing between the basic amino group and the nitrogen of the phenothiazine nucleus. This requirement of a three-atom alkyl side chain has been rationalized as being optimal because it permits overlap of the basic amino group and other essential structural features of the phenothiazine antipsychotics with those of the conformationally preferred form of dopamine (133). As can be noted from data in Table 56.2, in all instances 10-(3-aminopropyl)phenothiazine derivatives are significantly more potent blockers of a CAR in rats than their lower aminoethyl side chain homologs; e.g., the lower side chain homolog is only about one-fifth as potent as chlorpromazine. The homolog of chlorpromazine in which the ring and amino nitrogens are separated by four methylene units does not produce catalepsy upon i.v. administration of 25 mg/kg to mice, whereas chlorpromazine has an ED_{50} of 4 mg/kg under the same conditions (193).

Substitution of the propylene bridge of 10-(3-aminopropyl)phenothiazines may also influence antipsychotic potency quantitatively, and even qualitatively. Thus introduction of a methyl group into position 1 of the 3-aminopropyl side chain decreases antipsychotic activity and may result in imipramine-like properties. The chemical constitution of several 1-methyl-substituted derivatives of this type (194, 195) is uncertain because they were prepared by alkylation of the phenothiazine with 3-chloro-3-methyl-N,N-alkylpropyl-amines (196, 197), a reaction that proceeds via an azetidinium intermediate (198), to give mainly 10-(3-methyl-3-dialkylamino-propyl)phenothiazines. More recently, a derivative 56.**13a** of chlorpromazine, bearing a methyl substituent in the 1 position of the 3-dimethylaminopropyl side chain, has been rigorously characterized. In rats, it induces stimulant, rather than depressive, effects. The corresponding trifluoromethyl derivative 56.**13b** decreases motor activity

56.**13**

a X = 2-Cl, R = CH(CH_3)(CH_2)_2N(CH_3)_2
b X = 2-CF_3, R = CH(CH_3)(CH_2)_2N(CH_3)_2
c X = 2-Cl, R = *trans*- ▽ CH_2N(CH_3)_2
d X = 2-Cl, R = *trans*- ▭ CH_2N(CH_3)_2
e X = 2-Cl, R = *cis, trans*- ◇ N(CH_3)_2
f X = 2-Cl, R = *cis*- ⬡ CH_2N(CH_3)_2

g X = H, R = ◇ N—C_2H_5
h X = 4·CH_3, R = ⬡ N—n-C_3H_7
i X = H, R = ◇ N—CH_3
j X = 2-Cl, R = CO(CH_2)_2N(C_2H_5)_2
k X = 2-CF_3, R = CO(CH_2)_2N(C_2H_5)_2
l X = 5 → O, R = CO(CH_2)_2N(CH_3)_2
m X = 2-Cl, R = CO_2(CH_2)_2N(CH_3)_2

Table 56.2 Phenothiazine Derivatives: Chlorpromazine Indexes[a] in a Conditioned Escape Response Test in Rats (181, 191, 192)

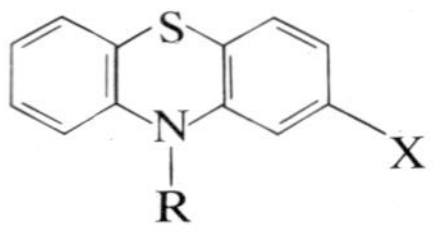

R	H	Cl	CH_3	CH_3O	CH_3S	CF_3	$COCH_3$	$C(=NOH)CH_3$	CN	SO_2CH_3	SO_2CF_3	SCF_3
$(CH_2)_2N(CH_3)_2$	0.1	0.22	—	—	—	0.7	—	—	—	—	—	—
$(CH_2)_3N(CH_3)_2$	0.4	1.0	2.2	0.5	1.0	2.4	0.6	0.83	—	0.7	2.4	1.0
$CH_2CH(CH_3)CH_2N(CH_3)_2$[b]	0.3	1.8	1.1	$(+) = 0.2$ $(-) = 0.8$	0.8	5.2	0.1	—	0.77	1.0	2.3	2.4
$(CH_2)_3N\underset{\text{piperazine}}{\bigcirc}NCH_3$	—	2.7	0.9	—	2.4	8.3	~2.1	1.0	—	—	5.8	3.5
$CH_2CH(CH_3)CH_2N\underset{\text{piperazine}}{\bigcirc}NCH_3$	—	2.0	—	—	1.4	9.9	1.1	—	—	—	—	—
$(CH_2)_3N\underset{\text{piperazine}}{\bigcirc}N(CH_2)_2OH$	—	9.0	2.5	—	—	21.0	—	—	6.6	—	—	—

[a] Chlorpromazine indexes (see text) were determined by dividing the ED_{50} (the oral dose of free base administered at time of peak activity effective in preventing 50% of rats from responding to a conditioned stimulus) for chlorpromazine, i.e., 9.9 mg/kg, in a conditioned escape response test (191, 192) by that of the indicated phenothiazine derivative.
[b] Racemate unless indicated otherwise.

in rats only slightly at an oral dose of 9 mg/kg (199).

In a series of phenothiazine derivatives, e.g., 56.**13c** (trans stereochemistry), in which position 1 of the side chain is incorporated into a cyclopropane ring, potent imipramine-like, rather than neuroleptic, actions are noted in animals. For example, 56.**13c** is approximately equipotent with imipramine in reversing reserpine-induced ptosis in rats. A trans-2-substituted cyclobutane derivative 56.**13d** also causes imipramine-like actions in rats, whereas the 3-substituted cyclobutane 56.**13e** (stereochemistry uncertain) and the cis-substituted cyclohexyl congener 56.**13f** lack significant ptosis-preventing activity, although they do produce stimulation in rats (200). 10-(N-Ethyl-4-piperidyl)phenothiazine (56.**13g**) is classed as a neuroleptic; however, low doses of several other piperidyl-substituted phenothiazines, e.g., 56.**13h** and 56.**13i**, antagonize chlorpromazine's ability to block a CAR in rats (201).

10 - (3 - Aminopropionyl)phenothiazines may be regarded as derivatives in which an oxygen is introduced into the 1 position of the 3-aminopropyl side chain. These compounds, as many others in which the alkyl chain is modified in the position adjacent to the phenothiazine nucleus, have predominantly antidepressant-like actions (see Chapter 58). Chloracizine (56.**13j**) has antidepressant (202), antihistaminic, local anesthetic, antispasmodic (203, 204), and anti-inflammatory activity (205). The related trifluoromethyl derivative, fluoracizine (56.**13k**), produces clinical antidepressant actions comparable to those of imipramine; it also causes anticholinergic effects (206, 207). In animals, the related sulfoxide 56.**13l** has anti-inflammatory activity similar to that of hydrocortisone (208). Only antispasmodic activity is noted for a series of aminoalkyl phenothiazine-10-carboxylates, e.g., 56.**13m** (209).

Introduction of a methyl group into position 2 of the 3-aminopropyl side chain, i.e.,

to give an isobutyl bridge, as can be noted from the data cited for trimeprazine and levomepromazine in Table 56.1 and the isobutyl series in Table 56.2, has only a minor and inconsistent influence on neuroleptic potency, although it often increases antipruritic and antihistaminic effects.

A promazine analog having an isobutyl bridge and a 2-COC_4H_9 substituent is a selective and more potent fusimotor depressant than chlorpromazine (210). As indicated in Table 56.2, in a CAR test in rats the (−) enantiomer, levomepromazine, is more potent than its (+) isomer. A similar observation has been made for trimeprazine; i.e., the (−) isomer is more potent than its (+) enantiomer (211). When groups larger than methyl, e.g., as in 56.**14a** and 56.**14b**, or ones capable of hydrogen bonding, e.g., as in 56.**14c**, are introduced in position 2 of the propylene bridge, potency in the rat avoidance test is decreased markedly (211). Neuroleptic potency is also decreased when the central carbon of the propylene bridge is incorporated into a ring system. Thus mepazine (56.**15a**) (212) and its 2-chloro derivative 56.**15b** (CI < 0.1 in a rat CAR test) are less potent neuroleptics than chlorpromazine (211). Both the cis and trans isomers of 56.**15c** are also practically without activity in the rat avoidance test (200). Methdilazine (56.**15d**), in which position 2 of the propylene bridge is incorporated into a pyrrolidine ring, has antihistaminic and antipruritic properties (213–215).

Introduction of a substituent into position 3 of the 3-aminopropyl side chain of antipsychotic phenothiazine derivatives apparently has little influence on activity. When this 3 carbon is incorporated into position 2 of an N-methylpiperidine neuroleptic potency is altered only slightly (216–218); e.g., 56.**15e** has a chlorpromazine index of 0.6 in a rat CAR test (211). The corresponding methylthio derivative thioridazine (56.**15f**), Table 56.1, is less potent

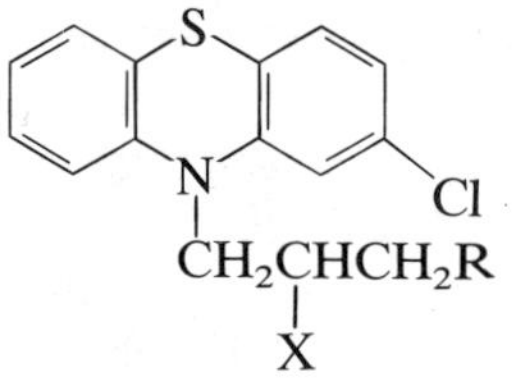

56.**14**

a X = C$_6$H$_5$, R = N(CH$_3$)$_2$
b X = CH$_2$N(CH$_3$)$_2$, R = N(CH$_3$)$_2$

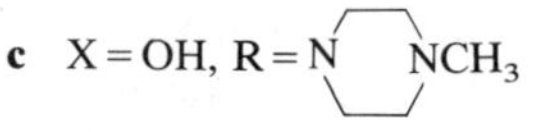

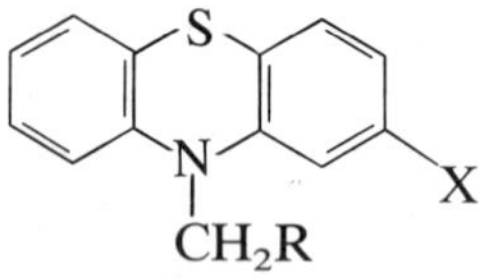

c X = OH, R = N⟩NCH$_3$

56.**15**

a X = H, R = ⟩N—CH$_3$

b X = Cl, R = ⟩N—CH$_3$

c X = Cl, R = ⟩—N(CH$_3$)$_2$

d X = H, R = ⟩N—CH$_3$

e X = Cl, R = CH$_2$—⟩N—CH$_3$

f X = SCH$_3$, R = CH$_2$—⟩N—CH$_3$

g X = S(O)CH$_3$, R = CH$_2$—⟩N—CH$_3$

h X = SO$_2$CH$_3$, R = CH$_2$—⟩N—CH$_3$

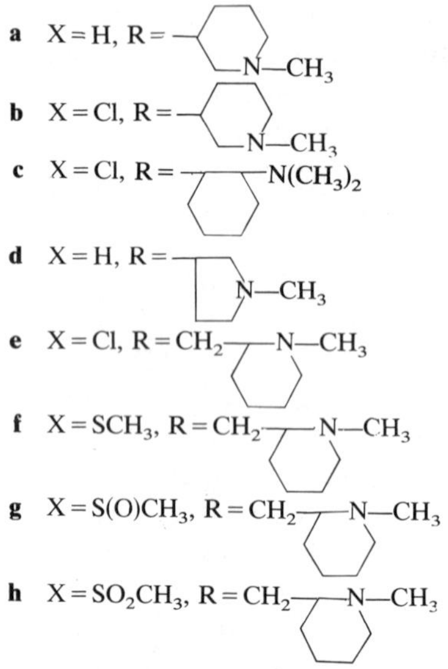

than chlorpromazine in most tests on s.c. administration. In a test for blockade of avoidance acquisition (63) the enantiomers of thioridazine showed only slight differences in potency. The (+) enantiomer had an AB$_{50}$ = 3.4 (2.2–4.6) mg/kg, i.p. whereas the (−) isomer was somewhat less potent, having an AB$_{50}$ = 5.9 (4.0–8.6) mg/kg i.p. in this test in which chlorpromazine has an AB$_{50}$ = 1.8 mg/kg i.p. (219). A metabolite

of thioridazine, the sulfoxide mesoridazine (56.**15g**), has a pharmacological profile similar to that of the parent, but with decreased cataleptogenic activity in rats (220). Clinically, mesoridazine is about twice as potent as chlorpromazine, but causes less intense side effects (221). The sulfone, inofal (56.**15h**), also produces improvement in schizophrenics (222).

Bridging of position 3 of the side chain to position 1 of the phenothiazine, e.g., as in 56.**16**, significantly reduces neuroleptic activity. In a CAR blocking test in rats, 56.**16** is less than one-fifth as potent as chlorpromazine and causes blockade only at doses that cause overt signs of stimulation (211).

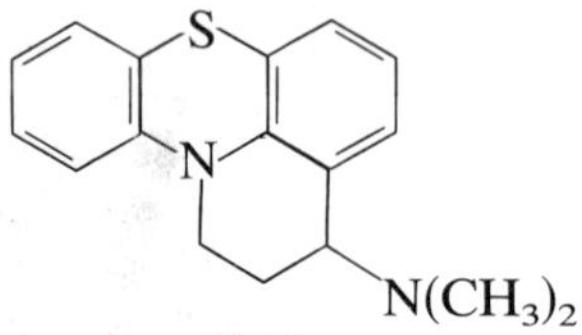

56.**16**

4.2.1.2 *Alteration of the Basic Amino Group.* Maximum neuroleptic potency is observed in aminoalkylated phenothiazines having a tertiary amino group. The primary amine didemethylchlorpromazine (56.**17a**) is much less potent than chlorpromazine as a depressant of behavioral reactivity (223), in several CAR tests, in a rotating-rod test, and as a potentiator of hexobarbital-induced sleeping time in mice (224). The related secondary amine, demethylchlorpromazine (56.**17b**) on the basis of brain concentrations in rats, is less than half as potent in depressing behavioral reactivity than is chlorpromazine (223). This and other secondary aminoalkylated phenothiazines, e.g., 56.**17c** (225) and 56.**17d**, are reported (172) to possess imipramine-like activity. The secondary amine 56.**17e** (110) is a major metabolite of prochlorphenazine (Table 56.1); however, it apparently has not been examined for neuropharmacological activity. A tertiary amine *N*-oxide

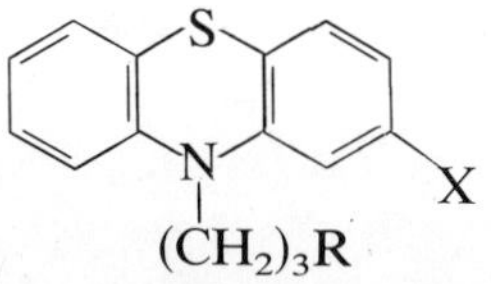

56.17

a   X = Cl, R = NH$_2$
b   X = Cl, R = NHCH$_3$
c   X = H, R = NHCH$_3$
d   X = CF$_3$, R = NHCH$_3$
e   X = Cl, R = NH(CH$_2$)$_2$NH$_2$
f   X = Cl, R = N(O)(CH$_3$)$_2$
g   X = Cl, R = N(CH$_3$)(CH$_2$)$_2$Cl
h   X = Cl, R = N(CH$_2$CH=CH$_2$)$_2$

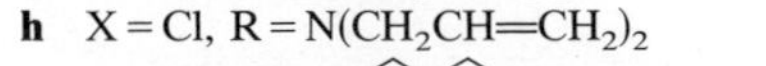

i   X = CF$_3$, R =

j   X = Cl, R =

k   X = Cl, R =

l   X = Cl, R =

m   X = Cl, R =

n   X = Cl, R =

o   X = Cl, R =

p   X = Cl, R =

q   X = CF$_3$, R =

56.**17f** is effective in some tests for neuroleptic activity, but its onset is slow and it is even less potent than the secondary amine 56.**17b** (224).

In general, alkylation of the basic amino group with groups larger than methyl decreases neuroleptic potency. Thus the *N*-methyl-*N*-(2-chloroethyl) relative 56.**17g** of chlorpromazine, a compound that might bind covalently at a neuroleptic site, is only one-fourth as potent as the parent in animal behavioral tests, although it does have prolonged action in an anti-amphetamine-induced motor activity test (226). The diethylamine 56.**18** (Table 56.3) is less potent than chlorpromazine in a conditioned es-

cape response test in rats (227). Similarly, the diallylamine 56.**17h** is significantly less effective than the prototype in prolonging pentobarbital-induced sleeping time in mice (228). In a rat CAR test, potency is also decreased by replacement of chlorpromazine's dimethylamino group with pyrrolidinyl, morpholinyl, or thiomorpholinyl groups 56.**19**, 56.**20**, and 56.**21**, respectively, Table 56.3.

In the 2-trifluoromethylphenothiazine series, the piperidinyl- and pyrrolidinylpropyl derivatives 56.**22** and 56.**23**, respectively (Table 56.3), are both somewhat less potent than the corresponding dimethylamine (Table 56.2, CI = 2.4). In contrast, introduction of a 4-methyl-1-piperazinyl group (Table 56.2) in place of chlorpromazine's dimethylamino group markedly increases potency. This compound, prochlorperazine, has a CI of 2.7.

These observations led to the suggestion (211) of a long, narrow receptor slot to accommodate the amino functionality. The concept was advanced that freely rotating alkyl groups larger than methyl swept a wider path and as a result had a greater effective width than that of piperazines, pyrrolidines, and piperidines in which the substituents are tied into a more narrow ring. This speculation is supported by the homopiperazinyl derivative, homophenazine (56.**17i**), a considerably less potent neuroleptic than its piperazinyl counterpart, fluphenazine (Table 56.1) (229), and by ring-carbon-substituted piperazines 56.**17j** which are less effective neuroleptics than their unsubstituted analogs (211).

Bridged piperidine derivatives such as an isoquinuclidine 56.**17k** (230), an 8-nortropanyl group, e.g., 56.**17l** (231), or even a diazobicyclononane, e.g., 56.**17m** (232), which are bulky but retain a sweep width comparable to that of the piperidine ring, retain a high degree of neuroleptic activity. The tropane series has been investigated most extensively (231). Neuroleptic activity in mice is greatly enhanced by introduction

Table 56.3 Influence of Modification of the Basic Amino Group on the Neuroleptic Potency of Some Phenothiazine Derivatives

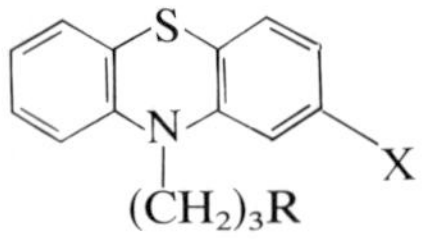

Structure Number	X	R	CI[a]
56.**18**	Cl	$N(C_2H_5)_2$	0.8
56.**19**	Cl	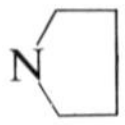	0.7
56.**20**	Cl	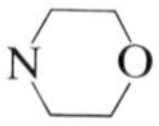	0.2
56.**21**	Cl	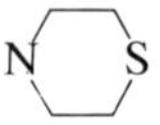	0.05
56.**22**	CF_3	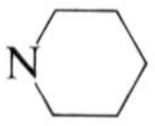	1.9
56.**23**	CF_3	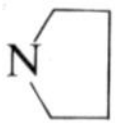	2.1
56.**24**	Cl	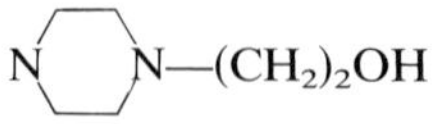 $N\!-\!N\!-\!(CH_2)_2OH$	9.0
56.**25**	CF_3	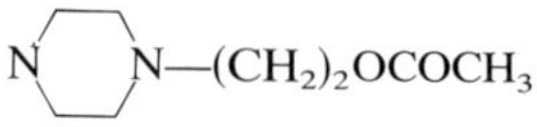 $N\!-\!N\!-\!(CH_2)_2OCOCH_3$	23.0
56.**26**	CF_3	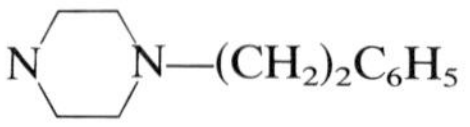 $N\!-\!N\!-\!(CH_2)_2C_6H_5$	3.0
56.**27**	CF_3	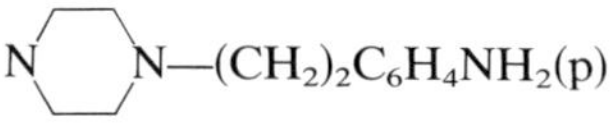 $N\!-\!N\!-\!(CH_2)_2C_6H_4NH_2(p)$	9.0
56.**28**	Cl	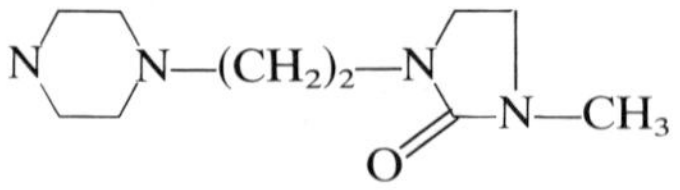 $N\!-\!N\!-\!(CH_2)_2\!-\!N$ ... $N\!-\!CH_3$	13.2[b,c]
56.**29**	CF_3	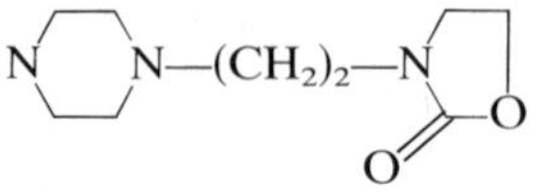 $N\!-\!N\!-\!(CH_2)_2\!-\!N$	24.8[b,d]
56.**30**	Cl	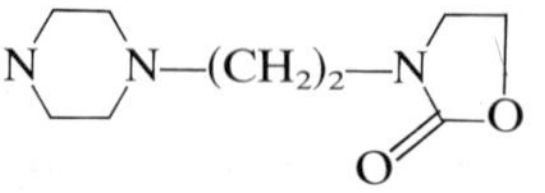 $N\!-\!N\!-\!(CH_2)_2\!-\!N$	23.1[b,e]

Table 56.3 (*Continued*)

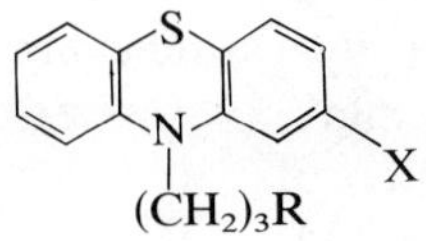

Structure Number	X	R	CI[a]
56.**31**	CF_3	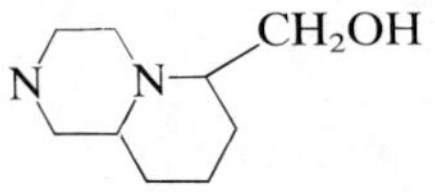	*ca.* 9[f]
56.**32**	Cl	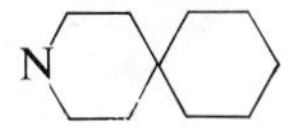	>5[g]
56.**33**	Cl	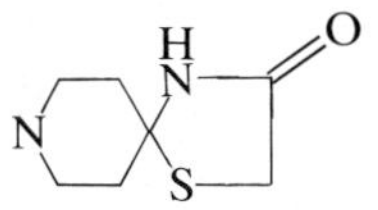	0.9[h]
56.**34**	Cl	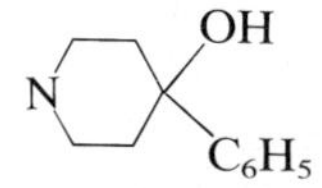	0.6[i]
56.**35**	Cl	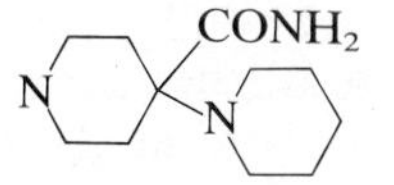	*ca.* 0.9[i]

[a] CI determined as described in footnote *a*, Table 56.2, unless indicated otherwise.
[b] CI derived from mouse antiaggression test, p.o. (192).
[c] Compound was 1.47 times as effective as perphenazine (56.**24**) (244).
[d] Compound was 2.75 times as effective as perphenazine (56.**24**) (244).
[e] Compound was 2.57 times as effective as perphenazine (56.**24**) (244).
[f] CI estimated from blockade of conditioned escape response in rats, s.c. (249).
[g] CI derived from sedation and decreased motor activity in rats (250).
[h] CI derived from conditioned avoidance response blockade in rats, p.o. (251).
[i] CI derived from antiaggression test (192) in mice, p.o. (251).

of a hydroxyl group to give 56.**17n**. Such derivatives 56.**17n**, in which the hydroxyl is trans to the tropane nitrogen, are almost three times more potent in mouse neuroleptic tests than are the pseudotropines, in which the hydroxyl is cis to the nitrogen. Conversion of either isomer to a 3,4,5-trimethoxybenzoate abolishes activity (231).

Substitution of position 4 of piperazinyl- or piperidinylpropyl-substituted phenothiazines has been studied comprehensively. The size of the terminal piperazine nitrogen substituent may be varied considerably with retention of significant neuroleptic activity. In a CAR test in rats the N-ethyl derivative 56.**17o** is slightly less effective than its N-methyl parent (prochlorperazine, Tables 56.1 and 56.2). The N-propyl homolog 56.**17p** is even less potent. In contrast, hydroxyethyl substitution of 56.**24** (233), perphenazine, substantially enhances potency relative to that of prochlorperazine, and the acetoxyethyl derivative 56.**25** (Table 56.3) (234) is even more potent.

A number of other esters of fluphenazine, the trifluoromethyl analog (Table 56.1) of 56.**24**, such as the enanthate and decanoate, find clinical utility in the maintenance therapy of schizophrenia (36, 235). Administered via s.c. or i.m. injection of a solution in an oil, such an ester forms a depot. The ester is then slowly released from this depot into the biophase, where it is hydrolyzed to the antipsychotic alcohol, to produce an effect (236) lasting for 1–6 weeks. In rats receiving i.m. injections of related labeled fatty acid esters of antipsychotic agents 95% of the remaining radioactivity resides in the region of the injection for as long as 80 days. These findings (237, 238) support the idea that the prolonged duration of these compounds results primarily from their slow release from an oily depot. Several factors affect the rate of absorption of some steroids from s.c. or i.m. depots. These are (1) the absorbing area, which is proportional to the amount of solvent injected, (2) the ability of the solvent to bind the compound, (3) the rate of release of the compound from the solvent, and (4) the rate at which the solvent itself is absorbed (239). In the case of fluphenazine esters in sesame oil it is not known which of these factors involve different rates of release from an oily depot (236). Fluphenazine itself, upon i.m. administration, has a rapid onset and prolonged duration (8.2 days) of antischizophrenic activity (240). A 1-adamantoate, following a single i.m. or s.c. injection of 25 mg/kg, is also a potent and long-acting inhibitor of CAR in rats (241).

Apparently bulk tolerance of terminal N-piperazine substituents at the site of antipsychotic action is considerable. As can be seen from the data in Table 56.3, significant potency is retained when these substituents are as large as phenethyl (56.**26**) or even p-aminophenethyl (56.**27**). The piperazinylethylimidazolone, imiclopazine (56.**28**) (Table 56.3) is more potent and longer acting than perphenazine (Table 56.1; 56.**24**, Table 56.3) as an inhibitor of CAR behavior in rats and in dogs (242). Clinically, imiclopazine is an effective antipsychotic (243). Several related oxazolidones, e.g., 56.**29** and 56.**30** (Table 56.3), are very potent in several tests for neuroleptic activity (244). Oxaflumazine (56.**17q**), another piperazine derivative having a large terminal nitrogen substituent, also presents a neuroleptic profile in animals (245) and is effective in schizophrenics (246). Another example of a phenothiazine derivative bearing a larger terminal piperazine nitrogen substituent and having potent neuroleptic (247) and clinical antipsychotic activity (248) is the hydroxyethoxyethyl derivative dixyrazine (see Table 56.1). In a series of phenothiazines having the basic nitrogen incorporated into a diazabicyclo[4.4.0]decane or diazabicyclo[4.3.0]nonane system (249) the hydroxymethyl derivative 56.**31** is the most potent blocker of a rat CAR.

Many modifications of position 4 of the piperidine ring of piperidinylpropylphenothiazines have been examined. Several of these, for example, the azaspirane 56.**32** (Table 56.3) (250) and chlorspirane (56.**33**) (Table 56.3), a clinically effective antipsychotic, retain a high degree of chlorpromazine-like activity (251). In a series of 4,4-disubstituted piperidine derivatives of this kind two of the most potent inhibitors of fighting behavior in mice are 56.**34** and 56.**35** (Table 56.3) (251). Various 4-monosubstituted piperidine derivatives also demonstrate antipsychotic properties. A 4-methoxypiperidine 56.**36a** has a CI of about 1.5 in a CAR blockade test in rats. Clinically, it is an effective antipsychotic

56.**36**

a	X = COCH$_3$, R = OCH$_3$
b	X = H, R = OH
c	X = CN, R = OH
d	X = SO$_2$CH$_3$, R = CONH$_2$
e	X = CF$_3$, R = COC$_6$H$_4$-4-F
f	X = Cl, R = COC$_6$H$_4$-4-F
g	X = SO$_2$N(CH$_3$)$_2$, R = (CH$_2$)$_2$OH
h	X = COCH$_3$, R = (CH$_2$)$_2$OH

with mild side effects (252). Many 4-hydroxyl- and hydroxyalkylpiperidines have neuroleptic (253) and antihistamic (254) actions. The 4-hydroxylated piperidine derivative 56.**36b** (255), as well as the related 2-cyanophenothiazine propericiazine (56.**36c**) (256), has clinical antipsychotic activity. A 4-carboxamidopiperidylpropyl derivative, pipamazine (Table 56.1), and its 2-methylsulfonyl congener 56.**36d** (257) have neuroleptic properties; however, their clinical application is primarily as antiemetics. Several 4-(4-fluorobenzoyl)piperidines, e.g., 56.**36e** and 56.**36f**, are potent and long-acting in anti-amphetamine and CAR blockade tests in mice (258–260).

Perhaps significant from a structure–activity standpoint, introduction of a hydroxyethyl substituent into the 4 position of appropriately substituted piperidinylpropylphenothiazines, as in the case of related piperazinyl compounds, enhances neuroleptic potency (253). Thus the 4-hydroxyethylpiperidine pipotiazine 56.**36g** has a pharmacological profile similar to that of fluphenazine (Table 56.1) (261) and the related 2-acetylphenothiazine, piperacetazine (56.**36h**), is about six times as potent (262) as chlorpromazine as a clinical antipsychotic (263, 264).

Palmitic and undecylenic acid esters of pipotiazine, like fatty acid esters of fluphenazine, have therapeutic utility in anti-

psychotic maintenance therapy (265). Neurological and pharmacological studies of pipotiazine palmitate (266) indicate a greater duration of action against apomorphine-induced emesis in dogs than that produced by fluphenazine decanoate. Consistent with this observation, a single i.m. injection of pipotiazine palmitate in oil controls schizophrenic symptoms for about 4 weeks as compared to 2 weeks for fluphenazine enanthate (267–269).

4.2.1.3 *Phenothiazine Ring Substituents.* The potency of antipsychotic phenothiazines is influenced both quantitatively and qualitatively by the location and the nature of substitution on the tricyclic nucleus. In Table 56.4 CI's for some ring-monosubstituted 10-(3-dimethylaminopropyl)phenothiazines (56.**37**–56.**62**) are listed in a very rough approximation of increasing neuroleptic potency. These comparative potencies, estimated from a variety of pharmacological test procedures, depend on a multitude of factors, including the nature of the side chain.

With the exception of the very weakly effective series of phenols (56.**37**–56.**40**), the data tabulated in Table 56.4 indicate convincingly that substitution of position 2 is optimal for neuroleptic potency. In general, potency increases in the following order of position of ring substitution: 1 < 4 < 3 < 2.

Substitution of position 1 has not been extensively studied. In rats, an oral dose of 90 mg/kg of 1-chloropromazine causes overt effects, e.g., mydriasis, piloerection, exophthalmia, and increased motor activity, similar to those seen with antidepressives. Like antidepressives, the 1-chloro derivative of promazine also prevents reserpine-induced ptosis in mice and rats. At comparatively large doses it is effective in a mouse rage test (192). 1-Hydroxypromazine (56.**37**) (Table 56.4) is only marginally effective in rotating-rod and hexobarbital-potentiation tests in mice (270).

Table 56.4 Chlorpromazine Indexes (CI's)^a for Ring-Monosubstituted Derivatives of 10-(3-Dimethylaminopropyl)phenothiazines

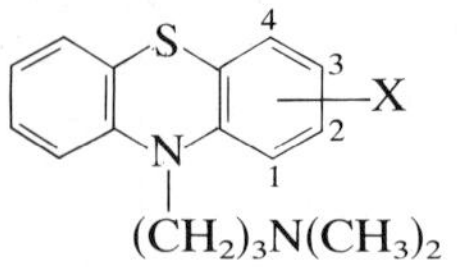

$(CH_2)_3N(CH_3)_2$

Structure Number	X	CI^a	Method^b
56.**37**	1-OH	0.02	c,d
56.**38**	2-OH	0.025	c,d
56.**39**	3-OH	0.13	d,e
56.**40**	4-OH	~0.4	d,e
56.**41**	4-CF$_3$	<0.06	f
56.**42**	4-Cl	<0.08	g
56.**43**	H	0.4 (0.07)^f (0.07)^h	d
56.**44**	2-CH$_3$O	0.5 (0.07^f (0.04)^h	d
56.**45**	2-CONHNH$_2$	0.07	f
56.**46**	3-Cl	0.18	f
56.**47**	2-CH(CH$_3$)$_2$	0.32 (≪0.5)^i	j
56.**48**	2-CH$_3$	0.28 (2.2)^d (<0.5)^i	j
56.**49**	3-C(CH$_3$)$_3$	—(~1)^i	j
56.**50**	2-C(CH$_3$)$_3$	0.18 (3–4)^i	j
56.**51**	3-CF$_3$	0.43	f
56.**52**	2-CO$_2$CH$_3$	0.49	f
56.**53**	2-n-C$_3$H$_7$CO	2.0^k	l
56.**54**	2-C$_2$H$_5$CO	~2.0^k (2.0)^h	l
56.**55**	2-CH$_3$CO	0.6 (0.49)^f (3.0)^h (3.5)^h	d
56.**56**	2-SO$_2$CH$_3$	0.7	d
56.**57**	2-C(=NOH)CH$_3$	0.83	d
56.**58**	2-Cl	1.0	d
56.**59**	2-CH$_3$S	1.0	d
56.**60**	2-CF$_3$S	1.0	d
56.**61**	2-CF$_3$	2.4 (1.7)^f(6.0)^h	d
56.**62**	2-CF$_3$SO$_2$	2.4	d

^{a} CI's were determined by dividing the ED value (mg/kg) for chlorpromazine in the indicated assay system by that of the test compound. In some instances CI's were estimated from literature data as indicated by footnote.

^{b} Test method used for derivation of CI not in parentheses. CI's in parentheses were derived via assay method indicated by footnote.

^{c} CI estimated by comparison with promazine (56.**43**) for which a CI value of 0.4 was used (see footnote d). A rotating-rod test in mice, i.v. (270), was used.

^{d} See footnote a, Table 56.2.

^{e} CI estimated by comparison with promazine (56.**43**) in a rotating-rod test, i.p., in mice (224). ^{f} CAR test in rats, i.p. (271). ^{g} Catalepsy test in mice, i.v. (193).

^{h} Jumping-box test in dogs, s.c., using ED$_{50}$ in μmoles/kg (278).

^{i} Tranquilization estimated in monkeys, p.o. (275).^{j} CAR test in rats, i.p. (275).

^{k} This compound was 0.67 as potent as 56.**51** and 2.3 times as potent as 56.**43** in the test indicated in footnote l (274).

^{l} Inclined plane test in mice, s.c. (274).

Based on the data presented in Tables 56.1–56.4, combined with other CAR blockade data (193, 231, 271–278), 2-substitution of the phenothiazine nucleus increases neuroleptic potency in approximately the following order: $OH < H \approx OCH_3 \approx CO-NHNH_2 < CN < CH(CH_3)_2 < CH_3 < C(CH_3)_3 \approx CO_2CH_3 \approx n\text{-}C_3H_7CO \approx C_2H_5CO < CH_3CO \approx SO_2CH_3 \approx C(=NOH)CH_3 < Cl \approx SCH_3 \approx S(O)CH_3(220) \approx Br \approx SCF_3 < SO_2N(CH_3)_2 < SO_2CF_3 \approx CF_3$. The influence of 2-substitution on the neuroleptic activity of some thioridazine congeners (279) and promazine derivatives having various acetylenic, ethylenic, and substituted carbinol groups in position 2 (280) has also been examined.

The role of the 2 substituent in influencing neuroleptic potency remains uncertain. It has been suggested (211) that this effect may be proportional to the electron withdrawing character of the 2 substituent provided it lacks ionic character that by non-specific binding might prohibit the molecule from reaching the site of action; however, several exceptions are apparent, e.g., the potency-enhancing influence of electron-releasing alkyl groups (56.47–56.50) (Table 56.4). On the basis of theoretical calculations and model building it has been suggested (281) that in some neuroleptics the 2 substituent is exerting a direct van der Waals force of attraction on the amino group of the side chain. This is considered unlikely because in crystal structures the distances involved are too great for this to occur. Additionally, it is unlikely that such a weak force of attraction between these two functions would be sufficient to determine the overall conformation of the molecule. It seems more likely that the potency-enhancing action is via a direct receptor effect (282).

In some instances the neuroleptic potency of phenothiazine derivatives may be enhanced somewhat by substitution of position 3. Thus 3-chloro- (56.46) (Table 56.4) and 3-trifluoromethylpromazine (56.51)

(Table 56.4) are more potent than the parent 56.43 (Table 56.4) in a CAR blockade test in rats (271). Also, the 3-*tert*-butyl derivative 56.49 (Table 56.4) is equipotent with chlorpromazine in a test for tranquilization of monkeys (275). In all cases, however, even though the 3 isomers are more potent than promazine they are considerably less potent than their 2-substituted counterparts.

Substitution of position 4 of promazine decreases neuroleptic potency. Thus 4-trifluoromethyl- (56.41) (Table 56.4) and 4-chloropromazine (56.42) (Table 56.4) are inactive at twice the ED_{50} of promazine in a mouse catalepsy test. The 4-trifluoromethyl derivative 56.41 (Table 56.4) is also less effective than promazine in a CAR blockade test in rats (271).

In general, disubstitution of even neuroleptically active 2-substituted phenothiazines has little effect or is detrimental to potency. Thus 1,2-dichloropromazine (56.63a), like 1-chloropromazine produces antidepressant, rather than neuroleptic, symptoms in rats. Introduction of a 4-chloro (56.63b) or 4-methyl (56.63c) substituent into chlorpromazine has little influence on activity; both compounds are qualitatively and quantitatively similar to chlorpromazine (283). A 2,3-methylenedioxy derivative 56.63d of promazine has a Cl < 0.1 in a CAR test in rats (284). Introduction of a second substituent into position 7 or 8 of chlorpromazine or triflupromazine markedly decreases CAR blocking activity. 7-

56.63

a	$X = 1,2\text{-}Cl_2$	h	$X = 2\text{-}CF_3, 8\text{-}Cl$
b	$X = 2,4\text{-}Cl_2$	i	$X = 2\text{-}CF_3, 8\text{-}CH_3$
c	$X = 2\text{-}Cl, 4\text{-}CH_3$	j	$X = 2,4,8\text{-}(Cl\ or\ CH_3)$
d	$X = 2,3\text{-}OCH_2O$	k	$X = 2\text{-}Cl, 7,8\text{-}(CH_3O)_2$
e	$X = 2\text{-}Cl, 7\text{-}CH_3O$	l	$X = 2\text{-}Cl, 7,8\text{-}OC(CH_3)_2O$
f	$X = 2\text{-}Cl, 7\text{-}HO$	m	$X = 2\text{-}Cl, 5\text{-}O$
g	$X = 2\text{-}CF_3, 7\text{-}CH_3O$	n	$X = 2\text{-}Cl, 5\text{-}O_2$

Methoxychlorpromazine (56.**63e**) is inactive in prolonging hexobarbital-induced sleep and is significantly less potent than chlorpromazine in a mouse rotating-rod test (270). The metabolism of chlorpromazine and tissue distribution of several of its metabolites (see Section 3.2) has been extensively studied (118, 119, 285, 286). 7-Hydroxychlorpromazine (56.**63f**) is less potent than chlorpromazine in behavioral studies (118) whereas 7-methoxytriflupromazine (56.**63g**) has a CI of about 0.3 in a rat CAR test. In the same test 8-chloro-(56.**63h**) and 8-methyltriflupromazine (56.**63i**) are less than one-fifth as potent as chlorpromazine (287, 288).

A series of 2,4,8-trisubstituted derivatives of promazine with various combinations of chloro and methyl groups 56.**63j** provides compounds that are generally less potent and less toxic than their 2,4-disubstituted counterparts (289). A 7,8-dimethoxy derivative 56.**63k** of chlorpromazine is slightly more potent than the related acetonide 56.**63l**. Although both compounds cause marked hypotensive and CNS-depressant effects in dogs, neither is as potent as chlorpromazine in tests for neuroleptic activity (290).

Oxidation of the 5 sulfur of antipsychotic phenothiazines invariably decreases neuroleptic potency (224, 270, 291). The sulfoxide metabolite 56.**63m** (292) of chlorpromazine has a CI of 0.14 in a rat CAR test (293). Sulfones derived from antipsychotic phenothiazines lack significant neuroleptic activity. For example, chlorpromazine sulfone (56.**63n**) does not block CAR in rats at an oral dose of 150 mg/kg.

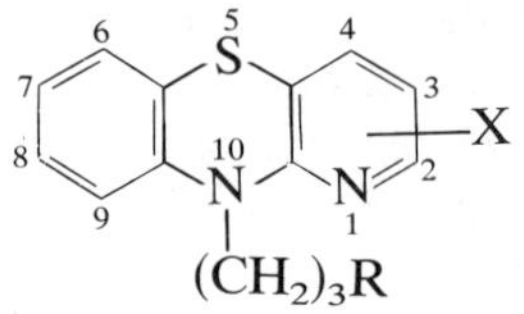

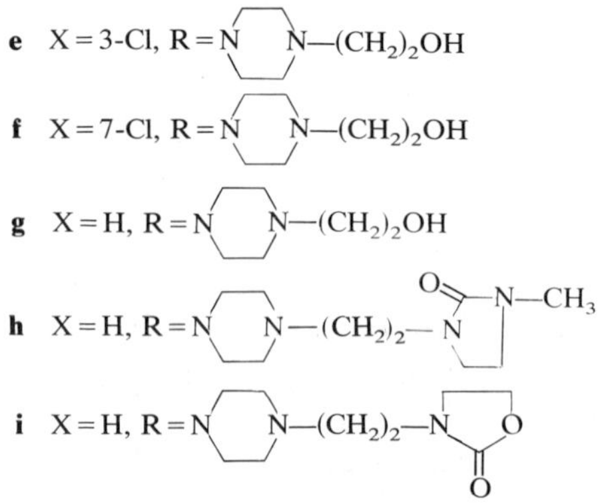

4.2.1.4 *Azaphenothiazine Derivatives.* Appropriately substituted 1-azaphenothiazines, e.g., prothipendyl (56.**64a**), apparently are more effective CNS depressants than corresponding 2-, 3-, and 4-azaphenothiazines. Prothipendyl (56.**64a**) (294) is more potent than the analogous phenothiazine, promazine in many tests for neuroleptic activity

56.**64**

a　X = H, R = N(CH$_3$)$_2$
b　X = 6-Cl, R = N(CH$_3$)$_2$
c　X = 8-Cl, R = N(CH$_3$)$_2$
d　X = 3-Cl, R = N(CH$_3$)$_2$
e　X = 3-Cl, R = N⟩N—(CH$_2$)$_2$OH
f　X = 7-Cl, R = N⟩N—(CH$_2$)$_2$OH
g　X = H, R = N⟩N—(CH$_2$)$_2$OH
h　X = H, R = N⟩N—(CH$_2$)$_2$—N(cyclic)—CH$_3$
i　X = H, R = N⟩N—(CH$_2$)$_2$—N(cyclic)

(164, 278, 295, 296). It is about one-fifth as potent as chlorpromazine in depressing motor activity in mice (295) and has a CI of about 0.4 in rat and dog CAR tests (278). Clinically, prothipendyl is a sedative–hypnotic (297) with possible antipsychotic activity (298). Aminoalkylated 1-azaphenothiazines are usually more potent than corresponding phenothiazines in potentiating narcosis in mice (295, 299). Potency is decreased by chloro substitution in the 6 (56.**64b**) and 8 (56.**64c**) positions; however, it is enhanced by chloro substitution in position 3; e.g., 56.**64d** has a CI of 0.8 on i.p. administration in a test for catalepsy production in mice. In this same test cloxypendyl (56.**64e**) has a CI of 3.5 and is effective in the treatment of schizophrenia. In contrast the 7-chloro isomer 56.**64f** of cloxypendyl is only a weak depressant in animals (300). The unsubstituted relative oxypendyl (56.**64g**) of cloxypendyl emphasizes the significance of the side chain on neuroleptic potency. Thus the hydroxyethylpiperazine 56.**64g** is considerably

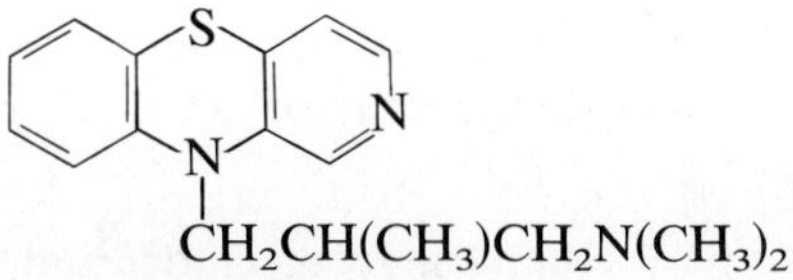

CH₂CH(CH₃)CH₂N(CH₃)₂

$\text{CH}_2\text{CH}(\text{CH}_3)\text{CH}_2\text{N}(\text{CH}_3)_2$

56.**65**

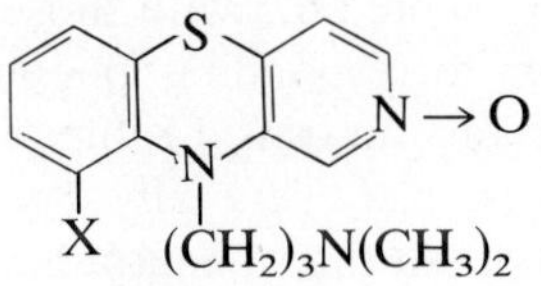

X $(\text{CH}_2)_3\text{N}(\text{CH}_3)_2$

56.**66a** X = H
56.**66b** X = Cl

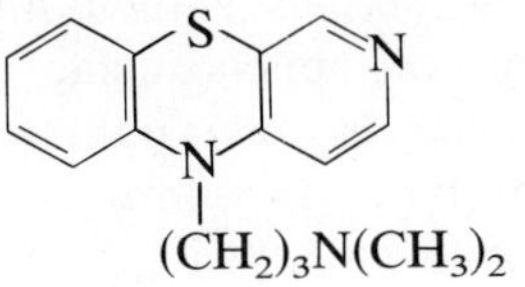

$(\text{CH}_2)_3\text{N}(\text{CH}_3)_2$

56.**67**

$(\text{CH}_2)_3\text{N}(\text{CH}_3)_2$

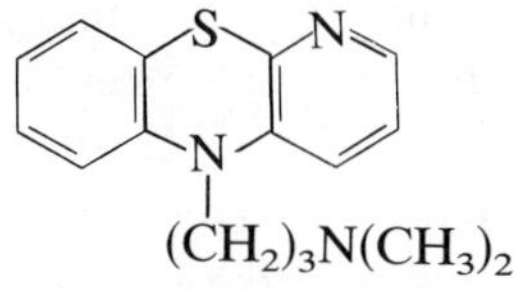

56.**68**

more potent than its dimethylamino counterpart prothipendyl (56.**64a**). Oxypendyl has antiemetic potency comparable to that of triflupromazine (301). Clinically, oxypendyl produces sedation with little improvement in disturbed behavior (302). On oral administration in a mouse antiaggression test, the imidazolone 56.**64h** is less than one-seventh as potent as its 2-chlorophenothiazine counterpart imiclopazine (56.**30**) (Table 56.3) and the related oxazolidone 56.**64i** is even less potent (244).

2-Azaphenothiazines (288, 303) are generally less potent neuroleptics than their 1-aza relatives, e.g., in a CAR test in rats 56.**65** has CI of 0.16 (181). However, several 2-azaphenothiazine N-oxides, e.g., 56.**66a** and 56.**66b**, are claimed (304) to have useful CNS properties. The 3-azaphenothiazine 56.**67** has only slight sedative and hypnotic properties in mice (305). Several 10-aminoalkyl-4-azapheno-

thiazines, e.g., 56.**68**, are reported; however, their neuropharmacological properties are not described (306–308).

4.2.1.5 *Thieno[1,4]benzothiazines.*

In a series of isomeric N-dimethylaminopropyl-thienobenzothiazines, 56.**69**–56.**71**, isosteres of promazine in which the thieno group replaces a benzo-fused ring of the phenothiazine, neuroleptic activity in rats and mice depends on the mode of annelation of the thiophene ring (309). Compounds bearing the same substituents and side chain with the thiophene moiety in 2,3 (56.**69**) and 3,4 (56.**70**) annelation have neuroleptic properties, whereas those with a 3,2 (56.**71**) annelation are without notable activity.

In an anti-apomorphine test in rats 56.**69c** is the most potent member of the series, having a CI of 0.5.

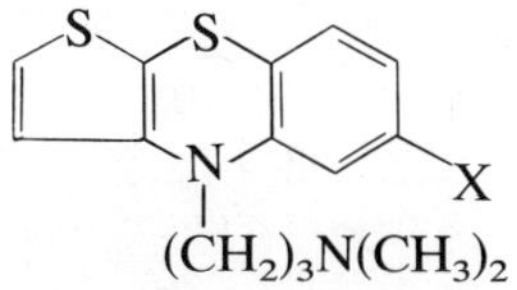

$(\text{CH}_2)_3\text{N}(\text{CH}_3)_2$

56.**69a** X = H
56.**69b** X = Cl
56.**69c** X = CF₃

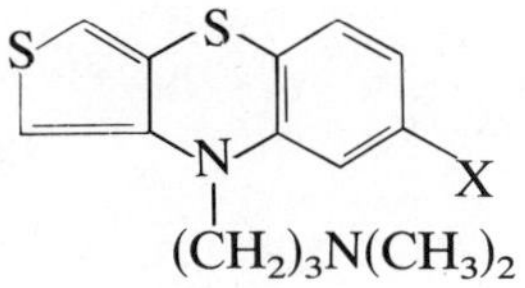

$(\text{CH}_2)_3\text{N}(\text{CH}_3)_2$

56.**70** X = H, Cl, CF₃

$(\text{CH}_2)_3\text{N}(\text{CH}_3)_2$

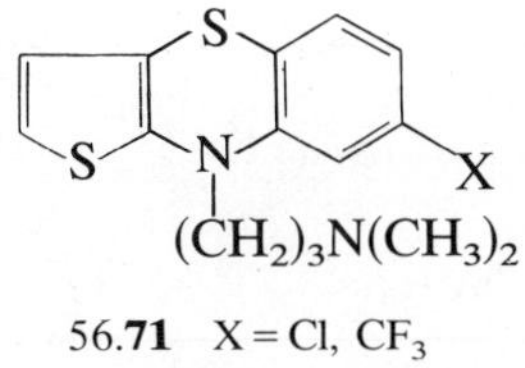

56.**71** X = Cl, CF₃

4.2.1.6 *"Ring-Opened" Analogs of Phenothiazines Retaining the Sulfur Atom.*

Diphenylamines, e.g., 56.**72a** (310), which may be regarded as ring-opened analogs of phenothiazines, are claimed to have

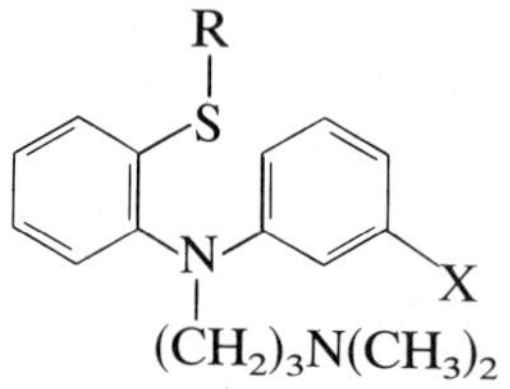

R
|
S
/   \
(benzene ring)   (benzene ring)
N   X
|
(CH₂)₃N(CH₃)₂

56.**72a** R = X = H
56.**72b** R = CH₃, X = Cl
56.**72c** R = CH₃, X = H

narcotic-potentiating actions (311). Derivatives, e.g., 56.**72b**, are claimed to have tranquilizing and antiemetic actions (312). The corresponding dechloro derivative 56.**72c,** however, has only marginal neuroleptic activity. It blocks CAR in 20% of rats treated with 200 mg/kg p.o. and has a CI of 0.04 in a test for depression of motor activity in mice.

4-Aminoalkyl-2-phenyl-1,4-benzothiazines, e.g., 56.**73** (313), and their 3-phenyl isomers, e.g., 56.**74** (314), which differ from antipsychotic phenothiazines only in that one ring instead of being fused to the benzothiazine is a freely rotat-

ing phenyl substituent, are essentially devoid of neuroleptic activity (314).

4.2.2 PHENOXAZINE DERIVATIVES. As can be seen by comparing the chlorpromazine indexes of various phenoxazine derivatives tabulated in Table 56.5 with those similarly derived for corresponding phenothiazines in a CAR test in rats (Table 56.2), the phenoxazines are generally less potent neuroleptics than their phenothiazine counterparts (315). The potency difference between the two series, however, depends on the nature of the 2 substituent and the side chain. Thus the phenoxazine analog of chlorpromazine is only 0.038 as potent as the prototype. In contrast, the phenoxazine [Table 56.5, X = CF₃; R = (CH₂)₃-NCH₂CH₂N(CH₂CH₂OH)CH₂CH₂] is about equipotent with its phenothiazine counterpart fluphenazine (Table 56.2) (316). Despite relative potency differences in the two series, structure–activity relationships are generally similar. Thus in the phenoxazine series, as in the phenothiazine series,

Table 56.5 Chlorpromazine Indexes (CI's)ᵃ for Phenoxazine Derivatives

(phenoxazine structure with O at top, N–R at bottom, X substituent)

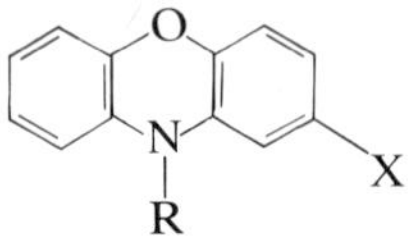

R	X				
	H	CH₃	Cl	SO₂N(CH₃)₂	CF₃
(CH₂)₃N(CH₃)₂	<0.02	—	0.038	<0.1	0.29
CH₂CH(CH₃)CH₂N(CH₃)₂	<0.05	—	<0.05	—	—
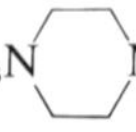 (CH₂)₃N⟨ring⟩NCH₃	—	<0.03	0.076	>0.5 (2.7)ᵇ	0.92 (1.8)ᵇ
(CH₂)₃N⟨ring⟩N(CH₂)₂OH	—	<0.03	—	0.79 (10.5)ᵇ	20.2 (10.0)ᵇ

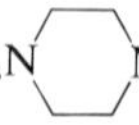

ᵃ Derived from CAR test data in rats; see footnote a, Table 56.2.
ᵇ CI obtained by dividing ED₅₀ (1.9 mg/kg, p.o.) of chlorpromazine in a dog anti-apomorphine test (317) by the ED₅₀ derived for the test compound in the same manner.

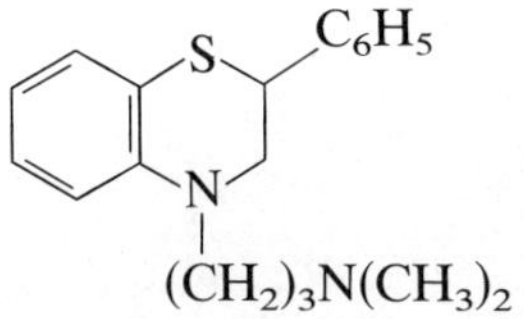

56.73

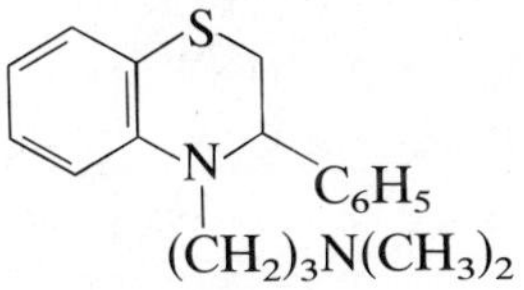

56.74

neuroleptic potency is increased by appropriate substitution of position 2 as follows: $H < Cl < SO_2N(CH_3)_2 < CF_3$. Also, side chain alterations in the two series have the same relative, but not necessarily parallel, order for increasing neuroleptic potency:

$$-(CH_2)_2N(CH_3)_2 < -(CH_2)_3N(CH_3)_2$$
$$\approx -CH_2CH(CH_3)CH_2N(CH_3)_2$$
$$< -(CH_2)_3\overline{NCH_2CH_2N(CH_3)CH_2CH_2}$$
$$< -(CH_2)_3\overline{NCH_2CH_2N(CH_2CH_2OH)CH_2CH_2}.$$

Several other studies have been directed toward phenoxazines having a modified aminoalkyl side chain. The pyrrolidinylpropylphenoxazines 56.**75** are about one-tenth as potent as chlorpromazine after i.p. administration in a CAR test in rats. In a test for prolonging hexobarbital-induced sleeping time in mice, 56.**75a** is as potent as promazine and 56.**75b** is somewhat more effective (318). In neuroleptic tests in rats and mice, all members of a series of piperidinylpropylphenoxazines 56.**76** are uniformly less potent than their phenothiazine

56.75a X = H
56.75b X = C₂H₅

counterparts. Potency of these compounds in a CAR test in rats (s.c.) is generally increased by introducing a 2-acetyl substituent and by substitution of position 4 of the piperidine ring in the following order: 56.**76**, $R = H \approx OC_2H_5 < OCH_3 < OH < (CH_2)_2OH$ (253).

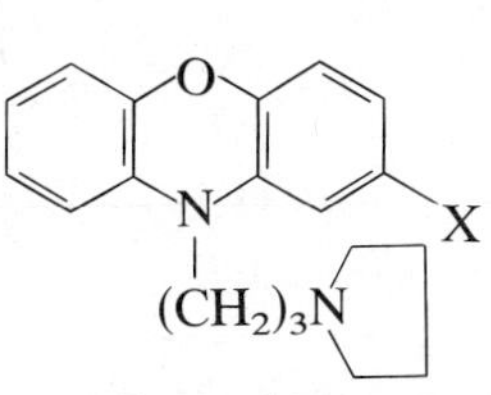

Like their phenothiazine relatives, two phenoxazines, 56.**77a** and 56.**77b**, having a *trans*-2-dimethylaminomethylcyclopropyl substituent in position 10 cause overt antidepressive-like effects in rats. In a test for prevention of reserpine-induced ptosis in rats these phenoxazines are less potent than the corresponding phenothiazines (200).

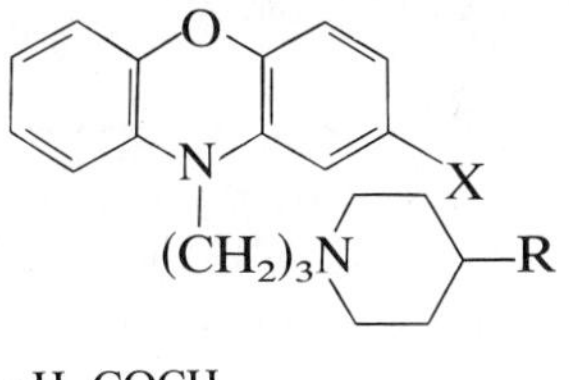

56.76   X = H, COCH₃
         R = H, OH, OCH₃, OC₂H₅, (CH₂)₂OH

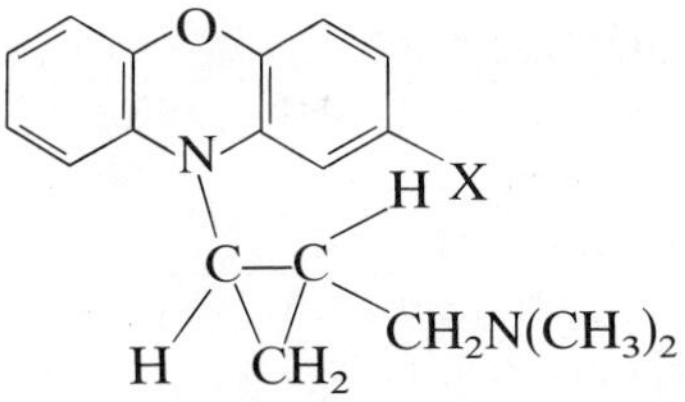

56.77a   X = H
56.77b   X = Cl

4.2.3 PHENOSELENAZINE DERIVATIVES. Although many 10-aminoalkylphenoselenazines have been prepared (288, 319, 320), relatively few pharmacological data (Table 56.6) are available. These data indicate that appropriately substituted phenoselenazines have neuroleptic potency intermediate between their counterparts in the phenothiazine and phenoxazine series. Once again, similar structure–activity relationships are noted. Potency is increased by substitution of position 2, and this increase is greater with a trifluoromethyl substituent than with

Table 56.6 Chlorpromazine Indexes (CI's)^a for Phenoselenazine Derivatives in a Conditioned Escape Response Test in Rats

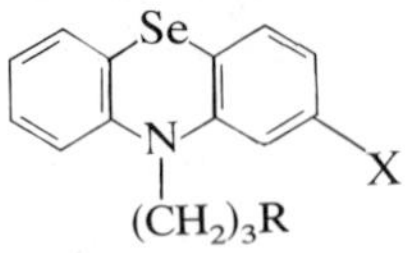

R	X		
	H	Cl	CF$_3$
N(CH$_3$)$_2$	ca. 0.06	0.1	1.2
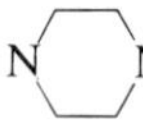 N⬡NCH$_3$	—	1.1	3.0

^{a} See footnote a, Table 56.2.

a chloro substituent. In common with related tricyclics, potency is additionally enhanced by replacing the dimethylamino group of the side chain by an *N*-methylpiperazinyl system.

4.2.4 ACRIDAN DERIVATIVES. Acridan analogs of neuroleptic phenothiazines fall into two categories depending on the position of attachment of the aminopropyl side chain, i.e., to positions 9 or 10 of the tricyclic nucleus. Potency and structure–activity relationships of 10-aminoalkylacridans generally are similar to those of corresponding phenoselenazines. Thus the 10-aminoalkylacridan counterpart 56.**78a** of promazine has a CI<0.03 in a rat CAR test. Potency is enhanced by introduction of appropriate substituents into position 3 of the acridan system, i.e., the position corresponding to the 2 position of a phenothiazine. Again, the chloro derivative 56.**78b** (CI of about 0.1 in a rat CAR) is more potent than the unsubstituted derivative and the trifluoromethyl relative 56.**78c** (CI = 2.1 in the same test) is still more potent. Side chain modification in the 10-acridan series has an effect on neuroleptic potency similar to that seen in the phenothiazine series. Thus the hydroxyethyl-

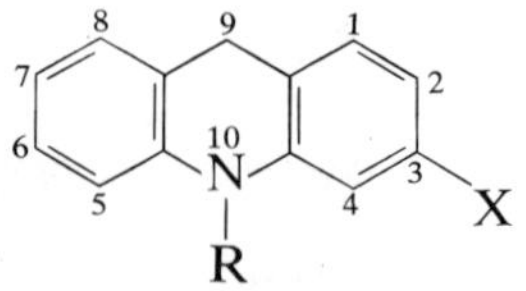

56.**78**

a   X = H, R = (CH$_2$)$_3$N(CH$_3$)$_2$
b   X = Cl, R = (CH$_2$)$_3$N(CH$_3$)$_2$
c   X = CF$_3$, R = (CH$_2$)$_3$N(CH$_3$)$_2$
d   X = H, R = (CH$_2$)$_3$—N◯N—(CH$_2$)$_2$OH
e   X = H, R = *trans*-△—CH$_2$N(CH$_3$)$_2$

piperazinylpropyl derivative 56.**78d** is about 16 times more potent than the corresponding dimethylaminopropyl compound 56.**78a** in a rat CAR test and a *trans*-2-dimethylaminomethylcyclopropyl substituent induces antidepressant-like effects in rats (200).

Substitution of position 9 of 10-aminoalkylacridans significantly decreases or abolishes neuroleptic activity. At 100 mg/kg p.o. in rats the 9-methyl derivative 56.**79a** causes antidepressant-like symptoms, whereas the corresponding 3-trifluoromethyl-substituted relative 56.**79b** causes only mild neuroleptic symptoms. 9,9-Disubstitution, e.g., the 9,9-dimethyl derivative dimethacrin (56.**79c**) (321), has potent antidepressant actions in animals (322) and in man (323). A 3-trifluoromethyl congener 56.**79d** of dimethacrin causes only mild antidepressant-like overt symptoms in rats treated with 100 mg/kg p.o. In a series of 9,9-dimethyl-10-(4,4-disubstituted

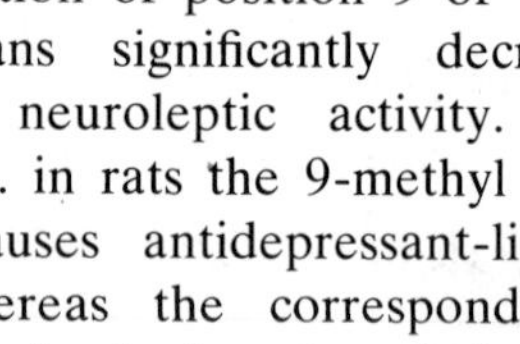

56.**79**

a   X = R = H, R′ = CH$_3$
b   X = CF$_3$, R = H, R′ = CH$_3$
c   X = H, R = R′ = CH$_3$
d   X = CF$_3$, R = R′ = CH$_3$

piperidylpropyl)acridans, the most potent compounds are 56.**80a** and 56.**80b**; however, they do not inhibit fighting behavior and decrease activity in mice only at oral doses of 100–150 mg/kg (251).

Planar 9-aminoalkylacridines, e.g., 56.**8** (see Section 4.2), are devoid of significant CNS effects; however, some related acridans are potent neuroleptic agents (324, 325). In general, the 9-aminopropylacridans are more potent than their 10-substituted isomers. Thus 56.**81a** is considerably more potent than its isomer 56.**78a**. In a mouse rage test the 9 isomer 56.**81a** has a CI of 0.15. As usual with neuroleptic aminoalkylated tricyclics, introduction of

56.**80a** R = CONH$_2$, R' = N⟨⟩

56.**80b** R = H, R' = N⟨⟩NCH$_3$

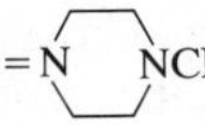

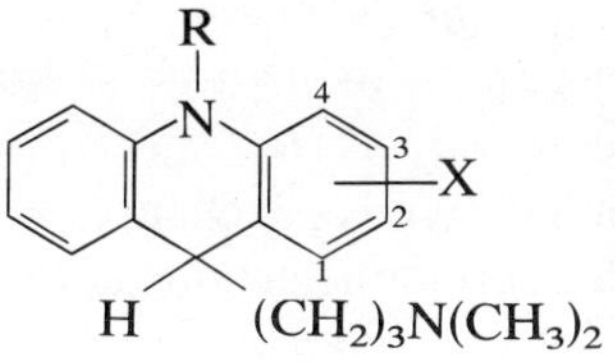

56.**81**

a   X = R = H
b   X = 2-Cl, R = H
c   X = 2-CF$_3$, R = H
d   X = H, R = CH$_3$
e   X = 2-Cl, R = CH$_3$
f   X = 2-CF$_3$, R = CH$_3$
g   X = 2-Cl, R = C$_2$H$_5$
h   X = H, R = CH$_2$CH = CH$_2$
i   X = CF$_3$, R = CH$_2$—▷

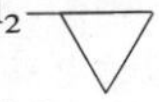

j   X = H, R = CH$_2$C$_6$H$_5$
k   X = 1-Cl, R = CH$_3$
l   X = 4-Cl, R = CH$_3$
m   X = 3-Cl, R = H

appropriate substituents into a position meta to the side chain, i.e., position 2 of 9-(3-aminopropyl)acridans, enhances potency. This is illustrated by the 2-chloro derivative clomacran (56.**81b**), a potent neuroleptic (326), which has a CI of 1.1 in a rat CAR test. Clinical studies indicate clomacran is about equipotent or somewhat more potent than chlorpromazine (327–334). As usual, the trifluoromethyl congener 56.**81c** is even more potent; it has a CI of 5.7 in a rat CAR test.

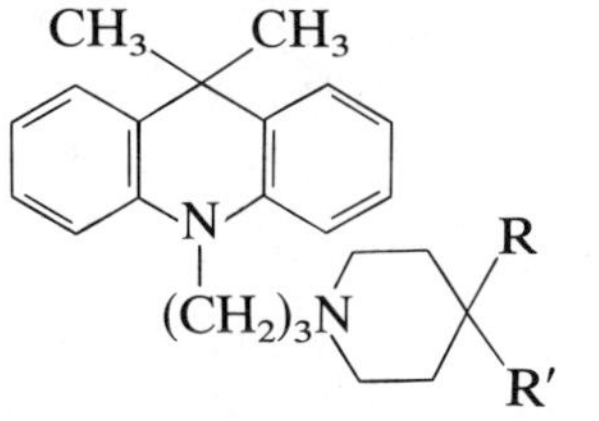

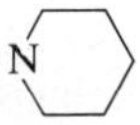

Introduction of 10-alkyl group into 9-aminoalkylacridans has a variable effect on neuroleptic potency. Alkylation of position 10 with a methyl group generally increases potency slightly. In a rat CAR test the 10-methylacridan 56.**81d** has a CI of <0.2, whereas the related 2-chloro-(56.**81e**) and 2-trifluoromethyl-10-methylacridans (56.**81f**) have CI's of about 1.3 and 8.5, respectively. The 2-chloro-10-ethylacridan 56.**81g** (CI = 2.8) is an even more potent neuroleptic than the homologous 10-methyl derivative. Antidepressant-like effects are also noted for 56.**81g**; it prevents reserpine-induced ptosis in rats at 14.4 mg/kg p.o. The 10-allyl derivative 56.**81h** (CI = 3.3) is effective in a test for prevention of mouse rage. In contrast, the 10-cyclopropylmethyl compound 56.**81i** (CI = 0.85), even though it bears a potency-enhancing 2-trifluoromethyl group, is less potent in the mouse test and the 10-benzyl analog 56.**81j** produces only overt symptoms of stimulation in rats treated with an oral dose of 200 mg/kg.

As noted with other 6-6-6 tricyclic antipsychotics, appropriate substitution of position 2 of 9-aminoalkylacridans generally increases potency. Only stimulation is observed in rats treated with oral doses of 100–200 mg/kg of 1-chloro- (56.**81k**) and 4-chloro-10-methyl-9-(3-dimethylaminopropyl)acridans (56.**81l**). A 3-chloroacridan (56.**81m**) produces no overt symptoms in rats given 50 mg/kg p.o.; however, higher doses produce ataxia and depression.

The influence on neuroleptic potency of modification of the 9-aminoalkyl side chain of acridans is somewhat different from that noted with many other tricyclic systems, e.g., phenothiazines and phenoxazines. In this series, methylpiperazinylpropyl substitution does not increase neuroleptic potency. Thus in a mouse rage test 56.**82a**–56.**82c** are significantly less potent than their dimethylaminopropyl analogs.

Introduction of an additional substituent, e.g., methyl (56.**83a**) or hydroxyl (56.**83b**), into position 9 of 9-(3-dimethylaminopropyl)acridans drastically decreases overt CNS-depressant properties in rats.

Some 2-substituted 9-(3-dimethylaminopropylidene)acridans, e.g., 56.**84a**, are potent neuroleptics (324, 335). This activity, as noted in other series of aminoalkylidene-substituted tricyclics, is associated almost exclusively with the isomers in which the side chain is oriented toward the substituted ring of the tricycle. In rats, an oral dose of 10 mg/kg of Z-56.**84a** decreases motor activity and causes ptosis and a characteristic hind limb spread. In contrast, the same dose of the E isomer increases motor activity and produces overt signs of

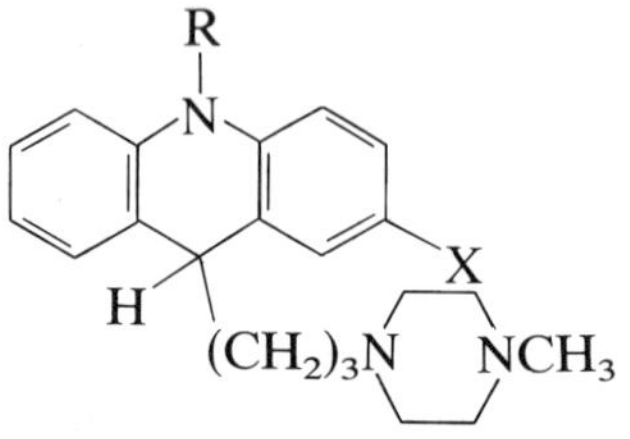

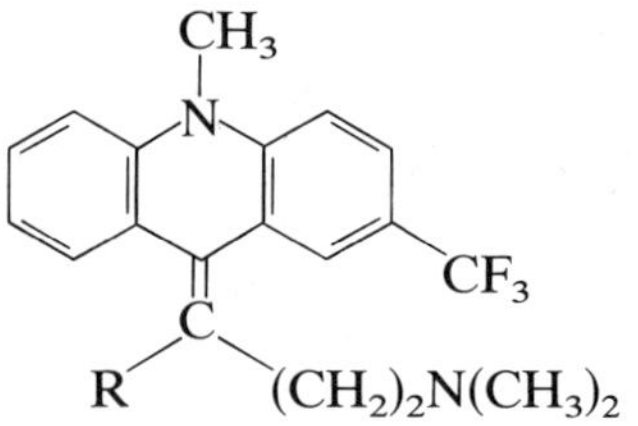

56.**84a**   R = H
56.**84b**   R = CH$_3$

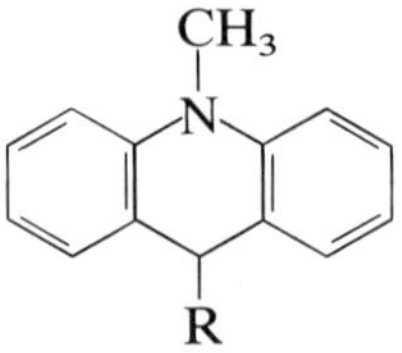

56.**85a**   R =

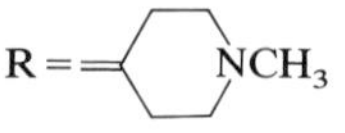

56.**85b**   R =

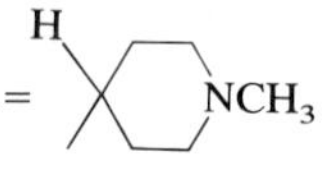

stimulation. Neither of the geometric isomers of the methyl-substituted olefin 56.**84b** causes overt neuroleptic effects in rats. Only mydriasis and exophthalmia are observed after administration of 25 mg/kg p.o. Several 9-(N-methyl-4-piperidylidene)-substituted acridans cause potent neuroleptic effects (336). For example, 56.**85a** has a CI of 8.3 in a ptosis-production test in rats (316). The corresponding piperidine derivative 56.**85b**, however, fails to cause neuroleptic actions at doses below 100 mg/kg p.o. (336).

4.2.5   PHENOTHIAPHOSPHINE   DERIVATIVES. Relatives of phenothiazine antipsychotics in which the ring nitrogen is replaced by phosphorus, e.g., 56.**86**, only weakly depress motor activity in mice at 30 mg/kg, i.p., that is, at about 30 times the dose required for promazine. An uncyclized analog 56.**87**, however, depresses motor activity of mice by 89% after a dose of 10 mg/kg i.p. (337).

4.2.6   THIOXANTHENE   DERIVATIVES.   In general, structure versus neuropharmacological activity studies suggest that the 9-

56.**82a**   X = R = H
56.**82b**   X = Cl, R = H
56.**82c**   X = H, R = CH$_3$

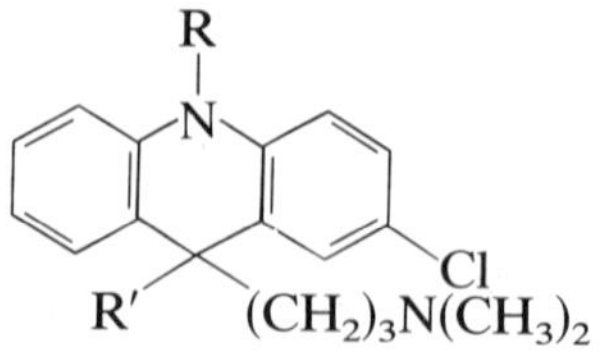

56.**83a**   R = H, R′ = CH$_3$
56.**83b**   R = CH$_3$, R′ = OH

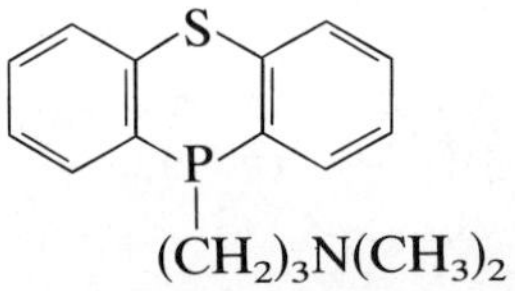

(CH$_2$)$_3$N(CH$_3$)$_2$

56.**86**

(CH$_2$)$_3$N(CH$_3$)$_2$

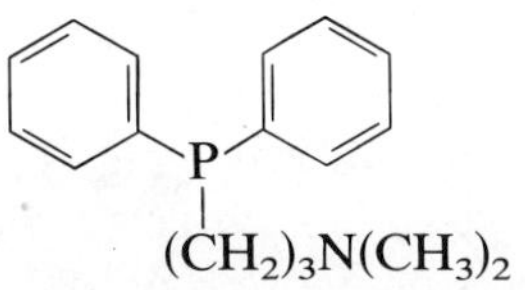

56.**87**

aminoalkylated thioxanthenes closely parallel their phenothiazine counterparts, although the thioxanthenes are usually less potent. For example, substitution of position 2 increases neuroleptic potency in both series in a similar fashion. Thus 9-(3-dimethylaminopropyl)thioxanthene (56.**88a**) has a CI of less than 0.03 in a rat CAR test. The 2-chloro analog 56.**88b** is only weakly depressant in mice and rats; however, the 2-methylthio derivative 56.**88c** is somewhat more potent (CI = 0.4) and the 2-trifluoromethyl derivative 56.**88d** is significantly more potent (CI *ca.* 1). As in the phenothiazine series, introduction of a methylpiperazinylpropyl side chain increases potency even more. Thus 56.**88e** has a CI of *ca.* 1.1 in a rat CAR test (175). A related 2-sulfonamide 56.**88f** blocks CAR in rats at a dose of 1 mg/kg i.p. and antagonizes apomorphine-induced emesis in dogs at 0.05 mg/kg i.v. Unlike its phenothiazine counterpart thioproperazine (Table 56.1), however, 56.**88f** does not cause tremors or

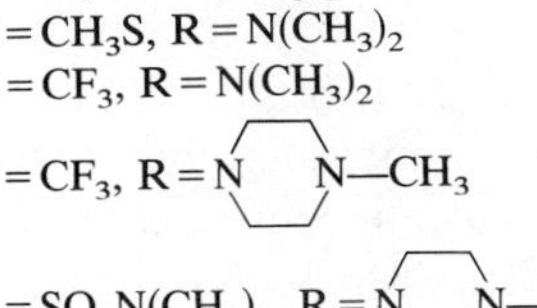

56.**88**

a   X = H, R = N(CH$_3$)$_2$

b   X = Cl, R = N(CH$_3$)$_2$

c   X = CH$_3$S, R = N(CH$_3$)$_2$

d   X = CF$_3$, R = N(CH$_3$)$_2$

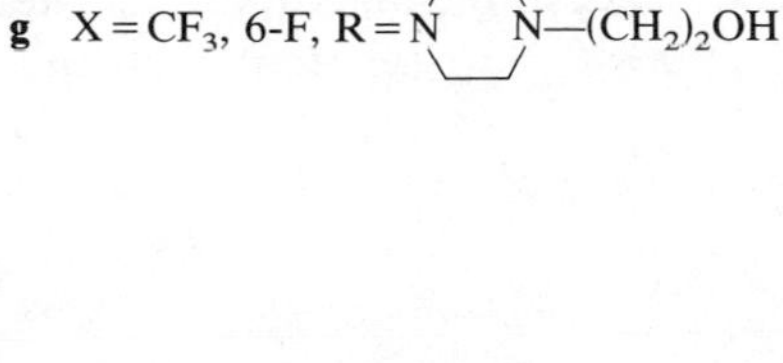

e   X = CF$_3$, R = N   N—CH$_3$

f   X = SO$_2$N(CH$_3$)$_2$, R = N   N—CH$_3$

g   X = CF$_3$, 6-F, R = N   N—(CH$_2$)$_2$OH

catalepsy in monkeys treated with 25 mg/kg p.o. for 6 days (338).

A 2,6-disubstituted thioxanthene bearing a 9-hydroxyethylpiperazinylpropyl side chain 56.**88g** resembles fluphenazine (Table 56.1) in its ability to increase the disappearance of [^{14}C]-dopamine in mouse brain, and its effects seem to be long lasting (339).

As in the case of 9-aminoalkylacridans, additional substitution of the 9 position of 9-aminoalkylthioxanthenes essentially abolishes neuroleptic activity. These effects are not observed in rats treated with 182 mg/kg p.o. of the 9-methyl derivatives 56.**89a** and 56.**89b** (175), and the 9-hydroxyl derivative 56.**89c** causes only a slight decrease in spontaneous motor activity of mice after i.p. administration (340).

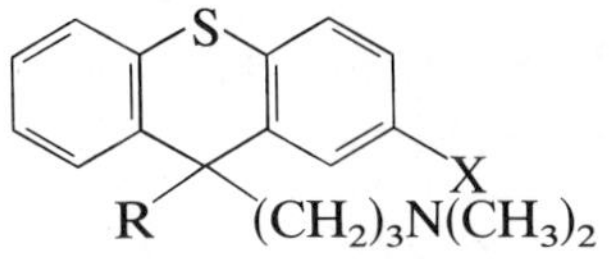

56.**89a**   X = H, R = CH$_3$

56.**89b**   X = CF$_3$, R = CH$_3$

56.**89c**   X = Cl, R = OH

Structure–activity relationships for 9-(3-aminopropylidene)-substituted thioxanthenes (thioxanthene-$\Delta^{9,\gamma}$-propylamines) are very similar to those for other 6–6–6 tricyclic antipsychotics. These compounds are usually more potent than their saturated relatives (175, 341–345). When the thioxanthene system is asymmetrically substituted these compounds exist as geometric isomers. In all instances, the neuroleptic potency of the *Z* (cisoid; i.e., with the aminoalkyl chain on the same side of the double bond as the substituted ring) isomer (344, 346–349) is 5–40 times that for the *E* isomer. As in the phenothiazine series, 2-substitution has a marked influence on neuroleptic potency, i.e., H < Cl < CF$_3$. 9 - (3 - Dimethylaminopropylidene)thioxanthene (prothixene, 56.**90a**) does not produce ptosis in rats given at a dose of 22

56.**90**

a   X = H, R = N(CH$_3$)$_2$
b   X = Cl, R = N(CH$_3$)$_2$
c   X = CF$_3$, R = N(CH$_3$)$_2$
d   X = OH, R = N(CH$_3$)$_2$
e   X = CH$_3$, R = N(CH$_3$)$_2$
f   X = i-C$_3$H$_7$, R = N(CH$_3$)$_2$
g   X = n-C$_5$H$_{11}$, R = N(CH$_3$)$_2$
h   X = C$_6$H$_5$CH$_2$O, R = N(CH$_3$)$_2$
i   X = Br, R = N(CH$_3$)$_2$
j   X = CH$_3$O, R = N(CH$_3$)$_2$
k   X = Cl, 6-F, R = N(CH$_3$)$_2$

l   X = SO$_2$N(CH$_3$)$_2$, R = N⎯N—CH$_3$

m   X = Cl, R = N⎯N—(CH$_2$)$_2$OH

n   X = CF$_3$, R = N⎯N—(CH$_2$)$_2$OH

o   X = CF$_3$, 6-F, R = N⎯N—(CH$_2$)$_2$OH

p   X = CF$_3$, R = N⎯N—(CH$_2$)$_2$OH

q   X = CF$_3$, 6-F, R = N⎯(CH$_2$)$_2$OH

mg/kg p.o. On oral administration in a rat CAR test, the Z isomer 56.**90b** (chlorprothixene) has a CI of 2.3 (175). Both compounds are effective in the treatment of schizophrenia (350–352). In contrast, the E isomers of 56.**90b** and 56.**90c** have low CI values of <0.2 and ca. 0.14, respectively. Generally, the nature of the 2 substituent of 9-(3-dimethylaminopropylidene)thioxanthenes influences neuroleptic potency in a manner very similar to that observed in the phenothiazine series (see Table 56.4). For example, the 2-hydroxyl derivative Z-56.**90d** is 100 times less potent than chlorprothixene upon i.p. administration to mice in a rotating-rod test (353). In the same test 2-alkyl derivatives, e.g., 56.**90e** and 56.**90f**, are nearly equipotent with chlorpromazine, whereas the E isomers are almost inactive.

The Z isomers of compounds having large 2-alkyl substituents, e.g., 56.**90g**, are inactive at 5 mg/kg i.v. (354). The benzyloxy derivative 56.**90h** causes CNS depression in rats at only high doses (300–500 mg/kg p.o.) (353). After i.p. administration to mice, the Z-2-bromo 56.**90i** and 2-methoxy 56.**90j** derivatives reduce spontaneous motor activity. They have CI values of 0.1–0.3, respectively. It is noteworthy that the 6-fluoro derivative 56.**90k** of chlorprothixene is about twice as potent as chlorprothixene in a cataleptic test in rats (355); however, the 6,7-difluoro derivative lacks significant neuroleptic actions in mice and rats (356). The 1-, 3-, and 4-halo- and trifluoromethylthioxanthene - $\Delta^{9,\gamma}$ - propyl - amines are significantly less potent than their 2 isomers (342).

Many side chain-modified aminopropylidene derivatives of thioxanthene have been studied (175, 342, 345); however, only a few 2-substituted isomeric pairs have been separated. In studies of purified Z isomers, side chain modification affects neuroleptic potency of thioxanthenes in much the same way that it influences phenothiazines. For example, thiothixene (56.**90l**) is approximately equipotent with its phenothiazine counterpart, thioproperazine (Table 56.1), as a neuroleptic (171, 338, 341, 342, 357). Thiothixene is effective in treating schizophrenia (358–361). The hydroxyethylpiperazine clopenthixol (56.**90m**), likewise has potency comparable to that of its phenothiazine relative, perphenazine (Table 56.1), in CAR tests in dogs and rats (362, 363) and is a clinically effective antipsychotic (364). The corresponding trifluoromethyl derivative 56.**90n** (flupentixol) is also a clinically effective antipsychotic (364, 365); it is four to eight times more potent than chlorprothixene in animal tests for neuroleptic activity (366). Flupentixol enanthate is useful in antipsychotic maintenance therapy (265). A 6-fluoro derivative of flupentixol, i.e., teflutixol (56.**90o**), is more potent than the par-

ent in blocking apomorphine- and amphetamine-induced stereotypy and in inducing
catalepsy. It is the most potent blocker
known for dopamine-sensitive adenylate
cyclase of striatum ($IC_{50} = 9.7 \times 19^{-10}$ M).
It increases dopamine turnover and ele-
vates HVA and DOPAC in rodent brain
(367, 368). The most potent member of
another series of amine-modified thioxanthenes having a propylidene bridge is
56.**90p**; its potency is similar to that of
chlorpromazine in blocking CAR in rats
and decreasing motor activity in mice
(345). Piflutixol (56.**90q**) is a 4-(2-hydroxy-
ethyl)piperidine relative of teflutixol
(56.**90o**).

9-(3-Dimethylaminopropyl)-1-azathio-
xanthene (56.**91**) is claimed to have only
spasmolytic and analgetic activity (369);
however, an aminopropylidene derivative,
the 1-azathioxanthene 56.**92** (370), and
several 4-aza derivatives, e.g., 56.**93** (371),
are claimed to have neuroleptic, antidepressant, and antiserotonin activity.

Appropriately substituted piperidylidene
derivatives of thioxanthenes (372) are potent neuroleptics (336). In some instances
these substances, in which the spatial relationship between the basic nitrogen and the

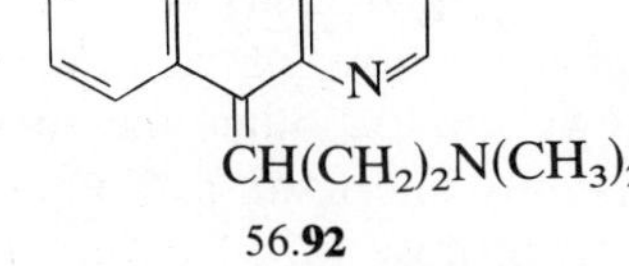

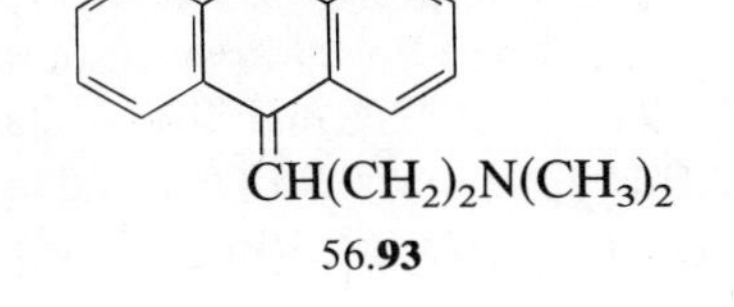

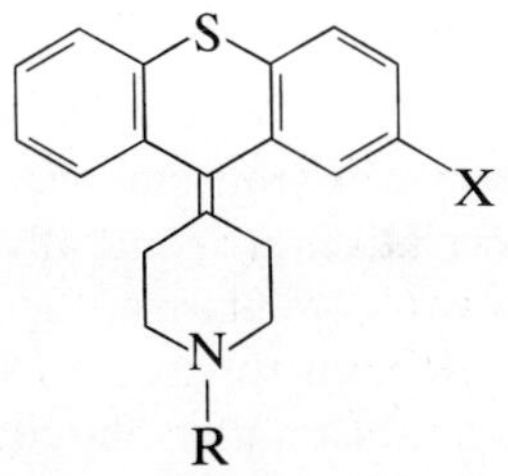

56.**94a**   X = Cl, R = CH$_3$
56.**94b**   X = CF$_3$, R = CH$_3$
56.**94c**   X = CF$_3$, R = CH$_2$—

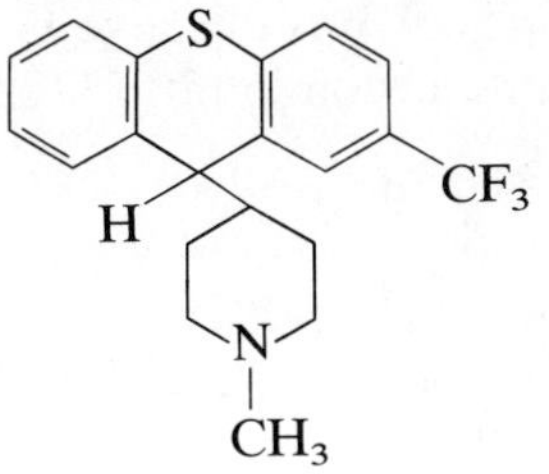

56.**95**

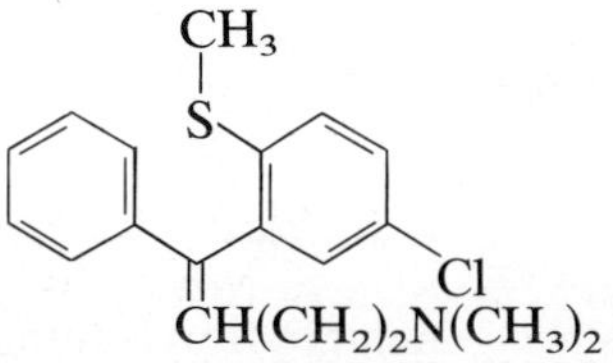

56.**96**

56.**91**

56.**92**

56.**93**

tricyclic system is more restricted than in
the case of more flexible side chains, are even
more potent than their Z-dimethylamino-
propylidene counterparts. For example, 2-
chloro (56.**94a**) and 2-trifluoromethyl
(56.**94b**) derivatives have CI values of 1.0
and 7.4, respectively, in a rat ptosis-
production test. Alteration of the piperidylidene nitrogen substituent may also enhance potency; e.g., the cyclobutylmethyl
derivative 56.**94c** has a CI of 16.8 in the
same test (336). Potential antipsychotic activity without EPS effects is claimed for
several of these compounds and some 1,2-
benzo-fused relatives (373–375). As is usually the case, reduction of the side chain
olefin, e.g., 56.**95**, significantly decreases
neuroleptic efficacy in rats (336).

Several ring-opened analogs, e.g., 56.**96**,
of chlorprothixene cause only mild depres-

sant, antihistaminic, and spasmolytic actions (376).

4.2.7 SELENOXANTHENE DERIVATIVES. Selenoxanthene derivatives are generally less potent than their neuroleptic thioxanthene counterparts. The selenium relative 56.**97a** of prothixene has antihistaminic activity in guinea pigs. The Z-2-chloro derivative 56.**97b** is less than one-half as potent as chlorprothixene in a mouse rotating-rod test and E-56.**97b** is even less effective. Neither 56.**97a** nor 56.**97b** is effective in a test for catalepsy production in rats (377).

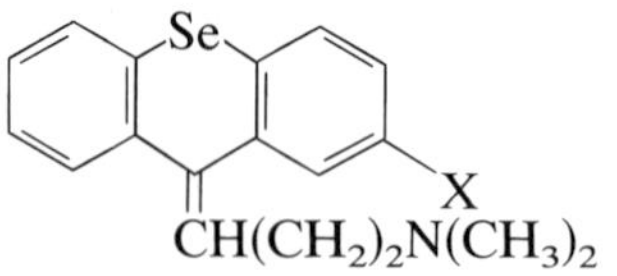

56.**97a**   X = H
56.**97b**   X = Cl

4.2.8 XANTHENE DERIVATIVES. In general, structure versus neuroleptic activity relationships are similar for xanthene and thioxanthene derivatives. As in the thioxanthene series, 9-aminopropylxanthenes are usually less potent than their olefinic xanthene-$\Delta^{9,\gamma}$-propylamine relatives; however, by introduction of proper 2 substituents and basic side chains potent neuroleptic 9-aminopropylxanthenes may be obtained. As in other series of antipsychotic 6–6–6 compounds, the unsubstituted compound 56.**98a** (CI < 0.04 in a rat CAR test) is only weakly active, the 2-chloro

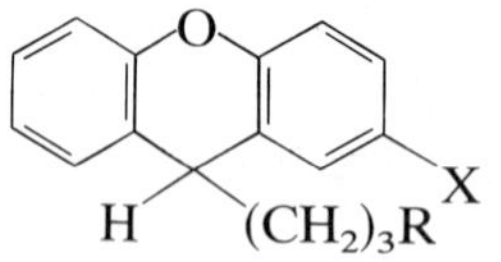

56.**98**

a   X = H, R = N(CH$_3$)$_2$
b   X = Cl, R = N(CH$_3$)$_2$
c   X = CF$_3$, R = N(CH$_3$)$_2$

d   X = CF$_3$, R = N⟍＿⟋N—CH$_3$

e   X = CF$_3$, R = N⟍＿⟋N—(CH$_2$)$_2$OH

derivative 56.**98b** (CI *ca.* 0.035) is marginally more effective, and the 2-trifluoromethyl derivative 56.**98c** (CI = 1.5) is decidedly more potent (175). In a clinical study, however, the latter compound had antidepressant actions (387). As in the corresponding acridan series, replacement of the dimethylamino group with a methylpiperazinyl moiety reduces neuroleptic potency; e.g., 56.**98d** has a CI of 0.5 in a rat CAR test. The hydroxyethylpiperazine 56.**98e** is somewhat more potent (CI = 2.2) (175).

Among xanthene-$\Delta^{9,\gamma}$-propylamines, as in related tricyclic series, neuroleptic activity of unsymmetrical derivatives is found predominantly in the Z isomers. Thus the Z isomer (349) of 2-chloro-N,N-dimethylxanthene-$\Delta^{9,\gamma}$-propylamine (56.**99a**) causes neuroleptic actions on oral administration of 5–50 mg/kg to rats whereas E-56.**99a** does not produce these effects even at 200 mg/kg p.o. Similarly, the Z-2-trifluoromethyl derivative 56.**99b** (349) has a CI of 1.3 in a rat CAR test, whereas E-56.**99b** causes no response at 23 mg/kg p.o. (336). One of the isomers (presumably Z) of the 2-methoxyxanthene 56.**99c** (dimeprozan) is equipotent with chlorpromazine in

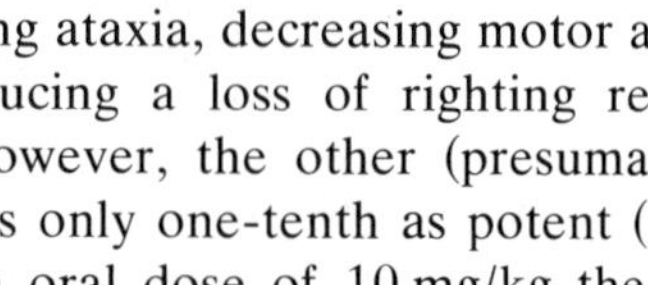

56.**99a**   X = Cl
56.**99b**   X = CF$_3$
56.**99c**   X = OCH$_3$

producing ataxia, decreasing motor activity, and inducing a loss of righting reflex in mice; however, the other (presumably E) isomer is only one-tenth as potent (171).

At an oral dose of 10 mg/kg the piperidylidene-substituted xanthene 56.**100a** produces overt neuroleptic-like symptoms in rats (175). Potential antipsychotic activity with decreased EPS liability is claimed for 56.**100b** (clopipazan) (373) and a 1,2-benzo-fused relative, 56.**100c** (375).

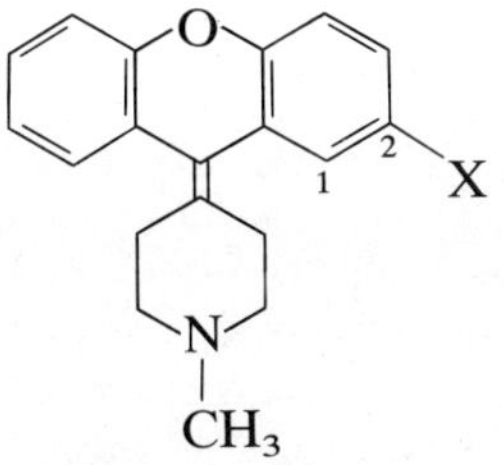

56.**100a**   X = CF₃
56.**100b**   X = Cl
56.**100c**   X = 1,2-(CH=CH)₂

4.2.9   ANTHRACENE AND DIHYDROANTHRACENE DERIVATIVES. Aminoalkyl derivatives of anthracene, e.g., 56.**9** (X = H) (379), including those with a substituent 56.**9** (X = Cl, CF₃) in position 2, cause only weak CNS effects. The corresponding 9,10-dihydroanthracenes (380), however, may be very potent neuroleptics. For example, in a test for production of ptosis in rats the 2-chloro derivative 56.**101a** has a CI of about 0.3, and the related trifluoromethyl compound 56.**101b** has a CI of 1.5 in a rat CAR test. Although the *cis*-10-methyl derivative 56.**101c** (fluotracen) has significantly less neuroleptic potency than 56.**101b**, it still retains a high degree of activity and in addition it displays striking antidepressive actions both in animals (381) and humans (382) (see Chapter 58). In mice, fluotracen shows much greater antidepressant activity than related 10,10-dimethyl-substituted compounds, e.g., 56.**101d** and 56.**101e** (383).

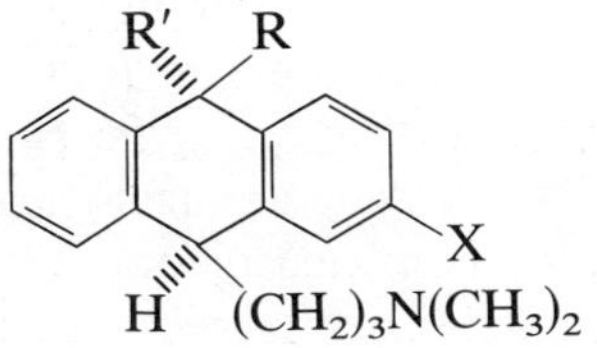

56.**101**

a   X = Cl, R = R′ = H
b   X = CF₃, R = R′ = H
c   X = CF₃, R = CH₃, R′ = H
d   X = H, R = R′ = CH₃
e   X = CF₃, R = R′ = CH₃

Several 9-aminoalkylated 9,10-ethano-bridged dihydroanthracenes (384, 385) have antihistaminic and neuropharmacological actions. The aminomethyl derivative 56.**102a**, benzoctamine (386), inhibits aggression in mice (387) and is a clinical anxiolytic equivalent to diazepam (388); however, it lacks antipsychotic activity (389, 390). Maprotiline, the aminopropyl homolog 56.**102b**, causes antidepressant effects in dogs (391) and inhibits synaptosomal uptake of norepinephrine (392).

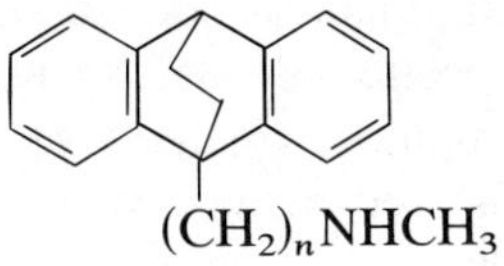

56.**102a**   *n* = 1
56.**102b**   *n* = 3

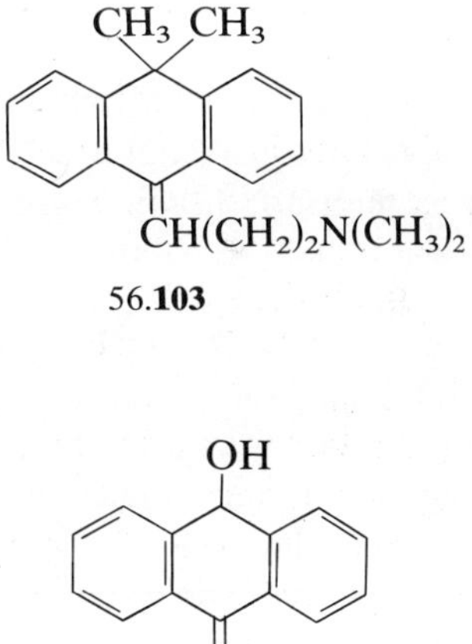

56.**103**

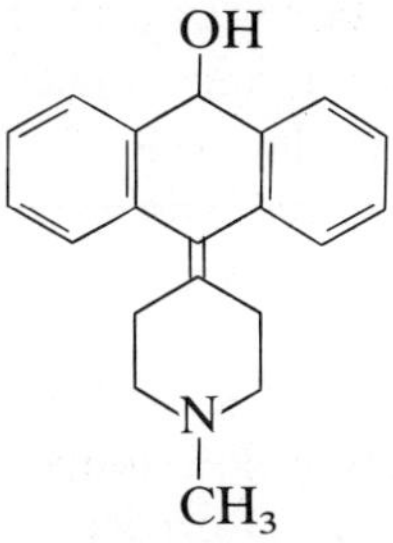

56.**104**

Some aminoalkylated dihydroanthracenes having a double bond at position 9, e.g., melitracene (56.**103**) (393) and danitracen (56.**104**) (394), have potent and clinically useful antidepressant activity (see Chapter 58).

4.3 Tricyclic Antipsychotic Agents with a Central Seven-Membered Ring (6–7–6 Compounds)

Many aminoalkylated 6–7–6 compounds have predominantly antidepressive actions and are discussed in Chapter 58. During the past 10 years, however, this class of compounds has been the subject of considerable antipsychotic investigation.

4.3.1 DIBENZ[b,e]OXEPINS AND RELATED COMPOUNDS. A series of Z- and E-amino-propylidenedibenz[b,e]oxepins 56.**105**, i.e., with the aminoalkyl side chain on the same or opposite side as the heteroatom, provide striking evidence of the importance of stereochemical factors in determining neuroleptic activity (395). 11-Aminopropylidene derivatives of dibenzoxepin lacking a substituent on a benzenoid ring, e.g., 56.**105** (X = H, doxepin), are predominantly antidepressant with concomitant anticholinergic and central effects (396). In the Z series, introduction of a 2 substituent results in compounds with significantly greater CNS-depressant potency than that of related E isomers. Among a number of 2-substituted Z isomers 56.**105** [X = Cl, CF_3, CH_3O, CH_3S, CH_3CO, $(CH_3)_2NSO_2$] maximum potency in a CAR test in rats is noted for the 2-chloro derivative, which is pharmacologically identical with chlorpromazine (395). Alteration of the aminoalkyl side chain also influences potency. The hydroxyethylpiperazinyl derivative pinoxepin (56.**106**) is effective at low doses in a rat CAR test, presents a pharmacological profile similar to that of its phenothiazine counterpart perphenazine

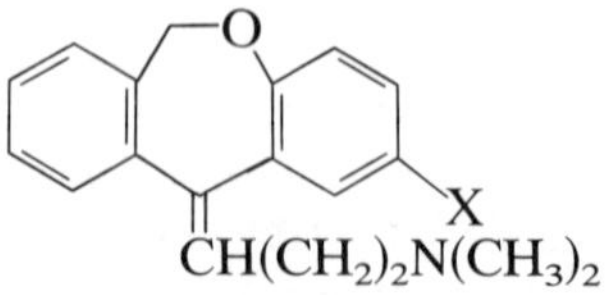

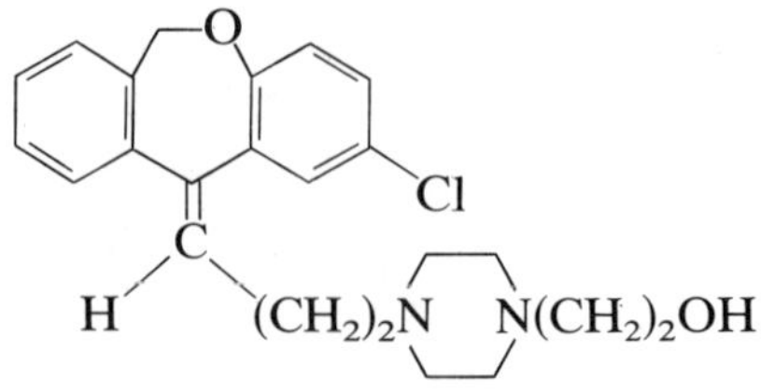

56.**106**

(Table 56.1), and is a potent antipsychotic-sedative in the clinic (397, 398). In contrast, the E isomer is devoid of CNS-depressant activity at the doses studied (395).

Additional evidence of the importance of the stereochemical relationship of the nuclear substituent to the side chain is provided by two series of geometric isomers with chlorine and methoxy groups in positions 2 and 9 (Table 56.7). Potency is maximal when both the heteroatom and ring substituent have a Z orientation. It appears that the relationship of the side chain to the nuclear substituent is of greater importance than its relationship to the nuclear heteroatom.

Several aminopropylidene-substituted tricyclic systems related to the dibenz[b,e]-oxepins, e.g., 56.**107a** (399–401), 56.**107b** (402, 403), 56.**107c** (404, 405), 56.**107d** (406), 56.**107e** (167), and 56.**108a** (407), cause mainly antidepressant-like effects. In several tests for neuroleptic activity, one of the geometric isomers (presumably Z) of 2-substituted derivatives 56.**108b** and 56.**108c** is significantly more potent (407). Generally, dibenzocycloheptatrienes, e.g., 56.**108c**, are more potent neuroleptics than their reduced analogs, e.g., 56.**108b** (399–401, 407, 408). A pharmacological profile suggestive of both neuroleptic and antidepressant actions is observed with the Z-2-methylsulfonyl derivative 56.**108d** (232). Clinically, 56.**108d** causes weak antipsychotic and antianxiety effects (409, 410). A related chloro-substituted morphanthridine 56.**108e** is moderately effective in schizophrenic patients (411–413).

56.**105**

X = H, Cl, CF_3, OCH_3, SCH_3, $COCH_3$, $SO_2N(CH_3)_2$

Table 56.7 Chlorpromazine Indexes (CI's)[a] for 2- and 9-Substituted *E*- and *Z*-Dimethylaminopropylidenedibenz[*b,e*]-oxepins (395)

X	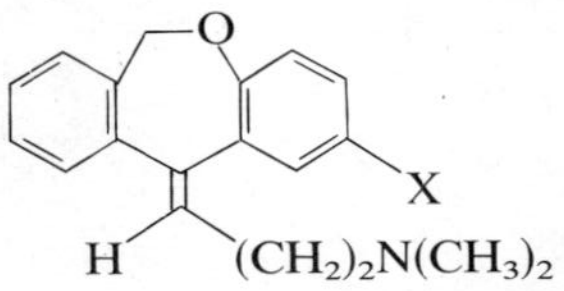 (CH$_2$)$_2$N(CH$_3$)$_2$	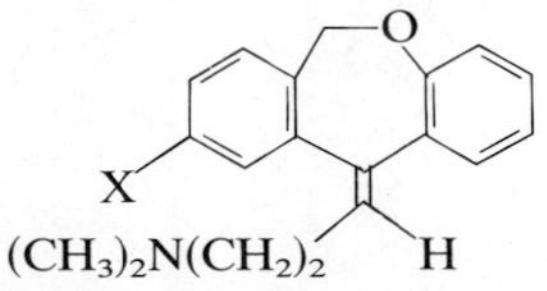 (CH$_3$)$_2$N(CH$_2$)$_2$	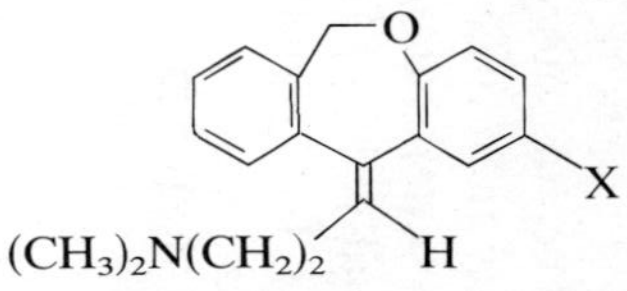 (CH$_3$)$_2$N(CH$_2$)$_2$	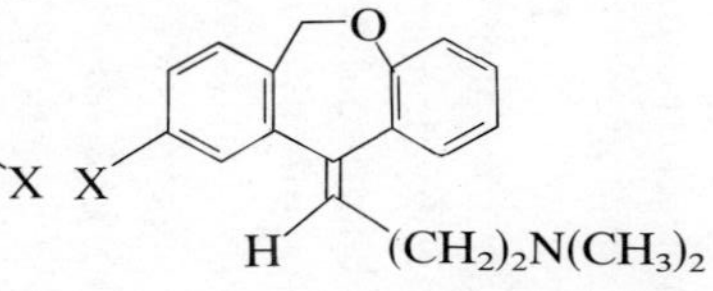 (CH$_2$)$_2$N(CH$_3$)$_2$
Cl	1.0[a]	0.27	0.10	<0.10
CH$_3$O	0.45	0.20	0.10	<0.10

[a] CI's were determined by dividing the ED$_{50}$ (4 mg/kg) in a rat CAR test for the *Z*-2-chloro derivative (equipotent with chlorpromazine) by the similarly derived value for the test compound.

901

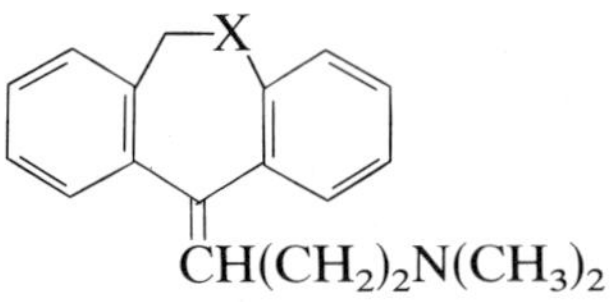

56.**107**

a X = CH$_2$
b X = S
c X = SO$_2$
d X = NH
e X = NCH$_2$

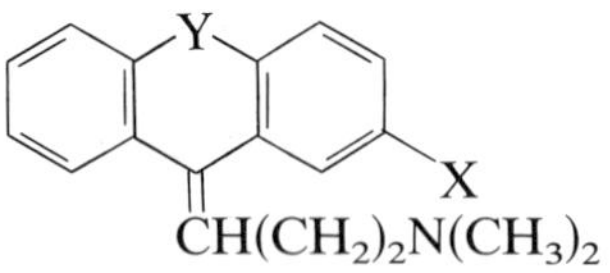

56.**108**

a X = H, Y = CH = CH
b X = Cl, Y = (CH$_2$)$_2$
c X = Cl, Y = CH = CH
d X = SO$_2$CH$_3$, Y = CH = CH
e X = Cl, Y = CH = N

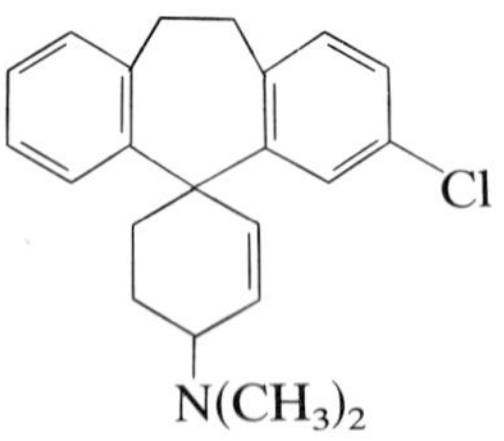

56.**109**

A spiro dibenzocycloheptadiene 56.**109** also displays stereospecificity. Although the stereochemistry has not been defined, only one of the diastereomers of 56.**109** (414) antagonizes apomorphine-induced stereotypy in rats, suggesting strict stereochemical requirements for potent and selective blockers of dopamine receptors (415). A striking example of stereoselectivity for antipsychotic activity is displayed by atropisomers of the piperidylidene-substituted dibenzocycloheptatrienes 56.**110a** and 56.**110b**. Although the absolute configurations of the isomers have not been determined, only (−)-56.**110a** and (−)-56.**110b** block CAR in squirrel monkeys (416, 417). CAR blocking activity is also noted with

(−)-56.**110c**, but not with the (+) atropisomer (418).

Aminopropylidene-substituted thienyl isoteres of the dibenzo[b,e]thiepin system, e.g., dithiaden (56.**111a**) and its 6-chloro derivative 56.**111b**, have significant neuroleptic activity (419). Unfortunately, the stereochemistry, which is so important in 11-aminoalkylated derivatives of dibenzoxepin and related compounds, is not reported for these substances.

The isomeric thienyl analogs, 56.**111c** and 56.**112**, of amitriptyline have different pharmacological properties. For example, 56.**111c** has more potent CNS-depressant activity than 56.**112**, whereas the latter has more potent antidepressant activity (420). Clinically, 56.**111c** produces antianxiety effects (421) and is useful in treating the manic phases of manic-depressive psychoses (422). The piperidylidene derivative

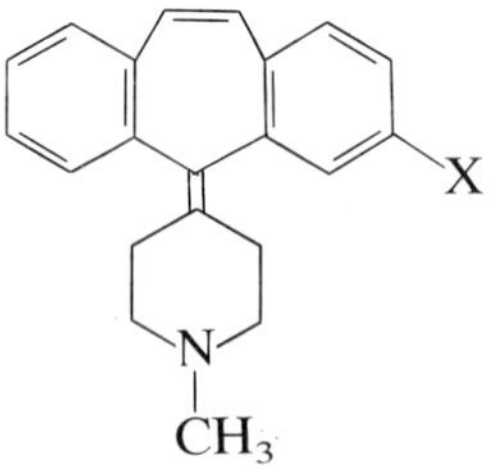

56.**110**

a X = SCF$_3$, R = CH$_3$
b X = SCF$_3$, R = CH$_2$⊲
c X = CN, R = CH$_3$

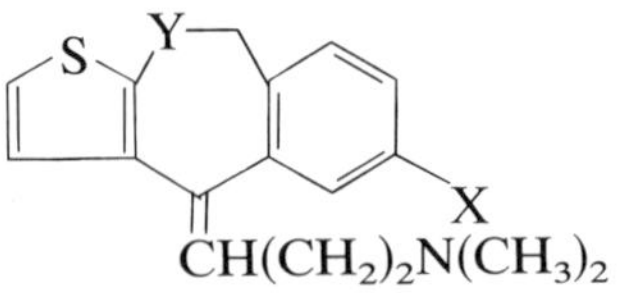

56.**111a**   X = H, Y = S
56.**111b**   X = Cl, Y = S
56.**111c**   X = H, Y = CH$_2$

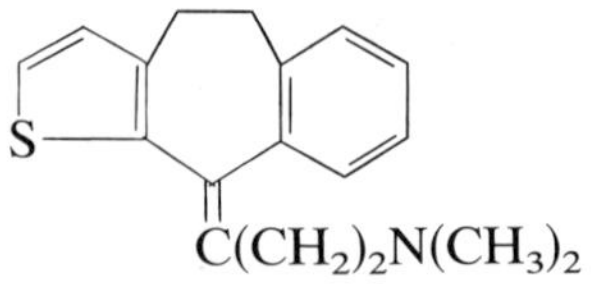

56.**112**

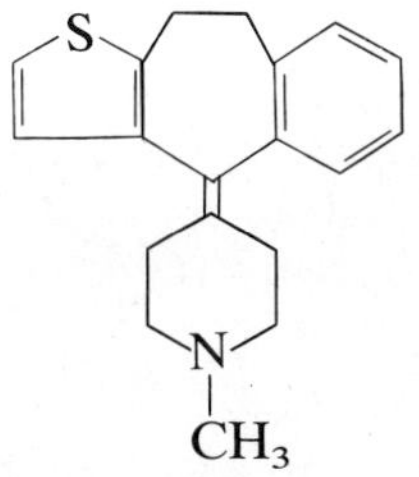

56.**113**

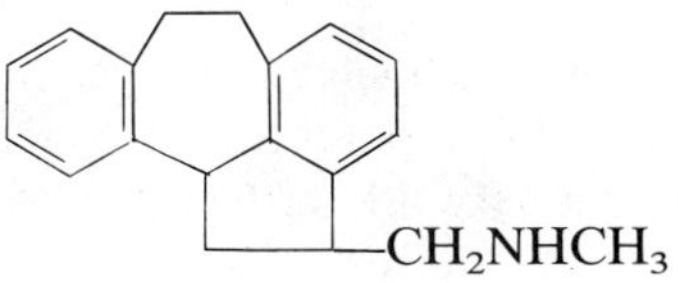

56.**114**

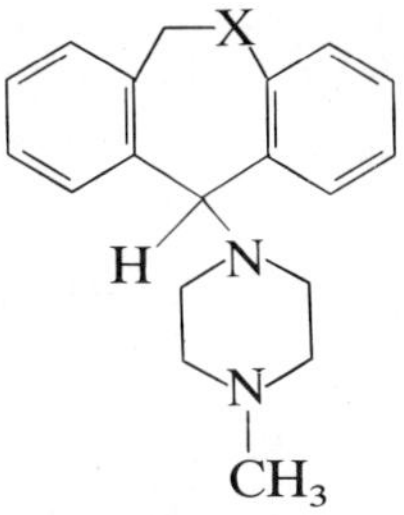

56.**115a** X = S
56.**115b** X = O
56.**115c** X = SO$_2$

56.**113** related to 56.**111c** produces sedation (423) and is effective in depressed schizophrenics (424).

In a series of bridged amitriptyline derivatives, both Z- and E-56.**114** produce CNS effects in a hexobarbital sleep reinduction test in mice (425).

An N-methylpiperazinyldibenzo[b,e]-thiepin, perazothin (56.**115a**), causes both antidepressant and CNS-depressant actions in animals (167, 426). Similar but less potent effects are noted for the oxygen isostere perazoxin (56.**115b**) (427); however, the sulfone 56.**115c** is practically inactive (405).

4.3.2 DIBENZ[b,e][1,4]OXAZEPINES AND RELATED COMPOUNDS. Many antipsychotics are 6–7–6 compounds in which the aminoalkyl side chain is attached to a nitrogen

atom that bridges the two outer rings. Illustrative of this class of compounds is a series 56.**116** of 5-aminoalkyl-5,11-dihydrodibenz[b,e][1,4]oxazepines and thiazepines that produce neuroleptic actions in several pharmacological tests (428). In both these series, irrespective of nuclear substitution, a 5-(3-dimethylaminopropyl) side chain affords compounds with only CNS-stimulant properties at relatively high doses (429). Dibenz[b,e][1,4]oxazepines bearing a hydroxyethylpiperazinylpropyl group in position 5 and a substituent, e.g., chloro or trifluoromethyl, in position 7 (e.g., 56.**116a**) or 3 (e.g., 56.**116b**) have antianxiety activity at low doses and potent neuroleptic activity at higher doses. Thus 56.**116a** and 56.**116b** are about three to four times as potent as chlordiazepoxide or chlorpromazine in a conflict behavior test in rats. Both compounds are effective in a rat CAR test at 0.5–1.0 mg/kg i.p., whereas chlorpromazine is not effective at these doses. In addition, both compounds are equivalent to, or more potent than, chlorpromazine in tests for decreasing motor activity and disrupting CAR in rats. In a rat muricide test 56.**116a** and 56.**116b** are more potent than the antianxiety agent chlordiazepoxide, but less effective than neuroleptics chlorpromazine and thioridazine or the antidepressant imipramine.

The 2-bromo-3-chlorooxazepine 56.**116c** has CNS-depressant potency equal to that

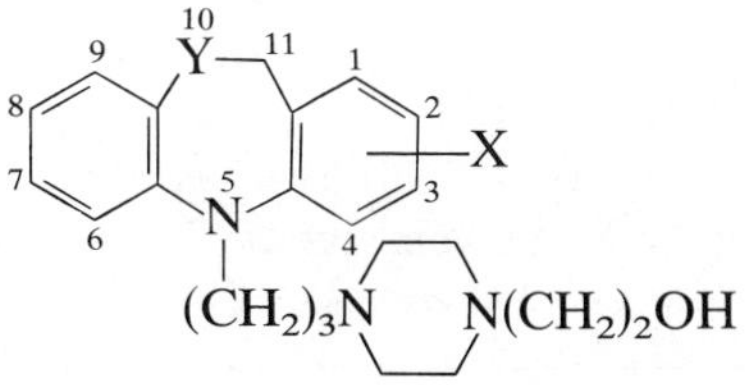

56.**116**

a X = 7-CF$_3$, Y = O
b X = 3-Cl, Y = O
c X = 2-Br, 3-Cl, Y = O
d X = 3,7-Cl$_2$, Y = O
e X = 7-CF$_3$, Y = S
f X = 3-Cl, Y = S

of the 3-chloro derivative 56.**116b**; however, the 3,7-dichloro analog 56.**116d** is significantly less potent. In general, dibenzthiazepines, e.g., 56.**116e** and 56.**116f**, are less effective than their related oxazepines in various neuropharmacological tests (428).

Many 4,4-disubstituted piperidinylpropyldibenzazepines, such as carpipramine (56.**117a**) and 3-chlorocarpipramine (56.**117b**), have been studied for neuropharmalogical activity (251). Although carpipramine does not cause marked neuroleptic activity in animals, it is effective in the treatment of chronic schizophrenics (430); it has combined antipsychotic and antidepressant actions (431). The 3-chloro derivative 56.**117b** has a CI of 0.2 in a rat CAR test and it is effective in various other neuropharmacological tests, although it does not produce catalepsy (432). It is marketed in Japan as a combination antipsychotic–antidepressant that activates behavioral and emotional function (433).

Opipramol (56.**118**), a dibenzazepine, decreases motor activity and inhibits fighting in mice; however, in chronic tests it has antidepressant-like actions (434). Another dibenzazepine derivative, an octahydropyridoindolobenzazepine 56.**119** has a CI of 0.63 in decreasing motor activity in

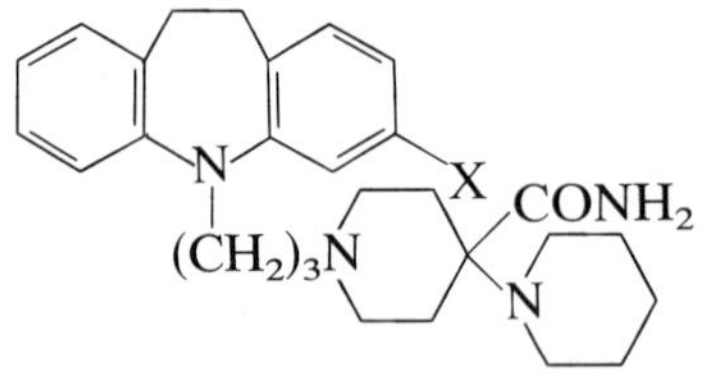

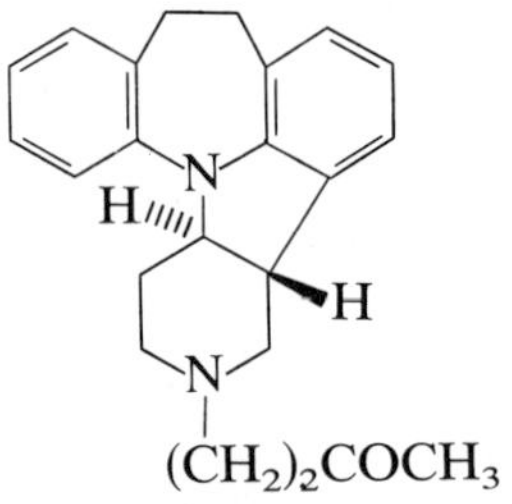

56.**119**

mice. It also has analgetic properties, being 15.2 times more potent than codeine in a phenylquinone writhing test in mice (435).

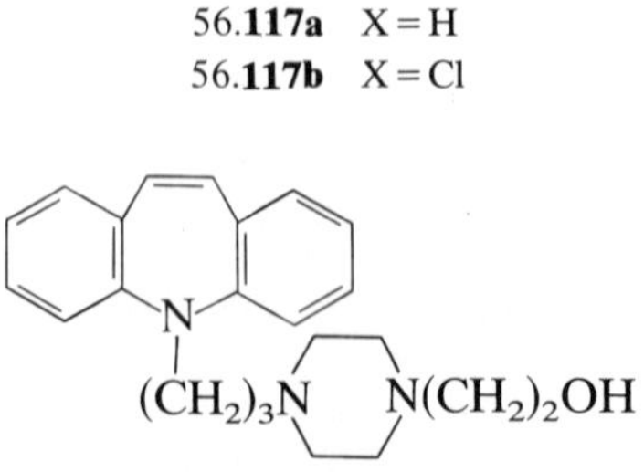

4.3.3 DIBENZO[b,f]THIEPINS AND RELATED COMPOUNDS. Potent neuroleptic activity is produced by a series of 10,11-dihydrodibenzo[b,f]thiepins, related dibenzoxepins, dibenzoselenepins, dibenzocyclo-

56.**120**

a	X = H, Y = S	f	X = 8-Cl, Y = Se
b	X = 8-Cl, Y = S	g	X = H, Y = CH$_2$
c	X = 8-Cl, Y = O	h	X = 8-Cl, Y = CH$_2$
d	X = 8-SCH$_3$, Y = O	i	X = H, Y = Si(CH$_3$)$_2$
e	X = H, Y = Se		

heptadienes, and dibenzosilepins (i.e., compounds having the tricyclic nucleus 56.**120**, where Y = S, O, Se, CH$_2$, Si(CH$_3$)$_2$, respectively) substituted with an appropriate basic group in the 10 position, i.e., one of the atoms of the ethylene bridge of the two outer rings. In these series (e.g., 167, 426, 436) an N-methylpiperazinyl group is most advantageous for neuroleptic potency.

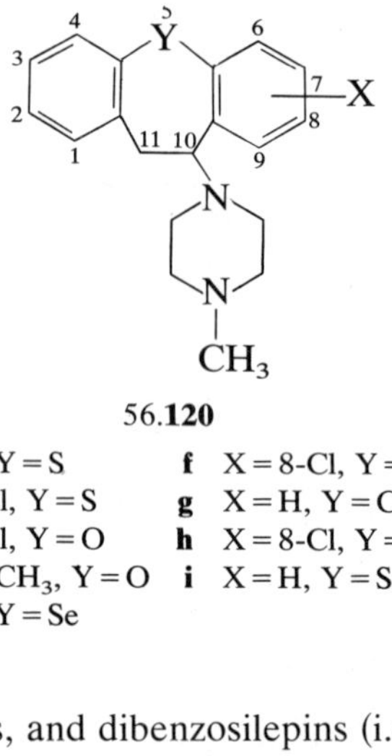

Next to aminoalkyl-substituted phenothiazines, 10-piperazinyldibenzo[b,f]thiepins are probably the most extensively studied series of tricyclic neuroleptics. The

56.**117a**   X = H
56.**117b**   X = Cl

56.**118**

parent of this series is perathiepin (56.**120a**). On i.v. administration to mice perathiepin has a CI of 3.1 in a rotating-rod test and on i.p. administration in a rat catalepsy test, it has a CI of 0.86 (cf. Table 56.8). As in other series of tricyclic antipsychotics, nuclear substitution of the position meta to the basic side chain significantly enhances potency. Thus the 8-chloro derivative octoclothepin (Clorotepin®, 56.**120b**) is three to four times more potent than perathiepin in both the rotating-rod and catalepsy tests. Interestingly, the enantiomers of these dibenzothiepins lack stereoselectivity in tests for CNS-depressant activity, e.g., the mouse rotating-rod and decreased motor activity tests (437, 438); however, their neuroleptic actions in causing catalepsy and in antagonizing apomorphine-induced chewing and agitation in rats are highly stereoselective. Almost all neuroleptic activity is noted in the

Table 56.8 Chlorpromazine Indexes (CI's) for Some 8-Substituted 10-(4-Methylpiperazinyl)-10,11-dihydrodibenzo[b,f]thiepins

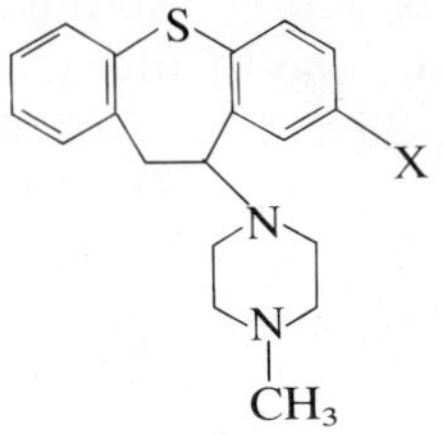

Structure Number	X	Rotating-Rod, Mice, i.v.[a]	Catalepsy, Rats, i.p.[b]	Ref.
56.**122**	H	3.1	0.86	443, 445
56.**123**	Cl	9.7	3.6	445
56.**124**	CF_3	6.8	12.7	446
56.**125**	OH	1.9	1.9	447
56.**126**	CN	14.3	3.0	445
56.**127**	NO_2	8.2[c]	—	448
56.**128**	SCH_3	6.5	4.3	449
56.**129**	OCH_3	11.9	6.6	447
56.**130**	$COCH_3$	36.6	9.2	450
56.**131**	CHO	50.9	3.2	450
56.**132**	F	5.0	3.2	451, 452
56.**133**	Br	5.3	3.4	451
56.**134**	I	1.5[c]	3.4	451
56.**135**	CH_3	4.3	—	453
56.**136**	$C(CH_3)_3$	0.84	—	453
56.**137**	C_2H_5	6.6	11.9	454
56.**138**	NH_2	2.8	—	448
56.**139**	$SeCH_3$	3.2	18.3	455
56.**140**	SC_2H_5	14.6	3.7	449
56.**141**	$SO_2N(CH_3)_2$	1.8	7.2	456

[a] Chlorpromazine has an $ED_{50} = 0.585$ mg/kg, i.v., and 8.2 mg/kg, p.o., in this test.
[b] Chlorpromazine has an $ED_{50} = 8.6$ mg/kg, i.p., and 16.0 mg/kg, p.o., in this test.
[c] Comparison of p.o. data.

56.**121**

(+) isomer (439–441). The absolute stereochemistry of the (+) isomer, determined by X-ray diffractometric methods, is (S)-56.**121** (442), a fact of possible importance in understanding the topography of the neuroleptic drug receptor.

The dibenzoxepin 56.**120c** is about one-fifth as potent as the corresponding thiepin in the mouse rotating-rod test i.v. (436, 443). Similarly, the 8-methylthio analog 56.**120d** is not as potent as its thiepin counterpart (see Table 56.8), although as a central sedative it has a CI of about 4 (426, 436).

10-Piperazinyldibenzoselenepins 56.**120e** and 56.**120f** are about one-half as potent as their thiepin relatives. Likewise, in the dibenzocycloheptadiene series the N-methyl-piperazine derivatives 56.**120g** and 56.**120h** are potent but less effective neuroleptics than the corresponding thiepins (441). The 5,5-dimethylsilepin 56.**120i** has only marginal activity in a mouse rotarod test (444).

An extraordinarily large number of nuclear-substituted derivatives of the dibenzothiepin perathiepin (56.**122**) (443, 445) has been studied in the mouse rotating-rod, the rat catalepsy, and several other tests. Representative examples of some 8-substituted 10-(4-methylpiperazinyl)-10,11-dihydrodibenzo[b,f]thiepins and their CI values are tabulated in Table 56.8. As can be discerned from these data, rank order of substituent effects on potency depends on the pharmacological test system. A quantitative structure–activity relationship (QSAR) study has been carried out with 18 of these 8-substituted derivatives

(446). Generally, in both tests 8-substitution correlates in a vague fashion with CAR data for 2-substituted 10-(3-dimethylaminopropyl)phenothiazines (Table 56.4); however, some discrepancies are apparent. For example, the 8-chloro derivative 56.**123** (octoclothepin) (445) is more potent in the mouse rotating-rod test than is the 8-trifluoromethyl analog 56.**124** (trifluthepin) (446) and 8-hydroxyl substitution 56.**125** of the dibenzothiepin decreases potency only slightly in both tests (447), whereas in the phenothiazine series similar substitution nearly abolishes activity in a CAR test (Table 56.4). Some other 8-substituted dibenzothiepins that are potent in the mouse rotating-rod test are the cyano (56.**126**) (cyanothepin) (445), nitro (56.**127**) (nitrothepin) (448), methylthio (56.**128**) (metiothepin) (449), methoxyl (56.**129**) (octometothepin) (447), acetyl (56.**130**), and formyl (56.**131**) derivatives (450) of perathiepin (56.**122**). Other 8-halogenated derivatives, e.g., fluoro 56.**132** (451, 452), bromo 56.**133** (451), and iodo 56.**134** (451), retain a high order of activity in the two pharmacological tests. The 8-fluoro analog 56.**132** (fluothepin) is noteworthy for its extraordinary potency in decreasing motor activity in mice (452). Representatives of other 8 substituents that permit retention of a high degree of potency are alkyl [56.**135** (453), 56.**136** (453), and 56.**137** (454)], amino (56.**138**) (448), methylseleno (56.**139**) (455), ethylthio (56.**140**) (449), and dimethylaminosulfonyl (56.**141**) (450) derivatives.

Apparently, the influence of the position of substitution of the dibenzothiepin system has been examined most extensively for the methoxyl group. In the mouse rotating-rod test p.o., the order of decreasing potency upon substitution of different positions (see 56.**116**, X = S) with methoxyl is 8 (56.**129**, CI = 11.9) (447) ≫ 2 (CI = 0.59) (457) ≈ 6 (CI = 0.55) (458) > 7 (CI = 0.23) (459). In the rat catalepsy test, only the 8-methoxyl derivative 56.**129** (octometothepin) has an

ED_{50} less than 50 mg/kg p.o. A marked decrease in potency is also observed on substitution of position 9 (460).

Substitution of position 2 of dibenzothiepins is of considerable interest because this presents a substituent–side chain orientation comparable to that in the prototype of antipsychotics without EPS liability, i.e., clozapine (56.**4**), which is potent in the mouse rotating-rod test, but does not produce catalepsy in rats. Most 2-substituted relatives of perathiepin (56.**122**) are also considerably more potent in the coordination test than in the catalepsy test. The halogen derivatives (461) are particularly noteworthy. Only the 2-fluoro derivative has an ED_{50} less than 50 mg/kg p.o. in the rat catalepsy procedure. CI values for 2-substituted perathiepin derivatives in the mouse rotarod test p.o. are F (2.3), Cl (6.8), Br (6.1), and I (6.8) (461). Other 2-substituted perathiepins include trifluoromethyl, methoxy, methylthio, and acetyl derivatives (462). Although these compounds are without significant cataleptic activity, they are only weakly effective in the rotarod test. Greater potency in this test (p.o.) is noted for 2-amino (CI = 6.6) and 2-acetamido (CI = 4.6) derivatives (462). The 2-nitro and 2-hydroxy derivatives are ineffective in producing catalepsy and are relatively weak depressants (463).

Disubstitution of perathiepin has been studied extensively. Metabolism of octoclothepin (56.**120b**), which is marketed as an antipsychotic in Czechoslovakia, involves ring hydroxylation (464). The urine of rats given octoclothepin gives two TLC spots corresponding to 2- and 3-hydroxy derivatives. Only the 2-hydroxylated product is found in the urine of octoclothepin-treated schizophrenic patients (464). 2-Hydroxyoctoclothepin (56.**120**: Y = S, X = 2-OH, 8-Cl) is only weakly effective in the mouse rotarod test (CI = 0.22) and lacks cataleptic activity. In contrast, the 3-hydroxy derivative is highly effective in both the mouse rotarod (CI = 9.8) and rat cataleptic (CI = 6.7) tests (464). 6-Methoxy and 6-hydroxy derivatives of octoclothepin have relatively potent CNS-depressant and cataleptic activity. Other metabolic processes, e.g., N-demethylation and S- and N-oxidation, result in loss of activity (465). A 2-acetoxy congener of octoclothepin lacks significant neuroleptic activity in animals (356). The 2-fluoro-3-hydroxy derivative of octoclothepin is a potent tranquilizer with slight cataleptogenic activity (466). Many dihalogenated derivatives have also been examined. 7,8-Dihalogenated derivatives (452, 467) are generally less potent than 2,8- or 3,8-dihalogenated isomers (355, 468) and their effect is usually less protracted (469). Although there are exceptions, e.g., the 3-fluoro-8-methylthio derivative (3-fluorometiothepin), which has striking potency in the mouse rotarod (CI = 15.2) and rat catalepsy (CI = 6.4) tests (470), 2,8- and 3,8-disubstituted dibenzothiepins are generally less potent than their 8-monosubstituted parents; however, some 3-fluorooctoclothepin derivatives have a prolonged duration of neuroleptic activity (471). 6,9-Dichloro substitution of perathiepin is particularly detrimental to activity. This compound (56.**120**: Y = S; X = 6,9-Cl$_2$) has no measurable activity in the mouse rotarod (i.v.) or catalepsy (i.p.) tests at 10 mg/kg. The 7,8-dichloro isomer has a CI of 0.5 in the former test and 3.0 in the latter one (472). A trihalogenated derivative 3,7-difluorooctoclothepin is an orally active cataleptic and blocks apomorphine-induced emesis. The compound is somewhat related to pimozide (see Section 4.4.2) (473). Benzo-fused derivatives of perathiepin have little CNS-depressant activity. The 6,7 (474) and 1,11 (475) benzo-fused compounds lack significant depressant activity. A 7,8-benzo-fused congener (476) is only weakly effective; it has a CI of about 0.4 in both the mouse rotarod and rat catalepsy tests. Comparable results are produced by a 7,8-trimethylene bridged analog (477).

56.**142**

a   X = R = H
b   X = 8-Cl, R = —△
c   X = 8-Cl, R = C$_6$H$_5$
d   X = 8-Cl, R = COCH$_3$
e   X = 8-Cl, R = SO$_2$CH$_3$
f   X = 8-Cl, R = (CH$_2$)$_2$OH
g   X = 8-Cl, R = (CH$_2$)$_3$OH
h   X = 8-CH$_3$O, R = (CH$_2$)$_3$OH
i   X = 8-CH$_3$S, R = (CH$_2$)$_3$OH
j   X = 3-F, 8-CH$_3$S, R = (CH$_2$)$_3$OH
k   X = 2-Cl, R = (CH$_2$)$_2$OH

Oxidation of antipsychotic dibenzothiepin derivatives generally has an adverse effect on activity (478). The 5-sulfoxide of octoclothepin is less potent and more toxic than its parent (437) and the sulfone is practically devoid of activity (426). Piperazinyl *N*-oxides also have markedly decreased CNS-depressant and cataleptogenic activity (478).

Many modifications of the piperazinyl methyl group ot perathiepin and its 2-substituted derivatives 56.**142** have been examined (444, 479). The demethyl homolog, norperathiepin (56.**142a**), is a less potent neuroleptic than its parent. Replacement of the methyl group with larger alkyl, unsaturated alkyl, cycloalkyl, cycloalkylalkyl, aralkyl, substituted aralkyl (480), pyridyl (480), aminoalkyl, amidoalkyl, cyanoalkyl, carboxyalkyl, cyclic acetalalkyl (481), and various other groups has an inconsistent influence on neuroleptic potency (479). For example, *N*-cyclopropylnorperathiepin (56.**142b**) is very potent, whereas *N*-aryl derivatives, e.g., 56.**142c**, are almost inactive. Acylation, e.g., 56.**142d**, or sulfonylation, e.g., 56.**142e**, of the terminal piperazine nitrogen abolishes activity in the

mouse rotating-rod and the rat catalepsy tests (437). Hydroxyalkyl derivatives (467) and their fatty acid esters, which have potential utility in antipsychotic maintenance therapy (447, 482), are the most comprehensively studied modifications of the terminal piperazinyl substituent (355, 447, 461, 467, 478, 479, 483). Among the most effective of these neuroleptic alcohols are noroxyclothepin (56.**142f**), oxyclothepin (56.**142g**), oxymetothepin (56.**142h**), and oxyprothepin (56.**142i**) (479). In the mouse rotating-rod test they have potency equal to, or greater than, that of octoclothepin (479). They are of special interest because their cataleptogenic activity is minimal. Oxyprothepin (56.**142i**) is effective in schizophrenic and manic syndromes (484–486). An especially prolonged duration of action is noted with its 3-fluoro derivative 56.**142j** (483). Separation of neuroleptic and cataleptic actions comparable to that of clozapine is observed with 56.**142k** (461, 487). Esters of these alcohols are of special interest for use in antipsychotic maintenance therapy (447). Oxyprothepin (56.**142i**) decanoate (448–490) is of special interest. It has a longer duration of action against apomorphine-induced emesis in dogs than does fluphenazine decanoate (490).

An oxazolidinone derivative 56.**143** related to perathiepin is of considerable interest because it appears to produce neuroleptic actions with minimal EPS liability. It has been resolved. In tests for increase in HVA in rats, inhibition of adenylate cyclase and blockade of apomorphine-induced emesis, activity was noted almost exclusively in the (*S*)-(+) isomer, 56.**143** (491); i.e., the isomer with the same configuration as the neuroleptically active antipode of octoclothepin. Whether some related dibenzothiepins are completely stereospecific in their biological activities is not certain (492–494).

Substitution of the methylpiperazine moiety with methyl in position 3, e.g.,

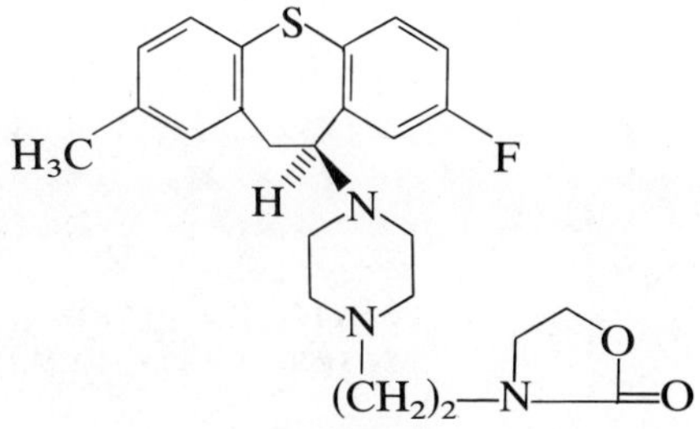

56.**143**

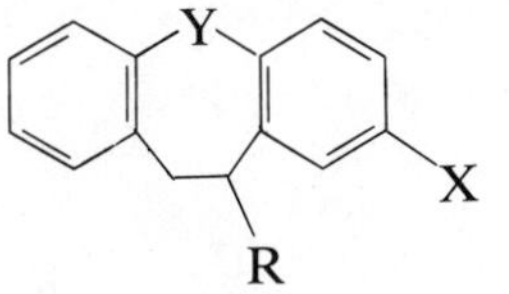

56.**144**

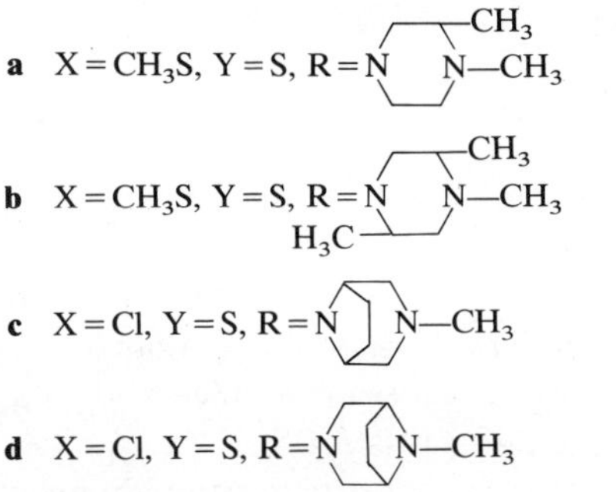

a X = CH₃S, Y = S, R = N⟩N—CH₃

b X = CH₃S, Y = S, R = N⟩N—CH₃, H₃C

c X = Cl, Y = S, R = N⟩N—CH₃

d X = Cl, Y = S, R = N⟩N—CH₃

e X = Cl, Y = S, R = NH₂

f X = CH₃O, Y = S, R = —⟨ ⟩N—CH₃

g X = Cl, Y = CH₂, R = N—⟨ ⟩N—CH₃

h X = H, Y = S, R = O(CH₂)₂N(CH₃)₂

i X = Cl, Y = S, R = O(CH₂)₂N(CH₃)₂

56.**144a**, or the 2,5 positions, e.g., 56.**144b**, reduces potency of the parent in both the mouse rotarod and rat cataleptic tests (444). Other modifications or replacement of the methylpiperazinyl group of perathiepin and its relatives generally results in a marked decrease in neuroleptic potency. Even ethylene-bridged piperazine analogs of octoclothepin are less effective neuroleptics than the parent. For example, in the mouse rotarod test 56.**144c** is two-thirds as potent as octoclothepin (CI = 1.8) and its

isomer 56.**144d** is less than one-half as potent as the parent (495). Replacement by amino (56.**144e**), methylamino, dimethylamino, diethylaminoethyl (496), piperidinyl, 4-hydroxypiperidinyl, 4-carbethoxy-4-phenylpiperidinyl, morpholinyl, or even a homopiperazinyl group results in loss of CNS activity. In contrast, the 4-(N-methylpiperidinyl) analog 56.**144f** has neuroleptic potency approximating that of its N-methylpiperazinyl counterpart (167, 453). Similar neuroleptic actions are seen with the related 10-(N-methylpiperidinyl)dibenzocycloheptadiene (56.**144g**) and the corresponding dibenzocycloheptadiene (497). A 10-dimethylaminoethyl ether of 10,11-dihydrodibenzo[b,f]thiepin, e.g., amethothepin (56.**144h**), has activity in the mouse rotarod test that is markedly enhanced by substitution of the 8 position, e.g., to give amethoclothepin (56.**144i**) (498). An extremely interesting replacement of the methylpiperazinyl moiety is represented by a 10-(3-methylethylaminopyrrolidinyl) group. This substitution is unique because two centers of asymmetry are introduced into the molecule. Surprisingly, little difference is noted in the ability of enantiomorphs to antagonize amphetamine-induced stereotypy in rats; however, differences in potency are observed between the diastereoisomers. Thus maximum potency is noted for the (3′S,10S) (56.**145**, CI = 6.8) and (3′R,10R) (56.**146**, CI = 3.3) enantiomers, whereas the diastereomers with the (3′S,10R) (CI = 0.5) and (3′R,10S) (CI = 0.4) configurations are much less potent (493).

Unlike the dibenzothiepins, in the dibenzocycloheptadiene series the 10-dimethylamino derivative 56.**147a**, as well as the corresponding primary and secondary monomethylamines, has CNS-depressant activity. The 10-dimethylaminoethoxy derivative 56.**147b** is a potent depressant (167).

The 11-keto analog 56.**148** of octoclothepin is more potent than chlorpromazine

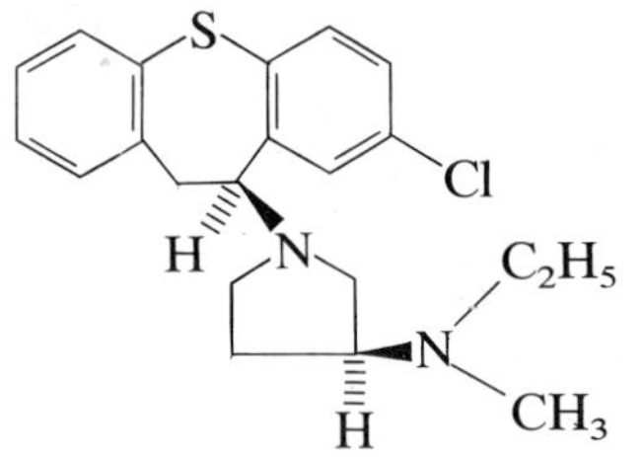

56.**145**

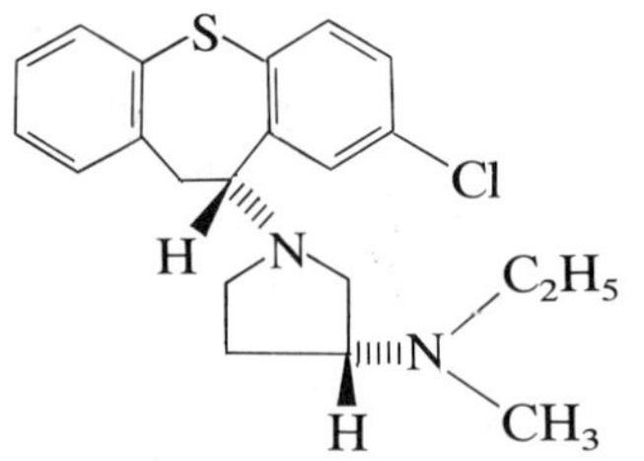

56.**146**

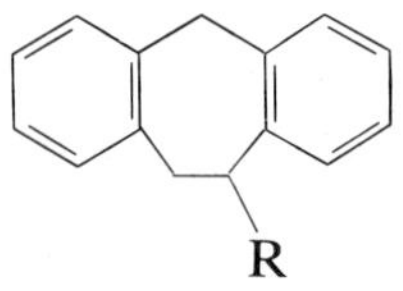

56.**147a** R = N(CH_3)_2
56.**147b** R = O(CH_2)_2N(CH_3)_2

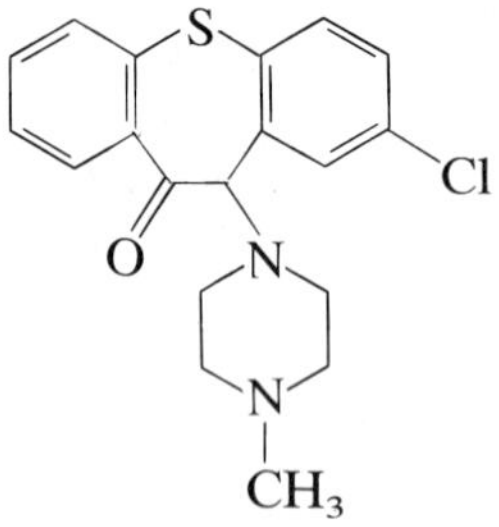

56.**148**

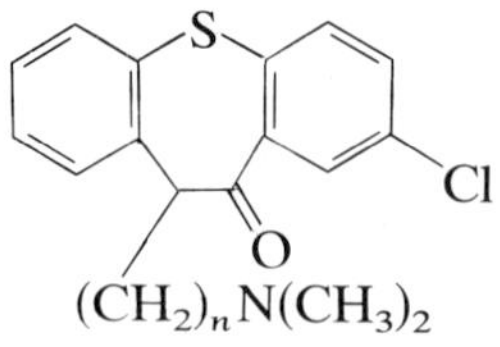

56.**149a** $n = 2$
56.**149b** $n = 3$

in various neuroleptic tests. In the clinic it has antidepressant (499) and antischizophrenic (500) activity. Several 11-dimethyl-aminoalkyl-10-keto relatives, 56.**149a** and 56.**149b**, of octoclothepin show CNS-depressant, antireserpine, and antihistamine actions (501). Peradithiepin (56.**150a**), a thienyl isostere of perathiepin, is a potent CNS depressant with relatively weak cataleptogenic activity. Its chloro derivative 56.**150b** is similar to octoclothepin in the rat catalepsy test but it is relatively weak in the mouse rotarod test (502–504). The related cycloheptane 56.**150c** has

chlorpromazine-like activity in both these tests (426).

A pyridyl isostere 56.**151a** of perathiepin is considerably less potent than the parent as a CNS depressant in mice and as a cataleptogenic in rats (505).

In general, 10-piperazinyldibenzo[*b,f*]-thiepins and related 6–7–6 compounds are equipotent or less potent than their 10,11-dihydro counterparts (355, 447, 449, 451, 455, 459, 477, 495, 506, 507). A notable exception is in the 7,8-dihalogenated series where the unsaturated dibenzothiepins are considerably more potent but shorter acting

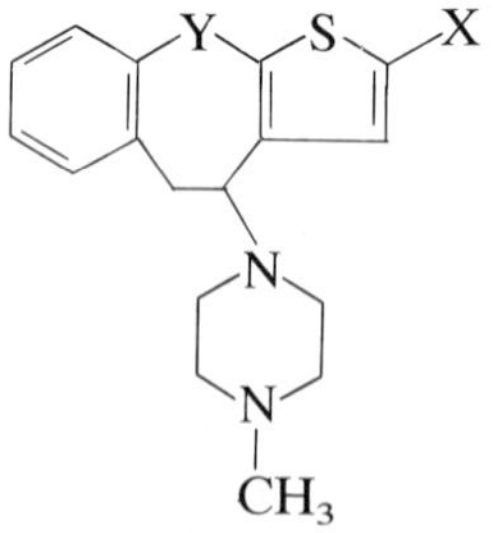

56.**150**
56.**150a** X = H, Y = S
56.**150b** X = Cl, Y = S
56.**150c** X = H, Y = CH_2

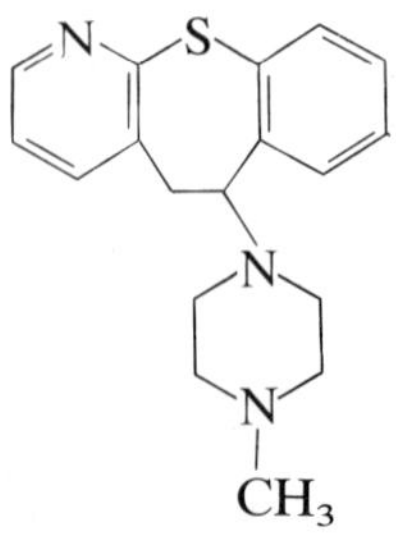

56.**151a**

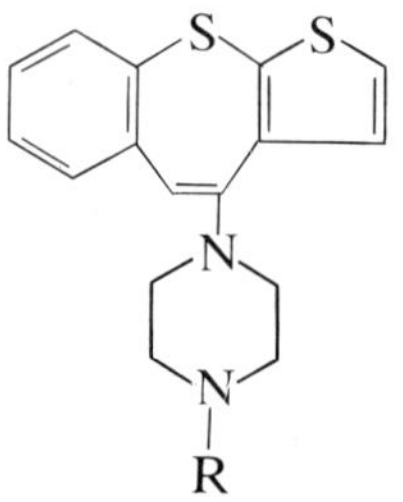

56.**151b** R = CH_3
56.**151c** R = (CH_2)_3OH

than their 10,11-dihydro analogs (452) in both the mouse rotarod and rat catalepsy tests. In both these tests, potency equal to or greater than that of perphenazine is noted for the pyrrolidine 56.**152a**, as well as for the *N*-methylpiperazine, dehydroclothepin (56.**152b**) (498, 508); however, the ether 56.**152c** is only weakly effective (426). The 10-(4-methylpiperazyl)dibenz[*b,f*]oxepin 56.**152d** is more potent than chlorpromazine in antagonizing amphetamine- or apomorphine-induced effects (509, 510). Two unsaturated thienyl isosteres 56.**151b** and 56.**151c** are about equipotent with their saturated parent, peradithiepin, in the mouse rotarod and rat catalepsy tests (506); however, stability in aqueous solution and perhaps toxicity are deterrents to clinical evaluation of these enamines.

Although 10-(3-dimethylaminopropyl)dibenzo[*b,f*]thiepin (56.**153a**) (511) produces only stimulation in rats given an oral dose of 300 mg/kg, cataleptic activity is observed with the chloro-substituted relatives 56.**153b** and 56.**153c** (501). An exocyclic

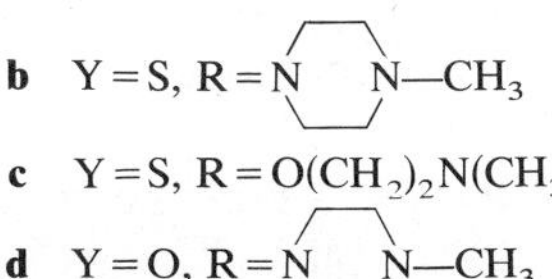

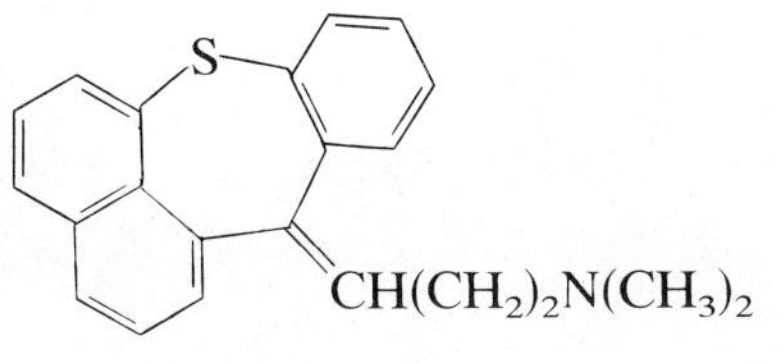

56.**154**

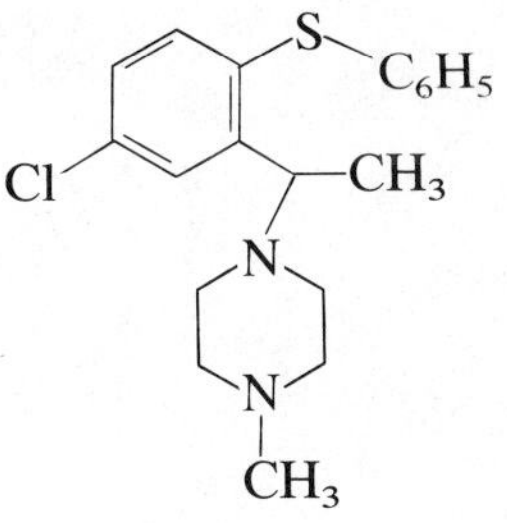

56.**155**

olefinic isomer of 56.**153a** has neither depressant nor antidepressant actions (167); however, a 1,11-benzo-fused derivative 56.**154** shows pronounced antireserpine and anticataleptic actions in animals (474). Ring-opened analogs $C_6H_5CH_2CH(C_6H_5)$-$N(CH_2CH_2)_2NCH_3$ (167) and 56.**155** (512) of perathiepin and octoclothepin are devoid of apparent CNS activity (167).

4.3.4 DIBENZO[*b,f*][1,4]THIAZEPINES AND RELATED COMPOUNDS. 11-Piperazinyl derivatives of dibenzo[*b,f*][1,4]thiazepines (56.**156**, Y = S), dibenz[*b,f*][1,4]oxazepines (56.**156**, Y = O), dibenzo[*b,e*][1,4]diazepines (56.**156**, Y = NH), and morphanthridines (56.**156**, Y = CH_2) have significant CNS activity (513–516).

Members of this series that have been studied in the clinic or marketed in some countries included the thiazepines clotiapine (56.**156a**) and metiapine (56.**156b**), the oxazepines loxapine (56.**156c**) and its *N*-demethyl derivative amoxepin, the diazepine clozapine (56.**4**, 56.**156d**), and the morphanthridine perlapine (56.**156e**). Clotiapine (517–519), metiapine (517, 520), and loxapine (517, 521–526) are classical antipsychotics with typical pharmacological profiles. In a rat

56.**152**

a   Y = S, R =

b   Y = S, R =

c   Y = S, R = $O(CH_2)_2N(CH_3)_2$

d   Y = O, R =

$(CH_2)_nN(CH_3)_2$

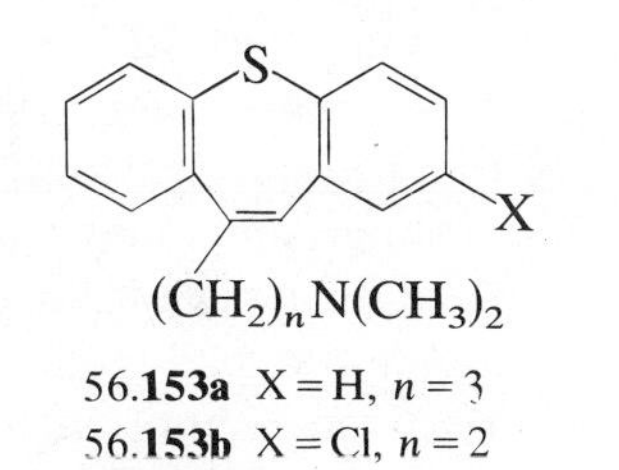

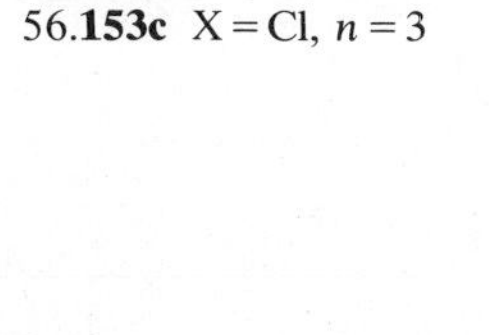

56.**153a** X = H, *n* = 3
56.**153b** X = Cl, *n* = 2
56.**153c** X = Cl, *n* = 3

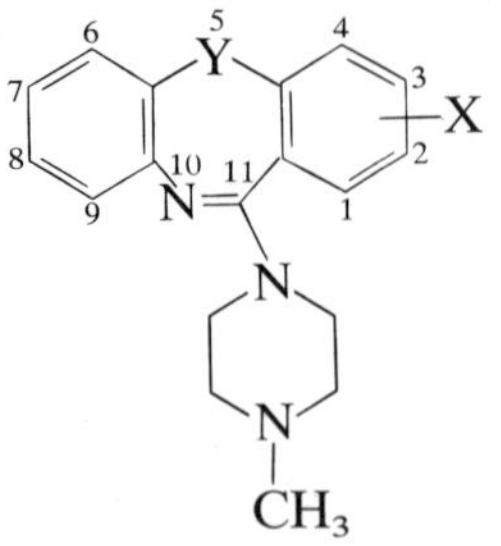

56.**156**

a	X = 2-Cl, Y = S	**g**	X = 8-Cl, Y = S
b	X = 2-CH$_3$, Y = S	**h**	X = 2-Cl, Y = CH$_2$
c	X = 2-Cl, Y = O	**i**	X = H, Y = NH
d	X = 8-Cl, Y = NH	**j**	X = H, Y = O
e	X = H, Y = CH$_2$	**k**	X = H, Y = S
f	X = 2-Cl, Y = NH		

catalepsy test s.c. the CI values for clotiapine, metiapine, and loxapine are 5.3, 0.76, and 10.9, respectively. Clozapine (527–529) is the first example of a new class of neuroleptics with a novel pharmacological profile. Amoxapine (516, 530), in which the piperazine nitrogen in position 4 is unsubstituted, has antidepressant properties. Perlapine (531, 532) is devoid of antipsychotic activity; it is an hypnotic agent.

In examining structure–activity relationships in these series of compounds cataleptic actions and antagonism of apomorphine-induced stereotypy following s.c. administration to rats have been used (515, 518). In the rat catalepsy test the order of decreasing potency in compounds of the general structure 56.**156** (X = Cl or CH$_3$) is Y = O > S > CH$_2$ > NH ≫ SO > SO$_2$.

Compounds without a bridging group, e.g., the phenanthridine 56.**157** and the

56.**157**

56.**158**

analogous "ring-opened" derivative 56.**158**, are devoid of significant neuroleptic activity.

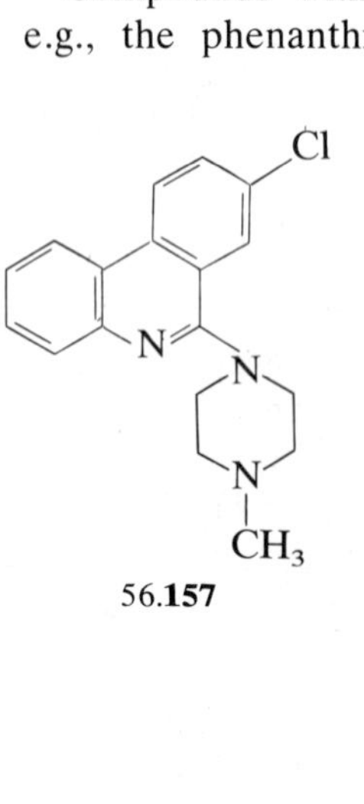

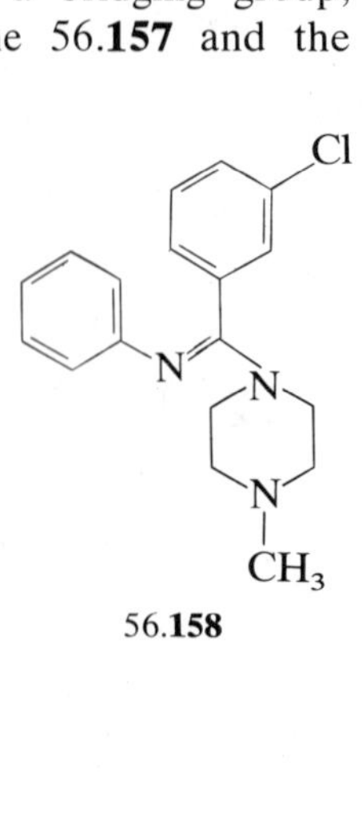

As in other series of tricyclic neuroleptics, some piperazinyldibenzoazepines 56.**156** that lack nuclear substitution may have some CNS-depressant properties, but they generally cause little, if any, activity in the rat catalepsy and apomorphine antagonism tests. For neuroleptic activity, a nuclear substituent, e.g., a chlorine atom in the 2 position, is essential. Substitution with chlorine in other positions gives compounds that are practically inactive in both of these tests. The influence of different substituents in position 2 of 11-(4-methylpiperazinyl)dibenz[b,f][1,4]oxazepines (56.**156**, X = O) in the rat apomorphine antagonism test is very much like that seen in other tricyclic series; i.e., SO$_2$N(CH$_3$)$_2$ > SO$_2$CF$_3$ ≈ NO$_2$ ≈ Cl ≈ CN ≈ SO$_2$CH$_3$ > Br > SO$_2$C$_2$H$_5$ ≈ SCH$_3$ ≈ F ≈ OCH$_3$ > CH$_3$ ≈ SCF$_3$ > SC$_2$H$_5$ > OCF$_3$ > SOCH$_3$ > NH$_2$ > H. A somewhat different order of potency of these 2-substituted oxazepines is observed in the rat catalepsy test. Here, the 2-nitro derivative is very potent. It is 1.25 times more potent in this test than in the apomorphine antagonism test. In contrast, the 2-methylsulfonyl derivative is only $\frac{1}{75}$ as potent in the rat catalepsy test as in the apomorphine antagonism test. Comparable separation of potencies in the two tests is also seen with different 2 substituents in the thiazepine series; however, in the diazepines a similar influence of 2 substituents on separation of potency in the two tests is not observed. Because catalepsy may correlate with EPS (533), compounds with comparatively low cataleptogenic potency might be expected to produce less EPS in man.

The 8-chloro-substituted dibenzodiazepine clozapine (56.**4**, 56.**156d**) is an extremely interesting compound. Although it is inactive in producing catalepsy or inhibiting apomorphine-induced stereotypies in rats, it is an effective antipsychotic agent with a very low propensity for causing EPS

(534). These most advantageous properties of clozapine are tempered somewhat by the observation that it may cause hematologic disturbances, such as agranulocytosis (535) and leukopenia (536). These properties, as well as the concomitant limitations, have made clozapine the subject of intense research in many laboratories. Its exceptional pharmacological and biochemical profile is strikingly illustrated by comparison of these data for clozapine with those of its isomeric 2-chloro derivative 56.**156f** (Table 56.9) (11, 537), a compound with very similar physicochemical properties (516) and molecular topography as determined by X-ray crystal structure analysis (538). Pharmacologically, it is most noteworthy that clozapine inhibits a CAR in mice only at doses that markedly decrease motor activity, whereas its 2-chloro isomer behaves as a conventional neuroleptic in these tests. In contrast, clozapine inhibits the electroencephalographic arousal reaction induced by electrical stimulation of the mesencephalic reticular formation and it exhibits central anticholinergic activity. The relative affinities of classical neuroleptics for muscarinic cholinergic receptor binding in rat brain correlate inversely with their ability to produce EPS. Clozapine has greatest affinity for this receptor (21, 72). Biochemical results, however, indicate that clozapine, unlike classical neuroleptics, apparently does not block dopamine receptors (539). The 2-chloro isomer 56.**156f** of clozapine, like classical neuroleptics, accelerates dopamine turnover in the brain, resulting in an increase in HVA and DOPAC content, an effect most probably related to blockade of dopamine receptors (651). Clozapine is considerably less potent in this test and, unlike the classical agents, enhances, rather than decreases, dopamine levels in the rat striatum. The dopamine-increasing effect of clozapine is also observed with the dibenzothiazepine 56.**156g** and compounds, e.g., 56.**159a** and 56.**159b**, in which the methyl group of the piperazinyl side chain is replaced by hydroxyalkyl groups, but is abolished by introduction of a second nuclear halogen in position 2, e.g., 56.**159c** and 56.**159d**. Dopamine is not elevated by 2-chloro-substituted dibenzothiazepines and related compounds [clotiapine (56.**156a**), loxapine (56.**156c**), the 2-chloro isomer of clozapine (56.**156f**), and the

Table 56.9   Comparison of the Pharmacological and Biochemical Effects of Clozapine (56.4, 56.156d) and its 2-Chloro Isomer (56.156f) (515)

Test	Clozapine	56.**156f**
Catalepsy, rat, ED_{50}, mg/kg, s.c.	I^a	1.8
Apomorphine antagonism, rat, ED_{50}, mg/kg, s.c.	I^a	1.7
CAR, mouse, ED_{50}, mg/kg, p.o.	20.0	2.0
Inhibition motor activity, mouse, ED_{50}, mg/kg, p.o.	2.5	3.0
Inhibition of EEG arousal reaction, rabbit, ED_{150}, mg/kg, i.v.	1.5	I^a
HVA, striatal, rat, ED_{300}, mg/kg, p.o.	56	9
Dopamine, striatal, rat, content	b	c
Dopamine, striatal, rat, turnover	b	b
Serotonin, whole brain, rat, content	b	I^a
Serotonin, whole brain, rat, turnover	I^a	I^a

[a] Inactive at doses tested.
[b] Increased.
[c] Decreased.

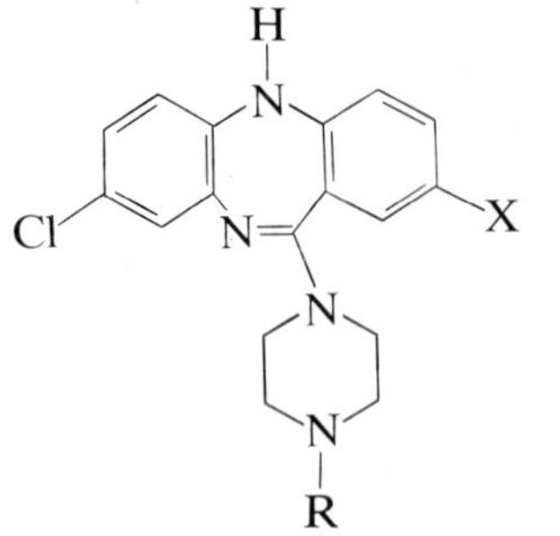

56.**159**

a	X = H, R = (CH$_2$)$_2$OH	**c**	X = Cl, R = CH$_3$
b	X = H, R = (CH$_2$)$_3$OH	**d**	X = F, R = CH$_3$

morphanthridine 56.**156h**], perlapine (56.**156e**) (540), 56.**156i**, 56.**156j**, 56.**156k**, or various butyrophenone and tricyclic antipsychotics (539). Serotonin content in the rat brain is increased by clozapine, whereas its 2-chloro isomer 56.**156f** does not affect serotonin content or turnover. Other procedures in which clozapine differs from classical neuroleptics include its weak action in increasing serum prolactin levels (541), its inability to sensitize striatal dopamine receptors to agonists (although this is controversial) (542), its failure to cause tardive dyskinesias, and its inability to reduce dopamine-induced impulse frequency of dopaminergic neurons of the substantia nigra (543). Although clozapine, like most neuroleptics, does inhibit dopamine-sensitive adenylate cyclase (544), this property is shared by nonantipsychotic agents, e.g., some antidepressants (545) and serotonin antagonists (546).

As a consequence of a comprehensive study of dibenzoazepines in various pharmacological and biochemical tests, the general conclusion is that the classical procedures for detecting neuroleptic activity in animals are poor predictors of potential antipsychotic activity (539).

The psychotropic activity of dibenzoazepines 56.**156** strongly depends on the nature of the side chain. Tricyclic compounds in this class with a dimethylamino-

propyl substituent in position 11 cause antidepressant actions (547). Piperazine "ring-opened" congeners, 56.**160a** and 56.**160b**, related to loxapine and clotiapine are without significant neuroleptic activity (548). The monobasic piperidinyl (56.**161a**), piperazinyl (56.**161b**), and N-acetylpiperazinyl (56.**161c**) derivatives are inactive in the rat anti-apomorphine and cataleptic tests. N-Oxidation of the distal nitrogen of the piperazine reduces potency. Thus 56.**161d** is about one-third as potent as loxapine in these tests. Compounds in which the piperazinyl methyl group is removed often display antidepressant-like actions. The activity pattern of these compounds, e.g., amoxapine (56.**161e**), combines properties of both neuroleptics and antidepressants (530).

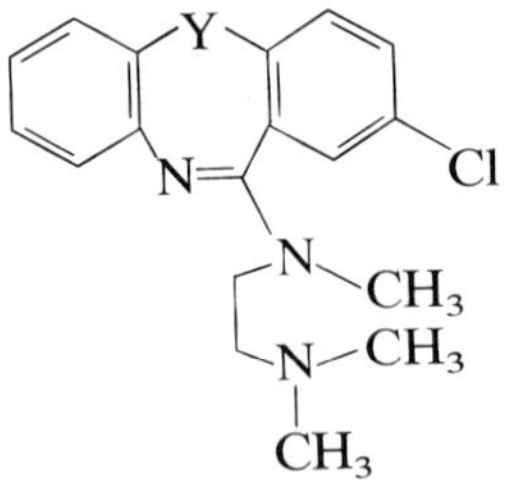

56.**160a** Y = O
56.**160b** Y = S

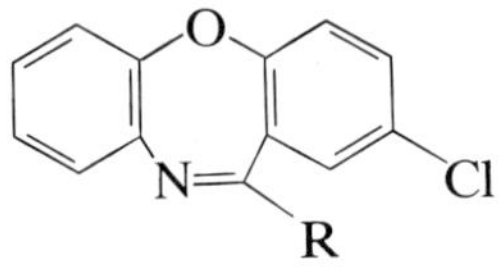

56.**161**

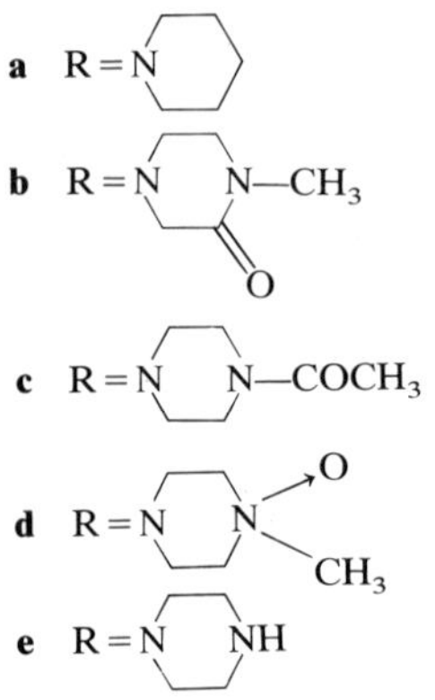

a R = N⟨piperidinyl⟩

b R = N⟨N—CH$_3$, =O⟩

c R = N⟨N—COCH$_3$⟩

d R = N⟨N→O, CH$_3$⟩

e R = N⟨NH⟩

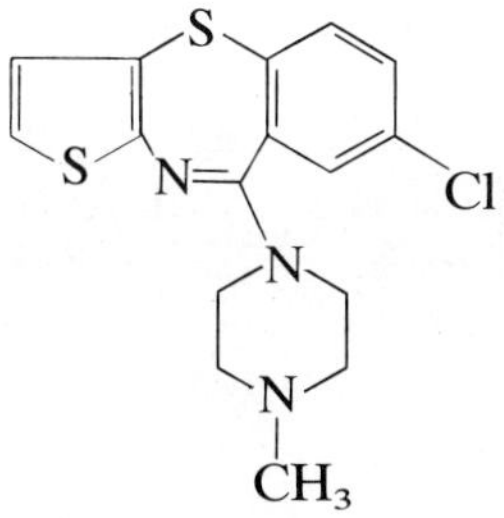

56.**162**

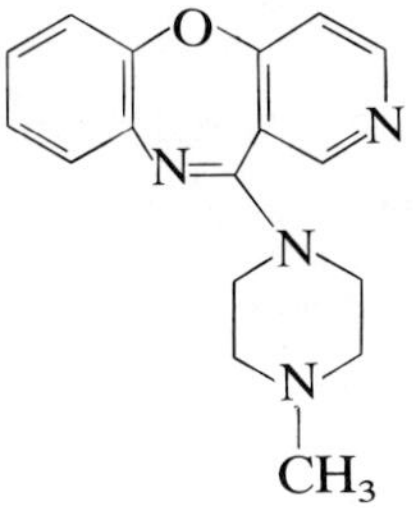

56.**163**

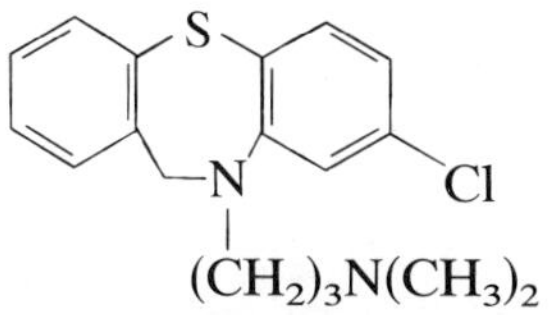

56.**164**

Exchange of one of the benzene rings of dibenzoazepines by a thiophene or pyridine ring generally results in nearly complete loss of neuroleptic potency. For example, the thiophene isostere of clotiapine, the thieno[3,2-*b*][1,4]benzothiazepine derivative 56.**162** (549), as well as the pyrido-[4,3-*b*][1,5]benzoxazepine 56.**163** (550), are practically devoid of neuroleptic activity.

An *N*-dimethylaminopropyl derivative of dihydrodibenzothiazepine, homochlorpromazine (56.**164**), lacks significant chlorpromazine-like activity (551).

4.3.5   BENZOCYCLOHEPTAPYRIDOISOQUINO-LINES.   Several benzocycloheptapyrido-isoquinolines have embedded in their framework a dibenzocycloheptadiene tricycle. These compounds, which are relatively rigid structures, have potent neuroleptic actions. They are of particular interest be-

cause their neuropharmacological potency depends greatly on strict stereochemical requirements. Thus they may provide excellent tools in an attempt to decipher the topographical requirements of the receptor site with which at least this class of neuroleptic agents interacts. The precursor to this family of neuroleptics is 1*H*-benzo-[6,7]cyclohepta[1,2,3-*de*]pyrido[2,1-*a*]iso-quinoline (taclamine, 56.**165**). The trans isomer exhibits actions characteristic of antianxiety drugs in laboratory animals (552, 553).

Many 3-tertiary carbinol derivatives (56.**166**) related to the parent 56.**165** have been examined for their ability to antagonize amphetamine-induced stereotypy in rats (554). The CI values for these compounds in an antagonism of (+)-amphetamine-induced stereotypy test in rats are tabulated in Table 56.10.

It is evident from these results that neuroleptic activity depends critically on the relative configurations at positions 3, 4a, and 13b. Thus of the four possible racemic pairs of ethyl carbinols 56.**166b–e**, only 56.**166b**, which has a 4a,13b-trans and 3(OH),13b(H)-trans configuration, has significant activity. Similarly, all other compounds lacking this trans,trans orientation,

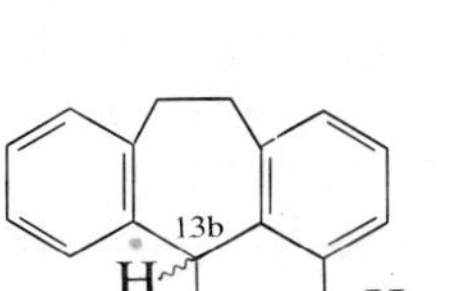

56.**165**

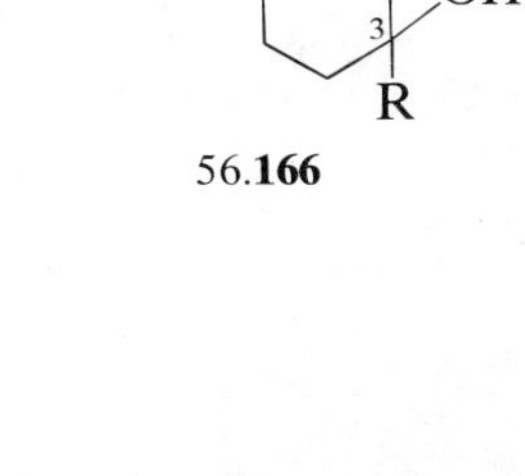

56.**166**

Table 56.10   CI Values for 3-Substituted Benzo[6,7]cyclohepta[1,2,3-*de*]pyrido[2,1-*a*]isoquinolin-3-ols (56.166) (554)

Structure Number	R	4a,13b Rel. Config.	3(OH),13b(H) Rel. Config.	CI, Amphetamine Antag., Rats, i.p.
56.**166a**	CH_3	trans	[a]	<0.38
56.**166b**	C_2H_5	trans	trans	0.75
56.**166c**	C_2H_5	cis	trans	[b]
56.**166d**	C_2H_5	trans	cis	[b]
56.**166e**	C_2H_5	cis	cis	[c]
56.**166f**	$C{\equiv}CH$	trans	cis	[c]
56.**166g**	$C{\equiv}CH$	cis	cis	[c]
56.**166h**	$n\text{-}C_3H_7$	trans	trans	0.5
56.**166i**	$c\text{-}C_3H_5$	trans	trans	6.0
56.**166j**	$i\text{-}C_3H_7$	trans	trans	6.0
56.**166k**	$CH_2CH{=}CH_2$	trans	[a]	<0.38
56.**166l**	$n\text{-}C_4H_9$	trans	trans	0.75
56.**166m**	$t\text{-}C_4H_9$	trans	trans	12.1
56.**166n**	$t\text{-}C_4H_9$	cis	trans	
56.**166o**	$n\text{-}C_6H_{13}$	trans	trans	1.5
56.**166p**	$c\text{-}C_6H_{11}$	trans	trans	6.0
56.**166q**	C_6H_5	trans	trans	3.0
56.**166r**	$2\text{-}CH_3OC_6H_4$	trans	trans	12.1

[a] Unknown relative configuration.
[b] Failed to protect aggregated mice against the lethal effect of amphetamine.
[c] No anti-amphetamine effect at 20 mg/kg, i.p.

i.e., 56.**166f**, 56.**166g**, and 56.**166n**, are inactive. In general, potency of the tertiary carbinols with the trans,trans stereochemistry increases with the size of *n*-alkyl substituent: *n*-hexyl   56.**166o** > *n*-butyl 56.**166l** ≈ ethyl 56.**166b** > *n*-propyl 56.**166h** > allyl 56.**166k** ≈ methyl 56.**166a**. Branching of the alkyl substituent in position 3 is particularly beneficial for potency. Thus phenyl- (56.**166q**), cyclohexyl- (56.**166p**), isopropyl- (dexaclamol) (56.**166j**), cyclopropyl- (56.**166i**), and *tert*-butyl-substituted (56.**166m**) derivatives have a high degree of activity. In fact, racemic 56.**166m** (butaclamol) is nearly as potent as fluphenazine in this test. Among a series of 4-(substituted phenyl) derivatives 56.**166r** is the most potent antagonist of amphetamine-induced stereotypy; it is equipotent with butaclamol (555). In addition to its activity in antagonizing amphetamine-induced stereotypy in mice, butacla-

mol also increases brain turnover of dopamine in animals (556, 557), inhibits the dopamine-stimulated increase in olfactory tubercle (556) and striatal (558) adenylate cyclase activity, increases the affinity of tyrosine hydroxylase for pteridine cofactor in striatum and nucleus accumbens *in vivo* (559), increases rat striatal HVA (560), and inhibits the electrically stimulated release of [^{3}H]-dopamine from rat striatal slices *in vitro* (147). Butaclamol is also effective in schizophrenic patients (561), although it does not seem to offer a striking advantage over other antipsychotics and causes a high incidence of EPS (562, 563). Further, pharmacological (564, 565) and biochemical (147, 556, 559, 560) studies demonstrate that the neuroleptic activity of butaclamol (56.**166m**) and some of its close congeners e.g., its isopropyl homolog (dexaclamol, 56 **166j**), resides exclusively in the (+) enantiomers. The (+) enantiomer of dexaclamol

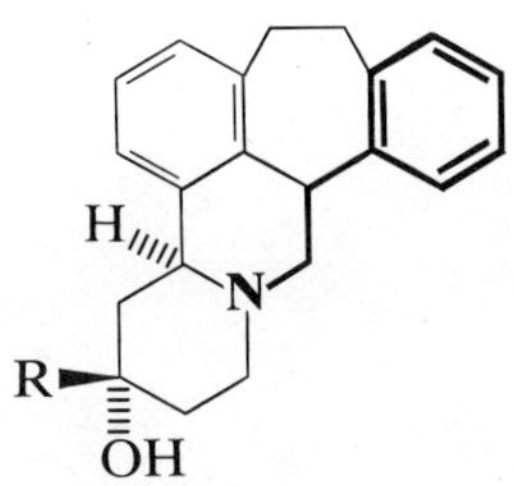

56.**167**

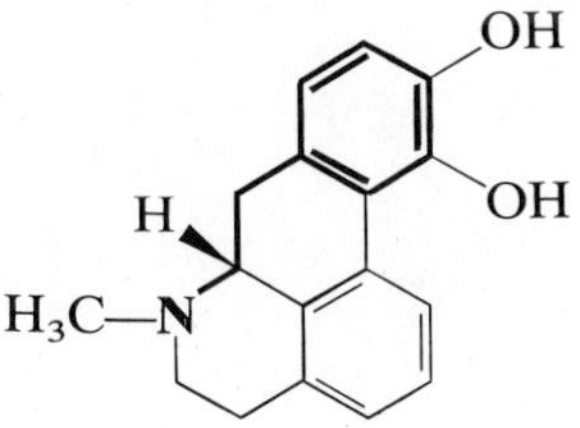

56.**168**

is equipotent with butaclamol in the anti-apomorphine test; (+)-butaclamol is twice as potent as its racemate. The active isomers have a (3*S*,4a*S*,13b*S*) absolute configuration. Quantitative conformational analyses reveal a striking similarity in the distances between the nitrogen and the phenyl ring plane of the extended phenethylamine moieties of (3*S*,4a*S*,13b*S*)-(+)-butaclamol (56.**167**) and (6a*R*)-(−)-apomorphine (56.**168**) (566), a dopaminergic agent with absolute optical specificity toward the receptor (567). This observation suggests a similar mode of interaction of these ligands with a common primary binding site on the dopamine receptor and the location of possible accessory binding sites (564). Using dexaclamol as a probe ligand to the receptor, the conformation of compounds covering several different classes of dopamine receptor antagonists has been studied (568).

4.4 Butyrophenones and Related Compounds

Haloperidol (56.**3a**) is the prototype of a group of butyrophenone derivatives having very potent and specific antipsychotic activ-

ity. The general class of butyrophenone antipsychotics has been the subject of several structure–activity relationship reviews (185, 452, 453). Two members of this class of neuroleptic compounds, spiroperidol and benperidol (Table 56.11), are the most potent agents of this kind presently known (571). Many of the more than 5000 compounds studied in this general class exhibit neuropharmacological properties typical of most neuroleptics (569). More than 20 of these compounds have been studied for antipsychotic properties in humans.

The CI values for some of these compounds are presented in Table 56.11 (569). Considerable variation in these values, as well as onset and duration of activity, is the result of different test methods, animal species, and routes of administration. One test in which major discrepancies are noted for the neuroleptic butyrophenones is the inhibition of dopamine-sensitive adenylate cyclase procedure (572, 573). Although butyrophenone neuroleptics, such as haloperidol, are weaker than chlorpromazine in inhibiting the dopamine-sensitive cyclase, *in vivo* behavioral and clinical data show them to be considerably more potent (569). This striking variation, so apparent in the discussion of structure–activity relationships of tricyclic antipsychotics, emphasizes that *it is critically important to understand the test method.* Some of the more generally employed pharmacological tests for this series of compounds are the jumping-box test in dogs and rats (574), inhibition of apomorphine-induced emesis in dogs (278), the anti-amphetamine test in rats (164), and an assay for α-adrenoreceptor blockade, an antinorepinephrine test in rats (279).

The most potent neuroleptics in this series are 4-aminobutyrophenones [ArCO(CH$_2$)$_3$NR] in which the aryl group (Ar) is optimally a 4-fluorophenyl, the bridge between the benzoyl and amino groups is an unbranched propylene, and NR is a 4-substituted piperidinyl, tetrahydropyridyl, or piperazinyl group. Greatest potency is noted for tertiary amines, but

Table 56.11 CI Values for Some Butyrophenones in Several Pharmacological Tests[a]

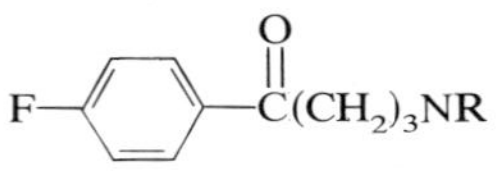

$$F-C_6H_4-\overset{\displaystyle O}{\overset{\|}{C}}-(CH_2)_3NR$$

| Compound | NR | Jumping-Box Test[b,c] | | Dog | | | | Rat | |
| | | | | Apomorphine Test[c,d] Peak Effect, hr | | | Jumping-Box Test[c,e] | Anti-amphetamine Test[c,f] | Antinor-epinephrine Test[c,g] |
		Oral[a]	Subcutaneous	Potency	Onset	Duration			
Haloperidol	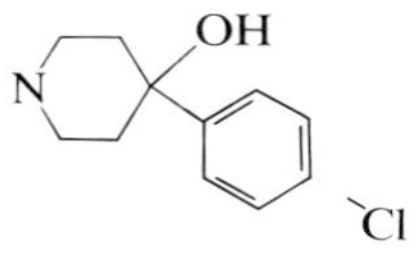	50	50	47	$<\frac{1}{2}$	6	17	35	$\frac{1}{4}$
Spiroperidol	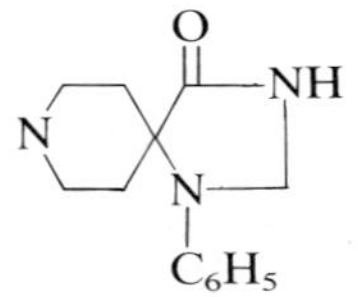	500	500	2800	4	8	100	33	$\frac{1}{2}$
Benperidol	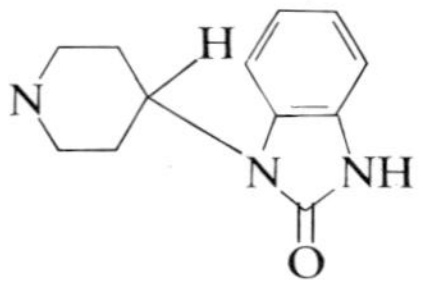	500	500	1400	$\frac{3}{4}$	2	33	33	1.6
Droperidol	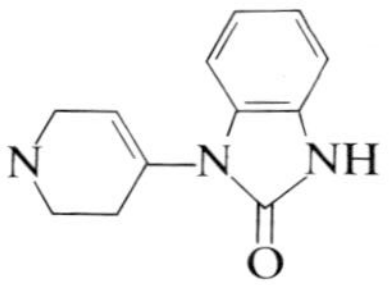	250	250	700	$<\frac{1}{2}$	2	33	33	5
Trifluperidol	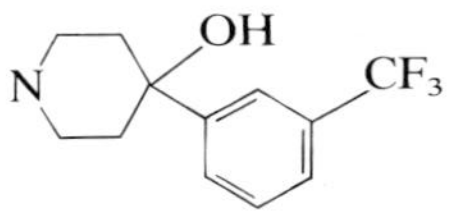	50	50	140	$\frac{3}{4}$	3	33	33	1.6

Compound								
Methylperidol	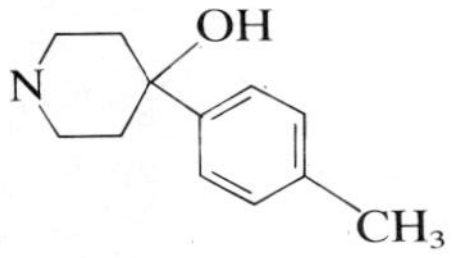 17	25	47	$\frac{3}{4}$	4	10	33	$\frac{1}{2}$
Paraperidide	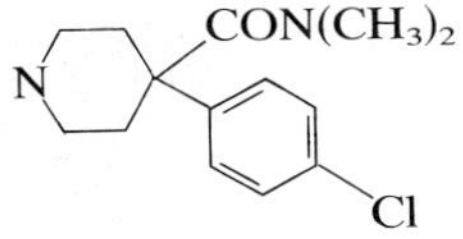 50	25	70	$<\frac{1}{2}$	6	5	10	$\frac{1}{14}$
Haloperidide	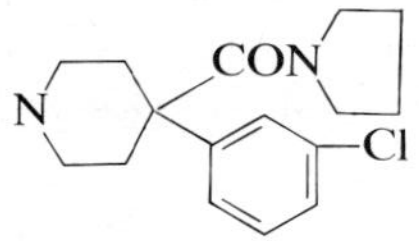 8	42	350	$<\frac{1}{2}$	12	5	10	$\frac{1}{20}$
Methylperidide	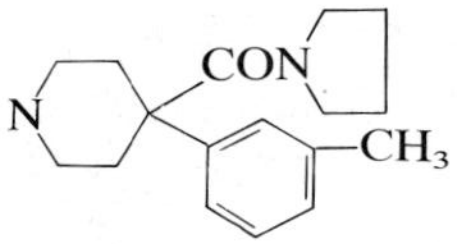 5	125	350	$<\frac{1}{2}$	6	10	10	$\frac{1}{10}$
Butropipazone	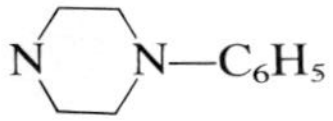 1.6	$\frac{5}{8}$	$\frac{1}{2}$	$\frac{3}{4}$	1.5	$\frac{1}{2}$	1	3
Fluanisone	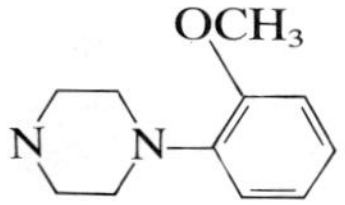 5	12	5	$<\frac{1}{2}$	2	3	3	8
Floropipamide	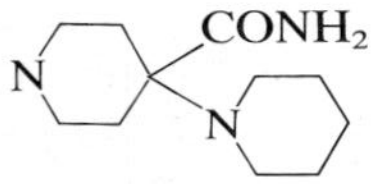 2.5	1.2	$\frac{1}{2}$	$<\frac{1}{2}$	4	$\frac{1}{10}$	$\frac{1}{5}$	$\frac{1}{5}$

Table 56.11 (*Continued*)

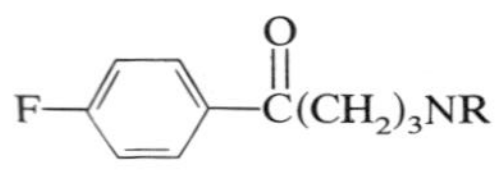

$$F{-}C_6H_4{-}\overset{\displaystyle O}{\overset{\|}{C}}(CH_2)_3NR$$

Compound	NR	Dog						Rat	
		Jumping-Box Test[b,c]		Apomorphine Test[c,d] Peak Effect, hr			Jumping-Box Test[c,e]	Anti-amphetamine Test[c,f]	Antinorepinephrine Test[c,g]
		Oral[a]	Subcutaneous	Potency	Onset	Duration			
Anisoperidone[h]	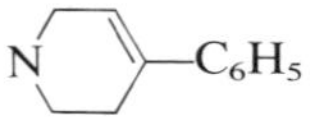 $N{-}C_6H_5$ (tetrahydropyridine)	$\frac{1}{8}$	$<\frac{1}{30}$	$\frac{1}{2}$	$<\frac{1}{2}$	$\frac{3}{4}$	$\frac{1}{2}$	1	1.5
Aceperone	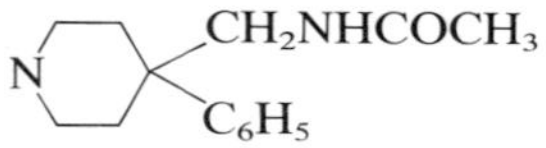 N (piperidine) $CH_2NHCOCH_3$, C_6H_5	$\frac{1}{2}$	$\frac{1}{8}$	1	$<\frac{1}{2}$	3	$\frac{1}{10}$	$\frac{1}{160}$	$\frac{1}{2}$
Chlorpromazine		1	1	1	$\frac{3}{4}$	1.5	1	1	1

[a] Data from Ref. 569.

[b] Trained dogs are required to cross a hurdle when presented with an auditory warning signal to avoid shock. The efficacy of compound in producing avoidance is determined (574).

[c] Relative potency compared (ED$_{50}$ mg/kg) with chlorpromazine, which is arbitrarily assigned a value of 1.

[d] Dogs administered subcutaneously doses of experimental compounds are challenged with an emetic dose of apomorphine at various time intervals thereafter. Inhibition of emesis, onset, and duration of effect are determined (278).

[e] Experimental compounds are administered subcutaneously to rats. The experimental procedure is the same for dogs.

[f] Ability of subcutaneously administered compounds to inhibit compulsory gnawing and chewing responses to in intravenous dose of 10 mg/kg of amphetamine is determined (164).

[g] Ability of subcutaneously administered compounds to prevent lethality of 1.25 mg/kg (i.v.) of norepinephrine 1 hr after drug is determined (278).

[h] The 4′-F substituent of the butyrophenone is replaced by CH$_3$O.

a few secondary amines are also active. Chemical modifications influencing antipsychotic potency are (1) the nature and substitution of the aryl group, (2) variation of the carbonyl functionality, (3) alteration of the propylene bridge, and (4) changes involving the basic amino group.

4.4.1 VARIATIONS INVOLVING THE ARYL

GROUP. All butyrophenones that have been studied clinically for antipsychotic activity, with the exception of anisoperidone (Table 56.11), bear a para-fluoro substituent on the benzoyl group. Significantly, in all tests except the rat anti-epinephrine test, anisoperidone is markedly less potent than haloperidol. The unsubstituted benzoyl derivative of anisoperidone, i.e., 4-(4-phenyl-1,2,3,6-tetrahydropyridyl)butyrophenone (peridol), is about 16 times more potent than anisoperidone, but 16 times less potent than haloperidol, in the rat jumping-box test (575).

Following the discovery that 4-(4-hydroxy-4-phenylpiperidinyl)butyrophenone (56.**169**, X = Y = H) is a powerful CNS depressant, a variety of congeners bearing substituents in the benzoyl and 4-phenylpiperidinyl groups was examined (576). In all instances the 4'-fluoro derivatives (56.**169**, X = 4'-F) are 2.3–3.3 times more potent than corresponding unsubstituted compounds in a pentobarbital-potentiation test in mice, a test in which haloperidol is 5.2 times more potent than chlorpromazine. Substitution of the piperidinyl phenyl group increases potency further in the following order: 56.**169**, Y = H < 4-F < 4-Cl < 4-CH$_3$ (576). Other substitutions of this kind that give compounds with potent neuroleptic actions are illustrated by

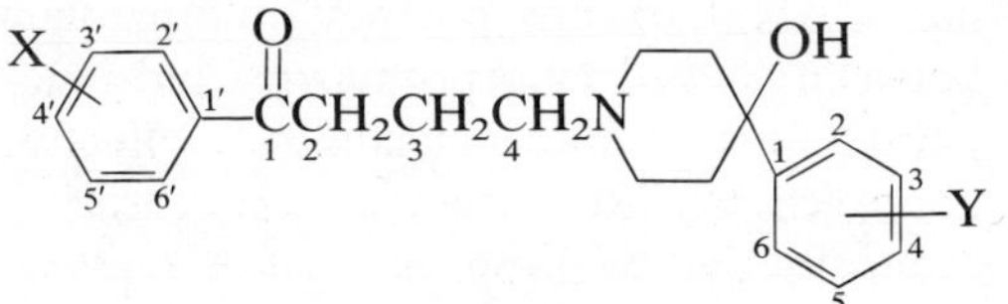

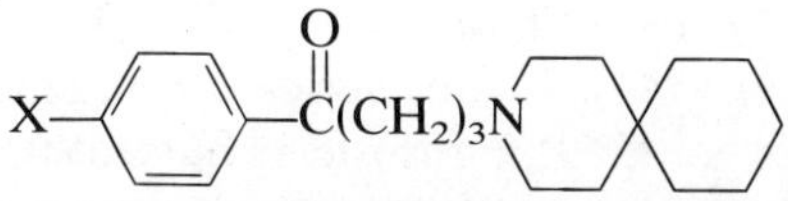

56.**170a** X = F
56.**170b** X = H
56.**170c** X = CH$_3$O

bromoperidol (56.**169**, X = 4'-F, Y = 4-Br) (577, 578), and trifluperidol (56.**169**, X = 4'-F, Y = 3-CF$_3$), both of which have CI values of 62.5 in the dog jumping-box test, s.c. Clofluperol (56.**169**, X = 4'-F, Y = 3-CF$_3$, 4-Cl) is 125 times more potent than chlorpromazine in this test (185). A compound of particular interest in that it involves additional substitution of the benzoyl group is 56.**169** (X = 2'-NH$_2$, 4'-F, Y = 3-CF$_3$); it is more potent than its 2'-unsubstituted counterpart, trifluperidol, in a number of neuroleptic tests (579).

Among a series of azaspiranylbutyrophenones (56.**170**) maximum neuroleptic potency is also noted for the 4'-fluoro derivative 56.**170a**, although the unsubstituted 56.**170b** and 4'-methoxy 56.**170c** derivatives retain some CNS-depressant activity (580).

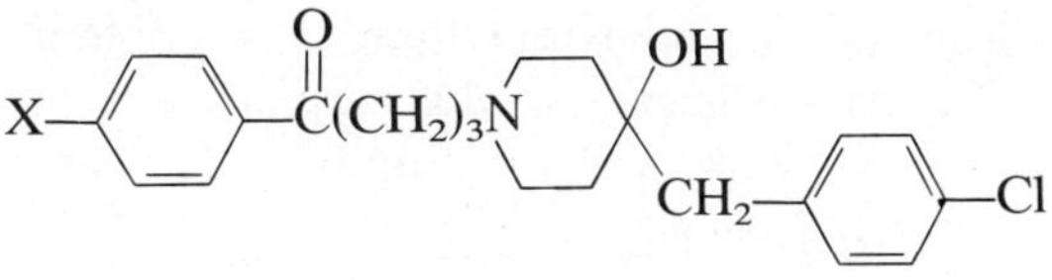

56.**171** X = H, F, Cl, Br, CH$_3$, CH$_3$O

In a series of 4-(4-benzyl-4-hydroxypiperidinyl)butyrophenones (56.**171**), a 4'-fluoro substituent is optimal for neuroleptic activity; 56.**171** (X = F) is intermediate in potency between haloperidol and chlorpromazine in blocking a CAR in rats and in protecting against amphetamine-induced toxicity in mice. Potency is significantly decreased in the unsubstituted derivative 56.**171** (X = H) as well as in the chloro, bromo, methyl, and methoxyl congeners

56.**169**

56.**171** (X = Cl, Br, CH$_3$, CH$_3$O, respectively) (581). In this series, as is generally observed (569), an isosteric butyrothienone is less potent than the corresponding butyrophenone (581).

The neuroleptic-potency-enhancing effect of a 4′-fluoro substituent is also noted in butyrophenone derivatives of 4-phenyl-1-substituted isonipecotic esters 56.**172**. Comparison of mydriatic versus analgetic data in mice (582) indicates that these compounds have a chlorpromazine-like profile (583); i.e., "analgesia" is produced at doses that do not cause mydriasis (584). In this test, the CI for "analgetic" potency of 4′-substituted derivatives (56.**172**) is X = F, 1,1; X = H, 0.62; X = Cl, CH$_3$, CH$_3$O < 0.04. A 2-thienyl congener has a CI of 0.77, but produces mydriasis at about three times the "analgetic" dose.

Even more comprehensive data relative to the influence of substitution of the benzoyl moiety on morphine-like analgesia are available for a corresponding series of lower homologous propiophenones 56.**173**. In this series, maximum analgetic potency is seen with the unsubstituted compound. The order of decreasing potency is as follows: H > F > CH$_3$ > Cl > NO$_2$ ≈ OCH$_3$ ≈ OH ≈ Br ≈ piperidine. In all cases meta isomers are about four times more potent than para isomers. Alkyl groups larger than methyl and polysubstitution decrease analgetic potency (585, 586).

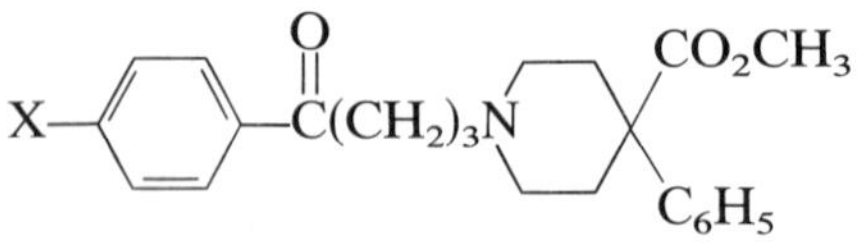

4.4.2 VARIATIONS INVOLVING THE CARBONYL GROUP. In general, modification of the carbonyl group of butyrophenones results in a marked decrease in neuroleptic potency. A series of diarylbutylamines, i.e., butyrophenones in which the carbonyl group is replaced by an aryl moiety, are an exception. A few members of this class are very potent and long-acting antipsychotics.

The CI values for several carbonyl-modified congeners of spiroperidol in jumping-box and anti-apomorphine tests in dogs (278) are summarized in Table 56.12.

Olefinic (spirilene), phenoxy (spiramide), and benzodioxanyl (spiroxatrine) congeners are all less potent than spiroperidol although they retain a high degree of activity with a rapid onset and relatively short duration. Spiroxatrine also has marked analgetic activity. The three spiroperidol congeners are unusually specific in blocking apomorphine- and amphetamine-induced effects as compared to norepinephrine antagonist activity (363).

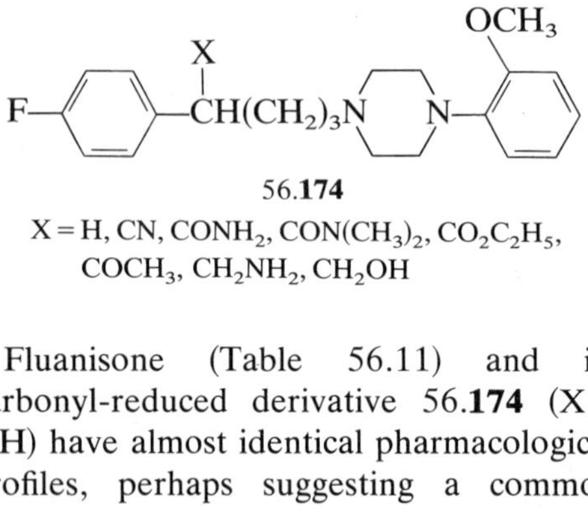

56.**174**

X = H, CN, CONH$_2$, CON(CH$_3$)$_2$, CO$_2$C$_2$H$_5$, COCH$_3$, CH$_2$NH$_2$, CH$_2$OH

Fluanisone (Table 56.11) and its carbonyl-reduced derivative 56.**174** (X = OH) have almost identical pharmacological profiles, perhaps suggesting a common metabolic product. In a series of related compounds maximum neuroleptic potency is seen with the nitrile 56.**174** (X = CN) (587).

The azaspiranylbutyrophenone 56.**175a** has CAR blocking potency intermediate between that of chlorpromazine and haloperidol in rats and is a clinically effective antipsychotic. Reduction of the carbonyl group to give 56.**175b**, as well as replacement by oxygen (56.**175c**) or sulfur

56.**172**   X = H, F, Cl, CH$_3$, CH$_3$O

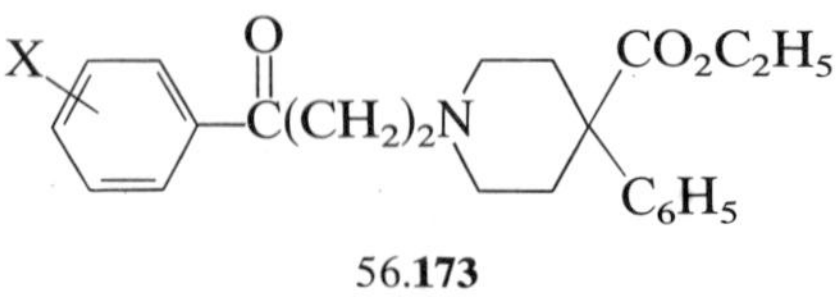

56.**173**

X = H, F, CH$_3$, Cl, NO$_2$, CH$_3$O, HO, Br, c-C$_5$H$_{10}$N

Table 56.12 CI Values for Spiroperidol and Some Carbonyl-Modified Congeners in Dogs (278)

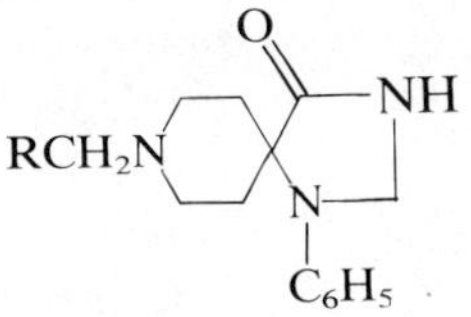

Compound	R	Anti-apomorphine Test[a]	Jumping-Box Test[b]
Spiroperidol	4-FC$_6$H$_4$CO(CH$_2$)$_2$	2800	500
Spirilene	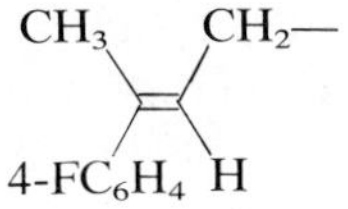 (CH$_3$, 4-FC$_6$H$_4$)C=CH(CH$_2$—)H	280	50
Spiramide	4-FC$_6$H$_4$O(CH$_2$)$_2$	280	167
Spiroxatrine	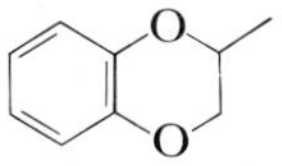 (benzodioxane structure)	140	83

[a] CI as antagonist of apomorphine-induced emesis in dogs, s.c. (278).
[b] CI of s.c. administered compound in a dog jumping-box test (574).

(56.**175d**), decreases neuroleptic potency, whereas replacement of the ketone by a sulfone (56.**175e**) results in a loss or CNS-depressant activity (580). Sulfoxides (588, 589) related to haloperidol and spiroperidol (Table 56.12) are claimed to have antipsychotic activity.

A thianaphthene derivative 56.**176**, in which the butyrophenone carbonyl group is replaced by the heterocyclic double bond, is claimed (590) to have neuroleptic potency equivalent to that of chlorpromazine. Another thianaphthene derivative 56.**177**

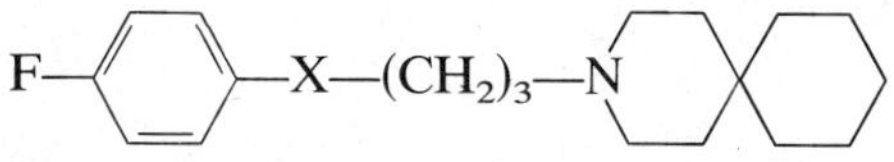

56.**175**

a X = C = O
b X = CHOH
c X = O
d X = S
e X = SO$_2$

has *in vitro* binding characteristics (calf caudate nuclei homogenate) and dopamine and haloperidol displacement properties similar to those of known neuroleptics, but it is inactive in a rat CAR test (591). Potent neuroleptic action is also claimed for 56.**178**, a compound bearing a structural relationship to 56.**176** and spiroxatrine (Table 56.12). This benzofuran derivative is a clinically effective antipsychotic (592, 593). Neuroleptic activity resides in the R-(−) isomer 56.**178** (594). Comparison of such chiral dopamine antagonists with each other and with chiral dopamine agonists may offer an improved understanding of the mode of interaction of these agents with their receptors (564).

The most effective members of a series of butyrophenone-related (ketone reduced) 8-azaspiro[4,5]decane-7,9-diones are 56.**179a–c**. These compounds are more potent than chlorpromazine in blocking a

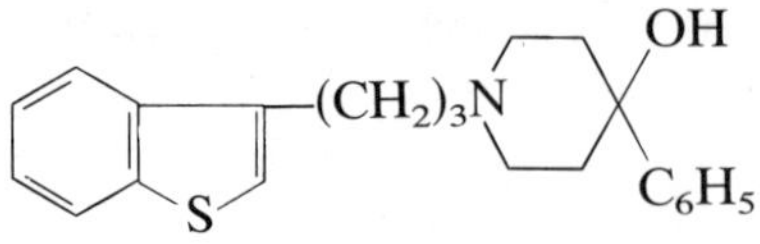

56.**176**

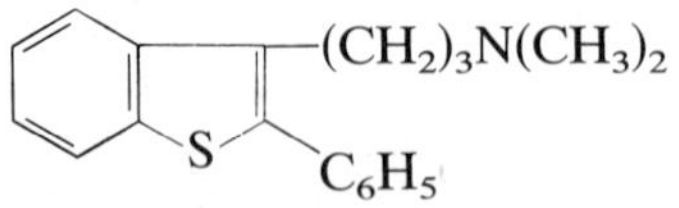

56.**177**

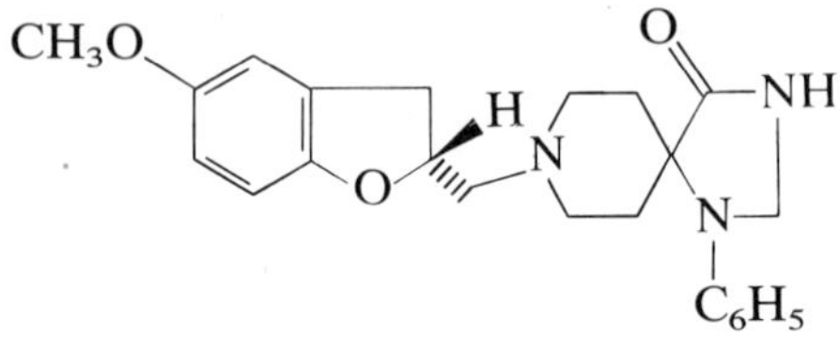

56.**178**

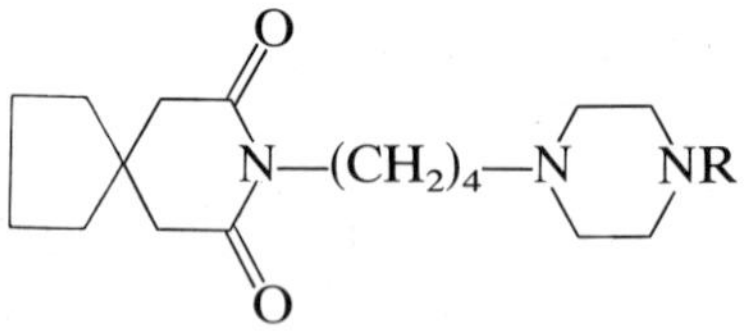

56.**179a** R =

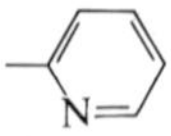

56.**179b** R =

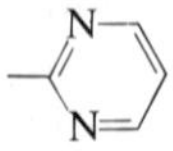

56.**179c** R =

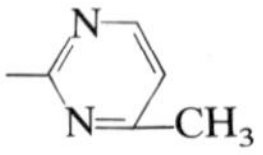

CAR in rats and causing tranquilizing effects in monkeys (595). The 2-pyrimidyl derivative 56.**179b** is of special interest because its potent neuroleptic actions are accompanied by only mild sedation, hypothermia, analgesia, and α-adrenoreceptor blocking effects (596). It produces short-lasting antipsychotic activity in the clinic (597).

Another distant butyrophenone analog 56.**180**, in which the keto group is replaced by an imidazolone moiety, displays clinical antipsychotic activity with a relatively high incidence of EPS (598). A somewhat related compound, in which the

butyrophenone carbonyl is incorporated into an oxazolone ring, is 56.**181**, which antagonizes amphetamine- and apomorphine-induced stereotypy and causes catalepsy (599). The benzimidazolone domperidone (56.**182**) is a potent antinauseant which, unlike many other antiemetics, does not provoke EPS or adverse adrenolytic effects (600, 601).

A particularly interesting class of butyrophenone derivatives is the diarylbutylamines. These may be viewed as butyrophenones in which the ketone is replaced by an aryl group. Thus pimozide (56.**183a**) may be regarded as an analog of benperidol (Table 56.11). It is the prototype of a series of diarylbutylamines which have many structure–activity relationships in common with the butyrophenones (184, 185). In general, structural requirements for a high order of neuroleptic potency in the diarylbutylamines are (1) the presence of a para-fluoro substituent on both phenyl rings, (2) an unbranched propylene bridge between the basic nitrogen and the benzhydryl moiety, and (3) a properly substituted piperidine ring (185). Pimozide (CI = 15.6 in dog CAR test s.c.) is less potent than benperidol in several neuroleptic tests. It is long-acting and relatively nontoxic (602). It is also a clinically effective antipsychotic (603); however, it offers no marked advantage over currently available agents (177). Some of the congeners 56.**183b–d** of pimozide (56.**183a**) are also potent, long-acting antipsychotics. They illustrate the similarity in structure–activity relationships between the diarylbutylamines and butyrophenones. For example, penfluridol

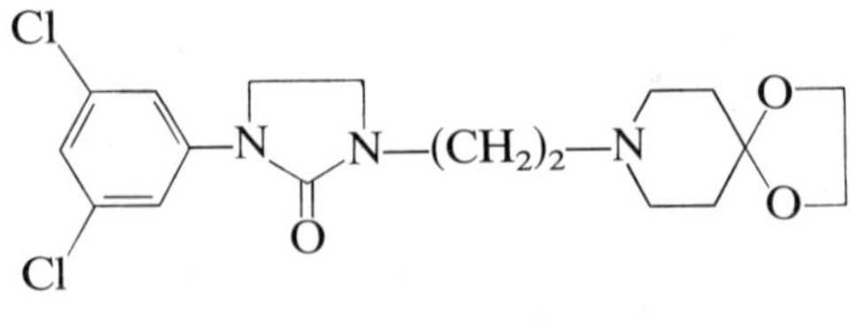

56.**180**

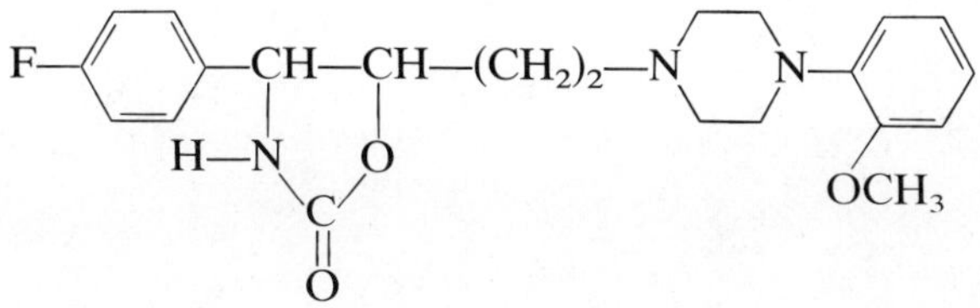

56.**181**

(56.**183b**), a congener of the butyrophenone clofluperol (56.**169**, X = 4'-F; Y = 4-CF$_3$, 4-Cl), is a potent long-acting neuroleptic effective clinically following a single weekly oral dose (604); it rarely causes extrapyramidal effects (605). Clopimozide (56.**183c**) has an even longer duration of action than pimozide (606). Fluspirilene (56.**183d**), an analog of the butyrophenone spiroperidol (Table 56.11), is an extremely potent neuroleptic (607). A single weekly dose of fluspirilene is equal to, or more effective than, a daily dose of haloperidol in schizophrenic patients (608).

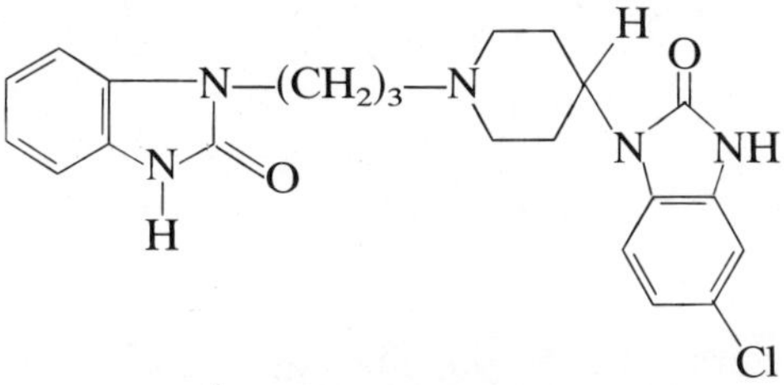

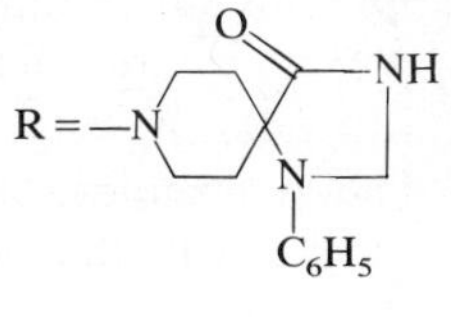

Cyclic analogs of the diarylbutylamines, e.g., 56.**184**, lack significant neuroleptic activity (609).

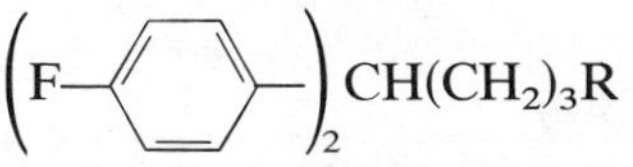

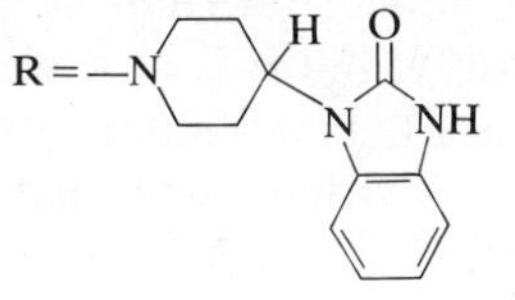

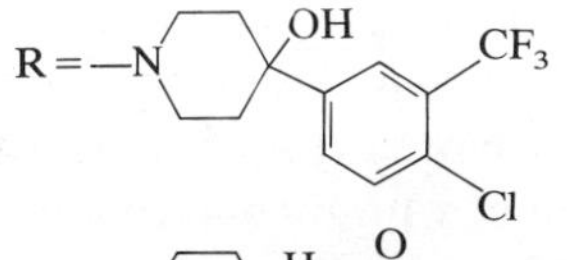

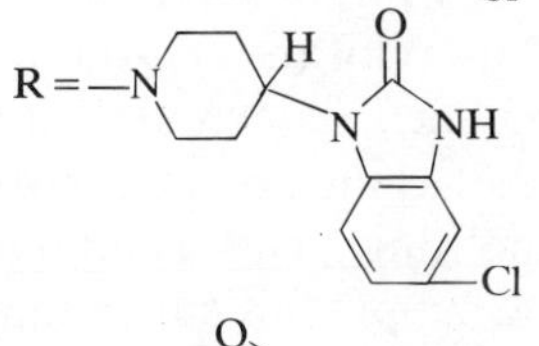

Structure–activity relationship studies indicate that in the diarylbutylamine series a benzhydrylic hydrogen is required for neuroleptic potency (184). A fully substituted benzhydrylic carbon coupled with a lower homologous side chain affords a potent analgetic bezitramide (56.**185**) (610).

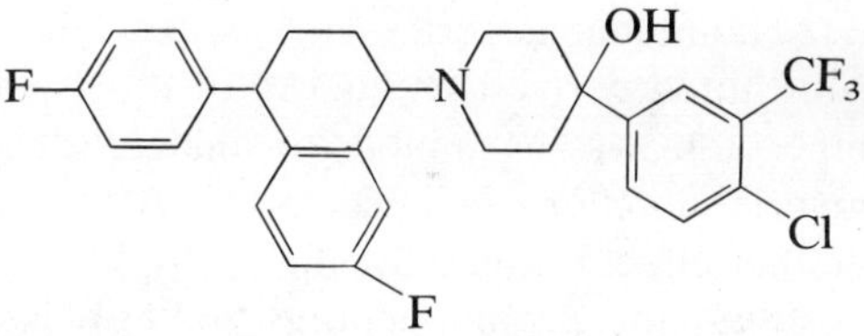

56.**182**

56.**183**

a   R =

b   R =

c   R =

d   R =

56.**184**

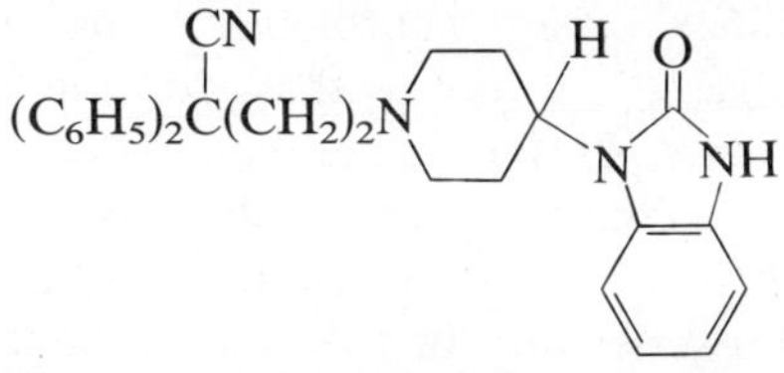

56.**185**

4.4.3 ALTERATION OF THE PROPYLENE CHAIN. As a rule, shortening, lengthening, or branching of the propylene chain of 4-aminobutyrophenones decreases neuroleptic potency (569). It has been suggested that the similarity of the butyrophenone system to γ-aminobutyric acid (GABA) may be significant (584).

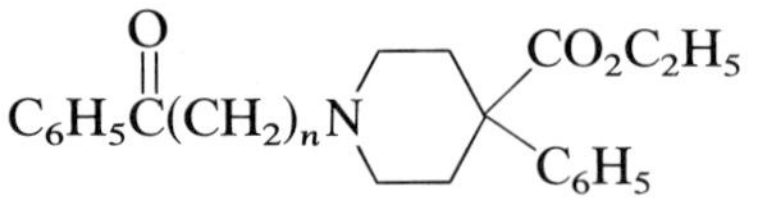

$$C_6H_5\overset{\overset{\displaystyle O}{\|}}{C}(CH_2)_n N \quad \text{(piperidine)} \quad \overset{CO_2C_2H_5}{\underset{C_6H_5}{}}$$

56.**186a** $n = 1$
56.**186b** $n = 2$
56.**186c** $n = 3$
56.**186d** $n = 4$

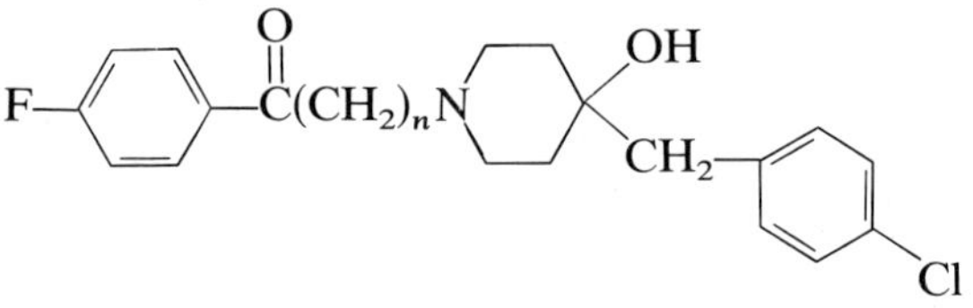

$$F\text{—}C_6H_4\text{—}\overset{\overset{\displaystyle O}{\|}}{C}(CH_2)_n N \quad \text{(piperidine)} \quad \overset{OH}{\underset{CH_2\text{—}C_6H_4\text{—}Cl}{}}$$

56.**187a** $n = 3$
56.**187b** $n = 2$

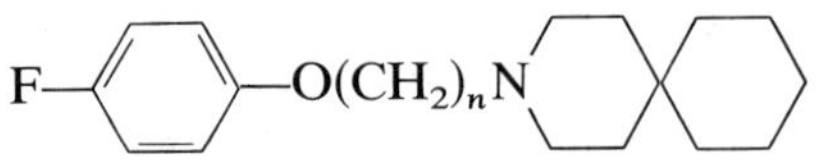

$$F\text{—}C_6H_4\text{—}O(CH_2)_n N \text{(azaspirane)}$$

56.**188** $n = 2\text{–}5$

$$F\text{—}C_6H_4\text{—}\overset{\overset{\displaystyle O}{\|}}{C}CH_2\overset{R}{\underset{}{C}}H\overset{R'}{\underset{}{C}}HCHN \text{(piperidine)}$$

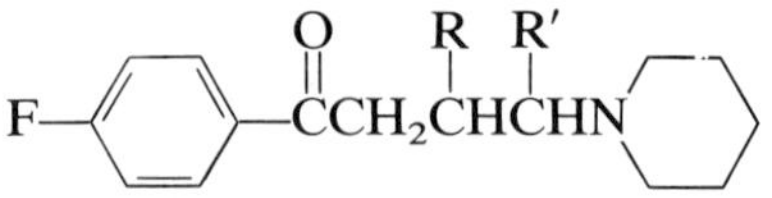

56.**189a**   R = CH$_3$, R′ = H
56.**189b**   R = H, R′ = CH$_3$

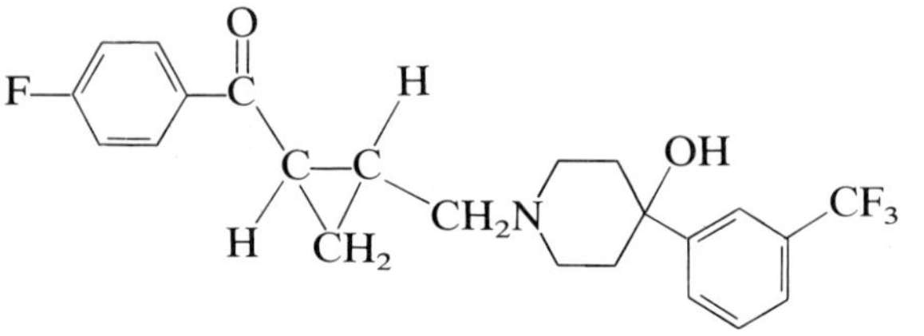

56.**190**

A homologous series of 1-benzoylalkyl-substituted derivatives 56.**186** of ethyl iso-nipecotate was examined for analgetic and mydriatic actions in mice (583). Although neither effect is noted for the acetophenone 56.**186a**, the propiophenone 56.**186b** is a potent analgetic and, depending on ring substitution, butyrophenones (e.g., 58.**186c**) are neuroleptic, producing "analgesia" at doses that do not cause mydriasis. Further lengthening of the alkylene chain 56.**186d** decreases both analgetic and mydriatic potency (583).

In a series of 1-benzoylalkyl-4-benzyl-4-hydroxypiperidines 56.**187**, maximum neuroleptic potency is also noted with a propylene bridge. Thus 56.**187a** has CAR blocking potency intermediate between that of haloperidol and chlorpromazine in rats, whereas the propiophenone 56.**187b** lacks significant activity (581).

Another illustration of the optimum four-atom spacing between the para-fluoro-phenyl and the piperidine nitrogen of

neuroleptics is provided by a homologous series of N-(phenoxyalkyl)azaspiranes 56.**188**. Most potent neuroleptic activity is noted for the propylene congener 56.**188** ($n = 3$) (580).

In a series of methyl-branched 4-amino-butyrophenones, 56.**189a** is more potent than 56.**189b**, but it is only weakly depressant in mice (611). Among analogs of antipsychotic butyrophenones having a cyclopropylmethyl in place of the usual propylene bridge, greatest potency (CI = 10) in a test for depression of motor activity in mice is noted for 56.**190** (trans); it is equipotent with its butyrophenone counterpart trifluperidol (612). Another propylene chain-modified compound is 56.**191**, in which the chain is incorporated into a piperidine ring. This compound blocks a CAR and suppresses amphetamine-induced lethality at doses intermediate between those of chlorpromazine and haloperidol (613, 614). The benzamide 56.**192** (halo-pemide), a side chain isostere of a butyro-

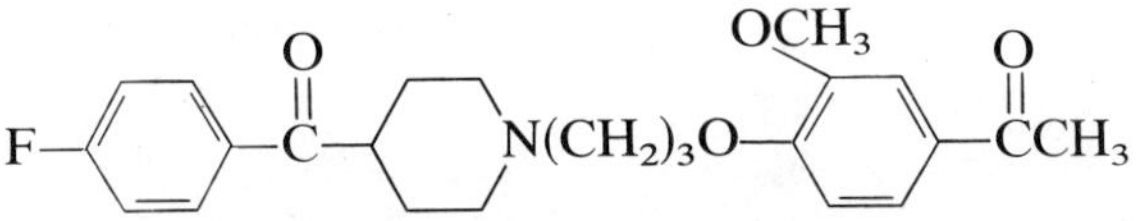

56.**191**

phenone, is a psychotropic agent with a unique clinical and pharmacological profile (615).

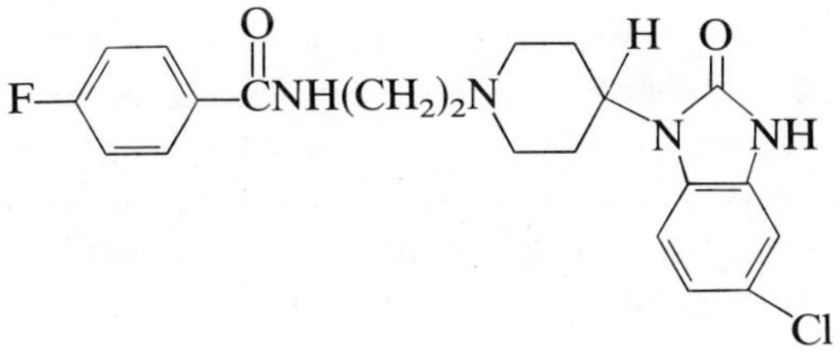

56.**192**

4.4.4   MODIFICATIONS INVOLVING THE BASIC AMINO GROUP.   The nature of amine substitution of a 4-aminobutyrophenone has a significant influence on antipsychotic potency; however, considerable variation is possible with retention of at least some activity. Generally, incorporation of the nitrogen in position 4 of butyrophenones into a six-membered ring, e.g., 4-substituted piperidinyl, 1,2,3,6-tetrahydropyridyl, or piperazinyl derivatives, is optimal for neuroleptic activity. Replacement of the six-membered basic heterocycle by uncyclized amines or by larger or smaller rings usually affords compounds with diminished neuroleptic potency (569).

Antipsychotic activity has been described for only a few 4-aminobutyrophenones in which the amino group is not part of a ring. Several of these are secondary amines. For example, 56.**193a** has a CI of 7–8 in several neuroleptic tests (616). Clinically, 56.**193a** is equally as effective an antipsychotic as haloperidol, but it produces a high incidence of EPS (617–619). Several other secondary 4-aminobutyrophenones, 56.**193b** and 56.**193c**, are considerably more potent than chlorpromazine in behavioral tests in mice (620). The para-fluoro deriva-

tive 56.**193b** resembles both reserpine and haloperidol in its [³H]-norepinephrine-releasing properties in mouse heart and HVA-elevating actions. It differs from reserpine in having only a weak effect on brain serotonin levels and from haloperidol in its effect on catecholamine levels (621). In a related cyclohexyl series, *trans*-56.**193d** is one of the most potent compounds in causing overt neuroleptic symptoms and in blocking norepinephrine and serotonin uptake by mouse heart and spleen preparations. This isomer is more potent than its counterpart *cis*-56.**193d** and about equipotent with 56.**193b** in most tests (620, 622). A related methoxylated compound 56.**193e** is more potent than haloperidol in several behavioral tests in mice and exhibits highly selective blockade of norepinephrine uptake (623).

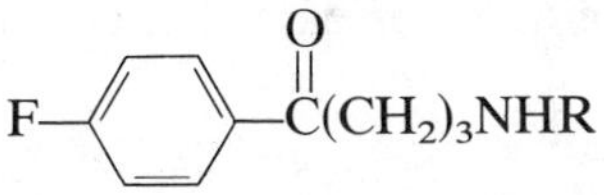

56.**193**

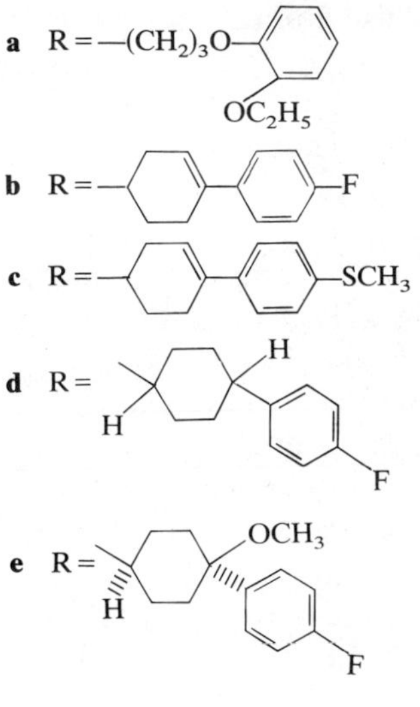

a   R = —(CH₂)₃O— ... OC₂H₅

b   R = ...

c   R = ...SCH₃

d   R = ...

e   R = ...

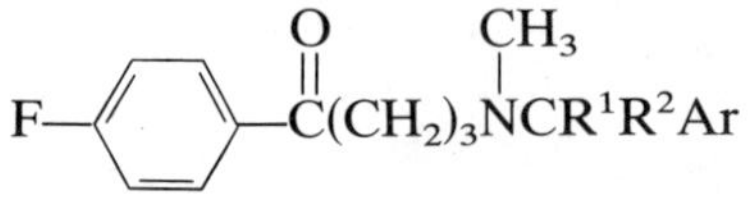

56.**194** $R^1, R^2 = H$ or CH_3
        $Ar = C_6H_5$ or $3,4\text{-}(CH_3O)_2C_6H_3$

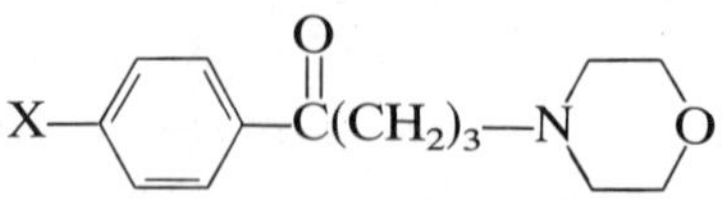

56.**195a** $X = H$
56.**195b** $X = F$

Useful CNS-depressant properties are claimed (624) for some uncyclized tertiary amine derivatives 56.**194** of 4′-fluorobutyrophenone. Although neuroleptic data are not available for simple 4-(dialkylamino)-butyrophenones, several morpholinyl derivatives 56.**195** have antidepressant-like, rather than neuroleptic, properties. Thus 56.**195a**, a monoamine oxidase inhibitor, reverses reserpine-induced actions in animals (625). The 4′-fluoro derivatives, e.g., 56.**195b**, lack CNS-depressant activity (626).

Several 4-aminobutyrophenones in which the basic nitrogen is part of a five-membered ring cause neuroleptic effects. A pyrrolidine 56.**196a** elicits haloperidol-like behavioral effects in mice, rats, and squirrel monkeys (627, 628); however, it is ineffective in schizophrenic patients (629). Some isoindoline derivatives, e.g., 56.**196b**, are very potent depressants of motor activity in mice (630). Another compound in which the basic nitrogen is incorporated into a fused five-membered ring system 56.**196c** produces gross behavioral changes in mice, suggesting CNS-depressant activity (631).

In a series of 4-aminobutyrophenones having the basic nitrogen as part of a seven-membered ring of indolo-fused azepines, 56.**196d** is the most potent in mouse behavioral studies; it is about twice as potent as thioridazine and has a greater therapeutic index (632). In the clinic, however, 56.**196d** is not an effective antipsychotic (633).

4.4.4.1 4-Piperidinylbutyrophenones.

Among 4-piperidinylbutyrophenones, maximum antipsychotic potency results from substitution of position 4 of the piperidine ring, whereas substitution of the 2 or 3 positions markedly decreases potency (569). Changes, such as amide formation or quaternization, that decrease the basicity of the piperidine nitrogen generally abolish activity (580).

Alkyl substitution of position 4 has little effect on potency. For example, the unsubstituted 56.**197a**, mono-, and dialkylated derivatives have comparable CNS-depressant properties. The monomethyl derivative 56.**197b** has neuroleptic potency similar to that of chlorpromazine; however, unlike the prototype, it antagonizes reserpine-induced actions in animals (634, 635). Incorporation of 4,4-dialkylpiperidinyl substituents into a carbocyclic system, e.g., the azaspirane 56.**170a**, significantly enhances potency (580). Several other spiropiperidine carbocyclic and spiropyrrolidine carbocyclic, as well as oxygenated heterocyclic (580) and azabicyclic analogs (630), are similar to 56.**170a**; they are intermediate between chlorprom-

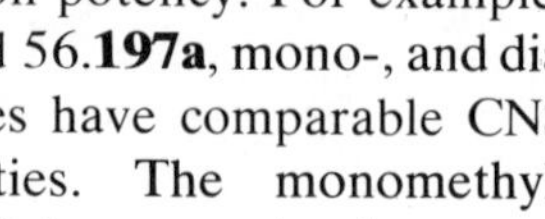

56.**196**

a $R = $

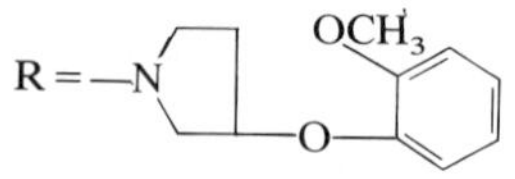

b $R = $

c $R = $

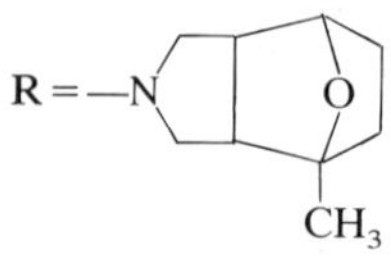

d $R = $

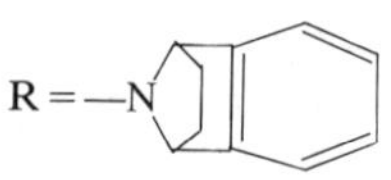

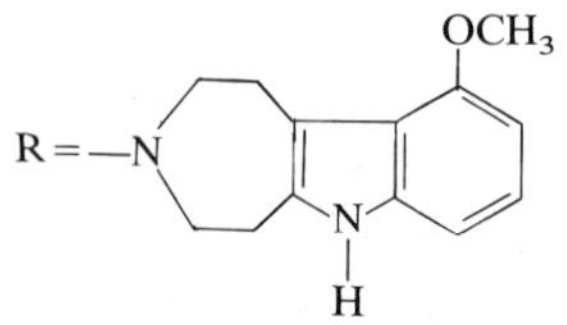

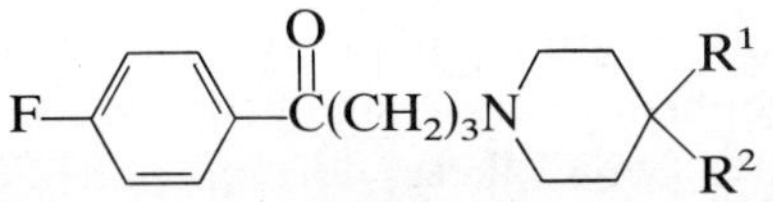

56.**197**

a $R^1 = R^2 = H$
b $R^1 = H$, $R^2 = CH_3$
c $R^1 = H$, $R^2 = OH$
d $R^1 = H$, $R^2 = OCONH-i-C_3H_7$
e $R^1 = H$, $R^2 = COC_6H_4-4-F$
f $R^1 = H$, $R^2 = COC_6H_4-4-Cl$
g $R^1 = H$, $R^2 = N(CH_2C_6H_5)COCH_3$

h $R^1 = H$, $R^2 =$

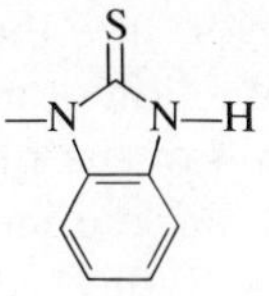

i $R^1 = H$, $R^2 =$

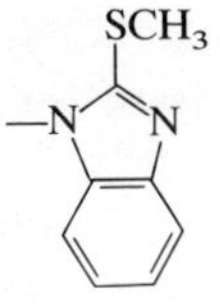

j $R^1 = C_6H_5$, $R^2 = CH_2NHCOCH_3$
k $R^1 = C_6H_5$, $R^2 = CH_2NHCO_2C_2H_5$

l $R^1 =$

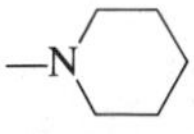

, $R^2 = COC_2H_5$

azine and haloperidol in suppressing a CAR in rats.

A number of other 4-(4-substituted piperidinyl)butyrophenones, particularly derivatives bearing an alcoholic hydroxyl, a substituted benzoyl, a tertiary carboxamide, or an amino group in position 4 of the piperidine ring, are very potent antipsychotic drugs. It is among these compounds that most clinically studied and commercially marketed butyrophenones are found.

Although neuroleptic potency is associated mainly with 4,4-disubstituted piperidines, several monosubstituted derivatives are active. For example, the 4-hydroxylated piperidine 56.**197c** produces overt neuroleptic symptoms in animals; however, it is effective in schizophrenic patients only at higher doses that cause side effects (636). The carbamate 56.**197d** is about one-tenth as potent as trifluperidol in blocking a CAR in mice (637); however, its clinical utility is questionable (638). Several

4-benzoylated piperidines, e.g., 56.**197e** (lenperone) (639) and 156.**197f** (cloperone) (640), have been studied extensively (614). Lenperone is more potent than chlorpromazine, but less potent than haloperidol in selectively blocking a CAR in mice and cats (641). Clinically, lenperone (56.**197e**) is effective in the treatment of schizophrenia (642, 643) and anxiety neurosis (644) with relatively minor side effects (645). The related para-chlorobenzoyl derivative 56.**197f** has antianxiety, antiemetic, analgetic, and β-adrenoreceptor blocking actions without causing side effects associated with many antipsychotics (646). Several acylaminopiperidines, e.g., 56.**197g**, are weak CNS depressants. In a rat CAR test 56.**197g** has a CI of about 0.25 (647). Other 4-(4-monosubstituted piperidinyl) derivatives of 4′-fluorobutyrophenone include the benzimidazolone benperidol (Table 56.11), which is an extremely potent neuroleptic. Neuroleptic actions are also claimed for the corresponding benzimidazoles, benzotriazoles, and benzimidazole-2-thiols, e.g., 56.**197h** (648) and 56.**197i** (649). Animal tests suggest potential neuroleptic activity with decreased EPS liability for 56.**197h** (650, 651).

A high degree of neuroleptic potency is associated with 4-(4-aryl-4-hydroxypiperidinyl)butyrophenones. Included in this category are haloperidol, trifluperidol, and methylperidol (Table 56.11) as well as several other substituted phenyl derivatives (56.**169**) (see Section 4.4.1) (185, 476–479). Only limited data are available regarding the CNS activity when the phenyl substituent of these compounds is replaced by other groups. In general, replacement by a benzyl group affords compounds about one-half as potent as their phenyl counterparts (581).

Some 4-carboxamido-4-phenylpiperidinyl-substituted butyrophenones, e.g., paraperidide, haloperidide, and methylperidide (Table 56.11), have neuroleptic potency comparable to that of corresponding 4-phenyl-4-piperidinols in a jumping-box test in dogs (362). The spirocarboxamido-piperidine derivative 56.**198a** is a potent anticholinergic agent that produces unique clinical antipsychotic actions (652). A related spirooxazolidinone 56.**198b** has a neuroleptic profile more akin to that of chlorpromazine than to that of the somewhat related spiroperidol (Table 56.11) (653), whereas the azaspirane 56.**198c** has CNS-depressant properties (580).

Several 4-phenyl-4-acylaminomethyl-piperidinyl derivatives of butyrophenone, e.g., 56.**197j** (aceperone, Table 56.11), have been studied clinically. Aceperone and its carbamate analog 56.**197k** are relatively weak neuroleptics that produce potent adrenolytic actions (654).

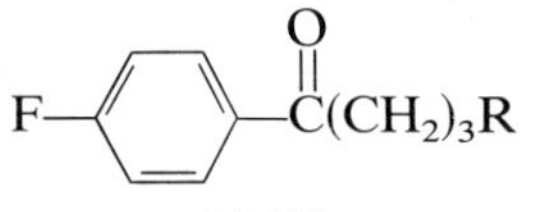

56.**198**

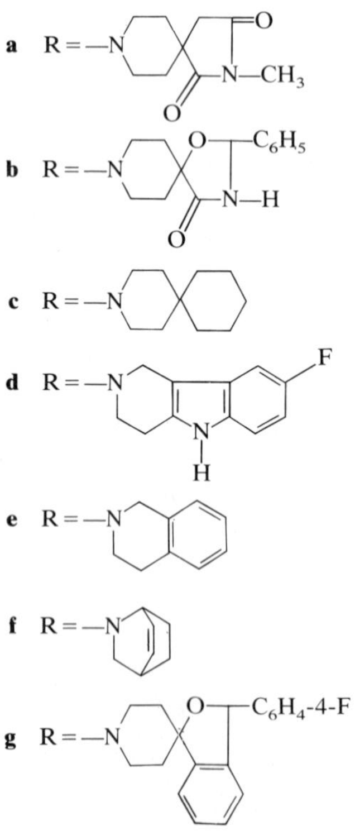

a   R = —N ...

b   R = —N ...

c   R = —N ...

d   R = —N ...

e   R = —N ...

f   R = —N ...

g   R = —N ...

Many 4-aminopiperidinyl derivatives of butyrophenone have significant neuroleptic activity. Two of these, floropipamide (Table 56.11) and floropipetone (56.**197l**), bear a 4-piperidinyl substituent in the piperidine ring. These compounds are less potent than haloperidol on oral administration in a dog jumping-box test (362). In cats, however, 56.**197l** and a series of congeners have CNS-depressant properties that are qualitatively superior to those of haloperidol (655). Introduction of an aniline substituent into position 4 of the piperidine ring generally causes a marked increase in neuroleptic potency. As indicated in Table 56.11, spiroperidol and benperidol, spiro derivatives incorporating an aniline moiety, are extremely potent neuroleptics (569). The carboline (i.e., indolo-fused) derivative 56.**198d** combines neuroleptic properties with analgetic potency approximately equal to that of morphine (656). In contrast, the isoquinoline (i.e., benzo-fused)-substituted butyrophenone 56.**198e** does not produce neuroleptic effects in animals (628). An ethylidene-bridged piperidine derivative 56.**198f** of 4′-fluorobutyrophenone causes CNS-depressant and moderate CAR blocking effects in mice (631). In a series of spiro[isobenzofuran-1(3*H*),4′-piperidines] 56.**198g** is a potent CAR blocker in rats and monkeys, but is ineffective in tests for nonselective dopamine blocking activity, perhaps indicating potential selective antipsychotic activity (657).

4.4.4.2   4-(1,2,3,6-Tetrahydropyridyl)-butyrophenones.

Many tetrahydropyridyl derivatives of butyrophenone have been studied (658) and several of these compounds, e.g., droperidol (569, 659) and anisoperidone (Table 56.11) (569), are clinically effective antipsychotics. Droperidol, the tetrahydropyridyl analog of benperidol, is about one-half as potent as the piperidine in several neuroleptic tests; however, it is somewhat more effective in a norepinephrine antagonism test in rats (569).

4.4.4.3 4-*Piperazinylbutyrophenones.*

High neuroleptic potency among derivatives of 4-piperazinylbutyrophenone generally requires an aromatic substituent in position 4 of the piperazine ring (569). Potency of phenyl-substituted derivatives is further enhanced by an ortho-methoxyl substituent. Thus fluanisone is three times more potent than butropipazone (Table 56.11) in the jumping-box test in dogs (362). A fluanisone homolog 56.**199** in which the 4′-fluoro substituent is replaced by a morpholinyl group is not effective as a clinical antipsychotic (660); however, it has highly potent tranquilizing and sedating properties in rats (661). Substitution of position 4 of the piperazine ring with a 2-pyridyl group (602) affords azaperone (56.**200a**), a compound projected to be a sedative–neuroleptic on the basis of its antiaggressive (CI = 5) and antishock properties in animals (662). A tetralin derivative 56.**200b** (663) has potent neuroleptic actions in mice and rats. A related cyclohexyl carbamate 56.**200c** has a typical neuroleptic profile in mice and rats, and it is equipotent with haloperidol in antagonizing epinephrine-induced mortality (664).

Several piperazine-fused derivatives of butyrophenone also possess significant antipsychotic activity. For example, **azabuperone (azabutirone, 56.201a)** is an effective

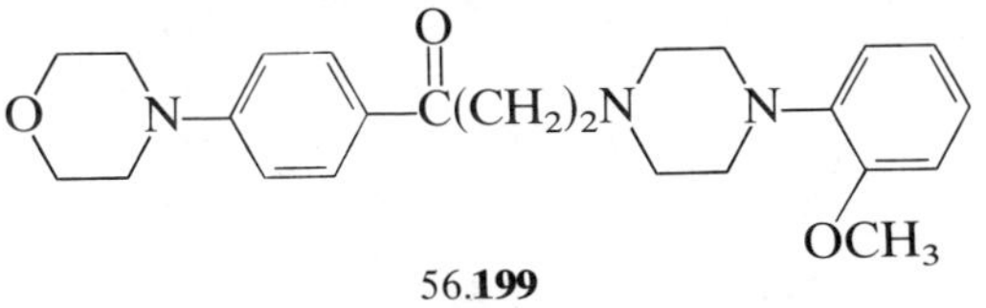

56.**201a** R = —N (bicyclic pyrrolizidine-fused piperazine)

56.**201b** R = —N (tetrahydroisoquinoline-fused piperazine)

56.**201c** R = —N (pyrazinopyridoindole)

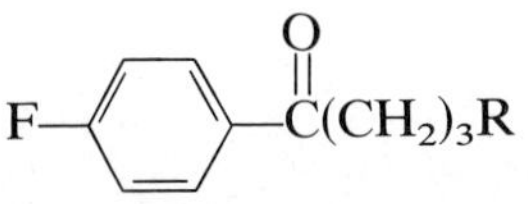

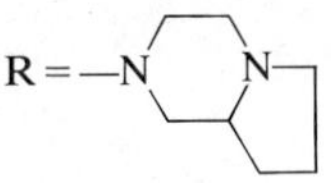

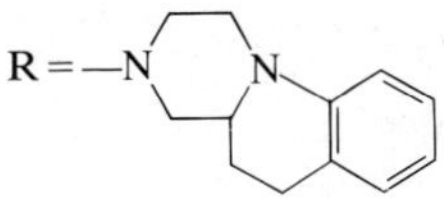

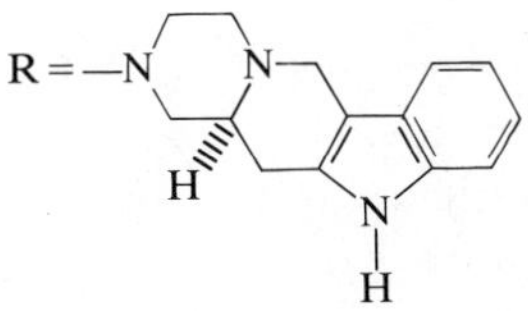

neuroleptic in animal tests and it is utilized clinically in Russia (665). Centpryaquin (56.**201b**) has neuroleptic activity approximately equivalent to that of chlorpromazine in a CAR blockade test. It also has significant hypotensive effects (666, 667). In a series of pyrazino [2′,1′:6,1]pyrido-[3,4-*b*]indoles, 66.**201c** is the most potent compound in a suppression of CAR test (CI = 15) with a prolonged duration of action and minor cardiovascular effects (668).

4.5 Reserpine and Related Compounds

l-Reserpine, or 11,17α-dimethoxy-16β-carbomethoxy-18β-(3,4,5-trimethoxy-benzoyl)-3β,20α-yohimbane, 56.**202** (3, 669, 670), is the principal alkaloid of *Rauwolfia serpentina* and is largely responsible for the neuroleptic and hypotensive properties of the crude extracts of this plant.

Reserpine is now mainly of historical interest in psychiatry and it serves as a pharmacological tool. It is less effective than many other antipsychotics and is generally not used for this purpose, although it may be employed in patients who cannot tolerate other classes of antipsychotics. Today, reserpine and related compounds are used mainly as antihypertensives. The rauwolfia

56.**199**

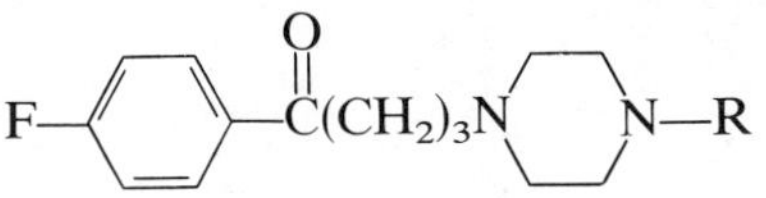

56.**200a** R = 2-pyridyl

56.**200b** R = (tetralin)

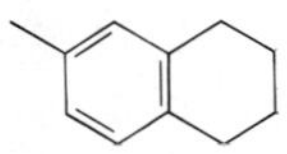

56.**200c** R = CO_2-*c*-C_6H_{11}

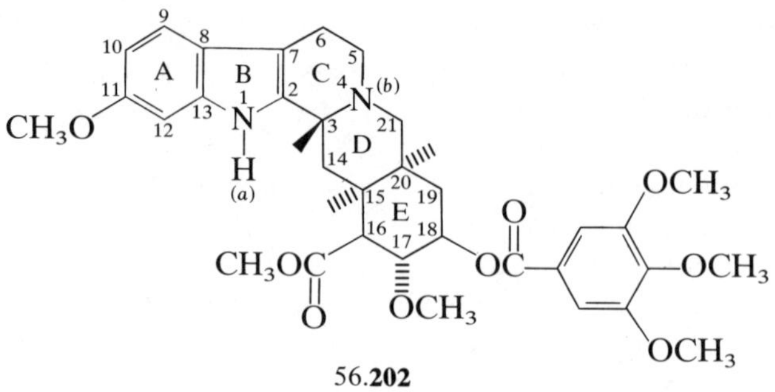

56.**202**

alkaloids and related structures produce their antipsychotic actions by a different mechanism than the neuroleptics discussed to this point. Apparently, these compounds owe their pharmacological actions to a release of biogenic amines from storage sites (771). Thus even structure–activity relationships in this series should be considered as distinct from those of many other classes of antipsychotics.

In a search for more effective and selective antipsychotics, many structural modifications of reserpine have been examined, although during the past decade virtually no research has been conducted in this area. For this reason, a general, rather than comprehensive, treatment of the numerous other rauwolfia alkaloids, synthetic yohimbane derivatives, and simpler compounds related to parts of the reserpine molecule, is presented. The subject is covered more comprehensively in several reviews (125,671–673).

4.5.1 RESERPINE AND OTHER RAUWOLFIA ALKALOIDS. The rauwolfia alkaloids have been classified into four groups; i.e., all yohimbane isomers 56.**203a**, reserpine-type alkaloids (e.g., 56.**203b** and derivatives), ring E heterocyclics (e.g., ajmalicine, 56.**204**) and their anhydronium analogs (e.g., serpentine, 56.**205**), and ajmaline-type alkaloids (56.**205**).

In this class, neuroleptic activity is noted only in the reserpine-type alkaloids, i.e., derivatives of 56.**203b**. Reserpine has six asymmetric centers and thus 64 possible stereoisomers. Only 56.**202** has appreciable neuroleptic activity (125). Even close congeners (674, 675) of 56.**203a** lack reserpine-like activity.

Seven additional rauwolfia alkaloids of the reserpine-type, i.e., derivatives of

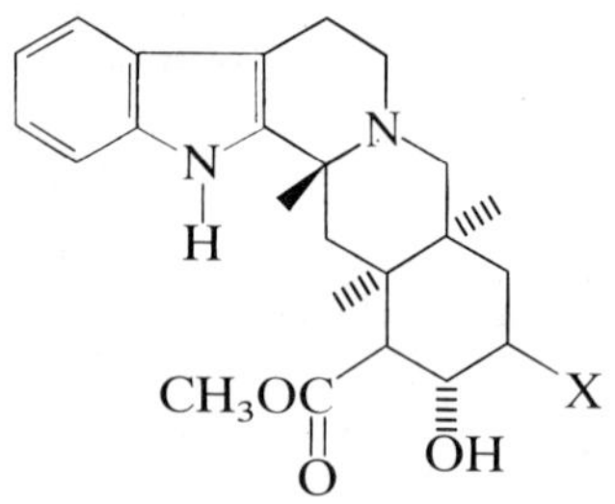

56.**203a**   X = H
56.**203b**   X = OH

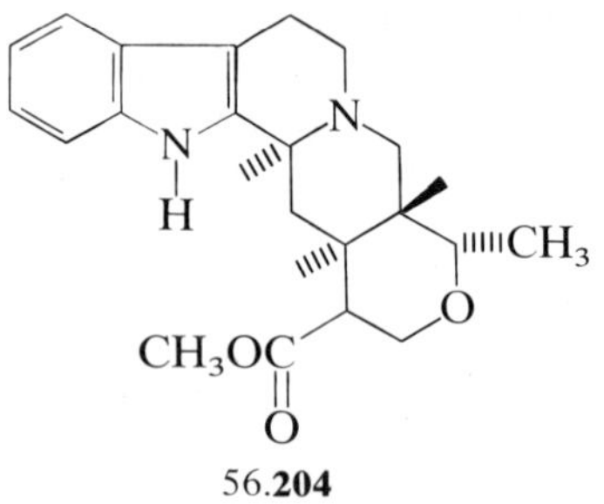

56.**204**

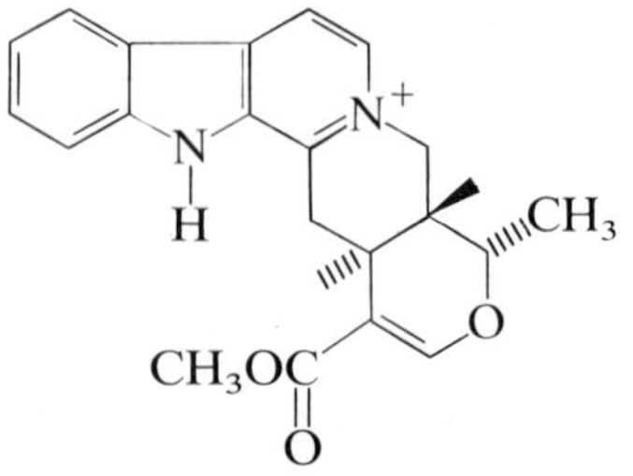

56.**205**

Table 56.13 Reserpine-Type Alkaloids

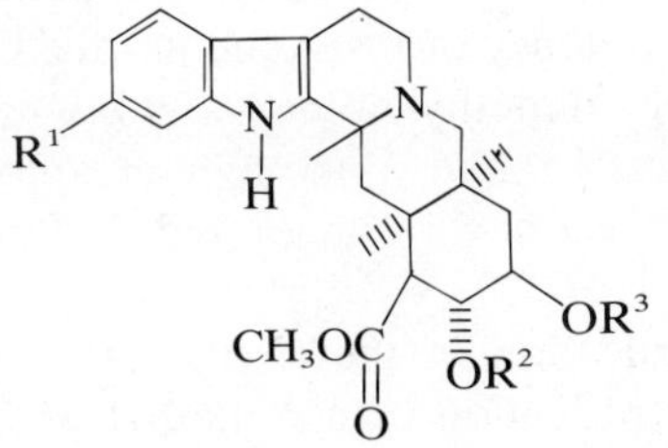

Alkaloid	R^1	R^2	R^3	Ref.
Deserpidine	H	CH_3	TMB^a	676
Raunescine	H	H	TMB^a	677
Isoraunescine	H	TMB^a	H	677
Pseudoreserpine	CH_3O	H	TMB^a	678
Raugustine	CH_3O	TMB^a	H	679
Rescinnamine	CH_3O	CH_3	TMC^b	680
Rescidine	CH_3O	H	TMC^b	681

^{a} TMB = $3,4,5\text{-}(CH_3O)_3C_6H_2CO-$.
^{b} TMC = $trans\text{-}3,4,5\text{-}(CH_3O)_3C_6H_2CH{=}CHCO-$.

56.**203b**, are listed in Table 56.13. Deserpidine is equipotent with reserpine, and rescinnamine is a somewhat less potent neuroleptic agent. Raunescine and pseudoreserpine retain weak neuroleptic activity (671). The other reserpine-type alkaloids (isoraunescine, raugustine, and rescidine) have little or no neuroleptic potency (125). These data suggest the 17-ether group, but not the 11-methoxyl, of reserpine is required for this kind of activity.

4.5.2 SYNTHETIC YOHIMBANE DERIVATIVES RELATED TO RESERPINE. Many synthetic yohimbane derivatives that are related to reserpine have been examined in attempts to separate, modify, or enhance the cardiovascular and neuroleptic actions of the alkaloid. Even minor modifications often significantly influence neuroleptic potency.

Quaternization of the basic (N_b) nitrogen of reserpine abolishes neuroleptic activity; however, reserpoxidine (reserpine N_b-oxide) and raujemidine ($\Delta^{19,20}$-reserpine) (682) retain significant ptosis-producing actions in mice (683). Substitution of the indole nitrogen (N_a) with methyl or allyl

groups eliminates activity. In fact, the former compound is a reserpine antagonist (684). The amide analog 56.**207a** of reserpine, as well as reserpic acid (56.**207b**), methyl reserpate (56.**207c**), and reserpic acid 18-O-trimethoxybenzoate (56.**207d**), also lack CNS-depressant properties (685), whereas methyl 18-ketoreserpate (56.**207e**) has about one-fifth the neuroleptic potency of reserpine (686).

Of the many reserpine analogs in which the esters in positions 16 and 18 are altered, none has greater neuroleptic potency than reserpine, although several have comparable potency (687) and in some instances a degree of selectivity is achieved. For example, syrosingopine (56.**207f**) causes antihypertensive actions at doses that produce minimal sedation, whereas 56.**207g**, 56.**207h** (688), and 56.**207i** (685)

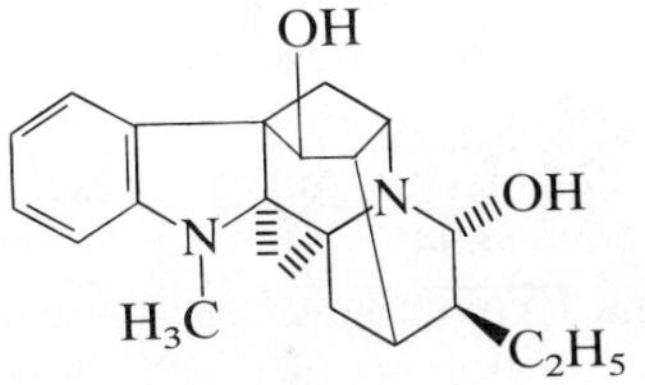

56.**206**

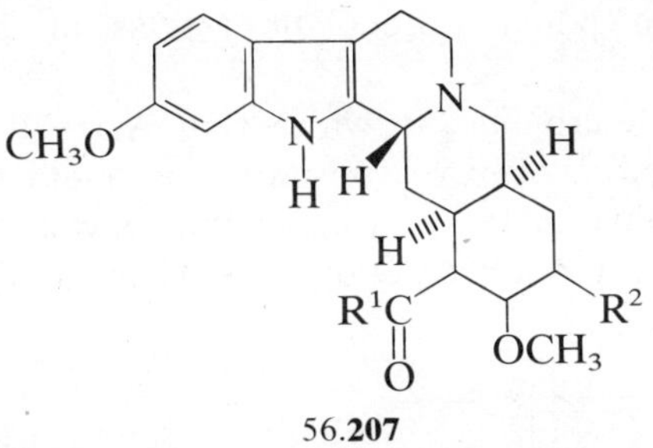

56.**207**

a $R^1 = NH_2$, $R^2 = 3,4,5\text{-}(CH_3O)_3C_6H_2CO_2$
b $R^1 = R^2 = OH$
c $R^1 = CH_3O$, $R^2 = OH$
d $R^1 = OH$, $R^2 = 3,4,5\text{-}(CH_3O)_3C_6H_2CO_2$
e $R^1 = CH_3O$, $R^2 = O$
f $R^1 = CH_3O$, $R^2 = 3,5\text{-}(CH_3O)_2\text{-}4\text{-}C_2H_5OCO_2C_6H_2CO_2$
g $R^1 = CH_3O$, $R^2 = 3\text{-}(CH_3)_2NC_6H_4CO_2$
h $R^1 = CH_3O$, $R^2 = (CH_3)_3CCO_2$
i $R^1 = CH_3O(CH_2)_2O$, $R^2 = 3,4,5\text{-}(CH_3O)_3C_6H_2CO_2$
j $R^1 = CH_3O$, $R^2 = C_2H_5O$

cause mainly sedative effects. Etherification of the 18-hydroxyl group of methyl reserpate (56.**207c**) with methyl or ethyl groups affords compounds having neuroleptic activity (689); however, groups larger than ethyl decrease potency. Both the normal 18β and isomeric 18α ethers have a rapid onset of activity after oral administration (671). Maximum potency, about half that of reserpine, is noted with the 18β-ethyl ether 56.**207j** (3).

Several other racemates related to reserpine (56.**202**), but having different E-ring substituents, include compounds in which the 17α-methoxyl group is replaced by ethoxyl, propoxyl, cyano, and N-methylacetamido groups (690). Demethoxydeserpidine, in which the 17-methoxyl group of reserpine is removed, causes reserpine-like effects in dogs, whereas the corresponding 16α epimer is inactive (691). Introduction of a 19-methyl substitutent decreases the sedative activity of deserpidine (692). Several ring-E unsaturated reserpine analogs, e.g., 56.**208**, lack significant reserpine-like activity (693, 694).

Among yohimbane derivatives with halogen substituents in ring E greatest potency is noted with 17α-halo derivatives; however, clinical evaluation is precluded by their potent adrenolytic actions in dogs (695).

Deserpidine, in which ring A is substituted at various positions by methoxyl, methyl, or benzo-fusion (696), as well as a 12-aza relative (690) have been studied.

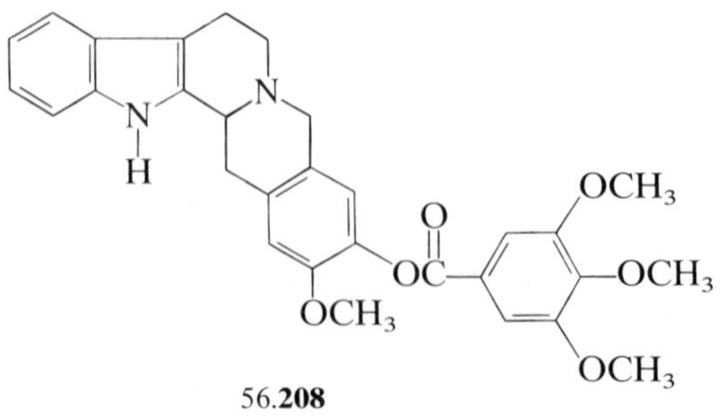

56.**208**

10-Chloro- (697) and 10-fluorodeserpidine (698) have about one-tenth the ptosis-producing potency of reserpine in rats. Corresponding dimethylamino- (690), methyl-, methoxy-, and methylmercaptodeserpidines also have reduced sedative potency (699).

Modification of the C ring of reserpine, e.g., introduction of a 6-methyl or 6-ethyl substituent, may increase potency (700). Other reserpine congeners having an altered tetrahydro-β-carboline (rings A, B, and C) system include a ring C homolog in which the fused piperidine ring is replaced by a saturated azepine (690), an analog in which the indolo bicycle (A, B rings) is replaced by a 3,4-dimethoxybenzo-fused system (701) to give a compound with reserpine-like activity (702), and analogs in which the indolo system is replaced by a 2,3-thianaphtheno-fused moiety. The thianaphthene related to 3-epideserpidine lacks neuroleptic activity (703). Pharmacological properties of the corresponding thianaphtheno relative (704) of deserpidine (Table 56.13) are not reported.

4.5.3 SIMPLER COMPOUNDS RELATED TO PARTS OF THE RESERPINE MOLECULE. Many examples illustrate the utility of simpler synthetic substitutes for therapeutically useful alkaloids; e.g., procaine is a simpler relative of the alkaloid cocaine, and quinacrine and other synthetic antimalarials are derived from the alkaloid quinine. Such synthetic materials often have the advantage of easier preparation, greater efficacy, and perhaps more selectivity than the natural product. Thus it is natural that many simpler fragments of reserpine, e.g., derivatives of β-carboline, indole, isoquinoline, cyclohexanol, and trimethoxybenzoic acid, have been the subject of considerable research. To date, this research, the subject of a previous review (673), has been directed toward antihypertensive activity and has been of limited success.

4.6   Benzoquinolizine Derivatives

Various derivatives of 1,3,4,6,7,11b-hexa-hydro-2*H*-benzo[*a*]quinolizine   (56.**209**) are included among the ipecac and proto-berberine alkaloids. A study of relatives of the principal ipecac alkaloid, emetine, re-sulted in the discovery of tetrabenazine (56.**210a**) (705), which like reserpine causes sedative effects and decreases levels of serotonin and norepinephrine in several animal species (706, 707). Examination of congeners of tetrabenazine resulted in the discovery of benzquinamide (56.**211**) (708, 709), which like reserpine and tetraben-azine blocks a CAR in rats and monkeys, but unlike these agents does not decrease the biogenic amines at doses that block CAR and does not produce overt sedative or cholinergic effects (710).

Several dibenzoquinolizines, including the protoberberine alkaloid norcoralydine

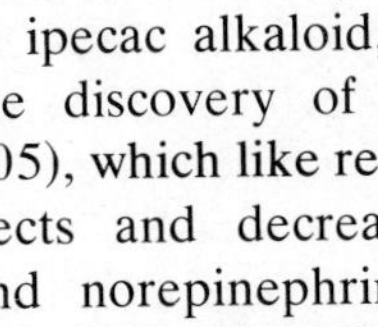

56.**209**

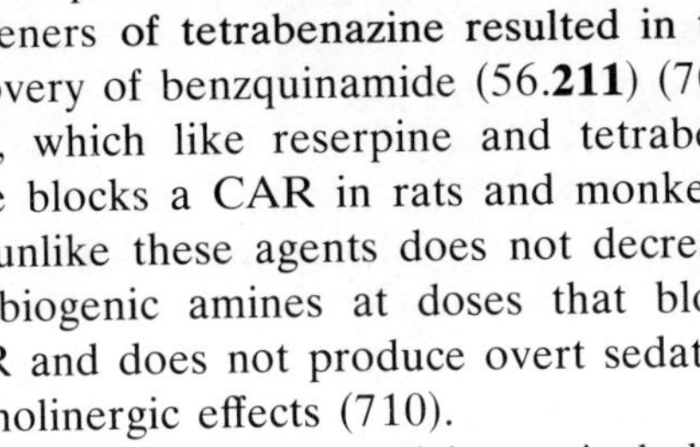

56.**210a**   R = CH$_3$
56.**210b**   R = C$_2$H$_5$

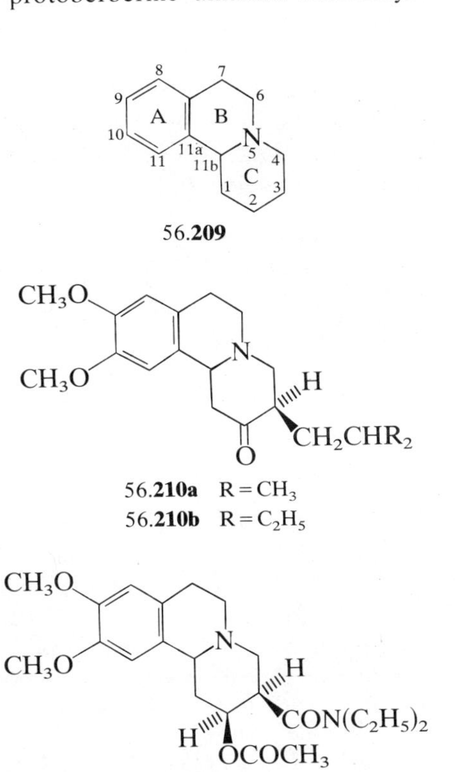

56.**211**

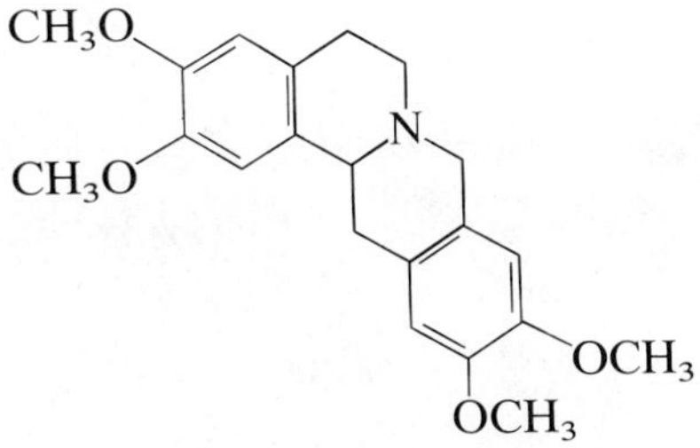

56.**212**

(xylopinine, 56.**212**) also produce neuroleptic effects in animals, but do not deplete brain catecholamines (711).

4.6.1   TETRABENAZINE   AND   RELATED COMPOUNDS.   Among a series of 3-substituted   1,3,4,6,7,11b-hexahydro-2*H*-benzo[*a*]quinolizinones (705) tetrabenazine (56.**210a**) has the longest duration of ac-tion; however, it is shorter-acting than, and has only one-tenth to one-twentieth the amine depleting potency of, reserpine in rabbits. However some analogs, e.g., 56.**210b**, are more potent than tetraben-azine. Quaternization of the quinolizine nitrogen, aromatization of ring C, or re-moval of the ketone decreases or eliminates activity (712); however, conversion of the ketone to a thioketone or to thioketals results in compounds that retain depressant effects in mice (713).

Relocation of the 3-alkyl substituent of tetrabenazine to position 1 eliminates seda-tive and biochemical activity (705). Modifi-cation of the dimethoxybenzo-fused ring A of tetrabenazine generally has a detrimen-tal influence on neuroleptic-like activity. For example, 9-methoxy-, 9,10,11-trimeth-oxy-, 9,10-methylenedioxy, 9,10-diethoxy-, and 9,10-dihydroxy relatives are less effec-tive than 56.**210a**, as is a congener in which the substituted A ring is replaced by a tetramethylene bridge. In contrast, replace-ment of the substituted A ring of tetraben-azine by a 2,3-indolo-fused system affords octahydroindoloquinolizines with sedative and hypotensive properties (174).

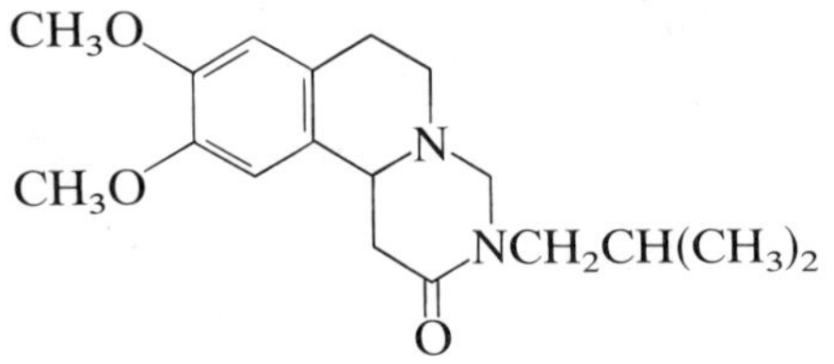

56.**213**

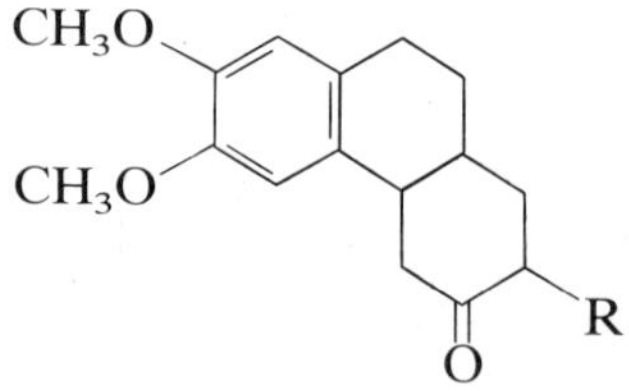

56.**214**   R = alkyl

In a series of 3-substituted 3-azabenzo-[*a*]quinolizin-2-ones greatest brain serotonin and norepinephrine depletion in rabbits is caused by the 3-isobutyl isostere 56.**213** of tetrabenazine; however, it is considerably less potent than the parent (715).

Apparently a basic nitrogen at position 5 of the benzoquinolizine is required for tetrabenazine-like activity. A series of octahydrophenanthrenes 56.**214** with either cis or trans fusion of the B and C ring does not block CAR or produce sedation (716).

Reduction of 3-substituted hexahydro-2*H*-benzo[*a*]quinolizin-2-ones gives alcohols 56.**215a** and 56.**215b** having weaker sedative and narcosis-producing actions

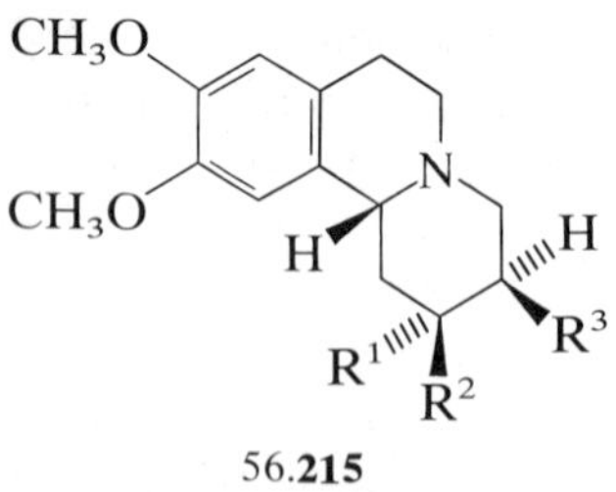

56.**215**

a   R^1 = OH, R^2 = H, R^3 = alkyl
b   R^1 = H, R^2 = OH, R^3 = alkyl
c   R^1 = C$_2$H$_5$, R^2 = OH, R^3 = CH$_2$CH(C$_2$H$_5$)$_2$
d   R^1 = C$_2$H$_5$, R^2 = OH, R^3 = CH$_2$CH(CH$_3$)$_2$
e   R^1 = OH, R^2 = C$_2$H$_5$, R^3 = C$_2$H$_5$
f   R^1 = OH, R^2 = C$_2$H$_5$, R^3 = CH$_2$CH(CH$_3$)$_2$

than those of corresponding ketones. Brain levels of serotonin and norepinephrine are also lowered for a shorter time. Alcohols in which the 2-hydroxyl is cis to the 3-alkyl group 56.**215b** are generally more potent and more toxic than related trans isomers 56.**215a**; however, a *trans*-10,11-methyl-enedioxy analog of 56.**215a** has neuroleptic-like effect on cerebral monoamine turnover (717). Esterification of the trans alcohols decreases potency; however, in the cis series acetylation enhances narcosis-potentiating and sedative effects, whereas toxicity is decreased (718). Among various secondary carbinols of this type, *N*-quaternization abolishes activity (712).

2α-Ethyl-2β-hydroxy-3α-alkylbenzo-quinolizines 56.**215c** and 56.**215d** are 7.2 and 3.6 times more potent, respectively, than tetrabenazine in a test for decreasing rat brain serotonin levels. In contrast, in the related series having a 2β-ethyl substituent, little or no activity is noted with 56.**215e** and only moderate amine depletion is caused by 56.**215f**. In a series of dehydrated analogs 56.**216** the isobutyl derivative 56.**216a** is somewhat more potent than the ethyl analog 56.**216b** (719).

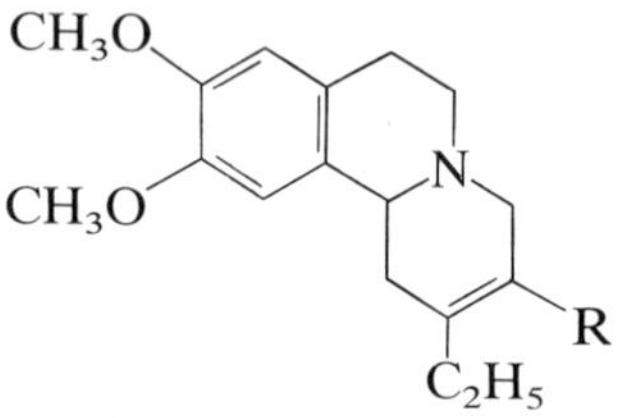

56.**216a**   R = CH$_2$CH(CH$_3$)$_2$
56.**216b**   R = C$_2$H$_5$

A relatively simpler benzoquinolizine, i.e., ($\pm$)-2-ethyl-2-hydroxy-1,3,4,6,7,11b-hexahydro-2*H*-benzo[*a*]quinolizine, 56.**209** (2-C$_2$H$_5$-2-HO) improves mood, drive, and social behavior in schizophrenic patients at well tolerated doses (720).

4.6.2 BENZQUINAMIDE   AND   RELATED COMPOUNDS. The keto amide 56.**217** [X = 9,10-(CH$_3$O)$_2$], an analog of tetrabenazine modified at position 3, causes release

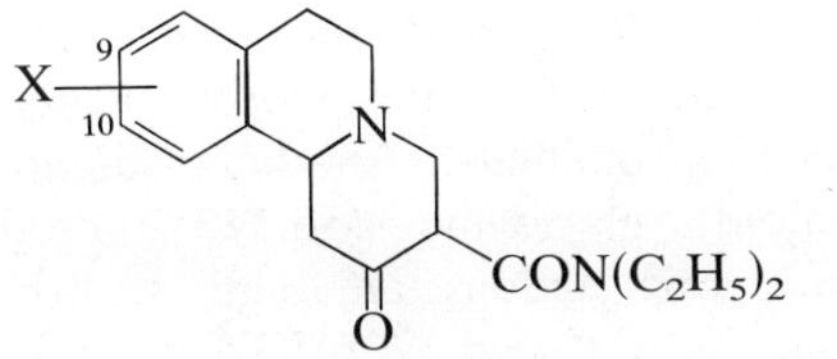

56.**217**

of cerebral amines and at relatively high doses it disrupts a CAR in animals (708, 709). The effect of modification of the amide functionality, the carbonyl group, and the aromatic ring substituents of 56.**217** on pharmacological activity has been examined. Maximum CAR blocking activity in rats is noted for the diethylamide 56.**217** [X = 9,10-$(CH_3O)_2$]. The corresponding diisopropylamide also retains a high degree of activity, but dimethyl and di-*n*-propyl derivatives are inactive at 30 mg/kg i.p. (708, 709).

Introduction of A ring substituents, e.g., 56.**217** (X = 10-Cl, 10-F, 10-NO_2), that might decrease the basicity of the tertiary amine markedly decrease CAR blocking potency in rats. In contrast, introduction of electron-releasing groups in ring A, e.g., 56.**217** (X = 9-CH_3O, 10-CH_3), as well as the unsubstituted congener 56.**217** (X = H), results in compounds with significant, but less potent, neuroleptic activity than 56.**217** [X = 9,10-$(CH_3O)_2$].

Reduction of the keto group of 56.**217** [X = 9,10-$(OCH_3)_2$] affords a mixture of axial 56.**218a** and equatorial 56.**218b** alcohols. The axial alcohol 56.**218a** is more

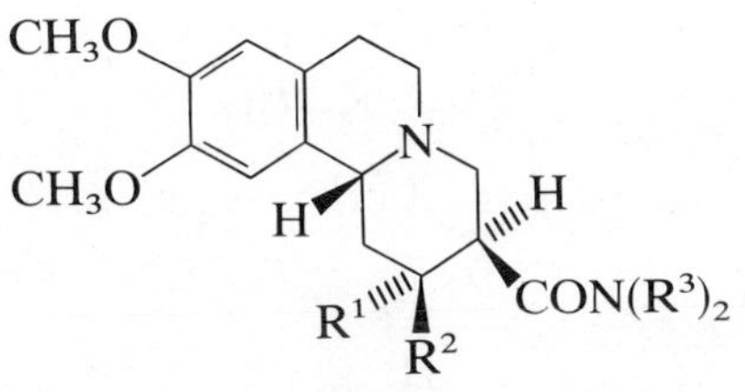

56.**218**

a R^1 = H, R^2 = OH, R^3 = C_2H_5
b R^1 = OH, R^2 = H, R^3 = C_2H_5
c R^1 = H, R^2 = OCOCH$_3$, R^3 = H

potent than 56.**218b**; it is almost equipotent with tetrabenazine in lowering brain amine levels and in blocking a CAR in animals (710).

Benzquinamide (56.**211**), the acetate derived from 56.**218a**, is about one-fourth as potent as chlorpromazine in blocking CAR behavior in rats and monkeys (721); however, unlike 56.**218a**, it has very little effect on brain amine levels. The primary amide 56.**218c**, a major metabolite of benzquinamide in several animal species, does not block CAR (722).

A hexahydro[1,4]oxazino[3,4-*a*]isoquinoline relative 56.**219** of benzquinamide, one of a series (723) in which the 2-substituted carbon is replaced by oxygen, elicits both chlorpromazine- and chlordiazepoxide-like effects (724).

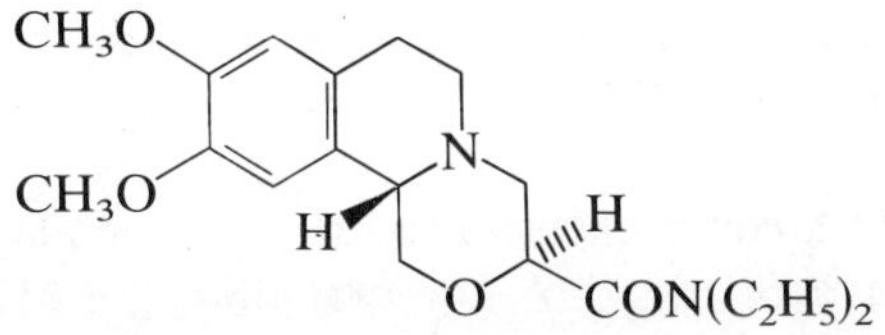

56.**219**

4.6.3 DIBENZOQUINOLIZINES. Norcoralydine (xylopinine, 56.**212**) a compound related to reserpine and tetrabenazine, produces pharmacological effects resembling those of chlorpromazine, but it does not decrease brain levels of norepinephrine. It may act by blocking central and peripheral α-adrenergic responses (725, 726). In several animal tests, e.g., prolongation of hexobarbital-induced sleep and antagonism of methamphetamine lethality in mice, (−)-56.**212** is more potent and less toxic that its (+) enantiomer (711).

Tetrahydropalmitine [gyndarin, 2,3,9,10-$(CH_3O)_4$-56.**220**] (727), tetrahydroberberine [2,3-OCH$_2$O-9,10-$(CH_3O)_2$-56.**220**], and some derivatives (728) have chlorpromazine-like effects in animals and humans (729, 730). In a test for decrease of activity in mice, (−)-tetrahydropalmitine is

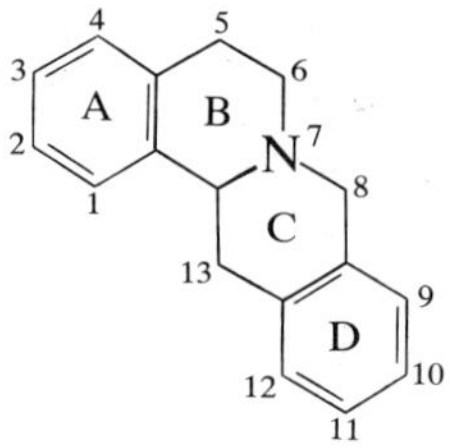

56.**220**

more potent than the (+) isomer which produces instead a transient excitation (730).

An ethoxy analog of tetrahydropalmitine [2,3,10,11-$(C_2H_5O)_4$-56.**220**] has little depressant activity on acute administration; however, it induces a cumulative central depression similar to that associated with long-term use of reserpine (731). The S-(−) isomer of 2,3,10,11-tetrahydroxy-berberine [2,3,10,11-$(HO)_4$-56.**220**] is more potent than its enantiomer as an antagonist of rat striatal dopamine-sensitive adenylate cyclase (732).

In a comprehensive study (733), analogs and derivatives of norcoralydine (56.**212**) were examined in a rat CAR test (191). On oral administration (±)-56.**212** is somewhat less potent than chlorpromazine in this test, whereas tetrahydropalmitine and tetrahydroberbine have CI values of about 0.5 and 0.3, respectively. Among a series of related compounds maximum potency in the CAR test is associated with norcoralydine (56.**212**). Potency is generally decreased by removal or relocation of one or more of the methoxy substituents, replacement of a methoxy group by hydroxy, ethoxy, or benzyloxy groups, replacement of the 10-methoxy substituent with a 3,4,5-trimethoxybenzoyloxy moiety, or introduction of methyl groups at positions 6 or 8 (733).

4.6.4 TETRAHYDROISOQUINOLINES AND RELATED COMPOUNDS. Some compounds that retain only the tetrahydroisoquinoline AB rings of benzoquinolizines have significant neuroleptic activity. For example, the aporphine alkaloids bulbocapnine

(56.**221**) (734) and nuciferine (56.**222**) (735) produce weak chlorpromazine-like effects in animals. Another isoquinoline alkaloid, glaziovine (56.**223**), produces neuroleptic actions although a dose response is not seen (736). To determine if the cisoid or transoid phenethylamine moieties are responsible for the neuroleptic effects of bulbocapnine, the rigid tricyclic phenethylamines 56.**224** and 56.**225** have

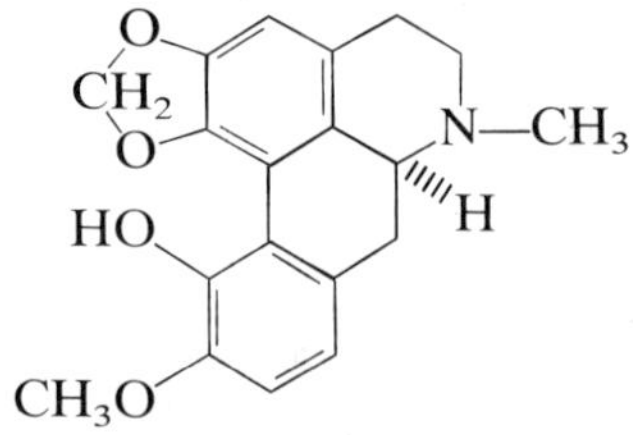

56.**221**

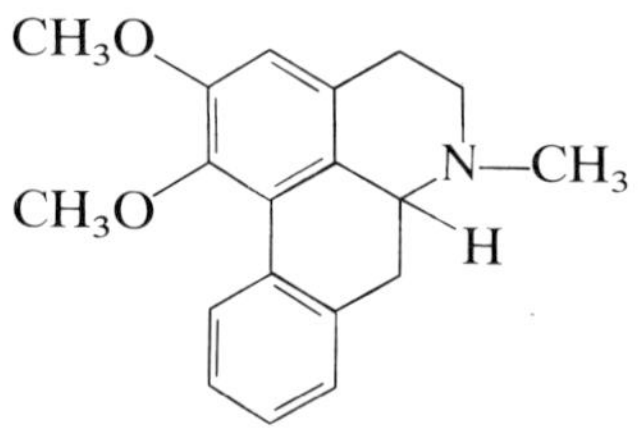

56.**222**

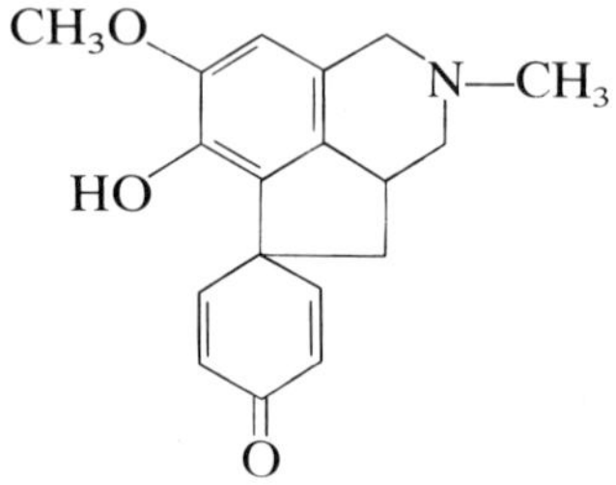

56.**223**

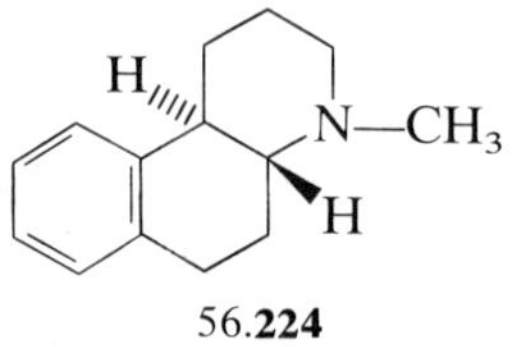

56.**224**

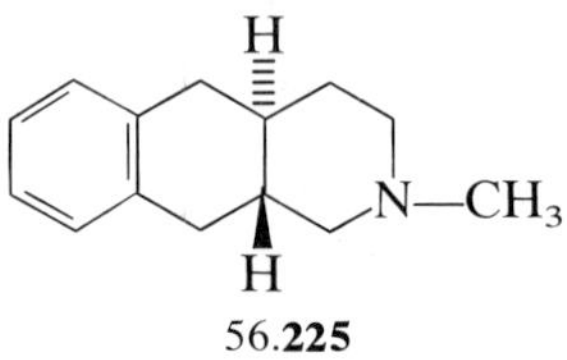

56.**225**

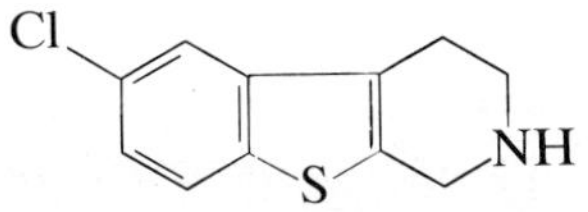

56.**226**

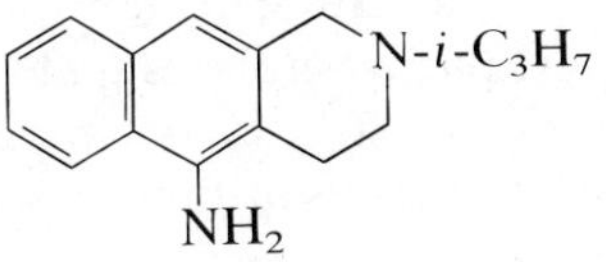

56.**227**

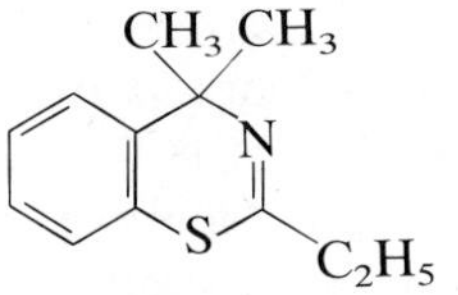

56.**228**

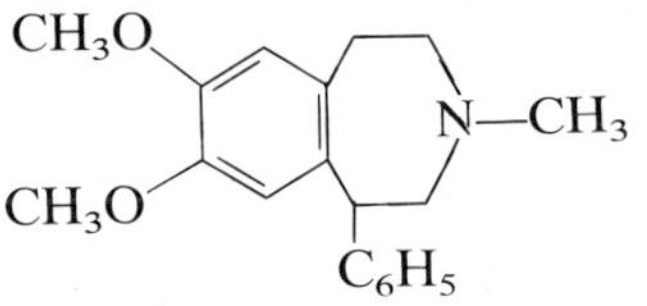

56.**229**

been examined. Potent cataleptic activity and blockade of the response of the rat vas deferens to dopamine are observed only for the transoid isomers (737).

Other isoquinoline-like compounds with neuroleptic-like effects include the thia-naphthenopyridine 56.**226**, which is effective in a mouse-fighting test (738), some benzisoquinolines, e.g., 56.**227**, that are claimed (739) to have antiaggressive and sedative properties, a more distantly related series of benzothiazines, e.g., 56.**228** (740), that decrease motor activity, potentiate barbiturate-induced effects, and antagonize amphetamine-induced effects, and an isoquinoline homolog, a tetrahydro-3-benzazepine trimonam (trimopam, 56.**229**), that reduces aggressive behavior in mice and monkeys (741) and presents a clinical profile that falls between perphenazine and diazepam (742).

4.7 Indole Derivatives

Interest in indole derivatives as potential psychotropic agents is enhanced by the suggestion that serotonin may be a central neurotransmitter (743, 744). Although some indoles and related compounds are potent antagonists of the peripheral actions of serotonin, most of these compounds have little effect on the CNS (745–748). Several indoles and related compounds, however, have significant neuroleptic activity.

4.7.1 OXYPERTINE AND RELATED COMPOUNDS. Oxypertine (56.**230**), which may be viewed as a butyrophenone relative, is the prototype of a group of indolylalkylphenylpiperazines that are potent CNS depressants (749, 750). In the clinic, oxypertine is of value in treating chronic schizophrenia (751). It is of particular benefit for its mood-elevating and stimulant properties in schizophrenics where apathy is a major problem (752).

In a jumping-box test in rats and dogs oxypertine is equipotent with chlorpromazine when administered subcutaneously and two to three times more potent when given orally (115). Among a series of compounds related to oxypertine, a number of analogs have neuroleptic-like activity in monkeys and adrenolytic activity in rats. They also prolong hexobarbital-induced sleep and inhibit a head-withdrawal reflex in mice (753). A cis-2,3-dihydro analog of oxypertine, on the basis of animal studies, appears to have potential neuroleptic activity without EPS liability (754).

Basic structural requirements for neuroleptic activity in this series are indicated

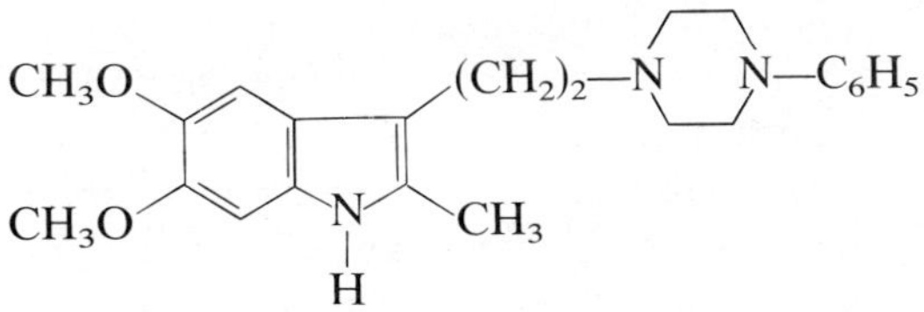

56.**230**

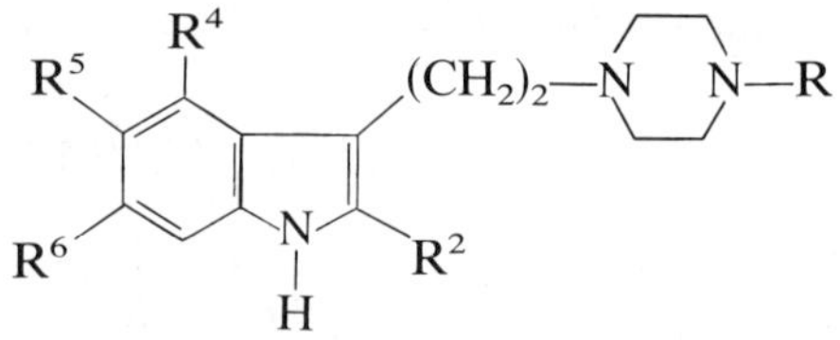

56.**231**

by the general formula 56.**231**. Substitution of the indole nucleus with alkyl or alkoxy groups causes a marked effect only in the head-withdrawal reflex test. Substitution with 6-methoxy or 5,6-dialkoxy groups significantly enhances potency, but 6-methyl or 6-ethoxy substitution decreases it. Several oxypertine relatives with 4-methyl-5-methoxy substitution, e.g., 56.**231** ($R^2 = R^4 = CH_3$; $R^5 = CH_3O$; $R = C_6H_5$) and the corresponding compound where $R = 2\text{-}CH_3OC_6H_4$, are about one-fourth as potent as diazepam in causing ataxia, decreasing motor activity, and antagonizing convulsions induced by electroshock or strychnine in mice (755). Among heterocyclic analogs of oxypertine, greatest hexobarbital-potentiating activity is claimed for the 7-aza analog (756).

2-Methyl substitution has an inconsistent effect on activity; however, oxypertine (56.**230**) has nearly twice the central, and only one-half the peripheral, adrenolytic potency of the 2-unsubstituted congener. Antipsychotic activity is cited (757) for alpertine, a congener of oxypertine in which the 2-methyl group is replaced by a carboethoxy moiety.

In compounds in which the ethylene bridge of 56.**231** is varied from one to four methylene units, maximum neuroleptic and adrenolytic potency is with a two- or three-carbon bridge. Generally, compounds having an ethylene bridge are more effective inhibitors of the head-withdrawal reflex, but in other tests the propylene homologs produce similar responses.

Aryl substitution of the terminal piperazine nitrogen of 56.**231** is essential for activity. Substitution with a phenyl or sub-stituted-phenyl ring results in maximum neuroleptic and adrenolytic potency. 2-Pyridyl, 2-pyrimidyl, or benzyl substitution generally decreases potency, whereas hydrogen or alkyl substituents abolish activity in all tests. The nature of substitution of the piperazinyl phenyl group is quite important relative to adrenolytic potency, which is enhanced by ortho substitution with alkoxy, alkyl, or halogen groups and decreased by para and meta substitution. In contrast, substitution of the phenyl ring has little effect on neuroleptic potency (749). Clinically, an ortho-chloro derivative melipertine (56.**231**, $R = 2\text{-}CH_3OC_6H_4$; $R^2 = CH_3$; $R^5 = R^6 = CH_3O$) causes EPS at doses below those that produce antipsychotic activity (758).

CNS-depressant properties are also observed for several other indoles that incorporate structural features of oxypertine and the neuroleptic butyrophenones (759). In a test for antagonism of isolation-induced aggressive behavior in mice (760) 56.**232a** is nearly equipotent with chlorpromazine, whereas 56.**232b** and 56.**232c** are about one-third and one-fifth as potent, respectively.

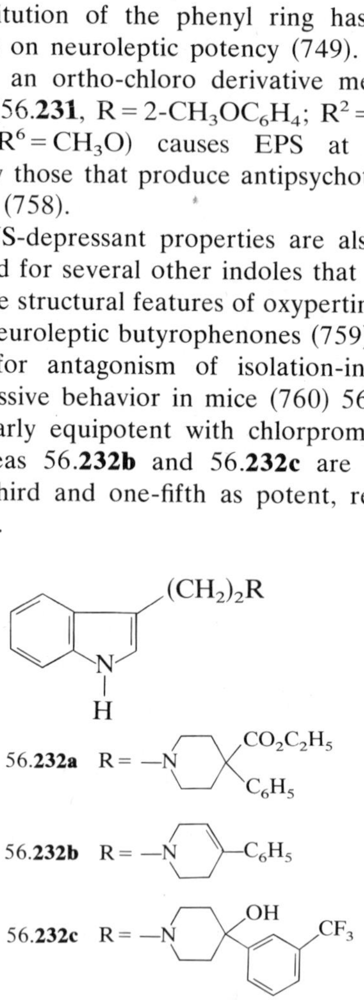

4.7.2 OTHER INDOLE DERIVATIVES. A series of indolylethylpyridines 56.**233** calm monkeys, prolong barbiturate-induced anesthesia, and antagonize amphetamine-stimulated motor activity in mice. Although

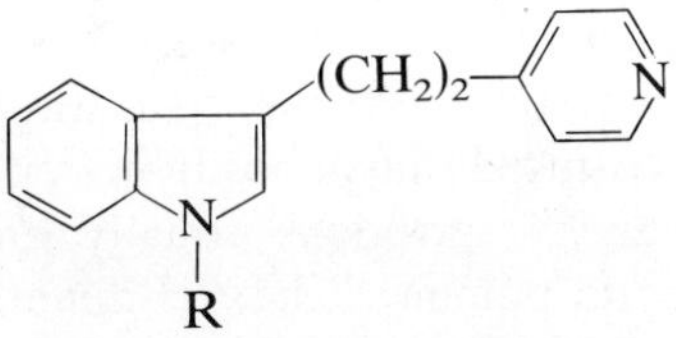

56.**233** R = H, CH$_3$, CH$_2$C$_6$H$_5$

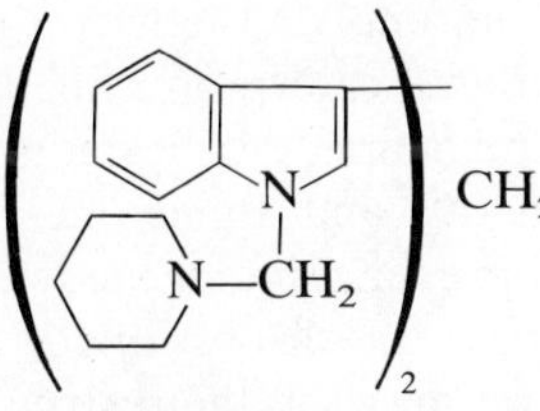

56.**234**

the *N*-benzyl derivative 56.**233** (R = C$_6$H$_5$CH$_2$) has little influence on motor activity, it is almost equipotent with chlorpromazine as an inhibitor of the amphetamine-induced response (761). Some *N*-pyridyltryptamines have CNS-depressant actions in mice (762).

Potent CNS-depressant, chlorpromazine-potentiating, and analgetic properties are caused by a bis(indolyl)methane 56.**234** (763).

Two other 3-substituted indoles, *N*-(2-hydroxyethyl)-3-indolylmethylamine and 1-methyl-3-(1-hydroxy-2-dimethylamino-ethyl)indole, protect mice against electroshock-induced convulsions and produce a chlorpromazine-like effect (764). Some carboline derivatives also have neuroleptic actions; e.g., a carboline congener, 56.**235**, related to 56.**234** is claimed to have tranquilizing and serotonin antagonist activity (765). The related tryptolines 56.**236** inhibit motor activity in rats, possibly by a serotonergic mechanism (766).

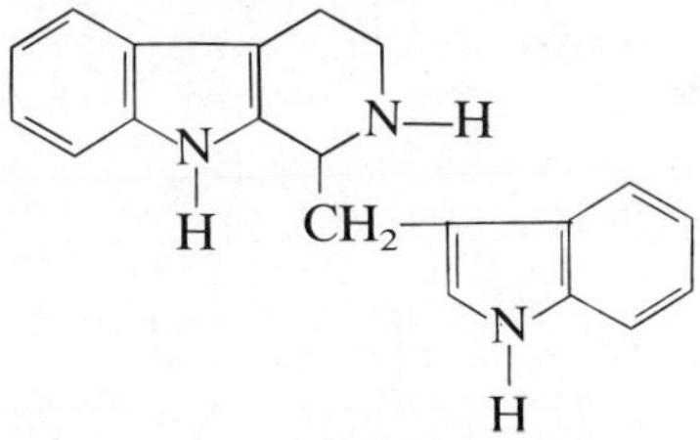

Clinical studies in Russia reveal antipsychotic activity combined with some stimulant actions for the carboline derivative, carbidin (56.**237**) (767).

3-Dimethylamino-1,2,3,4-tetrahydrocarbazole (56.**238**), another tryptamine derivative, prevents amphetamine-induced stereotyped behavior in rats and blocks reserpine-induced ptosis in mice, suggesting both antipsychotic and antidepressant actions. Some derivatives, e.g., a 6,8-difluoro derivative, are selective in the amphetamine-antagonism test, having a CI of 6.0. Other congeners, e.g., a 5-methyl derivative, are selective antidepressants (768). An indolo-3-azepine derivative, 56.**239**, blocks a CAR, is hypothermic, and inhibits the aggression of fighting mice (769); however, it is not effective in chronic schizophrenic patients (770). Some 3-chloro-6-amino-7*H*-indolo[3,2-*b*][1,5]benzoxazepines, e.g., 56.**240**, are claimed (771) to have useful neuroleptic activity.

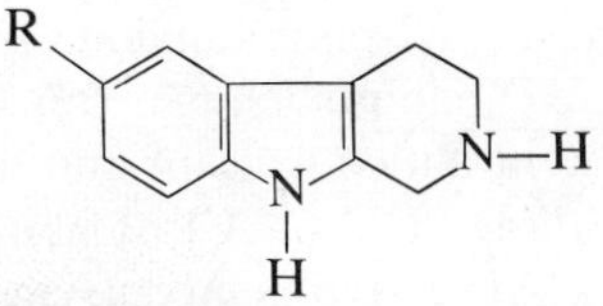

56.**236**

R = H, HO, CH$_3$O

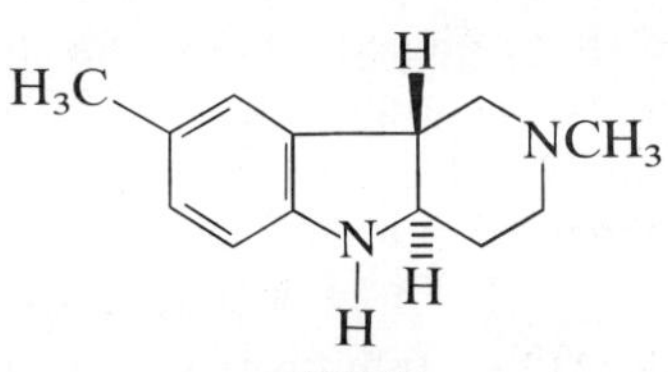

56.**237**

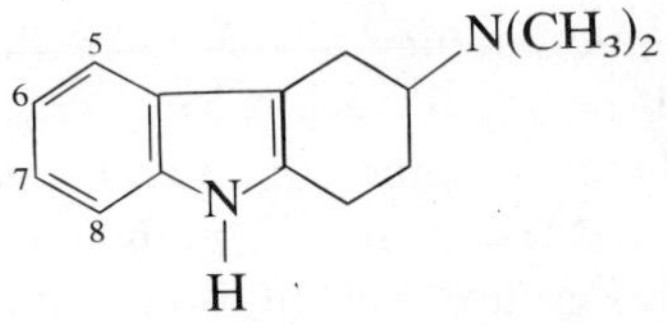

56.**235**

56.**238**

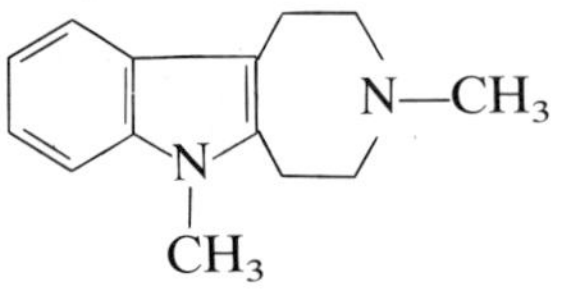

56.**239**

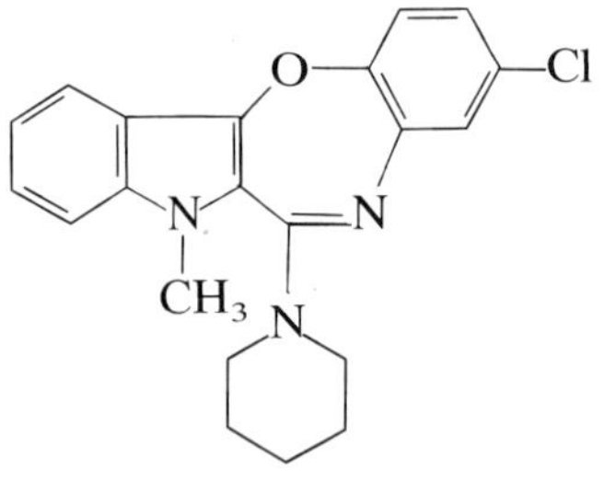

56.**240**

4.8 β-Aminoketones

Certain compounds related to the alkaloidal respiratory analeptic lobeline, a β-aminoketone, have potent α-adrenoreceptor blocking activity (772). One of these compounds, 2-piperidinylmethyl-3,4-dihydro-1(2H)-naphthalenone (56.**241a**), is also a potent anticonvulsant and neuroleptic (773, 774); it has a CI of about 0.3 in blocking CAR and in antagonizing amphetamine-induced effects in rodents (775). The need for the aromatic portion in molecules of this type is evidenced by the lack of α-adrenolytic activity by the corresponding benzene-ring reduced analog, which causes only modest nicotinic actions (772).

Examination of aminomethylnaphthalenones for neuroleptic and adrenolytic activity (775) reveals 56.**241a** is about one-third to one-fourth as potent as chlorpromazine in a CAR blocking test in rats. Substitution of a pyrrolidinyl group (56.**241b**) for the piperidine of 56.**241a** has little effect on neuroleptic potency in this test, whereas a marked decrease results on replacement with dimethylamino (56.**241c**), morpholinyl (56.**241d**), or N-methylpiperazinyl (56.**241e**) groups. Substitution of position 4 of 2-aminomethyltetralones generally in-

creases toxicity and decreases CNS-depressant properties; however, substitution of the benzo-fused ring in position 7 or in both the 6 and 7 positions usually enhances neuroleptic potency. The 6,7-dimethyl derivative 56.**242a** is the most potent neuroleptic agent in this series, although it lacks significant adrenolytic activity. It is almost equipotent with chlorpromazine in blocking a CAR and amphetamine-induced hypermotility in rats and about one-half as potent in depressing motor activity in mice (775). Some 5,8-disubstituted tetralones, designed because of their structural relationship to tricyclic antipsychotics, exhibit neuroleptic activity. In a CAR blockade test in rats, one of these, 56.**242b**, has a CI value of 10 (776). Moderate activity in producing hypothermia and antagonizing amphetamine-induced hypermobility is noted for a 2-piperazinylmethyl-substituted tetralone 56.**241f** (777). A secondary aminomethyl-substituted tetralone 56.**241g** is nearly equipotent with chlorpromazine in blocking central norepinephrine receptors,

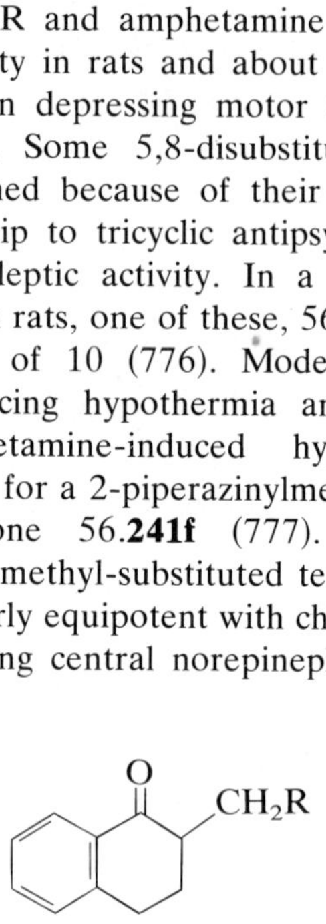

56.**241a**   R = —N⟨piperidine⟩

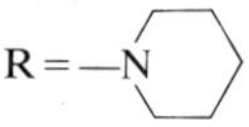

56.**241b**   R = —N⟨pyrrolidine⟩

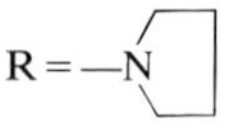

56.**241c**   R = —N(CH₃)₂

56.**241d**   R = —N⟨morpholine⟩O

56.**241e**   R = —N⟨piperazine⟩NCH₃

56.**241f**   R = —N⟨piperazine⟩N—⟨aryl⟩OCH₃

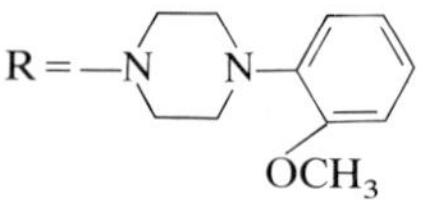

56.**241g**   R = —NH(CH₂)₂—⟨aryl⟩—OH

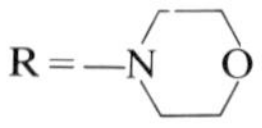

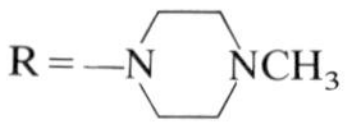

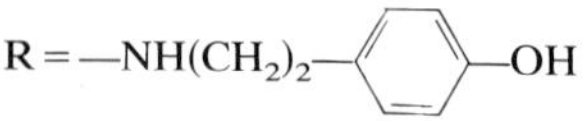

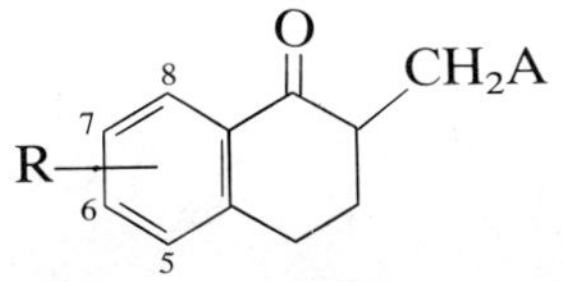

56.242a   R = 6,7-$(CH_3)_2$, A = N(piperidine)

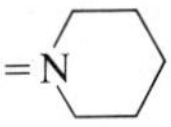

56.242b   R = 5-CH_3O, 8-Cl

but it is much less effective in blocking dopamine receptors (778).

Several Mannich bases of pyrrole ketones also cause marked neuroleptic-like actions. One of the most potent compounds of this kind is molindone (56.**243a**) (779). In animals molindone is a more potent antagonist of apomorphine-induced emesis than is chlorpromazine. It blocks CAR and has a typical neuroleptic profile. Unlike typical neuroleptics, however, molindone antagonizes tetrabenazine-induced ptosis and potentiates the stimulant effects of 5-hydroxytryptophan (780, 781). Molindone is a clinically effective antipsychotic, about equipotent with trifluoperazine (782, 783). It causes some stimulation (784), is less sedating, and produces less weight gain than many other antipsychotics (785). Molindone was marketed as an antipsychotic in the United States in 1974.

A molindone analog 56.**243b** has antiemetic and neuroleptic properties in animals (786); however, clinical antipsychotic activity is accompanied by a high incidence of EPS (787). Another structural relative 56.**244** of molindone is the most potent

56.243a   R = —N(morpholine)

56.243b   R = —N(spiro-dioxolane piperidine)

member of a series in decreasing motor activity in mice (788). Other β-aminoketones with neuroleptic-like effects include 56.**245** (789, 790) and the piperazine derivatives 56.**246a** (791) and 56.**246b** (792).

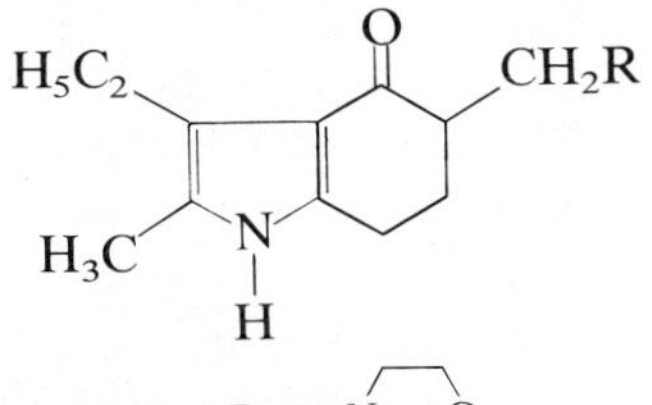

56.**244**

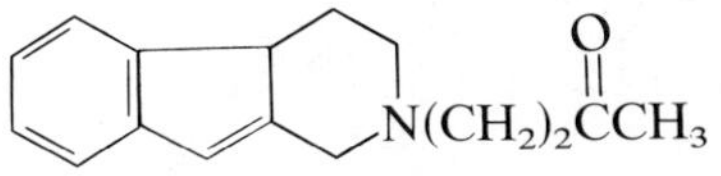

56.**245**

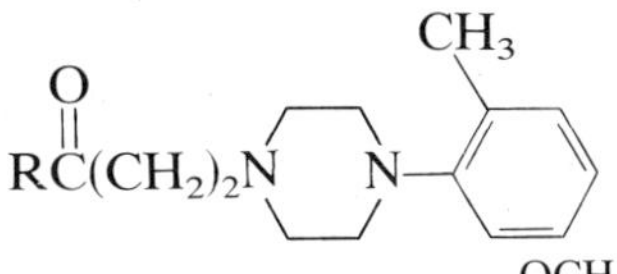

56.**246a**   R = —CH=CH—(3,4,5-trimethoxyphenyl)

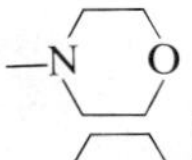

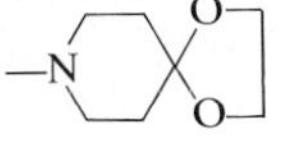

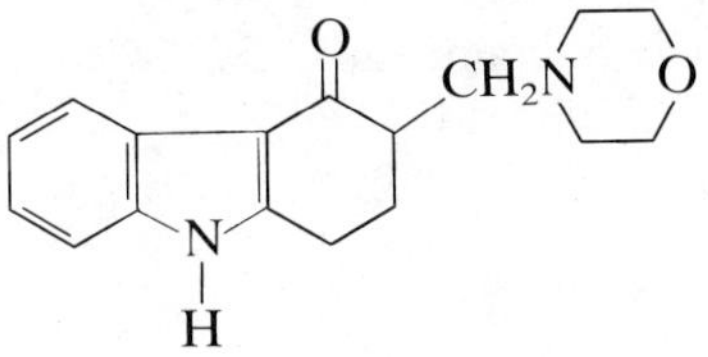

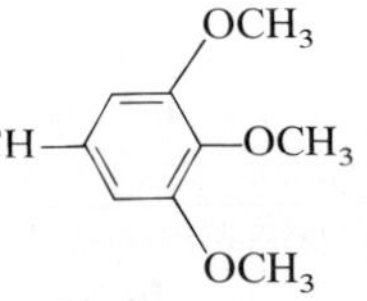

56.**246b**   R = (3-methyl-1-phenylpyrazol-5-yl)

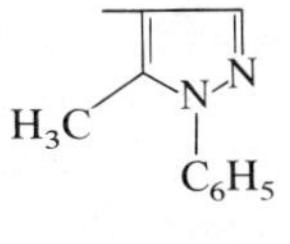

4.9   Benzodioxan Derivatives

Because most antipsychotics have α-adrenoreceptor blocking activity and most α-adrenolytics at high, near toxic doses produce chlorpromazine-like effects in animals, the potent peripheral α-adrenergic blocking agent piperoxan (56.**247a**) (793) has been modified chemically in an effort to enhance its central effects (794, 795). Examination of these compounds in a CAR blockade test in rats (796) indicates that replacement of the piperidinyl substituent of piperoxan with other tertiary amino groups affords compounds with little CNS activity. Replacement with secondary amino groups, however, gives compounds with potency of the same order as that of chlorpromazine. In the CAR test in rats maximum potency is noted with lower alkylamino substituents 56.**247b** ($n = 1$–4). The n-amyl derivative pentamoxane (56.**247b**) ($n = 4$) has a CI of about 0.5 (797).

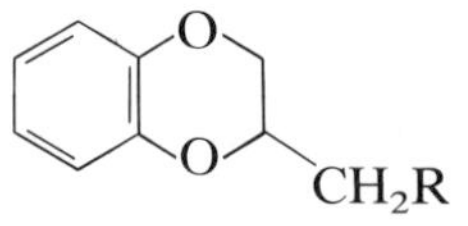

56.**247a**   R $=$ —N⟨⟩

56.**247b**   R $=$ —NH(CH$_2$)$_n$CH$_3$

Substitution of position 8 of 56.**247b** with a small alkoxyl group increases neuroleptic potency as much as tenfold. In a CAR blocking test ethoxybutamoxane (56.**248a**) has a CI of 10–15 (798). In dogs 80 μg/kg of 56.**248a** is the median effective dose for antagonizing the response to twice the threshold emetic dose of apomorphine. Stereospecificity is also observed in this class of neuroleptics. In a variety of tests (−)-ethoxybutamoxane is twice as potent as the racemate, whereas the (+) isomer is markedly less potent (799).

Additional ring chlorination generally decreases potency, but prolongs neuroleptic activity. Thus the 7-chloro derivative of ethoxybutamoxane, i.e., chloroethoxybutamoxane (56.**248b**), is about one-half as potent but twice as long-acting as its non-chlorinated parent (798).

Noteworthy CNS-depressant actions are also produced by several other benzodioxan derivatives. A pentamoxane isostere,

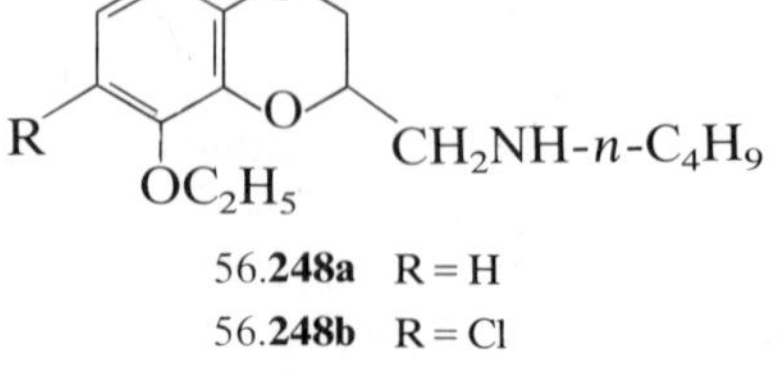

56.**248a**   R $=$ H

56.**248b**   R $=$ Cl

quiloflex (56.**249a**), is a central muscle relaxant that has been studied clinically (800). A methoxybutyl-substituted benzodioxanylethanolamine 56.**249b** blocks a CAR at low doses (801) and the sulfoxide 56.**249c** retains CNS-depressant properties, but is less toxic than the corresponding amine, butamoxane (56.**247b**, $n = 3$) (802). A benzodioxan isostere, trebenzomine (56.**250**), is predicted to have short-acting antipsychotic activity on the basis of electroencephalographic studies (803). A related tetralin 56.**251** is a potent inhibitor of many apomorphine-induced effects in animals (804).

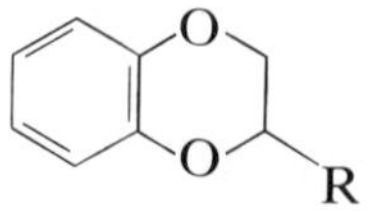

56.**249a**   R $=$ CH$_2$NH(CH$_2$)$_3$OCH$_3$
56.**249b**   R $=$ CHOHCH$_2$NH(CH$_2$)$_4$OCH$_3$
56.**249c**   R $=$ CH$_2$S(O)(CH$_2$)$_3$CH$_3$

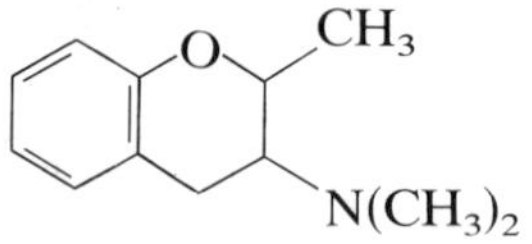

56.**250**

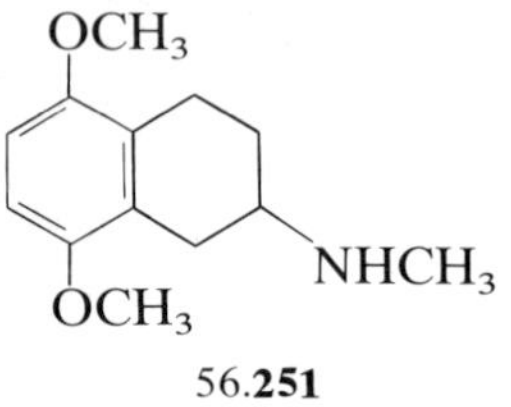

56.**251**

4.10   Benzamides and Related Compounds

A derivative of procainamide, metoclopramide (56.**252a**), has antiemetic activity, and at much higher doses it produces neuroleptic actions (521). Clinically, metoclopramide is used in gastrointestinal diagnostics, and in treating various types of vomiting and a variety of functional organic gastrointestinal disorders. Side effects of EPS

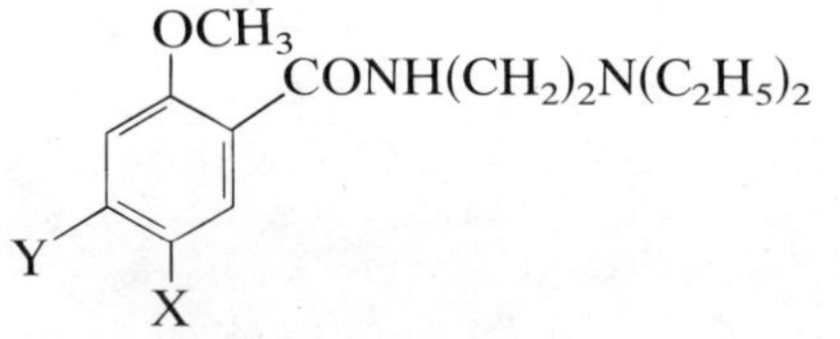

OCH₃

$\text{CONH(CH}_2)_2\text{N(C}_2\text{H}_5)_2$

Y

X

56.**252a** X = Cl, Y = NH₂
56.**252b** X = Br, Y = NH₂
56.**252c** X = SO₂CH₃, Y = H

occur in a few patients (805). Pharmacologically, metoclopramide exhibits a number of actions, e.g., antagonism of amphetamine- and apomorphine-induced effects in rodents (806–808), generally associated with neuroleptics (809). In the clinic, however, the antipsychotic activity of metoclopramide is negligible (810).

Many other benzamides have been prepared in an effort to accentuate the neuroleptic actions of metoclopramide. The bromo analog of metoclopramide, i.e., bromopride (56.**252b**), has similar actions (811). Clebropride (56.**253a**) is the most potent member of a series of piperidyl benzamides (812) in tests related to blockade of central dopamine receptors. A comprehensive structure–activity relationship study of this series reveals that the *N*-

OCH₃

CONH—⟨ ⟩—N—R

H₂N

Cl

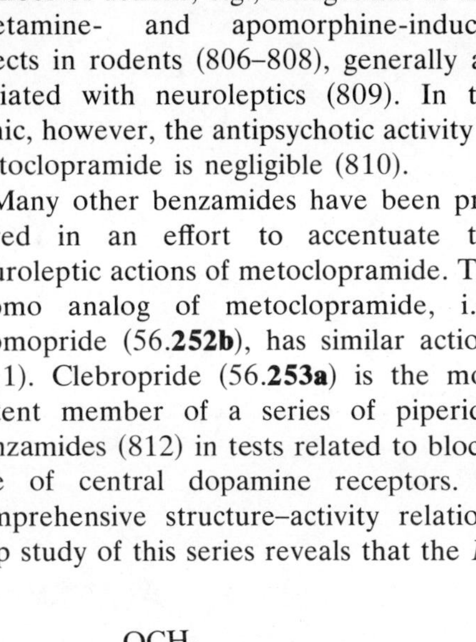

56.**253a** R = CH₂C₆H₅
56.**253b** R = H

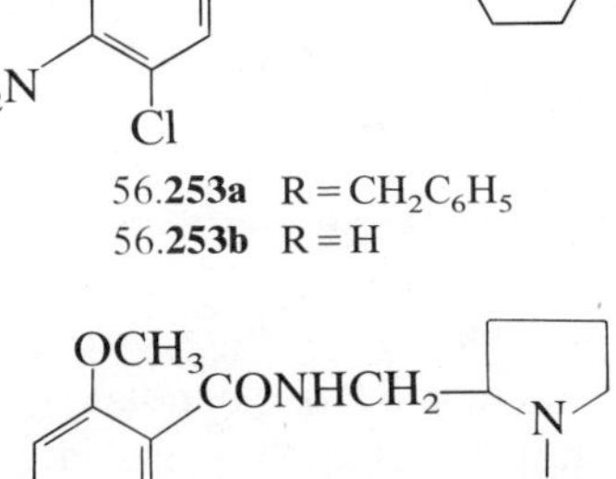

OCH₃

CONHCH₂—⟨N⟩

X |
           R

56.**254**

a X = SO₂NH₂, R = C₂H₅
b X = SO₂C₂H₅, R = C₂H₅
c X = CONH₂, R = C₂H₅
d X = SO₂NH₂, R = CH₃
e X = SO₂NH₂, R = n-C₃H₇

debenzylated product 56.**253b**, the major metabolite of clebropride, is inactive in an anti-apomorphine test in rats at a dose of 100 mg/kg p.o. (812). Sulpiride (56.**254a**), another benzamide, is also a potent antiemetic (813). It inhibits apomorphine-induced stereotypy (814) and increases CNS dopamine turnover (815) via receptor blockade (816). Clinically, sulpiride is an effective antipsychotic (817, 818). It is effective in patients without elevating serum prolactin levels and causes relatively few adverse side effects (819). It is marketed in Europe as an antipsychotic. Neuroleptic and antiemetic actions are also produced by an analog of sulpiride, i.e., sultopride (56.**254b**), a clinically effective antipsychotic that causes EPS (820). Practical endocrinologic use of sulpiride is described (821). Sultopride has clinical application in treatment of delirium tremens (822). A related carboxamide 56.**254c** also antagonizes amphetamine-induced effects in animals (823). Tigan (56.**255**), another benzamide, like metoclopramide is a clinically effective antipsychotic that produces some EPS; however, neuroleptic data are not available (824).

Metoclopramide (56.**252a**), clebropride (56.**253a**) and its debenzylated metabolite 56.**253b**, sulpiride (56.**254a**), and tigan (56.**255**) all inhibit apomorphine-induced circling in rats with unilateral nigro-striatal lesions, induce some catalepsy, and elevate striatal and mesolimbic HVA. The order of potency is clebropride > metoclopramide > sulpiride > 56.**253b** (824). All compounds, except clebropride, do not affect rat striatal dopamine-sensitive adenylate cyclase (824–827). Clebropride blocks this enzyme only at high concentrations. These data suggest that substituted benzamides are pharmacologically distinct group of dopamine receptor antagonists having a mechanism of action different from that of classical neuroleptics. Differences in the modes of action of various benzamides may explain their varying clinical potencies (824, 828). The

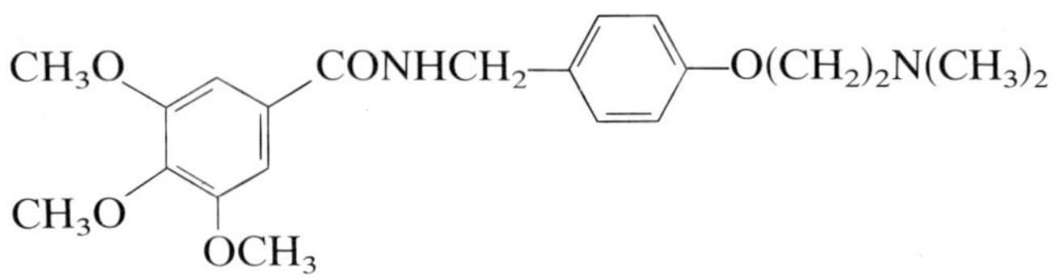

$$CH_3O \quad \text{—} \quad CONHCH_2\text{—} \quad \text{—} O(CH_2)_2N(CH_3)_2$$

$$CH_3O$$
$$OCH_3$$

56.**255**

differences in anti-apomorphine actions of various sulfonyl-substituted benzamide neuroleptics, e.g., 56.**252c** (tiapride) and 56.**254a–e** (829), may be explained by a two dopamine receptor hypothesis (830).

Two other 3,4,5-trimethoxybenzamides, i.e., the oxazolidine (56.**256a**) and trioxazine (56.**256b**), have CNS-depressant properties. The former is weakly effective as a cataleptogenic in blocking a CAR and in a rotarod test in rats (831). Trioxazine has sedative and antianxiety actions, but is not effective in chronic schizophrenic patients (832).

Additional analogs of metoclopramide and sulpiride include sulfonamides, e.g., 56.**257** (833), pyridines, e.g., 56.**258** (834), a 3-aminopyrrolidine, 56.**259** (835), some oxadiazoles, e.g., 56.**260** (836), and a vinylogous amide 56.**261** (837). All these compounds have significant anti-apomorphine, CAR blocking, or other neuroleptic actions in animals.

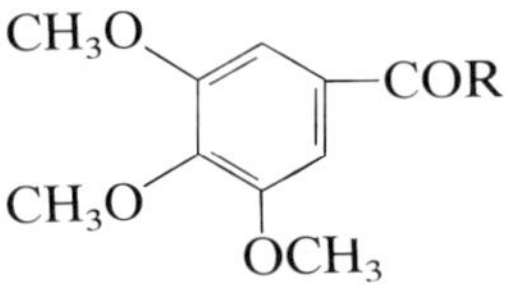

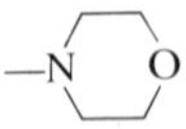

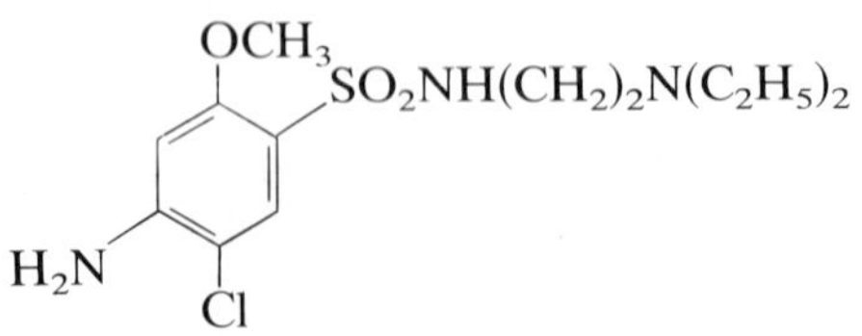

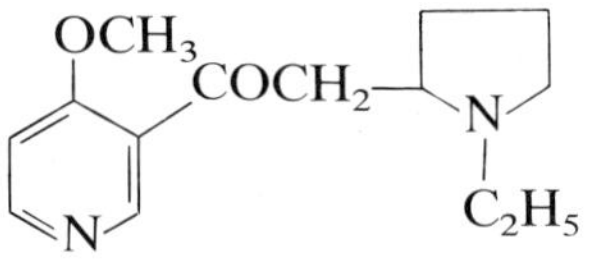

56.**258**

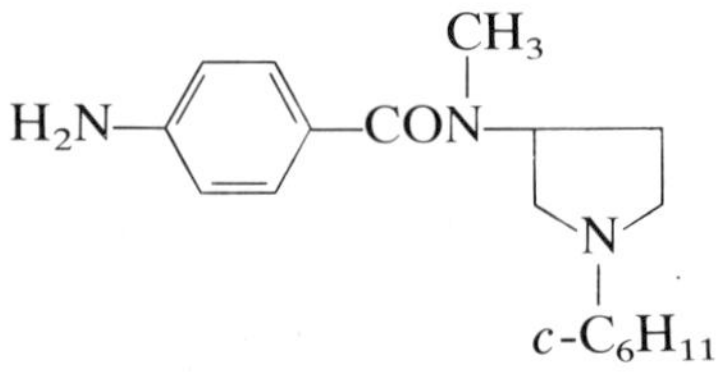

56.**259**

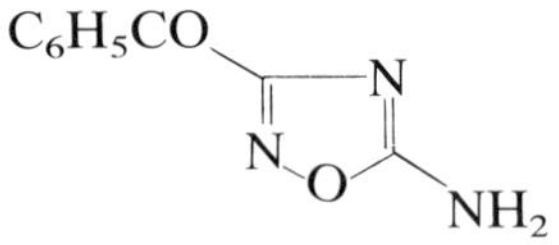

56.**260**

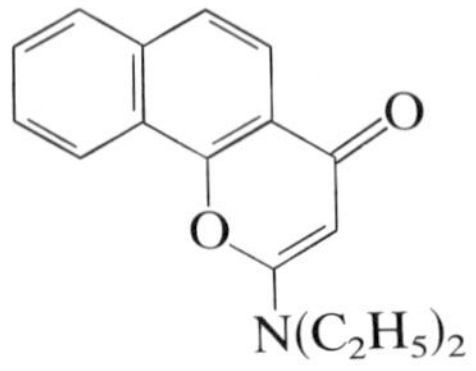

56.**261**

$$CH_3O \quad \text{—} \quad COR$$
$$CH_3O$$
$$OCH_3$$

56.**256a**   R = —N (oxazolidine)

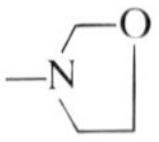

56.**256b**   R = —N (morpholine)

$$OCH_3$$
$$SO_2NH(CH_2)_2N(C_2H_5)_2$$
$$H_2N \quad Cl$$

4.11   Arylpiperazine Derivatives

Many piperazine derivatives, particularly in the tricyclic and butyrophenone series, are potent antipsychotics that are included in previous sections of this chapter. Other piperazines, with a variety of pharmacological actions, are reviewed elsewhere (838). In addition, many 1-arylpiperazines bearing a large variety of substituents in position 4 have distinct CNS-depressant, and in some instances typical neuroleptic, actions.

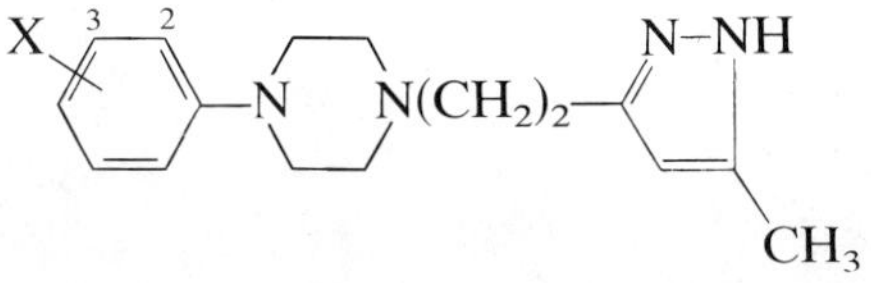

56.**262a**   X = 3-Cl
56.**262b**   X = 2-Cl
56.**262c**   X = 3-CH₃

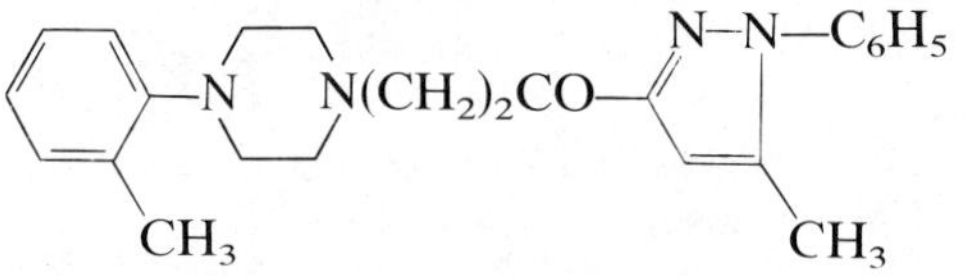

56.**263**

Some of these 1-arylpiperazines bear a heterocyclic-alkyl substituent in position 4. For example, several 1-phenyl-4-[2-(5-methyl-3-pyrazolyl)ethylpiperazines], e.g., mepiprazol (56.**262a**) (839), emiprazol (56.**262b**) (840), and toliprazol (56.**262c**) (481) have significant neuroleptic actions in animals. Mepiprazol is of modest clinical benefit in schizophrenic patients. Potent α-adrenolytic actions are noted with a related pyrazolyl Mannich base 56.**263** (842). Many series of 1-arylpiperazines having a heterocyclic-alkyl substituent in position 4 have distinct CNS-depressant actions. Only a representative sampling of the more potent members of these series is presented here. Several spiro-cyclopentane-glutarimides, e.g., 56.**264a** and 56.**264b**, are selective CNS depressants in mice and have CI values of about 0.2 and 2.0, respectively, in a CAR blockade test in rats (843). A 3-pyridyloxypropyl derivative toprilidine (56.**264c**) has significant sedative and α-adrenolytic actions (844). Triazolonylalkyl derivatives of 1-phenylpiperazine include triazolinone (56.**264d**), which abolishes aggression and blocks a CAR in rats (845), and trazodone (56.**264e**), which has chlordiazepoxide-like clinical actions (846), and is a CNS depressant with a distinctive pharmacological profile (847). Other examples of 1-phenyl-piperazines with a heterocyclic substituent in position 4 include the ox-

azolidinone 56.**264f**, which has a CI of 0.5 in blocking isolation-induced aggression in mice (848), the quinazolinedione derivative 56.**264g**, a potent serotonin antagonist (849), and the benzosulfonimide 56.**264h**, which has chlorpromazine-like activity in several animal tests (850).

Some 1-phenylpiperazines that also incorporate a β-aminoketone system are exemp-

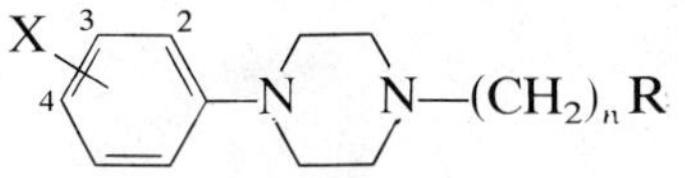

56.**264**

a   X = 2-CH₃O, n = 2, R =

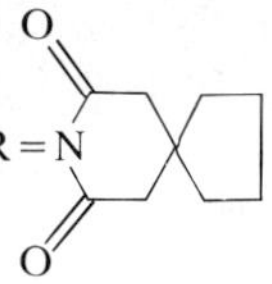

b   X = 2-Cl, n = 4, R =

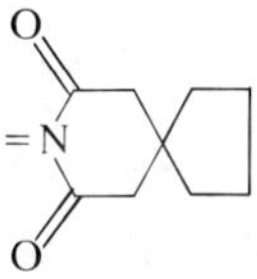

c   X = 2-CH₃, n = 3, R =

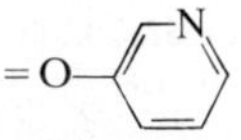

d   X = 3-Cl, n = 3, R =

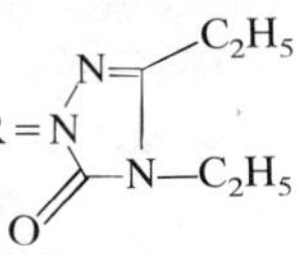

e   X = 3-Cl, n = 3, R =

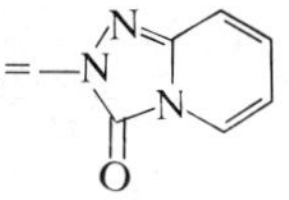

f   X = H, n = 2, R =

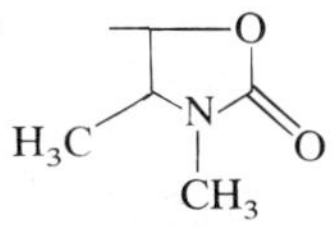

g   X = H, n = 3, R =

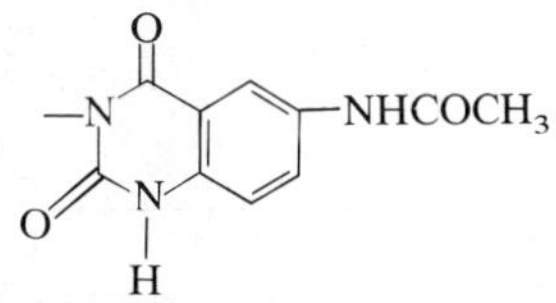

h   X = 4-F, n = 3, R =

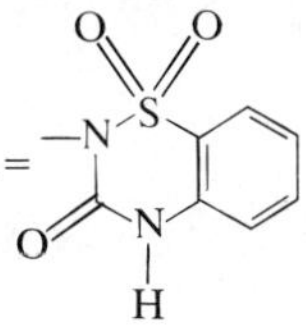

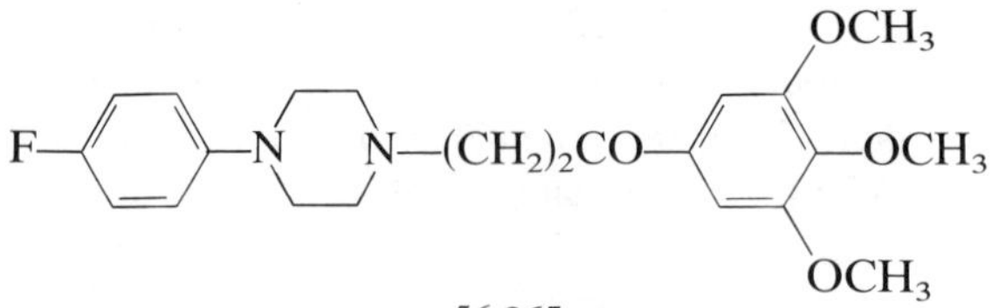

56.**265**

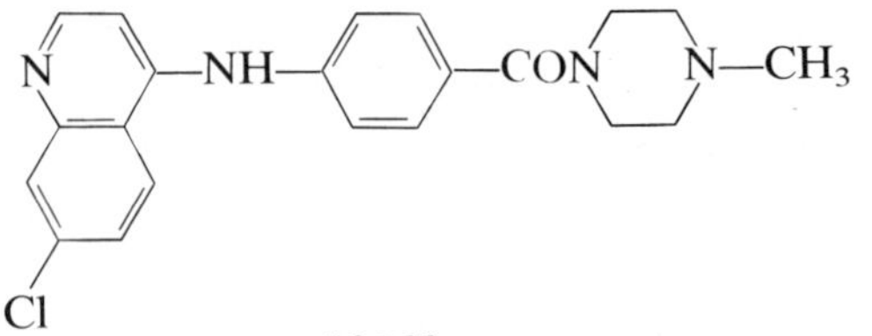

56.**266**

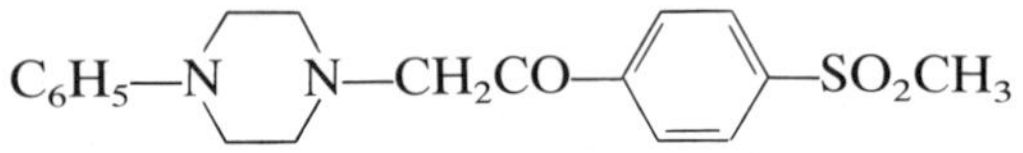

56.**267**

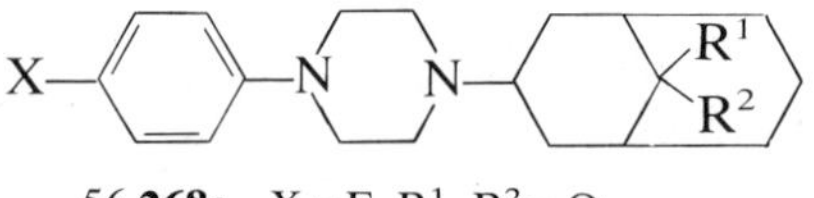

56.**268a**   X = F, R^1, R^2 = O
56.**268b**   X = R^1 = H, R^2 = OH
56.**268c**   X = H, R^1 = OH, R^2 = C$_6$H$_5$

lified by 56.**265**, which has a higher order of CNS-depressant activity with comparatively low toxicity in mice (851). Other piperazines with a carbonyl-containing substituent include a benzoyl derivative 56.**266**, which is a short-acting reserpine-like depletor of catecholamines that causes neuroleptic effects (852), several 1-phenyl-4-(4-alkylsulfonyl)phenacylpiperazines, e.g., mesylphenacryzine (56.**267**), which produce typical neuroleptic effects in mice and antagonize amphetamine-induced agitation in rats (853), and a δ-aminoketone 56.**268a** that has a CI of 0.3–0.5 in decreasing motor activity and inhibiting fighting behavior in mice and in a CAR blockade test in rats. In general, alcoholic de-

rivatives of 56.**268a**, e.g., 56.**268b** and 56.**268c**, are more potent than the ketone; in similar tests the alcohols are nearly equipotent with chlorpromazine (854).

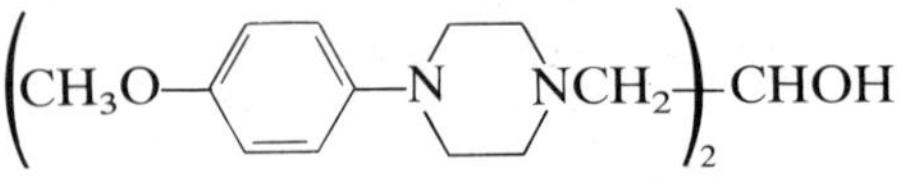

56.**271**

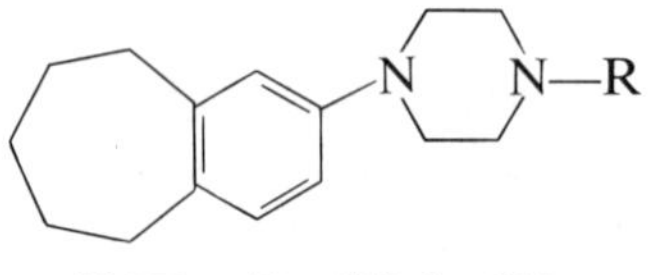

56.**272a**   R = CH$_2$C≡CH
56.**272b**   R = C$_6$H$_5$

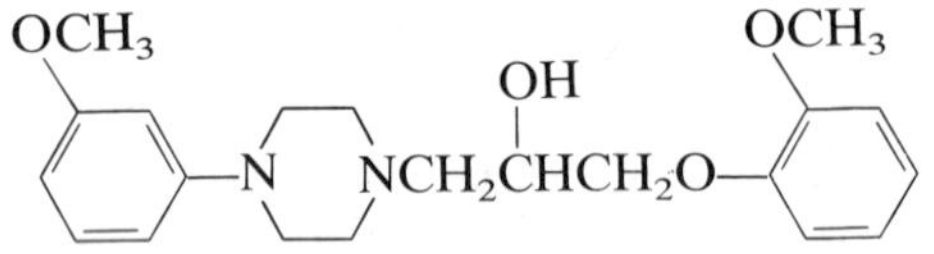

56.**269**

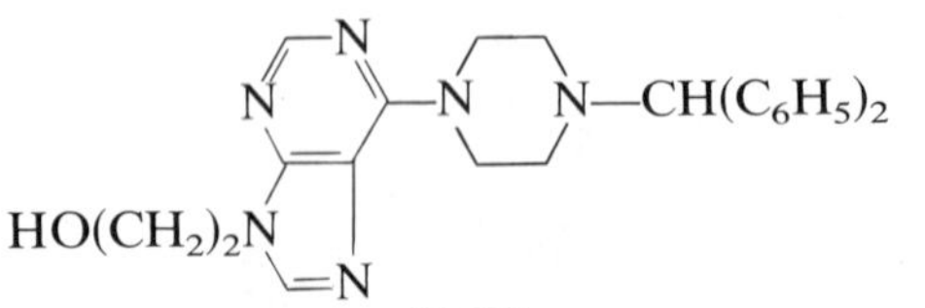

56.**270**

A phenylpiperazine 56.**269** bearing a β-adrenoreceptor blocking-type substituent in position 4 has CNS-depressant potency comparable to that of chlorpromazine (855). A xanthine-substituted piperazine 56.**270** presents a CNS-depressant profile suggestive of chlordiazepoxide-like activity (856), whereas the bis-piperazinyl derivative 56.**271** causes short-acting tetrabenazine-like actions (857). Several benzocycloheptanes, e.g., 56.**272a** (858) and 56.**272b** (859), also produce marked CNS depression in mice.

4.12   Miscellaneous Compounds with Neuroleptic Activity

Neuroleptic properties have been ascribed to many compounds that are not conveniently classed in Sections 4.1–4.11. Description of all these compounds in this section is not possible. For this reason, only a somewhat arbitrarily selected sampling of such agents is presented here. An attempt is made to include some of the more speculative findings that may stimulate future neuroleptic research.

Prenylamine $[(C_6H_5)_2CH(CH_2)_2NHCH-(CH_3)CH_2C_6H_5]$, an amphetamine derivative, lowers brain norepinephrine levels. Like tetrabenazine it partially protects against the behavioral and norepinephrine-depleting effects of reserpine, perhaps suggesting that it competes with the same site that reserpine does (860, 861). Neuroleptic activity is also produced by certain benzimidazole derivatives of amphetamine (862). Some other aralkylamines that produce neuroleptic actions in animals include the triazolopyridine 56.**273** (863) and the indene 56.**274** (864) which block a CAR in rats. Neuroleptic-like effects are also caused by the cis, but not the trans, amino alcohol 56.**275** (865), the aminoacetophenone 56.**276** (866), and a phenyl-substituted bicyclic amine 56.**277**. The latter compound, however, is not effective in chronic withdrawn schizophrenic patients (770). It

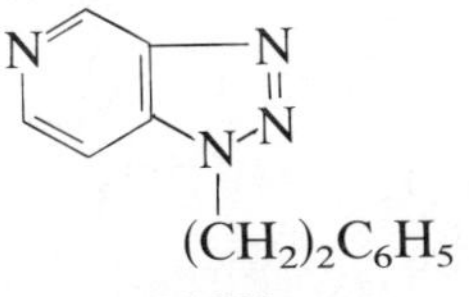

56.**275**

$HO-\!\!\!\!\!\bigcirc\!\!\!\!\!-COCH_2NH-n-C_4H_9$

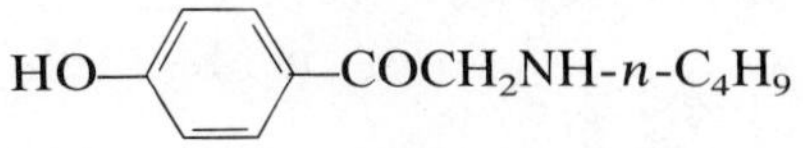

56.**276**

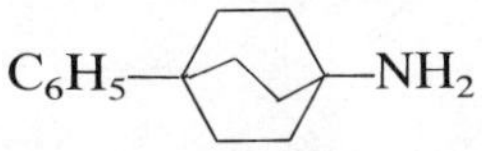

56.**277**

does have antidepressant-like effects (see Chapter 58).

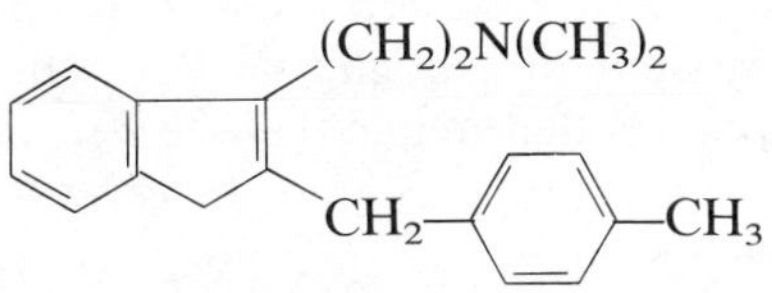

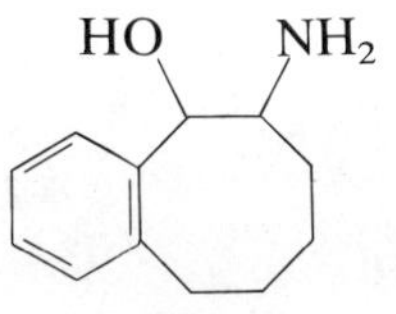

Potent CNS-depressant activity is produced by the dihydroquinolinecarbamates 56.**278** and 56.**279**. In a cataleptogenic test in rats 56.**278** ($R = C_2H_5O$) has a CI of 1.5.

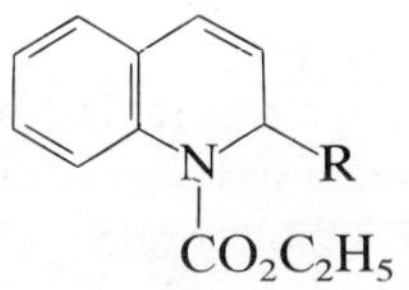

56.**278**   R = H, OCH$_3$, OC$_2$H$_5$, SCH$_3$

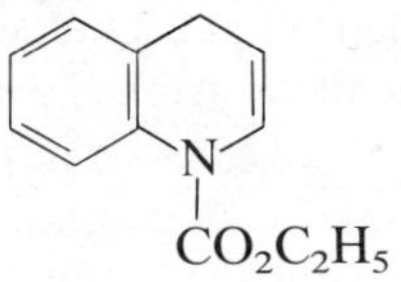

56.**279**

As an α-adrenergic antagonist in cats, it has a CI of 6 (867). In chronic schizophrenics, however, this compound is only weakly effective and produces troublesome side effects (868). Various other structures related to 56.**278** cause neuroleptic actions, e.g., amphetamine antagonism and CAR blockade, in mice and rats (869).

Triazine derivatives, 56.**280a** (870, 871) and 56.**280b** (872), produce clinical improvement in schizophrenic patients.

$(CH_2)_2C_6H_5$

56.**273**

$(CH_2)_2N(CH_3)_2$

$CH_2-\!\!\!\!\!\bigcirc\!\!\!\!\!-CH_3$

56.**274**

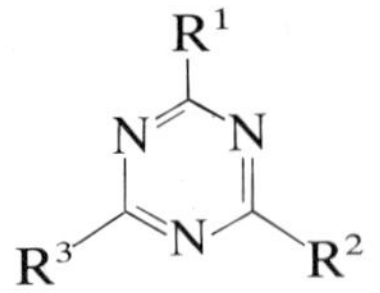

56.**280a** R^1 = NH$_2$, R^2 = OCH$_3$, R^3 = CH$_3$
56.**280b** R^1 = C$_2$H$_5$, R^2 = OCH$_3$, R^3 = NHC$_2$H$_5$

56.**280c** R^1 = NH$_2$, R^2 = CF$_3$, R^3 = N⟩⟨N(CH$_2$)$_2$OH

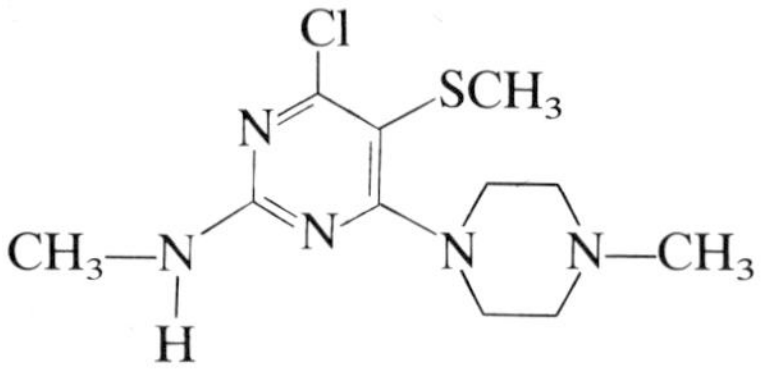

56.**281**

Another triazine 56.**280c** has a chlorpromazine-like neuroleptic profile in mice and rats (873). A somewhat related pyrimidine, mezilamine (56.**281**), inhibits dopamine-sensitive adenylate cyclase from rat brain. As with clozapine, it produces a dose-dependent increase in HVA that is more marked in the limbic system than in the striatum of rabbit brain, whereas the reverse is true in rats (874).

Other miscellaneous compounds with significant neuroleptic-like activity include some aminoalkyl trimethoxyphenyl sulfones, e.g., 56.**282**, that have chlorpromazine-like activity in a number of animal tests (875), and the cannabinoids (876), both synthetic and natural, one of the few classes of CNS agents lacking a basic nitrogen atom. Several of the latter type of compounds, e.g., 56.**283**, have CI values of 3–15 in decreasing motor activity and blocking fighting behavior in mice (877). A related compound 56.**284** has pharmaco

logical properties resembling those of both chlorpromazine and chlordiazepoxide (878). Some benzoxocins, e.g., 56.**285**, and benzoxonins, e.g., 56.**286**, produce overt neuroleptic symptoms, such as decreased motor activity, low body posture, ptosis, hypothermia, and catalepsy, in rats at doses equal to, or less than, those required for natural Δ^2 and Δ^6 tetrahydrocannabinols (879).

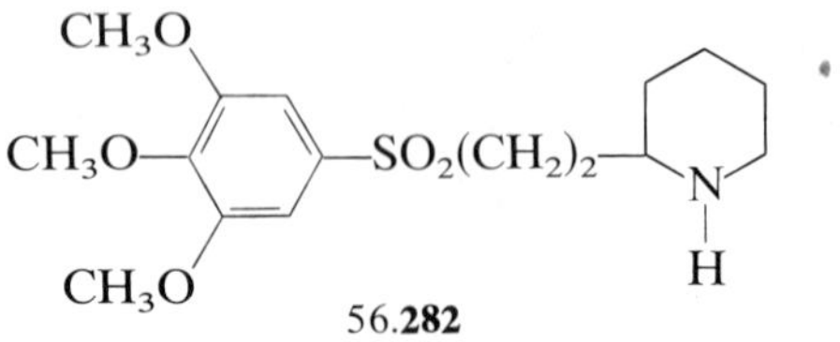

Another area of antipsychotic research involves agents that may affect a putative depressant central neurotransmitter, γ-aminobutyric acid (GABA), which may compete with the putative excitatory neurotransmitter, glutamic acid. It is postulated that potent neuroleptics may act by

56.**283**

56.**284**

56.**285**

occupying GABA receptors, making them inaccessible to glutamic acid (880). Thus compounds that mimic the effect of GABA on postsynaptic receptors in certain areas of the brain are of particular interest in human neurological disorders (881). Support for this notion is afforded by the ob-

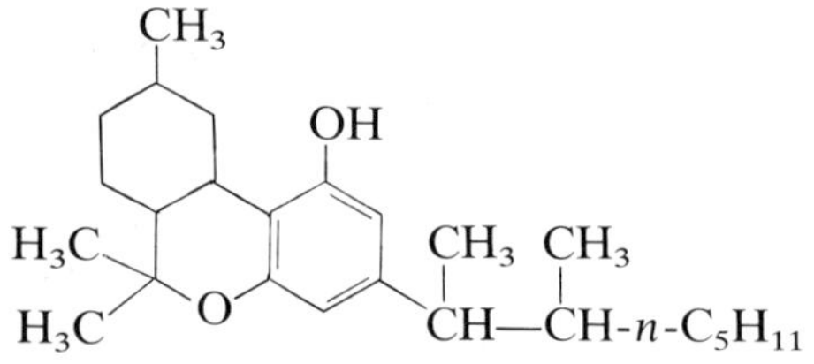

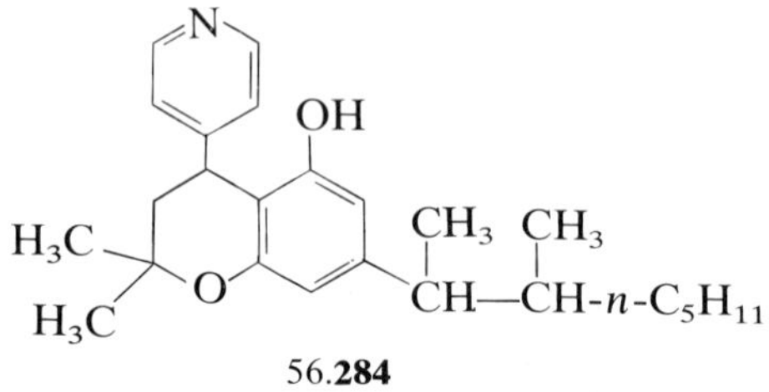

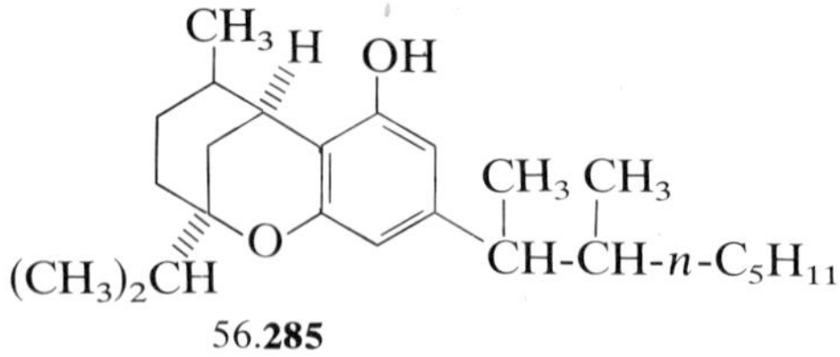

56.**282**

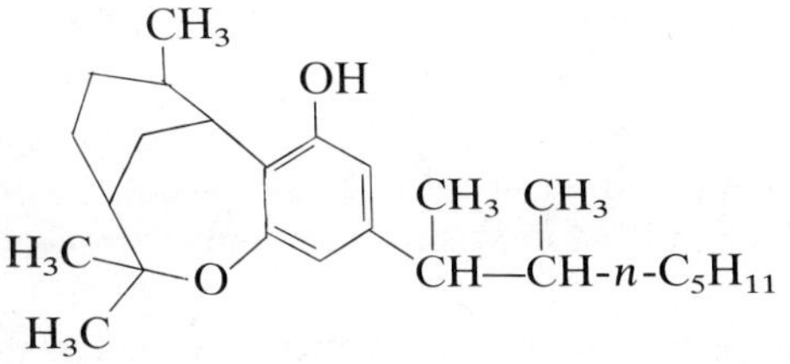

56.**286**

servation that antipsychotic butyrophenones are effective inhibitors of rat brain synaptosomal GABA uptake with relative potencies that correlate with their clinical effectiveness (882) (see Section 5). It is also conceivable that GABA-like agents could enhance the antipsychotic actions of dopamine antagonists, perhaps to permit lower doses of antipsychotics with concomitantly reduced EPS (883). GABA deficiency is implicated in two diseases of the brain, i.e., Huntington's disease (884) and epilepsy (885).

No attempt is made to review all agents affecting central GABA levels. Instead, a few selected compounds that may increase these levels are described. For example, the anticonvulsant and antiepileptic actions of sodium dipropylacetate [(n-$C_3H_7)_2CHCO_2Na$] are mediated via an increase in brain levels of GABA (886). (R)-(−)-Nipecotic acid (piperidine-3-carboxylic acid) (887) and guvacine (1,2,3,6-tetrahydropyridine-3-carboxylic acid) (888) may increase GABA levels by inhibiting uptake; however, these polar compounds do not penetrate into the brain. Some related compounds, 3-azabicyclohexanecarboxylic acid derivatives, e.g., 56.**287**, are claimed (889) to be of value in the treatment of schizophrenia, Huntington's chorea, cerebral insufficiency, and epilepsy.

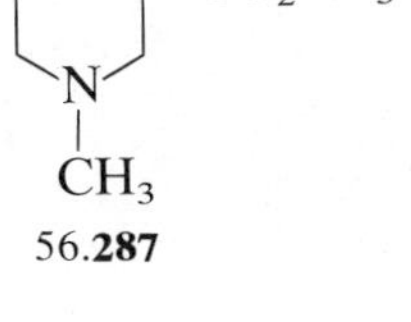

56.**287**

Some direct-acting GABA receptor agonists include *trans*-4-aminocrotonic acid ($HO_2CCH{=}CHCH_2NH_2$) (890), muscimol 56.**288** (891), isonipecotic acid (piperidine-4-carboxylic acid), isoguvacine (1,2,3,6-tetrahydropyridine-4-carboxylic acid), and a bicyclic isoxazole 56.**289** (881). A tranquilizing effect is produced by low doses of muscimol; however, it does not produce antipsychotic effects (892). Baclofen (56.**290**), a structural congener of GABA

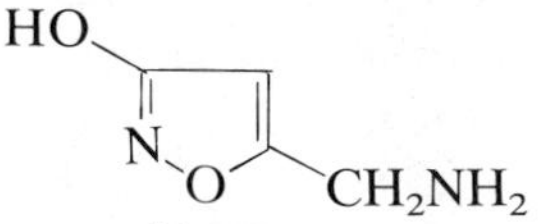

56.**288** 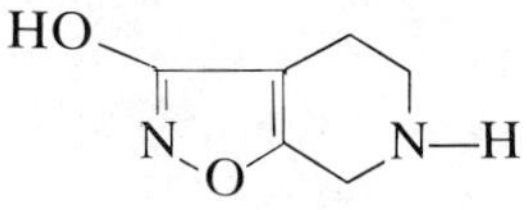   56.**289**

that is widely used in Europe for the treatment of spasticity, was once thought to be a GABA agonist. On this basis, it was examined in schizophrenic patients. Although preliminary studies were favorable (893), more recent evidence indicates it is not of significant value in the treatment of chronic schizophrenia (894). It has since been established that baclofen is not a GABA agonist (895, 896), but it inhibits postsynaptic receptors of substance

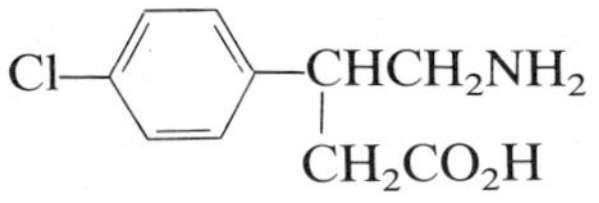

56.**290** 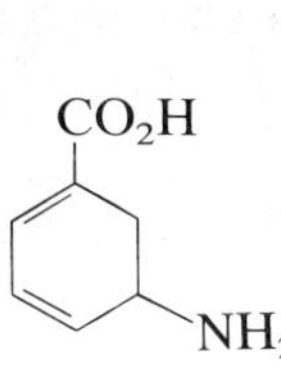   56.**291**

P probably by a general depressant effect on spinal units (897). Brain levels of dopamine and norepinephrine are decreased by baclofen (898). Anti-dopaminergic activity is also produced by another GABA analog, γ-hydroxybutyric acid [$HO(CH_2)_3COOH$] (899).

Gabaculine (56.**291**) inhibits the enzyme GABA transaminase, responsible for

metabolic degradation of GABA (900). 3-Isoxazolidinone also inhibits GABA metabolism (901).

Because GABA is present in relatively large amounts in the brain and because GABA and many of the simpler analogs, with the exception of muscimol (56.**288**), are not able to penetrate the CNS, it is difficult to assess the ultimate therapeutic utility of agents influencing central levels of GABA.

Other lines of research of possible broad implication include the suggestion that schizophrenia may be a prostaglandin deficiency disease (902). Prostaglandin E_2, like chlorpromazine, blocks a CAR in both naïve and trained rats (903). Substance P, a polypeptide with a molecular weight of about 1670, exhibits CNS-depressant effects and is proposed as a transmitter substance in sensory pathways (904). D-Penicillamine produces improvement in schizophrenic patients (905). Catechol estrogens, e.g., 2-hydroxyestradiol and 2-hydroxyestrone, are found in rat brain where they may have an important function in neuroendocrine regulation (906). Finally, it is observed that injections of β-endorphin, i.e., β-lipotropin residues 61–91, into the brains of rats elicit a cataleptic state similar to that produced by most antipsychotics, suggesting that this polypeptide might be an endogenous neuroleptic whose levels may be significant in certain forms of psychopathology (907). The spectrum of effects elicited by β-endorphin, however, contrasts significantly with those produced by haloperidol, an observation that contradicts the notion that β-endorphin may be a naturally occurring neuroleptic (908). At present it is not possible to assess the significance of these miscellaneous observations in the course of antipsychotic research. Antipsychotic efficacy has not yet been demonstrated in any opioids, although the history of morphine as a nineteenth-century antipsychotic has been traced (909) and its current status reviewed (910).

5 GENERAL CONSIDERATIONS OF ANTIPSYCHOTIC ACTIONS

The preceding section describes many types of chemicals that produce neuroleptic actions. This diversity of the structures of antipsychotic drugs presents a serious problem in trying to identify the precise structural requirements for neuroleptic activity. Before attempting to determine such structural requisites it is obviously important to establish the capability of these agents to reach the reactive site (see Section 3.2) and that they are acting by the same mechanism.

Reserpine and related compounds, such as tetrabenazine and benzquinamide, apparently act by different mechanisms than many other classes of antipsychotics. It is not established, however, that neuroleptics, such as tricyclics, indole derivatives, β-aminoketones, benzodioxans, benzamides, and arylpiperazines, act in a common fashion.

Many biochemical mechanisms have been advanced to rationalize the action of neuroleptics. These hypotheses range from the view that such drugs interact nonspecifically with neuronal and subcellular membranes to the concept that they specifically block postsynaptic receptors of neurotransmitters. Like local anesthetics many of these drugs are membrane stabilizers and could block nerve transmission by changing the permeability of a membrane to ions (911). They are potent surface-active agents that might prevent the access of neurotransmitters to their receptors by coating the postsynaptic membrane (912). Conversely, the very stringent stereostructural requirements for antipsychotic activity suggest that many of these drugs act at specific macromolecular receptor sites. Thus on the basis of the superimposability of the solid-state structures of dopamine and norepinephrine on a portion of that of chlorpromazine, it has been suggested that the antipsychotics might selectively interact with catecholamine receptors (133).

The concept that neuroleptic agents interfere with central dopaminergic mechanisms is firmly established. Such interference may be the consequence of blockade of dopamine-sensitive adenylate cyclase, inhibition of synaptic release of dopamine, or blockade of postsynaptic dopamine receptors (913). Of the three possibilities, the last seems most likely. It is difficult to relate consistently antipsychotic activity with the ability of a neuroleptic to block dopamine-sensitive adenylate cyclase in dopamine-rich areas of the brain (69, 914). Inhibition of synaptic release finds support in the excellent correlation of this effect of neuroleptics on rat striatal slices and their clinical potency as illustrated in Fig. 56.1. However, this might occur by various mechanisms; e.g., it may be related to the efficacy of these agents in stabilizing all membranes of sensitive brain dopaminergic neurons (147). These presynaptic blocking concentrations are too high to be observed clinically in the patient's serum water (75). Also, neuroleptics generally produce an increase instead of a decrease in the release of dopamine within striatal and limbic structures (915).

It seems plausible that neuroleptics bind to receptor sites in the brain to trigger an antipsychotic effect. Tritiated dopamine, haloperidol (155, 916), and spiroperidol (917) label binding (receptor) sites in mammalian brain. Further, butyrophenones, phenothiazines, and several related drugs, as illustrated in Fig. 56.2 (75) and by the data presented in Table 56.14 (156), block the binding of tritiated haloperidol (at postsynaptic receptor sites) at concentrations that correlate with clinical potencies (156, 918). Unfortunately, there is little correlation between labeled neuroleptic binding sites and the density of central dopamine-containing terminals (919), and antipsychotic potency does not correlate with affinity for tritiated dopamine binding sites as suggested by the data presented in Table 56.14 (156, 913).

Thus despite the acknowledged interference of neuroleptic agents with dopaminergic mechanisms, it is not clear exactly what receptors are involved and how this is related to antipsychotic activity. Using tritiated spiroperidol two specific neuroleptic binding sites have been identified in rat striatal homogenates (917). Clarification of the importance of these two kinds of sites might advance our understanding of the role of neuroleptics in schizophrenia. Different sites seem to be involved for dopamine agonists and antagonists (156). The sites may be located pre- and postsynaptically (920). Dopamine receptors in glial cells may differ from neuronal postsynaptic dopamine receptors (921). There is also evidence for the existence of excitation- and inhibition-mediating dopamine receptors that are affected differently by various

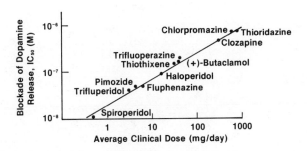

Fig. 56.1 Concentrations of neuroleptics causing 50% inhibition of electrically stimulated release of [^{3}H]-dopamine from rat striatal slices compared to average clinical dose for controlling schizophrenia (147).

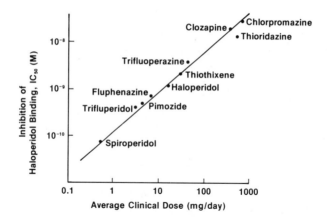

Fig. 56.2 Correlation between concentrations of neuroleptics causing 50% inhibition of butaclamol-specific [³H]-haloperidol binding on either rat or calf caudate homogenate and clinical potencies (75).

agonists and antagonists (922, 923). In another classification, dopamine receptors are subtyped as alpha or D-2, which are unrelated to adenylate cyclase, and beta or D-1, which are linked to adenylate cyclase (924). The concept of such multiple receptors, which may have important implications for therapeutic medicine, has been reviewed (925). Agonists or antagonists with specificity for certain populations of dopamine receptors may offer significant therapeutic benefit.

Even if antipsychotic activity is the consequence of interaction with dopamine sites in the brain, however, the precise mechanism of the interaction is difficult to define. This is further complicated by several other factors. Initially, blockade of dopamine receptors in the brain might incite a cascade of events that modify other central neuronal paths to counter the primary change (923). In this case, even agents that selectively interact with a specific receptor may provoke a number of nonspecific

Table 56.14 Comparison of Affinities of Neuroleptics for [³H]-Haloperidol and [³H]-Dopamine Binding Sites of Calf Striatal Membranes with Average Clinical Dose (156)

Compound	Inhibition of [³H]-Haloperidol Binding, K_i, nM	Inhibition of [³H]-Dopamine Binding, K_i, nM	Average Clinical Dose, μmol/kg/day
Spiroperidol	0.25	1400	0.058
(+)-Butaclamol	0.55	70	2.14
Pimozide	0.80	4100	0.108
Trifluperidol	0.95	880	—
Fluphenazine	1.2	180	0.168
Thiothixene	1.4	540	0.393
Haloperidol	1.5	650	0.152
Trifluoperazine	2.1	740	0.297
Chlorpromazine	10.3	900	12.0
Thioridazine	14.0	1780	12.6
Clozapine	100.0	1890	24.6

biologic responses (926). Secondly, neuroleptic binding sites in the microsomal fraction of the striatum are heterogeneous and are related not only to the action of dopamine, but also to that of serotonin and norepinephrine (927, 928). The occurrence of other neurohumoral agents, e.g., acetylcholine, γ-aminobutyric acid (GABA), and substance P, in the striatum and limbic forebrain, brain areas associated with the pathophysiology of schizophrenia, suggest that these substances might also play a role in schizophrenia (913). The correlation between inhibition of GABA uptake into rat brain synaptosomes and clinical potency of neuroleptics, particularly butyrophenones (Table 56.15), indicates a possible involvement of this neurotransmitter in antipsychotic activity (882). Another alternative possibility for the mode of action of anti-

psychotic drugs (929) is that they owe their therapeutic efficacy to a suppressing action on reticular activating systems that involve norepinephrine as the neurotransmitter (930, 931).

The multiplicity of possible modes of action of antipsychotics coupled with the demonstration of various dopaminergic pathways in the brain (932) and different kinds of dopamine receptors permits the rationalization of differences in activity even within a class of neuroleptics (830). Factors such as these, however, seriously complicate efforts to understand neuroleptic structure–activity relationships and the mode of interaction of these substances with receptors.

Some general structure–activity relationship considerations for antipsychotics have been advanced. In most neuroleptics an

Table 56.15   Inhibition of GABA Uptake into Rat Brain Synaptosomes by Antipsychotic Agents (882)

Compound	Inhibition of GABA Uptake, IC_{50}, μM^a	Average Clinical Dose, $\mu mol/kg/day^b$
Butyrophenones		
Fluspirilene	3	0.066
Pimozide	10	0.108
Benperidol	30	0.060
Spiroperidol	40	0.058
Trifuperidol	65	0.096
Haloperidol	75	0.152
Moperone	100	0.802
Fluanisone	500	3.44
Tricyclic antipsychotics		
Trifluoperazine	17	0.297
Fluphenazine	18	0.168
Triflupromazine	20	4.59
Chlorpromazine	21	12.00
Promazine	30	33.10
Flupenthixol	35	0.099
Thiothixene	38	0.393

[a] Concentrations that inhibit $[^3H]$-GABA uptake into rat brain synaptosomes by 50%.
[b] Midpoint values of daily dose ranges assuming a human weight of 70 kg (882).

56.**292**

aromatic ring is separated from a tertiary nitrogen by a four-atom spacing (185) in an "S-shaped" conformation 56.**292** (933).

Certain structure–activity considerations for antipsychotics are reminiscent of those noted for the opioids (934). In both these drug types there is a diversity of structural classes combined with strict stereochemical requirements for activity within the individual classes. In both cases, this apparent paradox might be rationalized by a multiple modality model (935), i.e., interaction of ligands with either a single type of receptor or a group of related but nonidentical receptors. In either case, multiple modes of interaction might result from association of different ligands with different recognition loci on the receptors. As with the opioids, two criteria might be used to distinguish between identical and different binding modes of neuroleptics. If identical modes are involved, structure–activity relationships and stereochemical requisites should be the same for the drugs being compared. Conversely, divergence of either of these requirements reflects different modes of ligand–receptor interaction.

Thus ligands that interact with the same receptor in the same way should exhibit similar incremental changes in potency when identically N-substituted derivatives in different series are compared. Also, stereochemical orientation of important groups, e.g., the aromatic ring and tertiary nitrogen, should be the same. Employing these criteria emphasizes the lack of meaningful biologic data for comparison of the different general classes of neuroleptics. For example, there is a general lack of data for consistent variation of the N-substituents of the various classes of neuroleptics in comparable test systems. Obviously, many

complications might be anticipated from gross comparison of *in vivo* results. Available data suggest that similar modification of the N-substituent(s) in, e.g., aminoalkylated tricyclics, butyrophenones, indole derivatives, β-aminoketones, benzamides, and arylpiperazines, generally affects neuroleptic potency in an inconsistent fashion. Even in the 6–6–6 tricyclics some differences in rank order of potency of substituted aminoalkyl derivatives are observed in different series. In most instances dimethylaminopropyl- or propylidene-substituted 6–6–6 tricyclics are less potent than their methylpiperazinyl counterparts; however, in the case of 9-substituted acridans (Section 4.2.4) the reverse appears to be true; 56.**81b** is more potent in a rat CAR test than is 56.**82b**. However, sufficient data are not available to substantiate the conclusion that the 9-aminoalkylacridans interact with (a) receptor(s) in a fashion different from that of other 6–6–6 tricyclics.

In most series of tricyclic neuroleptics modification of the N-substituent generally seems to affect potency in a uniform manner, suggestive of similar receptor–ligand interaction. In many members of these series, however, the flexible molecules do not permit discernment of the active conformation. Thus the many X-ray diffractometric, NMR, and quantum chemical methods employed to determine preferred conformations of these molecules are of limited value (936).

More meaningful attempts to identify the neuroleptic pharmacophore might be achieved by comparison of various agents with conformationally rigid and stereoselective neuroleptics. Geometric comparison of dexaclamol [(+)-56.**166j**], a rigid and stereoselective neuroleptic, with several other classes of neuroleptics suggests conformations of the flexible molecules that may be preferred for receptor interaction (568), although it is not established that all these agents act in the same way.

The use of stereoisomeric neuroleptic ligands as receptor probes has been the subject of relatively little study and has been confined almost exclusively to the dibenzo[*b,f*]thiepin series (Section 4.3.3). Of those compounds studied, e.g., octoclothepin (56.**121**), and several derivatives (56.**143** and 56.**145**), neuroleptic activity resides predominantly in those isomers with (10*S*) stereochemistry. Thus these agents could reasonably be expected to interact with the same receptor in the same manner. That the (10*R*) enantiomer 56.**146** is almost one-half as potent as 56.**145** in neuroleptic tests is perhaps a significant observation. Clearly, the topographical characteristics of neuroleptic receptors remain obscure. Definition of the chemical components that make up the neuroleptic pharmacophore awaits further study. A thorough analysis of the structural, especially configurational and conformational, features of the tricyclics necessary for antipsychotic activity may help considerably in determining the mode(s) of action of these drugs.

Formulas 56.**293**, 56.**294**, and 56.**295** illustrate the structural features so far iden-

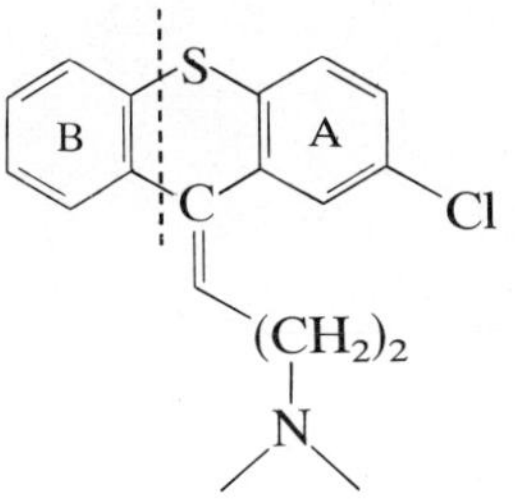

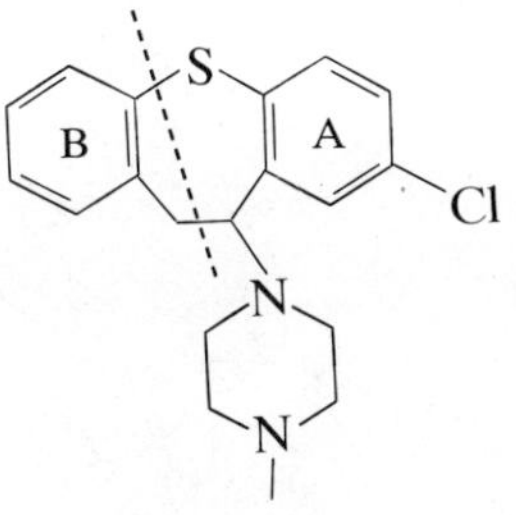

56.**295**

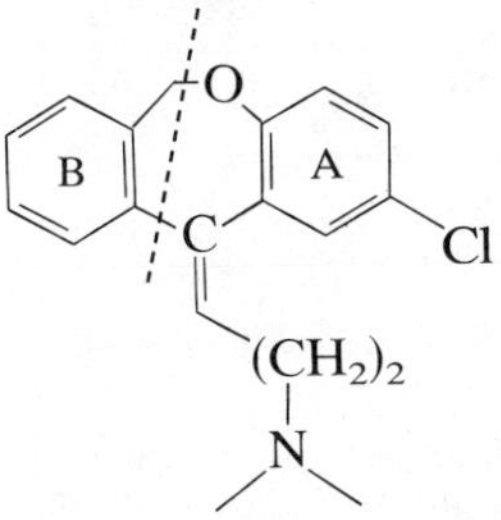

tified as being necessary for potent neuroleptic activity in the tricyclic series. They are a tricyclic ring system with a six- or seven-membered central ring, a chain of three atoms joining a terminal amino group to the central ring, and a substituent such as chloro at a position meta to the atom of the central ring from which the side chain projects. The loss in potency when the 2 substituent is relocated or if the side chain is lengthened or shortened appears to be the result of receptor-related events rather than to changes in physical properties. There is no significant change in surface activity, ionization constant, or water solubility of these analogs, and all four isomers of chloro-10-(3-dimethylaminopropyl)-phenothiazine accumulate in the brain of the mouse to the same extent (193).

These observations coupled with the requirement that aminopropylidene derivatives, e.g., 56.**293** and 56.**294**, must have the *Z* orientation for a significant degree of neuroleptic activity suggest a critical spatial relationship between the substituted A ring and the amino group. The common structural features of 56.**293**, 56.**294**, and 56.**295** are to the right of the dashed lines. In the three structures ring B is oriented differently with respect to ring A, suggesting that it may play a less specific role in binding. That the piperidylidenes, e.g., 56.**296**, are at least as potent as the *Z*-aminopropylidenes 56.**293** and 56.**294** in most tests for neuroleptic activity indicates that when bound to the receptor, rings A and B are equidistant from the amino

56.**293**

56.**294**

56.**296**

group. Thus the requirement of a *Z* orientation between ring A and the amino group in 56.**293** and 56.**294** may suggest that in these isomers initial binding of the amino group places ring A in a location that favors its interaction with appropriate receptor locus.

As indicated in Section 4, planar tricyclic derivatives lack significant neuroleptic activity. A somewhat folded conformation appears important for antipsychotic activity (936). The dihedral angle between the planes of the two benzene rings of chlorpromazine is 139.4° (937). The ability to attain such a nonplanar conformation may be important to place ring B in a position for supplemental binding or to remove this ring from a site that would interfere with the receptor interaction of ring A. In binding with serum albumin only one of the rings of a phenothiazine seems to be involved (938).

The role of the ring substituent, especially in a position meta to that from which the side chain projects, is uncertain. It may provide supplemental binding, facilitate conformational changes at the receptor site to induce an optimal fit, or facilitate transport by increasing lipophilicity. The latter suggestion implies that substitution at other ring positions may introduce steric factors that are detrimental to optimum drug–receptor interaction.

It is established that phenothiazines are able to donate an electron to form a relatively stable radical cation. This has led to the suggestion that this class of antipsychotics may owe their activity to their ability to form charge-transfer complexes with cellular constituents (939). A study of free radicals derived from many phenothiazine derivatives, however, reveals no correlation between the stability of the radicals and antipsychotic activity (940). That the radical cation might be the active drug species (101, 941) seems improbable. Although phenothiazine radical species interact with NADH, melanin, and enzymes (101), many other potent tricyclic neuroleptics are poor electron donors. The dihydroanthracenes, for example, should lose an electron only with difficulty and a radical, if generated, would be much less stable than those derived from the phenothiazines.

In conclusion, despite the wealth of pharmacological, biochemical, physical, and structure–activity relationship data accumulated for many neuroleptic agents, the mode of action of these substances and the precise structural requirements needed for activity remain to be defined. Identification of the pharmacophore(s) required for activity and determination of the mode(s) of action of this class of drugs promises to offer a challenge for even the most sophisticated biologic and chemical techniques for many years to come.

REFERENCES

1. G. Sen and K. C. Bose, *Indian Med. World*, **2**, 194 (1931).

2. J. M. Mueller, E. Schlittler, and H. Bein, *Experientia*, **8**, 338 (1952).

3. L. Dorfman, A. Furlenmeier, C. F. Huebner, R. Lucas, H. B. MacPhillamy, J. M. Meuller, E. Schlittler, R. Schwyzer, and A. F. St. André, *Helv. Chim. Acta*, **37**, 59 (1954),

4. H. J. Bein, *Experientia*, **9**, 107 (1953).

5. N. S. Kline, *Ann. N.Y. Acad. Sci.*, **59**, 107, (1954).

6. C. A. Winter, *J. Pharmacol. Exp. Ther.*, **94**, 7 (1948).

7. S. Courvoisier, J. Fournel, R. Ducrot, M. Kolsky, and P. Koetchet, *Arch. Int. Pharmacodyn. Ther.*, **92**, 305 (1952).

8. J. Delay, T. Deniker, and J. M. Harl, *Ann. Med. Psychol. Fr.*, **110,** 112 (1952).

9. H. E. Lehmann and G. E. Hanrahan, *Arch. Neurol. Psychiatr.*, **71,** 227 (1954).

10. P. A. Janssen, in *Discoveries in Biological Psychiatry*, F. J. Ayd and B. Blackwell, Eds., Lippincott, Philadelphia, 1970, p. 165.

11. G. Stille and H. Hippius, *Pharmakopsychiatr. Neuropsychopharm.*, **4,** 182 (1971).

12. H. E. Lehmann, in *Comprehensive Textbook of Psychiatry*, 2nd ed., Vol. 1, A. M. Freedman, H. I. Kaplan, and B. J. Sadock, Eds., Williams and Wilkins, Baltimore, 1975, p. 851.

13. H. E. Lehmann, in *Contemporary Standards for the Pharmacotherapy of Mental Disorders*, J. Levine, Ed., Futura Pub. Co., Mount Kisco, N.Y., 1978, p. 41.

14. S. S. Kety, in *Treatment of Schizophrenia: Progress and Prospects*, L. J. West and D. E. Flinn, Eds., Grune & Strattan, New York, 1976, p. 35.

15. H. M. Babigian, in *Comprehensive Textbook of Psychiatry*, 2nd ed., Vol. 1, A. M. Freedman, H. I. Kaplan, and B. J. Sadock, Eds., Williams and Wilkins Co., Baltimore, Md., 1975, p. 860.

16. A. Hoffer, H. Osmond, and J. Smythies, *J. Ment. Sci.*, **100,** 29 (1954).

17. A. Hoffer, in *International Review of Neurobiology*, Vol. 4, C. C. Pfeiffer and J. R. Smythies, Eds., Academic, New York-London, 1962, p. 307.

18. H. Osmond and J. Smythies, *J. Ment. Sci.*, **98,** 309 (1952).

19. M. Morgan and A. J. Mandell, *Science*, **165,** 442 (1969).

20. S. H. Snyder, *Am. J. Psychiatr.*, **130,** 61 (1973).

21. S. H. Snyder, S. P. Banerjee, H. I. Yamamura, and D. Greenberg, *Science*, **184,** 1243 (1974).

22. S. Gershon, B. Angrist, and B. Shopsin, in *Biology of the Major Psychoses* (*Res. Publ. Assoc. Res. Nerve Ment. Dis.*, **54**), D. X. Freedman, Ed., Raven Press, New York, 1975, p. 85.

23. T. Lee, P. Seeman, W. W. Tourtellotte, I. J. Farley, and O. Hornykeiwicz, *Nature*, **274,** 897 (1978).

24. F. Owen, T. J. Crow, M. Poulter, A. J. Cross, A. Longden, and G. J. Riley, *Lancet*, **1978-II,** 223.

25. J. M. Davis and R. Casper, *Drugs*, **14,** 260 (1977).

26. J. O. Cole and J. M. Davis, in *Psychopharmacology: A Review of Progress 1957–1967*, USPHS Publication, 1836, Washington, D.C., 1968, p. 1057.

27. H. L. Klawans, C. Goetz, and R. Westheimer, in *Clinical Neuropharmacology*, H. Klawans, Ed., Raven Press, New York, 1976, p. 1.

28. M. Tansella and A. Balestrieri, *Arzneim.-Forsch.*, **26,** 943 (1976).

29. R. Quitkin, A. Rifkin, and D. F. Klein, *Arch. Gen. Psychiatr.*, **32,** 1276 (1975).

30. H. Wijsenbeek, M. Steiner, and S. C. Goldberg, *Psychopharmacologia*, **36,** 147 (1974).

31. S. E. Ericksen, S. W. Hurt, S. Chang, and J. M. Davis, *Psychopharm. Bull.*, **14**:2, 15 (1978).

32. T. Itil, A. Keskiner, L. Heinemann, T. Han, P. Gannon, and W. Hsu, *Psychosomatics*, **11,** 456 (1970).

33. M. L. Clark, H. P. Ramsey, R. E. Ragland, D. K. Rahhal, E. A. Serafetinides, and J. P. Costiloe, *Psychopharmacologia*, **18,** 260 (1970).

34. B. Blackwell, in *The Future of Pharmacotherapy New Drug Delivery Systems*, F. J. Ayd, Ed., International Drug Therapy Newsletter, Baltimore, 1973, p. 17.

35. C. J. Klett, in *The Future of Pharmacotherapy New Drug Delivery Systems*, F. J. Ayd, Ed., International Drug Therapy Newsletter, Baltimore, 1973, p. 11.

36. J. E. Groves and M. R. Mandel, *Arch. Gen. Psychiatr.*, **32,** 893 (1975).

37. G. E. Hogarty and S. C. Goldberg, *Arch. Gen. Psychiatr.*, **28,** 54 (1973).

38. J. P. Leff, *Brit. J. Hosp. Med.*, **8,** 377 (1972).

39. J. Delay and P. Deniker, in *Psychotropic Drugs*, S. Garattini and V. Ghetti, Eds., Elsevier, Amsterdam, 1957, p. 485.

40. M. Shepherd and D. C. Walt, in *Current Developments in Psychopharmacology*, Vol. 4, Spectrum Publications, Los Angeles, 1977, p. 217.

41. P. F. Kennedy, H. I. Hershon, and F. J. McGuire, *Brit. J. Pyschiatr.*, **118,** 509 (1971).

42. D. F. Klein and J. M. Davis, *Diagnosis and Drug Treatment of Psychiatric Disorders*, Williams and Wilkins, Baltimore, 1969, p. 52.

43. C. J. Klett and E. Caffey, *Arch. Gen. Psychiatr.*, **26,** 374 (1972).

44. H. Kazamatsuri, C.-P. Chien, and J. O. Cole, *Arch. Gen. Psychiatr.*, **27,** 491 (1972).

45. G. C. Crane, *Brit. J. Psychiatr.*, **122,** 395 (1973).

46. J. P. Curran, *Am. J. Psychiatr.*, **130,** 406 (1973).

47. R. J. Baldessarini, *Can. Psychiatr. Assoc. J.*, **19,** 551 (1974).

48. R. M. Kobayashi, *New Engl. J. Med.*, **296,** 257 (1977).

49. A. Villeneuve and Z. Böszörményi, *Lancet*, **1970-I,** 353.

50. B. Carroll, G. C. Curtis, and E. Kokmen, *Am. J. Psychiatr.*, **134,** 785 (1977).

51. W. E. Fann, C. R. Lake, and C. J. Gerber, *Psychopharmacologia*, **37,** 101 (1974).

52. H. L. Klawans and R. Rubovits, *J. Neurol. Neurosurg. Psychiatr.*, **27,** 941 (1974).

53. P. M. O'Flanagan, *Brit. J. Med.*, **1,** 269 (1975).

54. F. A. Reda, J. M. Scanlan, and K. Kemp, *New Engl. J. Med.*, **291,** 280 (1974).

55. S. Merlis and P. A. Carone, in *Psychopharmacological Treatment: Theory and Practice*, H. Denber, Ed., Dekker, New York, 1975, p. 81.

56. R. F. Prien, C. J. Klett, and E. M. Coffey, *Arch. Gen. Psychiatr.*, **29,** 420 (1973).

57. D. P. Bobon, P. A. Janssen, and J. Bobon, Eds., *Modern Problems of Pharmacopsychiatry, The Neuroleptics*, Karger, Basel, 1970.

58. B. K. Koe, in *Neuroleptics*, S. Fielding and H. Lal, Eds., Futura Publishing Co., Mount Kisco, N.Y., 1974, p. 143.

59. C. J. E. Niemegeers, in *Neuroleptics*, S. Fielding and H. Lal, Eds., Futura Publishing Co., Mount Kisco, N.Y., 1974, p. 98.

60. G. Sedvall, B. Uvnäs, and Y. Zotterman, Eds., *Antipsychotic Drugs: Pharmacodynamics and Pharmacokinetcis*, Pergamon, New York, 1976.

61. I. Creese, D. R. Burt, and S. H. Snyder, in *Handbook of Psychopharmacology*, Vol. 10, *Neuroleptcis and Schizophrenia*, L. L. Iversen, S. D. Iversen, and S. H. Snyder, Eds., Plenum, New York, 1978, p. 37.

62. S. Fielding and H. Lal, in *Handbook of Psychopharmacology*, Vol. 10, *Neuroleptics and Schizophrenia*, L. L. Iversen, S. D. Iversen, and S. H. Snyder, Eds., Plenum, New York, 1978, p. 91.

63. A. Davidson and E. Weidley, *Life Sci.*, **18,** 1279 (1976).

64. H. Y. Meltzer and V. S. Fang, *Arch. Gen. Psychiatr.*, **33,** 279 (1976).

65. A. Carlsson and M. Lindqvist, *Acta Pharmacol. Toxicol.*, **20,** 140 (1963).

66. G. Sedvall, in *Handbook of Psychopharmacology*, Vol. 6, L. L. Iversen, S. D. Iversen, and S. H. Snyder, Eds., Plenum, New York, 1977, p. 127.

67. B. S. Bunney and G. K. Aghajanian, in *Frontiers in Catecholamine Research*, S. H. Snyder and E. Usdin, Eds., Pergamon, New York, 1973, p. 957.

68. R. H. Roth, V. H. Morgenroth, and L. C. Murrin, in *Antipsychotic Drugs: Pharmacodynamics and Pharmacokinetics*, G. Sedvall, B. Uvnäs, and Y. Zotterman, Eds., Pergamon, New York, 1976, p. 133.

69. Y. C. Clement-Cormier, J. W. Kebabian, G. L. Petzold, and P. Greengard, *Proc. Natl. Acad. Sci. U.S.*, **71,** 1113 (1974).

70. A. S. Horn and O. T. Phillipson, *Eur. J. Pharmacol.*, **37,** 1 (1976).

71. S. J. Peroutka, D. C. U'Prichard, D. A. Greenberg, and S. H. Snyder, *Neuropharmacol.*, **16,** 549 (1977).

72. R. J. Miller and C. R. Hiley, *Nature*, **248,** 596 (1974).

73. I. Creese, A. P. Feinberg, and S. H. Snyder, *Eur. J. Pharmacol.*, **36,** 231 (1976).

74. S. H. Snyder, *Am. J. Psychiatr.*, **133,** 197 (1976).

75. P. Seeman, *Biochem. Pharmacol.*, **26,** 1741 (1977).

76. A. Carlsson, *Am. J. Psychiatr.*, **135,** 164 (1978).

77. R. Byck, in *The Pharmacological Basis of Therapeutics*, 5th ed., L. S. Goodman and A. Gilman, Eds., Macmillan, New York, 1975, p. 152.

78. S. H. Curry, J. M. Davis, J. H. L. Marshall, and D. S. Janowsky, *Arch. Gen. Psychiatr.*, **22,** 209 (1970).

79. S. H. Curry, A. D'Mello, and G. P. Mould, *Brit. J. Pharmacol.*, **42,** 403 (1971).

80. S. H. Curry, J. E. Derr, and H. M. Maling, *Proc. Soc. Exp. Biol. Med.*, **134,** 314 (1970).

81. S. E. Sjöstrand, G. B. Cassano, and E. Hansson, *Arch. Int. Pharmacodyn. Ther.*, **156,** 34 (1965).

82. G. B. Cassano, S. E. Sjöstrand, and E. Hansson, *Arch. Int. Pharmacodyn. Ther.*, **156,** 48 (1965).

83. W. O. Kwant and P. Seeman, *Biochem. Pharmacol.*, **20,** 2089 (1971).

84. A. L. Green, *J. Pharm. Pharmacol.*, **19,** 207 (1967).

85. P. A. J. Janssen and F. T. N. Allewijn, *Arzneim.-Forsch.*, **19,** 199 (1969).

86. G. A. V. deJaramillo and P. S. Guth, *Biochem. Pharmacol.*, **12,** 525 (1963).

87. L. E. Hollister, *Clinical Pharmacology of Psychotherapeutic Drugs*, Churchill Livingstone, New York, 1978, p. 131.

88. S. H. Curry, *J. Pharm. Pharmacol.*, **22,** 193 (1970).

89. S. H. Curry, *J. Pharm. Pharmacol.*, **22,** 753 (1970).

90. A. A. Manian, L. H. Piette, D. Holland, T. Grover, and F. Leterrier, in *Advances in Biochemical Psychopharmacology*, Vol. 9, I. S. Forrest, C. J. Carr, and E. Usdin, Eds., Raven Press, New York, 1974, p. 149.

91. S. H. Curry, *Anal. Chem.*, **40,** 1251 (1968).

92. S. H. Curry, J. H. L. Marshall, J. M. Davis, and D. S. Janowsky, *Arch. Gen. Psychiatr.*, **22,** 289 (1970).

93. L. Rivera-Calimlim, L. Castañeda, and L. Lasagna, *Clin. Pharmacol. Ther.*, **14,** 978 (1973).

94. S. F. Cooper, J.-M. Albert, J. Hillel, and G. Caille, *Curr. Ther. Res., Clin. Exp.*, **15,** 73 (1973).

95. G. Sakalis, S. H. Curry, G. P. Mould, and M. H. Lader, *Clin. Pharmacol. Ther.*, **13,** 931 (1972).

96. J. M. Davis, D. B. Bettis, H. Dekirmenjian, S. E. Ericksen, and D. L. Garver, in *Clinical Pharmacology*, Vol. 3, H. L. Klawans, Ed., Raven Press, New York, 1978, p. 85.

97. G. Alfredsson, B. Wade-Helgodt, and G. Sedvall, *Psychopharmacol.*, **48,** 123 (1976).

98. L. Rivera-Calimlin, H. Nasrallah, J. Strauss, and L. Lasagna, *Am. J. Psychiatr.*, **133,** 646 (1976).

99. D. L. Garver, H. Dekirmenjian, J. M. Davis, R. Casper, and S. E. Ericksen, *Am. J. Psychiatr.*, **134,** 304 (1977).

100. M. E. Jarvik, in *The Pharmacological Basis of Therapeutics*, L. S. Goodman and A. Gilman, Eds., Macmillan, New York, 1965, Chap. 12.

101. E. F. Domino, R. D. Hudson, and G. Zografi, in *Drugs Affecting the Central Nervous System*, Vol. 2, A. Burger, Ed., Dekker, New York, 1968.

102. M. Gordon, Ed., *Psychopharmacological Agents*, Vol. 2, Academic, New York-London, 1967.

103. I. S. Forrest, F. M. Forrest, A. G. Bolt, and M. T. Serra, in *Neuropharmacology*, H. Brill, J. O. Cole, P. Deniker, H. Hippius, and P. B. Bradley, Eds., Excerpta Medica, Amsterdam, 1967, p. 1182.

104. J. W. Daly and A. A. Manian, *Biochem. Pharmacol.*, **16,** 2131 (1967).

105. P. F. Coccia and W. W. Westerfeld, *J. Pharmacol. Exp. Ther.*, **157,** 446 (1967).

106. A. H. Beckett and E. E. Essien, *J. Pharm. Pharmacol.*, **25,** 188 (1973).

107. A. DeLeenheer, in *Proc. Eur. Soc. for Study of Drug Toxicity, Toxicological Problems of Drug Combinations*, Vol. 13, S. B. De C. Baker and G. A. Neuhaus, Eds., 1972, p. 63.

108. A. DeLeenheer and A. Heyndrickx, *J. Pharm. Sci.*, **61,** 914 (1972).

109. K. Zehnder, K. Kalberer, W. Kries, and J. Rutschmann, *Biochem. Pharmacol.*, **11,** 535 (1962).

110. H. J. Gaertner and U. Breyer, *Arzneim.-Forsch.*, **22,** 1084 (1972).

111. U. Breyer, H. J. Gaertner, and A. Prox, *Biochem. Pharmacol.*, **23,** 313 (1974).

112. A. P. Melikian and I. S. Forrest, *Proc. West. Pharmacol. Soc.*, **15,** 78 (1972).

113. C. L. Huang and K. G. Bhansali, *J. Pharm. Sci.*, **57,** 1511 (1968).

114. J. Dreyfuss and E. C. Schreiber, *Annu. Rep. Med. Chem.*, **5,** 246 (1970).

115. A.-H. M. Afifi and E. L. Way, *J. Pharm. Sci.*, **56,** 720 (1967).

116. A. A. Manian, D. H. Efron, and D. E. Goldbert, *Life Sci.*, **4,** 2425 (1965).

117. A. A. Manian, D. H. Efron, and S. R. Harris, *Life Sci.*, **10,** 679 (1971).

118. B. S. Bunney and G. K. Aghajanian, *Life Sci.*, **15,** 309 (1974).

119. A. V. P. MacKay and A. Healy, *J. Pharmacol.* (Paris), **5:** Suppl. 2, 63 (1974).

120. A. G. Bolt and I. S. Forrest, *Life Sci.*, **6,** 1285 (1967).

121. I. Huus and A. R. Khan, *Acta Pharmacol. Toxicol.*, **25,** 397 (1967).

122. D. C. Hobbs, *J. Pharm. Sci.*, **57,** 105 (1968).

123. W. Sundijn, I. Van Wijngaarden, and F. Allewijn, *Eur. J. Pharmacol.*, **1,** 47 (1967).

124. G. A. Braun and G. I. Poos, *Eur. J. Pharmacol.*, **1,** 58 (1967).

125. E. Schlittler and A. J. Plummer, in *Psychopharmacological Agents*, Vol. 1, M. Gordon, Ed., Academic, New York-London, 1964, p. 9.

126. A. Pletscher, A. Brossi, and K. F. Gey, in *International Review of Neurobiology*, Vol. 4, C. C. Pfeiffer and J. R. Smythies, Eds., Academic, New York-London, 1962, p. 275.

127. D. E. Schwartz, H. Bruderer, J. Rieder, and A. Brossi, *Biochem. Pharmacol.*, **15,** 645 (1966).

128. E. H. Wiseman, E. C. Schreiber, and R. Pinson, Jr., *Biochem. Pharmacol.*, **13,** 1421 (1964).

129. B. K. Koe and R. Pinson, Jr., *J. Med. Chem.*, **7,** 635 (1964).

130. L. E. Hollister, *Drugs*, **4,** 321 (1972).

131. P. A. J. Janssen and W. F. VanBever, in *Current Developments in Psychopharmacology*, Vol. 2, W. E. Essman and L. Valzelli, Eds., Spectrum Publications, New York, 1975, p. 165.

132. J. M. van Rossum, *Arch. Int. Pharmacodyn. Ther.*, **160,** 492 (1966).

133. A. S. Horn and S. H. Snyder, *Proc. Natl. Acad. Sci. U.S.*, **68,** 2325 (1971).

134. R. J. Miller and L. L. Iversen, *J. Pharm. Pharmacol.*, **26,** 142 (1974).

135. H. Leblanc, G. C. L. Lachelin, S. Abu-Fadil, and S. S. Yen, *J. Clin. Endocrin. Metab.*, **43,** 668 (1976).

136. N.-E. Andén, B.-E. Roos, and B. Werdinius, *Life Sci.*, **3**, 149 (1964).

137. R. Laverty and D. F. Sharman, *Brit. J. Pharmacol. Chemother.*, **24**, 759 (1965).

138. B.-E. Roos, *J. Pharm. Pharmacol.*, **17**, 820 (1965).

139. M. DaPrada and A. Pletscher, *Experientia*, **22**, 465 (1966).

140. D. F. Sharman, *Brit. J. Pharmacol. Chemother.*, **28**, 153 (1966).

141. N.-E. Andén, H. Corrodi, K. Fuxe, and T. Hökfelt, *Eur. J. Pharmacol.*, **2**, 59 (1967).

142. H. Corrodi, K. Fuxe, and T. Hökfelt, *Life Sci.*, **6**, 767 (1967).

143. K. F. Gey and A. Pletscher, *Experientia*, **24**, 335 (1968).

144. H. Nybäck and G. Sedvall, *J. Pharmacol. Exp. Ther.*, **162**, 294 (1968).

145. N.-E. Andén, S. G. Butcher, H. Corrodi, K. Fuxe, and U. Ungerstedt, *Eur. J. Pharmacol.*, **11**, 303 (1970).

146. R. J. Miller, A. S. Horn, and L. L. Iversen, *Mol. Pharmacol.*, **10**, 759 (1974).

147. P. Seeman and T. Lee, *Science*, **188**, 1217 (1975).

148. N.-E. Andén, *Arch. Pharmacol.*, **283**, 419 (1974).

149. R. M. MacLeod, in *Frontiers of Neuroendocrinology*, L. Martini and W. F. Ganong, Eds., Raven Press, New York, 1976, p. 169.

151. R. Horowski and K. J. Graf, *Neuroendocrinol.*, **22**, 273 (1976).

152. G. Langer, E. J. Sachar, P. H. Gruen, and F. S. Halpern, *Nature*, **266**, 639 (1977).

153. H. Y. Meltzer, R. G. Fessler, and V. S. Fang, *Psychopharmacol.*, **54**, 183 (1977).

154. I. Creese, D. R. Burt, and S. H. Snyder, *Life Sci.*, **17**, 993 (1975).

155. P. Seeman, M. Chau-Wong, J. Tedesco, and K. Wong, *Proc. Natl. Acad. Sci. U.S.*, **72**, 4376 (1975).

156. I. Creese, D. R. Burt, and S. H. Snyder, *Science*, **192**, 481 (1976).

157. P. M. Seeman and H. S. Bialy, *Biochem. Pharmacol.*, **12**, 1181 (1963).

158. P. Seeman and W. O. Kwant, *Biochim. Biophys. Acta*, **183**, 512 (1969).

159. P. Seeman, in *International Review of Neurobiology*, Vol. 9, C. C. Pfeiffer and J. R. Smythies, Eds., Academic, New York-London, 1966, p. 145.

160. W. O. Kwant and P. Seeman, *Biochim. Biophys. Acta*, **193**, 338 (1969).

161. P. Seeman and T. Lee, *J. Pharmacol. Exp. Ther.*, **190**, 131 (1974).

162. D. M. Quastel, J. T. Hackett, and K. Okamoto, *Can. J. Physiol. Pharmacol.*, **50**, 279 (1972).

163. T. M. Itil, *Dis. Nerv. System*, **33**, 557 (1972).

164. P. A. J. Janssen, C. J. E. Niemegeers, and K. H. L. Schellekens, *Arzneim.-Forsch.*, **15**, 104 (1965).

165. K. Stach, M. Thiel, and F. Bickelhaupt, *Monatsh. Chem.*, **93**, 1090 (1962).

166. S. O. Winthrop, M. A. Davis, F. Herr, J. Stewart, and R. Gaudry, *J. Med. Chem.*, **6**, 130 (1963).

167. M. Protiva, *Farm. Ed. Sci.*, **21**, 76 (1966).

168. T. Ohgoh, S. Tanaka, M. Fujimoto, and A. Kitahara, *J. Pharm. Soc., Japan*, **97**, 24 (1977).

169. W. Pöldinger, *Schweiz. Arch. Neurol. Psychiatr.*, **94**, 440 (1964).

170. M. Ferrari and C. Lanzani, *Arch. Ital. Sci. Farmacol.*, **12**, 141 (1962).

171. G. E. Bonivicino, H. G. Arlt, Jr., K. M. Pearson, and R. A. Hardy, Jr., *J. Org., Chem.*, **26**, 2383 (1961).

172. M. H. Bickel and B. B. Brodie, *Int. J. Neuropharmacol.*, **3**, 611 (1964).

173. C. Van der Stelt, H. M. Tersteege, and W. T. Nauta, *Arzneim.-Forsch.*, **14**, 1324 (1964).

174. V. Seidlová, J. Metyšová, F. Hradil, Z. Votava, and M. Protiva, *Česk. Farm.*, **14**, 75 (1965).

175. C. Kaiser, A. M. Pavloff, E. Garvey, P. J. Fowler, D. H. Tedeschi, C. L. Zirkle, E. A. Nodiff, and A. J. Saggiomo, *J. Med. Chem.*, **15**, 665 (1972).

176. P. A. J. Janssen, C. J. E. Niemegeers, K. H. L. Schellekens, A. Dresse, F. M. Lenaerts, A. Pinchard, W. K. A. Schaper, J. M. VanNeuten, and F. J. Verbruggen, *Arzneim.-Forsch.*, **18**, 261 (1968).

177. R. M. Pinder, R. N. Brogden, P. R. Sawyer, T. M. Speight, R. Spencer, and G. S. Avery, *Drugs*, **12**, 1 (1976).

178. D. J. Vadodaria, C. V. Deliwala, S. S. Mandrekar, and U. K. Sheth, *J. Med. Chem.*, **12**, 860 (1969).

179. D. N. Johnson, W. H. Funderburk, and J. W. Ward, *Curr. Ther. Res., Clin. Exp.*, **12**, 402 (1970).

180. E. Schenker and H. Herbst, in *Progress in Drug Research*, Vol. 5, E. Jucker, Ed., Birkhaüser, Basel-Stuttgart, 1963, p. 269.

181. C. L. Zirkle and C. Kaiser, in *Medicinal Chemistry*, 3rd ed., Part II, A. Burger, Ed., Wiley-Interscience, New York, 1970, pp. 1410–1469.

182. C. L. Zirkle and C. Kaiser, in *Psychopharmacological Agents*, Vol. 3, M. Gordon, Ed., Academic, New York, 1974, p. 39.

184. H. W. Gschwend, in *Industrial Pharmacology, A Monograph Series, Neuroleptics*, Vol. 1, S. Fielding and H. Lal, Eds., Futura Publishing Co., Mt. Kisco, N.Y., 1974, p. 1.

185. P. A. J. Janssen, in *Industrial Encyclopedia of Pharmacology and Therapeutics*, Vol. 1, Section 5, C. J. Cavallito, Ed., Pergamon, New York, 1973, p. 37.

186. E. Usdin and D. H. Efron, *Psychotropic Drugs and Related Compounds*, 2nd ed., *Dep. Health Educ. Walfare Publ. No.* (*HSM*) *72-9074*, U.S. Government Printing Office, Washington, D.C., Stock No. 1724-0194, 1972.

187. I. S. Forrest, C. J. Carr, and E. Usdin, Eds., *Phenothiazines and Structurally Related Drugs*, Vol. 9, *Advances in Biochemical Psychopharmacology*, Raven Press, New York, 1974.

188. M. W. Parkes, in *Progress in Medicinal Chemistry*, Vol. 1, G. P. Ellis and G. B. West, Eds., Butterworths, London, 1961, p. 72.

189. P. B. Bradley, in *Physiological Pharmacology*, Vol. 1, W. S. Root and F. G. Hofmann, Eds., Academic, New York, 1963, p. 417.

190. E. F. Domino, *Clin. Pharmacol. Ther.*, **3**, 599 (1962).

191. L. Cook and E. Weidley, *Ann. N.Y. Acad. Sci.*, **66**, 740 (1957).

192. D. H. Tedeschi, R. E. Tedeschi, A. Mucha, L. Cook, P. A. Mattis, and E. J. Fellows, *J. Pharmacol. Exp. Ther.*, **125**, 28 (1959).

193. A. L. Green, *J. Pharm. Pharmacol.*, **19**, 207 (1967).

194. D. Lenke, *Arzneim.-Forsch.*, **11**, 874 (1961).

195. Rhône-Poulenc, Fr. Pat. 1,167,661 (1958); through *Chem. Abstr.*, **55**, 9436h (1961).

196. P. Charpentier, *C. R. Acad. Sci.*, **225**, 306 (1947).

197. P. Gaillot and J. Gaudichon, U.S. Pat. 2,892,839 (1959); through *Chem. Abstr.*, **53**, 15103c (1959).

198. R. C. Fuson and C. L. Zirkle, *J. Am. Chem. Soc.*, **70**, 2760 (1948).

199. C. Kaiser, P. J. Fowler, and C. L. Zirkle, unpublished results.

200. C. Kaiser, D. H. Tedeschi, P. J. Fowler, A. M. Pavloff, B. M. Lester, and C. L. Zirkle, *J. Med. Chem.*, **14**, 179 (1971).

201. O. Neischulz, I. Hoffman, and K. Popendiker, *Med. Exp.*, **1**, 246 (1959); through *Chem. Abstr.*, **54**, 15672 (1960).

202. I. P. Lapin, *Zh. Neuropathol. Psikhiat. S. S. Korsakova*, **64**, 281 (1964).

203. R. Dahlbom, *Acta Chem. Scand.*, **7**, 873 (1953).

204. R. Dahlbom and T. Ekstrand, *Acta Chem. Scand.*, **5**, 102 (1951).

205. J. Weinstock, A. R. Maass, V. D. Wiebelhaus, G. Sosnowski, and J. P. Rosenbloom, *3rd Middle Atlantic Reg. Meet., Am. Chem. Soc.. Philadelphia*, 1968.

206. A. N. Gritsenko, Z. I. Ermakova, S. V. Zhuravlev, T. A. Vikhlyaev, T. A. Klygul, and O. V. Ul'yanova, *Khim.-Farm. Zh.*, **5**, 18 (1971); through *Chem. Abstr.*, **75**, 140776f (1971).

207. A. L. Ekonomov, A. N. Gritsenko, and A. E. Vasilev, *Khim.-Farm. Zh.*, **11**, 76 (1977).

208. A. R. Maass, G. Sosnowski, V. D. Wiebelhaus, and J. Weinstock, *J. Pharmacol. Exp. Ther.*, **163**, 239 (1968).

209. A. W. Weston, R. W. DeNet, and R. J. Michaels, Jr., *J. Am. Chem. Soc.*, **75**, 4006 (1953).

210. D. R. Maxwell, M. A. Read, K. F. Rhodes, and E. A. Sumpter, *Abstr. Volunteer Papers, 5th Congr. Pharmacol., San Francisco*, 1972, p. 152.

211. M. Gordon, L. Cook, D. H. Tedeschi, and R. E. Tedeschi, *Arzneim.-Forsch.*, **13**, 318 (1963).

212. O. Nieschulz, K. Popendiker, and K.-H. Sack, *Arzneim.-Forsch.*, **4**, 232 (1954).

213. L. Buchel and J. Levy, *Thérapie*, **15**, 1064 (1960).

214. I. S. Epstein, *Ann. Allergy*, **18**, 754 (1960).

215. Y.-H. Wu and R. F. Feldcamp, *J. Org. Chem.*, **26**, 1529 (1961).

216. S. L. Shapiro, H. Soloway, and L. Freedman, *J. Am. Pharm. Assoc., Sci. Ed.*, **46**, 333 (1957).

217. J.-P. Bourquin, G. Schwarb, G. Gamboni, R. Fischer, L. Ruesch, S. Guldimann, V. Theus, E. Schenker, and J. Renz, *Helv. Chim. Acta*, **41**, 1072 (1958).

218. O. Nieschulz, I. Hoffmann, and K. Popendiker, *Arzneim.-Forsch.*, **10**, 156 (1960).

219. P. E. Setler, unpublished results.

220. D. M. Gallant, M. P. Bishop, and D. Sprehe, *Curr. Ther. Res., Clin. Exp.*, **7**, 102 (1965).

221. H. Freeman, M. Rivera Oktem, and N. Oktem, *Curr. Ther. Res., Clin. Exp.*, **11**, 263 (1969).

222. J. Glatzel, *Med. Welt*, **23**, 62 (1972).

223. G. G. Brune, H. H. Kohl, W. G. Steiner, and H. E. Himwich, *Biochem. Pharmacol.*, **12**, 679 (1963).

224. H. S. Posner, E. Hearst, W. L. Taylor, and G. J. Cosmides, *J. Pharmacol. Exp. Ther.*, **137**, 84 (1962).

225. J. R. Geigy, A.-G., Belg. Pat. 670,541; through *Chem. Abstr.*, **59**, 7537 (1963).

226. P. Seeman, H. Machleidt, J. Kahling, and S. Sengupta, *Can. J. Physiol. Pharmacol.*, **52**, 558 (1974).

227. P. Viaud, *J. Pharm. Pharmacol.*, **6**, 361 (1954).

228. G. J. Martin, R. Brendel, and J. M. Beiler, *Arzneim.-Forsch.*, **6**, 408 (1956).

229. T. M. Itil, *Arzneim.-Forsch.*, **15**, 817 (1965).

230. F. J. Villani and C. A. Ellis, *J. Med. Chem.*, **9**, 185 (1966).

231. J. P. Long, A. M. Lands, and B. L. Zenitz, *J. Pharmacol. Exp. Ther.*, **119**, 479 (1957).

232. G. A. Medvedev and M. D. Mashkovskii, *Farmakol. Toksikol.* (Moscow), **35**, 401 (1972).

233. J. W. Cusic, U.S. Pat. 2,766,235 (1956); through *Chem. Abstr.*, **51**, 7442 (1957).

234. H. L. Yale, A. I. Cohen, and F. Sowinski, *J. Med. Chem.*, **6**, 347 (1963).

235. F. J. Ayd, Jr., *Am. J. Psychiatr.*, **132**, 491 (1975).

236. J. Dreyfuss, J. J. Ross, Jr., J. M. Shaw, I. MIller, and E. C. Schreiber, *J. Pharm. Sci.*, **65**, 502 (1976).

237. L. Julou, G. Bourat, R. Ducrot, J. Fournel, and C. Garret, *Acta Psychiatr. Scand. Suppl.*, **241**, 9 (1973).

238. A. Jørgensen, K. F. Overø, and V. Hansen, *Acta Pharmacol. Toxicol.*, **29**, 339 (1971).

239. W. L. Honrath, A. Wolff, and A. Meli, *Steroids*, **2**, 425 (1963).

240. A. J. Levenson, *Curr. Ther. Res., Clin. Exp.*, **19**, 320 (1976).

241. H. L. Yale, *J. Med. Chem.*, **20**, 302 (1977).

242. D. Lenke, N. Brock, and B. Neteler, *Arzneim.-Forsch.*, **17**, 317 (1967).

243. H. Berzewski and H. Hippius, *Arzneim.-Forsch.*, **17**, 329 (1967).

244. D. Lenke, B. Neteler, and N. Brock, *Arzneim.-Forsch.*, **21**, 288 (1971).

245. J. R. Boissier and C. Dumont, *Thérapie*, **26**, 481 (1971).

246. P. Deniker, D. Ginestet, P. Peron-Magnan, L. Colonna, and H. Loo, *Thérapie*, **26**, 227 (1971).

247. T. V. Mikhailova, A. I. Terekhina, and A. P. Gilev, *Farmakol. Toksikol.* (Moscow), **32**, 31 (1969).

248. T. Fokstuen, *Int. J. Neuropsychiatr.*, **1**, 294 (1965).

249. C. Casagrande, A. Galli, R. Ferrini, and G. Miragoli, *Arzneim.-Forsch.*, **21**, 808 (1971).

250. C. H. Grogan, R. Kelly, and L. M. Rice, *J. Med. Chem.*, **9**, 654 (1966).

251. M. Nakanishi, C. Tashiro, T. Munakata, K. Araki, T. Tsumagari, and H. Imamura, *J. Med. Chem.*, **13**, 644 (1970).

252. H. Berzewski, H. Hippius, H. Petri, and R. Schiffter, *Arzneim.-Forsch.*, **20**, 949 (1970).

253. A. Ribbentrop and W. Schaumann, *Arch. Int. Pharmacodyn. Ther.*, **149**, 374 (1964).

254. W. B. McKeon, Jr., *Arch. Int. Pharmacodyn. Ther.*, **146**, 374 (1963).

255. C. Barchewitz and H. Helmchen, *Pharmako-psychiatr./Neuro-Psychopharmakol.*, **3**, 293 (1970).

256. J. Bobon, J. M. Gernay, J. Collard, F. Goffioril, and M. Breulet, *Acta Neurol. Belg.*, **68**, 154 (1968).

257. P. Populaire, B. Decouvelaere, G. Lebreton, S. Pascal, and B. Terlain, *Arch. Int. Pharmacodyn. Ther.*, **173**, 281 (1968).

258. R. F. Boswell, Jr., W. J. Welstead, Jr., R. L. Duncan, D. N. Johnson, and W. H. Funderburk, *J. Med. Chem.*, **21**, 136 (1978).

259. D. N. Johnson, B. C. Turley, C. B. Coffin, M. R. Jones, and W. H. Funderburk, *Fed. Proc.*, **37**, 480 (1978).

260. D. N. Johnson, C. A. Leonard, B. C. Turley, M. R. Jones, and W. H. Funderburk, *Drugs, Exp. Clin. Res.*, **4**: 2, 1 (1978).

261. M. M. P. Broussolle, J. Grambert, and M. Hodam, *Ann. Med.-Psychol.*, **129**: 2, 436 (1971).

262. D. M. Gallant and M. P. Bishop, *Curr. Ther. Res., Clin. Exp.*, **12**, 387 (1970).

263. K. Haworth, L. M. Jones, and W. Mandel, *Am. J. Psychiatr.*, **117**, 749 (1961).

264. Y. LaPierre and M. Lee, *Curr. Ther. Res., Clin. Exp.*, **19**, 105 (1976).

265. F. J. Ayd, Jr., *Int. Drug Ther. Newslett.*, **7**, 1 (1972).

266. R. Guerrero-Figueroa, E. Guerrero-Figueroa, D. M. Gallant, and H. Deha Vega, *Curr. Ther. Res., Clin. Exp.*, **16**, 659 (1974).

267. D. M. Gallant, *Psychopharm. Bull.*, **11**: 1, 11 (1975).

268. D. M. Gallant, D. Mielke, G. Bishop, T. Oelsner, and R. Guerrero-Figueroa, *Dis. Nerv. Syst.*, **36**, 193 (1975).

269. J. V. Ananth, R. C. Jain, H. E. Lehmann, and T. A. Ban, *Curr. Ther. Res., Clin. Exp.*, **18**, 585 (1975).

270. H. S. Posner and E. Hearst, *Int. J. Neuropharmacol.*, **3**, 635 (1964).

271. J. C. Burke, G. L. Hassert, Jr., and J. P. High, *Meet. Soc. Pharmacol. Exp. Ther., French Lick, Indiana, November 8–10, 1956.*

272. J. C. Burke, G. L. Hassert, Jr., and J. P. High, *J. Pharmacol. Exp. Ther.*, **119**, 136 (1957).

273. E. A. Nodiff, S. Lipschutz, P. N. Craig, and M. Gordon, *J. Org. Chem.*, **25**, 60 (1960).

274. W. Wirth, R. Grösswald, U. Hörlein, Kl.-H. Risse, and H. Kreiskott, *Arch. Int. Pharmacodyn. Ther.*, **115**, 1 (1958).

275. F. Sowinski and H. L. Yale, *J. Med. Pharm. Chem.*, **5**, 54 (1962).

276. K. P. Bhargava and O. Chandra, *Brit. J. Pharmacol. Chemother.*, **22**, 154 (1964).

277. D. M. Gallant, M. P. Bishop, and W. Shelton, *Curr. Ther. Res., Clin. Exp.*, **7**, 204 (1965).

278. P. A. J. Janssen, C. J. E. Niemegeers, and K. H. L. Schellekens, *Arzneim.-Forsch.*, **15**, 1196 (1965).

279. M. Remy, in *Psychopharmacology Frontiers*, N. S. Kline, Ed., Little, Brown, Boston, 1959, p. 85.

280. J. Schmitt, M. Suquet, M. Brunaud, and G. Callet, *Bull. Soc. Chim. Fr.* [5], **1961**, 1140.

281. A. P. Feinberg and S. H. Snyder, *Proc. Natl. Acad. Sci. U.S.*, **72**, 1899 (1975).

282. A. S. Horn, M. L. Post, and O. Kennard, *J. Pharm. Pharmacol.*, **27**, 553 (1975).

283. J. Hebký, O. Rádek, and J. Kejha, *Collect. Czech. Chem. Commun.*, **24**, 3988 (1959).

284. P. N. Craig, M. Gordon, J. J. Lafferty, B. M. Lester, A. J. Saggiomo, and C. L. Zirkle, *J. Org. Chem.*, **26**, 1138 (1961).

285. R. P. Maickel, F. M. Fedynskj, W. Z. Potter, and A. A. Manian, *Toxicol. Appl. Pharmacol.*, **28**, 8 (1974).

286. H. Barry, III, M. L. Steenberg, A. A. Manian, and J. P. Buckley, *Psychopharmacologia*, **34**, 351 (1974).

287. P. N. Craig, E. A. Nodiff, J. J. Lafferty, and G. E. Ullyot, *J. Org. Chem.*, **22**, 709 (1957).

288. P. N. Craig, M. Gordon, J. J. Lafferty, B. M. Lester, A. M. Pavloff, and C. L. Zirkle, *J. Org. Chem.*, **25**, 944 (1960).

289. J. Hebký, J. Kejha, and M. Karásek, *Collect. Czech. Chem. Commun.*, **26**, 1559 (1961).

290. A. A. Manian, N. Watzman, M. L. Steenberg, and J. P. Buckley, *Life Sci.*, **7**, 731 (1968).

291. R. B. Moffett and B. D. Aspergren, *J. Am. Chem. Soc.*, **82**, 1600 (1960).

292. R. J. Warren, W. E. Thompson, J. E. Zarembo, and I. B. Eisdorfer, *J. Pharm. Sci.*, **56**, 1496 (1967).

293. K. P. Bhargava and O. Chandra, *Brit. J. Pharmacol. Chemother.*, **22**, 154 (1964).

294. H. L. Yale and F. Sowinski, *J. Am. Chem. Soc.*, **80**, 1651 (1958).

295. A. von Schlichtegroll, *Arzneim.-Forsch.*, **8**, 489 (1958).

296. P. A. J. Janssen, C. J. E. Niemegeers, and K. H. L. Schellekens, *Arzneim.-Forsch.*, **16**, 339 (1966).

297. G. M. Simpson and J. W. S. Angus, *Curr. Ther. Res., Clin. Exp.*, **9**, 265 (1967).

298. H. Linke, *Muench. Med. Wochenschr.*, **100:** 25, 969 (1958).

299. A. von Schlichtegroll, *Arzneim.-Forsch.*, **7**, 237 (1957).

300. A. Gross, K. Thiele, W. A. Schuler, and A. von Schlichtegroll, *Arzneim.-Forsch.*, **18**, 435 (1968).

301. H. Goethe, *Arzneim.-Forsch.*, **12**, 321 (1962).

302. G. M. Simpson and J. W. S. Angus, *Curr. Ther. Res., Clin. Exp.*, **9**, 225 (1967).

303. A. J. Saggiomo, P. N. Craig, and M. Gordon, *J. Org. Chem.*, **23**, 1906 (1958).

304. S. Umio and T. Kishimoto, Jap. Pat. 6809228 (1968); through *Chem. Abstr.*, **69**, 106724d (1968).

305. F. H. Clarke, G. B. Silverman, C. M. Watnick, and N. Sperber, *J. Org. Chem.*, **26**, 1126 (1961).

306. Rhône-Poulenc, Fr. Pat. 1,167,657 (1958); through *Chem. Abstr.*, **55**, 9436 (1961).

307. Rhône-Poulenc, Brit. Pat. 797,061 (1958); through *Chem. Abstr.*, **53**, 2261 (1959).

308. A. Gross and K. Thiele, U.S. Pat. 3,299,057 (1967); through *Chem. Abstr.*, **61**, 4382 (1967).

309. C. J. Grol and H. Rollema, *J. Med. Chem.*, **18**, 857 (1975).

310. M. Suquet and J. Schmitt, *Bull. Soc. Chim. Fr.* [5], **1961**, 2113.

311. J. Schmitt, Fr. Pat. 1,229,643 (1960); through *Chem. Abstr.*, **55**, 23443 (1961).

312. M. H. Sherlock, N. Sperber, and D. Papa, U.S. Pat. 2,889,328 (1959); through *Chem. Abstr.*, **54**, 411 (1960).

313. A. Funke, G. Funke, and B. Millet, *Bull. Soc. Chim. Fr.* [5], **1961**, 1524.

314. M. Wilhelm and P. Schmidt, *J. Heterocycl. Chem.*, **6**, 635 (1969).

315. U. Hoerlein, Kl. H. Risse, and W. Wirth, *Med. Chem. Abh. Med.-Chem. Forschungsstaetten Farbenfabriken Bayer*, **7**, 79 (1963); through *Chem. Abstr.*, **61**, 1128 (1964).

316. T. Fujita and D. H. Tedeschi, *Pharmacologist*, **7**, 155 (1965).

317. C. A. Leonard, T. Fujita, D. H. Tedeschi, C. L. Zirkle, and E. J. Fellows, *J. Pharmacol. Exp. Ther.*, **154**, 339 (1966).

318. H. Vanderhaeghe and L. Verlooy, *J. Org. Chem.*, **26**, 3827 (1961).

319. M. P. Olmsted, P. N. Craig, J. J. Lafferty, A. M. Pavloff, and C. L. Zirkle, *J. Org. Chem.*, **26**, 1901 (1961).

320. G. Cordella and F. Sparatore, *Farm. Ed. Sci.*, **20**, 446 (1965).

321. I. Molnar and T. Wagner-Jauregg, *Helv. Chim. Acta*, **48**, 1782 (1965).

322. U. Jahn, *Naunyn-Schmiedebergs Arch. Pharmakol. Exp. Pathol.*, **253**, 48 (1966).

323. E. Guth and G. Hoffman, *Wien. Klin. Wochenschr.*, **78**, 14 (1966).

324. C. L. Zirkle, U.S. Pat. 3,449,334 (1969); through *Chem. Abstr.*, **71**, 49800r (1969).

325. Smith Kline & French Laboratories, Fr. Pat. 1,530,413 (1968); through *Chem. Abstr.*, **72**, 3397g (1970).

326. P. J. Fowler, C. L. Zirkle, E. Macko, C. Kaiser, H. Sarau, and D. H. Tedeschi, *Arzneim.-Forsch.*, **27**, 866 (1977).

327. H. Freeman and M. Rivera Oktem, *Curr. Ther. Res., Clin. Exp.*, **8**, 395 (1966).

328. G. M. Simpson, J. Iqbal, and F. Iqbal, *Curr. Ther. Res., Clin. Exp.*, **8**, 447 (1966).

329. W. G. Case and K. Rickels, *Curr. Ther. Res., Clin. Exp.*, **9**, 477 (1967).

330. L. J. Hekimian, A. Floyd, and S. Gershon, *Curr. Ther. Res., Clin. Exp.*, **9**, 17 (1967).

331. C.-P. Chien and M.-M. Tsuang, *Curr. Ther. Res., Clin. Exp.*, **10**, 223 (1968).

332. H. Freeman, N. Oktem, and M. Rivera Oktem, *Curr. Ther. Res., Clin. Exp.*, **10**, 537 (1968).

333. M. P. Bishop, L. B. Mason, D. M. Gallant, and G. Bishop, *Curr. Ther. Res., Clin. Exp.*, **11**, 447 (1969).

334. W. T. Lampe, II, *Curr. Ther. Res., Clin. Exp.*, **11**, 300 (1969).

335. C. L. Zirkle, U.S. Pat. 3,131,190 (1964); through *Chem. Abstr.*, **61**, 4326 (1964).

336. C. Kaiser, P. J. Fowler, D. H. Tedeschi, B. M. Lester, E. Garvey, C. L. Zirkle, E. A. Nodiff, and A. J. Saggiomo, *J. Med. Chem.*, **17**, 57 (1974).

337. R. A. Wiley and J. H. Collins, *J. Med. Chem.*, **12**, 146 (1969).

338. J. F. Muren and B. M. Bloom, *J. Med. Chem.*, **13**, 14 (1970).

339. J. Hyttel, *J. Pharm. Pharmacol.*, **26**, 588 (1974).

340. I. Møller Nielsen, B. Fjalland, V. Pedersen, and M. Nymark, *Psychopharmacologia*, **26**, Suppl. 100 (1972).

341. P. V. Petersen, N. Lassen, T. Holm, R. Kopf, and I. Møller Nielsen, *Arzneim.-Forsch.*, **8**, 395 (1958).

342. I. Møller Nielsen, W. Hougs, N. Lassen, T. Holm, and P. V. Petersen, *Acta Pharmacol. Toxicol.*, **19**, 87 (1962).

343. J. F. Muren and B. M. Bloom, *J. Med. Chem.*, **13**, 17 (1970).

344. K. Pelz, E. Svátek, J. Metyšová, F. Hradil, and M. Protiva, *Collect. Czech. Chem. Commun.*, **35**, 2623 (1970).

345. L. Fontanella, L. Mariani, E. Occelli, B. Rosselli del Turco, and A. Diena, *Farm. Ed. Sci.*, **26**, 489 (1971).

346. J. D. Dunitz, H. Eser, and P. Strickler, *Helv. Chim. Acta*, **47**, 1897 (1964).

347. J. P. Schaefer, *Chem. Commun.*, **743**, (1967).

348. D. C. Remy and W. A. Van Saun, Jr., *Tetrahedron Lett.*, **27**, 2463 (1971).

349. C. Kaiser, R. J. Warren, and C. L. Zirkle, *J. Med. Chem.*, **17**, 131 (1974).

350. P. V. Petersen and I. M. Møller Nielsen, in *Psychopharmacological Agents*, Vol. 1, M. Gordon, Ed., Academic, New York, 1964, p. 301.

351. D. M. Gallant, M. P. Bishop, and W. Shelton, *Curr. Ther. Res., Clin. Exp.*, **7**, 415 (1965).

352. A. A. Sugerman and F. J. Lichtigfeld, *Curr. Ther. Res., Clin. Exp.*, **7**, 707 (1965).

353. K. Pelz, E. Svátek, J. Metyšová, F. Hradil, and M. Protiva, *Collect. Czech. Chem. Commun.*, **35**, 2623 (1970).

354. K. Pelz and M. Protiva, *Collect. Czech. Chem. Commun.*, **32**, 2161 (1967).

355. M. Rajšner, J. Metyšová, E. Svátek, F. Mitšík, and M. Protiva, *Collect. Czech. Chem. Commun.*, **40**, 719 (1975).

356. I. Cervená, K. Sindelář, Z. Kopicová, J. Holubek, E. Svátek, J. Metyšová, M. Hrubantová, and M. Protiva, *Collect. Czech. Chem. Commun*, **42**, 2001 (1977).

357. A. Weissman, *Psychopharmacologia*, **12**, 142 (1968).

358. M. P. Bishop, T. E. Fulmer, and D. M. Gallant, *Curr. Ther. Res., Clin. Exp.*, **8**, 509 (1966).

359. D. M. Gallant, M. P. Bishop, E. Timmons, and A. Gould, *Curr. Ther. Res., Clin. Exp.*, **8**, 153 (1966).

360. A. A. Kurland, A. Pinto, B. H. Dim, and C. A. Johnson, *Curr. Ther. Res., Clin. Exp.*, **9**, 298 (1967).

361. J. Simeon, A. Keskiner, D. Ponce, T. Itil, and M. Fink, *Curr. Ther. Res., Clin. Exp.*, **9**, 10 (1967).

362. P. A. J. Janssen, C. J. E. Niemegeers, and K. H. L. Schellekens, *Arzneim.-Forsch.*, **16**, 339 (1966).

363. P. A. J. Janssen, C. J. E. Niemegeers, K. H. L.

Schellekens, and F. M. Lenaerts, *Arzneim.-Forsch.*, **17,** 841 (1967).

364. W. Poeldinger, *Arzneim.-Forsch.*, **17,** 1133 (1967).

365. T. J. Crow and E. C. Johnstone, *Brit. J. Pharmacol.*, **59,** P466 (1977).

366. H. Gross and E. Kaltenbäck, *Acta Psychiatr. Scand.*, **41,** 42 (1965).

367. I. Møller-Nielsen, V. Boeck, A. V. Christensen, P. Danneskiold-Samsoe, J. Hyttel, J. Langeland, V. Pedersen, and O. Svendsen, *Acta Pharmacol. Toxicol.*, **41,** 369 (1977).

368. J. Hyttel, *Acta Pharmacol. Toxicol.*, **41,** 449 (1977).

369. Rhône-Poulenc, Belg. Pat. 622,072 (1963); through *Chem. Abstr.*, **60,** 1758 (1964).

370. E. Jucker and A. Ebnoether, U.S. Pat. 3,086,972 (1963); through *Chem. Abstr.*, **59,** 10057f (1963).

371. E. Jucker and A. Ebnoether, Belg. Pat. 638,971 (1964); through *Chem. Abstr.*, **62,** 9138b (1965).

372. E. L. Engelhardt, H. C. Zell, W. S. Saari, M. E. Christy, C. D. Colton, C. A. Stone, J. M. Stavorski, H. C. Wenger, and C. T. Ludden, *J. Med. Chem.*, **8,** 829 (1965).

373. SmithKline Corporation, U.S. Pat. 4,086,350 (1978).

374. B. K. Koe, *Pharmacologist*, **20,** 273 (1978).

375. SmithKline Corporation, U.S. Pat. 4,073,912 (1978).

376. V. Seidlová, J. Metyšová, F. Hadril, Z. Votava, and M. Protiva, *Cesk. Farm.*, **14,** 75 (1965).

377. K. Sindelář, E. Svátek, J. Metyšová, J. Metyš, and M. Protiva, *Collect. Czech. Chem. Commun.*, **34,** 3792 (1969).

378. J. Janecek and B. C. Schiele, *Psychopharmacologia*, **6,** 462 (1964).

379. S. Lecolier, *Chim. Ther.*, **3,** 193 (1968); through *Chem. Abstr.*, **70,** 77149h (1969).

380. P. N. Craig and C. L. Zirkle, Belg. Pat. 694,036 (1967).

381. P. J. Fowler, C. L. Zirkle, E. Macko, P. E. Setler, H. M. Sarau, A. Misher, and D. H. Tedeschi, *Arzneim.-Forsch.*, **27,** 1589 (1977).

382. T. M. Itil, N. Polvan, L. Engin, M. B. Guthrie, and M. F. Huque, *Curr. Ther. Res., Clin. Exp.*, **21,** 343 (1977).

383. P. V. Petersen, N. Lassen, V. Hansen, T. Huld, J. Hjortkjaer, J. Holmblad, I. Møller Nielsen, M. Nymark, V. Pedersen, A. Jørgensen, and W. Hougs, *Acta Pharmacol. Toxicol.*, **24,** 121 (1966).

384. J. R. Boissier, C. Dumont, and R. Ratouis, *Chim. Ther.*, **5,** 323 (1967); through *Chem. Abstr.*, **69,** 27094v (1968).

385. J. R. Boissier, R. Ratouis, C. Dumont, L. Taliani, and J. Forest, *J. Med. Chem.*, **10,** 86 (1967).

386. M. Wilhelm and P. Schmidt, *Helv. Chim. Acta*, **52,** 1385 (1969).

387. L. Maître, M. Staehelin, and H. J. Bein, *Biochem. Pharmacol.*, **19,** 2875 (1970).

388. R. L. Biddy, R. S. Smith, and G. S. Magrinat, *J. Clin. Pharmacol. J. New Drugs*, **10,** 29 (1970).

389. J. Henisz, A. Kubacki, W. Szelenberger, and I. Wtosinska, *Psychiatr. Pol.*, **3,** 675 (1969).

390. L. Geisler and H.-D. Rost, *Arzneim.-Forsch.*, **20,** 957 (1970).

391. H. Brunner, P. R. Hedwall, M. Meier, and H. J. Bein, *Agents Actions*, **2,** 69 (1971); through *Chem. Abstr.*, **76,** 10334v (1972).

392. L. Maître, M. Staehelin, and H. J. Bein, *Biochem. Pharmacol.*, **20,** 2169 (1971).

393. H. Bratlund, *Acta Psychiatr. Scand.*, **37,** 295 (1961).

394. B. Saletu, J. Grünsberger, R. Flener, L. Linzmayer, and H. Sieroslawski, *Curr. Ther. Res., Clin. Exp.*, **20,** 810 (1976).

395. J. R. Tretter, J. F. Muren, B. M. Bloom, and A. Weissman, *Am. Chem. Soc. Med. Chem. Symp.*, *Bloomington, Indiana*, June 1966.

396. A. Ribbentrop and W. Schaumann, *Arzneim.-Forsch.*, **15,** 863 (1965).

397. D. M. Gallant, M. P. Bishop, and W. Shelton, *Curr. Ther. Res., Clin. Exp.*, **8,** 241 (1966).

398. A. A. Sugerman and F. J. Lichtigfeld, *Curr. Ther. Res., Clin. Exp.*, **8,** 244 (1966).

399. M. Protiva, V. Hněvsová-Seidlová, Z. J. Vejdélek, I. Jirkovsky, Z. Votava, and J. Metyšová, *J. Med. Pharm. Chem.*, **4,** 411 (1961).

400. M. Protiva, V. Hněvsová-Seidlová, I. Jirkovsky, L. Novak, and Z. J. Vejdélek, *Cesk. Farm.*, **10,** 506 (1962); through *Chem. Abstr.*, **57,** 7196e (1962).

401. S. O. Winthrop, M. A. Davis, G. S. Meyers, J. G. Gavin, R. Thomas, and R. Barber, *J. Org. Chem.*, **27,** 230 (1962).

402. J. Metyšová, J. Metyš, and Z. Votava, *Arzneim.-Forsch.*, **13,** 1039 (1963).

403. J. Metyšová, J. Metyš, and Z. Votava, *Arzneim.-Forsch.*, **15,** 524 (1965).

404. S. O. Winthrop, M. A. Davis, F. Herr, J. Stewart, and R. Gaudry, *J. Med. Pharm. Chem.*, **5,** 1207 (1962).

405. M. Rajšner, E. Svátek, V. Seidlová, E. Adlerová,

and M. Protiva, *Collect. Czech. Chem. Commun.,* **34,** 1278 (1969).

406. A. E. Drukker, E. I. Judd, J. M. Spoerl, and F. Kaminski, *J. Heterocycl. Chem.,* **2,** 276 (1965).

407. E. L. Engelhardt, M. E. Christy, C. D. Colton, M. B. Freedman, C. C. Boland, L. M. Halpern, V. G. Vernier, and C. A. Stone, *J. Med. Chem.,* **11,** 325 (1968).

408. F. J. Villani, C. A. Ellis, C. Teichman, and C. Bigos, *J. Med. Pharm. Chem.,* **5,** 373 (1962).

409. G. M. Simpson and J. W. S. Angus, *Curr. Ther. Res., Clin. Exp.,* **9,** 24 (1967).

410. A. A. Sugerman, *Curr. Ther. Res., Clin. Exp.,* **8,** 479 (1966).

411. B. Angrist, J. Rotrosen, M. Aaronson, and S. Gershon, *Curr. Ther. Res., Clin. Exp.,* **20,** 94 (1976).

412. H. E. Lehmann, T. A. Ban, and M. Deutsch, *Psychopharmacol. Bull.,* **13,** 7 (1977).

413. G. M. Simpson, B. Zoubok, and J. H. Lee, *Curr. Ther. Res., Clin. Exp.,* **19,** 87 (1976).

414. J. Castañer and P. Thorpe, *Drugs Future,* **3,** 251 (1978).

415. B. Carnmalm, L. Johansson, S. Ramsby, N. E. Stjernström, S. B. Ross, and S.-O. Ogren, *Nature,* **263,** 519 (1976).

416. D. C. Remy, K. E. Rittle, C. A. Hunt, P. S. Anderson, B. H. Arison, E. L. Engelhardt, R. Hirshmann, B. V. Clineschmidt, V. J. Lotti, P. R. Bunting, R. J. Ballentine, N. L. Papp, L. Flataker, J. J. Witoslawski, and C. A. Stone, *J. Med. Chem.,* **20,** 1013 (1977).

417. M. Williams and B. V. Clineschmidt, *Fed. Proc.,* **37,** 856 (1978).

418. S. E. Robinson, V. J. Lotti, and F. Sulser, *J. Pharm. Pharmacol.,* **29,** 564 (1977).

419. M. Rajšner, J. Metyš, and M. Protiva, *Collect. Czech. Chem. Commun.,* **32,** 2854 (1967).

420. J. M. Bastian, A. Ebnöther, E. Jucker, E. Rissi, and A. P. Stoll, *Helv. Chim. Acta,* **54,** 277 (1971).

421. E. Messmer, *Arzneim.-Forsch.,* **19,** 735 (1969).

422. E. Venecovský, Vl. Šedivec, E. Peterová, and P. Baudis, *Arzneim.-Forsch.,* **19,** 491 (1969).

423. A. Gehring, P. Blaser, R. Spiegel, and W. Pöldinger, *Arzneim.-Forsch.,* **21,** 15 (1971).

424. W. V. Krumholz, J. A. Yaryura-Tobias, and L. White, *Curr. Ther. Res., Clin. Exp.,* **10,** 342 (1968).

425. E. Galantay, C. Hoffman, N. Paolella, J. Gogerty, L. Iorio, G. Leslie, and J. H. Trapold, *J. Med. Chem.,* **12,** 444 (1969).

426. M. Protiva, *Pharm. Ind.,* **2,** 923 (1970).

427. I. Jirkovský, J. Metyš, and M. Protiva, *Collect. Czech. Chem. Commun.,* **32,** 3448 (1967).

428. H. L. Yale, B. Beer, J. Pluscec, and E. R. Spitzmiller, *J. Med. Chem.,* **13,** 713 (1970).

429. M. Protiva, M. Borovička, V. Hach, Z. Votava, J. Šrámková, and J. Horáková, *Experientia,* **13,** 291 (1957).

430. M. Nakanishi, T. Tsumagari, T. Okada, and Y. Kase, *Arzneim.-Forsch.,* **18,** 1435 (1968).

431. P. Deniker, H. Lôo, E. Zarifian, G. Garreau, A. Benyacoub, and J. M. Roux, *Ann. Med. Psychol.,* **136:**9, 1069 (1978).

432. M. Nakanishi, T. Tsumagari, and A. Nakanishi, *Arzneim.-Forsch.,* **21,** 391 (1971).

433. Yoshitomi Pharm. Ind., Ltd., *Jap. Med. Gaz.,* **12:**Feb. 20, 7 (1975).

434. W. Theobald, O. Buch, H. A. Kunz, C. Morpurgo, E. G. Stenger, and G. Wilhelmi, *Arch. Int. Pharmacodyn. Ther.,* **148,** 560 (1964).

435. Endo Labs, Inc., Belg. Pat. 140,177 (1977).

436. V. Seidlová, K. Pelz, E. Adlerová, I. Jirkovský, J. Metyšová, and M. Protiva, *Collect. Czech. Chem. Commun.,* **34,** 2258 (1969).

437. J. O. Jílek, E. Svátek, J. Metyšová, J. Pomykáček, and M. Protiva, *Collect. Czech. Chem. Commun.,* **32,** 3186 (1967).

438. J. O. Jílek, K. Sindelar, J. Pomykáček, O. Horešovsky, K. Pelz, E. Svátek, B. Kakác, J. Holubek, J. Metyšova, and M. Protiva, *Collect. Czech. Chem. Commun.,* **38,** 115 (1973).

439. J. Metyšová and M. Protiva, *Act. Nerv. Super.,* **17,** 218 (1975).

440. T. J. Petcher, J. Schmutz, H. P. Weber, and T. G. White, *Experientia,* **31,** 1389 (1975).

441. V. Seidlová and M. Protiva, *Collect. Czech. Chem. Commun.,* **32,** 1747 (1967).

442. A. Jaunin, T. J. Petcher, and H. P. Weber, *J. Chem. Soc., Perkin II,* 186 (**1977**).

443. M. Protiva, J. O. Jílek, J. Metyšová, V. Seidlová, I. Jirkovský, J. Metys, E. Adlerová, I. Ernest, K. Pelz, and J. Pomykáček, *Farm., Ed. Sci.,* **20,** 721 (1965).

444. K. Sindelář, J. O. Jílek, V. Bártl, J. Metyšová, B. Kakác, J. Holubek, E. Svátek, J. Pomykáček, and M. Protiva, *Collect. Czech. Chem. Commun.,* **41,** 910 (1976).

445. J. O. Jílek, J. Pomykácek, J. Metyšová, and M. Protiva, *Collect. Czech. Chem. Commun.,* **35,** 276 (1970).

446. (a) J. P. Tollenaere, H. Moereels, and M. Protiva, *Eur. J. Med. Chem.,* **11,** 293 (1976); (b) K. Pelz, I. Jirkovský, J. Metyšová, and M. Protiva, *Collect. Czech. Chem. Commun.,* **34,** 3936 (1969).

447. J. O. Jílek, K. Sindelář, A. Dlabač, E. Kazdová, J. Pomykáček, Z. Šedivý, and M. Protiva, *Collect. Czech. Chem. Commun.*, **38**, 1190 (1973).

448. E. Adlerová, I. Ernest, J. Metyšová, and M. Protiva, *Collect. Czech. Chem. Commun.*, **33**, 2666 (1969).

449. J. O. Jílek, J. Metyšová, J. Pomykáček, and M. Protiva, *Collect. Czech. Chem. Commun.*, **39**, 3338 (1974).

450. K. Sindelář, J. Metyšová, B. Kakáč, J. Holubek, E. Svátek, J. O. Jílek, J. Pomykáček, and M. Protiva, *Collect. Czech. Chem. Commun.*, **39**, 2099 (1974).

451. K. Šindelář, J. Metyšová, and M. Protiva, *Collect. Czech. Chem. Commun.*, **38**, 2484 (1973).

452. I. Cervená, J. Metyšová, E. Svátek, B. Kakáč, J. Holubek, M. Hrubantová and M. Protiva, *Collect. Czech. Chem. Commun.*, **41**, 881 (1976).

453. K. Pelz, I. Jirkovský, E. Adlerová, J. Metyšová, and M. Protiva, *Collect. Czech. Chem. Commun.*, **33**, 1895 (1968).

454. V. Valenta, J. Metyšová, Z. Šedivý, and M. Protiva, *Collect. Czech. Chem. Commun.*, **39**, 783 (1974).

455. K. Šindelář, J. Metyšová, and M. Protiva, *Collect. Czech. Chem. Commun.*, **37**, 1734 (1972).

456. K. Šindelář, J. Metyšová, and M. Protiva, *Collect. Czech. Chem. Commun.*, **38**, 2137 (1973).

457. K. Šindelář, A. Dlabač, J. Metyšová, B. Kakáč, J. Holubek, E. Svátek, Z. Šedivý, and M. Protiva, *Collect. Czech. Chem. Commun.*, **40**, 1940 (1975).

458. M. Protiva, Z. Šedivý, and J. Metyšová, *Collect. Czech. Chem. Commun.*, **40**, 2667 (1975).

459. V. Bártl, J. Metyšová, J. Metyš, J. Nemec, and M. Protiva, *Collect. Czech. Chem. Commun.*, **38**, 2301 (1973).

460. K. Šindelář, B. Kakáč, J. Metyšová, and M. Protiva, *Farm. Ed. Sci.*, **28**, 256 (1973).

461. J. O. Jílek, K. Šindelář, M. Rajšner, A. Dlabač, J. Metyšová, Z. Votava, J. Pomykáček, and M. Protiva, *Collect. Czech. Chem. Commun.*, **40**, 2887 (1975).

426. K. Šindelář, A. Dlabač, B. Kakác, E. Svátek, J. Holubek, Z. Šedivý, E. Princová, and M. Protiva, *Collect. Czech. Chem. Commun.*, **40**, 2649 (1975).

463. J. O. Jílek, J. Pomykáček, J. Metyšová, M. Bartosova, and M. Protiva, *Collect. Czech. Chem. Commun.*, **43**, 1741 (1978).

464. K. Šindelář, J. O. Jílek, J. Metyšová, J. Pomykáček, and M. Protiva, *Collect. Czech. Chem. Commun.*, **39**, 3548 (1974).

465. K. Šindelář, J. Holubek, A. Dlabač, M. Bartosova, and M. Protiva, *Collect. Czech. Chem. Commun.*, **42**, 2231 (1977).

466. K. Šindelář, J. O. Jílek, J. Pomykáček, Z. Šedivý, and M. Protiva, *Collect. Czech. Chem. Commun.*, **43**, 471 (1978).

467. J. O. Jílek, I. Červená, Z. Kopicová, K. Šindelář, E. Svátek, J. Metyšová, A. Dlabać, J. Pomykáček, and M. Protiva, *Collect. Czech. Chem. Commun.*, **41**, 443 (1976).

468. K. Šindelář, Z. Kopicová, J. Metyšová, and M. Protiva, *Collect. Czech. Chem. Commun.*, **40**, 3530 (1975).

469. I. Červená, K. Šindelář, J. Metyšová, E. Svátek, M. Ryska, M. Hrubantová, and M. Protiva, *Collect. Czech. Chem. Commun.*, **42**, 1705 (1977).

470. Z. Kopicová, J. Metyšová, and M. Protiva, *Collect. Czech. Chem. Commun.*, **40**, 3519 (1975).

471. M. Rajšner, E. Svátek, J. Metyšová, M. Bartosova, F. Miksik, and M. Protiva, *Collect. Czech. Chem. Commun.*, **42**, 3079 (1977).

472. K. Šindelář, B. Kakáč, E. Svátek, J. Holubek, J. Metyšová, M. Hrubantová, and M. Protiva, *Collect. Czech. Chem. Commun.*, **38**, 3321 (1973).

473. K. Šindelář, J. Metyšová, J. Holubek, Z. Šedivý, and M. Protiva, *Collect. Czech. Chem. Commun.*, **42**, 1179 (1977).

474. M. Rajšner, E. Svátek, J. Metyšová, and M. Protiva, *Collect. Czech. Chem. Commun.*, **40**, 1604 (1975).

475. Z. Kopicová and M. Protiva, *Collect. Czech. Chem. Commun.*, **39**, 3147 (1974).

476. Z. Kopicová, E. Svátek, and M. Protiva, *Collect. Czech. Chem. Commun.*, **40**, 1960 (1975).

477. I. Červená, E. Svátek, J. Metyšová, and M. Protiva, *Collect. Czech. Chem. Commun.*, **39**, 3733 (1974).

478. J. O. Jílek, J. Metyšová, E. Svátek, F. Jančik, J. Pomykáček, and M. Protiva, *Collect. Czech. Chem. Commun.*, **38**, 599 (1973).

479. J. O. Jílek, J. Pomykáček, J. Metyšová, and M. Protiva, *Collect. Czech. Chem. Commun.*, **36**, 2226 (1971).

480. J. O. Jílek, J. Metyšová, J. Němec, Z. Šedivý, J. Pomykáček, and M. Protiva, *Collect. Czech. Chem. Commun.*, **40**, 3386 (1975).

481. J. O. Jílek, J. Metyšová, and M. Protiva, *Collect. Czech. Chem. Commun.*, **39**, 3153 (1974).

482. I. Červená, J. O. Jílek, A. Dlabač, and M. Protiva, *Collect. Czech. Chem. Commun.*, **41**, 3437 (1976).

483. Z. Kopicová, J. Metyšová, and M. Protiva, *Collect. Czech. Chem. Commun.*, **40**, 3519 (1975).

484. J. Švestka, A. Rodová, and K. Náhunek, *Act. Nerv. Super.*, **15**, 103 (1973).

485. J. Švestka, K. Náhunek, and A. Rodová, *Act. Nerv. Super.*, **16**, 162 (1974).

486. D. Taussigová, O. Vinař. amd J. Baštecký, *Act. Nerv. Super.*, **16**, 163 (1974).

487. A. Dlabač, J. Metyšová, E. Kazdová, and J. Metyś, *Act. Nerv. Super.*, **17**, 217 (1975).

488. A. Dlabač, *Psychopharmacologia*, **26**:Suppl., 106 (1972).

489. A. Dlabač and E. Kazdová, *Act. Nerv. Super.*, **16**, 166 (1974).

490. A. Dlabač, *J. Pharmacol.* (Paris), **5**:Suppl. 2, 26 (1974).

491. W. Aschwanden, E. Kyburz, and P. Schönholzer, *Helv. Chim. Acta*, **59**, 1245 (1976).

492. T. G. White and J. Schmutz, *Experientia*, **33**, 1399 (1977).

493. T. K. Gupta, B. R. Vishnuvajjala, D. T. Witiak, and M. C. Gerald, *Experientia*, **33**, 65 (1977).

494. M. Protiva, *Drugs Future*, **2**, 250 (1977).

495. J. O. Jílek, J. Metyšová, and M. Protiva, *Collect. Czech. Chem. Commun.*, **36**, 4074 (1971).

496. J. O. Jílek, V. Seidlová, E. Svátek, and M. Protiva, *Monatsh. Chem.*, **96**, 182 (1965).

497. J. Fouche, J. C. Blondel, R. Horclois, C. James, A. Leger, and G. Poiget, *Bull. Soc. Chim. Fr.* [2], **1973**, 2697.

498. J. O. Jílek, K. Šindelář, J. Metyšová, J. Metyś, J. Pomykáček, and M. Protiva, *Collect. Czech. Chem. Commun.*, **35**, 3721 (1970).

499. A. A. Sugerman, *Curr. Ther. Res., Clin. Exp.*, **13**, 549 (1971).

500. D. M. Gallant, R. Guerrero-Figueroa, and M. P. Bishop, *Curr. Ther. Res., Clin. Exp.*, **13**, 469 (1971).

501. R. Smrž, J. O. Jílek, B. Kakáč, J. Holubek, E. Svátek, M. Bartošová, and M. Protiva, *Collect. Czech. Chem. Commun.*, **41**, 3420 (1976).

502. M. Rajšner, J. Metyšová, and M. Protiva, *Farm. Ed. Sci.*, **23**, 140 (1968).

503. M. Rajšner, J. Metyšová, and M. Protiva, *Collect. Czech. Chem. Commun.*, **34**, 468 (1969).

504. M. Rajšner, J. Metyšová, and M. Protiva, *Collect. Czech. Chem. Commun.*, **35**, 378 (1970).

505. V. Bártl, J. Metyšová, and M. Protiva, *Collect. Czech. Chem. Commun.*, **38**, 1693 (1973).

506. K. Šindelář, J. Metyšová, and M. Protiva, *Collect. Czech. Chem. Commun.*, **36**, 3404 (1971).

507. V. Bártl, J. Metyšová, and M. Protiva, *Collect. Czech. Chem. Commun.*, **38**, 2778 (1973).

508. K. Šindelář, J. Metyšová, J. Metyš, and M. Protiva, *Naturwissenschaften*, **56**, 374 (1969).

509. L. Coscia, P. Causa, E. Giuliani, and A. Nunziata, *Arzneim. Forsch.*, **25**, 1436 (1975).

510. L. Coscia, P. Causa, and E. Giuliani, *Arzneim.-Forsch.*, **25**, 1261 (1975).

511. C. L. Zirkle, U.S. Pat. 3,100,307 (1963).

512. M. Rajšner, F. Mikšik, and M. Protiva, *Collect. Czech. Chem. Commun.*, **43**, 1276 (1978).

513. G. Stille, H. Lauener, E. Eichenberger, F. Hunziker, and J. Schmutz, *Arzneim.-Forsch.*, **15**, 841 (1965).

514. J. Schmutz, F. Hunziker, G. Stille, and H. Lauener, *Chim. Ther.*, 424 (1967).

515. J. Schmutz, *Arzneim.-Forsch.*, **25**, 712 (1975).

516. J. Schmutz, *Pharmacol. Acta Helv.*, **48**, 117 (1973).

517. J. Schmutz, F. Künzle, F. Hunziker, and R. Gauch, *Helv. Chim. Acta*, **50**, 245 (1967).

518. G. Stille, H. Ackermann, E. Eichenberger, and H. Lauener, *Int. J. Neuropharmacol.*, **4**, 375 (1965).

519. J. Delay, P. Deniker, D. Gineslet, and P. Péron-Magnan, *Ann. Med. Psychol.*, **122**, 402 (1964).

520. D. M. Gallant, M. P. Bishop, and R. Guerrero-Figueroa, *Curr. Ther. Res., Clin. Exp.*, **12**, 794 (1970).

521. J. R. Boissier, P. Simon, J. Fichelle-Pagny, and J. M. Lwoff, *Encéphale*, **54**, 517 (1965).

522. M. P. Bishop, G. M. Simpson, C. W. Dunnett, and H. Kiltie, *J. Pharmacol.* (Paris), **5**:Suppl. 2, 8 (1974).

523. R. A. O'Connell, M. Jeewa, and K. Allen, *Curr. Ther. Res., Clin. Exp.*, **21**, 101 (1977).

524. J. Paprocki and M. Versiani, *Curr. Ther. Res., Clin. Exp.*, **21**, 80 (1977).

525. R. C. Heel, R. N. Brogden, T. M. Speight, and G. S. Avery, *Drugs*, **15**, 198 (1978).

526. F. J. Ayd, Jr., *Dis. Nerv. Syst.*, **38**, 883 (1977).

527. F. Hunziker, E. Fischer, and J. Schmutz, *Helv. Chim. Acta*, **50**, 1588 (1967).

528. G. Stille, H. Lauener, and E. Eichenberger, *Farm. Ed. Prat.*, **26**, 603 (1971).

529. H. Gross and E. Langner, *Wien. Med. Wochenschr.*, **116**, 814 (1966).

530. D. M. Gallant, W. C. Swanson, D. H. Mielke, R. Guerrero-Figueroa, and H. Collins, *Curr. Ther. Res., Clin. Exp.*, **15**, 56 (1973).

531. F. Hunziker, F. Künzle, and J. Schmutz, *Helv. Chim. Acta*, **49**, 1433 (1966).

532. G. Stille, A. Sayers, H. Lauener, and E. Eichenberger, *Psychopharmacologia*, **28**, 325 (1973).

533. J. M. van Rossum, P. A. J. Janssen, J. R. Boissier, L. Julou, D. M. Loew, I. Møller-Nielsen, I. Munkvad, A. Randrup, G. Stille, and D. H. Tedeschi, in *The Neuroleptics*, D. P. Bobon, P. A. J. Janssen, and J. Bobon, Eds., Karger, Basel, 1970, p. 23.

534. F. J. Ayd, Jr., *Int. Drug Ther. Newslett.*, **9,** 5 (1974).

535. H. A. Amsler, L. Teerenhovi, E. Barth, K. Harjula, and P. Vuopio, *Acta Psychiatr. Scand.*, **56,** 241 (1977).

536. R. Battegay, B. Cotar, and J. Fleischhauer, *Compr. Psychiatr.*, **18,** 423 (1977).

537. H. R. Bürki, W. Ruch, H. Asper, M. Baggiolini, and G. Stille, *Schweiz. Med. Wochenschr.*, **103,** 1716 (1973); *Eur. J. Pharmacol.*, **27,** 180 (1974).

538. T. J. Petcher and H.-P. Weber, *J. Chem. Soc., Perkin II*, **1976** 1415.

539. H. R. Bürki, A. C. Sayers, W. Ruch, and H. Asper, *Arzneim.-Forsch.*, **27,** 1561 (1977).

540. S. Wilk and M. Stanley, *Eur. J. Pharmacol.*, **41,** 65 (1977).

541. H. R. Bürki, E. Eichenberger, A. C. Sayers, and T. G. White, *Pharmakopschiatr.*, **8,** 115 (1975).

542. (a) A. C. Sayers, H. R. Bürki, W. Ruch, and H. Asper, *Psychopharmacologia*, **41,** 97 (1975); (b) G. Gianutsos and K. E. Moore, *Life Sci.*, **20,** 1585 (1977).

543. B. S. Bunney and G. K. Aghajanian, in *Modern Pharmacology-Toxicology, Pre- and Postsynaptic Receptors*, Vol. 3, E. Usdin and W. E. Bunney, Jr., Eds., Dekker, New York, 1975, p. 89.

544. R. J. Miller and L. L. Iversen, *Trans. Biochem. Soc.* (554th Meet. London) **2,** 256 (1974).

545. M. E. Karobath, *Eur. J. Pharmacol.*, **30,** 159 (1975).

546. K. Von Hungen, S. Roberts, and D. F. Hill, *Brain Res.*, **94,** 57 (1975).

547. F. Hunziker, F. Künzle, and J. Schmutz, *Helv. Chim. Acta*, **49,** 244 (1966).

548. G. Stille, H. Lauener, E. Eichenberger, F. Hunziker, and J. Schmutz, *Arzneim.-Forsch.*, **15,** 841 (1965).

549. G. Schwarb, unpublished results, cf. Ref. 515.

550. F. Hunziker, unpublished results; cf. Ref. 515.

551. Z. Votava, J. Metyšová, and Z. Horáková, *Cesk. Farm.*, **7,** 125 (1958).

552. F. Bruderlein, L. Humber, and K. Pelz, *Can. J. Chem.*, **52,** 2119 (1974).

553. K. Voith and F. Her, *Abstr. Pap., 5th Int. Congr. Pharmacol., San Francisco, 1972*, Abstract No. 1457, p. 243.

554. F. T. Bruderlein, L. G. Humber, and K. Voith, *J. Med. Chem.*, **18,** 185 (1975).

555. K. Voith, F. T. Bruderlein, and L. G. Humber, *J. Med. Chem.*, **21,** 694 (1978).

556. W. Lippmann, T. Pugsley, and J. Merker, *Life Sci.*, **16,** 213 (1975).

557. W. Lippmann and T. Pugsley, *Pharmacol. Res. Commun.*, **7,** 371 (1975).

558. R. J. Miller, A. S. Horn, and L. L. Iversen, *J. Pharm. Pharmacol.*, **27,** 212 (1975).

559. B. Zirkovic, A. Guidotti, and E. Costa, *J. Pharm. Pharmacol.*, **27,** 359 (1975).

560. T. A. Pugsley, J. Merker, and W. Lippmann, *Can. J. Physiol. Pharmacol.*, **54,** 510 (1976).

561. D. H. Mielke, D. M. Gallant, T. Oelsner, C. M. Kessler, W. K. Tomlinson, and G. H. Cohen, *Dis. Nerv. Syst.*, **36,** 7 (1975).

562. L. E. Hollister, K. L. Davis, and P. A. Berger, *Psychopharm. Commun.*, **1,** 493 (1975).

563. M. L. Clark, L. P. Costiloe, F. Wood, A. Paredes, and F. G. Fulkerson, *Dis. Nerv. Syst.*, **38,** 943 (1977).

564. L. G. Humber, F. Bruderlein, and K. Voith, *Mol. Pharmacol.*, **11,** 833 (1975).

565. K. Voith and J. R. Cummings, *6th Int. Pharmacol. Congr., Helsinki, July 20–25*, Abstr. No. 1186 (1975).

566. J. Giesecke, *Acta Crystallogr., Sect. B*, **29,** 1785 (1973).

567. W. S. Saari, S. W. King, and V. J. Lotti, *J. Med. Chem.*, **16,** 171 (1973).

568. M. Moereels and J. P. Tollenaere, *Life Sci.*, **23,** 459 (1978).

569. P. A. J. Janssen, in *Psychopharmacological Agents, Medicinal Chemistry, A Series of Monographs*, Vol. 4, Part II, M. Gordon, Ed., Academic, New York, 1967, p. 199.

570. P. A. J. Janssen, in *Psychopharmacological Agents, Medicinal Chemistry, A Series of Monographs*, Vol. 4, Part III, M. Gordon, Ed., Academic, New York, 1974, p. 129.

571. H. J. Haase and P. A. J. Janssen, Eds., *The Action of Neuroleptic Drugs*, Year Book Chicago, 1965.

572. B. K. Krueger, J. Forn, and P. Greengard, in *Pre- and Postsynaptic Receptors*, E. Usdin and W. E. Bunney, Eds., Dekker, New York, 1975, p. 123.

573. L. L. Iversen, A. S. Horn, and R. J. Miller, in *Pre- and Postsynaptic Receptors*, E. Usdin and W. E. Bunney, Eds., Dekker, New York, 1975, p. 207.

574. C. J. E. Niemegeers and P. A. J. Janssen, *J. Pharm. Pharmacol.*, **12,** 744 (1960).

575. P. A. J. Janssen and C. J. E. Niemegeers, *Arzneim.-Forsch.*, **11,** 1037 (1961).

576. P. A. J. Janssen, C. van de Westeringh, A. H. M. Jageneau, P. J. A. Demoen, B. K. F. Hermans, G. H. P. van Daele, K. H. L. Schellekens, C. A. M. van der Eycken, and C. J. E. Niemegeers, *J. Med. Pharm. Chem.*, **1,** 281 (1959).

577. C. J. E. Niemegeers and P. A. J. Janssen, *Arzneim.-Forsch.*, **24,** 45 (1974).

578. A. Wauquier and C. J. E. Niemegeers, *Arzneim.-Forsch.*, **26,** 1356 (1976).

579. T. Honma, K. Sasajima, K. Ona, S. Kitagawa, Sh. Inaba, and H. Yamamoto, *Arzneim.-Forsch.*, **24,** 1248 (1974).

580. C. H. Grogan, C. F. Geschickter, M. E. Freed, and L. M. Rice, *J. Med. Chem.*, **8,** 62 (1965).

581. N. J. Harper, A. B. Simmonds, W. T. Wakama, G. H. Hall, and D. K. Vallance, *J. Pharm. Pharmacol.*, **18,** 150 (1966).

582. A. H. M. Jageneau and P. A. J. Janssen, *Arch. Int. Pharmacodyn. Ther.*, **106,** 199 (1956).

583. P. A. J. Janssen, A. H. M. Jageneau, P. J. A. Demoen, C. van de Westeringh, J. H. M. de Canniere, A. H. M. Raeymaekers, M. S. J. Wouters, S. Sanczuk, and B. K. F. Hermans, *J. Med. Pharm. Chem.*, **2,** 271 (1960).

584. P. A. J. Janssen, in *International Review of Neurobiology*, Vol. 8, C. C. Pfeiffer and J. R. Smythies, Eds., Academic, New York-London, 1965, p. 221.

585. P. A. J. Janssen, A. H. M. Jageneau, P. J. A. Demoen, C. van de Westeringh, A. H. M. Raeymaekers, M. S. J. Wouters, S. Sanczuk, B. K. F. Hermans, and J. L. M. Loomans, *J. Med. Pharm. Chem.*, **1,** 105 (1959).

586. P. A. J. Janssen, A. H. M. Jageneau, P. J. A. Demoen, C. van de Westeringh, J. H. M. de Cannière, A. H. M. Raeymaekers, M. S. J. Wouters, S. Sanczuk, and B. K. F. Hermans, *J. Med. Pharm. Chem.*, **1,** 309 (1959).

587. H. Morren, D. Zivkovic, R. Linz, H. Strubbe, and L. Marchal, *Ind. Chim. Belge*, **28,** 123 (1963); through *Chem. Abstr.*, **59,** 8732 (1963).

588. Sumitomo Chemical Co., Ltd., Jap. Pat. 059300 (1974).

589. Sumitomo Chemical Co., Ltd., Jap. Pat. 067079 (1974).

590. C. Kaiser and C. L. Zirkle, U.S. Pat. 3,558,637 (1971).

591. M. J. Kukla, C. M. Woo, J. R. Kehr, and A. Miller, *J. Med. Chem.*, **21,** 348 (1978).

592. D. H. Mielke, *Psychopharmacol. Commun.*, **1,** 117 (1975).

593. B. M. Angrist, G. Sathananthan, H. Thompson, and S. Gershon, *Curr. Ther. Res., Clin. Exp.*, **18,** 359 (1975).

594. N. K. Chandhuri, T. J. Ball, and N. Finch. *Experientia*, **33,** 575 (1977).

595. Y.-H. Wu, J. W. Rayburn, L. E. Allen, H. C. Ferguson, and J. W. Kissel, *J. Med. Chem.*, **15,** 477 (1972).

596. L. E. Allen, H. C. Ferguson, R. H. Cox, J. W. Kissel, and J. W. Rayburn, *Fed. Proc.*, **31,** 529 Abs. (1972).

597. G. L. Sathananthan, I. Sanghvi, N. Phillips, and S. Gershon, *Curr. Ther. Res., Clin. Exp.*, **18,** 701 (1975).

598. G. Sathananthan, P. Mir, and S. Gershon, *Curr. Ther. Res., Clin. Exp.*, **19,** 516 (1976).

599. G. B. Fregmen, M. Vidali, T. Chieli, and I. Bussoleron, *6th Int. Congr. Pharmacol.*, *Helsinki*, July 20–25, Abstr. No. 336 (1975).

600. G. B. Fregman and M. Vidali, *Pharmacology*, **15,** 485 (1977).

601. A. J. Reyntjens, C. J. E. Niemegeers, J. M. Van Neuten, P. Laduron, J. Heykants, K. H. L. Schellekens, R. Marsboom, A. Jageneau, A. Broekaert, and P. A. J. Janssen, *Arzneim.-Forsch.*, **28,** 1194 (1978).

602. P. A. J. Janssen, C. J. E. Niemegeers, K. H. L. Schellekens, A. Dresse, F. M. Lenaerts, A. Pinchard, W. K. A. Schaper, J. M. Van Nueten, and F. J. Verbruggen, *Arzneim.-Forsch.*, **18,** 261 (1968).

603. G. Chouinard, H. E. Lehmann, and T. A. Ban, *Curr. Ther. Res., Clin. Exp.*, **12,** 598 (1970).

604. (a) P. A. J. Janssen, C. J. E. Niemegeers, K. H. L. Schellekens, F. M. Lenaerts, F. J. Verbruggen, J. M. Van Nueten, and W. K. A. Schaper, *Eur. J. Pharmacol.*, **11,** 139 (1970); (b) F. Baro, J. Brugmans, R. Dom, and R. Van Lommel, *J. Clin. Pharmacol.*, **10,** 330 (1970).

605. K. Y. Ota, A. A. Kurland, and V. B. Slotnick, *J. Clin. Pharmacol.*, **14,** 202 (1974).

606. P. A. J. Janssen, C. J. E. Niemegeers, K. H. L. Schellekens, F. M. Lenaerts, and A. Wauquier, *Arzneim.-Forsch.*, **25,** 1287 (1975).

607. P. A. J. Janssen, C. J. E. Niemegeers, K. H. L. Schellekens, F. M. Lenaerts, F. J. Verbruggen, J. M. Van Nueten, R. H. M. Marsboom, V. V. Herin, and W. K. G. Schaper, *Arzneim.-Forsch.*, **20,** 1689 (1970).

608. H. Immich, F. Eckmann, H. Neumann, O. Schäppenle, H. Schwarz, and H. Tempel, *Arzneim.-Forsch.*, **20,** 1699 (1970).

609. M. Rajšner, Z. Kapicová, J. Holubek, E. Svátek, J. Metys, M. Bartošová, F. Mikšík, and M. Protiva, *Collect. Czech. Chem. Commun.*, **43,** 1760 (1978).

610. H. Knape, *Brit. J. Anesth.*, **42,** 325 (1970).

611. S. J. Dominianni, R. P. Pioch, R. L. Young, and P. J. Stimart, *J. Med. Chem.*, **14,** 1009 (1971).

612. M. Baboulène, G. Sturtz, and J. Hache, *Chim. Ther.*, **7,** 493 (1972).

613. D. N. Johnson, W. H. Funderburk, and J. D. Ward, *Arch. Int. Pharmacodyn. Ther.*, **211,** 326 (1974).

614. R. L. Duncan, Jr., G. C. Helsley, W. J. Welstead, Jr., J. P. DaVanzo, W. H. Funderburk,

and C. D. Lunsford, *J. Med. Chem.*, **13**, 1 (1970).

615. A. J. M. Loonen, I. Van Wijngaarden, P. A. J. Janssen, and W. Soudijn, *Eur. J. Pharmacol.*, **50**, 403 (1978).

616. G. M. Simpson, J. W. S. Angus, and J. G. Edwards, *Curr. Ther. Res., Clin. Exp.*, **9**, 486 (1967).

617. J. G. Edwards and G. M. Simpson, *Curr. Ther. Res., Clin. Exp.*, **10**, 520 (1968).

618. A. A. Sugerman, J. Herrmann, and M. O'Hara, *Curr. Ther. Res., Clin. Exp.*, **10**, 529 (1968).

619. C. Villeneuve, J. V. Ananth, T. A. Ban, and H. E. Lehmann, *Curr. Ther. Res., Clin. Exp.*, **12**, 223 (1970).

620. D. Lednicer, D. E. Emmert, R. Lahti, and A. D. Rudzik, *J. Med. Chem.*, **15**, 1235 (1972).

621. R. A. Lahti and D. Lednicer, *Biochem. Pharmacol.*, **23**, 1701 (1974).

622. D. Lednicer, D. E. Emmert, R. Lahti, and A. D. Rudzik, *J. Med. Chem.*, **15**, 1239 (1972).

623. D. Lednicer, D. E. Emmert, R. Lahti, and A. D. Rudzik, *J. Med. Chem.*, **16**, 1251 (1973).

624. M. E. Freed and S. J. Childress, U.S. Pat. 3,197,507 (1965); through *Chem. Abstr.*, **64**, 8091 (1966).

625. R. F. Squires and J. B. Lassen, *Biochem. Pharmacol.*, **17**, 369 (1968).

626. D. Jack, N. J. Harper, A. C. Ritchie, and N. F. Hayes, Belg. Pat. 653,093 (1964); through *Chem. Abstr.*, **64**, 9738 (1966).

627. M. Bleiberg and J. W. Ward, *Fed. Proc.*, **30**, 390 Abs. (1971).

628. W. J. Welstead, G. C. Helsley, R. L. Duncan, A. D. Cale, C. R. Taylor, J. P. DaVanzo, B. V. Franko, and C. Lunsford, *J. Med. Chem.*, **12**, 435, 442 (1969).

629. A. A. Sugerman, J. Herrman, and M. O'Hara, *Curr. Ther. Res., Clin. Exp.*, **12**, 234 (1970).

630. C. H. Grogan and L. M. Rice, *J. Med. Chem.*, **10**, 621 (1967).

631. S. J. Dominianni, R. P. Pioch, and R. L. Young, *J. Med. Chem.*, **14**, 1008 (1971).

632. J. B. Hester, A. D. Rudzik, H. H. Keasling, and W. Veldkamp, *J. Med. Chem.*, **13**, 23 (1970).

633. L. O'Meallie, D. M. Gallant, M. P. Bishop, G. Bishop, and C. A. Steele, *Curr. Ther. Res., Clin. Exp.*, **11**, 460 (1969).

634. F. Schulsinger, *Nord. Med.*, **73**, 605 (1965).

635. J. A. Christensen, S. Herenstam, J. B. Lassen, and N. Sterner, *Acta Pharmacol. Toxicol.*, **23**, 109 (1965).

636. A. A. Sugerman, *Curr. Ther. Res., Clin. Exp.*, **10**, 533 (1968).

637. J. P. Li, R. G. Stein, J. Biel, J. A. Gylys, and S. A. Ridlon, *J. Med. Chem.*, **13**, 1230 (1970).

638. J. L. Gendron, R. L. Zimmerman, and B. C. Schiele, *Curr. Ther. Res., Clin. Exp.*, **15**, 333 (1973).

639. R. M. Quock and R. A. Louie, *7th Ann. Meet. Soc. Neurosci., Anaheim, Calif., Nov. 6, 1977*, Abstr., Vol. 3, No. 813.

640. J. Castañer and P. Thorpe, *Drugs Future*, **3**, 445 (1978).

641. D. N. Johnson, W. H. Funderburk, and J. W. Ward, *Arch. Int. Pharmacodyn. Ther.*, **194**, 197 (1971).

642. (a) H. C. B. Denber, *Ann. Med. Psychol.*, **131**, 131 (1973); (b) K. Sandler, J. Digiacomo, and J. Mendels, *Curr. Ther. Res., Clin. Exp.*, **20**, 549 (1976).

643. B. R. S. Nakra, *Curr. Med. Res. Opin.*, **4**, 529 (1977).

644. L. F. Fabre, Jr. and R. T. Harris, *Curr. Ther. Res., Clin. Exp.*, **19**, 328 (1976).

645. B. Woggon, A. Franke, H. Hucker, E. Reuther, D. Athen, J. Angst, and H. Hippius, *Int. Pharmacol.*, **12**, 113 (1977).

646. H. Feldmann and H. C. B. Denber, *Ann. Med. Psychol.*, **134**:2, 269 (1976).

647. N. J. Harper and C. F. Chignell, *J. Med. Chem.*, **7**, 729 (1964).

648. J. Castañer and P. Blancafort, *Drugs Future*, **3**, 451 (1978).

649. Daüchi Seiyaku, Jap. Pat. 070497 (1976).

650. M. Sato, M. Arimoto, K. Ueno, H. Kojima, T. Yamasaki, T. Sakurai, and A. Kasahara, *J. Med. Chem.*, **21**, 1116 (1978).

651. T. Yamasaki, T. Sakurai, H. Kojima, and A. Kasahara, *Jap. J. Pharmacol.*, **27**:S, 124P (1977).

652. E. Jucker, *Angew. Chem., Int. Ed.*, **2**, 493 (1963).

653. S. Lecolier and G. Trouiller, *Chim. Ther.*, **4**, 437 (1969).

654. P. A. J. Janssen, Belg. Pat. 606,849 (1961); through *Chem. Abstr.*, **56**, 12861 (1962).

655. B. Hermans, P. Van Daele, C. van de Westeringh, C. Van der Eycken, J. Boey, and P. A. J. Janssen, *J. Med. Chem.*, **8**, 851 (1965).

656. E. T. Kumura, P. W. Dodge, P. R. Young, and R. P. Johnson, *Arch. Int. Pharmacodyn. Ther.*, **190**, 124 (1971).

657. R. C. Allen, V. J. Bauer, R. W. Kosley, Jr., A. R. McFadden, G. M. Shutske, M. L. Cornfeldt, S. Fielding, H. M. Geyer, III, and J. C. Wilkes, *J. Med. Chem.*, **21**, 1149 (1978).

658. P. A. J. Janssen, U.S. Pat. 2,973,365 (1961); through *Chem. Abstr.*, **55**, 15515 (1961); Belg.

Pat. 577,977 (1959); through *Chem. Abstr.*, **54,** 4629 (1960).

659. E. Cocito, G. Ambrosini, A. Arata, P. Bevilacqua, and E. Tortora, *Arzneim.-Forsch.*, **20,** 1119 (1970).

660. I. S. Turek, K. Ota, R. Machado, P. Ferro-Diaz, and A. Kurland, *Curr. Ther. Res., Clin. Exp.*, **12,** 532 (1970).

661. D. E. Wilson, H. I. Chernov, P. S. Bernard, D. A. Partyka, B. S. Barbaz, and G. DeStevens, *Arch. Int. Pharmcodyn. Ther.*, **191,** 15 (1971).

662. C. J. E. Niemegeers, J. M. Van Nueten, and P. A. J. Janssen, *Arzneim.-Forsch.*, **24,** 1798 (1974).

663. I. Červena, A. Dlabač, J. Němec, and M. Protiva, *Collect. Czech. Chem. Commun.*, **40,** 1612 (1975).

664. C. Gouret, P. Bouvet, and G. Raynaud, *C. R. Soc. Biol.*, **167,** 1366 (1974).

665. K. S. Raevsky, V. V. Marcovich, L. K. Murakhina, L. S. Nazarova, A. M. Likhosherstov, and A. P. Skoldinov, *Khim.-Farm. Zh.*, **10,** 55 (1976).

666. G. B. Singh, S. Nityanand, R. C. Srimal, V. A. Rao, P. C. Jain, and B. N. Dhawan, *Experientia*, **29,** 1529 (1973).

667. G. B. Singh, R. C. Srimal, S. Nityanand, and B. N. Dhawan, *Arzneim.-Forsch.*, **28,** 1087 (1978).

668. A. K. Saxena, P. C. Jain, N. Anand, and P. R. Dua, *J. Med. Chem.*, **16,** 560 (1973).

669. R. B. Woodward, F. E. Bader, H. Bickle, A. J. Frey, and R. W. Kierstead, *J. Am. Chem. Soc.*, **78,** 2025 (1956).

670. R. Pepinski, J. W. Turley, U. Okaya, T. Doyne, V. Vand, A. Shimada, F. M. Lovell, and Y. Sogo, *Acta Crystallogr.*, **10,** 813 (1957).

671. E. Schlittler, J. Druey, and A. Marxer, in *Progress in Drug Research*, Vol. 4, E. Jucker, Ed., Birkhauser, Basel-Stuttgart, 1962, p. 326.

672. R. E. Woodson, Jr., H. W. Youngken, E. Schlittler, and J. A. Schneider, *Rauwolfia: Botany, Pharmacognosy, Chemistry and Pharmacology*, Little, Brown, Boston-Toronto, 1957.

673. S. G. Agbalyan, *Russ. Chem. Rev.*, **30,** 526 (1961).

674. P. A. Diassi, F. L. Weisenborn, C. M. Dylion, and O. Wintersteiner, *J. Am. Chem. Soc.*, **77,** 4687 (1955).

675. C. F. Huebner, R. Lucas, H. B. MacPhillamy, and H. A. Troxell, *J. Am. Chem. Soc.*, **77,** 469 (1955).

676. E. Schlittler, P. R. Ulshafer, M. L. Pandow, R. Hunt, and L. Dorfman, *Experientia*, **11,** 64 (1955).

677. N. Hosansky and E. Smith, *J. Am. Pharm. Assoc., Sci. Ed.*, **44,** 639 (1955).

678. M. W. Klohs, F. Keller, R. E. Williams, and G. W. Kusserow, *J. Am. Chem. Soc.*, **79,** 3763 (1957).

679. J. M. Mueller, *Experientia*, **13,** 479 (1957).

680. E. Haack, A. Popelak, H. Spingler, and F. Kaiser, *Naturwissenschaften*, **41,** 214, 428 (1954).

681. A. Popelak, E. Haack, G. Lettenbauer, and H. Spingler, *Naturwissenschaften*, **48,** 73 (1961).

682. M. Shamma and R. J. Shine, *Tetrahedron Lett.*, **33,** 2277 (1964).

683. M. Shamma and E. F. Walker, Jr., *Chem. Ind.* (London), **1962,** 1866.

684. C. F. Huebner, *J. Am. Chem. Soc.*, **76,** 5792 (1954).

685. R. A. Lucas, R. J. Kiesel, and M. J. Ceglowski, *J. Am. Chem. Soc.*, **82,** 493 (1960).

686. M. M. Robison, W. G. Pierson, R. A. Lucas, I. Hsu, and R. L. Dziemian, *J. Org. Chem.*, **28,** 768 (1963).

687. R. A. Lucas, M. E. Kuehne, M. J. Ceglowski, R. L. Dziemian, and H. B. MacPhillamy, *J. Am. Chem. Soc.*, **81,** 1928 (1959).

688. T. Petrzilka, A. Frey, A. Hofmann, H. Ott, H. Schenk, and F. Troxler, U.S. Pat. 2,959,591 (1960); through *Chem. Abstr.* **55,** 7444 (1961).

689. M. M. Robison, R. A. Lucas, H. B. MacPhillamy, W. Barrett, and A. J. Plummer, *Experientia*, **17,** 14 (1961).

690. G. Müller and A. Allais, *Naturwissenschaften*, **47,** 82 (1960).

691. F. L. Weisenborn, *J. Am. Chem. Soc.*, **79,** 4818 (1957).

692. L. Bláha, B. Kakáč, and J. Weichet, *Collect. Czech. Chem. Commun.*, **27,** 857 (1962).

693. W. Logemann, L. Almirante, L. Caprio, and A. Meli, *Chem. Ber.*, **88,** 1952 (1955).

694. W. Logemann, L. Caprio, L. Almirante, and A. Meli, *Chem. Ber.*, **89,** 1043 (1956).

695. M. von Strandtmann, G. Bobowski, and J. Shavel, Jr., *J. Med. Chem.*, **8,** 338 (1965).

696. L. Velluz, G. Müller, R. Joly, G. Nominé, J. Mathieu, A. Allais, J. Warnant, J. Valls, R. Bucourt, and J. Jolly, *Bull. Soc. Chim. Fr.*, **1958,** 673.

697. L. Velluz, M. Peterfalvi, and R. Jequier, *Compt. Rend.*, **247,** 1905 (1958).

698. L. Novák and M. Protiva, *Collect. Czech. Chem. Commun.*, **26,** 681 (1961).

699. M. Protiva, M. Rajšner, and J. O. Jílek, *Monatsh. Chem.*, **91,** 703 (1960).

700. L. Velluz, G. Müller, and A. Allais, *Compt. Rend.*, **247**, 1746 (1958).

701. J. O. Jílek, J. Pomykáček, and M. Protiva, *Collect. Czech. Chem. Commun.*, **26**, 1145 (1961).

702. K. Pelz, L. Bláha, and J. Weichet, *Collect. Czech. Chem. Commun.*, **26**, 1160 (1961).

703. I. Jirkovsky and M. Protiva, *Collect. Czech. Chem. Commun.*, **28**, 2582 (1963).

704. R. D. Schuetz, G. P. Nilles, and R. L. Titus, *J. Org. Chem.*, **33**, 1556 (1968).

705. A. Brossi, H. Lindlar, M. Walter, and O. Schnider, *Helv. Chim. Acta*, **41**, 119 (1958).

706. A. Pletscher, *Science*, **126**, 507 (1957).

707. A. Pletscher, H. Besendorf, and H. P. Bachtold, *Arch. Exp. Pathol. Pharmakol.*, **232**, 499 (1958).

708. J. R. Tretter, U.S. Pat. 3,053,845 (1962).

709. J. R. Tretter, J. G. Lombardino, K. F. Finger, and A. Weissman, *Abstr. Pap., 140th Meet. Am. Chem. Soc., Chicago, September 1961*, p. 4-0.

710. A. Weissman and K. F. Finger, *Biochem. Pharmacol.*, **11**, 871 (1962).

711. H. Nakanishi, T. Owega, and K. Shimamoto, *Jap. J. Pharmacol.*, **16**, 10 (1966).

712. A. Pletscher, A. Brossi, and K. F. Gey, in *International Review of Neurobiology*, Vol. 4, C. C. Pfeiffer and J. R. Smythies, Eds., Academic, New York-London, 1962, p. 275.

713. M. R. Harnden and J. H. Short, *J. Med. Chem.*, **10**, 1183 (1967).

714. A. Cohen and P. G. Philpott, U.S. Pat. 2,908,686 (1959).

715. J. G. Lombardino, J. I. Bodin, C. F. Gerber, W. M. McLamore, and G. D. Laubach, *J. Med. Pharm. Chem.*, **3**, 505 (1961).

716. K. E. Fahrenholtz, A. Capomaggi, M. Lurie, M. W. Goldberg, and R. W. Kierstead, *J. Med. Chem.*, **9**, 304 (1966).

717. A. Saner and A. Pletscher, *J. Pharmacol. Exp. Ther.*, **203**, 556 (1977).

718. A. Brossi, L. H. Chopard-dit-Jean, and O. Schnider, *Helv. Chim. Acta*, **41**, 1793 (1958).

719. A. Brossi, H. Bruderer, M. DaPrada, F. A. Steiner, and A. Pletscher, *Arzneim.-Forsch.*, **15**, 670 (1965).

720. N. Goncalves, *Int. Pharmacopsychiatr.*, **11**, 65 (1976).

721. A. Scriabine, A. Weissman, K. F. Finger, C. S. Delahunt, J. W. Constantine, and J. A. Schneider, *J. Am. Med. Assoc.*, **184**, 276 (1963).

722. J. W. Daly and A. A. Manian, *Biochem. Pharmacol.*, **16**, 2131 (1967).

723. F. H. Clarke, R. T. Hill, J. Koo, R. M. Lopano, M. A. Maseda, M. Smith, S. Soled, G. Von Veh, and I. Vlattas, *J. Med. Chem.*, **21**, 785 (1978).

724. R. Kellner, M. L. Freese, R. T. Rada, and F. J. Wall, *J. Clin. Pharmacol.*, **16**, 194 (1976).

725. H. Nakanishi, *Jap. J. Pharmacol.*, **12**, 208 (1962); *ibid.*, **14**, 317 (1964).

726. H. Yamamoto, *Jap. J. Pharmacol.*, **13**, 230 (1963).

727. C. Horig, M. Klotzbach, H. Koch, E. Mayer, and J. Richter, *Pharmazie*, **31**, 499 (1976).

728. J. Yamahara, T. Konishima, Y. Sakakibara, M. Ishigura, T. Sawada, and H. Fujimara, *Chem. Pharm. Bull.* (Japan), **24**, 1909 (1976).

729. B. Hsu and K. C. Kin, *Arch. Int. Pharmacodyn. Ther.*, **139**, 318 (1962).

730. B. Hsu and K. C. Kin, *Biochem. Pharmacol.*, **12**:Suppl., 101 (1963).

731. J. Knoll, in *Animal and Clinical Pharmacologic Techniques in Drug Evaluation*, Vol. 2, P. E. Siegler and J. H. Moyer, III, Eds., Year Book, Chicago, 1964, p. 305.

732. Y. C. Clement-Cormier, H. Phillips, L. R. Myerson, and V. E. Davis, *Pharmacologist*, **20**, 232 (1978).

733. C. Kaiser, B. M. Lester, D. H. Tedeschi, and C. L. Zirkle, unpublished results.

734. F. Lipparini, A. Loizzo, A. Scotti de Carolis, and V. G. Longo, *Naunyn-Schmiedebergs Arch. Pharmakol. Exp. Pathol.*, **269**, 475 (1971).

735. E. Macko, B. Douglas, J. A. Weisbach, and D. T. Walz, *Arch. Int. Pharmacodyn. Ther.*, **197**, 261 (1972).

736. G. Ferrari and C. Casagrande, *Farm. Ed. Sci.*, **25**, 449 (1970).

737. E. E. Smissman, S. El-Antably, L. W. Hedrich, E. J. Walaszek, and L.-F. Tseng, *J. Med. Chem.*, **16**, 109 (1973).

738. F. P. Miller, G. Garske, and D. Gauger, *Pharmacologist*, **13**, 207 (1971).

739. Sandoz, Belg. Pat. 824,884 (1976).

740. T. V. Sokolova, K. I. Lopatina, I. V. Zaitseva, R. M. Salimov, N. P. Speranski, and V. A. Zagorevs, *Khim.-Farm. Zh.*, **10**:9, 42 (1976).

741. A. Keskiner, T. M. Itil, T. H. Han, B. Saletu, and W. Hsu, *Curr. Ther. Res., Clin. Exp.*, **13**, 714 (1971).

742. I. Huston, C. Swett, Jr., and J. O. Cole, *Curr. Ther. Res., Clin. Exp.*, **21**, 70 (1977).

743. J. H. Gaddum and K. A. Hameed, *Brit. J. Pharmacol.*, **9**, 240 (1954).

744. B. B. Brodie and P. A. Shore, *Ann. N.Y. Acad. Sci.*, **66**, 631 (1957).

745. E. N. Shaw and D. W. Woolley, *J. Pharmacol. Exp. Ther.*, **116**, 164 (1956).

746. G. Ehrhart and I. Hennig, *Arch. Pharm.* (Berlin), **294**, 550 (1961).

747. C. W. Whittle and R. N. Castle, *J. Pharm. Sci.*, **52**, 645 (1963).

748. L. S. Harris and F. C. Uhle, *J. Pharmacol. Exp. Ther.*, **128**, 358 (1960).

749. D. W. Wylie and S. Archer, *J. Med. Pharm. Chem.*, **5**, 932 (1962).

750. S. Archer, D. W. Wylie, L. S. Harris, T. R. Lewis, J. W. Shulenberg, M. R. Bell, R. K. Kullnig, and A. Arnold, *J. Am. Chem. Soc.*, **84**, 1306 (1962).

751. C. D. Neal, M. P. Collis, and N. W. Imrah, *Curr. Ther. Res., Clin. Exp.*, **11**, 367 (1969).

752. D. U. Uaili, *Zh. Neuropat. Psikhiatr. Korsakov*, **69**, 589 (1969).

753. D. W. Wylie, *J. Pharmacol. Exp. Ther.*, **127**, 276 (1959).

754. E. N. Greenblatt, J. Coupet, C. E. Rauh, and V. S. Myers, *Abstr., 7th Int. Congr. Pharmacol., Paris, 1978*, p. 493.

755. G. R. Allen, Jr., V. G. DeVries, E. N. Greenblatt, R. Littell, F. J. McEvoy, and D. B. Moran, *J. Med. Chem.*, **16**, 949 (1973).

756. S. Archer, U.S. Pat. 3,362,956 (1968).

757. Anonymous, *J. Am. Med. Assoc.*, **235**, 1370 (1976).

758. D. Mielke, D. M. Gallant, and M. P. Bishop, *Curr. Ther. Res., Clin. Exp.*, **15**, 324 (1973).

759. W. J. Welstead, Jr., J. P. DaVanzo, G. C. Helsley, C. D. Lunsford, and C. R. Taylor, Jr., *J. Med. Chem.*, **10**, 1015 (1967).

760. J. P. DaVanzo, M. Daugherty, R. Ruckart, and L. Kang, *Psychopharmacologia*, **9**, 210 (1966).

761. J. H. Mirsky, H. D. White, and T. B. O'Dell, *J. Pharmacol. Exp. Ther.*, **125**, 122 (1959).

762. S. Misztal and M. Grabowska, *Dissert. Pharm. Pharmacol.*, **22**, 313 (1970).

763. J. Pórszász, K. Gibiszer-Pórszász, S. Földeák, and B. Matkovics, *Experientia*, **21**, 93 (1965).

764. K. P. Singh and D. S. Bhandari, *Arzneim.-Forsch.*, **23**, 973 (1973).

765. Roussel UCLAF, U.S. Pat. 4,005,206 (1977).

766. R. A. Green, J. D. Barchas, G. R. Elliott, J. S. Carman, and R. J. Wyatt, *Pharmacol. Biochem. Behav.*, **5**, 383 (1976).

767. W. M. Herrmann and J. Fabricius, *Dis. Nerv. Syst.*, **35**:7, 28 (1974).

768. A. Mooradian, P. E. Dupont, A. G. Hlavac, M. D. Aceto, and J. Pearl, *J. Med. Chem.*, **20**, 487 (1977).

769. J. B. Hester, A. H. Tang, H. H. Keasling, and W. Veldkamp, *J. Med. Chem.*, **11**, 101 (1968).

770. H. E. Lehmann, T. A. Ban, and S. L. Debow, *Curr. Ther. Res., Clin. Exp.*, **9**, 306 (1967).

771. Warner-Lambert Co., U.S. Pat. 4,073,789 (1978).

772. K. Nádor and J. Pórszász, *Arzneim.-Forsch.*, **8**, 313 (1958).

773. J. Knoll, *Arch. Exp. Pathol. Pharmakol.*, **236**, 92 (1959).

774. J. Knoll, *Arch. Exp. Pathol. Pharmakol.*, **238**, 114 (1960).

775. J. Knoll, K. Nádor, B. Knoll, H. Heidt, and J. G. Nievel, *Arch. Int. Pharmacodyn. Ther.*, **130**, 155 (1961).

776. W. M. Welch, C. A. Harbert, R. Sarges, W. P. Stratten, and A. Weissman, *J. Med. Chem.*, **20**, 699 (1977).

777. A. M. Eirin, E. Ravina, J. M. Montanes, and J. M. Calleja, *Eur. J. Med. Chem.*, **11**, 29 (1976).

778. M. Williams, J. A. Totaro, and B. V. Clineschmidt, *J. Pharm. Pharmacol.*, **30**, 390 (1978).

779. K. Schoen, I. J. Pachter, and A. Rubin, *Abstr. Pap. 153rd Meet. Am. Chem. Soc., Miami Beach, Fla., April 1967*, p. M-46.

780. A. A. Rubin, H. C. Yen, and M. Pfeffer, *Nature*, **216**, 578 (1967).

781. A. A. Sugerman and J. Herrmann, *Clin. Pharmacol. Ther.*, **8**, 261 (1967).

782. J. L. Claghorn, *Curr. Ther. Res., Clin. Exp.*, **11**, 524 (1969).

783. H. Freeman and A. N. D. Frederick, *Curr Ther. Res., Clin. Exp.*, **11**, 670 (1969).

784. D. M. Gallant and M. P. Bishop, *Curr. Ther. Res., Clin. Exp.*, **10**, 441 (1968).

785. R. Kellner, R. T. Rada, A. Egelman, and B. Macaluso, *Curr. Ther. Res., Clin. Exp.*, **20**, 686 (1976).

786. S. W. Holmes and J. A. Gylys, *Fed. Proc.*, **30**, 598 Abs. (1971).

787. A. Elizur and S. Gershon, *Curr. Ther. Res., Clin. Exp.*, **13**, 584 (1971).

788. R. Littell, E. N. Greenblatt, and G. R. Allen, Jr., *J. Med. Chem.*, **15**, 875 (1972).

789. D. M. Loew and P. Zwirner, *Psychopharmacologia*, **26**:Suppl., 54 (1972).

790. J. Roubicek, J. Klos, and A. Tschudin, *Psychopharmacologia*, **26**:Suppl., 71 (1972).

791. J. A. Fernandez, R. A. Bellare, C. V. Deliwala, N. K. Dadkar, and U. K. Sheth, *J. Med. Chem.*, **15**, 417 (1972).

792. V. P. Arya, R. S. Grewal, J. David, and C. L. Kaul, *Experientia*, **23**, 514 (1967).

793. E. Fourneau and D. Bovet, *Arch. Int. Pharmacodyn. Ther.*, **46**, 178 (1933).

794. J. Mills, R. C. Rathbun, and I. H. Slater, *Abstr. Pap. 132nd Meet. Am. Chem. Soc., New York, September 1957*, p. 6-0.

795. J. Mills, M. M. Boren, W. E. Buting, W. N. Cannon, and Q. F. Soper, *Abstr. Pap., 132nd Meet. Am. Chem. Soc., New York, September 1957*, p. 7-0.

796. T. Verhave, J. E. Owen, Jr., D. Fadely, and J. R. Clark, *J. Pharmacol. Exp. Ther.*, **122**, 78A (1958).

797. F. G. Henderson, B. L. Martz, and I. H. Slater, *J. Pharmacol. Exp. Ther.*, **122**, 30A (1958).

798. R. C. Rathbun, J. K. Henderson, R. W. Kattau, and C. E. Keller, *J. Pharmacol. Exp. Ther.*, **122**, 64A (1958).

799. I. H. Slater and G. T. Jones, *J. Pharmacol. Exp. Ther.*, **122**, 69A (1958).

800. H. Klupp and .I. Streller, *Arzneim.-Forsch.*, **9**, 604 (1959).

801. V. G. Longo and V. Rosnati, *Psychopharmacologia*, **8**, 145 (1965).

802. V. Daukas and A. Lastauskas, *Chem. Abstr.*, **64**, 12662 (1966).

803. T. M. Itil, J. Marasa, A. Bigelow, and B. Saletu, *Curr. Ther. Res., Clin. Exp.*, **16**, 80 (1974).

804. D. B. Rusterholz, J. P. Long, J. R. Flynn, J. R. Glyn, C. F. Barftnecht, R. W. Lind, and A. K. Johnson, *Arch. Int. Pharmacodyn. Ther.*, **232**, 246 (1978).

805. R. M. Pinder, R. N. Brogden, P. R. Sawyer, T. M. Speight, and G. S. Avery, *Drugs*, **12**, 81 (1976).

806. B. Costall and R. J. Naylor, *Psychopharmacologia*, **32**, 161 (1973).

807. L. Ahtee and G. Buncombe, *Acta Pharmacol. Toxicol.*, **35**, 429 (1974).

808. A. Dolphin, P. Jenner, C. D. Marsden, C. Pycock, and D. Tarsy, *Pyschopharmacologia*, **41**, 133 (1975).

809. R. O'Keefe, D. F. Sharman, and M. Vogt, *Brit. J. Pharmacol.*, **38**, 287 (1970).

810. B. R. S. Nakra, A. J. Bond, and M. H. Lader, *J. Clin. Pharmacol.*, **15**, 449 (1975).

811. P. Mouille, G. Cheynol, and C. Gadhin, *Ann. Pharm. Fr.*, **35**, 53 (1977); *Chem. Abstr.*, **87**, 78363m (1977).

812. J. Prieto, J. Moragues, R. G. Spickett, A. Vega, M. Columbo, W. Salazar, and D. J. Roberts, *J. Pharm. Pharmacol.*, **29**, 147 (1977).

813. R. Kato, Y. Sato, and K. Shimomura, *J. Pharmacol. (Paris)*, **5**:Suppl. 2, Abstract CM1, 48 (1974).

814. B. Costall and R. J. Naylor, *Psychopharmacologia*, **43**, 69 (1975).

815. A. Tagliamonti, G. DeMontis, M. Olianis, L. Vargiu, G. U. Corsini, and G. L. Gessa, *J. Neurochem.*, **24**, 707 (1975).

816. F. Honda, Y. Satoh, K. Shimomura, H. Satoh, H. Noguchi, S. I. Uchida, and R. Kato, *Jap. J. Pharmacol.*, **27**, 397 (1977).

817. P. Castrogiovanni, C. B. Cassano, L. Conti, C. Maggini, L. Bonollo, and B. Sarteschi, *Int. Pharmacopsychiatr.*, **11**, 74 (1976).

818. M. Nishiuia, *Curr. Ther. Res., Clin. Exp.*, **20**, 164 (1976).

819. D. H. Mielke, D. M. Gallant, and C. Kessler, *Am. J. Psychiatr.*, **134**, 1371 (1977).

820. H. Dufour, J. Costelli, H. Luecioni, J. C. Scotto, and J. M. Suter, *J. Pharmacol. (Paris)*, **5**:2, 26 (1974).

821. M. Lanzo, D. Picard, and N. Carlon, *Thérapie*, **30**, 231 (1975).

822. R. Planche, *Sem. Hop-The.*, **52**, 261 (1976).

823. G. Orzalesi, R. Salleri, I. Valpato, and A. Fravolini, *Boll. Chim. Farm.*, **115**, 317 (1976); *Chem. Abstr.*, **85**, 177207d (1976).

824. P. N. C. Elliott, P. Jenner, G. Huizing, C. D. Marsden, and R. Miller, *Neuropharmacol.*, **16**, 333 (1977).

825. E. Peringer, P. Jenner, I. M. Donaldson, C. D. Marsden, and R. Miller, *Neuropharmacol.*, **15**, 463 (1976).

826. B. D. Roufogalis, M. Thornton, and D. N. Wade, *Life Sci.*, **19**, 927 (1976).

827. N. Trabucchi, R. Longoni, P. Fresia, and P. F. Spano, *Life Sci.*, **17**, 1551 (1976).

828. P. N. C. Elliott, G. Huizing, P. Jenner, C. D. Marsden, and R. Miller, *Brit. J. Pharmacol.*, **57**, 472P (1976).

829. L. Justin-Besancon, C. Laville, M. J. Margarit, and M. M. Thominet, *Compt. Rend. Acad. Sci. (Paris)*, **279**, 375 (1974).

830. A. J. Puech, P. Simon, and J. R. Boissier, *Eur. J. Pharmacol.*, **50**, 291 (1978).

831. F. Parravicini, M. Pinza, P. Ventura, S. Banfi, and G. Pifferi, *Farm. Ed. Sci.*, **31**, 49 (1976).

832. W. V. Krumholz, H. I. Chipps, and S. Merlis, *J. Clin. Pharmacol.*, **7**, 108 (1967).

833. Choay SA, Belg. Pat. 842,753 (1976).

834. Ciba Geigy AG, Belg. Pat. 846,542 (1977).

835. G. Narcisse, F. Hubert, G. Ucnida-Ernouf, and J. Perdriau, *Thérapie*, **32**, 121 (1977).

836. B. Cavalerri, G. Volpe, B. Rosselli Del Turco, and A. Diena, *Farm. Ed. Sci.*, **31**, 393 (1976).

837. A. Ermili, A. Balbi, G. Roma, A. Ambrosini, and N. Passerini, *Farm. Ed. Sci.*, **31**, 627 (1976).

838. H. G. Morren, V. Bienfet, and A. M. Reyntjens,

in *Psychopharmacological Agents*, Vol. 1, M. Gordon, Ed., Academic, New York, 1964, p. 251.

839. N. Goncalves, *Psychopharmacologia*, **25**, 281 (1972).

840. E. Merck A.-G., Neth. Pat. Appl. 6,514,242 (1966); through *Chem. Abstr.*, **65**, 13722 (1966).

841. V. Koppe, K. Schulte, S. Sommer, and H. Muller-Calgan (E. Merck A.-G.), Brit. Pat. 1,124,710 (1966); through *Chem. Abstr.*, **69**, 106747 (1968).

842. R. S. Grewal, C. L. Kaul, and J. David, *J. Pharmacol. Exp. Ther.*, **160**, 268 (1968).

843. Y.-H. Wu, K. R. Smith, J. W. Rayburn, and J. W. Kissel, *J. Med. Chem.*, **12**, 876 (1969).

844. E. Lindner, *Arzneim.-Forsch.*, **22**, 1445 (1972).

845. M. T. Ramacci, P. Sale, and L. Angelucci, *J. Pharmacol.* (Paris), **5**:2, 82 (1974).

846. D. Wheatley, *Curr. Ther. Res., Clin. Exp.*, **20**, 74 (1976).

847. B. Silvestrini, V. Cioli, S. Burberi, and B. Catanese, *Int. J. Neuropharmacol.*, **7**, 587 (1968).

848. M. Fielden, W. J. Welstead, Jr., N. D. Dawson, Y.-H. Chen, R. P. Mays, J. P. DaVanzo, and C. D. Lunsford, *J. Med. Chem.*, **16**, 1124 (1973).

849. E. Hong, *Arzneim.-Forsch.*, **23**, 1726 (1973).

850. S. Hayao, W. G. Strycker, B. M. Phillips, H. Fujimori, and H. Vidrio, *J. Med. Chem.*, **11**, 1246 (1968).

851. R. B. Petigara, C. V. Deliwala, S. S. Mandrekar, N. K. Dadkar, and U. K. Sheth, *J. Med. Chem.*, **12**, 865 (1969).

852. G. A. R. Johnson and A. D. Rudzik, *Pharmacologist*, **12**, 218 (1970).

853. Z. J. Vejdelĕk, J. Metyš, F. Hradil, and M. Protiva, *Collect. Czech. Chem. Commun.*, **40**, 1204 (1975).

854. R. N. Schut, F. E. Ward, and R. Rodriguez, *J. Med. Chem.*, **15**, 301 (1972).

855. S. N. Rastogi, N. Anand, P. P. Gupta, and J. N. Sharma, *J. Med. Chem.*, **16**, 797 (1973).

856. S. Consolo, H. Ladinsky, G. Peri, and S. Garattini, *Biochem. Pharmacol.*, **26**, 1517 (1977).

857. W. P. Burkard, M. Jalfre, J. E. Blum, and W. Haefely, *J. Pharm. Pharmacol.*, **23**, 646 (1971).

858. Z. J. Vejdělek, B. Kakáč, J. Němec, and M. Protiva, *Collect. Czech. Chem. Commun.*, **38**, 2989 (1973).

859. Z. J. Vejdělek, J. Němec, Z. Šedivý, L. Tuma, and M. Protiva, *Collect. Czech. Chem. Commun.*, **39**, 2276 (1974).

860. A. Carlsson and M. Lindqvist, *Acta Pharmacol. Toxicol.*, **24**, 112 (1966).

861. J. Vieth and D. Preiss, *Arch. Int. Pharmacodyn. Ther.*, **162**, 283 (1966).

862. L. B. Piotrovskii and O. I. Kiselev, *Khim.-Farm. Zh.*, **9**, 3 (1975).

863. A. Ahmad, M. M. Vohra, and G. Archari, *Jap. J. Pharmacol.*, **17**, 622 (1967).

864. C. R. Ganellin, J. M. Loynes, H. F. Ridley, and R. G. Spickett, *J. Med. Chem.*, **10**, 826 (1967).

865. B. Lal, J. M. Khanna, and N. Anand, *J. Med. Chem.*, **15**, 23 (1972).

866. E. Holm. H. Weidinger, F. Kirchner, and F. Boettinger, *Arzneim.-Forsch.*, **20**, 1671 (1970).

867. B. Belleau, R. Martel, G. Lacasse, M. Menard, N. L. Weinberg, and Y. G. Perron, *J. Am. Chem. Soc.*, **90**, 823 (1968).

868. G. M. Simpson, J. W. S. Angus, A. A. Sugerman, and H. Stolberg, *J. Clin. Pharmacol.*, **8**, 196 (1968).

869. J. F. Muren and A. Weissman, *J. Med. Chem.*, **14**, 49 (471).

870. T. Yui and Y. Takeo, U.S. Pat. 3,296,074 (1967).

871. G. M. Simpson, E. Kunz-Bartholini, and T. P. S. Watts, *J. Clin. Pharmacol.*, **7**, 221 (1967).

872. S. Chiba, Y. Saji, H. Hibino, Y. Takeo, and T. Yui, *Arzneim.-Forsch.*, **18**, 303 (1968).

873. A. Tobe and T. Kobayashi, *Jap. J. Pharmacol.*, **26**, 559 (1976).

874. A. Uzan, G. LeFur, N. Mitrani, M. Kabouche, and A.-M. Danadieu, *Life Sci.*, **23**, 261 (1978).

875. R. C. Moreau, Y. Adam, and O. Foussard-Blanpin, *Eur. J. Med. Chem.*, **10**, 247 (1975).

876. R. Mechoulam, Ed., *Marijuana Chemistry, Pharmacology, Metabolism and Clinical Effects*, Academic, New York, 1973.

877. B. Loev, P. E. Bender, F. Dowalo, E. Macko, and P. J. Fowler, *J. Med. Chem.*, **16**, 1200 (1973).

878. J. A. Clark, M. S. G. Clark, and A. Cook, *Abstr. Pap. 168th Natl. Meet. Am. Chem. Soc., Atlantic City, N.J., Sept. 8–13, 1974*, MEDI 10.

879. S. Houry, R. Mechoulam, P. J. Fowler, E. Macko, and B. Loev, *J. Med. Chem.*, **17**, 287 (1974).

880. P. A. J. Janssen, in *International Review of Neurobiology*, Vol. 8, C. C. Pfeiffer and J. R. Smythies, Eds., Academic, New York-London, 1965, p. 221.

881. P. Krogsgaard-Larsen, G. A. R. Johnston, D. Lodge, and D. R. Curtis, *Nature*, **268**, 53 (1977).

882. S. J. Enna, J. P. Bennett, Jr., D. R. Burt, I. Creese, and S. H. Snyder, *Nature*, **263**, 338 (1976).

883. D. D. Van Kammen, *Am. J. Psychiatr.*, **134,** 138 (1977).

884. T. L. Perry, S. Hansen, and M. Kloster, *New Engl. J. Med.*, **288,** 337 (1973).

885. D. W. Straughan, in *Biochemistry and Neurology*, H. F. Bradford and C. D. Marsden, Eds., Academic, London, 1975, p. 213.

886. S. Simler, L. Ciesielski, M. Maitre, H. Randrianarisoa, and P. Mandel, *Biochem. Pharmacol.*, **22,** 1701 (1973).

887. P. Krogsgaard-Larsen and G. A. R. Johnston, *J. Neurochem.*, **25,** 797 (1975).

888. G. A. R. Johnston, P. Krogsgaard-Larsen, and A. Stephanson, *Nature*, **258,** 627 (1975).

889. Sandoz, SA, Belg. Pat. 848,936 (1977).

890. G. A. R. Johnston, D. R. Curtis, P. M. Beart, C. J. A. Game, R. M. McCulloch, and B. Twitchin, *J. Neurochem.*, **24,** 157 (1975).

891. D. R. Curtis, A. W. Duggan, D. Felix, and G. A. R. Johnston, *Brain Res.*, **32,** 69 (1971).

892. C. A. Tamminga, J. W. Crayton, and T. N. Chase, *Am. J. Psychiatr.*, **136,** 746 (1978).

893. P. K. Frederiksen, *Lancet*, **1,** 702 (1975).

894. L. B. Bigelow, H. Nasrallah, J. Carman, J. C. Gillin, and R. J. Wyatt, *Am. J. Psychiatr.*, **134,** 318 (1977).

895. S. R. Naik, A. Guidotti, and E. Costa, *Neuropharmacol.*, **15,** 479 (1976).

896. J. Davies and J. C. Watkins, *Brain Res.*, **70,** 501 (1974).

897. (a) K. Saito, S. Konishi, and M. Otsuka, *Brain Res.*, **97,** 177 (1975); (b) J. L. Henry and Y. Ben-Ari, *Brain Res.*, **117,** 540 (1976).

898. N. E. Anden and H. Wachtel, *Acta Pharmacol. Toxicol.*, **40,** 310 (1977).

899. K. Menon, D. Bieger, and O. Hornykiewicz, *J. Neural Transm.*, **39,** 177 (1976).

900. K. Kobayashi, S. Miyazawa, A. Terahara, H. Mishima, and H. Kurihara, *Tetrahedron Lett.*, **7,** 537 (1976).

901. D. K. J. Goricki, S. J. Peesker, and J. D. Wood, *Biochem. Pharmacol.*, **25,** 1653 (1976).

902. D. F. Horrobin, *Lancet*, **1977-I,** 936.

903. W. J. Potts and P. F. East, *Arch. Int. Pharmacodyn. Ther.*, **191,** 74 (1971).

904. P. Stern, *J. Neural Transm.*, **32,** 236 (1969).

905. D. J. Mattke and M. Adler, *Dis. Nerv. Syst.*, **32,** 388 (1971).

906. S. M. Paul and J. Axelrod, *Science*, **197,** 657 (1977).

907. Y. F. Jacquet and N. Marks, *Science*, **194,** 632 (1976).

908. D. S. Segal, R. G. Browne, F. Bloom, N. Ling, and R. Guillemin, *Science*, **198,** 411 (1977).

909. E. T. Carlson and M. M. Simpson, *Am. J. Psychiatr.*, **120,** 112 (1963).

910. A. Comfort, *Clin. Toxicol.*, **11,** 383 (1977).

911. P. Seeman, *Pharmacol. Rev.*, **24,** 583 (1972).

912. P. A. J. Janssen, *Int. J. Neuropsychiat.*, **3**:Suppl. 1, S10 (1967).

913. O. Hornykiewicz, *Neuroscience*, **3,** 773 (1978).

914. J. W. Kebabian, G. L. Petzold, and P. Greengard, *Proc. Natl. Acad. Sci. U.S.*, **69,** 2145 (1972).

915. K. F. Lloyd and G. Bartholini, *Experientia*, **31,** 560 (1975).

916. D. R. Burt, S. Enna, I. Creese, and S. H. Snyder, *Proc. Natl. Acad. Sci., U.S.*, **72,** 4655 (1975).

917. M. Briley and S. Z. Langer, *Eur. J. Pharmacol.*, **50,** 283 (1978).

918. P. Seeman, T. Lee, M. Chau-Wong, and K. Wong, *Nature*, **261,** 717 (1976).

919. S. J. Enna, J. P. Bennett, Jr., D. B. Bylund, I. Creese, D. R. Burt, M. E. Charness, H. I. Yamamura, R. Simantov, and S. H. Snyder, *J. Neurochem.*, **28,** 233 (1977).

920. M. C. Nowycky and R. H. Roth, *Progr. Neuropsychopharmacol.*, **2,** 139 (1978).

921. F. A. Henn, D. J. Anderson, and A. Sellström, *Nature*, **266,** 637 (1977).

922. A. R. Cools, H. A. J. Struyker-Boudier, and J. M. van Rossum, *Eur. J. Pharmacol.*, **37,** 283 (1976).

923. J. M. van Rossum, *Fed. Proc.*, **37,** 2415 (1978).

924. J. W. Kebabian, *Life Sci.*, **23,** 479 (1978).

925. J. W. Kebabian and D. B. Calne, *Nature*, **277,** 93 (1979).

926. A. R. Cools, G. Hendriks, and J. Korten, *J. Neural Transm.*, **36,** 91 (1975).

927. J. E. Leysen, W. Gommeren, and P. M. Laduron, *Biochem. Pharmacol.*, **27,** 307 (1978).

928. J. E. Leysen, C. J. E. Niemegeers, J. P. Tollenaere, and P. M. Laduron, *Nature*, **272,** 168 (1978).

929. C. Kornetsky and R. Markowitz, in *Model Systems in Biological Psychiatry*, D. J. Ingle and H. Schein, Eds., M.I.T. Press, Cambridge, Mass., 1975, p. 26.

930. P. B. Bradley and B. J. Key, *Electroenceph. Clin. Neurophysiol.*, **10,** 560 (1968).

931. J. Boakes, P. B. Bradley, and J. M. Candy, *Brit. J. Pharmacol.*, **45,** 391 (1972).

932. U. Ungerstedt, *Acta Physiol. Scand.*, Suppl. 367 (1971).

933. P. A. J. Janssen, in *Modern Problems in Pharmacopsychiatry; The Neuroleptics*, Vol. 5, D. P. Bobon, J. A. J. Janssen, and J. Bobon, Eds., S. Karger, Basel, 1970, p. 33.

934. P. S. Portoghese, *Acc. Chem. Res.*, **11**, 21 (1978).

935. P. S. Portoghese, *J. Med. Chem.*, **8**, 609 (1965).

936. J. P. Tollenaere, H. Moereels, and M. H. J. Koch, *Eur. J. Med. Chem.*, **12**, 199 (1977).

937. J. J. H. McDowell, *Acta Crystallogr.*, **25B**, 2175 (1969).

938. J. Krieglstein, W. Meiler, and J. Staab, *Biochem. Pharmacol.*, **21**, 985 (1972).

939. E. F. Domino, *U.S. Public Health Serv., Publ.*, **1836**, 1045 (1968).

940. J. Levy, T. N. Tozer, L. D. Tuck, and D. B. Loveland, *J. Med. Chem.*, **15**, 898 (1972).

941. P. S. Guth and M. A. Spirtes, in *International Review of Neurobiology*, Vol. 9, C. C. Pfeiffer and J. R. Smythies, Eds., Academic, New York-London, 1966, p. 145.

CHAPTER FIFTY-SEVEN

Antianxiety Agents

SCOTT J. CHILDRESS

Research and Development
Wyeth Laboratories
Philadelphia, Pennsylvania 19101, USA

CONTENTS

1 ANXIETY

A humorous, although functional, definition of anxiety is the condition for which everyone is taking Valium! Anxiety is so widespread that, in a 12-month period, diazepam is estimated to be taken by 20% of American women and 14% of American men (1). Anxiety is an emotional state characterized by a disquietude of mind and a fearful anticipation of untoward events which may be brought on by stressful events in normal life. The antecedent stress may be readily apparent as, for example, a death in the family. There are many gradations between anxiety that can be recognized as appropriate to surrounding events and pathological anxiety, which rises to a degree inappropriate to any recognizable cause, or for which no cause at all can be perceived. The more severe condition can be recognized by its intensity, pervasiveness, persistence, and interference with normal life (2). In addition to the disturbance of mood, high levels of anxiety usually involve changes in bodily functions such as sleep and autonomic nervous and gastrointestinal systems. Anxiety can be mixed with depression and is not always easily diagnosed.

The neurophysiological basis of anxiety is not well-understood. The limbic system of the brain is believed to be the seat of the emotions. It is located in the most primitive part of the cortex and in the hypothalamus. Electrical stimulation through electrodes implanted in certain parts of the limbic system can overcome conditioned fear in animals. The reticular formation of the brain is involved in anxiety states. The reticular system is believed to be a normalizing control system acting through feedback. A weakening of its inhibitory action leads to overstimulation and anxiety.

Knowledge of the biochemistry of anxiety is quite primitive despite an enormous amount of investigative work. Padjen and Bloom (3) have pointed out that virtually every known neurotransmitter as well as both cyclic AMP and cyclic GMP have been implicated as playing roles. Medicinal chemists have fully developed the two principal classes of antianxiety drugs, the propanediols and the benzodiazepines, by empirical procedures but have not as yet been able to employ the wealth of available biochemical information in the rational design of antianxiety agents.

2 TESTS FOR ANTIANXIETY AGENTS

Pharmacologists resort to a spectrum of animal tests in order to evaluate the antianxiety potential of new compounds. Since physical tension is a prominent symptom in anxiety states, it is not surprising that tests to measure muscle-relaxant effects should be employed in antianxiety testing. Many laboratories simply measure the dose required to deprive an animal of the ability to right itself when placed on its back. The result is expressed as PD_{50}, the dose that deprives 50% of an animal group of the righting reflex. Other laboratories estimate the activity by measuring the dose causing mice to slide down a screen inclined at 70°. This test provides an estimate of muscle relaxation and incoordination.

Almost all the present-day antianxiety agents have anticonvulsant activity as measured in tests against the effects of pentylenetetrazole and electroshock (see Chapter 55). Such activity is a consequence of depression above the spinal level. Anticonvulsant activity has not been very helpful in elucidating the mechanism of action of antianxiety drugs—not all anticonvulsants are effective against anxiety—but it has provided useful and reproducible screening tests for possible antianxiety activity.

Behavioral tests form the second line of screening methods (4). To a trained observer the alteration in normal animal behavior after drug treatment may be quite profound and is useful in screening and classifying new chemical compounds. Alterations in the sociability, alertness, and gait of the cat are particularly informative. Certain unusual behavior patterns, such as aggression, can be elicited from animals in various ways—mice are made aggressive by foot shock—and the effect of a drug in modifying this behavior can be determined.

The disruption of conditioned behavior at doses that do not interfere severely with consciousness or instinctual behavior is characteristic of the antipsychotic drugs such as chlorpromazine (Chapter 56). Although the antianxiety drugs are usually said not to interfere with conditioned behavior (5), it is possible to set up experimental models of conditioned behavior that permit evaluation of these agents. Basically these tests involve training an animal to perform an action, such as pressing a lever, to avoid a painful stimulus (e.g., an electric shock) that may be given with or without warning. If the animal fails to avoid the shock, a further action, such as pressing the same lever, must be taken to escape from the painful stimulus. Myriad variations of this basic situation have been devised, and the changes in approach, avoidance, and escape behavior patterns after drug treatment have been observed (6).

One such variation is a conflict test developed by Geller and Seifter (7). In this test a trained rat is given food rewards at random intervals in response to lever pressing. Each rat exhibits a characteristic and rather stable rate of lever pressing when not under drug treatment. The rat has learned that during an audible signal of a few minutes' duration that is occasionally presented each press of the lever will provide a food reward but will be accompanied by a punishing shock. The force of the shock is adjusted so that the conflict between the rat's desire for food and its fear of the shock is not well resolved. Each rat develops a characteristic response pattern during the conflict period. Under treatment with an effective antianxiety agent a rat's responses during the conflict period rise—food is chosen over fear. Lack of side effects is indicated by the preservation of the characteristic rate of lever pressing during the nonconflict portion of the test. More powerful central depressants—barbiturates—lower the overall rate of lever pressing. Neuroleptics such as promazine and analgesics such as morphine are not effective in this test. Indeed, removal of the punishing shock does not cause an immediate recovery of the rate of lever pressing. Hence it is not the shock itself that deters the rat but rather the threat of it (8). To the extent that a rat's brain mimics the human brain, this test has the elegance of appearing to simulate the clinical situation of anxiety.

A third line of study of the antianxiety agents is at the neurophysiological level.

As measured by electroencephalography, differential depression of the various areas of the brain occurs. As expected in view of the theories about the neurophysiological basis of anxiety, the limbic system and, less readily, the reticular system are depressed before the cortex is affected. The depression of reflexes is a good measure of the muscle-relaxing ability of the antianxiety agents which is associated with depression of interneuronal circuits. The greater the number of interneurons involved in the reflex, the greater the sensitivity of that reflex to the effects of the tranquilizers. For a more detailed discussion of the muscle-relaxant aspects of these agents consult Chapter 47.

The clinical study of antianxiety drugs in a well-controlled manner is difficult (9). Patients respond to the therapeutic environment; there is a considerable interaction with the physician. Studies are usually done with physician evaluations of multiple psychological and somatic factors and changes over time are recorded. Because of the shifts in base levels with time and the difficulty of proper patient selection, an appreciable number of patients may be required to establish activity.

3 TREATMENT OF ANXIETY

It is fair to say that anxiety has been treatable since the discovery of alcohol. Other sedatives have also been used. The barbiturates, for example, have a genuine antianxiety action but cause a depression of the central nervous system extending into the cortex. The newer antianxiety agents are able to exert their effects without producing generalized depression. Berger (5) has pointed out that this ability is related to dose. Excessive doses of tranquilizers do cause extensive depression of the central nervous system, and it is important in treating anxiety not to exceed the useful dosage.

Although some neuroleptics, particularly

thioridazine (10) and dixyrazine (11), may be used in low dosage for anxiety, these agents are not considered here; neither are the sedatives of the antihistamine type such as hydroxyzine (Chapter 54). Doxepin has been established to have antianxiety activity but it is used almost exclusively in depression and is discussed in Chapter 58. β-Adrenergic blocking agents can be shown to be effective in clinical antianxiety studies, but there is skepticism that the effect is other than a somatic one (12). Anxious patients usually have several physical symptoms—palpitations, trembling, dizziness—mediated by sympathetic activity and susceptible to reversal by β-adrenergic blockade (Chapter 42). There can, of course, be value to a patient in relieving his overt problems, and β-blockers have been called drugs of choice for anxiety in which somatic complaints are predominant (13).

There are two principal classes of agents now in use, central muscle relaxants and benzodiazepines, the antianxiety action of which can be attributed to unrelated pharmacological effects only in part.

4   CENTRAL MUSCLE RELAXANTS

The introduction of meprobamate (57.1) in 1955 provided the first generally useful replacement for the overly sedating barbiturates in the treatment of anxiety (14). Meprobamate resulted from a classical medicinal chemistry investigation of relatives of mephenesin (57.2). The latter compound had been introduced as a muscle relaxant with sedative properties. The association of these properties had suggested its possible value in treating anxiety characterized by physical stress (15). Its effective-

$$H_2NCO_2CH_2\underset{\underset{CH_2CH_2CH_3}{|}}{\overset{\overset{CH_3}{|}}{C}}CH_2OCONH_2$$

57.1

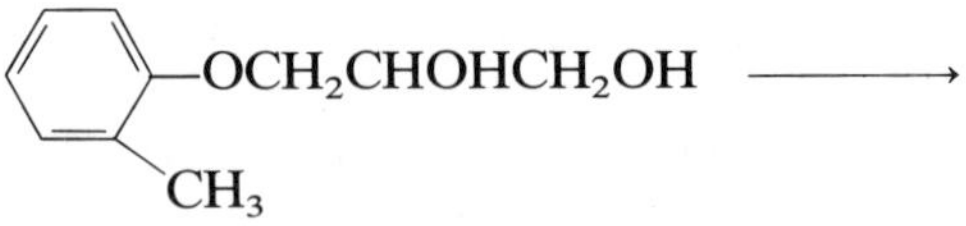

OCH₂CHOHCH₂OH structure:

—OCH$_2$CHOHCH$_2$OH ⟶

57.2

HO— —OCH$_2$CHOHCO$_2$H

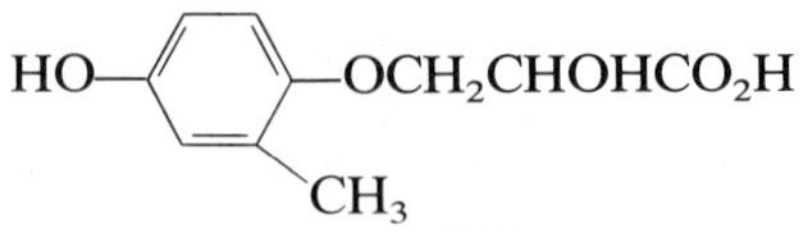

57.3

ness was sufficient to set off a search for better compounds since its low potency and short duration of action resulting from its rapid conversion into 2-hydroxy-3-(4-hydroxy-2-methylphenoxy)propionic acid (57.3) limited its clinical usefulness.

Esterification of mephenesin was studied extensively as a means of hindering the rapid metabolism. Mephenesin carbamate was the ultimate product of this work. Animal tests, however, showed it to be not longer in action than mephenesin but of somewhat higher potency. It was marketed for oral use, but its principal therapeutic indication remained muscle relaxation. It is of interest that the dicarbamate ester of mephenesin is inactive.

Variation in the general structure of mephenesin was carried on in parallel to the work on its esters. 2,2-Diethyl-1,3-propanediol was found in screens to have anticonvulsant activity of limited duration. Esterification of both hydroxyl groups increased the duration of action. Examination of the isomeric 1,3-propanediol dicarbamates having 2-substitution totaling four carbon atoms revealed the methyl-propyl isomer to be the most potent. This compound was marketed as meprobamate and was later followed by its N-butyl analog, tybamate (57.4). In the meprobamate series it was found that replacement of the propyl group by a phenyl group increased the anticonvulsant activity but did not improve the muscle-relaxant potency (16).

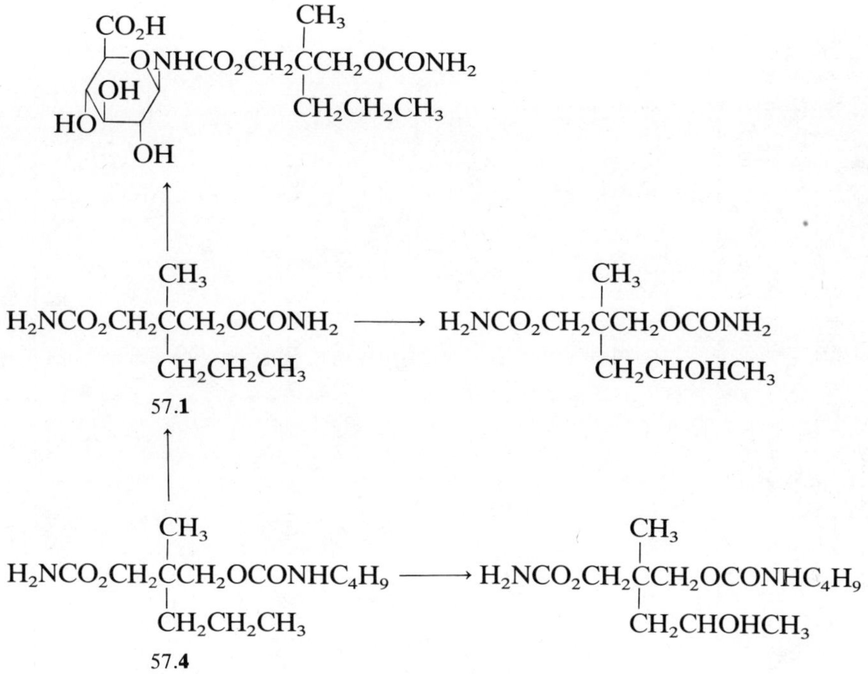

$$\text{CO}_2\text{H}$$

$$\underset{\substack{\\ \text{O}\text{NHCO}_2\text{CH}_2\overset{\overset{\displaystyle\text{CH}_3}{|}}{\underset{\underset{\displaystyle\text{CH}_2\text{CH}_2\text{CH}_3}{|}}{\text{C}}}\text{CH}_2\text{OCONH}_2}}{}$$

$$\overset{\text{CH}_3}{\underset{\text{CH}_2\text{CH}_2\text{CH}_3}{\text{H}_2\text{NCO}_2\text{CH}_2\overset{|}{\underset{|}{\text{C}}}\text{CH}_2\text{OCONH}_2}} \longrightarrow \overset{\text{CH}_3}{\underset{\text{CH}_2\text{CHOHCH}_3}{\text{H}_2\text{NCO}_2\text{CH}_2\overset{|}{\underset{|}{\text{C}}}\text{CH}_2\text{OCONH}_2}}$$

57.**1**

$$\overset{\text{CH}_3}{\underset{\text{CH}_2\text{CH}_2\text{CH}_3}{\text{H}_2\text{NCO}_2\text{CH}_2\overset{|}{\underset{|}{\text{C}}}\text{CH}_2\text{OCONHC}_4\text{H}_9}} \longrightarrow \overset{\text{CH}_3}{\underset{\text{CH}_2\text{CHOHCH}_3}{\text{H}_2\text{NCO}_2\text{CH}_2\overset{|}{\underset{|}{\text{C}}}\text{CH}_2\text{OCONHC}_4\text{H}_9}}$$

57.**4**

Fig. 57.1 Metabolism of meprobamate and tybamate.

The interneuronal blockade produced by meprobamate is greater than that produced by mephenesin. Although meprobamate depresses the flexor and other complex spinal reflexes it does not depress the ascending reticular activating system. It lowers the spontaneous electrical potential of the thalamus without affecting the cortex. It also shortens the duration of seizures consequent to stimulation of the limbic system. It is not active against the autonomic nervous system. Meprobamate has the taming effect that is characteristic of antianxiety compounds. Its muscle-relaxant effect (relief of tension) probably accounts for some, but not all, of its clinical action.

Many attempts have been made to find an improvement on meprobamate. Several

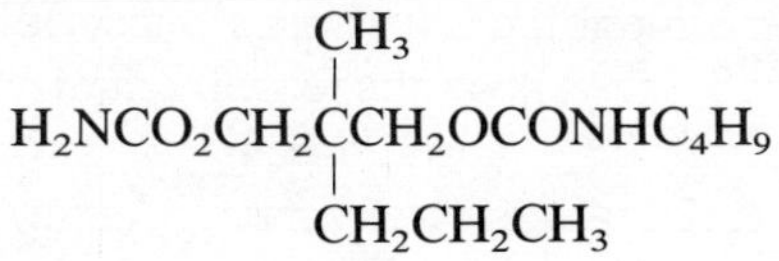

$$\overset{\text{CH}_3}{\underset{\text{CH}_2\text{CH}_2\text{CH}_3}{\text{H}_2\text{NCO}_2\text{CH}_2\overset{|}{\underset{|}{\text{C}}}\text{CH}_2\text{OCONHC}_4\text{H}_9}}$$

57.**4**

such compounds are marketed as shown in Table 57.1. Claims of greater potency, lower sedation, and fewer side effects were made for these products. Several other related compounds have been withdrawn from the U.S. market in response to regulatory pressure from the Food and Drug Administration, but they were already market failures. There are many possible reasons for failure, e.g., ineffective sponsorship, aside from a lack of the requisite activity.

The surviving compounds in the table are fairly close in potency. Tybamate is the most recent of the compounds and appears to have certain pharmacological advantages. It antagonizes the pressor effect of serotonin and the EEG activation caused by lysergic acid diethylamide. In further contrast to meprobamate, convulsions do not follow its withdrawal from chronic use. Emylcamate and phenprobamate are available in Europe.

Insofar as it has been reported, the

Table 57.1 Key Pharmacological Properties of Antianxiety Agents of the Central Muscle-Relaxant Type[a]

Compound	Structure	Median Effective Dose (ED$_{50}$), mg/kg			Toxicity (LD$_{50}$), mg/kg	Ref.
		Activity Against				
		PD$_{50}$,[b] mg/kg	Maximum Electro-shock	Pentylene-tetrazole		
Meprobamate	$H_2NCO_2CH_2\text{—}\overset{\text{CH}_3}{\underset{\text{C}_3\text{H}_7}{C}}\text{—}CH_2OCONH_2$	300 175 i.v.	165	67 102 i.p.	1000 482 i.v.	17
Tybamate	$H_2NCO_2CH_2\text{—}\overset{\text{CH}_3}{\underset{\text{C}_3\text{H}_7}{C}}\text{—}CH_2OCONHC_4H_9$	235 68 i.v.	198	120	830 254 i.v.	17
Phenprobamate	$C_6H_5CH_2CH_2CH_2OCONH_2$	400	48	95	840	18
Emylcamate	$(C_2H_5)_2\underset{\text{CH}_3}{C}COCONH_2$	125	100–150	60–75	550	19
Chlormezanone	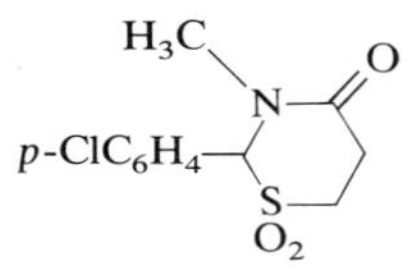	133 i.p.	45 i.p.	120 i.p.	1380 650 i.p.	20

[a] Except where indicated, data are for mice treated orally.
[b] Paralyzing dose.

metabolism of these agents leads to inactivation, with the partial exception of tybamate (Fig. 57.1). Meprobamate is excreted by the rat and by man partly unchanged and partly in the form of a glucuronide. Hydroxylation of the propyl group of meprobamate to a 2-hydroxypropyl group also takes place. Hydroxylation of tybamate in the rat is accompanied by debutylation, and both meprobamate and hydroxymeprobamate are found in the urine. That hydroxytybamate greatly exceeds in amount the meprobamate and hydroxymeprobamate supports the thesis that the activity of tybamate is independent of the partial conversion to meprobamate. The metabolism of phenprobamate is certainly an inactivating one, since man converts 67% of an oral dose into hippuric acid (21). Some hydroxylation of the phenyl group also occurs.

Although structurally quite dissimilar, chlormezanone is pharmacologically similar to meprobamate. A small amount of this compound is excreted in man unchanged, but most of the p-chlorobenzaldehyde available by simple hydrolysis is converted into p-chlorohippuric acid (22).

5 BENZODIAZEPINES

The development of the benzodiazepines was directly responsible for the decline in importance of the propanedioldicarbamates. These newer compounds appear to be more specific in their antianxiety action and less sedative at effective doses.

5.1 Mode of Action

Every conceivable mode of action has been suggested as the basis of the effect of benzodiazepines. The most attractive hypothesis at present relates to action on systems involving γ-aminobutyric acid (GABA). Benzodiazepines give protection against the convulsant effects of GABA

antagonists, picrotoxin and bicuculline, and have thus been proposed as facilitators of GABA-mediated inhibitory synapses. Others have shown benzodiazepines to antagonize GABA-mediated inhibition of cerebellar Purkinje cells. Haefely (23) has reviewed the synaptic pharmacology of benzodiazepines and finds the effects on GABA-mediated inhibition to reach maximum at about 10 times the threshold doses. In contrast to barbiturates there is no depression of synaptic excitation at reasonable doses.

Benzodiazepines have been found to bind to specific receptors on rat forebrain cell membranes that do not bind meprobamate, barbiturates, or ethanol (24). GABA receptor agonists increase and antagonists decrease the benzodiazepine binding affinity (25). The influence of GABA may be through conformational changes in the receptor. Convulsive doses of pentylenetetrazole and electroshock increase the number of receptors without affecting the binding affinity (25a). The most startling aspect of the benzodiazepine receptors is the correlation of the affinities of various compounds with their potencies in relevant pharmacological tests. There are reports (25b–25d) of a natural ligand for the benzodiazepine receptor—an endogenous antianxiety agent—but the interaction between GABA and benzodiazepines offers a modulating system for a known neurotransmitter which may be a sufficient explanation of benzodiazepine activity.

5.2 Structure–Activity Relationships

In the course of follow-up work related to his doctoral dissertation Sternbach discovered chlordiazepoxide in 1955 (26). Pharmacological test data for the most important benzodiazepines among the several thousand that have been made subsequently are given in Table 57.2. Since the important ones are quite active the table

Table 57.2 Key Pharmacological Properties of 1,4-Benzodiazepines[a]

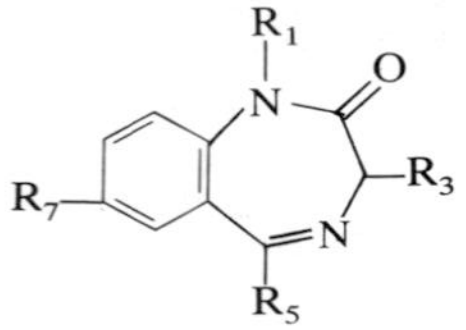

Compound	R_1	R_3	R_5	R_7	Pentylenetetrazole	Maximum Electroshock	Inclined Screen	Cat Behavior MED[b] mg/kg	Toxicity (LD_{50}), mg/kg
					Median Effective Dose (ED_{50}), mg/kg — Activity Against				
Nordiazepam	H	H	C_6H_5	Cl	6.0	25	75	1.0	2750
Nitrazepam	H	H	C_6H_5	NO_2	0.7	30	15	0.1	1550
Diazepam	CH_3	H	C_6H_5	Cl	1.4	6.4	30	0.2	720
Oxazepam	H	OH	C_6H_5	Cl	0.6	3.1	225	1.0	>5000
Oxazepam Hemisuccinate	H	$-OCOCH_2CH_2CO_2H$	C_6H_5	Cl	1.0	17			1148
Temazepam	CH_3	OH	C_6H_5	Cl	0.7	2.6	20	0.5	1160
Camazepam	CH_3	$-OCON(C_2H_5)_2$	C_6H_5	Cl	5.8	60			970
Lorazepam	H	OH	$o\text{-}ClC_6H_4$	Cl	0.07	2.0			>3000
Clonazepam	H	H	$o\text{-}ClC_6H_4$	NO_2	0.2	400	250	0.1	>4000
Bromazepam	H	H	2-Pyridyl	Br	0.7	34	30	0.2	2350
Prazepam	$-CH_2C_3H_5$	H	C_6H_5	Cl	4.1	62	100	0.5	>2000
Flurazepam	$-CH_2CH_2N(C_2H_5)_2$	H	$o\text{-}FC_6H_4$	Cl	1.6	82	200	2.0	870
Chlordiazepoxide	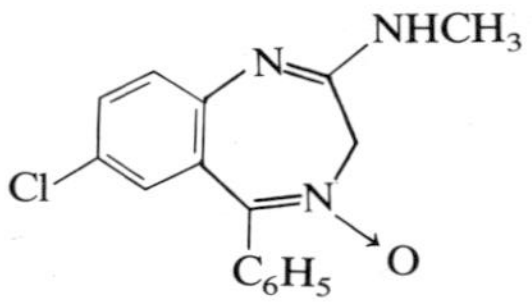				8.0	30	100	2.0	720
Demoxepam	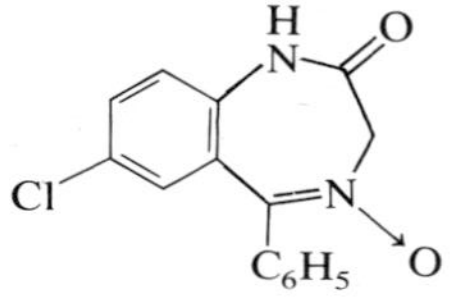				6.1	52	100	5.0	1950

Table 57.2 (Continued)

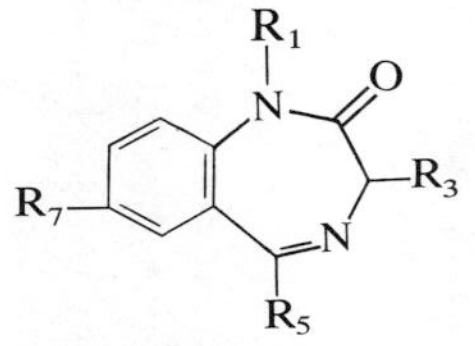

| Compound | R_1 | R_3 | R_5 | R_7 | Median Effective Dose (ED_{50}), mg/kg | | | Cat Behavior MED^b mg/kg | Toxicity (LD_{50}), mg/kg |
| | | | | | Activity Against | | Inclined Screen | | |
					Pentyl-enetetrazole	Maximum Electroshock			
Clorazepate dipotassium	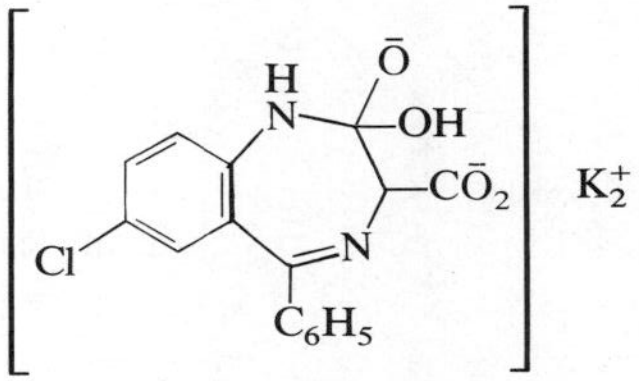				1.7	5.0			700
Medazepam	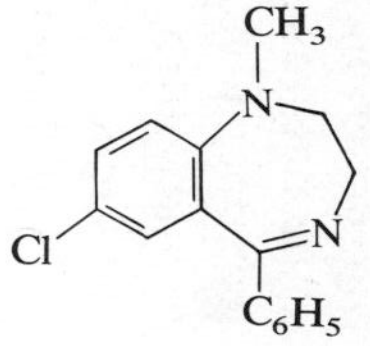				1.6	38	150	4.0	1070
Triazolam	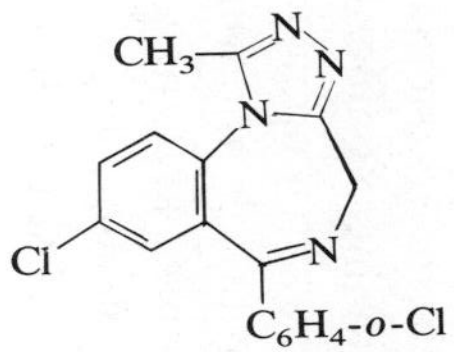				0.07	23			>800 i.p.

[a] Except where indicated the data are for mice treated orally (1, 26–30).
[b] Minimal effective dose.

does not fully reveal the structure–activity requirements.

For the singular compound chlordiazepoxide, there is only a limited number of analogs. The greater importance of the benzodiazepinones is illustrated by the absence from the market of other 2-aminobenzodiazepines. It has been shown, nevertheless, that both the N-methyl group and the 4-oxide function can be removed from chlordiazepoxide with the retention of good activity. The 2-dimethylamino analog is of comparable potency. The 7-chloro substituent may be replaced by other electronegative groups to afford compounds of good activity, and replacement of the 5-phenyl substituent by a 2-heteroaryl group permits retention of some activity. Introduction of a 3-methyl group causes a drop in potency. The compound 2-amino-7-chloro-3-hydroxy-5-phenyl-3H-1,4-benzodiazepine has good activity.

Interest in benzodiazepinones has been greater not only because of their easier synthesis but also because of the metabolic conversion of chlordiazepoxide into benzodiazepinones, principally demoxepam and oxazepam. Generalizations on structural requirements similar to those made about the amino compounds can be given. The paramount importance of the nature of the 7 position is apparent. Electronegative substituents are necessary and nitro and trifluoromethyl groups give highest potencies. Substitution in the 6, 8, or 9 positions reduces activity. An aryl group is required in the 5 position. The prototype 5-phenyl substituent can be replaced by a phenyl group containing an electronegative substituent in the ortho position with an increase in potency. Substitution in both ortho positions also enhances activity. A 2-pyridyl group is effective as shown by bromazepam, but para-substituted phenyl groups greatly lower potency.

The introduction of alkyl groups into the 3 position reduces potency but 3-hydroxy groups afford compounds of comparable potency to that of the nonhydroxy analogs (31). Compounds bearing 3-hydroxy groups are characterized by low toxicity, probably owing to ready conjugation and excretion (32). Esterification of 3-hydroxy groups gives compounds of similar potency. Camazepam is a carbamate ester that is marketed in Europe (33) and it is said to be found unaltered in brain tissue (34). 3-Alkoxy groups as well give compounds of good potency. Although esters of 3-carboxy compounds exhibit considerable activity (28), intermediary metabolism may be involved since the 3-carboxy group of clorazepate dipotassium, for example, is rapidly lost upon acidification to afford nordiazepam.

3-Substitution can give rise to asymmetry. Oxazepam hemisuccinate has been resolved into its enantiomers and the dextrorotatory isomer has been shown to be the more potent enantiomer in the clinic (35). The steric stability of 3-hydroxybenzodiazepinones has not been established, and the different potencies of the isomers may reflect different rates of conversion into oxazepam.

The principal difference between 2-aminobenzodiazepines and benzodiazepinones in terms of structural manipulation lies in the possibility of alkylation of the latter at the 1 position. Methylation frequently results in an increase in potency, but the value of alkylation insofar as potency is concerned is limited to the lower groups. A startling variety of alkyl groups, from vinyl groups (36) to those bearing functional substituents, has been examined with predictably variable results. Among the substituted alkyl groups are cyclopropylmethyl (e.g., prazepam) (37), 2,2,2-trifluoroethyl (e.g., halazepam) (38), and 2-methylsulfonylethyl (39). Many such compounds have found their way to the clinic.

A change of the 2-carbonyl group of benzodiazepinones into a thione is accompanied by a decrease in potency, but in some cases [e.g., 7-chloro-5-(*o*-chloro-phenyl)-1,3-dihydro-1-methyl-2*H*-1,4-ben-zodiazepine-2-thione] the antipentylene-tetrazole potency $(ED_{50} = 0.7 \text{ mg/kg})$ is nevertheless quite high. Replacement of 2-carbonyl groups by methylene groups also affords compounds of high potency. One such compound, medazepam, has been marketed. Oxidation of the 4-nitrogen atom has an erratic effect but is usually deleterious. Saturation of the 4,5 double bond reduces potency, as does a shift of the unsaturation into the 3,4 position.

With the passage of time the simpler transformations of the benzodiazepines have become fully exploited. Although the potential for more complicated changes such as ring bridging was seen rather early, recent work has been concentrated on the fusion of additional rings onto the system or the use of heterocyclic rings to replace the benzo portion. Cloxazolam (57.**5**) is an example of a compound carrying an additional fused ring (40); it is more sedative than diazepam (41). Ripazepam (57.**6**) has the benzo portion of the system replaced by a pyrazole (42). As illustrations of the hazard of extrapolating structure–activity

57.**7**

relationships, alkylation of the amide nitrogen in this series reduces activity, and the *s*-triazolo[4,3-*a*]1,4-benzodiazepines do not require for high activity an electronegative substituent in the position corresponding to the 7 position of benzodiazepines (30).

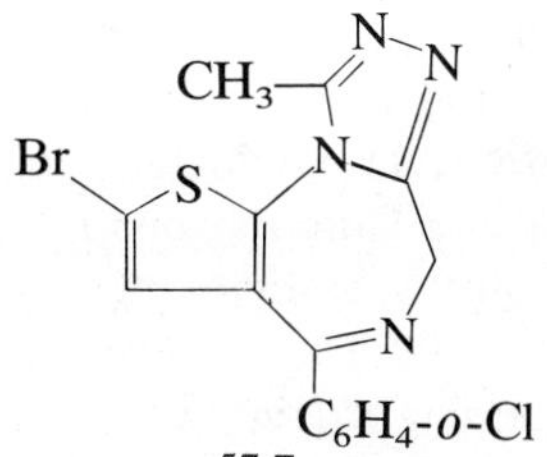

Chemists have begun to fuse rings onto already substantially modified structures, and the preparation of 57.**7** has recently been described (43). Some of the compounds bearing additional fused rings may be considered to be derived from 2-aminobenzodiazepines, e.g., triazolam. Triazolam is marketed as a hypnotic (Chapter 54), but a glance at Table 57.2 shows that its expected antianxiety effects are great. Similar views, of course, obtain for the hypnotics nitrazepam and flurazepam as well as for the anticonvulsant clonazepam.

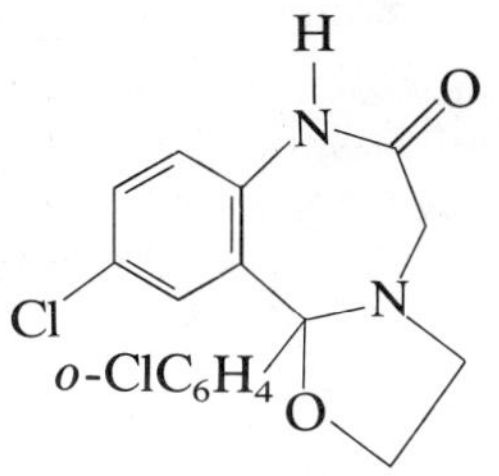

57.**5**

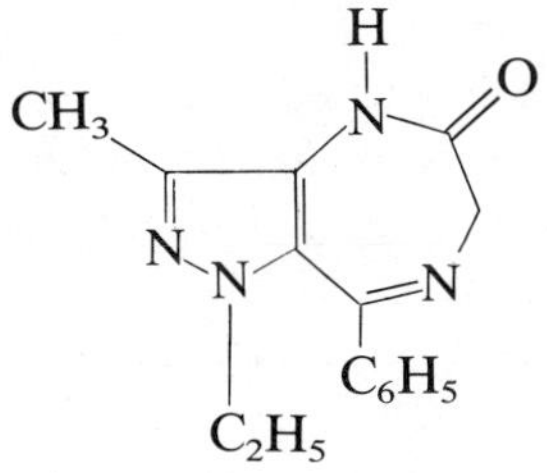

57.**6**

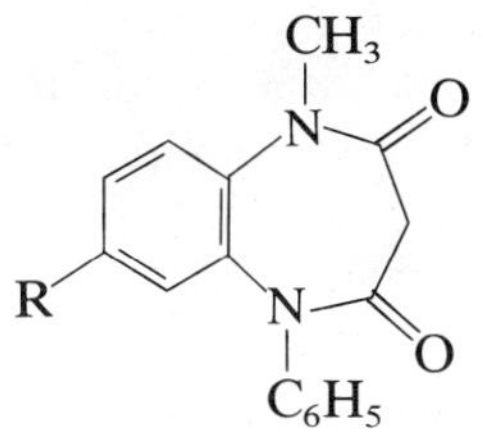

57.**8**   R = Cl
57.**9**   R = CF$_3$

The greatest structural changes that have allowed retention of an antianxiety profile have been made in the preparation of 1,5-benzodiazepinediones. The activity of clobazam (57.**8**) lies between that of chlordiazepoxide and diazepam (44). The compound is marketed and triflubazam (57.**9**) has been studied in the clinic.

An attempt was made to relate the activity of benzodiazepines to the molecular conformation as revealed in crystallographic work. Thus diazepam was seen as having a strong resemblance to diphenylhydantoin (45). The superficial attractiveness of finding a similarity between two anticonvulsants of different chemical types vanished when it was pointed out that dechlorodiazepam was essentially superimposable on diazepam yet was almost inactive (46). It is readily apparent, of course, that the conformation assumed at a receptor is not necessarily that occurring in the crystal.

5.3   Metabolism

The metabolism of the older benzodiazepines (Fig. 57.2) has been extensively studied (47). Because of the close structural relationship of several important compounds there are a number of common metabolites. In man and dog demoxepam (57.**10**), arising from hydrolysis of the 2-methylamino substituent or more probably the 2-amino substituent that results from demethylation, is a metabolite of chlordiazepoxide (57.**11**). It becomes more prominent upon chronic administration. Further metabolism of demoxepam provides a host of excretion products, not all of which are yet identified. Many are conjugates of aromatic hydroxylated products, but 3-hydroxylation with retention of the 2-amino function has not been observed. Demoxepam is in part hydrolyzed to the derivative (57.**12**). Nordiazepam (57.**13**) from reduction of demoxepam has recently been confirmed in man to be a chlordiazepoxide metabolite, thus giving a crossing into the metabolic pathway of diazepam (47a).

Diazepam (57.**14**) is rapidly converted in man and dog to nordiazepam, with the intact drug having a dose-dependent half-life as short as 1 hr (48). Nordiazepam is very persistent—the shortest half-life quoted by various authors is about 2 days; more than 7 days pass before its disappearance from circulating serum. 3-Hydroxylation of diazepam and nordiazepam takes place to afford temazepam (57.**15**) and oxazepam (57.**16**), which are excreted in the urine as glucuronide conjugates. In the rat 4-hydroxylation of the 5-phenyl substituent in diazepam is a major conversion of the intact drug and its other metabolites.

In contrast to nordiazepam the analogous nonmethylated bromazepam (57.**17**) is rapidly 3-hydroxylated and has a half-life of about 12 hr (49). The benzodiazepine ring is extensively opened and the conjugate of 2-(2-amino-3-hydroxy-5-bromobenzoyl)pyridine is the main excretion product in human urine.

Dealkylation at the 1 position of benzodiazepinones is observed in prazepam (57.**18**) and temazepam, but the latter is not extensively demethylated, probably owing in part to its rapid conversion into the conjugate. Oxazepam is also quickly converted into its glucuronide and urinary excretion is substantially complete in this form. The biotransformation half-life in healthy subjects ranges from 3 to 21 hr. Lorazepam is similarly metabolized with a half-life of about 16 hr (50). Medazepam (57.**19**) is both oxidized and demethylated, in either order, to 2-ones (diazepam and nordiazepam).

Metabolism of 1,5-benzodiazepines is characterized by 1-dealkylation and aromatic hydroxylation (51).

The importance of the pharmacological effects of the metabolites of the benzodiazepines in their clinical action is clear, and efforts have been made to relate the antianxiety effects to the observed serum concentrations (52). These attempts have not been very successful. With diazepam the presence of so many active metabolites is a confounding effect, but Dasberg was able to correlate certain anxiety factors with plasma levels following administration of nordiazepam (53). The impossibility of making instantaneous assessments of anxiety and the unpredictable course of anxiety over time make very difficult the task of relating activity to concentrations in the body. It is, after all, the concentration at some CNS site that counts. Thus serum concentrations of diazepam weakly correlated, although those of bromazepam did not correlate, with electroencephalographic measurements (54). In mice, it was possible to relate the brain concentrations of diazepam and nordiazepam respectively following diazepam administration to the duration of

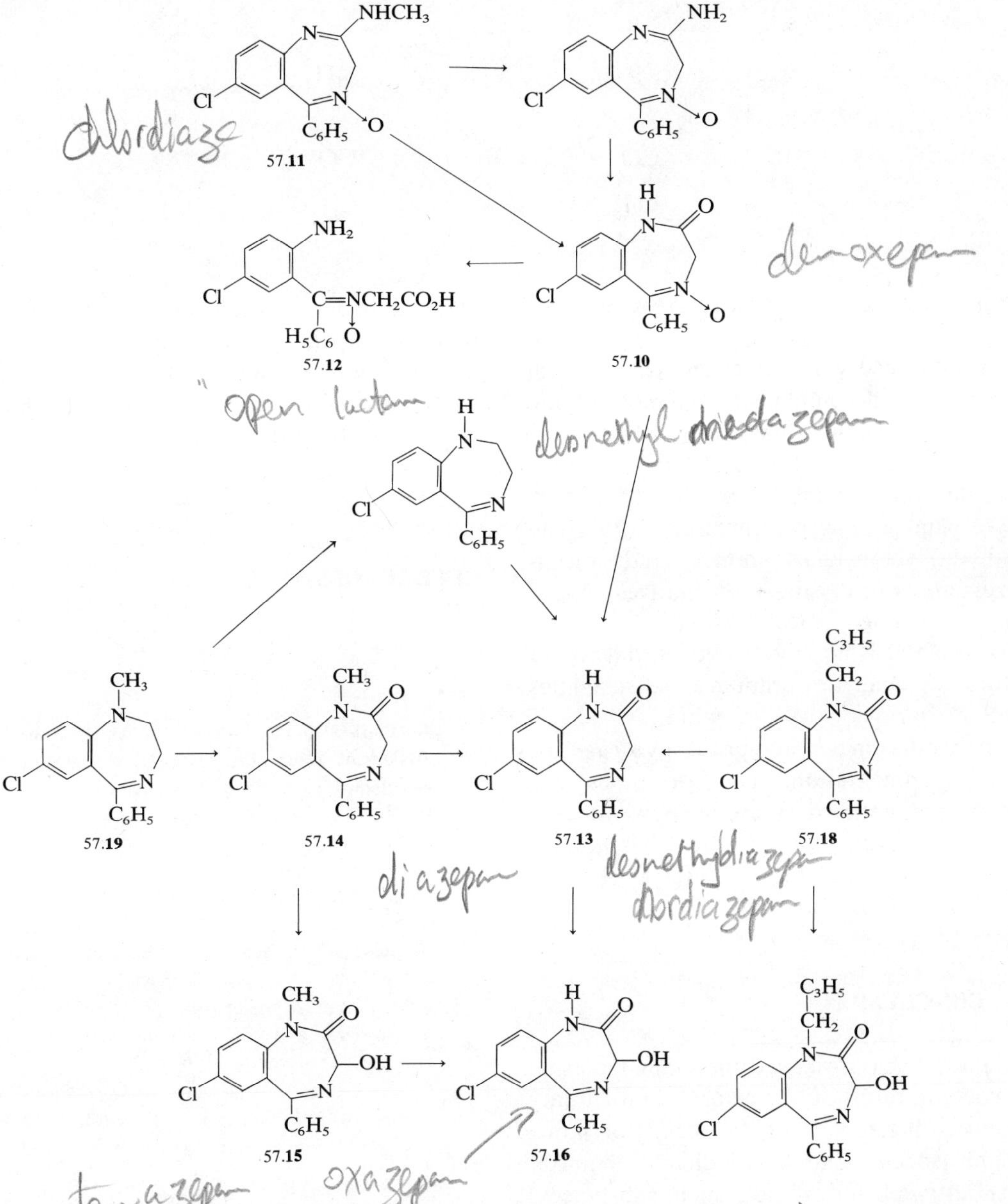

Fig. 57.2 Simplified metabolism of benzodiazepines.

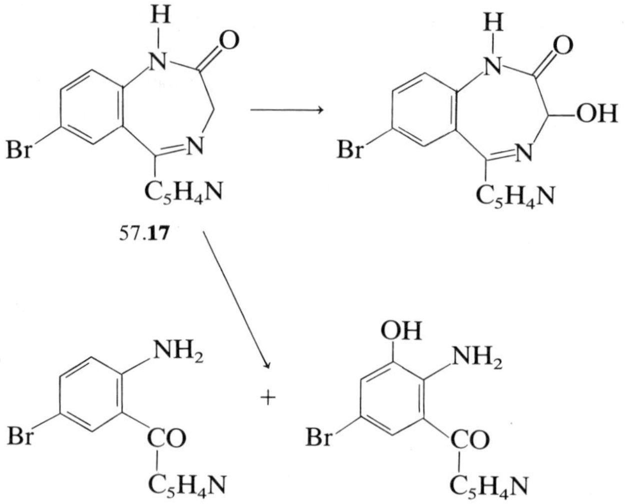

57.**17**

muscle relaxation and antiaggressive activity (55).

The necessity for frequent dosing with agents that accumulate as do most of the benzodiazepinones has been challenged, and once-daily administration of clorazepate dipotassium, a prodrug for nordiazepam, is now recommended (56). The 3-hydroxybenzodiazepinones and bromazepam afford the alternative therapeutic regimen since these drugs do not accumulate. It may be expected that future work will lead to optimum dose schedules for the various benzodiazepines.

Benzodiazepines are primarily drugs for oral administration, and occasions for parenteral antianxiety use are few. Indeed, a stable, water-soluble product has not yet been made available. Future work may provide such a compound.

6 CONCLUSION

Klein (57) has discussed the many facets of anxiety in terms of choice of drug for treatment, which points up the need for more highly specific agents. Medicinal chemists will attempt to provide such substances. Two practical problems obstruct the post-

laboratory development of candidate compounds: (1) the great difficulty in clinical testing, and (2) the regulatory move toward class labeling of compounds, which tends to obtund differences that exist.

REFERENCES

1. S. Edmiston, *Family Health*, **10;** 1, 25 (1978).
2. G. L. Kierman, *Med. World News*, **17;** 23, 26 (1976).
3. A. Padjen and F. Bloom, in *Mechanisms of Action of Benzodiazepines*, E. Costa and P. Greengard, Eds., Raven Press, New York, 1975, p. 93.
4. P. Soubrie, P. Simon, and J. R. Boissier, in *Neuropsychopharmacology, Proceedings IX Congress Collegium Internationale Neuropsychopharmacologicum, Paris, 1974*, J. R. Boissier, H. Hippius, and P. Pichot, Eds., Excerpta Medica, Amsterdam, 1975, p. 720.
5. F. M. Berger, in *Methods in Drug Evaluation*, P. Mantegazza and F. Piccinini, Eds., North-Holland, Amsterdam, 1966, p. 218.
6. L. Cook and J. Sepinwall, in *Mechanisms of Action of Benzodiazepines*, E. Costa and P. Greengard, Eds., Raven Press, New York, 1975, p. 1.
7. I. Geller and J. Seifter, *Psychopharmacologia*, **1,** 482 (1960).

8. D. L. Margules and L. Stein, in *Neuropsychopharmacology, Proceedings V Congress Collegium Internationale Neuropsychopharmacologicum, Washington, 1966,* H. Brill, Ed., Excerpta Medica, Amsterdam, 1967, p. 108.

9. E. H. Uhlenhuth, D. A. Turner, G. Purchatzke, T. Gift, and J. Chassan, *Psychopharmacology,* **52,** 79 (1977).

10. D. B. Smith, *Dis. Nerv. Syst.,* **28,** 455 (1967).

11. M.-L. Hakola and P. Hakola, *Int. J. Neuropsychiatr.,* **3,** 219 (1967).

12. P. Tyrer, *The Role of Bodily Feelings in Anxiety,* Oxford University Press, London, 1976.

13. Anon., *Lancet,* **1976–II,** 611.

14. B. J. Ludwig and J. R. Potterfield, *Advan. Pharmacol. Chemother.,* **9,** 173 (1971).

15. L. S. Schlan and K. R. Unna, *J. Am. Med. Assoc.,* **140,** 672 (1949).

16. B. J. Ludwig, L. S. Powell, and F. M. Berger, *J. Med. Chem.,* **12,** 462 (1969).

17. F. M. Berger, M. Kletzkin, and S. Margolin, *Med. Exp.,* **10,** 327 (1964).

18. G. Stille, *Arzneim.-Forsch.,* **12,** 340 (1962).

19. B. Melander, *J. Med. Pharm. Chem.,* **1,** 443 (1959).

20. R. M. Gesler and A. R. Surrey, *J. Pharmacol. Exp. Ther.,* **122,** 517 (1958).

21. F. Schatz and U. Jahn, *Arzneim.-Forsch.,* **16,** 866 (1966).

22. E. W. McChesney, W. F. Banks, Jr., G. A. Portmann, and A. V. R. Crain, *Biochem. Pharmacol.,* **16,** 813 (1967).

23. W. F. Haefely, *Agents Action,* **7,** 353 (1977).

24. R. F. Squires and C. Braestrup, *Nature,* **266,** 732 (1977).

25. J. F. Tallman, J. W. Thomas, and D. W. Gallagher, *Nature,* **274,** 383 (1978).

25a. S. M. Paul and P. Skolnick, *Science,* **202,** 892 (1978).

25b. P. J. Marangos, S. M. Paul, P. Greenlaw, F. K. Goodwin, and P. Skolnick, *Life Sci.,* **22,** 1893 (1978).

25c. M. Karobath, G. Sperk, and G. Schönbeck, *Eur. J. Pharmacol.,* **49,** 323 (1978).

25d. A. Guidotti, G. Toffano, and E. Costa, *Nature,* **275,** 553 (1978).

26. L. H. Sternbach, in *The Benzodiazepines,* S. Garattini, E. Mussini, and L. D. Randall, Eds., Raven Press, New York, 1973, p. 1.

27. S. J. Childress and M. I. Gluckman, *J. Pharm. Sci.,* **53,** 577 (1964).

28. S. C. Bell, R. J. McCaully, C. Gochman, S. J. Childress, and M. I. Gluckman, *J. Med. Chem.,* **11,** 457 (1968).

29. P. Duchene-Marullaz, C. Lakatos, F. De Marchi, and M. V. Torrielli, *Farm. Ed. Prat.,* **22,** 506 (1967).

30. A. D. Rudzik, J. B. Hester, A. H. Tang, R. N. Straw, and W. Friis, in *The Benzodiazepines,* S. Garattini, E. Mussini, and L. O. Randall, Eds., Raven Press, New York, 1973, p. 285.

31. S. C. Bell and S. J. Childress, *J. Org. Chem.,* **27,** 1691 (1962).

32. M. Wretlind, Å. Pilbraat, A. Sunderwall, and J. Vessman, *Acta Pharmacol. Toxicol.,* **40,** Suppl. I, 28 (1977).

33. R. Ferrini, G. Miragoli, and B. Taccardi, *Arzneim.-Forsch.,* **24,** 2029 (1974).

34. M. Cesa-Bianchi, P. Ghirardi, and F. Ravaccia, *Arzneim.-Forsch.,* **24,** 2032 (1974).

35. M. Lescovelli, A. Castellani, and D. Perbellini, *Arzneim.-Forsch.,* **26,** 1623 (1976).

36. A. Walser and R. I. Fryer, *J. Med. Chem.,* **17,** 1228 (1974).

37. R. C. Robichaud, J. A. Gylys, K. L. Sledge, and I. W. Hillyard, *Arch. Int. Pharmacodyn. Ther.,* **185,** 213 (1970).

38. M. Steinman, J. G. Topliss, R. Alekel, Y.-S. Wong, and E. E. York, *J. Med. Chem.,* **16,** 1354 (1973).

39. Y. Asami, M. Otsuka, M. Akatsu, S. Kitagawa, S. Inaba, and H. Yamamoto, *Arzneim.-Forsch.,* **25,** 534 (1975).

40. T. Kamioka, H. Takagi, S. Kobayashi, and Y. Suzuki, *Arzneim.-Forsch.,* **22,** 884 (1972).

41. B. Saletu, M. Matejcek, K. Knor, U. Ferner, and U. Schneewind, *Curr. Ther. Res. Clin. Exp.,* **20,** 510 (1976).

42. H. A. DeWald, I. C. Nordin, Y. J. L'Italien, and R. F. Parcell, *J. Med. Chem.,* **16,** 1346 (1973).

43. C. H. Boehringer Sohn, Ger. Pat. 2,533,924 (1978).

44. K. Sandler, D. Brunswick, J. Digiacomo, and J. Mendels, *Curr. Ther. Res. Clin. Exp.,* **21,** 114 (1977).

45. A. Camerman and N. Camerman, *Science,* **168,** 1457 (1970).

46. L. H. Sternbach, F. D. Sancilio, and J. F. Blount, *J. Med. Chem.,* **17,** 374 (1974).

47. D. J. Greenblatt and R. I. Shader, *Benzodiazepines in Clinical Practice,* Raven Press, New York, 1974.

47a. R. Dixon, M. A. Brooks, E. Postma, M. R. Hackman, S. Spector, J. D. Moore, and M. A.

Schwartz, *Clin. Pharmacol. Ther.*, **20,** 450 (1976).

48. M. A. Schwartz, B. A. Koechlin, E. Postma, S. Palmer, and G. Krol, *J. Pharmacol. Exp. Ther.*, **149,** 423 (1965).

49. S. A. Kaplan, M. L. Jack, R. E. Weinfeld, W. Glover, L. Weissman, and S. Cotler, *J. Pharmacokinet. Biopharm.*, **4,** 1 (1976).

50. D. J. Greenblatt, R. T. Schillings, A. A. Kyriakopoulos, R. I. Shader, S. F. Sisenwine, J. A. Knowles, and H. W. Ruelius, *Clin. Pharmacol. Ther.*, **20,** 329 (1976).

51. K. B. Alton, R. M. Grimes, C. Shaw, J. E. Patrick, and J. L. McGuire, *Drug Metab. Dispos.*, **3,** 352 (1975).

52. R. C. Smith, H. Dekirmenjian, J. Davis, R. Casper, L. Gosenfeld, and C. Tsai, in *Pharmacokinetics of Psychoactive Drugs: Blood Levels and Clinical Response*, L. A. Gottschalk and S. Merlis, Eds., Spectrum Publications, New York, 1976, p. 141.

53. H. H. Dasberg, *Psychopharmacologia*, **43,** 191 (1975).

54. M. Fink, P. Irwin, R. E. Weinfeld, M. A. Schwartz, and A. H. Conney, *Clin. Pharmacol. Ther.*, **20,** 184 (1976).

55. S. Garattini, E. Mussini, F. Marcucci, and A. Guaitani, in *The Benzodiazepines*, S. Garattini, E. Mussini, and L. O. Randall, Eds., Raven Press, New York, 1973, p. 75.

56. P. J. Carrigan, G. C. Chao, W. M. Barker, D. J. Hoffman, and A. H. C. Chun, *J. Clin. Pharmacol.*, **17,** 18 (1977).

57. D. F. Klein, in *Drug Treatment of Mental Disorders*, L. L. Simpson, Ed., Raven Press, New York, 1976, p. 61.

CHAPTER FIFTY-EIGHT

Antidepressant Agents

CARL KAISER

and

PAULETTE E. SETLER

Research and Development Division
Smith Kline & French Laboratories
1500 Spring Garden Street
Philadelphia, Pennsylvania 19101, USA

CONTENTS

997

1   INTRODUCTION

Depression is an occasional component of daily life, but it may also be a symptom of primary affective illness. Descriptions of depression are found even in ancient literature; physicians as early as Galen associated melancholy with brain function. Until recently, however, treatment of depression was only supportive, limited largely to treatment of the accompanying sleeplessness, removing the patient from an unsympathetic environment, and isolation of suicidal cases. Twentieth-century advances in therapy began with the use of psychoanalytic techniques and electroconvulsion therapy. The modern era in the treatment of depression began with the introduction of antidepressant drugs in the late 1950's. These were the monoamine oxidase (MAO) inhibitors and the tricyclic antidepressants.

The first of the MAO inhibitors was iproniazid (58.**1**; see Section 4.1.1). During clinical studies of iproniazid as an antituberculosis agent a mood-elevating effect was observed. The significance of this observation was not apparent. In 1952 Zeller et al. (1) discovered that iproniazid was a potent inhibitor of MAO, and subsequently observed that iproniazid potentiated certain pharmacological effects of some sympathomimetic amines (2, 3). It was found to elevate amine levels in the brain and to prevent the reduction of amine levels induced by reserpine. Brodie and Shore (1957) (4) showed that iproniazid, especially in conjunction with reserpine, could cause excitement in animals. Based on these observations Kline and co-workers (5) tested iproniazid in depressed patients with favorable results.

Because of serious side effects associated with iproniazid and other hydrazine derivatives, a widespread search for less toxic MAO inhibitors extended to nonhydrazine compounds such as tranylcypromine (see Section 4.1.2.4).

The first of the tricyclic antidepressants was imipramine (58.**2**; see Section 4.2.1), which is a member of a group of aminoalkyl derivatives of iminodibenzyl synthesized by Häfliger and Schindler (6) in 1951 as potential antihistaminics, sedatives, analgetics, or antiparkinsonism agents. During clinical studies of a few of the dibenzazepine derivatives, Kuhn in 1957 (7) observed that imipramine appeared to be of specific therapeutic value in the treatment of depressive states. Since the discovery of imipramine, many related compounds have been developed and are employed in the treatment of depression.

More recently, newer antidepressants have been developed, many of which differ

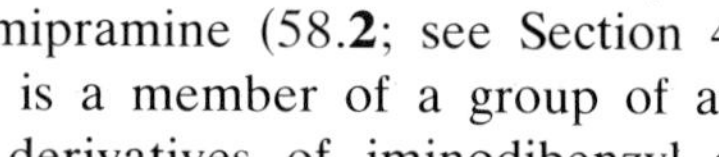

$CONHNHCH(CH_3)_2$

58.**1**

$(CH_2)_3N(CH_3)_2$

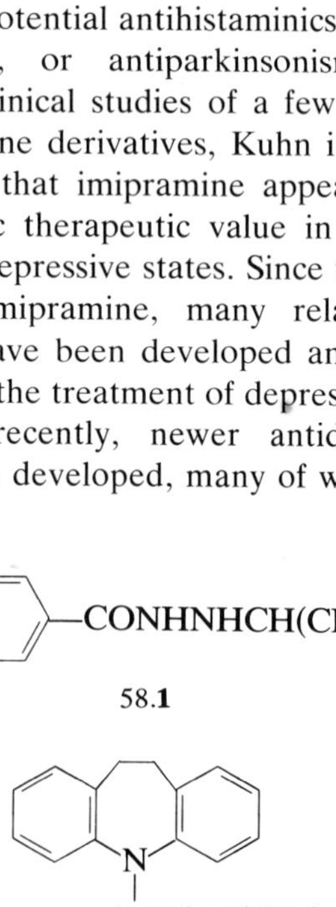

58.**2**

chemically and/or in biological activity from the original group of imipramine-like tricyclic antidepressants.

2 CLINICAL ASPECTS

2.1 Depression

Depression is a normal response to loss and disappointment; it is a sadness which, though possibly intense, is usually of relatively brief duration. Depression is also a prominent feature of several clinical syndromes classified as mood disorders or affective disorders.

Affective disorders include unipolar depressive illness, unipolar manic disorder, and bipolar affective disorder. Bipolar affective disorder is a recurrent depression with manic or hypomanic phases. Unipolar depressive disorders are usually subdivided into endogenous or vital depression and reactive or psychoneurotic depression. The latter usually responds poorly to pharmacotherapy (8).

Endogenous depression, whether unipolar or bipolar, has as its dominant feature intense sadness or despondency. This dysphoric state is usually accompanied by a loss of interest, inability to feel pleasure, and feelings of inadequacy, worthlessness, and guilt. Psychomotor retardation or agitation are usually present, as are somatic disturbances (9). The most characteristic somatic feature of endogenous depression is sleep disturbance, with early morning wakening and inability to return to sleep. Anorexia and weight loss are common, as is disproportionate fatigue. Another common and difficult feature is thoughts of death and suicide. This constellation of signs and symptoms results in at least temporary disruption of the patient's life. As expressed by Lehmann (10), depressed patients may be characterized by their inability to be productive, to enjoy, to love.

Unipolar and bipolar illnesses are apparently discrete entities with distinct genetic predisposition (11), differences in age of onset, duration of symptom-free periods, and premorbid history (12).

Several lines of evidence point to the possibility that unipolar depression may itself be a heterogeneous group of disease states, "... several discrete psychiatric illnesses that share a common core pathological phenomenon—the depressive mood" (8, p. 174). Unfortunately, there are, as yet no adequate means to distinguish these discrete subgroups, nor is the underlying biochemical pathophysiology known for any.

The heterogeneity of depressive states poses a serious problem for those interested in pharmacotherapy for depression. The importance of differentiating among types of depressive syndromes when choosing treatment was pointed out by Kuhn (13) in one of his original reports of the therapeutic efficacy of imipramine.

The combined forces of biologic psychiatry and clinical pharmacology have attempted two approaches to the problem. One approach is the monitoring of biologic variables in depressed patients to search for biochemical abnormalities. An understanding of the underlying pathophysiology of depressive illnesses would increase the possibility of designing therapeutic agents to selectively compensate for the biologic deficit. Conversely, the second approach attempts to understand the mechanisms of action of drugs which are effective in the treatment of depression in order to find the key to the biochemical/physiological basis of depressive illness. To a large extent both approaches have concentrated on the biogenic monoamines in the central nervous system and the catecholamine hypothesis of affective disorders.

The catecholamine hypothesis, in its simplest form, proposes that "... some, if not all, depressions are associated with an absolute or relative deficiency of catecholamines, particularly norepinephrine, at functionally important adrenergic receptor sites in the brain. Elation, conversely, may be associated with an excess of such amines" (14, p. 509). The foundation on which this theory of depression rested was the observation that (1) reserpine, which reduces the catecholamine content of the central nervous system, produces behavioral depression in animals and was shown in a study by Harris (15) to cause depression in a significant number of patients taking reserpine for hypertension; and (2) the MAO inhibitor iproniazid, which increases brain monoamine levels, blocks reserpine-induced depression in animals and alleviates depression in man. Also consistent with the catecholamine hypothesis was the subsequent finding that the tricyclic antidepressants inhibit the uptake of norepinephrine into neurons, thus impairing the degradation of norepinephrine and potentiating its effect. The drugs whose actions provided the basis for the catecholamine hypothesis of depression are not, however, without effect on other neurotransmitter systems in the brain. Reserpine depletes the brain of serotonin and dopamine as well as norepinephrine, and tricyclic antidepressants, which have little effect on dopamine uptake, do inhibit the uptake of serotonin, although to a lesser extent than that of norepinephrine. Consideration of these factors led to modifications of the original hypothesis to include a primary or contributory role for a serotonin deficit in the etiology of depression (16, 17).

Since the initial formulation of the catecholamine hypothesis of affective disorders, psychiatric investigators have attempted to find the absolute or relative deficiency of monoamines predicted in the brains of depressed patients. This is obviously a nearly impossible task. Biologic psychiatry has necessarily relied on indirect measures of central monoamine function, such as urinary excretion of catecholamine metabolites, levels of amine metabolites in cerebrospinal fluid, and content of

monoamines in postmortem brain tissue from depressed patients, especially suicides. Alterations in monoamine metabolism have been described, but these controversial differences have not convincingly characterized any depressive condition (17–22). Paradoxically, when alterations in amine metabolism were demonstrated, the apparent changes were not reversed by treatment, but were often exacerbated; treatments effective in depression tended to alter amine metabolism in the manner hypothesized to be an indication of the disease state (23).

Although many years of research have elapsed since the initial formulation of the monoamine hypothesis of depression, it remains an intriguing hypothesis, of heuristic value, neither proved nor disproved, nor supplanted by any more promising theory. The biochemical substrate(s) of depression(s) has remained elusive and we are as yet unable to select or design pharmacotherapy for depression on other than empirical or hypothetical grounds.

2.2 Treatment of Depression

In many patients, especially those hospitalized for neurotic or reactive depression, depression is a self-limiting disorder with a high rate of response to placebo (24, 25). Endogenous unipolar depression is, however, a clear indication for antidepressant drug therapy (8, 26) and successful treatment can be achieved in 70–80% of the patients (27, 28). Patients with bipolar affective disorder are frequently treated with lithium and an antidepressant drug. Patients with reactive or neurotic depression may respond to antidepressant drugs, but psychotherapy is usually especially beneficial in neurotic depression (26, 28). Antidepressants may be given in combination with antipsychotics in psychotic depression.

Among the antidepressant drugs, the MAO inhibitors are generally reserved for those patients who fail to respond to other drug therapy and in cases of high suicide risk. It has been reported that MAO inhibitors are also particularly effective in treating phobic anxiety (26, 29). Because of the relatively high risk of serious side effects, MAO inhibitors must be used with caution and the patients must be carefully instructed and monitored.

The response to the tricyclic antidepressant drugs is often fairly slow; therapeutic effects may not be seen for 1–4 weeks (8, 26). After amelioration of depressive symptoms, maintenance doses of antidepressants are required for a variable period depending on the past history of recurrence of depression. Continuation studies show that in patients on maintenance therapy, there is a lower frequency of recurrence (30).

Electroshock therapy may be used to obtain a rapid effect in cases of high suicide risk or after failure of drug therapy, or concomitantly with antidepressant drugs. The use of electroshock therapy is controversial. Electroconvulsive shock has been shown to be as effective as antidepressant drugs and the effect is more rapid in onset. The relapse rate, however, is high in patients treated with electroshock and therefore maintenance drug therapy is usually advised (8). Electroshock has many disadvantages, including production of temporary confusion and amnesia. The possibility of subtle long-term damage also exists.

2.3   Side Effects and Adverse Reactions

The use of MAO inhibitors mainly as drugs of last resort is due to the risk of hypertensive crisis and hepatotoxicity. The latter is a problem associated with the hydrazine drugs and may not be related to MAO. Hypertension brought on in patients taking MAO inhibitors by ingestion of foods, beverages, or drugs containing pressor amines is related to MAO inhibition. Degradation of the pressor amines by MAO is blocked in these patients, and severe and occasion-

ally fatal hypertensive crises may occur. Patients and families of patients taking MAO inhibitors must be instructed about the potential dangers of cheeses and other foods that are incompatible with MAO inhibitors. Hypertensive crises may also result from combination of MAO inhibitors with drug preparations containing pressor amines or their precursors and from combination of MAO inhibitors with tricyclic antidepressants which inhibit amine uptake. An adequate washout period is required before patients are switched from MAO inhibitors to other types of antidepressants or vice versa.

At therapeutic doses imipramine-like tricyclic antidepressants produce a number of autonomic side effects as a result of muscarinic receptor antagonism and norepinephrine potentiation. Most common among these are dry mouth, blurred vision, constipation, and tachycardia or palpitations. Postural hypotension, ECG abnormalities, urinary retention, and paralytic ileus are less common but of greater concern. Development of some tolerance to autonomic effects is not uncommon. Central effects include sedation, which may be desirable in agitated patients, if not in others, and central anticholinergic effects such as confusion and delirium. High doses may sometimes produce grand mal seizures. Hypomanic states such as schizophrenic excitement may be induced in bipolar or psychotic depressed patients. Jaundice or agranulocytosis may be seen in a small number of patients.

Although tricyclic antidepressants are not contraindicated in patients with cardiac disease, they should be employed cautiously in these patients. Tricyclic antidepressants often cause nonspecific T wave changes. Patients receiving high doses may also show prolongation of the PR interval and widening of the QRS complex (31). Cardiac effects may be fatal in cases of overdosage (32, 33). Reports of sudden death in patients with cardiac disease taking tricyclic antidepressants emphasize the need for surveillance of cardiac patients (32, 33).

Overdosage with tricyclic antidepressants can be fatal and provides a potential means of suicide in severely depressed patients.

2.4 Absorption, Metabolism, and Plasma Levels

The tricyclic antidepressants are readily absorbed from the gastrointestinal tract and are widely distributed in tissues. Highest concentrations are generally found in the lungs and liver (34–36). Autoradiographic examination of the distribution of several tricyclic antidepressants in cat and mouse brain reveals similar distribution patterns. Only low levels remain in the brain after 4 hr (37). Most of the dose of a tricyclic antidepressant is excreted as metabolic products in the urine (34–36, 38–40).

Metabolism of imipramine involves mainly *N*-demethylation, *N*-oxidation, aromatic ring hydroxylation, and conjugation of the resulting hydroxyl derivatives with glucuronic acid. Hydroxylation of the central ring also appears to occur (34, 35, 38, 39, 41, 42). Metabolism of other tricyclic antidepressants seems to follow a very similar path (36, 40).

As a result of the chemical diversity of nontricyclic inhibitors of brain uptake of biogenic amines no generalization relative to their metabolic fate is possible. It does not appear that metabolism is an important factor for the biological action of these substances.

Some inhibitors of MAO are inactive *in vitro* and owe their *in vivo* activity to biotransformation products (see Section 4.1.1); however, in most instances metabolic products are not implicated in the action of these compounds. Information concerning the metabolism of some drugs of this class has been compiled in reviews of MAO inhibitors (43–45).

Among the commonly used tricyclic antidepressants there is a marked interpatient variability in response to a fixed dose. There is also considerable variation in steady-state plasma levels of drug in patients taking the same dose. The relationship between clinical response and plasma level of drug is a matter of controversy and concern as is the relationship between plasma level of drug and incidence of side effects.

Although some studies have shown that plasma level and clinical response are highly correlated (46, 47), others found no correlation (48), and still others detected a U-shaped relationship between plasma level and response with poor response at lowest and highest plasma levels (49, 50). In general, however, patients with unusually low plasma levels failed to show favorable clinical response to drug. Rapid metabolism in some patients may underlie drug failure (47). In most studies there was little correlation between plasma level of drug and side effects, which led to speculations that many subjective side effects were not, in fact, drug related.

The secondary amine metabolites of tricyclic antidepressants are also effective. They are highly but variably bound to plasma protein (51). In addition to variability in plasma levels of drug among patients taking a fixed dose, there is also a wide variation in the ratio of tertiary to secondary amine. Also, the ratio of tertiary to secondary amine in cerebrospinal fluid may differ from that in plasma (52), although in general, the levels of drug in plasma and cerebrospinal fluid are highly correlated.

3 BIOLOGIC ACTIONS

3.1 Pharmacological and Biochemical Effects: Mechanism of Action

3.1.1 MAO INHIBITORS. MAO inhibitors presumably act by inhibiting the enzyme, MAO, that deaminates the catecholamines and serotonin. As a consequence, these transmitter amines accumulate in nerve terminals, and the degradation of synaptically released transmitter is probably retarded, thus effecting an enhancement of, or prolongation of, the postsynaptic event. The evidence supporting this mechanism includes the observation that clinically effective MAO inhibitors do significantly reduce MAO activity in the human brain. Data also show that patients treated with MAO inhibitors have elevated levels of brain monoamines and that the time of maximum elevation after the onset of treatment approximates the time of onset of the antidepressant effect (53). MAO inhibitors also inhibit the uptake of norepinephrine, but the extent to which this contributes to the clinical effect is not known (54, 55).

Recently, multiple forms of MAO have been identified *in vitro* and *in vivo*. These enzymes, which have been divided into two classes, A and B, are localized in specific tissues, have preferred substrates, and may be differentially affected by drugs. MAO inhibitory antidepressants, however, are mainly nonspecific inhibitors; they inhibit both A and B types of MAO (56).

3.1.2 IMIPRAMINE-LIKE DRUGS. Imipramine-like tricyclic antidepressants, which include desipramine, amitryptyline, nortriptyline, protriptyline chlorimipramine, and doxepin (see Sections 4.2.1 and 4.2.2), as well as imipramine itself, block the accumulation of norepinephrine into synaptosomes (57) and brain slices (58) *in vitro* and into whole brain *in vivo* (59). Secondary amines are more potent than tertiary amines, whereas tertiary amines are more effective inhibitors of serotonin accumulation. This reduction of monoamine accumulation is primarily a reflection of inhibition of the uptake mechanism of the neuronal membrane, but, at least *in vitro*, most of these agents also cause release of stored neurotransmitter from the nerve terminals (58). Imipramine-like drugs also block the uptake of norepinephrine and serotonin into platelets.

The turnover of norepinephrine and serotonin is reduced after acute administration of imipramine-like drugs, (60, 61). After chronic administration of drug, which more closely resembles the clinical situation, the turnover of norepinephrine tends to increase (62).

The imipramine-like drugs produce few overt effects in animals at nontoxic doses, but do interact at low doses with monoamines and with drugs that affect monoamines. In the brain, imipramine-like drugs enhance the effects of exogenously applied norepinephrine and of synaptically released norepinephrine (63). These tricyclics also potentiate the pressor effect of exogenous norepinephrine. Imipramine-like drugs reverse the behavioral and autonomic effects of reserpine, tetrabenazine, and other short-term monoamine-depleting drugs. They also reduce the long-term depletion of norepinephrine by 6-hydroxydopamine; serotonin uptake inhibitors in this group reduce the long-term depletion of brain serotonin by drugs such as fenfluramine or *p*-chloroamphetamine (64) (see Section 4.3.1). Imipramine-like drugs enhance the behavioral effects of amphetamine, apomorphine, and L-dopa. Amphetamine enhancement may be due, wholly or in part, to inhibition of amphetamine metabolism rather than an effect on catecholamines (65).

The imipramine-like drugs, especially the secondary amines, have cholinolytic actions which can be considered the cause of many of the side effects in depressed patients. Whether central antimuscarinic activity contributes to the therapeutic effect is unknown.

Fluotracen (see Section 4.2.4) is an effective antidepressant similar to the imipramine-like drugs in structure and in some animal tests, such as reserpine antagonism, that predict antidepressant activity. It differs from imipramine-like drugs in that it is also an effective dopamine receptor antagonist *in vivo* and *in vitro* (66).

3.1.3 OTHER ANTIDEPRESSANTS. Newer antidepressants and potential antidepressants have been developed that have pharmacological and biochemical effects that differ from those discussed above. Drugs have been developed that are relatively selective inhibitors of the uptake of norepinephrine or of serotonin. At least two relatively selective norepinephrine uptake inhibitors, viloxazine (Section 4.3.2) and maprotiline (Section 4.2.4), have shown clinical efficacy (67, 68), whereas most of the selective inhibitors of serotonin uptake are still in the early stages of clinical trial and early results are equivocal (69, 70).

Nomifensine (see Section 4.2.6), a clinically effective antidepressant, differs from the imipramine-type drugs in that it is an effective inhibitor of dopamine uptake as well as norepinephrine uptake but has little effect on serotonin. Nomifensine produces overt amphetamine-like effects in animals (71).

Mianserin (Section 4.2.3) and danitracen (Section 4.2.4) are two examples of clinically effective antidepressants which are exceptionally weak inhibitors of amine uptake and whose clinical effectiveness cannot be ascribed to this traditional mechanism. Both compounds are potent antagonists of serotonin and histamine and one or both of these actions may be related to clinical activity (72, 73). A recent report indicates that amitriptyline and nortriptyline also have significant serotonin receptor blocking activity which may contribute to their clinical actions (74). In addition to effects on serotonin and histamine, mianserin increases the release of norepinephrine induced by field stimulation and antagonizes the reduction of norepinephrine release by clonidine, suggesting that mianserin may block presynaptic α-receptors (75). Block of presynaptic α-receptors could lead to enhanced noradrenergic function analogous to that which presumably results from uptake inhibition.

Iprindole (see Section 4.2.5) is another type of clinically active antidepressant that does not inhibit the uptake of monoamines *in vivo* or *in vitro* (76, 77). Iprindole is a weak antagonist of reserpine (77), and although it does potentiate the effects of amphetamine it does so by prevention of hydroxylation of amphetamine (78). Chronic administration of iprindole reduces the sensitivity of the norepinephrine receptor-coupled adenylate cyclase in the forebrain, a property shared by chronic administration of desmethylimipramine, imipramine, chlorpromazine, some MAO inhibitors, and electroconvulsive shock. This property has been suggested as the mechanism of the antidepressant effect of iprindole and perhaps other antidepressants (79).

The emergence of many new antidepressants with differing profiles of biochemical and behavioral activity makes it increasingly difficult to determine which effects are correlated with clinical activity. In addition to the effects described above for the various antidepressants, a large group of antidepressants as well as other psychoactive drugs inhibit a histamine-sensitive adenylate cyclase from guinea pig hippocampus (80, 81). Selected tricyclic antidepressants, both secondary and tertiary amines, were even more potent inhibitors of histamine-sensitive guanylate cyclase from mouse neuroblastoma cells than of histamine-sensitive adenylate cyclase (82). These interesting data point to the diversity of the biochemical effects of the antidepressants.

3.2 Test Procedures

MAO inhibition is usually measured *in vitro*. Brain or liver homogenates may be used as the enzyme source. The amount of enzymatic degradation of substrate is determined in the presence and absence of the inhibitor. *In vivo*, the accumulation of monoamines and deaminated metabolites is measured after systemic administration of drug. Pharmacological tests for assessing MAO inhibition are reserpine reversal and tryptamine-potentiation tests. The latter measures the ability of a compound to potentiate the convulsant action of tryptamine, a substrate for MAO.

Imipramine-like drugs may be identified by their ability to block uptake of norepinephrine and/or serotonin *in vitro* using brain slices or homogenates, as discussed above. Pharmacological procedures used to identify imipramine-like activity are antireserpine activity in rodents, potentiation of the behavioral effects of amphetamine, and potentiation of hyperthermia induced by sympathomimetics (34, 35, 83). The most frequently used tests are those in which compounds are tested for their ability to prevent or reverse the behavioral effects of reserpine, tetrabenazine, and other short-term depletors of monoamines.

Since many of the newer antidepressants are inactive in these traditional tests for imipramine-like compounds, there has been a search for test procedures that will identify all antidepressant drugs irrespective of mechanism of action. At the same time, interest has developed in creating animal models of depression in which to study drug effects; models such as separation despair and induced behavioral helplessness have been recommended (84), but whether antidepressants reverse the "depression" in these tests has not been studied. The one such test in which a number of antidepressants are active is that of Porsolt et al. (85), in which rats are placed in individual containers of water, in which they fairly quickly assume a quiet, floating, balancing posture. This period of immobility is referred to, perhaps incorrectly, as behavioral despair. Clinically active antidepressants of several types, at fairly high doses, shorten

the "despair" period. Whether this test has predictive value for identifying new antidepressants is not known. The same is true for antagonism of histamine-sensitive cyclases, antagonism of serotonin, and reduction of the sensitivity of norepinephrine receptor-coupled adenylate cyclase.

4 EFFECT OF CHEMICAL STRUCTURE ON ANTIDEPRESSANT ACTIVITY

In this section, the relationship between chemical structure and antidepressant potency is considered for various classes of antidepressant agents. Although the subject of numerous studies, the precise structural requirements for MAO inhibitors with antidepressant activity have not been defined. Many different chemical classes are potent inhibitors, with varying degrees of selectivity for the different forms of MAO. A similar situation exists with other antidepressants with imipramine-like activity. Especially during the past decade, a number of chemical classes having profiles of pharmacological and biochemical activities resembling those of imipramine have been described. In these classes, too, structural requirements for antidepressant activity are very difficult to define. Even within the various chemical classes, which are themselves difficult to categorize, as will be appreciated by the very arbitrary classification employed in this section, differences in activity are frequently noted. For example, compounds within a chemically related group may show differences in selectivity as inhibitors of uptake of biogenic amines, e.g., norepinephrine, serotonin, and dopamine. The problem is further confused by the clinical antidepressant activity of a few compounds that do not appear to act by an MAO-inhibitory or imipramine-like mechanism. Clinical observation and quantitative pharmaco-EEG have uncovered several compounds of this kind that are not predicted by pharmacological tests (86).

As a result of the difficulties in classifying antidepressants either by a precise mechanism or chemical classification, in considering the influence of chemical structure on antidepressant activity, those agents that appear to act by inhibiting MAO are described first. All remaining antidepressants, which may act by a variety of other mechanisms, are described according to a somewhat arbitrary classification according to chemical structure.

4.1 Inhibitors of Monoamine Oxidase

Although inhibitors of MAO have been used for the treatment of depression for about 25 years, their precise mechanism of action is still not established with certainty. Presumably, these compounds act by inhibiting the MAO-catalyzed oxidation of neurotransmitter amines. The resulting increased levels of norepinephrine, serotonin, or dopamine may underlie the antidepressant effects. Interest in these agents has declined because of concomitant side effects and drug interactions. Nevertheless, this class of antidepressants may represent a preferred therapy for certain depressed patients (87, 88). Advances in our knowledge of MAO justify a reevaluation of its inhibitors as drugs (89). Multiple forms of the enzyme are established (90, 91). Although the arbitrary designation of A and B forms probably is an oversimplification, it is useful in considering substrate and inhibitor selectivity. Neurotransmitter monoamines, e.g., norepinephrine, dopamine, and serotonin, are deaminated mainly by type A MAO (92). Phenethylamine and benzylamine are deaminated mainly by type B MAO (93). Tyramine and tryptamine are substrates for both type A and B MAO.

Marketed MAO inhibitors are nonselective (tranylcypromine, phenelzine) or pre-ferential type B inhibitors (pargyline), although some selective inhibitors of type A MAO are known (94, 95).

Because side effects of MAO inhibitors include potentiation of pressor responses to ingested amines, selectivity with respect to tissue, enzyme form, and substrate may enhance clinical benefit and circumvent certain side effects. Thus research toward clinically superior selective MAO inhibitors based on current knowledge of the enzyme might be fruitful (89). Several reviews of MAO inhibitors are available (90, 96–98).

Where possible, in this section potencies of the various MAO inhibitors are related to iproniazid (58.**1**) either in tests for *in vitro* or *in vivo* inhibition of MAO or in other test procedures employed to identify antidepressant drugs (Section 3.2).

4.1.1 HYDRAZINE INHIBITORS OF MAO. Many hydrazines and hydrazides have MAO-inhibitory activity; however, precise SAR are difficult to discern. Further, some hydrazines with little *in vitro* activity are metabolized *in vivo* to produce potent MAO inhibitors. Tissue penetration and specificity may also play an important part in defining the potency of these compounds (99, 100). Because comprehensive reviews (43, 99) and quantitative SAR studies (101) on the MAO-inhibitory action of hydrazine derivatives are available, the subject is considered only generally in this section.

4.1.1.1 *Substituted Hydrazines.* Although hydrazine lacks significant MAO-inhibitory properties, alkyl substitution may confer significant activity. *In vitro* MAO-inhibitory data for some alkyl-, cycloalkyl-, and aralkyl-substituted hydrazines are presented in Table 58.1 (102). Among alkylhydrazines maximum potency is noted with ethylhydrazine. Increasing the size of the alkyl group beyond ethyl decreases potency. *n*-Octylhydrazine is almost devoid of MAO-inhibitory activity (99). Isopropylhydrazine is more effective than its straight chain isomer; it is equipotent with

Table 58.1   *In Vitro* MAO-Inhibitory Activity of Some Substituted Hydrazines RNHNH$_2$ (102)

R	I_{50}^a	R	I_{50}^a
CH_3	1.25×10^{-6}	$c\text{-}C_5H_{11}$	2.5×10^{-5}
CH_3CH_2	4.0×10^{-7}	C_6H_5	7.9×10^{-5}
$CH_3(CH_2)_2$	5.0×10^{-7}	$C_6H_5CH_2$	6.3×10^{-7}
$CH_3(CH_2)_3$	6.3×10^{-6}	$C_6H_5(CH_2)_2$	2.5×10^{-6}
$CH_3(CH_2)_4$	2.0×10^{-5}	$C_6H_5(CH_2)_3$	2.0×10^{-5}
$CH_3(CH_2)_5$	2.5×10^{-5}	$C_6H_5CH_2CH(CH_3)$	4.0×10^{-4}
$HO(CH_2)_3$	1×10^{-5}	$C_6H_5CH_2CH(COOH)$	$\gg 1 \times 10^{-3}$
$(CH_3)_2N(CH_2)_2$	2×10^{-4}	$C_6H_5CH=CHCH_2$	3.1×10^{-4}
$c\text{-}C_5H_9$	1×10^{-5}	Iproniazid	5.0×10^{-6}

^{a} Beef liver mitochondrial MAO was employed with a $1 \times 10^{-2} M$ tyramine substrate. Inhibition of oxygen uptake was measured manometrically. I_{50} is the molar concentration of inhibitor that produces a 50% decrease in MAO activity.

ethylhydrazine as an inhibitor of *in vitro* oxidation of serotonin by rat liver homogenate (43). In a similar system, employing guinea pig liver as the MAO source, 2-pentylhydrazine is about 100 times more potent than iproniazid (103).

In general, cycloalkyl-substituted hydrazines are about equipotent with their *n*-alkyl counterparts (Table 58.1); however, they are less effective than related simple branched alkyl derivatives. To illustrate, the *in vivo* MAO-inhibitory potency of cyclohexylhydrazine ($C_6H_{11}NHNH_2$) is only one-fourth that of 3-pentylhydrazine [$(C_2H_5)_2CHNHNH_2$] (103).

A hydrogen atom on the hydrazine nitrogen bearing the alkyl group is essential for MAO-inhibitory activity. Unsymmetrical dialkyl-substituted hydrazines, R^1R^2-NNH$_2$, are generally less potent than related monoalkyl derivatives. Possibly this observation is a consequence of differences in lipophilicity. Inspection of the data in Table 58.1 suggests a strong correlation between lipophilicity and *in vitro* MAO-inhibitory activity. In some cases, this decrease is pronounced. For example, 1,2-diisopropylhydrazine is 300 times less potent than isopropylhydrazine in an *in vitro* test for MAO inhibition (104), whereas the

isomeric *n*-hexylhydrazine (Table 58.1) is comparably less potent. In contrast, the disubstituted compound is nearly 13 times more potent than isopropylhydrazine as an enhancer of rat brain serotonin levels (99). N-Benzyl-N'-isopropylhydrazine and N-(β-methylphenethyl)-N'-isopropylhydrazine produce similar *in vivo* results. Apparently these disubstituted hydrazines are cleaved metabolically to release the potent monosubstituted derivative. Possibly the second N-substituent serves as a transporting moiety and prevents premature chemical interaction of the free hydrazine group prior to reaching the target sites in the brain (43).

Hydroxyalkylhydrazines are usually less potent MAO inhibitors than related alkylhydrazines. Thus β-hydroxyethylhydrazine, $HO(CH_2)_2NHNH_2$, is less potent than ethylhydrazine as an *in vitro* inhibitor of beef liver mitochondrial MAO (Table 58.1) (102); however, in a reserpine-reversal test in mice the alcohol is more effective than iproniazid (103). Etherification of the alcohol may significantly enhance potency. In a series of aryloxyalkylhydrazines maximum inhibition of the activity of rat liver homogenate is produced by 58.**3a,** which is also 10–20 times more potent than iproniazid in reversing reserpine-induced sedation in mice. Sulfur (58.**3b**) and amino (58.**3c**) analogs are about one-half as potent as 58.**3a** in this test (105).

Many related aminoalkylhydrazines are MAO inhibitors (106, 107). *In vitro*, *N,N*-disubstituted aminoethyl- and aminopropylhydrazines are weak inhibitors of MAO (106). As indicated in Table 58.1, $(CH_3)_2N(CH_2)_2NHNH_2$ is only $\frac{1}{40}$ as potent as iproniazid as an MAO inhibitor *in vitro*. Amino-substituted derivatives of larger alkylhydrazines sometimes are more potent. For example, $(C_2H_5)_2N(CH_2)_3CH$-$(CH_3)NHNH_2$ is equipotent with iproniazid in a reserpine-reversal test in mice (103). Some arylaminoalkylhydrazines, e.g., 58.**3d**, which is 40 times more potent than iproniazid, are likewise very effective in this test. Potent MAO inhibition is also caused by homologous benzylaminoalkyl derivatives, e.g., $C_6H_5CH_2N(CH_3)(CH_2)_2NHNH_2$ (106).

Although phenylhydrazine is a relatively weak MAO inhibitor *in vitro* (Table 58.1) and lacks significant *in vivo* activity, benzylhydrazine is effective both *in vitro* and *in vivo*. It is about 40 times more potent than iproniazid in a test for reversal of reserpine-induced sedation in mice. Additional lengthening of the straight chain alkylene bridge, however, decreases potency. Thus phenelzine (58.**4a**), which is in clinical use, is only one-tenth as potent as benzylhydrazine in the reserpine antagonism test, and the propylene homolog 58.**4b** is markedly less effective. These results are paralleled *in vitro* (Table 58.1). Simple branching of the alkylene bridge of aralkylhydrazines often enhances potency significantly. α-Methylbenzylhydrazine (mebanazine, 58.**4c**) readily reverses reserpine-induced depression in mice (108); however, additional branching (e.g., 58.**4d**) abolishes activity (109). Another branched chain aralkylhydrazine, pheniprazine (58.**5a**), inhibits MAO both *in vitro* and *in vivo*, and it is an effective clinical antidepressant. Pheniprazine is 40 times more potent than iproniazid in antagonizing reserpine-induced effects in mice. It resembles amphetamine in its ability to arouse mice from reserpine-induced stupor.

Replacement of the phenyl ring of pheniprazine (58.**5a**) with heterocyclic groups, e.g., pyridyl, thienyl, furyl, or benzodioxanyl, decreases MAO-inhibitory potency (110). Nuclear substitution with polar groups, e.g., hydroxy, amino, (111), nitro, or alkoxy, generally decreases potency (110); however, butoxy-(58.**5b**) and phenoxy-substituted (58.**5c**) derivatives are almost equipotent with 58.**5a** in a test for reversal of reserpine-induced sedation in mice, and they are less toxic (112). Hydrogenation of the phenyl group, *N*-alkylation, and *N*-acylation of pheniperazine generally decrease MAO-inhibitory potency (110, 113). A quaternary salt, $C_6H_5CH_2CH(CH_3)NHN^+(CH_3)_3$-$X^-$, and a carboxylic acid congener, C_6H_5-$CH_2CH(COOH)NHNH_2$, lack significant MAO-inhibitory activity (110). A sydnonimine relative, sydnophene (58.**6**), of pheniprazine has MAO-inhibitory activity (114). Clinical studies demonstrate antidepressant and mild stimulant activity (115).

An *N*-aralkylated hydroxylamine congener, $C_6H_5CH_2CH(CH_3)NHOH$, of pheniprazine weakly inhibits deamination of tyramine by rabbit-liver MAO (116);

$$X-\text{⟨benzene ring⟩}-\underset{\overset{|}{CH_3}}{CH_2CH}NHNH_2$$

58.5a X = H
58.5b X = *n*-C_4H_9O
58.5c X = C_6H_5O

$$C_6H_5XCH_2\underset{\overset{|}{CH_3}}{CH}NHNH_2 \qquad C_6H_5XNHNH_2$$

58.3a X = O	**58.4a** X = $(CH_2)_2$
58.3b X = S	**58.4b** X = $(CH_2)_3$
58.3c X = NH	**58.4c** X = CH_3CH
58.3d X = NCH$_3$	**58.4d** X = $(CH_3)_2C$

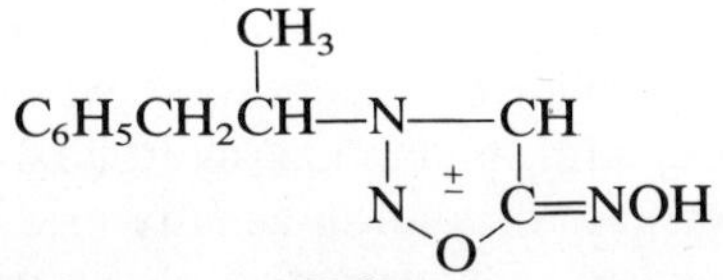

$$\begin{array}{c} CH_3 \\ | \\ C_6H_5CH_2CH-N-\!\!-CH \\ \underset{O}{\overset{N}{\underset{|}{\underset{\pm}{}}}}\;\;C{=}NOH \end{array}$$

58.**6**

however, the *O*-substituted congener, $C_6H_5CH_2CH(CH_3)ONH_2$, does not inhibit the oxidation of serotonin by guinea pig liver MAO (117).

4.1.1.2 *Hydrazide Derivatives.* Unsubstituted hydrazides, $RCONHNH_2$, do not significantly inhibit the *in vitro* action of beef liver mitochondrial MAO on a tyramine substrate (102). Thus the hydrazides of isonicotinic acid (4-pyridyl-$CONHNH_2$), picolinic acid (2-pyridyl-$CONHNH_2$), benzoic acid (C_6H_5-$CONHNH_2$), and various substituted β-phenylpropionic acids lack significant MAO-inhibitory activity (102). Monosubstitution of the amino group of the hydrazide, however, may introduce potent MAO-inhibitory properties (118). The efficacy of a substituted hydrazide depends on the nature of both the acyl group and the N' substituent, although potency generally parallels that of the nonacylated hydrazine. To illustrate, the relative order of *in vivo* MAO-inhibitory potency for a series of N'-alkylated serine hydrazides (Table 58.2) is similar to that determined *in vitro* for a corresponding series of alkylhydrazines (Table 58.1). An exception is noted in the case of ethyl- and propylhydrazines. These are the most potent alkylhydrazines (Table 58.1). In contrast, among the homologous series of N'-alkyl-substituted hydrazides, maximum potency is produced by propyl or butyl substitution (Table 58.2). A potency rank comparable to that observed in N'-substituted serine hydrazides is observed upon similar substitution of other acylhydrazides (118).

Some *in vivo* MAO-inhibitory data for N'-aralkyl-substituted *p*-chlorobenzhydrazides are presented in Table 58.3. As with

Table 58.2   Relative *in Vivo* MAO-Inhibitory Potency of *N'*-Alkylated Serine Hydrazides (118)

RNHNHCOCH(NH₂)CH₂OH	
R	Relative Potency[a]
CH_3	0.3
CH_3CH_2	1.28
$CH_3(CH_2)_2$	0.97
$(CH_3)_2CH$	1.89
$CH_3(CH_2)_3$	1.87
$CH_3(CH_2)_4$	1.48
$CH_3(CH_2)_5$	0.95
$CH_3(CH_2)_6$	0.33
$(CH_3(CH_2)_7$	0.00

[a] Potency relative to iproniazid. This was obtained by comparing increase of rat brain serotonin produced by 100 mg/kg of iproniazid with that produced by an equimolar amount of compound 16 hr after administration.

N'-alkyl hydrazides, in this series again potency depends on the N' substituent. Thus the N'-benzyl- and N'-α-methylbenzylhydrazides are potent MAO inhibitors. In contrast to related aralkylhydrazines, however, N'-α-methylphenethyl-*p*-chlorobenzhydrazide is markedly less potent than its

Table 58.3   Relative *in Vivo* MAO-Inhibitory Potency of *N'*-Aralkyl *p*-Chlorobenzhydrazides (118)

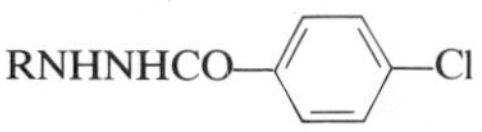

RNHNHCO—⟨benzene ring⟩—Cl

R	Relative Potency[a]
$(CH_3)_2CH$	1.36
$C_6H_5CH_2$	2.19
$C_6H_5CH(CH_3)$	2.03
$C_6H_5(CH_2)_2$	1.06
$C_6H_5CH_2CH(CH_3)$	0.54
$4\text{-}ClC_6H_4CH_2$	0.68
$3,4\text{-}(CH_3O)_2C_6H_3CH_2$	0.27

[a] See footnote *a* in Table 58.2.

N'-benzyl counterpart. An N'-α-methyl-phenethyl-substituted pivalic acid hydrazide likewise is less potent than its N'-benzyl relative (118).

That the nature of acyl substitution influences *in vivo* MAO-inhibitory potency is indicated by the data presented in Table 58.4 for some acyl-modified isopropylhydrazides (118). Apparently the main function of the acyl group is that of a "carrier"; it is hydrolyzed metabolically to release the MAO-inhibitory alkylhydrazine at the target organ. Modification of the acyl group may afford MAO inhibitors with selective affinities for specific organs. For example, α-glutamylisopropylhydrazide exerts a preferential action on brain MAO, whereas palmitylisopropylhydrazide acts preferentially on MAO in the heart (118, 119).

Generally α-amino substitution of the acyl group of N'-substituted hydrazides en-hances *in vivo* MAO-inhibitory potency, whereas α-hydroxy substitution, which may interfere with metabolic hydrolysis (43), may decrease or abolish activity (see Table 58.4). Isopropylhydrazides of natural L-amino acids are significantly more potent MAO inhibitors than those derived from the D isomers. This may reflect facile metabolic hydrolysis of the L enantiomers compared with the relatively difficult cleavage of the unnatural derivatives.

As can be seen from the data listed in Table 58.4, isopropyl substitution of the acylated nitrogen has a variable influence on MAO-inhibitory potency (118). The potency of these derivatives is somewhat surprising because the hydrazine metabolite, i.e., 1,2-diisopropylhydrazine, is much less potent than isopropylhydrazine (104).

The difference in MAO-inhibitory potency of heterocyclic carboxylic acid hyd-

Table 58.4 Relative *in Vivo* MAO-Inhibitory Potency of Some Isopropyl-hydrazides (118)

$R^1CONR^2NHCH(CH_3)_2$		
R^1	R^2	Relative Potency[a]
CH_3	H	0.74
CH_3	$(CH_3)_2CH$	2.56
$(CH_3)_3C$	H	1.52
$(CH_3)_3C$	$(CH_3)_2CH$	1.12
$CH_3CH(OH)$	H	0.83
$CH_3CH(OH)$	$(CH_3)_2CH$	1.96
$HOCH_2C(CH_3)_2CH(OH)$	H	0.02
$4\text{-}ClC_6H_4$	H	1.36
$4\text{-}ClC_6H_4$	$(CH_3)_2CH$	0.70
L-$CH_3CH(NH_2)$	H	2.53
D-$CH_3CH(NH_2)$	H	0.22
$H_2N(CH_2)_2$	H	0.21
L-$HOCH_2CH(NH_2)$	H	2.13
D-$HOCH_2CH(NH_2)$	H	1.33
L-$C_6H_5CH_2CH(NH_2)$	H	1.71
L-$HOOC(CH_2)_2CH(NH_2)$	H	2.50
D-$HOOC(CH_2)_2CH(NH_2)$	H	0.00
L-$CH_3CH(NHCOCH_3)$	H	2.10
D-$CH_3CH(NHCOCH_3)$	H	0.00

[a] See footnote *a* in Table 58.2.

razides is noteworthy. Several of these compounds are potent MAO inhibitors with antidepressant activity in humans. Isocarboxazide (58.**7**), which is used clinically, is 7–33 times more potent than iproniazid in various tests for MAO inhibition (120, 121). In contrast, the structurally related isoxazole 58.**8** lacks MAO-inhibitory activity. Depending on the test method, nialamide (58.**9**) is 3–12 times more potent than iproniazid, but it produces less liver toxicity (122). The *cis*-(−)-oxadiazinone 58.**10,** but not its enantiomer, is an effective *in vivo* inhibitor of MAO (123).

Several sulfonic acid hydrazides inhibit MAO. *In vitro* studies employing guinea pig liver MAO indicate N-(p-tosyl)-N-benzylhydrazine (58.**11a**), as well as the corresponding *p*-chlorobenzenesulfonyl 58.**11b** and methanesulfonyl 58.**11c** derivatives, has about one-half the inhibitory potency of pheniprazine (124). Corresponding N-sulfonyl-N'-benzylhydrazines (RSO$_2$-NHNHCH$_2$C$_6$H$_5$) are generally less potent (124).

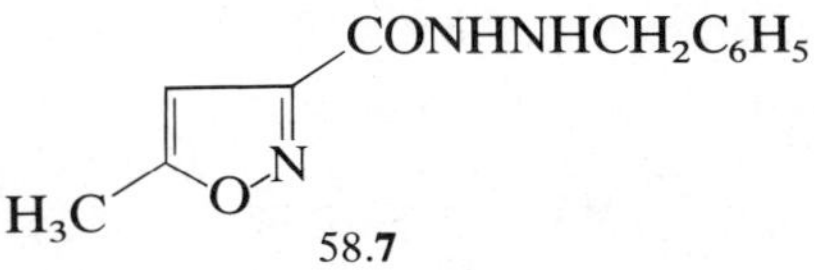

$$RSO_2NNH_2 \mid CH_2C_6H_5$$

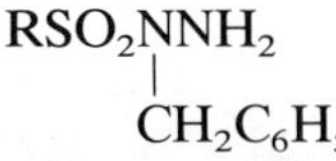

58.**11a**   R = 4-CH$_3$C$_6$H$_4$
58.**11b**   R = 4-ClC$_6$H$_4$
58.**11c**   R = CH$_3$

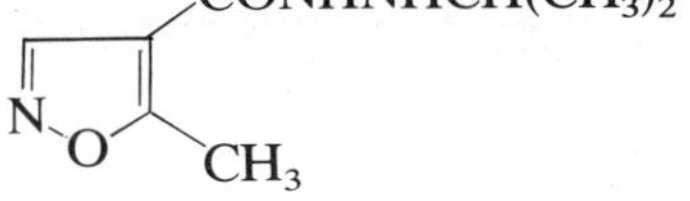

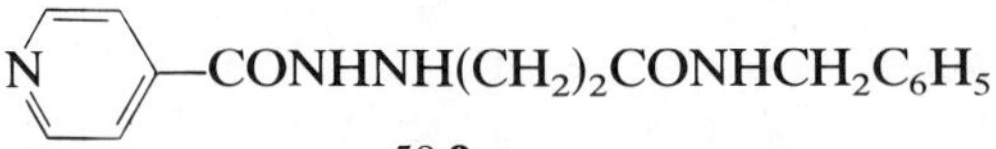

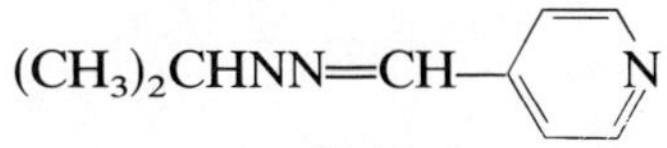

$$(CH_3)_2CHNN{=}CH-\text{(pyridine)}$$

58.**12**

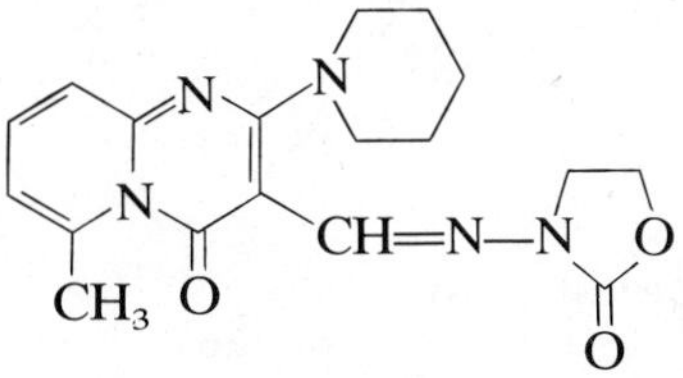

56.**13**

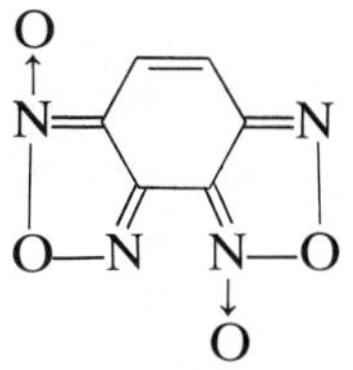

58.**14**

Hydrazones, like hydrazides, apparently must be hydrolyzed metabolically to produce an inhibitor of MAO. Thus C$_6$H$_5$CH$_2$C(CH$_3$)=NNH$_2$, a precursor of hydrazine, is inactive; however, 58.**12,** a potential precursor of isopropylhydrazine, is a potent MAO inhibitor. A novel hydrazone derivative, 58.**13,** as well as its pyrido-reduced analog, is a long-acting, potent, and irreversible inhibitor of rat liver and brain MAO *in vivo*, but not *in vitro* (125). The furoxanobenzofuroxan 58.**14,** which is vaguely similar to a hydrazone, is a very potent inhibitor of MAO (126).

4.1.2 NONHYDRAZINE INHIBITORS OF MONO-AMINE OXIDASE.   A large variety of chemicals, e.g., alcohols, amidines, guanidines, isothioureas, xanthines, amphetamines, and choline phenyl ethers, inhibit MAO.

Since the discovery of iproniazid's clinical antidepressant properties and MAO-

CONHNHCH$_2$C$_6$H$_5$

58.**7**

CONHNHCH(CH$_3$)$_2$

58.**8**

CONHNH(CH$_2$)$_2$CONHCH$_2$C$_6$H$_5$

58.**9**

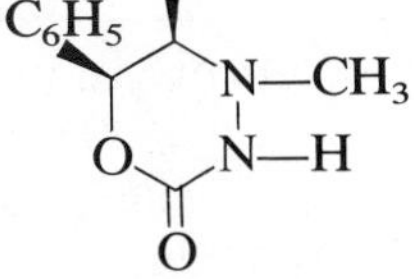

58.**10**

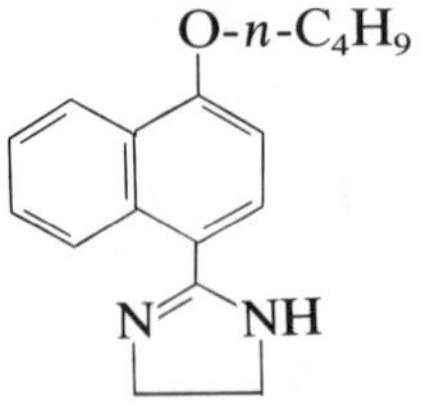

$O-n-C_4H_9$

58.15

$(CH_3)_3C$ — $\overset{S}{C}NH(CH_2)_2$ — N O

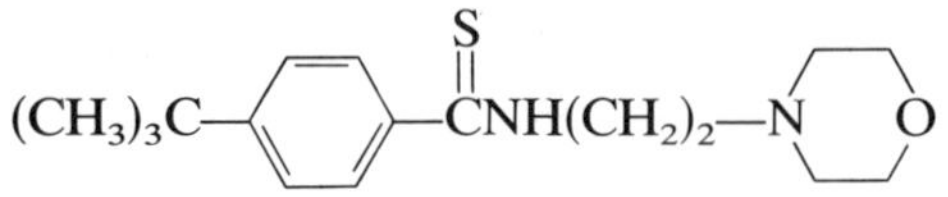

58.16

inhibitory activity, many nonhydrazine inhibitors of the enzyme have been discovered. The most significant compounds of this type are harmala alkaloids and related β-carbolines, indolealkylamines, propargylamines, 2-phenylcyclopropylamine and related compounds, and aminopyrazines (44). Two other prototypic compounds, not conveniently categorized in these classes, are the 2-(alkoxynaphthyl)-2-imidazoline 58.**15,** a potent *in vivo* and *in vitro* inhibitor of MAO (127), and the morpholinoethylthiobenzamide 58.**16,** which is effective in a mouse test for antidepressant activity (128).

4.1.2.1 *Harmala Alkaloids and Related Carbolines.* The harmala alkaloids harmine (58.**17**) and harmaline (3,4-dihydroharmine) and some related β-carboline derivatives, e.g., tryptoline (58.**18**) (129), are

58.17

58.18

potent *in vivo* and *in vitro* inhibitors of MAO (130).

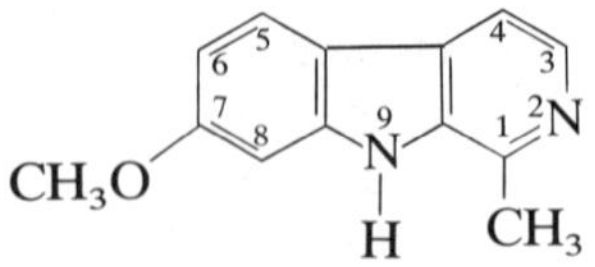

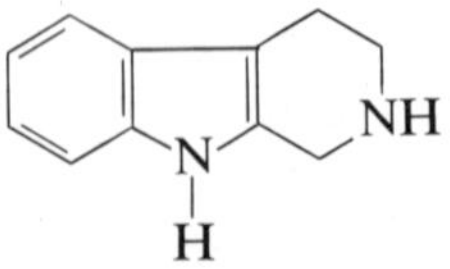

Generally, β-carbolines and their 3,4-dihydro counterparts are about equipotent, whereas 1,2,3,4-tetrahydro derivatives are much less effective. Thus harmine and harmaline are nearly equipotent and both are considerably more potent than tetrahydroharmine (1,2,3,4-tetrahydro-58.**17**) in several *in vitro* tests for MAO inhibition (130–132). Harmine is more than 100 times more potent than iproniazid in preventing oxidation of serotonin in the presence of rat liver homogenate (130). Unexpectedly, harmine and harmaline are 10^3–10^4 times less potent inhibitors of oxidation of several substrates in a test utilizing highly purified beef liver mitochondrial MAO than in similar tests with rat or guinea pig liver homogenates (133). MAO from human and rat liver mitochondria, however, is strongly inhibited (134).

The 7-methoxyl group of harmine is not required for MAO-inhibitory activity; the corresponding unsubstituted β-carboline is nearly equipotent with harmine *in vitro* (130). In contrast, relocation of the methoxy to position 6 results in a compound with only one-fifth the *in vitro* MAO-inhibitory potency of harmine (132). Phenolic analogs of harmine (i.e., harmol) (131), harmaline (i.e., harmalol) (131), and tetrahydroharmine (i.e., tetrahydroharmol) (132), are less than $\frac{1}{100}$ as potent as their methoxy counterparts as *in vitro* inhibitors of MAO.

The presence of the 1-methyl substituent apparently is not needed for the MAO-inhibitory activity of a β-carboline. Thus the 1-unsubstituted compounds tetrahydronorharman and its 2-methyl derivative are effective inhibitors of MAO *in vitro* (135).

α-Carboline is a comparatively weak inhibitor of MAO *in vitro* (130). γ-Carbolines are generally considerably less potent MAO inhibitors than are β-carbolines (132).

4.1.2.2 *Indolealkylamines.* Although tryptamine is a substrate for MAO, introduction of alkyl substituents alpha to the amino group provides compounds with inhibitory activity (136–138). Both α-methyltryptamine (58.**19a**) and α-ethyltryptamine (etryptamine, 58.**19b**) inhibit tyramine oxidation in the presence of guinea pig liver MAO (139). In this system α-methyltryptamine is more potent than the α-ethyl homolog, which is equipotent with iproniazid. Conversely, using beef liver MAO, a series of α-alkyltryptamines is less potent than iproniazid. In this procedure the optical isomers of 58.**19a** and 58.**19b** are nearly equipotent and MAO-inhibitory activity increases with increasing size of the α-alkyl substituent: propyl> ethyl>methyl (102). Only the (+) isomer of 58.**19b** antagonizes reserpine-induced depression in mice (138). Several aza analogs of etryptamine are less effective (2 and 8-aza) than the indole or inactive (3a-aza) (140). Another α-substituted tryptamine, the carbazole 58.**20,** is more potent than iproniazid as an inhibitor rat liver homogenate-catalyzed oxidation of serotonin (132).

Disubstitution of the α position of the aminoethyl side chain of tryptamine decreases MAO-inhibitory potency. α,α-Dimethyltryptamine is considerably less effective than α-methyltryptamine in in-

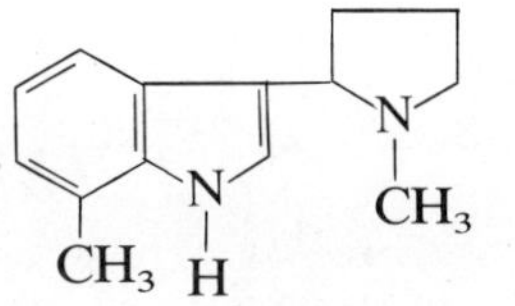

58.21

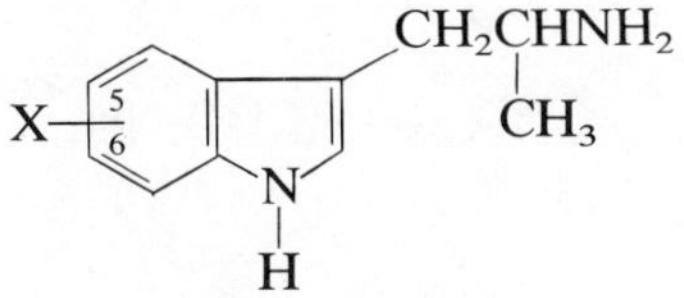

58.**22a**   X = 5-OH
58.**22b**   X = 5-OCH₃
58.**22c**   X = 6-Cl

creasing levels of serotonin in rat brain (141).

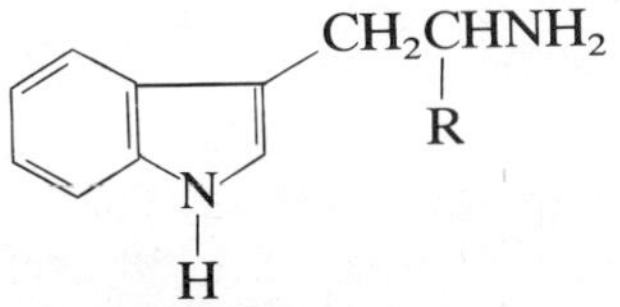

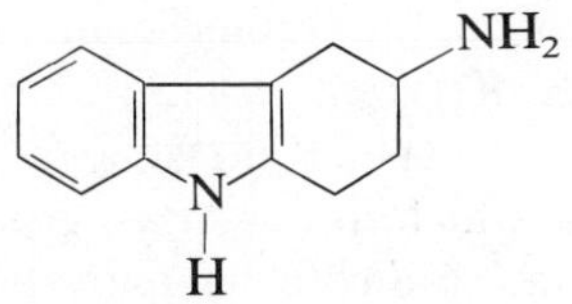

Several 3-(2-pyrrolidinyl)indoles, e.g., 58.**21,** are potent *in vitro* inhibitors of MAO. In addition, some of these compounds are effective in tests for neuroleptic activity, such as blockade of conditioned behavior in rats and inhibition of isolation-induced aggression in mice (142).

Substitution of the indole nucleus of α-alkyltryptamines has a variable influence on MAO-inhibitory potency. *In vitro*, 5-hydroxy-58.**22a** (139), 5-methoxy-58.**22b** (143), and 6-chloro-α-methyltryptamine (58.**22c**) (144) are less potent inhibitors of MAO than the parent 58.**19a**. In contrast, substitution of positions 4, 5, or 7 with chlorine (144) or position 4 with methyl (145) enhances potency. The 7-methyl derivative of 58.**19b** is about 10 times more potent than the parent as an inhibitor of MAO *in vitro* (146).

Methyl substitution of the amino group of tryptamine may also introduce MAO-inhibitory activity. Several N,N-dimethyltryptamine derivatives inhibit the action of guinea pig MAO on a tryptamine substrate (147).

Significant *in vitro* inhibition of MAO is also caused by isotryptamine (53.**23a**) and isoserotonin (58.**23b**). The tryptamine isomer is somewhat more potent than its

58.**19a**   R = CH₃
58.**19b**   R = C₂H₅

58.**20**

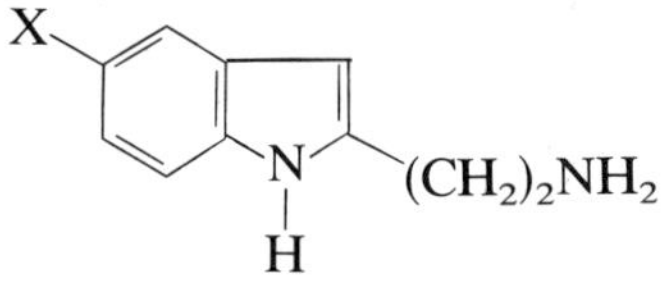

1014 Antidepressant Agents**

58.**23a** X = H
58.**23b** X = OH

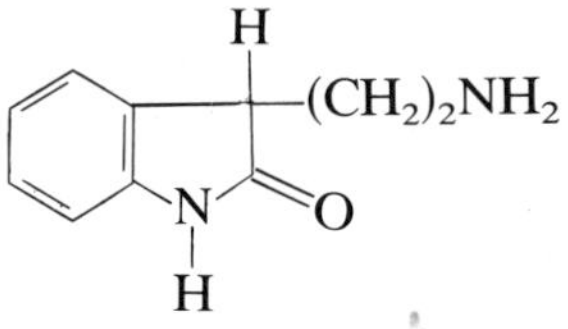

58.**24**

5-hydroxylated derivative. The oxindole analog 58.**24** of tryptamine also induces modest *in vitro* MAO inhibition (135).

4.1.2.3 Propargylamines and Related Compounds.

N-Benzyl-N-methyl-2-propynylamine (pargyline, 58.**25a**) is a potent inhibitor of MAO. It is about eight times more potent than iproniazid as an inhibitor of the oxidation of serotonin in the presence of rat liver mitochondrial MAO (148). It is also effective in a dopa-potentiation test in mice (149). Pargyline is employed clinically as an antihypertensive drug. Substitution of the benzene ring of pargyline has a variable influence on MAO-inhibitory potency. Several ortho-substituted derivatives, such as 58.**25b–e**, are more potent than the parent *in vitro*. The 1-naphthyl analog 58.**26** is more potent than pargyline both *in vivo* and in *in vitro* (149). The indanamine 58.**27a** is nearly 20 times more potent than pargyline both *in vivo* and in

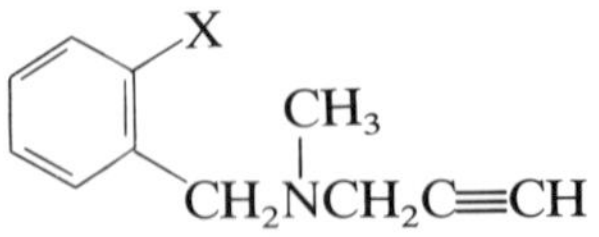

58.**25**

a X = H
b X = Cl
c X = Br
d X = OCH₃
e X = CH₃

vitro (150). It has a marked selectivity for brain MAO (151). The tetralin 58.**27b** is even more potent than the indan (152). The benzothiepin 58.**27c** is also an MAO inhibitor. It antagonizes the effects of reserpine and causes excitation in mice (152).

Replacement of the benzyl group of pargyline with β-phenethyl (58.**28a**) or 3-phenylpropyl (58.**28b**) does not significantly alter potency; however, additional lengthening of this alkyl bridge markedly

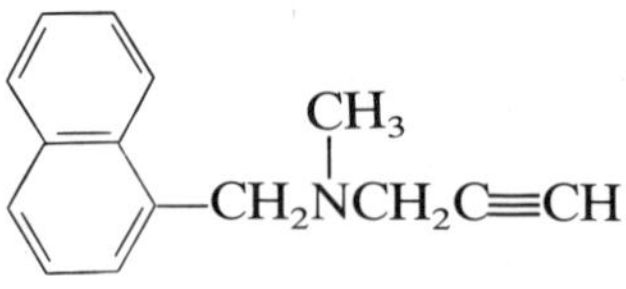

58.**26**

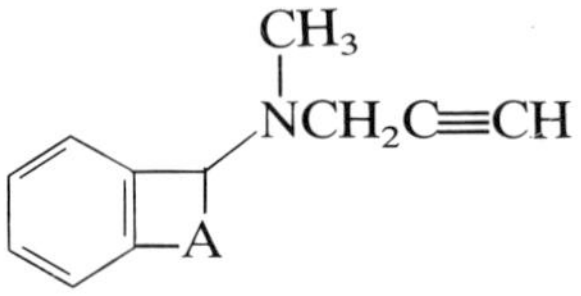

58.**27a** A = (CH₂)₂
58.**27b** A = (CH₂)₃
58.**27c** A = (CH₂)₃S

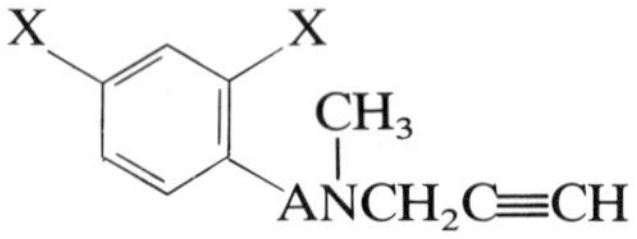

58.**28a** X = H, A = (CH₂)₂
58.**28b** X = H, A = (CH₂)₃
58.**28c** X = H, A = CH₂CH(CH₃)
58.**28d** X = Cl, A = O(CH₂)₃

decreases potency (149). The phenylisopropyl homolog deprenyl (58.**28c**) is a potent inhibitor of MAO *in vitro*. It also causes amphetamine-like CNS stimulation (153), is effective in the clinic, and is claimed to inhibit, rather than potentiate, the effects of tyramine (154). Deprenyl is selective for type B MAO. A pargyline analog in which the benzyl group is replaced by a 2,4-dichlorophenoxypropyl system, i.e., clorgyline (58.**28d**) (155), is of particular interest. It appears to be relatively specific for type A MAO which is predominant in sympathetic nerves (94). In humans, clorgyline has antidepressant activity comparable to that of imipramine (156). It increases levels of norepinephrine, serotonin, and dopamine in various brain areas (157).

The N-methyl group of pargyline is required for maximum potency. Removal of this group decreases potency only slightly; however, replacement with ethyl, phenyl, or carbethoxy groups practically abolishes MAO-inhibitory activity. The propynyl group is also important for activity. Replacement with a propyl or allyl substituent results in loss of MAO-inhibitory activity, but the 2-butynyl homolog of pargyline retains some *in vitro* activity (149).

Replacement of the propynyl group of pargyline with a cyclopropyl substituent provides some potent MAO inhibitors. One such compound is encyprate (58.**29**), which significantly inhibits MAO *in vivo* although it is relatively ineffective *in vitro* (149). Other compounds of this type include some aryloxyalkyl derivatives. Some of these, e.g., 58.**30a**, cause *in vivo* actions that are greater than those that would be predicted from their *in vitro* effect on MAO. In mice, 58.**30a** is more potent than pargyline in a dopa-potentiation test. It is also a potent inhibitor of the oxidation of kynuramine by rat liver mitochondrial MAO (158). Additionally, 58.**30a** seems to be a selective *in vivo* inhibitor of type A MAO (159). The

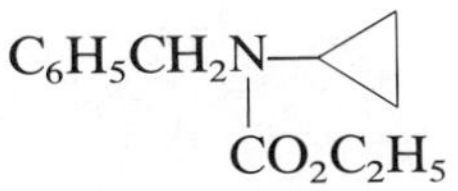

related monochloro derivative 58.**30b,** like harmaline, preferentially blocks MAO oxidation of serotonin (160).

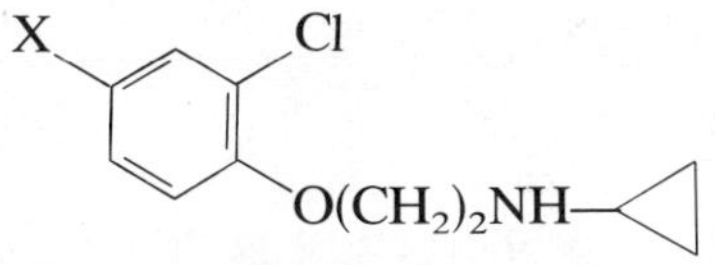

MAO-Inhibitory properties are retained by analogs of 58.**30** in which the ether oxygen is replaced by a sulfur, as well as those in which the ethylene chain is replaced by an isopropyl bridge. The α-methylphenethyl congener 58.**31** also retains potent *in vivo* and *in vitro* MAO-inhibitory activity (158).

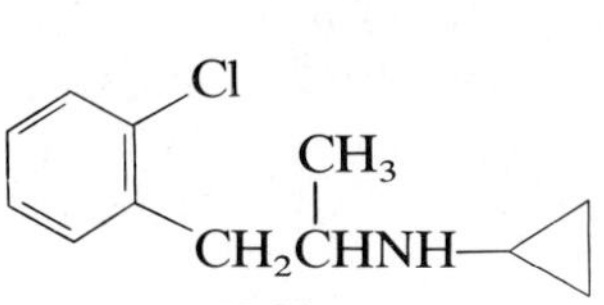

58.**31** 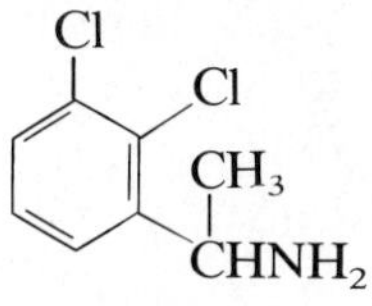   58.**32**

Removal of the propynyl group of pargyline, i.e., to afford benzylamines, permits retention of MAO-inhibitory actions. 2,3-Dichloro-α-methylbenzylamine (58.**32**) is particularly interesting. The (+) isomer inhibits oxidation of serotonin (a substrate of type A MAO) by rat mitochondrial MAO more effectively than it inhibits phenethylamine (a substrate for type B MAO). The (−) isomer has an opposite selectivity for types A and B MAO (161).

4.1.2.4 *Cyclopropylamines. trans*-2-Phenylcyclopropylamine (tranylcypromine, 58.**33**) is a very potent inhibitor of MAO both *in vivo* and *in vitro.* Many derivatives and other compounds related to tranylcypromine are potent *in vivo* inhibitors of MAO as determined pharmacologically by their ability to potentiate tryptamine-induced convulsions in rats (162).

No generalization can be drawn regarding the influence of geometric or optical isomerism on MAO-inhibitory activity among substituted cyclopropylamines. (±)-*trans*-2-Phenylcylopropylamine (58.**33**) is about two to three times more potent than the cis isomer in a tryptamine-potentiation test (162). These isomers are both about 40

58.**29**

58.**30a** X = Cl
58.**30b** X = H

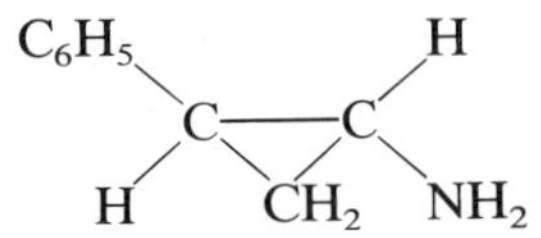

58.**33**

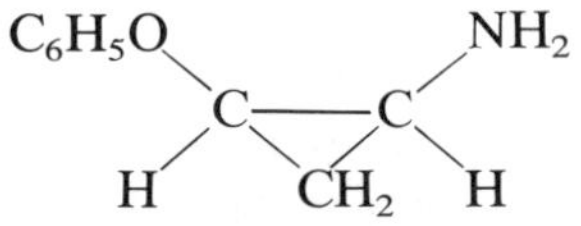

58.**34**

times more potent than iproniazid as inhibitors of beef mitochondrial MAO oxidation of tyramine (102). Pharmacologically, the (+)-trans isomer is approximately equipotent with the trans racemate, but it is about four times more potent than the (−)-trans isomer. Comparable *in vitro* results are obtained with the (+)- and (−)-trans isomers in several systems (133, 163). Interestingly, the (−) isomer is a more potent inhibitor of catecholamine uptake into brain synaptosomes than is the (+) isomer (164). In accordance with this observation, greater clinical antidepressant activity is noted for the (−) enantiomer (165); however, this conclusion is not supported by a clinical study of the effect of tranylcypromine on platelet MAO or amine uptake in normal subjects (166).

In contrast to the geometric isomers of 2-phenylcyclopropylamine, in a series of 2-phenoxycyclopropylamines the cis isomers, e.g., 58.**34,** usually are more potent inhibitors of MAO than the trans isomers; however, no consistent difference is observed in various *in vitro* tests (167).

Apparently a cyclopropane ring is required for potent MAO-inhibitory activity in this series. Both trans and cis isomers of 2-phenylcyclobutyl-, 2-phenylcyclopentyl-, 2-phenylcyclohexyl-, and 2-phenylcycloheptylamines are essentially inactive as tryptamine potentiators (162) and in other tests for antidepressant activity (168).

Substitution of the benzene ring of tranylcypromine generally decreases, or has little influence on, tryptamine-potentiating activity. Usually potency increases with position substitution in the order: para > meta > ortho. For example, the 4-chloro derivative 58.**35a** is about two-thirds as potent as tranylcypromine, whereas the meta congener 58.**35b** is only one-fifth as potent as the parent, and the ortho isomer 58.**35c** is even less potent. Whether the substituent is electron-withdrawing or electron-donating is of little importance. Thus 4-trifluoromethyl (58.**35d**) and 4-methoxy (58.**35e**) congeners are essentially equipotent with tranylcypromine in a tryptamine-potentiation test (162).

Substitution at position 2 of cyclopropylamine enhances MAO-inhibitory potency. Cyclopropylamine does not potentiate tryptamine-induced convulsions in rats and lacks *in vitro* activity (102, 169). Introduction of a 2-methyl substituent affords 58.**36a**, which is about $\frac{1}{1000}$ as potent as tranylcypromine (170). 2-Amyl- (58.**36b**) and 2-cyclohexylcyclopropylamine (58.**36c**) are about one-fifth as potent as tranylcypromine.

Introduction of naphthyl or thianaphthenyl substituents into position 2 of cyc-

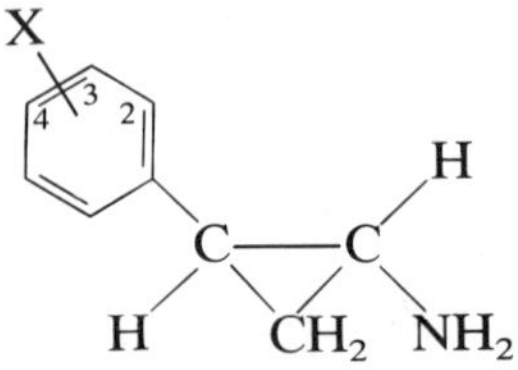

58.**35**

a X = 4-Cl
b X = 3-Cl
c X = 2-Cl
d X = 4-CF$_3$
e X = 4-OCH$_3$

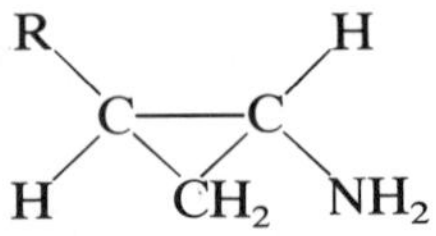

58.**36a** R = CH$_3$
58.**36b** R = *n*-C$_5$H$_{11}$
58.**36c** R = *c*-C$_6$H$_{11}$

lopropylamine affords compounds with significant MAO-inhibitory activity. *trans*-2-Phenoxy- (162, 167), 2-phenylthio- (162), and cyclohexyloxycyclopropylamine (171) are nearly equipotent with tranylcypromine in a variety of tests for MAO inhibition. 2-Benzyl- and 2-phenethylcyclopropyl-amines, however, are only $\frac{1}{10}$ and $\frac{1}{100}$ as potent, respectively, as tranylcypromine in a tryptamine-potentiation test (162).

Substitution of the amino group of tranylcypromine generally decreases MAO-inhibitory potency. Nonetheless, both *N*-methyl (58.**37a**) and *N,N*-dimethyl (57.**37b**) derivatives are at least one-half as effective as the parent in the tryptamine-potentiation test. Alkylation or aralkylation with larger groups results in a marked decrease in MAO-inhibitory potency. For example, the isopropyl derivative 58.**37c** is about $\frac{1}{100}$ as potent as tranylcypromine. Acylation also generally decreases or abolishes activity. The carbobenzoxy derivative 58.**37d** is an exception; it is nearly twice as potent as tranylcypromine as a tryptamine potentiator.

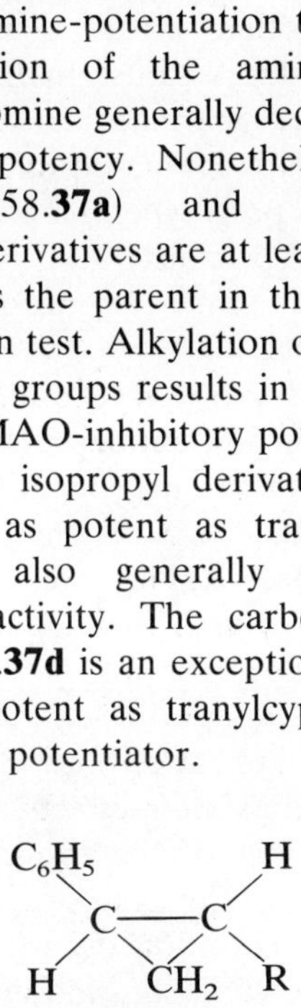

58.**37**

a R = NHCH$_3$
b R = N(CH$_3$)$_2$
c R = NHCH(CH$_3$)$_2$
d R = NHCO$_2$CH$_2$C$_6$H$_5$
e R = CH$_2$NH$_2$

Substitution of position 1 of 2-phenyl-cyclopropylamine with a methyl group has little effect on MAO-inhibitory potency. Both *trans*- and *cis*-1-methyl-2-phenyl-cyclopropylamine are equipotent with tranylcypromine in a tryptamine-potentiation test (162). In contrast, introduction of methyl or phenyl substituents into positions 2 or 3 (172) markedly decreases potency. Two fused-ring congeners

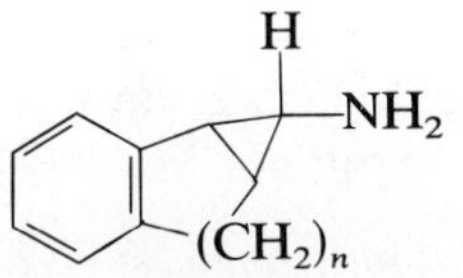

58.**38a** $n = 1$
58.**38b** $n = 2$

that are 2,3-disubstituted cyclopropyl-amines are of particular interest because of the conformational restraints imposed upon them. The *trans*-indan 58.**38a** is about one-fifth as potent as tranylcypromine; however, the related tetralin 58.**38b** is practically inactive in a tryptamine-potentiation test (162).

Separation of the amino group from the cyclopropane ring by a methylene bridge, e.g., 58.**37e**, abolishes MAO-inhibitory activity. Nonetheless, antidepressant-like actions, e.g., reversal of reserpine-induced sedation in rabbits, are produced by the trans, but not by the cis, isomer of 58.**37e** (173).

Other tranylcypromine analogs include a positional isomer, 1-phenylcyclopropyl-amine, which is about $\frac{1}{25}$ as potent as tranylcypromine *in vivo*, arylaziridines, e.g., 58.**39** (163, 174), and aryldiaziridines, e.g., 58.**40** (175). *In vitro* MAO-inhibitory potency of 1-alkyl-2-phenylaziridines increases with increased alkyl chain length. Thus the phenethyl derivative 58.**39** significantly inhibits oxidation of tryptamine by rat liver homogenate (174). In a similar

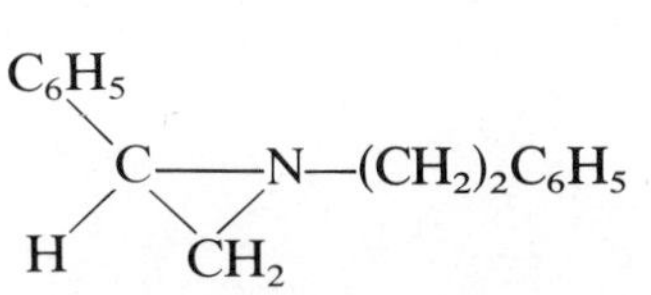

58.**39**

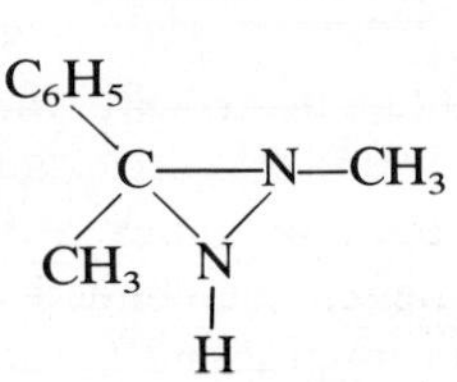

58.**40**

in vitro test, 58.**40** is almost equipotent with iproniazid (175) as an inhibitor of the oxidation of serotonin.

4.1.2.5 *Aminopyrazines.* 2-Methyl-3-piperidinylpyrazine (58.**41**) and several related compounds are potent *in vivo* inhibitors of MAO (176, 177). 58.**41** is only marginally active *in vitro*, so it may be a metabolic product that is responsible for its *in vivo* activity.

For maximum potency in a test for antagonism of reserpine-induced depression in mice a disubstituted pyrazine must bear adjacent alkyl and tertiary amino groups in positions 2 and 3. Considerable variation in the tertiary amino group is possible without loss of efficacy. Maximum reserpine-antagonist potency is observed with a homopiperidinyl substituent. The alkyl substituent may be methyl or ethyl; however, activity is lost if an alkyl group is not present.

Substitution of positions 5 or 6 of 2-alkyl-3-piperidinylpyrazines abolishes activity; however, several substituted 2-alkyl-3-dimethylaminopyrazines, e.g., 58.**42,** retain significant MAO-inhibitory activity (178). Various *N*-oxides and several other potential metabolic products of 58.**41** are ineffective as *in vitro* inhibitors of MAO in mouse liver or brain homogenates (177).

58.41

58.42

4.2 Tricyclic Antidepressants

Almost simultaneously with the discovery that iproniazid (58.**1**) and other inhibitors of MAO have useful clinical antidepressant properties, the clinical effectiveness of a tricyclic agent imipramine (58.**2**) in human depression was observed. This finding led

to the investigation of a large number of aminoalkylated tricyclic compounds in the treatment of this variegated disease complex. Some of the biological tests used to examine these substances for antidepressant activity are described in Section 3.2.

Because of the diversity of these screening methods and the disease complex itself it is often impossible to compare the many tricyclic and other types of non-MAO-inhibitory antidepressants. In this section, where possible, pharmacological activities of compounds are compared to the tricyclic antidepressant prototypes imipramine and amitriptyline, primarily in reserpine-, tetrabenazine-, and benzoquinolizine-antagonism tests.

As in the case of tricyclic antipsychotic agents (Chapter 56), antidepressant activity of tricyclic compounds depends on the tricyclic system, the side chain, and the nature of the basic amino group. Studies of the molecular features affecting the potency of tricyclic antidepressants as inhibitors of uptake of norepinephrine by rabbit aortic strips (174) or into rat cerebral cortex slices (180) indicate maximum effectiveness when the aromatic rings of the tricyclic nucleus are at appreciable angles to one another. In general, weak inhibition occurs with compounds that are coplanar, and intermediate potency is observed in compounds in which the aromatic rings are not bridged. These studies also indicate the primary amine and the tertiary dimethylamine derivatives are equipotent in series where inhibition is marked. The secondary methylamines of some tricyclics, e.g., dihydrodibenzazepine, dibenzocycloheptadiene, and diphenylmethanes, are more potent in these tests than their respective primary or tertiary derivatives. In contrast, in the dibenzocycloheptatriene series all three amines are equipotent in a test employing cerebral cortex slices. The molecular geometry of inhibitors of the uptake of catecholamines and serotonin in synaptosomal preparations of rat brain has been studied by comparison with relatively rigid molecules, e.g., (1*R*, 4*S*)-*N*-methyl-4-phenyl-1,2,3,4-tetrahydro-1-naphthyl-amine and 4-phenylbicyclo[2.2.2]octan-1-amine. The well-defined molecular geometry of these rigid uptake inhibitors suggests the relative separation and orientation of an aromatic ring and the amino nitrogen is a fundamental structural/-conformational requirement for uptake blocking activity of a large family of such inhibitors including the tricyclic antidepressants, with potency being modulated by additional structural and stereochemical factors (57).

In agreement with the observation that most potent inhibitors of amine uptake are ones in which the rings of the tricyclic nucleus are at appreciable angles, most antidepressant tricyclics have a seven-(or eight) membered central ring. Unlike the tricyclic antipsychotics, which require a tertiary amino group, some potent antidepressants, as suggested by the brain synaptosomal uptake studies, have a secondary amino group. Also in contrast to the tricyclic antipsychotics, substitution of the position meta to the bridging atom that bears the aminoalkyl side chain usually does not produce a profound effect on antidepressant activity. In some instances antidepressants, unlike the tricyclic antipyschotics, may have a two-, rather than a three-carbon atom side chain.

4.2.1   DIBENZAZEPINES AND RELATED COMPOUNDS. Despite the large number of aminoalkylated dihydrodibenzazepines (iminodibenzyls), dibenzazepines (iminostilbenes), and related compounds that have been prepared (34), comparative pharmacological data for these compounds are relatively sparse. The prototype of this class of antidepressants is imipramine (58.**2**), which currently is in clinical use. At least in part the action of imipramine results from one of its metabolites, desipramine (58.**43a**). Desipramine is more potent and

has a quicker onset of action than its metabolic precursor in a test for antagonism of reserpine-induced sedation in rats. The clinical utility of desipramine in treating endogenous depression is well established (183).

A series of analogs of imipramine has been examined for prevention or reversal of the characteristic depressant syndrome produced in rats by a tetrabenazine-related compound (184). In this test, activity in reversing the depressant actions is confined to methyl-substituted secondary amines. Thus desipramine (58.**43a**) reverses the actions induced by the depressant. It produces excitation, whereas imipramine even at a significantly higher dose does not reverse, but only prevents, the actions of the depressant. In a related tetrabenazine-antagonist test in rats 58.**43a** is five to six times more potent than 58.**2** (185). Also, in a test that measures the ability of a compound to enhance the response of the cat nictitating membrane to norepinephrine, secondary aminopropyl derivatives of dihydrodibenzazepines are more potent than corresponding tertiary amines (186). The primary amine 58.**43b** is slightly less

58.**43**

a   R = (CH$_2$)$_3$NHCH$_3$
b   R = (CH$_2$)$_3$NH$_2$
c   R = (CH$_2$)$_3$NHC$_2$H$_5$
d   R = (CH$_2$)$_3$NH-*i*-C$_3$H$_7$
e   R = (CH$_2$)$_3$NH-*n*-C$_4$H$_9$
f   R = (CH$_2$)$_3$N(O)(CH$_3$)$_2$
g   R = (CH$_2$)$_3$N(CH$_3$)CH$_2$COC$_6$H$_4$-4-Cl
h   R = (CH$_2$)$_3$N

i   R = (CH$_2$)$_2$NHCH$_3$
j   R = (CH$_2$)$_4$NHCH$_3$
k   R = CH$_2$CH(CH$_3$)CH$_2$N(CH$_3$)$_2$
l   R = CO(CH$_2$)$_2$N(CH$_3$)$_2$
m   R = CO(CH$_2$)$_2$NHCH$_3$

potent than imipramine as a tetrabenazine antagonist in rats (185). Substitution of the amino group with alkyl groups larger than methyl, i.e., 58.**43c–e,** abolishes a benzoquinolizine-antagonist effect and introduces toxicity (184). An *N*-oxide 58.**43f** of imipramine is only one-third as potent as the parent in a tetrabenazine-antagonist test in rats (185). A tertiary amine lofepramine (58.**43g**) bearing a 4-chlorophenacyl substituent is rapidly metabolized to 58.**43a** in man (187). This compound is very similar to 58.**43a** in its ability to suppress norepinephrine and serotonin uptake into rat brain monoaminergic neurons (188). Its pharmacological profile, which suggests similarity to imipramine but with fewer side effects (189), is borne out in clinical studies (190, 191). Another tertiary amine carpipramine (58.**43h**) causes some of the pharmacological actions of imipramine and is effective in the depressive state in schizophrenic patients (192).

As with tricyclic antipsychotics (Chapter 56), maximum potency of antidepressant dihydrobenzazepine derivatives occurs when the basic nitrogen is separated from the tricyclic nucleus by a propylene bridge. Significant activity is retained, however, by the ethylene bridged homolog. Thus 58.**43i** is about one-half as effective as desipramine in reversing sedation induced by a tetrabenazine-related compound. Compounds with chain lengths exceeding propylene, e.g., 59.**43j,** are comparatively ineffective in this test. Branching of the propylene chain, e.g., trimipramine (58.**43k**), has little effect on antidepressant activity (35, 193, 194). Analogs 58.**43l** and 58.**43m** bearing a carbonyl functionality in position 1 of the propyl side chain of imipramine or desipramine have antidepressant-like biological actions; e.g., they potentiate reserpine-induced effects in frogs and inhibit uptake of serotonin by human thrombocytes (195).

Several antidepressant dihydrodibenzazepines with more strikingly modified side chains are the quinuclidine 58.**44** (196), the tetracyclic compounds 58.**45** (197), in which the side chain is incorporated into position 4 of the dibenzazepine nucleus, and a 10–methylaminodihydrodibenzazepine, metapramine (58.**46**) (198). The tetracyclic 58.**45a** is comparable to imipramine in reversing reserpine-induced ptosis and in causing anticholinergic effects, whereas the *N*-benzyl relative azipramine (58.**45b**) lacks anticholinergic and antihistaminic actions (197). Metapramine (58.**46**) combines clinical antidepressant and psychostimulant actions with a rapid onset of action (198).

Nuclear substitution of aminopropyl derivatives of dihydrodibenzazepines has a variable influence on antidepressant potency. Introduction of substituents into a position meta to the tricycle's bridging atom bearing the aminoalkyl side chain, i.e., the 3 position, has little effect. Thus

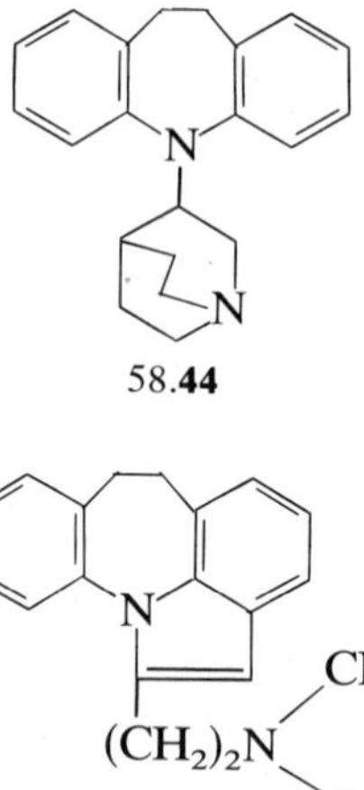

58.**44**

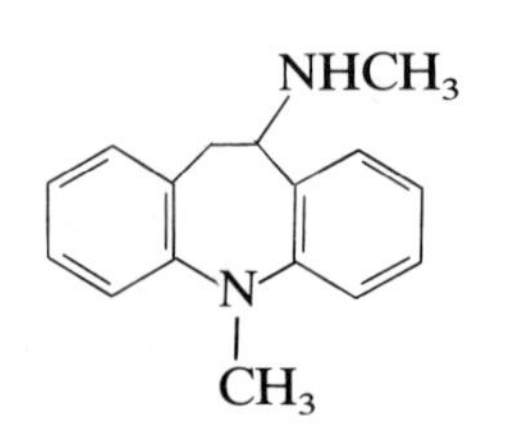

58.**45a** R = CH₃
58.**45b** R = CH₂C₆H₅

58.**46**

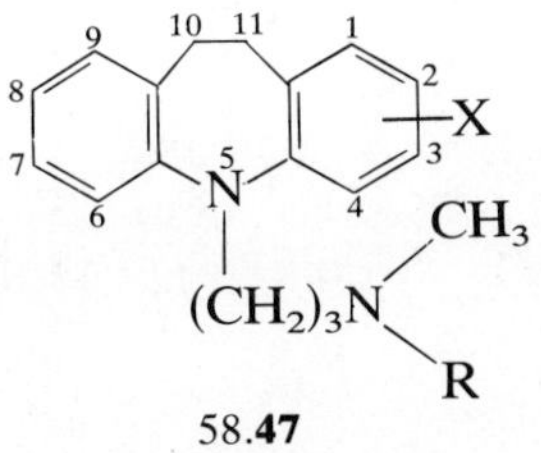

58.**47**

a   X = 3-Cl, R = CH$_3$
b   X = 10 = O, R = CH$_3$
c   X = 10-CH$_3$, R = H
d   X = 2-OH, R = H
e   X = 2,8-(CH$_3$)$_2$, R = H
f   X = 3,7-Cl$_2$, R = CH$_3$

chlorimipramine (58.**47a**) is somewhat less potent than imipramine in reversing sedation caused by a tetrabenazine-like compound in rats (184); it is significantly less effective than desipramine in potentiating norepinephrine- and serotonin-induced contractions of cat nictitating membrane (186) and in antagonizing reduction of reserpine-induced locomotor activity in mice (199). Clinically, chlorimipramine is similar to imipramine with regard to effectiveness, onset of action, and nature of side effects (200). The 10-keto derivative 58.**47b** has clinical potency comparable to that of imipramine (201, 202); however, it apparently lacks pronounced pharmacological properties (203). A 10-methyl derivative 58.**47c** is nearly equipotent with desipramine whereas the 2-hydroxy derivative 58.**47d** lacks significant activity in reversing the actions of a tetrabenazine-like compound in rats (184).

Nuclear disubstitution generally decreases antidepressant properties greatly. For example, the 2,8-dimethyl derivative 58.**47e** does not prevent sedation induced in rats by a tetrabenazine-related compound (184), and a 3,7-dichloro derivative 58.**47f** is practically inactive as an antidepressant (193).

Replacement of one of the benzo-fused rings in the imipramine tricyclic nucleus with a pyrido-fused system, i.e., 58.**48**, results in decreased tetrabenazine antagonist potency and increased toxicity (204).

Antidepressant structure–activity relationships of aminoalkylated dibenzazepines closely parallel those of their 10,11-dihydro counterparts. Clinically, 58.**49** has antianxiety and sedative properties in addition to moderate antidepressive actions. In dogs 58.**49** has about one-seventh the antiemetic potency of chlorpromazine, but it is essentially inactive in a conditioned escape response test in rats (205). It is as effective as desipramine in antagonizing reserpine-induced sedation in mice (199) and in potentiating the effects of norepinephrine and serotonin on the cat nictitating membrane (35). The secondary amine 58.**50a** and its 3-chloro derivative 58.**50b** reverse the effects of a tetrabenazine-related compound at slightly lower intraperitoneal doses than are required for their 10,11-dihydro counterparts, 58.**43a** and 58.**47a**. Unlike its 10,11-dihydro derivative, the 10-methyldibenzazepine 58.**50c** blocks, but does not reverse, benzoquinolizine-induced effects in rats; however, the 10,11-dimethyl congener 58.**50d** causes significant reversal.

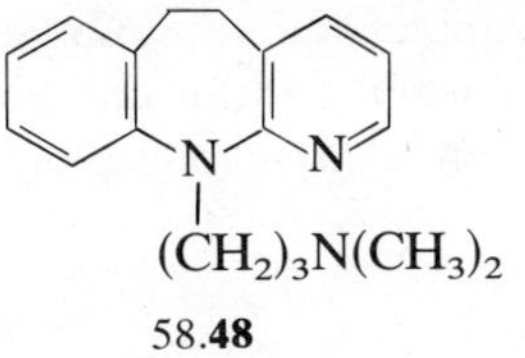

58.**48**

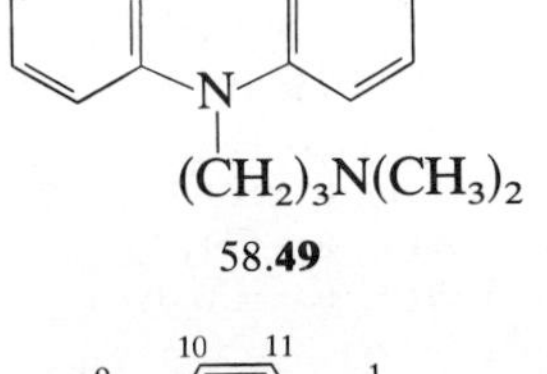

58.**49**

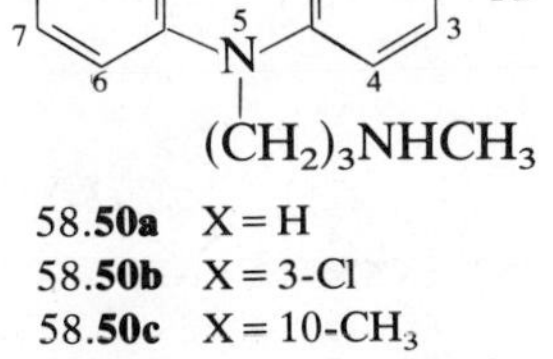

58.**50a**   X = H
58.**50b**   X = 3-Cl
58.**50c**   X = 10-CH$_3$
58.**50d**   X = 10,11-(CH$_3$)$_2$

Several piperazinylpropyl derivatives 58.**51** of dibenzazepine at intraperitoneal doses as high as 60 mg/kg are ineffective in preventing or reversing sedation induced in rats by a tetrabenazine-related compound (184). Opipramol (58.**51c**) slightly depresses motor activity and fighting behavior in mice. In acute tests it does not antagonize reserpine-induced ptosis or tetrabenazine-induced sedation; however, in chronic tests 58.**51c** antagonizes the reserpine-induced effect (206). In man, opipramol produces antianxiety and antidepressive actions (207).

Included among imipramine analogs of the type 58.**52** are various dibenzo[b, e][1,-4]diazepines (208–210), such as 58.**52a,** which is approximately equal in potency to imipramine as an antagonist of reserpine-induced effects in several animal species (210). Dibenzothiazepines, e.g., 58.**52b,** are also claimed (211) to have antidepressant properties. A benzothiazepinone 58.**53,** related to 58.**52b,** has an imipramine-like activity in animals; however, it is not effective in depressed patients (212). Several dibenzoxazepines, e.g., 58.**52c** and 58.**54a,** have significant antihistaminic actions (213); 58.**54a** also increases spontaneous

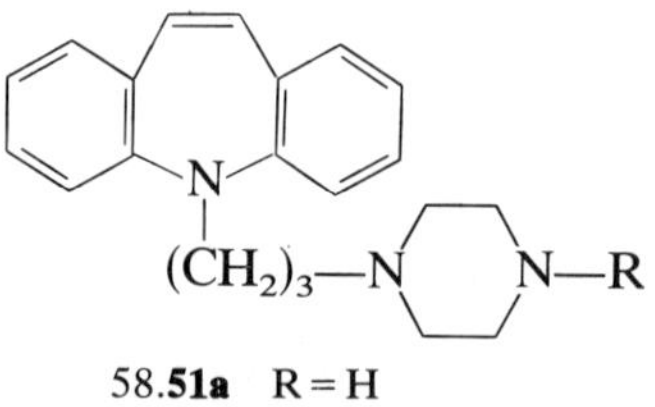

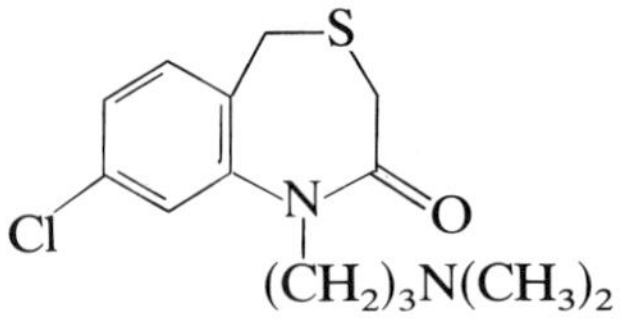

58.**53**

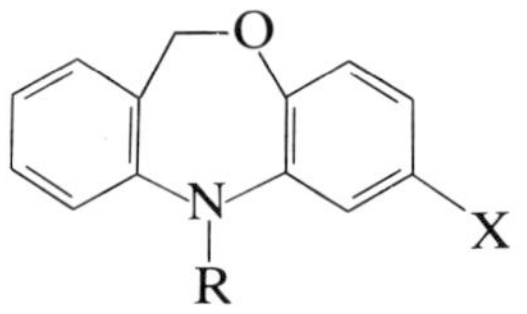

58.**54a**   X = H, R = $(CH_2)_2N(CH_3)_2$
58.**54b**   X = Cl, R = $CONH_2$

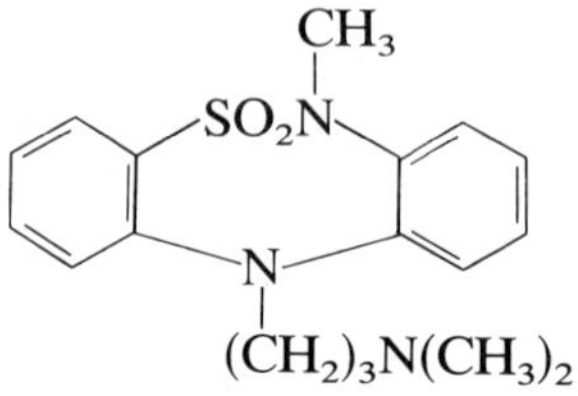

58.**55**

motor activity in rats (214). The related carbamide 58.**54b,** which causes imipramine-like effects in animals (215, 216), was well tolerated in preliminary clinical testing (217). Several dibenzothiadiazepines, e.g., 58.**55,** cause imipramine-like actions in animals (218).

4.2.2 DIBENZOCYCLOHEPTANES AND RELATED COMPOUNDS. Amitriptyline (58.**56a**) is the prototype of a group of aminoalkylated dibenzocycloheptanes (dibenzocycloheptadienes) with therapeutically useful antidepressant activity. The major pharmacological and clinical actions of amitriptyline are similar to those of imipramine (58.**2**) (219). On oral administration to mice, this clinically used antidepressant is about 1.6 times more potent than imipramine as a tetrabenazine antagonist, whereas it is somewhat less potent as a reserpine antagonist (66).

The secondary amine nortriptyline (58.**56b**), a metabolic product (221) of amitriptyline, retains the antibenzo-

58.**51a**   R = H
58.**51b**   R = CH_3
58.**51c**   R = $(CH_2)_2OH$

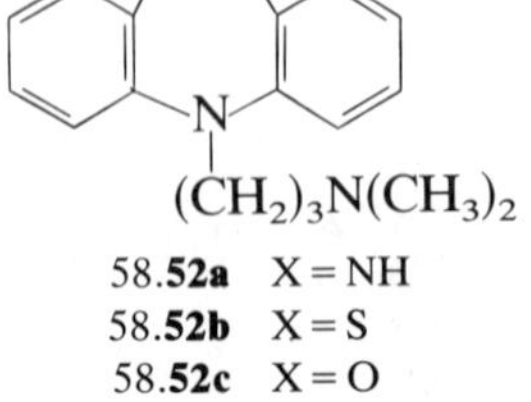

58.**52a**   X = NH
58.**52b**   X = S
58.**52c**   X = O

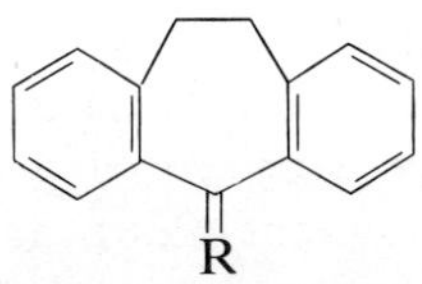

58.56

a R = CH(CH$_2$)$_2$N(CH$_3$)$_2$
b R = CH(CH$_2$)$_2$NHCH$_3$
c R = CHCH$_2$—N—CH$_3$

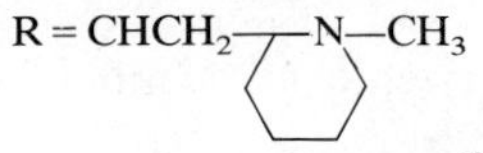

d R = CH(CH$_2$)$_2$N( )(C$_6$H$_5$)(CO$_2$C$_2$H$_5$)

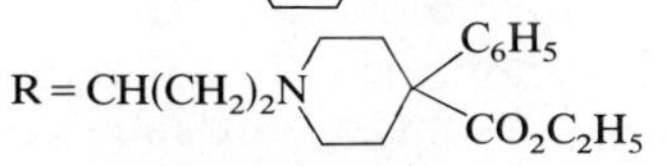

e R = CHCOCH$_2$N(CH$_3$)$_2$
f R = CHCOCH$_2$NHCH$_3$
g R = CHCH(OH)CH$_2$NHCH$_3$

h R = CH—( )(N—CH$_3$)(O)

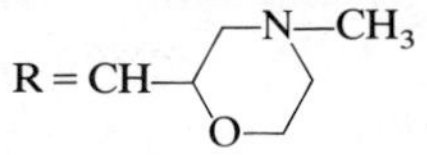

i R = ( )—N(CH$_3$)$_2$

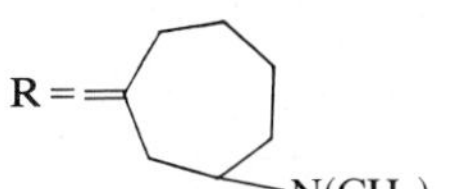

j R = NO(CH$_2$)$_2$N(CH$_3$)$_2$
k R = NO(CH$_2$)$_2$NHCH$_3$

quinolizine action of the parent (222) and is two to five times more potent as a clinical antidepressant (35). Nortriptyline is currently used as an antidepressant in the United States.

A number of amitriptyline derivatives having a modified side chain cause significant antidepressant actions. Thus 58.**56c** is a more potent antidepressant than amitriptyline (186) and 58.**56d** produces imipramine-like effects and analgesia in mice (223). Introduction of a carbonyl functionality into position 2 of the side chain of amitriptyline, i.e., 58.**56e,** has little influence on the pharmacological profile (224), whereas similar modification of nortriptyline affords a congener 58.**56f** having both antidepressant and antianxiety properties. The corresponding alcohol 58.**56g** has similar properties (225). Incorporation of the side chain into a morpholine ring, e.g., 58.**56h,** affords compounds claimed (226) to have potent antitetrabenazine activity. The dimethylaminocycloheptane de-

rivative 58.**56i** is less potent than imipramine in an L-dopa-potentiation test (227). The aminoethyloximino derivative noxiptiline (58.**56j**) is the most potent member of a series having pharmacological properties similar to those of amitriptyline, with perhaps a more favorable influence on mood (228). Surprisingly, the demethyl analog 58.**56k** of noxiptiline is less potent than its parent in reserpine antagonist tests and in depressed patients (229).

Amitriptyline also evokes CNS-depressant effects. It prolongs duration of thiopental-induced sleep, causes incoordination of muscle activity on a rotating rod, and produces hypothermia in mice. Several nuclear-substituted derivatives have been compared with amitriptyline in these tests. 3-Chloro substitution 58.**57a** enhances potency, whereas similar methyl substitution 58.**57b** decreases CNS-depressant actions (230). Also, the geometric isomers of 58.**57a** differ significantly in their ability to reduce spontaneous motor activity, to produce narcosis, and to block conditioned behavioral responses in animals (231). A series of partially hydrogenated analogs of amitriptyline, e.g., 58.**58,** antagonizes central benzoquinolizine-induced effects in rats (232). Several other amitriptyline analogs, 58.**59a** and 58.**59b**, benzothienocycloheptanes bearing an unsaturated piperidylidene side chain, have pharmacological properties

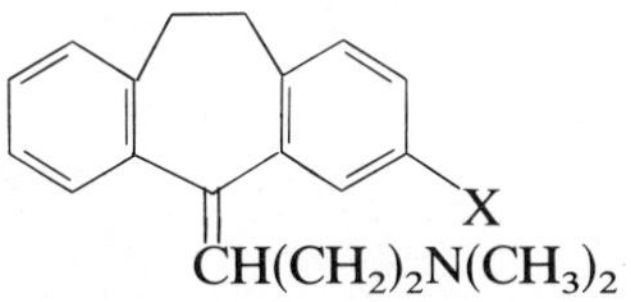

CH(CH$_2$)$_2$N(CH$_3$)$_2$
58.**57a**   X = Cl
58.**57b**   X = CH$_3$

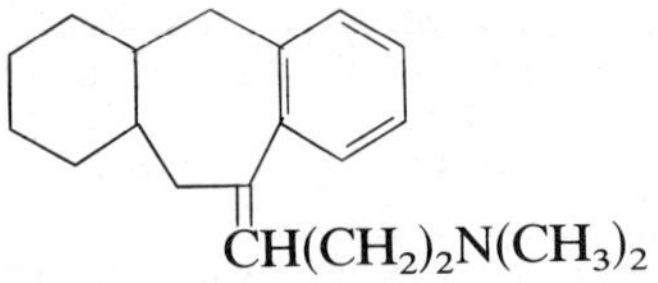

CH(CH$_2$)$_2$N(CH$_3$)$_2$
58.**58**

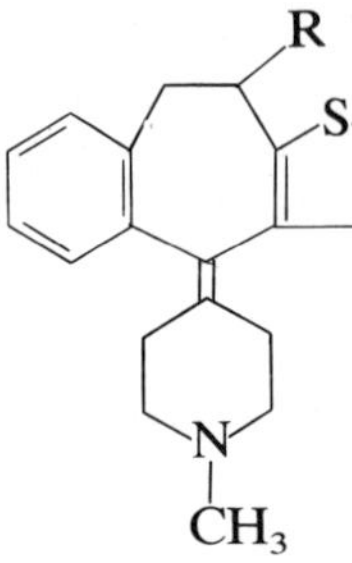

58.**59a** R = H
58.**59b** R = CH₃

shared by other antidepressants. Thus pizotifen (58.**59a**) produces imipramine-like effects (233); however, it is a potent central antagonist of serotonin and fails to inhibit norepinephrine reuptake *in vivo* (234, 235). The related 10-methyl derivative 58.**59b** shares some pharmacological properties with the serotonin antagonist cyproheptadine and the antidepressant mianserin (236).

Aminopropyl derivatives 58.**60** are generally less effective CNS depressants than their unsaturated counterparts (230, 237). For example, the analog 58.**60a** of amitriptyline is less potent than the parent (238). A related branched chain derivative butriptyline (58.**60b**) has a psychopharmacological profile similar to that of imipramine (239). In the clinic butriptyline has antianxiety and sedative properties in addition to antidepressant activity (240, 241). The side chain reduced analog 58.**60c** of nortrip-

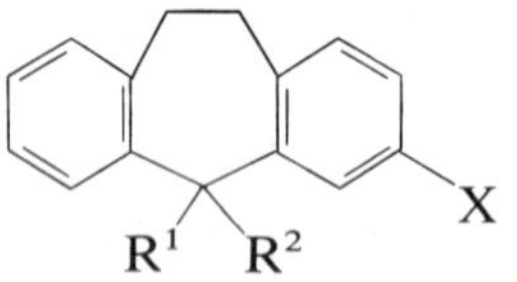

58.**60**

a X = R¹ = H, R² = (CH₂)₃N(CH₃)₂
b X = R¹ = H, R² = CH₂CH(CH₃)CH₂N(CH₃)₂
c X = R¹ = H, R² = (CH₂)₃NHCH₃
d X = Cl, R¹ = H, R² = (CH₂)₃NHCH₃
e X = R¹ = H, R² = O⟨ring⟩NCH₃
f X = H, R¹ = OH, R² = (CH₂)₃NHCH₃
g X = R¹ = H, R² = NH(CH₂)₆CO₂H

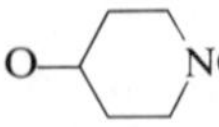

tyline is about 0.37 times as potent as its parent in a tetrabenazine-antagonism test in mice. The 3-chloro congener 58.**60d** is slightly less potent (238). The ether hepzidine (58.**60e**) is moderately effective in an antireserpine test in mice (242). A benzopyridocycloheptane tropanyl ether somewhat related to hepzidine inhibits the uptake of biogenic catecholamines by rat brain synaptosomes (243). 5-Hydroxyl dibenzocycloheptane derivatives, e.g., 58.**60f,** uniformly lack significant CNS activity (230). The amino acid 58.**60g** increases locomotor activity in mice, competitively inhibits dopamine uptake, and causes a release at low concentrations. At higher concentrations it has similar effects on norepinephrine and serotonin uptake and release mechanisms (244).

Several novel bridged-ring ether derivatives of amitriptyline cause very powerful antidepressant actions (220). The potencies of these compounds relative to that of amitriptyline in a tetrabenazine-antagonism test are presented in Table 58.5. The stereochemical configuration of the 11 substituent is very important. Maximum activity is observed when the substituent (Table 58.5, R = OH or NH₂) is trans to the ether bridge. Preliminary clinical studies indicate depressed patients receiving 8–24 mg of the trans-hydroxyl derivative (Table 58.5, R = *trans*-OH; R¹ = H) are improved and are more stimulated than patients receiving a daily dose of 150 mg of amitriptyline (245). The corresponding cis isomers, although still more potent than amitriptyline, are many times less effective than the trans compounds. An 11-keto derivative and the corresponding oxime are also potent antagonists of tetrabenazine-induced depression in mice (220).

Several amitriptyline congeners, e.g., 58.**61** (246), 58.**62** (247), and 58.**63** (248), involving substitution of position 4 of the dibenzocycloheptane system have insignificant activity in reserpine-antagonism tests in mice.

Table 58.5 Antitetrabenazine Potency of Bridged-Ring Ether Derivatives in the Dibenzo-cycloheptane Series (220)

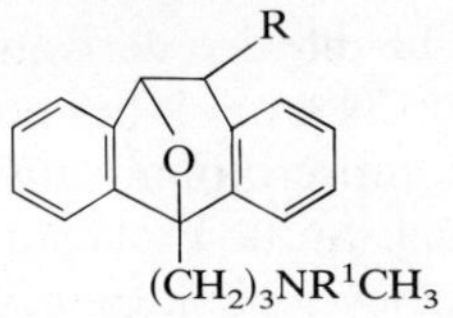

R

O

$(CH_2)_3NR^1CH_3$

R	R^1	Relative Amitriptyline Potency[a]
cis-OH	CH_3	2
trans-OH	CH_3	26
cis-OH	H	1.1
trans-OH	H	110
=O	CH_3	7.2
=NOH	CH_3	60
trans-NH_2	CH_3	31

[a] Relative amitriptyline potency was calculated by dividing the ED_{50}(mg/kg, p.o.) for amitriptyline in the tetrabenazine-antagonism test (238) in mice by the corresponding value for the indicated compound.

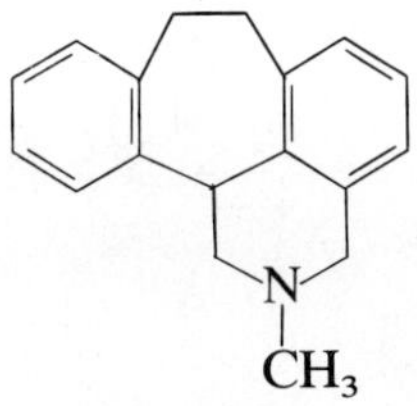

CH_3

58.**63**

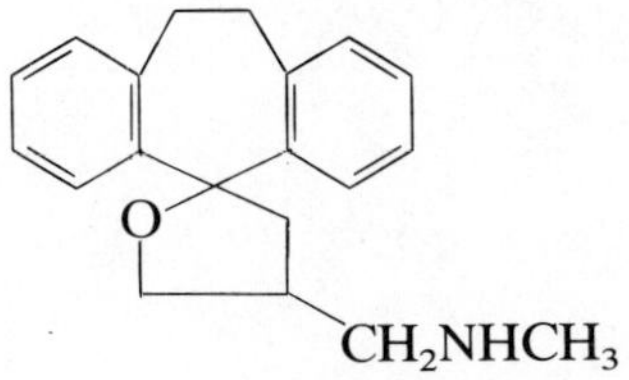

O

CH_2NHCH_3

58.**64**

Cl

N

CH_3

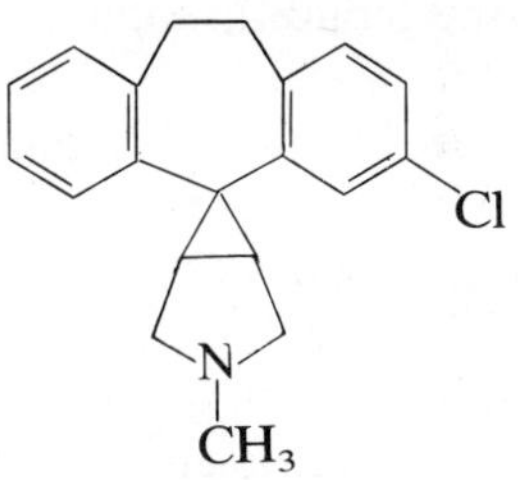

58.**65**

Other amitriptyline derivatives in which the dibenzocycloheptane nucleus and the side chain are joined in a spiro fashion have significant antidepressant properties. The tetrahydrofurfurylamine 58.**64,** one of a series, has potency comparable to that of

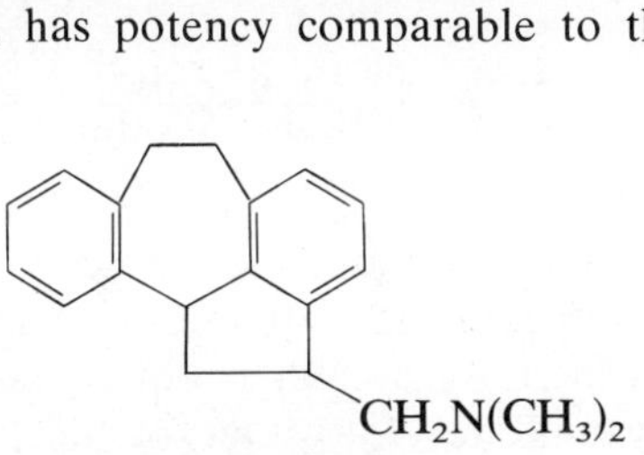

$CH_2N(CH_3)_2$

58.**61**

CH_2

$CH_2N(CH_3)_2$

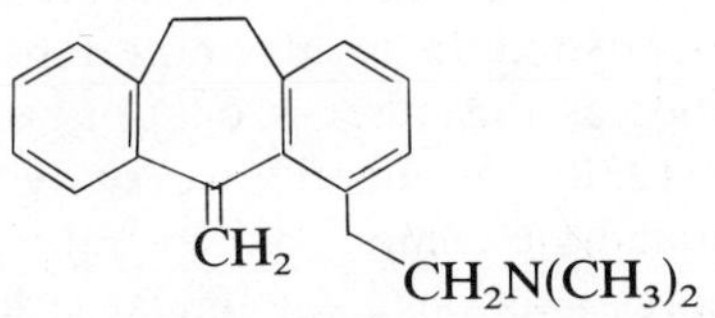

58.**62**

desipramine in tests for prevention of reserpine-induced ptosis in mice and tetrabenazine-induced depression in rats, but it is less effective in preventing oxotremorine-induced hypothermia in mice (249). A novel spirocyclopropyl derivative 58.**65** (stereochemistry not established) has marked imipramine-like activity in dopa and serotonin interaction tests in mice (227).

Two other amitriptyline relatives in which the side chain is incorporated into a bridge between positions 5 and 10 of the dibenzocycloheptane system have been examined for antidepressant activity. One of these, 58.**66,** has a pharmacological profile (250, 251) similar to that of imipramine and is effective in some patients with endogenous depression (252). Another, 58.**67,** inhibits norepinephrine uptake by rat vas deferens. It also increases motor

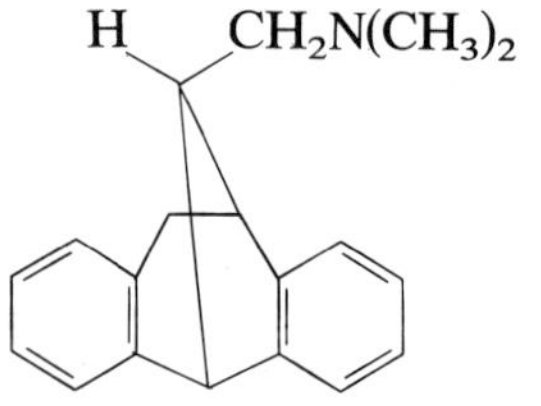

58.**66**

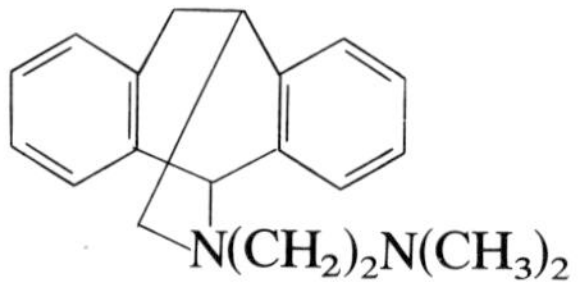

N(CH$_2$)$_2$N(CH$_3$)$_2$

58.**67**

activity, but does not prevent tetrabenazine-induced catalepsy in mice (253).

The dibenzocycloheptene analog 58.**68a** of amitriptyline has clinical antidepressant and sedative activities (254). This introduction of a 10,11 double bond into nortriptyline enhances antidepressant potency as measured in a tetrabenazine antagonism test in mice (238). In this test 58.**68b** is about 1.4 times as effective as nortriptyline whereas the primary amine 58.**68c** is practically equipotent. Conversely, the piperazine 58.**68d** is less than $\frac{1}{45}$ as potent in the same test. An allenic derivative 58.**68e,** whose conformation has been studied by X-ray crystallographic methods (255), has both CNS-depressant and antidepressant properties in animal tests,

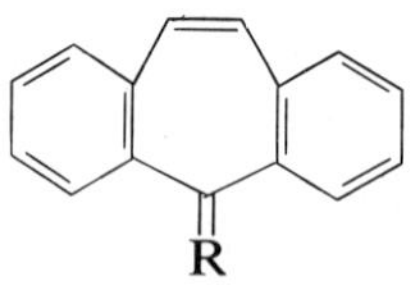

58.**68**

a   R = CH(CH$_2$)$_2$N(CH$_3$)$_2$
b   R = CH(CH$_2$)$_2$NHCH$_3$
c   R = CH(CH$_2$)$_2$NH$_2$
d   R = CH(CH$_2$)$_2$N□NH
e   R = C = CHCH$_2$N(CH$_3$)$_2$
f   R = =□NCH$_3$

thereby suggesting potential clinical utility for the treatment of anxiety and depression (256). A piperidylidene derivative cyproheptadine (58.**68f**), as well as the corresponding 10,11-dihydro derivative, has little effect on the CNS, but it has potent antihistaminic and antiserotonin activity (257).

Nuclear substitution of the antidepressant dibenzocycloheptatrienes decreases their effectiveness. The difference in potency of the resulting geometrical isomers, however, is noteworthy. Thus, in an antitetrabenazine test the cis isomer (258) of 58.**69a** is about 0.6 times as potent as the unsubstituted compound, whereas the trans isomer is less than $\frac{1}{60}$ as potent. The nuclear-substituted tertiary amine 58.**69b** has a pharmacological profile suggestive of combined antidepressant and neuroleptic properties. Its potency in reserpine and tetrabenazine antagonist tests is approximately equivalent to that of amitriptyline.

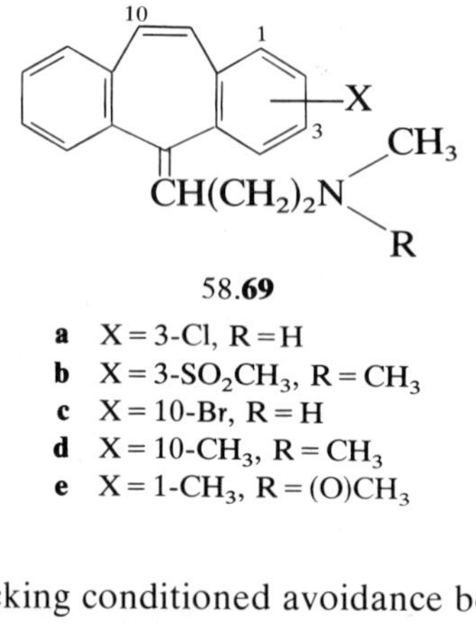

58.**69**

a   X = 3-Cl, R = H
b   X = 3-SO$_2$CH$_3$, R = CH$_3$
c   X = 10-Br, R = H
d   X = 10-CH$_3$, R = CH$_3$
e   X = 1-CH$_3$, R = (O)CH$_3$

In blocking conditioned avoidance behavior and antagonizing apomorphine-induced emesis in dogs, 58.**69b** is equipotent with chlorpromazine (259). One of the isomers of the 10-bromo derivative 58.**69c** is about two-thirds as potent as the unsubstituted compound 58.**68b** in an antitetrabenazine test whereas the other is only one-sixth as potent (238). A quantitative study of the anticholinergic action of several tricyclic antidepressants on a rat fundal strip indicates the 10-methyl derivative 58.**69d** is most potent (260). The 1-methyl *N*-oxide (58.**69e**) is at least as effective as imipramine in depressed patients (261, 262).

In this series of dibenzocycloheptene (dibenzocycloheptatriene) derivatives, reduction of the olefinic side chain often enhances antidepressant activity. Thus protriptyline (58.**70a**), the side chain-reduced counterpart of 58.**68b,** is 9–10 times more potent than amitriptyline as a tetrabenazine antagonist in mice (238), and it has enhanced clinical activity without causing as much sedation (263). Protriptyline is currently used clinically. The corresponding primary amine is nearly equipotent with nortriptyline. 3-Substitution of protriptyline generally decreases antitetrabenazine actions. The 3-sulfonamide 58.**70b** is about 0.6 times as effective as protriptyline, whereas the chlorine- (58.**70c**) and sulfone-substituted (58.**70d**) congeners are considerably less potent (238).

A 3-aminocyclohexenyl-substituted dibenzocycloheptene 58.**71** is equipotent with imipramine in an L-dopa-potentiation test (227). A spiro-4-aminocyclohexenyl derivative 58.**72** inhibits uptake of norepinephrine and serotonin and lacks anticholinergic activity in animals (264).

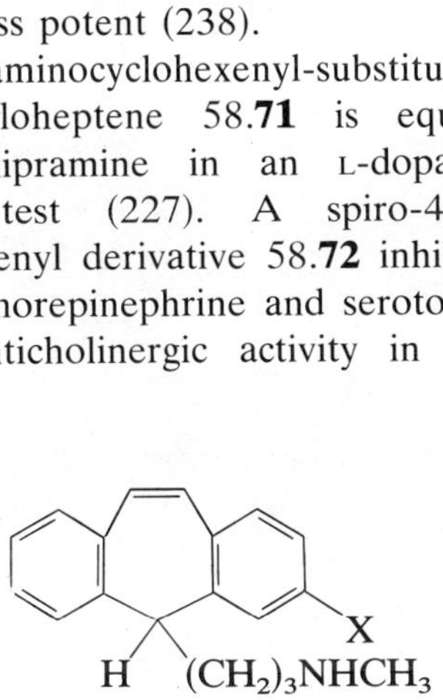

NH$_2$

58.**72**

CH(CH$_2$)$_2$NHCH$_3$

58.**73**

CH(CH$_2$)$_2$N(CH$_3$)$_2$

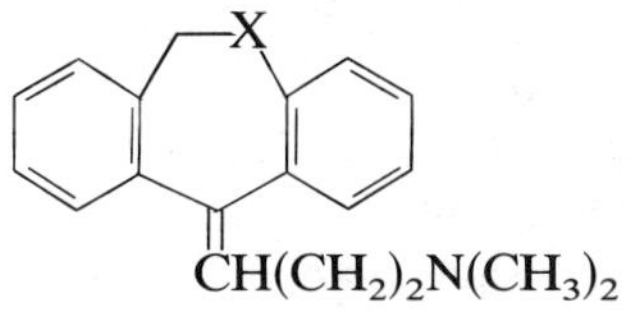

58.**74**

a	X = O	**d**	X = SO$_2$
b	X = S	**e**	X = NH
c	X = SO	**f**	X = NCH$_3$

Incorporation of the 9,10-ethylene bridge of nortriptyline into a cyclopropane affords octriptyline (58.**73**), which has amitriptyline-like properties in animals (265).

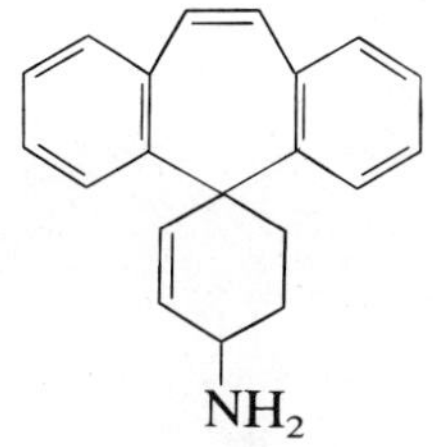

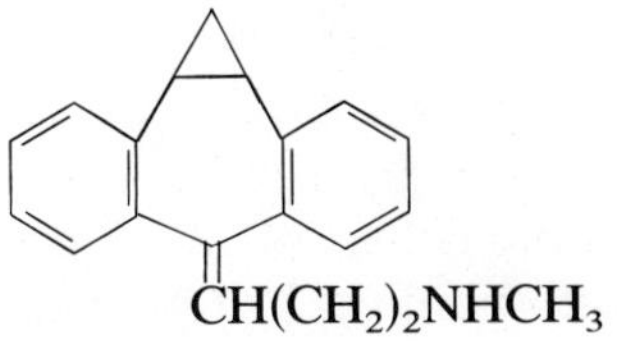

Several amitriptyline analogs with the general structure 58.**74** are clinically effective antidepressants. Doxepin (58.**74a**), a mixture of geometric isomers, has antidepressant activity comparable to that of amitripytline, but it is more sedating. It is particularly useful in the treatment of agitated depressed patients (266–268) and is currently in clinical use. Both the trans (269) and cis isomers have antidepressant actions in animals (270). Doxepin is somewhat less effective than amitriptyline in a test for stimulant activity in pigeons, whereas the corresponding secondary amine is approximately equipotent with the parent (271). The cis isomer 58.**74a** potentiates amphetamine-induced responses and produces neuroleptic effects in animals. It

H   (CH$_2$)$_3$NHCH$_3$

58.**70a** X = H
58.**70b** X = SO$_2$N(CH$_3$)$_2$
58.**70c** X = Cl
58.**70d** X = SO$_2$CH$_3$

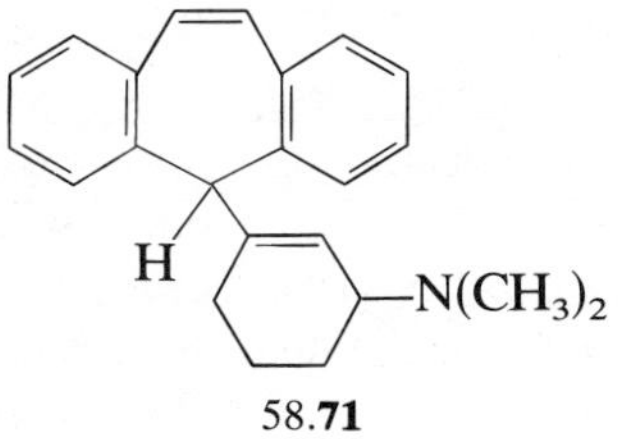

H   —N(CH$_3$)$_2$

58.**71**

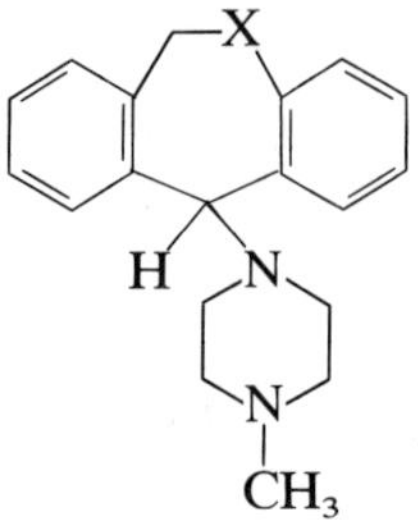

58.**75a** X = O
58.**75b** X = S

also has antidepressant activity in man (272). Introduction of a chlorine substituent into position 2 of 58.**74a**, particularly in the cis isomer, affords compounds with marked neuroleptic activity (270).

The piperazinyl-substituted dibenzoxepin 58.**75a** is somewhat less potent than amitriptyline upon oral administration to rats in an antireserpine test (273).

Antidepressant activity is also produced by dibenzo[b, e]thiepins, e.g., prothiadene (58.**74b**), related to amitriptyline. In animals, prothiadene causes weak depression of the CNS, inhibits the action of reserpine, and has marked antihistaminic properties. Nuclear substitution of prothiadene with halogen or alkyl groups decreases antireserpine potency in rats (274). A 3,8-difluoro congener retains the depressant properties of prothiadene but lacks significant antireserpine activity (275). CNS depression, prothiadene-like antireserpine actions, potent antihistaminic, and antiserotonergic properties are produced by the piperidylidenyl dibenzothiepin perithiadene (58.**76**) (274). The secondary amine (northiadene) derived from prothiadene, as

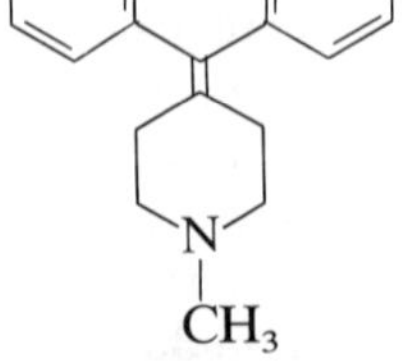

58.**76**

well as the dihydro derivative (hydrothiadene, 58.**77a**), the corresponding 2-bromo compound 58.**77b**, and a diethylaminoethyl ether of dibenzothiepin 58.**77c** are prothiadene-like antagonists of reserpine-induced ptosis in mice. The piperazinyldibenzothiepin 58.**75b** is also a potent central depressant and antagonist of reserpine-induced effects (254).

The dibenzothiepin S-oxide 58.**74c** has weaker antireserpine activity than prothiadene (58.**74b**) and lacks significant sedative properties, but it is a potent antihistaminic (276). The sulfone 58.**74d** potentiates subhypnotic doses of ethanol and blocks conditioned avoidance response behavior in mice and rats although less effectively than does amitriptyline (277). One of a series of morphanthridines (278, 279) related to 58.**74e** and 58.**74f**, i.e., 58.**78**, produces stimulant, rather than antidepressant, actions in the clinic (280). The tertiary amine 58.**74f** also causes stimulation in depressed patients (281).

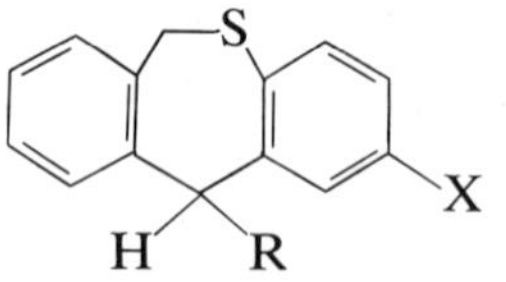

58.**77a** X = H, R = (CH$_2$)$_3$N(CH$_3$)$_2$
58.**77b** X = Br, R = (CH$_2$)$_3$N(CH$_3$)$_2$
58.**77c** X = H, R = O(CH$_2$)$_2$N(C$_2$H$_5$)$_2$

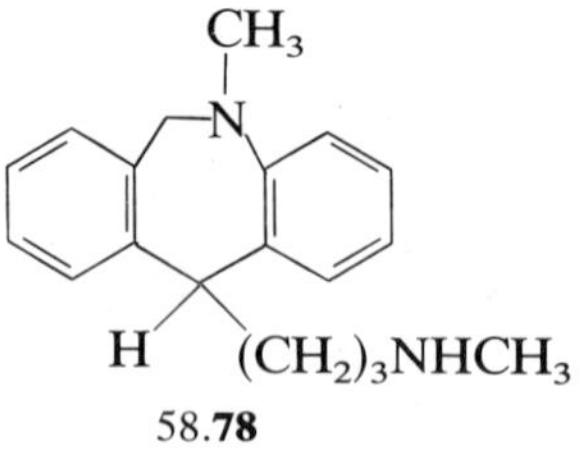

58.**78**

4.2.3 OTHER TRICYCLIC ANTIDEPRESSANTS WITH A SEVEN-MEMBERED CENTRAL RING. In this general classification are considered antidepressant 6–7–6 compounds in which the basic side chain is attached to the two- or, in rare instances, a three- atom bridge of the seven-membered central ring. This includes a group of 10-aminoalkyl derivatives of 10,11-dihydrodibenz[*b, e*]azepine, e.g., 58.**79a** and related diazepines, 58.**79b** and 58.**79c**, thiazepines, 58.**79d**, and oxazepines, 58.**79e**.

A large number of azepines, e.g., propazepine (58.**79a**), has been synthesized and studied pharmacologically (254, 282–285). Propazepine has potent antihistaminic and local anesthetic activity in guinea pigs (282). In other tests this compound resembles imipramine. In man, propazepine is better tolerated, but only one-half as potent as imipramine (254).

The prototype of a novel class of antidepressant dibenzazepines, in which a side chain is incorporated into an additional ring, is mianserin (58.**80a**). Originally selected for clinical study on the basis of its electroencephalographic profile in normal volunteers (86), mianserin is especially effective in endogenous depression (286–291). Subsequent clinical and pharmacological studies indicate mianserin has a different profile from that of conventional tricyclic antidepressants (292). It seems to lack anticholinergic and cardiotoxic proper-

ties, and causes unusual effects on monoamine metabolism. Mianersin increases, whereas imipramine-like antidepressants reduce, brain norepinephrine (293). More recent *in vitro* studies, however, reveal antidepressant actions, e.g., potentiation of norepinephrine, and blockade of norepinephrine and serotonin uptake (75, 294, 295). *In vivo*, mianserin has little effect on catecholamine and serotonin uptake, which is consistent with its inability to block tyramine-induced effects in humans (296). An increase in turnover of catecholamines appears to be a specific action of 58.**80a** (61).

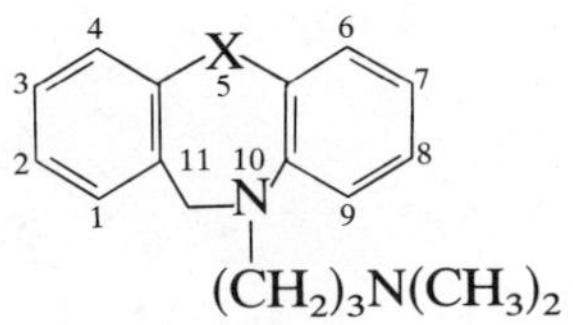

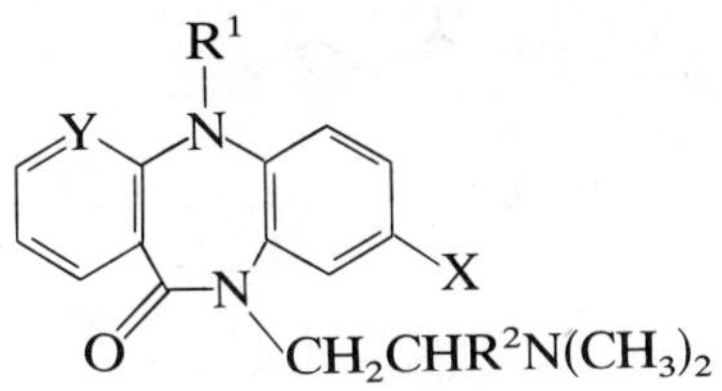

58.**81**

a $R^1 = R^2 = X = H$, $Y = CH$
b $R^1 = CH_3$, $R^2 = X = H$, $Y = CH$
c $R^1 = CH_3$, $R^2 = H$, $X = SO_2C_2H_5$, $Y = CH$
d $R^1 = X = H$, $R^2 = CH_3$, $Y = N$

The oxazepine congeners, 58.**80b** and 58.**80c**, of mianserin (58.**80a**) also produce EEG profiles suggestive of antidepressant activity in normal volunteers (86). In depressed patients 58.**80b** has antidepressant efficacy equivalent to that of amitriptyline (297).

Several dibenzodiazepines, e.g., 58.**79b** and 58.**79c**, are inhibitors of pseudocholinesterase (209). Related aminoethyl derivatives of 11-diazepinones, e.g., 58.**81a**, are potent antihistaminic agents with antianaphylactic properties (298). Dibenzepine (58.**81b**) has gained clinical acceptance in Europe as a selective antidepressant with mood-elevating actions (299, 300). It is noteworthy that in this series antidepressant properties are associated with a two-carbon spacing between the tricycle and the basic amino

$(CH_2)_3N(CH_3)_2$
58.**79**

a $X = CH_2$ d $X = S$
b $X = NH$ e $X = O$
c $X = NCH_3$

CH_3

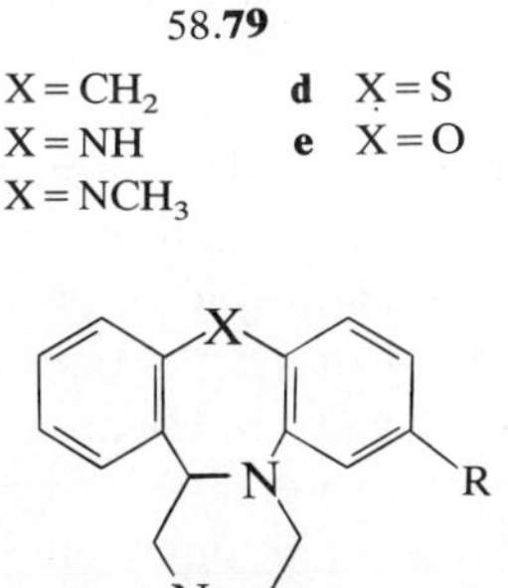

58.**80a** $X = CH_2$, $R = H$
58.**80b** $X = O$, $R = CH_3$
58.**80c** $X = O$, $R = H$

group instead of the usual propylene bridge (301). An ethylsulfonyl analog 58.**81c** of dibenzepine also causes imipramine-like effects in animals (302). A pyridobenzo-diazepine relative propizepine (58.**81d**) of dibenzepine is effective in various animal tests for antidepressants; it has clinical activity (303).

Two aminopropyl derivatives of dibenzo-[d, f][1, 3]diazepin-6-one, 58.**82a** and 58.**82b**, produce an EEG pattern suggestive of antidepressant activity in normal volunteers (304).

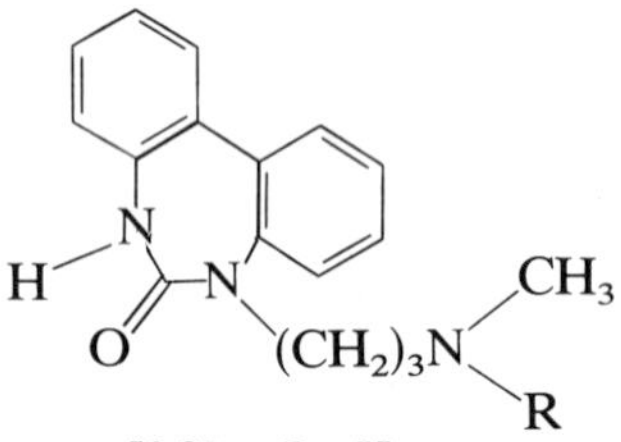

58.**82a**　R = H
58.**82b**　R = CH₃

Several dibenzo[b,f][1,4]thiazepines (254, 305), e.g., 58.**79d** and 58.**83a**, have neurotropic properties. In mice, reserpine-induced hypothermia and ptosis are antagonized in a comparable manner by 58.**83a**, imipramine, and desipramine; however, unlike the dibenzazepines 58.**83a** does not augment amphetamine effects (306). The related tertiary amine 58.**83b** has little activity on the CNS (254). Several 11-substituted congeners, 58.**84a** and 58.**84b**, are antagonists of serotonin; 58.**84a** antagonizes the ulcerogenic effect of reserpine in rats (307).

Dibenz[b, f][1, 4]oxazepines, e.g. 58.**79e**, generally have little effect on the CNS,

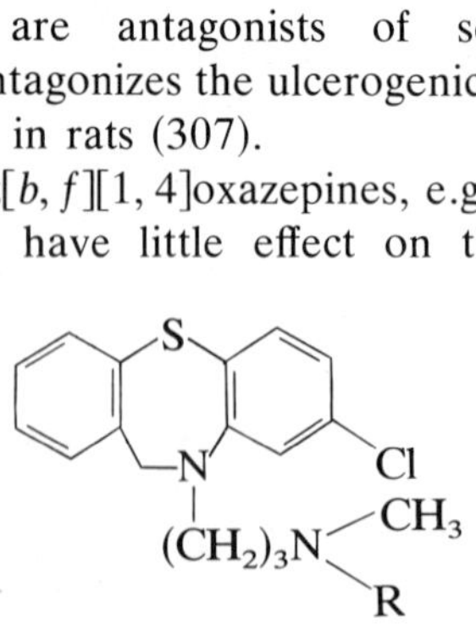

58.**83a**　R = H
58.**83b**　R = CH₃

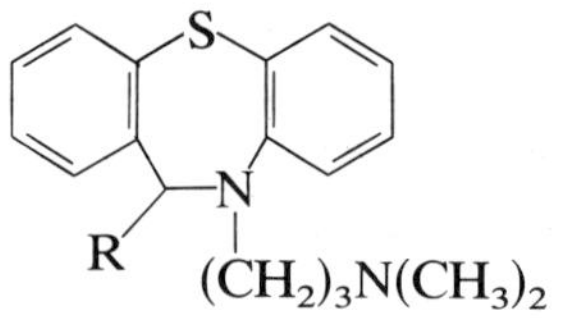

58.**84a**　R = CH₃
58.**84b**　R = C₆H₅

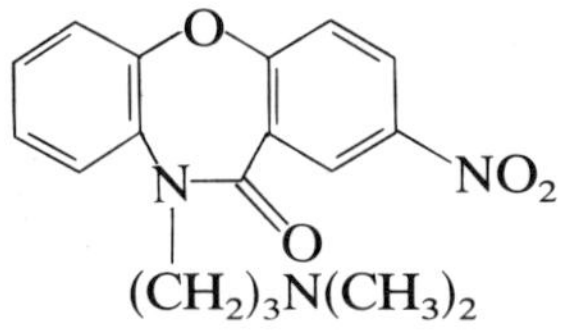

58.**85**

although some of these compounds have slight CNS-depressant, antiserotonin, antihistaminic, and antispasmodic properties (254, 308). Antidepressant activity comparable to that of imipramine is observed with the oxazepinone sintamil (58.**85**) (309).

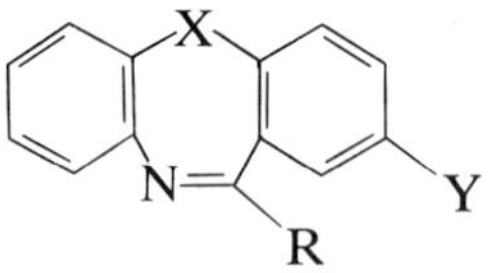

58.**86**　X = NCH₃, S, O

a　Y = H, R = N‾‾NCH₃

b　X = O, Y = Cl, R = N‾‾NH

c　Y = H, R = (CH₂)₃N(CH₃)₂

Various 11-substituted derivatives of 5H-dibenzo[b, e][1, 4]diazepines, as well as related thiazepines and oxazepines, have significant psychotropic actions. N-Methyl-piperazinyl-substituted compounds, e.g., 58.**86a** (X = NCH₃, S, O), are potent neuroleptics (see Chapter 56); however, the related unsubstituted piperazine amoxapine (58.**86b**, X = O) is an effective antidepressant in the clinic (310, 311).

Some related 11-dimethylaminopropyl-substituted derivatives, 58.**86c**, and corresponding 10,11-dihydro analogs, 58.**87**, pro-

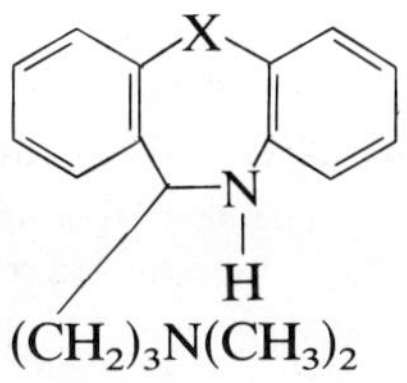

58.**87**   X = NCH₃, S, O

duce characteristic antidepressant responses, such as norepinephrine potentiation and increased motor activity, in mice.

In rats, 58.**86a** (X = S), has potency comparable to that of imipramine as an antagonist of tetrabenazine-induced ptosis and catalepsy (312).

CNS-depressant effects are produced by 10-substituted dibenzo[b, f]thiepins and the oxepins 58.**88** (254). Thiepinone (58.**89**) is not only a depressant, but also has antireserpine activity (313).

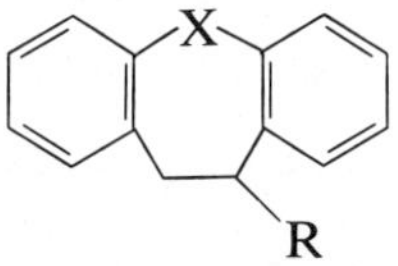

58.**88**   X = S, O

R = NCH₃, O(CH₂)₂N(CH₃)₂

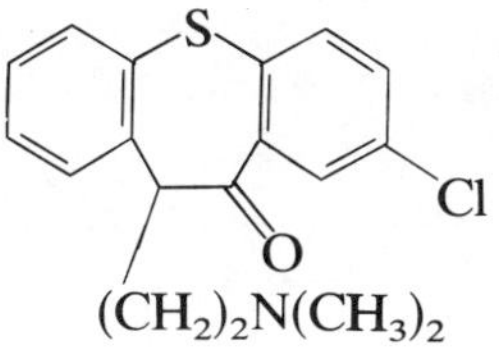

58.**89**

4.2.4 TRICYCLIC ANTIDEPRESSANTS WITH A SIX-MEMBERED CENTRAL RING. In general, antidepressant action among tricyclic compounds with a six-membered central ring is associated with structural modifications that may hinder the ring system (or perhaps only a vital portion of the nucleus) from attaining a planar stereochemical conformation.

For example, melitracene (58.**90**) (314–316), a 9,9-dimethyldihydroanthracene,

and the corresponding dimethylacridan (dimethacrin) 58.**91a** (317) are clinically effective antidepressants. Dimethacrin is equipotent with imipramine as a reserpine or benzoquinolizine antagonist in mice and rats (318). A related dimethylaminoethyl-thiocarbamate 58.**91b** has combined anti-parkinsonian and antidepressant properties (319). In these molecules the methyl groups in position 9 prevent interaction of the tricyclic nucleus with a planar surface.

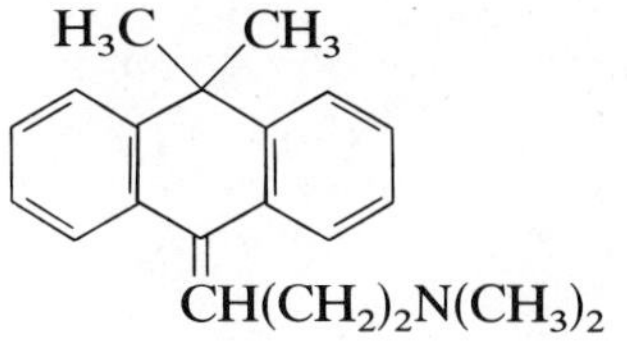

58.**90**

Some other 9-substituted 6–6–6 tricyclic compounds also possess significant antidepressant activity, although it is not clear that all these structures are prohibited from attaining a planar conformation. Thus a series of acridones 58.**92a–c** produces imipramine-like activity in animals (320). The influence of 58.**92c** on central biogenic amine levels (321), as well as its absorption, distribution, and excretion (322), was investigated in mice and rats. It has a stimulant action in animals and is a clinically effective antidepressant (323).

Comprehensive pharmacological examination of a 9-methyldihydroanthracene fluotracen (58.**93a**) suggests a combination of antidepressant and antipsychotic actions (66). Based on quantitative pharmaco-EEG studies in humans, low doses of fluotracen cause neuroleptic-like actions, whereas at

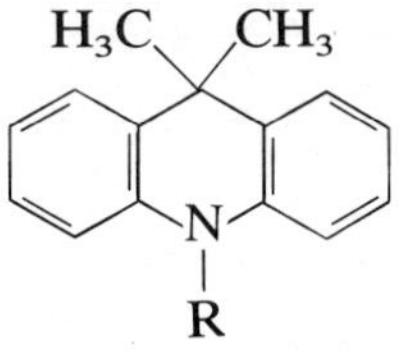

58.**91a**   R = (CH₂)₃N(CH₃)₂
58.**91b**   R = COS(CH₂)₂N(CH₃)₂

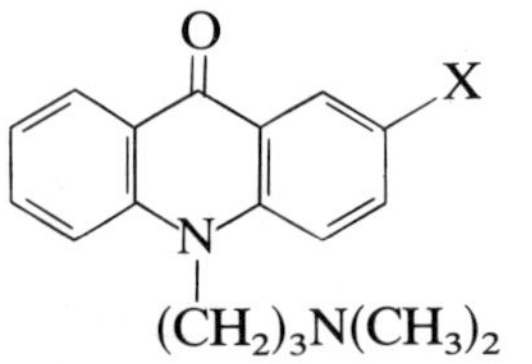

58.**92a**   X = H
58.**92b**   X = OCH$_3$
58.**92c**   X = Cl

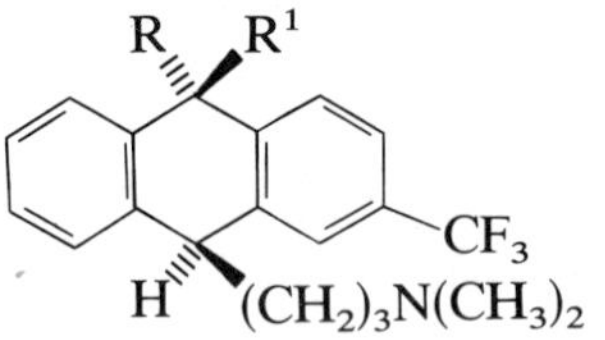

58.**93a**   R = H, R^1 = CH$_3$
58.**93b**   R = R^1 = H
58.**93c**   R = R^1 = CH$_3$

higher doses antidepressant type effects are seen. Clinically, fluotracen has a particularly rapid onset of action with relatively minor side effects (324, 325). From a SAR standpoint the pharmacological profile of fluotracen is of particular interest. The related 10-demethyl derivative 58.**93b** has a full range of neuroleptic properties and is considerably more potent than chlorpromazine in many tests used to assess this type of activity. Conversely, the 10,10-dimethylated dihydroanthracene 58.**93c** only weakly antagonizes reserpine-induced ptosis in mice and apparently has little or no neuroleptic activity (326). Another 9-substituted dihydroanthracene, danitracen (58.**94**), is a very potent, clinically effective

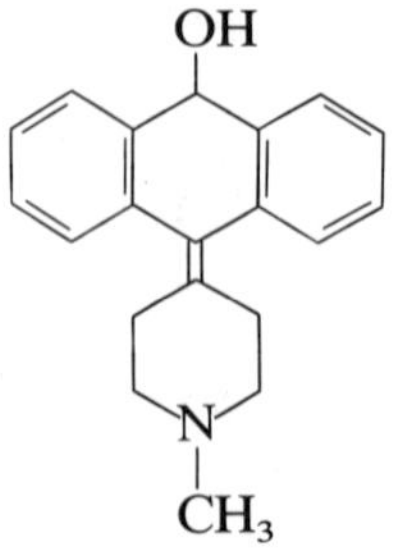

58.**94**

antidepressant (327, 328). In animal experiments it has pronounced sedative, anti-aggressive, anxiolytic (329), antihistaminic, antiserotonergic, and anticholinergic actions (330). Danitracen also antagonizes the action of oxotremorine (331) and a 5-hydroxytryptophan-induced syndrome (72).

A number of 9,10-alkylene bridged derivatives of 9,10-dihydroanthracene have meaningful antidepressant activity. The ethano-bridged compound maprotiline (58.**95a**) produces imipramine-like effects in dogs (332); it also blocks rat synaptosomal uptake of norepinephrine (333), but has little effect on serotonin systems (334). Extensive pharmacological and clinical examination of maprotiline (335) supports its antidepressant efficacy (336–339). A related methano-bridged derivative 58.**95b** has the characteristic pharmacological profile of an antidepressant (340). Side chain-modified congeners of 58.**95a** and 58.**95b** produce antidepressant-like actions.

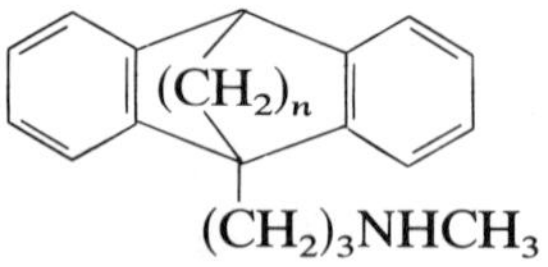

58.**95a**   n = 2
58.**95b**   n = 1

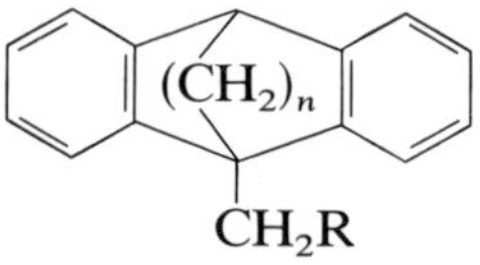

58.**96a**   n = 2, R = CHOHCH$_2$NHCH$_3$

58.**96b**   n = 2, R =

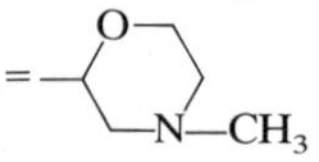

58.**96c**   n = 1, R = CH$_2$NHCH$_3$

Thus the side chain-hydroxylated derivative 58.**96a** of maprotiline is a potent and selective inhibitor of norepinephrine in rat brain; it has no effect on serotonin uptake (341). Tetrabenazine-antagonist and norepinephrine-potentiating actions are claimed for a related morpholine 55.**96b** (342), whereas antihistaminic, antiserotonergic, and anticholinergic properties are claimed for 58.**96c** (343).

Alterations of antipsychotic phenothiazine derivatives so that attainment of a conformation capable of interacting with a planar surface is hindered or prohibited often transforms activity from neuroleptic to antidepressant. Substitution of position 1 of the 3-dimethylaminopropyl side chain of chlorpromazine, a modification inducing a steric interaction with the *peri* hydrogens in positions 1 and 9 of the nucleus to deter a planar conformation of the tricycle, invariably decreases neuroleptic activity and sometimes affords antidepressant compounds. For example, incorporation of position 1 of the side chain into a cyclopropane ring results in 58.**97**, a compound without significant conditioned avoidance blocking activity in rats, but which has marked imipramine-like activity. It prevents reserpine-induced ptosis in rats at about one-fifth the dose required for amitriptyline (344). Related cyclopropyl-substituted phenoxazines and acridans likewise are antagonists of reserpine-induced effects in rats. The *trans*-cyclobutyl congener 58.**98** is less potent than 58.**97**, but it does prevent reserpine-induced ptosis

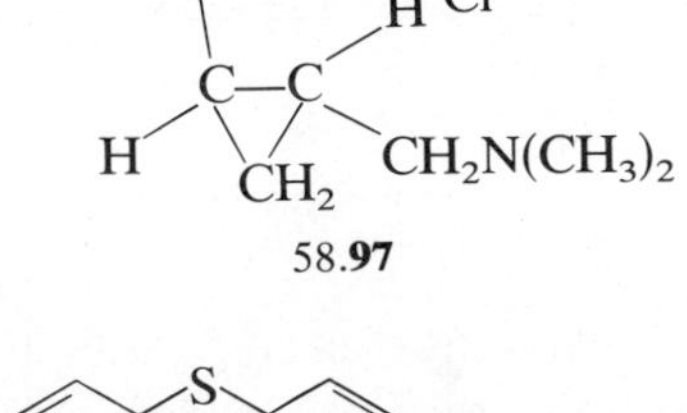

58.**99a**   X = H, R = —⟨ ⟩NCH$_3$

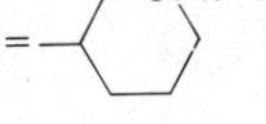

58.**99b**   X = CH$_3$, R = —⟨ ⟩N-n-C$_3$H$_7$

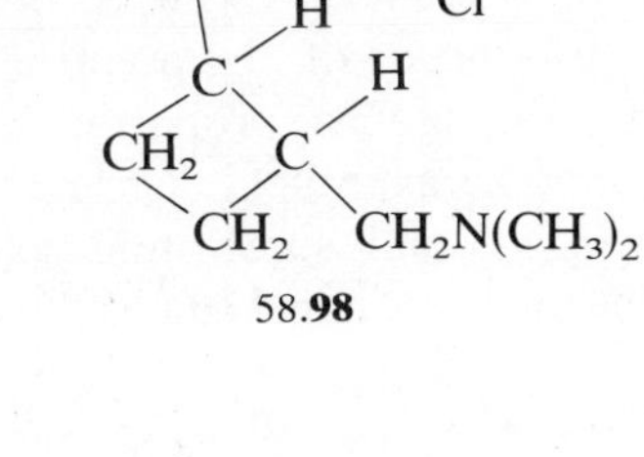

CO(CH$_2$)$_2$N(C$_2$H$_5$)$_2$

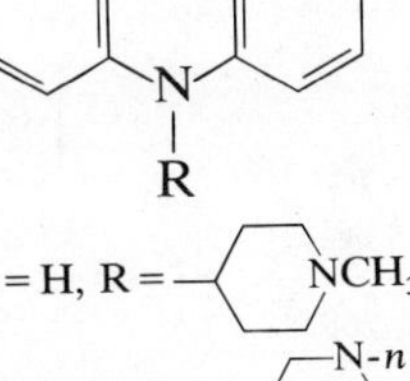

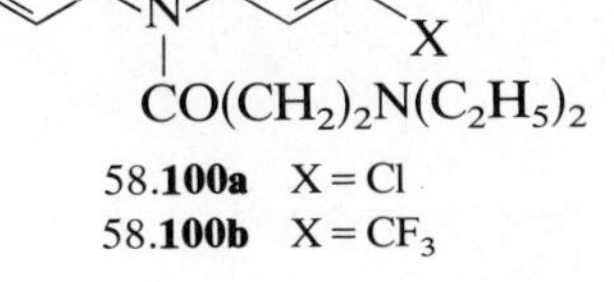

58.**100a**   X = Cl
58.**100b**   X = CF$_3$

COS(CH$_2$)$_2$N(i-C$_3$H$_7$)$_2$

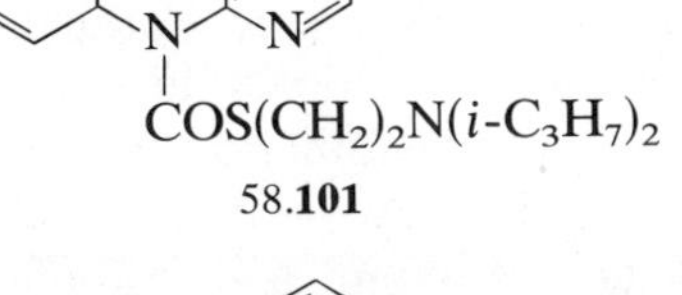

58.**101**

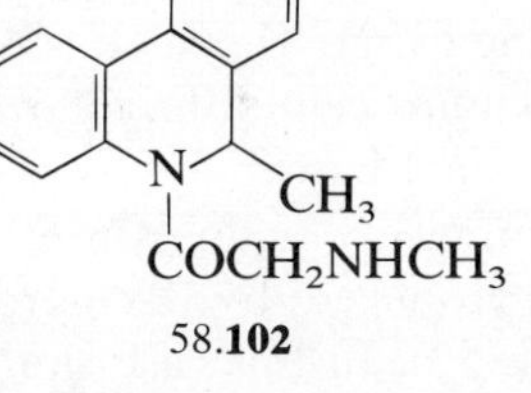

58.**102**

in rats (344). Chlorpromazine-blocking activity is caused by some piperidinyl-substituted phenothiazines, e.g., 58.**99a** and 58.**99b** (345). Clinical antidepressant activity is produced by chlorpromazine analogs bearing a carbonyl group in position 1 of the side chain. For example, both chloracizine (58.**100a**) (346) and its trifluoromethyl analog fluoracizine (58.**100b**) (347, 348) are therapeutically effective antidepressants. An azaphenothiazine-10-thiocarboxylate 58.**101** also induces antidepressant-like symptoms, e.g., mydriasis and increased sensitivity to touch, in mice (349). The aminoacyl-substituted phenanthridine 58.**102**, selected for clinical study

58.**97**

58.**98**

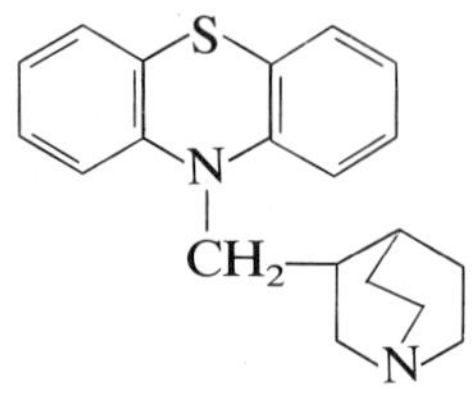

58.**103**

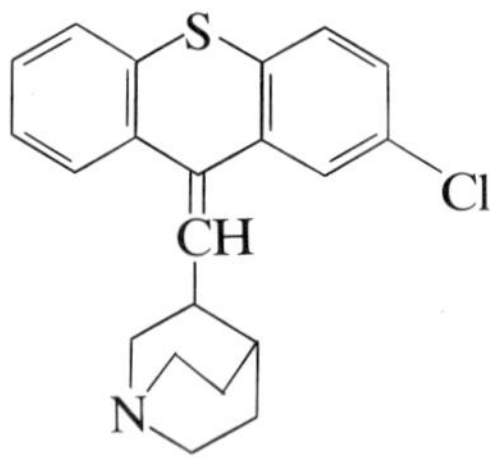

58.**104**

on the basis of quantitative EEG studies, is effective in depressed patients (350). Antidepressant, antihistaminic, antitussive, and antiserotonergic actions are also produced by the phenothiazine metaquitazine (58.**103**) (351). A related thioxanthene 58.**104** has serotonin and norepinephrine antagonist actions approximating those of desipramine (352). The actions of the latter two compounds cannot be interpreted on a conformational basis.

Imipramine-like actions in mice and rats are also produced by 1-chloropromazine (58.**105**) (353). In this case the substituent in position 1 of the phenothiazine nucleus may interact sterically with the side chain

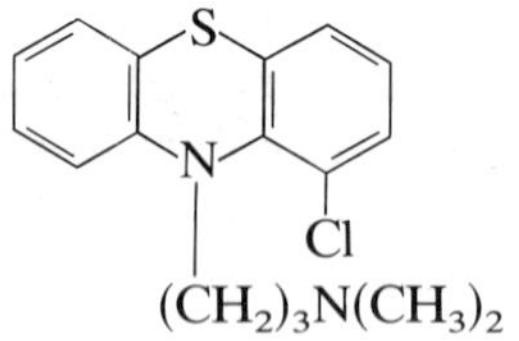

58.**105**

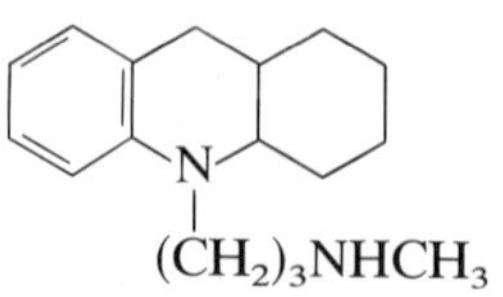

58.**106**

to hinder attainment of planarity by the tricyclic nucleus.

Several tricyclics with a six-membered central ring, having a reduced flanking ring that prohibits attainment of a conformation that can undergo complementary interaction with a planar surface, have imipramine-like properties. The partially hydrogenated acridan 58.**106** has weak imipramine-like activity (354). Similarly, cyclohepta[b]quinolines, e.g., 58.**107a**, are effective in a dopa-potentiation test in mice (355). Several other cycloheptaquinolines 58.**107b** have imipramine-like activity in various animal tests, including antagonism of tetrabenazine-induced depression in mice (356).

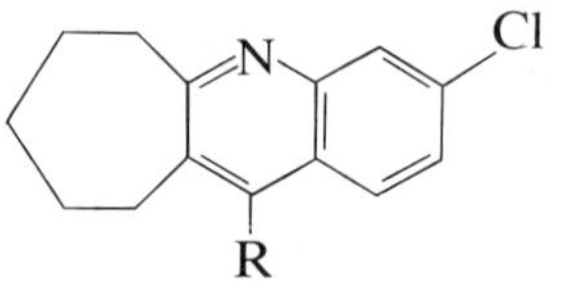

58.**107a**   R = OCH$_2$CH(CH$_3$)CH$_2$N(CH$_3$)$_2$
58.**107b**   R = NH$_2$, OH, Cl

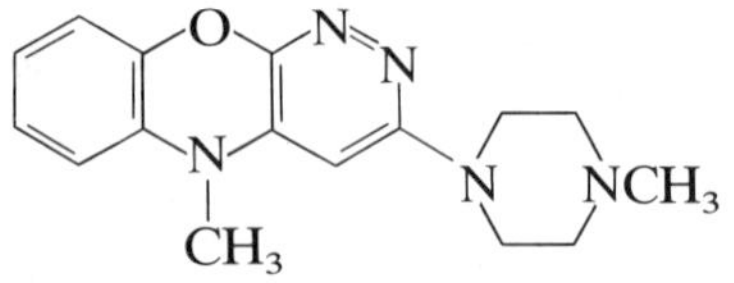

58.**108**

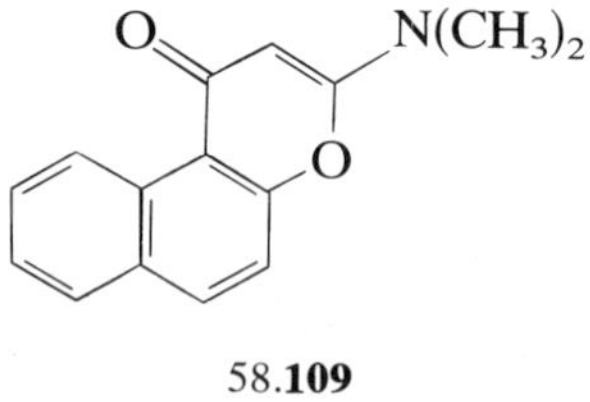

58.**109**

A structurally diverse tricyclic antidepressant with a six-membered central ring is azaphen (58.**108**), a clinically effective antidepressant (357) with properties similar to those of imipramine (358). Reserpine antagonist properties are also noted for some naphtho[1, 2-b]pyrans, e.g., 58.**109** (359), and some imidazo[4, 5-g]-benzothiazoles, e.g., 58.**110** (360).

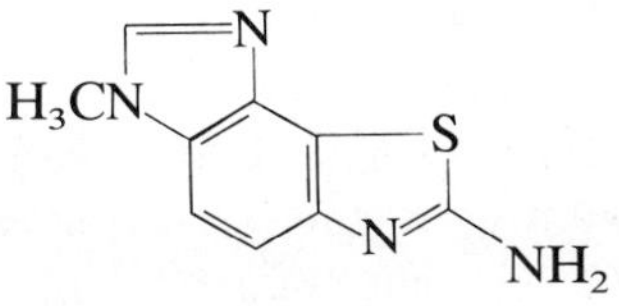

58.**110**

4.2.5 TRICYCLIC ANTIDEPRESSANTS WITH FIVE- AND EIGHT-MEMBERED CENTRAL RINGS.

Aminoalkylated tricyclic compounds having a five- or eight-membered central ring are generally less important as psychotropic agents than related compounds with six- or seven-membered central rings; however, several members of this series do have significant antidepressant activity.

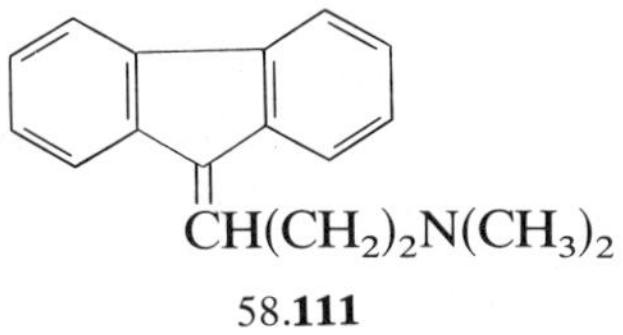

CH(CH$_2$)$_2$N(CH$_3$)$_2$

58.**111**

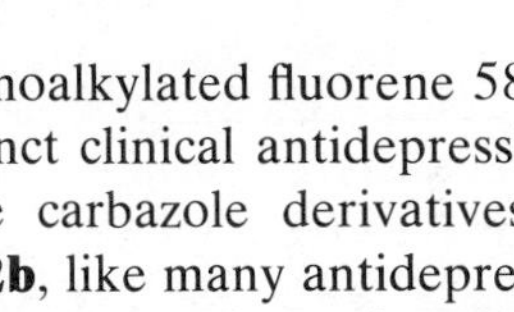

(CH$_2$)$_3$NR^{1}R^2

58.**112a**   R^1 = R^2 = H
58.**112b**   R^1 = H, R^2 = CH$_3$
58.**112c**   R^1 = R^2 = CH$_3$

The aminoalkylated fluorene 58.**111** produces distinct clinical antidepressive effects (361). The carbazole derivatives 58.**112a** and 58.**112b**, like many antidepressants, inhibit uptake of catecholamines by rat brain synaptosomes; 58.**112b** is a highly specific inhibitor of dopamine uptake (243). The related tertiary amine 58.**112c** also has a pharmacological profile suggestive of antidepressant activity (362). Among a series of related 2,3-polymethyleneindoles and similar compounds (363), several are particularly noteworthy. The antidepressant pentamethylene derivative iprindole (58.**113**) is marketed in a number of coun-

tries. This is a somewhat unique antidepressant having a biological profile distinct from that of conventional tricyclic antidepressants (see Section 3.1). Unlike imipramine and amitriptyline, iprindole does not block REM sleep in cats (364) nor does it antagonize benzoquinolizine-induced effects in rodents. It also fails to

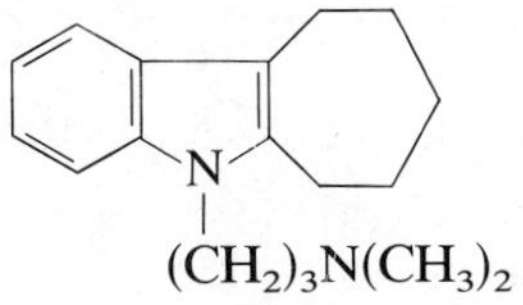

(CH$_2$)$_3$N(CH$_3$)$_2$

58.**113**

inhibit uptake of norepinephrine by rat heart or brain tissue (77). Iprindole does potentiate the central actions of amphetamine, probably by inhibiting metabolism (78). In the clinic, iprindole is a well tolerated antidepressant (365). It may be of particular benefit in treating depressed patients with cardiac problems (366). A compound that is chemically related to iprindole, the tetrahydrothiopyranoindole 58.**114** is nearly three times as potent as imipramine on oral administration in an antireserpine test in mice (363).

A number of tricyclic compounds having a five-membered central ring and a flanking saturated heterocyclic or carbocyclic ring to which is attached an amino or aminoalkyl side chain produce actions characteristic of antidepressant drugs. Tetrahydrocarbazoles bearing an amine substituent at one of the saturated ring positions are claimed to have antidepressant properties (367, 368). This activity has been confirmed in man for the 3-dimethylaminotetrahydrocarbazole ciclindole (58.**115**) (369–372). This compound, which is not an MAO inhibitor

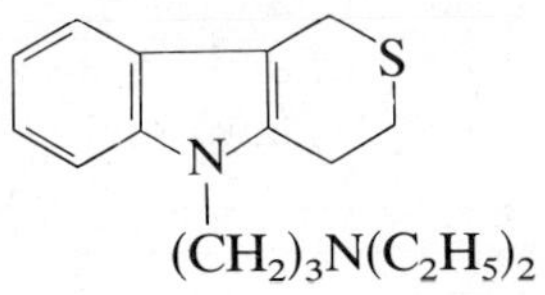

(CH$_2$)$_3$N(C$_2$H$_5$)$_2$

58.**114**

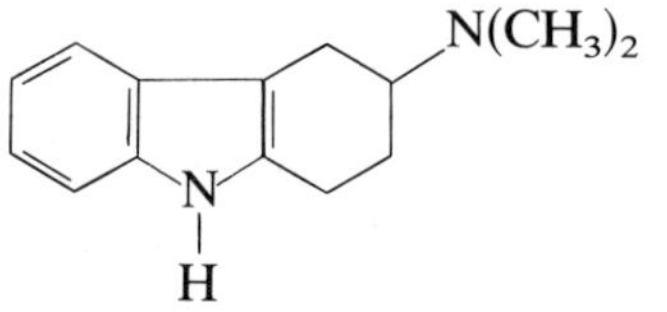

58.**115**

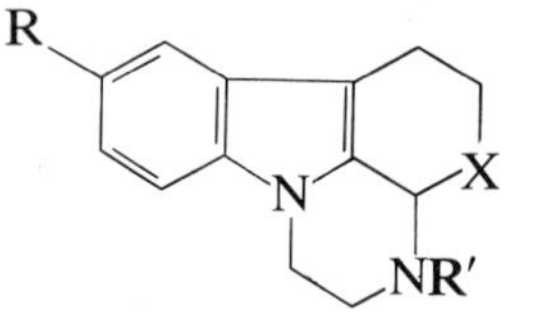

58.**116a** R = CH$_3$, R′ = H, X = CH$_2$
58.**116b** R = CH$_3$O, R′ = CH$_3$, X = NCH$_3$

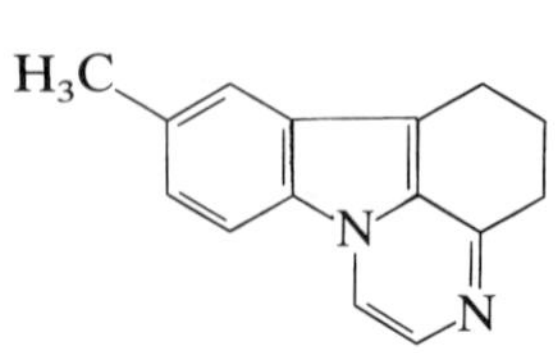

58.**117**

(372), and several nuclear-substituted derivatives are effective in preventing reserpine-induced ptosis and amphetamine-induced stereotypy in rats (373). A 6,8-difluoro derivative has chlorpromazine-like properties. Several related substances in which the amine substituent is incorporated into a ring also have antidepressant actions. Both pirazidol (58.**116a**) (374) and its unsaturated relative 58.**117** (375) have imipramine-like actions in animals. Although less potent than imipramine as an inhibitor of brain norepinephrine uptake, 58.**116a** inhibits GABA uptake (376). Pirazidol is a clinically effective antidepressant (377). Several halogenated relatives 58.**116** (R = Cl, Br; X = CH$_2$, R = C$_2$H$_5$) have been studied (378). A carboline analog incazene (58.**116b**) is about one-half as potent as imipramine in depressed patients but causes fewer side effects (379).

A somewhat related tetrahydrothiopyrano[3,4-b]indole, tandamine (58.**118a**), is a potent antidepressant as demonstrated in various test systems. In drug interaction studies with reserpine, tetrabenazine, and

tremorine, tandamine is more potent than imipramine and related clinically effective antidepressant drugs. Its activity resides predominantly in the (−) isomer (380). Tandamine is an effective blocker of norepinephrine uptake but has no effect on serotonin uptake (381) and only weakly potentiates the effects of 5-hydroxytryptophan (382). The N-demethyl analog of tandamine, a major metabolite, is less potent than the parent as a reserpine antagonist (380). Clinical pharmacology of tandamine is also suggestive of potential antidepressant efficacy (383, 384). An oxygen analog 58.**118b** also has antidepressant properties as indicated by a test for prevention of reserpine-induced ptosis in rats (385), inhibition of norepinephrine uptake, and potentiation of 5-hydroxytryptophan-induced effects (381). A related 1,4-oxazino[4,3-a]indole 58.**119a** is about 12 times more potent than imipramine upon intraperitoneal administration in a test for prevention of reserpine-induced ptosis in rats (386). A lower homolog 58.**119b** is about one-fourth as potent as desipramine as an inhibitor of uptake of norepinephrine

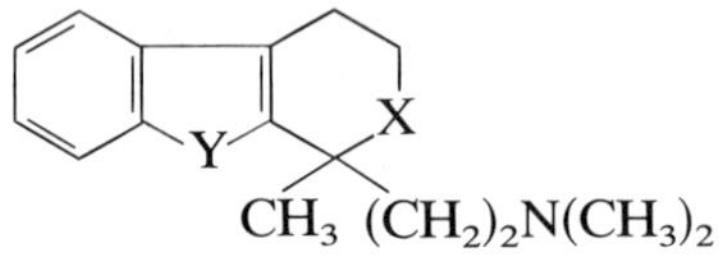

58.**118**

a X = S, Y = NC$_2$H$_5$
b X = O, Y = NCH$_3$
c X = CH$_2$, Y = NC$_2$H$_5$
d X = (CH$_2$)$_2$, Y = NC$_2$H$_5$
e X = —(5-membered ring),
   Y = NC$_2$H$_5$
f X = O, Y = CH$_2$

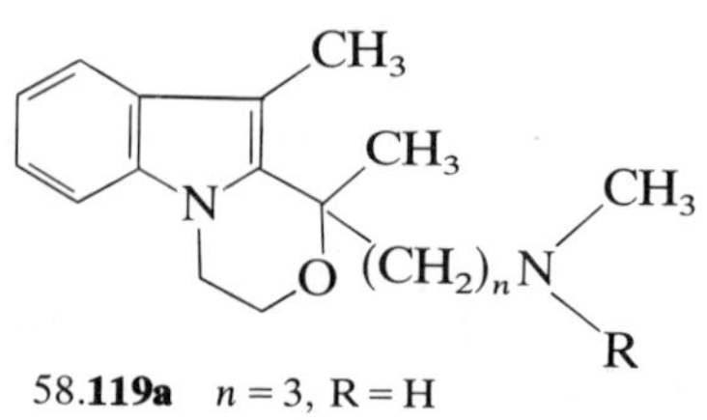

58.**119a** n = 3, R = H
58.**119b** n = 2, R = CH$_3$

by mouse heart (387). Tandamine relatives with a flanking carbocyclic ring, e.g., 58.**118c–e**, are also more potent than imipramine and amitriptyline in reversing reserpine-induced ptosis in rats. The order of potency is cyclohexyl (58.**118c**) > cycloheptyl (58.**118d**) > cyclopentyl (58.**118e**) (388). This same order of potency is noted in tests for inhibition of norepinephrine uptake and potentiation of 5-hydroxytryptophan-induced effects (389).

Among a series of indeno[2, 1-*c*]pyrans and thiopyrans (390) the greatest potency as a potentiator of behavioral effects induced by 5-hydroxytryptophan in mice is produced by pirandamine (58.**118f**); however, it is very selective, but less potent than imipramine in blocking serotonin uptake into cortical synaptosomes of rat brain and does not prevent reserpine-induced hypothermia. The (−) enantiomer of pirandamine retains the potency of the racemate whereas the (+) isomer is much less effective (391).

Reversed annelation of the thiopyrano and indole rings of tandamine, i.e., 58.**120a**, greatly alters biological potency (380, 382); however, a similar annelation of rings of pirandamine, i.e., 58.**120b**, only slightly alters activity (390, 391).

Antidepressant properties are produced by several aminoalkylated tricyclics having an eight-membered central ring. For example, the dibenzocyclooctane 58.**121a** is more potent than its dibenzocycloheptane analog 58.**60a**; it is about 0.64 times as potent as nortriptyline as an antagonist of tetrabenazine-induced effects in mice (238). A pyridine isostere 58.**121b** has an oral ED_{50} of 20 mg/kg in a test for antagonism

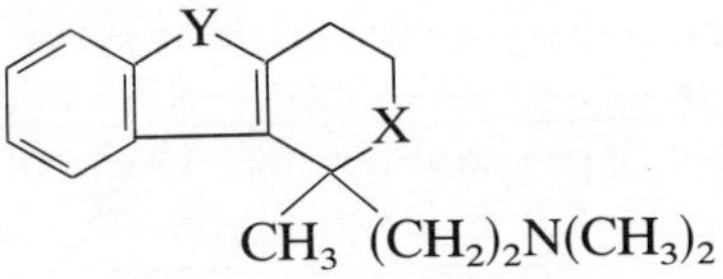

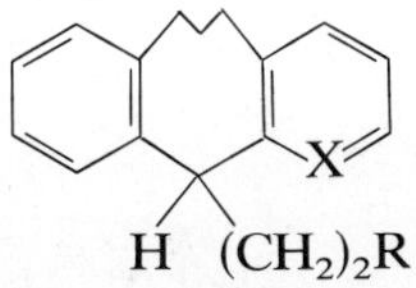

58.**121a** X = CH, R = CH₂NHCH₃
58.**121b** X = N, R = N(CH₃)₂

58.**121c** X = CH, R =

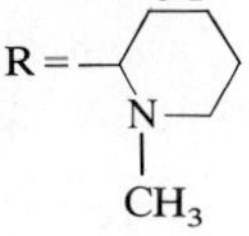

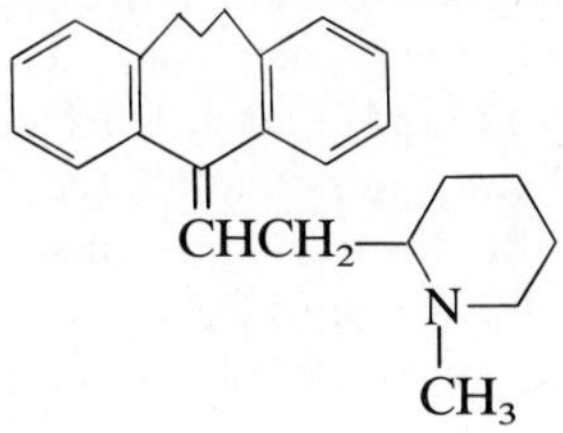

58.**122**

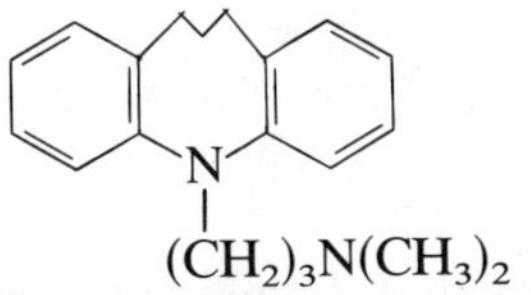

(CH₂)₃N(CH₃)₂
58.**123**

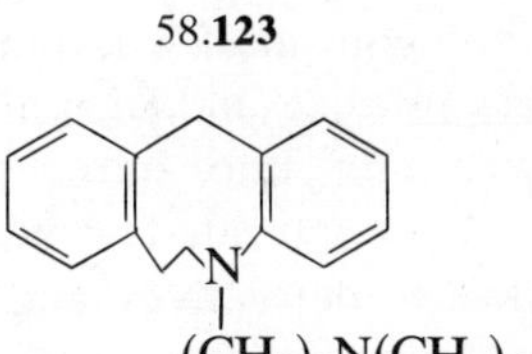

(CH₂)₃N(CH₃)₂
58.**124**

CH₃ (CH₂)₂N(CH₃)₂

58.**120a**   X = S, Y = NC₂H₅
58.**120b**   X = O, Y = CH₂

of tetrabenazine-induced ptosis in mice (392). More generally, the dibenzocyclooctanes are less effective antidepressant-like compounds than related dibenzocycloheptanes; however, in a conditioned response test in rats and as a mydriatic in mice 58.**121c** and 58.**122** have potency comparable to that of amitriptyline (393).

The dibenz[*b*, g]azocine homolog 58.**123** of imipramine is claimed to have antiemetic and antidepressant utility (394). Also, the isomeric dibenz[*b*, *e*]azocine 58.**124** (propazocine) has significant antireserpine activity (254); however, the dibenz[*b*, *f*]azocine 58.**125** is considerably less effective than

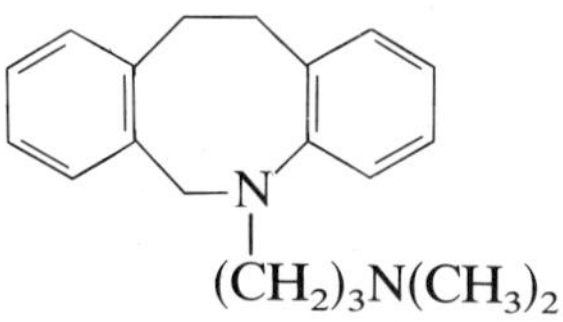

58.**125**

imipramine as an antagonist of reserpine-induced responses in mice, rats, and rabbits (210).

4.2.6 AMINOALKYL DERIVATIVES OF DIPHE-NYLMETHANE AND RELATED COMPOUNDS. Several compounds that at least superfically resemble an aminoalkylated tricyclic in which the third ring is absent or not bridged have antidepressant actions comparable to those of classical tricyclic antidepressants. Among a series of substituted 1,1-diphenyl-3-amino-1-propenes and 1,1-diphenyl-3-aminopropanes, most potent antidepressant properties are observed with compounds with the structure 58.**126** (395). These compounds 58.**126** are more potent than desipramine in causing antagonism of reserpine-induced hypothermia in mice and in inhibiting uptake of serotonin into human platelets. Generally, the saturated analogs, side chain-substituted derivatives, and homologous butenyl compounds are less effective than 58.**126** in these tests. The corresponding unsubstituted compound 58.**126** (R = X = H) is being studied for potential antidepressant activity (396). In another series (397), zimelidine (58.**127**) is a selective inhibitor of serotonin uptake by homogenates and slices of rat hypothalamus, whereas geometric isomers are selective inhibitors of neuronal uptake of norepi-

58.**126** X = F, Cl
R = H, CH$_3$

nephrine. Zimelidine (398) is more potent than chlorimipramine in reducing blood serotonin. The N-demethyl metabolite of 58.**127** is 10 times as potent as the parent in inhibiting serotonin uptake (399). Initial studies indicate useful antidepressant activity (400–402). A related compound 58.**128**, having the basic side chain incorporated into pyrrolidine ring, has therapeutic effects comparable to those of amitriptyline (403). A somewhat related 3-aminopropylidenyl benzocyclooctane, 58.**129**, has antireserpine actions in animals (404).

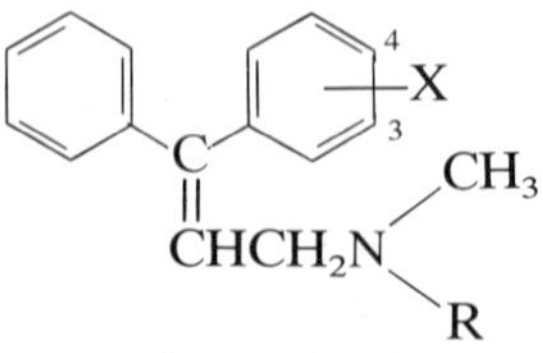

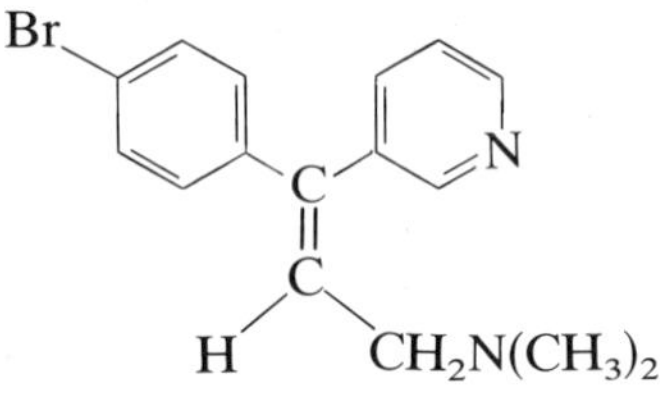

58.**127**

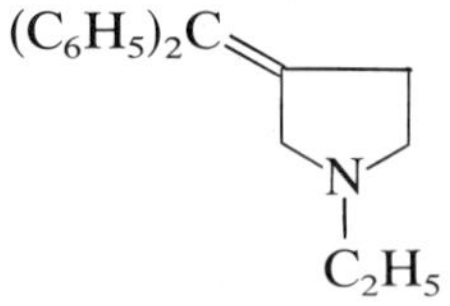

58.**128**

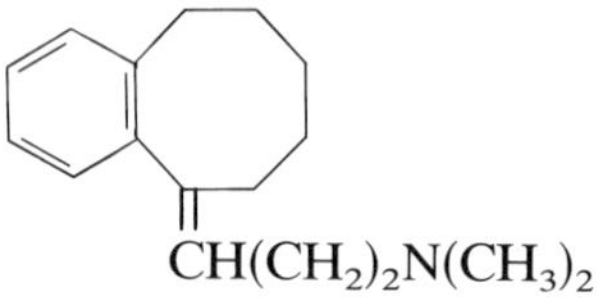

58.**129**

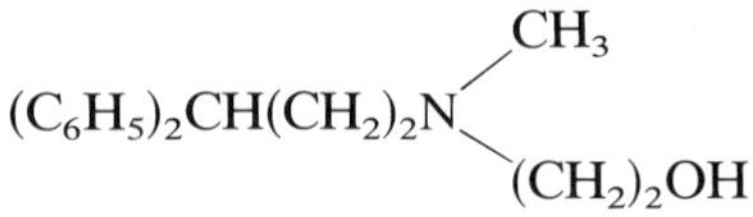

58.**130**

Several diarylmethane derivatives bearing a saturated aminoalkyl side chain also have antidepressant actions. Thus 58.**130** is more potent than amitriptyline in tests for reserpine antagonism. It blocks norepinephrine uptake and in general has a pharmacological and biochemical profile similar to that of imipramine (405). Among many other diphenylmethane derivatives 58.**131** is notable as an inhibitor of neuronal uptake of norepinephrine and serotonin, although it is somewhat less potent than desipramine. It also potentiates L-dopa-induced responses and causes motor stimulation in animals (406). Another diphenylmethane derivative 58.**132** in which the aminoalkyl side chain is incorporated in a hexahydroindenopyridine moiety has an antidepressant profile comparable to that of desipramine in rodents. The epimer of 58.**132** has similar activity (407).

$$(C_6H_5)_2CHC(CH_3)_2NH_2$$

58.**131**

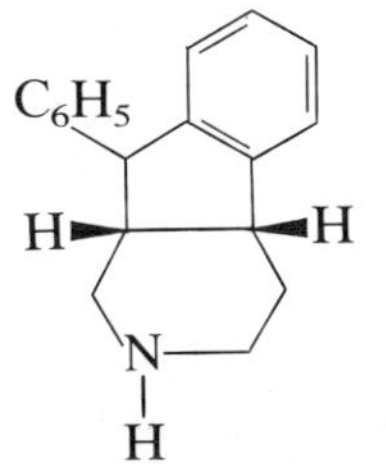

58.**132**

Some novel antidepressants are phenyl-substituted tetrahydroisoquinolines that incorporate a diphenylmethyl moiety in their structure. Nomifensine 58.**135** (408, 409) blocks norepinephrine, dopamine, and serotonin (very weakly) uptake, potentiates norepinephrine-induced actions, and has antireserpine effects (410–412). Clinical studies indicate nomifensine is an effective antidepressant (413–415). Metabolism of this drug, marketed as an antidepressant in various parts of the world (408), results in extensive hydroxylation of the 4-phenyl group (416). Although these metabolites are less effective uptake inhibitors than the parent (416), 3′,4′-dihydroxynomifensine is a potent dopamine receptor agonist (417).

Another 4-phenyltetrahydroisoquinoline 58.**134** is equipotent with imipramine in preventing reserpine-induced ptosis in mice

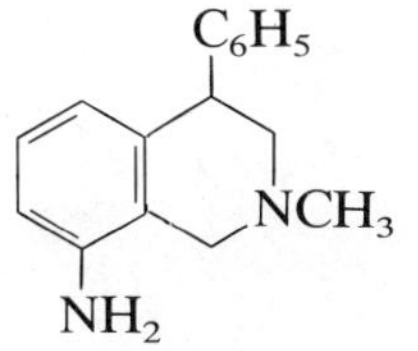

56.**133**

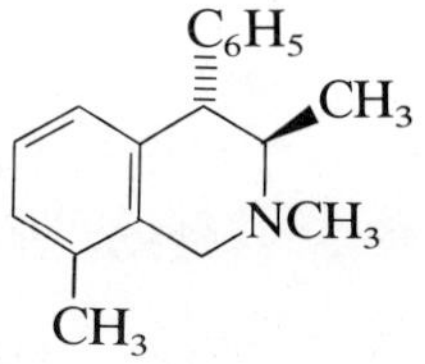

58.**134**

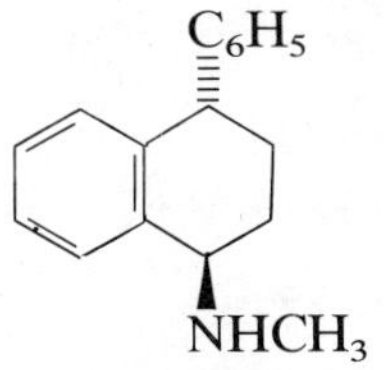

58.**135**

(418). The aminotetralin 58.**135** is an inhibitor of norepinephrine, serotonin, and dopamine uptake in rat brain tissue (419).

A benzhydrol ether, tofenacine (58.**136**), has pharmacological, biochemical, and clinical properties of an antidepressant (420–422). Fenazoxine (58.**137**), a cyclic benzhydrol ether, inhibits neuronal uptake of norepinephrine and tyramine (423).

The (−) isomer of a benzhydrol derivative $[(C_6H_5)_2C(OH)CH(CH_3)CH_2NH_2]$ causes clinical antidepressant actions; however, concomitant side effects are produced (424, 425). A somewhat related carbinol, the imidazoline 58.**138**, prevents tetrabenazine-induced ptosis and reverses reserpine-induced hypothermia in mice; it

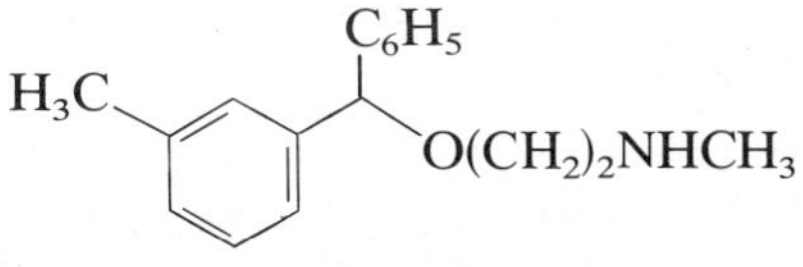

58.**136**

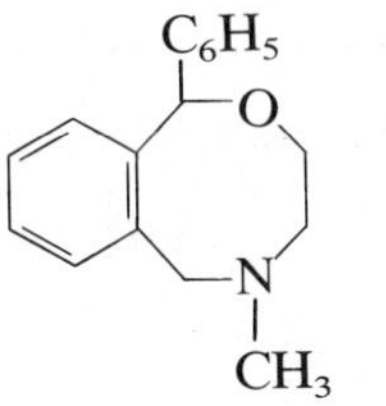

58.**137**

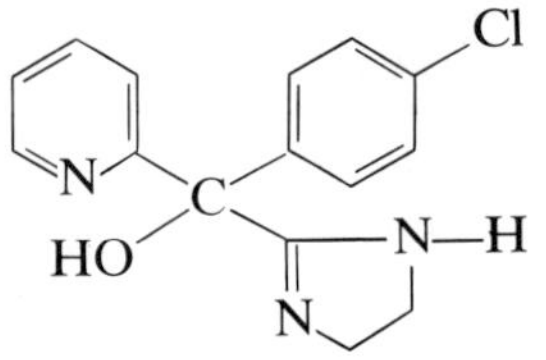

58.**138**

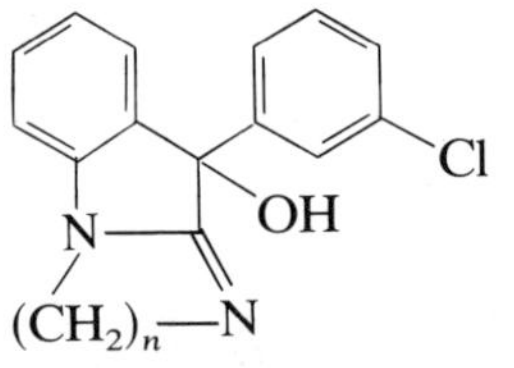

58.**139a** $n = 3$
58.**139b** $n = 4$

does not antagonize acetylcholine or norepinephrine (426). Several benzhydrol derivatives closely related to 58.**138** present biologic profiles suggestive of antidepressant activity. One of these, ciclazindol (58.**139a**), is more potent than desipramine as an inhibitor of norepinephrine uptake; however, it is less effective in blocking serotonin uptake (427–429). It also reverses reserpine-induced hypothermia and potentiates methamphetamine-induced effects in mice (430). Clinical pharmacology indicates antidepressant activity of the amitriptyline-type, but with fewer side effects. At 100 mg/day ciclazindol is a peripheral norepinephrine reuptake blocker (431). A relative of ciclazindol, i.e., mazindol (158.**140**), has antireserpine, antitetrabenazine, antimuricidal, and stimulant actions in animals (432). The mechanism of action is apparently similar to that of classical tricyclic antidepressants (433). A diazepine homolog 58.**139b** is

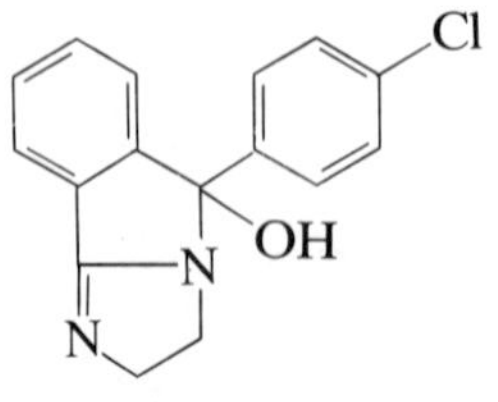

58.**140**

claimed (434) to be a more potent antidepressant than imipramine.

Another interesting benzhydrol derivative is cyprolidol (58.**141**) (435). This trans pyridyl-substituted cyclopropane increases voluntary motor activity in mice and antagonizes reserpine-induced ptosis and depression in rabbits (436, 437). Cyprolidol has insignificant MAO-inhibitory activity (435) but it is an effective antidepressant in man (438). The cis isomer lacks the effects of cyprolidol on behavioral responses in dogs (435). Antidepressant-like actions are caused in animals by a group of somewhat related pyridine-containing cyclopropanes 58.**142** (439).

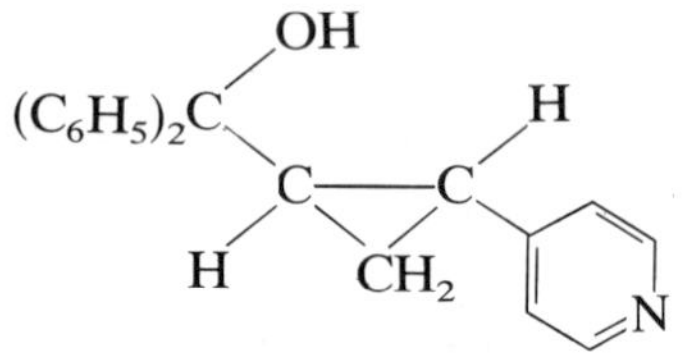

58.**141**

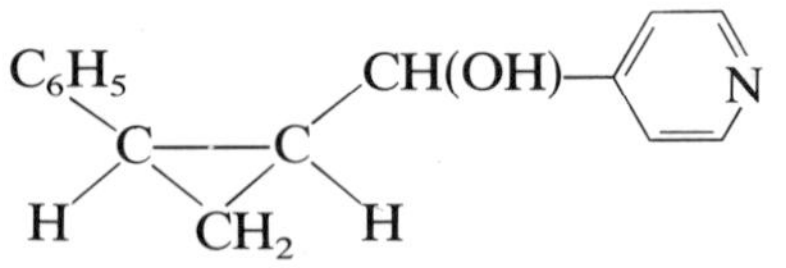

58.**142**

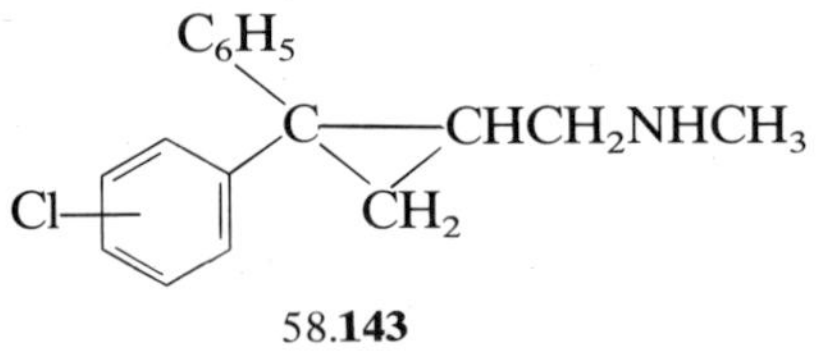

58.**143**

Antidepressant actions are also claimed (440, 441) for a series of diarylcyclopropylmethylamines, e.g., 58.**143**. Of a number of phenylcycloalkylamines, 58.**144a** and 58.**145a** have similar activity in blocking norepinephrine and serotonin uptake and in potentiating the behavioral effects of dopa and serotonin. Similar actions are also produced by 58.**145b**; however, 58.**144b** is effective only in the dopa-potentiation test (442). A homolog of

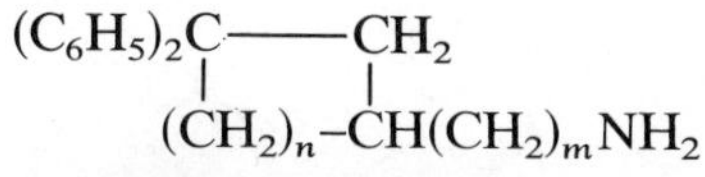

$(C_6H_5)_2C$———CH_2
$(CH_2)_n$–$CH(CH_2)_m NH_2$

58.**144a** $n = 2, m = 0$
58.**144b** $n = 3, m = 0$
58.**144c** $n = 3, m = 1$

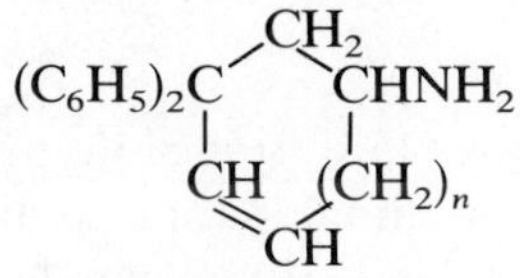

$(C_6H_5)_2C$ $\overset{CH_2}{\underset{CH}{\diagdown}}$ CHNH₂ $(CH_2)_n$

58.**145a** $n = 0$
58.**145b** $n = 1$

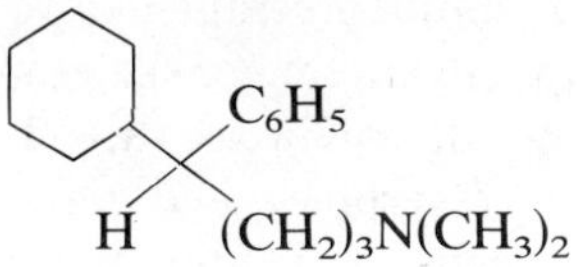

58.**146**

58.**144a**, i.e., 58.**144c**, is a potent inhibitor of norepinephrine uptake (443).

Clinical antidepressant actions are produced by a diphenylmethane analog in which one of the phenyl rings has been hydrogenated. This compound, gamfexine (58.**146**), antagonizes reserpine-induced ptosis in mice. In cats and monkeys it interferes with reserpine-induced depression. It also potentiates the pressor response to norepinephrine in dogs and cats (444). A number of somewhat related phthalans, indenes, indans, and other bicyclic alkylamines that incorporate a diphenylmethyl grouping have significant antidepressant actions (326, 445, 446). One of these compounds, the phthalan 58.**147a**, is about 30 times more potent than amitriptyline as an antagonist of reserpine-induced ptosis in mice. It also potentiates norepinephrine effects in rats; however, it lacks appreciable anticholinergic, MAO-inhibitory, or amphetamine-like CNS-stimulating activity. Among a series of related compounds, reserpine-antagonist potency is decreased by shortening the aminoalkyl chain or by converting the secondary amine to a ter-

tiary amine (326). Like protriptyline and desipramine, 58.**147a** strongly inhibits uptake of norepinephrine by mouse hearts (447). A derivative of 58.**147a**, i.e., nitalapram (citalopram, 58.**148**), is a specific serotonin potentiating agent (448–450); it inhibits serotonin uptake both *in vivo* and *in vitro*. The compound does not have norepinephrine-potentiating, anticholinergic, or antihistaminic properties characteristic of many tricyclic antidepressants (448).

Nitralapram *N*-oxide, a metabolic product, is less potent than the parent in animals (451). A quantitative structure–activity relationship study of nitalapram-related compounds is reported (452). A vinylogous relative of 58.**147a**, i.e., 58.**149**, is the most potent of a series of such compounds in a mouse test for tetrabenazine antagonism (453). Other congeners of 58.**147a** with significant antidepressant-like properties include a sulfur counterpart

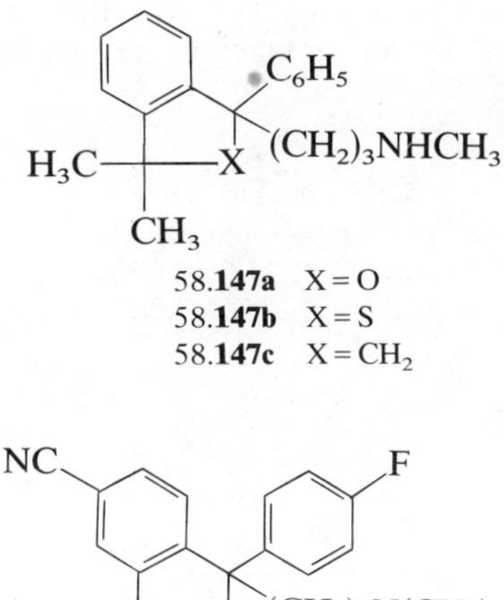

58.**147a**   X = O
58.**147b**   X = S
58.**147c**   X = CH₂

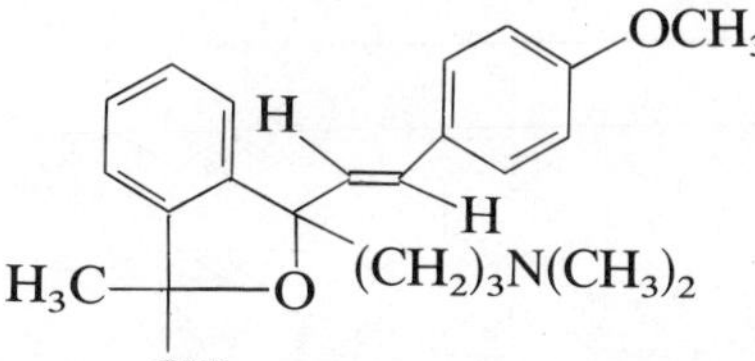

58.**148**

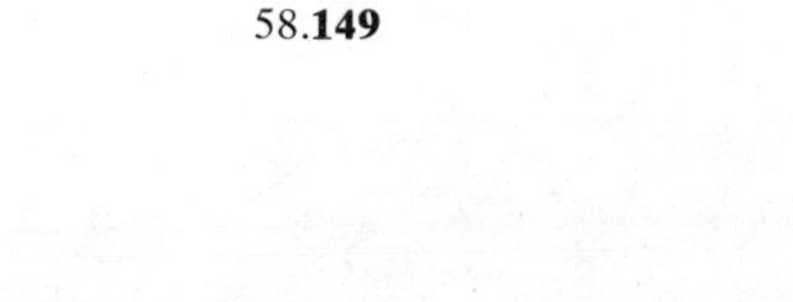

58.**149**

58.**147b** and an indan analog 58.**147c**. Biochemical and histochemical data for 58.**147b** and a number of analogs show that these compounds have a selective action on the membrane pump of central and peripheral neurons and practically no anticholinergic activity (454). The indan 58.**147c** is a potent and selective inhibitor of norepinephrine uptake, whereas it only weakly inhibits serotonin uptake (455). Compounds of the general structure 58.**147** inhibit mitochondrial activity in intact yeast cells, a test that generally correlates with clinical antidepressant potency (445, 446). A related indene 58.**150** is about one-fifth as potent as imipramine in preventing reserpine-induced ptosis in mice (456). The phthalide 58.**151** increases turnover of rat brain norepinephrine, but not serotonin or dopamine (457).

Additional phthalan derivatives incorporating a diphenylmethane framework include some spiroisobenzofuran piperidines, e.g., 58.**152**, which is more potent than imipramine in reversing tetrabenazine-

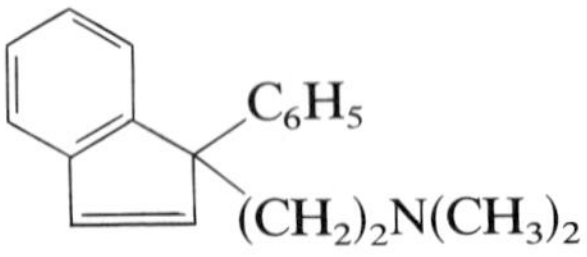

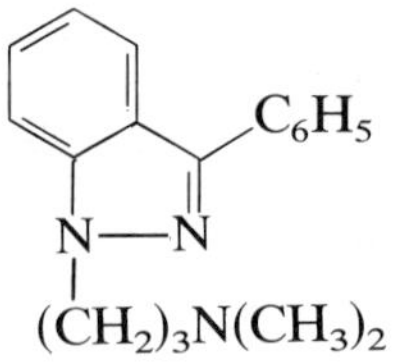

58.**153**

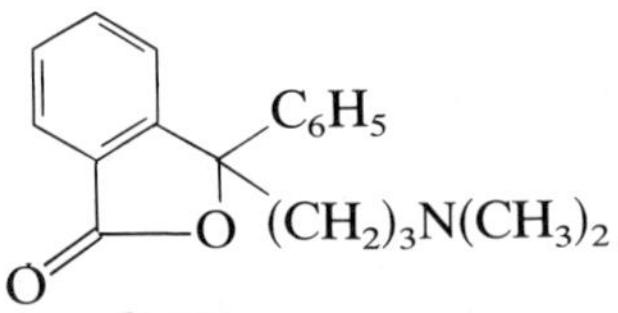

induced ptosis (458). It is more potent than desipramine as an inhibitor of brain norepinephrine uptake (459). Some N-hydroxylated derivatives of 58.**152** are also very effective tetrabenazine antagonists (460).

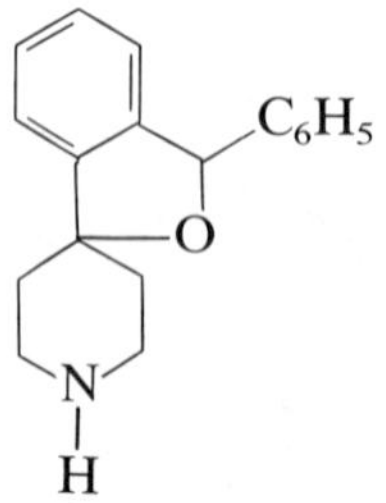

Another antidepressant-like compound with a diphenylmethane skeleton and an aminoalkyl side chain is 58.**153** (461); it antagonizes reserpine- and tetrabenazine-induced effects, and potentiates amphetamine-induced self-stimulation and L-dopa-induced increase in motor activity.

Several other compounds with biologic actions suggestive of antidepressant potential incorporate in their structure a diphenylamine or diphenylsulfide moiety together with a basic side chain. For example, amedalin (58.**154a**) and daledalin

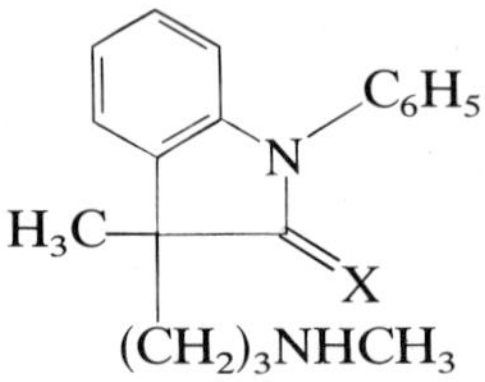

58.**150**

58.**151**

58.**152**

58.**154a**   X = O
58.**154b**   X = H$_2$

(58.**154b**), diphenylamine derivatives, have a profile of pharmacological action similar to that of the tricyclic antidepressants (462). Amedalin (58.**154a**) has clinical antidepressant properties (463). A related chloro-substituted benzimidazolone 58.**155** has similar pharmacological properties with little sedative or anticholinergic action; it is a clinically effective antidepressant (464, 465).

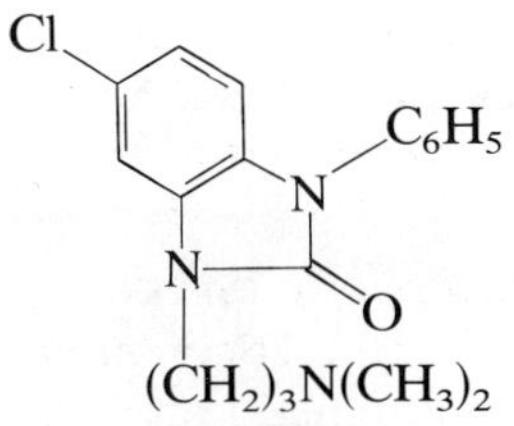

58.**155**

4.2.7   AMINOALKYL DERIVATIVES OF DICARBO-
CYCLICS JOINED BY A TWO-ATOM BRIDGE (RING-
OPENED ANALOGS OF TRICYCLIC COMPOUNDS).
Antidepressant-like actions are produced
by several aminoalkylated compounds in
which two carbocyclic groups are attached
to adjacent atoms.

Fluoxetine (58.**156a**) is an example of
this type of compound. It is a specific inhibitor of serotonin uptake both *in vivo*
and *in vitro* (466–469). It causes an inhibition of serotonin uptake into platelets of
human volunteers (470). A closely related
compound, nisoxetine (58.**156b**), is a potent
and specific inhibitor of norepinephrine uptake (471, 472). It suppresses REM sleep in
cats in a fashion very similar to that of
classical tricyclic antidepressants (473).

A tetrahydrotriazine derivative 58.**157a**
of 1,2-diphenylethane represents an example of an aminoalkyl substituted derivative
in which aryl groups are attached to adjacent carbons. The pharmacological profile

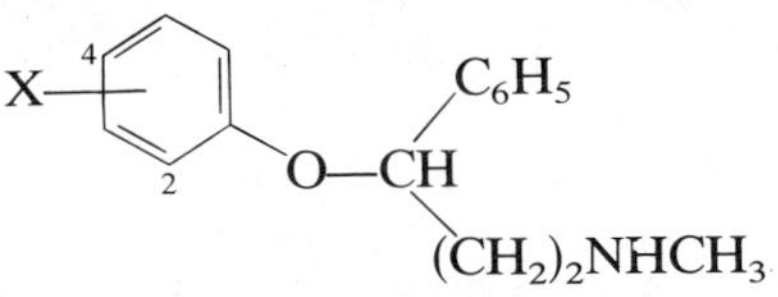

58.**156a**   X = 4-CF$_3$
58.**156b**   X = 2-CH$_3$O

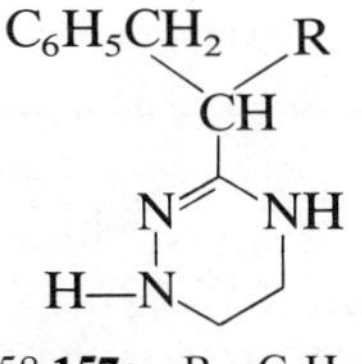

58.**157a**   R = C$_6$H$_5$
58.**157b**   R = CH$_3$

of 58.**157a** in mice and rats is similar to
that of tricyclic antidepressants. It blocks
reserpine-induced   ptosis,   potentiates
amphetamine-induced effects, and inhibits
amine uptake into brain slices (474, 475).

Several other compounds with antidepressant-like properties incorporate into
their molecular framework aryl groups attached to adjoining carbon and sulfur
atoms. For example, 58.**158** has antidepressant activity in the clinic (476).

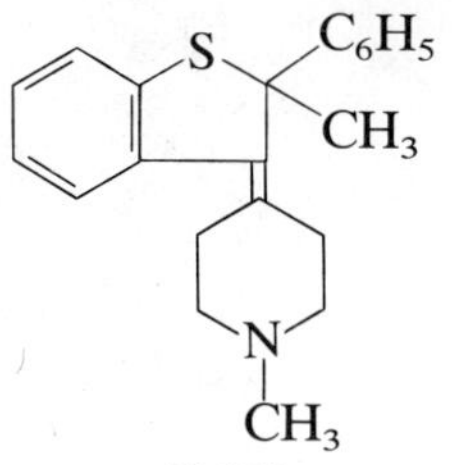

58.**158**

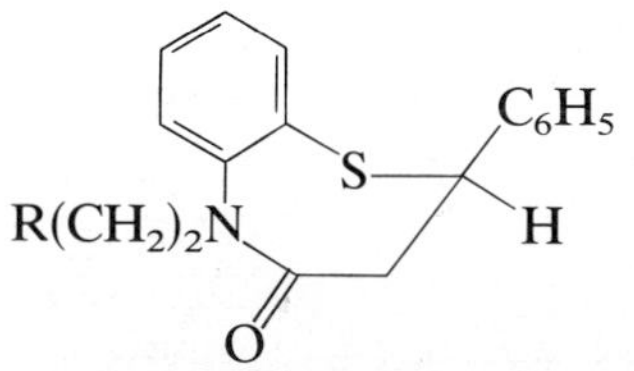

58.**159a**   R = N(CH$_3$)$_2$
58.**159b**   R = CH$_2$N(CH$_3$)$_2$

58.**159c**   R = CH$_2$N⟨   ⟩NCH$_3$

Thiazesim (58.**159a**) has potent clinical
antidepressant properties (477–479). It is
effective in calming septally lesioned rats
(480); however, it has insignificant reserpine antagonist activity (481). Thiazesim
specifically affects the amygdala area of the
brain in cats (482). Like imipramine and
amitriptyline it blocks the instinctive response of rats to kill mice (483) at about
one-half the dose that impairs mobility of
rats in a rotating rod procedure. In these
procedures the (+) and (−) enantiomers of
thiazesim are about equipotent with the
racemate. Of several other relatives of
thiazesim (484, 485) examined in these
tests the propylene side chain congeners

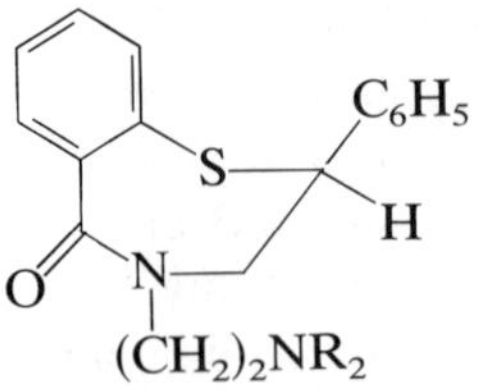

58.**160a**　R = CH$_3$
58.**160b**　R = C$_2$H$_5$

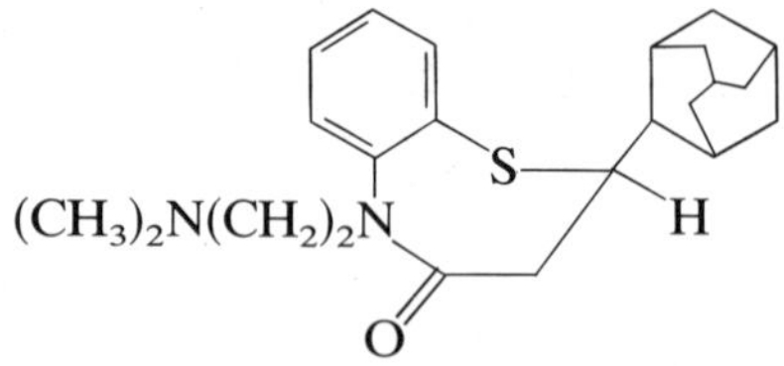

58.**161**

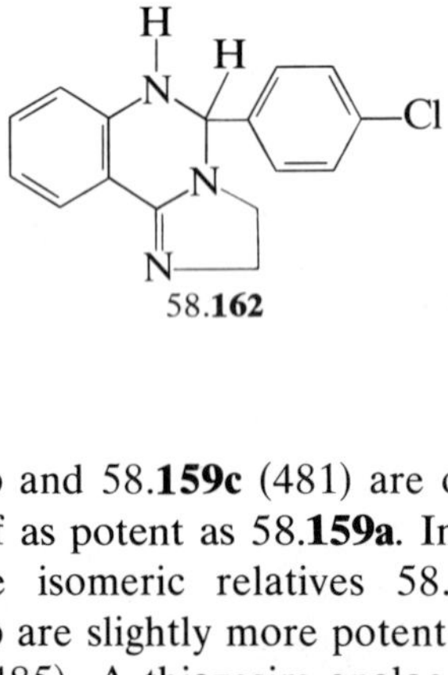

58.**162**

58.**159b** and 58.**159c** (481) are only about one-half as potent as 58.**159a**. In the same test the isomeric relatives 58.**160a** and 58.**160b** are slightly more potent than thiazesim (485). A thiazesim analog 58.**161** in which the phenyl group is replaced by a 2-adamantyl substituent is 1.5 times more potent than the parent in a rat muricidal test (486).

The imidazo[1,2-*c*]quinazoline 58.**162**, which incorporates within its molecular framework phenyl groups attached to adjoining carbon and nitrogen atoms, causes pharmacological actions typical of tricyclic antidepressants. In clinical studies it increases the duration of non-REM sleep (487).

4.3　Antidepressant Mono- and Bicyclic Compounds Bearing an Amine-containing Side Chain

Many members of a diverse group of compounds having the common structural feature of an aromatic mono- or bicyclic system to which an amine is attached directly or by a variety of bridges have antidepressant-like properties. Included in this very general classification are various aralkylamines, aryloxy- and aryloxyalkylamines, tetrahydroisoquinolines, aminotetralins, aminoalkylindoles, and piperazine derivatives. Although it is clear that these structurally diverse compounds may act in different fashions to induce an antidepressant effect, it is convenient to group them into a single section.

4.3.1　ARALKYLAMINE DERIVATIVES. According to the catecholamine hypothesis of affective disorders, depression may be a manifestation of a functional deficiency of a biogenic amine at critical central synapses. L-Dopa, which is readily decarboxylated in the brain to afford dopamine, is effective in depressed patients; however, it is of little therapeutic utility because the patients quickly become refractory (488). That other antidepressant aralkylamines may act with the same pre- or postsynaptic receptors as dopamine or related biogenic amines seems plausible. Among various ring- and side chain-substituted phenethylamines, 4-chloro-phenethylamine [4-ClC$_6$H$_4$(CH$_2$)$_2$NH$_2$] is particularly effective; it is a potent inhibitor of norepinephrine and serotonin uptake by brain tissue (489). α-Methyl-4-chloro-phenethylamine (parachloroamphetamine, 58.**163a**) (490, 491) and its N-methyl derivative 58.**163b** (492) have antidepressant actions in the clinic and in animals. Amide derivatives of α,α-dimethyl-N-chloro-phenethylamine 58.**164** are claimed (493) to be antidepressants that inhibit serotonin

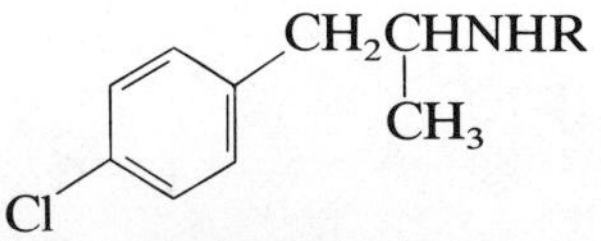

58.**163a**   R = H
58.**163b**   R = CH₃

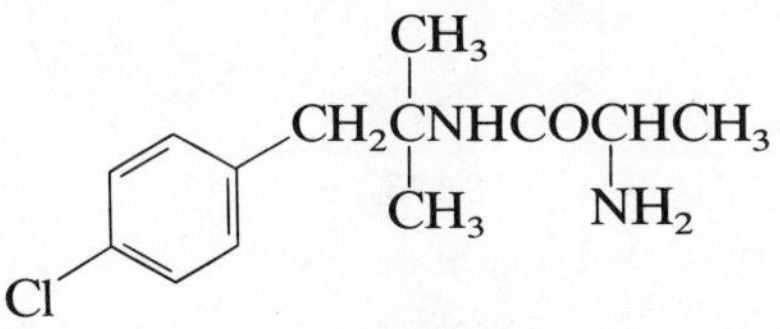

58.**164**

uptake. The (−) isomer is a highly selective inhibitor of serotonin accumulation in mouse and rat brain slices (494). Structure–activity relationships among halogenated amphetamines have been reviewed (495).

Another amphetamine derivative, fenfluramine (58.**165**), an anorectic drug, causes imipramine-like activity in various pharmacological tests in mice (496).

Bupropion (58.**166a**) (497) represents a new kind of antidepressant drug. Like imipramine, bupropion reverses tetrabenazine-induced sedation in mice, but it does not affect various conditioned avoidance responses in rats. It is a relatively weak inhibitor of norepinephrine (498) and serotonin uptake and is devoid of significant sympathomimetic and MAO-inhibitory ac-

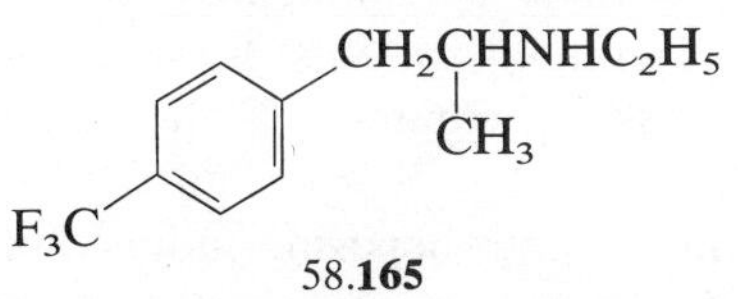

58.**165**

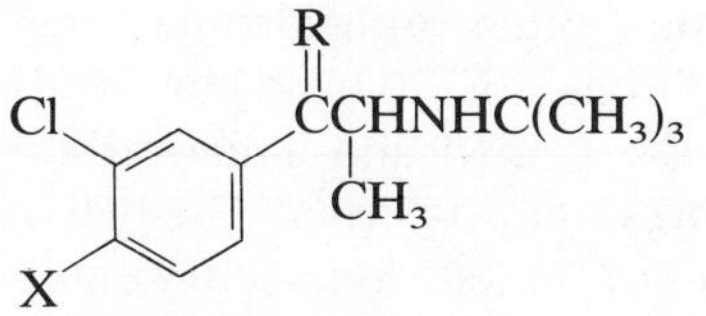

58.**166a**   X = H, R = O
58.**166b**   X = Cl, R = (H, OH)

tivities (499, 500). Bupropion is effective in the treatment of depression in man (501, 502). A phenylpropanolamine 58.**166b** related to bupropion also displays antidepressant-like actions in animals (503). α-Allylphenethylamine [aletamine, C₆H₅CH₂CH(CH₂CH = CH₂)NH₂] has a general pharmacological profile similar to that of the tricyclic antidepressants. It decreases motor activity and is more potent than imipramine in an antireserpine test in mice (504). Clinically, it induces a relaxed feeling blended with stimulation, but it is ineffective in schizophrenic patients (505). An amidine derivative 58.**167** antagonizes reserpine-induced ptosis and hypothermia in animals (506).

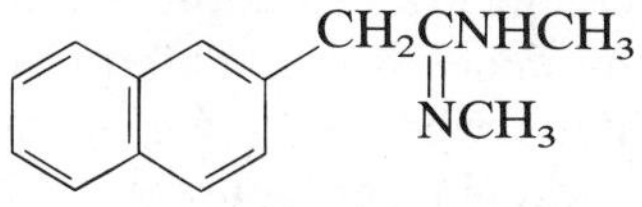

58.**167**

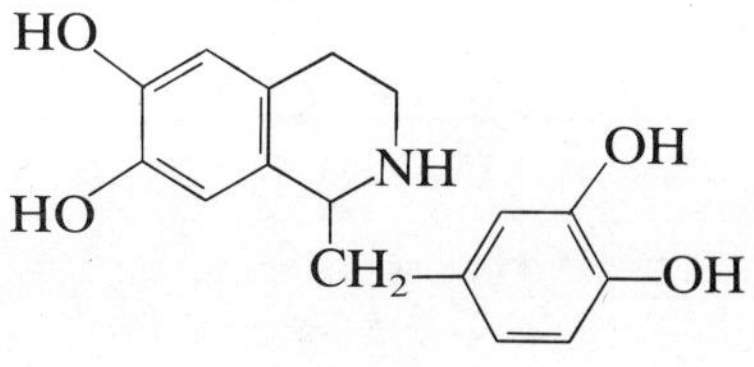

58.**168**

Several other compounds having a phenethylamine moiety incorporated into a cyclic framework cause antidepressant-like actions. The tetrahydroisoquinoline tetrahydropapaveroline (58.**168**), a possible dopamine metabolite, antagonizes reserpine- and oxotremorine-induced effects, but unlike many antidepressants, it does not potentiate the responses of animals to amphetamine (507). A cis azetidine 58.**169** is seven times more potent than the trans isomer as an inhibitor of norepinephrine uptake by rat vas deferens. Also in this test, *trans*-2-phenylcyclopropylamine (tranylcypromine, see Section 4.1.2.4) is about 600 times more potent than its cis isomer (508). These results (54) suggest a partially eclipsed conformation of phenethylamines may be preferred for inhibition of norepinephrine uptake by both peripheral and brain tissue. Other antidepressants having a phenethylamine grouping incorporated into a ring include 58.**170**–58.**175**. The arylquinolizidines, 58.**170a** and 58.**170b**, are at least as potent as imipramine in a dopa-potentiation test (509, 510). Some morpholines, e.g., flumexadol (58.**171a**), act as mixed serotonin agonists and antagonists on isolated tissue (511). The homolog oxaflozane (58.**171b**) has clinical antidepressant activity (512, 513); it antagonizes reserpine and oxotremorine effects in animals (514).

A rigid analog of parachloroamphetamine (58.**163a**), the benzobicyclononadiene 58.**172**, is five times more potent than chlorimipramine as an inhibitor of serotonin uptake whereas it has no apparent effect on norepinephrine uptake (515–517).

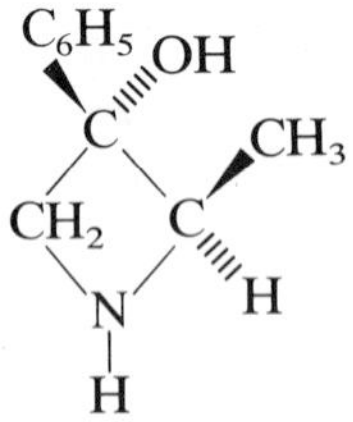

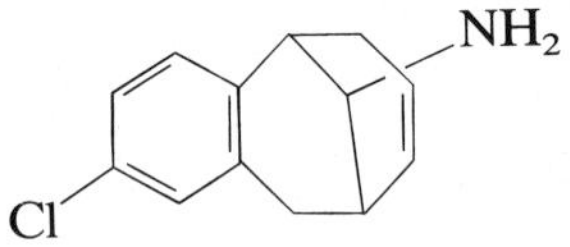

58.**172**

58.**173**

58.**174**

58.**175**

58.**169**

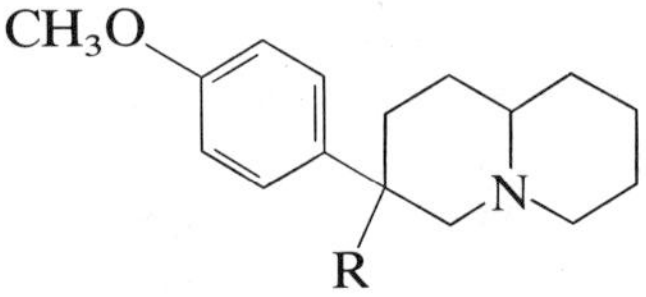

58.**170a** R = OH
58.**170b** R = H

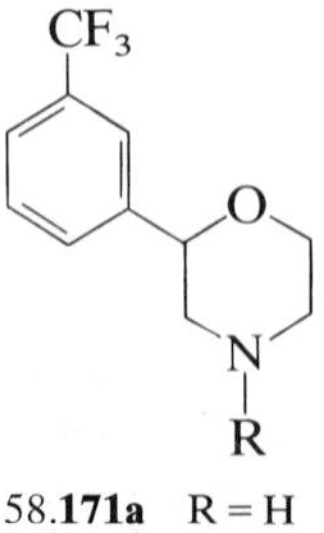

58.**171a** R = H
58.**171b** R = i-C$_3$H$_7$

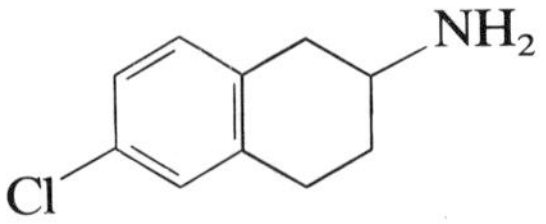

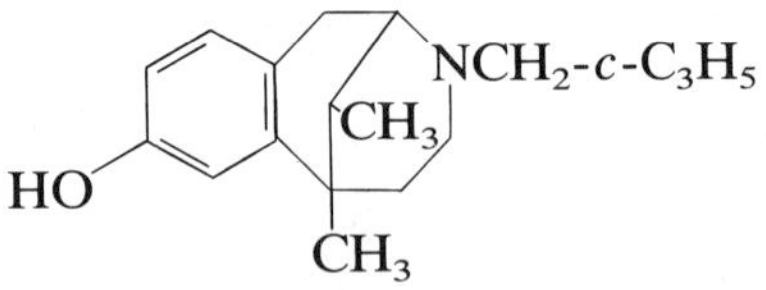

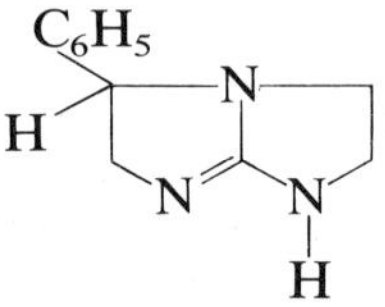

A structurally related 2-aminotetralin 58.**173**, like parachloroamphetamine, lowers brain levels of tryptophan hydroxylase and serotonin, but is a much weaker inhibitor of serotonin uptake than is 58.**172** (518). The analgetic benzazocine, cyclazocine (58.**174**), produces EEG patterns similar to those of antidepressants. It improves depressed patients; however, secondary effects are common (519). Deximafen (58.**175**) is a potent antagonist of reserpine- or tetrabenazine-induced effects, but it causes only minor overt symptoms in animals (520).

Various other aralkylamines having a one-, three-, or four-carbon bridge between the phenyl and amino groups have antidepressant properties. The benzylamine 58.**176** is a potent long-acting inhibitor of norepinephrine uptake by mouse brain (521). An aminotetralin derivative 58.**177** also causes antidepressant actions in ani-

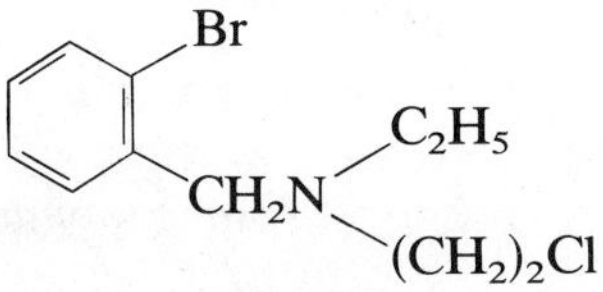

58.176

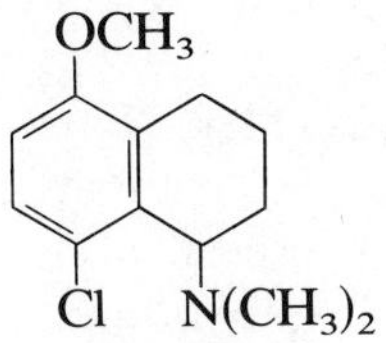

58.177

mals, but it is of doubtful benefit to depressed patients (522).

A three-carbon bridge is noted in the antidepressants 58.**178**–58.**183a**. The cyclopropylmethylamine 58.**178** fails to inhibit MAO, but it reverses reserpine-induced depression in rabbits (173). The bicyclooctane 58.**179** is claimed to have both antidepressant and antipsychotic actions. Some members of a series (524) of triazines, e.g., 58.**157b** (see 58.**157a**, Section 4.2.7), are more potent than imipramine in reversing reserpine-induced ptosis, potentiating amphetamine toxicity, and prolonging hexobarbital-induced sleeping time in mice. A phenethylpiperidine 58.**180**, one of a series (525), is approximately equipotent with amitriptyline in a dopa-potentiation test in mice. The 4-substituted piperidine 58.**181** is a potent and selective inhibitor of serotonin uptake; however, it does not inhibit norepinephrine

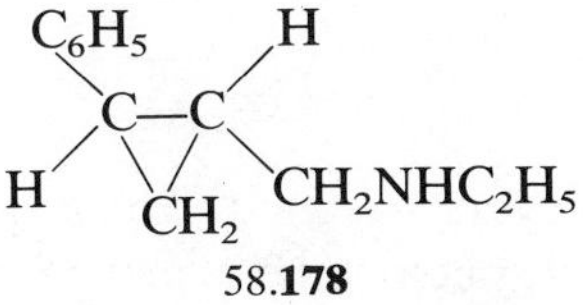

58.178

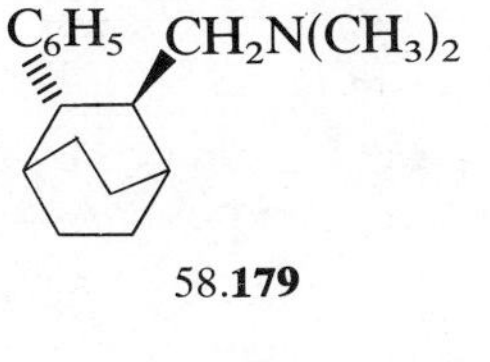

58.179

uptake in rat brain (341, 526). An aminopiperidinol 58.**182** lacks MAO-inhibitory activity but antagonizes reserpine-induced ptosis in mice (527). Antidepressant activity is claimed (528) for some 7-amino-benzocycloheptene derivatives, e.g., 58.**183a**. The homologous 55.**183b** is also claimed (529) to have antidepressant activity.

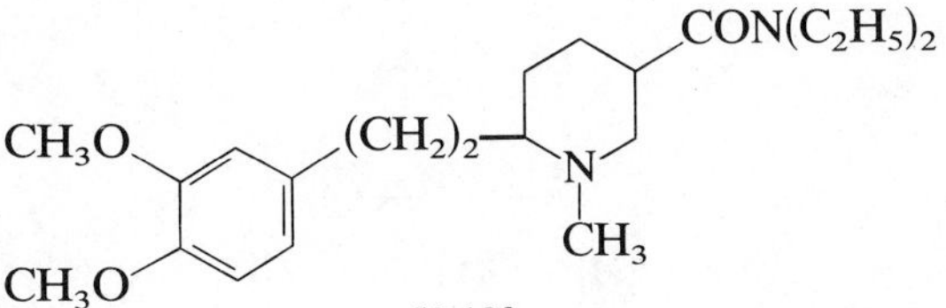

58.180

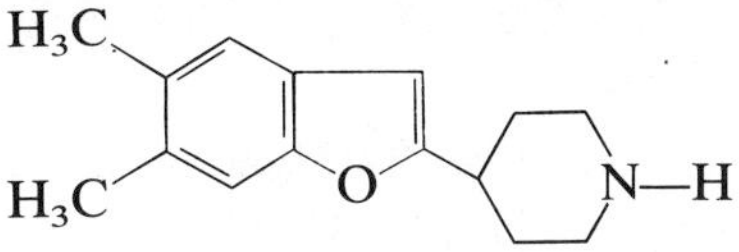

58.181

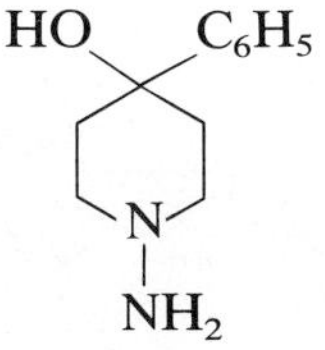

58.182

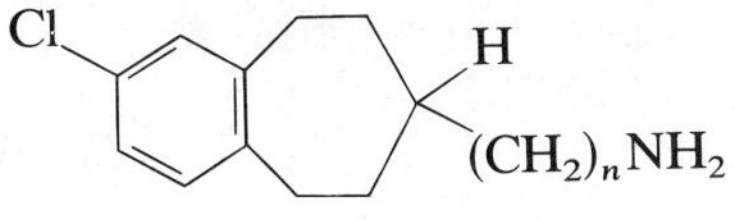

58.183a $n = 0$
58.183b $n = 1$

Antidepressant-like compounds with a four-carbon bridge between a phenyl ring and a basic amino group include 58.**184**–58.**185**. The bicyclooctane 55.**184** has a pharmacological profile similar to that of imipramine; however, it is not effective in patients suffering from endogenous depression (530). An adamantyl derivative 58.**185** weakly antagonizes reserpine-induced re-

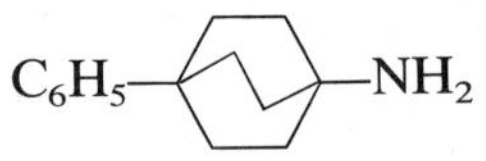

58.**184**

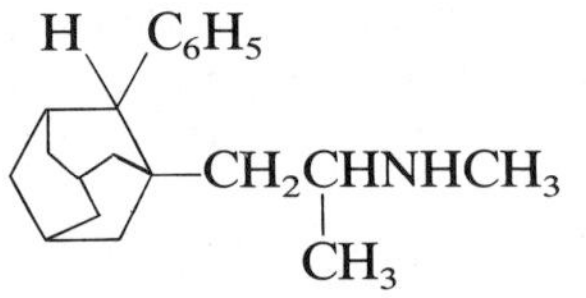

58.**185**

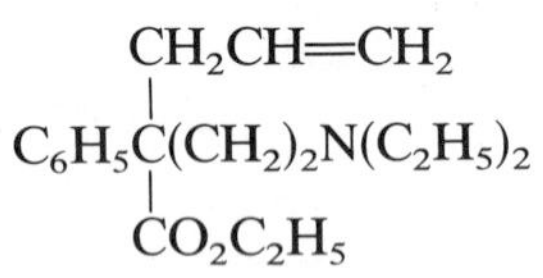

$$CH_2CH{=}CH_2$$
$$C_6H_5\overset{|}{\underset{|}{C}}(CH_2)_2N(C_2H_5)_2$$
$$CO_2C_2H_5$$

58.**186**

sponses and potentiates norepinephrine-induced effects in animals (531).

An analog 58.**186** of γ-aminobutyric acid has antidepressant-like properties in animals, but it is not effective in depressed patients (532).

4.3.2 ARYLOXYALKYLAMINES AND RELATED COMPOUNDS. Several aryloxyalkylamine derivatives have significant imipramine-like activity *in vivo* and *in vitro*.

Viloxazine (58.**187**) apparently has anti-depressant activity (533); however, a more rapid onset of action (534) than imipramine and even clinical efficacy have been questioned (535). Pharmacological studies indicate that viloxazine antagonizes reserpine-induced effects, potentiates norepi-nephrine-induced responses, and blocks norepinephrine and serotonin uptake (536). A *p*-methoxyphenoxymethylpiperidine, fe-moxetine (58.**188**), is a potent inhibitor

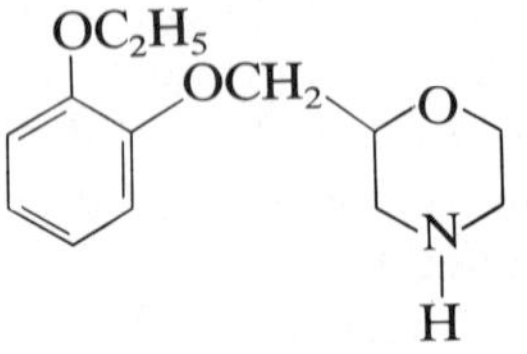

58.**187**

of serotonin uptake (537). It is a relatively weak blocker of norepinephrine uptake and potentiates serotonin *in vivo* (538); however, it is inferior to amitriptyline in depressed patients (69). A close relative 58.**189** produces hypermotility and anticonvulsant actions in combination with 5-hydroxytryptophan (539). Mefexamide [4-$CH_3OC_6H_4OCONH(CH_2)_2N(C_2H_5)_2$] has imipramine-like activity at doses that do not cause side effects in animals (540). A naphthyloxyalkylpiperidine 58.**190** is a potent and selective inhibitor of neuronal serotonin uptake. It is a potential antidepressant that may be of value in determining the uptake mechanism and functional significance of serotonin (541).

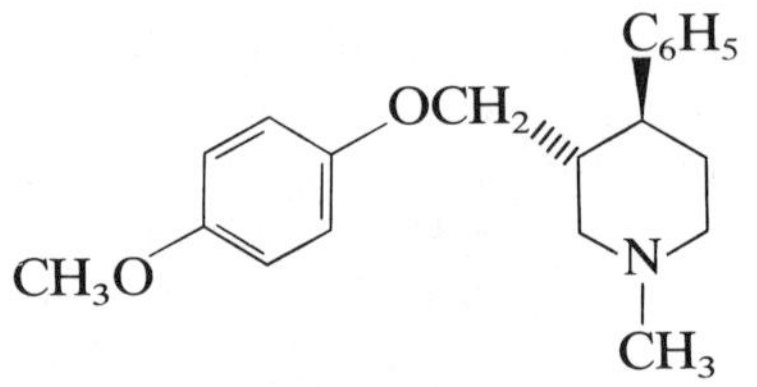

58.**188**

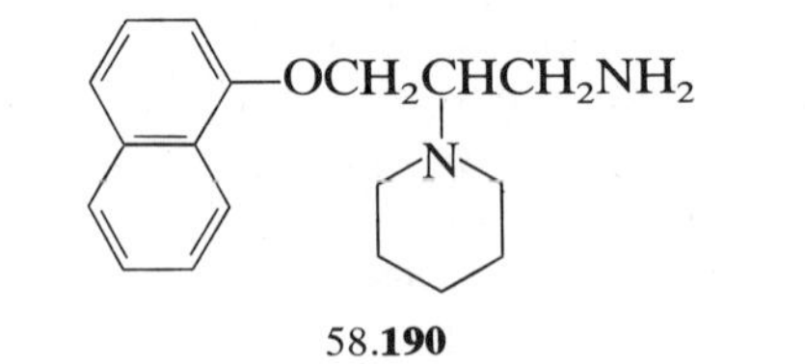

58.**189**

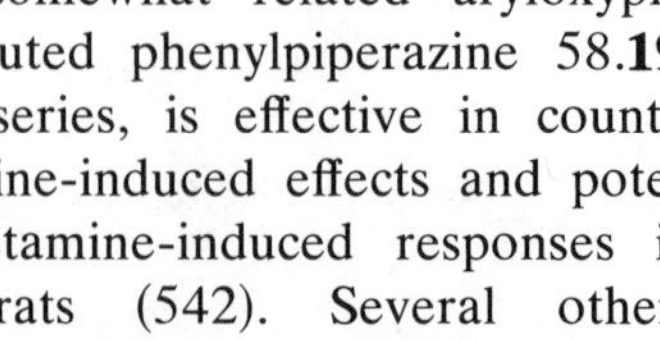

58.**190**

A somewhat related aryloxypropanol-substituted phenylpiperazine 58.**191**, one of a series, is effective in counteracting reserpine-induced effects and potentiating amphetamine-induced responses in mice and rats (542). Several other anti-depressant-like compounds with a three-carbon atom bridge between the oxygen and basic nitrogen include the aryloxy-propylamine 58.**192**, a serotonin blocker that decreases prolactin levels in ovariec-tomized estrogen-treated rats (543), and the tropanes 58.**193** (544) and 58.**194** (545), which antagonize reserpine-induced effects in rats. Another acetal derivative 58.**195** has imipramine-like activity without anti-cholinergic properties (546). It also pre-vents synaptosomal reuptake of norepi-nephrine (547).

Other compounds having an aryloxy-ethylamine framework are 58.**196**–58.**198**. The imidazoline 58.**196** (fenmetazole) has imipramine-like properties in animals; it decreases accumulation of norepinephrine, dopamine, and serotonin by rat forebrain synaptosomes (548). Initial studies in de-pressed patients are promising (549). Aryloxyethylpyrrolidines 58.**197** are twice

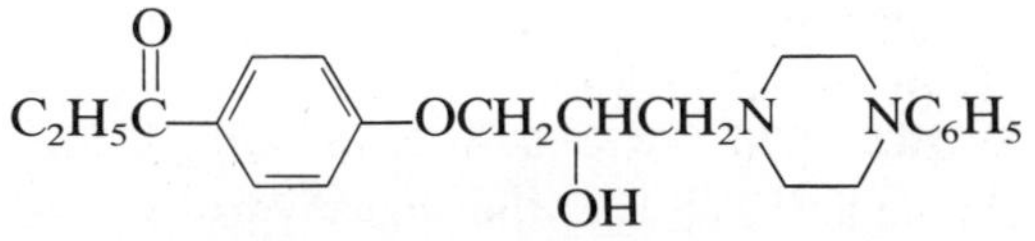

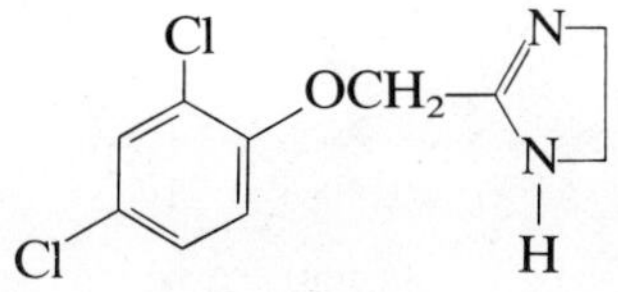

58.**196**

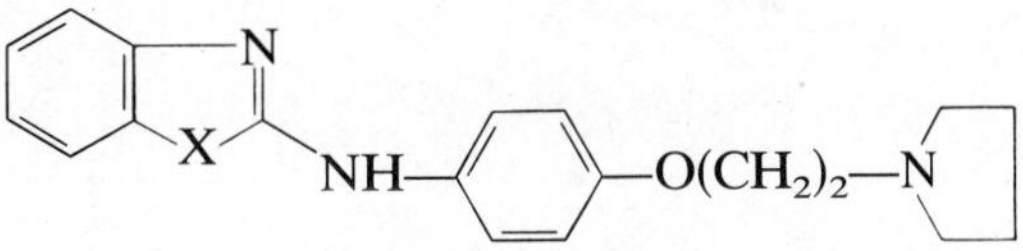

58.**197**   X = O, S

58.**198**   X = Cl, CH_3O

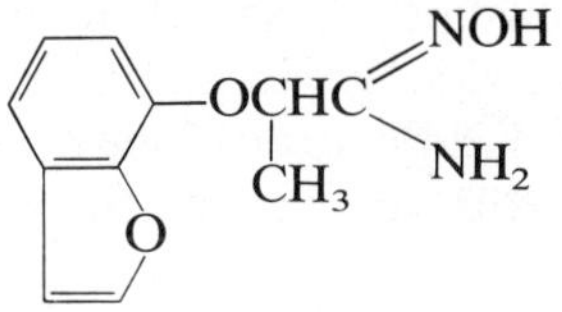

58.**199**

58.**191**

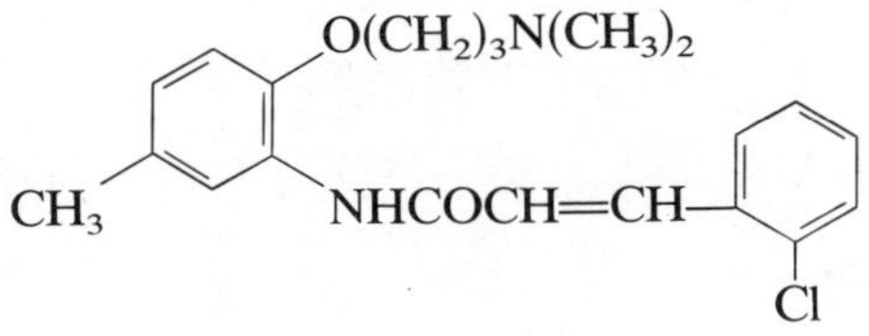

58.**192**

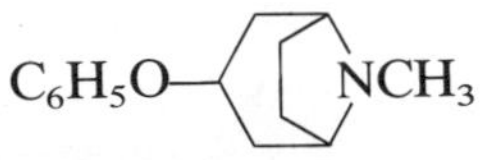

58.**193**

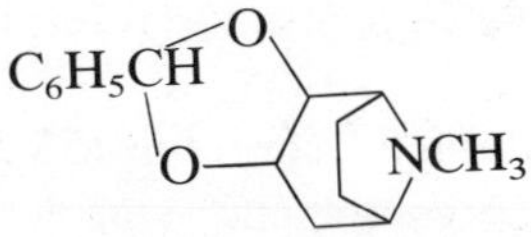

58.**194**

$(C_6H_5O)_2CHCH_2N(CH_3)_2$

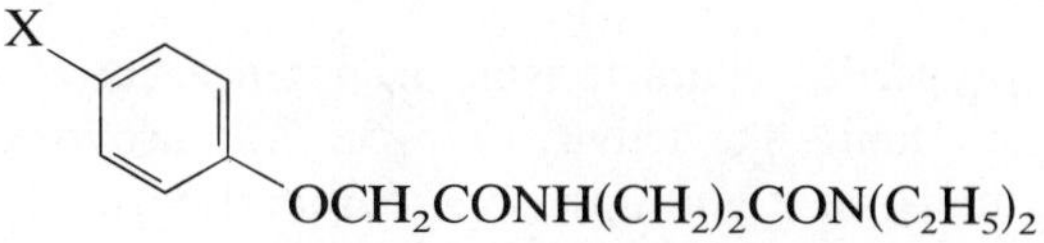

58.**195**

as potent as imipramine in causing a rever-sal of reserpine-induced hyperthermia in mice (550). Unique clinical antidepressant activity is produced by 58.**198** (551). The amidoxime 58.**199** has imipramine-like ac-tivity. It inhibits reserpine-induced effects and aggressive behavior and potentiates the effects of amphetamine in rats (552).

4.3.3 ARYL- AND ARALKYLPIPERAZINE DERI-VATIVES. Aryl- and benzylpiperazines having antidepressant properties are exemplified by quipazine (58.**200**), the pyrazine derivative 58.**201**, trazodone (58.**202**), and befuraline (58.**203a**). Qui-pazine has a pharmacological profile similar to that of tricyclic antidepressants (553). It is a serotonin-like drug that increases acetylcholine in the striatum of rats, sug-gesting inhibitory control of cholinergic interneurons by serotonergic neurons pro-jecting to the striatum (554). The pyrazine derivative 58.**201** has pharmacological

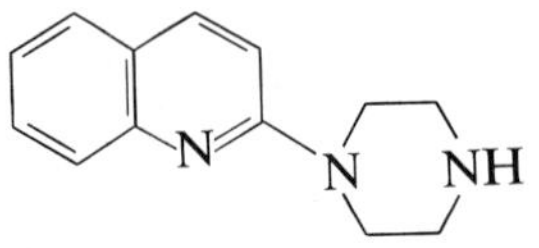

58.**200**

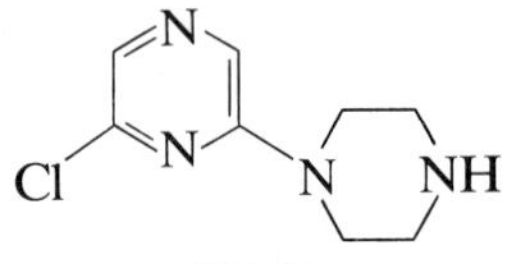

58.**201**

properties characteristic of potent central serotonin-like activity (555, 556). It also inhibits serotonin uptake in cerebral cortical tissue with no appreciable effect on norepinephrine uptake (557). Its urinary metabolites, including an *N*-benzoyl derivative, have been characterized (558). Quinoxaline (559) and 1,2,4-benzotriazine (560), relatives of 58.**201**, are claimed to have similar activity.

Trazodone (58.**202**) has a novel and complex pharmacological profile suggestive of antidepressant activity (561). It is slightly less potent, but more selective, than chlorimipramine in blocking serotonin uptake into rat brain synaptosomes (562). It also inhibits the hypotensive effect of clonidine, a central α-adrenergic receptor agonist (563). Befuraline (58.**203a**) is a phosphodiesterase inhibitor with little anticholinergic activity. It antagonizes the ac-

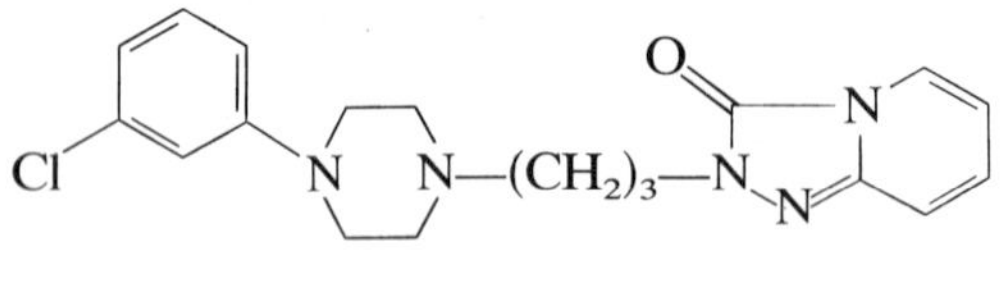

58.**202**

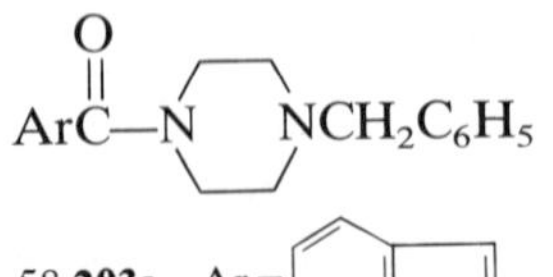

58.**203a**   Ar =

58.**203b**   Ar = 2-pyridyl

tions of reserpine and potentiates the effects of norepinephrine (564). Unlike imipramine, befuraline lacks a cardiodepressive action in dogs (565). In an open study befuraline was effective in about 50% of depressed patients (566, 567). A pyridyl relative 58.**203b** of befuraline appears more potent than imipramine. It is less toxic than amitriptyline with no apparent cholinergic or cardiotoxic properties (568).

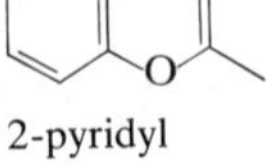

4.3.4 CARBOLINES AND OTHER INDOLE DERIVATIVES. A number of indole derivatives, especially carbolines, have antidepressant properties that are not necessarily or entirely associated with MAO inhibition.

The β-carboline 5-hydroxytryptoline (6-HO-58.**18**), an inhibitor of MAO, is equipotent with imipramine as an inhibitor of serotonin uptake by brain tissue (569). Imipramine-like actions, combined with sedation and analgesia, are noted for a series of pyridyl-substituted β-carbolines, e.g., 58.**204** (570). Antidepressant actions are claimed (571) for the hexahydro-β-carboline 58.**205**. Pentacyclic β-carbolines

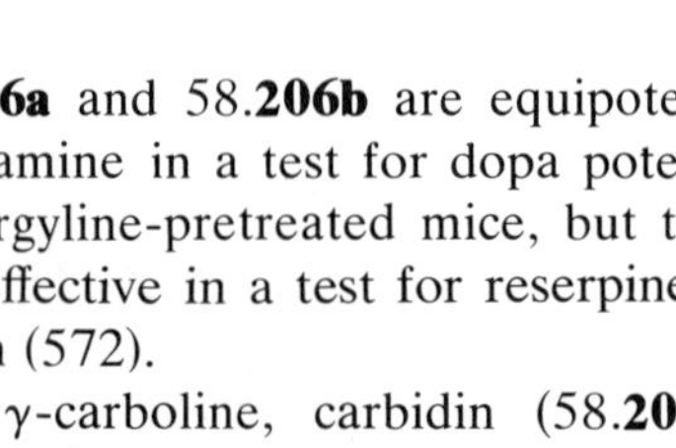

58.**204**

58.**206a** and 58.**206b** are equipotent with imipramine in a test for dopa potentiation in pargyline-pretreated mice, but they are less effective in a test for reserpine antagonism (572).

A γ-carboline, carbidin (58.**207**), has both antidepressant and neuroleptic properties in animals and man (573).

Other indole derivatives with antidepressant properties include 58.**208**–58.**211**. The piperidylindole 58.**208** is claimed (574) to have antidepressant activ-

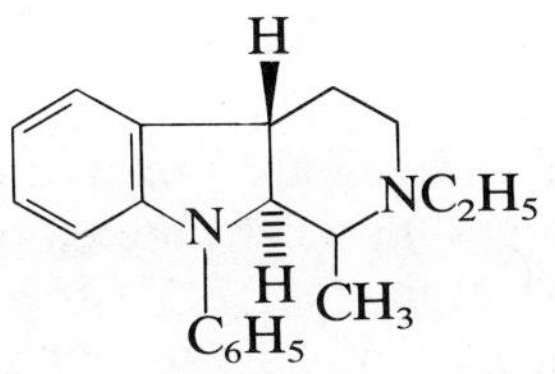

58.**205**

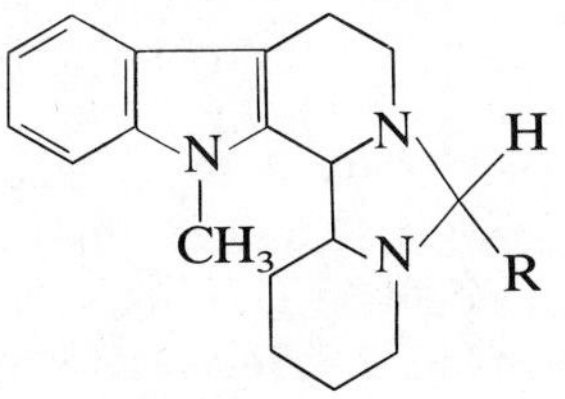

58.**206a**   R = C$_6$H$_5$
58.**206b**   R = C$_2$H$_5$

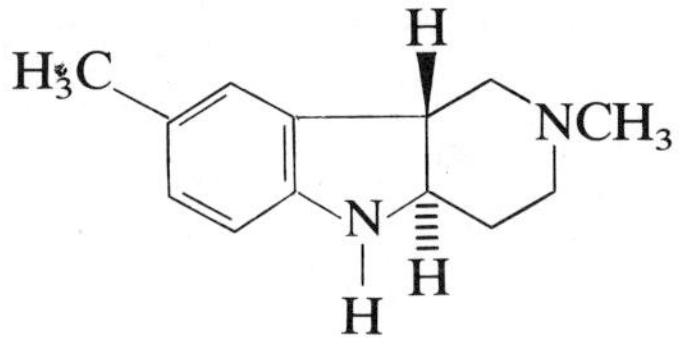

58.**207**

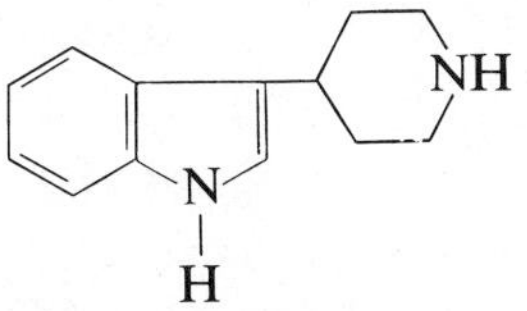

58.**208**

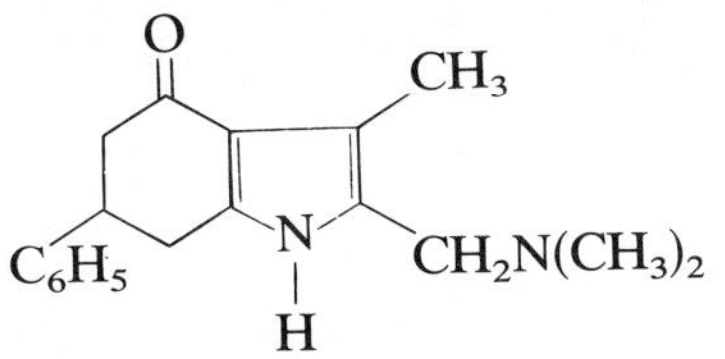

58.**209**

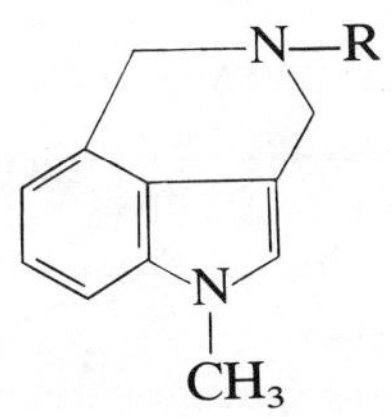

58.**210**   R = H, C$_2$H$_5$

ity whereas 58.**209** antagonizes tetrabenazine-induced ptosis in mice and potentiates the pressor response to norepinephrine in dogs (575). Several pyrrolo[4,3,2-*de*]isoquinolines, e.g., 58.**210**, are more potent than amitriptyline in preventing reserpine-induced ptosis in mice (576). The indolylmethyleneimidazolidinone 58.**211** has an oral ED$_{50}$ of 5 mg/kg against ptosis induced by 100 mg/kg of tetrabenazine in mice (577). Antidepressant actions are also produced by the reduction product of strychnine (578) and several ergoline derivatives (579).

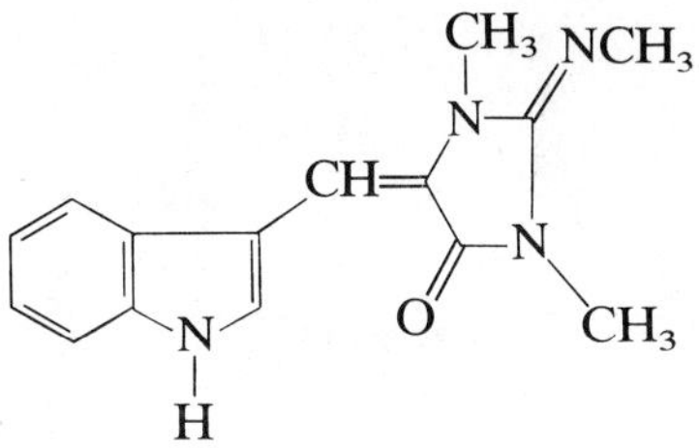

58.**211**

4.4   Miscellaneous Antidepressant Agents

Several compounds that cannot be categorized as a tricyclic or related compound or as an inhibitor of MAO have substantial antidepressant activity.

Some amide derivatives have antidepressant properties. The trimethoxycinnamamide 58.**212** produces clinical antidepressant effects (580). Another trimethoxybenzamide 58.**213** has pharmacological properties that resemble those of the tricyclic antidepressants (581). It antagonizes reserpine-induced effects in rats and potentiates amphetamine-induced hypermotility in mice (582). An acetamide derivative (caroxazone, 58.**214**) of benzoxazinone prevents the effects of reserpine in various animal species (583–585). It elevates norepinephrine, serotonin, and dopamine levels in rat brain (586) and pro-

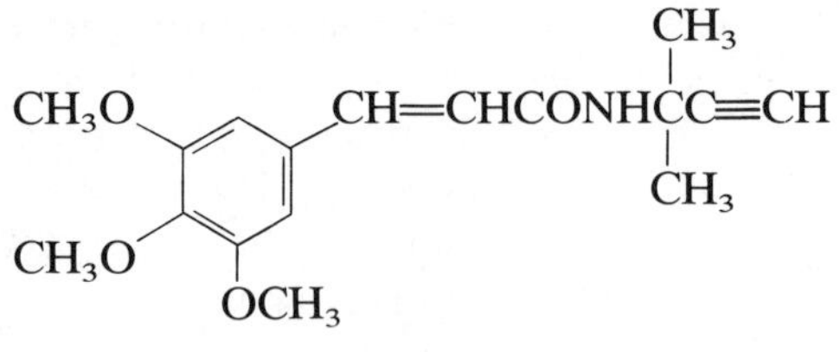

58.**212**

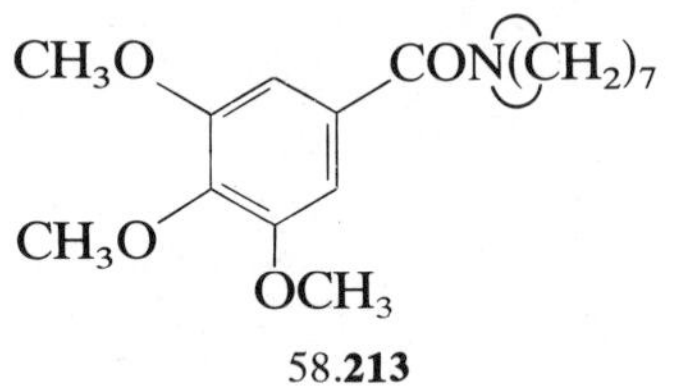

58.**213**

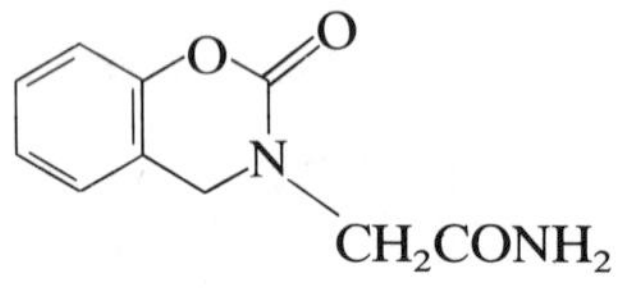

58.**214**

duces antidepressant effects in the clinic (587). These effects are apparently the consequence of weak MAO-inhibitory activity which is slightly greater for the type B than type A enzyme (588).

Certain centrally acting phosphodiesterase inhibitors also have antidepressant properties. For example, cartazolate (58.**215**) is effective in patients suffering from psychotic depression (589); however, its antianxiety actions are doubtful (590).

Potent antidepressant, hallucinogenic, and psychotomimetic actions are produced by some anticholinergic agents (591); although they are effective antidepressants, tachyphylaxis and psychotomimetic effects

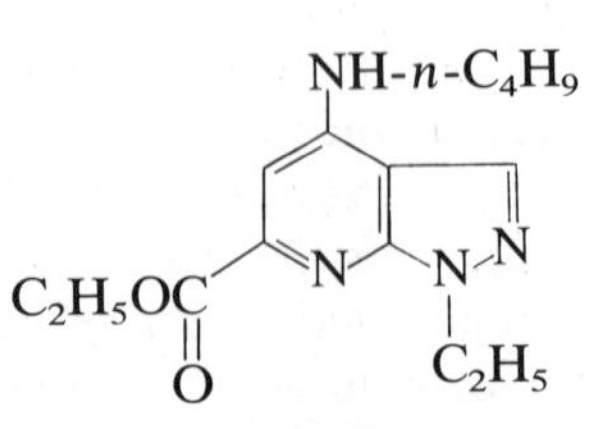

58.**215**

interfere with the clinical utility of some of these drugs (592).

Several *O*-aminoalkyl oximes of phenylalkyl ketones produce antidepressant actions. For example, 58.**216a** is a potent antagonist of tetrabenazine-induced ptosis (593). A closely related compound fluvoxamine (58.**216b**) is a clinically effective antidepressant (594, 595); it is a specific inhibitor of serotonin uptake (596, 597).

Toloxatone (58.**217**) is an antidepressant characterized by its ability to activate tryptophan hydroxylase and to inhibit serotonin catabolism (598). It weakly antagonizes reserpine-induced effects and potentiates responses to amphetamine (599). In a series of phenacylthioimidazolines, most potent reserpine antagonist properties in mice are produced by 58.**218**, which is 12 times more potent than imipramine in this test (600). Another 2-substituted imidazoline 58.**219** blocks norepinephrine uptake by neurons; however, toxic side effects preclude clinical study (601).

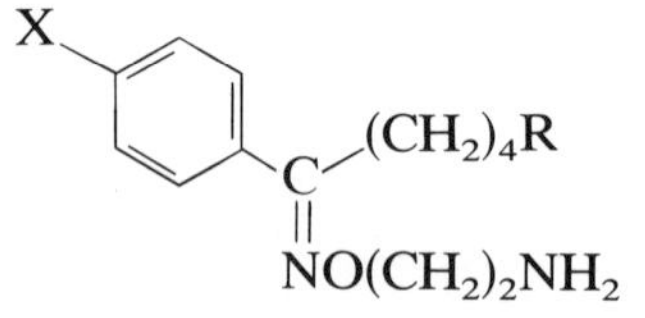

58.**216a**   X = H, R = CH_3
58.**216b**   X = CF_3, R = OCH_3

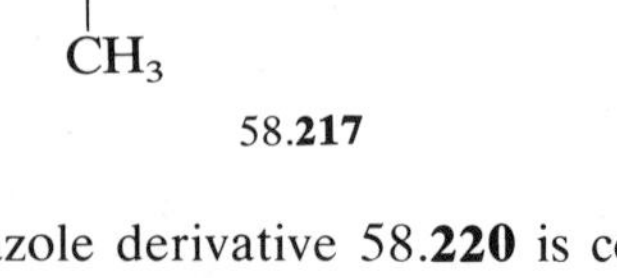

58.**217**

A urazole derivative 58.**220** is comparable to amitriptyline in a dopa-potentiation test in mice (602). Clinically, it is as effective as imipramine in the treatment of depression (603, 604).

Rubidium and cesium salts produce antidepressant actions in animals; they cause

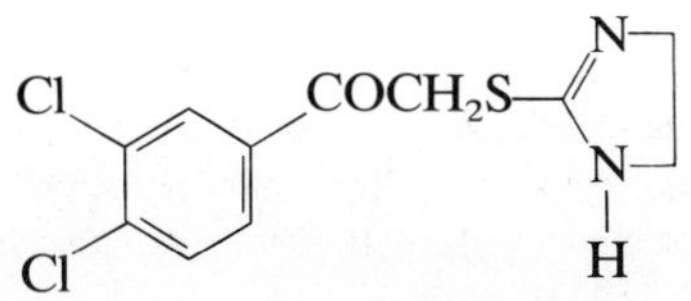

Cl—[ring]—COCH₂S—[imidazoline with N, N-H]

58.218

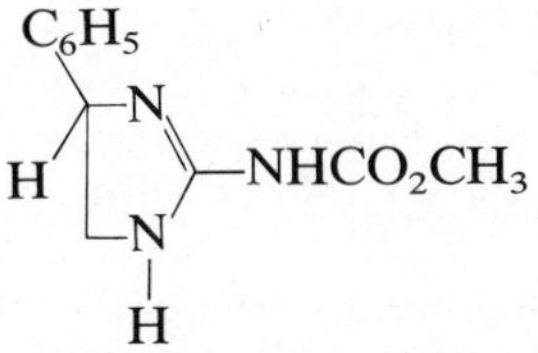

C₆H₅—[imidazoline ring]—NHCO₂CH₃ (H on ring)

58.219

$(CH_3)_2CH—N—N—CH(CH_3)_2$
O=[ring with N-H]=O

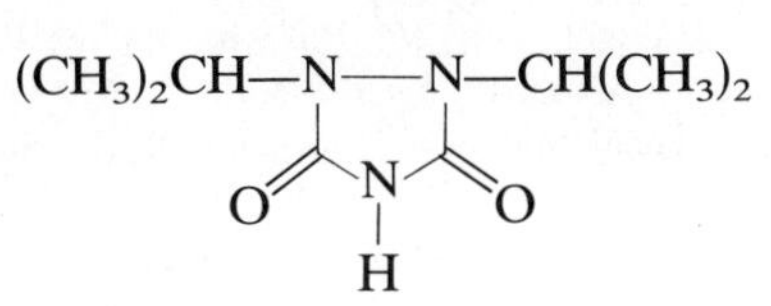

58.220

increased motor activity when administered for prolonged periods (605). In rats, cesium specifically increases serotonin turnover, whereas rubidium is more specific for norepinephrine. Also, rubidium increases shock-induced aggression in rats, but cesium does not (606). Clinically, rubidium improves depressed patients (607, 608). Although no toxic effects are noted, the 50–60 day half-life of rubidium may present safety problems in its clinical utility (609). Results of an extensive study confirm the effectiveness of lithium in preventing broad swings in mood in patients with manic depression (610).

Some natural body chemicals may be of benefit in treating depression. Thyroid-releasing hormone (TRH, protirelin) produces some clinical antidepressant actions (611–613). Although its efficacy is questionable (614), specific depressed subgroups may respond (615). The mechanism of action is not known; however, it apparently does not involve release of thyroid-stimulating hormone from the pituitary gland (616). *S*-Adenosyl-L-methionine also has clinical antidepressant activity (617). Melanocyte-stimulating hormone release inhibiting factor, MIF-I [H-Pro-Leu-Gly-NH₂(L, L)], produced marked improvement in endogenously depressed patients (618, 619). Some analogs (620) of MIF-I potentiate dopa-induced behavior in mice. The most effective synthetic analog in this test is H-Pro-MeLeu-Gly-NH₂(L, D) (621).

Several steroids cause antidepressant effects. Preliminary studies indicate that prednisone is of benefit in depressed patients (622). Mesterolone (17β-hydroxy-1α-methyl-5α-androstane-3-one), predicted to have imipramine-like activity on the basis of quantitative pharmaco-EEG studies, also appears to have clinical merit (623). Combined administration of dexamethasone with various antidepressants gives a rapid onset of action in depressed patients (624).

Other miscellaneous compounds for which antidepressant properties have been reported include the β-adrenoreceptor agonist salbutamol (625), 5-hydroxy-L-tryptophan (626), D-phenylalanine (627–629), and procaine (630). The utility of procaine, however, could not be confirmed in subsequent studies (631).

REFERENCES

1. E. A. Zeller, J. Barsky, J. P. Fouts, W. F. Kirchheimer, and L. S. VanOrden, *Experientia*, **8,** 349 (1952).

2. E. C. Greismer, J. Barsky, C. A. Dragstedt, J. A. Wells, and E. A. Zeller, *Proc. Soc. Exp. Biol. Med.*, **84,** 699 (1953).

3. J. Rebhun, S. M. Feinberg, and E. A. Zeller, *Proc. Soc. Exp. Biol. Med.*, **87,** 218 (1954).

4. B. B. Brodie and P. A. Shore, *Ann. N.Y. Acad. Sci.*, **66,** 631 (1957).

5. H. P. Loomer, J. C. Saunders, and N. S. Kline, *Am. Psychiatr. Assoc. Rep.*, **8,** 129 (1957).

6. F. Häfliger and W. Schindler, U.S. Pat. 2,554,736 (1951).

7. R. Kuhn, *Schweiz. Med. Wochenschr.*, **87,** 1135 (1957).

8. D. F. Klein and J. M. Davis, *Diagnosis and Drug Treatment of Psychiatric Disorders*, Williams and Wilkins, Baltimore, 1969.

9. R. L. Spitzer, J. Endicott, R. A. Woodruff, and N. Anderson, in *Depression, Clinical, Biological and Psychological Perspectives*, G. Usdin, Ed., Brunner/Mazel Pub., New York, 1977 p. 73.

10. H. E. Lehmann, in *Pharmacotherapy of Depression*, J. O. Cole and J. R. Wittenborn, Eds., Charles C Thomas, Springfield, Ill., 1966, p. 3.

11. M. T. Tsuang, in *Biology of the Major Psychoses, Res. Publ. Assoc. Res. Nerv. Ment. Dis.*, Vol. 54, D. X. Freedman, Ed., Raven Press, New York, 1975, p. 27.

12. C. Perris, *Acta Psychiatr. Scand.*, **42:** Suppl. 194 (1966).

13. R. Kuhn, *Am. J. Psychiatr.*, **115,** 459 (1958).

14. J. J. Schildkraut, *Am. J. Psychiatr.*, **122,** 509 (1965).

15. T. H. Harris, *Am. J. Psychiatr.*, **113,** 950 (1957).

16. A. Coppen, A. J. Prange, P. G. Whybrow, and R. Noguera, *Arch. Gen. Psychiatr.*, **26,** 474 (1972).

17. D. L. Murphy, I. C. Campbell, and J. L. Costa, *Progr. Neuro-Psychopharmacol.*, **2,** 1 (1978).

18. J. J. Schildkraut, *Ann. Rev. Pharmacol.*, **13,** 427 (1973).

19. J. J. Schildkraut, *Psychopharmacol. Bull.*, **10,** 5 (1974).

20. F. K. Goodwin and R. M. Post, in *Biology of the Major Psychoses, Res. Publ. Assoc. Res. Nerv. Ment. Dis.*, Vol. 54, D. X. Freedman, Ed., Raven Press, New York, 1975, p. 289.

21. B. J. Carroll, in *The Psychobiology of Depression*, J. Mendels, Ed., Spectrum Publications, New York, 1975, p. 143.

22. R. J. Baldessarini, in *The Psychobiology of Depression*, J. Mendels, Ed., Spectrum Publications, New York, 1975, p. 69.

23. R. M. Post and F. K. Goodwin, in *The Psychobiology of Depression*, J. Mendels, Ed., Spectrum Publications, New York, 1975, p. 47.

24. F. A. Jenner, *Brit. J. Clin. Pharmacol.*, **4,** 1995 (1977).

25. A. Raskin, *Am. J. Psychiatr.*, **131,** 181 (1974).

26. L. E. Hollister, *Clinical Use of Psychotherapeutic Drugs*, Charles C Thomas, Springfield, Ill., 1973.

27. J. M. Davis, in *Drug Treatment of Mental Disorders*, L. L. Simpson, Ed., Raven Press, New York, 1975, p. 127.

28. A. J. Gelenberg and G. L. Klerman, *Rational Drug Ther.*, **12,** 1 (1978).

29. C. L. Ravaris, D. S. Robinson, A. Nies, J. O. Ives, and D. Bartlett, *Am. Fam. Physician*, **18,** 105 (1978).

30. F. Quitkin, A. Rifkin, and D. F. Klein, *Arch. Gen. Psychiatr.*, **33,** 337 (1976).

31. D. S. Robinson and E. Barker, *J. Am. Med. Assoc.*, **236,** 2089 (1976).

32. M. J. Antonaccio and R. D. Robson, in *Antidepressants*, S. Fielding and H. Lal, Eds., Futura Publishing Co., Mount Kisco, N.Y., 1975, p. 191.

33. G. D. Burrows, J. Vohra, D. Hunt, J. G. Sloman, B. A. Scoggins, and B. Davies, *Brit. J. Psychiatr.*, **129,** 335 (1976).

34. F. Häfliger and V. Burckhardt, in *Psychopharmacological Agents*, Vol. 1, M. Gordon, Ed., Academic, New York-London, 1964, Chap. 3.

35. L. Gyermek, in *International Review of Neurobiology*, Vol. 9, C. C. Pfeiffer and J. R. Smythies, Eds., Academic, New York, 1966.

36. R. E. McMahon, F. J. Marshall, H. W. Culp, and W. M. Miller, *Biochem. Pharmacol.*, **12,** 1207 (1963).

37. G. B. Cassano and E. Hansson, in *Neuropsychopharmacology*, H. Brill, Ed., Excerpta Medica, New York-London, 1967, p. 1191.

38. J. L. Crammer and B. Scott, *Psychopharmacologia*, **8,** 461 (1966).

39. J. Christiansen, L. F. Gram, B. Kofod, and O. J. Rafaelsen, *Psychopharmacologia*, **11,** 255 (1967).

40. M. E. Amundson and J. A. Manthey, *J. Pharm. Sci.*, **55,** 277 (1966).

41. M. H. Bickel and M. Baggiolini, *Biochem. Pharmacol.*, **15,** 1155 (1966).

42. W. Hammer and F. Sjöqvist, *Life Sci.*, **6,** 1895 (1967).

43. J. H. Biel, A. Horita, and A. E. Drukker, in *Psychopharmacological Agents*, Vol. 1, M. Gordon, Ed., Academic, New York-London, 1964, Chapter 11.

44. C. L. Zirkle and C. Kaiser, in *Psychopharmacological Agents*, Vol. 1, M. Gordon, Ed., Academic, New York-London, 1964, Chapter 12.

45. G. R. Pscheit, in *International Review of Neurobiology*, Vol. 7, C. C. Pfeiffer and J. R. Smythies, Eds., Academic, New York-London, 1964, p. 191.

46. R. A. Braithwaite, R. Goulding, G. Theano, J. Bailey, and A. Coppen, *Lancet*, **1972–I,** 1297.

47. J. M. Perel, M. Shostak, E. Gann, S. J. Kantor, and A. H. Glassman, in *Pharmacokinetics of Psycho-Active Drugs*, L. A. Gottschalk and S. Meiles, Eds., Spectrum Publications, New York, 1976.

48. G. D. Burrows, B. Davies, and B. A. Scoggins, *Lancet*, **1972–II,** 619.

49. M. Åshberg, B. Crönholm, F. Sjoqvist, and D. Tuck, *Brit. Med. J.*, **3,** 331 (1971).

50. P. Kragh-Sorensen, C. Eggert-Hansen, P. C. Baastrup, and E. F. Hvidberg, *Psychopharmacologia*, **45,** 305 (1976).

51. A. H. Glassman and J. M. Perel, *Arch. Gen. Psychiatr.*, **28,** 649 (1973).

52. G. Muscettola, F. K. Goodwin, W. Z. Potter, M. M. Claeys, and S. Markey, *Arch. Gen. Psychiatr.*, **35,** 621 (1975).

53. P. O. Ganrot, E. Rosengren, and C. G. Gottfries, *Experientia*, **18,** 260 (1962).

54. A. S. Horn and S. H. Snyder, *J. Pharmacol. Exp. Ther.*, **180,** 523 (1972).

55. R. J. Ziance, J. Moxley, M. Mullis, and W. Gray, *Arch. Int. Pharmacodyn. Ther.*, **228,** 30 (1977).

56. N. H. Neff and H. Y. T. Yang, *Life Sci.*, **14,** 2061 (1974).

57. B. K. Koe, *J. Pharmacol. Exp. Ther.*, **199,** 649 (1976).

58. R. E. Heikkila, S. S. Goldfinger, and H. Orlansky, *Res. Commun. Chem. Pathol. Pharmacol.*, **13,** 237 (1976).

59. F. Sulser, M. W. Owens, S. J. Strada, and J. V. Dingel, *J. Pharmacol. Exp. Ther.*, **168,** 272 (1969).

60. J. Schubert, H. Nybäck, and G. Sedvall, *J. Pharm. Pharmacol.*, **22,** 136 (1970).

61. B. E. Leonard and W. F. Kafoe, *Biochem. Pharmacol.*, **25,** 1939 (1976).

62. J. J. Schildkraut, M. Roffman, P. J. Orsulak, A. F. Schatzberg, M. A. Kling, and Th. G. Reigle, *Pharmakopsychiat./Neuropsychopharmacol.*, **9,** 193 (1976).

63. M. Segal and F. E. Bloom, *Brain Res.*, **72,** 99 (1974).

64. D. Ghezzi, R. Samanin, S. Bernasconi, G. Tognani, M. Gerna, and S. Garattini, *Eur. J. Pharmacol.*, **24,** 205 (1973).

65. F. Sulser, M. W. Owens, and J. V. Dingell, *Life Sci.*, **5,** 2005 (1966).

66. P. J. Fowler, C. L. Zirkle, E. Macko, P. E. Setler, H. M. Sarau, A. Misher, and D. H. Tedeschi, *Arzneim.-Forsch.*, **27,** 1589 (1977).

67. G. Molnar, *Can. Psychiatr. Assoc. J.*, **22,** 19 (1977).

68. R. M. Pinder, R. N. Brogden, T. M. Speight, and G. S. Avery, *Drugs*, **13,** 401 (1977).

69. K. Ghose, R. Gupta, A. Coppen, and J. Lund, *Eur. J. Pharmacol.*, **42,** 31 (1977).

70. T. Itil, A. Bhattachyaryya, I. V. Polvan, M. Hugue, and G. N. Menon, *Progr. Neuro-Psychopharmacol.*, **1,** 309 (1977).

71. P. A. Nicholson and P. Turner, Eds., *Proceedings of a Symposium on Nomifensine, Brit. J. Clin. Pharmacol.*, **4:** Suppl. 2 (1977).

72. J. Maj, L. Baran, A. Rawlow, and H. Sowinska, *Pol. J. Pharmacol. Pharm.*, **29,** 213 (1977).

73. J. Kähling, H. Ziegler, and H. Balhause, *Arzneim.-Forsch.*, **25,** 1737 (1975).

74. K. Fuxe, S. O. Ögren, L. Agnati, J. Å. Gustáfsson, and G. Jonsson, *Neurosci. Lett.*, **6,** 339 (1977).

75. P. A. Baumann and L. Maître, *Naunyn-Schmiedebergs Arch. Pharmacol.*, **300,** 31 (1977).

76. B. Rosloff and J. M. Davis, *Psychopharmacol.*, **40,** 53 (1974).

77. M. I. Gluckman and T. Baum, *Psychopharmacol.*, **15,** 169 (1969).

78. J. J. Freeman and F. J. Sulser, *J. Pharmacol. Exp. Ther.*, **183,** 307 (1972).

79. F. Sulser, J. Vetulani, and P. Mobley, *Biochem. Pharmacol.*, **27,** 257 (1978).

80. J. P. Green and S. Maayani, *Nature*, **269,** 163 (1977).

81. P. O. Kanof and P. Greengard, *Nature*, **212,** 329 (1978).

82. E. Richelson, *Nature*, **274,** 176 (1978).

83. W. J. Kinnard, H. Barry, 3rd, N. Watzman, and J. P. Buckley, in *Antidepressant Drugs*, S. Garattini and M. N. G. Dukes, Eds., Excerpta Medica, New York-London, 1967, p. 89.

84. G. Klerman, in *Preclinical and Clinical Correlations*, A. Sudilovsky, S. Gershon, and B. Beer, Eds., Raven Press, New York, 1975, p. 159.

85. R. D. Porsolt, G. Anton, N. Blavet, and M. Jalfre, *Eur. J. Pharmacol.*, **47,** 379 (1978).

86. T. M. Itil, *Dis. Nerv. Syst.*, **33,** 557 (1972).

87. P. Tyrer, *Brit. J. Psychiatr.*, **128,** 354 (1976).

88. F. J. Ayd, Jr., Ed., *Int. Drug Ther. Newslett.*, **12:** 1, 1 (1977).

89. R. W. Fuller, *Abstr. Pap. 174th Am. Chem. Soc. Natl. Meet., Chicago, Ill., August 29–September 1, 1977*, p. MEDI-14.

90. M. Sandler and M. B. H. Youdim, *Pharmacol. Rev.*, **24,** 331 (1972).

91. R. McCauley and E. Racker, *Mol. Cell. Biochem.*, **1,** 73 (1973).

92. R. F. Squires, in *Advan. Biochem. Psycho-*

pharmacol., Vol. 5, E. Costa and M. Sandler, Eds., Raven Press, New York, 1972, p. 355.

93. H.-Y. T. Yang and N. H. Neff, *J. Pharmacol. Exp. Ther.*, **187**, 365 (1973).

94. C. Goridis and N. H. Neff, *Neuropharmacol.*, **10**, 557 (1971).

95. J. A. Roth, *Gen. Pharmacol.*, **7**, 381 (1976).

96. E. Costa and M. Sandler, Eds., *Monoamine Oxidases—New Vistas, Advan. Biochem. Psychopharmacol.*, Vol. 5, Raven Press, New York, 1972.

97. B. T. Ho, *J. Pharm. Sci.*, **61**, 821 (1972).

98. T. Fujita, *J. Med. Chem.*, **16**, 923 (1973).

99. A. Pletscher, K. F. Gey, and P. Zeller, in *Progress in Drug Research*, Vol. 2, E. Jucker, Ed., Birkhäuser, Basel-Stuttgart, 1960, pp. 471–590.

100. W. R. McGrath and A. Horita, *Toxicol. Appl. Pharmacol.*, **4**, 178 (1962).

101. C. L. Johnson, *J. Med. Chem.*, **19**, 600 (1976).

102. S. Sarkar, Ph.D. thesis, Northwestern University, Evanston, Ill., 1961.

103. W. Schuler and E. Wyss, *Arch. Int. Pharmacodyn. Ther.*, **128**, 431 (1960).

104. J. A. Carbon, W. P. Burkard, and E. A. Zeller, *Helv. Chim. Acta*, **41**, 1883 (1958).

105. D. J. Drain, J. G. B. Howes, R. Lazare, A. M. Salaman, R. Shadbolt, and H. W. R. Williams, *J. Med. Chem.*, **6**, 63 (1963).

106. J. H. Biel, P. A. Nuhfer, A. E. Drukker, T. F. Mitchell, Jr., A. C. Conway, and A. Horita, *J. Org. Chem.*, **26**, 3338 (1961).

107. J. H. Biel, A. E. Drukker, and T. F. Mitchell, *J. Am. Chem. Soc.*, **82**, 2204 (1960).

108. A. Spinks and B. A. Whittle, *Int. J. Neuropharmacol.*, **5**, 125 (1966).

109. A. Spinks and E. H. P. Young, *Proc. First Int. Pharmacol. Meet. 1961*, p. 303.

110. J. H. Biel, A. E. Drukker, T. F. Mitchell, E. P. Sprengeler, P. A. Nuhfer, A. C. Conway, and A. Horita, *J. Am. Chem. Soc.*, **81**, 2805 (1959).

111. J. Finkelstein, J. A. Romano, E. Chiang, and J. Lee, *J. Med. Chem.*, **6**, 153 (1963).

112. F. E. Anderson, D. Kaminsky, B. Dubnick, S. R. Klutchko, W. A. Cetenko, J. Gylys, and J. A. Hart, *J. Med. Pharm. Chem.*, **5**, 221 (1962).

113. J. H. Biel, P. A. Nuhfer, and A. C. Conway, *Ann. N.Y. Acad. Sci.*, **80**, 568 (1959).

114. V. G. Yashunskii, V. Z. Gorkin, M. D. Mashkovskii, R. A. Altshuler, I. V. Veryovkina, and L. E. Kholodov, *J. Med. Chem.*, **14**, 1013 (1971).

115. R. A. Altshuler and B. I. Kochelaev, *Khim.-Farm. Zh.*, **4**, 59 (1971).

116. F. Bennington, R. D. Morin, and L. C. Clarke, Jr., *J. Med. Chem.*, **8**, 100 (1965).

117. E. L. Schumann, R. V. Heinzelman, M. E. Greig, and W. Veldkamp, *J. Med. Chem.*, **7**, 329 (1964).

118. P. Zeller, A. Pletscher, K. F. Gey, H. Gutmann, B. Hegedus, and O. Straub, *Ann. N.Y. Acad. Sci.*, **80**, 555 (1959).

119. A. Pletscher and K. F. Gey, *Helv. Physiol. Pharmacol. Acta*, **16**, 26C (1958).

120. T. S. Gardner, E. Wenis, and J. Lee, *J. Med. Pharm. Chem.*, **2**, 133 (1960).

121. D. R. Maxwell, W. R. Gray, and E. M. Taylor, *Brit. J. Pharmacol.*, **17**, 310 (1961).

122. R. P. Rowe, B. M. Bloom, S. Y. P'an, and K. F. Finger, *Proc. Soc. Exp. Biol. Med.*, **101**, 832 (1959).

123. D. L. Trepanier, J. N. Eble, and G. H. Harris, *J. Med. Chem.*, **11**, 357 (1968).

124. C. S. Rooney, E. J. Cragoe, Jr., C. C. Porter, and J. M. Sprague, *J. Med. Pharm. Chem.*, **5**, 155 (1962).

125. K. Magyar, E. Satory, Z. Meszaros, and J. Knoll, *Med. Biol.*, **52**, 384 (1974).

126. A. G. Bolt and M. J. Sleigh, *Biochem. Pharmacol.*, **23**, 1969 (1974).

127. M. Harfenist, F. E. Soroko, and G. M. McKenzie, *J. Med. Chem.*, **21**, 405 (1978).

128. Hoffmann-LaRoche AG, Belg. Pat. 852,144 (1977); Derwent 64940Y/37.

129. J. Castañer and D. M. Paton, *Drugs Future*, **3**, 156 (1978).

130. S. Udenfriend, B. Witkop, R. G. Redfield, and H. Weissbach, *Biochem. Pharmacol.*, **1**, 160 (1958).

131. A. Pletscher, H. Besendorf, H. P. Bächtold, and K. F. Gey, *Helv. Physiol. Pharmacol. Acta*, **17**, 202 (1959).

132. M. Ozaki, H. Weissbach, A. Ozaki, B. Witkop, and S. Udenfriend, *J. Med. Pharm. Chem.*, **2**, 591 (1960).

133. A. Burger and S. Nara, *J. Med. Chem.*, **8**, 859 (1965).

134. V. Z. Gorkin and L. V. Tatyanenko, *Life Sci.*, **6**, 791 (1967).

135. K. Freter, H. Weissbach, B. Redfield, S. Udenfriend, and B. Witkop, *J. Am. Chem. Soc.*, **80**, 983 (1958).

136. J. R. Vane, *Brit. J. Pharmacol.*, **14**, 87 (1959).

137. W. M. Govier, B. G. Howes, and A. J. Gibbons, *Science*, **118**, 596 (1953).

138. K. P. Sing and S. K. Gautam, *Arzneim.-Forsch.*, **27**, 2002 (1977).

139. M. E. Greig, R. A. Walk, and A. J. Gibbons, *J. Pharmacol. Exp. Ther.*, **127,** 110 (1959).

140. B. Carnmalm, A. Misiorny, S. B. Ross, and N. E. Stjernström, *Acta Pharm. Suec.*, **11,** 196 (1974).

141. K. F. Gey and A. Pletscher, *Brit. J. Pharmacol.*, **19,** 161 (1962).

142. G. A. Youngdale, D. G. Anger, W. C. Anthony, J. P. DaVanzo, M. E. Greig, R. V. Heinzelman, H. H. Keasling, and J. Szmuszkovicz, *J. Med. Chem.*, **7,** 415 (1964).

143. A. G. Terzian, R. R. Safrasbekian, R. S. Sukasian, and G. T. Tatevosian, *Experientia*, **17,** 493 (1961).

144. B. A. Whittle and E. H. P. Young, *J. Med. Chem.*, **6,** 378 (1963).

145. H. Azima, D. Arthurs, A. Silver, and F. J. Azima, *Am. J. Psychiatr.*, **119,** 573 (1962).

146. J. B. Hester, M. E. Greig, W. C. Anthony, R. V. Heinzelman, and J. Szmuszkovicz, *J. Med. Chem.*, **7,** 274 (1964).

147. R. B. Barlow, *Brit. J. Pharmacol.*, **16,** 153 (1961).

148. J. D. Taylor, A. A. Wykes, Y. C. Gladish, and W. B. Martin, *Nature*, **187,** 941 (1960).

149. L. R. Swett, W. B. Martin, J. D. Taylor, G. M. Everett, A. A. Wykes, and Y. C. Gladish, *Ann. N.Y. Acad. Sci.*, **107,** 891 (1963).

150. C. F. Huebner, E. M. Donoghue, A. J. Plummer, and P. A. Furness, *J. Med. Chem.*, **9,** 830 (1966).

151. L. Mâitre, *J. Pharmacol. Exp. Ther.*, **157,** 81 (1967).

152. K. Šindelář and M. Protiva, *Collect. Czech. Chem. Commun.*, **33,** 4315 (1968).

153. J. Knoll, Z. Ecseri, K. Kelenen, J. Nievel, and B. Knoll, *Arch. Int. Pharmacodyn. Ther.*, **155,** 154 (1965).

154. J. Knoll, E. Sz. Vizi, and Gy. Somogyi, *Arzneim.-Forsch.*, **18,** 109 (1968).

155. J. P. Johnston, *Biochem. Pharmacol.*, **17,** 1285 (1968).

156. D. Wheatley, *Brit. J. Psychiatr.*, **117,** 573 (1970).

157. A. B. Bevan Jones, C. M. B. Pare, W. J. Nicholson, K. Price, and R. S. Stacey, *Brit. Med. J.*, **5791,** 17 (1972).

158. J. Mills, R. Katau, I. H. Slater, and R. W. Fuller, *J. Med. Chem.*, **11,** 95 (1968).

159. R. W. Fuller and S. K. Hemrick, *Proc. Soc. Exp. Biol. Med.*, **158,** 323 (1978).

160. R. W. Fuller, B. J. Warren, and B. B. Molloy, *Biochem. Pharmacol.*, **19,** 2934 (1970).

161. R. W. Fuller and S. K. Hemrick, *Res. Commun. Chem. Pathol. Pharmacol.*, **20,** 199 (1978).

162. C. L. Zirkle, C. Kaiser, D. H. Tedeschi, R. E. Tedeschi, and A. Burger, *J. Med. Pharm. Chem.*, **5,** 1265 (1962).

163. J. F. Mcran, Ph.D. thesis, University of Ottawa, Ottawa, Canada, 1961.

164. A. S. Horn and S. H. Snyder, *J. Pharmacol. Exp. Ther.*, **180,** 523 (1972).

165. J. I. Escobar, B. C. Schiele, and R. Zimmerman, *Am. J. Psychiatr.*, **131,** 1025 (1974).

166. V. Gentil, B. Alevizos, and M. Lader, *Biochem. Pharmacol.*, **27,** 1197 (1978).

167. J. Finkelstein, E. Chiang, and J. Lee, *J. Med. Chem.*, **8,** 432 (1965).

168. W. R. McGrath and W. L. Kuhn, *Arch. Int. Pharmacodyn. Ther.*, **172,** 405 (1968).

169. E. A. Zeller and S. Sarkar, *J. Biol. Chem.*, **237,** 2333 (1962).

170. S. Sarkar, R. Banerjee, M. S. Ise, and E. A. Zeller, *Helv. Chim. Acta*, **43,** 439 (1960).

171. J. Finkelstein, E. Chiang, F. M. Vane, and J. Lee, *J. Med. Chem.*, **9,** 319 (1966).

172. C. Kaiser, B. M. Lester, C. L. Zirkle, A. Burger, C. S. Davis, T. J. Delia, and L. Zirngibl, *J. Med. Pharm. Chem.*, **5,** 1243 (1962).

173. U. M. Teotino, D. Della Bella, A. Gandini, and G. Benelli, *J. Med. Chem.*, **10,** 1091 (1967).

174. J. N. Wells, A. V. Shirodkar, and A. M. Knevel, *J. Med. Chem.*, **9,** 195 (1966).

175. C. J. Paget and C. S. Davis, *J. Med. Chem.*, **7,** 626 (1964).

176. J. A. Gylys, P. M. R. Muccia, and M. K. Taylor, *Ann. N.Y. Acad. Sci.*, **107,** 899 (1963).

177. B. Dubnick, D. F. Morgan, and G. E. Phillips, *Ann. N.Y. Acad. Sci.*, **107,** 914 (1963).

178. W. B. Lutz, S. Lazarus, S. Klutchko, and R. I. Meltzer, *Abstr. Pap., 144th Meet. Am. Chem. Soc., Los Angeles, 1963,* p. 25-L.

179. R. A. Maxwell, P. D. Keenan, E. Chaplin, B. Roth, and S. Batmanglidj Eckhardt, *J. Pharmacol. Exp. Ther.*, **166,** 320 (1969).

180. A. I. Salama, J. R. Insalaco, and R. A. Maxwell, *J. Pharmacol. Exp. Ther.*, **178,** 474 (1971).

181. F. Sulser, J. Watts, and B. B. Brodie, *Ann. N.Y. Acad. Sci.*, **96,** 279 (1962).

182. J. R. Gillette, J. V. Dingell, F. Sulser, R. Kuntzman, and B. B. Brodie, *Experientia*, **17,** 417 (1961).

183. A. Lapolla and H. Jones, *Am. J. Psychiatr.*, **127,** 335 (1970).

184. M. H. Bickel and B. B. Brodie, *Int. J. Neuropharmacol.*, **3,** 611 (1964).

185. W. Theobald, O. Büch, H. A. Kunz, and G. Morpurgo, *Med. Pharmacol. Exp.*, **15,** 187 (1966).

186. E. B. Sigg, L. Soffer, and L. Gyermek, *J. Pharmacol. Exp. Ther.*, **142**, 13 (1963).

187. G. P. Forshell, B. Siwers, and J. R. Tuck, *Eur. J. Clin. Pharmacol.*, **9**, 291 (1976).

188. T. Segawa, Y. Nomura, A. Tanaka, and H. Murakami, *J. Pharm. Pharmacol.*, **29**, 139 (1977).

189. E. Ericksoo and O. Rohte, *Arzneim.-Forsch.*, **20**, 1561 (1970).

190. W. Obermair and W. Pöldinger, *Int. Pharmacopsychiatr.*, **12**, 65 (1977).

191. K. Opitz and U. Borchert, *Arzneim.-Forsch.*, **18**, 316 (1968).

192. M. Nakanishi, T. Tsumagari, T. Okada, and Y. Kasé, *Arzneim.-Forsch.*, **18**, 1435 (1968).

193. D. Bente, H. Hippius, W. Pöldinger, and K. Stach, *Arzneim.-Forsch.*, **14**, 486 (1964).

194. K. Rickels, P. E. Gordon, C. C. Weise, S. E. Bazilian, H. S. Feldman, and D. A. Wilson, *Am. J. Psychiatr.*, **127**, 208 (1970).

195. G. F. Oxenkrug, *Farmakol. Toxsikol.*, **38**, 23 (1975).

196. A. Uzan and G. Le Fur, *Ann. Pharm. Fr.*, **33**, 345 (1975).

197. L. Toscano, G. Grisanti, G. Fioriello, E. Seghetti, A. Bianchetti, G. Bossoni, and M. Riva, *J. Med. Chem.*, **19**, 208 (1976).

198. M. Bonierbale, H. Dufour, J. C. Scotto, and J. M. Sutter, *L'Encéphale*, **2**, 219 (1976).

199. E. B. Sigg, L. Gyermek, and R. T. Hill, *Psychopharmacologia*, **7**, 144 (1965).

200. M. H. Symes, *Brit. J. Psychiatr.*, **113**, 671 (1967).

201. W. Pöldinger, A. Gehring, A. Schäublin, and R. Thilges, *Arzneim.-Forsch.*, **19**, 492 (1969).

202. J. Simeon, M. Fuchs, O. Nikolovski, and L. Bucci, *Psychosomatics*, **11**, 342 (1970).

203. S. Garattini and M. N. G. Dukes, Eds., *Antidepressant Drugs*, Excerpta Medica, Amsterdam, 1967, p. 205, 397.

204. F. J. Villani and T. A. Mann, *J. Med. Chem.*, **11**, 894 (1968).

205. P. N. Craig, B. M. Lester, A. J. Saggiomo, C. Kaiser, and C. L. Zirkle, *J. Org. Chem.*, **26**, 135 (1961).

206. W. Theobald, O. Büch, H. A. Kunz, G. Morpurgo, G. Wilhelmi, and E. G. Stenger, *Arch. Int. Pharmacodyn. Ther.*, **148**, 560 (1964).

207. J. E. Murphy, J. F. Donald, and G. Beaumont, *Clin. Trials J.*, **8**, 28 (1971).

208. F. Hunziker, F. Künzle, and J. Schmutz, *Helv. Chim. Acta*, **46**, 2337 (1963).

209. A. R. Hanze, R. E. Strube, and M. E. Greig, *J. Med. Chem.*, **6**, 767 (1963).

210. A. M. Monro, R. M. Quinton, and T. I. Wrigley, *J. Med. Chem.*, **6**, 255 (1963).

211. Rhône-Poulenc, Belg. Pat. 617,554 (1962); through *Chem. Abstr.*, **58**, 13973 (1963).

212. A. L. Leon, W. B. Abrams, M. Markowitz, and E. C. Meisner, *J. Clin. Pharmacol.*, **9**, 399 (1969).

213. H. L. Yale and F. Sowinski, *J. Med. Chem.*, **7**, 609 (1964).

214. A. R. Furgiuele, J. P. High, Z. P. Horovitz, and J. C. Burke, *Arch. Int. Pharmacodyn. Ther.*, **160**, 4 (1966).

215. I. S. Gibbs, A. Heald, H. Jacobson, D. Wadke, and I. Weliky, *J. Pharm. Sci.*, **65**, 1380 (1976).

216. R. G. Babington and Z. P. Horovitz, *Arch. Int. Pharmacodyn. Ther.*, **202**, 106 (1973).

217. I. Weliky and E. S. Neiss, *Int. J. Clin. Pharmacol. Biopharm.*, **12**, 252 (1975).

218. A. Weber and J. Frossard, *Ann. Pharm. Fr.*, **24**, 445 (1966).

219. G. L. Klerman and J. O. Cole, *Pharmacol. Rev.*, **17**, 101 (1965).

220. M. E. Christy, C. C. Boland, J. G. Williams, and E. L. Engelhardt, *Am. Chem. Soc. Med. Chem. Symp., Bloomington, Ind., 1966*.

221. H. B. Hucker and C. C. Porter, *Fed. Proc.*, **20**, 172 (1961).

222. V. G. Vernier, F. R. Alleva, H. M. Hanson, and C. A. Stone, *Fed. Proc.*, **21**, 419 (1962).

223. M. A. Davis, F. Herr, R. A. Thomas, and M.-P. Charest, *J. Med. Chem.*, **10**, 627 (1967).

224. J.-R. Boissier, C. Dumont, and R. Ratouis, *Therapie*, **26**, 459 (1971).

225. W. B. Lacefield, *J. Med. Chem.*, **14**, 82 (1971).

226. Sumitomo Chemical KK, Jap. Pat. 52062283 (1977); Derwent No. 47630Y/27.

227. K. E. Eichstadt, J. C. Reepmeyer, R. B. Cook, P. G. Riley, D. P. Davis, and R. A. Wiley, *J. Med. Chem.*, **19**, 47 (1976).

228. H. Coper, H. Hippius, and H. Selbach, *Arzneim.-Forsch.*, **19**, 835 (1969).

229. D. Bente, J. Feder, H. Helmchen, H. Hippius, and L. Rosenberg, *Arzneim.-Forsch.*, **23**, 247 (1973).

230. M. Protiva, V. Hnévsová-Seidlová, Z. J. Vejdélek, I. Jirkovský, Z. Votava, and J. Metyšová, *J. Med. Pharm. Chem.*, **4**, 411 (1961).

231. S. O. Winthrop, M. A. Davis, G. S. Myers, J. G. Gavin, R. Thomas, and R. Barber, *J. Org. Chem.*, **27**, 230 (1962).

232. P. Dostert and E. Kyburz, *Helv. Chim. Acta*, **53**, 882 (1970).

233. W. V. Krumholz, J. A. Yaryura-Tobias, and L.

White, *Curr. Ther. Res. Clin. Exp.*, **10**, 342 (1968).

234. A. K. Dixon, R. C. Hill, D. Roemer, and G. Scholtysik, *Arzneim.-Forsch.*, **27**, 1968 (1977).

235. J. E. Standal, *Acta Psychiatr. Scand.*, **56**, 276 (1977).

236. M. Markó and E. Flückiger, *Experientia*, **32**, 491 (1976).

237. F. J. Villani, C. A. Ellis, C. Teichman, and C. Bigos, *J. Med. Pharm. Chem.*, **5**, 373 (1962).

238. E. L. Engelhardt, M. E. Christy, C. D. Colton, M. B. Freedman, C. C. Boland, L. M. Halpern, V. G. Vernier, and C. A. Stone, *J. Med. Chem.*, **11**, 325 (1968).

239. K. Voith and F. Herr, *Arch. Int. Pharmacodyn. Ther.*, **182**, 318 (1969).

240. W. Lippmann, Ayerst Symposium, *J. Med.*, **2**, 250 (1971).

241. J. Cox and L. E. J. Evans, *Med. J. Aust.*, **2**, 878 (1977).

242. D. Mulder and C. J. van Eeken, *Arch. Int. Pharmacodyn. Ther.*, **162**, 497 (1966).

243. S. H. Snyder, A. S. Horn, K. M. Taylor, and J. T. Coyle, in *L-Dopa and Behavior*, S. Malitz, Ed., Raven Press, New York, 1972, p. 35.

244. J. Offermoier, B. Potgieter, H. G. DuPreez, and P. J. Meiring, *S. Afr. Med. J.*, **51**, 62 (1977).

245. P. Gannon, T. Itil, A. Keskiner, and B. Hsu, *Arzneim.-Forsch.*, **20**, 971 (1970).

246. E. Galantay, C. Hoffman, N. Paolella, J. Gogerty, L. Iorio, G. Leslie, and J. H. Trapold, *J. Med. Chem.*, **12**, 444 (1969).

247. L. G. Humber, F. Herr, and M.-P. Charest, *J. Med. Chem.*, **14**, 982 (1971).

248. L. G. Humber, M. A. Davis, G. Beaulieu, and M.-P. Charest, *Can. J. Chem.*, **46**, 2981 (1968).

249. I. Monkovic, Y. G. Perron, R. Martel, W. J. Simpson, and J. A. Gylys, *J. Med. Chem.*, **16**, 403 (1973).

250. J. Castañer and K. Hillier, *Drugs Future*, **3**, 142 (1978).

251. C. L. Mitchell, A. C. Conway, N. J. Tresnak, and W. J. Hammar, *Fed. Proc.*, **35**, 784 (1976).

252. G. Pinard, *Curr. Ther. Res., Clin. Exp.*, **21**, 368 (1977).

253. J. Gootjes, A. B. H. Funcke, and H. Timmerman, *Arzneim.-Forsch.*, **22**, 632 (1972).

254. M. Protiva, *Farm. Ed. Sci.*, **21**, 76 (1966).

255. P. G. Jones, O. Kennard, and A. S. Horn, *Acta Crystallogr.*, **34**, B2027 (1978).

256. A. P. Roszkowski, M. E. Schuler, M. Marx, and J. A. Edwards, *Experientia*, **31**, 960 (1975).

257. E. L. Engelhardt, M. E. Christy, H. C. Zell, C. M. Cylion, M. B. Freedman, and J. M. Sprague, *Abstr. Pap. 141st Meet. Am. Chem. Soc.*, *Washington, D.C. 1962*, p. 4-N.

258. K. Hoogsteen, *Acta Crystallogr.*, **21**, A116 (1966).

259. A. A. Sugerman, *Curr. Ther. Res., Clin. Exp.*, **8**, 479 (1966).

260. J. Atkinson and H. Ladinsky, *Brit. J. Pharmacol.*, **45**, 519 (1972).

261. B. Woggon and J. Angst, *Int. Pharmacopsychiatr.*, **12**, 38 (1977).

262. J. Castañer and K. Hillier, *Drugs Future*, **3**, 318 (1978).

263. E. A. Daneman, *Psychosomatics*, **6**, 342 (1965).

264. N. Finch, in *Industrial Pharmacology, A Monograph Series, Antidepressants*, S. Fielding and H. Lal, Eds., Futura, New York, 1975, p. 9.

265. W. E. Coyne and J. W. Cusic, *J. Med. Chem.*, **17**, 72 (1974).

266. I. Gomez-Martinez, *Curr. Ther. Res., Clin. Exp.*, **10**, 116 (1968).

267. B. J. Goldstein and D. G. Pinosky, *Curr. Ther. Res., Clin. Exp.*, **11**, 169 (1969).

268. G. Bauer and H. Nowak, *Arzneim.-Forsch.*, **19**, 1642 (1969).

269. K. Stach and F. Bickelhaupt, *Monatsh. Chem.*, **93**, 896 (1962).

270. J. R. Tretter, J. F. Muren, B. M. Bloom, and A. Weissman, *Am. Chem. Soc. Med. Chem. Symposium, Bloomington, Ind., 1966*.

271. A. Ribbentrop and W. Schaumann, *Arzneim.-Forsch.*, **15**, 863 (1965).

272. G. M. Simpson and T. Salim, *Curr. Ther. Res., Clin. Exp.*, **7**, 661 (1965).

273. I. Jirkovský, J. Metyš, and M. Protiva, *Collect. Czech. Chem. Commun.*, **32**, 3448 (1967).

274. J. Metyšová, J. Metyš, and Z. Votava, *Arzneim.-Forsch.*, **13**, 1039 (1963).

275. M. Rajsner and M. Protiva, *Collect. Czech. Chem. Commun.*, **32**, 2021 (1967).

276. J. Metyšová, J. Metyš, and Z. Votava, *Arzneim.-Forsch.*, **15**, 524 (1965).

277. S. O. Winthrop, M. A. Davis, F. Herr, J. Stewart, and R. Gaudry, *J. Med. Chem.*, **5**, 1207 (1962).

278. A. E. Drukker, C. I. Judd, J. M. Spoerl, and F. E. Kaminski, *J. Heterocycl. Chem.*, **2**, 276, 283 (1965).

279. S. O. Winthrop, M. A. Davis, F. Herr, J. Stewart, and R. Gaudry, *J. Med. Chem.*, **5**, 1199 (1962).

280. G. M. Simpson and A. Siegler, *Curr. Ther. Res., Clin. Exp.*, **8**, 406 (1966).

281. R. A. Yeary, M. Finkelstein, N. Cant, and S. B. Kennedy, *Am. J. Proctology*, **16**, 376 (1965).

282. M. Protiva, M. Borovička, V. Hach, Z. Votava, J. Srámková, and Z. Horáková, *Experientia*, **13**, 291 (1957).

283. M. Borovička and M. Protiva, *Collect. Czech. Chem. Commun.*, **23**, 1330 (1958).

284. J. O. Jílek, J. Pomykáček, E. Svátek, V. Seidlová, M. Rajšner, K. Pelz, B. Hoch, and M. Protiva, *Collect. Czech. Chem. Commun.*, **30**, 445 (1965).

285. L. H. Werner, S. Ricca, E. Mohacsi, A. Rossi, and V. P. Arya, *J. Med. Chem.*, **8**, 74 (1965).

286. A. J. Coppen and K. Ghose, *Arzneim.-Forsch.*, **26**, 1166 (1976).

287. M. O. Jaskari, U. G. Ahlfors, L. Ginman, K. Lydekcne, and P. Tienari, *Pharmakopsychiatr. Neuro-Psychopharmakol.*, **10**, 101 (1977).

288. A. Coppen, R. Gupta, S. Mongtomery, K. Ghose, J. Bailey, B. Burns, and J. J. DeRidder, *Brit. J. Psychiatr.*, **129**, 342 (1976).

289. D. Wheatley, *Curr. Ther. Res., Clin. Exp.*, **18**, 849 (1975).

290. F. J. Ayd, Jr., *Int. Drug Ther. Newslett.*, **8**: 3, 9, (1973).

291. K. Okamoto, T. Nakomo, and K. Inanaga, *Fol. Psychol. Neurol. Japon.*, **32**, 171 (1978).

292. M. Peet and H. Behagel, *Brit. J. Clin. Pharmacol.*, **5**: Suppl. 1, 5S (1978).

293. W. F. Kafoe, J. J. DeRidder, and B. E. Leonard, *Biochem. Pharmacol.*, **25**, 2455 (1976).

294. I. Goodlet, S. E. Mireylees, and M. F. Sugrue, *Brit. J. Pharmacol.*, **61**, 307 (1977).

295. P. F. Von Voightlander and E. G. Losey, *Res. Commun. Chem. Pathol. Pharmacol.*, **13**, 389 (1976).

296. K. Ghose, A. Coppen, and P. Turner, *Psychopharmacology*, **49**, 201 (1976).

297. T. M. Itil, N. Polvan, and W. Hsu, *Curr. Ther. Res., Clin. Exp.*, **14**, 395 (1972).

298. F. Hunziker, H. Lauener, and J. Schmutz, *Arzneim.-Forsch.*, **13**, 324 (1963).

299. R. Battegay and W. Poeldinger, *Arzneim.-Forsch.*, **17**, 481 (1967).

300. A. Baron, *Med. Welt*, 388 (1967).

301. G. Stille, H. Lauener, and E. Eichenbe, *Schweiz. Med. Wochenschr.*, **95**, 366 (1965).

302. T. Nose and Y. Kowa, *Jap. J. Pharmacol.*, **21**, 47 (1971).

303. J.-M. Lwoff, C. Larousse, P. Simon, and J. R. Boissier, *Therapie*, **26**, 451 (1971).

304. T. M. Itil, in *Psychotropic Drugs and the Human EEG*, T. M. Itil, Ed., S. Karger, Basel, 1974, p. 59.

305. H. L. Yale and F. Sowinski, *Arzneim.-Forsch.*, **16**, 550 (1966).

306. Z. P. Horovitz, A. R. Furgiuele, J. P. High, and J. C. Burke, *Arch. Int. Pharmacodyn. Ther.*, **151**, 180 (1964).

307. J. O. Jílek, K. Pelz, D. Pavičková, and M. Protiva, *Collect. Czech. Chem. Commun.*, **30**, 1676 (1965).

308. J. O. Jílek, J. Pomykácek, J. Metyšová, J. Metyš, and M. Protiva, *Collect. Czech. Chem. Commun.*, **30**, 463 (1965).

309. J. David and R. S. Grewal, *Indian J. Exp. Biol.*, **12**, 225 (1974).

310. D. M. Gallant, M. P. Bishop, and R. Guerrero-Figueroa, *Curr. Ther. Res., Clin. Exp.*, **13**, 364 (1971).

311. A. Åberg and G. Holmberg, *Curr. Ther. Res., Clin. Exp.*, **22**, 304 (1977).

312. F. Hunziker, F. Künzle, and J. Schmutz, *Helv. Chim. Acta*, **49**, 244 (1966).

313. R. Smrž, J. O. Jílek, B. Kakáč, J. Holubek, E. Svátek, M. Bartošová, and M. Protiva, *Collect. Czech. Chem. Commun.*, **41**, 3420 (1976).

314. H. Bratlund, *Acta Psychiatr. Neurol. Scand.*, **37**, 295 (1961).

315. D. Biros, B. C. Schiele, and D. Ferguson, *Curr. Ther. Res., Clin. Exp.*, **11**, 289 (1969).

316. G. Francesconi, A. LoCascio, S. Mellina, F. Fici, M. Bagnoli, and R. Lepore, *Curr. Ther. Res., Clin. Exp.*, **20**, 529 (1976).

317. E. Guth and G. Hoffman, *Wien. Klin. Wochenschr.*, **78**, 14 (1966).

318. U. Jahn, *Arch. Exp. Pathol./Pharmakol.*, **253**, 48 (1966).

319. D. S. Farrier, *Arzneim.-Forsch.*, **27**, 575 (1977).

320. M. Filczewski, K. Oledzka, I. Malecki, and T. Paszek, *Diss. Pharm. Pharmacol.*, **22**, 263 (1970); through *Chem. Abstr.*, **74**, 74797q (1971).

321. J. Wysokowski, *Diss. Pharm. Pharmacol.*, **23**, 646 (1971).

322. B. Szukalski and M. Kobylinska, *Diss. Pharm. Pharmacol.*, **23**, 640 (1971).

323. L. Krzywosiński, M. Bogdal, and H. Kierylowicz, *Pol. J. Pharmacol. Pharm.*, **27**, 471 (1975).

324. T. M. Itil, N. Polvan, L. Engin, M. B. Guthrie, and M. F. Huque, *Curr. Ther. Res., Clin. Exp.*, **21**, 343 (1977).

325. J. Castañer and H. Bundgaard, *Drugs Future*, **2**, 523 (1977).

326. P. V. Petersen, N. Lassen, V. Hansen, H. Huld, J. Hjortkjaer, J. Holmblad, I. Møller Nielsen, M. Nymark, V. Pedersen, A. Jørgensen, and W.

Hougs, *Acta Pharmacol. Toxicol.*, **24,** 121 (1966).

327. S. Kaumeier, J. Dohren, and D. Flach, *Curr. Ther. Res., Clin. Exp.*, **21,** 108 (1977).

328. B. Saletu, J. Grünberger, R. Flener, L. Linzmayer, and H. Sieroslawski, *Curr. Ther. Res., Clin. Exp.*, **20,** 810 (1976).

329. G. Engelhardt, *Arzneim.-Forsch.*, **25,** 1723 (1975).

330. J. Kähling, H. Ziegler, and H. Ballhause, *Arzneim.-Forsch.*, **25,** 1737 (1975).

331. B. Oderfeld-Nowak, A. Wieraszko, and, B. Heiler, *Pol. J. Pharmacol. Pharm.*, **29,** 215 (1977).

332. H. Brunner, P. R. Hedwall, M. Meier, and H. J. Bein, *Agents Actions*, **2,** 69 (1971); through *Chem. Abstr.*, **76,** 10334v (1972).

333. L. Maître, M. Staehelin, and H. J. Bein, *Biochem. Pharmacol.*, **20,** 2169 (1971).

334. L. Maître, *J. Int. Med. Res.*, **3:** Suppl. 2, 2, (1975).

335. R. M. Pinder, R. N. Brogden, T. M. Speight, and G. S. Avery, *Drugs*, **13,** 321 (1977).

336. H. E. Lehmann, J. C. Pecknold, T. A. Ban, and L. Orbach, *Curr. Ther. Res., Clin. Exp.*, **19,** 463 (1976).

337. A. N. Singh, B. Saxena, M. Gent, and H. L. Nelsen, *Curr. Ther. Res., Clin. Exp.*, **19,** 451 (1976).

338. M. Amin, E. Brahm, L. A. Bronheim, A. Klingner, T. A. Ban, and H. E. Lehmann, *Curr. Ther. Res., Clin. Exp.*, **15,** 691 (1973).

339. W. Rieger, K. Rickels, N. Norstad, and J. Johnson, *J. Int. Med. Res.*, **3,** 413 (1975).

340. H. Fukushima, M. Nakamura, and H. Yamamoto, *Arch. Int. Pharmacodyn. Ther.*, **229,** 163 (1977).

341. P. C. Waldmeier, P. A. Baumann, M. Wilhelm, R. Bernasconi, and L. Maître, *Eur. J. Pharmacol.*, **46,** 387 (1977).

342. Sumitomo Chemical KK, Belg. Pat. 843,875 (1975); Derwent No. 05619Y/04.

343. Sumitomo Chemical KK, Jap. Pat. 52068170 (1975); Derwent No. 51145Y/29.

344. C. Kaiser, D. H. Tedeschi, P. J. Fowler, A. M. Pavloff, B. M. Lester, and C. L. Zirkle, *J. Med. Chem.*, **14,** 179 (1971).

345. O. Nieschulz, I. Hoffmann, and K. Popendiker, *Med. Exp.*, **1,** 246 (1959).

346. I. P. Lapin, *Zh. Nevropat. Psikhiat. Korsakov.*, **64,** 281 (1964).

347. A. N. Gritsenko, Z. I. Ermakova, S. V. Zhuravlev, T. A. Vikhlyaev, T. A. Klygul, and O. V.

Ul'yanova, *Khim.-Farm. Zh.*, **5,** 18 (1971); through *Chem. Abstr.*, **75,** 140776f (1971).

348. G. N. Lakoza, *Farmakol. Toksikol.* **34,** 397 (1971); through *Chem. Abstr.*, **75,** 139223s (1971).

349. E. R. Atkinson, P. L. Russ, M. A. Tucker, and F. J. Rosenberg, *J. Med. Chem.*, **14,** 1005 (1971).

350. T. M. Itil, R. Cora, W. Hsu, E. Cig, and B. Saletu, *Arzneim.-Forsch.*, **22,** 2063 (1972).

351. R. DeBeule, *Ars. Medici*, **29,** 2463 (1974).

352. A. Uzon and G. LeFur, *Ann. Pharm. Fr.*, **33,** 350 (1975).

353. D. H. Tedeschi, C. L. Zirkle, and C. Kaiser, to be published.

354. V. G. Ermolaeva, V. G. Yashunskii, A. I. Polezhaeva, and M. D. Mashkovskii, *Khim.-Farm. Zh.*, **2,** 20 (1968); through *Chem. Abstr.*, **69,** 106517p (1968).

355. C.-M. Lee, *J. Med. Chem.*, **11,** 388 (1968).

356. N. Plotnikoff, J. Keith, M. Heimann, W. Keith, and C. Perry, *Arch. Int. Pharmacodyn. Ther.*, **146,** 406 (1963).

357. A. I. Polezhaeva, O. P. Vertogradova, and M. R. Bagreeva, *Khim.-Farm. Zh.*, **4,** 59 (1970); through *Chem. Abstr.*, **73,** 2459n (1970).

358. M. D. Mashkovskii and L. F. Roshchina, *Farmakol. Toksikol.*, **34,** 144 (1971); through *Chem. Abstr.*, **75,** 18396s (1971).

359. A. Ermili, B. Balbi, G. Roma, A. Ambrosini, and N. Passerini, *Farm. Ed. Sci.*, **31,** 627 (1976).

360. E. A. Kuznetsova, N. T. Pryanishnikova, L. I. Gaidukova, I. V. Fedina, and S. V. Zhuravlev, *Khim.-Farm. Zh.*, **12,** 11 (1975).

361. W. Pöldinger, *Schweiz. Arch. Neurol. Psychiatr.*, **94,** 440 (1964).

362. M. Ferrari and C. Lanzani, *Ital. Sci. Farmacol.*, **12,** 141 (1962).

363. M. E. Fried, E. Hertz, and L. M. Rice, *J. Med. Chem.*, **7,** 313 628 (1964).

364. B. L. Baxter and M. I. Gluckman, *Nature*, **223,** 750 (1969).

365. F. J. Ayd, Jr., *Dis. Nerv. Syst.*, **30,** 818 (1969).

366. W. E. Fann, J. M. Davis, D. S. Janowsky, J. S. Kaufmann, J. D. Griffith, and J. A. Oates, *Arch. Gen. Psychiatr.*, **26,** 158 (1972).

367. Belg. Pat. 793,493 (1972).

368. Ger. Pat. 2,240,211 (1973).

369. D. M. Gallant, M. P. Bishop, and R. Guerrero-Figueroa, *Curr. Ther. Res., Clin. Exp.*, **14,** 61 (1972).

370. E. D. Eckert, R. Zimmermann, L. Dehnel, and

B. C. Schiele, *Curr. Ther. Res., Clin. Exp.*, **22,** 644 (1977).

371. J. N. Nestoros, T. A. Ban, and H. E. Lehmann, *Int. Pharmacopsychiatr.*, **12,** 86 (1977).

372. A. A. Sugerman, *Curr. Ther. Res., Clin. Exp.*, **24,** 227 (1978).

373. A. Mooradian, P. E. Dupont, A. G. Hlavac, M. D. Aceto, and J. Pearl, *J. Med. Chem.*, **20,** 487 (1977).

374. B. Z. Askinazi, M. I. Vlasova, and N. A. Kogan, *Khim.-Farm. Zh.*, **10:** 4, 19 (1976).

375. M. D. Mashkovskii, A. N. Grinev, N. I. Andreeva, V. I. Shvedov, and L. B. Altukhova, *Farmakol. Toxsikol.*, **34,** 387 (1971).

376. M. D. Mashkovskii, K. S. Raevsky, N. I. Maisov, Yu. G. Sandalov, and N. I. Andreeva, *Khim.-Farm. Zh.*, **10,** 3 (1976).

377. K. Ju. Novitskij, *Pharmazie*, **30,** 819 (1975).

378. V. I. Shvedov, E. S. Krichevskii, O. B. Romanova, A. N. Grinev, N. I. Andreeva, and M. D. Mashkovskii, *Khim.-Farm. Zh.*, **12,** 85 (1978).

379. N. I. Andreeva, *Abstr. 7th Int. Congr. Pharmacol., Paris, 1978*, p. 248.

380. I. Jirkovksy, L. G. Humber, K. Voith, and M.-P. Charest, *Arzneim.-Forsch.*, **27,** 1642 (1977).

381. T. Pugsley and W. Lippmann, *Psychopharmacologia*, **47,** 33 (1976).

382. W. Lippmann and T. Pugsley, *Biochem. Pharmacol.*, **25,** 1179 (1976).

383. R. S. B. Ehsanullah, K. Ghose, M. J. Kirby, and D. Witts, *Brit. J. Clin. Pharmacol.*, **3,** 950P (1976).

384. B. Saletu, P. Krieger, J. Grünberger, H. Schanda, and I. Sletten, *Int. Pharmacopsychiatr.*, **12,** 137 (1977).

385. L. G. Humber, C. A. Demerson, A. A. Asselin, M.-P. Charest, and K. Pelz, *Eur. J. Med. Chem.*, **10,** 215 (1975).

386. C. A. Demerson, G. Santroch, L. G. Humber, and M.-P. Charest, *J. Med. Chem.*, **18,** 577 (1975).

387. W. Lippmann and T. Pugsley, *Arch. Int. Pharmacodyn. Ther.*, **227,** 324 (1977).

388. A. A. Asselin, L. G. Humber, J. Komlossy, and M.-P. Charest, *J. Med. Chem.*, **19,** 792 (1976).

389. T. Pugsley and W. Lippmann, *Experientia*, **33,** 57 (1977).

390. I. Jirkovsky, L. G. Humber, and R. Noureldin, *Eur. J. Med. Chem.*, **11,** 571 (1976).

391. W. Lippmann and T. Pugsley, *Pharmacol. Res. Commun.*, **8,** 387 (1976).

392. F. J. Villani, C. A. Ellis, and T. A. Mann, *J. Pharm. Sci.*, **60,** 1586 (1971).

393. S. O. Winthrop, M. A. Davis, F. Herr, J. Stewart, and R. Gaudry, *J. Med. Chem.*, **6,** 130 (1963).

394. Rhône-Poulenc, Fr. Pat. 1,403,603 (1960).

395. G. Jones, R. F. Maisey, A. R. Somerville, and B. A. Whittle, *J. Med. Chem.*, **14,** 161 (1971).

396. A. W. Peck and R. M. Pigache, *Brit. J. Clin. Pharmacol.*, **2:** 2, 178P (1975).

397. S. B. Ross and A. L. Renyi, *Neuropharmacology*, **16,** 57 (1977).

398. J. Castañer and K. Hillier, *Drugs Future*, **3,** 71 (1978).

399. B. Siwers, V.-A. Ringberger, J. R. Tuck, and F. Sjoqvist, *Clin. Pharmacol. Ther.*, **21,** 194 (1977).

400. S. B. Ross, S. Jansa, L. Wetterberg, B. Fyrö, and B. Hellner, *Life Sci.*, **19,** 205 (1976).

401. O. Benkert, G. Laakmann, L. Ott, A. Strauss, and R. Zimmer, *Arzneim.-Forsch.*, **27,** 2421 (1977).

402. S. A. Montgomery, R. McAwley, G. Rani, and D. B. Montgomery, *Abstr. 7th Int. Congr. Pharmacol., Paris, 1978*, p. 246.

403. J. Carranza, H. Saldana, and R. Ramirez, *Curr. Ther. Res., Clin. Exp.*, **20,** 552 (1976).

404. E. Adlerová and M. Protiva, *Collect. Czech. Chem. Commun.*, **32,** 3177 (1967).

405. B. Carnmalm, M.-L. Persson, S. B. Ross, N. E. Stjernström, and S. O. Ögren, *Acta Pharm. Suec.*, **12,** 173 (1975).

406. M. Shimizu, T. Hirooka, T. Karasawa, Y. Masuda, M. Oka, T. Ito, C. Kamei, Y. Sohji, M. Hori, K. Yoshida, and H. Kaneko, *Arzneim.-Forsch.*, **24,** 166 (1974).

407. J. Augstein, A. L. Ham, and P. R. Leeming, *J. Med. Chem.*, **15,** 466 (1972).

408. Anonymous, *Scrip*, **240,** 18 (1977).

409. I. Hoffmann, G. Ehrhart, and K. Schmitt, *Arzneim.-Forsch.*, **21,** 1045 (1971).

410. P. F. Teychenne, D. M. Park, L. J. Findley, F. C. Rose, and D. B. Calne, *J. Neurol. Neurosurg. Psychiatr.*, **39,** 1219 (1976).

411. U. Schacht and W. Heptner, *Biochem. Pharmacol.*, **23,** 3413 (1974).

412. I. Hoffmann, *Arzneim.-Forsch.*, **23,** 45 (1973).

413. J. Ananth and N. Van Den Steen, *Curr. Ther. Res., Clin. Exp.*, **23,** 213 (1978).

414. J. C. Pecknold, T. A. Ban, H. E. Lehmann, and A. Klingner, *Int. J. Clin. Pharmacol.*, **11,** 304 (1975).

415. C. Braestrup and J. Scheel-Krüger, *Eur. J. Pharmacol.*, **38,** 305 (1976).

416. H. Kruse, I. Hoffmann, H. J. Gerhards, M. Leven, and U. Schacht, *Psychopharmacologia*, **51,** 117 (1977).

417. J. A. Poat, G. N. Woodruff, and K. J. Watling, *J. Pharm. Pharmacol.*, **30**, 495 (1978).

418. D. Trepanier and S. Sunder, *J. Med. Chem.*, **16**, 342 (1973).

419. B. K. Koe, *Fed. Proc.*, **35**, 427 (1976).

420. W. Hespe and J. Beem, *Arzneim.-Forsch.*, **25**, 1911 (1975).

421. G. Bram and N. Shanmuganathan, *Curr. Ther. Res., Clin. Exp.*, **13**, 625 (1971).

422. R. Brasseur, *L'Encéphale*, **60**, 265 (1971).

423. J. R. Bassett, K. D. Cairncross, N. B. Hackett, and M. Story, *Brit. J. Pharmacol.*, **37**, 69 (1969).

424. H. H. Keasling and R. B. Moffett, *J. Med. Chem.*, **14**, 1106 (1971).

425. R. B. Moffett and T. L. Pickering, *J. Med. Chem.*, **14**, 1100 (1971).

426. R. I. Taber, A. Barnett, and F. E. Roth, *Pharmacologist*, **11**, 247 (1969).

427. A. J. Swaisland, R. A. Franklin, P. J. Southgate, and A. J. Coleman, *Brit. J. Clin. Pharmacol.*, **4**, 61 (1977).

428. R. F. Sugden, *Brit. J. Pharmacol.*, **51**, 467 (1974).

429. J. Castañer and L. de Angelis, *Drugs Future*, **3**, 508 (1978).

430. E. S. Johnson, P. J. Southgate, R. F. Sugden, and A. C. White, *Abstr. Volunteer Pap., 5th Int. Congr. Pharmacol., San Francisco, Calif., 1972*, p. 116.

431. K. Ghose, V. A. Rama Rao, J. Bailey, and A. Coppen, *Psychopharmacology*, **57**, 109 (1978).

432. J. H. Gogerty, W. Houlihan, M. Galen, P. Eden, and C. Penberthy, *Fed. Proc.*, **27**, 501 (1968).

433. M. Babbini, M. Gaiardi, and M. Bartoletti, *Pharmacology*, **15**, 46 (1977).

434. Wyeth Ltd., Brit. Pat. 1,464,288 (1977).

435. A. P. Gray and H. Kraus, *Abstr. Pap. 150th Meet. Am. Chem. Soc., Atlantic City, N.J.*, 1965, p. 15-P.

436. I. W. Sletten, X. Pichardo, and S. Gershon, *Curr. Ther. Res., Clin. Exp.*, **7**, 609 (1965).

437. B. Korol, M. L. Brown, and I. W. Sletten, *Curr. Ther. Res., Clin. Exp.*, **8**, 543 (1966).

438. A. Nagy and S. Gershon, *Dis. Nerv. Syst.*, **27**, 257 (1966).

439. M. Cussac, A. Boucherle, and J. Hache, *Eur. J. Med. Chem.*, **12**, 177 (1977).

440. Sumitomo Chemical KK, Jap. Pat. 52091845 (1976); Derwent No. 65655Y/37.

441. Sumitomo Chemical KK, Jap. Pat. 52062245 (1975); Derwent No. 47615Y/27.

442. B. Carnmalm, T. DePaulis, E. Jakupovic, L. Johansson, U. H. Lindberg, B. Ulff, N. E. Stjernström, A. L. Renyi, S. B. Ross, and S.-O. Ögren, *Acta Pharm. Suec.*, **12**, 149 (1975).

443. B. Carnmalm, T. DePaulis, E. Jakupovic, A. L. Renyi, S. B. Ross, S.-O. Ögren, and N. E. Stjernström, *Acta Pharm. Suec.*, **14**, 377 (1977).

444. B. C. Schiele, L. M. Tredici, and R. L. Zimmermann, *Curr. Ther. Res., Clin. Exp.*, **8**, 565 (1966).

445. D. Linstead and D. Wilkie, *Biochem. Pharmacol.*, **20**, 839 (1971).

446. B. Dubinsky, K. Karpowicz, and M. E. Goldberg, *Pharmacologist*, **13**, 255 (1971).

447. B. Waldeck, *J. Pharm. Pharmacol.*, **20**, 111 (1968).

448. J. Hyttel, *Psychopharmacology*, **51**, 225 (1977).

449. B. Fjalland and A. V. Christensen, *Acta Physiol. Scand., Suppl.* **440**, 145 (1976).

450. J. Hyttel, *Acta Pharmacol. Toxicol.*, **40**, 439 (1977).

451. A. V. Christensen, B. Fjalland, V. Pedersen, P. Danneskiold-Samsøe, and O. Svendsen, *Eur. J. Pharmacol.*, **41**, 153 (1977).

452. A. J. Bigler, K. P. Bøgesø, A. Toft, and V. Hansen, *Eur. J. Med. Chem.*, **12**, 289 (1977).

453. F. J. McEvoy, R. F. R. Church, E. N. Greenblatt, and G. R. Allen, Jr., *J. Med. Chem.*, **15**, 1111 (1972).

454. A. Carlsson, K. Fuxe, B. Hamberger, and T. Malmfors, *Brit. J. Pharmacol.*, **36**, 18 (1969).

455. A. I. Salama and M. E. Goldberg, *Arch. Int. Pharmacodyn. Ther.*, **225**, 317 (1977).

456. S. J. Dykstra, K. N. Campbell, D. G. Lankin, and D. Rivard, *Abstr. Pap. 149th Meet. Am. Chem. Soc., Detroit, 1965*, p. 17-N.

457. B. E. Leonard, *Arch. Int. Pharmacodyn. Ther.*, **199**, 94 (1972).

458. V. J. Bauer, B. J. Duffy, D. Hoffman, S. S. Klioze, R. W. Kosley, Jr., A. R. McFadden, L. L. Martin, and H. H. Ong, *J. Med. Chem.*, **19**, 1315 (1976).

459. H. M. Geyer, S. A. Ridlon, V. Schacht, and W. J. Novick, Jr., *Fed. Proc.*, **35**, 784 (1976).

460. S. S. Klioze, V. J. Bauer, and H. M. Geyer III, *J. Med. Chem.*, **20**, 610 (1977).

461. T. Iwasaki, Y. Ikeda, and N. Takano, *Jap. J. Pharmacol.*, **25**: Suppl., 93P (1975).

462. A. Cañas-Rodriguez and P. R. Leeming, *Nature*, **223**, 75 (1969); *J. Med. Chem.*, **15**, 762 (1972).

463. D. M. Gallant, M. P. Bishop, R. Guerrero-Figueroa, L. O'Meallie, and B. Moore, *Curr. Ther. Res., Clin. Exp.*, **11**, 296 (1969).

464. O. H. Arnold and H. Guss, *Arzneim.-Forsch.*, **19**, 490 (1969).

465. O. H. Arnold and H. Guss, *Wien. Klin. Wochenschr.*, **51,** 913 (1968).

466. R. W. Fuller, K. W. Perry, and B. B. Molloy, *J. Pharmacol. Exp. Ther.*, **193,** 796 (1975).

467. D. T. Wong, F. P. Bymaster, J. S. Horng, and B. B. Molloy, *J. Pharmacol. Exp. Ther.*, **193,** 804 (1975).

468. R. J. Katz and B. J. Carroll, *Psychopharmacol.*, **51,** 189 (1977).

469. L. Lemberger, H. Rowe, R. Carmichael, R. Crabtree, J. S. Horng, F. Bymaster, and D. Wong, *Clin. Pharmacol.*, **23,** 421 (1978).

470. L. Lemberger, H. Rowe, R. Carmichael, S. Oldham, J. S. Horng, F. P. Bymaster, and D. T. Wong, *Science*, **199,** 436 (1978).

471. D. T. Wong, J. S. Horng, and F. P. Bymaster, *Life Sci.*, **17,** 755 (1975).

472. S. Terman, L. Lemberger, and H. Rowe, *Fed. Proc.*, **34,** 295 (1975).

473. I. H. Slater, G. T. Jones, and R. A. Moore, *Psychopharmacol. Commun.*, **2,** 181 (1976).

474. A. H. Abdallah and D. M. Roby, *Fed. Proc.*, **36,** 1044 (1977).

475. M. Namima and M. V. Aylott, *Abstr. 7th Int. Congr. Pharmacol. Paris, 1978*, p. 189.

476. C. Barchewitz and H. Helmchen, *Pharmakopsychiat./Neuro-Psychopharmacol.*, **3,** 293 (1970).

477. Z. P. Horovitz, *Psychosomatics*, **6,** 281 (1965).

478. Y. I. J. Mapp, R. Dykyj, C. K. Corbey, and J. H. Nodine, *Pharmacologist*, **5,** 234 (1963).

479. H. Freeman, M. R. Oktem, M. W. Kristofferson, and C. K. Gorby, *Curr. Ther. Res., Clin. Exp.*, **7,** 655 (1965).

480. J. Krapcho, E. R. Spitzmiller, and C. F. Turk, *J. Med. Chem.*, **6,** 544 (1963).

481. Z. P. Horovitz, A. R. Furgiuele, E. Uczen, and P. W. Ragozzino, *Fed. Proc.*, **24,** 134 (1965).

482. Z. P. Horovitz, A. R. Furgiuele, L. J. Brannick, J. C. Burke, and B. N. Craver, *Nature*, **200,** 369 (1963).

483. Z. P. Horovitz, J. J. Piala, J. P. High, J. C. Burke, and R. C. Leaf, *Int. J. Neuropharmacol.*, **5,** 405 (1966).

484. J. Krapcho and C. F. Turk, *J. Med. Chem.*, **9,** 191 (1966).

485. J. Krapcho, C. F. Turk, and J. J. Piala, *J. Med. Chem.*, **11,** 361 (1968).

486. V. L. Narayanan, *J. Med. Chem.*, **15,** 682 (1972).

487. B. Roth, J. Faber, and S. Nevšímalová, *Act. Nerv. Super.*, **14,** 35 (1972).

488. T. Persson and J. Wålinder, *Brit. J. Psychiatr.*, **119,** 277 (1971).

489. S. B. Ross, A. L. Renyi, and S. Ögren, *First Congr. Hung. Pharmacol. Soc., Oct. 18–22,* 1971.

490. H. M. van Praag, J. Korf, and F. van Woudenberg, *Psychopharmacologia*, **18,** 412 (1970); H. M. van Praag, J. Korf, F. van Woudenberg, and T. P. Kits, *ibid.*, **13,** 145 (1968).

491. W. Lippmann, *J. Pharm. Pharmacol.*, **20,** 385 (1968).

492. P. Deniker, P. Peron-Magnan, C. Eliet-LeGuillou, and M. Hanus, *Therapie*, **26,** 219 (1971).

493. Astra Lakemedel AB, Belg. Pat. 854,804 (1977); Derwent No. 16439Y/10.

494. U. H. Lindberg, S.-O. Thorberg, A. L. Renyi, S. B. Ross, and S.-O. Ögren, *Acta Pharm. Suec.*, **15,** 87 (1978).

495. R. W. Fuller, *Ann. N.Y. Acad. Sci.*, **305,** 147 (1978).

496. R. C. Srimal, H. K. Singh, and B. N. Dhawan, *Arch. Int. Pharmacodyn. Ther.*, **188,** 320 (1970).

497. N. B. Mehta, *Abstr. Papers, 175th Am. Chem. Soc. Meet., Ahaheim, Calif., March 13–17, 1978*, p. MEDI-5.

498. C. Hörig, M. Klotzbach, H. Koch, E. Mayr, and J. Richter, *Pharmazie*, **31,** 499 (1976).

499. F. E. Soroko, N. B. Mehta, R. A. Maxwell, R. M. Ferris, and D. H. Schroeder, *J. Pharm. Pharmacol.*, **29,** 767 (1977).

500. F. E. Soroko and R. A. Maxwell, *Fed. Proc.*, **37,** 481 (1978).

501. L. F. Fabre, Jr., D. McLendon, and A. Mallette, *Clin. Pharmacol. Ther.*, **21,** 102 Abstr. (1977).

502. W. E. Fann, D. H. Schroeder, N. B. Mehta, F. E. Soroko, and R. A. Maxwell, *Curr. Ther. Res., Clin. Exp.*, **23,** 222 (1978).

503. L. Lemberger, E. Sernatinger, and R. Kuntzman, *Biochem. Pharmacol.*, **19,** 3021 (1970).

504. J. T. Hitchens, R. Orzechowski, S. Goldstein, and I. Shemano, *Toxicol. Appl. Pharmacol.*, **21,** 302 (1972).

505. D. W. Nachand, A. A. Kurland, and T. E. Hanlon, *J. Clin. Pharmacol.*, **7,** 116 (1967).

506. M. Namima and M. V. Aylott, *Fed. Proc.*, **36,** 1006 (1977).

507. P. Simon, M. A. Goujet, R. Chermat, and J. R. Boissier, *Therapie*, **26,** 1175 (1971).

508. D. D. Miller, J. Fowble, and P. N. Patil, *J. Med. Chem.*, **16,** 177 (1973).

509. M. E. Rogers, J. Sam, and N. P. Plotnikoff, *J. Med. Chem.*, **17,** 726 (1974).

510. M. E. Rogers and J. Sam, *J. Med. Chem.*, **18,** 1126 (1975).

511. R. Daudel, L. Esnault, C. Labrid, N. Busch, J. Moleyre, and J. Lambert, *Eur. J. Med. Chem.*, **11**, 443 (1976).

512. A. Rascol, H. Maurel, J. David, and M. Layani, *Therapie*, **29**, 95 (1974).

513. H. C. B. Denber, *Ann. Med. Psychol.*, **1**, 138 (1973).

514. J. Hache, P. Duchêne-Marullaz, and G. Streichenberger, *Therapie*, **29**, 81 (1974).

515. I. Goodlet, S. E. Mireyless, and M. F. Surgue, *Brit. J. Pharmacol.*, **59**, 481P (1977).

516. M. R. Sugrue, I. Goodlet, and S. E. Mireylees, *Eur. J. Pharmacol.*, **40**, 121 (1976).

517. J. Castañer and K. Hillier, *Drugs Future*, **3**, 315 (1978).

518. R. W. Fuller, D. T. Wong, H. D. Snoddy, and F. P. Bymaster, *Biochem. Pharmacol.*, **26**, 1323 (1977).

519. M. Fink, J. Simeon, T. M. Itil, and A. M. Freedman, *Clin. Pharmacol. Ther.*, **11**, 41 (1970).

520. F. C. Colpaert, F. M. Lenaerts, C. J. E. Niemegeers, and P. A. J. Janssen, *Arch. Int. Pharmacodyn. Ther.*, **215**, 40 (1975).

521. S. B. Ross and A. L. Renyi, *J. Pharm. Pharmacol.*, **28**, 458 (1976).

522. S. Park, S. Gershon, B. Angrist, and A. Floyd, *Curr. Ther. Res., Clin. Exp.*, **14**, 65 (1972).

523. Lilly Ind. Ltd., Belg. Pat. 844,429 (1977); Derwent No. 07532Y/05.

524. D. L. Trepanier, K. L. Shriver, and J. N. Eble, *J. Med. Chem.*, **12**, 257 (1969).

525. M. N. Aboul-Enein, L. Morgan, and J. Sam, *J. Pharm. Sci.*, **61**, 127 (1972).

526. J. Castañer and S. J. Hopkins, *Drugs Future*, **3**, 430 (1978).

527. N. J. Harper, C. W. T. Hussey, M. E. Peel, A. C. Ritchie, and J. M. Waring, *J. Med. Chem.*, **10**, 819 (1967).

528. Roussel UCLAF, Belg. Pat. 844,556 (1977); Derwent No. 07574Y/05.

529. Roussel UCLAF, Belg. Pat. 845,189 (1977); Derwent No. 11153Y/07.

530. S. Gershon, L. J. Hekimian, and A. Floyd, *Arzneim.-Forsch.*, **18**, 243 (1968).

531. J. K. Chakrabarti, M. J. Foulis, T. M. Hotten, S. S. Szinai, and A. Todd, *J. Med. Chem.*, **17**, 602 (1974).

532. C. Giurgea, J. Dauby, F. Moeyersoons, and F. Mouravieff-Lesuisse, in *Antidepressant Drugs*, S. Garattini and M. N. G. Dukes, Eds., Excerpta Medica Foundation, Amsterdam, 1967, p. 222.

533. D. P. Wheatley, *J. Int. Med. Res.*, **3**: Suppl. 3, 105 (1975).

534. F. J. Bereen, *Lancet*, **1973–I**, 379.

535. J. Guy Edwards, *Brit. Med. J.*, **2**, 1327 (1977).

536. K. B. Mallion, A. H. Todd, R. W. Turner, J. G. Bainbridge, D. T. Greenwood, J. Madinaveitia, A. R. Somerville, and B. A. Whittle, *Nature*, **238**, 157 (1972).

537. J. Buus Lassen, R. F. Squires, J. A. Christensen, and L. Molander, *Psychopharmacologia*, **42**, 21 (1975).

538. J. Buus Lassen, E. Peterson, B. Kjellberg, and S. O. Olsson, *Eur. J. Pharmacol.*, **32**, 108 (1975).

539. J. Buus Lassen, *Acta Pharmacol. Toxicol.*, **41**: Suppl. 4, 43 (1977).

540. J. Thuiller, in *Antidepressant Drugs*, S. Garattini and M. N. G. Dukes, Eds., Excerpta Medica Foundation, Amsterdam, 1967, p. 208.

541. T. A. Pugsley and W. Lippmann, *Arch. Int. Pharmacodyn. Ther.*, **228**, 322 (1977).

542. S. N. Rastogi, N. Amand, and C. R. Prasad, *J. Med. Chem.*, **15**, 286 (1972).

543. M. G. Subramanian and R. R. Gala, *I.R.C.S. Med. Sci.*, **4**, 529 (1976).

544. L. György, A. K. Pfeifer, M. Dóda, É. Galambos, J. Molnár, G. Kraiss, and K. Nádor, *Arzneim.-Forsch.*, **18**, 517 (1968).

545. S. J. Daum, A. J. Gambino, M. D. Aceto, and R. L. Clarke, *J. Med. Chem.*, **15**, 509 (1972).

546. A. Vagne, M. Manier, M. A. Brunet, and A. Boucherle, *Therapie*, **26**, 553 (1971); through *Chem. Abstr.*, **75**, 97163q (1971).

547. A. Vagne, O. A. Nedergaard, M. A. Brunet, and A. Boucherle, *Compt. Rend. Soc. Biol.*, **164**, 1769 (1970).

548. M. Namima and M. V. Aylott, *Pharmacologist*, **18**, 134 (1976).

549. C.-P. Chien and R. M. Kaplan, *Curr. Ther. Res., Clin. Exp.*, **11**, 471 (1969).

550. C. J. Sharpe, P. J. Palmer, D. E. Evans, G. R. Brown, G. King, R. S. Shadbolt, R. B. Trigg, R. J. Ward, A. Ashford, and J. W. Ross, *J. Med. Chem.*, **15**, 523 (1972).

551. P. G. Thuiller and J. Thuiller, *Arzneim.-Forsch.*, **14**, 556 (1964).

552. A. Areschka, J.-M. Mahaux, F. Verbruggen, C. Houben, M. Descamps, M. Broll, J.-P. Werbenec, R. Charlier, J. Simiand, and P. Eymard, *Eur. J. Med. Chem.*, **10**, 398 (1975).

553. R. Rodríguez and E. G. Pardo, *Pharmacologia*, **21**, 89 (1971).

554. C. Euvrard, F. Javoy, A. Herbet, and J. Glowinski, *Eur. J. Pharmacol.*, **41**, 281 (1977).

555. W. C. Lumma, Jr., R. D. Hartman, W. S. Saari, E. L. Engelhardt, R. Hirshmann, B. V. Cline-

schmidt, M. L. Torchiana, and C. A. Stone, *J. Med. Chem.*, **21,** 536 (1978).

556. B. V. Clineschmidt, J. C. McGuffin, and A. B. Pflueger, *Eur. J. Pharmacol.*, **44,** 65 (1977).

557. B. V. Clineschmidt, J. A. Totaro, A. B. Pflueger, and J. C. McGuffin, *Pharmacol. Res. Commun.*, **10,** 219 (1978).

558. A. G. Zacchei, T. I. Wishousky, and L. Weidner, *Fed. Proc.*, **37,** 814 (1978).

559. Merck and Co., Inc., U.S. Pat. 4,091,101 (June 15, 1977).

560. Merck and Co., Inc., U.S. Pat. 4,091,098 (April 25, 1977).

561. B. Silvestrini, V. Cioli, S. Burberi, and B. Catanese, *Int. J. Neuropharmacol.*, **7,** 587 (1968).

562. E. Stefanini, F. Fadda, L. Medda, and G. L. Gessa, *Life Sci.*, **18,** 1459 (1976).

563. P. A. vanZwieten, *Pharmacol.*, **15,** 331 (1977).

564. I. J. E. Boksay and R.-O. Weber, *Arch. Pharmacol.*, **293:** Suppl., R12 (1976).

565. J. Komarek and F. N. Neumann, *Arzneim.-Forsch.*, **27,** 2066 (1977).

566. R. Clemens and U. Clemens, *Arzneim.-Forsch.*, **27,** 2416 (1977).

567. B. Unterhalt, *Drugs Future*, **3,** 426 (1978).

568. I. Kosóczky, K. Grasser, E. Kiszelly, É. Toncsev, and L. Petöcz, *Abstr. 7th Int. Congr. Pharmacol.*, *Paris, 1978*, p. 187.

569. K. J. Kellar, G. R. Elliott, R. B. Holman, J. L. Madrid, M. L. Bernstein, J. D. Barchas, and J. Vernikos-Danellis, *Pharmacologist*, **17,** 258 (1975).

570. M. Grabowska, L. Antiewicz, and J. Michaluk, *Diss. Pharm. Pharmacol.*, **24,** 423 (1971).

571. Endo Laboratories, Inc., Belg. Pat. 845,368 (1976); Derwent No. 00043Y/01.

572. M. Grabowska and L. Gajda, *Diss. Pharm. Pharmacol.*, **23,** 309 (1971).

573. N. Barkov, A. Geller, and M. E. Jarvik, *Psychopharmacologia*, **21,** 82 (1971).

574. Roussel UCLAF, Belg. Pat. 858,101 (1978); Derwent No. 15899A/09.

575. M. Cohen, P. Milonas, Z. Weisberger, J. Thompson, and A. A. Rubin, *Pharmacologist*, **13,** 255 (1971).

576. C. A. Demerson, A. H. Philipp, L. G. Humber, M. J. Kraml, M.-P. Charest, H. Tom, and I. Vávra, *J. Med. Chem.*, **17,** 1140 (1974).

577. Hoffmann-LaRoche SA, Belg. Pat. 858,424 (1978); Derwent No. 17679A/10.

578. R. Rees and H. Smith, *J. Med. Chem.*, **10,** 624 (1967).

579. A. L. Jaton, D. M. Loew, and J. M. Vigouret, *Brit. J. Pharmacol.*, **56,** 371P (1976).

580. A. Flemenbaum and B. C. Schiele, *Curr. Ther. Res., Clin. Exp.*, **13,** 53 (1971).

581. E. Pálosi, L. Szporny, and K. Nádor, *J. Pharm. Sci.*, **57,** 709 (1968).

582. E. Pálosi, C. Mészáros, and L. Szporny, *Arzneim.-Forsch.*, **19,** 1882 (1969).

583. G. K. Suchowsky and L. Pegrassi, *Arzneim.-Forsch.*, **19,** 643 (1969).

584. G. K. Suchowsky, L. Pegrassi, A. Bonsignori, C. Bertazzoli, and T. Chieli, *Eur. J. Pharmacol.*, **6,** 327 (1969).

585. L. Bernardi, S. Coda, L. Pegrassi, and G. K. Suchowsky, *Experientia*, **24,** 774 (1968).

586. A. Moretti, L. Pegrassi, A. H. Glässer, and G. K. Suchowsky, *Boll. Chim. Farm.*, **113,** 36 (1974).

587. G. K. Suchowsky and L. Pegrassi, *Arzneim.-Forsch.*, **19,** 643 (1969).

588. A. Moretti, C. Caccia, A. Martini, and A. Amico, *Abstr. 7th Int. Congr. Pharmacol.*, *Paris, 1978*, p. 247.

589. G. Sathananthan, P. Mir, F. L. Minn, and S. Gershon, *Curr. Ther. Res., Clin. Exp.*, **19,** 475 (1976).

590. P. Collins, G. Sakalis, and F. L. Minn, *Curr. Ther. Res., Clin. Exp.*, **19,** 512 (1976).

591. J. H. Biel, in *Advances in Chemistry Series*, Vol. 45, F. W. Schueler, Ed., American Chemical Society, Washington, D. C., 1964, p. 114.

592. H. K. Davis, H. F. Ford, J. P. Tupin, and A. Colvin, *Dis. Nerv. Syst.*, **25,** 179 (1964).

593. H. B. A. Welle, J. van Dijk, J. E. Davies, V. Claassen, and Th. A. C. Boschman, *Chim. Ther.*, **5,** 367 (1970).

594. T. M. Itil, A. Bhattachyaryya, N. Polvan, M. Huque, and G. N. Menon, *Progr. Neuro-Psychopharmacol.*, **1,** 309 (1977).

595. J. H. Wright and H. C. B. Denber, *Curr. Ther. Res., Clin. Exp.*, **23,** 83 (1978).

596. V. Claassen, J. E. Davies, G. Hertting, and P. Placheta, *Brit. J. Pharmacol.*, **60,** 505 (1977).

597. J. Castañer and P. J. Thorpe, *Drugs Future*, **3,** 288 (1978).

598. J.-P. Kan, J.-F. Pujol, A. Malnoe, M. Strolin-Benedetti, C. Gouret, and G. Raynaud, *Eur. J. Med. Chem.*, **12,** 13 (1977).

599. G. B. Fregman, M. Vidali, T. Chieli, and I. Bussoleron, *6th Int. Congr. Pharmacol.*, *Helsinki, July 20–25*, Abstr. No. 336 (1975).

600. C. J. Sharpe, R. S. Shadbolt, A. Ashford, and J. W. Ross, *J. Med. Chem.*, **14,** 977 (1971).

601. M. B. Wallach, A. P. Roszkowski, and L. D.

Waterbury, *Abstr. 7th Int. Congr. Pharmacol.*, *Paris, 1978*, p. 247.

602. S. Gershon, L. J. Hekimian, and A. Floyd, Jr., *J. Clin. Pharmacol.*, **7**, 348 (1967).

603. T. F. Burke and D. I. Templar, *Curr. Ther. Res., Clin. Exp.*, **10**, 335 (1968).

604. A. M. Simopoulos, A. Pinto, P. W. Babikow, and A. A. Kurland, *Curr. Ther. Res., Clin. Exp.*, **10**, 570 (1968).

605. Y. Yamauchi, M. Nakamura, and K. Koketsu, *Kurume Med. J.*, **19**, 175 (1972); through *Chem. Abstr.*, **78**, 314r (1973).

606. B. Eichelman, N. B. Thoa, and J. Perez-Cruet, *Fed. Proc.*, **31**, 289 Abs (1972).

607. B. J. Carroll and P. T. Sharp, *Science*, **172**, 1355 (1971).

608. S. R. Platman, *Dis. Nerv. Syst.*, **32**, 604 (1971).

609. R. R. Fieve, H. Meltzer, D. L. Dunner, M. Levitt, J. Mendlewicz, and A. Thomas, *Am. J. Psychiatr.*, **130**, 55 (1973).

610. Anonymous, *Chem. Week*, **110**: 10, 41 (March 8, 1972).

611. J. Arehart-Treichel, *Sci. News*, **102**, 315 (1972).

612. A. J. Prange, Jr., I. C. Wilson, P. P. Lara, L. B. Allrop, and G. R. Breese, *Lancet*, **2**, 999 (1972).

613. M. J. E. van der Vis-Melsen and J. D. Wiener, *Lancet*, **1972–II**, 1415.

614. A. A. Sugerman, M. Swartzburg, P. S. Mueller, and J. Rochford, *Curr. Ther. Res., Clin. Exp.*, **19**, 94 (1976).

615. F. W. Furlong, G. M. Brown, and M. F. Beeching, *Am. J. Psychiatr.*, **133**, 1187 (1976).

616. N. P. Plotnikoff, A. J. Prange, Jr., G. R. Breese, M. S. Anderson, and I. C. Wilson, *Science*, **178**, 417 (1972).

617. A. Agnoli, V. Andreoli, M. Casacchia, and R. Cerbo, *J. Psychiatr. Res.*, **13**, 43 (1976).

618. R. H. Ehrensing and A. J. Kastin, *Arch. Gen. Psychiatr.*, **30**, 63 (1974).

619. A. Barbeau, M. Roy, and A. J. Kastin, *Can. Med. Assoc. J.*, **114**, 120 (1976).

620. A. Failli, K. Sestanj, H. U. Immer, and M. Götz, *Arzneim.-Forsch.*, **27**, 2286 (1977).

621. K. Voith, *Arzneim.-Forsch.*, **27**, 2290 (1977).

622. H. D. Kurland, *Am. J. Psychiatr.*, **122**, 457 (1965).

623. W. M. Herrman and R. C. Beach, *Pharmakopsychiatr.*, **11**, 164 (1978).

624. F. J. Ayd, Jr., *Int. Drug Ther. Newslett.*, **3**, 27 (1968).

625. D. Widlöcher, Y. Lecrubier, R. Jouvent, A. J. Puech, and P. Simon, *Lancet*, **1977–II**, 767 (1977).

626. T. Nakajima, Y. Kudo, and Z. Kaneko, *Folia Psychiatr. Neurol. Japon.*, **32**, 223 (1978).

627. E. Fischer, B. Heller, M. Nachon, and H. Spatz, *Arzneim.-Forsch.*, **25**, 132 (1975).

628. R. L. Borison, P. J. Maple, H. S. Havdala, and B. I. Diamond, *Res. Commun. Chem. Pathol. Pharmacol.*, **21**, 363 (1978).

629. H. Beckman and E. Ludolph, *Arzneim.-Forsch.*, **28**, 1283 (1978).

630. W. W. K. Zung, D. Gianturco, E. Pfeiffer, H. W. Wang, A. Whanger, T. P. Bridge, and S. G. Potkin, *Psychosomatics*, **15**, 127 (1974).

631. E. J. Olsen, L. Bank, and L. F. Jarvik, *J. Gerontol.*, **33**, 514 (1978).

CHAPTER FIFTY-NINE

Anorexigenics

WILLIAM J. HOULIHAN

and

RONALD G. BABINGTON

Pharmaceutical Research and Development
Division
Sandoz, Inc.
East Hanover, New Jersey 07936, USA

CONTENTS

1   INTRODUCTION

In the affluent nations of the world, obesity is a prevalent and growing concern, both medically and socially (1–10). Obesity is a chronic nutritional disease that is difficult to treat, and in most cases it is impossible to achieve total remission. It is a state wherein caloric intake exceeds expenditure. The excess calories are converted to fat and then ultimately to useless weight. The solution is simple enough—to reverse the caloric balance until the excess fat is eliminated. Unfortunately, getting the overweight patient to comply with such a regimen is one of the most frustrating challenges facing the physician.

Unhealthy eating patterns are established early in life and by adulthood most individuals reject the idea of being obese in favor of being overweight. Obesity cannot be judged in terms of body weight alone; it depends on skeletal frame and muscular development. The crucial factor is the percentage of body fat; statistically most of the affluent population are obese. An optimal percentage of body fat, for mature males would be 15–18% and for females 22–25%; in actuality, at the peak of body maturity the average individual has already reached 35% body fat (5). This accumulation may continue until serious medical complications arise or vanity intercedes and an effort is undertaken to reduce.

Once the patient has decided to shed excess weight, the physician must rely on average charts (11) or clinical judgment to determine the amount of weight to be lost. Since each kilogram of adipose tissue is equivalent to 7000 cal, a shift in the caloric

balance of 1000 cal/day would result in the loss of 1 kg/week (4, 5). Thus the patient's caloric requirements should be established, taking into account possible changes in intake as well as increased expenditure.

The treatment of obesity can be categorized into four basic approaches. The most drastic and least common is surgical intervention to shorten intestinal length, thereby decreasing exposure time of ingested calories to absorption. Bypass surgery is used only in cases of morbid obesity and is a heroic measure. The patient must be emotionally stable and physically capable of withstanding the trauma.

The second approach is to increase caloric expenditure via exercise. Although exercise utilizes excess calories, the extra physical exertion required to make a substantial difference in the caloric balance is in itself not practical for most individuals. Moreover, overweight persons tend to be hypoactive and are difficult to motivate to begin an efficient exercise program; if successful, the consequence is increased appetite.

The foundation for any program to lose weight involves reduction of the caloric substrate, i.e., dieting. For long-term success, it is important that a well-balanced but restricted diet be developed and adhered to, even after the desired weight is attained. Fad diets may show striking results but they should be discouraged because they can be detrimental to health and the relapse rate is nearly 100%.

Because so many patients find dieting difficult and seek some support measure, the use of drugs in a reducing program as an adjunct to diet and exercise is well established. Because a pharmacological entity to control fat regulation *per se* does not exist, the current treatment of choice involves appetite suppression. The available agents leave much to be desired. With few exceptions all clinically proved drugs possess the phenethylamine nucleus, with the associated disadvantages. Tolerance and overt CNS excitation are the two main concerns, with cardiovascular, gastrointestinal, and interaction problems occurring frequently. Abuse liability with the anorectic class of drugs is exceptionally high because of the profound CNS-stimulatory effects of the phenethylamines; all are currently controlled by the United States government.

At best, even with pharmacological support, prognosis for maintaining a desirable weight level is only good, never excellent; relapse occurs routinely. The fatter the patient and the longer the history of obesity, the worse the prognosis. The best chance of success is with patients with mild obesity of short duration, a good initial response, and no emotional problems. Prognosis is also good in patients with medical complications that are relieved by weight loss.

Of the four basic approaches, the pharmacological category offers a real chance to improve the treatment of obesity. An ideal agent would have anorexia as its sole pharmacological effect and would be efficacious without dietary restrictions. It would be potent with a large therapeutic index and should be inexpensive. There should be minimal biodegradation. Certainly the compound would not produce tolerance and would lack abuse liability.

Obviously, the current state of the art leaves much to be desired. But the search continues and as the knowledge of the physiology and psychology of hyperphagia increases so will the chances of finding better anorexigenics.

2 TECHNIQUES FOR EVALUATING ANOREXIGENICS

2.1 Animal Testing

Two fundamental approaches are used extensively to study anorexic effects in animals: free feeding and operant behavioral paradigms (12). Both measure the ability of a compound to reduce food consumption in animals made hungry by dietary restrictions.

For screening purposes, the preferred method involves some aspect of free feeding wherein food intake is measured over a specified period of time (13–16). Usually, the subjects have limited access to food during which the daily rations must be consumed. Once the animals become familiar with the experimental situation, daily intake quickly stabilizes and drug effects can be accurately compared to base-line consumption.

A more sophisticated modification (17) utilizes an "eatometer" (18) to monitor feeding over extended periods of time as well as selected short intervals. This technique provides additional information on eating patterns and the qualitative effects of pharmacologic agents but has limited utility for the initial screening of test compounds.

The major criticism of free feeding studies is the difficulty in distinguishing true anorectic effects from conflicting pharmacological properties such as overt behavioral depression. Thus several operant tests based on food-motivated behavior have been tried with mixed results.

Consistent with the original thought that careful monitoring of ongoing behavior would be more informative than free feeding *per se*, studies involving lever pressing on fixed ratio schedules (19–21), runway performance (22), or response in appetitive–shock combination paradigms (23) can distinguish between overt and appetitive behavioral effects. However, careful analysis of the data indicates a high correlation between the effective dose for suppressing appetite in the free feeding and operant situations. Moreover, studies utilizing other operant schedules demonstrate an opposite effect of amphetamine on food-motivated behavior (23–25). Apparently motivation is not a critical factor in determining anorexigenic activity in animals.

A universal problem in the screening of drugs that operate through an action on the central nervous system is the absence of animal models that replicate human pathologies. The situation is no different in the area of obesity, in that most studies examine effects on appetitive behavior in animals made hungry by dietary restrictions rather than in obese subjects. A stronger effort is needed to develop appropriate models at the preclinical level. For example, the models that have evolved are capable of verifying anorectic efficacy in a number of phenethylamine derivatives but have been less successful in identifying unique compounds with confirmed activity in man (12, 26).

2.2 Human Testing

Anorectic clinical trials differ drastically from animal tests. The human subjects are at least 15–20% overweight whereas experimental animals are on a restricted diet and underweight. Clinical and preclinical studies are also quite different in that the main parameter for determining drug effects in man is decreases in body weight whereas in animals diminished food consumption is measured.

The amount of information obtained in therapeutic trials directly related to antiobesity effects is meager. Despite a large literature on the clinical testing of anorectic agents, a standard protocol has not yet been documented (27). Aside from weight loss, the only other objective measurement in man to gain acceptance has been skinfold thickness (28, 29), and subjective information is limited to the occasional clinical report containing comments as to the effect of drug on appetite.

Needless to say, several important criteria should be considered for every clinical protocol (30, 31). The patient population should be as homogeneous as possible, and ideally the daily caloric intake should be equivalent for each subject, a difficult assignment in outpatient trials. A crossover design is usually employed to compensate for the relatively large weight loss during the early stages of dietary programs. The test drug should be compared to a standard agent as well as placebo, and multiple dose levels are desirable. The study should be of sufficient length to garner information on peak effect, duration of activity, development of tolerance, and incidence of side effects. Individuals with medical complications associated with obesity, currently on medication or previously treated with anorectic agents, should be excluded. Motivation and a realistic comprehension of the objectives must not be ignored when selecting subjects for an anorectic study.

3 APPETITE SUPPRESSION

3.1 Neuroanatomic Substrates

Current concepts regarding the control of feeding derive from animal experiments wherein it has been possible to identify several intimately involved CNS structures (Figs. 59.1, 59.2). Similarly, neurochemical studies have implicated norepinephrine, dopamine, and serotonin in some aspect of appetitive control. Less clear is the interrelationship between the neuroanatomic and neurochemical evidence as well as the relevance of the animal findings to appetite processes in man.

In several animal species, bilateral electrolytic lesions or knife cuts of the lateral hypothalamic (LH) nucleus (Fig. 59.2) cause anorexia, aphagia, and dramatic loss of body weight (32, 33). Initially, feeding behavior is completely destroyed and starvation is inevitable unless the animal is force-fed. If intragastric feeding is continued long enough, the subject regains the ability to sustain itself; but marked deficits in feeding responses persist. Conversely, electrical stimulation of the LH nucleus produces hyperphagia and obesity (34, 35).

The gross behavioral effects of lesions or

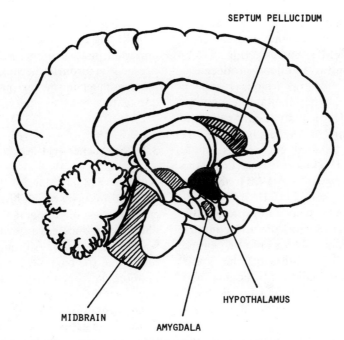

Fig. 59.1 Diagram of a medial sagittal section through a brain to demonstrate the relative positions of several structures thought to be involved in the control of feeding behavior.

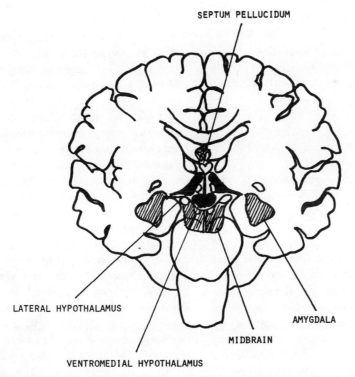

Fig. 59.2 Diagram of a frontal section through a brain at the level of the hypothalamus to further illustrate the locations of those neuroanatomic substrates implicated in hunger and satiety.

electrical stimulation of a second hypothalamic nucleus, the ventromedial hypothalamic (VMH) nucleus, (Fig. 59. 2) are in direct contrast to effects produced in the LH. Thus bilateral lesions result in hyperphagia and experimental obesity (36–38), whereas electrical stimulation inhibits feeding behavior (39). When both the LH and VMH are lesioned, the results mimic lesioning the LH alone (35); severing the connections between the VMH and LH produces hyperphagia and obesity (40).

These findings have been interpreted (32, 35, 41) to mean that (a) the LH contains mechanisms responsible for initiating eating and is the feeding center; (b) the VMH controls the termination of feeding and thus is the satiety center; and (c) the feeding center (LH) dominates the satiety center (VMH).

It has long been known, however, that several extrahypothalamic structures profoundly influence feeding behavior (Figs. 59.1, 59.2). Lesions or electrical stimulation in the amygdala, septum, or midbrain tegmentum can produce ingestive alterations similar to, but less intense than, those at the hypothalamic level (42–50). Because all are linked anatomically to the hypothalamus, they have been implicated in a complex feeding regulatory system with the integrative mechanisms residing in the hypothalamus.

Recent evidence suggests that extrahypothalamic influence is even more extensive than originally appreciated (51–53). Numerous fiber tracts originating in widespread brain areas have been shown to transverse the hypothalamus; interruption of those tracts appears to be more important in the etiology of lesion effects than destruction of hypothalamic nuclei *per se.* Considering that feeding in animals is affected by habit, circadian rhythms, and environmental cues, the influence of higher levels of neural integration cannot be ignored. For example, the body weight of rats fed the usual laboratory chow is quite stable, but they can be enticed to obesity by substituting more palatable diets (54). It is important that such lines of investigation be pursued vigorously because hypothalamic feeding mechanisms in man are certainly dominated by higher nervous functions.

3.2 Neurochemical Mechanisms

At the cellular level, the biochemical mechanisms subserving the pharmacological activities of amphetamine and related phenethylamines have been extensively investigated (55–56). Although there is little doubt that the biogenic amines are involved in anorexia, conclusive evidence to confirm one or the other as the preeminent neuroregulator is lacking. Numerous conflicting studies exist, and by selective citation of the literature, neurochemical documentation can be presented to attack or defend the role of each candidate (55b, 56–59).

Many of the inconsistencies can be attributed to methodological differences, including such fundamental considerations as differences in species, dose, and brain tissue. Extremes in dosages have been used, often with no apparent appreciation of the behavioral consequences. Results obtained with whole brain are compared to drug effects at the regional level. Acute and chronic studies have been treated as equivalent, and not enough attention is paid to the time interval from the time of dosing to response measurement (56).

Despite the incongruities, it is probable that the majority of the anorectic agents influence the catecholamine system; but the relative roles of norepinephrine (NE) and dopamine (DA) are controversial (55–56, 60–65). Most of the active appetite suppressant drugs have the phenethylamine nucleus, and thus are structurally related to the catecholamines; although regional differences in the endogenous levels of NE and DA exist, each has substantial concentrations in areas thought to be involved with feeding behavior (66–68).

Catecholaminergic transmission in the brain involves several processes; drugs might alter any of these to exert an anorectic effect (55–59). Drug-induced shifts in the steady-state levels of NE or DA are considered to reflect a change in neurochemical regulation. The effect of amphetamine and similar compounds on the concentrations of NE and DA has been measured both in whole brain and at selected neuroanatomic sites with equivocal findings (56). In general, the level of both amines is decreased but the magnitude varies widely for each amine. Similarly, there is conflicting evidence for the effects of the amphetamine-like drugs on each of the processes contributing to catecholamine turnover (55b, 56). The anorectic agents have been shown to influence all the major mechanisms (Figs. 59.3, 59.4):

1. Biosynthesis: amphetamine appears to inhibit both NE and DA synthesis but the evidence is far from conclusive, especially at the regional level.

2. Metabolism: enzymatic degradation can occur by extraneuronal O-methylation (catechol O-methyltransferase) or intraneuronal deamination (monoamine oxidase). Amphetamine produces a shift to O-methylation but the evidence, favors an increased availability of synaptic amines rather than inhibition of monoamine oxidase.

3. Reuptake: a second, more important mechanism for terminating the effects of the catecholamines is reuptake into the presynaptic terminals. The phenethylamine drugs apparently block the reuptake process for both transmitters.

4. Release: NE and DA are stored in granules as well as cytoplasm at the

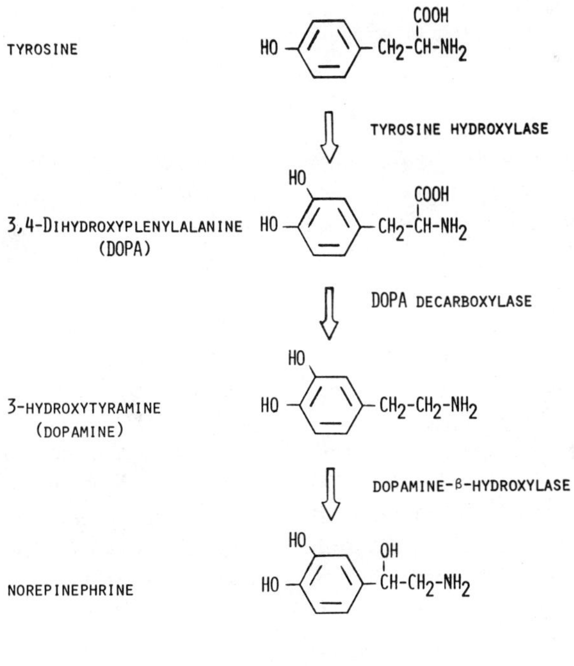

Fig. 59.3 Schematic outline of norepinephrine biosynthesis, including dopamine.

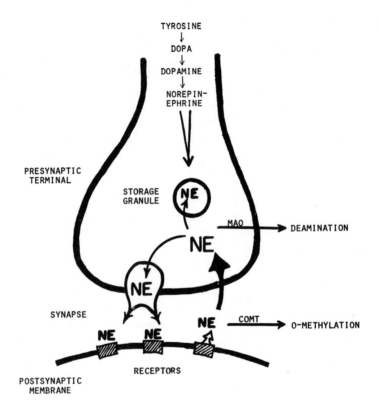

TYROSINE
↓
DOPA
↓
DOPAMINE
↓
NOREPIN-
EPHRINE

PRESYNAPTIC
TERMINAL

STORAGE
GRANULE   NE

MAO → DEAMINATION

NE

SYNAPSE   NE

NE   NE   NE   COMT → O-METHYLATION

RECEPTORS

POSTSYNAPTIC
MEMBRANE

Fig. 59.4 Hypothetical norepinephrine synapse depicting biosynthesis, storage and release, reuptake, and metabolism. The basic scheme would be the same for dopamine.

synaptic cleft. The effect of the amphetamine drugs is to stimulate the release of the catecholamines at both sites.

Current thoughts are that the predominant effect of the anorectic phenethylamines is on the reuptake and release mechanisms (26, 56) but the synthetic and metabolic influence cannot yet be ruled out.

The importance of the catecholaminergic system as the principal neurochemical mediator for anorexia has been challenged by findings with fenfluramine. Fenfluramine contains the phenethylamine nucleus and is an active anorexigenic agent (69), but it differs from the other phenethylamine compounds in two significant modes. First, fenfluramine causes CNS depression rather

than excitation (55–56b, 70); and second, it is believed that the anorectic effect is mediated by a serotoninergic system (71–73). Even with fenfluramine, however, the results for a tryptaminergic system are not conclusive (74); there is further controversy whether the anorexia results from a direct or indirect action on serotonin neurons (64, 71, 73, 75).

As with the neuroanatomic substrates, extrapolation of the neurochemical findings from animal to man is tenuous at best. The tedious effort of carefully correlating the complex interrelationships between anatomy, neurochemistry, and feeding behavior is just beginning and must be completed before valid conclusions can be drawn regarding anorectic mechanisms in man.

4 PHENETHYLAMINE DERIVATIVES

The basic skeleton found in the majority of clinically useful anoretic agents is the β-phenethylamine unit 59.**1**. Modification of this framework by the introduction of one or two methyl groups in the α-position or an oxygen function in the β-position has led to the useful β-phenylisopropylamines (59.**2**), β-phenyl-*tert*-butyl amines (59.**3**), phenylpropanolamines (59.**4**), phenylaminopropanones (59.**5**), and the 2-methyl-1-phenylmorpholines (59.**6**).

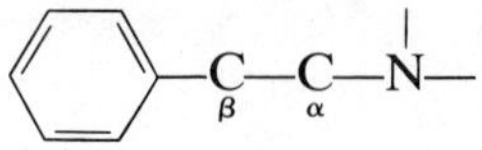

59.1

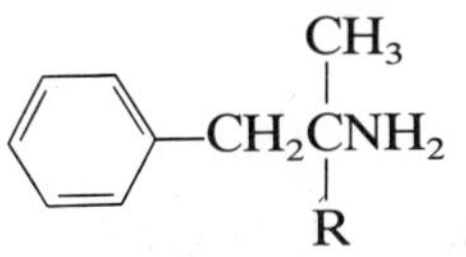

59.2 R = H
59.3 R = CH₃

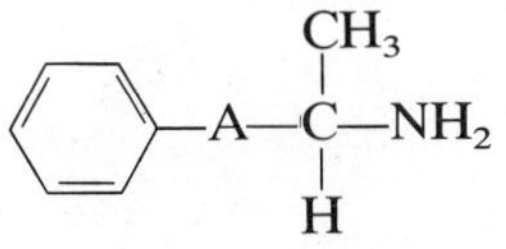

59.4 A = CHOH
59.5 A = C=O

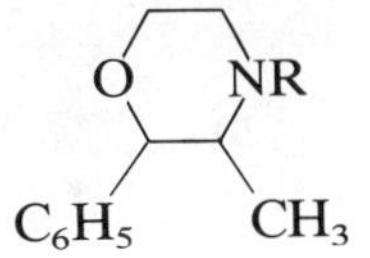

59.6

4.1 β-Phenylisopropylamines

Anorectic agents on the United States market that are β-phenylisopropylamine (59.**2**) derivatives are amphetamine (59.**2**), dextroamphetamine, the (+) isomer of amphetamine, methamphetamine (59.**7**), benzphetamine (59.**8**), and fenfluramine (59.**9**). The recommended adult dosage and prescription scheduling (BNDD) for these substances are given in Table 59.1.

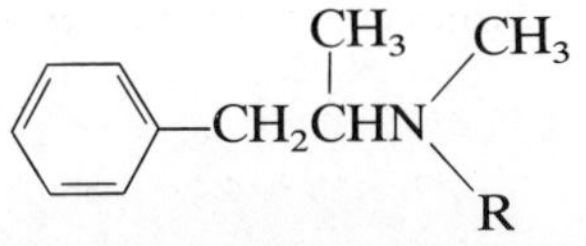

59.7 R = H
59.8 R = CH₂C₆H₅

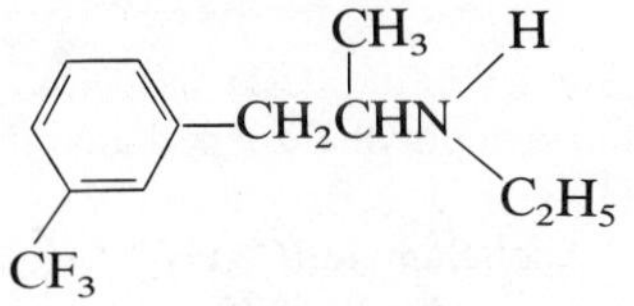

59.9

4.1.1 AMPHETAMINE, DEXTROAMPHETAMINE, METHAMPHETAMINE, AND BENZPHETAMINE.

Amphetamine (59.**2**), first prepared by Edeleano in 1887 (76), was recognized by Alles (77), in a series of papers starting in 1927, to possess a variety of CNS activities. The use of *dl*-amphetamine as an aid in the control of obesity in humans was reported about a decade later by Lesses and Meyerson (78) and Nathanson (79). Subsequent studies revealed that the (+) isomer, dextroamphetamine, has fewer side effects than the (±) mixture; it is more widely used as an anoretic agent. The (−) isomer, levamfetamine, has more central-stimulant and cardiovascular effects and is no longer available as a clinical agent in the United States.

In an attempt to alleviate some of the undesirable stimulant effects, amphetamines has been combined with sedatives and tranquilizers such as amobarbital and prochlorperazine (cf. Table 59.1). Various cation resins, in particular the sulfonated styrene copolymers, have been complexed with amphetamines to prolong effectiveness and minimize stimulant effects; such preparations are available on the U.S. market (cf. Table 59.1).

The N-alkylated analogs, methamphetamine (59.**7**) and benzphetamine (59.**8**), both possess anorectic and central-stimulant properties in the range of *d*-

Table 59.1 Anorectics Marketed in the United States

No.	USAN Name,[a] CA Name (Date on U.S. Market)	Trade Name (Salt Form)[b]	Recommended Daily Adult Dosage[b] Mg/dose	Number of doses	BNDD[c] Schedule
59.2	Amphetamine ($C_9H_{13}N$), (±)-α-methylbenzeneethanamine (1944)	Benzedrine® (H_2SO_4)	15 5–10	1 3	II
59.8	Benzphetamine ($C_{17}H_{21}N$), (+)-N,α-dimethyl-N-(phenylmethyl)-benzeneethanamine (1960)	Didrex® (HCl)	25–50	1–3	III
59.24	Chlorphentermine ($C_{10}N_{14}ClN$), 4-chloro-α,α-dimethyl-benzeneethanamine (1965)	Pre-State® (HCl)	65	1	III
59.25	Chlortermine ($C_{10}H_{14}ClN$), 2-chloro-α,α-dimethyl-benzeneethanamine (1973)	Voranil® (HCl)	50	1	III
59.2	Dextroamphetamine ($C_9H_{13}N$), (+)-α-methylbenzeneethanamine (1944)	Dexedrine® (H_2SO_4) Obotan® (tannate)	10–15 5–10	1 3	II
	Cation resin complex with 1:1 dextroamphetamine and amphetamine	Biphetamine®, Delcobese®, Obetrol® (H_2SO_4)	7.5–20	1	II
	Combined with: 97 mg amobarbital 7.5 mg prochlorperazine	Dexamyl® (H_2SO_4) Eskatrol® (H_2SO_4)	15 15	2–3 1	II II
59.28	Diethylpropion ($C_{13}H_{19}NO$), α-(diethylamino)phenyl-1-propanone (1959)	Tenuate® Tepanil® (HCl)	25 75	3 1	IV
59.9	Fenfluramine ($C_{12}H_{16}F_3N$), N-ethyl-α-methyl-3-(trifluoromethyl)benzeneethanamine (1973)	Pondimin® (HCL)	20	1–3	III
59.63	Mazindol ($C_{16}H_{13}ClN_2O$), 5-(4-chlorophenyl)-2,5-dihydro-3H-imidazo[2,1-a]isoindol-5-ol (1973)	Sanorex® (Base)	1	3	III
59.7	Metamphetamine ($C_{10}H_{15}N$), (S)-N,α-dimethyl-benzeneethanamine (1944)	Desoxyn®, Fetamin® (HCl)	2.5–5.0	2–3	II
59.35	Phendimetrazine ($C_{12}H_{17}NO$), (3R)-trans-3,4-dimethyl-2-phenylmorpholine (1961)	Bacarate®, Bontril®, Melfiat®, Plegine® Statobex®, Tanorex® (tartrate)	35	2–3	III
59.36	Phenmetrazine ($C_{11}H_{15}NO$), trans-3-methyl-2-morpholinephenyl (1956)	Preludin® (HCl)	25 50–75	2–3 1	II

Table 59.1 (*Continued*)

No.	USAN Name,[a] CA Name (Date on U.S. Market)	Trade Name (Salt Form)[b]	Recommended Daily Adult Dosage[b]		BNDD[c] Schedule
			Mg/dose	Number of doses	
59.**3**	Phentermine ($C_{10}H_{15}N$), α,α-dimethylbenzene-ethanamine (1959)	Fastin®, Wilpo® (HCl)	8	3	IV
		Ionamin® (resin)	15–30	1	IV

[a] *USAN and the USP Dictionary of Drug Names*, M.C. Griffiths, Ed., United States Pharmacopeial Convention, Inc., Rockville, Md., 1975.
[b] *Physicians Desk Reference*, 37th ed., Medical Economics Co., Litton Industries, Oradell, N. J., 1977.
[c] *Controlled Substances Manual*, American Druggist "Blue Book," The Hearst Corp., New York, 1976, pp. 11–60.

amphetamine and are clinically used in the (+) isomer form (cf. Table 59.1).

Side effects with this class of compounds can be grouped into four major categories; CNS, cardiovascular, gastrointestinal, and abuse dependence. All the anorectic drugs except fenfluramine excite the central nervous system and exhibit a common profile of clinical signs including restlessness, insomnia, tremor, euphoria, and headache. Cardiovascular side effects include elevated blood pressure, palpitations, and tachycardia. Nausea, vomiting, dry mouth, unpleasant taste, diarrhea, and constipation are all symptoms associated with gastrointestinal irritation or sympathetic nervous system stimulation.

Abuse and dependence—both physiological and psychological—are a particular problem with the amphetamine group. Liability fluctuates among the various drugs but can usually be directly correlated with the intensity of CNS excitability produced. Tachyphylaxsis and tolerance are associated problems, and massive dose levels may be achieved upon prolonged usage. Symptoms of chronic abuse include insomnia, severe dermatoses, alopecia, and dramatic personality changes which at the extreme result in schizophrenic-like behavior. Withdrawal is characterized by profound fatigue and mental depression.

Because of the powerful central-stimulant properties of the amphetamine-like agents, there has been a tendency to experiment surreptitiously for every imaginable disease entity. Most drugs in this group are dangerous, as indicated by their relegation to Schedule III by the U.S. Department of Justice. Thus proper restraints should be observed against the indiscriminate use of these agents.

Current concepts regarding the neurochemical mechanisms subserving anorexia have been discussed in Section 3.2. A detailed critique of the literature is beyond the scope of this chapter, but for the interested reader there are several excellent reviews available (3, 55, 56–59).

To resolve the precise neuromechanisms responsible for the anorectic effects of the amphetamines, an integrated theory involving fundamental mechanisms at three stages is needed: neuroanatomic loci, the relative roles of the various putative neurotransmitters, and the particular neurotransmission process altered. If taken separately, more than one plausible explanation of anorexigenesis is defensible for each of the individual facets. Understandably, a single unified concept that encompasses the experimental data for the overall process has not evolved.

There is little doubt that the anorectic effect is primarily exerted through an action on the central nervous system (80). Similarly, there is strong evidence that the hypothalamus is intimately involved (81, 82). Now it appears that extrahypothalamic influence is far more complex than originally appreciated (83, 84) and any comprehensive theory of action cannot ignore both direct and indirect effects at ubiquitous CNS sites.

Simply from structural analogy, it is reasonable to suspect that the pharmacological actions of amphetamine involve catecholaminergic mechanisms. Because of the diversity of CNS effects, the determination whether a single neurotransmitter mediates anorexia—and if so, which one—has been difficult. Beginning with the finding by Weissman et al. (85) that the inhibition of catecholamine synthesis with α-methyltyrosine would suppress feeding behavior, numerous investigators (63, 64, 75, 86, 87) have tried to manipulate noradrenaline and dopamine pharmacologically in an attempt to definitively establish one or the other as preeminent—with equivocal success.

Despite general agreement that amphetamine enhances the availability of neurotransmitter to postsynaptic receptors, again there is disagreement as to exactly how that enhancement is accomplished. Although numerous authors favor stimulation of release of functional catecholamine (88–92), others feel that the predominant action is a blockade of reuptake (93–96). In either case, the ultimate consequences would be the same (97, 98).

4.1.1.1 *Analogs.* Propylhexedrine (59.**10**; cyclexedrine) is a symphathomimetic agent widely used as an inhalant for nasal con-

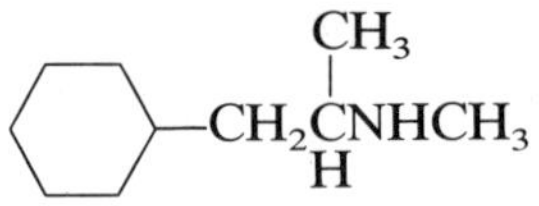

59.**10**

gestion (99). In several European countries the substance is available as an anorectic agent and used at doses of 75–100 mg daily for effective appetite control (100, 101).

A variety of *N*-substituted amphetamines have been investigated in man and found to have appetite suppressing properties. Since these substances are extensively metabolized to amphetamine they exhibit a profile of activity similar to the parent drug. The more widely studied derivatives are mefenorex (RO 4-5282; 59.**11**) (102–106) fenproporex (59.**12**) (107, 108), and furfenorex (59.**13**) (109–113).

The (−) isomer of 2,4-dichloroamphetamine (59.**14**) was evaluated in obese patients and found to be poorly tolerated and exhibited erratic appetite control (114). In man A-31960 (59.**15**) at 50 mg daily gave an anorectic effect similar to 5 mg of methamphetamine (59.**7**) (115, 116).

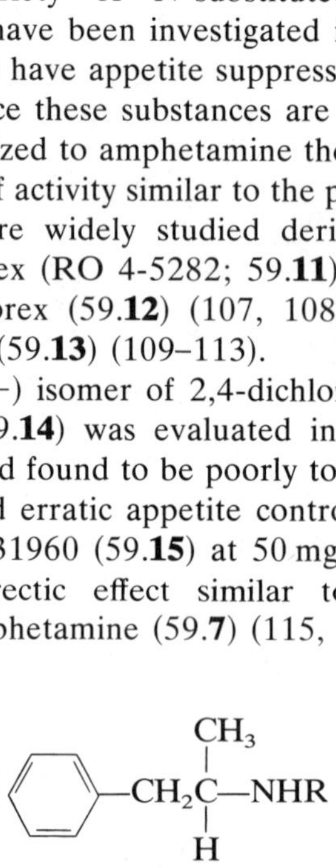

59.**11**   R = CH₂CH₂CH₂Cl
59.**12**   R = CH₂CH₂CN

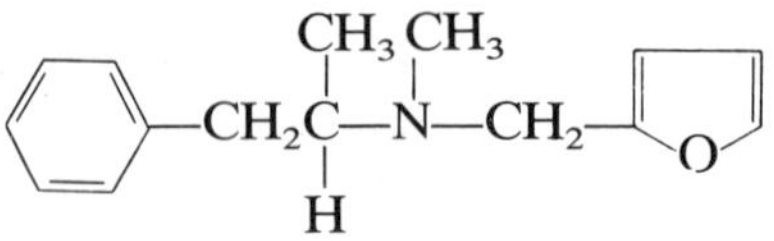

59.**13**

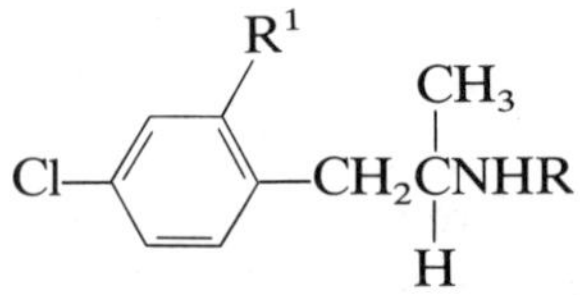

59.**14**   R = H, R¹ = Cl
59.**15**   R = CH₂—△ , R¹ = H

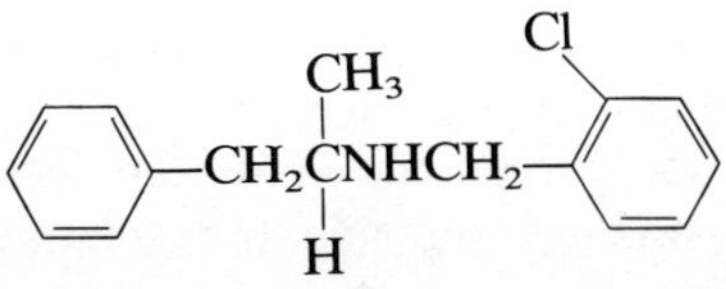

59.**16**

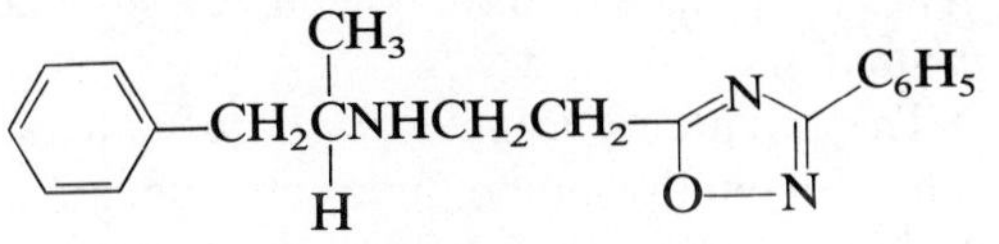

59.**17**

When evaluated for anorectic activity at 1.5 mg/kg in man, 2- and 3-methylamphetamine had little effect, the 3,4-dimethyl analog gave apparent but transient activity, and the 4-methyl gave apparent activity (117).

Other *N*-substituted amphetamines that have received extensive pharmacological studies in animals are clobenzorex (59.**16**) (111, 118, 119) and WD 67/2 (59.**17**) (120).

4.1.2 FENFLURAMINE. The only FDA-approved indication for the use of fenfluramine (59.**9**) is adult obesity. Unlike the rest of the anorectic drugs, fenfluramine produces CNS depression rather than excitation. In general, the drug is well tolerated and with careful management side effects are mild to moderate and disappear with continued use. When side effects are produced they are described as drowsiness, light-headedness, and dizziness. Postural hypotension has been reported. Gastrointestinal and autonomic symptoms include diarrhea, nausea, vomiting, and micturation. Paradoxically, adult anorectic doses are excessive in children and can produce amphetamine-like excitation which can be fatal. At present, fenfluramine is the drug of choice as an anorectic in Europe.

Dependence liability is less obvious with fenfluramine than the amphetamine-like anorectic drugs, probably due to the absence of CNS stimulation.

Among the anorectic agents, only fenfluramine causes behavioral depression rather than excitation; this has been attributed to its unique involvement with serotonin rather than catecholamines. Similarly, fenfluramine anorexia is thought to be involved with tryptaminergic mechanisms (64, 71, 73, 75). In fact, Shoulson and Chase (121) have obtained evidence in humans that fenfluramine-induced anorexia is related to serotonergic function in the brain.

There is evidence that the behavioral anorectic activities of fenfluramine might be indirectly mediated through the metabolite, norfenfluramine (121–123). Fenfluramine is dealkylated to norfenfluramine in several species (124–126), and both the metabolite and parent compound can be isolated from brain tissue up to 24 hr after a systemic injection (126). A thorough review of the pharmacological and therapeutic properties of fenfluramine has been published recently (69).

4.1.2.1 *Analogs.* The fenfluramine derivatives flucetorex (59.**18**) (126–128), fenfluramine glycinate (59.**19**) (129–131), S992 or SE780 (59.**20**), flutiorex (59.**21**) (132), and the α-methoxy-substituted SK & F 1-39728-A (59.**22**) have undergone advanced studies as anorectic agents.

The *N*-hydroxyethylbenzoate S992 or SE780 is reported to be more useful than fenfluramine as an anoretic agent because it lacks stimulation after chronic administra-

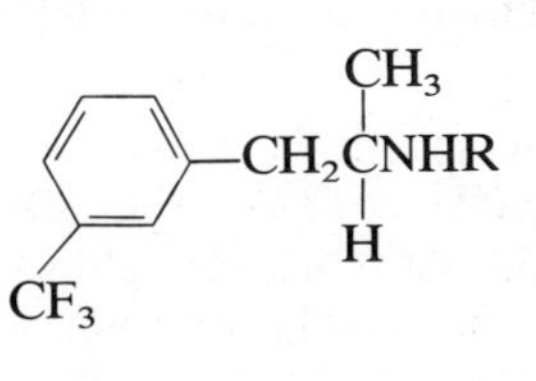

59.**18** R = $\overset{O}{\overset{\|}{C}}CH_2$O—⟨benzene⟩—$\overset{H}{\overset{|}{N}}$COCH$_3$

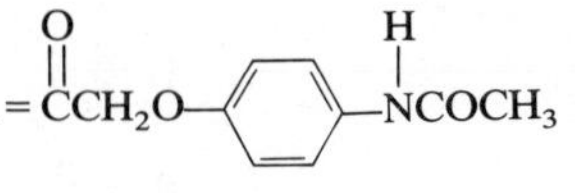

59.**19** R = CH$_2$CO$_2$H

59.**20** R = CH$_2$CH$_2$O$\overset{}{\underset{\overset{\|}{O}}{C}}C_6H_5$

CH₃ structure image (59.21):

$$\text{(aryl, SCF}_3)\text{-CH}_2\overset{\underset{\mid}{H}}{\underset{\mid}{C}}\text{CH}_3\text{NHC}_2\text{H}_5$$

59.21

OCH₃ structure (59.22, 59.23):

$$\text{(aryl, CF}_3)\text{-}\overset{\underset{\mid}{H}}{\underset{\mid}{C}}\text{OCH}_3\text{-CH}_2\text{NHR}$$

59.22 R = CH₂C₆H₅
59.23 R = H

tion and is active over a longer time period (133, 134). Clinical studies at 150–600 mg daily showed 59.**20** caused significant weight loss in obese adults (135–137).

Flutiorex (138) has been evaluated in humans as an appetite suppressant at 20 mg and found to be more effective in men than in women (139, 140). In man 59.**22** is extensively metabolized to the norbenzyl derivative 59.**23** and various acidic substances (141).

Oral evaluation of SK & F 1-39728-A in rats has shown it to be equipotent to fenfluramine as an anorectic agent, but without as much sedative or hypotensive activity (142–144). Several N-acyl (145–148), N-aminoethyl (149), and N-hydroxyethyl (150) analogs of fenfluramine are claimed to possess useful anorectic activity in animals.

4.2 β-Phenyl-*tert*-butylamines

Anorectic agents available in the United States that contain the β-phenyl-*tert*-butylamine structure are chlorphentermine (59.**24**), chlortermine (59.**25**), and phentermine (59.**3**).

structure image (59.24, 59.25):

$$\text{(R-aryl)}\text{-CH}_2\overset{\underset{\mid}{CH_3}}{\underset{\mid}{C}}\text{CH}_3\text{-NH}_2$$

59.24   R = 4-Cl
59.25   R = 2-Cl

4.2.1 CHLORPHENTERMINE, CHLORTERMINE, AND PHENTERMINE.

The basic therapeutic indication for phentermine and its chlorinated analogs remains the treatment of adult obesity. Controlled clinical trials have verified anorectic activity although results in general practice have been less than dramatic.

The phentermine analogs share with the other phenethylamine anorectic agents a variety of CNS, GI, and autonomic side effects. A particular disadvantage with phentermine is the high incidence of drug-related insomnia (6, 151). Although chlorphentermine is claimed to cause minimal CNS excitation at anorectic dose levels, the implications are misleading. The biologic half-life is exceptionally long and continued use quickly leads to plasma levels sufficient to exert overt stimulatory effects (6). Abuse liability with phentermine and its derivatives is apparently substantially lower than with the amphetamine-like agents (7). To date, no neurochemical or neuropharmacological evidence is available that describes for phentermine or chlorphentermine a unique mechanism of action.

4.2.1.1 *Analogs.* Cloferex (59.**26**), the N-carboethoxy analog of chlorphentermine, is an effective anorectic devoid of stimulation in children (152) and adults (153). The patent literature contains a variety of dichloro (154, 155), di-, tri-, and tetramethyl (156, 157), and X-chloro-Y-methyl (158) ring-substituted analogs of phentermine as well as the N-2-cyanoethyl (159), N-glycinamide (160), and di-N-substituted (161) derivatives that are claimed to possess anorectic activity. MJ 9184 (59.**27**), an interesting combination of phentermine and a substituted norephedrine, is a weakly toxic substance that is

structure image (59.26):

$$\text{Cl-}\text{(aryl)}\text{-CH}_2\overset{\underset{\mid}{CH_3}}{\underset{\mid}{C}}\text{CH}_3\text{NHCO}_2\text{C}_2\text{H}_5$$

59.26

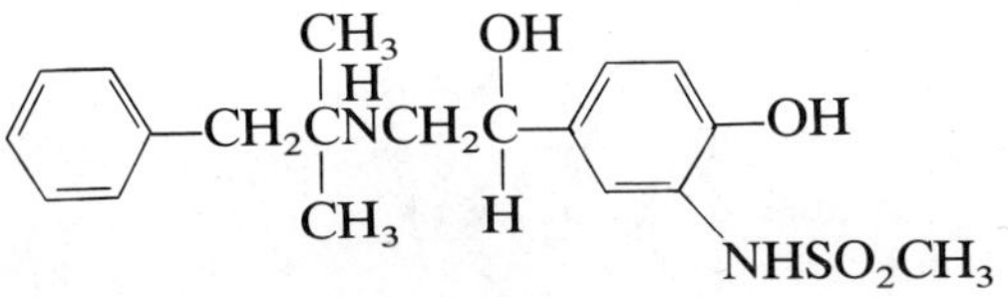

59.**27**

about 10 times as potent as amphetamine as an appetite suppressant when evaluated intraperitoneally in rats (162).

4.3   β-Phenyl-β-oxyisopropylamines

The β-phenyl-β-oxyisopropylamine system is found in one anorectic agent available in the United States, namely, diethylpropion (59.**28**).

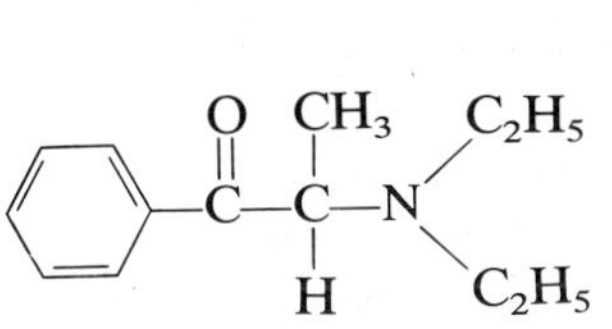

59.**28**

4.3.1   DIETHYLPROPION. Diethylpropion is chemically related to amphetamine and as might be expected, any differences in pharmacological profiles are quantitative rather than qualitative (6, 7, 163). However, diethylpropion has emerged as the drug of choice in the United States as an anorectic agent because it is efficacious and stimulatory side effects are substantially less than with the amphetamines, phentermines, and phenmetrazines. In addition, it is more effective, has fewer side effects, and is less expensive than fenfluramine.

Adverse effects include a mild spectrum of the usual CNS excitatory symptoms: dryness of the mouth, nausea, constipation, and headache. Hemodynamic side effects are also weak and diethylpropion can be used in patients with mild to moderate cardiovascular problems but is prescribed with caution in more severe cases. Drug abuse is recognized, but abuse and dependence liability are considered low in comparison to the more potent stimulants.

Because of the chemical and pharmacological relationships, there is no reason to suspect that diethylpropion and amphetamine are acting through different mechanisms of action. Even so, diethylpropion is more potent by the oral than by the subcutaneous route of administration (163), suggesting that a hepatic metabolite is the active substance. This is consistent with the finding that diethylpropion is rapidly metabolized to a complex mixture of ephedrine and pseudoephedrine stereoisomers (164–168).

4.3.1.1   *Analogs.* The *p*-chloro derivative SK & F 70948 (59.**29**) has anorectic activity in man and is devoid of central stimulation when given at a daily dose of 75–150 mg (169, 170). Unchanged drug and reduced ketone are the major metabolites found in humans after oral administration of 59.**29** (171).

A large number of substituted analogs of diethylpropion containing a Cl (172), OCH_3 (173, 174), CH_3 (173), CF_3 (175), or CN (176) group in the phenyl ring or various *N*-alkyl (177), NCO_2R (178), or piperidino derivative (179) and the cyclohexyl (180) and 2-thienyl (181) analogs (59.**30**), respectively, are reported in the patent literature to be useful anorectic agents.

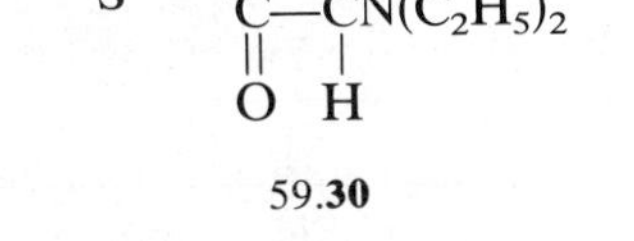

59.**29**

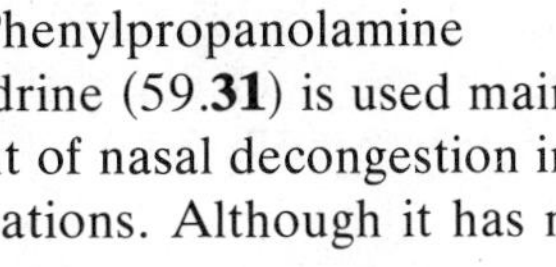

59.**30**

4.3.2   PHENYLPROPANOLAMINE AND ANALOGS. Phenylpropanolamine or *dl*-norephedrine (59.**31**) is used mainly for the treatment of nasal decongestion in a variety of medications. Although it has never adequately been proved effective as an anorectic in man it has been accepted as safe by the U.S. Food and Drug Administration and is therefore available without prescription in the United States (182). Clinical trials in man have demonstrated that phenylpropanolamine decreases food intake and leads to weight loss (183, 185). The most common anorectic formulations contain 25 mg of phenylpropanolamine and a mild stimulant such as caffeine. In animals phenylpropanolamine causes decreased food intake (183) and does not give rise to any overt activity changes (184).

Anorectic activity in rats of about 1.5 times that of phenmetrazine (59.**36**) has been reported for L-ephedrine (59.**32**). Placement of a second methyl group on the nitrogen atom (59.**33**) decreased the activity tenfold (186). Addition of an NH_2, OH, or OCH_3 on the phenyl ring of norephedrine gives rise to useful appetite supressants (187) and isoephedrine (59.**34**) containing various substituents on the phenyl ring is also reported to be anorexigenic (188).

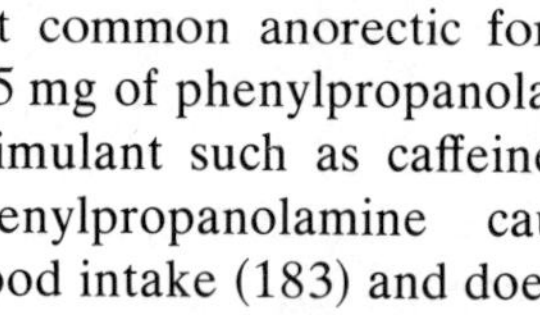

59.**31** R = R$_1$ = H
59.**32** R = CH$_3$ R$_1$ = H
59.**33** R = R$_1$ = CH$_3$

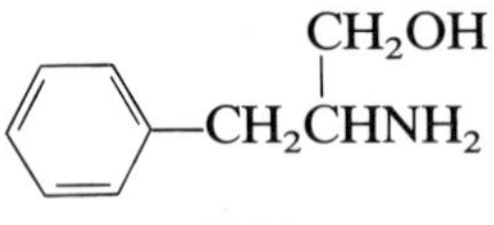

59.**34**

4.4 1-Methyl-2-phenylmorpholines

Substances marketed in the United States that possess a 1-methyl-2-phenyl-morpholine framework are phendimetrazine (59.**35**) and phenmetrazine (59.**36**); both are marketed as the (+) form of the respective *threo* isomer (59.**37**) (189, 190).

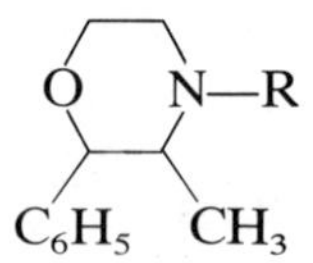

59.**35** R = CH$_3$
59.**36** R = H

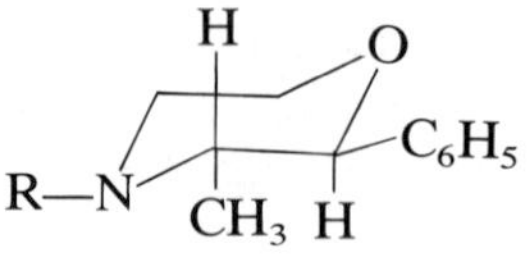

59.**37** R = H, CH$_3$

4.4.1 PHENDIMETRAZINE AND PHENMETRAZINE. There are no unusual pharmacological properties to distinguish phenmetrazine or phendimetrazine from the amphetamine-like phenethylamines. Likewise, the pattern of side effects is analogous to that produced by the amphetamines and the probability of drug abuse is quite high. Two reports of toxic psychosis from phenmetrazine have been documented (191, 192).

4.4.1.1 *Analogs.* Fenbrutrazate (59.**38**) is available in Germany and is used to control appetite at doses up to 800 mg/day (193). The N–N combined phenmetrazine–amphetamine 59.**39** is more active than phenmetrazine in animal testing (194). Several *N*-methyleneamide (195), *N*-acyl (196), and *N*-arylalkyl (197) analogs of phenmetrazine are reported to be useful appetite supressants.

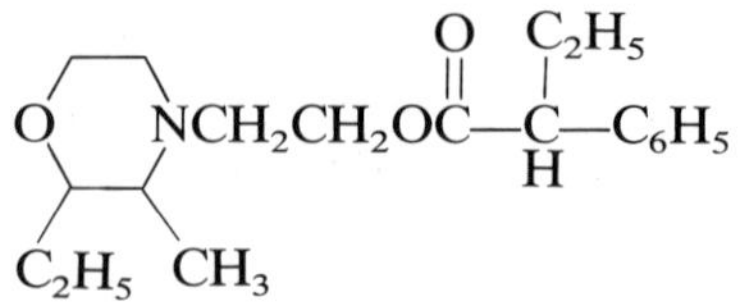

59.**38**

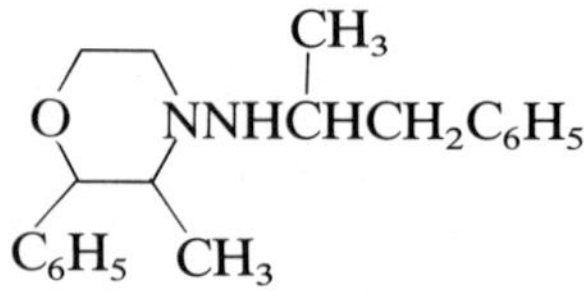

59.**39**

4.5   Structure–Activity Relationships

Amphetamine or dextroamphetamine have served as the standards for most of the structure–activity relationships (SAR) studies on anorectic agents reported in the literature and are used here as the reference substances when possible. The effect of structural changes on other properties, such as central stimulation and cardiovascular effects, of phenethylamines are not correlated with anorectic activity. Excellent SAR studies on the pressor effects (198) and locomotor activity (199) of phenethylamines are available.

Quantitative differences in the appetite suppressant activity of several β-phenylisopropylamine stereoisomers have been described. It is well documented that the (+) isomer of amphetamine is more active than the (−) isomer in suppressing food intake in man and a variety of animals (55). Other stereoisomers that have been compared in the rat are given in Table 59.2. For these substances the absolute configuration of amphetamine (200), 4-chloroamphetamine (200, 201), and fenfluramine (202) has been established as (S) for the (+) isomer and (R) for the (−) isomer, but those of 2,4- and 3,4-

dichloroamphetamines have not been determined. If one assumes that the dichloro compounds follow the same relationship of optical rotation and absolute configuration, it appears that mono-N-alkylated or ring-substituted β-phenylisopropylamines have maximum activity in the (+) or (S) configuration, whereas di-substituted phenyl derivatives are more potent anorectic agents in the (−) or (R) configuration. Additional studies are needed to clarify this point.

The α-methyl group in the β-phenylisopropylamines plays a key role in the anorectic activity of the molecule. Replacement of the α-methyl by hydrogen or any other group results in a marked or complete loss of anorectic activity (203–205). Strong electron-withdrawing groups such as CF_3 or CN in the α-position (59.**40,** 59.**41**) have a particularly negative effect on the activity of amphetamine (206–208).

Shifting the α-methyl to the β-position (59.**42**) or binding it to the nitrogen atom to form the aziridine 59.**43** abolishes essentially all of the central and anorectic effects (209–210).

Addition of a second methyl group on the α-carbon of amphetamine gives phentermine (59.**3**), a substance of about equal anorectic activity in animals and humans.

Table 59.2 Oral Rat Anorectic Activity of Some Amphetamine Stereoisomers

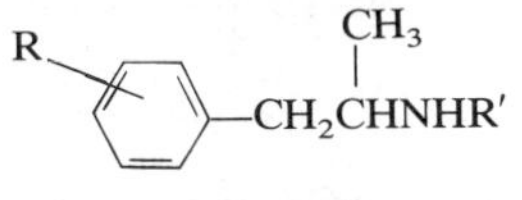

| R | R' | ED$_{50}$, mg/kg | | | |
		(+)	(±)	(−)	Ref.
H	H	2.8	4.3	6.4	201
4-Cl	H	1.3	2.1	2.6	201
2,4-Cl$_2$	H	10.0	4.1	2.6	114
3,4-Cl$_2$	H	4.0	2.9	1.8	114
3-CF$_3$	C$_2$H$_5$	2.8	5.2	10.0	205
3-CF$_3$	CH$_2$CH$_2$OH	4.0	5.2	15.0	205

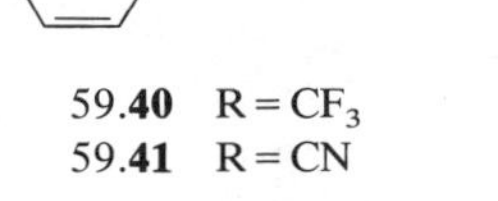

59.**40**   R = CF$_3$
59.**41**   R = CN

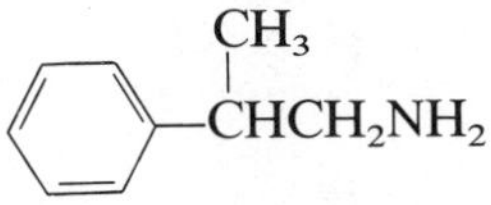

59.**42**

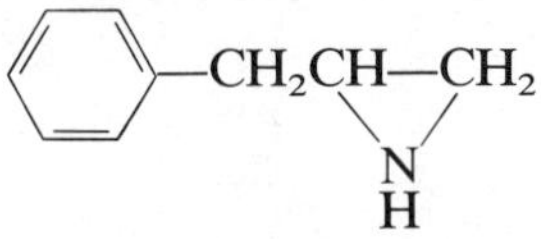

59.**43**

Alkyl groups larger than methyl, cycloalkyl (203) or aralkyl groups (204) all lower or abolish the anorectic activity. Combining the two α-methyl groups of phentermine into the cyclopropyl analog 59.**44** decreases the activity to about 0.3 of amphetamine (211).

Addition of a methyl, ethyl, or propyl group on the β-carbon of amphetamines results in a decrease of anorectic activity (212). Placement of a hydroxyl group on the β-carbon of amphetamine results in phenylpropanolamine (59.**31**), a substance about half as active as d-amphetamine (cf. Section 4.3.2), whereas addition of β-hydroxyl in phentermine (59.**3**) gives an inactive compound (213).

Recent studies with fenfluramine (59.**9**) have shown that addition of a methoxy group in the β-position gave more active derivative 59.**45**, whereas replacement with a hydroxyl (59.**46**) resulted in a substantial loss of activity (214).

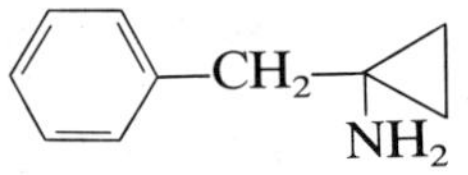

59.**44**

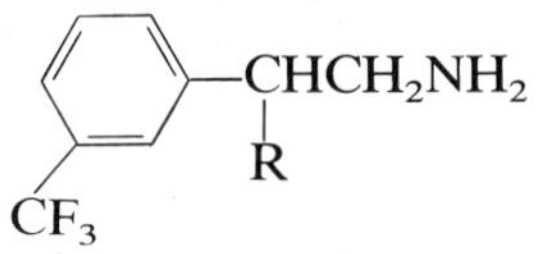

59.**45**   R = OCH$_3$
59.**46**   R = OH

With few exceptions introduction of a substituent on the phenyl ring of amphetamine or phentermine results in diminished or total loss of anorectic activity. From the relative anorectic potency data given in Table 59.3 substituents in the meta and para positions of amphetamine offer the best chance for retaining or possibly improving activity. Lipophilic groups such as Cl, F, CF$_3$, and, somewhat surprisingly,

Table 59.3 Relative Oral Anorectic Potency of Ring-Substituted Amphetamines in Rats

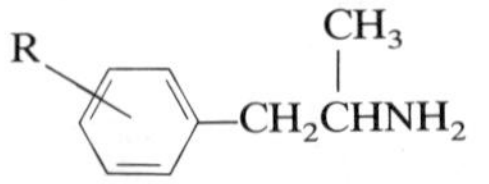

R	Relative Potency	R	Relative Potency
H	1.0^a	o-SCH$_3$	0.2^b
p-N(CH$_3$)$_2$	1.0^b	o-SCH$_2$C$_6$H$_5$	0.2^b
m-CF$_3$	$1.0^b, 0.7^c$	p-SO$_2$CH$_3$	0.2^b
p-F	0.9^c	p-i-C$_3$H$_7$	0.2^b
p-Cl	0.5^d	p-SO$_2$N(CH$_3$)$_2$	0.2^b
p-SCH$_3$	0.5^b	p-NH$_2$	0.2^b
p-CF$_3$	$0.5^b, 0.3^c$	o-CF$_3$	$0.2^b, 0.1^c$
m-F	0.4^c	p-SCH$_2$C$_6$H$_5$	$0^{b,e}$
o-F	0.3^c	p-SO$_2$NH$_2$	$0^{b,e}$
m-SCH$_3$	0.2^b	p-SO$_2$NHCH$_3$	$0^{b,e}$

[a] ED$_{50}$ 1.7–2.8 mg/kg.
[b] Ref. 215.
[c] Ref. 217.
[d] Ref. 216.
[e] Inactive at 30 mg/kg.

$N(CH_3)_2$ are the better substituents to place on the phenyl ring. Recent studies with m-SCF_3 analogs of fenfluramine (59.**9**) indicate that this may be active in the range of a m-CF_3 group (144).

The effect of ring substituents on the anorectic activity of phentermines is given in Table 59.4. Halogens such as Cl and Br but not F are the better substituents to maintain activity. In contrast to amphetamine the location of the Cl or Br atom on the phenyl group does not have as great an effect on activity.

Addition of one or more groups such as alkyl, cycloalkyl, acyl, or others on the nitrogen atom of amphetamines or phentermines results in loss of anorectic activity relative to the parent NH_2 compound (15, 220–223). Nitrogen-substituted compounds that have activity in the range of the parent NH_2 are those that have alkyl or acyl groups easily metabolized *in vivo* to the parent substance (cf. Section 4.6).

The most thorough study of N-substituents on anorectic activity has been

Table 59.4 Relative Oral Anorectic Potency of Ring-Substituted Phentermines in Rats d-Amphetamine = 1.0

R— (phenyl ring) —CH_2CNH_2 with CH_3 groups above and below the central carbon

R	Relative Potency	R	Relative Potency
H	1.0^a, 0.5^b	o-F	$0^{a,d}$
m-Cl	0.9^a	o-CH_3	$0^{a,d}$
p-Br	0.9^a	m-CH_3	$0^{a,d}$
o-Br	0.9^a	p-CH_3	$0^{a,d}$
o-Cl	0.8^a	p-OCH_3	$0^{a,d}$
p-F	0.05^c	p-OH	$0^{a,d}$
m-F	0.05^c		

[a] Ref. 213.
[b] Ref. 218.
[c] Ref. 219.
[d] Inactive at 30 mg/kg.

carried out on fenfluramine (59.**9**) by Beregi and co-workers (220). A listing of some of the substituents used in their work is given in Table 59.5.

4.6 Metabolism

The major metabolic pathways for ring-unsubstituted and N-alkylated β-phenylisopropylamines in animals and man are (1) aromatic hydroxylation at the para position; (2) hydroxylation at the benzylic carbon atom; (3) N-dealkylation; (4) oxidative deamination to the ketone followed by reduction to an alcohol or oxidation to benzoic acid; and (5) unchanged β-phenylisopropylamine. Excretion of the products from the first two pathways can occur as the free hydroxyl or as an O-conjugated glucoronide or sulfate, whereas benzoic acid is frequently found conjugated as hippuric acid. The metabolic profile exhibited by a particular β-phenylisopropylamine may contribute significantly to the overall pharmacological effects since processes like p-hydroxylation or N-dealkylation can lead to biologically active metabolites.

The metabolic pattern exhibited by amphetamines is markedly influenced by the urinary pH. Basic urine favors tubular absorption and further metabolism, whereas acidic urine favors excretion of the amphetamines. The most reproducible metabolic studies are those carried out with an acidic urine in the range of 4.8–5.0 pH (224).

Detailed studies of dl- and d-amphetamine in man and numerous animal species have been reviewed (225). The major metabolites for d-amphetamine are given in Fig. 59.5. In rats the p-hydroxylated derivative norephedrine (59.**48**) is the major metabolite, whereas the deaminated oxidized metabolite benzoic acid constitutes the major metabolite in man (224). Formation of the oxidized

Table 59.5 Oral Rat Anorectic Activity of Some N-Substituted Fenfluramines

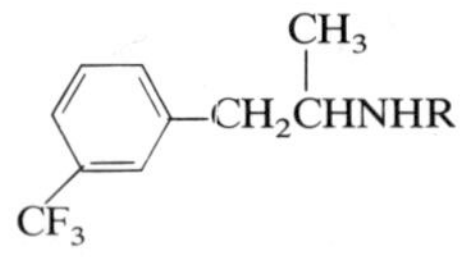

R	ED$_{50}$, mg/kg	R	ED$_{50}$, mg/kg
H	2	n-C$_4$H$_9$	10
CH$_2$CO$_2$H	4	CH$_2$CH$_2$Cl	10
COC$_2$H$_5$	4.3	CH$_2$C$_6$H$_5$	10
CH$_2$CO$_2$C$_2$H$_5$	5	CH$_2$CCH$_3$=CH$_2$	10
C$_2$H$_5$	5.2	(CH$_2$)$_3$C≡CH	10
CH$_2$CH$_2$OH	5.2	n-C$_3$H$_7$	10
CH$_3$	6.8	CH$_2$CH=CHC$_6$H$_5$	>20
CH$_2$CONH$_2$	7.5	CH$_2$CH=C(CH$_3$)$_2$	>20
CH$_2$C≡CH	7.6	CH$_2$CH=CHCH$_3$	>20
CH$_2$CH=CH$_2$	8.4	(CH$_2$)$_3$OH	35
HC(CH$_3$)$_2$	8.7	CH$_2$CH$_2$CO$_2$H	>15
CH$_2$CH$_2$OC$_2$H$_5$	10		

metabolites from amphetamine is believed to occur either through N-hydroxyamphetamine (59.**49**) or the carbinolamine (59.**51**) to form phenylacetone (59.**52**) (226). This substance then undergoes further oxidation to benzoic acid, which may be excreted in the conjugated form as hippuric acid (59.**55**). The oxidation probably occurs directly at the methylene group since phenylpyruvic or phenyllactic acids, products of oxidation at the methyl group, do not appear as metabolites (225). A secondary metabolic pathway of minor importance for phenylacetone is the stereospecific reduction to d-phenylisopropanol (59.**53**) (225).

Introduction of a N-alkyl group or an N-alkyl group plus a lipophilic group such as CF$_3$ or Cl on the phenyl ring of amphetamine leads to an increase in the total metabolism of the drug in man. In a comparative study the percent of recovered unchanged drug in acidic human urine for d-amphetamine, methamphetamine, and d-N-ethylamphetamine was $ca.$ 60, 50, and 30%, respectively (224). In one human

study 18–29% of fenfluramine (59.**9**) was excreted unchanged and 12–22% was found as the N-deethylated norfenfluramine (137). A separate study in man found that 66–93% of fenfluramine was recovered in the urine as 3-trifluoromethylhippuric acid, indicating that extensive metabolism of the side chain had occurred (136). Methamphetamine (59.**7**) is metabolized in man and several animal species primarily by oxidation on the nitrogen atom to give a secondary hydroxylamine and on the two α-carbons to cause demethylation to amphetamine and oxidative deamination to phenylacetone (227, 228). An additional effect of N-alkyl groups is the increasing stereoselectivity on the metabolism of one stereoisomer in man. For instance, there is a much greater difference in the dealkylation of d- and l-ethylamphetamine than for d- and l-methamphetamine (224).

The metabolic pathway for β-phenyl-$tert$-butylamines (59.**3**) is less complex than that of their isopropylamine analogs since

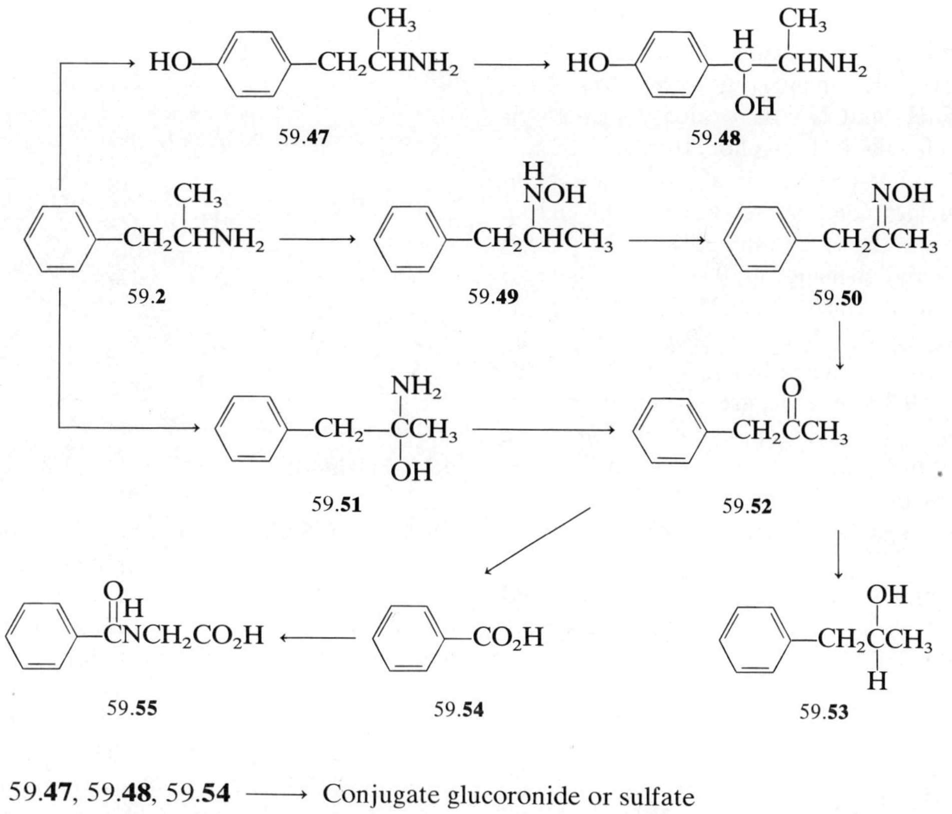

59.**47**, 59.**48**, 59.**54** $\longrightarrow$ Conjugate glucoronide or sulfate

Fig. 59.5 Major metabolic pathways for amphetamine.

the oxidative deamination pathway is blocked by the presence of the second methyl group on the α-carbon atom and the benzylic carbon is impeded, presumably by steric crowding, from hydroxylation (225).

In the rat the major metabolic pathway for phentermine (59.**3**) is aromatic p-hydroxylation (225). When this position is blocked as in chlorphentermine (59.**18**), 60–90% of the drug is found in the urine as unchanged drug (229, 230). In man several N-oxidized metabolites have also been found. After oral administration and extraction of a weakly basic urine (pH 7.4) *ca.* 10% of chlorphentermine and 5% of phentermine was found as the N-oxidized products 59.**56** (231).

The metabolism of diethylpropion in man proceeds through an extremely com-

plex pathway involving sequential N-deethylation, reduction of the carbonyl group, aromatic hydroxylation, conjugate formation, and oxidative cleavage. In one human study 23 metabolites were isolated. These consisted of ketones (10%), p-hydroxylated ketones (8.3%), alcohols (4.1%), p-hydroxylated alcohols (7.1%), hippuric acid (26.5%), dl-mandelic acid (0.3%), benzoic acid (3.4%), 3,4-dihydroxybenzoic acid (3.4%), and two basic compounds of unknown structure (25%) (164).

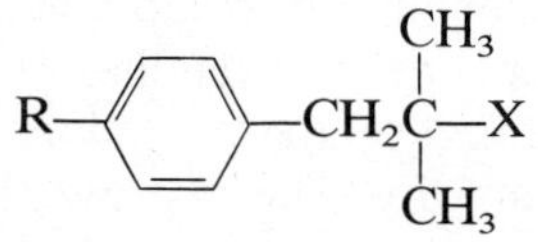

59.**56** R = H, Cl
X = NHOH, NO, NO$_2$

The stereochemistry of the alcohols (59.**57**) obtained in man from acidic urine extracts is mainly (+)-*threo* for the NHC$_2$H$_5$ and N(C$_2$H$_5$)$_2$ alcohols and (−)-*threo* for the NH$_2$ alcohol (164, 166, 232).

Phendimetrazine (59.**35**), in contrast to diethylpropion, is metabolized through a simple pathway. In man 30% of the dose is recovered unchanged, 30% is demethylated to phenmetrazine (59.**36**), and 20% is found as the N-oxide 59.**58** (233). The major metabolic pathways for propylhexedrine (59.**10**) in man are N-demethylation, p- or 4-hydroxylation, and oxidation of the nitrogen atom. Metabolic products observed in the neutral and basic urine extracts of male subjects given propylhexedrine orally were norpropylhexedrine (59.**59**), cyclohexylacetoxime (59.**61**), and *cis*- and *trans*-4-hydroxypropylhexedrine (59.**60**) (234).

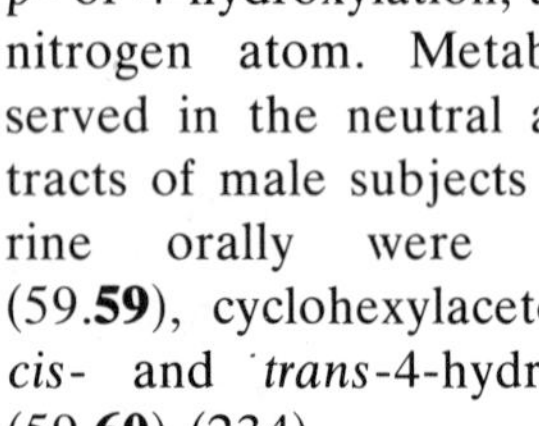

59.**57**   R$_1$, R$_2$ = H or C$_2$H$_5$

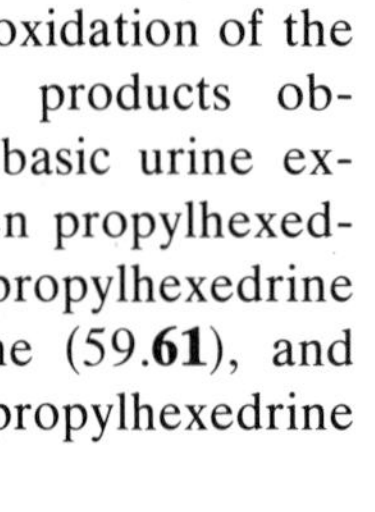

59.**58**

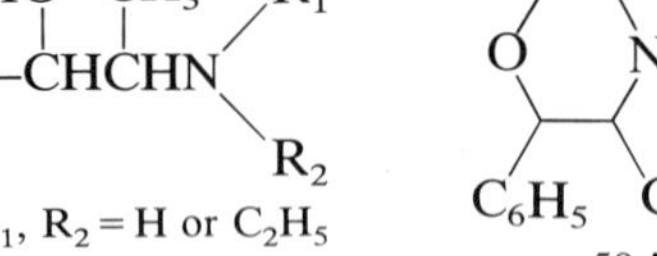

59.**59**   R = R^1 = H
59.**60**   R = CH$_3$, R^1 = OH

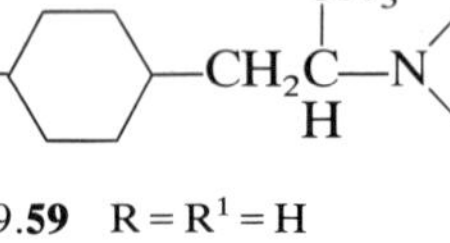

59.**61**

5   DIPHENYLMETHYLAMINO AND DIPHENYLMETHYLOXY DERIVATIVES

A growing number of compounds that contain the diphenylmethylamino or diphenylmethyloxy unit 59.**62** are reported to have anorectic activity. The first member of this class to reach the market is mazindol (59.**63**).

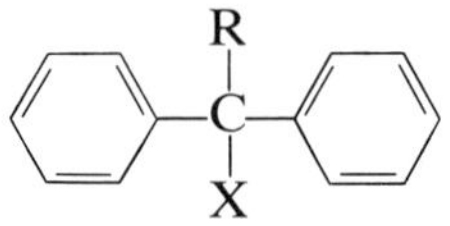

59.**62**   X = O or N

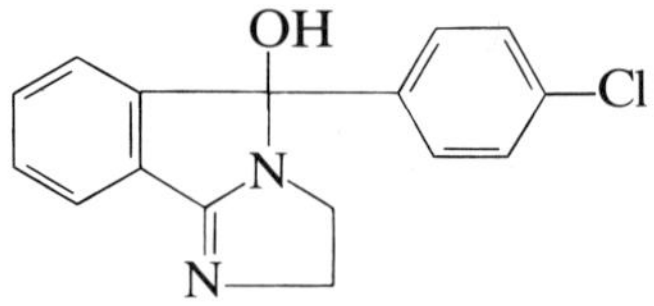

59.**63**

5.1   Mazindol

Mazindol (59.**63**) is the only prescription anorectic agent on the United States market that does not contain a phenethylamine framework (Table 59.1) (235, 236). In neutral or basic media mazindol exists in the cyclic imidazo[2,1-*a*]isoindole form (59.**63**) whereas in acidic media the protonated imidazoline form 59.**64** dominates (237). Reflectance ultraviolet (237) and X-ray (238) studies on mazindol in the solid state reveal that the substance exists in the cyclic tautomer form 59.**63**.

Mazindol is *ca.* five to seven times more active than *d*-amphetamine on a milligram basis in causing appetite suppression in humans. The main side effects include dry mouth, tachycardia, constipation, nervousness, and insomnia. To date, the only pharmacological effect of mazindol that has been exploited in man is appetite suppression. Clinical citations have appeared, suggesting several other potential therapeutic applications including treatment of depression (16, 239, 240), hyperlipidemia (241–

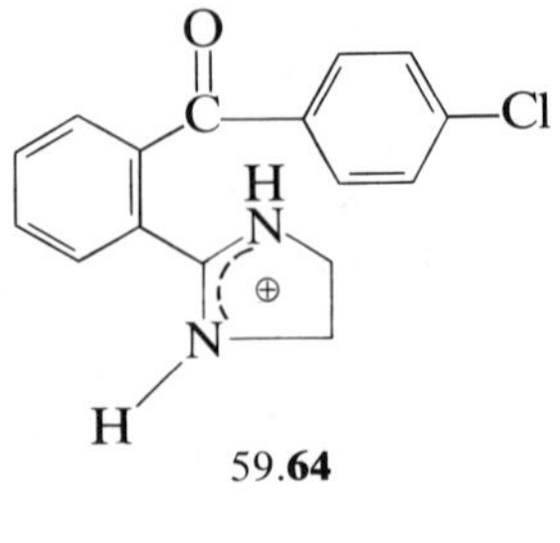

59.**64**

243), and hyperglycemia (244, 245). In addition, mazindol causes minimal adverse cardiovascular reactions and might have a particular applicability in obese patients with a history of cardiovascular problems.

The mechanism responsible for the anorectic effects of mazindol has not yet been resolved. It was originally reported (246) that mazindol differs from amphetamine in that the basic neurochemical effect is to block the reuptake of norepinephrine into presynaptic nerve terminals. That concept has been challenged by several authors (247–252), who demonstrated an amphetamine-like effect on dopamine neuromechanisms. The latter studies, however, were carried out using rat brain striatal tissues and probably reflect the basis for motor stimulatory properties rather than anorexia. In fact, the blockade of norepinephrine reuptake originally reported for whole brain has been corroborated in hypothalamic tissue (252–255), a site more intimately involved with feeding behavior. Apparently mazindol causes profound changes in more than one neurochemical system, but which effect is anorectic-related remains a source of debate.

SAR studies on mazindol in rats have shown that the most active anorectic agents are unsubstituted phenyl of those that contain a Cl or F atom in the meta or para position of the phenyl ring (256). Introduction of a double bond in the imidazoline ring or changing this ring to a pyrimidine (257) or diazepine (258) system results in substantial loss of anorectic activity (259). Expansion of the isoindole ring to the imidazo[1,2-*a*]isoquinolols 59.**65** results in substances with anorectic actively similar to mazindol (260). The alcohol analog of the

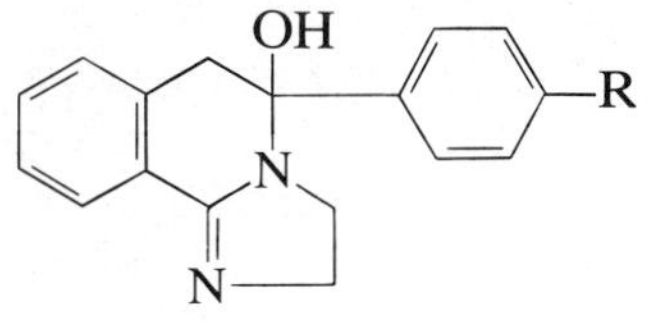

59.**65**   R = H, Cl, F

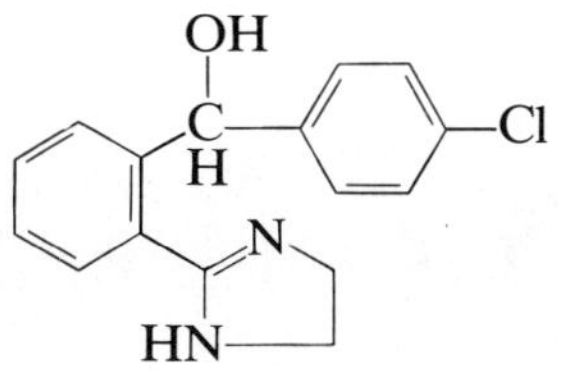

59.**66**

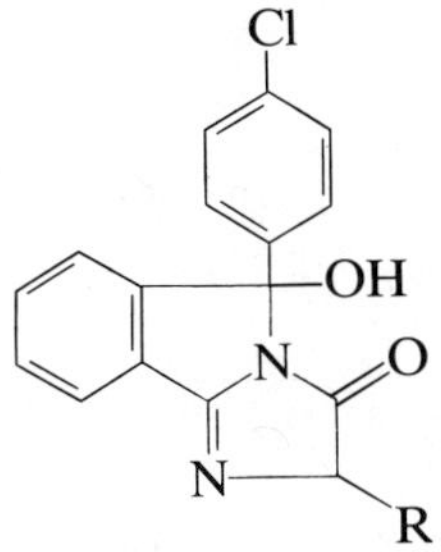

59.**67**   R = H
59.**68**   R = OH

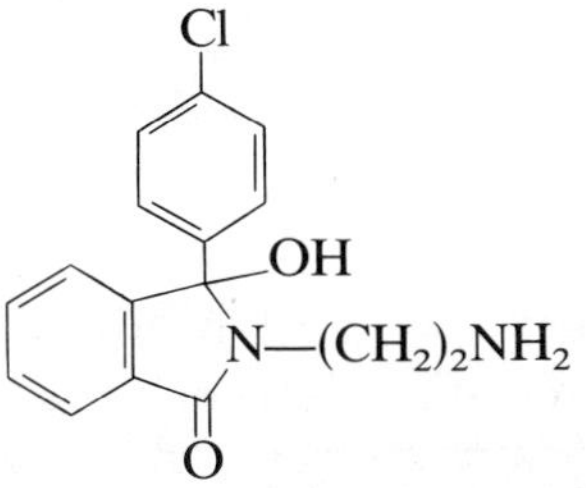

59.**69**

imidazoline tautomer (59.**66**) of mazindol retains *ca.* $\frac{1}{10}$ the activity (261).

Metabolic studies of mazindol in rats has led to the identification of the oxidized imidazoline compounds 59.**67** and 59.**68** and the phthalimidine 59.**69** (262).

5.2 Others

The 2,5-benzodiazecine derivative WY-5244 (59.**70**) was one of the most potent appetite suppressants found in the study of a number of related compounds (263–265). The effect of WY-5244 on cardiovascular activity and adrenergic mechanisms has been reported (266, 267). The closely related 2,6-benzodiazonine is also reported to be useful as an anorectic agent (59.**71**) (268).

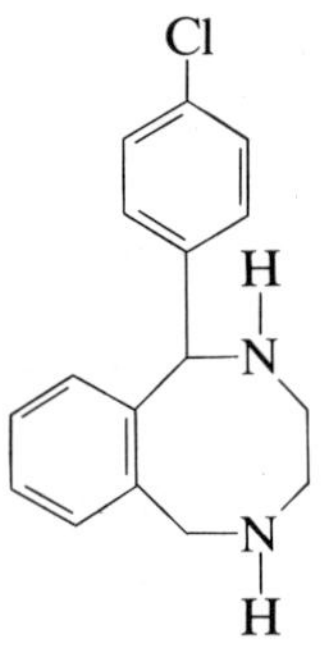

59.**70**

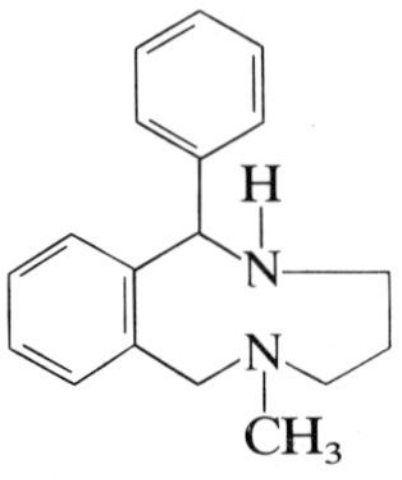

59.**71**

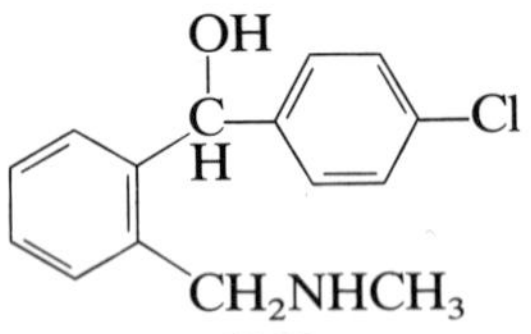

59.**72**

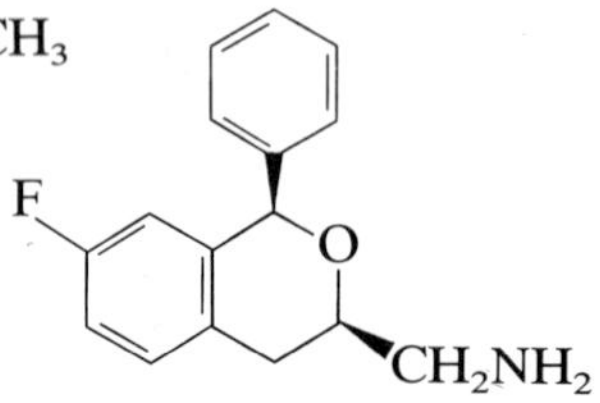

59.**73**

The benzhydrol derivative PR-F-36-Cl (59.**72**) was the most active anorectic agent prepared in a series of related compounds (269, 270). Oral appetite-suppressant testing in rats revealed that 59.**72** was about equal to phenmetrazine (59.**36**) and the (+) isomer was about twice as active as the (−) isomer (269). The compound is a weak stimulant in rats, has no effects on the cardiovascular system, and prevents the uptake of norepinephrine by adrenergic tissue (271).

The *cis*-1*H*-2-benzopyran R-800 (59.**73**) and several analogous compounds have an oral anorectic activity of *ca.* 40 mg/kg in rats (272). R-800 causes a strong vasconstriction in rat perfused lung (273).

The benzohydrolamine derivatives 59.**74** and 59.**75** are claimed to be useful anorectics with activity about equal to amphetamine in the dog (274, 275). Several imidazobenzhydrols, particularly the *p*-chloro derivative 59.**76**, are anorectic agents (276).

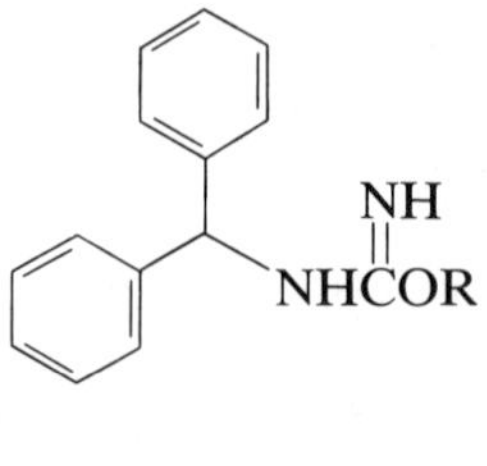

59.**77**   R = lower alkyl

Pseudoureas of benzhydrylamine (59.**77**) (277), various isoindolines, and isoindoles such as 59.**78** (278) and 59.**79** (279) are reported to possess useful levels of anorectic activity in rats.

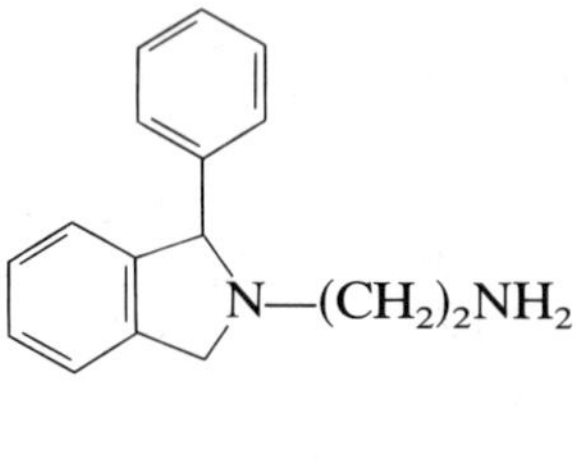

59.**78**

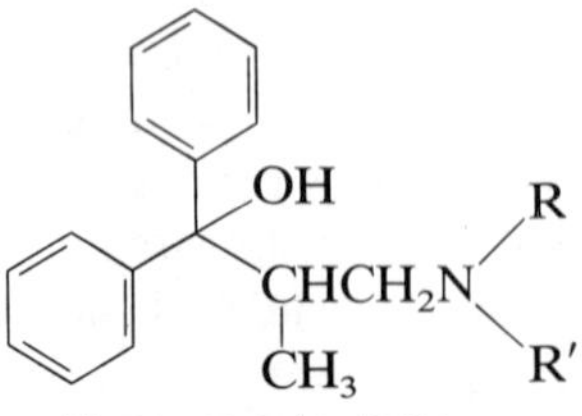

59.**74**   R, R¹ = (CH₂)₄
59.**75**   R = H, R¹ = C₂H₅

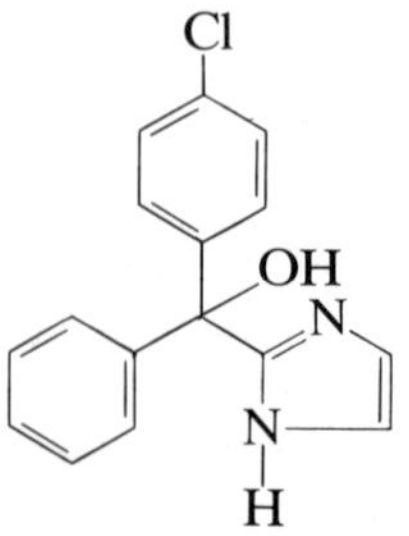

59.**76**

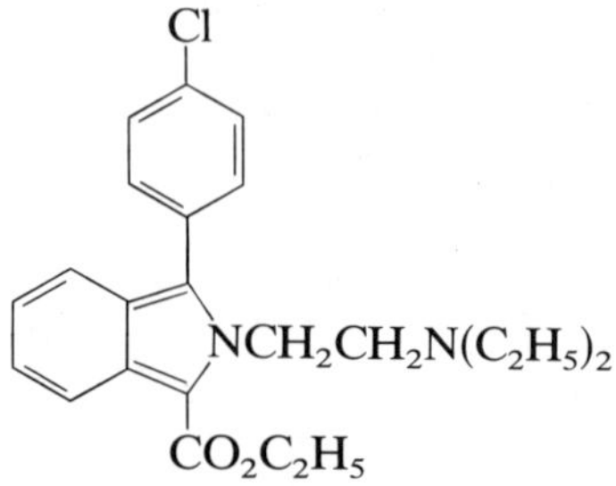

59.**79**

6 OXAZOLINES AND THIOIMIDAZOLINES

6.1 Oxazolines

Studies on the incorporation of phenylethanolamine and phenylpropanolamine into the 2-amino-5-aryl-2-oxazoline structure 59.**80** led to the development of aminorex (59.**81**) as an anorectic agent (280). Clinical evaluation of aminorex showed it to be an effective anorexigen at 22 mg with a profile of side effects similar to other marketed agents (281, 282). After the substance had been marketed in Europe evidence was accumulated that it caused pulmonary hypertension in humans (283) and animals (282). As a result of these findings further development of aminorex and its analogs clominorex (59.**82**) and fluminorex (59.**83**) were curtailed.

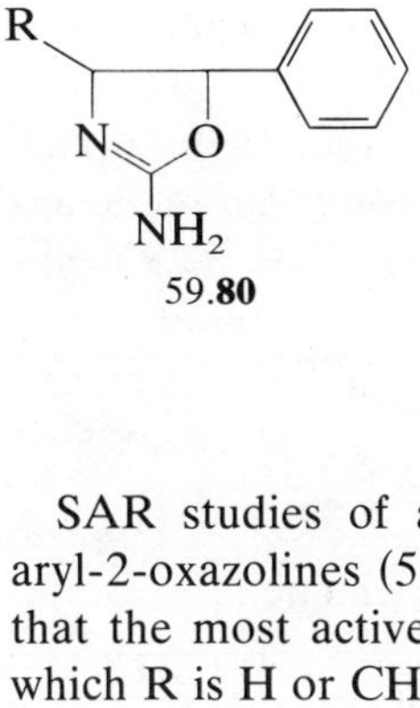

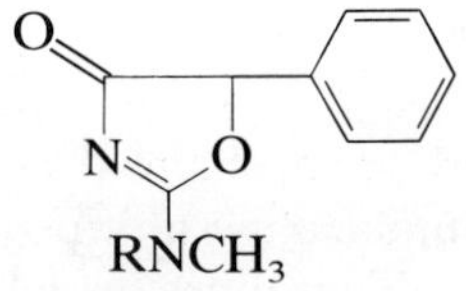

59.**84** R = CH₃, ▽

59.**85**

59.**86**

59.**87**

59.**80**

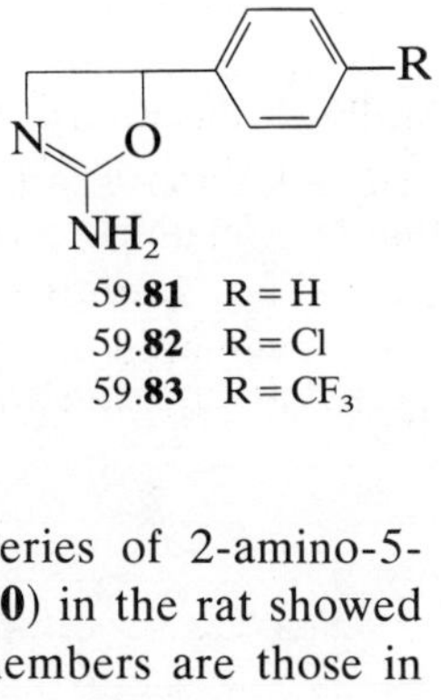

59.**81** R = H
59.**82** R = Cl
59.**83** R = CF₃

SAR studies of a series of 2-amino-5-aryl-2-oxazolines (59.**80**) in the rat showed that the most active members are those in which R is H or CH₃, and a hydrogen atom or an electron-withdrawing group such as F, Cl, CF₃, or Br is in the para position of the phenyl ring. Substitution on the nitrogen with alkyl or phenyl groups or introduction of a second double bond in the ring resulted in less active analogs. In contrast to the amphetamines the *dl* and *d* isomers of 59.**80** (R = CH₃) had about the same potency (283, 285).

The 4-one analogs 59.**84,** where R is CH₃ (286–288) or cyclopropyl (289), are active in the range of aminorex. Pondex (59.**85**) has been evaluated in obese women

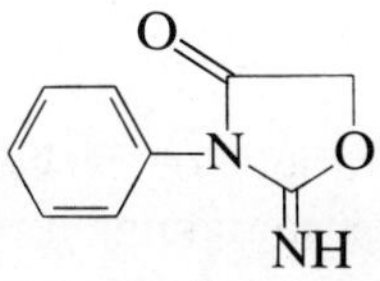

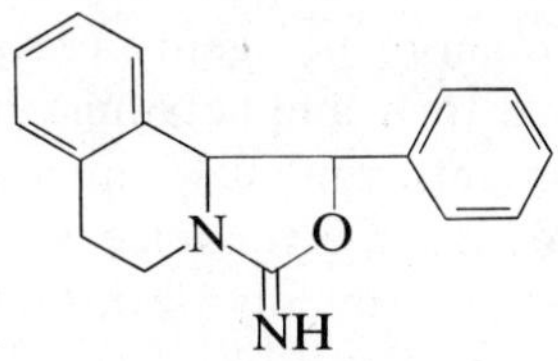

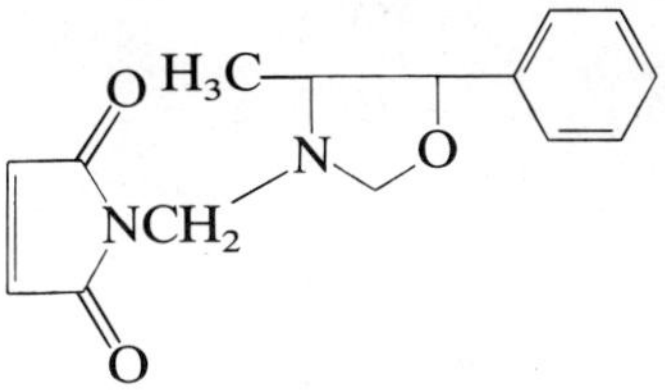

and found to be comparable to phenmetrazine (59.**36**) as an anorectic agent (290).

The β-isomers of the fused isoquinoline analog (59.**86**) of aminorex and the 3-imidomethyl derivative 59.**87** are reported to have anorectic activity in rats (291, 292).

AMPO (59.**88**) is about one-fifth as active as *d*-amphetamine in suppressing food intake in rats and *ca.* $\frac{1}{11}$ as active in mice, cats, and dogs. It acts on the feeding center in the lateral-hypothalamic area (293) and is weaker than aminorex in the pulmonary dog study (294). The thio analog (59.**89**) of AMPO is *ca.* one-fifth as active when evaluated in mice (295).

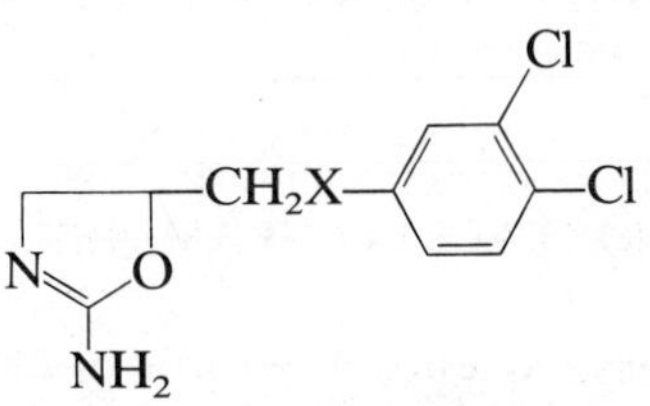

59.**88** X = O
59.**89** X = S

6.2 Thioimidazolines

A variety of cyclic and open chain structures containing a thioimidazoline unit possess anorectic activity. The most widely studied member is the acetophenone analog DITA (59.**90**) (296). DITA is an orally active anorectic agent possessing activity relative to *d*-amphetamine of 0.7 in mice, 0.2 in rats, and 0.15 in dogs (297, 298). Anorectic activity in mice is thought to be mediated mainly through the dopaminergic system (298).

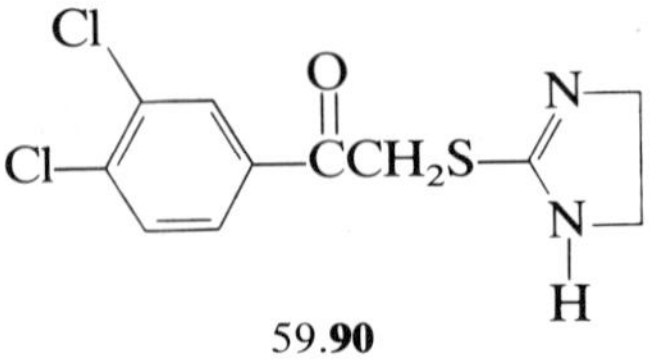

59.**90**

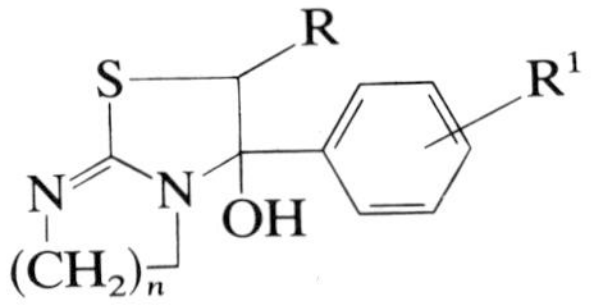

59.**91**   *n* = 1, 2, 3

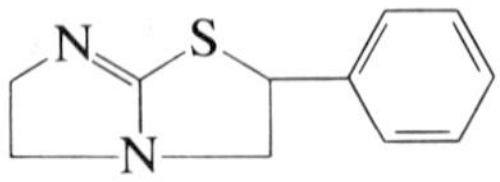

59.**92**

Several 3-hydroxy-3-arylimidazo[2,1-*b*]-thiazoles (299), thiazolo[3,2-*a*]pyrimidines (299, 300), and thiazolo[3,2-*a*][1,3]diazepines (301) (59.**91**) are claimed to have anorectic activity in rats. These compounds are cyclic tautomeric analogs of DITA.

Levamisole (59.**92**), an anthelminthic, and some substituted analogs also possess anorectic activity (302).

7 PHENOXYALKYLENEAMINES

A phenoxyalkyleneamine unit of the general formula 59.**93** can be recognized in a number of anorexigenic substances. In an

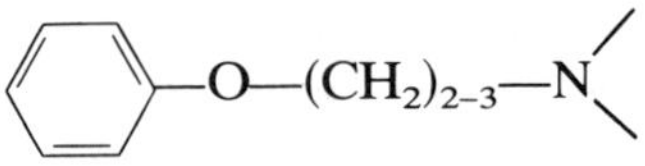

59.**93**

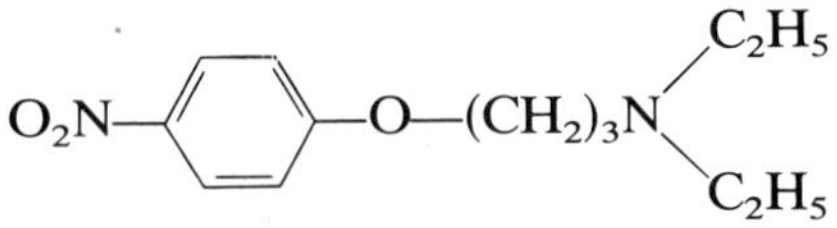

59.**94**

extensive SAR study of the anorectic activity of aryloxyalkyleneamines in rats it was found that electron-withdrawing groups such as NO_2, CN, and 3-sydnonyl located in the para position gave rise to the most active analogs. The *p*-nitro (59.**94**) and the *p*-cyano (59.**95**) derivatives were slightly more active than *d*-amphetamine (303). Analogs of 59.**94** where the NO_2 group is replaced by H (304) or Cl (305) are also reported to be useful anorectics, with activity in the range of phendimetrazine (59.**35**).

The imidazole derivative 59.**96** is about $\frac{1}{10}$ as active as *d*-amphetamine when tested orally in the mouse (306).

A number of 2-phenoxymethylmorpholines are claimed to be useful anorectic agents. The 2-ethoxy derivative 59.**97** has been evaluated in man and found to be active at 240–300 mg/day (307).

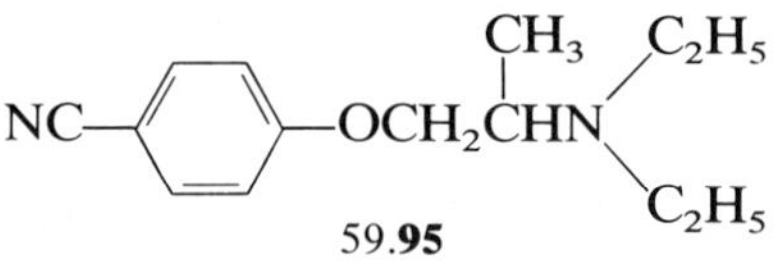

59.**95**

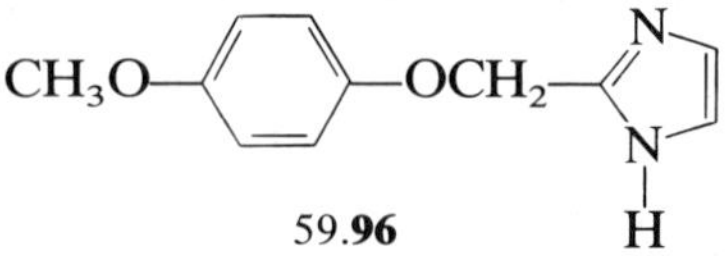

59.**96**

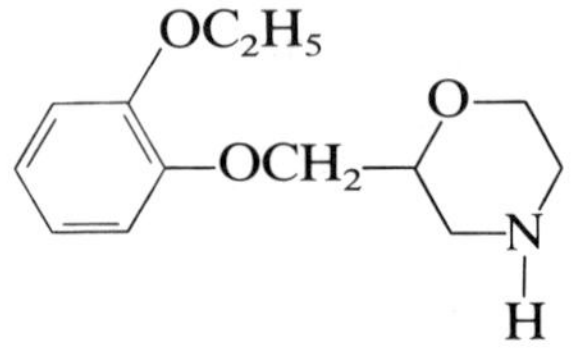

59.**97**

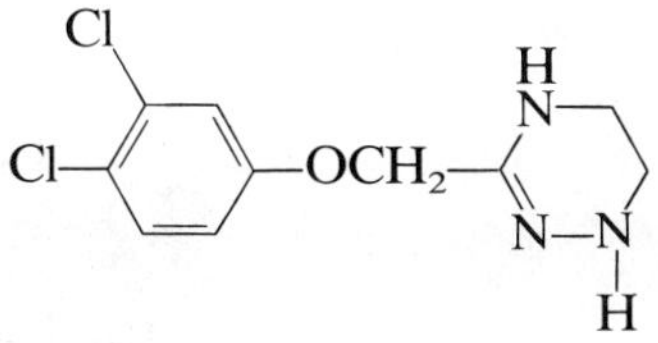

59.**98**

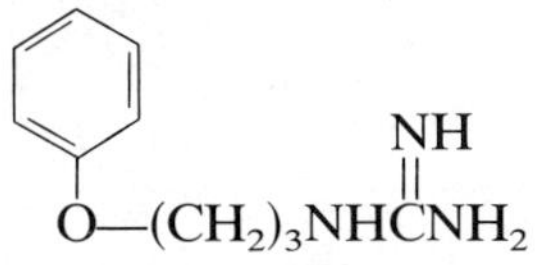

59.**99**

Both the triazine 59.**98** (308) and the guanidine 59.**99** (309) were found to be useful anorectics in rats.

A variety of phenthioalkyleneamines and the S-oxide analogs such as those given in 59.**100** are claimed to be anorectic agents (310).

Several phenylalkyloxyguanidines (59.**101**) exert appetite suppression in dogs and rats by a mechanism that may not involve sympathomimetic amines (311). The 3-phenylpropyloxy analog U-16,178F was about half as active as amphetamine in suppressing food intake in rats but only about one-fifth as active in causing body weight loss (312).

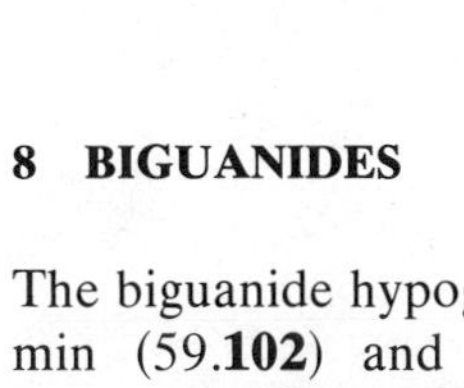

59.**100** $n = 2$–5
R = alkyl

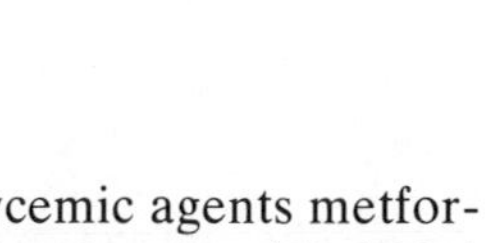

59.**101** $n = 1, 2, 3$

8 BIGUANIDES

The biguanide hypoglycemic agents metformin (59.**102**) and phenformin (59.**102a**) have periodically been reported to be useful as weight control agents (313).

Clinical studies of phenformin in obese women showed it produced weight loss in excess of the degree of anorexia caused by the drug (314). In obese diabetic patients phenformin was useful in producing weight loss, although the mechanism of action may not involve a true anorectic effect (313, 315).

Metformin has also been found to cause weight loss in obese normal and diabetic patients (313, 316). Because of the large doses of drug needed to effect weight loss, it was concluded that metformin was not suitable for the treatment of simple obesity, although valuable in the management of obese diabetics (317).

The biguanide derivative 59.**103** has a level of anorectic activity similar to d-amphetamine when tested orally in rats (318, 319).

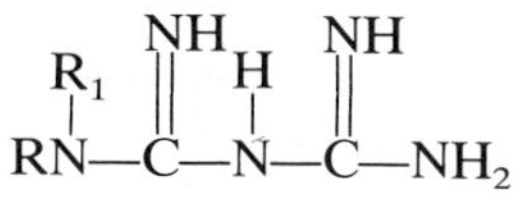

59.**102** $R = C_6H_5CH_2CH_2$, $R^1 = H$
59.**102a** $R = R^1 = CH_3$

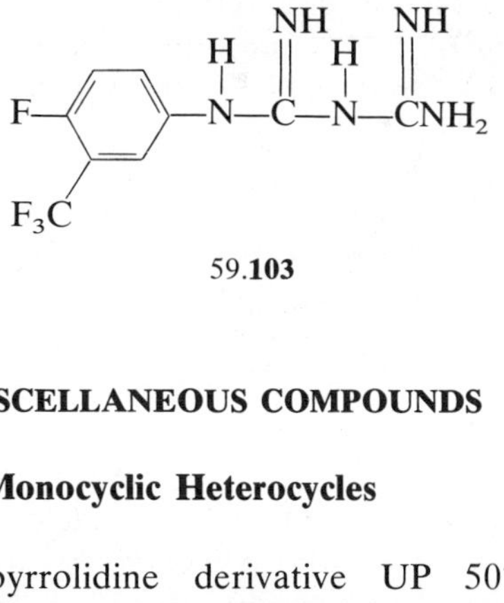

59.**103**

9 MISCELLANEOUS COMPOUNDS

9.1 Monocyclic Heterocycles

The pyrrolidine derivative UP 507-04 (59.**104**) is about half as active as amphetamine when tested orally in rats (320), and the pyrrole 59.**105** is reported to be ca. one-tenth as active as d-amphetamine in the dog (321). L-Histidine (59.**106**) given at 16 g daily in man caused loss of appetite after 6 days of administration by a mechanism of action that may in part be due to binding of zinc in the plasma (322). A

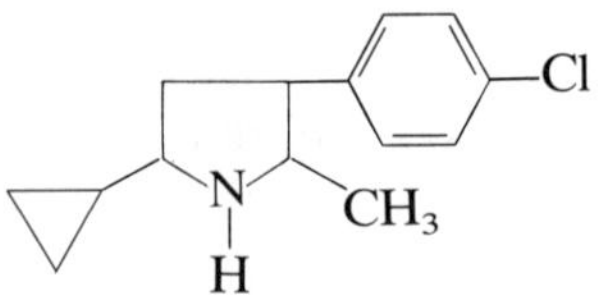

59.**104**

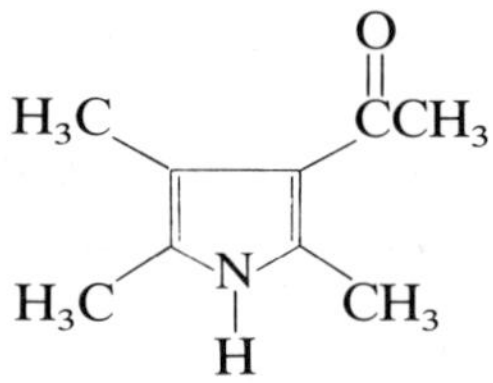

59.**105**

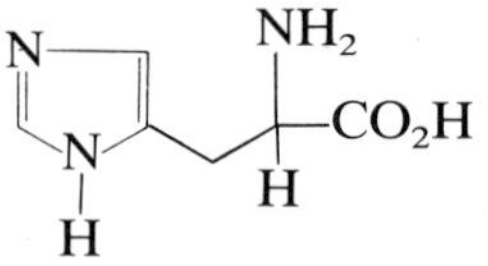

59.**106**

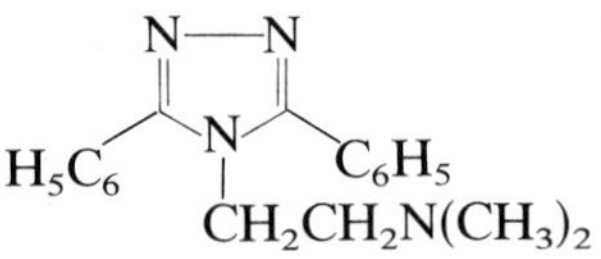

59.**107**

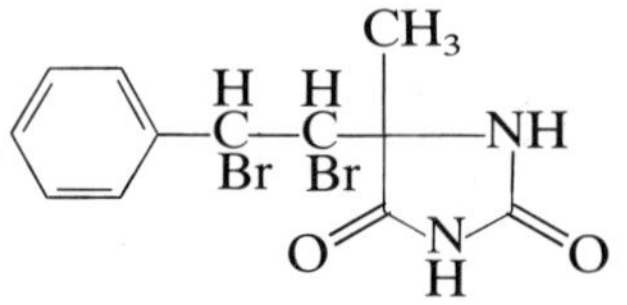

59.**108**

series of 1,2,4-triazoles such as 59.**107** have anorectic activity in the rat (323). The hydantoin 59.**108** (pesomin) showed an anticonvulsive profile in animals (324) but displayed a good level of appetite depressant activity in man (325, 326).

The l-aryl-substituted piperazines containing a Cl (327–329), CH₃ (328, 329), CF₃ (328, 329), or SCF₃ (330–332) in the meta position or a F or CF₃ group (333) in the para position of the phenyl ring (59.**109**) or a substituted 1,3-thiazole (59.**110**) (334) are orally active anorexigens

in the rat. The 6-chloropiperazine (59.**111**) is *ca.* 10 times more active orally in the cat than fenfluramine (59.**9**) (335).

Among a series of 1-arylcycloalkyloxy-butynamino ether derivatives of piperazine the 2,4-dichlorophenyl derivative 59.**112** was the most active member in suppressing food intake in rats (336). Several enamine analogs of piperazine such as 59.**113** and 59.**114** are claimed to be useful anorectics (337, 338). A number of 1,3,5-triazenes such as 59.**115** are active anorectics in the rat (339).

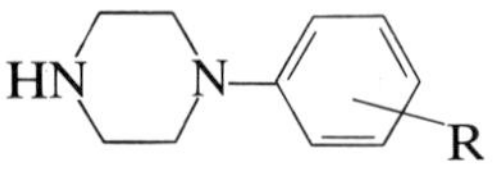

59.**109**

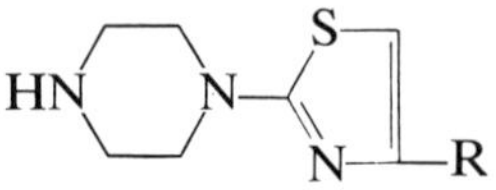

59.**110**

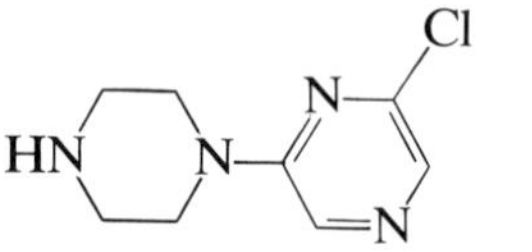

59.**111**

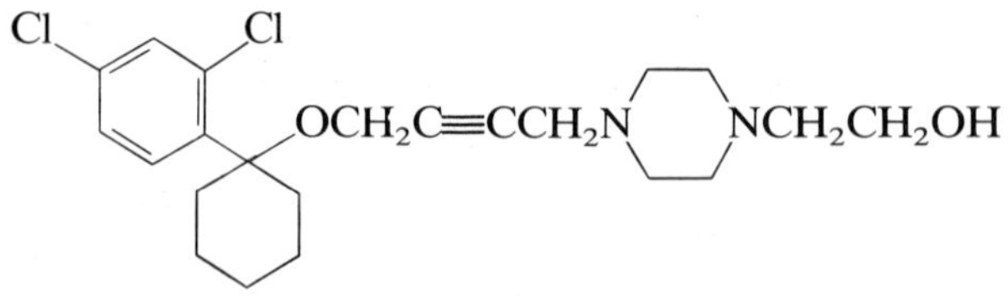

59.**112**

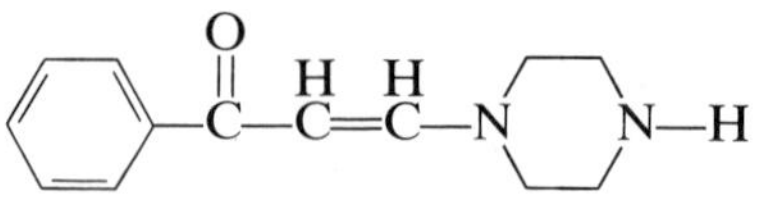

59.**113**

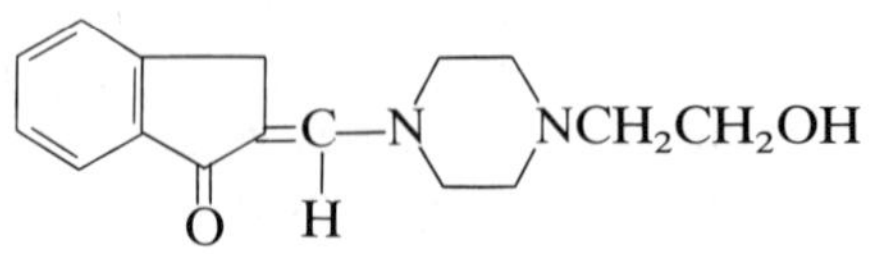

59.**114**

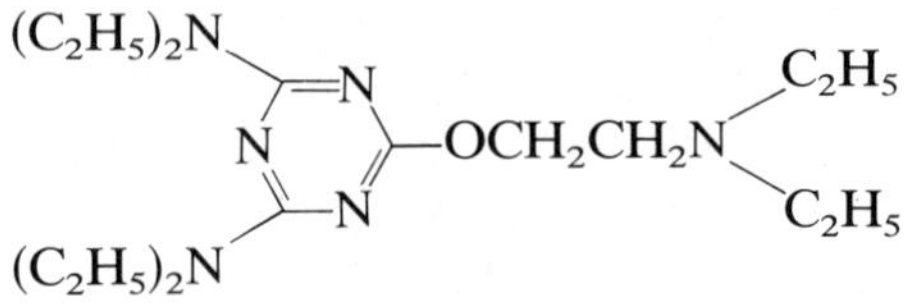

59.**115**

9.2 Bicyclic Heterocycles

Tryptamine derivatives 59.**116** substituted in the 5 (340) or 8 (341) position and containing an α-alkyl or phenyl group are useful anorectics. The α-methyl-α-ethyl analog 59.**116** has an oral ED_{50} of 15 mg/kg in the rat and is relatively non-toxic (342). Benzofuran-2-carboxamide 59.**117** (L4035) is about one-fifth as active as d-amphetamine in rats in depressing food intake and is thought to exert sympathomimetic effects similar to the phenethylamines (343).

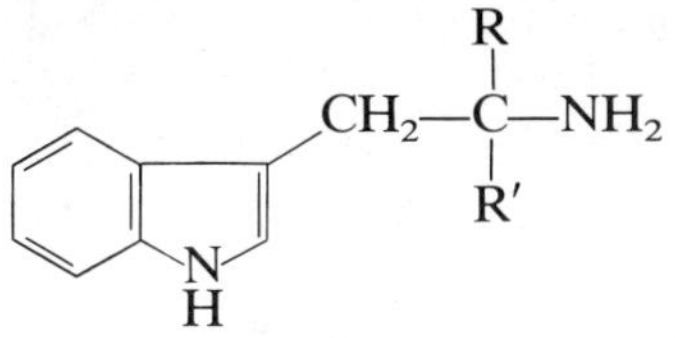

59.**116**

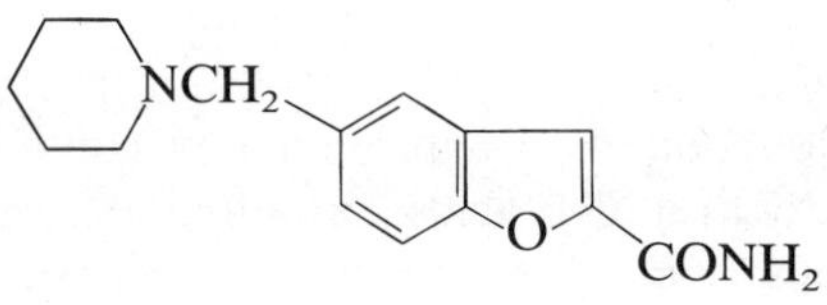

59.**117**

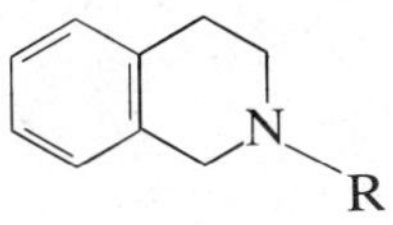

59.**118**

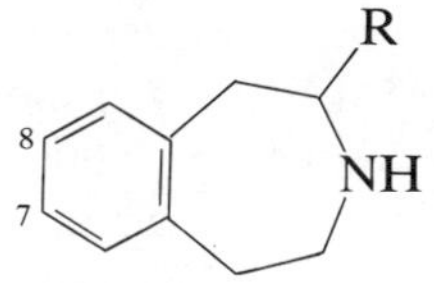

59.**119** R = H, CH$_3$

The 1H-3-benzazepines 59.**119** containing a 7-chloro (344), 7-acyloxy (345), or 7,8-methylenedioxy (346) substituent have appetite suppressing activity in rats. The benzimidazole 59.**120** has anorectic activity similar to flenfluramine (59.**9**) in oral rat testing (347). Several 1-alkyl-4-aminotetrahydroquinolines (59.**121**) (348) and 2-alkyl-isoquinolines (59.**118**) (349) are appetite suppressants.

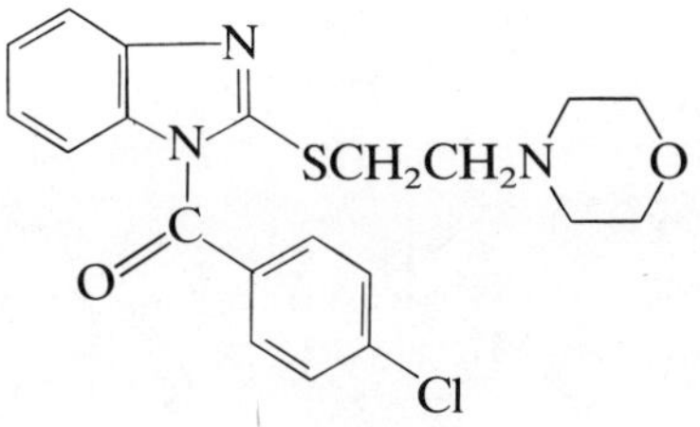

59.**120**

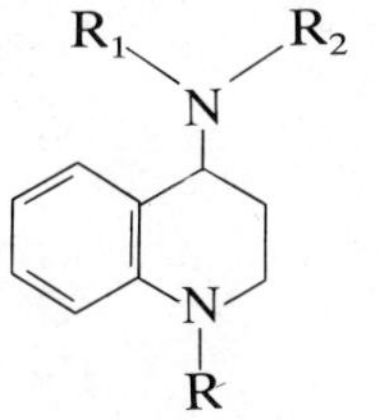

59.**121**

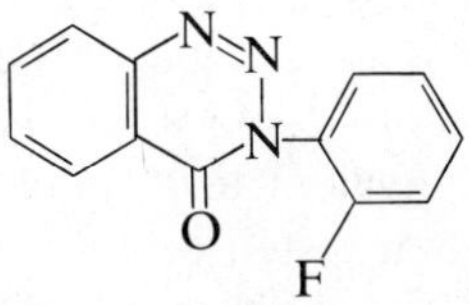

59.**122**

The benzotriazolinone 59.**122** (350), the purine amide 59.**123** (351), and the phthalazine 59.**124** (352) are claimed to possess appetite suppressant activity in rodents. Amphetamine-like anorectic activity was found in ($-$)-n- (59.**125**) but not ($+$)-ψ-cocaine when given intraperitoneally, intramuscularly, intravenously, or orally to rats (353).

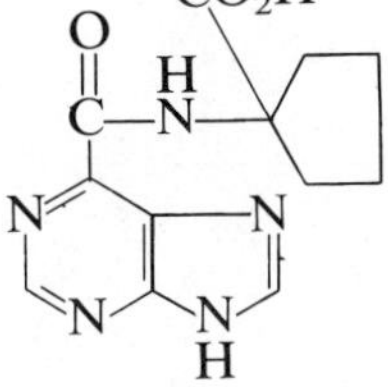

59.**123**

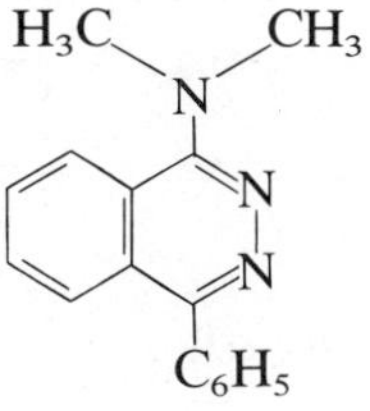

59.**124**

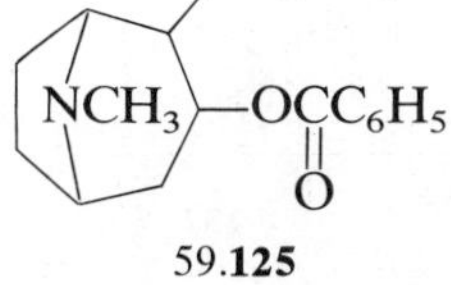

59.**125**

9.3 Tri- and Polycyclic Heterocycles

The quinolinoazepine 59.**126** evaluated subcutaneously in rats had an anorectic ED_{50} of 0.2 mg/kg and the isomeric 59.**127**

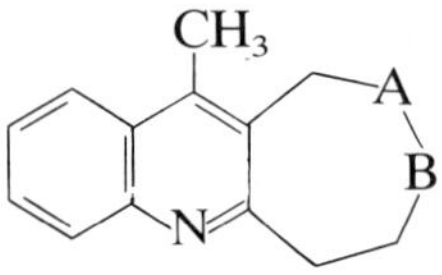

59.**126**   A = CH$_2$ B = NH
59.**127**   A = NH   B = CH$_2$

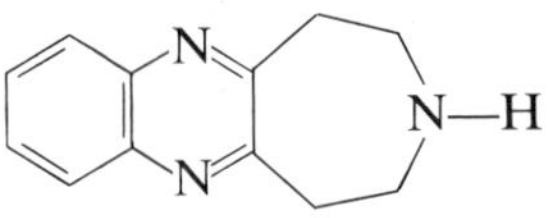

59.**128**

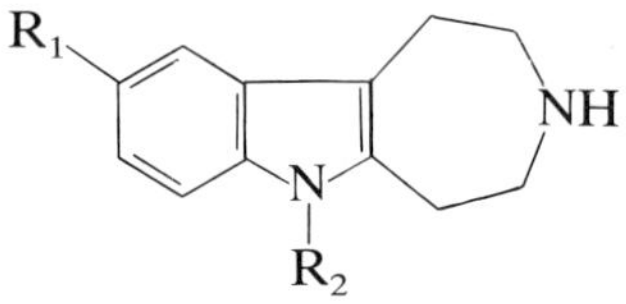

59.**129**   R$_1$ = H   R$_2$ = CH$_3$
59.**130**   R$_1$ = CH$_3$ R$_2$ = H

had an ED$_{50}$ of 1.1 mg/kg (354, 355). The related azepino[4,5-*b*]quinoxaline (59.**128**) is also claimed to be an anorectic (356). Indoloazepines 59.**129** and 59.**130** are equivalent to *d*-amphetamine as anorectics when tested orally in mice (357).

The dibenzo-1,2,5-triazepine 59.**131** is a potent anorectic when given intraperitoneally to rats (358). Apomorphine (59.**132**) showed a short-lasting anorexia when administered intraperitoneally to rats with an activity level *ca.* 2.5 times that of *d*-amphetamine (359). The pentacyclic systems 59.**133** are reported to possess anorectic activity (360).

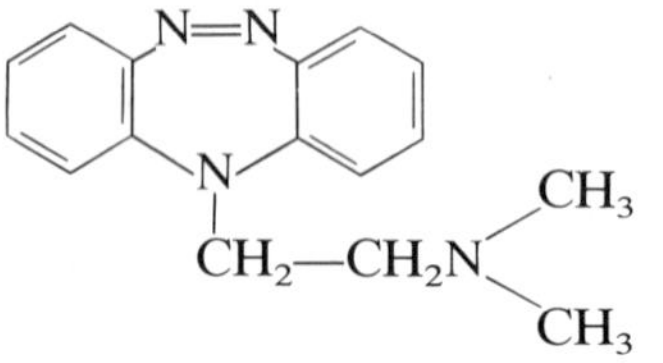

59.**131**

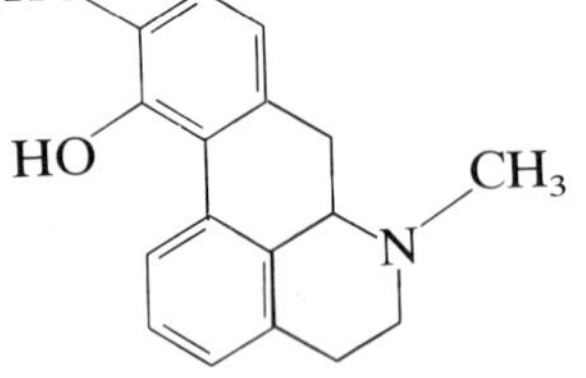

59.**132**

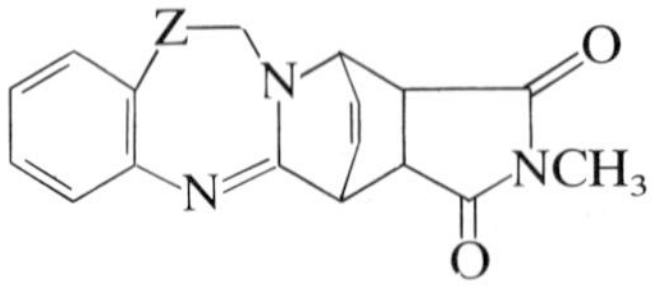

59.**133**   Z = CH$_2$, O, S

9.4   Natural Substances

Depressed food intake in the rat and other animal species has been observed when the amino acid composition of the diet is unbalanced or when dietary protein is excessively high or low (361–363). The significance of such responses in day-to-day regulation of food intake has not been completely clarified (364). A combination of carrageenins and proteins in a ratio of 2 : 1 given by oral or rectal application suppresses food intake in humans (365).

A series of compounds referred to as fat-mobilizing substances (FMS) have been isolated from the urine of fasting rats (366). They are possibly polypeptides of mol wt > 50,000 bound to a protein and contain a variety of amino acids, carbohydrates, hexosamine, and cholesterol or a cholesterol-like substance (367, 368). One of these, FMS I, when administered subcutaneously to rats, decreased the uptake of food (368). Trypsin digestion of FMS I afforded FMSIA, a lower molecular weight fragment of mol wt > 10,000 that reduced food uptake in rats when administered subcutaneously (368) or intraperitoneally (369).

The fat-mobilizing substance (FMS) isolated from the urine of healthy fasted humans (367) when given 25–100 mg intravenously to healthy humans did not cause a loss of appetite, but did cause weight loss (370). A similar result was observed when human FMS was injected into mice. An acceleration of fat catabolism is believed to have caused the weight loss (371).

Enterogastrone, a gastric hormone isolated from dog duodenum, when administered intravenously or subcutaneously to mice gave a short reduction in food uptake, possibly by a humoral interaction on the CNS system (372). Prostaglandins E_1 and E_2 given 0.1 mg/kg subcutaneously to rats resulted in a sustained decrease in food uptake. It is speculated that this effect may be due to interaction with the hypothalamus (373). Bile acids, especially those substituted at positions, 3,7 or 3,12 with hydroxyl groups and a carboxyl at position 24 suppress food intake in rodents and humans (374).

9.5   Others

The $(-)$ isomer of the keto-acid 59.**134** possesses anorectic activity in dogs approximately equal to that of diethylpropion (59.**28**) (375, 375a). In rats at 100 mg/kg oral it caused a good reduction of food intake and body weight gain and was devoid of sympathomimetic properties (376). Reduction of food intake and no CNS effects were obtained when 2-propenyl-2-cyclohexen-1-one (59.**135**) was given orally to rats (377). Sulfone 59.**136** is claimed to be a more potent anorectic than fenfluramine (59.**9**) in rats (347).

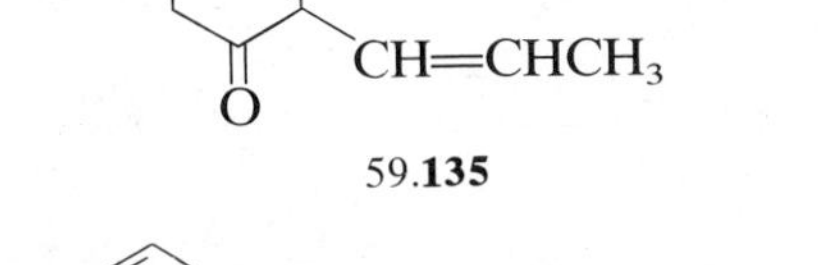

59.**134**

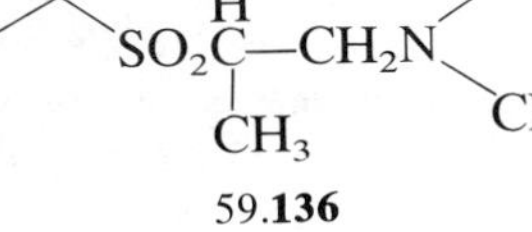

59.**135**

59.**136**

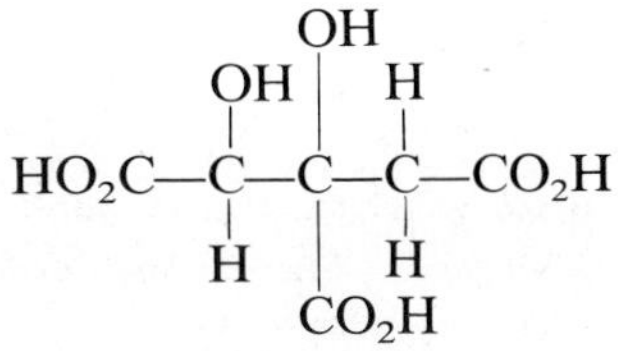

59.**137**

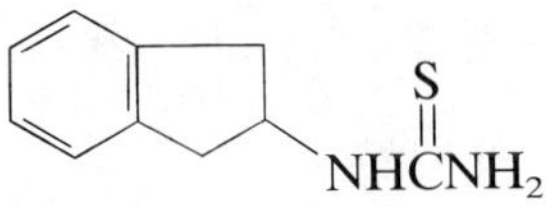

59.**138**

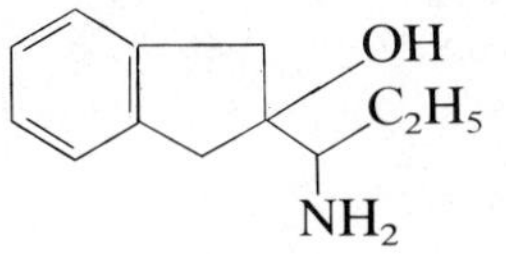

59.**139**

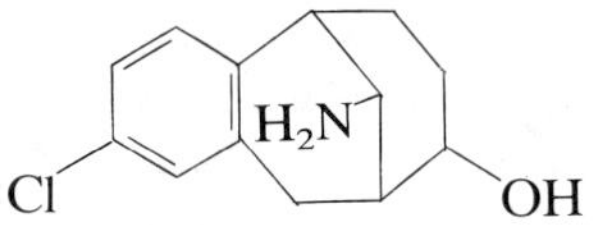

59.**140**

Food intake and weight gain were reduced when $(-)$-*threo*-hydroxycitric acid (59.**137**) was given orally to rats or mice. Suppression of appetite by 59.**137** is possibly due to the alternation of metabolite flux in the central nervous system (378). The indanylthiourea 59.**138** (379) and amino alcohols 59.**139** (380) and 59.**140** (381) are claimed to be useful as anorectic agents in animals.

REFERENCES

1. T. Silverstone, Ed., *Obesity: Its Pathogenesis and Management*, Publishing Sciences Group, Inc., Acton, Mass., 1975.

2. A. Howard, Ed., *Recent Advances in Obesity Research*, Newan Publishing Ltd., London, 1975.

3. D. Novin, W. Wyrwicka, and G. A. Bray, Eds., *Hunger—Basic Mechanisms and clinical Implications*, Raven Press, New York, 1976.

4. J. Mayer, *Postgrad Med.*, **51,** 66 (1972).

5. *Am. Druggist,* **57,** (1974).

6. D. Craddock, *Drugs,* **11,** 378 (1976); *Curr. Ther.,* 71 (1976).

7. J. Anderson, *Practitioner,* **212,** 536 (1974).

8. A. C. Sullivan, L. Cheng, and J. G. Hamilton, *Ann. Rep. Med. Chem.,* **11,** 200 (1976).

9. B. Colesnick, *Am. Fam. Physician,* **10,** 192 (1974).

10. W. Modell "Drugs for Overeating," in *Drugs of Choice 1976–1977,* W. Modell, Ed., C. B. Mosby, St. Louis, 1976, pp. 300–309.

11. *Stat. Bull. Metropolitan Life Insur. Co.* **47,** 1 (1966).

12. G. A. Heise, "Animal Techniques for Evaluating Anorexigenic Agents", in *Pharmacologic Techniques in Drug Evaluation,* J. H. Nodine and P. E. Siegler, Eds., Year Book Medical Publishers, Chicago, 1964, pp. 279–282.

13. J. Spengler and P. Waser, *Naunyn–Schmiedeberg's Arch. Pharmacol.,* **237** 171 (1959).

14. A. Abdallah and H. D. White, *Arch. Int. Pharmacodyn. Ther.,* **188,** 271 (1970).

15. R. H. Cox, Jr. and R. P. Maickel, *J. Pharmacol. Exp. Ther.,* **181,** 1 (1972).

16. J. H. Gogerty, C. Penberthy, L. C. Iorio, and J. H. Trapold, *Arch. Int. Pharmacodyn. Ther.,* **214,** 285 (1975).

17. J. E. Blundell, C. J. Latham, and M. B. Leshem, *J. Pharm. Pharmacol.,* **28,** 471 (1976).

18. H. R. Kissileff, *Physiol. Behav.,* **5,** 163 (1970).

19. J. E. Owen, Jr., *J. Exp. Anal. Behav.,* **3,** 293 (1960).

20. P. L. Carlton, *J. Exp. Anal. Behav.,* **4,** 379 (1961).

21. B. P. H. Poschel, *J. Comp. Physiol. Psychol.,* **56,** 968 (1963).

22. N. J. Carlson, G. A. Doyle, and T. G. Bidder, *Psychopharmacologia,* **8,** 157 (1965).

22a. O. S. Ray and L. Stein, *J. Exp. Anal. Behav.,* **2,** 363 (1959).

23. R. T. Kelleher and L. Cook, *J. Exp. Anal. Behav.,* **2,** 267 (1959).

24. R. T. Kelleher, W. Fry, J. Deegan, and L. Cook, *J. Pharmacol. Exp. Ther.,* **133,** 271 (1961).

25. C. B. Ferster, J. B. Appel, and R. A. Hiss, *J. Exp. Anal. Behav.,* **5,** 73 (1962).

26. R. P. Maickel and J. E. Zabik, *Life Sci.,* **21,** 173 (1977).

27. H. A. Levy and G. Faludi, "Clinical Techniques for Evaluating Anorexigenic Agents", in *Pharmacologic Techniques in Drug Evaluation,*

J. H. Nodine and P. E. Siegler, Eds., Year Book Medical Publishers, Chicago, 1964, pp. 283–290.

28. J. Brozek and A. Keys, *Physiol. Rev.,* **33,** 245 (1953).

29. H. J. Monotye, F. H. Epstein, and M. O. Kjelsberg, *Am. J. Clin. Nutr.,* **16,** 417 (1965).

30. S. L. Halpern, *Med. Clin. North Am.,* **48,** 1335 (1964).

31. B. W. Elliott, *Curr. Ther. Res.,* **12,** 502 (1970).

32. B. K. Anand and J. R. Brobeck, *Yale J. Biol Med.,* **24,** 123 (1951).

33. A. F. Debons and I. Krimsky, *Postgrad. Med.,* **51,** 74 (1972).

34. B. K. Anand and S. Dua, *Ind. J. Med. Res.,* **43,** 113 (1955).

35. H. D. Patton, "Higher Controls of Autonomic Outflows: The Hypothalamus," in *Physiology and Biophysics,* 19th ed., T. C. Ruch and H. D. Patton, Eds., W. B. Saunders, Philadelphia, 1966, pp. 247–249.

36. A. W. Hetherington and S. W. Ranson, *Proc. Soc. Exp. Biol. Med.,* **41,** 465 (1939).

37. A. W. Hetherington and S. W. Ranson, *Anat. Rec.,* **78,** 149 (1940).

38. A. W. Hetherington and S. W. Ranson, *J. Comp. Neurol.,* **76,** 475 (1942).

39. B. G. Hoebel, *Ann. N. Y. Acad. Sci.,* **157,** 758 (1969).

40. D. J. Albert and L. H. Storlien, *Science,* **165,** 599 (1969).

41. J. A. F. Stevenson, *Ann. N. Y. Acad. Sci.,* **157,** 1069 (1969).

42. C. D. Wood, *Neurology,* **8,** 215 (1958).

43. P. J. Morgane and A. J. Kosman, *Am. J. Physiol.,* **197,** 158 (1959).

44. F. M. Skultety, *Ann. N. Y. Acad. Sci.,* **157,** 861 (1969).

45. F. M. Skultety and T. M. Gary, *Neurology,* **12,** 394 (1962).

46. S. A. Lorens and C. Y. Kondo, *Physiol. Behav.,* **4,** 729 (1969).

47. S. P. Grossman, *Advan. Psychosom. Med.,* **7,** 49 (1972).

48. B. W. Robinson and M. Mishkin, *Science,* **136,** 260 (1962).

49. D. Singh and D. R. Meyer, *J. Comp. Physiol. Psychol.,* **65,** 163 (1968).

50. J. F. Lubar, C. F. Schaefer, and D. G. Wells, *Ann. N. Y. Acad. Sci.,* **157,** 875 (1969).

51. E. M. Stricker and M. J. Zigmond, "Brain Catecholanimes and the Lateral Hypothalamic Syndrome," in Ref. 3, pp. 19–32.

52. B. G. Hoebel, "Satiety: Hypothalamic Stimulation Anorectic Drugs, and Neurochemical Substrates," in Ref. 3, pp. 33–50.

53. S. P. Grossman, "Neuroanatomy of Food and Water Intake," in Ref. 3, pp. 51–60.

54. A. Sclafani, "Appetite and Hunger in Experimental Obesity Syndromes," in Ref. 3, pp. 281–295.

55. E. Costa and S. Garattini, Eds., *Amphetamines and Related Compounds*, Raven Press, New York, 1970.

55a. L. D. Lytle, "Control of Eating Behavior," in *Nutrition and the Brain*, Vol. 2, R. J. Wurtman and J. J. Wurtman, Eds., Raven Press, New York, 1977, pp. 1–143.

55b. Garattini, S. and Samanin, R., Eds., *Central Mechanisms of Anoretic Drugs*, Raven Press, New York, 1978.

56. C. J. Estler, *Advan. Pharmacol. Chemother.*, **13**, 305 (1975).

57. R. J. Baldessarini, *Ann. Rev. Med.*, **23**, 343 (1972).

58. P. A. Shore, *Ann. Rev. Pharmacol.*, **12**, 209 (1972).

59. M. Vogt, *Brit. Med. Bull.*, **29**, 168 (1973).

60. J. Glowinski, J. Axelrod, and L. L. Ivergen, *J. Pharmacol. Exp. Ther.*, **153**, 30 (1966).

61. R. Laverty and D. F. Sharman, *Brit. J. Pharmacol.*, **24**, 759 (1965).

62. B. E. Leonard, *Biochem. Pharmacol.*, **21**, 1289 (1972).

63. S. G. Holtzman and R. E. Jewett, *Psychopharmacologia*, **22**, 151 (1971).

64. B. V. Clineschmidt, J. C. McGuffin, and A. B. Werner, *Eur. J. Pharmacol.*, **27**, 313 (1974).

65. L. A. Baez, *Psychopharmacologia*, **35**, 91 (1974).

66. M. Vogt, *J. Physiol.*, **123**, 451 (1954).

67. O. Hornykiewicz, *Pharmacol. Rev.*, **18**, 925 (1966).

68. J. Glowinski and R. J. Baldessarini, *Pharmacol. Rev.*, **18**, 1201 (1966).

69. R. M. Pinder, R. N. Grogden, P. R. Sawyer, T. M. Speight, and G. S. Avery, *Drugs*, **10**, 241 (1975).

70. J. P. Colmore and J. D. Moore, *J. New Drugs*, **6**, 123 (1966).

71. W. H. Funderbunk, J. C. Hazelwood, R. T. Ruckart, and J. W. Ward, *J. Pharmacol.*, **23**, 468 (1971).

72. F. Cattabani, A. Reveulta, and E. Costa, *Neuropharmacology*, **11**, 753 (1972).

73. S. Jespersen and J. Scheel-Kruger, *J. Pharm. Pharmacol.*, **25**, 49 (1973).

74. M. F. Sugrue, I. Goodlet, and I. MacIndewar, *J. Pharm. Pharmacol.*, **27**, 950 (1975).

75. R. Samanin, D. Ghezzi, L. Valzelli, and S. Garattini, *Eur. J. Pharmacol.*, **19**, 318 (1972).

76. E. Edeleano, *Chem. Ber.*, **20**, 616 (1887).

77. G. A. Alles, *J. Pharmacol. Exp. Ther.*, **32**, 121 (1927); **47**, 339 (1933); G. A. Alles and M. Prinzmetal, *ibid.*, **48**, 161 (1933).

78. M. F. Lesses and a. Meyerson, *New Engl. J. Med.*, **218**, 119 (1938).

79. M. H. Nathanson, *J. Am. Med. Assoc.*, **108**, 528 (1939).

80. S. O. Cole, *Psychol. Bull.*, **68**, 81 (1967).

81. S. F. Leibowitz, *Brain Res.*, **84**, 160 (1975).

82. S. F. Leibowitz, *Brain Res.*, **98**, 529 (1975).

83. J. E. Ahlskog, *Brain Res.*, **82**, 211 (1974).

84. R. J. Carey, *Pharm. Biochem. Behav.*, **5**, 519 (1976).

85. A. Weissman, B. K. Koe, and S. S. Tenen, *J. Pharmacol. Exp. Ther.*, **151**, 339 (1966).

86. H. H. Frey and R. Schulz, *Biochem. Pharm.*, **22**, 3041 (1973).

87. K. B. J. Franklin and L. J. Herberg, *Nemopharmacol.*, **16**, 45 (1977).

88. L. A. Carr and K. E. Moore, *Science*, **64**, 322 (1969).

89. K. Y. Ng, T. N. Chase, and I. J. Kipin, *Nature*, **228**, 468 (1970).

90. A. Carlsson, "Amphetamine and Brain Catecholamines," in Ref. 55, p. 289.

91. R. J. Boakes, P. B. Bradley, and J. M. Candy, *Brit. J. Pharmacol.*, **45**, 391 (1922).

92. R. J. Ziance, A. J. Azzaro, and C. O. Rutledge, *J. Pharmacol. Exp. Ther.*, **182**, 284 (1972).

93. J. Glowinski and J. Axelrod, *J. Pharmacol. Exp. Ther.*, **149**, 43 (1965).

94. M. R. Ferris, F. L. M. Tang, and R. A. Maxwell, *J. Pharmacol. Exp. Ther.*, **181**, 407 (1972).

95. S. H. Snyder, M. J. Kuhar, A. I. Green, J. T. Coyle, and E. G. Shaskan, *Int. Rev. Neurobiol.*, **13**, 127 (1970).

96. P. F. Von Voightlander and K. E. Moore, *J. Pharmacol. Exp. Ther.*, **184**, 542 (1973).

97. K. E. Moore, *Biol. Psychiatr.*, **12**, 451 (1977).

98. M. Raiteri, A. Bertollini, F. Angelini, and G. Levi, *Eur. J. Pharmacol.*, **3**, 189 (1975).

99. N. W. Blacow and A. Wade, Eds., *Martindale The Extra Pharmacopoeia*, The Pharmaceutical Press, London, 26th ed., 1972, p. 124.

100. Approved Names, *Brit. Med. J.*, 1335 (1962); *Unlisted Drugs*, **19**, 70 (1967).

101. J. Gonzalez Barranco, J. A. Rull, and O.

Lozano Castaneda, *Prensa Med. Mex.*, **39,** 298 (1974).

102. J. E. Blum, *Arzneim.-Forsch.*, **19,** 748 (1969).

103. H. Bricaire and M. Philbert, *La Presse Med.*, **74,** 2695 (1966).

104. M. Demole and R. E. Elgin, *Cah. Nutr. Diet,* **2,** 63 (1967).

105. M. Fey and H. P. Gurtner, *Arzneim.-Forsch.*, **22,** 2090 (1972).

106. H. Bruder, Swiss Pat. 493, 462 (1970); through *Chem. Abstr.,* **73,** 120289 (1070).

107. P. Tognoni, P. L. Morselli, and S. Garattini, *Eur. J. Pharmacol.*, **20,** 125 (1972).

108. Manufactures J. R. Bottu, Fr. Pat. M5,375 (1967); through *Chem. Abstr.,* **71,** 80906 (1969).

109. Societe Industrielle pour la Fabrication des Antibiotiques, Fr. Pat. M 3,332 (1965); *Chem. Abstr.,* **63,** 13214 (1965).

110. J. R. Boissier, C. R. Dumont, R. Ratouis, and D. Moisy, *Arch. Int. Pharmacodyn.*, **167,** 150 (1967).

111. J. R. Boissier, R. Ratouis, and C. Dumont, *Ann. Pharm. Fr.*, **24,** 57 (1966).

112. J. R. Boisser, J. Hirtz, C. Dumont, and A. Gierardin, *Ann. Pharm. Fr.*, **26,** 215 (1968).

113. J. Marsel, G. Doering, G. Remberg, and G. Spiteller, *Z. Rechtsmed.*, **70,** 245 (1952).

114. J. E. Owen, Jr., *J. Pharm. Sci.*, **52,** 679 (1963).

115. R. L. Herting, R. J. Powers, and G. Dillon, *Pharmacologist,* **11,** 264 (1969).

116. B. W. Horrom, U.S. Pat. 3,689,504 (1972); *Chem. Abstr.,* 140019 (1972).

117. D. F. Marsh and D. A. Herring, *J. Pharmacol. Exp. Ther.*, **100,** 298 (1958).

118. H. Wieduwilt, K. H. Haendel, and E. Jassmann, Ger. (East) Pat. 117,066 (1975); through *Chem. Abstr.,* **85,** 20817 (1976).

119. B. Glasson, A. Benakis, and M. Thomasset, *Arzneim.-Forsch.*, **21** 1985 (1971).

120. R. Dalla Vedova and G. D'Alo, *Boll. Chim. Farm.*, **112,** 273 (1973).

121. I. Shoulson and T. N. Chase, *Clin. Pharmacol. Ther.*, **17,** 616 (1975).

122. A. J. Goudie, M. Raylor, and R. J. Wheeler, *Psychopharmocologia,* **38,** 67 (1974).

123. C. L. E. Broekkamp, A. J. M. Weemaes, and J. M. van Rossum, *J. Pharm. Pharmacol.*, **27,** 129 (1975).

124. R. B. Bruce, and W. R. Maynard, *J. Pharm. Sci.*, **57,** 1173 (1968).

125. A. H. Beckett and L. G. Brookes, *J. Pharm. Pharmacol.*, *19 Suppl.*, 415 (1967).

126. C. D. Morgan, F. Cattabeni, and E. Costa, *J. Pharmacol. Exp. Ther.*, **180,** 127 (1972).

127. *Int. Congr. Pharmacol., 6th, Helsinki, 1975 Abstr.* p. 357.

128. A. Buzas, Jap. Pat. 75:89,335 (1975); through *Chem. Abstr.,* **86,** 55182 (1977).

129. Ref. 3, p. 354.

130. L. Beregi, P. Hugon, and J. C. Le Douarec, U.S. Pat. 3,760,009 (1974); *Chem. Abstr.,* **83,** 10866 (1975).

131. L. Beregi, C. Malon, P. Hugon, and J. Duhalt, Ger. Pat. 2,437,883 (1975); through *Chem. Abstr.,* **83,** 10866 (1975).

132. Snythelabs, Netherlands Pat. Appl. 7,307,572 (1977).

133. M. Taylor and A. J. Aoudie, *Psychopharmacologia,* **35,** 13 (1974).

134. L. G. Beregi, P. Hugon, J. C. LeDouarec, M. Laubie, and J. Duhault, in Ref. 55, pp. 39–45.

135. *Postgrad. Med. J.*, *Suppl. 1,* 159 (1975).

136. J. C. Guilland, J. Kleeping, A. Escousse, J. P. Didier, G. Rucart, and J. Mounie, *Therapie,* **30,** 117 (1975).

137. G. L. S. Pawan, P. M. Payne, and E. L. Sheldrick, *Brit. J. Pharmacol.*, **41,** 416P (1971).

138. J. F. Giudicelli and H. Najer, Ger. Pat. 2,325,328 (1974); through *Chem. Abstr.,* **80,** 82378 (1974).

139. J. F. Giudicelli, C. Richer, and A. Berdeaux, *Brit. J. Clin. Pharmacol.*, **3,** 113 (1976).

140. J. G. Giudicelli, C. Richer, A. Berdeaux, and N. Guessons, *Eur. J. Clin. Pharm.*, **10,** 325 (1976).

141. A. P. Intoccia, B. Hwang, G. Joseph, G. Konicki, and S. S. Walkenstein, *Neuropharmacology,* **11,** 761 (1972).

142. E. Macko, H. Saunders, G. Heil, P. Fowler, and G. Reichard, *Arch. Int. Pharmacodyn. Ther.*, **200,** 102 (1972).

143. F. Cattabeni, A. Revuelta, and E. Costa, *Neuropharmacology,* **11,** 753 (1972).

144. J. J. Lafferty and C. Kaiser, Ger. Pat. 2,137,807 (1972); through *Chem. Abstr.,* **76,** 153322 (1972).

145. Union et Cie.-Societe Francais de Recherche Medicale, Brit. Pat. 1,182,557 (1970); through *Chem. Abstr.,* **72,** 90120 (1970).

146. L. Beregi, P. Hugon, and J. C. LeDouarec, U.S. Pat. 3,663,595 (1972); *Chem. Abstr.,* **77,** 61613 (1972).

147. A. Buzas and J. Bruneau, Ger. Pat. 2,613,328 (1976).

148. K. H. Boltze and D. Lorenz, U.S. Pat.

3,769,319 (1973); *Chem. Abstr.*, **80,** 3286 (1974).

149. Societe Nogentaise de Produits Chimiques, Fr. Pat. M 4,288 (1966); through *Chem. Abstr.*, **68,** 59250 (1968).

150. L. Beregi, P. Hugon, J. C. LeDouarec, and J. Duhault, Ger. Pat. 2,003,353 (1970); through *Chem. Abstr.* **73,** 66249 (1970).

151. J. M. Steel, J. F. Munro, and L. J. P. Duncan, *Practitioner*, **211,** 232 (1973).

152. P. Bjurrlf, S. Carlstrom, and G. Rorsman, *Acta Med. Scand.*, **182,** 273 (1967).

153. J. Spranger and J. Dorken, *Med. Wochenschr.*, **21,** 105 (1967).

154. Troponwerke Dinklage & Co., Ger. Pat. 1,248,033 (1967); through *Chem. Abstr.*, **68,** 68657 (1968).

155. Troponwerke Dinklage & Co., Ger. Pat. 1,216,881 (1966); through *Chem. Abstr.*, **65,** 3789 (1966).

156. CIBA Ltd., Bel. Pat. 633,761 (1963); through *Chem. Abstr.*, **61,** 3020 (1964).

157. CIBA Ltd., Fr. Pat. M 5,332 (1967); through *Chem. Abstr.*, **71,** 123886 (1969).

158. CIBA Ltd., Bel. Pat. 633,760 (1963); through *Chem. Abstr.*, **61,** 3021 (1964).

159. J. R. Bottu, Fr. Pat. M 7,351 (1968).

160. M. C. E. Carron and C. L. C. Carron, Fr. Pat. M 7,628; through *Chem. Abstr.*, **76,** 126634 (1972).

161. Dr. A. Wander A.-G., Swiss Pat. 393,306 (1965); through *Chem. Abstr.*, **64,** 2004 (1966).

162. W. T. Comer and H. R. Roth, U.S. Pat. 3,993,776 (1976).

163. D. R. Jasinski, J. G. Nutt, and J. D. Griffith, *Clin. Pharmacol. Ther.*, **16,** 645 (1974).

164. E. C. Schreiber, B. H. Min, A. V. Zeiger, and J. F. Lang, *J. Pharmacol. Exp. Ther.*, **159,** 372 (1967).

165. F. Banci, G. P. Cartoni, A. Cavalli, and A. Monai, *Arzneim.-Forsch.*, **21,** 1616 (1971).

166. B. Testa, *Acta Pharm. Suec.* **10,** 441 (1973).

167. B. Testa and A. H. Beckett, *Pharm. Acta Helv.*, **49,** 21 (1974).

168. D. Mihailova, A. Rosen, B. Testa, and A. H. Beclott, *J. Pharm. Pharmacol.*, **26,** 711 (1974).

169. F. Alexander, P. J. Tannenbaum, and A. P. Crosley, Jr., *Fed. Proc.*, **26,** 290 (1967).

170. E. Rosen, S. M. Free, and G. C. Heil, *J. Pharm. Sci.*, **60,** 1900 (1971).

171. A. H. Beckett and R. D. Hossie, *J. Pharm. Pharmacol.*, **21,** 157S (1969).

172. A. J. Rottendorf Chemische Fabrik, Belg. Pat. 622,585 (1963); through *Chem. Abstr.*, **59,** 2723 (1963).

173. Boehringer Ingelheim G.m.b.H., Brit. Pat. 1,069,797 (1967); through *Chem. Abstr.*, **68,** 95537 (1968).

174. H. Koeppe and K. Zeile, S. Afr. Pat. 6704448 (1968); through *Chem. Abstr.*, **70,** 57433 (1969).

175. Richardson-Merrell Inc., Fr. Pat. M 3,590 (1965); through *Chem. Abstr.*, **64,** 5002 (1966).

176. Boehringer Ingelheim G.m.b.H., Brit. Pat. 1,069,797 (1971); through *Chem. Abstr.*, **75,** 151534 (1971).

177. E. J. Warawa and J. H. Biel, U.S. Pat. 3,577,461 (1971).

178. A. A. Carr and D. R. Meyer, Ger. Pat. 2,030,686 (1971); through *Chem. Abstr.*, **74,** 76198 (1971).

179. Temmler-Werke Vereinigte Chemische Fabriken, Ger. Pat. 1,195,329 (1965); through *Chem. Abstr.*, **63,** 11268 (1965).

180. C. H. Boehringer Sohn, Bel. Pat. 621,456, (1963); through *Chem. Abstr.*, **59,** 9835 (1963).

181. Laboratoire Roger Bellon, Fr. Pat. M 3,414 (1965); through *Chem. Abstr.*, **64,** 701 (1966).

182. B. G. Hoebel, in *Handbook of Psychopharmacology*, L. L. Iversen, S. D. Iversen, and S. H. Snyder, Eds., 1975.

183. B. G. Hoebel, in Ref. 3, pp. 33–50.

184. A. N. Edpstein, *J. Comp. Physiol. Psychol.*, **52,** 37 (1959).

185. S. I. Griboff, R. Berman, and H. I. Silverman, *Curr. Ther. Res.*, **17,** 535 (1975); H. I. Silverman, *Am. J. Pharm.*, **135,** 45 (1963).

186. H. Hoffman, *Arch. Int. Pharmacodyn.*, **160,** 180 (1966).

187. Commercial Solvents Corp., Jap. Pat. 75,160,231; through *Chem. Abstr.*, **85,** 159630 (1976).

188. E. Sandrin and St. Guttmann, Ger. Pat. 2,206,961 (1971); through *Chem. Abstr.*, **77,** 151659 (1972).

189. D. Dvornik and G. Schilling, *J. Med. Chem.*, **8,** 466 (1965).

190. F. H. Clarke, *J. Org. Chem.*, **27,** 3251 (1962).

191. M. F. Bethel, *Brit. Med. J.*, **1,** 30 (1957).

192. J. Evans, *Lancet*, **2,** 1306 (1969).

193. D. Craddock, *Obesity and Its Management*, 2nd ed., Churchill and Livingstone, Edinburgh, 1973.

194. M. J. Kalm, *J. Med. Chem.*, **7,** 427 (1964); D. L. Knapp, *ibid.*, **7,** 433 (1964).

195. G. D. Searle & Co., Brit. Pat. 831,933 (1960); through *Chem. Abstr.*, **55,** 2697 (1961).

196. Dynachim S.a.r.l., Fr. Pat. 2,168,139 (1973); through *Chem. Abstr.*, **80,** 48010 (1974).

197. P. E. Cross and R. P. Dickinson, Ger. Pat. 2,361,824 (1974); through *Chem. Abstr.*, **81,** 130718 (1974).

198. W. H. Hartung, *Ind. Eng. Chem.*, **37,** 126 (1945).

199. J. B. van der Schoot, E. J. Ariens, J. M. van Rossum, and J. A. Th. Horkmans, *Arzneim.-Forsch.*, **12,** 902 (1962).

200. P. Karrer and K. Ehrhardt, *Helv. Chim. Acta*, **34,** 2202 (1951).

201. P. W. Feit and H. Bruun in C. Kaergaard Nielsen, M. P. Magnussen, E. Kampmann, and H.-H. Frey, *Arch. Int. Pharmacodyn. Ther.*, **170,** 428 (1967).

202. A. H. Beckett and L. G. Brookes, *Tetrahedron*, **24,** 1283 (1968).

203. M. Cussac, A. Bouherle, and J. Hache, *Eur. J. Med. Chem.*, **10,** 112 (1975).

204. O. Nieschulz and G. Schneider, *Arzneim.-Forsch.*, **14,** 104 (1964).

205. B. W. Horron, S. Afr. Pat. 68,04,291; through *Chem. Abstr.*, **71,** 12786 (1969).

206. R. M. Pinder and A. Burger, *J. Pharm. Sci.*, **56,** 970 (1967).

207. R. M. Pinder, R. W. Brimblecombe, and D. W. Green, *J. Med. Chem.*, **12,** 322. (1969).

208. R. M. Pinder and A. Burger, *Arzneim.-Forsch.*, **20,** 245 (1970).

209. J. W. Daly, C. R. Creveling, and B. Witkop, *J. Med. Chem.*, **9,** 276 (1966).

210. K. Brewster and R. M. Pinder, *J. Med. Chem.*, **15,** 1078 (1972).

211. C. Kaiser, C. A. Leonard, G. C. Heil, B. M. Lester, B. H. Tedeschi, and C. L. Zirkle, *J. Med. Chem.*, **13,** 820 (1970).

212. K. Binovic and S. Vrancea, *Chim. Ther.*, **3,** 313 (1968).

213. T. Holm, I. Huus, R. Kopf, I. Moller Nielsen, and P. V. Petersen, *Acta Pharmacol.*, **17,** 121 (1960).

214. S. L. Beregi and J. Duhault, *Arzneim.-Forsch.*, **27,** 116 (1977).

215. G. F. Holland, C. J. Buck, and A. Weissman, *J. Med. Chem.*, **6,** 519 (1963).

216. H.-H. Frey, in Ref. 55, p. 343.

217. J. C. Le Douarec and L. Beregi, *Conf. Hung. Ther. Invest. Pharmacol., 2nd, Budapest, 1962*, pp. 115–125.

218. R. B. Lawlor, M. C. Trivedi, and J. Yelnosky, *Arch. Int. Pharmacodyn. Ther.*, **179,** 401 (1969).

219. E. D. Bergmann and Z. Goldschmidt, *J. Med. Chem.*, **11,** 1242 (1968).

220. L. G. Beregi, P. Hugon, J. C. LeDouarec, M. Laubic, and J. Duhault, in Ref. 55, pp. 21–61.

221. M. Freifelder, *J. Med. Chem.*, **6,** 813 (1963).

222. A. Gemignani, P. Versace, F. Cugurra, and A. Vaccari, *Arch. Int. Pharmacodyn.*, **200,** 88 (1972).

223. J.-R. Bossier, R. Ratouis, and C. Dumont, *Ann. Pharm. Fr.*, **24,** 57 (1966).

224. A. H. Beckett and L. G. Brookes, in Ref. 3, pp. 109–120.

225. R. L. Smith and L. G. Dring, in Ref. 3, pp. 121–140.

226. J. Wright, A. K. Cho and J. Gal, *Life Sci.*, **20,** 467 (1977).

227. A. H. Beckett, *Xenobiotica*, **1,** 365 (1971).

228. A. H. Beckett, M. Mitchard, and A. A. Shihab, *J. Pharm. Pharmacol.*, **23,** 347 (1971).

229. K. Opitz and M. L. Weischer, *Arzneim.-Forsch.*, **16,** 1311 (1966).

230. U. Koester, J. Caldwell, and R. L. Smith, *Biochem. Soc. Trans.*, **2,** 881 (1974).

231. A. H. Beckett and P. M. Belanger, *J. Pharm. Pharmacol.*, **26,** 205 (1974).

232. B. Testa and A. H. Beckett, *J. Pharm. Pharmacol.*, **25,** 119 (1973).

233. A. H. Beckett and A. Raisi, *J. Pharm. Pharmacol.*, **28,** 40P (1976).

234. K. K. Midha, A. H. Beckett, and A. Saunders, *Xenobiotica*, **4,** 627 (1974).

235. W. J. Houlihan, Ger. Pat. 1,1814,540; *Chem. Abstr.*, **71,** 81368 (1969).

236. T. S. Sulkowski, U.S. Pat. 3,768,178 (1975); *Chem. Abstr.*, **84,** 4993 (1976).

237. S. Barcza and W. J. Houlihan, *J. Pharm. Sci.*, **64,** 829 (1975).

238. H. P. Weber, unpublished results, Sandoz Ltd., Basel.

239. M. Babbini, M. Gaiardi, and M. Bartoletti, *Pharmacology*, **15,** 46 (1977).

240. A. Kornhaber, *Psychosomatics*, **14,** 162 (1973).

241. R. Dolecek and M. Zavada, *Cas. Lek. Ces.*, **112,** 144 (1973).

242. R. Dolecek, *Cas. Lek. Ces.*, **114,** 249 (1975).

243. S. P. Woodhouse, E. R. Nye, K. Anderson, and J. Rawlings, *N. Z. Med. J.*, **81,** 546 (1975).

244. C. Sirtori, A. Hurwitz, and D. L. Azarnoff, *Am. J. Med. Sci.*, **261,** 341 (1971).

245. L. C. Harrison, A. P. King-Roach, and K. C. Sandy, *Metabolism*, **24,** 1353 (1975).

246. R. G. Engstrom, L. A. Kelly, and J. H. Go-

gerty, *Arch. Int. Pharmacodyn.*, **214,** 308 (1975).

247. M. O. Carruba, A. Groppetti, P. Mantegazza, L. Vicentini, and F. Zarnbotti, *Brit. J. Pharm.*, **56,** 431 (1976).

248. Z. L. Kruk and M. R. Zarrindast, *Brit. J. Pharm.*, **58,** 367 (1976).

249. F. Zambotti, M. O. Carruba, F. Barzaghi, L. Vicentini, A. Groppetti, and P. Mantegazza, *Eur. J. Pharmacol.*, **36,** 405 (1976).

250. A. Jori and E. Dolfini, *Eur. J. Pharmacol.*, **41,** 443 (1977).

251. M. O. Carruba, G. B. Picotti, F. Zambotti, and P. Mantegazza, *Arch. Pharmacol.*, **298,** 1 (1977).

252. M. F. Sugrue, G. Shaw, and K. G. Charlton, *Eur. J. Pharmacol.*, **42,** 379 (1977).

253. B. K. Koe, *J. Pharmacol. Exp. Ther.*, **199,** 649 (1976).

254. R. E. Heikkila, F. S. Cabbat, and K. Mytilineou, *Fed. Proc.*, **36,** 381 (1977).

255. R. Samanin, C. Bendotti, S. Bernasconi, E. Borroni, and S. Garattini, *Eur. J. Pharmacol.*, **43,** 117 (1977).

256. P. Aeberli, P. Eden, J. H. Gogerty, W. J. Houlihan, and C. Penberthy, *J. Med. Chem.* **18,** 177 (1975).

257. T. S. Sulkowski, U.S. Pat. 3,900,494 (1975); *Chem. Abstr.*, **84,** 4993 (1976).

258. W. J. Houlihan, U.S. Pat. 3,755,360 (1973); *Chem. Abstr.*, **79,** 115651 (1973).

259. P. Aeberli, P. Eden, J. H. Gogerty, W. J. Houlihan, and C. Penberthy, *J. Med. Chem.*, **18,** 182 (1975).

260. W. J. Houlihan, Ger. Pat. 2,460,527, (1975); *Chem. Abstr.*, **83,** 164180 (1975).

261. W. J. Houlihan, Fr. Pat. 2,100,576 (1972); *Chem. Abstr.*, **77,** 164703 (1972).

262. H. A. Dugger, R. A. Coombs, H. J. Schwarz, B. H. Migdalof, and B. A. Orwig, *Drug Metab. Dispos.*, **4,** 262 (1976).

263. M. I. Gluckman, *Pharmacologist*, **7,** 146 (1965).

264. T. S. Sulkowski, U.S. Pat. 3,499,806 (1970); *Chem. Abstr.*, **72,** 111532 (1970).

265. T. S. Sulkowski, M. A. Wille, A. Masciti, and J. L. Diebold, *J. Org. Chem.*, **32,** 2180 (1967).

266. T. Baum and M. I. Gluckman, *J. Pharmacol. Exp. Ther.*, **158,** 510 (1967).

267. *Ibid.*, **157,** 32 (1967).

268. W. J. Houlihan, Fr. Pat. 1,530,074 (1968); *Chem. Abstr.*, **71,** 61434 (1969).

269. K. Freter, M. Götz, and J. T. Oliver, *J. Med. Chem.*, **13,** 1228 (1970).

270. K. Freter, M. Goetz, J. T. Oliver, and K. Zeile, S. Afr. Pat. 69,02707 (1969); through *Chem. Abstr.*, **72,** 111005 (1970).

271. J. T. Oliver, *Arch. Int. Pharmacodyn.*, **211,** 253 (1974).

272. M. K. Klohs, F. J. Petracek and N. Sugisaka, U.S. Pat. 3,851,062 (1974); *Chem. Abstr.*, **82,** 133170 (1975).

273. K.-U. Seiler, O. Wassermann, and H. Wensky, *Clin. Exp. Pharmacol. Physiol.*, **3,** 323 (1976).

274. W. Veldkamp, U.S. Pat. 3,317,380 (1967); *Chem. Abstr.*, **67,** 54035 (1967).

275. H. H. Keasling and R. B. Moffett, *J. Med. Chem.*, **14,** 1106 (1971).

276. C. van der Stelt and P. S. Hofman, Ger. Pat. 2,305,212 (1973); through *Chem. Abstr.*, **79,** 115591 (1973).

277. S. O. Winthrop, U.S. Pat. 2,971,973 (1961).

278. R. S. Sulkowski, Ger. Pat. 1,926,477 (1970); through *Chem. Abstr.*, **72,** 66920 (1970).

279. R. Jaunin, Ger. Pat. 2,553,595 (1976); through *Chem. Abstr.*, **86,** 29623 (1977).

280. McNeil Laboratories Inc., Belg. Pat. 628,803 (1963); through *Chem. Abstr.*, **61,** 9501 (1964).

281. A. J. Hadley, *J. Clin. Pharmacol.*, **7,** 296 (1967); J. Gürtler, *Praxis*, **55,** 410 (1966); H. Carlstrum and P. Reizenstein, *Acta Med. Scand.*, **181,** 291 (1967).

282. L. Peters and J. I. Gourzisin, *Adipositas, Kreislauf und Anorektika*, R. Blankart, Ed., Huber, Bern, Switzerland, 1974, pp. 61–77.

283. H. P. Gurtner, M. Gertsch, C. Salzman, H. Scherrer, P. Stucki, and F. Wyss, *Schweiz. Med. Wochenschr.*, **98,** 1965 (1968); W. Schweizer, *Praxis*, **58,** 701 (1969); E. Lang, E. J. Haupt, J. A. Koehler, and J. Schmidt, *Muench. Med. Wochenschr.*, **111,** 405 (1969).

284. G. I. Poos, J. R. Carson, J. D. Rosenau, A. P. Roszkowski, N. M. Kelley, and J. McGowin, *J. Med. Chem.*, **6,** 266 (1963).

285. A. P. Roszkowski and N. M. Kelley, *J. Pharmacol. Exp. Ther.*, **40,** 367 (1963).

286. R. A. Hardy, Jr., C. F. Howell, and N. Q. Quinones, U.S. Pat. 3,313,688 (1967); *Chem. Abstr.*, **67,** 90791 (1967).

287. Laboratories Dausse, S. A., Netherlands Pat. Appl. 6,613,484 (1967); through *Chem. Abstr.*, **67,** 90792 (1967).

288. C. F. Howell, N. Q. Quinones, and R. A. Hardy, Jr., *J. Org. Chem.*, **27,** 1697 (1962).

289. R. Giudicelli, H. Najer, J. Menin, and M. Proteau, *Compt. Rend. Acad. Sci. Ser. D*, **265,** 165 (1967).

290. A. Krese and J. Kisela, *Ther. Hung.*, **16,** 89 (1968).

291. Sandoz, Ltd., Belg. Pat. 719,921 (1969).

292. M. J. Kalm, U.S. Pat. 3,081,308 (1963); *Chem. Abstr.*, **59,** 6412 (1963).

293. A. H. Abdallah, *Toxicol. Appl. Pharm.*, **25,** 344 (1973).

294. A. H. Abdallah, *Eur. J. Pharmacol.*, **27,** 249 (1974).

295. E. R. Freiter, A. H. Abdallah, and S. J. Strycker, *J. Med. Chem.*, **16,** 510 (1973).

296. H. C. White, S. J. Strycker, and V. C. Wysong, U.S. Pat. 3,715,367 (1973); *Chem. Abstr.*, **78,** 136295 (1973).

297. A. H. Abdallah and H. D. White, *Fed. Proc.*, **33,** 564 (1974).

298. D. A. Downs and J. H. Woods, *Psychopharmacologia*, **43,** 13 (1975).

299. W. J. Houlihan and R. E. Manning, Ger. Pat. 1,938,674 (1970); *Chem. Abstr.*, **72,** 11502 (1970).

300. R. E. Manning, Ger. Pat. 1,805,948 (1969); through *Chem. Abstr.*, **71,** 81401 (1969).

301. R. E. Manning, Ger. Pat. 2,160,655 (1973); through *Chem. Abstr.*, **79,** 66413 (1973).

302. F. Debarre, C. Jeanmart, P. E. Simon, Ger. Pat. 2,359,864 (1974); through *Chem. Abstr.*, **81,** 91520 (1974).

303. R. S. Shadbolt, C. J. Sharpe, G. R. Brown, A. Ashford, and J. W. Ross, *J. Med. Chem.*, **14,** 836 (1971).

304. Boehringer Ingelheim Ltd., Brit. Pat. 937,721 (1963); through *Chem. Abstr.*, **60,** 2728 (1964).

305. C. H. Boehringer Sohn, Fr. Pat. 1,529,480 (1968); through *Chem. Abstr.*, **71,** 12806 (1969).

306. E. R. Freiter, L. E. Begin, and A. Abdallah, *J. Heterocyclic Chem.*, **10,** 391 (1973).

307. S. E. Jaggers, J. L. Madinaveitta, and R. F. Maisey, U.S. Pat. 3,806,595 (1974); *Chem. Abstr.*, **83,** 940 (1975).

308. A. H. Abdallah, U.S. Pat. 3,646,204 (1972); *Chem. Abstr.*, **77,** 884 (1972).

309. Upjohn Co., Ger. Pat. 1,219,927 (1966); through *Chem. Abstr.*, **65,** 13609 (1966).

310. V. Lafon, Ger. Pat. 2,543,184 (1976); through *Chem. Abstr.*, **84,** 180241 (1976).

311. D. G. Martin, E. L. Schumann, M. Veldkamp, and H. Keasling, *J. Med. Chem.*, **8,** 456 (1965).

312. W. Veldkamp, H. H. Keasling, G. A. Johnson, W. A. Freyburger, and R. J. Collins, *J. Pharm. Sci.*, **56,** 829 (1967).

313. T. S. Danowski, *Ann. N.Y. Acad. Sci.*, **148,** 573–962 (1968).

314. J. M. Stowers and P. D. Bewsher, *Postgrad. Med. J.*, **45,** 13 (1969).

315. D. P. Patel and J. M. Stowers, *Lancet*, **2,** 282 (1964).

316. J. Peterson, *Acta Endocrinol.* **49,** 479 (1965).

317. J. A. Stron and A. A. H. Lawson, *Ann. N.Y. Acad. Sci.*, 673–683 (1968).

318. N. P. Buu-Hoï, S. Béranger, P. Jacquignon, A. Krikorian-Manoukian, and D. Courmarcel, *C. R. Acad. Sci. Ser. D*, **265,** 930 (1967).

319. N. P. Buu-Hoï, S. Béranger, and P. Jacquignon, Fr. Pat. M 6,786 (1971); through *Chem. Abstr.*, **75,** 20003 (1971).

320. G. Dumeur, N. Hüe, J. M. Lwoff, M. A. Mouries, and D. Tremblay, *Brit. J. Pharmacol.*, **58,** 437P (1976).

321. R. B. Moffett, *J. Med. Chem.*, **11,** 1251 (1968).

322. R. I. Henkin, U.S. Pat. 3,867,539 (1975); *Chem. Abstr.*, **83,** 37922 (1975).

323. Haco A.-G. Fr. Pat. M 2,723 (1964); through *Chem. Abstr.*, **62,** 11829d (1965); Brit. Pat. 970,480 (1964); through *Chem. Abstr.*, **62,** 568 (1965).

324. H. Feer and P. G. Waser, *Helv. Physiol. Pharmacol. Acta*, **14,** 29 and 36 (1956).

325. H. Tramer and H. Walter-Büel, *Deut. Med. Wochenschr.*, **81,** 1610 (1956).

326. D. Janz and F. Bahner, *Deut. Med. Wochenschr.* **79,** 845 (1954).

327. H. Najer, J. F. Giudicelli, Ger. Pat. 2,245,826 (1973); *Chem. Abstr.*, **79,** 13694 (1973).

328. L. R. Moser, J. A. Kaiser, and R. A. Hardy, Jr., U.S. Pat. 3,253,989, (1966); *Chem. Abstr.*, **65,** 5311 (1966).

329. Miles Laboratories Inc., Brit. Pat. 869,460 (1961); through *Chem. Abstr.*, **56,** 1463 (1962).

330. P. R. L. Giudicelli and H. Najer, Ger. Pat. 2,322,070 (1973); through *Chem. Abstr.*, **80,** 27293 (1974).

331. H. Najer, R. Dupont, and P. R. L. Giudicelli, Ger. Pat. 2,609,574 (1976); through *Chem. Abstr.*, **85,** 192769 (1976).

332. Synthelabo, F. Pat. 2,179,491 (1973); through *Chem. Abstr.*, **80,** 121001 (1974).

333. B. W. Horrom and H. B. Wright, Jr., U.S. Pat. 3,637,705 (1972); *Chem. Abstr.*, **76,** 113256 (1972).

334. P. E. Cross, Ger. Pat. 2,242,382, (1973); through *Chem. Abstr.*, **78,** 159666 (1973).

335. Merck and Co., Inc. Belg. Pat. 840,904 (1976).

336. A. Bodai, L. Paallos, L. E. Petocz, and I. Kosoczky, U.S. Pat. 3,904,628 (1975); *Chem. Abstr.*, **84**, 31126 (1976).

337. T. Raabe, K. Resag, and R. E. Nitz, Ger. Pat. 2,021,470 (1971); through *Chem. Abstr.*, **76**, 62552 (1972).

338. T. Raabe, S. Piesch, K. Resag, and R. E. Nitz, Ger. Pat. 2,021,262 (1971); through *Chem. Abstr.*, **76**, 72549 (1972).

339. Haco A.-G., Netherlands Pat. Appl. 6,410,685; through *Chem. Abstr.*, **65**, 12220 (1966).

340. Parke Davis & Co., Brit. Pat. 974,894, (1964); through *Chem. Abstr.*, **62**, 9110 (1965).

341. Parke Davis & Co., Brit. Pats. 974,893 and 974,894 (1974).

342. L. Zirngibl, R. Adrian, and U. Jahn, U.S. Pat. 3,947,584 (1976).

343. F. Chaillet, R. Charlier, A. Christiaens, and G. Deltour, *Arch. Int. Pharmacodyn.*, **164**, 451 (1966).

344. K. Hoegerle and E. Habicht, S. Afr. Pat. 69 07,046 (1970); through *Chem. Abstr.*, **73**, 120525 (1970).

345. A. Mentrup, K. Schromm, E. O. Renth, and E. Reichl, Ger. Pat. 2,016,136; through *Chem. Abstr.*, **76**, 34136 (1972).

346. A. Brossi, B. Pecherer, and R. Sunbury, U.S. Pat. 3,906,006, (1975); *Chem. Abstr.*, **84**, 59432 (1976).

347. Lab Lafon, Belg. Pat. 833,580 (1977).

348. J. R. Geigy A.-G., Swiss Pat. 476, 731 (1969).

349. C. H. Boehringer Sohn, Belg. Pat. 632,520 (1963); through *Chem. Abstr.*, **60**, 15688 (1964).

350. G. Satzinger, Ger. Pat. 1,271,118 (1968); through *Chem. Abstr.*, **69**, 77283 (1968).

351. H. E. Alburn and W. Dronch, U.S. Pat. 3,325,495 (1967); *Chem. Abstr.*, **68**, 49656 (1968).

352. H. M. Holava, Jr. and R: A. Partyka, *J. Med. Chem.*, **12**, 555 (1969).

353. G. Schmidt, *Arch. Int. Pharmcodyn.*, **156**, 87 (1965).

354. Dr. Karl Thomae G.m.b.H., Netherlands *Pat. Appl.* 74 14720; through *Chem. Abstr.*, **84**, 31038 (1976).

355. G. Griss, R. Hurnaus, W. Grell, and R. Reichl, Ger. Pat. 2,357,253 (1975); through *Chem. Abstr.*, **83**, 97254 (1975).

356. 356. R. Hurnaus, G. Griss, W. Grell, R. Sauter, R. Reichl, and M. Leitold, Ger. Pat.

357. 2,519,258 (1976); through *Chem. Abstr.*, **86**, 89889 (1977).

357. J. B. Hester, A. H. Tang, H. H. Keasling, and W. Veldkamp, *J. Med. Chem.*, **11**, 101 (1968).

358. J. R. Boissier and R. Ratouis, Fr. Pat. M5,850 (1968); through *Chem. Abstr.*, **71**, 13151 (1969).

359. F. Barzaghi, A. Groppetti, P. Mantegazza, and E. Müller, *J. Pharm. Pharmacol.*, **25**, 909 (1973).

360. H. L. Yale and J. A. Bristol, U.S. Pat. 4,003,905 (1977).

361. Q. R. Rogers and P. M.-B. Leung, *Fed. Proc.*, **32**, 1709 (1973).

362. A. E. Harper, N. J. Benevenga, and R. M. Wohlhueter, *Physiol. Rev.*, **50**, 428 (1970).

363. P. Leung and Q. R. Rogers, *Life Sci.*, **8**, 1 (1969).

364. A. E. Harper, in Ref. 3, pp. 103–113.

365. E. E. Rosenberg, Ger. Pat. 1,914,304 (1969); through *Chem. Abstr.*, **72**, 15758 (1970).

366. Canadian Patents and Development Ltd., Netherlands Pat. Appl. 6,507,333 (1965); through *Chem. Abstr.*, **65**, 9466 (1966).

367. J. R. Beaton, A. J. Szlavko, and J. A. F. Stevenson, *Can. J. Physiol. Pharmacol.*, **42**, 647 (1964).

368. J. R. Beaton and P. S. Uehara, *Can. J. Physiol. Pharmacol.*, **47**, 291 (1969).

369. M. Russek, J. A. F. Stevenson, and G. J. Mogenson, *Can. J. Physiol. Pharmacol.*, *ibid.*, **46**, 635 (1968).

370. A. Kekwick and G. L. S. Pawan, *Lancet*, **1968-II**, 198.

371. T. M. Chalmers, A. Kekwick, and G. L. S. Pawan, *Lancet*, **1958-I**, 866.

372. A. V. Schally, T. W. Redding, H. W. Lucien, and J. Meyer, *Science*, **157**, 219 (1967).

373. O. E. Scaramuzzi, C. A. Baile, and J. Mayer, *Experientia*, **27**, 256 (1971).

374. G. A. Bray, U.S. Pat. 3,591,687 (1971); *Chem. Abstr.*, **75**, 101283 (1971).

375. S.C.R.E.E.N. Paris, Ger. Pat. 2,501,834 (1975); S.C.R.E.E.N., Ger. Pat. 2,632,114 (1977); through *Chem. Abstr.*, **87**, 22787 (1977).

375a. H. Orzalesi, P. Chevallet, G. Berge, M. Boucard, J. J. Serrano, G. Privat, and C. Andray, *Eur. J. Med. Chem.-Chim. Ther.*, **13**, 259 (1978).

376. H. Orzalesi, P. Chevallet, M. Boucard, J. J.

Serrano, G. Privat, and C. Andary, *C. R. Acad. Sci., Ser. C,* **283,** 421 (1976).

377. G. R. Jansen and E. E. Howe, U.S. Pat. 3,529,064 (1970); through *Chem. Abstr.,* **73,** 120193 (1970).

378. A. C. Sullivan and J. Triscare, in Ref. 3, pp. 115–125.

379. J. L. Jackson, U.S. Pat. 3,985,898 (1976); *Chem. Abstr.,* **86,** 43444 (1977).

380. C. L. Hewett, D. S. Savage, J. Redpath, T. Sleigh, and D. R. Rae, Ger. Pat. 2,618,721 (1976); through *Chem. Abstr.,* **86,** 89479 (1977).

381. J. G. Maillard, Ger. Pat. 2,422,879 (1975); through *Chem. Abstr.,* **82,** 155958 (1975).

CHAPTER SIXTY

Hallucinogens

ALEXANDER T. SHULGIN

1483 Shulgin Road
Lafayette, California 94549, USA

CONTENTS

1 INTRODUCTION

Hallucinogens constitute a unique class of compounds in medicinal chemistry for a number of reasons. First, most pharmaceutical agents are designed to either recognize or repair an abnormal state, or to maintain a normal one. Some, such as anesthetics, are used to disrupt normalcy intentionally, but always with the goal of eventually cor-

1109

recting some deficiency. The use of hallucinogenic drugs, however, usually leads to a disorganization and reorganization of the intellectual and sensory integrity of the experimental subject. Although the process is relatively short-lived and reversible, it has not been considered beneficial in the treatment of recognized pathological states, and thus it has no generally accepted medical application.

Second, unlike most of the other pharmaceutical agents discussed in this text, these drugs produce effects that can be recognized only in human subjects. Animal studies have been used to compare specific pharmacological properties within related families of the hallucinogens, but these properties have not yet been extrapolated in any rational way to the CNS effects that are produced in man.

Third, the absence of any recognized medical utility of these materials, coupled with a small but real potential for abuse in society, has led to the enactment of stringent legislation. The intent of these legal steps was to curtail paramedical exploration with these drugs, but the realized effect has been the discouragement of most research that might involve them.

Despite these limitations, there is a continuing interest in these "psychotomimetic" drugs. As this name implies, their use can lead to the generation of a toxic state which bears some resemblance to psychosis (psychotomimetic = the mimicking of psychosis). The value of generating a "model psychosis" in a reversible manner, in an otherwise healthy individual, lies in the opportunity to observe and study any transient biochemical or physiological changes that might accompany it. It is hoped that any insight provided by these reversible changes may be applied to an understanding of spontaneous psychosis, and may also provide experimental subjects for the evaluation of antipsychotic medication.

These drugs have also been called "psychedelics," a name suggesting the frequently observed property of an enhancement of personal insight and awareness. This quality of amplification of both sensory and interpretive capacity is felt, subjectively, to be of great value by the user. The "altered state of consciousness" that results has, besides a purely hedonistic value, a potential for enhancing creativity and self-analysis.

These two properties, the one as prosaic as the other is audacious, would seem to guarantee a continuing fascination with these drugs in the research community.

2 HISTORY

There has always been a need in man for procedures that modify sensory and intellectual integrity. Many mechanisms are completely nonpharmacological and have, within each culture that uses them, become generally accepted and often encouraged. Religion is perhaps the best-known example. In those cultures that allow theology, there is always the creation of some form of a church which provides both a mechanism for the consumption of emotional energy and a framework of acceptability for the altered states of consciousness that result from this output. All individuals within each religious society are allowed the opportunity to participate to any desired degree, and excessive participation is usually tolerated. The forms that this expression can take vary widely. Capitulation to compulsive prayer, ritual mutilation, physical exhaustion resulting from starvation, dancing, or extended isolation—all can lead to some form of consciousness alteration. The sincerity and devastating effectiveness of voodoo cult magic, or of psychological murder, are well documented even though little understood mechanistically.

Very frequently artifacts, usually of botanical origin, are employed in this ubiquitous drive for sensory modification. In our society, alcohol, caffeine, and tobacco constitute the most frequently employed, and the most acceptable drugs. Their general acceptance makes them rarely considered as sensory-modifying botanical products, but pharmacologically each should be considered as a drug that is employed, ultimately, only for the changes in perception and state of consciousness that result from their use. A discussion of these is inappropriate for this chapter. Other drugs have found use and acceptability in other cultures but are used only rarely in our society; they are the origins of many of our so-called abuse drugs.

In the Old World, the use of opium and of cannabis is prehistoric. Opium probably originated in Asia Minor and was translocated both westward to Africa and eastward to the Orient. Cannabis had its origins in western China and its spread was first southward to India and then westward to Africa and the Mediterranean. All this occurred centuries before Christ. Various of the *Solanaceae* (belladonna, henbane, mandrake) have been widely employed in Europe as brews, as drugs, and as medicines. The record of the Western Hemisphere is even richer and more extensive. Many of the New World Indian cultures were built around the sacramental use of intoxicating plants such as datura, the morning glory seeds of the *Ipomoea*, the magic mushrooms of the *Psilocybe* spp., the peyote cactus, and the many snuffs of the Caribbean area. Tobacco, which had its origins in the New World, has contributed to the rest of the world the technique of smoking, a procedure that was quickly adapted to both opium and cannabis. Virtually all our present-day hallucinogenic drugs are either these plants themselves in one form or another, the chemicals isolated from them, or synthetic analogs of these isolates.

3 DETERMINATION OF POTENCY

3.1 Physical Models

A number of approaches have been made to correlate, and even explain, the relative potencies within a given family of hallucinogens by the measurement or calculation of molecular properties. In this way the use of living systems is avoided, but axiomatically such correlations still depend completely on the knowledge of the quantitative potency of the drugs in question, and these latter values, in turn, depend on some form of pharmacological titration.

A number of studies have involved the calculation of molecular parameters. Interatomic separations within a molecule can influence intermolecular hydrogen bonding to other molecules or to potential sites of action (1, 2). Intramolecular conformations are possible that might allow one active hallucinogen to resemble another (3). A number of studies have been made of energy calculations at various orbital sites within groups of known hallucinogenics (4, 5), but in the one case where such studies were directed to a very narrow chemical class (LSD analogs) there was poor correlation (6).

A number of molecular properties have been studied that are amenable to experimental measurement. Studies of crystal lattice geometry of active compounds (7, 8) have provided three-dimensional portraits of molecular conformation, but extrapolation to an *in vivo* solution environment leaves such results difficult to interpret. Three physicochemical approaches have overcome this theoretical difficulty by employing solutions in their analyses. Estimates have been made of the pi-bonding potential of a number of known active hallucinogens through a spectroscopic measurement of the strengths of the charge transfer complexes formed with *p*-dinitrobenzene (9). An extensive partition coefficient study has shown a fair correlation between the values of octanol : water partition (either measured or calculated) and human activity (10). They have suggested that a partition of about 1400 : 1 (at pH 7.4) is optimum for members of the phenylisopropylamine family of hallucinogens, with a loss of potency with change in either direction. The native fluorescence of dilute solutions of several known active drugs has been determined and correlated with human activity (11).

3.2 Animal Models

A closer approach to an understanding of the mechanism of action of the hallucinogens has been made by the development of animal models, but there is still no satisfactory system that duplicates human psychopharmacological intoxication. None of these systems has been widely accepted as a screening procedure for the prediction of hallucinogenic activity.

Several of the hallucinogens are effective agonists or antagonists in biologic *in vitro* systems, and these have been explored as potential screening tools. The close biochemical relationship between LSD and serotonin has been exploited to offer proposed mechanisms of action of LSD, but efforts to extrapolate these relationships to structural analogs have led to disappointing correlations with human effectiveness. A constant stumbling block, as an example, is 2-bromo-LSD (BOL), which is as active an antiserotonin agent as LSD but is substantially without hallucinogenic activity in man. Within small chemical families, a promising correlation between *in vitro* titration and *in vivo* effectiveness can be found: the anticholinergic activity of a family of gylcolate esters (12), the sympathetic stimulation such as mydriasis and hyperthermia in a family of amide variations of lysergic acid (13), and serotonin agonist potency in a homologous series related to DOM (14).

A number of promising assays have been explored based on the physiological responses of the intact test animal. One of these involves the study of hyperthermia. Rabbits are very responsive to small quantities of LSD (0.5 μg/kg), showing a rise in body temperature apparently of central origin (15). A reasonably good parallel, in rabbits, between this hyperthermia response and the known "excitatory syndrome" of LSD was found throughout the family of hallucinogenic lysergic acid amides and matched quite closely the reported human psychopharmacological potencies (16–18). These responses have been extended to the hallucinogenic tryptamines (19, 20). Aldous et al. (21) have shown the applicability of this response to the phenethylamine hallucinogens, and it is felt that this is probably the best animal test at present for estimating hallucinogenic potential.

Several behavioral approaches have been studied. The use of unrestrained or untrained rats was the basis of Hall's open-field test (22) in which animal activity patterns (rearing, preening, defecation, ranging) were found to be influenced to a degree proportionate to a drug's potency in man. This test has been applied to both the piperidinoglycolates (23) and the tryptamines (20, 24). Behavioral studies in other animals [head-twitch (25) and interference with nest-building (26) in mice, the sham rage response in cats (27), behavior disruption in monkeys (19)] have usually been restricted to a small group of closely related compounds. One behavioral response assay (the Bovet–Gatti profile) has been restructured to allow for the evaluation of hallucinogenic drugs (28). A recent review (29) has analyzed the extensive literature concerning these correlates. A failing with most of these assays is the need to employ large doses of the drug. In most cases these are approaching the lethal dose, and are certainly well above the dose–weight equivalent in man. Several specific assays have been critically analyzed (30) and it has been shown that not all families of drugs are validly detected, and that certain CNS agents that are not hallucinogenic respond as if they were. In general it was concluded that these models are of limited value.

3.3   Human Titration

The most reliable source of information concerning the qualitative and the quantititative nature of the hallucinogenic drugs must come from experimentation with human subjects. But these studies, by their very nature, are both ethically and legally difficult to perform. In the area of medical ethics it must be borne in mind that the study of such drugs employs the use of normal, healthy, and sane subjects, and involves the disruption of sensory and intellectual integrity in a way that some consider to be to the subject's disadvantage. Many research groups feel that the rewards to be gained from such studies do not warrant the inherent risks, and choose not to participate in this area of inquiry. Most medical institutions believe that no academic study is justified that does not produce information that can bear directly upon a problem of medical practice. As mentioned earlier, the classical approach employing animal experimentation cannot be followed fruitfully in studies with this class of drugs. And since there is a small but admittedly real risk that some of the psychological changes may not be rapidly reversible or may be recurrent, experiments must be conducted with the subject's advance knowledge of the nature of the responses that are to be expected. The double-blind study, in other words, is not possible.

There are other complications in the use of normal subjects in the study of hallucinogenic drugs. Qualitatively, the psychological changes that result can be extremely variable, both from drug to drug and from person to person. The visual sense can be amplified or distorted to varying degrees. Reports of changes in perspective, depth perception, and contrasts of light and dark are expressed by some but not by others. Some drugs frequently lead to a remarkable sensitivity to color shades and color contrasts. Edge effects (the apparent moving and redrawing of the outlines of physical objects) and creeping effects (the apparent movement of the objects themselves) may be the nuclei of perceptual distortions that can, in rare instances, give rise to actual hallucinations. More common, however, are interpretive distortions (faces that look like masks, inanimate objects that take on living characteristics) that are a blend of sensory and intellectual distortion. It is in this latter area, involving interpretive and cognitive capacities, that the most dramatic and disruptive indications of intoxication appear. There can be remarkable changes in self-perception, the reliving of past events, and the generation of states of intense emotion. With most of the hallucinogenic drugs, these events are readily recalled.

Any attempt to reduce these many qualitative variables to a single quantitative value of potency is subject to uncertainty. The development of some measure of tolerance to a drug's effects makes the repeated use of an experienced subject a properly questioned procedure. Yet the use of only naïve subjects can be criticized on the ethical grounds mentioned earlier. There is also a problem of agreement on the level of intoxication that should be accepted as the proper measure of "effective dose." The use of a threshold dosage as a measure of potency (the dose that provides the first suggestion of CNS intoxication) is compromised by the strong influence of the experimental setting and the expectations of the subject. And there can be a wide dose–response curve exhibited by some individuals to some drugs, in that increasing levels of the drug being tested can lead to a subjective report of a variety of increasingly complex events, suggesting a polyphasic nature of effect.

The distillation of these many uncertainties into a single number for quantitative comparisons in any structure–activity relationship study requires the acceptance of a large uncertainty factor in this number. But because the human animal alone can provide these data, these limitations must be accepted in any correlations between structure and potency.

4　MECHANISMS OF ACTION

4.1　Neurological Aspects

There is an immediately apparent chemical resemblance between the families of the hallucinogens and the major neurotransmitters. This relationship is the basis for much of the neuroanatomic research with these drugs and has led to an appealing explanation for the functional mechanisms of their action. The two principal catecholamine transmitters, dopamine (60.**1**) and norepinephrine (60.**2**) carry the exact carbon skeleton and an oxygenation pattern similar to the hallucinogen mescaline (60.**3**). Serotonin (60.**4**) is the major indolic

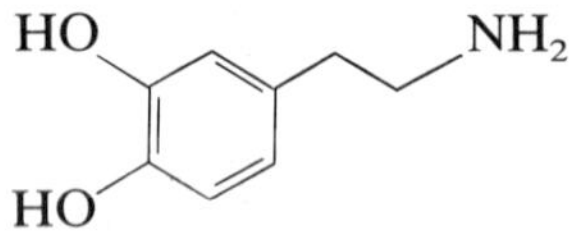

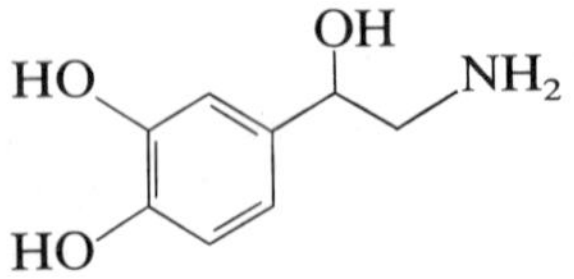

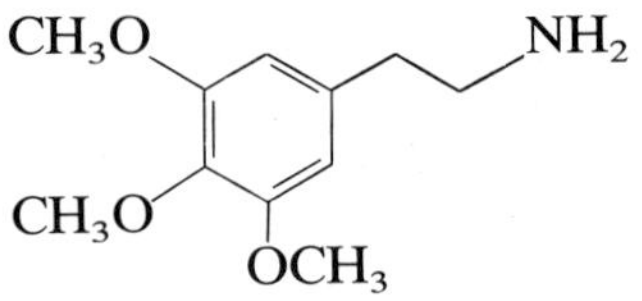

60.**3**

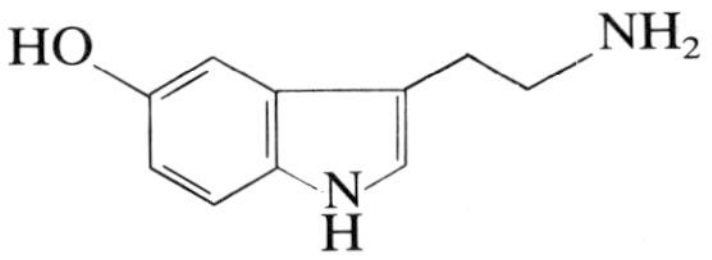

60.**4**

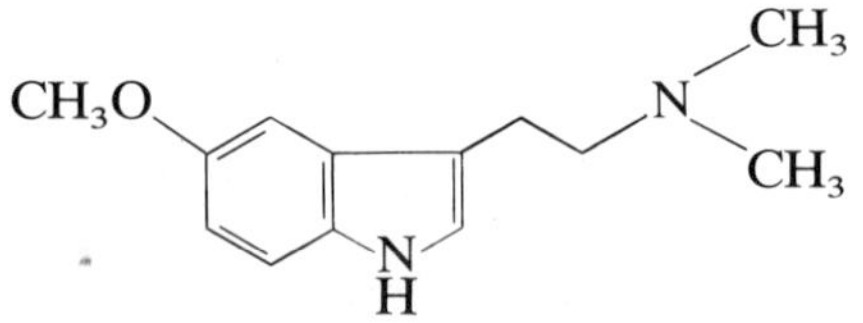

60.**5**

60.**6**

transmitter and is closely analogous to the potent hallucinogen 5-methoxy-*N,N*-dimethyltryptamine (60.**5**). The neurotransmitter acetylcholine (60.**6**) is a simple aliphatic ester which is separated by two carbon atoms from a nitrogen atom. By means of the fixed three-dimensional geometry found in the alkaloid atropine (60.**7**) this spatial separation is maintained. Atropine is the structural prototype of the class of anticholinergic hallucinogens, some of the more potent examples of which again display the actual two-carbon separation (i.e., quinuclidinyl benzilate, 60.**8**). The neurotransmitter γ-aminobutyric acid (60.**9**) is a close structural analog of the active component of the mushroom *Amanita muscaria*, muscimol (60.**10**). Although the remaining families of hallucinogenic drugs are more complex in structure than these prototypes, most still maintain within their structures the nucleus of one of these endogenous transmitters.

60.**1**

60.**2**

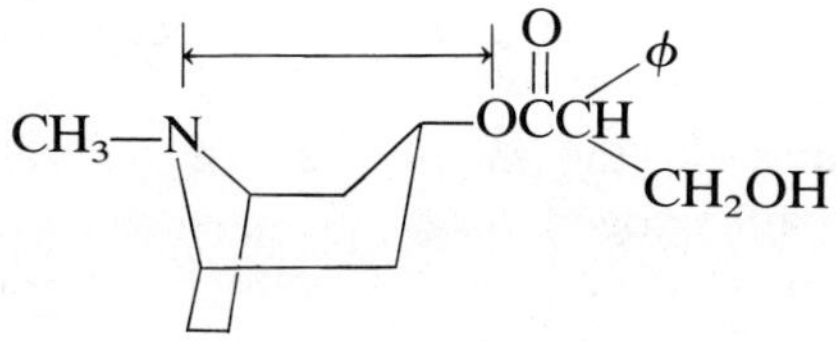

CH$_3$—N

60.7

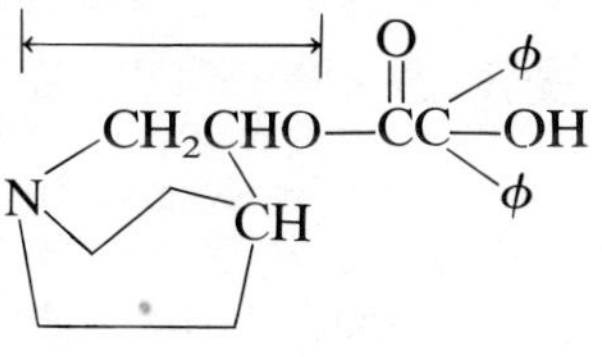

60.8

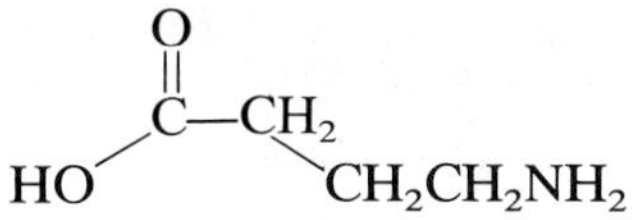

HO O C—CH$_2$ CH$_2$CH$_2$NH$_2$

60.9

HN O C—CH C—CH$_2$NH$_2$ O

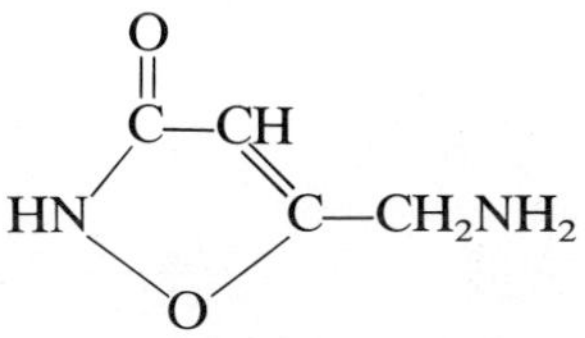

60.10

Another close connection between the hallucinogenic drugs and endogenous chemistry is apparent from the increasingly frequent reports of the ability of the body to generate them in the course of apparently normal metabolism. As an example, the simplest of the tryptamine hallucinogens, N,N-dimethyltryptamine (DMT, 60.11) has been found repeatedly in the blood and urine of humans (see Ref. 31 for a recent review). However, the levels observed are extremely low, and a causal role in problems of mental health is questionable, there being no consistent difference in normal and psychotic patients. Moreover, there is no evidence that 60.11 is endogenously produced; it might be a product of diet or of incidental bacterial

synthesis. The 5-hydroxy analog of DMT is bufotenine (60.12), an alkaloid found widely in nature and a known animal toxin. It was originally claimed to be a hallucinogen (32) but now the responses following its administration are considered largely cardiovascular, mediated by serotonin release (33–35). It, like DMT, appears in human urine at extremely low levels (36, 37). 3,4-Dimethoxyphenethylamine (60.19d) is the O,O-dimethyl ether of the neurotransmitter dopamine (60.1), and is responsible for the "pink spot" in the urinanalyses of schizophrenic patients (38). It is believed to be present in varying amounts in all individuals (39) and may appear only periodically (40). There is no indication that it is formed from dopamine, and it is apparently not active per se as a hallucinogen (41, 42). Still another close connection exists between neurotransmitters and alleged hallucinogens: epinephrine (60.13) is readily oxidized to an indolic species, adrenochrome (60.14) in the presence of air in vitro or enzymatically

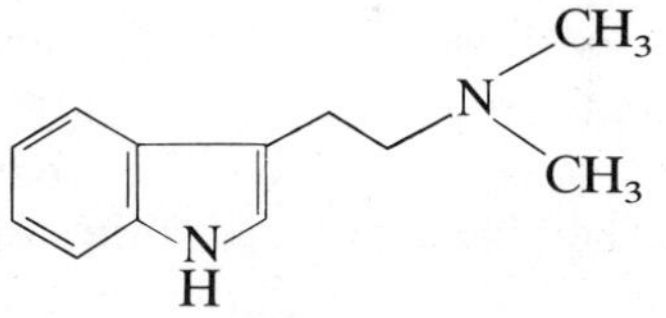

60.11

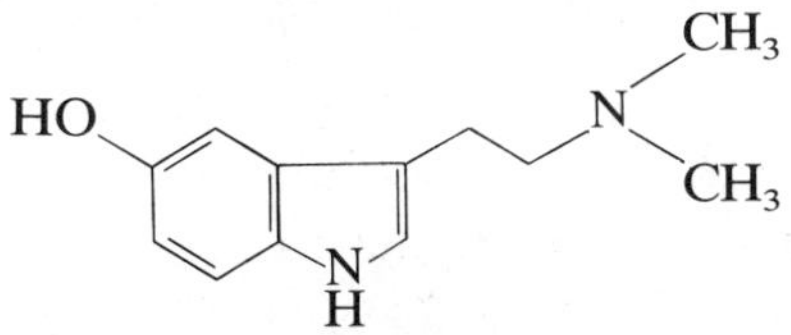

60.12

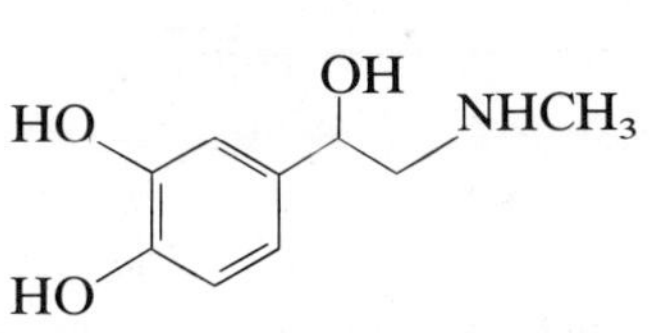

60.13

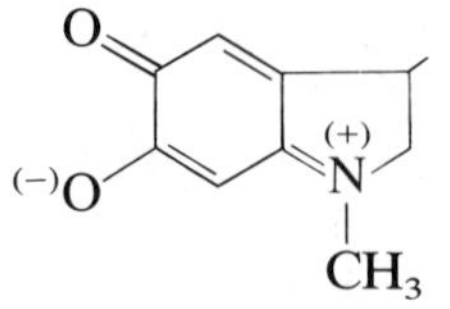

60.**14**

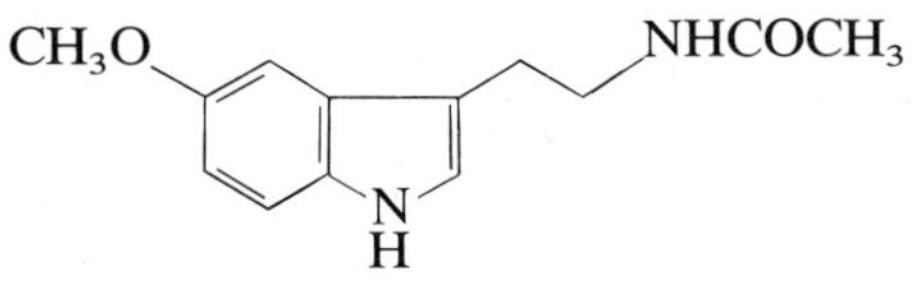

60.**15**

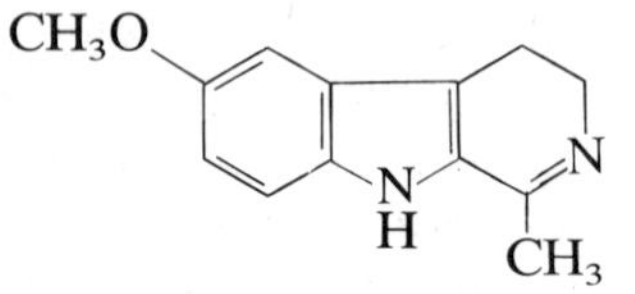

60.**16**

in vivo (43). Originally proposed as a hypothetical endogenous factor in mental illness, it has been reported to produce mood and perceptual changes (44); these properties have not been confirmed by other workers and the question remains unresolved (45). Again, little or none of this chemical is found in normal human serum (46). Finally, the hormone melatonin (60.**15**), associated with the pineal gland, can undergo facile cyclization to 60.**16** *in vitro* under physiological conditions (47), and there is a single report (48) that it has central activity in man. However, all attempts to identify it in body fluids or tissue extracts have failed.

Thus although potentially a number of naturally occurring factors can give rise to possible hallucinogens in the intact organism, none of these products has been satisfactorily incorporated into a lasting hypothesis concerning endogenous origins of mental illness.

4.2 Biotransformations of Hallucinogens

Studies on the metabolism of several of the hallucinogen drugs may shed some light on their mechanism of action within the body.

Oxidative deamination is one of the most frequently reported biotransformation routes among the hallucinogenic drugs. In amines located on a primary carbon, the usual products are the corresponding acid or the reduced alcohol; with amines attached to a secondary carbon, the product is usually the ketone (see Fig. 60.1). although most primary amines are deaminated by the enzyme monoamine oxidase (MAO) (49), mescaline (60.**3**), the best studied of the phenethylamine hallucinogenics, is uniquely refractory to this enzyme (50). Yet the oxidation product 3,4,5-trimethoxyphenylacetic acid is the major metabolite in the five species studied (including man) and appears to be produced enzymatically by an enzyme similar to diamine oxidase (51, 52). The α-methyl group that is found on most of the phenethylamine hallucinogenics provides a carbon skeleton identical to that of amphetamine, and structurally precludes MAO-induced conversion to the phenylacetic acid. However, oxidative deamination does occur in three of these materials, PMA (60.**22g**), MDA (60.**22o**), and DOM (60.**22aa**), to form the corresponding phenylacetone (53–55). Because none of these metabolites has been demonstrated to show biologic activity, this manner of biotransformation must be considered to be largely detoxifying.

A second major metabolic process encountered is *O*-demethylation or dealkylation. Five mono- or di-dimethylated metabolites of mescaline (60.**3**) are known (56), the three possible demethylation products of DOM (60.**22aa**) have been characterized and identified (57), and each of the three methoxyl group carbons of TMA-2 (60.**22b**) can appear separately as expired

$$ArCH_2CH_2NR_2 \longrightarrow ArCH_2COOH \quad (ArCH_2CH_2OH)$$

$$ArCH_2\underset{\underset{R'}{|}}{C}HNR_2 \longrightarrow ArCH_2\overset{\overset{O}{\|}}{C}R'$$

Fig. 60.1 Oxidative deamination of amines.

CO_2 (58). MDA (60.**22o**) contains a methylenedioxy ring rather than methoxyl groups, but this too has been demonstrated to be dealkylated metabolically (59). In each case a phenol, a catechol, or a hydroquinone is generated. These species are highly reactive chemically, and at least one product of known pharmacological efficacy (α-methyldopamine) (60) is formed.

The third principal metabolic route common to the hallucinogenic drugs is oxidation. Benzylic oxidation had been reported with both DOM (60.**22aa**) and DOET (60.**22bb**) (61, 62). Of greater theoretical interest is oxidative cyclization to form an indole species, reminiscent of the conversion of epinephrine to adrenochrome. Many of the hallucinogens are in fact indoles, and since the phenethylamine chain has the exact atom composition of indole itself, there has been frequent speculation that there might be some metabolic conversion from one family to the other. It has been shown (63) that one of the metabolites of DOM (2,5-dihydroxyphenylisopropylamine, 60.**17**), which bears a close chemical and pharmacological resemblance to the potent neurodegenerative agent 6-hydroxydopamine (60.**18**) (64), can undergo a facile oxidative cyclization to form a 5-hydroxyindole. The intermediate iminoquinone is potentially very reactive with nucleophilic agents found in normal body chemistry, and may be important in any explanation of biological activity.

In the following sections, the several known families of hallucinogens are presented in a format that allows correlation between their structures and their relative potencies in man. Synthetic compounds reported as hallucinogenic, based solely on animal screening, are not included.

5 β-PHENETHYLAMINES

The oldest known hallucinogen, and one of the most thoroughly studied, is mescaline (3,4,5-trimethoxyphenethylamine, 60.**3**). It was originally isolated from the peyote cactus of the southwestern United States and northern Mexico at the end of the last century (65) and its structure was verified by synthesis some 20 years later (66). Al-

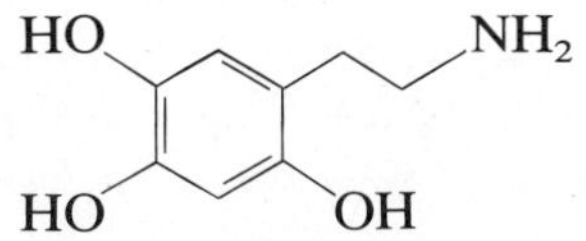

60.**18**

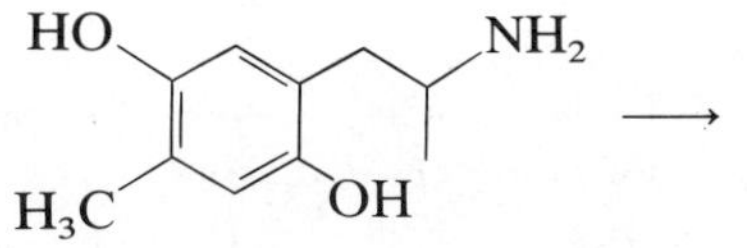

60.**17**

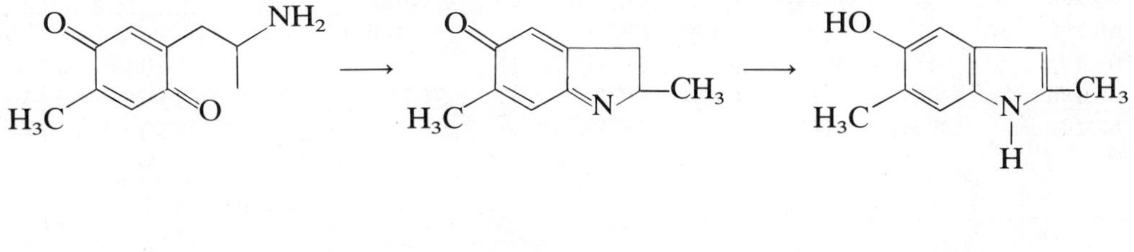

though it is one of the least potent of all of the hallucinogens known, it has been explored clinically in a large number of studies. The varied symptoms of central intoxication that it can elicit have provided a basic qualitative vocabulary for the description of other hallucinogenic drugs. Quantitatively, mescaline also can serve as a standard; the majority of studies have claimed consistent intoxication following an orally administered dose of 300–500 mg of the sulfate salt (67, 68) (equivalent to 225–375 mg of the free base), and an effective acute dosage has been accepted as 350 mg. Dividing this value by the observed effective level of a structurally related drug gives the potency relative to mescaline (Tables 60.1 and 60.2). These values, being derived from activity ranges, are only approximate (±25%, Ref. 75). Those analogs that have been assayed in human subjects are listed in Table 60.1, along with their relative potencies.

Several mescaline analogs require special comment. The vicinal 2,3,4 isomer (60.**19a**) has been studied in schizophrenic patients wherein it has appeared to be more effective than mescaline itself (69). This is a reversal of the effects reported in normal subjects; dosages are not given, but they must be presumed to be similar to those of mescaline. The 2,4,5 isomer is reported to be inactive by itself, although it appears to potentiate the action of mescaline when used as a pretreatment (71). DMPEA (60.**19d**) has already been discussed as the pink spot component in the urinanalyses of schizophrenic patients. At mescaline-like dosages 60.**19d** appears to be without action; it has been reported to have a mild stimulant action at the relatively high level of 1500 mg (76).

Modifications on the chain portion of the mescaline molecule are known. The insertion of an oxygen atom between the chain and the aromatic ring to give 60.**20** elimi-

Table 60.1 Hallucinogenic β-Phenethylamines

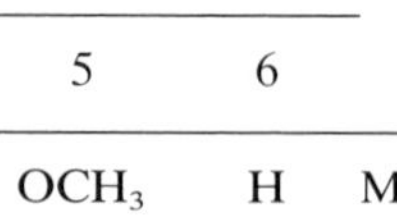

60.**19**

Structure No.	Substitution Position of R: 2	3	4	5	6	Name	Potency Relative to Mescaline	Ref.
60.**3**	H	OCH_3	OCH_3	OCH_3	H	Mescaline	1	67, 68
60.**19a**	OCH_3	OCH_3	OCH_3	H	H	—	~1	69
60.**19b**	OCH_3	H	OCH_3	OCH_3	H	—	<1	70, 71
60.**19c**	H	H	OCH_3	H	H	—	<1	72
60.**19d**	H	OCH_3	OCH_3	H	H	DMPEA	<1	41, 42
60.**19e**	H	OCH_3	OEt	OCH_3	H	Escaline	6	73
60.**19f**	H	OCH_3	OPr	OCH_3	H	Proscaline	6	73
60.**19g**	H	OCH_3	SCH_3	OCH_3	H	—	10	73
60.**19h**	OCH_3	H	CH_3	OCH_3	H	2-CD	20	74
60.**19i**	OCH_3	H	Br	OCH_3	H	2-CB	30	74

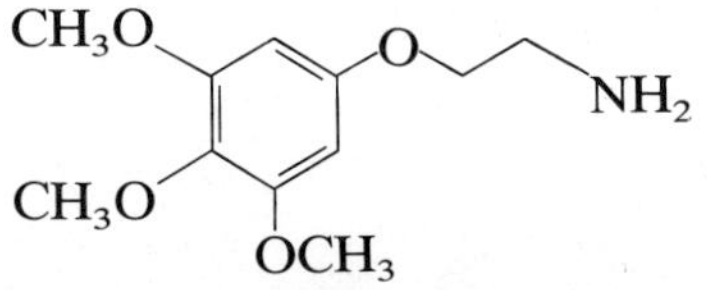

60.**20**

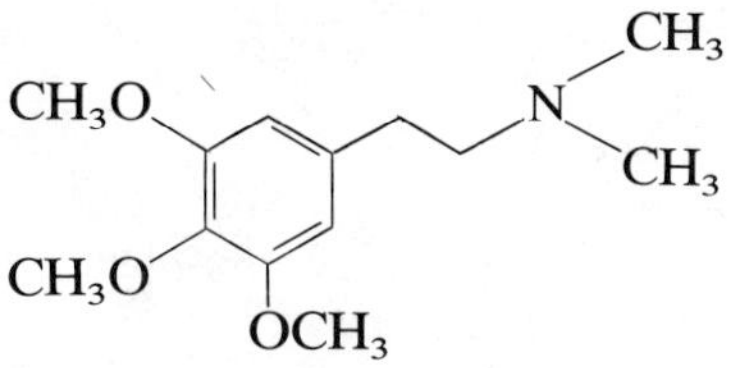

60.**21**

nates the hallucinogenic activity (77), as does the homologation at the nitrogen either to the monomethyl (78) or to the dimethyl homolog trichocerine (60.**21**; 76, 79, 80). Similarly, the neutral *N*-acetyl analog is not active (81). Only the addition of a methyl group at the α-carbon (next to the primary amino group) affords maintenance and extension of hallucinogenic activity; such compounds are discussed in the following section.

6 PHENYLISOPROPYLAMINES

The largest known family of hallucinogens is the group of substitution derivatives of phenylisopropylamine (2-amino-1-phenyl-propane, amphetamine). The several compounds in this family are listed in Table 60.2, arranged by chemical subgroup rather than by potency. They are frequently referred to in the literature by the code initials given.

The exact homolog to mescaline is TMA (60.**22a**), which was prepared as representing an amalgamation of the structures of two well-established centrally active drugs, mescaline and amphetamine (82). The material proved to be an effective hallucinogen (83) about twice as potent as mescaline (84). The remaining five positional isomers have been prepared and

evaluated, and with the exception of TMA-3 (60.**22c**), all have proved to be active hallucinogens in man. The 2,4,5-trisubstituted isomer TMA-2 (60.**22b**) is the most potent of these six, and this substitution pattern frequently emerges in the structures of active hallucinogenic agents.

Compounds with fewer methoxyl groups are known to be active, although their properties are sometimes a blend of the hallucinogen and the stimulant. The 4-monomethoxyanalog PMA (60.**22g**) is an active hallucinogen at 60–80 mg, but even at this level precipitous hypertension and cardiovascular stimulation have been observed. A number of deaths have been associated with the use of this drug (98). Two of the dimethoxy analogs that have been studied (60.**22h**, 60.**22i**) are active at the 1 mg/kg level in man but both are difficult to titrate quantitatively because they demonstrate extensive amphetamine-like CNS stimulation at hallucinogenically marginal dosages. The isomer corresponding to dopamine (3,4-DMA, 60.**22j**) when administered intravenously at dosages similar to those employed with mescaline elicited extensive visual distortions, but there were complications of gross body tremor (86). Only one of the three possible tetramethoxy analogs has been reported to be hallucinogenic. Of the several ether homologs that have been studied, the 4-ethoxy homolog of TMA-2 (MEM, 60.**22m**) is noteworthy because it maintains the potency of the parent compound. Homologation at the 2 or the 5 position leads to decreased effectiveness as hallucinogens (99).

A number of hallucinogenic drugs are known with a methylenedioxy group located in place in two adjacent methoxyl groups. The simplest of these and one of the best studied is MDA (60.**22o**). Unlike the open ring dimethoxy analog, MDA is active in the 80–120 mg range. It is unusual among the hallucinogens in that it leads not to the usual mescaline-like state of

Table 60.2 Hallucinogenic Derivatives of Phenylisopropylamine

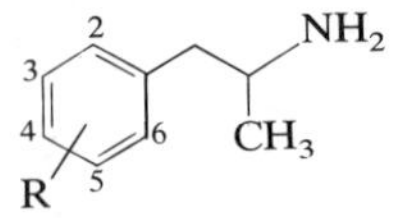

60.**22**

Structure No.	Substitution Position of R					Name	Potency Relative to Mescaline	Ref.
	2	3	4	5	6			
60.**22a**	H	OCH_3	OCH_3	OCH_3	H	TMA	2	83, 84
60.**22b**	OCH_3	H	OCH_3	OCH_3	H	TMA-2	20	85
60.**22c**	OCH_3	OCH_3	OCH_3	H	H	TMA-3	<2	85
60.**22d**	OCH_3	OCH_3	H	OCH_3	H	TMA-4	4	75
60.**22e**	OCH_3	OCH_3	H	H	OCH_3	TMA-5	10	75
60.**22f**	OCH_3	H	OCH_3	H	OCH_3	TMA-6	10	75
60.**22g**	H	H	OCH_3	H	H	PMA	6	75
60.**22h**	OCH_3	H	OCH_3	H	H	2,4-DMA	6	78
60.**22i**	OCH_3	H	H	OCH_3	H	2,5-DMA	6	78
60.**22j**	H	OCH_3	OCH_3	H	H	3,4-DMA	~1	86
60.**22k**	OCH_3	OCH_3	OCH_3	OCH_3	H	—	6	75
60.**22l**	H	OCH_3	$OCH_2\phi$	OCH_3	H	—	2	78
60.**22m**	OCH_3	H	OEt	OCH_3	H	MEM	20	78
60.**22o**	H	O—CH_2—O		H	H	MDA	3	87–89
60.**22p**	H	OCH_3	O—CH_2—O		H	MMDA	3	90, 91
60.**22q**	OCH_3	H	O—CH_2—O		H	MMDA-2	10	85
60.**22r**	OCH_3	O—CH_2O		H	OCH_3	MMDA-3a	10	85
60.**22s**	O—CH_2—O		OCH_3	H	H	MMDA-3b	3	85
60.**22t**	O—CH_2—O		H	H	OCH_3	MMDA-5	10	78
60.**22u**	OCH_3	O—CH_2—O		OCH_3	H	DMMDA	12	92
60.**22v**	OCH_3	OCH_3	O—CH_2—O		H	DMMDA-2	5	92
60.**22w**	OCH_3	H	SCH_3	OCH_3	H	p-DOT (Aleph-1)	40	93
60.**22x**	OCH_3	H	SEt	OCH_3	H	Aleph-2	80	78
60.**22y**	OCH_3	H	SPr(i)	OCH_3	H	Aleph-4	40	94
60.**22z**	OCH_3	H	SPr(n)	OCH_3	H	Aleph-7	60	94
60.**22aa**	OCH_3	H	CH_3	OCH_3	H	DOM (STP)	80	78, 95
60.**22bb**	OCH_3	H	Et	OCH_3	H	DOET	100	78, 96
60.**22cc**	OCH_3	H	Pr(n)	OCH_3	H	DOPR	80	14
60.**22dd**	OCH_3	H	Bu(n)	OCH_3	H	DOBU	40	14
60.**22ee**	OCH_3	H	Am(n)	OCH_3	H	DOAM	10	14
60.**22ff**	OCH_3	H	Br	OCH_3	H	DOB	400	97
60.**22gg**	OCH_3	H	I	OCH_3	H	DOI	400	78

visual and sensory distortion, but rather to a state of sensory amplification and enhancement without appreciable sympathomimetic stimulation. This property has led to extensive studies of this material in conjunction with psychotherapy, where there is usually seen an easy communication between subject and observer, or between subjects (87–89). This affective interaction is even more clearly evident in the N-methyl homolog of MDA, MDMA (60.**23a**) which is substantially free of per-

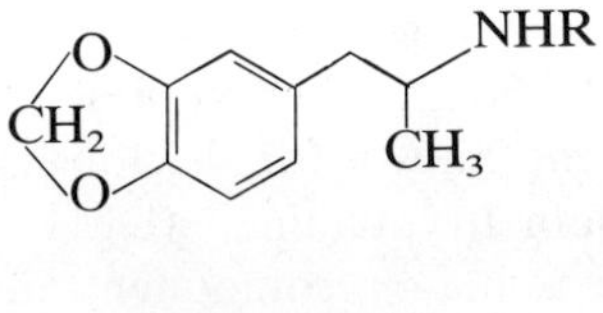

60.**23a**   R = CH$_3$
60.**23b**   R = C$_2$H$_5$

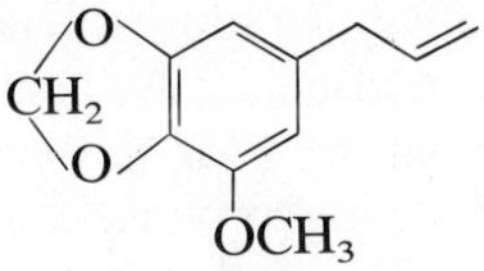

60.**24**

ceptual distortion at effective dosages (75–150 mg, Ref. 93). The N-ethyl counterpart (MDE, 60.**23b**) is similar in action except that it is about 25% less potent. Of all the variously substituted phenylisopropylamines that have been N-methylated and titrated in man (including the homologs of TMA-2, 2,5-DMA, DOM, and DOB: 60.**22b**, 60.**22i**, 60.**22aa**, and 60.**22ff**, respectively), it is only the methylenedioxy compound 60.**23a** that has maintained quantitative potency (94). As with mescaline itself, dimethylation of this compound eliminates any central action. There are six monomethoxy analogs of MDA possible, and five of them have been synthesized and reported. The isomer most closely related to natural products (to both mescaline and to the major essential oil of the intoxicant nutmeg, myristicin 60.**24**) is MMDA (60.**22p**). This base has been extensively explored in psychotherapy (100). The four additional isomers are listed in Table 60.2; it should be noted that the code employed is consistent with the oxygen placement of the TMA series. Thus there are two possible vicinal 2,3,4 isomers and no 2,4,6 isomer is possible. The 2,3,5 isomer is presently unknown. Two dimethoxymethylenedioxyphenylisopropylamines (of six possible isomers) are known to be active in man; these (60.**22u**, 60.**22v**) have the above correspondence to the two essential oils apiole and dill-apiole. Other isomers

are known chemically but are unexplored pharmacologically (101).

The 4 position of the 2,4,5 trisubstitution pattern has a profound influence on the quantitative potency of the molecule as can be seen in the parent 2,5-dimethoxyphenylisopropylamine as the group substituted at this position is varied (60.**25**).

The replacement of the 4-methoxyl group with a 4-thiomethyl group provides a doubling of potency, and a change in the qualitative nature of the induced intoxication with a minimum of the perceptual distortion and reality loss that are characteristic of mescaline and LSD, but rather with an enhanced intellectual integrative capacity that has been named an "aleph" effect. The ethyl and n-propyl analogs of this sulfur compound are of increased potency over the methyl prototype. The substitution of an aliphatic alkyl group at this 4 position doubles the potency again, and qualitatively produces effects that more closely resemble LSD. Again the ethyl homolog (60.**22bb**) is the highest in potency. The fifth class of 4 substitutents that has been studied is the halogens. Both the 4-bromo and the 4-iodo analogs (60.**22ff**, 60.**22gg**) are effective in man at about 1 mg total dose and are relatively long-lived in duration. Their qualitative effects closely resemble the methylenedioxy analogs already discussed but at somewhat increased dosages display a true hallucinogenic syndrome (102).

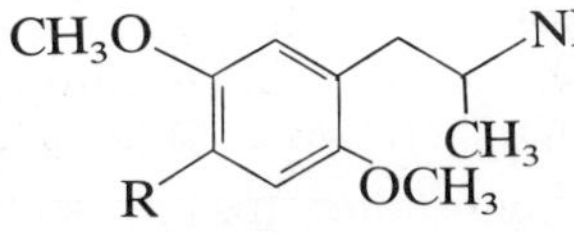

60.**25**

	R	Name	Potency (Mescaline = 1)
60.**22i**	H	DMA	8
60.**22b**	OCH$_3$	TMA-2	20
60.**22w**	SCH$_3$	para-DOT	40
60.**22aa**	CH$_3$	DOM (STP)	80
60.**22ff**	Br	DOB	400

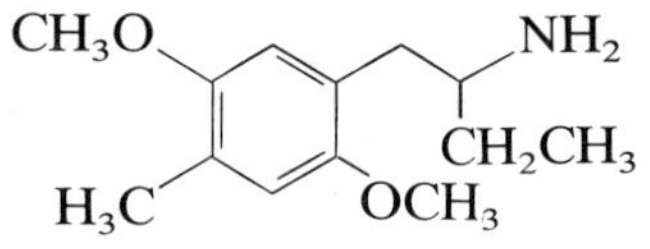

60.**26**

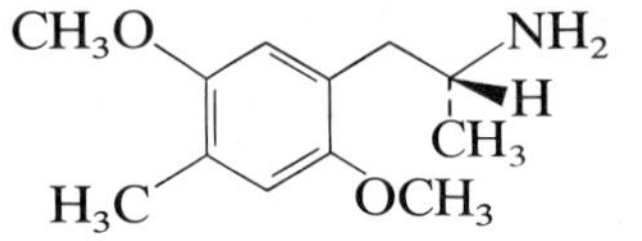

60.**27**

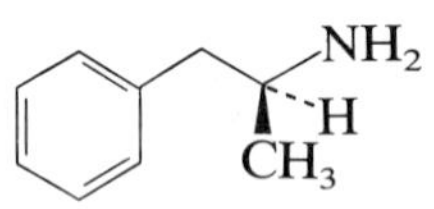

60.**28**

The homologation of the three-carbon amphetamine chain to the corresponding secondary butyl counterpart completely eradicates the hallucinogenic effects of the molecule. The α-ethyl homolog of DOM (60.**22aa**) is 60.**26,** which is an effective antidepressant (103, 104) that is undergoing clinical trials.

Studies of the optically active isomers of these racemic hallucinogens have shown that in most cases [MDA, 60.**22o** (105); DOM, 60.**22aa** (107); DOET, 60.**22bb** (108); and DOB, 60.**22ff** (94)] the hallucinogenic potency is associated with the absolute (R) configuration. This orientation is shown in the case of DOM (see 60.**27**) and is opposite to that possessed by dextroamphetamine (60.**28**). An exception to this generality is seen in the case of N-methyl-3,4 - methylenedioxyphenylisopropylamine (60.**23a**) wherein the (S) configuration is the major contributor to the activity reported for the racemate (109).

7 TRYPTAMINES

A large family of hallucinogens is known that contains the parent indole ring and carries various substitutions on the aromatic ring and/or on the primary amine nitrogen (see Table 60.3). The simplest compound and the one known for the longest time is N,N-dimethyltryptamine (DMT, 60.**11**), which is a major component of various New World snuffs and psychotropic drug decoctions. It is of relatively low potency, and in man is biologically active only by parenteral administration. It has been extensively studied clinically, and has served as a prototypal drug for this entire family. Dosages of 25 mg produce only a vague restlessness (33), the threshold being about 50 mg; the usual clinically effective dose is 75 mg. Orally, five times this amount is without effect. It is of extremely rapid onset by either injection or inhalation, with the first effects of central activity being apparent within a minute or two following administration. The effects are largely dissipated within the hour. The N,N-diethyl homolog of DMT is DET (60.**29a**), which is a little more potent and is of a more prolonged chronology of action. Following intramuscular administration, the onset is noticed in about 45 min, and the effects persist for 3 hr (123). The N,N-dipropyl counterpart (60.**29b**) is comparable in potency, effect, and duration, except that the termination of the intoxication is quite abrupt, a potentially useful clinical property (113, 124). This latter compound is, as are the diallyl and the diisopropyl analogs, orally active in man.

The substitution of an oxygen atom at the 4 position of the indole ring leads to compounds of increased potency, which are all orally active. The simplest of these is 4-hydroxyl-N,N-dimethyltryptamine (psilocin, 60.**29e**), which is the naturally occurring hallucinogenic component (along with its phosphate ester psilocybin, 60.**29f**) of the many "magic" mushrooms of the Western Hemisphere (125). Because the two drugs appear to be symptomatically and stoichiometrically identical in man, it is reasonable to assume 60.**29f** is converted to 60.**29e** *in vivo*. Psilocybin is the more stable

Table 60.3 Hallucinogenic Tryptamines

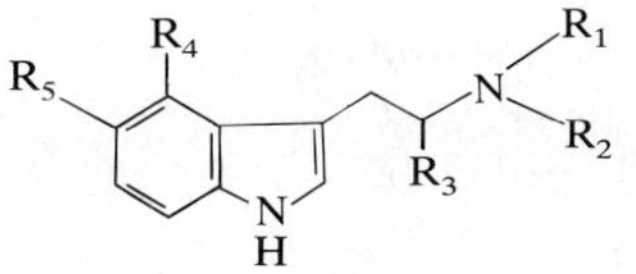

60.**29**

Structure No.	Substitution Position of R					Name	Potency Relative to DMT(=1)	Ref.
	1	2	3	4	5			
60.**11**	CH_3	CH_3	H	H	H	DMT	1	110
60.**29a**	C_2H_5	C_2H_5	H	H	H	DET	1	111
60.**29b**	n-C_3H_7	n-C_3H_7	H	H	H	DPT	1	112, 113
60.**29c**	i-C_3H_7	i-C_3H_7	H	H	H	DIPT	1.5	114
60.**29d**	Allyl	Allyl	H	H	H	—	1	115
60.**29e**	CH_3	CH_3	H	OH	H	Psilocin	8	116
60.**29f**	CH_3	CH_3	H	OPO_3H_2	H	Psilocybin	6	117, 118
60.**29g**	C_2H_5	C_2H_5	H	OH	H	CZ-74	8	119
60.**29h**	C_2H_5	C_2H_5	H	OPO_3H_2	H	CEY-19	6	119
60.**5**	CH_3	CH_3	H	H	OCH_3	5-MeO-DMT	10	93
60.**29i**	i-C_3H_7	i-C_3H_7	H	H	OCH_3	5-MeO-DIPT	10	120
60.**29j**	H	H	CH_3	H	H	Monase-M	3	121, 122
60.**29k**	H	H	CH_3	H	OCH_3	DMS	20	93

of the two alkaloids and has been studied very widely, both from the viewpoint of its transcendental and psychedelic properties (in emulation of its religious use in native Mexican populations) as well as neurologically (in search for physiological explanations of the observed sensory properties). A single dosage of 4–8 mg of 60.**29f** as a pure chemical duplicates a 2 g ingestion of dried *Psilocybe mexicana* constituting a score of more individual plants. Most experimental studies have employed the drug in the 5–15 mg range, although 30 mg levels have been reported (126). The diethyl homologs of both psilocin and psilocybin have been evaluated psychopharmacologically; they are of comparable potency quantitatively, but are of shorter duration and may be preferred for this reason in psychiatric practice (119). The *N*-demethylated homologs of psilocybin (*N*-monode-

methyl = baeocystin; *N*-didemethyl = norbaeocystin) have been established as occasional major components in several of the biologically active mushroom species (127, 128), but they are as yet unexplored pharmacologically.

Substitution at the indolic 5 position leads to compounds that are structurally similar to the neurotransmitter serotonin (60.**4**). The simplest structure is 5-hydroxy-*N,N*-dimethyltryptamine(bufotenine, 60.**12**), which has already been discussed as a cardiovascular stimulant that has been misassigned as a hallucinogen. Methylation of the 5-hydroxy group leads to the formation of the parenterally active hallucinogenic 5-MeO-DMT (60.**5**) effective in the 6–10 mg range. It has been reported as a natural component of several snuff mixtures used by the Indians in the New World. It is of exceptionally short duration of action, the initial intoxication occurring within seconds of administration, and the entire recovery completed usually within 15 min. The replacement of the methyl groups on the basic nitrogen with groups of increased steric bulk (as seen in the *N,N*-diisopropyl compound 60.**29i** and the mono-*tert*-butyl counterpart) results in hallucinogenic drugs that have similar potency but are active orally.

The addition of an α-methyl group to the ethylamine side chain produces a structure that superficially resembles the amphetamine molecule. In an apparently similar manner, the resulting products are refractory to metabolism, and are orally active as hallucinogens as the primary amines. α-Methyltryptamine (60.**29j**), at dosages of 20 mg, produces an intoxication that has been equated to 50 μg of LSD in intensity, although there is a slow onset and an unusually long duration of action (to 24 hr) (129, 130). The addition of a methoxy group at the 5 position results in 60.**29k,** of greatly increased potency but still of an unusually long duration of action (93).

A number of isomers and homologs of these alkylated tryptamines have been evaluated in clinical studies. The homologation of the α-methyl group of 60.**29j** to an ethyl radical results in a drug that has been employed experimentally as an antidepressant under the trade name of Monase (60.**30**, 129). It is considerably less potent than 60.**29j**, with dosages of 150 mg needed to produce a talkative intoxication. The addition of a methyl group at the 4 position yields α,4-dimethyltryptamine, 60.**31**, which has also been reported to have antidepressant properties, but there are no experimental details given (131). The lengthening of the side chain of DMT

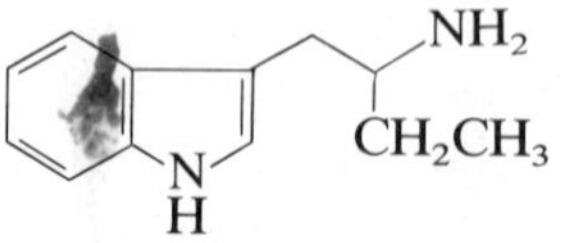

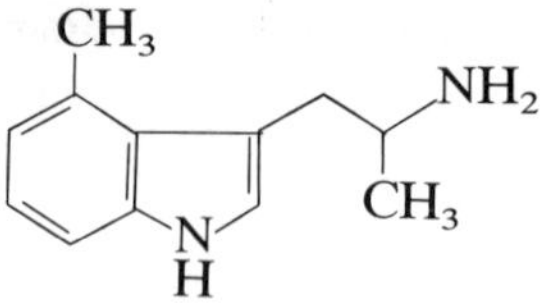

60.**31**

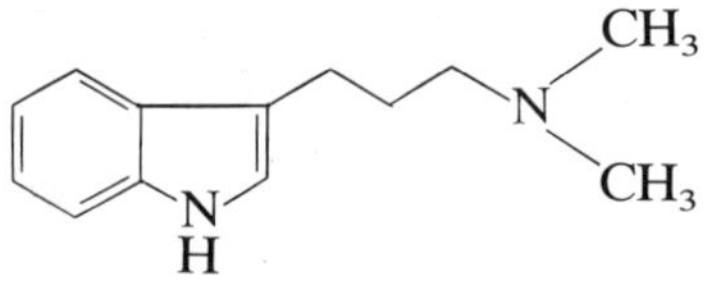

60.**32**

to three carbon atoms results in 60.**32,** which was without central effects following parenteral administration of 80 mg (33).

8   LYSERGIC ACID AMIDES

It was the discovery by Hofmann of the extraordinary potency and psychopharmacological complexity of lysergic acid diethylamide (60.**33a**) that literally ushered in the intense popular interest in the hallucinogenic drugs. The compound was first synthesized in 1938 as one of a large series of amides of lysergic acid to be studied for potential ergot-like potential (132). Its central activity was uncovered by accident in 1943 and has led to an extraordinary volume of research and publication in both the scientific and the paramedical world.

The lysergic acid four-ring nucleus possesses two asymmetric centers requiring four isomeric forms. All have been prepared and the hallucinogenic action is uniquely ascribable to the stereoisomer 60.**33a**. The 8-substituent, lying between two unsaturated systems, is easily epimerized with base. Thus a common synthetic contaminant in syntheses involving the lysergic acid ring system is the pharmacologically inert iso form as shown in 60.**33b**. A second position of exceptional chemical sensitivity is the double bond located at the 9,10 position. In either water or alcohol

60.**30**

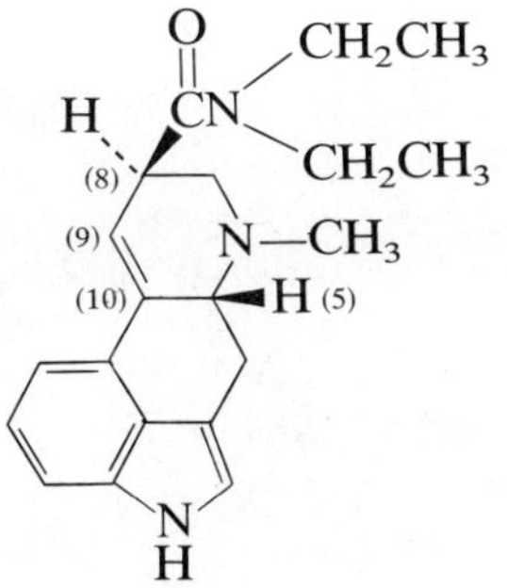

60.33

	5	8	Name
a	◀H	⫽⫽⫽H	*d*-LSD
b	◀H	◀H	*d*-isoLSD
c	⫽⫽⫽H	◀H	*l*-LSD
d	⫽⫽⫽H	⫽⫽⫽H	*l*-isoLSD

solution, a molecule of solvent is readily added, especially under the influence of UV irradiation. The products formed are presumably largely devoid of LSD-like action.

Many variations of the LSD molecule have been made in studies designed to account for the high activity and the qualitative nature of the LSD intoxication. Most modifications have involved variations of the alkyl groups on the amide nitrogen, or substitution on the indolic neutral nitrogen atom. Those that have been studied in man are listed in Table 60.4, and their comparative potencies are listed with the structures. None of these isomers is more potent than LSD itself, although the acetyl analog 60.**34b,** probably very labile *in vivo*, is equally potent. LSD is active in man, following oral administration, at threshold levels as low as 15 μg, of the tartrate salt. The nominally effective dosage is accepted as 50–100 μg. The 2-bromo analog of LSD (BOL-148) represents a challenging compound in that it is of similar intense serotonin antagonism pharmacologically, but is largely devoid of hallucinogenic activity. The explicit requirement for the intact *N,N*-diethyl structure of the amide portion

of LSD remains an unresolved enigma in this family of compounds.

The seeds of three species of plants have had a long-known reputation for being hallucinogenic, and have been found to contain ergot-like alkaloids. A morning glory plant known by the Aztec name of ololiuqui has been identified botanically as *Rivea corymbosa* (139). A second plant with seeds known to the Zapotec as badoh negro is a closely related *Convolvulacea* with the binomial *Ipomoea violacea* (140). The third source is the Hawaiian baby woodrose, *Argyreia nervosa*, which has been used historically in India. The alkaloid composition of these seeds is a fraction of a percent of their dry weight, but is made up largely of lysergic acid amide (60.**34o**) and the epimer isoergine (60.**35**). The labile acetaldehyde adducts lysergic acid-α-hydroxyethylamide (60.**36**) and the iso-counterpart (60.**37**) are apparently present in some samples, as are five additional minor alkaloids, ergometrine (60.**38**), elymoclavine (60.**39**), chanoclavine (60.**40**), lysergol (60.**41**) and agroclavine (60.**42**). The structures of the D ring portion of these several ergot-like alkaloids are illustrated, and the relative composition of the various morning glory seeds are listed in Table 60.5.

Several studies of contradictory nature have been reported concerning the human psychopharmacology of these seeds; the consumption of 100 or more seeds can lead to a state of apathy and listlessness (146) or to no effects at all, whereas effects have been reported from as few as six seeds (148). These discrepancies may be due to the extremely hard coat that these seeds have (149), which allows them to pass intact through the digestive system. Human studies on ergine (60.**34o**) (150–152) and isoergine (60.**35**) (150) would indicate that these two alkaloids may account for much of the effects of the total seed, either directly or via the hydroxyethylamide precursors.

Table 60.4 Hallucinogenic Lysergic Acid Amides

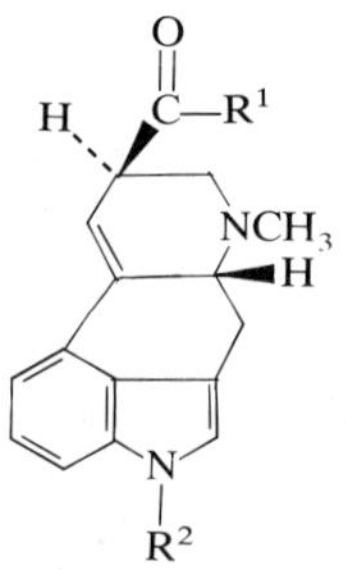

60.34

Structure No.	R^1	R^2	Name	Potency Relative to LSD^a	Ref.
60.**33a**	$N(CH_2CH_3)_2$	H	LSD-25	++++	
60.**34a**	$N(CH_2CH_3)_2$	CH_3	MLD-41	+++	13, 133
60.**34b**	$N(CH_2CH_3)_2$	$COCH_3$	ALD-52	++++	134
60.**34c**	$N(CH_2CH_3)_2$	CH_2OH	OML-632	+++	13, 133
60.**34d**	$NHCH_2CH_3$	H	LAE-32	++	134
60.**34e**	$NHCH_2CH_3$	CH_3	MLA-74	+	13
60.**34f**	$NHCH_2CH_3$	$COCH_3$	ALA-10	+	13
60.**34g**	$N(CH_2)_4$	H	LPD-824	++	13, 135
60.**34h**	$N(CH_2)_4$	CH_3	MPD-75	+	13
60.**34i**	$N(CH_2)_2O(CH_2)_2$	H	LSM-775	+++	13, 135
60.**34j**	$N(CH_3)_2$	H	DAM-57	++	13, 133
60.**34k**	$N(CH_3)CH_2CH_3$	H	LME	+	136
60.**34l**	$N(CH_3)CH_2CH_2CH_3$	H	LMP, LAMP	+	136
60.**34m**	$N(CH_2CH_3)CH_2CH_2CH_3$	H	LEP	+++	136
60.**34n**	$N(CH_2CH_2CH_3)_2$	H	—	++	137
60.**34o**	NH_2	H	LA-111	+	138

^{a} LSD = ++++; +++ = one-third the potency; ++ = one-tenth the potency; + = less than one-tenth the potency.

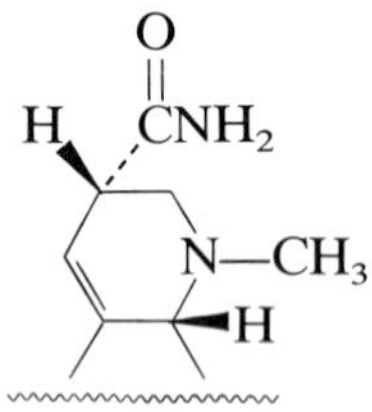

60.**35**

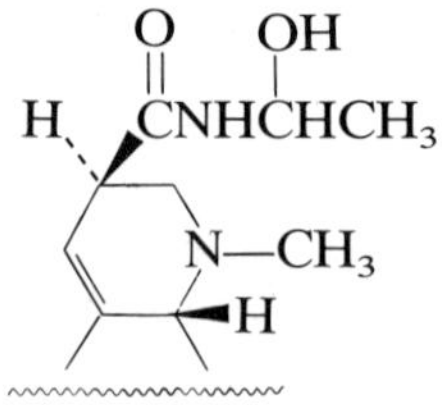

60.**36**

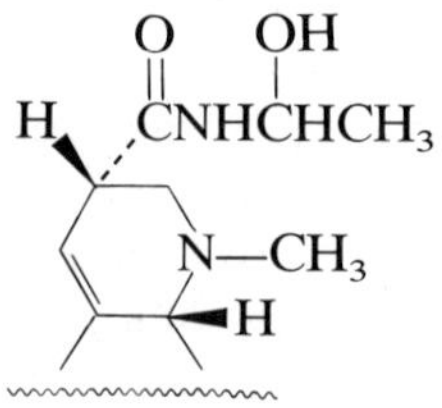

60.**37**

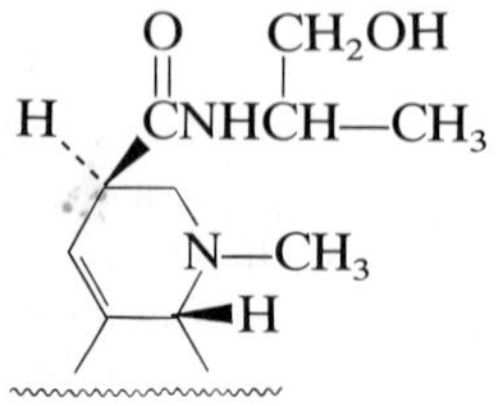

60.**38**

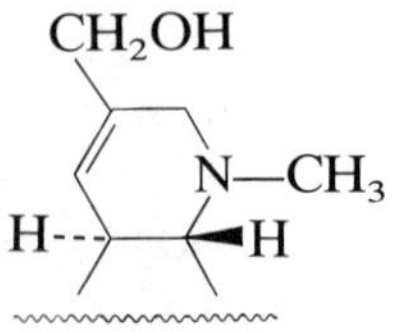

60.**39**

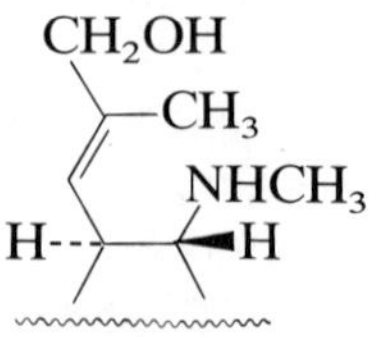

60.**40**

Table 60.5 Modifications of LSD

Compound	Composition, % of total alkaloids present		
	A. nervosa	*R. corymbosa*	*I. violacea*
60.**34o**	23 (141)	54 (142)	58 (142)
	25 (143)	48 (144)	10–16 (143)
			5–50 (144)
60.**35**	31 (141)	17 (142)	8 (142)
	18 (143)	35 (144)	18–26 (143)
			9–17 (144)
60.**36**	6 (141)		
60.**37**	4 (141)		
60.**38**	8 (141)		8 (142)
60.**39**	4 (141)	4 (142)	4 (142)
60.**40**	3 (141)	4 (142)	4 (142)
60.**41**	tr (141)	4 (142)	
60.**42**	1 (141)		
Total alkaloids	0.3 (143)	0.012 (142)	0.06 (142, 144)
(% of dry weight	0.6 (141)	0.04 (144)	0.04–0.08 (143)
of seeds)			0.02–0.04 (145)

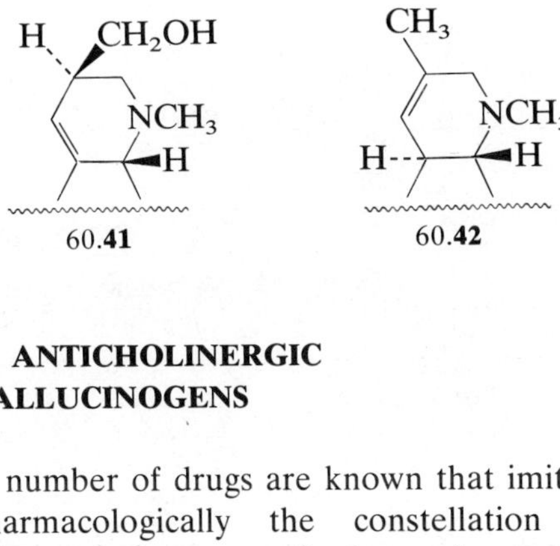

60.**41**

60.**42**

9 ANTICHOLINERGIC HALLUCINOGENS

A number of drugs are known that imitate pharmacologically the constellation of effects that are ascribed to the potent natural alkaloid, scopolamine, the ether analog of atropine (60.**7**). These materials are found as the active components in a large number of plants found around the world, and have been used for centuries for their magic and mystical powers. The belladonna plant, *Atropa belladonna*, was used in Europe in the Middle Ages as a witches' brew. Henbane, *Hyoscyamus niger*, was also widely cultivated throughout Europe as a hallucinogenic contribution to these brews, as has been mandrake, *Mandragora officinarum*. Pituri, *Duboisia hopwoodii*, has been broadly used by the Australian aborigines, and many species of *Datura* are known toxic plants and have been used, mainly in the New World, for centuries for religious purposes and as stupefacients. These plants, and the many drugs that have been synthesized in imitation of their principal active components, are somewhat different in their action for the other hallucinogens discussed in this chapter. With most of the hallucinogens, there may be distortions and synthesis in the sensory and intellectual areas, but there is usually the retention of insight (one knows that the effects are drug induced) and a good recall. With the anticholinergics, these properties are often lost, and delusion and loss of memory for the vivid visions and illusions are frequently experienced.

Most of the drugs discussed here have a constant chemical feature, the ethanolamine group that imitates the separation of heteroatoms of atropine and scopolamine as discussed earlier. The major drugs that have been studied in human subjects are listed in Table 60.6. The compound JB-329 (60.**43h**) has been investigated under the name Ditran. In this form it is a mixture of 30% piperidine and 70% ring-contracted pyrrolidine. An immense volume of research has been conducted, including human testing, on many additional analogs of these materials in connection with the search by the Chemical Warfare group for incapacitating agents useful in the military area. Most of this work has not been published and is not available for comparison. One of these compounds (BZ, 60.**43m**) has been recently studied in many animal models, and it is known to produce central

effects in man at dosages as little as 0.2 mg s.c. (158). The corresponding diphenylacetate at dosages of 4 mg produces drowsiness, confusion, and disorientation (158).

10 MISCELLANEOUS HALLUCINOGENS

Many compounds are known to be effective in man as hallucinogenic agents, but have not yet given rise to families of compounds allowing any structure–activity relationships to be determined. Some of these are discussed as single items and future research will certainly throw light on their molecular features that allow them to be hallucinogenic in action.

Table 60.6 Anticholinergic Hallucinogens

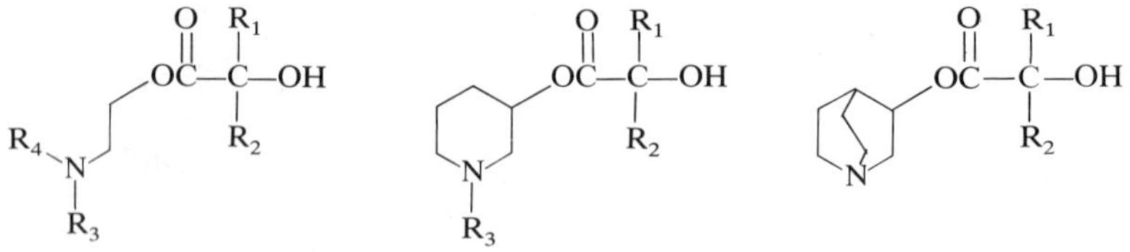

(a) Open chain   (b) Cyclic   (c) Bicyclic

60.**43**

Structure No.	Name	R_1	R_2	R_3	R_4	Ring System	Effective Dose Range, mg	Ref.
60.**43a**	Benactyzine	Phenyl	Phenyl	Et	Et	a	50–200	153
60.**43b**	JB-841	Phenyl	Phenyl	H		b	>100	154
							>20	155
60.**43c**	JB-18	Phenyl	Phenyl	Allyl		b	>20	155
60.**43d**	JB-868	Phenyl	Phenyl	$(CH_2)_2NHN(CH_3)_2$		b	>20	155
60.**43e**	JB-344	Phenyl	Thionyl	CH_3		b	10–20	154
60.**43f**	JB-318	Phenyl	Phenyl	Et		b	10–20	12, 156
60.**43g**	JB-851	Phenyl	Phenyl	$(CH_2)_2N(CH_3)_2$		b	>10	154
60.**43h**	JB-329[a]	Phenyl	Cyclopentyl	Et		b	10	154
60.**43i**	JB-840	Phenyl	Cyclohexyl	Me		b	10	154
60.**43j**	Win-2299	Thionyl	Cyclohexyl	Et	Et	a	5–10	157
60.**43k**	JB-328	Phenyl	Cyclohexyl	Et		b	5–10	154
60.**43l**	JB-336	Phenyl	Phenyl	Me		b	5–10	12
60.**43m**	QB; BZ	Phenyl	Phenyl			c	<1	158

[a] Ditran; a mixture containing the pyrrolidylmethyl isomer.

10.1   Harmaline

For many years there has been an intoxicating drink used in South America under any of several names, principally ayahuasca, caapi, or yaje. It is well established to have come from some of the many species of the plant genus *Banisteriopsis* and to contain alkaloids based on the carboline ring system. The principal alkaloid present is harmaline (60.**44**), which in man at dosages of about 4 mg/kg (orally) leads to a profound hallucinogenic state, with intense visual aspects. It has been studied clinically (48, 100). The methoxy group is located in the indolic 6 position, in marked contrast to the orientation found in serotonin and the related tryptamines. β-Carbolines with the more "natural" substitution orientation have been synthesized, but there are insufficient studies of their action to allow quantitative comparisons. The product with complete reduction in the pyridine ring (tetrahydroharmine) appears to be less active in man than harmaline (48).

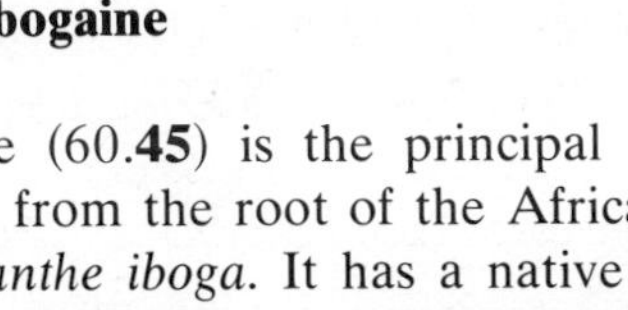

60.**44**

10.2   Ibogaine

Ibogaine (60.**45**) is the principal alkaloid isolated from the root of the African plant *Tabernanthe iboga*. It has a native reputation as a stimulant, and recent animal tests (159, 160) have shown behavior patterns that suggest it might be hallucinogenic in man. This has not been borne out in several clinical studies. In the range of 10–100 mg (161), there appears to be a mild intoxication state coupled with sedation; oral administration of 300 mg is reported (162) to produce a "fantasy enhancement" similar to lower dosages of harmaline.

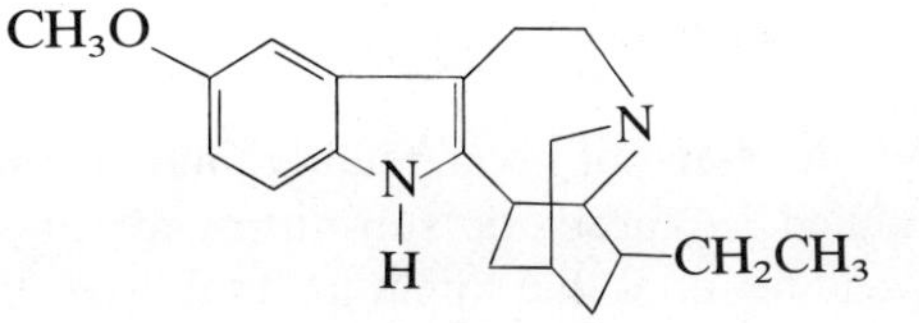

60.**45**

10.3   Phencyclidine

Phencyclidine (60.**46**) was initially introduced as a surgical anesthetic (163–165) but a few years later (in 1967) emerged as a drug of abuse in street use. Despite efforts to control its distribution and use by legislation, it has reappeared in recent years as a major pharmacological and social problem. Two properties, its remarkably high potency (5–10 mg) and its ease of synthesis, have made it one of the major drugs currently encountered in illicit transactions. An added complication is the fact that many of the slight modifications of either the amine function (such as 60.**47**) or the aromatic function (such as 60.**48**) present no synthetic challenge, but allow a simple circumvention of the law. The pharmacological spectrum of action of this group of compounds is very similar to that of the anticholinergics, including intense (and often not remembered) hallucinations and a catatonic state of affectless intoxication. It has been discontinued in legitimate clinical practice.

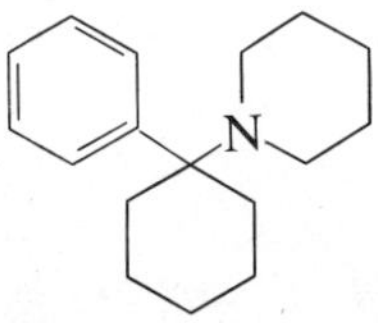

60.**46**

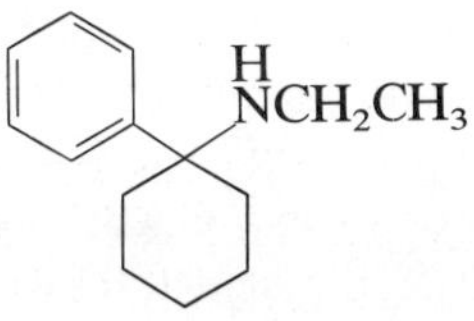

60.**47**

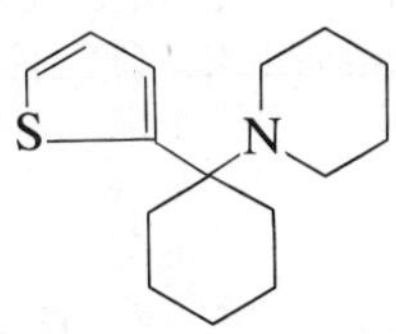

60.**48**

10.4 Ketamine

A number of compounds have been studied as anesthetic substitutes for phencyclidine, ones that might maintain the clinically useful dissociative state but that might minimize the postanesthetic recovery problems of hallucination that have faulted related products. Ketamine (60.**49**) is a recent example of a drug that, although only $\frac{1}{10}$ as potent as phencyclidine, produces a rapid onset of surgical anesthesia and has a short duration (166). This drug itself has recently become broadly abused, exploiting commercially prepared material improperly imported into the country. At subanesthetic levels, employed parenterally, it appears to produce a dissociated state and a mental loosening that is similar to several aspects of phencyclidine intoxication.

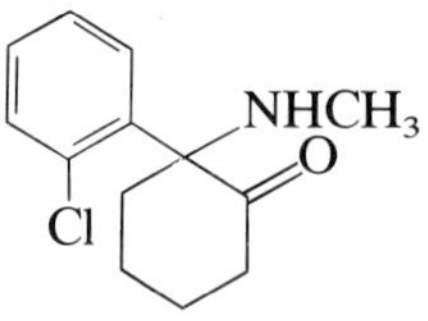

60.**49**

10.5 Ibotenic Acid

The *Amanita muscaria* mushroom has had a legendary reputation as an intoxicant, and the principal alkaloid that had been associated with it, muscarine, is known not to be present in amounts sufficient to account for the symptoms of poisoning by the intact mushroom. The isolation and characterization of two GABA agonists from the plant, ibotenic acid (60.**50**) and the decarboxylation product muscimol (60.**10**) appear to have shed light on the plant's action. At low levels [20 mg orally (167)] there was only facial flushing, and at 75 mg the action was still described as being weak and unlike that of the source mushroom. Another study at 90 mg (168) has described a motor discoordination and a narrowing of the field

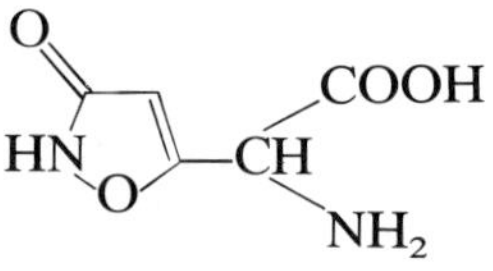

60.**50** 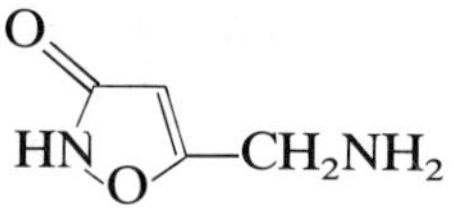   60.**10**

of vision. There were no effects that could be called hallucinations. Muscimol (60.**10**), on the other hand, seems to elicit a feeling of lassitude at 5 mg, with intoxication, dizziness, and mood elevation at twice this dose (167). With dosage levels of 15 mg there were visual distortions but none of the psychic reactions that would be observed with LSD. No structural analogs of these compounds have yet been tested in man.

10.6 Kawain

Another botanical binomial known in psychotropic pharmacology is *Piper methysticum*, the source of the drug kavakava. This plant is the source of a broadly used social intoxicant employed throughout the South Pacific. Two of the principal components have been shown to be the nitrogen-free compounds methysticin (60.**51**) and kawain (60.**52**). Research has centered around the pharmacological properties of these individual compounds and their simple homologs. The results have been largely disappointing, with subjective responses

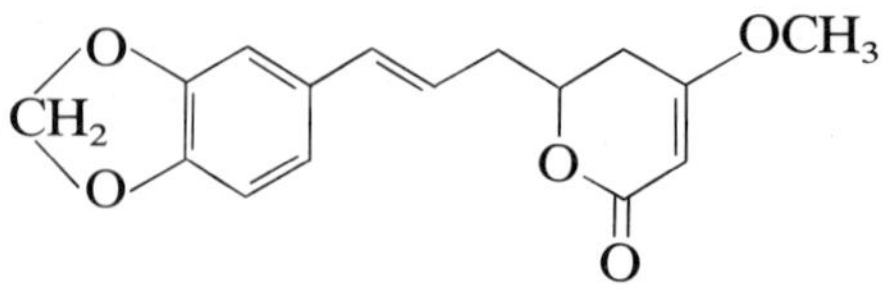

60.**51**

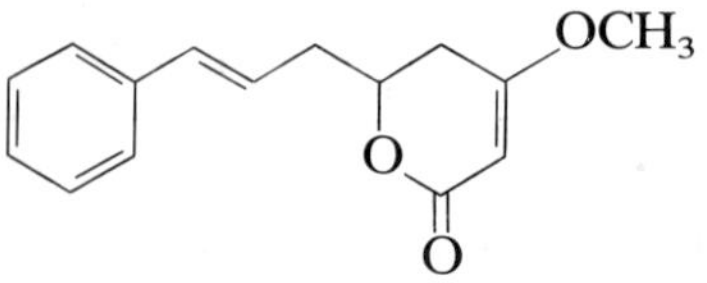

60.**52**

equally divided among reports of stimulation, sedation, and no activity whatsoever (169).

11   CANNABINOIDS

A unique group of centrally active chemicals occurs in the plant *Cannabis sativa*, known in our culture by the common name marihuana. This material has been known from antiquity and, although difficult to class as a hallucinogen, has been employed in many forms as an intoxicant, as a therapeutic agent, and as a subtle disinhibitor of sensory stimuli. The principal active components are nitrogen-free and result from union of a terpene with an alkyl-substituted resorcinol. Two major systems of structural nomenclature are frequently encountered in the literature, neither one completely satisfactory. One reflects this biosynthetic origin (60.**53a**) and numbers the carbons of the principal active component tetrahydrocannabinol in accord with the classical terpene convention, with the ring carbon carrying the methyl group being C_1, increasing about the ring past the nearer substituent to C_6, the methyl being C_7, and the isopropyl group being C_8–C_{10}. An advantage to this assignment is that there is consistency in the naming of analogs and congeners in which the pyran ring is opened. A second convention demands the intact dibenzopyran system 60.**53b**. The current Chemical Abstracts name, 3-pentyl-6a,7,8,10a-tetrahydro 6,6,9-trimethyl-6*H*-dibenzo[*b,d*]pyran-1-ol, is in accord with this second convention.

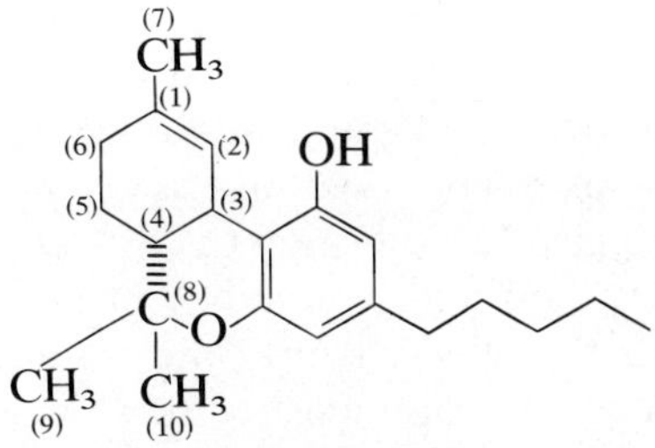

Although several dozen cannabinoid compounds are now known to be components of the intoxicating resinous extracts of the marihuana plant, only three (other than the principal active ingredient Δ^1-THC, 60.**53**) have been seriously considered as contributors to the overall pharmacological syndrome of intoxication. Two of these, the positional isomer Δ^6-THC

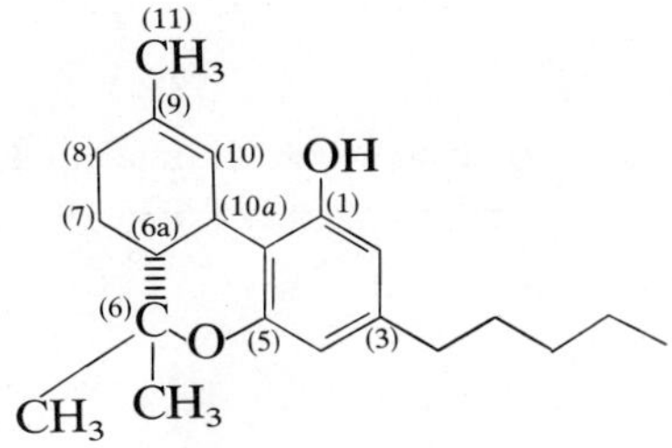

60.**53a** Δ^1-THC

60.**53b** Δ^9-THC

(60.**54**) and the aromatic counterpart cannabinol (CBN, 60.**55**) have both been shown to have some central action in man. The open ring counterpart cannabidiol (CBD, 60.**56**) has been found to be centrally inactive regardless of the route of administration [oral (170–171), smoking (172), i.v. (173)].

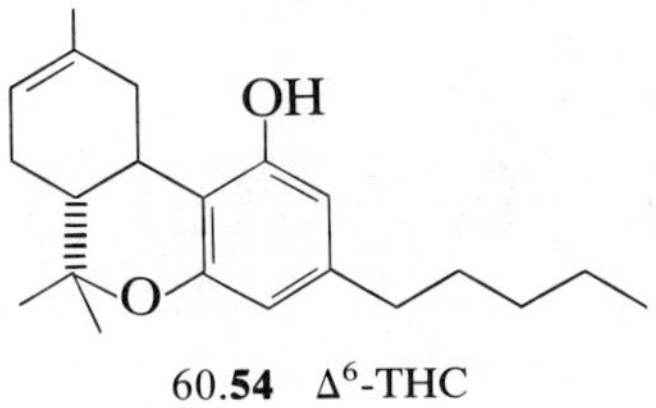

60.**54** Δ^6-THC

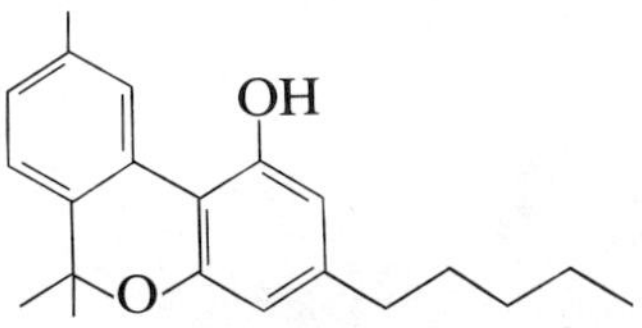

60.**55**   CBN

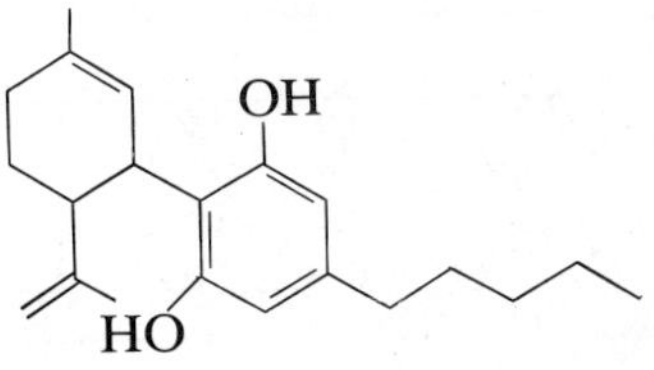

60.**56**   CBD

A large number of synthetic variants of THC have been prepared and studied pharmacologically. Most of these have the terpenacious double bond in the synthetically more logical $\Delta^{3,4}$ position ($\Delta^{6a,10a}$) and have concentrated upon variations in the structure of the alkyl chain at the resorcinol 5 position. Although most of these materials were assayed pharmacologically either by dog ataxia or by rabbit corneal areflexia

responses, a number of the more potent analogs have been found to be active in man. Table 60.7 compiles the cannabinoid compounds that are reported to have central action in man. A structural variant with a ketone function at the terpene methyl position (Nabilone, 60.**57**) is currently being studied clinically as a sedative (174).

Studies on the metabolic fate of THC have shown that hydroxylation is a major

Table 60.7 Hallucinogenic Cannabinoids

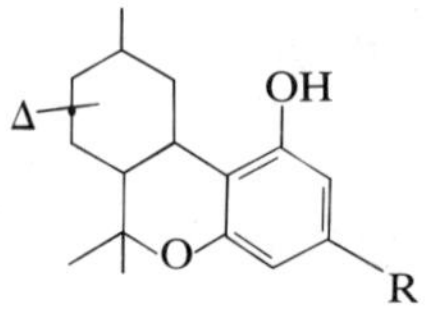

Structure No.	Name	Double Bond Position	R	Effective Dosage Range,[a] mg	Ref.
Natural Products					
60.**53**	Δ^1-THC	1,2	$n\text{-}C_5H_{11}$	20 (o)	170, 175
				5 (p)	170, 172
60.**54**	Δ^6-THC	6,1	$n\text{-}C_5H_{11}$	20 (o)	176
60.**55**	CBN	Aromatic	$n\text{-}C_5H_{11}$	>400 (o)	170
				15 (p)	173
Synthetic analogs					
	Δ^3-THC	3,4	$n\text{-}C_5H_{11}$	120 (o)	177, 178
				15 (p)	179
	Pyrahexyl	3,4	$n\text{-}C_6H_{13}$	60 (o)	177, 180
	DMHP	3,4	$CH(CH_3)CH(CH_3)C_5H_{11}$	5 (o)	181, 182
60.**57**	Nabilone	3,4 carbonyl at C_1	$C(CH_3)_2C_6H_{13}$	5 (o)	174
Human Metabolites					
	7-OH-Δ^1-THC	1,2 (7-OH)	$n\text{-}C_5H_{11}$	3 (p)	183
	6(β)OH-Δ^1-THC	1,2 (6-OH)	$n\text{-}C_5H_{11}$	4 (p)	184

[a] o = oral; p = parenteral.

60.**57**

pathway. This can occur on the amyl chain of the resorcinol moiety, or throughout the terpene ring. Two of the known metabolites in humans are terpenacious in nature, and because they have intrinsic central action they have been implicated in the mechanism of action of THC itself.

Because of the growing recognition of the extent and breadth of the use of marihuana in western society there has been an unprecedented effort invested in the study of its pharmacology and chemistry. Recent reviews (185–186) should be consulted to be abreast of current developments.

REFERENCES

1. J. R. Smythies, F. Benington, and R. Morin, *Int. Rev. Neurobiol.* **12,** 207 (1970).

2. J. M. Kelly and R. H. Adamson, *Pharmacology,* **10,** 28 (1973).

3. S. H. Snyder and E. Richelson, *Proc. Natl. Acad. Sci. U.S.,* **60,** 206 (1968).

4. S. H. Synder and C. R. Merril, *Proc. Natl. Acad. Sci. U.S.,* **54,** 258 (1965).

5. S. Kang and J. P. Green, *Nature,* **226,** 645 (1970).

6. M. Kumbar and D. V. Siva Sankar, *Res. Commun. Chem. Pathol. Pharm.,* **6,** 65 (1973).

7. R. W. Baker, C. Chothia, P. Pauling, and H. P. Weber, *Mol. Pharmacol.,* **9,** 23 (1973).

8. C. Chothia and P. Pauling, *Proc. Natl. Acad. Sci. U.S.,* **63,** 1063 (1969).

9. M-T. Sung and J. A. Parker, *Proc. Natl., Acad. Sci. U.S.,* **69,** 1346 (1972).

10. C. F. Barfknecht, D. E. Nichols, and W. J. Dunn, *J. Med. Chem.,* **18,** 208 (1975).

11. F. Antun, J. R. Smythies, F. Benington, R. D. Morin, C. F. Barfknecht, and D. E. Nichols, *Experientia,* **27,** 62 (1971).

12. L. G. Abood, *Drugs Affecting the Central Nervous System,* A. Burger, Ed., Dekker, New York, 1968, pp. 127–167.

13. A. Cerletti, *Neuro-Psychopharmacology,* P. B. Bradley, P. Deniker, and C. Radouco-Thomas, Eds., Elsevier, Amsterdam, (1959).

14. A. T. Shulgin and D. C. Dyer, *J. Med. Chem.,* **18,** 1201 (1975).

15. A. Horita and J. M. Dille, *Science* **120,** 1100 (1954).

16. A. Hofmann, *Svensk. Kem. Tidskr.* **72,** 723 (1960).

17. J. Jacob, G. Loiseau, P. Echinard-Garin, and C. Barthelemy, *Med. Exp.,* **7,** 296 (1962).

18. J. Jacob and C. Lafille, *Arch. Int. Pharmacodyn.* **145,** 528 (1963).

19. R. W. Brimblecombe, D. F. Downing, D. M. Green, and R. R. Hunt, *Brit. J. Pharmacol.,* **23,** 43 (1964).

20. R. W. Brimblecombe, *Int. J. Neuropharm.,* **6,** 423 (1967).

21. F. A. B. Aldous, B. C. Barrass, K. Brewster, D. A. Buxton, D. M. Green, R. M. Pinder, P. Rich, M. Skeels, and H. J. Tutt, *J. Med. Chem.* **17,** 1100 (1974).

22. C. S. Hall, *J. Comp. Psych.* **18,** 385 (1934).

23. V. C. Lipman, P. S. Shurrager, and L. G. Abood, *Arch. Int. Pharmacodyn.* **146,** 174 (1963).

24. R. W. Brimblecombe, *Psychopharmacologia,* **4,** 139 (1963).

25. S. J. Corne and R. W. Pickering, *Psychopharmacologia,* **11,** 65 (1967).

26. C. W. Schneider and M. B. Chenoweth, *Nature,* **225,** 1262 (1970).

27. F. Benington, R. D. Morin, L. C. Clark, and R. P. Fox, *J. Org. Chem.,* **23,** 1979 (1958).

28. J. R. Smythies, V. S. Johnson, and R. J. Bradley, *Brit. J. Psychiat.,* **115,** 55 (1969).

29. P. Brawley and J. C. Duffield, *Pharm. Rev.,* **24,** 31 (1972).

30. M. T. A. Silva and H. M. Calil, *Psychopharmacologia,* **42,** 163 (1975).

31. J. C. Gillin, J. Kaplan, R. Stillman, and R. J. Wyatt, *Am. J. Psychiatr.,* **133,** 203 (1976).

32. H. D. Fabing and J. R. Hawkins, *Science,* **123,** 886 (1956).

33. W. J. Turner and S. Merlis, *Arch. Neurol. Psychiatr.* **81,** 121 (1959).

34. H. Isbell, *Ethnopharmacologic Search for Psychoactive Drugs* D. Efron, Ed., U.S. Govern-

ment Printing Office, Washington, D.C. 1967, p. 377.

35. R. Fischer, *Nature*, **220,** 411 (1968).

36. H. Tanimukai, R. Ginther, J. Spaide, and H. E. Himwich, *Nature*, **216,** 490 (1967).

37. N. Narasimhachari and H. E. Himwich, *J. Psychiat. Res.*, **9,** 113 (1972).

38. A. J. Friedhoff and E. Van Winkle, *Nature*, **194,** 867 (1962).

39. E. Knoll and H. Wisser, *Clin. Chim. Acta*, **68,** 327 (1976).

40. D. A. Kalbhen and G. Braun, *Pharmacology*, **9,** 52 (1973).

41. L. E. Hollister and A. J. Friedhoff, *Nature*, **210** 1377 (1966).

42. A. T. Shulgin, T. Sargent, and C. Naranjo, *Nature*, **212,** 1606 (1966).

43. J. Axelrod, *Biochim. Biophys. Acta*, **85,** 247 (1964).

44. A. Hoffer, H. Osmond, and J. Smythies, *J. Ment. Sci.*, **100,** 29 (1954).

45. H. Blaschko, *Catecholamines*, H. Blaschko and E. Muscholl, Eds., Springer-Verlag, Berlin, 1972, p. 8.

46. S. Szara, J. Axelrod, and S. Perlin, *Am. J. Psychiat.*, **115,** 162 (1958).

47. W. M. McIssac, *Biochim. Biophys. Acta*, **52,** 607 (1961).

48. C. Naranjo, *Ethnopharmacologic Search for Psychoactive Drugs* D. Efron, Ed., U.S. Government Printing Office, Washington, D. C., 1967, p. 385.

49. H. Blaschko, *Pharmacol Rev.* **4,** 415 (1952).

50. L. C. Clark, F. Benington, and R. D. Morin, *J. Med. Chem.*, **8,** 353 (1965).

51. E. A. Zeller, J. Barsky, E. R. Berman, M. S. Cherkas, and J. R. Fouts, *J. Pharmacol. Exp. Ther.* **124,** 282 (1958).

52. Z. Huszti and J. Borsy, *Biochem. Pharmacol.*, **15,** 475 (1966).

53. A. H. Beckett and K. K. Midha, *Xenobiotica*, **4,** 297 (1974).

54. K. K. Midha, *J. Chromatogr.*, **101,** 210 (1974).

55. R. J. Weinkam, J. Gal, P. Callery, and N. Castagnoli, Jr., *Anal. Chem.*, **48,** 203 (1976).

56. J. Daly, J. Axelrod, and B. Witkop, *Ann. N.Y. Acad. Sci.*, **96,** 37 (1962).

57. J. S. Zweig and N. Castagnoli, Jr., *J. Med. Chem.*, **20,** 414 (1977).

58. T. Sargent III, A. T. Shulgin, and N. Kusubov, *Psychopharmacol. Commun.* **2,** 199 (1976).

59. G. M. Marquardt and V. DiStefano, *Life Sci.*, **15,** 1603 (1974).

60. E. Muscholl, *Catecholamines*, H. Blaschko and E. Muscholl, Eds., Springer-Verlag, 1972 p. 618.

61. J. E. Idänpään-Heikkilä and W. M. McIsaac, *Biochem. Pharmacol.*, **19,** 935 (1970).

62. L. W. Tansey, V. S. Estevez, and B. T. Ho, *Proc. West. Pharmacol. Soc.*, **18,** 132 (1975).

63. J. S. Zweig and N. Castagnoli, Jr., *J. Med. Chem.*, **17,** 747 (1974).

64. L. L. Butcher, *Neural Transmission*, **37,** 189 (1975).

65. A. Heffter, *Chem. Ber.*, **29,** 216 (1896).

66. E. Späth, *Monatsh. Chem.*, **40,** 129 (1919).

67. A. Rouhier, *Monographie du Peyotl Echinocactus williamsii Lem.* Lucien Decluma, Lonsle-Sauner, 1926.

68. K. Beringer, *Der Meskalinrauche. Seine Geschichte und Erscheinungsweise*, Julius Springer, Berlin, 1927.

69. K. H. Slotta and J. Müller, *Z. Physiol. Chem.*, **238,** 14 (1936).

70. M. P. J. M. Jansen, *Rec. Trav. Chim.*, **50,** 291 (1931).

71. A. Dittrich, *Psychopharmacologia*, **21,** 229 (1971).

72. W. T. Brown, P. L. McGeer, and I. Moser, *Can. Psychiat. J.*, **13,** 91 (1968).

73. U. Braun, G. Braun, P. Jacob III, D. E. Nichols, and A. T. Shulgin, N.I.D.A. Res. Monogr. Ser; **22,** 27 (1978).

74. A. T. Shulgin and M. F. Carter, *Psychopharm. Commun.* **1,** 93 (1975).

75. A. T. Shulgin, T. Sargent, and C. Naranjo, *Nature*, **221,** 537 (1969).

76. M. Vojtechovsky and D. Krus, *Acta Nerv. Sup.* 381 (1967).

77. A. Carlsson, H. Corrodi, and T. Magnusson, *Helv. Chim. Acta*, **46,** 1231 (1963).

78. A. T. Shulgin, *Handbook of Psychopharmacology*, Vol. 11, L. L. Iversen, S. D. Iversen, and S. H. Snyder, Eds., Plenum Press, New York, 1978 p. 243.

79. F. P. Ludueña, *Rev. Soc. Agric. Biol.*, **11,** 604 (1935).

80. F. P. Ludueña, *C.T.S. Biol.* **121,** 368 (1936).

81. K. D. Charalampous, K. E. Walker, and J. Kinross-Wright, *Psychopharmacologia*, **9,** 48 (1966).

82. P. Hey, *Quart. J. Pharm. Pharmacol.*, **20,** 129 (1947).

83. D. I. Peretz, J. R. Smythies, and W. C. Gibson, *J. Mental Sci.*, **101,** 317 (1955).

84. A. T. Shulgin, S. Bunnell, and T. Sargent, *Nature* **189,** 1011 (1961).

85. A. T. Shulgin, *Experientia*, **20**, 366 (1964).

86. M. D. Fairchild, *Some Central Nervous System Effects of Four Phenylsubstituted Amphetamine Derivatives*, PhD thesis, University of California at Los Angeles, 1963.

87. C. Naranjo, A. T. Shulgin, and T. Sargent, *Med. Pharmacol. Exp.* **17**, 359 (1967).

88. I. S. Turek, R. A. Soskin, and A. A. Kurland, *J. Psychedelic Drugs*, **6**, 7 (1974).

89. R. Yensen, F. B. DiLeo, J. C. Rhead, W. A. Richards, R. A. Soskin, B. Turek, and A. A. Kurland, *J. Nerv. Mental Dis.*, **163**, 233 (1976).

90. A. T. Shulgin, *Nature*, **201**, 1120 (1964).

91. A. T. Shulgin, T. Sargent, and C. Naranjo, *Pharmacology*, **10**, 12 (1973).

92. A. T. Shulgin and T. Sargent, *Nature*, **215**, 1494 (1967).

93. A. T. Shulgin and D. E. Nichols, in *The Psychopharmacology of Hallucinogens*, R. C. Stillman and R. E. Willette, Eds., Pergamon, 1978, p. 74.

94. A. T. Shulgin, unpublished data, 1978.

95. S. H. Snyder, L. A. Faillace, and L. E. Hollister, *Science*, **158**, 669 (1967).

96. S. H. Synder, L. A. Faillace, and H. Weingartner, *Am. J. Psychiat.*, **125**, 357 (1968).

97. A. T. Shulgin, T. Sargent, and C. Naranjo, *Pharmacology*, **5**, 103 (1971).

98. G. Cimbura, *J. Can. Med. Assoc.*, **110**, 1263 (1974).

99. A. T. Shulgin, *J. Med. Chem.*, **11**, 186 (1968).

100. C. Naranjo, *The Healing Journey: New Approaches to Consciousness*, Pantheon, New York, 1973.

101. F. Dallacker, *Monatsh. Chem.* **100**, 742 (1969).

102. M. Trampota, personal communication, 1978.

103. R. T. Standridge, H. G. Howell, J. A. Gylys, R. A. Partyka, and A. T. Shulgin, *J. Med. Chem.* **19**, 1400 (1976).

104. H. A. Tilson, J. H. Chamberlain, and J. A. Gylys, *Psychopharmacologia*, **51**, 169 (1977).

105. G. Marquardt, in Ref. 106.

106. A. T. Shulgin, *Handbook of Psychopharmacology*, Vol. 11, L. L. Iversen, S. D. Iversen, and S. H. Snyder, Eds., Plenum, New York, 1978.

107. A. T. Shulgin, *J. Pharm. Pharmacol.* **25**, 271 (1973).

108. S. H. Snyder, S. Unger, R. Blatchley, and C. F. Barfknecht, *Arch. Gen. Psychiat.*, **31**, 103 (1974).

109. G. M. Anderson, G. Braun, U. Braun, D. E. Nichols, and A. T. Shulgin, *N.I.D.A. Res. Monogr. Ser*; **22**, 8 (1978).

110. S. Szara, *Experientia*, **12**, 441 (1956).

111. S. Szara, in *Psychotropic Drugs*, S. Garattini and V. Ghetti, Eds., Elsevier, Amsterdam, 1957, p. 460.

112. L. A. Faillace, A. Vourlekis, and S. Szara, *J. Nerv. Ment. Dis.*, **145**, 306 (1967).

113. R. A. Soskin, S. Grof, and W. A. Richards, *Arch. Gen. Psychiatr.*, **28**, 817 (1973).

114. A. T. Shulgin, in *Psychopharmacological Agents*, Vol. 4, M. E. Gordon, Ed., Academic, 1976.

115. S. Szara and E. Hearst, *Ann. N.Y. Acad. Sci.*, **96**, 134 (1962).

116. A. B. Wolbach, E. J. Miner, and H. Isbell, *Psychopharmacologia*, **3**, 219 (1962).

117. J. Delay, P. Pichot, and P. J. Nicholas-Charles, *C. R. Acad. Sci.*, **247**, 1235 (1959).

118. M. Rinkel, C. R. Atwell, A. DiMascio, and J. Brown, *New Engl. J. Med.*, **262**, 295 (1960).

119. H. Leunder and G. Baer, *Neuropsychopharmacology*, **4**, 471 (1965).

120. A. T. Shulgin and M. F. Carter, unpublished data, 1977.

121. L. E. Hollister, J. M. Prusmack, J. A. Paulsen, and N. Rosenquist, *J. Nerv. Ment. Dis.*, **131**, 428 (1960).

122. H. B. Murphree, E. H. Jenner, and C. C. Pfeiffer, *Pharmacologist*, **2**, 64 (1960).

123. Z. Boszormenyi, P. Der, and T. Nagy, *J. Ment. Sci.*, **105**, 171 (1959).

124. S. Grof, R. A. Soskin, W. A. Richards, and A. A. Kurland, *Int. Pharmacopsychiat.*, **8**, 104 (1973).

125. R. Heim and R. G. Wasson, *Les Champignons Hallucinogènes du Mexique*, Muséum d'Histoire Naturelle, Paris, 1959.

126. S. Malitz, H. Esecover, B. Wilkens, and P. H. Hoch, *Compr. Psychiatr.*, **1**, 1 (1960).

127. A. Y. Leung and A. G. Paul, *J. Pharm. Sci.*, **56**, 146 (1967).

128. A. Y. Leung and A. G. Paul, *J. Pharm. Sci.*, **57**, 1667 (1968).

129. H. B. Murphree, R. H. Dippy, E. H. Jenney, and C. C. Pfeiffer, *Clin. Pharmacol. Ther.* **2**, 722 (1961).

130. S. Szara, *Experientia*, **17**, 76 (1961).

131. A. Hoffer and H. Osmond, *The Hallucinogens*, Academic, New York, 1967, p. 468.

132. A. Stoll and A. Hofmann, *Z. Phys. Chem.*, **251**, 155 (1938).

133. H. A. Abramson, in *Neuropsychopharmacology*, P. B. Bradley, P. Deniker, and C. Radouco-Thomas, Eds., Elsevier, Amsterdam, 1959, p. 71.

134. E. Rothlin, *Ann. N.Y. Acad. Sci.*, **66**, 668 (1957).

135. J. H. Gogerty and J. M. Dille, *J. Pharmacol. Exp. Ther.*, **120**, 340 (1957).

136. H. A. Abramson and A. Rolo, in *The Use of LSD in Psychotherapy and Alcoholism*, H. A. Abramson, Ed., Bobbs Merrill, New York, 1967.

137. A. Hofmann, *Acta Physiol. Pharmacol. Neerl.* **8**, 240 (1959).

138. A. Hofmann, *Bot. Mus. Leafl. Harvard Univ.*, **20**, 194 (1963).

139. R. E. Schultes, *A Contribution to our Knowledge of Rivea corymbosa, the Narcotic Ololiuqui of the Aztecs*, Botanical Museum, Harvard University, Cambridge, Mass., 1941, p. 15.

140. T. MacDougall, *Bol. Cent. Invest. Anthropol. Mex.*, **6** (1960).

141. J. Chao and A. H. der Marderosian, *J. Pharm. Sci*, **62**, 588 (1973).

142. A. Hofmann, *Bull. Narcotics*, **23**, 3 (1971).

143. J. W. Hylin and D. P. Watson, *Science*, **148**, 499 (1965).

144. K. Genest, *J. Chromatogr.*, **19**, 531 (1965).

145. W. A. Taber, L. C. Vining, and R. A. Heacock, *Phytochemistry*, **2**, 65 (1963).

146. H. Osmond, *J. Ment. Sci.*, **101**, 526 (1955).

147. V. J. Kinross-Wright, in *Neuropsychopharmacology* P. B. Bradley, P. Deniker, and C. Radouco-Thomas, Eds., Elsevier, Amsterdam, 1959, p. 453.

148. H. Isbell and C. W. Gorodetsky, *Psychopharmacologia*, **8**, 331 (1966).

149. R. G. Wasson, *Bot. Mus. Leafl. Harv. Univ.*, **20**, 161 (1963).

150. A. Hofmann, *Bot. Mus. Leafl. Harv. Univ.*, **20**, 194 (1963).

151. H. Solms, *J. Clin. Exp. Psychopath.*, **17**, 429 (1956).

152. H. Solms, *Praxis*, **45**, 746 (1956).

153. M. Vojtěchovský, V. Vitec, K. Ryšánek, and H. Bultasová, *Experientia*, **14**, 422 (1958).

154. L. G. Abood, A. M. Osfeld, and J. Biel, *Arch. Int. Pharmacodyn. Ther.*, **120**, 186 (1959).

155. L. G. Abood, J. H. Biel, and A. M. Ostfeld, in *Neuropsychopharmacology*, P. B. Bradley, P. Deniker, and C. Radouco-Thomas, Eds., Elsevier, Amsterdam, 1959, pp. 433.

156. A. M. Ostfeld, L. G. Abood, and D. A. Marcus, *Arch. Neurol. Psychiatr.*, **79**, 317 (1958).

157. H. H. Pennes and P. H. Hoch, *Am. J. Psychiatr.* **113**, 885 (1957).

158. W. Schallek and T. H. F. Smith, *J. Pharm. Exp.*

159. J. A. Schneider and E. B. Sigg, *Ann. N.Y. Acad. Sci.*, **66** 765 (1957).

160. W. Kostwoski, W. Rewerski, and T. Piechocki, *Pharmacology*, **7**, 259 (1972).

161. P. B. Schmid, *Arzneim.-Forsch.*, **17**, 485 (1967).

162. C. Naranjo, *Clin. Tox.*, **2**, 209 (1969).

163. M. Shepard and L. Wing, *Advan. Pharmacol.* **1** 250 (1962).

164. F. E. Greifenstein, J. Yoshitake, M. DeVault, and J. E. Gajewski, *Anaes. Analg.* **37**, 283 (1958).

165. G. Rosenbaum, B. D. Cohen, E. D. Luby, J. S. Gottlieb, and D. Yellen, *Arch. Gen. Psychiatr.*, **1**, 651 (1959).

166. E. F. Domino, P. Chodoff, and G. Corssen, *Clin. Pharmacol. Ther.*, **6**, 279 (1965).

167. P. G. Waser, in *The Ethnopharmacologic Search for Psychoactive Drugs*, D. Efron, Ed., U.S. Government Printing Office, Washington, D.C., 1967, p. 419.

168. W. S. Chilton, *McIlvania*, **2**, 17 (1975).

169. C. C. Pfeiffer, H. B. Murphree, and L. Goldstein, in *Ethnopharmacologic Search for Psychoactive Drugs*, D. Efron, Ed., U.S. Government Printing Office, Washington, D.C., 1967, p. 155.

170. L. E. Hollister, *Experientia*, **29**, 825 (1973).

171. I. G. Karnoil, I. Shirakawa, R. N. Takahashi, E. Knobel, and R. E. Musty, *Pharmacology*, **13**, 502 (1975).

172. H. Isbell, C. W. Gorodetzsky, D. Jasinski, U. Claussen, F. vom Spulak, and F. Korte, *Psychopharmacologia*, **11**, 184 (1967).

173. M. Perez-Reyes, M. C. Timmons, K. H. Davis, and E. M. Wall, *Experientia*, **29**, 1368 (1973).

174. L. Lemberger and H. Rowe, *Clin. Pharm. Ther.*, **18**, 720 (1975).

175. L. E. Hollister, and J. R. Tinklenberg, *Psychopharmacologia*, **29**, 247 (1973).

176. L. E. Hollister and H. K. Gillespie, see Ref. 170.

177. R. Adams, *Harvey Lect.*, **37**, 168 (1942).

178. S. Allentuck and K. M. Bowman, *Am. J. Psychiatr.*, **99**, 248 (1942).

179. L. E. Hollister, *Nature*, **227**, 968 (1970).

180. E. G. Williams, C. K. Himmelsbach, A. Wikler, D. C. Ruble, and B. J. Lloyd, Jr., *Public Health Rep.*, **61**, 1059 (1946).

181. H. Isbell, in *Proceedings of the Meeting of the Committee on the Problems of Drug Dependence, Addendum 1*, National Academy of Sciences 1968.

182. V. Sim, in *Psychotomimetic Drugs*, D. Efron, Ed.

Ther., **104**, 291 (1952).

Raven Press, New York, 1970 p. 332.

183. M. Perez-Reyes, M. C. Timmons, M. A. Lipton, K. H. Davis, and M. E. Wall, *Science*, **177,** 633 (1972).

184. M. E. Wall, D. R. Brine, and M. Perez-Reyes, *The Pharmacology of Marijuana*, M. C. Braude and S. Szara, Eds., Raven Press, New York, 1976, p. 93.

185. *Pharmacology of Marihuana*, M. C. Braude and S. Szara, Eds., Raven Press, New York, 1976.

186. R. Mechoulam, Ed. *Marijuana*, Academic, New York, 1973.

CHAPTER SIXTY-ONE

Radiopaques

C. T. PENG

Department of Pharmaceutical Chemistry
School of Pharmacy
University of California
San Francisco, California 94143, USA

CONTENTS

1 INTRODUCTION

Radiocontrast agents aid in the delineation of body organs and tissues against their immediate environment during fluoroscopic or roentgenographic examination. They function by rendering the spaces or cavities occupied or the surfaces adhered to by them either lucent or opaque, in contrast to their immediate surrounding tissues in the path of X-rays, and are accordingly classified as negative and positive contrast agents [1, 2]. Positive contrast agents absorb X-rays and produce a darker shadow on the fluoroscopic screen and lighter or whiter shadows on the X-ray film, of the organ to be visualized against the surrounding tissues (2). Radiopaques fall in this category. Negative contrast media are more transparent to X-rays than water or body tissue, and give a lighter shadow on the fluoroscopic screen and a darker or blacker shadow on the X-ray film. Fats, lipoid substances, and gases such as air, oxygen, nitrogen, carbon dioxide, helium, and nitrous oxide which absorb less X-ray radiation than the body tissue belong to this category.

Radiopaques have in common the property of opacity to X-ray radiation and comprise many substances which, although dissimilar in chemical form, structure, and pharmacological properties, consist of elements of high atomic number. To understand the unique dependence of radiopacity upon atomic number a brief discussion of the properties of X-rays is necessary.

2 PROPERTIES OF X-RAYS

X-Rays, also known as Roentgen rays, were discovered by W. C. Roentgen in 1895 (3, 4). Within a month of the discovery, medical examinations were being made using the newly discovered mysterious rays. X-Rays are penetrating electromagnetic radiations with quantum energies of a few thousand to several million electron volts, generated by transitions of either bound electrons within an atom or free electrons between two positive energy levels in the field of an atomic nucleus (5). The former is the atomic transition and consists of the filling of a hole or vacancy in an inner shell by an electron from an outer shell. The difference in binding energies between the two shells involved is emitted as electromagnetic radiation in the form of monochromatic (i.e., monoenergetic) X-rays, typical of the element and the transition. Transitions of free electrons between energy states give rise to continuous X-rays; these are produced when electrons accelerated to high kinetic energy are allowed to impinge on a metal target. The slowing down of fast electrons in the vicinity of the target nucleus is essentially an electron transition between two positive energy states in the field of a target nucleus and leads to the formation of bremsstrahlung, meaning "braking radiation," composed of polychromic X-rays.

X-Rays for medical use, produced by impinging fast electrons on a tungsten target in an X-ray tube, are polychromic. The diagnostic X-rays have an energy range of 30–100 kVp (kilovolts at the peak). The energy of X-rays produced in this manner depends on the kinetic energy of the accelerated electrons (5).

In traversing through matter, X-rays are attenuated by coherent (Rayleigh) and incoherent (Compton) scattering and absorbed by photoelectric process (6, 7). X-Rays of energy below 100 keV are mainly absorbed by the photoelectric process with a cross section (i.e., the probability for absorption) proportional to $Z^5/E^{7/2}$ (6), where E is the X-ray energy and Z is the atomic number of the absorber. Energy and wavelength of X-rays are related by the formula $\lambda = 12.40/E$, where λ is in angstroms and E in kiloelectron volts (8). As X-ray energy is increased, absorption by the photoelectric process diminishes, and Compton scattering becomes important. At energies above 1.02 MeV the X-rays are predominantly attenuated by pair production; this process does not play a role in the attenuation of medical diagnostic X-rays.

The attenuation of a collimated beam of monoenergetic X-rays is an exponential function of the depth of penetration (7). The relation may be expressed as

$$I = I_0 \, d^{-\mu d} \qquad (61.1)$$

where I_0 is the intensity of the initial X-ray beam, I the intensity of the transmitted X-ray beam, μ the mass absorption coefficient, and d the mass of the material penetrated. The mass absorption coefficient is a function of the X-ray energy and the atomic number Z of the absorber and is equal to the total cross section, expressed in square centimeters per gram, of the interactions mentioned above. In Table 61.1 are listed the atomic number, density, and total cross section of elements that either have been used or have potential use in contrast media. The total cross sections given are calculated for the absorption of mono-

chromatic X-rays of 40, 60, and 80 keV in energy (8); for the absorption of polychromic X-rays of the same energy designation, the values differ somewhat. The total cross section decreases monotonically as the X-ray energy is increased. At the K and L absorption edges, sharp discontinuities appear, and the total cross sections jump to higher values owing to enhanced absorption.

In roentgenography, the energy of X-rays is optimized according to the depth of penetration desired as determined by the size and density of the object under examination (1, 9–11). Depending on the operational energy range, a large fraction of the polychromatic X-rays may fall in the region where absorption by the radiopaque elements is small or may fall in the region of enhanced absorption near the K-edge. The fact that iodine and bromine have higher total cross sections for 40 keV X-rays than tantalum or tungsten, for example, is due to the proximity of the X-ray energy to the K-edges, which occur at 33.169 and 37.441 keV, respectively. Increasing the iodine content of an iodinated contrast medium from 28.7 to 37.5% doubles the contrast of the radiographic image at X-ray

Table 61.1   Physical Characteristics of Some Radiopaque Elements

Isotope	Atomic Number Z	Density g/cm^3	Total Cross Section for X-Rays of Several Energies,[a] cm^2/g		
			40 keV	60 keV	80 keV
Ca	20	1.55	1.792	0.6487	0.3630
Fe	26	7.85	3.559	1.174	0.5806
Br	35	3.12	8.061	2.607	1.200
I	53	4.93	22.40	7.696	3.549
Ba	56	3.5	24.53	8.627	3.997
Ta	73	16.6	10.25	3.581	7.482
W	74	19.3	10.73	3.686	7.788
Pt	78	21.37	12.35	4.254	8.778
Au	79	19.32	12.81	4.442	2.111
Pb	82	11.32	14.05	4.893	2.335
Bi	83	9.78	14.98	5.267	2.520
Th	90	11.38	18.36	6.450	3.106

[a] Taken from Ref. 8.

energy of 70 kVp but increases the contrast only by 60% at 90 kVp (9).

Substances in medical radiography are classified into five categories (2) according to their opacity to X-rays:

1. Radiolucent: gases.
2. Moderately radiolucent: fatty tissues.
3. Intermediate: connective tissue, muscle, blood cartilage, cholestrol stones, uric acid stones.
4. Moderately radiopaque: bone, calcium salts.
5. Very radiopaque: heavy metals and their salts.

3 CLASSIFICATION OF RADIOPAQUES

The basic characteristics desirable for a contrast medium are (1) satisfactory radiopacity (related to atomic number, material density, and concentration), (2) stability, (3) pharmacological inertness, and (4) minimum sensitizing properties (12). Radiopaques comprise heavy metals and their salts, iodized oils, organic iodine compounds, and miscellaneous agents.

Roentgenographic procedures requiring the use of radiopaques are listed in Table 61.10.

4 HEAVY METALS AND THEIR SALTS

4.1 Heavy Metals

Heavy metals with their high atomic numbers have satisfactory radiopacity and are potentially useful radiopaques. Powdered metals such as tantalum, gold, and lead have been used for experimental bronchography in dogs (13–15). Tantalum elicits no unfavorable tissue reaction and is widely used in surgery (16–19). The cost of its application as a radiopaque is minimal. Inhaled tantalum dust induces no acute or chronic inflammatory response in the airways or pulmonary tissue (20). Ingested tantalum powder produces no untoward effects on the gastrointestinal tract and is excreted. Injected tantalum powder is engulfed by the Kupffers cells without visible damage or pericellular reaction (21). The toxicity of tantalum powder is extremely low, for as much as 8000 mg/kg can be administered orally without systemic toxicity (14, 19).

Nadel et al. (14, 22) were the first to use tantalum dust for bronchography in canine and human lungs. Tantalum dust, with an average particle size of 2.5 μm in diameter, has been administered by insufflation in bronchography, esophagography (22), and gastrography (23). Tantalum dust adheres tenaciously to bronchial and esophagal mucosa to yield bronchograms and esophagrams of excellent detail over a prolonged period (14, 20, 22, 24). Experimental double contrast cystography has also been carried out (25). An aerosol preparation containing 2.4% tantalum dust (particle size, 2–50 μm), 5% lecithin (as surfactant), and 55% dichlorodifluoromethane has been introduced in order to simplify the preparation for the roentgenographic procedure and to shorten the preparation for examination (26). Commercial tantalum powders are nonporous (27) and must be fractionated before use in bronchography (28). Because of its high density and high atomic number, tantalum compares favorably with other contrast agents and yields superior bronchograms to those obtained with propylidone (63.**12d**) (14). Tantalum provides equal attenuation to an X-ray beam with 1/5–1/10 as much as the amount required of barium or iodine and about 1/20 the amount required of iodized oils (14–15). The metal is removed from the bronchi within a few days by the ciliary activity and by coughing (14, 20, 29) and from the lung in a much shorter time (20). The clearance of tantalum is slower, however, than barium sulfate under similar conditions (20); this may be attributed to its high density which prevents the transport of particles by the flow of body fluid. The clearance half-time ranges from 105 to 817 days when determined with the use of radioactive ^{182}Ta (29).

Powdered tantalum (average particle size 3 μm in diameter) has been given intravenously as suspensions to dogs and rabbits for splenohepatography (21). Although good splenohepatograms have been obtained, the aggregation of tantalum powder has caused fatal pulmonary embolism (21).

The usefulness of tantalum dust for bronchography has recently been reviewed (30, 31).

4.2   Heavy Metal Salts

Soluble heavy metal salts are in general highly toxic because of the presence of free metal ions, but many insoluble ones including oxides have been applied in roentgenography (32–38). Barium sulfate has been successfully used as a contrast agent for visualization of the alimentary tract for about 70 years (32). The use of ferrites as radiopaque agents has recently gained attention because the magnetism of this class of iron oxide allows the movement of the ingested material to be controlled by an external magnetic field (39–40). Attempts to sequester heavy metals by chelation for contrast use have not been successful (12, 33).

4.2.1 BARIUM SULFATE. Barium sulfate was introduced by Bachem and Gunter (41) in 1910 to replace insoluble and toxic bismuth salts for clinical visualization of the alimentary tract. Its nontoxicity, effectiveness, and low cost has made barium sulfate the most widely used radiocontrast agent for gastrointestinal roentgenographic examination since that time (42, 43).

Colloidal barium sulfate preparations are available from numerous commercial sources. Information about their exact composition has not been freely available because of proprietary interest (42, 44). Preparations may differ in their effectiveness for coating mucosal surface as determined by (1) particle size (2) ionic charge on suspended particles, (3) pH, (4) resistance to flocculation, (5) suspension aid, and (6) viscosity or osmotic toxicity (45).

The particle size of barium sulfate may vary from a fraction of a micron to several microns or more (43). Ultrafine grain size by itself may give inferior visualization of the gastric mucosa but the particles can be more easily held in suspension. On the other hand, particles larger than 1 μ may offer better contrast provided that they can be made to stay in suspension. An electron micrography of barium sulfate particles of less than 1 μm in diameter shows that they are of irregular shape (46). The influence of microcrystalline shape on the coating property of the suspension is not well known.

The viscosity of barium sulfate suspension is determined by the quantity and size of particles and can be modified by added peptizing agents (45). A thick paste of barium sulfate in water can be peptized or thinned by the addition of sodium citrate and sorbitol. The function of the citrate is to stabilize the colloidal preparation and that of the sorbitol is to enhance that function. The use of a polybasic acid and sugar alcohol combination can lead to the incorporation of so much barium sulfate in a liquid suspension as to obtain a preparation with a specific gravity close to 3 (47, 48). Other polybasic acids such as tartaric acid and ethylenediaminetetraacetic acid (edetic acid) may also be used.

Particles in unprotected barium sulfate suspensions have a tendency to aggregate, resulting in flocculation. Such suspensions may be stabilized by the use of a dispersing agent or by placing an electric charge on the particle (45). The surface of barium sulfate particles is either positively or negatively charged depending on the residual lattice ions present. It is also affected by the nature of the material added to coat the particles. The coated particles are uniformly charged and flow easily on account of the like charge on their surface which resists aggregation and increases the colloidal stability.

Additives for coating barium sulfate particles include methylcullulose (42, 45, 46, 49–54), carboxymethylcellulose (46, 47), hydroxypropylcellulose (46, 47, 55), chondroitin sulfate (56), heparin (45), and sodium dextran sulfate (45). Dispersing agents used for stabilization and peptization of the colloidal suspension include agar (43, 47, 48), acacia (42, 49), alginates (47, 49, 52, 57, 58), alginic acid–propylene glycol mixtures (59), anionic galactanes (59), betonite (42, 53), casein (42), erythrobic acid (51, 52, 60, 61), gelatin (42, 53), glycerol (53, 62), gum arabic (46, 48, 55), hexametaphosphate (50, 51, 55), lecithin (42, 58), mannitol (62), pectins (42, 47, 48, 55), polyalkylaryl sulfonates (59), polyethylene glycol 400 (57, 62, 63), polymetaphosphate (64), nonionic poly(oxyethylene)glycol stearate (58), polysorbate 80 (42, 62), poly(vinyl alcohol) (47, 48, 63), poly(vinylpyrrolidone) (47, 48, 55, 64), pyrophosphate (48), sodium ascorbate (51, 52, 60–62), sodium dioctylsulfosuccinate (62), sodium lauryl sulfoacetate (57, 62), sorbic acid (57, 62), sorbitol (47, 48, 57, 62), and trisodium citrate hydrate (48, 57, 59, 62). Classification of these agents by their function is only superficial since many have dual functions.

The mobility of the particles depends on the pH of the suspension, the ionic strength, the age, and the method of preparation. Adherence of barium sulfate particles to mucosal membrane is pH dependent, since the pH affects not only the electrokinetic charge on the barium sulfate particles but also the charge on the mucosal lining which is composed of glycoprotein mucopolysaccharide and capable of carrying charges (45). Coating of mucosal surfaces by commercial barium sulfate preparations has been studied by Schwartz et al. (65), who found that an optimal viscosity is important for satisfactory coating; at low viscosities the coating is too thin, and at high viscosities, the preparation is too viscid for use.

Many different preparations of colloidal barium sulfate for roentgenography are available commercially. The so-called "barium meals" are not limited to liquid suspensions; they also appear as tablets (66). Recently, barium sulfate suspensions containing an effervescent agent have been introduced for use in double contrast studies (67, 68). Barium sulfate coated with Fe_2O_3, MgO, and Al_2O_3 has been introduced (56, 69). The coated material has good dispersibility and very low viscosity in acidic media.

Barium sulfate is used not only in roentgenographic examination of gastrointestinal tract (44) but also in inhalation bronchography (54). The earlier experiments were made on dogs in 1920 by Bullowa and Gottlieb (70). More recently, barium sulfate was used for bronchography in infants and children (71). According to Clement (54), satisfactory bronchograms can be obtained with less barium sulfate if the bronchial surface is previously exposed to methylcellulose. Methylcellulose improves the bronchogram by forming a viscous film on the bronchial mucosa to which barium sulfate adheres easily, thus reducing considerably the amount of contrast agent required for an examination.

When used in bronchography, barium sulfate is nonallergenic and nontoxic. It induces only a mild, benign, foreign body reaction and causes no pulmonary fibrosis or bronchial spasms. It is cleared from the normal lung by ciliary action, coughing, and phagocytosis at a rate similar to that of tantalum (54). When the bronchial surface is precoated with methylcellulose, the clearance of barium sulfate is usually complete within 24–48 hr (54). Any residual amount that may remain trapped in the alveoli is usually located within the macrophages in tiny intra-alveolar granuloma. When used in roentgenography of gastrointestinal tract, barium sulfate has the inherent danger of inspissation and impaction when water is reabsorbed, particularly in the colon (43, 72, 43).

4.2.2 BISMUTH SUBNITRATE. Bismuth subnitrate was the first contrast agent used clinically to visualize the alimentary tract (32). It was found to be toxic in man through the reduction from nitrate to nitrite; as a result, bismuth subcarbonate was substituted (47). When the toxic action was traced to the metal itself, the use of bismuth salts was discontinued.

4.2.3 FERRITES. Novel materials such as ferrites have more recently been introduced as experimental radiocontrast agents (39, 40). Ferrites are iron oxide (Fe_2O_3) in solid solution with one or more metallic oxides. They possess about 80% of the radiopacity of barium sulfate and a higher percentage if oxides of high atomic number are incorporated. The ferrites are magnetic, a property that allows their movement within the body to be controlled by an external magnet.

Frei et al. (39) reported the use of magnesium ferrite as contrast material for X-ray diagnosis. Sugimoto et al. (40) studied the suitability of four ferrites containing Mg, Zn, Cu, Ni and Mn as radiopaques with respect to toxicity, solubility in the gastric juice, X-ray absorption, and effective magnetic field strength necessary for controlling the ferrite powder. These ferrites can be prepared to yield low solubility in acid or stimulated gastric juice. They are nonallergenic and have no acute toxicity (75). On prolonged daily oral administration (30 days), the ferrites cause a slight decrease in body weight, hematocrit, and the enzyme glutamic–pyruvic transaminase in rats and mice (76). The LD_{50} for rats and mice is >20 and >10 g/kg, respectively

(76). When fed to experimental animals, the ferrites are cleared entirely from the body within a week as shown in absorption studies using ^{55}Fe, ^{54}Mn, or ^{65}Zn labeled ferrites (75). Only soft ferrites, which do not coalesce in the absence of the applied magnetic field, are used as contrast media. Satisfactory roentgenograms of esophagus, stomach, bronchus, and small intestines have been obtained with these ferrites (40). The particle size of the ferrite powder may range from less than 1 μ to several microns in diameter, and a stable suspension of the particles may be obtained using stabilizing and peptizing agents (77–82) similar to those mentioned in Section 4.2.1.

4.2.4 METAL CHELATES. Chelating agents capable of combining with metals of high atomic number are potentially useful contrast media (12, 33, 34). Chelation may significantly reduce the toxicity of metal ions—the toxicity of Ca, Ni, Co, and Pb salts of ethylenediaminetetraacetic acid (EDTA or edetic acid) is many times lower than the toxicity of the metal ions. On the other hand, Cr, Cu, and Hg edetates and their metal ions have comparable toxicity, as indicated by the LD_{50} (7-day mortality) values. Since the binding between metal ions and the ligands is reversible, the sequestered metal ions in the latter group of chelates may have become free *in vivo*.

In addition to edetic acid, multidentate chelating agents such as 1,2-diaminocyclohexane-*N*,*N*′-tetraacetic acid, diethylenetriaminepentaacetic acid (DPTA), *N*,*N*′-(2-hydroxycyclohexyl)ethylenediaminediacetic acid, 2-hydroxycyclohexylethylenediaminetriacetic acid, and β-hydroxyethylethylenediaminetriacetic acid have been used to sequester heavy metal ions for roentgenographic purposes (33). Eight percent solutions of Bi–DTPA and Pb–EDTA were used in experimental bronchography and angiography in dogs (33) but the margin of safety between a useful dose and the minimum lethal dose is so narrow as to render them hazardous for clinical trials.

4.2.5 TANTALUM OXIDE. Although tantalum oxide is less radiopaque than tantalum powder by a factor of 0.5 per volume or 0.8 per mass, its chemical and biologic inertness and toxicity are very similar to that of tantalum (36). The technical advantages and safety in handling and storage of the oxide make it superior to use in roentgenography to metallic tantalum, which presents an explosion hazard. The oxide is formed as β-Ta_2O_5 with a particle size of about $1\,\mu$m or less by burning metallic tantalum powder in air. It is used in bronchography and esophagography by topical application. When injected intravenously in dogs and rabbits in experimental splenohepatography, the oxide forms microscopic emboli in the liver and kidney. Injected particles of the oxide are engulfed by the reticuloendothelial cells without appreciable cellular or pericellular reaction.

4.2.6 THORIUM DIOXIDE. The use of thorium dioxide as a contrast agent began in 1928–1929 (83); it has been used under the name of "Thorotrast" (Fellows-Testager Division, Detroit, Michigan) for angiography and cerebral arteriography. Thorotrast is a colloidal suspension of 25% by weight of thorium dioxide of particle size less than $0.15\,\mu$ in diameter, prepared by oxidation of thorium oxalate at 550°C (84). The high atomic number, high density, and the lack of acute toxicity makes thorium dioxide an ideal radiopaque for use in large quantities in roentgenography (85). Thorium dioxide gives excellent contrast and has proved of value in studies where other contrast media would fail.

The drawback of using thorium dioxide as a contrast agent is its radioactivity and indefinite retention in the body (86, 87). Thorium-232 is the longest-lived parent radionuclide in the thorium series (88). A considerable amount of work has been done regarding the disposition and fate of thorium dioxide following its systemic and local use in man for roentgenography (89–97). The dioxide when administered intravenously is engulfed by the phagocytic cells of the reticuloendothelial system and is permanently localized in these cells (89). The long-term effects of radiation are fibrosis and neoplastic growth in the liver and spleen and fibrosis of their efferent lymph nodes (35, 96). Localization of thorium and its daughter nuclides in the bone may result in leukemia and other blood dyscrasias (94). Locally injected thorium dioxide, if in contact with epithelium for long periods, induces carcinoma (35, 98).

When colloidal thorium dioxide was applied within the lumen of the gastrointestinal tract, no deleterious late effects were observed (35). The continuous shedding of the intestinal epithelium can remove the deposited dioxide and excrete it together with the intestinal content.

Because of the radiation effects of thorium, the use of thorium dioxide is limited only to the procedures approved by the U.S. Food and Drug Administration, such as hepatolienography in patients with metastatic cancer (35).

4.2.7 OTHER METALLIC SALTS. In addition to the heavy metal salts mentioned above, barium titanate and barium metatitanate have been used for visualization of hypopharynx, esophagus, stomach, and small intestine (37, 99). Barium metatitanate is used as a powder with grains measuring from 0.8 to $1.0\,\mu$. It is insoluble in water and has a density of 6 as compared to barium sulfate with a density of 4.5. In addition, the metatitanate adheres better to the intestinal mucosa than barium sulfate, a property considered favorable for visualization. Powdered calcium tungstate can also be used to opacify airways but was found ineffective for filling airways smaller than 2 mm in diameter (38).

5 IODIZED OILS

Radiopaque iodine atoms can be introduced into vegetable oils to form iodized oils by reaction with hydroiodic acid. This converts unsaturated fatty acid moieties into iodinated saturated ones, such as linoleic acid to diiodostearic acid and oleic acid to monoiodostearic acid (100). Commercial preparations of iodized oils are glyceryl esters (Lipiodol) and ethyl esters (Ethiodol) of iodinated fatty acids derived from the natural oils of poppy seeds. Lipiodol and Ethiodol contain approximately 38–42% and 37% of organically bound iodine, respectively. Ethyl diiodostearate (45.0% I) and ethyl triiodostearate (55.2% I) have higher iodine content than Ethiodol and are available as emulsions (108). The iodized oils are yellow or amber and decompose with liberation of iodine upon exposure to air or light. Ethiodol has a lower viscosity than Lipiodol. The toxicity or tolerance of iodized oils is determined by their viscosity (100, 101).

Iodinated oils are emulsified for injection with surfactants such as polyoxyethylene sorbitan monooleate (Tween-80) and sorbitan monooleate (Span-80) (102), polyethylene glycol-400 stearate (103, 104), soya lecithin (105), or ethylene oxide and castor oil (106), and stabilized with polyhydric alcohols such as glycerol and glucose. The toxicity of iodized oils administered intralymphatically is between one and two times that administered intravenously (100, 107). Ethiodol has an average lethal dose in the dog of 3.62 ml/kg for intralymphatic injection as compared to 1.58 ml/kg for intravenous injection (107). Iodized oils are injected slowly into the peripheral lymphatic; an 8 ml dose is usually given over a period of 40–80 min at a pressure of 0.4 atm. High injection speeds and pressure may cause rupture of the lymph trunk and extravasation.

Intralymphatically injected oil contrast medium may remain in the lymph nodes for months or even more than a year (100). The excess of that retained in the lymphatic system will enter the systemic veins via the thoracic duct or by way of lymphaticovenous communications and eventually pass into the pulmonary artery and its branches to be distributed in the lung capillaries. Experiments in the dog showed that 50% of the injected Ethiodol was found in the lung and about 23% of the dose in the nodes at 3 days post-lymphography. The concentration of iodized oil in the nodes remained essentially the same but that in the lung had decreased to about 13% of the dose at 17 days post-injection (100, 109).

Metabolic studies with ^{131}I-labeled Ethiodol indicated that the iodized oil was rapidly deiodinated by enzymes in tissues with the iodine appearing as inorganic iodide which was excreted by the kidney. In man, no more than 0.5% of the injected iodized oil was found in the blood at any one time, and the urinary excretion was less than 2.5% of the dose per day (110). The most serious side effect of the iodized oils is pulmonary or systemic embolization, which is related to the particle size of the oily droplets (100, 107).

Iodized oils are used in lymphography (100, 107), intra-arterial hepatography (104), and intravenous hepatosplenography (111). The oily contrast medium allows the detection of small avascular masses in the liver or spleen by tomography which is superior to both contrast angiography with water-soluble contrast media and scanning with radiopharmaceuticals; the former is too transient for tomographic imaging and the latter inadequate in resolution (111).

6 ORGANIC IODINE COMPOUNDS

Organic iodine compounds make up the largest group of radiopaque agents used in roentgenographic examination. They may be classified according to their intended application as angiographic, cholegraphic, urographic, and myelographic agents, or according to their route of administration as oral or intravascular agents. Chemically, they may be ionic or nonionic in nature.

The first iodinated organic compound

ever used as a contrast agent was tetra-iodophenolphthalein, introduced by Graham et al. (112) in 1926 for intravenous cholecystography. This compound was widely used for gall bladder visualization until 1940 when Dohrn and Diedrich (113) introduced iodoalphionic acid which produced a better roentgenogram of the gall bladder and fewer adverse reactions and was the agent of choice until the early 1950s; at this time a large variety of iodinated organic radiocontrast agents were introduced, most of which gave even better visualization and fewer side effects.

The historical development of organic iodine compounds as radiopaque agents was reviewed by Strain (32). The chemical aspects of some cholecystographic agents developed up to 1959, including iopanoic acid, were discussed by Archer (114). A more comprehensive review of the organic iodine compounds as X-ray contrast agents with emphasis on the structure–activity relationship and an extensive list of iodinated compounds synthesized in search of improved agents was compiled by Hoey et al. (115). The subject was discussed by Hoppe (116, 117), and Ackerman (118) and has more recently been reviewed from the point of view of drug design by Herms and Taenzer (119). Numerous reviews on the pharmacology and clinical application of iodinated contrast agents have also appeared (10, 120–129). Almén (130) has compared the advantages of nonionic versus ionic contrast agents and postulated from theoretical consideration that the nonionic contrast agents will be less toxic than the ionic ones because of lower osmolality. This theory has stimulated the synthesis and testing of dimers (9, 131–134), polymers (135–136), and nonionic iodinated compounds (137–140) for improved radiopaques. Metrizamide (137–138) and a number of dimers and polymers are the outcome of these studies.

In subsequent sections, the iodinated radiopaques are discussed with respect to their classification, synthesis, structure–activity relationships, analysis, pharmacology, and uses. The section on pharmacology includes the topics of cations, hyperosmolality, toxicity, neurotoxicity, protein binding, histamine release, pharmacokinetics, excretion, and biotransformation.

6.1 Classification

In general, iodinated contrast agents contain either the pyridone or benzene nucleus as the iodine-carrying moiety. With few exceptions, the newer contrast agents are derivatives of 2,4,6-triiodobenzoic acid and its congeners (61.**1**). The adoption of benzene ring as the iodine carrier originated from the observation by Wallingford et al. (141–142) that iodobenzoic acids have very low toxicity and the substituent groups determine the molecular and pharmacological properties. Thus R may be a functional subunit containing a substituent which may be strongly hydrophilic, such as carboxyl, or a group with both lipophilic and hydrophilic properties, such as alkyl, aralkyl, or alkoxyalkylcarboxyl. The substituents X and Y may affect protein binding, toxicity, or biotransformation, for example.

In the following, contrast agents that have been accepted for clinical use are listed by their United States Accepted Names (USAN) or by their International Nonproprietary Names (INN). No proprietary names for contrast agents are given. For a listing of the proprietary names, chemical formulas, and recommended use,

R (solubility)

(opacity) | | (opacity)

(solubilizing, X   Y (solubilizing,
detoxifying)   detoxifying)

| (opacity)

61.**1**

the compilations by Knoefel (143) and by Strain and Rogoff (144) should be consulted.

1. Triiodobenzoates (61.**2**)
    Acetrizoate (**a**)
    Diatrizoate (**b**)
    Diprotrizoate (**c**)
    Iodamide (**d**)
    Metrizoate (**e**)
2. Triiodoisophthalamates (61.**3**)
    Ioglicic acid (**a**)
    Ioseric acid (**b**)
    Iothalamic acid (**c**)
    Ioxitalamic acid (**d**)
3. Triiodophenyl alkanoates (61.**4**)
    Bunamiodyl (**a**)
    Iopanoic acid (**b**)
    Iophenoxic acid (**c**)
    Ipodate (**d**)
    Tyropanoic acid (**e**)
    Iolidonic acid (**f**)
4. Triiodophenoxy alkanoates (61.**4**)
    Iopronic acid (**g**)
5. Triiodobenzamides (61.**5**)
    Iobenzamic acid (**a**)
    Metrizamide (**b**)
6. Triiodoanilides (61.**6**)
    Iocetamic acid (**a**)
    Iomeglamic acid (**b**)
    Iosumetic acid (**c**)
7. Dimeric triiodobenzoates (61.**7**)

Iodipamide (**a**)
Ioglycamic acid (**b**)
Iotroxic acid (**c**)
Iodoxamic acid (**d**)
B-9720 (**e**)
8. Dimeric triiodoisophthalamates (61.**7**)
    Iocarmic acid (**f**)
    Iosefamic acid (**g**)
9. Other dimers and polymers
    Iozomic acid (Ph Zd 59A) (61.**8a**)
    Tris(iothalamic acid) (61.**9**)
10. Diiodophenyl alkanoate
    Iodoalphionic acid (61.**10**)
11. Iodophenyl alkanoate
    Iodophendylate (61.**11**)
12. Diiodopyridones (61.**12**)
    Iopydone (**a**)
    Iodopyracet (**b**)
    Iopydol (**c**)
    Propylidone (**d**)
    Sodium iodomethamate (**e**)
    Iopax (61.**13**)
13. Iodophthaleins (61.**14**)
    Iodophthalein
14. Miscellaneous
    Methiodal sodium (61.**15**)
    Dimethiodal sodium (61.**16**)
    Iodohippurate sodium (61.**17**)

The formulas of these agents are given in Scheme 61.1 and their characteristics in Table 61.2.

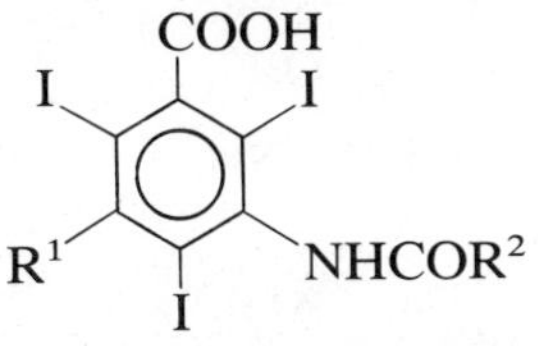

	R^1	R^2
a	H	CH_3
b	$NHCOCH_3$	CH_3
c	$NHCOCH_2CH_3$	CH_2CH_3
d	$CH_2NHCOCH_3$	CH_3
e	$N(CH_3)COCH_3$	CH_3

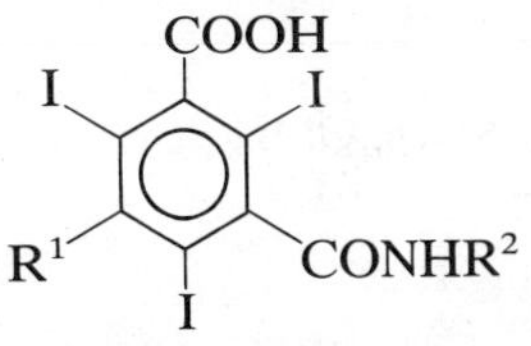

	R^1	R^2
a	$NHCOCH_3$	$CH_2CONHCH_3$
b	$NHCOCH_2OCH_3$	$CH(CH_2OH)CONHCH_3$
c	$NHCOCH_3$	CH_3
d	$NHCOCH_3$	CH_2CH_2OH

Scheme 61.1 Formulas of radiopaques.

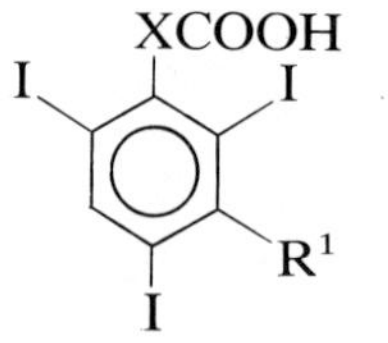

61.4

	X	R^1
a	—CH=C(CH$_2$CH$_3$)—	NHCOCH$_2$CH$_2$CH$_3$
b	—CH$_2$CH(CH$_2$CH$_3$)—	NH$_2$
c	—CH$_2$CH(CH$_2$CH$_3$)—	OH
d	—CH$_2$CH$_2$—	N=CHN(CH$_3$)$_2$
e	—CH$_2$CH(CH$_2$CH$_3$)—	NHCOCH$_2$CH$_2$CH$_3$
f	—CH$_2$CH(CH$_2$CH$_3$)—	NCOCH$_2$CH$_2$CH$_2$
g	—OCH$_2$CH$_2$OCH$_2$C(CH$_2$CH$_3$)COOH	NHCOCH$_3$

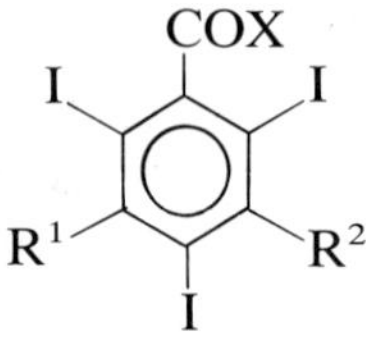

	X	R^1	R^2
61.**5a**	N(C$_6$H$_5$)CH$_2$CH$_2$COOH	H	NH$_2$
61.**5b**	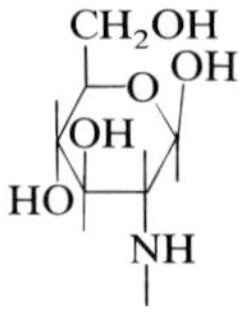 CH$_2$OH ...	NHCOCH$_3$	N(CH$_3$)COCH$_3$

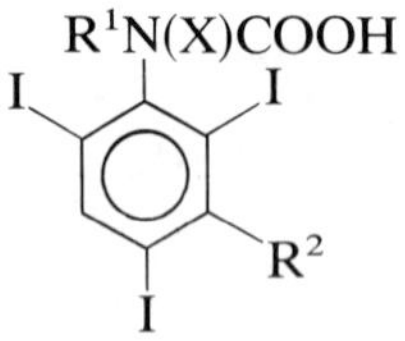

	X	R^1	R^2
61.**6a**	—CH$_2$CH(CH$_3$)—	COCH$_3$	NH$_2$
61.**6b**	—CO(CH$_2$)$_3$—	CH$_3$	NH$_2$
61.**6c**	—CO(CH$_2$)$_2$—	CH$_2$CH$_3$	NHCH$_3$

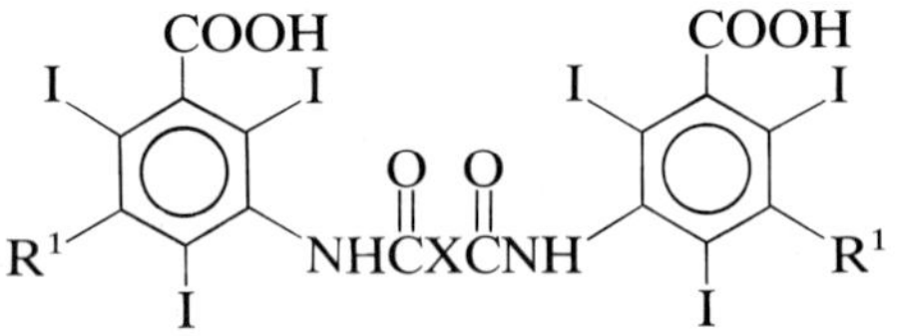

61.7

	X	R^1
a	—(CH$_2$)$_4$—	H
b	—CH$_2$OCH$_2$—	H
c	—(CH$_2$OCH$_2$)$_3$—	H
d	—CH$_2$(CH$_2$OCH$_2$)$_4$CH$_2$—	H
e	—(CH$_2$)$_7$—	CH$_2$NHCOCH$_3$
f	—(CH$_2$)$_4$—	CONHCH$_3$
g	—(CH$_2$)$_8$—	CONHCH$_3$

Scheme 61.1 (*Continued*)

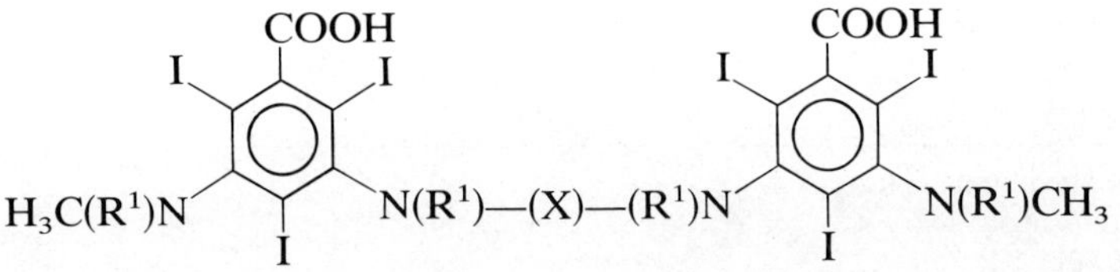

61.**8** X = —CH$_2$CH(OH)CH$_2$O(CH$_2$)$_4$OCH$_2$CH(OH)CH$_2$—, R^1 = COCH$_3$

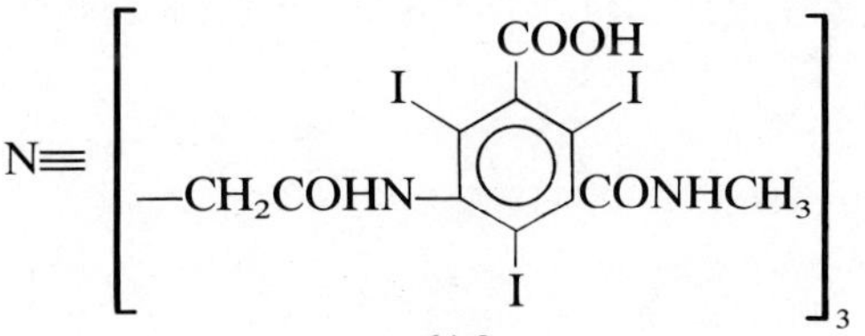

N≡ [—CH$_2$COHN— ... CONHCH$_3$]$_3$

61.**9**

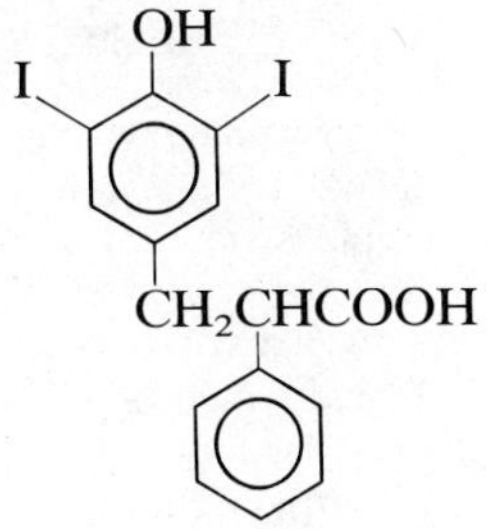

61.**10**

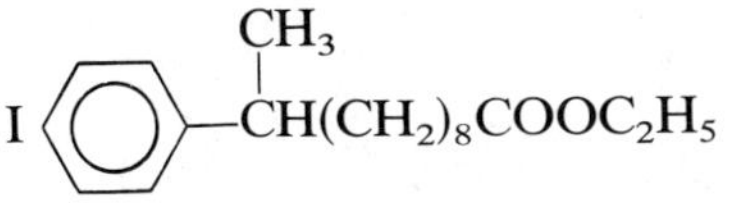

61.**11**

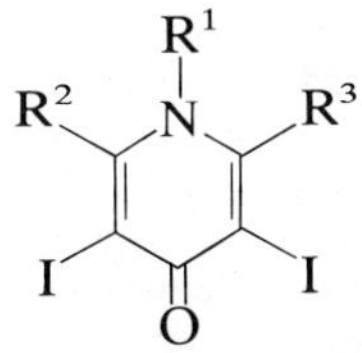

61.**12**

	R^1	R^2	R^3
a	H	H	H
b	CH$_2$COOH	H	H
c	CH$_2$CH(OH)CH$_2$OH	H	H
d	CH$_2$COOC$_3$H$_7$	H	H
e	CH$_3$	COONa	COONa

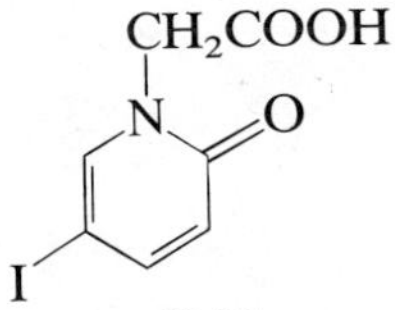

61.**13**

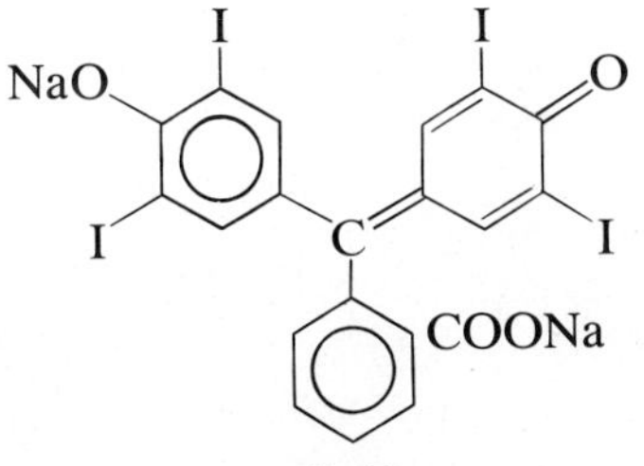

61.**14**

ICH$_2$SO$_3$Na
61.**15**

I$_2$CHSO$_3$Na
61.**16**

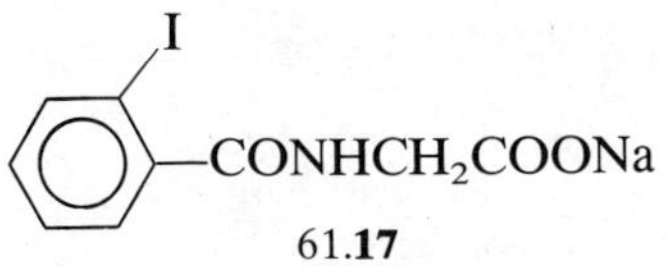

61.**17**

Scheme 61.1   (*Continued*)

Table 61.2 Characteristics of Iodine-containing Contrast Agents

USAN or INN Name	Chemical Name	Iodine Content, %	M.p., °C	LD_{50}, g/kg	Solubility, g/100 ml H_2O at 20°C	$pK_{H_2O}^{25}$	Ref.
Acetrizoate (61.**2a**)	3-(Acetylamino)-2,4,6-triiodobenzoic acid		278–283(d)	9.56	94.2	2.08	
	Sodium salt,	65.77			Freely		
	Meglumine salt	50.62			soluble		145
Diatrizoate (61.**2b**)	3,5-Diacetamido-2,4,6-triiodobenzoic acid		>300	11.0[a]		2.05	
	Sodium salt	59.87	261–262	11.4[a]	60	2.7	146,
	Meglumine salt	47.05	189–193(d)	13.8[a]	89		206, 207
Diprotrizoate (61.**2c**)	2,4,6-Triiodo-3,5,-di propionamidobenzoic acid		>300	0.0118[b]			
	Sodium salt	57.34			~50		146
Iodamide (61.**2d**)	3-(Acetylamino)-5-[(acetylamino)methyl]-2,4,6-triiodobenzoic acid	60.63	255–257	10.8[b]	0.3(22°C)	1.88	147, 148
	Sodium salt				>75		
Metrizoate (61.**2d**)	3-(Acetylamino)-5-(acetylmethylamino)-2,4,6-triiodobenzoic acid	60.63	281–282				149
	Sodium salt				86		
Ioglicic acid (61.**3a**)	5-Acetamido-2,4,6-triiodo-N-[(methylcarbamoyl)-methyl]isophthalamic acid	65.78					150
Ioseric acid (61.**3b**)	5(2-Methoxyacetamido)-2,4,6-triiodo-N-[2-hy-droxy-1-(methylcarbamoyl)-ethyl]isophthalamic acid	52.12					150
Iothalamic Acid (61.**3c**)	5-Acetamido-2,4,6-tri-iodo-N-methylisoph-thalamic acid	62.01	285(d)			1.74	
	Sodium salt				85		151
	Meglumine salt						
Ioxitalamic Acid (61.**3d**)	5-Acetamido-2,4,6-tri-iodo-N-(2-hydroxy-ethyl)isophthalamic acid	59.12	349				152
Bunamiodyl (61.**4a**)	2[[2,4,6-Triiodo-3-[(1-oxobutyl)amino]phenyl]methylene]butanoic acid		105–20	0.57[b]	Sl. sol.		153, 154
	Monosodium salt	57.60					
Iopanoic acid (61.**4b**)	3-Amino-α-ethyl-2,4,6-triiodobenzenepro-panoic acid	66.69	155.2–157(d-l form)		Insol.	5.06	155, 156
Iophenoxic acid (61.**4c**)	3-Ethyl-3-hydroxy-2,4,6-triiodobenzenepro-panoic acid	66.57	143–144			(pK_1) 4.66	157, 158
Ipodate (61.**4d**)	3-[[(Dimethylamino)-methylene]amino]-2,4,6-					(pK_2)	

Table 61.2 (*Continued*)

USAN or INN Name	Chemical Name	Iodine Content, %	M.p., °C	LD_{50}, g/kg	Solubility, g/100 ml H_2O at 20°C	$pK_{H_2O}^{25}$	Ref.
	triiodobenzenepropanoic acid	63.67	168–169		Insol.	6.11 / 5–5.5	159, 160
	Sodium salt		303–304(d)		Freely sol.		
	Calcium salt		298–302		0.1		
Tyropanoate (61.**4e**)	α-Ethyl-2,4,6-triiodo-3-[(1-oxobutyl)amino]benzenepropanoic acid		172–185.5		Sol.		157
	Monosodium salt	57.42					
Iolidonic acid (61.**4f**)	α-Ethyl-2,4,6-triiodo-3-(2-oxo-1-pyrrolindinyl)benzenepropanoic acid	59.58				4.89	161
Iopronic acid (61.**4g**)	(±)-2-{2-[3-(Acetylamino)-2,4,6-triiodophenoxy]ethoxymethyl}butanoic acid	56.57	130	1.09[b] / 1.95[c]		4.89	162, 163
Iobenzamic acid (61.**5a**)	N-(3-Amino-2,4,6-triiodobenzoyl)-N-phenyl-β-aminopropanoic acid	57.51	133–134.5	2.87[c]	Insol.	4.38	164, 165
Metrizamide (61.**5b**)	2-{[3-(Acetylamino)-5-(acetymethylamino)-2,4,-6-triiodobenzoyl]amino}-2-deoxy-D-glucose	48.2	230–240(d)	17.5[b]	>80		137, 138
Iocetamic acid (61.**6a**)	3-[Acetyl-(3-amino-2,4,6-triiodophenyl)amino]-2-methylpropanoic acid	62.01	224–225; 191–212 (Korver)	0.7[a] / 2.21[d]	Insol.	4.89	166, 167
Iomeglamic acid (61.**6b**)	5-[3-Amino-2,4,6-triiodophenyl)methylamino]-5-oxypentanoic acid	62.01	169	6.35[c]	Insol.		168–171
Iosumetic acid (61.**6c**)	4-{Ethyl[2,4,6-triiodo-3-(methylamino)phenyl]amino}-4-oxobutanoic acid	60.62					172, 173
Iodipamide (63.**7c**)	3,3′-[(1,6-Dioxo-1,6-hexanediyl)diimino]bis(2,4,6-triiodobenzoic acid)	66.81	306–308(d)		Insol.	1.74 (pK_1)	174–177
	Disodium salt			3.4[a]	Sol.	2.76 (pK_2)	
Ioglycamic acid (61.**7b**)	3,3′-{Oxybis[(1-oxo-2,1-ethanediyl)imino]}bis(2,4,6-triiodobenzoic acid)	67.55	222			1.67 (pK_1)	174, 175
	Meglumine salt		281(d) (three crystalline modifications)		Sol.	2.68 (pK_2)	
Iotroxic acid (61.**7c**)	3,3′-{Oxybis[2,1-ethanediyloxy(1-oxo-2,1-ethanediyl)imino]}bis(2,4,6-triiodobenzoic acid)						178
Iodoxamic acid (61.**7d**)	4,7,10,13-Tetraoxahexadecane-1,16-dioyl-bis(3-carboxy-2,4,6-tri-						

Table 61.2 (*Continued*)

USAN or INN Name	Chemical Name	Iodine Content, %	M.p., °C	LD$_{50}$, g/kg	Solubility, g/100 ml H$_2$O at 20°C	pK$_{H_2O}^{25}$	Ref.
	iodoanilide)	59.12	125	5.2^b	0.0364 (20°C)	1.8 (pK$_1$)	133, 179
B-9720 (61.**7e**)	5,5'-(Azelaoyldiimino)-bis[2,4,6-triiodo-3-(acetylamino)methyl-benzoic acid]	205–210		6.5^b	14(20°C, pH4.70)	2.8 (pK$_2$)	133
Iocarmic acid (61.**7f**)	5,5'-(Adipoyldiimino)bis (2,4,6-triiodo-*N*-methyl-isophthalamic acid)	60.72	302(d)				
	Dimeglumine salt			14–17.5^b	65(25°C)		180, 181
Iosefamic acid (61.**7g**)	5,5'-(Sebacoyldiimino)-bis(2,4,6-triiodo-*N*-methylisophthalamic acid)	58.17	279	13.1^b			180, 182
Iozomic acid (61.**8a**)	5,5'-[*N,N'*-Diacetyl-(4,9-dioxy-2,11-dihydroxy-1,12-dodecanediyl)di-imino]bis-(2,4,6-tri-iodo-*N*-methyl-isoph-thalamic acid)	52.25					183, 184
	Dimeglumine salt	41.22					
Tris(iothalamic acid) (61.**9**)	5,5',5''-(Nitrilotri-acetyltriimino)tris (2,4,6-triiodo-*N*-methyl-isophthalamic acid)	61.67					185
Iodoalphionic acid (61.**10**)	4-Hydroxy-3,5-diiodo-α-phenylbenzenepropanoic acid	51.38	157–162(d)		Insol.		186
	Disodium salt		>230				
Iophendylate (61.**11**)	Ethyl 10-(*p*-iodophenyl) undecylate	30.48			Sl. sol.		187–189
Iopydone (61.**12a**)	3,5-Diiodo-4(1*H*)-pyridinone	73.17	321 (d)		Insol.		190
Iodopyracet (61.**12b**)	3,5-Diiodo-4-oxo-1(4*H*)-pyridine acetic acid	62.50	245–249	6.3^b		2.15	120, 191
	2,2'-Iminodiethanol salt	49.76	155–157	2 (i.v. in dogs)	60		
Iopydol (61.**12c**)	1-(2,3-Dihydroxy-propyl)-3,5-diiodo-4–1*H*)-pyridinone	60.29	161				192
Propylidone (61.**12d**)	3,5-Diiodo-4-oxo-1(4*H*)-pyridineacetic acid propyl ester	56.78	186–187	0.3^b	0.014 (15°)		193, 194
Sodium iodo-methamate (61.**12e**)	1,4-Dihydro-3,5-diiodo-1-methyl-4-oxo-2,6-pyridinedicarboxylic acid, disodium salt	51.50	200(d)	4.60^b	Freely sol.		120, 190
Iopax (61.**13**)	5-Iodo-2-oxo-1(2*H*)-pyridine acetic acid, sodium salt	42.16		8^a	Very sol.		195, 196

^{a} I.v. in rats. ^{b} I.v. in mice. ^{c} Oral in mice. ^{d} Oral in rats.

6.2 Synthesis

The synthesis of iodinated contrast agents containing the phenyl ring as the carrier for radiopaque iodine atoms usually follows a general pattern which includes (1) the selection and synthesis of an intermediate containing the ring nucleus, (2) introduction of an activating group, such as nitro, amino, or hydroxyl, (3) iodination, (4) acylation, and finally (5) N-alkylation (197, 198), if necessary.

The activating groups are usually introduced by nitration as nitro groups which may be reduced to amino groups either before or after iodination. Reduction of the nitro group is effected by catalytic reduction using 5–10% palladium on charcoal or Raney nickel as catalyst (199, 200). The latter gives a high yield and a cleaner product than other reduction methods. Ammonium or sodium sulfide may also be used as a reductant (140, 152, 201, 202). The phenolic hydroxyl group is derived from diazotization of an amino group.

The phenyl ring, in the presence of an activating group, can accept three iodine atoms upon iodination with iodine mono-chloride (146). Iodination is usually carried out with iodine monochloride in dilute hydrochloric acid or dilute acetic acid or in potassium chloride solution (115, 146, 203). Acetylation reduces the toxicity and increases the solubility of iodinated aminobenzoic acids. Acetylation may also be effected by using ketene in the presence of sulfuric acid (202). A general method of acylation is the dissolution of the amine in dimethylformamide or dimethylacetamide (204) followed by addition of appropriate acyl chloride.

The effect of N-alkylation is bilitropic, increasing the contrast distribution in the liver as compared with the corresponding nonalkylated compound (179, 205). Houterman et al., in an attempt to prepare diatrizoate by a new procedure involving the hydrolysis of methyl diatrizoate in aqueous potassium hydroxide, found unexpectedly that the ester methyl group had methylated the acetamido group to metrizoic acid (cf. 118).

To illustrate the synthetic steps involved the synthesis of iocetamic acid (61.**6a**), an oral cholecystographic agent (166), is given below:

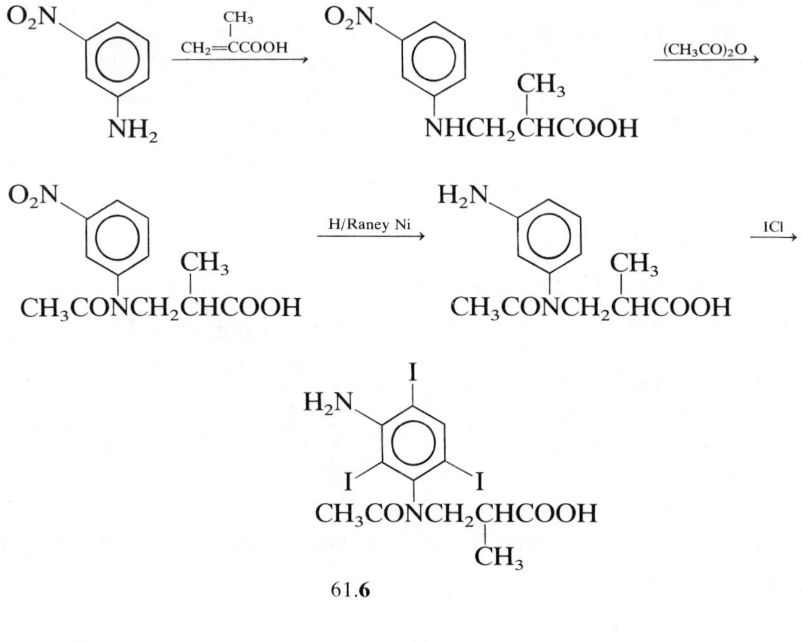

61.**6**

Hexaiodinated dimers are synthesized by condensing two iodine-carrying monomers of substituted 3-amino-2,4,6-triiodobenzoic acid with one molecule of a dicarboxylic acid chloride (133, 174, 204):

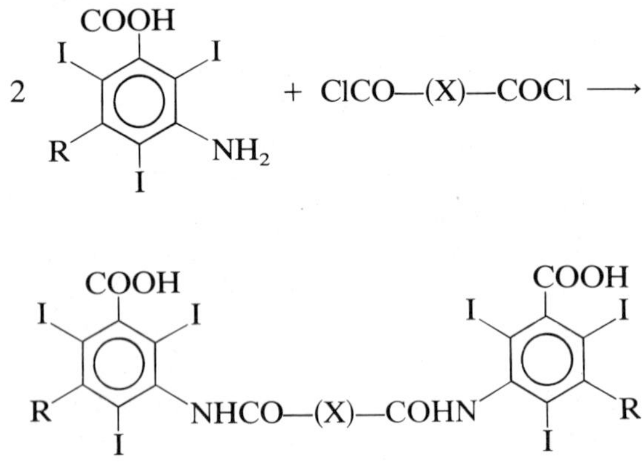

61.7

6.2.1 DIASTEREOISOMERS. Iodinated radiopaque compounds that contain a chiral center or chiral centers in the molecule form optical isomers or diastereoisomers. The presence of an asymmetric carbon atom in iopanoic acid (155), iophenoxic acid, or iodoalphionic acid (159), for example, leads to the formation of d and l forms. In iocetamic acid, free rotation around the axis connecting the iodinated benzene ring with the tertiary nitrogen atom is impeded by the bulky ortho-substituted iodine atoms, creating d and l forms (166). The molecule also contains an asymmetric carbon atom which gives rise to d' and l' forms. The racemates contain d,d' and l,l' as well as d,l' and d',l forms which are mutually diastereoisomeric and have different melting points and solubilities. Mixtures of diastereoisomers exhibit a wide melting range over many degrees.

Besides diastereoisomerism, iodinated radiopaques may show polymorphism; crystals formed under different conditions show identical infrared absorption bands but with different intensities (177, 179).

6.2.2 POTENTIAL RADIOPAQUES. A large number of organic iodine compounds synthesized in search of improved contrast agents are described in the patent literature; limitation of space does not allow a full tabulation of these compounds here. Since information concerning them may prove to be of value in the design and synthesis of new potential contrast agents, these compounds are listed in Tables 61.3 and 61.4 according to their ionic character and substitution in the triiodinated benzene ring. The hexaiodinated dimers are listed in Table 61.5, and other derivatives that have a different form of iodine-carrying moiety in Tables 61.6–61.9. Toxicity and proposed use are given when available. Many of these compounds have been evaluated clinically; some have been adopted for diagnostic use abroad. Many have lower toxicities and may prove to be better radiopaques than those in current use.

6.3 Structure–Activity Relationship

With few exceptions organic iodine compounds for X-ray diagnostic use contain an iodinated benzene ring or an iodinated pyridone nucleus. For reasons of low toxicity and high tolerance, modern contrast agents are variations of structures based on the triiodophenyl moiety as the iodine carrier. According to Hoey et al. (115) the desirable properties of intravascular contrast agents should include the following:

1. Maximum opacity to X-rays.
2. Pharmacological inertness.
3. High water solubility.
4. Chemical stability.
5. Selective excretion.
6. Low viscosity.
7. Minimum osmotic effect.

Contrast agents intended for oral cholecystography should possess, in addition,

Table 61.3   Potential Radiopaques: 1,3-Disubstituted 2,4,6-Triiodobenzene Derivatives

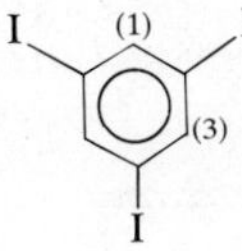

Substituent at (1)	Substituent at (3)	Uses	Comments	Ref.
		1. Ionic		
$C_nH_{2n} = COOH$ ($n = 0, 1$)	NRR^1 or $N = CHRR^1$ ($R, R^1 = H$, Me, Et, Ac)			205
$CH_2CHEtCO_2H$	$NAcR (R = Me$ or Et)	Oral cholecystography	Synthesis	206
CH_2CHRCO_2H ($R = H$, Me, or Et)	$-N=CR^1NR^2R^3$ ($R^1 = H$, Me, or Et; $R^2R^3 = H$ or Me, $R^2R^3 = (CH_2)_4$]	Oral cholecystography	Synthesis (8 compounds prepared)	207
CH_2CHRCO_2H ($R = Et$ or Ph)	NR^2COR^1 ($R^1 = H$, Me, or Pr; $R^2 = H$, Me, Et, or Pr)	Cholecystography	Synthesis	208
QCO_2H ($Q = (CH_2)_2$, CH_2CHEt, or $CH=CEt$)	NR^2COR^1 ($R^1 = Me$, Et, or Pr; $R^1 = H$, Me, iso-Pr, Bu, or allyl)	Oral cholecystography	Synthesis, toxicity studies	209
$QYCO_2H$	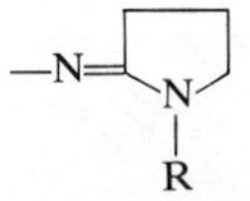 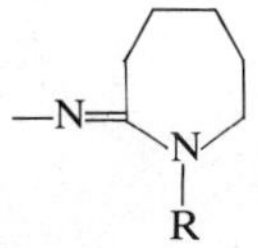		Synthesis (low toxicity and rapid clearance)	210
($Q = CONR^1$, $Y = $ a straight or branched alkylene or $QY = Y$)	($R, R^1 = H$, alkyl, hydroxyalkyl, methoxyalkyl, cycloalkyl, aryl, or aralkyl)			
QCO_2H ($Q = CH_2$, CHMe, CHEt, CH_2CHEt, CHPh, CH_2CHPh, or OCHPh)	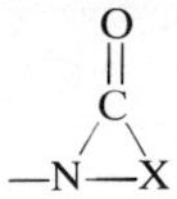 [$X = (CH_2)_2$, $(CH_2)_3$, or CH_2OCH_2]	Oral cholecystography	Synthesis (good organ specificity)	161, 211
$QCHRCO_2H$	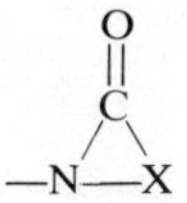 [$X = (CH_2)_2$, $(CH_2)_3$, or CH_2OCH_2]	Oral cholecystography	Synthesis (15 compounds prepared)	197
($Q = $ bond, CH_2, or O; $R = H$, Me, Et, or Ph)				
$(CH_2)_n CONRC_6H_4R^1$ [$n = 0$ or 1; $R = H$ or Me; $R^1 = 4\text{-}CH_2CO_2H$, 3- or $4\text{-}CH_2CH_2CO_2H$,	R^2 ($R^2 = NH_2$, NEtAc, or $N = CHNMe_2$)		Synthesis	205

Table 61.3 (*Continued*)

Substituent at (1)	Substituent at (3)	Uses	Comments	Ref.
3-$(CH_2)_3CO_2H$, 3-OCH_2CO_2H, 3-$OCHMeCO_2H$, 3-or 4-$OCHEtCO_2H$, 3-$OCHPrCO_2H$, or 3-$OCHBuCO_2H$]				
$CONHC_6H_4R$ [R = $O(CH_2)_nCO_2H$ or $(CH_2)_nCO_2H$]	NH_2	Oral or i.v. cholecystography	Synthesis	212
$CONRXCO_2H$ [X = H, $CH_2(CH_2)_2$, CH_2CHMe, or $CHEtCH_2$; R = H, Me, Et, Pr, iso-Pr, allyl, Bu, 2-hydroxyethyl, 3-methoxypropyl, $MeO(CH_2)_3$, furfuryl, or Ph]	$CONR^1R^2$ [R^1 = H, Me, Et; R^2 = H, Me, Et, CH_2CH_2OH, or $(CH_2)_3OMe$]	i.v. cholangiography and cholecystography	Synthesis	213–214
$CONRXCO_2H$ [X = $CH_2(CH_2)_2$, $MeCHCH_2$ or CH_2CHMe; R = H, lower alkyl, allyl, benzyl, 3-methoxypropyl, or 2-furanomethyl)	NR^1R^2 (R^1 = Ac or COEt; R^2 = alkyl or allyl)	Oral or i.v. cholecystography	Synthesis	212
$CONRC_6H_4X(CH_2)_n$ CO_2H [X = (o, p, m) a direct chemical bond or 0; R = H or alkyl]	NR^1R^2 (R^1 = H, acyl, or alkyl; R^2 = H or alkyl)		Synthesis	215
$NRCOCH_2XCO_2H$ (R = H or Me; X = CHMe or CHEt)	NH_2	Oral cholecystography	Synthesis	199
$NRCOXCH_2CO_2H$ [R = H, Me, or Et; X = CH_2, $(CH_2)_2$, or CH_2CHMe]	NH_2	Oral cholecystography	Synthesis, oral LD_{50} values in mice given	200
$NRCOQCO_2H$ [R = H, C_{1-4} alkyl; Q = $(CH_2)_2$, $(CH_2)_3$, CHEt, CH_2CHMe, CH_2CHEt]	H, OH, OMe, OEt, OPr, NH_2, I	Cholecystography	Synthesis (21 compounds prepared)	216
$NAcC(Me)_2CO_2H$	NH_2	Oral cholecystography	Synthesis (lower toxicity than iopanoic acid)	217
$OCH_2CH_2OCH_2$ $CHRCO_2H$ (R = Me or Et)	$CONR^1R^2$ (R^1 = H, R^2 = Me or Et, NR^1R^2 = morpholino)	Cholecystography	Synthesis; LD_{50} in mice: oral; 2.8–>4.0 g/kg; i.v.; ~0.55–1.4 g/kg	218

Table 61.3 (*Continued*)

Substituent at (1)	Substituent at (3)	Uses	Comments	Ref.
O(CH$_2$)$_n$(CH$_2$)$_m$ CHR^{1}CO$_2$H ($n = 2$–4; $m = 0, 1$; R^1 = H, Me, Et, Pr, C$_6$H$_5$, o-CH$_3$C$_6$H$_4$, p-CH$_3$C$_6$H$_4$)	NHCOMe, NR^2 (R^2 = H, Me, Et, C$_6$H$_5$)	Oral cholecysto-graphy	Synthesis, toxicity studies	163
OCHRCO$_2$H (R = H, Me, Et, Pr, or Bu)	NR^{1}COR^2 (R^1 = Me, Et, or Pr; R^2 = Me, Et, Pr, Bu, or CH$_2$C$_6$H$_5$)	Oral cholecysto-graphy	Synthesis (22 compounds prepared), toxicity, and excretion studies	198
O(C$_n$H$_{2n}$)CO$_2$H	NH$_2$, NHAc, N(Et)Ac, —N=CHNRR^1 (R, R^1 = H, Me, Et, or Ac)			205
O(CH$_2$)$_n$OCH$_2$CHRCO$_2$H ($n = 2$–4; R = Me or Et)	NHCOR^1 (R^1 = Me or Et)	Cholecystography	Synthesis (11 compounds prepared)	219
OCHRCO$_2$H (R = H, Me, Et, Pr, or Bu)	NR^{2}COR^1 (R^1 = Me, Et, or Pr; R^2 = Me, Et, Pr, Bu, or CH$_2$Ph)		Synthesis (22 compounds prepared)	198
OYCO$_2$H (Y = (CH$_2$)$_3$, CHEt, or CHPh)	CONR^{1}R^2 (R^1 = H or Me, R^2 = Me or Et, NR^{1}R^2 = morpholino)	Cholecystography	Synthesis	220
OC$_6$H$_4$CH$_2$CH(NH$_2$)CO$_2$H	OH	Bronchography, lymphography, encephalography, myelography	Synthesis	221
OCH(PhR)CO$_2$H (R = H, Me, or I)	NR^{1}COR^2 (R^1 = Me or Et; R^2 = H, Me, or Et)	Oral cholecys-tography	Synthesis	222

2. Nonionic

CHEtCO$_2$R (R = CH$_2$CCl$_3$, Bu, CH$_2$Ph, or CH$_2$OCOMe)	H		Synthesis	223
CH$_2$CHEtCO$_2$R (R = alkyl, CH$_2$Ph, CH$_2$OAc, CH$_2$O$_2$CMe, CH$_2$O$_2$CMe, or CH$_2$CCl$_3$)	NH$_2$		Synthesis	223, 224
CH$_2$X [X = N(CH$_2$OH)$_3$, NHC(CH$_2$OH)$_3$, NHCMe(CH$_2$OH)$_2$,	R (R = NH$_2$, NHAc, NAc$_2$, or I)	Pelviscopy	Synthesis	225

Table 61.3 (*Continued*)

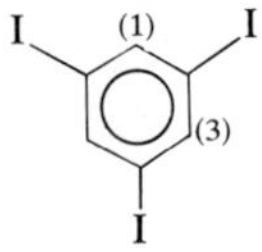

Substituent at (1)	Substituent at (3)	Uses	Comments	Ref.
NHCH$_2$CH$_2$OH, NH(CH$_2$)$_3$OH, NHC$_6$H$_{11}$, NHCH$_2$Ph, morpholino, piperidino, piperazino, *N*-methylglucaminyl, or *N*-(1-amino-1-deoxy-D-arabitol) residue]				
CH$_2$N(CH$_2$CH$_2$OH)$_2$	N(Ac)CH$_2$CH(OH)CH$_2$OH	Cholangiography	Synthesis, toxicity studies	226
CH$_2$X [X = Cl, Br, N(CH$_2$CH$_2$OH)$_2$, NHC(CH$_2$OH)$_3$, or *N*-methylglucamino]	N=CHNMe$_2$	Skiagraphy of gall bladder	Synthesis	227, 228
CHRR^1 [R = H, CH$_2$CO$_2$H; R^1 = CH$_2$CO$_2$H, N(CH$_2$CO$_2$H)$_2$, N(CH$_2$CO$_2$Me)$_2$]	NH$_2$, NHAc, NAc$_2$	Cholangiography	Synthesis (inactive)	229
CH$_2$NRR^1 [R = H, Me, or CH$_2$CHCH; R^1 = CH$_2$CH$_2$OH C(CH$_2$OH)$_3$, or CH$_2$(CHOH)$_4$CH$_2$OH]	N=CHNMe$_2$	Cholecystography	Synthesis	230
CON(CH$_2$CH=CH$_2$) CH$_2$CH$_2$CO$_2$Me	N=CHNMe$_2$	Cholecystography	Synthesis	231
CONRR^1 (R = H, Me, or Et; R^1 = Me, Et, Bu, iso-Bu, or CH$_2$CH$_2$OH; NRR^1 = morpholino or piperidino)	OH	Cholecystography	Synthesis	232
CONRXCO$_2$Me [X = CH$_2$, (CH$_2$)$_2$, or CH$_2$CHMe; R = H, allyl, (CH$_2$)$_3$, or (CH$_2$)$_3$OMe]	CONR^{1}R^2 (R^1, R^2 = H or Me)	I.v. cholangiography and cholecysto-graphy	Synthesis	233, 234
CONRXCO$_2$R^1 [X = CH$_2$, (CH$_2$)$_2$, CH(Me)CH$_2$, or CH$_2$CHMe; R = H, lower alkyl, allyl-benzyl, 3-methoxypropyl, or 2-furanomethyl; R^1 = Me, Et, nontoxic	NR^{2}R^3 (R^2 = Ac or COEt R^3 = alkyl or allyl)	Oral or i.v. chole-cystography	Synthesis	235

Table 61.3 (*Continued*)

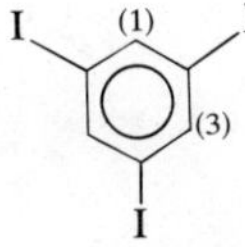

Substituent at (1)	Substituent at (3)	Uses	Comments	Ref.
inorganic or organic base residue]				
CONRCH$_2$CHR^{1}CO$_2$R^2 [R = H, Me, CHMe$_2$Et, (CH$_2$)$_3$OME, allyl; R^1 = H, Me, Et; R^2 = H, Me]	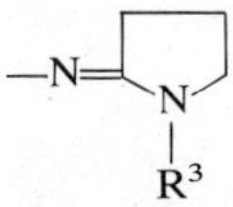 —N= structure with R^3 [R^3 = H, Me, Et, (CH$_2$)$_2$OH, (CH$_2$)$_2$OME, (CH$_2$)$_3$OME, cyclohexyl, Ph, OME]		Synthesis (30 compounds prepared	236
O(CH$_2$)$_3$CO$_2$Et	CONHMe	Cholecystography	Synthesis	232
OCHEtCO$_2$R (R = alkyl, CH$_2$Ph, CH$_2$OAc, CH$_2$O$_2$CCMe$_3$, or CH$_2$CCl$_3$)	H		Synthesis	224

hydrophilic and lipophilic properties. Because each of these properties is associated with certain molecular features and not all of them are structurally compatible, the best radiopaques represent a compromise in obtaining a maximum of these desirable qualities.

Relations between structure–dependent properties and characteristics of radiopaques are given below.

6.3.1 RADIOPACITY. This property is generally determined by the number of iodine atoms in the molecule, with more iodine atoms per molecule yielding better images provided that other properties are equal (130). Dimers, trimers, and polymers contain more iodine atoms per molecule than the monomers and are therefore more desirable for contrast use. Opacity is a physical property, affected not only by the atomic number but also by the localization

and concentration of contrast medium in the organ.

6.3.2 ACIDITY. The inductive effect of the iodine atoms in the molecule makes the substituted 2,4,6-triiodobenzoic acids stronger acids than the substituted 2,4,6-triiodophenyl or triiodophenoxy alkanoic acids. The pK_as of many contrast agents were measured by Felder et al. (179).

6.3.3 SOLUBILITY. Contrast agents for angiography are by necessity administered intravascularly in large doses, and for this a high water solubility is required. Agents for oral cholecystography need an optimum oil-and-water solubility so that upon ingestion, the molecule can be absorbed and transported across the intestinal cell membrane, transferred from blood to the liver, and concentrated in the gall bladder. Agents for myelography may be oils or water-

Table 61.4 Potential Radiopaques: 3,5-Disubstituted 2,4,6-Triiodobenzoic Acids and Derivatives

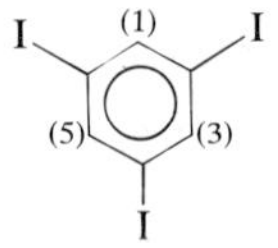

	Substituent				
(1)	(3)	(5)	Uses	Comments	Ref.
		1. Ionic			
CO_2H	CH_2NAc	$NAcCH_2CH$ $(OH)CH_2OH$	Angiography	Synthesis	237, 238
CO_2H	CH_2NHCO_2R [R = lower alkyl, hydroxyl alkyl, dihydroxyalkyl, alkoxyalkyl, mono-, di-, or poly(oxyalkylene)]	$NHCOR^1$ (R^1 = lower alkyl, hydroxyalkyl, or alkoxyalkyl)	Cholecysto-graphy	Synthesis (some compounds are well tole-rated at 45–500 mg/ml)	239
CO_2H	CH_2NHCO CHROH (R = H, Me)	$NHCOCHR^1R^2$ (R^1 = H, Me; R^2 = H, OH)		Synthesis	240
CO_2H	$CH(R)OR^1$ (R, R^1 = H or Me)	NR^2COR^3 (R^2 = H, Me, CH_2CH_2OH, $CH_2CH(OH)CH_2OH$, $CH_2CH_2OCH_2CH_2OH$, or $CH_2CONHMe$; R^3 = Me, Et, Pr, or CH_2OMe)		Synthesis (14 acids pre-pared)	241
CO_2H	CONHMe	NRAc (R = H, Mt, Et or CH_2CH_2OH)	Urography, angiography, myelography	Synthesis, toxicity studies	242, 243
CO_2H	$CONHCH_2CH_2OH$	NMeAc		Intracerebral LD_{50} in mice: 0.79 g/kg	244
CO_2H	CONMeR (R = H or Et)	$NHCONR^1R^2$ (R^1 = H or Me; R^2 = Me or Et)		Synthesis	245
CO_2H	$CONRCR^1(CH_2OH)_2$ (R = H, Me; R^1 = H, CH_2OH)	NHR^2 (R^2 = H, Ac, or $COCH_2OMe$)			246
CO_2H	$COANRR^1$ (A = amino acid residue; R = H; R^1 = H, Me, or CH_2CH_2OH; NRR^1 = morpholino)	$NHCOR^2$ (R^2 = Me, CH_2OMe, CH_2OH, or $(CH_2)_3Me$)	Urography, angiography, myelography	Synthesis	150, 247
CO_2H	NHR (R = H, Ac, or COEt)	NR^1R^2 (R^1 = H or Me; R^2 = Ac or COEt)	Angiography	Synthesis	248
CO_2H	NHR (R = H or Ac)	$NAcCH_2CONMe_2$		Synthesis	249
CO_2H	NHR (R = H, or Ac)	NMeAc		Synthesis	250
CO_2H	NHAc	R (R = H, NHAc, NMeAc, or CONHMe)		As hydrophilic water-insoluble polymers	251

Table 61.4 (*Continued*)

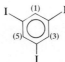

	Substituent				
(1)	(3)	(5)	Uses	Comments	Ref.

1. Ionic

(1)	(3)	(5)	Uses	Comments	Ref.
CO_2H	NHAc	$CONHCH_2CH_2OH$	Angiography, urography	Synthesis	152, 201
CO_2H	NHAc	NHR (R = H or Ac)		Synthesis	202, 252, 253
CO_2H	NHAc	CH_2CONHR (R = H, Me, CH_2CH_2OH)		Synthesis	254, 255
CO_2H	NHAc	$COCH_2OR$ (R = H or Me)		Synthesis and formulation	256
CO_2H	NHCOR (R = Me or Et)	R^1 (R^1 = H, NHAc, NHCOEt, CONHMe, NAcMe, CH_2NHAc, or $CONHCH_2CH_2OH$)	Angiography	Synthesis and formulation	257
CO_2H	$NHCOCH_2NHR$ (R = metrizoyl)	$CONHCH_2CH_2OH$		Synthesis, toxicity studies	258
CO_2H	NHCOR (R = H, Me, or Et)	CH_2NHCOR^1 (R^1 = H, Me, or Et)	Urography	Synthesis, toxicity studies	259
CO_2H	$NHCOCH_2OR$ (R = Me or Et)	CH_2NHAc	Angiography, urography	Synthesis	260
CO_2H	NRAc (R = Pr, Bu, or Am)	NR^1COR^2 (R^1 = H or Pr; R^2 = Me or Et)	I.v. cholecys-tography	Synthesis (60–80% of the dose excreted in the bile 4 hr after injection in rats)	261
CO_2H	R [R = $NAcCH_2CH_2OH$, $NAcCH_2CH(OH)$ $CH_2OH, N(COEt)$ CH_2CH_2OH, CONHMe, or $CONH(CH_2CH_2OH)$]	NR^1R^2 (R^1 = Me or CH_2CH_2OH; R^2 = Ac, EtCO)	Angiography encephalography	Synthesis (lower intracerebral toxicity than meth-iodal and iotha-lamic acid)	262
CO_2H	R [R = NH_2, NHAc, N(Me)Ac, NHCOEt, or N(Me)COEt]	R^1 [R^1 = CH_2NHAc, $NAc(CH_2CH_2OH)$, $N(COPr)(CH_2CH_2OH)$, $CONMe(CH_2CH_2OH)$]	Ventriculography, radiculography, lumbar myelo-graphy, angiography	Synthesis, toxicity studies	263
CO_2H	NRAc (R = Me, Et, or CH_2CH_2OH)	$CHNR^1Ac$ (R = H, Me, or CH_2CH_2OH)		Synthesis	264
CO_2H	OH	Me		Synthesis	265
CO_2CHRCO_2H (R = H or Et)	NHAc	NHAc	Angiography	Synthesis	248
CO_2CHRCO_2H (R = H or C_{1-4} alkyl)	NHR^1 (R^1 = H or C_{1-6} alkyl)	R^2 (R^2 = H or C_{1-6} alkylamino)	Cholecystography	Synthesis	266
$OCHRCO_2H$ (R = H or Et)	$CONHR^1$ (R^1 = H or Me)	$CONHR^2$ (R^2 = H or Me)		Synthesis	267

Table 61.4 (*Continued*)

Substituent (1)	(3)	(5)	Uses	Comments	Ref.
			1. Ionic		
OCHRCO$_2$H (R = H, Me, Et, n-Pr, n-C$_{4-8}$, or Ph)	CONHR^1	CONHR^2	Cholecystography	Synthesis (14 compounds prepared)	268
			2. Nonionic		
CO$_2$R (R = alkyl, CH$_2$Ph, CH$_2$OAc, CH$_2$OCO CMe$_3$, or CH$_2$CCl$_3$)	NHAc	CONHAc		Synthesis	224
CO$_2$R (R = C$_{1-12}$ alkyl)	NHAc	CONHCH$_2$CH$_2$OH		Synthesis	152, 201
CO$_2$R (R = phthalidyl, C$_{5-8}$ alkyl, CH$_2$Ph, CHMeOAc, CHMeO$_2$CCMe$_3$ CH$_2$O$_2$CCMe$_3$, or CH$_2$CH$_2$NMe$_2$)	NHAc	R^1 (R^1 = NMeAc or CONHMe)		Synthesis (13 esters prepared)	269
CO$_2$CH$_2$O$_2$CR (R = Me or CMe$_3$)	NHAc	CONHMe	Bronchography, hepatography, or salinography	Synthesis	270
CONHMe	NRAc (R = CH$_2$CO$_2$H or CH$_2$CONH$_2$)	COR^1 (R^1 = OH or NHMe)	Urography, arteriography, myelography	Synthesis, toxicity studies	271
CONHMe	NHAc	OR (R = β-D-glucopyranosyl, β-D-2,3,4,6-tetra-acetylglucopyranosyl)		Synthesis	140
CONHR (R = Me or CH$_2$CH$_2$OH)	R^1 (R^1 = CONHMe or NMeAc)	NR^2-gluconoyl (R^2 = H or Me)		Synthesis	272
CONRR^1 (NR^{1}R^2 = gluco-simino or N-methylgluco-simino)	R^2 (R^2 = NHAc or NAc$_2$)	R^3 (R^3 = NHAc or NMeAc)	Angiography, myelography	Synthesis	273
CONRR^1 [R = H, Me, Et, Pr, CHMe$_2$, CH$_2$ CH=CH$_2$, (CH$_2$)$_3$OMe, Ph, CH$_2$Ph; R^1 = Me, Et, CH$_2$CH=CH$_2$, or QCO$_2$H Q = CH$_2$CHMe]	N=CR^{2}NR^{3}R^4 [R^2 = H, Me, Et, CH$_2$CO$_2$H, or (CH$_2$)$_2$CO$_2$H; R^3 = H, Me, or Et; R^4 = Me, Et, or Ph]	R^5 (R^5 = H, CO$_2$H, or CONHMe)		Synthesis (60 compounds prepared)	274, 275

Table 61.4   (*Continued*)

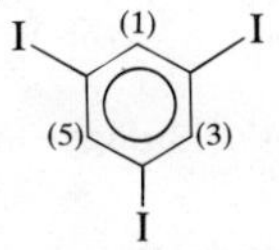

	Substituent				
(1)	(3)	(5)	Uses	Comments	Ref.
		1. Ionic			
CONRR^1 (R = H; R^1 = H, Me, or CH$_2$CH$_2$OH; NRR^1 = morpholino)	COXOH (X = amino acid residue	NHCOR^2 (R^2 = Me, CH$_2$OMe, or CH$_2$OH)		Synthesis	247
CH$_2$X (X = OH or Cl)	R (R = NH$_2$, NHAc, NAc$_2$ or I)	R^1 (R^1 = NH$_2$, NHAc, NAc$_2$, NHCOPr, OMe, or I)		Synthesis (11 compounds prepared)	276
QCO$_2$R (X = OH or Cl)	R^1 (R = NH$_2$, NHAc, NAc$_2$, or I)	R^2 (R^1 = NH$_2$, NHAc, NAc$_2$, NHCOPr, OMe, or I)		Synthesis (11 compounds prepared)	276
QCO$_2$R [Q = chemical bond, (CH$_2$)$_2$, or OCHEt; R = CH$_2$ CCl$_3$, Bu, CH$_2$CO$_2$Me, or CH$_2$CMe$_2$COMe]	R^1 (R^1 = H, NH$_2$, or NHAc)	R^2 (R^2 = H or CONHMe)		Synthesis	277
COX (X, Y = OH or NRR^1 with R = H, Me, or CH$_2$CHOH; R^1 = H or Me; NRR^1 = morpholino	COAY (A = residue of an amino acid, e.g., glycine, DL-serine, DL-alanine, sarcosine, proline, or glycyl-L-leucine)	NHZ (Z = H or COR with R = Ac, COCH$_2$OMe, COBu, or COCH$_2$OH)		Synthesis	278
CO$_2$R (R = alkyl, CH$_2$Ph, CH$_2$OAc, CH$_2$ OCOCMe$_3$, or CH$_2$CCl$_3$)	NHAc	CONHMe		Synthesis	224

soluble compounds. The molecular requirements for different contrast agents differ and do not necessarily focus on the same substituent groups.

Solubility of contrast agents is determined mainly by the presence of hydrophilic groups (115–116). The substitution of R in 61.**1** with carboxyl and X and Y with acylamino, alkylcarbamoyl, and hydroxylated alkylamino groups confers a high water solubility to the molecule. Thus the triiodobenzoates and triiodoisophthalamates are highly water-soluble compounds. Solutions with concentrations as high as 90% can be achieved with iothalamates and metrizoates. These highly soluble contrast agents are also strong acids with pK_a values less than 3.

Table 61.5 Potential Radiopaques: Dimers of Substituted 2,4,6-triiodobenzoic Acid

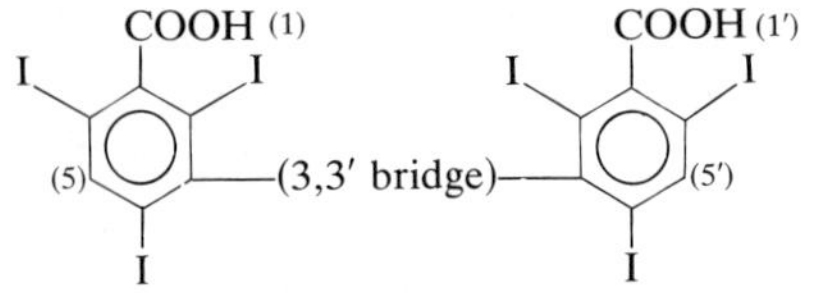

(3,3' Bridge)	(5), (5')	Uses	Comments	Ref.
		1. Ionic		
CONH(CH$_2$)$_3$NHCO	NHCONHMe	Urography	Synthesis	279
NMeCO(CH$_2$)$_4$COMeN	CONHMe	I.v. cholangiography	Synthesis, LD$_{50}$: 14.5 g/kg (mice, i.v.)	280
NHCO(CH$_2$)$_2$CONH	NHAc	Urography	LD$_{50}$: 18.1 g/kg (rat) (less toxic than diatrizoate and iothalamate)	281
NHCO(CH$_2$)$_4$CONH	H		Synthesis	282
NHCOCH$_2$OCH$_2$CONH	H		Synthesis	282
NHCO(CH$_2$OCH$_2$)$_3$CONH	H		Synthesis	283
NHCO(CH$_2$)$_2$(OCH$_2$CH$_2$)$_3$ CONH	H	I.v. cholangiography	Synthesis LD$_{50}$: 4.35 g/kg (bile/urine excretion ratio 3:1)	284
NHCO(CH$_2$)$_2$(OCH$_2$CH$_2$)$_4$ CONH	H	I.v. cholangiography	Synthesis	285, 286
NHCOXCONH (X = polymethylene or polyalkoxy)	CH$_2$NHAc		Synthesis (19 compounds prepared)	287
NHCOXCONH [X = (CH$_2$)$_n$, n = 4–8; MeCH(CH$_2$)$_3$, CH$_2$CH$_2$ (OCH$_2$CH$_2$)$_n$, n = 2–4, CH$_2$CH$_2$O(CH$_2$)$_3$OCH$_2$CH$_2$]	R (R = H, CH$_2$NHAc, CH$_2$NHCOEt, CH$_2$NHCOPr, CH$_2$NCOCH$_2$CH$_2$CH$_2$)		Synthesis (40 compounds prepared)	133
NHCO(CH$_2$)$_n$X(CH$_2$)$_n$CONH [X = S, O, SO, SO$_2$, S(CH$_2$)$_4$S, S(CH$_2$)$_2$O(CH$_2$)$_2$S, SO$_2$(CH$_2$)$_4$SO$_2$; n = 1 or 2]	R (R = NMeAc, NEtAc, NPrAc, NBuAc, CONHMe, NMeCOEt, NMeCOPr, or NMeCOCH$_2$OMe]	I.f. cholecystography	Synthesis	288
NAcCH$_2$CH(OH)CH$_2$OCH$_2$ CH(OH)CH$_2$AcN	CH$_2$NHAc	Angiography, urography, oral agent for GI tract	Synthesis	289
NAcCH$_2$(OH)CH$_2$O(CH$_2$)$_4$ OCH$_2$CH(OH)CH$_2$AcN	NMeAc	Arthrography, angiography	Synthesis	290, 291
NAcXAcN [X = CH$_2$CH(OH)CH$_2$OCH$_2$ CH(OH)CH$_2$, CH$_2$CH(OH)(CH$_2$)$_2$ CH(OH)CH$_2$, or CH$_2$CH(OH)(CH$_2$)$_4$ CH(OH)CH$_2$]	H		Synthesis	292
NAc(CH$_2$)$_n$AcN (n = 3–6)	CH$_2$NHAc	Arteriography, angiocardiography, urography	Synthesis	293

Table 61.5 (*Continued*)

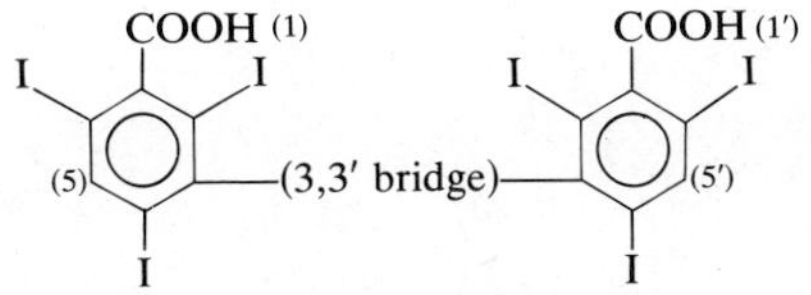

(3,3′ Bridge)	(5), (5′)		Uses	Comments	Ref.
N(R)XN(R) (X = C$_{3-15}$ alkylene or polyalkoxy; R = C$_{1-5}$ acyl)	NR^{1}R^2 (R^1 = C$_{1-5}$ alkyl; R^2 = C$_{1-5}$ acyl)		Synthesis		294, 295
CO(CH$_2$)$_n$CO (n = 4–8)	R [R = CH$_2$NHAc, CH$_2$NHCOEt, CH$_2$NHCOPr, or CH$_2$N(CH$_2$)$_3$CO]		Synthesis, toxicity studies		296
CO(X)CO [X = –CH$_2$CH$_2$O(CH$_2$)$_3$ OCH$_2$CH$_2$–, –CH$_2$CH$_2$ (OCH$_2$CH$_2$)$_n$–, with n = 2–4]	R (R = H, CH$_2$NHAc, CH$_2$NHCOEt, CH$_2$NHCOPr, CONHMe, CH(CH$_2$)$_3$CO)		Synthesis toxicity studies		296
	2. Nonionic				
NHCOXCONH [X = (CH$_2$)$_4$, CH$_2$OCH$_2$CH$_2$OCH$_2$, CH$_2$CH$_2$SCH$_2$CH$_2$, CH$_2$(OCH$_2$CH$_2$)$_2$OCH$_2$]	CONR^{1}R^2 [R^1 = CH(CONHMe) CH$_2$OMe, CHMeCONHMe, CH$_2$CONHMe, Me, H; R^2 = H, Me]	CONR^{3}R^4 (R^3 = H, Me; R^4 = H, CHMeCO$_2$H, CH$_2$CO$_2$H)	19 compounds prepared		204

Asymmetry in the substitution of the contrast molecule also influences the solubility (9). The sodium salt of diatrizoic acid with a symmetrical 3,5-diacetamido substitution has relatively low water solubility and concentrations greater than 50% cannot be obtained. The solubility is increased when one of the acetamido group is replaced with N-methylcarbamoyl, N-methylacetamido, or acetamidomethyl group, as in iothalamate, metrizoate, or iodamide.

Oral cholecystographic agents must possess an optimum oil-and-water solubility for duodenal absorption. Substituents such as a carboxyl and an alkyl or aralkyl groups can impart both hydrophilicity and lipophilicity to the molecule. Iopanoate, ipo-date, and tyropanoate, for example, being substituted triiodophenyl alkanoic acids, meet this requirement. The chain length of the substituent can affect the quality of the image. Epstein et al. (311) observed that in a series of iodinated p-hydroxyphenyl-alkanoic acids, optimal visualization of dog bladder was achieved with five to eight carbon atoms in the alkanoic acid chain. Felder et al. (312) reported that the insertion of a methyl group between the oxygen and the α-carbon in the series of substituted triiodophenoxyalkoxyalkanoic acids can improve oral absorption, biliary excretion, and gall bladder visualization.

6.3.4 CHEMOTOXICITY. The development of modern contrast agents began with the

Table 61.6 Potential Radiopaques: Polymeric Substituted 2,4,6-triiodobenzoic Acids

Compound	Uses	Comment	Ref.
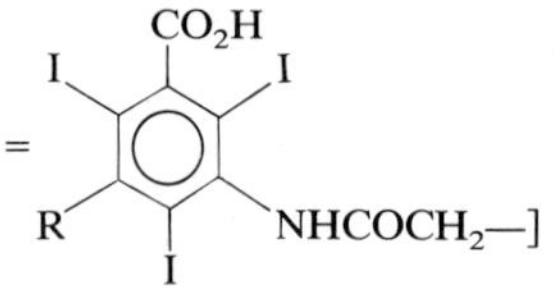 1. N≡(A, B, C)	Angiography	Synthesis	185

[A, B, C =

CO_2H and I, I, I substituents on ring, with R and NHCOCH$_2$—]

| 2. ----A–B–A–B–A–B---- | Roentgenography of gastrointestinal tract | | 135, 136 |

[A = —(Ac)N—(ring with CO_2H, I, I, I)—(X)— , where X = –N(Ac)–
or –CO(N(Me)–;

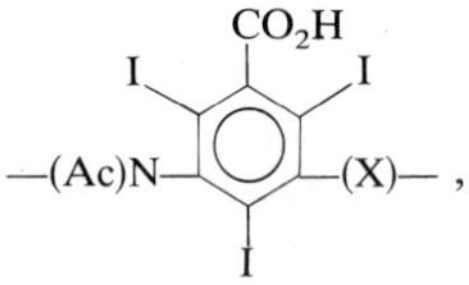

B = —(CH$_2$CH—CH$_2$O)$_2$(CH$_2$)$_4$(OCH$_2$CHCH$_2$)$_2$—, with OR groups,

where R = H or glyceryl]

Table 61.7 Potential Radiopaques: Substituted 3,5-diiodo-4(1H)-pyridones

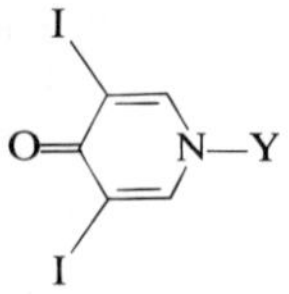

(structure: pyridone ring with O=, two I, and N—Y)

Y	Uses	Comment	Ref.
CH$_2$CO$_2$R (R = Bu, CH$_2$Ph, C$_4$–C$_{10}$ alkyl, CH$_2$OAc, CH$_2$OCOCMe$_3$, CH$_2$CCl$_3$)		Synthesis	223, 224, 277
(CH$_2$)$_n$CO$_2$R (R = H, Me, Et, Bu, Am, octyl, CH$_2$CH$_2$NMe$_2$, CH$_2$CH$_2$OH, NH$_2$)	Urography, lymphography	Synthesis (18 compounds prepared)	297
CH$_2$CONH(CH$_2$)$_n$NR^{1}R^2 [n = 2, 3; R^1 = R^2 = Me, Et, R^{1}R^2 = CH$_2$CH$_2$OCH$_2$CH$_2$]		Synthesis (high toxicity)	298
CH$_2$CH$_2$R [R = NMe$_2$, NEt$_2$, —N͡͡O , and their (CH$_3$)$_2$SO$_4$ salts, N$^+$(Et)$_2$CH$_2$CH$_2$OH·Cl$^-$] 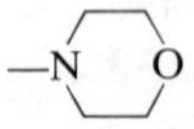		Synthesis (high toxicity)	298

Table 61.8   Potential Radiopaques: Monoiodophenyl Derivatives

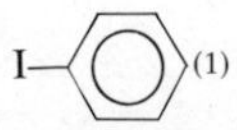

$$I—\bigotimes\text{(1)}$$

(1)	Uses	Comment	Ref.

CO$_2$XO$_2$CR
[X = (CH$_2$)$_2$, (CH$_2$)$_3$,
    CH$_2$CHMe, or (CH$_2$)$_4$;
R = Me, Et, Pr, i-Pr, Bu
    (CH$_2$)$_4$Me, (CH$_2$)$_5$Me, or CH$_2$OMe]
	Myelography	Synthesis	299

CO$_2$(CH$_2$)$_n$O$_2$CR
    [n = 2–4,
    R = Me, Et, Pr, i-Pr,
    (CH$_2$)$_3$Me, (CH$_2$)$_4$Me,
    (CH$_2$)$_5$Me, CH$_2$CHMe,
    or CH$_2$OMe]
	Myelography	Synthesis	300

–X–OCO$_2$R
[X = (CH$_2$)$_2$, (CH$_2$)$_3$,
    CHMeCH$_2$CH$_2$, CH$_2$CHEtCH$_2$,
    or CH$_2$CHBuCH$_2$;
R = Et, i-Pr, Bu, i-Bu,
    pentyl, hexyl, octyl, decyl,
    CHMeC$_6$H$_{13}$, CH$_2$CH(Et)Bu,
    CHMeCH$_2$CH(CH$_3$)$_2$, CH(Et)Pr,
    or CH$_2$CH$_2$OMe]
	Myelography, lym-
	    phography, broncho-
	    graphy, salpingo-
	    graphy
		Synthesis	301

observation by Wallingford et al. (141) that iodobenzoic acids have very low toxicity. Chemotoxicity refers to acute toxicity that, for substituted benzoic acids, can be modified by substitution, iodination, and acetylation (116–117). For example, amination of sodium benzoate decreases toxicity; the intravenous LD$_{50}$ values of 3-amino-benzoate and 3,5-diaminobenzoate (i.e., 3270 and 2600 mg/kg) in mice are higher than that of benzoate (1440 mg/kg). Acetylation decreases toxicity, as is evidenced by the even higher LD$_{50}$s of 3-acetamido-benzoate and 3,5-diacetamidobenzoate (3400 and 5580 mg/kg) than those of the corresponding amines. The detoxifying effect of acylation reaches a maximum of two carbon atoms in the actyl group in the series of 3-acylamino-2-,4,6-triiodo-benzoates, and further lengthening of the acyl chain causes an increase in toxicity (141).

Iodination may decrease or increase the toxicity depending on whether the parent compound is acetylated or unacetylated. Both 3-acetamido-2,4,6-triiodobenzoate and 3,5-diacetamido-2,4,6-triiodobenzoate (8300 and 14,000 mg/kg) have lower toxicities than the corresponding noniodinated parent compounds. The last member is the least toxic of the series and is available commercially as diatrizoate sodium and meglumine salts for clinical use in angiography, pyelography, urography, and other related roentgenographic procedures.

In hexaiodinated dimers, toxicity increases with increasing length of the dicarboxylic acid chain and also with increasing length of the substituent group in position 5 of the benzoic acid moiety (133, 313). Dimers with open positions in benzene rings linked by polymethylene polyoxadicarboxylic acid chain have higher intravenous toxicity in mice than those with

Table 61.9   Miscellaneous Potential Radiopaques

Compounds	Uses	Comments	Ref.
$ICH_2SO_2NRR^1$ [R = H, Me; $R^1 = CH_2CH(OH)CH_2OH$, $CH(CH_2OH)_2$, CH_2CH_2OH, $CH_2CH_2OCH_2CH_2OH$]	Myelography	Synthesis	302, 303
$\overset{\text{I}}{\underset{\text{I}}{RCOC}}$=CCOR [R = OH, $O(CH_2)_2OMe$, $O(CH_2)_2OEt$, $(OCH_2CH_2)OMe$, $(OCH_2CH_2)_2OEt$, $O(CH_2)_3Me$, $O(CH_2)_2CHMe$, $NH(CH_2)_2OH$, $NHCH_2CH(OH)Me$, $NHC(CH_2OH)_2Me$, $N(CH_2CHOH)_2$, $NHCHCO_2H$, or $NMeCH_2CO_2H$]		Synthesis (high toxi- city)	304
BuNHCONHR (R = 2,3,5,6-tetraiodo-*p*-tolysulfonyl)	Radiography of pancreas and prostate gland	Synthesis	305
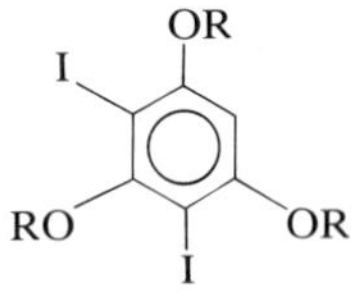 (R = glycosyl)	Urography		139
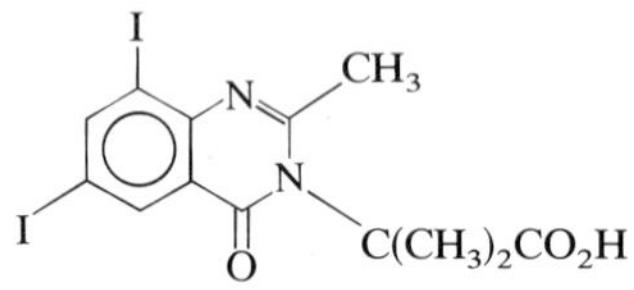		Synthesis toxicity studies	306
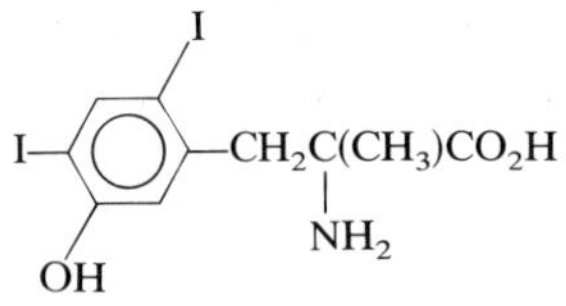	Cholecystography	Synthesis	307
	Cholecystography	Synthesis	308

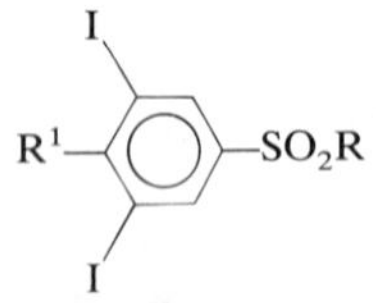

[$R^1 = NH_2$, N=CHNMe$_2$;
 R = NH_2, OH, NMe$_2$, NEt$_2$,
 NBu$_2$, morpholino, piperidino,
 NHCH$_2$CH$_2$OH, N(CH$_2$CH$_2$OH)$_2$, or
 NMeCH$_2$(CHOH)$_4$CH$_2$OH]

Table 61.9   (*Continued*)

Compounds	Uses	Comments	Ref.
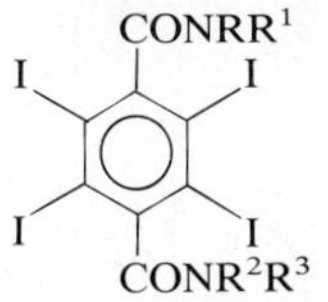 [NRR^1, NR^{2}R^3 = NHMe, NHCH$_2$CO$_2$H, NHCH(Pr)CO$_2$H, morpholino, 2-carboxy-1-pyrrolidinyl, NHCHEtCH$_2$CO$_2$H, NMeCH$_2$CO$_2$H, NEtCH$_2$CO$_2$H]		Synthesis	309
Me$_2\overset{+}{N}$(CH$_2$)$_n\overset{+}{N}$Me$_2$2X$^-$ $\quad\quad$R$\quad\quad$R^1 (n = 2, 4, 6, or 10; R, R^1 = H, ethylacetyl, 3-iodobenzyl, 2,4,5-triiodobenzyl, 5-amino-2,4-diiodobenzyl, 3-amino-2,4,6-triiodobenzyl; X = Cl, I)	Binding to cartilage	Synthesis	310

fully substituted benzene rings. Replacement of the *n*-butyramido group with a butyrolactamyl group decreases the toxicity of dimers linked by short dicarboxylic acid chain but increases the toxicity of those linked by long dicarboxylic acid chain. Introduction of one or more oxygen atoms into the dicarboxylic acid chain greatly reduces the toxicity. For this series of dimers, optimum tolerability was achieved in the compound formed by joining two molecules of 3-amino-5-acetylamino-methyl-2,4,6-triiodobenzoic acid with tetraoxahexadecanedicarboxylic acid (133).

In general, dimers have lower toxicity than the corresponding monomers.

6.3.5   PROTEIN BINDING AND EXCRETION. The capacity of contrast agents to bind serum proteins is related to certain structural features (313–315). Contrast agents with a fully substituted benzene ring show little or no protein binding and those having the ring open at position 5 bind readily with serum protein. Protein binding favors bilitropism (i.e., being hepatotrophic, excreted via the liver) rather than urotropism (i.e., being nephrotrophic, excreted via the kidney). The relative magnitude of biliary and urinary excretion of the contrast agent, also known as the B/U ratio, is determined by the structural features of the molecule, the dose, and the pathological state of the patient. Fumagalli et al. (197, 198) observed that *N*-alkylation promotes bilitropism.

According to Hansch (316, 317), protein binding is nonspecific and occurs with many sufficiently lipophilic compounds. The structural requirements for bilitropic agents are sufficient hydrophobicity and an open position 5 in the iodine-carrying benzene ring. Knoefel and Huang (318) observed that protein binding correlates with increasing toxicity in a series of substituted iodinated benzoic acids.

In hexaiodinated dimers, increasing the length of substituents in the benzene ring and the length of the dicarboxylic acid chain enhances hydrophobicity and increases the protein binding and the biliary-to-urinary excretion ratio (B/U) (319). Higher B/U excretion ratios are observed in dimers with open position 5 in the benzene ring than in those that are fully substituted. Introduction of one or more oxygen atoms into the dicarboxylic acid chain increases water solubility and reduces toxicity (133). Many hexaiodinated dimers are currently used as intravenous cholegraphic agents (320–322).

6.3.6 OSMOLALITY AND VISCOSITY. Osmolality and viscosity depend on the ionic character and structure of the contrast molecule (10, 11, 123, 130). Both osmolality and viscosity of a contrast medium can be reduced if spherical polymers and nonionic molecules are involved. Almén (130) has arrived at these conclusions from physicochemical principles. Because polymers contain more iodine atoms per molecule than monomers, for equal iodine content, the polymers will yield a small electrolyte concentration in solution and lower osmolality. Spherical molecules show less resistance to flow than linear molecules. Nonionic molecules make no contribution to electrolyte concentration and can reduce the toxicity markedly as compared to ionic ones. For example, the LD_{50} for the ionic metrizoic acid meglumine salt is 130 mg I/kg, if injected suboccipitally; but in the form of non-dissociable molecule metrizoic acid meglumide [1–(3-acetamido-5-N-methyl-acetamido-2,4,6-trioiodobenz-N-methyl-amido)-1-dexoy-D-glucitol], it is higher than 1000 mg I/kg (131). Based on this rationale, the search for improved contrast agents has been centered on dimers, trimers, polymers, and nonionic compounds. Dimers such as iocarmic acid (180–181) and iodoxamic acid (133, 179) and nonionic contrast agents such as metrizamide (138), triglycosyldiiodobenzene, and 2,4,6-triiodo-3-acetamido-5-N-methylcarbox-amido-phenyl-D-glycopyranoside (140) have been synthesized for clinical tests. Metrizamide has an extremely low toxicity and a wide spectrum of application.

6.4 Analysis

A contrast medium may be analyzed by its functionality or by its iodine content. *In vitro* analysis of iodine content of contrast media has been carried out by the Sandell–Kolthoff reaction (133). Contrast media in plasma may be determined by spectrophotomeric procedures (323–324) or by radiotracer techniques using ^{131}I labeled materials (325–328). Felder et al. (329) measured the concentration of water-soluble radiopaques by colorimetric determination of free aromatic amine function using the Bratten–Marshall reaction. Hartmann and Roepke (330) reported methods for determining the purity and stability of iodine-containing contrast agents of the aminobenzoic acid series. Kaufman et al. (331, 332) reported the use of fluorescent excitation method for determining iodine concentration in tissue samples by the K_α and K_β characteristic X-rays generated from irradiation with an [241]Am source. Koehler et al. (333) extended this method to *in vivo* measurement of hepatic iodine concentration after administration of radiopaque. The range of iodine determination is 0.05 to 40 mg/ml with an accuracy of approximately ±10%.

6.5 Pharmacology

Contrast media by necessity are relatively nontoxic. Adverse reactions accompanying their use vary and usually decrease in intensity and complexity in the order intracerebral > intravascular > oral route of administration > topical application (334–338). Many have intravenous LD_{50}s in the rat and mice in the range of tens of grams per kilogram body weight. The opacifying atom iodine has an intravenous LD_{50} in animals of 0.8–1.0 g/kg; yet the LD_{50}s of modern urographic contrast agents such as diatrizoate and iothalamate are in the range of 10–20 g/kg, which is of the same order of magnitude as the toxicity of glucose. The oral cholecystographic agents have considerably higher toxicity but the side reactions are generally restricted to gastrointestinal symptoms.

The pharmacological aspects and toxic reactions of contrast agents have been comprehensively reviewed by Hoppe (121), Almén (338), Ansell (339), and Berk and Loeb (340).

6.5.1 THE CATIONS. Iodinated contrast agents used in angiography, urography, and intravenous cholangiography, for example, are mostly substituted 2,4,6-triiodobenzoic acids that are formulated for intravenous administration as solutions of salts and are ionized at physiological pH. In high concentrations, these contrast media shows toxicities attributable to cations as well as the anion (9, 10, 34–42). The cations in regular use in contrast media are *N*-methylglucamine, sodium, calcium, and magnesium.

N-Methylglucamine (meglumine) ion has the following structure:

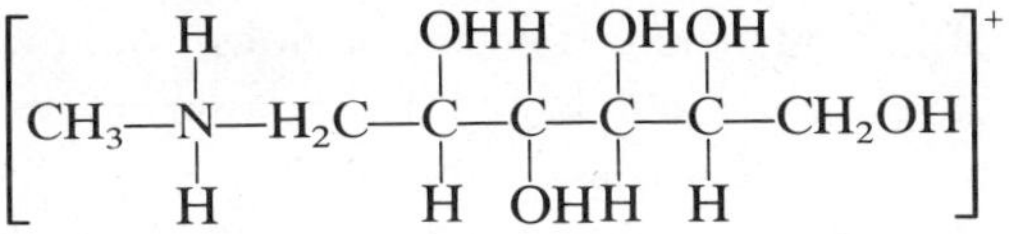

$$\left[\begin{array}{c} \quad\;\; H \qquad\quad OH\,H \;\; OH\,OH \\ CH_3{-}N{-}H_2C{-}C{-}C{-}C{-}C{-}CH_2OH \\ \quad\;\; H \qquad\quad H \;\; OH\,H \;\; H \end{array} \right]^+$$

Meglumine salts of contrast media such as diatrizoic, iothalamic, and metrizoic acid have higher viscosities than the corresponding sodium salts but are better tolerated and less toxic. High viscosity is a cause of toxicity of the meglumine salts and may be reduced by mixing with the sodium salt of the corresponding acid (341). Other organic bases, such as diethylamine, monoethanolamine, diethanolamine, triethanolamine (Tris), and morpholine, that have low toxicity are also used for cations (9, 144). The monoethanolamine salt of ioxitalamic acid shows a toxicity intermediate between those of sodium and meglumine salts (9). Diethanolamine and morpholine form 1:1 salts with 3,5-diiodo-4-oxo-1(4*H*)-pyridine acetic acid, named iodopyracet (Diodrast) and "Joduron" (144), respectively. The Tris molecule is spherical in shape and forms salts with diatrizoate, iothalamate, and metrizoate, for example, which yield solutions of lower viscosity than the corresponding meglumine salts. Other cations such as basic amino acids also form salts with the acid form of contrast agents and afford reduced toxicity (343).

Sodium salts of substituted 2,4,6-triiodobenzoic acids have high water solubility and solutions of 50–90% concentration corresponding to an iodine content of about 300 to more than 400 mg I/ml can thus be prepared for angiographic use (10, 11). An exception is sodium diatrizoate, which has a relatively low solubility in water, and solution concentrations exceeding 50% cannot be obtained. For high concentrations, the more soluble meglumine salts of diatrizoate are used instead. Sodium ions in excess amount are cardiotoxic (344); their concentration in contrast medium is many times higher than the ion concentration in plasma.

In normal blood, sodium, potassium, calcium, and magnesium ions are present in concentrations of 330, 20, 5–6, and 2–2.5 mg/100 ml plasma, respectively (345). The physiological functions of the cations are both antagonostic and complementary to one another. Sodium ions tend to increase the permeability of cell membrane whereas calcium ions act to counteract this effect. Calcium and magnesium ions are physiological antagonists. Magnesium ions can exert a deleterious effect on the nervous system if unaccompanied by the reversible antagonistic effects of calcium ions. The physiological interaction between these ions suggests that the toxicity of sodium ions in contrast medium can be modified by the addition of small concentrations of calcium and magnesium. Incorporation of potassium ions affords no beneficial effect. To minimize the toxicity, an optimum concentration of calcium and magnesium ions in the contrast medium is essential and should be 2.5 times their concentration ratio in plasma. Concentration ratio refers to the ratio of concentration of calcium or magnesium ions to that of sodium ions. Incorporation of optimal amounts of calcium and magnesium ions in solutions of sodium metrizoate can increase the LD_{50} values by 80–100% in the rabbit. Calcium ions alone lower the toxicity of methylglucamine metrizoate in LD_{50} tests in mice but not in the rabbit, whereas magnesium ions alone cause an increase in toxicity (345). A small amount of calcium ions in methylglucamine metrizoate causes less blood–brain barrier damage than when pure methylglucamine metrizoate of identical iodine content is given alone (342).

A combination of sodium, magnesium, and methylglucamine salts is referred to as the quad salts and is used to reduce the toxicity of ionic contrast media.

6.5.2 HYPEROSMOLALITY. Ionic contrast media for angiographic use are hyperosmotic relative to plasma. The osmolalities of the substituted triiodobenzoate anions diatrizoate, iothalamate, and metrizoate are approximately the same on the basis of equal iodine content (346). Injection of hyperosmolar contrast media causes hemodynamic responses which vary according to the rate and site of injection (341). Slow injection into the peripheral veins as in urography and intravenous cholangiography produces hypotension owing to a lowering of peripheral vascular resistance (347). Acute intravenous toxicity of contrast medium is increased with the rate of injection (138, 348–350). A large volume of hypertonic contrast medium, when rapidly injected into veins, arteries, and ventricles in selective angiography causes an elevation of the plasma osmolality and a shift of water out of red blood cells and from extravascular spaces to the blood, thereby increasing the circulating blood volume and peripheral blood flow which affect various aspects of circulation (10, 121, 128, 341, 344, 351–355). The more concentrated the injectate, the more intense the vascular reactions, and the more precipitous the onset (341, 351).

Systemic hypotension, changes in the activity of the smooth muscle cells in vessel walls, aggregation and crenation of red blood cells, and hypervolemia are examples of vascular reactions induced by the administration of ionic contrast media. Agglutination and crenation of red blood cells cause blood sludging and reduce the cells' ability to undergo deformation, thus blocking the blood flow to capillaries and leading to pulmonary hypertension and related physiological responses (356–361). The hypervolemia resulting from a shift of water elevates the ventricular filling pressure and increases the cardiac output from increased ventricular stroke work. The potassium ions released from shrinking and crenating red blood cells contribute to the lowering of systematic vascular resistance and blood pressure (362).

That osmolality is a major determinant of hemodynamic effects is obvious from the experiments conducted by Kloster et al. (363), who injected equiosmolar solutions of mannitol, sodium, and meglumine salts of diatrizoate and iothalamate, with an osmolality corresponding to 4.5 to almost 8 times the osmolality of blood serum, directly into the left ventricle of a dog and observed approximately similar hemodynamic responses. Hilal (354) reported that the bradycardia and hypertension due to intracarotid injection of contrast media and accompanying vascular reactions could be reproduced by injection of hypertonic solutions of sodium chloride of similar osmolarities. By comparing the hemo-dynamic effects from intracarotid injection of 50% sodium diatrizoate, 80% sodium iothalamate, and equiosmolar solutions of sodium chloride and dextrose, Cornell (364) concluded that the sodium ions may play a greater role than hypertonicity in causing these effects.

Toxic effects of sodium ions and hyperos-molality associated with monomeric ionic contrast agents are lessened when dimeric and trimeric contrast agents containing, respectively, six and nine iodine atoms per molecule are used. Both bis(iothalamic acid), i.e., iocarmic acid, and tris(iothalamic acid) produce less peripheral vasodilatation and reflex responses than the monomer iothalamic acid (9).

Nonionic contrast agents such as metri-zamide form nondissociable molecular solutions in water (365), thus circumventing the toxic effects due to hyperosmolality. Metrizamide has an extremely low cellular toxicity and can be injected at an iodine concentration of 380 mg I/ml into the common carotid artery of guinea pig without damage to the blood–brain barrier. The low intravenous toxicity has allowed metri-zamide to be widely used for angiography, myelography, and other procedures.

6.5.3 ADVERSE REACTIONS AND TOXICITY. In man, adverse reactions to contrast media vary greatly in type and severity from slight nausea or mild "hot flush" through a broad spectrum of increasingly severe cutaneous, respiratory, neurological, and cardiovascular disturbances that may, in extreme cases, result in the sudden death of the patient (335–340).

Ansari and Baldwin (366) reported acute renal failure following urography with meglumine diatrizoate, angiography with meglumine and sodium diatrizoate, oral cholecystography with iopanoic acid, and cholangiography with iodipamide. Roylance et al. (367, 368) reported the incidence of reactions to urographic agents.

The incidence and severity of adverse reactions from contrast media have gained greater attention recently, and a committee on contrast media was formed under the auspices of the International Society of Radiology in 1969 (369). Based on the analysis of a total of 112,003 cases of adverse reactions toward contrast media from Australia, Belgium, Canada, Norway, and the United States, Shehadi (334) reported the nonfatal incidence of reactions to be 2.3% for vascular studies, 5.65% for intravenous urography, and 10.11% for intravenous cholangiography. The incidence of reactions for total intravenous and intra-arterial examinations was 4.95%, and the incidence of fatal reactions was about 1/10,000, which is higher than the 1/60,000 reported earlier on the basis of retrospective studies. The contrast agents used in the cases studied were meglumine, diatrizoate, meglumine iothalamate, sodium diatrizoate, and sodium metrizoate.

In intravenous cholangiography, toxic symptoms occurred with a frequency of 12.6% for single-dose medication and 8.16% for drip infusion (334). Rapid injection of iodipamide resulted in a high reaction incidence and considerable toxicity whereas the slower injection led to a lower incidence of reaction and a greater margin of safety. The optimal injection time was reported to be 10 min for both single-dose and drip infusion.

In intravenous urography, the incidence of reactions was 5.38% for single bolus injection and 7.06% for drip infusion which required a higher dose of contrast medium (334). The incidence was higher with slow injection over a period of 3–10 min than with rapid injection performed in less than 2 min. This is a reversal of the hitherto widespread practice of administration of contrast media. Although the cause of this low incidence of reactions with rapid injection is not explained, it is not unreasonable to assume that less histamine is released (350).

In hypersensitive or allergic patients, idiosyncratic reactions may occur from a dose of contrast medium, and the overall incidence of adverse reactions in patients with allergy is about twice that in the general population (334–336, 370). Pretesting the patient by intradermal, subcutaneous, or intravenous injection of small doses has no value in predicting adverse reactions (334–336, 368, 371) but testing by *in vitro* leukocyte challenge has been reported to be of some predictive value (372). Premedication with antihistamines, anticholinergics, and diazepam (373) is less effective than with corticosteroids (335, 368).

6.5.4 NEUROTOXICITY. Contrast agents are toxic to the central nervous system (374). Their presence there is brought about either by direct injection into the cerebrospinal fluid or by leakage through the blood–brain barrier. Contrast agents are more toxic when administered intracisternally than intravenously (129). The ratio between intravenous and intracisternal LD_{50}s in the rabbit can be as high as 1450:1 for diatrizoate sodium (120).

The blood–brain barrier refers to the tight junctions between the cerebrovascular endothelial cells in cerebral blood vessels and is a physical barrier to the exchange of ions and large molecules between blood and brain (375–377). Concentrated solutions of electrolytes and relatively insoluble nonelectrolytes such as urea can reversibly open the barrier by separating the tight junctions through osmotically shrinking the endothelial cells (378–381). Barrier opening may be evaluated by the entry of dyes (e.g., trypan blue, Evans blue) (375, 383) or radioactive ions (e.g., ^{99m}Tc, ^{32}P) (384) into the brain parenchyma. This method together with those of induced convulsions (383–385) and damage to tissue cultures of neurons (386) have been used to determine the neurotoxicity of contrast agents. It should be pointed out that these methods

may not necessarily measure the same molecular property causing neurotoxicity.

Sodium, calcium, and meglumine salts of iothalamate, diatrizoate, and metrizoate as well as sodium chloride, at hyperosmolar concentrations, can damage the blood–brain barrier and cause it to open, thereby allowing passage of material between endothelial cells; but hyperosmolality alone is not sufficient to account for the difference in neurotoxicity among the contrast agents. Sodium salts of acetrizoate, iodamide, and metrizoate, for example, on intracarotid injection, cause an increase in capillary permeability, provoking cerebral edema (387).

According to Rapoport and Levitan (374), lipid solubility or the partition coefficient determines the neurotoxicity of contrast media. Lipid solubility regulates the passage of these agents through the unaltered blood–brain barrier. Neurons are very sensitive to chemicals, and minute concentrations of contrast medium in the brain can induce neurotoxicity (388). McClennan and Becker (389) reported that after intravenous injection of a contrast medium, as much as 1.5% of the plasma concentration may reach the cerebrospinal fluid. Tuohimaa and Melartin (385), using historadioautographic techniques, showed that the percent penetration of ^{131}I-tagged iothalamate and diatrizoate in the rat cerebral cortex correlates well with the degree of severity of neurotoxicity. When there was little or no penetration of contrast medium into the brain tissue, no convulsions were observed. Among the contrast agents studied, sodium diatrizoate was found to be more penetrating in the cerebral cortex than meglumine iothalamate. Also, the toxicity of small concentrations of diatrizoate, ioglycamide, and iopanoic acid on cultured neurons was related to their lipid solubility.

Using Hansch's rule for additive constitutive properties (390–393), Rapoport and Levitan (374) calculated the partition coefficients of iothalamate, ioxitalamate, diatrizoate, metrizoate, iodamide, diprotrizoate, and 2,4,6-triiodobenzoate. This study showed that the neurotoxicity of these agents increases with increase in the combined partition coefficient P and is related to the brain uptake index. The relation is similar to that observed by Oldendorf (394) between the chain length of short chain monocarboxylic acids and their transport across the blood–brain barrier, which reaffirms the dependence of neurotoxicity on lipid solubility.

In addition to osmolality and lipid solubility, neurotoxicity may also be caused by the presence of cations and contrast anions. Melartin et al. (395) studied the relative neurotoxicity of sodium and meglumine salts of diatrizoate and iothalamate in rats by intracisternal application and found that the sodium salts were about three times more neurotoxic than the meglumine salts when compared at comparable doses and that the diatrizoate anion was about 10 times more neurotoxic than the iothalamate anion. In both hypertonic and hypotonic ranges, neurotoxicity increases with increasing concentration of contrast medium. In comparing the neurotoxicity, not only the molal concentration of the contrast medium but also the brain weight of the experimental animals should be considered.

Damage to the spinal cord by contrast medium also causes neurotoxicity (337, 338, 396). Spinal cord damage was first observed by Antoni and Lindgren (397) following aortography. A survey conducted by Killen and co-workers (398, 399) showed that 90% of the reported spinal cord injuries was caused by acetrizoate, especially at high concentrations. Others (400–404) have shown that all water-soluble angiographic agents can inflict damage on the spinal cord. Contrast agents such as sodium iodide, acetrizoate, iodomethamate, diprotrizoate, diodone, diatrizoate, and thorium oxide have neurotoxicity decreasing in that order (404). Foster et al. (405) found that diodone, acetri-

zoate, and diprotrizoate have higher toxic effects on kidney and spinal cord following aortography than thorium dioxide, diatrizoate, and iothalamate. Damage to the spinal cord is highly likely in any procedure that concentrates the contrast agent in this region.

The damage may be modified by injection of vasodilators, vasoconstrictors, or other agents that change the relative flow of blood and contrast medium toward or away from the spinal cord or alter its reponse to the contrast medium (400, 406). Following intraaortic injection, the neurotoxicity of contrast agents may be increased by the presence of chemicals such as heparin (407), which increase the permeability of the blood–brain barrier. Hypothermia, procaine (prior-injected), 20% glucose, and low molecular weight dextran can exert a protective effect against spinal cord damage (405, 408–409). Diazepam can prevent clonic convulsions and muscular twitchings following myelography with iocarmic acid (410). The mechanism of these protective effects is not fully understood.

6.5.5   PROTEIN BINDING.   Protein binding is reputed to affect the toxicity and selective excretion of contrast media (313, 315, 411). Contrast media were shown by equilibrium dialysis to combine with serum albumin at a number of strong and weak binding sites on the protein (313–315, 412). Acetrizoate, iodipamide, and iopanoate with an open position 5 in the substituted benzene nucleus combine strongly with albumin, whereas the fully substituted triiodobenzoates such as diatrizoate and iothalamate bind only weakly. Acetrizoate and iodipamide bind to bovine serum albumin strongly at one site and weakly at several other sites whereas iopanoate binds strongly to three sites of the protein. The difference in the strength of protein binding sites may account for the species specificity of the toxicity of acetrizoate observed in 15 species of animals. According to Lang and Lasser (412, 413), the binding between the contrast material and protein is due to hydrophobic interaction.

Protein binding may affect the selective excretion by the kidney or liver of a contrast medium (315, 414, 415). The cholegraphic agents iodipamide and iopanoic acid show strong binding to serum protein. Although the relationship between the affinity for protein binding and the preferential uptake and excretion by the liver of contrast agents has not been clearly defined, two hypotheses were forwarded to explain the phenomenon. One hypothesis is that the binding with albumin prevents glomerular filtration of the contrast medium, thus providing a continuing concentration to liver parenchymal cells (415, 416), and the other hypothesis is based on the free penetration of serum albumin in the Disse's space which allows preferential access of the bound contrast medium to liver cells (417). Neither of these hypotheses is tenable because (1) it is not possible to force greater quantities of acetrizoate into the bile by increasing the serum binding capacity of acetrizoate to the level of iodipamide by priming with serum albumin (418), and (2) some substances such as Evans blue that are extensively bound to serum albumin are not excreted in the bile to any significant extent, whereas other poorly bound compounds such as p-aminohippuric acid are efficiently excreted by the liver (315). These findings point to the involvement of additional mechanisms besides serum protein binding in determining the biliary excretion of contrast medium.

Recently, Sokoloff et al. (419) showed that iopanoic acid and iodipamide but not iothalamate bind to the Y and Z proteins found in the liver and the mucosa in the small intestine. Song et al. (420) studied the role of serum albumin in the hepatic excretion of iodipamide and found that the contrast agent establishes an equilibrium between serum protein and the intrahepatic anion-binding Y protein, also known as ligandin, with the latter controlling the process of hepatic uptake and excretion in which serum albumin plays no role. Goldstein and Arias (421) have studied the interaction of ligandin with iopanoic acid, diatrizoate, iodipamide, and iodopyracet. It is apparent that the role of ligandin in the transfer of contrast medium from blood to liver is to bind the contrast material in the liver cell for intracellular accumulation.

Contrast media inhibit enzyme activity, and the degree of inhibition parallels their binding affinity to serum albumin. Iopanoate, iodipamide, acetrizoate and isofamic acid, and diatriazoate and iothalamate exert in a descending order, and inhibitory effect on the following enzymes: lysozyme, β-glucuronidase (two types), alcohol dehydrogenase, glucose-6-phosphate dehydrogenase (413, 422), adenosine triphosphatase, carbonic anhydrase (423), and cholinesterases of human red blood cells and plasma (424, 425). The glucuronidation of p-nitrophenol was more adversely affected by cholecystographic agents than urographic agents (426). Sodium ipodate strongly inhibits the microsomal p-nitroanisole demethylase and aniline hydroxylase activity (427). Metrizamide binds reversibly with catalase (428) and exhibits weaker inhibition of cholinesterase, glutamic–oxalacetic transaminase, and glucose-6-phosphate than diatrizoate and iothalamate (429).

Cholegraphic agents such as iodipamide and iopanoic acid are about 10–100 times more potent inhibitors of cholinesterases than the angiographic agent diatrizoate (424). Toxic reactions manifested as gastrointestinal symptoms and hypertonicity of bladder from the use of oral cholecystographic agents may be attributed to their anticholinesterase activities. The hypotensive effects induced in experimental animals by ioglycamic acid and iodipamide are not completely blocked by atropine sulfate, indicating that not all the toxic effects of cholegraphic agents are due to inhibition of acetylcholinesterase activities (430).

Contrast media produce morphological changes of red blood cells by altering their size and shape and also increase their tendencies for agglomeration and agglutination (431–434). The morphological changes brought about by different contrast agents are not related to osmolarity nor can they be correlated with viscosity or pH differences. The contrast media that produce greater changes in red blood cell morphology are those showing a higher protein binding capacity.

The deformation of RBC by acetrizoate may be protected by chlorpromazine and dibucaine (432). These drugs are known to stabilize the cell membrane and may bind to the same sites as acetrizoate, thus blocking its action on the cells. Treatment with colchicine causes damage to microtubules but provides inadequate protection against the action of acetrizoate, indicating no involvement of microtubules in the deformation.

Contrast media induce serum complement activation (435). The degree of activation is a function of concentration and chemical structure of the contrast agent. The order of serum complement activation by contrast agents is metrizamide < iothalamate < diatrizoate < acetrizoate < iodipamide and iopanoic acid, which is also the order of enzyme inhibition. Activation of serum complement results in structural and functional alterations of cell membranes owing to the release of small active peptides such as the anaphylatoxins, bringing about a wide variety of reactions including contraction of smooth muscle, increased capillary permeability, release of histamine from mast cells, directed attraction of polymorphonuclear leukocytes, and release of hydrolases from these cells. Contrast media affect the normal process of fibrin and plasma formation in the coagulation mechanism by changing the fibrin fiber diameter and increasing the size of

protein aggregates with an altered spatial arrangement of the clots (436).

6.5.6 HISTAMINE RELEASE. Contrast media administered to laboratory animals by either intravenous injection or infusion or local application caused histamine-like reactions: endothelial injury (437), changes in vascular permeability (438, 439), and perivascular edema (440). These agents release histamine from tissue mast cells by degranulation (441, 442). Leite et al. (443) reported that meglumine iodipamide and a mixture of sodium and meglumine salts of acetrizoate were more effective in histamine release in the rat than iodamide, and diatrizoate was ineffective. Others have reported the release of histamine from rat peritoneal mast cells by acetrizoate, diatrizoate, and iothalamate (444, 445). Histamine was found in the plasma of dogs following pulmonary artery injection of meglumine iodipamide (444) and in the perfusion of canine lung with meglumine salts of acetrizoate, diatrizoate, iothalamate, and iodipamide, or meglumine chloride alone (370). The ability or inability of diatrizoate to release histamine reported in these experiments is probably caused by the difference in injection rate. Meglumine salts of contrast media with the exception of diatrizoate release much greater quantities of histamine than the sodium salts. Histamine release is not caused by hyperosmolarity, for the injection of isosmotic sodium chloride (443) or dextrose (446) solutions produces negligible effects. Administration of diphenhydramine hydrochloride and burimamide (i.e., N-methyl-N'-[4-[4(5)-imidazolyl]butyl]thiourea), which are H_1- and H_2-receptor antagonists, respectively (447), abolishes the histamine release properties of the contrast agents *in vivo* (443).

In man, the allergic reactions from contrast media resemble those elicited by histamine injection, and the unpleasant side effects are rarer after fast injection than after slow injection of the same dose of contrast medium (350). Seidel et al. (446) showed that usual doses of chemically different contrast media were able to affect the plasma histamine levels in venous blood of healthy persons. Histamine release is stopped when the dose rate is reduced to 0.17 g/kg/min. This may explain the advantage of administering urographic agents by infusion to avoid reactions.

Patients with a history of allergy react more frequently to intravascular injection of contrast media than those with no history of hypersensitivity (336, 337). Reactions to contrast media are in some cases precipitous, resembling anaphylactoid reactions of immunologic nature. A major obstacle to the acceptance of an immunologic mechanism for reactions to contrast agents was the inability to demonstrate antibody formation by these agents (372, 411, 448). Using keyhole-limpet hemocyanin, bovine serum albumin, and bovine gamma globulin as carrier proteins, and 3-azo-2,4,6-triiodobenzoate, 3-azo-5-acetamido-2,4,6-triiodobenzoate, 3-acetamido-2,4,6-triiodobenzyl, and 4-acetamido-3,5-diiodobenzyl groups as haptens, Brasch et al. (449) were able to demonstrate antibody formation in the rabbit, thus establishing the link between immunologic responses and reactions to contrast media.

6.5.7 PHARMACOKINETICS. The quality of roentgenograms in cholangio-cholecystography and urography is determined by the localization of the contrast media applied. In oral cholecystography, the radiographic quality is determined by the absorption and excretion of contrast medium, which is controlled by many factors (450, 451). In intravenous cholangiography and urography, the excretion of contrast medium alone determines the opacification of the organ under examination (320, 452–454).

Absorption of oral cholecystographic agents occurs by passive diffusion of the non-ionized compound across the lipoidal barrier of intestinal mucosa (450) and is determined by the rate of solubilization of contrast medium which is affected by pH, the presence of bile salts, mixing, the effective surface area, and the physical state of the compound (451). The rate of absorption of iopanoic acid and iosumetic acid is increased if the contrast agent is administered concomitantly with sodium bicarbonate (173, 455, 456). Bile salts or a fatty meal have been recommended with the administration of iopanoic acid to ensure its solubilization and absorption in the duodenum and to improve gall bladder visualization (451, 458, 459). The fatty meal releases cholecystokinin, which promotes the enterohepatic circulation of bile salts, thus enhancing both intestinal absorption and hepatic excretion (450). The ability of bile salts to increase the excretion of iopanoic acid is attributed to an allosteric interaction between the bile salts and a carrier for the contrast medium in the canalicular membrane (460, 461).

Mixing and the physical state of the crystals affect the surface area which controls the solubilization of iopanoic acid (451, 457). The "amorphous" form of iopanoic acid formed by recent precipitation following reaction of sodium iopanoate with gastric acid is more soluble than the dried "crystalline" form found in commercial products.

The dose regimen is of great interest in pharmacokinetics studies because it can provide input to a proposed kinetic model. The advantage and disadvantage of a large single dose versus a fractionated dose of sodium tyropanoate have been evaluated (462). A large single dose yields a superior radiographic quality whereas the fractionated dose containing the quantity of the contrast medium has a less toxic effect on the kidney.

Because of the often incomplete absorption of oral cholecystographic agents, detailed analytical approaches to pharmacokinetics studies have not been available. Goldberg et al. (451) studied the biopharmaceutical factors influencing the intestinal absorption of iopanoic acid and attributed the frequent failure of the first dose of the agent to afford diagnostic visualization of gall bladder to impaired intestinal absorption. Uncertainty in absorption is avoided when intravenous agents are used.

Water-soluble dimers as iodipamide, ioglycamide, iodoxamate, and iotroxic acid are intravenous cholangiographic agents and can be injected to achieve a desired plasma concentration. Following injection, the pharmacokinetics of these contrast media including dilution and mixing with body fluid, uptake by the liver, and excretion into the bile and urine can be fitted to multicompartmental kinetic models. A logical kinetic model for the transfer of a substance through a secreting cell may consist of three phases: uptake (passage from the plasma into the cell); passage through the cell (with or without accumulation); and passage from the cell to the tubular lumen (excretion) (463, 464). Corman et al. (464) have proposed several pharmacokinetic models for ioglycamate. Although a simple, two-compartment model can account for approximately 90% of the administered drug, the experimental data are better fitted to three-compartment models. The introduction of an extravascular space with which the plasma contrast medium can rapidly exchange would avoid this difficulty of requiring a considerably larger initial volume of dilution for the contrast medium than the plasma volume in a two-compartment model (465) and is based on the observation that the distribution volume of iodipamide in the dog is similar to the extravascular fluid volume in size (466). Pharmacokinetic models involving three compartments have been proposed for ioglycamic acid by Corman et al. (464), for iodipamide by Shames et al. (465), and for iodoxamic acid by Strata et al. (467). Segre

and Rosati (468) have proposed nonlinear kinetic models for the disposition of iodipamide, ioglycamide acid, and iodoxamic acid in dogs. These models are shown in Fig. 61.1. In the nonlinear kinetic model, the contrast medium is excreted into the bile through the liver compartment 3, which is not in direct communication with the plasma compartment 1. For ioglycamic acid at doses above 175.5 μmol/kg, an alternative model has been proposed in which the passage of the contrast medium from blood to the liver is irreversible.

The relationship between infusion rate or plasma concentration on the one hand and biliary concentration (B), urinary concentration (U), B/U excretion ratio, and excretory deficit (i.e., the amount of contrast medium retained in the body) on the other have been studied in the case of iodoxamate and iodipamide by Berk et al. (469) in unanesthetized dogs. Biliary excretion depended on bile flow and erythritol clearance (which serves as an index of canalicular bile flow). The rate of biliary excretion and the concentration of iodine in the bile increased according to first-order kinetics at low plasma concentration of the contrast agents and leveled off when the plasma concentration reached 0.4 mol/ml. A reasonable fit of these data to equations for hyperbolas can be made, indicating saturation kinetics, which is characteristic of an active transport process presumably occurring at the biliary canaliculus. The rate of urinary excretion of these contrast agents varied linearly with the plasma concentration, indicating a passive transport process. The B/U excretion ratio decreased sharply with increasing plasma concentration, i.e., above 0.4 mol/ml. At an infusion rate of approximately 1 μmol/kg min, a biliary concentration of about 25 and 28 μmol/ml has been achieved for iodipamide and iodoxamate, respectively, which exceeds the concentration (approximately 13–16μ mol/ml) required for visualization of the biliary tree. From these data,

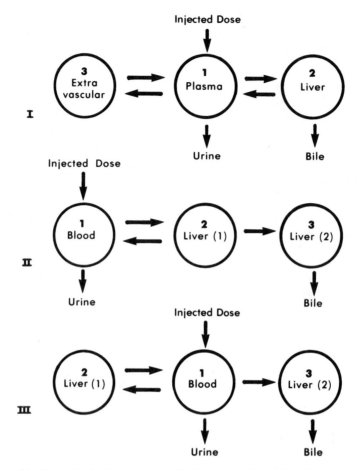

Fig. 61.1 Pharmacokinetic models for the excretion of iodipamide, iodipamide, iodoxamic acid, and ioglycamide in the dog (464–468).

Berk et al. suggested that iodoxamate is a better agent than iodipamide in patients with impaired biliary excretion, high basal bile flow, or when a small dose of the contrast medium is infused. Recently, Lin et al. (470) have investigated the saturation kinetics of iodipamide.

Drugs that may affect biliary excretion, such as phenobarbital, also exert an effect on the pharmacokinetics of iopanoate (471).

Pharmacokinetic studies of urographic agents such as water-soluble derivatives of 2,4,6-triiodobenzoic acid and 2,6-diiodopyridone showed that the renal excretion of these agents proceeds through glomerular filtration, active excretion in the proximal tubules, and passive reabsorption in the distal tubules of the nephron (471). Iodopyracet and acetrizoate are largely excreted by the proximal tubules in the dog whereas iodamide is only moderately excreted, and diatrizoate, iothalamate, and metrizoate are not excreted at all by the tubules but are eliminated by glomerular filtration. Studies with aglomerular fish or ureterally obstructed dog confirmed that there is no tubular excretion or reabsorption of sodium iothalamate (472).

The plasma concentration curve obtained following a single injection of sodium diatrizoate reflects the initial mixing in the vascular compartment, equilibration in the fluid space, and concomitant excretion via the kidneys. The initial volume of mixing is of a size comparable to the measured extracellular space. Based on the excretion data of ^{131}I-labeled sodium and meglumine diatrizoate, a three-compartment kinetic model, analogous to that proposed for iodipamide less the biliary exit has been developed using analog computer simulation. The model comprises a blood compartment, a tissue compartment, and a "deep" tissue compartment (452). The "deep" tissue compartment corresponds to the extracellular fluid space and is characterized by a very small entry constant and a large entry-to-elimination constants ratio, usually exceeding 10. This ratio was found to be 9.4 ± 4.5 with a half-time of elimination of 11.7 ± 1.15 hr for sodium diatrizoate as compared to 17 ± 4.5 and 14.5 ± 1.5 hr for the meglumine salt. These values show that the pharmacokinetic model for the diatrizoic acid remains the same, unaffected by its salt form.

Absorption and excretion of water soluble metrizamide and diatrizoate after suboccipital injection in the cat seems to follow first-order kinetics. The rate constants for absorption and excretion were determined by Golman and Dahl (473), who observed that 99% of the absorbed dose disappeared from cerebrospinal fluid during the 3 hr after suboccipital injection. The difference in the total amount of metrizamide excreted during 48 hr after intravenous and suboccipital injection in the rabbit is negligible, indicating the rapid removal of the agent from cerebrospinal fluid to blood (474).

6.5.8   EXCRETION.   Contrast media are excreted in both the bile and urine; the route that predominates is determined by their chemical structure and route of administration. Recently, hepatic and urinary excretions of contrast agents and their rates of excretion have been reviewed by Cattell

(414), Knoefel and Carrasquer (475), McChesney (476), and Sperber and Sperber (466).

Oral contrast agents bind serum protein at physiological pH (315, 414). Protein binding prevents glomerular filtration but does not impair hepatic excretion. Transport of these agents from the blood to the liver is an active saturable process (477) and involves the Y and Z proteins found in the liver as hepatic acceptors (419, 420). These acceptors show affinity for cholegraphic agents such as iopanoic acid and iodipamide, but exhibit little or no affinity for urographic agents such as iothalamate. The liver transport capacity of contrast medium, expressed as maximum transport rate or velocity T_m, is defined as the amount of compound going into the bile per unit time, which cannot be influenced by additional increases of dose (134). Rosati et al. (134) reported the T_ms for ioglycamic acid, iodipamide, and iodoxamic acid after rapid intravenous injection in the dog to be 0.768 ± 0.101, 0.530 ± 0.072, and 1.226 ± 0.109 μmol/kg min, respectively. These values remain essentially the same for slow infusion (453, 478). Iopanoate has a T_m value varying from 0.16 to 0.74 mol/kg min, depending on the presence of bile salts (479). In bile salt-depleted dog, less contrast agent is excreted. Maximum transport rates of iodipamide and iodoxamic acid in man have been reported by Julian et al. (480).

Contrast agents with strong affinity for serum protein show a threshold plasma value below which little or no excretion through the liver or the kidney occurs (478), and, in addition, a species difference exists in the excretion of cholegraphic agents (481). The threshold values of ioglycamic acid and iodipamide in the dog were shown to be 0.16 and 0.6 μmol/ml, respectively. Iodoxamic acid, iodipamide, and ioglycamic acid were excreted in the rabbit at higher concentrations to the extent of about 77, 38, and 42% of the dose in the bile and about 17, 38, and 35% of the dose in the urine, respectively (134). Iocetamic acid is excreted in the rat predominantly in the intestine but in human subjects, 41 and 62% of the administered dose appear in the urine in the first 24 and 48 hr (481). Distribution and excretion of iodipamide in mice and man have been studied by Kiyono et al. (482), using ^{131}I-labeled material. Earlier Fischer (483) derived from biliary and urinary excretion studies an optimal dose of 205 μmol/kg for iodipamide.

Biliary excretion of contrast medium is affected by the bile flow (414, 450, 460, 484, 485). Bile is isosmotic with plasma and is produced from the transport of water from the liver cell into the bile canaliculi (canalicular bile flow) and from the excretion and reabsorption of water and electrolytes in the bile ductules (ductular bile flow). Bile flow is increased by taurocholate and dehydrocholate; their presence in the canaliculi creates an osmotic gradient that produces the flow of water and solute. There is a positive correlation between the canalicular bile flow stimulated by taurocholate and the amount of iopanoic acid excreted by the liver. Feeding the patient a fatty meal or taurocholate at the time that iopanoic acid is administered can improve the quality of cholecystograms (450).

In addition to bile salts, contrast media (486) and other agents (469, 484) may also increase bile flow and cause choleresis. Iodipamide produces 0.025 ml bile/μmol excreted as compared with 0.009 ml bile/mol for ipodate, but both agents are able to achieve similar maximum bile iodine concentration. The reason for this phenomenon is that ipodate is excreted as glucuronide conjugate, incorporated in the bile salt micelles which exert a small choleretic effect, whereas iodipamide is excreted unchanged (487).

Other agents such as phenobarbital and cinchophen alter the bile flow and the biliary excretion of cholegraphic agents.

Pretreatment with phenobarbital decreases iodipamide bile excretion and increases iopanoate bile excretion (469). Cinchophen increases both biliary and urinary excretion of iophenoxic acid but has no effect on iopanoic acid (484). It has been reported recently that a high level of prostaglandin-like substance in the mucosa and muscle wall of gall bladder caused nonvisualization of the gall bladder in cholecystography (488).

Urinary excretion is a principal means of elimination for diatrizoate, iothalamate, metrizoate, metrizamide, and other urographic agents (414, 474, 489, 491). Diatrizoate, iothalamate, and metrizamide were excreted in the urine of the rabbit to the extent of greater than 80% 24 hr after injection (474, 489–491). The total recovery including the amount excreted in feces 96 hr after injection was about 91.5% of the dose for metrizamide, 93.8% for diatrizoate, and 86.0% for iothalamate (489).

These water-soluble contrast agents are excreted as rapidly as glomerular filtrate can be formed (414). Their elimination may be impaired by primary and secondary glomerular dysfunction or reduced renal blood flow which diminishes the filtration rate (492). After clearing the blood, the contrast medium in its passage down the nephron can affect the salt and water reabsorption in the proximal tubule and water reabsorption in the distal tubule. The osmotically active contrast medium can produce salt and water diuresis, and its presence in the nephron may still cause renal toxicity (493). In experimental animals (494) and in man (414), the sodium salt of diatrizoic acid produces less diuresis than the meglumine salt. The renal extraction of p-aminohippurate is reduced by the contrast anion and the meglumine cation (495).

The excretion of contrast agent by the liver or the kidney is not exclusive; when either of these organs is in dysfunction or diseased state, heterotopic excretion by the other organ will occur to compensate for the impediment (414, 488, 491). In patients with renal failure or advanced renal disease, contrast media may still be used to produce nephrograms (414); if the tubular obstruction prevents the passage of urine along the nephron, back-diffusion of the contrast medium into the interstitial volume will occur (495–497). During the periods of ureteric stasis, metrizamide is excreted faster than diatrizoate, thus producing a higher urinary iodine concentration (491, 498).

When suboccipitally injected, metrizamide was recovered in the urine and feces of rabbit, rat, and cat to the extent of more than 90% of the dose (489), similar to the recovery of iothalamate (499) and iocarmate (500) in dogs.

In peroral administration, metrizamide and diatrizoate are not well absorbed from the gastrointestinal tract; the urinary recovery of both agents in the rabbit was below 5% of the administered dose, 24 hours post-administration (474). Iophendylate, when given to rats, guinea pigs, or rabbits, was eliminated from the body in 5 hrs (501). It was transported along the lymph system.

6.5.9 BIOTRANSFORMATION. Contrast media may be excreted either metabolized or unchanged depending upon their molecular properties. The subject of biotransformation of contrast media has recently been reviewed by McChesney (502).

The fully substituted 2,4,6-triiodobenzoic acids used for angiography and urography have high water solubility and are stable chemically. Because of their low pK_as, they are highly ionized at physiological pH. These contrast agents are poorly absorbed from the gastrointestinal tract and rapidly excreted unchanged within 5–6 hr after intravenous injection (476). Their metabolic inertness is attributed to their inability to cross cell membranes and to penetrate liver microsomes to undergo biotransformation

(502). Their rapid excretion is caused by the absence of tubular reabsorption, thus allowing as rapid an excretion as the glomerular filtrate can be formed. Although evidence of formation of metabolites of acetrizoate, diatrizoate, and diprotrizoate has been reported, their evidence remains doubtful since they have not been isolated or chemically characterized.

In contrast to the 2,4,6-triiodobenzoic acids, substituted alkanoic and alkoxyalkanoic acids containing 2,4,6-triiodophenyl or 2,4,6-triiodophenoxy group with open position 5, such as iopanoic acid, tyropanoate, ioglycamic acid, and iopronic acid, have both lipophilic and hydrophilic properties. These contrast acids have an acidity constant about two units higher than the water-soluble, fully substituted 2,4,6-triiodobenzoic acids (179) and are not completely ionized at the physiological pH. In the nonionized form, the contrast molecules can be absorbed and transported across cell membranes after oral administration.

The oral cholecystographic agents are in general more toxic than angiographic and urographic agents. Detoxification of the former may involve glucuronidation, N-acetylation, O-acetylation, esterification, deiodination, and hydrolysis. These metabolites appear in the bile and urine. The metabolites of many cholegraphic agents have been characterized to some degree but are not chemically identified.

Conjugation with glucuronic acid occurs with most oral cholecystographic agents before excretion. Bunamiodyl (503, 504), iodoalphionate (505, 506), iolidonic acid (507), iophenoxic acid (508–510), and tyropanoate (503, 504) are excreted as glucuronides. McChesney and Banks (504) showed that 90% of the contrast agents in the urine appeared as glucuronides. Since glucuronides are usually poorly reabsorbed from the intestine, glucuronidation can thus circumvent extensive enterohepatic recirculation of the contrast medium.

The fate of iophenoxic acid (510) and the efficacy of iopanoate (502, 503) are uniquely linked to glucuronidation. Iophenoxic acid is retained in the body over a period of many years after administration and is slowly excreted. It forms acyl and ethereal monoglucuronides and the diglucuronide. These glucuronides have the uncommon property of being freely lipid-soluble and can undergo hepatic, intestinal, and renal tubular reabsorption. Wade et al. (510) pointed out that the rate of formation of glucuronide conjugates may be an important factor in the persistence of iophenoxic acid in the body. Iopanoate glucuronide when administered orally gave no visualization of gall bladder but when injected intravenously yielded an excellent cholecystogram 1 hr after administration, whereas an equivalent dose of iopanoate when injected required a delay of 8–24 hr for an image of diagnostic quality to become apparent, indicating that the iopanoate was converted to glucuronide before being excreted in the bile (502, 503).

Bornschein et al. (171, 511) reported the appearance of the unchanged iomeglamic acid, the methyl ester, the deiodinated derivative, the N-desmethyl derivative, the methyl ester of the latter derivative, the N-acetylated derivative, and the deiodinated methyl ester of iomeglamic acid in the urine of man 72 hr after a 3 g dose. Lindner et al. (164) showed evidence of biotransformation of iobenzamate in the mouse, rat, and man which involved conjugation with glucuronic acid, hydroxylation of the unsubstituted phenyl ring, or hydrolysis of the amide linkage, for example, but isolation and identification of the metabolic products were not carried out. Harwart et al. (160) studied the metabolic fate of ipodate and found that there was unchanged ipodate in the bile, and the major product excreted in urine was soluble in butanol. One of the metabolites was identified as 3-amino-2,4,6-triiodohydrocinnamic acid, a reduction product of ipodate.

The hexaiodinated dimeric intravenous cholangio-cholecystographic agents, such as iodipamide, ioglycamide, iodoxamate, and iotroxic acid, are excreted mainly unchanged (464, 483, 512–515). Strickler et al. (516) reported an unidentified metabolite of iodipamide, probably formed from hydrolysis of the amide linkage. Mützel et al. (517), using ^{131}I-labeled tracers, found that ioglycamide, iodoxamate, and iotroxic acid each yielded two urinary metabolites, one of which was more polar and the other less polar than the parent molecule. It was shown that neither of these two metabolites was a deiodinated product, and that the bile and plasma contained no metabolites. Pitre and Felder (518) reported three metabolites of iodoxamic acid in human urine; one of which was identified as 3-[3-(α-hydroxyethoxy)propionamido]2,4,6-triiodobenzoic acid, a product formed from symmetrical scission of the dimer.

Deiodination is not an important reaction in the biotransformation of contrast media in spite of the presence of deiodase in the mammalian liver (519). The rat and pig liver, however, can convert 2,3,5-triiodobenzoic acid into 2,5- and 3,5-diiodobenzoic acids (520–522). Iodoalphionate (523, 524), iothalamate (525), iodipamide, and ioglycamide (512) were reported to undergo deiodination to a small degree, never to exceed 1% of the dose. Since most organic iodine compounds are sensitive to light, the observed deiodination may be a result of both enzymatic reaction (522) and photolytic degradation (526).

Deiodination of contrast agents may affect the thyroid ^{131}I uptake. Iodoalphionate (527, 528), iodipamide (527, 529), and iodopyracet (530) affect the thyroid uptake by a slow release of the iodide. In thyroid patients, the thyroid uptake returns to normal 4 days after the administration of acetrizoate, 58 days after iopanoic acid (531), and many years after iophenoxate (532). Iophenoxate binds avidly to plasma protein and is transported across the placental barrier as long as 5 years after administration.

The cholecystographic agents may have a direct effect on the thyroid. Iodide-induced hyperthyroidism may result from ipodate administered for cholecystography (533) or from iophendylate injected for myelography (534). Intravenous administration of ioxitalamic acid to euthyroid patients increased their protein-bound iodine (PBI) and hormonal iodine levels, which returned to normal between 2 and 8 days (535).

6.6 Uses

In Table 63.10, major uses of contrast media are listed.

6.6.1 ANGIOGRAPHY. Methiodal sodium, sodium iodomethamate, and iodopyracet were the earliest water-soluble organic iodine compounds available for angiography (10). From the incidence of patient reactions and from laboratory investigations, it became known that these compounds were not entirely suitable for angiography use. In about 1950, substituted triiodobenzoic acid derivatives were beginning to be introduced as contrast agents (128, 141). Acetrizoate was the first of the series introduced followed by diprotrizoate and then by diatrizoate, iothalamate, metrizoate, iodamide, and ioxitalamic acid. Acetrizoate and diprotrizoate were found to have certain toxic effects but diatrizoate, iothalamate, and metrizoate were better tolerated and have found extensive use in angiography (128). Iodamide and ioxitalamic acid are widely used in Europe. Benton et al. (536) found that meglumine calcium diatrizoate is superior to meglumine diatrizoate and meglumine sodium diatrizoate. More recently, dimers and trimers of contrast agents and nondissociable compounds were introduced for angiographic use (9). Newer agents such as iocarmic acid (bisiothalamate), iozomic acid, and tris(iothalamate), as well as the

Table 61.10 Uses of Contrast Agents: Radiographic Procedures for Visualizing Organs Following Administration of Contrast Agents

Procedure	Organs Visualized
Angiography	Blood vessels
Arteriography	Arteries
Aortography	Aortas
Arthrography	Joints
Bronchography	Lungs
Cholangiography	Gall bladder and bile ducts
Cholecystography	Gall bladder
Esophagography	Esophagus
Hepatography	Liver
Hepatolienography	Liver and spleen
Hysterosalpingography	Uterus and oviducts
Lymphography	Lymph nodes and vessels
Lymphadenography	Lymph nodes
Lymphangiography	Lymph vessels
Myelography	Spinal cord, subarachnoid space
Pelviagraphy	Pelvis
Pyelography	Kidney and ureter
Splenography	Spleen
Splenohepatography	Liver and spleen
Urography	Urinary tract
Ventriculography	Ventricles of the brain

nondissociable metrizamide, have fewer side effects and are better tolerated. Almén (537) reported that metrizamide is the contrast medium of choice for cardioangiography and coronary angiography.

6.6.2 CHOLANGIOGRAPHY. Intravenous cholangiography was introduced in 1954 as a radiographic technique in the diagnosis of biliary tract disease and is practiced in cases in which conditions causing obstruction to passage and resorption are present and prevent the use of oral cholecystography (320). The sole contrast agent used in the procedure in the United States is iodipamide, which is available as sodium and meglumine salts. The difference between the two salt forms is in the volume of the dosage required for examination, with the volume of meglumine salt less than that of sodium salt. Adverse reactions following a single bolus injection are reduced if the contrast medium is administered by slow-infusion technique.

Many other cholangiographic agents are available. Ioglycamide or ioglycamic acid has been studied in relation to iodipamide by Brismar et al. (312). Ioglycamide is widely used in Europe and has an excellent contrast property for examinations of bile ducts after intravenous injection but offers no advantage over iodipamide in examinations of gall bladder. A new intravenous cholangiographic agent, iodoxamic acid, introduced in 1973, has apparently lower toxicity and is currently being studied (134, 538).

Newer cholangiography agents are mostly dimers of triiodobenzoates and triiodoisophthalamates with high water solubility and high biliary excretion.

6.6.3 CHOLECYSTOGRAPHY. The first cholecystogram was obtained in dogs with tetrabromophenolphthalein by Graham et al. in 1924 (539). Tetraiodophenolphthalein was used for cholecystography until 1943, when iodoalphionic acid was introduced (540), which produced better radio-

graphic visualization of the gall bladder with fewer toxic reactions. Its use was superseded by iopanoic acid, a substituted triiodobenzoic acid introduced in 1951 (541). Iopanoic acid is better tolerated and has a greater opacity than iodoalphionic acid. The N-butyryl derivative of iopanoic acid, tyropanoate, was introduced in 1963 and was found to be more readily absorbed from the gastrointestinal tract than iopanoic acid. This compound, in addition to rapid oral absorption, gives excellent opacification of the gall bladder under conditions of clinical use and has a low incidence of side effects. Opacification with tyropanoate occurs with diagnostic quality on the 4 hr film and the 8 hr film in 64% and 78% of the patients examined, respectively (542, 543).

A number of substituted 2,4,6-triiodobenzoic acid derivatives were introduced as cholecystographic agents. Among them, bunamiodyl and iophenoxic acid were later withdrawn by the manufacturers because bunamiodyl caused renal shutdown and iophenoxic acid caused high protein-bound iodine values persisting over many years.

Ipodate, introduced in 1961, can yield visualization of both gall bladder and bile ducts. Tyropanoate, iopanoic acid, and ipodate are widely used in oral cholecystography. They show about the same efficacy but differ in the intensity of opacification, the frequency of dim and absent shadows, and the frequency of side effects. Russell and Frederick (544) have compared these three agents but failed to demonstrate the superiority of any one contrast agent.

Iocetamic acid is a recently introduced cholecystographic agent (481). According to Parks (545), it is favorably compared with and preferred to the above three agents, but skin reactions were reported (546) in a few cases.

6.6.4 MYELOGRAPHY. Oil-soluble and water-soluble contrast agents have been used in myelography. These agents are administered intracisternally. The absorption of oily and water-soluble contrast media from the subarachnoid space is completely different. The oily media remain in the subarachnoid space for years after injection, whereas the water-soluble media are eliminated within a few days (500).

The water-soluble iodopyracet was introduced for myelography in 1931 (547). Because of the extreme irritant effects as well as occasional production of some long-term disabilities, it never gained wide use. Iodized oil Lipiodol had been used for myelography with less irritation. Its aftereffects were avoided if the oily medium was removed by aspiration from the spinal canal (548). Iophendylate was introduced by Ramsey et al. (549) for myelography in 1944 and proved to be an excellent contrast medium for the entire spinal canal and the basal cisterns. Like the iodized oil, it had to be aspirated to avoid aftereffects (550). Arachnoiditis did develop in some cases in the subarachnoid space, owing to the presence of residual iophendylate.

Iothalamate meglumine was used for myelography in 1964. Melartin et al. (395) showed that meglumine and iothalamate ions are less neurotoxic than sodium and diatrizoate ions. The irritating effect of meglumine iothalamate is so slight that its use in myelography requires no spinal anesthesia (410). Iocarmic acid (i.e., dimerized iothalamate) with a higher iodine content and a lower toxicity than iothalamate has been used in myelography and lumbosacral radioculography (129, 551). Both iocarmic acid and iothalamate tend to be spasmogenic, causing clonic convulsions or muscular twitchings in the leg (552). Nonionic, water-soluble metrizamide was introduced for myelography in 1973 (553). It is less irritating than available myelographic agents and is capable of visualizing small structures such as nerve roots, root pockets, and blood vessels. Metrizamide appears to be a superior myelographic agent.

The search for improved contrast agents for myelography continues. Iodine-containing organic carbonates (301) and iodinated phenyl glucoside (139) have recently been synthesized as potential myelographic agents.

6.6.5 UROGRAPHY. Contrast agents rapidly excreted by the kidney are used in excretion urography. Iopax or Uroselectan was first introduced for urography in Germany in 1929. Many other agents such as methiodal sodium, hippuran (sodium *o*-iodohippurate), sodium iodomethamate, and iodopyracet were also introduced. These agents were the earliest available, and iodopyracet was the most widely used (128).

With the introduction of modern contrast agents beginning in about 1950, urography has been conducted using the water-soluble, acetrizoate, diatrizoate, iodamide, iodipamide, iothalamate, and metrizoate. These agents, because of their higher radiopacity and better tolerance, have superseded the earlier agents although their individual toxicities vary. Among these, the diatrizoate is the least toxic and the most favored in urography (128).

Contrast agents cause osmotic diuresis. Studies show that sodium diatrizoate is excreted in higher concentration in the urine than is meglumine diatrizoate, owing to resorption of sodium ions in the renal tubules. Benness (494, 554) reported a difference in roentgenographic quality in pyelograms in favor of sodium contrast agents.

Dimeric and trimeric contrast agents with more iodine atoms per molecule improve the opacity of urine by their high iodine concentration and lessening of the osmotic diuresis. In sheep, these new large molecules produced less urinary solute output, less diuresis, and higher urinary concentration (322, 555). These agents are not yet available for clinical use.

The urine iodine concentration, after the

injection of nonionic metrazamide, is about twice as high as after sodium diatrizoate injection. Golman et al. (498) reported that during the periods of ureteric stasis, metrizamide was excreted faster than diatrizoate.

7 MISCELLANEOUS AGENTS

In addition to organic iodinated compounds, perfluorocarbons are also potential contrast agents. The least toxic one among them is perfluoroctyl bromide ($C_8F_{17}Br$), which has been introduced by Long et al. (556–559) for bronchography, myelography, splenography, lymphangiography, and special gastrointestinal studies requiring small volumes of nontoxic radiopaques.

Perfluoroctyl bromide has a high degree of chemical and physical stability and nonreactivity, a biologic inertness comparable to that of Teflon, a high oxygen solubility, and a low surface tension. Liquids with low surface tension wet surfaces readily and flow freely into tiny folds and orifices. This property in a contrast agent improves the quality of the roentgenogram. Perfluoroctyl bromide has a radiopacity about 50% of that of iothalamate, and may be administered as neat liquid or emulsions. Emulsions in normal saline can be prepared with the aid of emulsifying agent Pluronic F-68. Perfluorocarbon emulsions have a non-Newtonian viscosity which can be varied over a very wide range by changing perfluorocarbon and surfactant concentrations and emulsifying technique (556, 557).

Perfluoroctyl bromide when given tracheally either as neat liquid or as 10:1 emulsion was cleared roentgenologically from the lung within 24 hr. Evaporation and mucociliary clearance play an important role in the elimination of the radiopaque from the lungs. When the tissue samples were analyzed by gas chromatography, approximately 1% of the neat liquid and 8% of the emulsion were found still remaining in the tissue. The lungs had the largest amount, followed by the intestine, adipose tissue, and lymph nodes. When injected intrathecally into the dog, a dose of 0.5–1.0 ml/kg caused no toxic manifestation. It is much less irritating to the arachnoid tissue than iodophendylate (558).

Perfluoroctyl bromide is especially useful roentgenographically for patients who are allergic to iodine compounds and who have had meningitis prior to myelography (558).

REFERENCES

1. F. W. Wright and G. M. Arden, in *Radiocontrast Agents*, Vol. II, P. K. Knoefel, Ed., Pergamon, Oxford, 1971, p. 551.

2. I. Meschan, *Analysis of Roentgen Signs in General Radiology*, Vol. I, W. B. Saunders, Philadelphia, 1973, pp. 16, 39.

3. W. C. Roentgen, *Radiology*, **45,** 428 (1945).

4. W. C. Roentgen, *Radiology*, **45,** 433 (1945).

5. E. U. Condon, in *Handbook of Physics*, E. U. Condon and H. Odishaw, Eds., McGraw-Hill, New York, 1958, pp. 7–118.

6. B. G. Harvey, *Introduction to Nuclear Physics and Chemistry*, Prentice-Hall, Englewood Cliffs, N.J., 1969, pp. 320–325.

7. R. D. Evans, *The Atomic Nucleus*, McGraw-Hill, New York, 1955, p. 710.

8. W. H. McMaster, N. K. DelGrande, J. H. Mallet, and J. W. Hubble, *Compilation of X-Ray Cross Sections*, U.C.R.L. 50174, Section 1.

9. S. K. Hilal, *Invest. Radiol.*, **5,** 458 (1970).

10. H. W. Fischer, *Med. Progr. Tech.*, **1,** 131 (1972).

11. E. C. Lasser, in *Alimentary Tract Roentgenology*, 2nd ed., A. R. Margulis and H. J. Burhenne, Eds., C. V. Mosby Co., St. Louis, 1973, p. 127.

12. R. Shapiro and D. Papa, *Ann. N.Y. Acad. Sci.*, **78,** 756 (1959).

13. J. A. Nadel, W. G. Wolfe, and P. D. Graf, *Invest. Radiol.*, **3,** 229 (1968).

14. J. A. Nadel, W. G. Wolfe, P. D. Graf, J. E. Youker, N. Zamel, J. H. M. Austin, W. A. Hinchchliffe, R. H. Greenspan, and R. R. Wright, *New Engl. J. Med.*, **283,** 281 (1970).

15. R. B. Dilley and J. A. Nadel, *Ann. Otol. Rhinol. Laryngol.*, **79,** 945 (1970).

16. G. L. Burke, *Can. Med. Assoc. J.*, **43,** 125 (1940).

17. A. R. Koontz and R. L. Kimberly, *Ann. Surg.,* **137,** 833 (1953).

18. G. W. H. Schepers, *Arch. Ind. Hyg. Occup. Med.,* **12,** 121 (1955).

19. R. G. Vieth, G. T. Tindall, and G. L. Odom, *J. Neurosurg.,* **24,** 514 (1966).

20. L. H. Edmunds, Jr., P. D. Graf, S. S. Sagel, and R. H. Greenspan, *Invest. Radiol.,* **5,** 131 (1970).

21. G. Gianturco, B. Ruskin, F. R. Steggerda, and T. Takeuchi, *Radiology,* **102,** 195 (1972).

22. J. A. Nadel, W. J. Dodds, H. Goldberg, and P. D. Graf, *Invest. Radiol.,* **4,** 57 (1969).

23. W. J. Dodds, H. I. Goldberg, S. Kohatsu, L. J. McCarthy, J. Nadel, and F. F. Zboralske, *Invest. Radiol.,* **5,** 30 (1970).

24. R. B. Schlesinger, R. D. Schweizer, T. L. Chan, A. F. Keegan, and M. Lippmann, *Invest. Radiol.,* **10,** 115 (1975).

25. N. K. Blank, E. W. L. Fletcher, R. J. Steckel, *Invest. Radiol.,* **5,** 250 (1970).

26. U. Cegla, Ger. Pat. 2,151,706 (May 3, 1973); through *Chem. Abstr.,* **79,** 45821r (1973).

27. D. A. Weyel, T. C. Lee, and M. Corn, *Invest. Radiol.,* **9,** 284 (1974).

28. D. A. Weyel and M. Corn, *Invest. Radiol.,* **10,** 500 (1975).

29. T. Upham, L. S. Graham, R. J. Steckel, and N. Poe, *Am. J. Roentgenol., Radium Ther. Nucl. Med.,* **111,** 690 (1971).

30. J. A. Nadel and S. W. Clarke, in *Inhalation Particles III,* Vol. 1, W. H. Walton, Ed., Unwin Bros., Surrey, England, 1971, p. 43.

31. F. P. Stitik, D. L. Swift and D. F. Proctor, in *Pulmonary Care,* R. F. Johnstone, Ed., Grune and Stratton, New York, 1973, p. 35.

32. W. H. Strain, in *Radiocontrast Agents,* Vol. 1, P. K. Knoefel, Ed., Pergamon, Oxford, 1971, p. 1.

33. M. Rubin and G. D. Chiro, *Ann. N.Y. Acad. Sci.,* **78,** 764 (1959).

34. R. M. Nalbandian, W. T. Rice, and W. O. Nickel, *Ann. N.Y. Acad. Sci.,* **78,** 779 (1959).

35. R. L. Swarm, in *Radiocontrast Agents,* Vol. II, P. K. Knoefel, Ed., Pergamon, Oxford, 1971, p. 431.

36. R. Georg, W. W. Roeck, and E. N. C. Milne, *Invest. Radiol.,* **8,** 333 (1973).

37. F. Heitz and L. Hoechstetter-Heitz, *J. Radiol. Electrol. Med. Nucl.,* **55,** 168 (1974).

38. E. N. Sargent and R. Sherwin, *Am. J. Roent-*genol., *Radium Ther. Nucl. Med.,* **113,** 660 (1971).

39. E. H. Frei, E. Gunders, M. Pajewsky, W. J. Alkan, and J. Eschar, *J. Appl. Phys.,* **39**:2, 999 (1968).

40. M. Sugimoto, T. Watari, N. Watanabe, M. Tobe, and H. Takizawa, *Jap. J. Appl. Phys.,* **13**:1, 63 (1974).

41. C. Bachem and H. Guenther, *Z. Roentgenk, Radiumforsch.,* **12,** 369 (1910).

42. R. E. Miller, *Radiology,* **84,** 241 (1965).

43. J. P. Revill, in *Radiocontrast Agents,* Vol. II, P. K. Knoefel, Ed., Pergamon, Oxford, 1971, p. 345.

44. R. E. Miller, J. Skucas, M. R. Violante, and M. E. Shapiro, *Radiology,* **117,** 527 (1975).

45. J. R. Brown, *Radiology,* **81,** 839 (1963).

46. A. M. James and G. H. Gaddard, *Pharm. Acta Helv.,* **46,** 708 (1971).

47. G. Embring and O. Mattsson, *Acta Radiol.,* **7,** 245 (1968).

48. P. G. Embring, and P. O. Mattsson, Swed. Pat. 216,066 (Oct. 17, 1967); through *Chem. Abstr.,* **70,** 60842f (1969).

49. A. Nagami and T. Takamatsu, Jap. Pat. 70:34,160 (Nov. 2, 1970); through *Chem. Abstr.,* **74,** 67704d (1971).

50. K. Daigo and S. Okuyama, Jap. Pat. 72:03,753 (Feb. 1, 1972); through *Chem. Abstr.,* **76,** 131497j (1972).

51. K. Kikuchi and K. Daigo, U.S. Pat. 3,689,630 (Sept. 5, 1972); through *Chem. Abstr.,* **77,** 168616u (1972).

52. Sakai Chemistry Industry Co., Fr. Pat. 2,200,020 (April 19, 1974); through *Chem. Abstr.,* **83,** 84851c (1975).

53. M. Lungeanu and V. Economu, *Oncol. Radiol.,* **9,** 511 (1970); through *Chem. Abstr.,* **76,** 90013c (1972).

54. J. G. Clement, *J. Can. Assoc. Radiol.,* **20,** 106 (1969).

55. K. Nishizawa and K. Umezawa, Jap. Pat. 73:28,045 (Aug. 29, 1973); through *Chem. Abstr.,* **80,** 52402d (1974).

56. N. Karasawa, *Nippon Igaku Hoshasan Gakkai Zasshi,* **30**:3, 237 (1970); through *Chem. Abstr.,* **74,** 34612u (1971).

57. M. Buffetant, Fr. Pat. CAM 0255, (April 21, 1969); through *Chem. Abstr.,* **77,** 9586t (1972).

58. H. Hagstam, Swed. Pat. 218,439 (Jan. 23, 1968); through *Chem. Abstr.,* **71,** 33392y (1969).

59. Aktiebolag Astra, Apotekarnes Kemiska Fab-

riker, Fr. Pat. M 3,723 (Jan. 10, 1966); through *Chem. Abstr.*, **66,** 88653m (1967).

60. K. Daigo, K. Oda, and S. Okuyama, Ger. Pat. 2,304,690 (Aug. 4, 1974); through *Chem. Abstr.*, **81,** 6274m (1974).

61. K. Daigo, S. Okuyama, Jap. Pat. 73:24,248 (July 19, 1968); through *Chem. Abstr.*, **80,** 52393b (1974).

62. M. Buffetaut, Fr. Pat. M 6,098 (July 22, 1968); through *Chem. Abstr.*, **71,** 128776r (1969).

63. A. Nagami, Jap. Pat. 74:38,816 (Oct. 21, 1974); through *Chem. Abstr.*, **83,** 33082v (1975).

64. T. Hirohashi and S. Takai, Jap. Pat. 73:07,763 (March 8, 1973); through *Chem. Abstr.*, **80,** 30724h (1974).

65. S. E. Schwartz, H. W. Fischer, and A. J. S. House, *Radiology*, **112,** 727 (1974).

66. Y. Naol, Jap. Pat. 74:30,526 (March 19, 1974); through *Chem. Abstr.*, **81,** 54466x (1974).

67. M. Pajewski, J. Eschar, and A. Manor, *Clin. Radiol.*, **26,** 491 (1975).

68. M. A. Ziervogel, G. T. McCreath, R. Weir, and O. P. Fitzgerald-Finch, *Clin. Radiol.*, **24**:3, 302 (1973).

69. N. Takai, Jap. Pat. 73:40,728 (Dec. 6, 1973); through *Chem. Abstr.*, **82,** 21833g (1975).

70. J. G. M. Bullowa and C. Gottlieb, *J. Med. Sci.*, **160,** 98 (1920).

71. C. M. Nice, W. W. Waring, D. E. Killelea, and L. Hurwitz, *Am. J. Roentgenol., Radium Ther. Nucl. Med.*, **91,** 564 (1964).

72. J. H. Shapiro and H. G. Jacobson, *Ann. N.Y. Acad. Sci.*, **78,** 966 (1959).

73. A. R. Margulis, in *Alimentary Tract Roentgenology*, 2nd ed., A. R. Margulis and H. J. Burhenne, Eds., C. V. Mosby Co., St. Louis, 1973, p. 271.

74. C. Kaestle, *Fortschr. Geb. Roentgenstrahl.*, **11,** 266 (1907).

75. S. Tanaka, Y. Mochizuki, T. Uchikawa, and T. Yamane, *Radioisotopes*, **20**:3, 127 (1971); through *Chem. Abstr.*, **75,** 72091b (1971).

76. S. Suzuki, Y. Kawasaki, H. Kobayashi, M. Tobe, and Y. Ikeda, *Eisei Shikenyo Hokoku*, **91,** 19 (1973); through *Chem. Abstr.*, **81,** 99386n (1974).

77. M. Sugimoto, K. Daigo, S. Okuyama, M. Harada, S. Hirota, M. Kuroda, and S. Fuijii, Jap. Pat. 73:61,623 (Aug. 29, 1973); through *Chem. Abstr.*, **80,** 19606a (1974).

78. S. Takai and N. Karasawa, Jap. Pat. 73:24,247 (July 19, 1973); through *Chem. Abstr.*, **80,** 52401c (1974); Jap. Pat. 73:24,246 (July 19,

1973); through *Chem. Abstr.*, **80,** 52392a (1974).

79. Yeda Research and Development Co., Brit. Pat. 1,174,366 (Dec. 17, 1969); through *Chem. Abstr.*, **72,** 59097b (1970).

80. M. Sugimoto, Ger. Pat. 2,065,532 (May 16, 1974); through *Chem. Abstr.*, **81,** 54439r (1974).

81. E. H. Frei, S. Yerushalmi, and Y. Benmair, Brit. Pat. 1,339,537, (Dec. 5, 1973); through *Chem. Abstr.*, **80,** 87530w (1974).

82. T. Hoshino, K. Daigo, S. Okuyama, M. Harada, S. Hirota, M. Kuroda, S. Fujii, M. Jotsuka, Jap. Pat. 74:132,226 (Dec. 18, 1974); through *Chem. Abstr.*, **82,** 145011g (1975); Jap. Pat. 74:132,227 (Dec. 18, 1974); through *Chem. Abstr.*, **83,** 84897x (1975)).

83. J. Casper, *Ann. N.Y. Acad. Sci.*, **145,** 527 (1967).

84. R. J. Carrigan, *Ann. N.Y. Acad. Sci.*, **145,** 530 (1967).

85. E. Moniz, *Die Cerebrale Arteriographic und Phlebographie*, Springer, Berlin, 1940, p. 413.

86. N. P. Leach (Council on Pharmacy and Chemistry), *J. Am. Med. Assoc.*, **99,** 2183 (1932).

87. W. T. Kabisch, *Ann. N.Y. Acad. Sci.*, **145,** 676 (1967).

88. R. D. Evans, *The Atomic Nucleus*, McGraw-Hill, New York, 1955, p. 518.

89. H. E. MacMahon, A. S. Murphy, and M. I. Bates, *Am. J. Pathol.*, **23,** 585 (1947).

90. J. D. Abbatt, *Ann. N.Y. Acad. Sci.*, **145,** 767 (1967).

91. S. Dahlgren, *Ann. N.Y. Acad. Sci.*, **145,** 718 (1967).

92. M. Faber and C. Johansen, *Ann. N.Y. Acad. Sci.*, **145,** 755 (1967).

93. J. B. Hurch, *Ann. N.Y. Acad. Sci.*, **145,** 634 (1967).

94. W. S. S. Jee, N. L. Dockum, R. S. Mical., J. S. Arnold, and W. B. Looney, *Ann. N.Y. Acad. Sci.*, **145,** 660 (1967).

95. H. L. Kahn, *Ann. N.Y. Acad. Sci.*, **145,** 700 (1967).

96. J. da S. Horta, *Ann. N.Y. Acad. Sci.*, **145,** 676, 776, 830, (1967).

97. W. Wenz, *Ann. N.Y. Acad. Sci.*, **145,** 806 (1967).

98. R. I. Swarm, E. Miller, and H. J. Michelitch, *Pathol. Microbiol.*, **25,** 27 (1962).

99. F. A. D. Heitz, Ger. Pat. 2,361,143 (June 20, 1974); through *Chem. Abstr.*, **81,** 82378p (1974).

100. H. W. Fischer, *Recent Results Cancer Res.*, **23,** 13 (1969).

101. S. Glasstone, *Textbook of Physical Chemistry*, 2nd ed., Van Nostrand, New York, 1946, p. 496.

102. F. S. Hom, J. Autian, A. N. Martin, J. E. Berk., and J. G. Teplick, *J. Am. Pharm. Assoc., Sci. Ed.*, **46,** 254 (1957).

103. M. Guerbet and G. Tilly, Fr. Pat. M 4,986 (June 21, 1968); through *Chem. Abstr.*, **71,** 33398e (1969).

104. M. Vermess, R. H. Adamson, J. L. Doppman, A. S. Rabson, J. R. Herdt, and C. L. McIntosh, *Radiology*, **110,** 705 (1974).

105. B. T. Arbaeus, O. B. Ferno, and T. O. E. Linderot, Ger. Pat. 1,617,275 (May 13, 1971); through *Chem. Abstr.*, **75,** 52800d (1971); U S. Pat. 3,356,575 (Dec. 5, 1967); through *Chem. Abstr.*, **68,** 33205c (1968).

106. G. Fritsch., R. Voigt, and M. Luening, *Pharmazie*, **25**:4, 248 (1970).

107. L. K. Thompson, III, and W. G. Anlyan, *Surg. Gynecol. Obstet.*, **121**:1, 107 (1965).

108. M. M. A. Guerbet, Fr. Pat. M 4,523 (Nov. 28, 1966); through *Chem. Abstr.*, **68,** 29266f (1968).

109. P. R. Koehler, W. A. Meyers, J. F. Skelley, and B. Schaffer, *Radiology*, **82,** 866 (1964).

110. D. M. Seitzman, R. Wright, F. A. Halaby, J. H. Freeman, *Am. J. Roentgenol., Radium Ther.*, **89,** 140 (1963).

111. M. Vermess, R. H. Adamson, J. L. Doppman, A. S. Rabson, and J. R. Herdt, *Radiology*, **119,** 31 (1976).

112. E. A. Graham, W. H. Cole, G. H. Copher, and S. Moore, *J. Am. Med. Assoc.*, **86,** 467 (1926).

113. M. Dohrn and P. Diedrich, *Deut. Med. Wochenschr.*, **66,** 1133 (1940).

114. S. Archer, *Ann. N.Y. Acad. Sci.*, **78,** 720 (1959).

115. G. B. Hoey, P. E. Wright, R. D. Rands, Jr., in *Radiocontrast Agents*, Vol. I, P. K. Knoefel, Ed., Pergamon, Oxford, 1971, p. 23.

116. J. O. Hoppe, in *Medicinal Chemistry*, Vol. VI, E. E. Campaigne and W. H. Hartung, Eds., Wiley, New York, 1963, p. 290.

117. J. Hoppe, A. A. Larsen, and F. Coulston, *J. Pharmacol. Exp. Ther.*, **116,** 394 (1956).

118. J. Ackerman, in *Medicinal Chemistry*, 3rd ed., A. Burger, Ed., Wiley-Interscience, New York, 1970, p. 1686.

119. H.-J. Herms and V. Taenzer, in *Drug Design*, E. J. Ariens, Ed., Academic, New York, 1975, p. 263.

120. J. Hoppe, *Ann. N.Y. Acad. Sci.*, **78,** 727 (1959).

121. J. Hoppe and S. Archer, *Angiography*, **11,** 244 (1960).

122. P. K. Knoefel, *Radiopaque Diagnostic Agents*, Charles C. Thomas, Springfield, Ill., 1961.

123. H. W. Fischer, *Angiology*, **16,** 759 (1965).

124. H. W. Fischer, *Radiol. Clin. North Am.*, **4,** 625 (1966).

125. E. C. Lasser, *Radiol. Clin. North Am.*, **4,** 511 (1966).

126. A. T. Shockman, in *Topics in Medicinal Chemistry*, Vol. 1, J. L. Rabinowitz and R. M. Myerson, Eds., Interscience, New York, 1967, p. 381.

127. E. G. Lasser, in *Alimentary Tract Roentgenology*, Vol. 1, 2nd ed., A. R. Margulis and H. J. Burhenne, Eds., C. V. Mosby Co., St. Louis, 1973, p. 127.

128. H. W. Fisher, in *Current Concepts in Radiology*, E. J. Potchen, Ed., C. V. Mosby Co, St. Louis, 1972, p. 210.

129. R. G. Grainger, in *Modern Trends in Diagnostic Radiology*, Vol. 4, J. W. McLaren, Ed., Butterworths, London, 1970, p. 254.

130. T. Almén, *J. Theor. Biol.*, **24,** 216 (1969).

131. R. E. Gonsette, *Acta Radiol. Suppl.*, **335,** 25 (1973).

132. L. Björk, J. Erikson, and B. Ingelman, *Am. J. Roentgenol., Radium Ther. Nucl. Med.*, **107,** 637 (1969).

133. E. Felder, D. Pitre, L. Fumagalli, and E. Lorenzotti, *Farm. Ed. Sci.*, **28,** 912 (1973).

134. J. Rosati, P. Schiantarelli, and P. Tirone, *Farm., Ed. Sci.*, **28,** 996 (1973).

135. L. Björk, U. Erikson, and B. Ingelman, *Invest. Radiol.*, **5,** 142 (1970).

136. L. Björk, U. Erikson, B. Ingelman, and B. Zaar, *Upsala J. Med. Sci.*, **79,** 103 (1974).

137. H. Holtermann, *Acta Radiol. Suppl.*, **335,** 1 (1973).

138. S. Salvesen, *Acta Radiol. Suppl.*, **335,** 5 (1973).

139. M. Sovak, B. Nahlovsky, J. H. Lang, and E. C. Lasser, *Radiology*, **117,** 717 (1975).

140. F. L. Weitl, M. Sovak, and M. Ohno, *J. Med. Chem.*, **19,** 333 (1976).

141. V. H. Wallingford, H. G. Decker, and M. Krutz, *J. Am. Chem. Soc.*, **74,** 4365 (1952).

142. V. H. Wallingford, *Ann. N.Y. Acad. Sci.*, **78,** 707 (1959).

143. P. K. Knoefel, in *Radiocontrast Agents*, Vol. I, P. K. Knoefel, Ed., Pergamon, New York, 1971, p. 299.

144. W. H. Strain, S. M. Rogoff, in *Angiography*, Vol. I, 2nd ed., H. L. Abrams, Ed., Little, Brown, Boston, 1971, p. 35.

145. V. H. Wallingford, *J. Am. Pharm. Assoc., Sci. Ed.*, **42,** 721 (1953).

146. A. A. Larsen, C. Moore, J. Sprague, B. Cloke, J. Moss, and J. O. Hope, *J. Am. Chem. Soc.*, **78,** 3210 (1956).

147. E. Felder, D. Pitre, and L. Fumagalli, *Helv. Chim. Acta*, **48,** 259 (1965).

148. E. Felder, D. Pitre, H. Zutter, Ger. Pat. 2,229,360 (July 11, 1974); through *Chem. Abstr.*, **81,** 135763 (1974).

149. D. Pitre and L. Fumagalli, *Farm. Ed. Sci.*, **17,** 340 (1962).

150. E. Klieger and E. Schroeder, *Arch. Pharm.* (Weinheim, Ger.), **306**:11, 834 (1973).

151. G. B. Hoey, R. D. Rands, G. De LaMater, D. W. Chapman, and P. E. Wiegert, *J. Med. Chem.*, **6,** 24 (1963).

152. M. Guerbet and G. Tilly, Fr. Pat. M 6,777 (April 21, 1969); through *Chem. Abstr.*, **74,** 125233j (1971).

153. H. Cassebaum and K. Dierbach, *Pharmazie*, **16,** 389 (1961).

154. A. Geffen, *Radiology*, **72,** 839 (1959).

155. S. Archer, U.S. Pat. 2,705,726 (April 5, 1955); through *Chem. Abstr.*, **50,** 5030i (1956).

156. D. Pitre and S. Boveri, *J. Med. Chem.*, **11,** 406 (1968).

157. S. Archer and J. O. Hoppe, U.S. Pat. 2,895,988 (1959); through *Chem. Abstr.*, **54,** 1445h (1960).

158. D. Papa, H. F. Ginsberg, I. Lederman, and V. DeCamp, *J. Am. Chem. Soc.*, **75,** 1107 (1953).

159. H. Priewe and A. Poljak, *Chem. Ber.*, **93,** 2347 (1960).

160. A. Harwart, K. H. Kimbel, H. Langecker, and J. Willenbrink, *Arch. Exp. Pathol. Pharmacol.*, **237,** 186 (1959).

161. E. Felder and D. Pitre, S. Afr. Pat. 68:01,614 (Aug. 9, 1968); through *Chem. Abstr.*, **70,** 87549c (1969).

162. G. Rosati, P. De Mitcheli, and P. Schiantarelli, *Acta Radiol.*, **12,** 882 (1972).

163. E. Felder, D. Pitre, L. Fumagalli, and E. Lorenzotti, *Farm. Ed. Sci.*, **31,** 349 (1976).

164. I. Lindner, H. Stormann, W. Obendorf, and R. Kilches, *Arzneim.-Forsch.*, **11,** 384 (1961).

165. Osterreichische Stickstoffwerke Akt.-Ges., Brit. Pat. 870,321 (June 14, 1961); through *Chem. Abstr.*, **55,** 24683e (1961).

166. J. A. Korver, *Rec. Trav. Chim.*, **87,** 308 (1968).

167. N. V. Dagra, Neth. Pat. Appl. 6,515,305 (May 26, 1967); through *Chem. Abstr.*, **67,** 108422m (1967); Neth. Pat. Appl. 6,607,275 (Nov. 27, 1967); through *Chem. Abstr.*, **69,** 10263b (1968).

168. S. Pfeifer, J. Schäffner, and I. Bornschein, *Pharmazie*, **27,** 396 (1972).

169. S. Pfeizer, J. Schäffner, I. Bornschein, and R. Kraft, *Pharmazie*, **27,** 403 (1972).

170. H. Cassebaum and K. Dierbach, Ger. (East) Pat. 67,209 (June 5, 1969); through *Chem. Abstr.*, **72,** 66654j (1970).

171. I. Bornschein, J. Schäffner, and S. Pfeifer, *Pharmazie*, **30**:3, 196 (1975).

172. H. Gries, Ger. Pat. 2,050,217 (April 6, 1972); through *Chem. Abstr.*, **77,** 34150d (1972).

173. U. Speck, W. Clauss, L. Blumenbach, and A. Albrecht, *Invest. Radiol.*, **11,** 315 (1976).

174. H. Priewe, R. Rutkowski, K. Pirner, and K. Junkmann, *Chem. Ber.*, **87,** 651 (1954).

175. H. Priewe and R. Rutkowski, U.S. Pat. 2,776,241 (Jan. 1, 1957); through *Chem. Abstr.*, **51,** 5831e (1957); U.S. Pat. 2,853,424 (Sept. 23, 1958); through *Chem. Abstr.*, **53,** 8077g (1959).

176. J. Kotler-Brajtburg, A. Swirska, and A. Raczka, *Rocz. Chem.*, **36,** 763 (1962); through *Chem. Abstr.*, **58,** 5568a (1963).

177. W. Neudert and H. Ropke, *Helv. Chim. Acta*, **41,** 851 (1958).

178. H. Pfeiffer, U. Speck, and K. H. Kolb, Ger. Pat. 2,405,652 (Aug. 21, 1975); through *Chem. Abstr.*, **83,** 192867w (1975).

179. E. Felder, D. Pitre, and M. Grandi, *Farm. Ed. Sci.*, **28,** 925 (1973).

180. C. B. Hoey, R. D. Rands, P. E. Wiegart, D. W. Chapman, R. L. Zey, and G. De La Mater, *J. Med. Chem.*, **9,** 964 (1966).

181. St. Kunze and W. Schiefer, *Deut. Med. Wochenschr.*, **97,** 245 (1972).

182. M. Kramer, *Arzneim.-Forsch.*, **14,** 451 (1964).

183. L. Bjork, U. Erickson, and B. Ingelman, *Upsala J. Med. Sci.*, **77,** 19 (1972).

184. L. Bjork, U. E. Erickson, and B. G. A. Ingelman, Swed. Pat. 344,166 (April 4, 1972); through *Chem. Abstr.*, **79,** 18398b (1973).

185. P. E. Wiegert, Brit. Pat. 1,346,795 (Feb. 13, 1974); through *Chem. Abstr.*, **81,** 3627t (1974).

186. B. F. Tullar and J. O. Hoppe, U.S. Pat. 2,551,696 (May 15, 1951); through *Chem. Abstr.*, **46,** 1592d (1952).

187. W. H. Strain, J. T. Plati, and L. Strafford, *J. Am. Chem. Soc.*, **64,** 1436 (1942).

188. W. H. Strain, J. T. Plati, and S. L. Warren, U.S. Pat. 2,348,231 (May 9, 1944); through *Chem. Abstr.*, **39,** 1515[4] (1945).

189. W. Baker, E. E. Cook, and W. G. Leeds, *J. Soc. Chem. Ind.*, **63,** 223 (1944).

190. M. Dohrn and P. Diedrich, *Ann.* **494,** 284 (1932); *Chem. Abstr.*, **26,** 3506 (1932).

191. J. Reitmann, U.S. Pat. 1,993,039 (March 5, 1935); through *Chem. Abstr.*, **29,** 2547[2] (1935).

192. J. Reitmann, Ger. Pat. 579,224 (June 22, 1933); through *Chem. Abstr.*, **27,** 4880 (1933).

193. D. J. Branscombe, Brit. Pat. 517,382 (Jan. 29, 1940); through *Chem. Abstr.*, **35,** 7124[3] (1941).

194. E. G. Tomich, B. Basil, and B. Davis, *Brit. J. Pharmacol.*, **8,** 166 (1953).

195. Y. Sugii, I. Shimoya, and H. Shindo, *J. Pharm. Soc.* (Japan), **50,** 727 (1930); through *Chem. Abstr.*, **24,** 5326 (1930).

196. A. Binz, C. Räth, and K. Junkmann, *Biochem. Z.*, **227,** 200 (1930).

197. L. Fumagalli, E. Felder, and D. Pitre, *Pharmazie*, **30,** 78 (1975).

198. L. Fumagalli and D. Pitre, *Farm. Ed. Sci.*, **24,** 568 (1969).

199. H. Cassebaum and K. Dierbach, Ger. (East) Pat. 67,435 (June 20, 1969); through *Chem. Abstr.*, **72,** 43166n (1970).

200. H. Cassebaum and K. Dierbach, Ger. (East) Pat. 67,209 (June 5, 1969); through *Chem. Abstr.*, **72,** 66654j (1970).

201. M. Guerbet and G. Tilly, Brit. Pat. 1,146,133 (March 19, 1969); through *Chem. Abstr.*, **71,** 30243q (1969).

202. T. Zdravil, Fr. Pat. 2,186,460 (Feb. 15, 1974); through *Chem. Abstr.*, **81,** 13278u (1974).

203. E. Berliner, *J. Chem. Educ.*, **43,** 124 (1966).

204. E. Klieger, U. Speck, and E. Schroeder, Ger. Pat. 2,505,320 (Aug. 5, 1976); through *Chem. Abstr.*, **85,** 159717r (1976).

205. E. Felder, D. Pitre, L. Fumagalli, H. Suter, and H. Zutter, *Helv. Chim. Acta*, **52,** 1339 (1969).

206. E. Felder and D. Pitre, Swiss Pat. 480,071 (Dec. 15, 1969); through *Chem. Abstr.*, **72,** 100292b (1970).

207. H. Pfeiffer, K. H. Kolb, A. Hartwart, and P. E. Schulze, Ger. Pat. 1,956,844 (Nov. 8, 1969); through *Chem. Abstr.*, **75,** 35474h (1971).

208. J. H. Ackerman, U.S. Pat. 3,452,084 (June 24, 1969); through *Chem. Abstr.*, **71,** 70346g (1969).

209. V. H. Wallingford, U.S. Pat. 3,446,837 (May 27, 1969); through *Chem. Abstr.*, **71,** 38602b (1969).

210. W. Obendorf, E. Schwarzinger, J. Kreiger, and I. Lindner, Austrian Pat. 319,463, (Dec. 27, 1974); through *Chem. Abstr.*, **82,** 16245e (1975).

211. E. Felder and D. Pitre, Ger. Pat. 1,922,615 (Nov. 20, 1969); through *Chem. Abstr.*, **72,** 66626b (1970).

212. W. Obendorf and I. Lindner, Ger. Pat. 1,467,996 (Nov. 12, 1970); through *Chem. Abstr.*, **74,** 141313u (1971).

213. Oesterreichische Stickstoffwerke A.-G., Brit. Pat. 1,087,840 (Oct. 18, 1967); through *Chem. Abstr.*, **68,** 95664c (1968).

214. Oesterreichische Stickstoffwerke A.-G., Austrian Pat. 258,464 (Nov. 27, 1967); through *Chem. Abstr.*, **68,** 62714y (1968).

215. H. Suter, D. Pitre, and L. Fumagalli, Swiss Pat. 490,090 (June 30, 1970); through *Chem. Abstr.*, **73,** 112947c (1970).

216. H. Cassebaum, K. Dierbach, and H. Bekker, *Pharmazie*, **27,** 391 (1972).

217. N. V. Dagra, Neth. Pat. Appl. 6,515,305 (May 26, 1967); through *Chem. Abstr.*, **67,** 108422m (1967).

218. E. Felder and D. Pitre, Ger. Pat. 2,212,741 (Dec. 28, 1972); through *Chem. Abstr.*, **78,** 71710c (1973).

219. E. Felder and D. Pitre, Ger. Pat. 2,128,902 (June 22, 1972); through *Chem. Abstr.*, **77,** 101109n (1972).

220. Laboratoires Andre Guerbet, Brit. Pat. 1,080,496 (Aug. 23, 1967); through *Chem. Abstr.*, **69,** 108457b (1968).

221. J. Bernstein and F. A. Sowinski, Ger. Pat. 2,321,498 (Nov. 15, 1973); through *Chem. Abstr.*, **80,** 26969z (1974).

222. D. Pitre, L. Fumagalli, and E. Lorenzotti, *Farm. Ed. Sci.*, **27**:5, 408 (1972).

223. Beecham Group Ltd., Fr. Pat. 2,180,568 (Jan. 4, 1974); through *Chem. Abstr.*, **81,** 63494g (1974).

224. M. J. Soulal and K. Utting, U.S. Pat. 3,795,698 (March 5, 1974); through *Chem. Abstr.*, **80,** 120582q (1974).

225. J. Hebky, V. Jelinek, B. First, and M. Karasek, Czech. Pat. 121,655 (Jan. 15, 1967); through *Chem. Abstr.*, **68,** 2696j (1968).

226. J. Hebky, *Pharm. Ind.*, **32,** (10A), 938 (1970); through *Chem. Abstr.*, **74,** 95084V (1971).

227. J. Hebky, V. Jelinek, and M. Karasek, Czech. Pat. 121,654 (Jan. 15, 1967); through *Chem. Abstr.*, **69,** 2698m (1968).

228. J. Hebky and M. Karasek, Czech. Pat 121,653

(Jan. 15, 1967); through *Chem. Abstr.*, **68**, 2697k (1968).

229. G. Shtacher, *J. Pharm. Sci.*, **57**, 1710 (1968).

230. SPOFA United Pharmaceutical Works, Neth. Pat. Appl. 6,516,673 (June 22, 1966); through *Chem. Abstr.*, **67**, 21607b (1967).

231. W. Obendorf, E. Schwarzinger, J. Kreiger, I. Lindner, Austrian Pat. 320,139 (July 31, 1972); through *Chem. Abstr.*, **83**, 65498b (1975).

232. Laboratoires Andre Guerbet, Brit. Pat. 1,080,496 (Aug. 23, 1967); through *Chem. Abstr.*, **69**, 108457b (1968).

233. Oesterreichische Stickstoffwerke A.-G., Brit. Pat. 1,087,840; through *Chem. Abstr.*, **68**, 95564c (1968).

234. Oesterreichische Stickstoffwerke A.-G., Austrian Pat. 258,464 (Nov. 27, 1967); through *Chem. Abstr.*, **68**, 62714g (1968).

235. W. Obendorf and I. Lindner, Ger. Pat. 1,467,996 (Nov. 12, 1970); through *Chem. Abstr.*, **74**, 141313u (1971).

236. W. Obendorf, E. Schwarzinger, J. Krieger, and I. Lindner, Austrian Pat. 319,226 (Dec. 10, 1974); through *Chem. Abstr.*, **83**, 9777e (1975).

237. E. Felder, D. Pitre, and H. Zutter, Ger. Pat. 2,229,360 (July 11, 1974); through *Chem. Abstr.*, **81**, 135763u (1974).

238. Bracco Industria Chemica S.P.A., Fr. Pat. 2,150,805 (May 18, 1973); through *Chem. Abstr.*, **80**, 112687n (1974).

239. E. Felder, D. Pitre, Ger. Pat. 2,422,718 (Feb. 13, 1975); through *Chem. Abstr.*, **83**, 96763p (1975).

240. E. Felder and D. Pitre, Ger. Pat. 2,425,912 (July 17, 1973); through *Chem. Abstr.*, **83**, 78877z (1975).

241. E. Felder and D. Pitre, Ger. Pat. 2,317,535 (May 30, 1974); through *Chem. Abstr.*, **81**, 91212g (1974).

242. G. Tilly, Ger. Pat. 2,117,250 (Oct. 28, 1971); through *Chem. Abstr.*, **76**, 33966s (1972).

243. G. Tilly, Fr. Pat. 2,085,636 (Feb. 4, 1972); through *Chem. Abstr.*, **77**, 92871a (1972).

244. G. Tilly, Fr. Pat. 2,074,734 (Nov. 12, 1971); through *Chem. Abstr.*, **77**, 92845v (1972).

245. J. Bernstein and L. A. Losee, U.S. Pat. 3,666,800 (May 30, 1972); through *Chem. Abstr.*, **77**, 88116r (1972).

246. P. E. Wiegert, Ger. Pat. 2,526,848 (Jan. 2, 1976); through *Chem. Abstr.*, **84**, 89851h (1976).

247. E. Klieger, B. Wolfgang, and E. Schroeder, U.S. Pat. 3,953,501 (April 27, 1976); through *Chem. Abstr.*, **85**, 177976d (1976).

248. H. Cassebaum and K. Dierbach, *Pharm.* **21**:3, 167 (1966).

249. V. H. Wallingford, U.S. Pat. 3,346,630 (Oct. 10, 1967); through *Chem. Abstr.*, **68**, 9555v (1968).

250. E. B. Akerblom, Ger. Pat. 2,033,525 (Jan. 21, 1971); through *Chem. Abstr.*, **74**, 87613f (1971).

251. B. G. A. Ingelman, Ger. Pat. 2,346,774 (March 28, 1974); through *Chem. Abstr.*, **81**, 68565r (1974).

252. T. Povse, P. Zupet, and M. Japelj, Ger. Pat., 2,319,985 (Nov. 8, 1973); through *Chem. Abstr.*, **80**, 26990z (1974).

253. K. T. Zdravail, Brit. Pat. 1,407,138 (April 24, 1972); through *Chem. Abstr.*, **83**, 205958d (1975).

254. N. V. Dagra, Neth. Pat. Appl. 69, 12, 10,102 (Feb. 10, 1971); through *Chem. Abstr.*, **75**, 35436x (1971).

255. E. Klieger, *Chim. Ther.*, **7**:6, 475 (1972).

256. H. Pfeiffer, G. Zoellner, and W. Beich, Ger. Pat. 2,118,219 (Oct. 26, 1972); through *Chem. Abstr.*, **78**, 20204h (1973).

257. M. Sovak, Ger. Pat. 2,028,595 (Dec. 17, 1970); through *Chem. Abstr.*, **74**, 57331r (1971).

258. G. Tilly, M. J. C. Hardouin, J. Lautrou, Ger. Pat. 2,523,567 (Dec. 11, 1975); through *Chem. Abstr.*, **84**, 184889k (1976).

259. E. Felder and D. Pitre, Ger. Pat. 1,273,747 (July 25, 1968); through *Chem. Abstr.*, **69**, 99405v (1968).

260. H. Pfeiffer, G. Zoellner, and W. Beich, Ger. Pat. 2,124,904 (Dec. 7, 1972); through *Chem. Abstr.*, **78**, 58076f (1973).

261. H. Holtermann, L. G. Haugen, and V. Nordal, Norw. Pat. 115,708 (Nov. 18, 1968); through *Chem. Abstr.*, **71**, 12783m (1969).

262. S. Salvesen, L. G. Haugen, J. Haavaldsen, V. Nordal, Norw. Pat. 122,430 (June 28, 1971); through *Chem. Abstr.*, **75**, 144023f (1971).

263. L. G. Haugen, S. Salvesen, J. Haavaldsen, and V. Nordal, Ger. Pat. 1,928,838 (Dec. 11, 1969); through *Chem. Abstr.*, **72**, 78695m (1970).

264. Bracco Industria Chimica S.p.A., Fr. Pat. 1,469,823 (Feb. 17, 1967); through *Chem. Abstr.*, **68**, 12715d (1968).

265. O. Radek, J. Kejha, O. Nemecek, and V. Jelinek, Czech. Pat. 120,776 (Dec. 15, 1966); through *Chem. Abstr.*, **68**, 12716e (1968).

266. A. A. Larsen, (to Sterling Drug Inc.) Ger. Pat. 1,229,679 (Dec. 1, 1966); through *Chem. Abstr.*, **66**, 40725j (1967).

267. T. Yoshikawa, T. Kotake, and T. Naito, Jap. Pat. 68:03,370 (Feb. 7, 1968); through *Chem. Abstr.*, **69,** 96273q (1968).

268. H. Cassebaum, K. Dierbach, and H. Bekker, *Pharmazie,* **22**:9, 470 (1967).

269. M. J. Soulal and K. Utting, Ger. Pat. 2,428,140 (Jan. 23, 1975); through *Chem. Abstr.*, **82,** 155890g (1975).

270. Beecham Group Ltd., Fr. Pat. 2,230,377 (Dec. 20, 1974); through *Chem. Abstr.*, **83,** 48224s (1975).

271. G. Tilly, Ger. Pat. 2,216,627 (Oct. 19, 1972); through *Chem. Abstr.*, **78,** 15837n (1973).

272. G. Tilly, M. J. C. Hardouin, and J. Lautron, Ger. Pat., 2,456,685 (Dec. 7, 1973); through *Chem. Abstr.*, **83,** 114021b (1975).

273. T. Almén and J. Haavaldsen, Ger. Pat. 2,031,724 (Jan. 7, 1971); through *Chem. Abstr.*, **74,** 99662e (1971).

274. W. Obendorf, E. Schwarzinger, J. Krieger, and I. Lindner, Austrian Pat. 317,867 (Sept. 25, 1974); through *Chem. Abstr.*, **82,** 16583w (1975).

275. W. Obendorf, I. Lindner, E. Schwarzinger, and J. Krieger, Ger. Pat. 2,235,935 (Feb. 7, 1974); through *Chem. Abstr.*, **80,** 108545x (1974).

276. J. Hebky, J. Polacek, *Collect. Czech. Chem. Commun.*, **35**:2, 664 (1970); *Chem. Abstr.*, **72,** 89938m (1970).

277. M. J. Soulal and K. Utting, Ger. Pat. 2,219,707 (Oct. 25, 1973); through *Chem. Abstr.*, **80,** 26978b (1974).

278. E. Klieger, W. Beich, and E. Schroeder, Ger. Pat. 2,207,950 (Aug. 23, 1973); through *Chem. Abstr.*, **79,** 136874v (1973).

279. J. Bernstein and L. A. Losee, Ger. Pat. 2,038,263 (Feb. 18, 1971); through *Chem. Abstr.*, **74,** 99665h (1971).

280. G. Tilly, Brit. Pat. 1,385,684 (Feb. 26, 1975); through *Chem. Abstr.*, **83,** 27930d (1975).

281. Schering, A.-G., Neth. Pat. App. 6,508,845 (Jan. 10, 1967); through *Chem. Abstr.*, **67,** 21688d (1967).

282. E. Hartmann and H. Roepke, *Fresenius' Z. Anal. Chem.*, **232**:4, 268 (1967); *Chem. Abstr.*, **68,** 16166y (1968).

283. H. Pfeiffer, U. Speck, and K. H. Kolb, Ger. Pat. 2,405,652 (Aug. 21, 1975); through *Chem. Abstr.*, **83,** 192867w (1975).

284. E. Felder and D. Pitre, Ger. Pat. 1,922,578 (Nov. 13, 1969); through *Chem. Abstr.*, **72,** 59099d (1970).

285. E. Felder and D. Pitre, Brit. Pat. 1,225,217 (March 17, 1971); through *Chem. Abstr.*, **75,** 11813v (1971).

286. E. Felder and D. Pitre, Ger. Pat. 1,937,211 (Feb. 4, 1971); through *Chem. Abstr.*, **74,** 99663f (1971).

287. E. Felder and D. Pitre, Ger. Pat. 1,922,606 (Nov. 13, 1969); through *Chem. Abstr.*, **72,** 66657n (1970).

288. J. H. Ackerman, S. Afr. Pat. 68:02,537 (Sept. 27, 1968); through *Chem. Abstr.*, **71,** 38603c (1969).

289. B. G. A. Ingelman, Ger. Pat. 1,816,894 (July 24, 1969); through *Chem. Abstr.*, **71,** 101558j (1969).

290. L. Bjork, U. Erikson, and B. Ingelman, *Upsala J. Med. Sci.*, **77**:1, 19 (1972).

291. L. Bjork, U. E. Erikson, and B. G. A. Ingelman, *Am. J. Roentgenol., Radium Ther. Nucl. Med.*, **109**:3, 606 (1970).

292. Pharmacia Aktiebolag, Brit. Pat. 1,207,975 (Oct. 7, 1970); through *Chem. Abstr.*, **74,** 42164q (1971).

293. T. K. I. V. Ekstrand, A. Ronlan, B. V. Wickberg, and A. H. Munksgaard, Ger. Pat. 2,236,429 (Feb. 22, 1973); through *Chem. Abstr.*, **78,** 1234308m (1973).

294. L. Bjork, U. E. Erikson, and B. G. A. Ingelman, Swed. Pat. 354,853 (March 26, 1973); through *Chem. Abstr.*, **80,** 26953q (1974).

295. L. Bjork, Fr. Pat. 7251 (Sept. 8, 1969); through *Chem. Abstr.*, **77,** 118198p (1972).

296. E. Felder, *Radiol. Electrol. Med. Nucl.*, **56**:Suppl. 1, 38 (1975).

297. J. Kejha, O. Radek, and O. Nemecek, *Cesk. Farm.*, **16**:2, 92 (1967); through *Chem. Abstr.*, **67,** 108535a (1967).

298. B. Carnmalm, J. Gyllander, N. A. Jonsson, and L. Mikiver, *Acta Pharm. Suec.*, **11,** 49 (1974).

299. J. E. Siggins and J. H. Ackerman, *J. Med. Chem.*, **9,** 973 (1966).

300. J. E. Siggins and J. H. Ackerman, U.S. Pat. 3,346,620 (Oct. 10, 1967); through *Chem. Abstr.*, **68,** 87025n (1968).

301. B. N. Newton, *J. Med. Chem.*, **19,** 1362 (1976).

302. Eprova, Ltd., Fr. Pat. 2,130,221 (Dec. 8, 1972); through *Chem. Abstr.*, **78,** 140405W (1973).

303. H. Suter, H. Zutter, and H. R. Mueller, Ger. Pat. 2,201,578, (Oct. 5, 1972); through *Chem. Abstr.*, **78,** 3694a (1973).

304. H. Suter and H. Zutter, *Pharm. Acta Helv.*, **50**:5, 152 (1975).

305. A. J. M. Bedford, Ger. Pat. 2,136,255 (March 22, 1972); through *Chem. Abstr.*, **78,** 151644z (1973).

306. B. Carnmalm, J. Gyllander, N. A. Jonsson, and L. Mikiver, *Acta Pharm. Suec.*, **11,** 167 (1974).

307. G. Shtacher and S. Dayigi, *J. Med. Chem.*, **15**:11, 1174 (1972).

308. O. Radek, J. Kejha, O. Nemecek, and B. Kakac, *Cesk. Farm.*, **16**:1, 34 (1967); through *Chem. Abstr.*, **68,** 114214g.

309. J. Zutter and J. Brunner, Ger. Pat. 1,958,333 (Aug. 27, 1970); through *Chem. Abstr.*, **78,** 151644g (1973).

310. S. V. P. Ootegham, R. G. Smith, and G. D. Daves, Jr., *J. Med. Chem.*, **19,** 1349 (1976).

311. B. S. Epstein, S. Natelson, and B. Kramer, *Am. J. Roentgenol., Radium Ther.*, **56,** 201 (1946).

312. E. Felder, D. Pitre, L. Fumagalli, and F. Lorenzotti, *Farm. Ed. Sci.*, **31,** 349 (1976).

313. E. C. Lasser and J. H. Lang, *Invest. Radiol.*, **5,** 446 (1970).

314. J. H. Lang and E. C. Lasser, *Invest. Radiol.*, **2,** 396 (1967).

315. P. K. Knoefel, in *Radiocontrast Agents*, Vol. I, P. K. Knoefel, Ed., Pergamon, Oxford, 1971, p. 133.

316. C. Hansch, *Farm. Ed. Sci.*, **23,** 293 (1968).

317. F. Helmer, K. Kiehs, and C. Hansch, *Biochemistry*, **7,** 2858 (1968).

318. P. K. Knoefel and K. C. Huang, *J. Pharmacol. Exp. Ther.*, **117**, 307 (1956).

317. F. Helmer and K. C. Huang, *J. Pharmacol. Exp. Ther.*, **117**, 307 (1956).

319. G. B. Hoey, *Invest. Radiol.*, **5,** 453 (1970) (discussion).

320. R. E. Wise, in *Alimentary Tract Roentgenology*, Vol. II, A. R. Margulis and H. J. Burhenne, Eds., C. V. Mosby Co., St. Louis, 1973, p. 1291.

321. J. Brismar, P. Lindgren, and G.-F. Saltzman, *Acta Radiol. Diag.*, **11,** 129 (1971).

322. G. T. Benness, *Aust. Radiol.*, **14,** 416 (1970).

323. P. Purkiss, R. D. Lane, W. R. Cattell, I. K. Fry, and A. G. Spencer, *Invest. Radiol.*, **3,** 271 (1968).

324. F. Medzihradsky, P. J. Dahlstrom, T. B. Hunter, J. R. Thornbury, and T. M. Silver, *Invest. Radiol.*, **10,** 532 (1975).

325. T. Dennenberg, *Acta Med. Scand. Suppl.*, **442,** 1 (1966).

326. J. Kutzner and K. H. Van de Weyer, *Fortschr. Geb. Roentgenstr. Nuklearmed.*, **114,** 74 (1971).

327. V. Taenzer, *Eur. J. Pharmacol.*, **6,** 137 (1973).

328. N. W. Tauxe, M. K. Burbank, F. T. Maher, and J. C. Hunt, *Proc. Mayo Clin.*, **39,** 761 (1964).

329. E. Felder, D. Pitre, and M. Grandi, *J. Pharm. Sci.*, **64,** 684 (1975).

330. E. Hartmann and H. Roepke, *Fresenius' Z. Anal. Chem.*, **232**:4, 268 (1968).

331. L. Kaufman, J. Nelson, D. Price, D. Shames, and C. J. Wilson, *IEEE Trans. Nucl. Sci.*, **NS-20,** 402 (1973).

332. L. Kaufman, F. Deconinck, D. C. Price, P. Guery, C. J. Wilson, B. Hruska, S. J. Swann, D. C. Camp, A. L. Voegele, R. D. Friesen, and J. A. Nelson, *Invest. Radiol.*, **11,** 210 (1976).

333. R. E. Koehler, L. Kaufman, A. Brito, and J. A. Nelson, *Invest. Radiol.*, **11,** 134 (1976).

334. W. H. Shehadi, *Am. J. Roentgenol., Radium Ther. Nucl. Med.*, **124,** 145 (1975).

335. D. M. Witten, *J. Am. Med. Assoc.*, **231,** 974 (1975).

336. D. M. Witten, F. D. Hirsch, and G. W. Hartman, *Am. J. Roentgenol., Radium Ther. Nucl. Med.*, **119,** 832 (1973).

337. G. Ansell, *Invest. Radiol.*, **5,** 374 (1970).

338. T. Almén, in *Radiocontrast Agents*, Vol. II, P. K. Knoefel, Ed., Pergamon, Oxford, 1971, p. 443.

339. G. Ansell, in *Recent Advances in Radiology*, T. Lodge and R. E. Steiner, Eds., Churchill Livingstone, Edinburgh, 1975, p. 335.

340. R. N. Berk and P. M. Loeb, *Semin. Roentgenol.*, **11,** 147 (1976).

341. H. W. Fischer, *Radiology*, **91,** 66 (1968).

342. H. W. Fischer, S. R. Reuter, and N. P. Moscow, *Invest. Radiol.*, **3,** 324 (1968).

343. F. Koehler, Ger. Pat. 2,261,584 (April 25, 1974); through *Chem. Abstr.*, **81,** 82400q (1974).

344. T. G. Brown, Jr., *Angiology*, **18,** 273 (1967).

345. S. Salvesen, P. L. Nilsen, and H. Holtermann, *Acta Radiol. Suppl.*, **270,** 17 (1967).

346. B. E. Bordalen, H. Wang, and H. Holtermann, *Invest. Radiol.*, **5,** 559 (1970).

347. G. F. Saltzman, and K. A. Sundstrom, *Acta Radiol.*, **54,** 353 (1960).

348. E. F. Bernstein, J. D. Palmer, T. A. Aaberg, and R. L. Davis, *Radiology*, **76,** 88 (1961).

349. D. Busfield, K. Child, and E. Tomich, *Brit. J. Radiol.*, **35,** 815 (1962).

350. P. Aspelin, and T. Almén, *Invest. Radiol.*, **11,** 309 (1976).

351. P. Lindgren, *Invest. Radiol.*, **5,** 24 (1970).

352. H. W. Fischer and J. W. Eckstein, *Am. J. Roentgenol.*, **86,** 166 (1961).

353. H. W. Fischer, *Angiology*, **16,** 759 (1965).

354. S. K. Hilal, *Acta Radiol. Diag.*, **5,** 211 (1966).

355. J. O. Hoppe, L. P. Duprey, W. A. Borisenok, and J. G. Bird, *Angiology*, **18,** 257 (1967).

356. R. C. Read and M. W. Meyer, *Surg. For.*, **10**, 472 (1959).

357. R. C. Read, J. A. Johnson, J. A. Vick, and M. W. Meyer, *Circ. Res.*, **8**, 538 (1960).

358. M. W. Meyer and R. C. Read, *Radiology*, **82**, 630 (1964).

359. H. Schmid-Schönbein and R. H. Wells, *Ergeb. Physiol.*, **63**, 146 (1971).

360. H. Schmid-Schönbein and R. H. Wells, *Arch. Ges. Physiol.*, **307**, 59 (1969).

361. R. Wells and H. Schmid-Schönbein, *J. Appl. Physiol.*, **27**, 213 (1969).

362. H. D. McIntosh, V. W. Hurst, H. K. Thompson, Jr., J. J. Morris, and R. E. Whalen, *Angiology*, **18**, 306 (1967).

363. F. E. Kloster, J. D. Bristow, G. A. Porter, M. P. Judkins, and H. E. Griswold, *Invest. Radiol.*, **2**, 353 (1967).

364. S. H. Cornell, *Invest. Radiol.*, **3**, 318 (1968).

365. T. Almén and B. Trägårdh, *Acta Radiol. Suppl.*, **335**, 197 (1973).

366. Z. Ansari and D. S. Baldwin, *Nephron*, **17**, 28 (1976).

367. J. Roylance, P. Davis, and M. B. Roberts, *Proc. Roy. Soc. Med.*, **67**, 44 (1974).

368. P. Davis, M. B. Roberts, and J. Roylance, *Brit. Med. J.*, **2**, 434 (1975).

369. W. H. Shehadi, *Radiology*, **113**, 219 (1974).

370. E. C. Lasser, A. J. Waters, and J. H. Lang, *Radiology*, **110**, 49 (1974).

371. H. W. Fischer and V. L. Doust, *Radiology*, **103**, 497 (1972).

372. K. N. Bhat, C. M. Arroyave, and R. Crown, *Ann. Allergy*, **37**, 169 (1976).

373. A. F. Lalli, *Radiology*, **112**, 267 (1974).

374. S. I. Rapoport and H. Levitan, *Am. J. Roentgenol., Radium Ther. Nucl. Med.*, **122**, 186 (1974).

375. S. I. Rapoport, H. K. Thompson, and J. M. Bidinger, *Acta Radiol. Diag.*, **15**, 21 (1974).

376. T. S. Reese and M. J. Karnovsky, *J. Cell Biol.*, **34**, 207 (1967).

377. M. J. Karnovsky, *J. Gen. Physiol.*, **52**, 64s (1968).

378. S. I. Rapoport, *Am. J. Physiol.*, **219**, 270 (1970).

379. S. I. Rapoport, in *Symposium on Small Vessel Angiography: Imaging, Morphology, Physiology and Clinical Application*, S. K. Hilal, Ed., C. V. Mosby Co., St. Louis, 1973, p. 137.

380. S. I. Rapoport, M. Hori, and I. Klatzo, *Am. J. Physiol.*, **223**, 323 (1972).

381. S. I. Rapoport, in *Pharmacology and Pharmacokinetics: Problems and Perspectives*, T. Teorell, P. L. Dedrick, and P. Condliffe, Eds., Plenum, New York, 1974, p. 241.

382. T. Broman and O. Olsson, *Acta Radiol.*, **30**, 326 (1948).

383. T. M. Farber, H. Sorer, N. B. Fizette, *Res. Comm. Chem. Pathol. Pharmacol.*, **8**:3, 431 (1974).

384. R. Gonsette and G. André-Balisaux, *Acta Radiol. Diag.*, **8**, 535 (1969).

385. P. J. Tuohimaa and E. Melartin, *Invest. Radiol.*, **5**, 22 (1970).

386. M. Kormano and H. Hervonen, *Radiology*, **120**, 727 (1976).

387. R. E. Gonsette, *Acta Radiol. Diag.*, **13**, 889 (1972).

388. K. F. Lampe, G. James, M. Erbesfeld, T. J. Mende, and M. Viamonte, *Invest. Radiol.*, **5**, 79 (1970).

389. B. L. McClennan and J. A. Becker, *Am. J. Roentgenol., Radium Ther. Nucl. Med.*, **113**, 427 (1971).

390. T. Fujita, J. Iwasa, and C. Hansch, *J. Am. Chem. Soc.*, **86**, 5175 (1964).

391. C. Hansch, in *Drug Design*, Vol. I, E. J. Ariens, Ed., Academic, New York, 1971, p. 271.

392. C. Hansch and W. R. Glave, *Mol. Pharmacol.*, **7**, 337 (1971).

393. A. Leo, C. Hansch, and D. Elkins, *Chem. Rev.*, **71**, 525 (1971).

394. W. H. Oldendorf, *Am. J. Physiol.*, **224**, 1450 (1973).

395. E. Melartin, P. J. Tuohimaa, and R. Dabb, *Invest. Radiol.*, **5**, 13 (1970).

396. L. Engevik, *Acta Chir. Scand. Suppl.*, **392**, 1 (1968).

397. N. Antoni and E. Lindgren, *Acta Chir. Scand.*, **98**, 230 (1949).

398. D. A. Killen and J. H. Foster, *Ann. Surg.*, **152**, 211 (1960).

399. E. M. Lance, D. Killen, and G. Owens, *Surg. Forum*, **9**, 728 (1959).

400. G. Margolis and T. G. Yerasimides, *Acta Radiol. Diag.*, **5**, 388 (1966).

401. D. A. Killen and J. H. Foster, *Surgery*, **59**, 969 (1966).

402. B. H. Stewart, R. L. Diamond, C. F. Ferguson, and P. H. Shepherd, *J. Urol.*, **94**, 695 (1965).

403. D. A. Killen and E. M. Lance, *Surgery*, **47**, 260 (1960).

404. E. M. Lance and D. A. Killen, *Surg. Forum*, **11**, 139 (1960).

405. J. H. Foster, D. A. Killen, P. T. Sessions, G. W.

Rhea, E. W. Winfrey, and H. A. Collins, *Vasc. Dis.*, **1,** 8 (1964).

406. G. Nylander, *Acta Radiol. Suppl.*, **266,** 7 (1967).

407. L. Szlavy and G. Vadon, *Radiol. Clin. Biol.*, **38,** 406 (1969).

408. P. G. Jeppson, *Acta Neurol. Scand.*, **38** : Suppl. 160 (1962).

409. P. D. Kenan, G. T. Tindall, G. Margolis, and R. S. Wood, *J. Neurosurg.*, **15,** 92 (1958).

410. L. Irstam, *Acta Radiol. Diag.*, **15,** 647 (1975).

411. E. C. Lasser, *Radiology*, **91,** 63 (1968).

412. J. H. Lang and E. C. Lasser, *J. Med. Chem.*, **14,** 233 (1971).

413. E. C. Lasser and J. H. Lang, *Invest. Radiol.*, **5,** 514 (1970).

414. W. R. Catell, *Invest. Radiol.*, **5,** 473 (1970).

415. H. O. Bang and J. Georg, *Acta Pharmacol. Toxicol.*, **4,** 87 (1948).

416. H. Bennhold, H. Ott, and M. Wiech, *Deut. Med. Wochenschr.*, **75,** 11 (1950).

417. R. N. Berk, P. M. Loeb, L. E. Goldberg, and J. Sokoloff, *New Engl. J. Med.*, **290,** 202 (1974).

418. E. C. Lasser, R. S. Farr, T. Fujimagari, and W. N. Tripp, *Am. J. Roentgenol., Radium Ther.*, **87,** 338 (1962).

419. J. Sokoloff, R. N. Berk, J. H. Lang, and E. C. Lasser, *Radiology*, **106,** 519 (1973).

420. C. S. Song, E. R. Beranbaum, and M. A. Rothschild, *Invest. Radiol.*, **11,** 39 (1976).

421. E. J. Goldstein and I. M. Arias, *Invest. Radiol.*, **9,** 594 (1974).

422. E. C. Lasser and J. H. Lang, *Invest. Radiol.*, **5,** 446 (1970).

423. J. Lang and E. C. Lasser, *Invest. Radiol.*, **10,** 314 (1975).

424. M. Kormano and M. Härkönen, *Invest. Radiol.*, **8,** 68 (1973).

425. E. C. Lasser and J. H. Lang, *Invest. Radiol.*, **1,** 237 (1966).

426. B. Hüthwohl and E. Truber, *Naunyn-Schmiedebergs Arch. Pharmacol.*, **282,** Suppl. P37 (1974).

427. B. Huthwohl, H. Hohage, and E. Truber, *Naunyn-Schmiedebergs Arch. Pharmacol.*, **287** : Suppl. R79 (1975).

428. D. Rickwood, A. Hell, G. D. Birnie, and C. Chr. Gilhuus-Moe, *Biochim. Biophys. Acta*, **342,** 367 (1974).

429. S. Salvesen and K. Fry, *Acta Radiol. Suppl.*, **335,** 247 (1973).

430. A. Livingston, T. Sooriyamoorthy, and J. Griffen, *Invest. Radiol.*, **9,** 282 (1974).

431. P. Schiantarelli, F. Peroni, P. Tirone, and G. Rosati, *Invest. Radiol.*, **8,** 199 (1973).

432. F. Peroni, P. Schiantarelli, G. Rosati, and P. Tirone, *Invest. Radiol.*, **8,** 205 (1973).

433. E. C. Lasser, *Invest. Radiol.*, **8,** 189 (1973).

434. M. A. Lichtman and M. S. Murphy, *Invest. Radiol.*, **9,** 588 (1974).

435. J. H. Lang, E. C. Lasser, and W. P. Kolb, *Invest. Radiol.*, **11,** 303 (1976).

436. K. Verebely, H. Kutt, R. M. Torack, and F. McDowell, *Blood*, **33,** 468 (1969).

437. W. A. Mersereau and H. R. Robertson, *J. Neurosurg.*, **18,** 289 (1961).

438. S. E. Sörensen, *Acta Radiol. Diag.*, **11,** 274 (1971).

439. P. I. Branemark, B. Jacobsson, and S. E. Sörensen, *Acta Radiol. Diag.*, **8,** 547 (1969).

440. G. J. Harrington and W. P. Wiedeman, *Radiology*, **84,** 1108 (1965).

441. A. M. Rothchild, *Brit. J. Pharmacol.*, **25,** 59 (1965).

442. W. D. M. Paton, *Pharmacol. Rev.*, **9,** 269 (1957).

443. M. P. Leite, C. R. Moraes, and J. G. Leme, *Acta Radiol. Diag.*, **15,** 172 (1975).

444. S. D. Rockoff and R. Brasch, *Invest. Radiol.*, **6,** 110 (1971).

445. S. D. Rockoff, C. Kuhn, and M. Charphyvy, *Invest. Radiol.*, **6,** 186 (1971).

446. G. Seidel, G. Groppe, and C. Meyer-Burgdorff, *Agents Actions*, **4** : 3, 143 (1974).

447. J. W. Black, W. A. M. Duncan, C. J. Durant, C. R. Ganellin, and E. M. Parsons, *Nature*, **236,** 385 (1972).

448. W. L. Miller, J. L. Doppman, and A. P. Kaplan, *J. Allerg. Clin. Immunol.*, **56,** 291 (1975).

449. R. C. Brasch, J. L. Caldwell, and H. H. Fudenberg, *Invest. Radiol.*, **11,** 1 (1976).

450. R. N. Berk, P. M. Loeb, L. E. Goldberger, and J. Sokoloff, *New Engl. J. Med.*, **290,** 204 (1974).

451. L. E. Goldberger, R. N. Berk, J. H. Lang, and P. M. Loeb, *Invest. Radiol.*, **9,** 16 (1974).

452. V. Tanenzer, P. Koeppe, K. F. Samwer, and G. H. Kolb, *Eur. J. Clin. Pharmacol.*, **6,** 137 (1973).

453. G. Rosati, *Radiol. Med.*, **56,** 808 (1970).

454. A. A. Moss, J. Nelson, and J. Amberg, *Am. J. Roentgenol., Radium Ther. Nucl. Med.*, **117,** 406 (1973).

455. R. M. Taketa, R. N. Berk, J. H. Lang, E. C. Lasser, and C. R. Dunn, *Am. J. Roentgenol., Radium Ther. Nucl. Med.*, **114,** 767 (1972).

456. J. A. Nelson, A. A. Moss, H. L. Goldberg, L. Z. Benet, and J. Amberg, *Invest. Radiol.*, **8,** 1 (1973).

457. J. Levy, *Am. J. Pharm.*, **135,** 78 (1963).

458. A. A. Moss, J. R. Amberg, and R. S. Jones, *Invest. Radiol.*, **7,** 11 (1972).

459. J. A. Nelson and A. E. Staubus, *Invest. Radiol.*, **10,** 371 (1975).

460. R. N. Berk, L. E. Goldberger, and P. M. Loeb, *Invest. Radiol.*, **9,** 7 (1974).

461. E. L. Forker and G. Gibson, in *The Liver*, G. Baumgartner and R. Preisig, Eds., S. Karger, New York, 1973, p. 326.

462. H. W. Fischer and F. A. Burgener, *Invest. Radiol.*, **9,** 24 (1974).

463. I. Sperber, *Pharmacol. Rev.*, **11,** 109 (1959).

464. L. A. Corman, I. M. Freundlich, J. S. Lehman, G. Onesti, P. E. Siegler, C. D. Swartz, and J. H. Nodine, *Curr. Ther. Res. Clin. Exp.*, **9,** 99 (1967).

465. D. M. Shames and A. A. Moss, *Invest. Radiol.*, **9,** 141 (1974).

466. I. Sperber, G. Sperber, in *Radiocontrast Agents*, Vol. I, P. K. Knoefel, Ed., Pergamon, Oxford, 1971, p. 179.

467. A. Strata, G. Magnani, F. Tirelli, and G. Rosati, *J. Radiol. Electrol. Med. Nucl.*, **56**: Suppl. 1, 40 (1975).

468. G. Segre and G. F. Rosati, *J. Radiol. Electrol. Med. Nucl.*, **56**: Suppl. 1, 44 (1975).

469. R. N. Berk, P. M. Loeb, A. Cobo-Frenkel, and J. L. Barnhart, *Radiology*, **119,** 529 (1976).

470. S. K. Lin, A. A. Moss, and S. Riegelman, *Invest. Radiol.*, **12,** 175 (1977).

471. J. A. Nelson, H. W. Pepper, H. I. Goldberg, A. A. Moss, and J. R. Amberg, *Invest. Radiol.*, **8,** 126 (1973).

472. R. J. Griep and W. B. Nelp, *Radiology*, **93,** 807 (1969).

473. K. Golman and S. G. Dahl, *Acta Radiol. Suppl.*, **335,** 276 (1973).

474. K. Golman, *Acta Radiol. Suppl.*, **335,** 258 (1973).

475. P. K. Knoefel and G. Carrasquer, in *Radiocontrast Agents*, Vol. I, P. K. Knoefel, Ed., Pergamon, Oxford, 1971, p. 261.

476. E. W. McChesney, in *Radiocontrast Agents*, Vol. I, P. K. Knoefel, Ed., Pergamon Press, Oxford, 1971, p. 336.

477. G. Miller, W. A. Fuchs, and R. Preisig, *Schweiz. Med. Wochenschr.*, **99,** 577 (1969).

478. G. Rosati and P. Schiantarelli, *Invest. Radiol.*, **5,** 232 (1976).

479. J. A. Nelson and A. E. Staubus, *Invest. Radiol.*, **11,** 63 (1976).

480. G. Juliani, E. Gaia, and E. Mariani, *J. Radiol. Electrol. Med. Nucl.*, **56**: Suppl. 1, 42 (1975).

481. J. M. Janbroers, J. C. Sanders, H. P. Til, V. J. Feron, and A. P. de Groot, *Toxicol. Appl. Pharmacol.*, **14,** 232 (1969).

482. K. Kiyono, T. Kasuya, and T. Kobayashi, *Radioisotopes*, **20**:2, 78 (1971); through *Chem. Abstr.*, **75,** 33659y (1971).

483. H. W. Fischer, *Radiology*, **84,** 483 (1965).

484. W. J. Cooke, G. H. Mudge, *Invest. Radiol.*, **10,** 189 (1975).

485. C. R. Dunn, R. N. Berk, *Am. J. Roentgenol., Radium Ther. Nucl. Med.*, **114,** 758 (1972).

486. J. A. Nelson, A. E. Staubus and J. R. Amberg, *Invest. Radiol.*, **9,** 438 (1974).

487. G. T. Benness, C. A. Evill, D. Varga, and M. Soschko, *Invest. Radiol.*, **10,** 526 (1975).

488. J. R. Wood and I. F. Stanford, *Brit. J. Radiol.*, **47,** 825 (1974).

489. K. Golman, *Acta Radiol. Suppl.*, **335,** 253 (1973).

490. K. Golman, *Acta Radiol. Suppl.*, **335,** 264 (1973).

491. K. Golman, *Acta Radiol. Suppl.*, **335,** 268 (1973).

492. L. B. Talner and A. J. Davidson, *Invest. Radiol.*, **3,** 310 (1968).

493. R. Hasson and T. Lindholm, *Acta Med. Scand.*, **174,** 611 (1963).

494. G. T. Benness, *Aust. Radiol.*, **12,** 245 (1968).

495. L. B. Talner and A. J. Davidson, *Invest. Radiol.*, **3,** 301 (1968).

496. N. Bank, B. F. Mutz, and H. S. Aynedjian, *J. Clin. Invest.*, **46,** 695 (1967).

497. J. R. Jaenike, *J. Lab. Clin. Med.*, **73,** 459 (1969).

498. K. Golman, T. Almén, and H. Förste, *Invest. Radiol.*, **11,** 80 (1976).

499. R. L. Campbell, J. A. Campbell, R. F. Heimburger, J. E. Kalsbeck, and J. Mealey, *Radiology*, **83,** 286 (1964).

500. H. Brabrand, H. D. Lessmann, and H. Wenker, *Radiologie*, **12,** 66 (1972).

501. N. K. Sviridov, *Farmacol. Toksikol.* (Moscow), **35** (3), 372 (1972); through *Chem. Abstr.*, **77,** 70854v (1972).

502. E. W. McChesney, in *Radiocontrast Agents*, Vol. I, P. K. Knoefel, Ed., Pergamon, Oxford, 1971, p. 147.

503. E. W. McChesney and J. O. Hoppe, *Arch. Int. Pharmacodyn. Ther.*, **105,** 306 (1956).

504. E. W. McChesney and W. F. Banks, Jr., *Proc. Soc. Exp. Biol. Med.*, **119,** 1027 (1965).

505. H. Langecker and C. Ertel, *Arch. Exp. Pathol. Pharmakol.*, **230,** 324 (1957).

506. D. W. Singerland, *J. Clin. Endocrinol. Metab.*, **17,** 82 (1957).

507. D. Pitre and L. Fumagalli, *Chim. Ther.*, **5** : 3, 185 (1970).

508. E. B. Astwood, *Trans. Ass. Am. Physicians* (Philadelphia), **70,** 183 (1957).

509. G. H. Mudge, G. J. Strewler, Jr., N. Desbiens, W. O. Berndt, and D. N. Wade, *J. Pharmacol. Exp. Ther.*, **178,** 159 (1971).

510. D. N. Wade, N. Desbiens, G. J. Strewler, Jr., W. O. Berndt, and G. H. Mudge, *J. Pharmacol. Exp. Ther.*, **178,** 173 (1971).

511. I. Bornschein, H. H. Borchert, and S. Pfeifer, *Pharmazie*, **29,** 730 (1974).

512. H. Langecker, A. Harwart, and K. Junkmann, *Arch. Exp. Pathol. Pharmakol.*, **220,** 195 (1953).

513. E. Clerc, *Aertzl. Wochenschr.*, **10,** 1156 (1955).

514. B. H. Billing, O. Maggiore, and M. A. Cartter, *Ann. N.Y. Acad. Sci.*, **111,** 319 (1963).

515. H. Langecker, A. Harwart, K. H. Kolb, and M. Kramer, *Arch. Exp. Pathol. Pharmakol.*, **247,** 493 (1964).

516. H. S. Strickler, E. L. Saier, E. Kelvington, J. Kempic, E. Campbell, and R. C. Graver, *J. Clin. Endocrinol. Metab.*, **24,** 15 (1964).

517. W. Mutzel, V. Taenzer, and R. Wolf, *Invest. Radiol.*, **11,** 598 (1976).

518. D. Pitre and E. Felder, *Farm. Ed. Sci.*, **29,** 793 (1974).

519. R. Barke, *Radiol. Diagn. Berlin*, **5,** 193 (1964).

520. W. M. Barker, D. J. Thompson, and J. H. Ware, *Fed. Proc. Fed. Am. Soc. Exp. Biol.*, **26,** 568 (1967).

521. P. Moy and A. G. Ebert, *Fed. Proc. Fed. Am. Soc. Exp. Biol.*, **26,** 567 (1967).

522. W. H. Gutenmann, C. A. Bache, and D. J. Lisk, *J. Agric. Food Chem.*, **15,** 600 (1967).

523. W. T. Salter, G. Karandikar, and P. Block, *J. Clin. Endocrinol.*, **9,** 1080 (1949).

524. D. W. Slingerland, *J. Clin. Endocrinol. Metab.*, **17,** 82 (1957).

525. R. Barke, *Radiol. Diagn. Berlin*, **6,** 197 (1965).

526. R. H. Jarboe, J. B. Data, and J. E. Christian, *J. Pharm. Sci.*, **57,** 323 (1968).

527. H. Billion, W. Frommhold, K. Oeff, and W. Shutz, *Ärtzl. Wochenschr.*, **10,** 574 (1955).

528. K. Oeff, W. Frommhold, F. A. Pezold, and O. Schuchter, *Klin. Wochenschr.*, **31,** 123 (1953).

529. K. H. Kimbel, W. Börner, and E. Heise, *Fortschr. Geb. Roentgenstr.*, **83,** (1955).

530. H. Billion and W. Schlungbaum, *Klin. Wochenschr.*, **33,** 1089 (1955).

531. H. S. Ogden and G. E. Sheline, *J. Lab. Clin. Med.*, **54,** 53 (1959).

532. J. J. Jankowski, M. Feingold, and S. S. Gellis, *J. Pediatr.*, **70,** 436 (1967).

533. R. L. Himsworth, M. Fischer, and M. J. Denham, *Brit. Med. J.*, **4,** 162 (C) (1975).

534. A. M. Silas and A. G. White, *Brit. Med. J.*, **4,** 162 C (1975).

535. R. Aquaron, *Clin. Chim. Acta*, **41,** 175 (1972).

536. J. R. Benton and G. H. Wilson, *Invest. Radiol.*, **11,** 602 (1976).

537. T. Almén, *Acta Radiol. Suppl.*, **335,** 216 (1973).

538. C. A. Evill and G. T. Benness, *Invest. Radiol.*, **11,** 459 (1976).

539. E. A. Graham, W. H. Cole, and G. H. Copher, *J. Am. Med. Assoc.*, **82,** 1777 (1924).

540. M. Dohrn and P. Diedrich, *Deut. Med. Wochenschr.*, **66,** 1133 (1940).

541. S. J. Archer, J. O. Hoppe, and T. R. Lewis, *J. Am. Pharm. Assoc.*, **40,** 617 (1951).

542. S. Y. Han and D. M. Witten, *Radiology*, **112,** 529 (1974).

543. M. Oliphant, J. P. Whalen, and J. A. Evans, *Radiology*, **112,** 531 (1974).

544. J. G. Russell and P. R. Frederick, *Radiology*, **112,** 519 (1974).

545. R. E. Parks, *Radiology*, **112,** 525 (1974).

546. M. L. Janower and M. A. Hannon, *Radiology*, **118,** 301 (1976).

547. S. Arnell and F. Lidström, *Acta Radiol.*, **12,** 287 (1931).

548. C. S. Kulik and A. O. Hampton, *New Engl. J. Med.*, **224,** 455 (1941).

549. G. H. Ramsey, J. D. French, and W. H. Strain, *Radiology*, **43,** 236 (1944).

550. J. K. Jakobsen, *Acta Radiol. Diagn.*, **14,** 638 (1973).

551. P. Ahlgren, *Acta Radiol.*, **13,** 753 (1972).

552. I. O. Skalpe, *Acta Radiol. Suppl.*, **335,** 57 (1973).

553. T. Hindmarsh, *Acta Radiol. Diagn.*, **16,** 417 (1975).

554. G. T. Benness, *Clin. Radiol.*, **21,** 157 (1970).

555. C. A. Evill and G. T. Benness, *Invest. Radiol.*, **10,** 552 (1975).

556. D. M. Long, M. S. Liu, P. S. Szanto, D. P. Alrenga, M. M. Patel, M. V. Rios, and L. M. Nyhus, *Radiology*, **105,** 323 (1972).

557. D. M. Long, M. S. Liu, P. S. Szanto, and P. Alrenga, *Rev. Surg.*, **29,** 71 (1972).

558. M. S. Liu and D. M. Long, *Invest. Radiol.*, **9,** 479 (1974).

559. M. S. Liu and D. M. Long, *Invest. Radiol.*, **11,** 479 (1976).

CHAPTER SIXTY TWO

Nonsteroidal Anti-inflammatory Agents

T. Y. SHEN

Merck Sharp & Dohme Research Laboratories
Rahway, New Jersey 07065, USA

CONTENTS

1   INTRODUCTION

Inflammation is a host defense mechanism in response to various infections or metabolic stimuli. The cardinal manifestations of inflammation were well recognized in early civilization and described by Celsus in the first century AD as *calor* (heat), *rubor* (redness), *tumor* (swelling), and *dolor* (pain). Loss of function, more critical in our industrious life, is also emphasized by contemporary researchers.

In biochemical and pharmaceutical terms, the complexity and dynamics of the inflammatory process may be analyzed in several ways: acute versus chronic, immunologic versus nonimmunologic, and cellular versus humoral aspects.

Briefly, the sequence of early events in inflammation may be summarized as follows:

1. Initial injury, release of inflammatory mediators.

2. Vasodilation.

3. Increased vascular permeability, exudation.

4. Leukocyte emigration, chemotaxis, and phagocytosis of the stimulus.

These are followed by either resolution and healing or, in case of persistent stimulation, chronic and degenerative inflammation.

An operational scheme of the generation and function of various humoral factors involved in inflammation is outlined in Fig. 62.1. Four principal and interacting cascades are the complement system, plasmin system, clotting system (kinins), and the emerging arachidonic acid cascade (e.g., prostaglandins) (1). Various metabolites or factors derived from these cascades serve to amplify or regulate vascular permeability, cellular infiltration, and tissue injury. Vasoactive amines (histamine and serotonin), lysosomal hydrolases, and mediators elaborated from the activated lymphocytes (lymphokines) and other monocytes are also involved.

The principal cellular events involved in both immune and nonimmune inflammations are shown in Fig. 62.2.

The three-way interaction of macrophages, subsets of T-lymphocytes (e.g., T suppressors, helpers, killers), and B-lymphocytes constitutes another dynamic system, which is mainly responsible for the pathological consequences in rheumatoid arthritis and other immunologic inflammatory diseases.

The superposition of these cellular and humoral events produces inflammation, pain, and tissue destruction in a variety of diseases. Among them, a family of arthritis disorders, which affect *ca.* 7% of the total population, is by far the most important area of drug application (2). The annual United States market for antiarthritic drugs, $0.3 billion in 1978, is expected to double by 1981. A group of nonsteroid anti-inflammatory–analgesic drugs de-

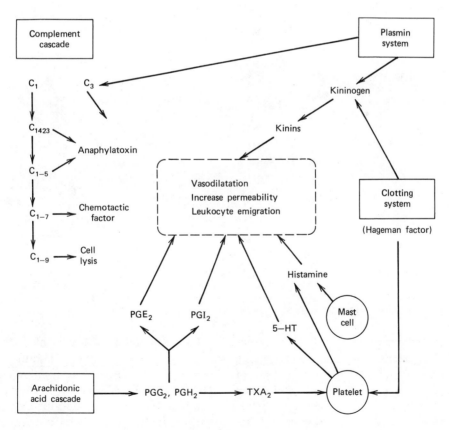

Fig. 62.1 Humoral factors in acute inflammation.

Acute Inflammation

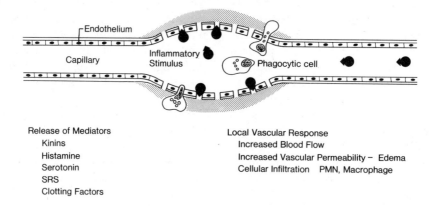

Release of Mediators
    Kinins
    Histamine
    Serotonin
    SRS
    Clotting Factors

Local Vascular Response
    Increased Blood Flow
    Increased Vascular Permeability – Edema
    Cellular Infiltration   PMN, Macrophage

Immune Inflammation

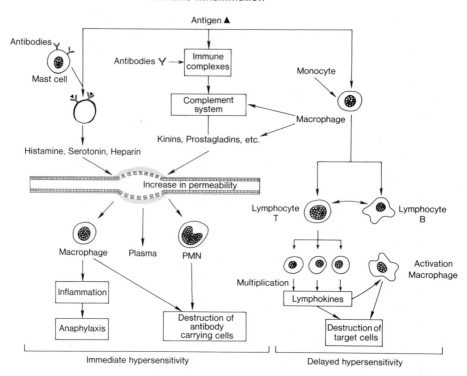

Fig. 62.2   Cellular events in acute and immune inflammation.

scribed below can provide only symptomatic relief by suppressing one or more key processes in inflammation. Ideally, of course, if the etiologic event or agent of the disease can be identified, one may hope to achieve more fundamental therapeutic actions. However, although many biochemical and immunologic aspects of arthritis are steadily being unraveled, identification of the most critical or rate-limiting ones as therapeutic targets remain elusive. The continued search for superior anti-inflammatory drugs still proceeds in a semiempirical, yet highly productive manner. As in the past, the interplay of clinical observations, immunopharmacological models, and new drugs, both as therapeutic agents and as research tools, will continue to bring forth breakthroughs in this field.

Synthetic aspirin was introduced nearly 100 years ago. In recent decades, there has been a steady progression of active compounds, from the pyrazolones in the 1940s, through corticosteroids in the 1950s, to a new family of "nonsteroidal" anti-inflammatory drugs (NSAIDS) developed in the 1960s. In the present decade, many new members of the aryl acidic family have emerged from various laboratories. Furthermore, reexamination of a group of slow-acting antirheumatic drugs (SAARDS), discovered previously in the clinic, has been stimulated by the current interest in immunopharmacological agents. Thus after two decades of NSAID development, anti-inflammatory research is in a transition state, exploring new directions for the next generation of antiarthritic agents.

The intensive worldwide effort in arthritic research is evidenced by a voluminous scientific literature. More than 35 journals are devoted to rheumatology and inflammation research. Periodic reviews, numerous monographs and proceedings of international meetings, and hundreds of patents on anti-inflammatory agents are in print (2–18). As convenient and comprehensive references, the following publications are particularly valuable: *Primer on the Rheumatic Diseases* (1973) (2), *Anti-inflammatory Agents* (1974) (3), *Inflammation* (1978) (4), and *Anti-inflammatory Drugs* (1978) (5). Among primary sources pertinent to medicinal chemical interests in arthritis research the following journals are commonly referred to: *Arthritis and Rheumatism, Agents and Actions, Prostaglandins, Prostaglandins and Medicine, Journal of Medicinal Chemistry, Biochemical Pharmacology*, and a new journal, *European Journal of Rheumatology and Inflammation*.

In the following sections a brief discussion of the pathogenesis of clinical diseases, current laboratory models, properties of many categories of anti-inflammatory agents, and possible future trends are presented. Because of the extensive literature on this subject, only some highlights and typical examples, often arbitrarily chosen, are included to illustrate various medicinal chemical aspects of anti-inflammatory research. Some comments on prostaglandins, immunoregulants, and uricosuric agents pertaining to anti-inflammatory therapy are included here, but readers should refer to other chapters on these topics in Part I and II for more information.

2 INFLAMMATORY DISEASES

Since the principal application of anti-inflammatory agents is in the realm of rheumatic diseases, a brief survey of clinical classifications, pathogenesis concepts, and biochemical mechanisms related to arthritic disorders is given below. Other inflammatory diseases, e.g., dermatitis, periodontitis, uveitis, and several prostaglandin-related symptoms are summarized in Section 11.

2.1 Clinical Classifications

Rheumatic diseases are comprised of a large family of clinical syndromes with a common involvement of the joints, chiefly the synovial joints, and/or para-articular structures. An estimated 16 million people in the United States are suffering from "arthritis." The prevalence in persons between 45 and 64 years old is more than 15%. The major rheumatic diseases are rheumatoid arthritis, osteoarthritis, ankylosing spondylitis (Bechterew's syndrome), gout, and systemic lupus erythematosus. In a broad survey, the Arthritis Foundation has classified more than 80 rheumatic diseases into 13 categories (2). Recent analysis indicates that heredity may predispose to most inflammatory rheumatic diseases and also determine the age of onset, sex ratio, and some clinical features (19).

2.2 Pathogenesis Concepts

If we treat inflammation as a host defense mechanism, the inflammatory response would normally produce a resolution of the stimulating event and be self-limiting. However, under conditions favoring a persistent or self-generating stimulus, the ensuing chronic inflammation may lead to metabolic derangement and tissue degeneration. Several pathogenesis concepts have been postulated, describing possible mechanisms which underlie the chronicity or vicious circle of rheumatic diseases, with

varying degrees of immunologic and metabolic characteristics.

2.2.1 GOUT. The primary event in acute gouty arthritis (20) is the local deposition of crystalline monosodium urate hydrate. Ingestion of the crystals by neutrophilic leukocytes leads to activation and release of lysosomal enzymes. The negatively charged urate crystals also activate complement and Hageman factor. The latter initiates the clotting mechanism and the kinin cascade (see Fig. 62.3) resulting in pain, increase of vascular permeability, and accumulation of leukocytes.

The recognition of this pathogenesis process has provided a rational basis in the treatment of gout. Allopurinol (62.**1**), a xanthine oxidase inhibitor, reduces the biosynthesis of uric acid from hypoxanthine and guanine. The uricosuric probenecid

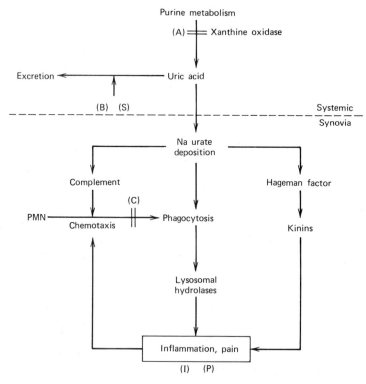

Fig. 62.3 Pathogenesis of gout. Inhibition by (A) allopurinol, (B) probenecid, (S) sulfinpyrazone, (C) colchicine, (I) indomethacin, (P) phenylbutazone.

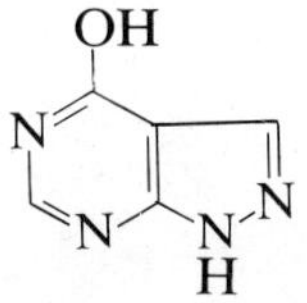

62.**1**   Allopurinol

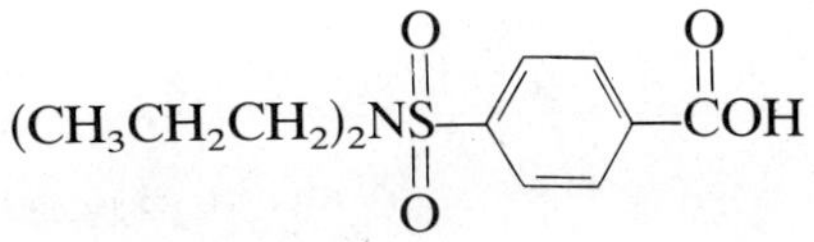

62.**2**   Probenecid

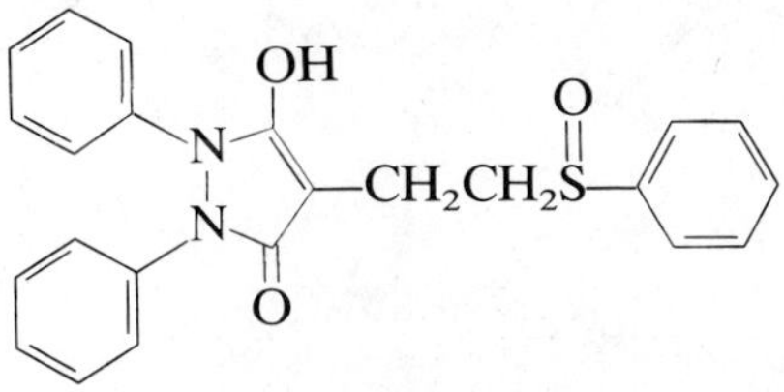

62.**3**   Sulfinpyrazone

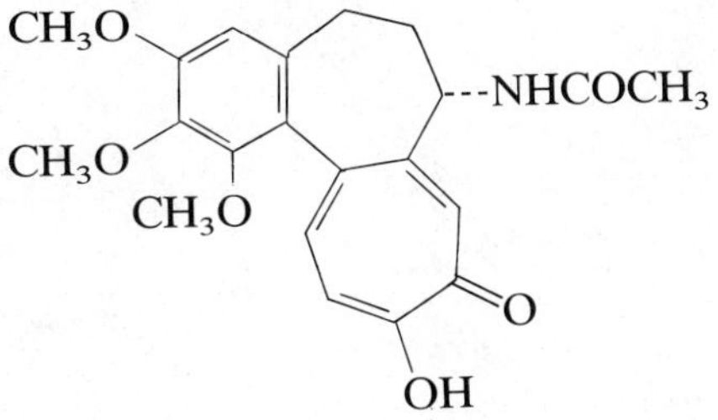

62.**4**   Colchicine

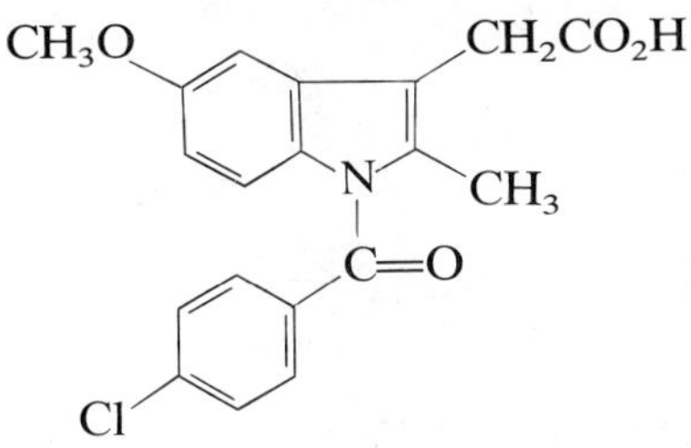

62.**5**   Indomethacin

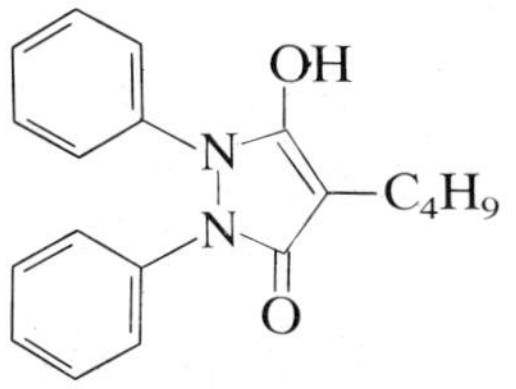

62.**6**   Phenylbutazone

(62.**2**) and sulfinpyrazone (62.**3**) promote the excretion of uric acid. The microtubule inhibitor colchicine (62.**4**) inhibits the chemotactic response of PMN. Anti-inflammatory drugs indomethacin (62.**5**) and phenylbutazone (62.**6**) are also very effective in relieving acute gouty attacks.

2.2.2   RHEUMATOID ARTHRITIS.   The etiology of rheumatoid arthritis is still not clear. Recent attempts to isolate infectious microorganisms, e.g., streptococci, mycoplasma (PPLO), and viruses, from rheumatoid joints have been inconclusive (21, 22). Some viruses are known to produce transient diseases (e.g., rubella infection) (23) and other chronic degenerative diseases (e.g., Aleutian mink disease). The association of rheumatoid arthritis with major histocompatibility antigens, e.g., D-4, sug-

gests that genetic disposition may also be contributory (24).

Immunologic reactions appear to play a major role in the perpetuation of rheumatoid inflammations (25). Clinical evidence supporting this concept follows:

1. Extensive infiltration and proliferation of lymphocytes in the synovium.
2. Active local synthesis of IgG and rheumatoid factor (RF).
3. Presence of antigen–antibody complexes in synovial fluids and leukocytes ("R.A. cells").

A pathogenesis cycle evolved from these observations is shown in Fig. 62.4. Following an unknown initiating factor, the production of abnormal and antigenic IgG

Pathogenesis Cycle of Rheumatoid Arthritis

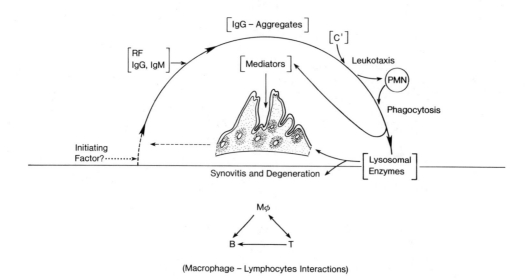

Fig. 62.4   Pathogenesis cycle of rheumatoid arthritis.

stimulates the synthesis of rheumatoid factors (IgM and IgG) and forms immune complexes, IgG aggregates. Activation of the complement system leads to the generation of chemotactic factors which attract polymorphonuclear leukocytes (PMN) into the articular cavity. PMNs are phagocytic cells which ingest the immune complexes to become "R.A. cells" and then discharge a variety of hydrolases from their lysosomal granules. These enzymes degrade extracellular tissue components, polysac-

charides, and collagens in the cartilage matrix, and also provoke an acute and proliferative inflammatory response in rheumatoid joints.

In chronic inflammation, macrophages, following PMNs, are believed to play a dominant role in joint degradation (Fig. 62.5).

To interrupt this vicious cycle, the ideal solution for removing the initiating factor or terminating the production of antigenic IgG is still being pursued. Drug interven-

Cartilage Destruction

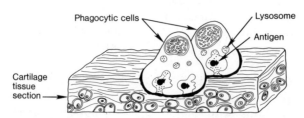

Fig. 62.5   Cartilage destruction.

tion at other sites in the cycle may also slow down the progression of the disease. The antirheumatic action of gold preparations (see Section 7.1 below) and chloroquine (see Section 7.2) are examples. Because prostaglandins are involved in various inflammatory and immunologic processes (see Section 2.3 below), inhibitors of prostaglandin synthesis may also moderate the clinical syndromes.

2.2.3 SYSTEMIC LUPUS ERYTHEMATOSUS. Systemic lupus erythematosus (SLE) is also a chronic inflammatory disease of unknown origin. It may affect many different organs with diverse manifestations, including fever, erythematosus rash, renal, neurological, and cardiac abnormalities. The pathogenesis of SLE probably starts with an immunologic abnormality, possibly of viral origin. The production of anti-DNA and antiribosomal antibodies leads to formation of immune complexes and complement fixation. The deposition of immune complexes in vessel walls and the basement membrane of glomeruli initiates a sequence of local inflammatory reactions analogous to those seen in the rheumatoid synovium: neutrophil infiltration, phagocytosis of immune complexes, release of lysosomal enzymes, and damage of basement membrane. Familial factors have also been implicated in pathogenesis.

2.2.4 OSTEOARTHRITIS. Osteoarthritis is an extremely common degenerative joint disease with a low degree of inflammation. It is characterized by progressive deterioration of articular cartilage and abnormal bony formation in the joint. Earlier histological studies and recent biochemical analysis have identified several possible pathogenic factors. Microcrystalline hydroxyapatite from faulty bone metabolism is an inflammatory substance (26). Lysosomal hydrolases are discharged by leukocytes and chondrocytes at the base of articular cartilage. Altered metabolic activities of chondrocytes, e.g., DNA repli-

cation and proteoglycan biosynthesis, are indicated by an initial increase in the repair phase of cartilage, followed by a marked decline. Finally the defective repair mechanism is overwhelmed by the degradative process leading to joint destruction. An imbalance of nutritional factors (e.g., vitamin D and calcitonin) and bone metabolism also contributes to the chronic degenerative disease. Much progress has been made in elucidating the structure and biochemical properties of connective tissue in recent years (27). Several surgically induced or genetically prone animal models are available (28–30).

3 LABORATORY MODELS AND BIOCHEMICAL ASSAYS

There is no single test *in vitro* or *in vivo* that correlates well with the complex clinical manifestations of arthritic diseases. The relative potency of different drugs, even with similar chemical structures, often varies in different assays. Some of the assays described below will become obsolete within a few years because of the rapid succession of new findings about arthritic diseases. Evaluation of the long-term efficacy of compounds in chronic degenerative models, which currently requires extensive time and effort, must be made more efficient. The need for new valid and reliable assays to bridge and gap between current concepts of arthritis and the realities of drug development in the laboratory is obvious.

New models are essential for discovering antiarthritic agents more effective than current anti-inflammatory–analgesic drugs, which provide mainly symptomatic relief. It is of interest to note that major advances in arthritis therapy were mostly made in the clinic through serendipity or medical reasoning. These clinical leads, aspirin, phenylbutazone, corticosteroids, gold, antimalarials, D-penicillamine, and levamisole, each in turn stimulated the further development of new laboratory models to mimic their clinical properties and, as hoped, to discover improved analogs. The recent endeavor in many laboratories to fashion new immunopharmacological assays for finding drugs with "antirheumatic action" like D-penicillamine is an example.

Detailed compilations of numerous *in vitro* and *in vivo* assays are given in Refs. 4 and 31. Some of the more commonly used models and some recently developed assays are outlined below.

3.1 Biochemical Assays *in Vitro*

Many *in vitro* assays, each based on a specific biochemical or cellular mechanism,

have been developed for the initial screening of anti-inflammatory compounds. These are listed in Table 62.1. Some of the earlier proposals turned out to be relatively nonspecific, with poor overall correlation with *in vivo* anti-inflammatory activity. In recent years, biochemical approaches based on the regulation of the arachidonic cascade and leukocyte functions have received greater attention.

3.1.1 THE ARACHIDONIC ACID CASCADE (Fig. 62.6). The inhibition of prostaglandin biosynthesis at the cyclooxygenase site became a popular *in vitro* approach to discover novel anti-inflammatory structures following Vane's observation that this is a plausible mechanism for the anti-inflammatory action of aspirin and indomethacin

Table 62.1   *In Vitro* Anti-Inflammatory Assays

  I. Earlier proposals
      Uncoupling oxidative phosphorylation
      Inhibition of protein denaturation
      Stabilization of erythrocyte membrane or isolated lysosome
      Acceleration of sulfhydryl exchange
      Fibrinolysis
      Inhibition of platelet aggregation
      Inhibition of mixed lymphocyte reaction
      Inhibition of chemotaxis (Boyden chamber)
      Complement inhibition
 II. Regulation of arachidonic acid cascade
      Inhibition of membrane phospholipase
      Inhibition of cyclooxygenase
      Inhibition of thromboxane synthetase
      Inhibition of lipoxygenase
      Neutralization of oxygen radicals ($\cdot[O_2^-]$, $\cdot[OH]$)
III. Regulation of leukocyte functions
      Inhibition of macrophage
          Phagocytosis
          Release of lysosomal hydrolases and prostaglandins
      Inhibition of leukocyte
          Chemotaxis
          Adherence
IV. Inhibition of tissue degeneration
      Inhibition of proteases
          Neutral proteases, elastase, cathepsin G
          Collagenase
          Cathepsin D
      Inhibition of the release of lysomal hydrolases

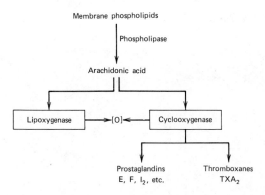

Fig. 62.6 Two major pathways of arachidonic acid cascade.

(32). Prostaglandins potentiate the early inflammatory response, causing vasodilation, increasing permeability, facilitating cellular infiltration, and sensitizing the pain receptor to bradykinin. PGE$_2$ (62.**7**) and PGI$_2$ (62.**8**) are particularly pro-inflammatory (33). Thromboxane A$_2$ (62.**9**) is a potent platelet aggregating agent and

62.**7** PGE$_2$

62.**8** PGI$_2$

62.**9** Thromboxane A$_2$

vasoconstrictor (34). In chronic inflammation, PGEs accumulate at inflamed sites and may play a homeostatic function by inhibiting lymphocyte activation and exerting a negative feedback control mechanism (35). Various prostaglandins and their differential effects on the cellular levels of cyclic AMP and cyclic GMP influence many vascular and tissue responses in a complex and dynamic manner (36). *In vivo*, the net effect of cyclooxygenase inhibitors is mainly anti-inflammatory. Their peripheral, as opposed to central, analgesic action may be attributed to the blockade of hypersensitization of the pain receptor by prostaglandins (37) (Fig. 62.7). However, because some side effects of these drugs, e.g., gastrointestinal and renal toxicities, are also associated with the nonspecific reduction of all prostaglandins controlled by cyclooxygenase, several alternative sites of inhibition have been considered (38). The suppression of thromboxane synthesis is one possible approach to more selective action. The lipoxygenase pathway also provides metabolites that are chemotactic, vasoactive, and platelet-aggregating factors. To achieve greater anti-inflammatory potency, the blockade of the release of arachidonic acid from its membrane-associated esters, thus inhibiting both the cyclooxygenase and lipoxygenase pathways, is another direction (39, 40).

3.1.2 LEUKOCYTE FUNCTIONS. Improved assay procedures to measure the inhibition of chemotaxis (40), adherence (42), and infiltration of leukocytes are continually being developed. With the growing interest in the pivotal roles of macrophages in inflammation, the inhibition of macrophage migration, phagocytosis, and the release of lysosomal hydrolases and prostaglandins have been investigated (43–45).

3.1.3 PROTEASES (46, 47). Proteases, particularly those functioning optimally at near neutral pH, are intimately involved in the initiating events, cellular recruitment, and degenerative aspects of inflammation. The

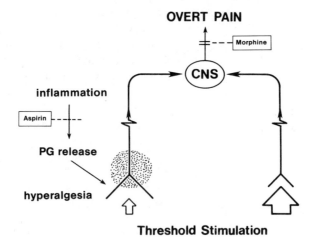

Fig. 62.7 Potentiation of pain receptor by prostaglandins and its blockade by cyclooxygenase inhibitors.

activation and propagation of inflammatory cascades, the complement, kinins, and plasmin system require proteolytic cleavage. Synovial cells, PMN, and macrophage are major sources of elastase, cathepsin G, collagenase, and plasminogen activator. Plasmin generated from plasminogen in turn activates latent collagenases in rheumatoid synovia. Selective modulation of propagating proteolytic activities in the joint is obviously desirable. The cooperative actions of various proteases are indicated by the nature of their substrates listed in Table 62.2. Cartilage preparations and acute inflammatory models, e.g., urate synovitis, UV or croton oil topical inflammation, have been used to evaluate the efficacy of *in vitro*

enzyme inhibitors. Many potent *in vitro* inhibitors of various proteases have been described (46). However, information about their *in vivo* anti-inflammatory and antidegenerative activities and potential systemic side effects, especially after chronic oral administration, is still insufficient to determine their antiarthritic applications.

3.2 *In Vivo* Models

Many *in vivo* inflammatory and immunologic models have been established (31, 48). Most of these involve nonspecific acute or semichronic responses to a variety

Table 62.2 Substrates of Neutral Proteases

Substrate	Enzyme		
	Collagenase	Cathepsin G	Elastase
Collagen	+	+	+
Proteoglycan		+	+
Elastin, basement membrane			+
Kininogen, complement C_5			+

Table 62.3   Commonly Used Anti-Inflammatory Models

Model	Species	Predominant Response	Time of Measurement
1. Carrageenin-induced paw edema	Rat	Exudation of fluid and leukocytes	3 hr
2. UV erythema	Guinea pig	Vascular dilatation and permeability	2–4 hr
3. Peritoneal and pleural irritation (carrageenin, Ca pyrophosphate)	Rat, guinea pig	Exudation of proteins mediators and cells	
4. Cotton pellet	Rat	Fibroblast proliferation, connective tissue repair	7 days
5. Adjuvant arthritis	Rat	Disseminated, immunologic, chronic polyarthritis	21 days or later
6. Urate crystal induced synovitis	Dog	Acute pain, loss of function	

of inflammatory stimuli (see Table 62.3). Some are particularly pertinent to specific applications such as urate crystal-induced synovitis (gout) and ocular and topical inflammation. Peripheral analgesic assays and antipyretic assays are useful in defining the overall pharmacological profile of active compounds (Table 62.4). Because gastrointestinal irritation is the most common side effect of anti-inflammatory drugs, a few acute models, in spite of their limited value in predicting long-term GI tolerance in man, are generally used. Different profiles of several current antiarthritic drugs are illustrated in Table 62.5 and Fig. 62.8.

Immunological assays, such as those listed in Table 25.1 in Chapter 25, are also useful in defining the immunoregulatory activities of antirheumatic agents.

Among the most commonly used primary and secondary *in vivo* assays are the following: similar experiments in adrenalectomized rats are often used to indicate that the anti-inflammatory effect of a "nonsteroidal" agent is not mediated by activation of the pituitary–adrenal system.

3.2.1 CARRAGEENIN-INDUCED PAW EDEMA IN RATS. A widely used technique in the development of NSAIDS is to measure

Table 62.4   Ancillary Tests for Anti-Inflammatory Agents

Method	Species	Response
1. Yeast-induced fever	Rat	Pyresis
2. Randall–Selitto	Rat	Pain threshold of inflamed paw
3. Peripheral analgesic assays (phenylquinone, acetylcholine, acetic acid, etc.)	Mouse	Abdominal constriction response induced by nociceptive agents
4. Gastric hemorrhage	Rat	Gastric irritation
5. Intestinal perforation	Rat	Ulcerogenic potential

Table 62.5　Pharmacological Profiles of Aspirin and Other NSAIDS—ED_{50} in mg/kg Given by Oral Route

Model	Aspirin	Diflunisal	Indomethacin
Analgesic to yeast-induced inflammation (rat)	87	4.6	2.2
Pain in dog knee joint	68	24	1.7
Antipyretic (rat)	40	27.8	1.8
Carrageenin-induced foot inflammation (rat)	89	9.8	2.7
Adjuvant arthritis (rat)	78	10.4	0.27
PG synthetase inhibition, μg/ml	13	0.6	0.1
Intestinal perforating ulcers (rat)	None at 1024	520	5.2
Gastric hemorrhage (rat)	81	None at 256	5.4

their ability to inhibit edema produced in the hind paw of the rat by injection of a phlogistic agent (49). Carrageenin, a sulfated mucopolysaccharide derived from Irish sea moss, *Chondrus*, was found to be a phlogistic agent of choice over others, e.g., brewer's yeast, formalin, dextran, and egg albumin, used previously.

The time course of developing edema is biphasic (50). The first phase is attributable to the release of histamine, serotonin, and kinins in the first hour after injection of

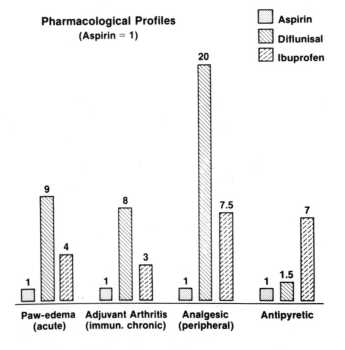

Fig. 62.8　Pharmacological profiles (aspirin = 1).

carrageenin. A more pronounced second phase is related to the release of prostaglandin-like substances in 2–3 hr. Leukocyte emigration also plays an important role in this model. Most NSAIDS have been found to be effective in this assay, with ED_{50} ranging from 1 to 100 mg/kg p.o. The dose–response relationship and reproducibility are generally satisfactory. The potency ceiling of most compounds ($\leqslant 70\%$ inhibition of foot volume increase) is imposed by their ability to inhibit the second prostaglandin phase only.

3.2.2   PERITONEAL AND PLEURAL IRRITATION.

Various irritants (carrageenin, bradykinin, calcium pyrophosphate, etc.) produce acute inflammation when placed in the pleural or peritoneal cavities of rats or guinea pigs (26, 50–52). The volume and contents of the exudate, such as polymorphonuclear leukocytes, monocytes, protein, histamine, prostaglandins, and other mediators, can easily be determined at different stages of the inflammatory process. Artificial cavities can also be produced in rats by the subcutaneous implantation of polyvinyl sponges in the abdominal region. Carrageenin-induced pleurisy in rats is responsive to inhibition by both steroidal and nonsteroidal anti-inflammatory drugs. Various versions of this model allow quantitations of the anti-inflammatory activity and are particularly versatile in mechanism of action studies.

3.2.3   GRANULOMA FORMATION.

The classical granuloma assay was developed initially to measure the anti-inflammatory effect of corticosteroids; it was later found to respond to NSAIDS like indomethacin analogs as well (53). Two sterilized cotton pellets are implanted beneath the abdominal skin of the rat through a single incision down the linea alba. In response to this persistent irritant, macrophages, tissue histocytes, and blood leukocytes migrate to the site of implantation, leading to the formation of fibrin strands and granulation tissue. Test compounds are given orally once daily from day 0 through day 6. On day 7, the rats are sacrificed and the increased weight of dried pellets is used to estimate the inhibitory effect of the compound. For most NSAIDS, the ceiling of the inhibition is around 25% with a flat dose-response curve. The body weight gain and the weight of thymus and adrenals of test animals are used to indicate any nonspecific toxicity or adrenal stimulation, which may also decrease the granuloma formation.

Some modifications of this assay have been made recently (48).

3.2.4   ADJUVANT-INDUCED ARTHRITIS.

Adjuvant arthritis in susceptible strains of rats has been extensively used as a model of chronic inflammation simulating rheumatoid arthritis (31, 48). This experimental disorder is induced by subcutaneous injection of Freund's complete adjuvant, which is a suspension of heat-killed *Mycobacterium butyricum* in mineral oil, in either the tail or the paw. Cell wall components and oligomeric muramyl dipeptide derivatives may also be used as better defined arthritogens. A localized primary inflammatory response at the injection site is followed by a disseminated immunologic disease which develops from day 7 to 26. The systemic disease is characterized by the swelling of the contralateral noninjected limb, local hyperpyrexia, nodules on the ears and tail, and multiple joint lesions. Various hematologic parameters, such as elevations of lysosomal enzymes and changes of serum proteins, have been observed in arthritic rats.

In assessing the efficacy of test compound on the severity of the disease on day 14 or later, three different dosing schedules have been used:

1. Preventive protocol: daily oral dosing on day $-1, 0, +1$ with readout on day 14–21, to inhibit the early immunologic events.

2. Regular protocol: daily oral dosing on day $-1, 0$, through day 13, to inhibit the development of the disease.

3. Therapeutic protocol: daily oral dosing on day 21 or later after the disease has fully developed, to reduce the severity of an established disease.

As expected, immunosuppressives are active in the preventive protocol whereas most NSAIDS are more effective in the regular protocol. Agents active in the therapeutic protocol may have greater efficacy in treating established rheumatoid arthritis in the clinic.

Induction of acute and chronic arthritis by various bacterial cell walls and their water-soluble peptidoglycan components (54), by preformed collagen–anticollagen complexes (55), and by a variety of other antigens (56, 57), has also been described.

3.2.5 CRYSTAL DEPOSIT SYNOVITIS. Injection of a suspension of microcrystalline sodium urate into one hind knee joint of a dog induces an acute painful synovitis similar to gout (58). The anti-inflammatory and analgesic effects of test compounds can be measured by the weight avoidance of the injected leg. This assay is more variable than rat models but does involve a nonrodent species in the preclinical evaluation of potential drug candidates.

Other inorganic crystals such as calcium pyrophosphate (59) and hydroxyapatite (51) have also been used to produce pseudogout and osteoarthritic lesions in the joint.

3.2.6 UV ERYTHEMA IN GUINEA PIGS. Inhibition of the erythema of depilated guinea pig skin after exposure to ultraviolet irradiation (60 sec) is a useful method for assessing topical and systemic anti-inflammatory drug activities (31).

Following irradiation, the initial increase in vascular permeability, inhibitable by antihistamines, is followed by leukocyte emigration into the site and development of erythema, which reaches maximum intensity in 2–4 hr. At 12–20 hr the second phase of increased vascular permeability and accumulation of polymorphonuclear leukocytes at injured sites reaches its maximum. The erythemas are scored subjectively at 2–4 hr on a blind basis. It is more variable and cumbersome than the rat paw edema methods, but has been used satisfactorily in some laboratories.

As a topical assay, the skin penetration of the compound being tested varies greatly with the solvent or pharmaceutical vehicles used in the application. Care should be taken in comparing the relative potency of compounds with different physical characteristics.

3.2.7 YEAST FEVER. As an antipyretic assay, rats are injected subcutaneously with a suspension of brewer's yeast in methylcellulose solution (31). A rise in rectal temperature of about 2°C or more occurs and persists for more than 24 hr. At 18 hr after injection, test compounds are given orally. Temperature is recorded at half-hour intervals. An ED_1 is used to indicate the dose causing 1° lowering, which is also approximately 50% alleviation of the fever. Excellent reliability has been observed.

4 CHEMICAL AND PHYSICAL PROPERTIES

A diversity of chemical structures, described in several hundred patents in the past decade alone, have been found to possess varying degrees of anti-inflammatory activities. In view of the complexity and multitude of cellular and humoral factors involved in inflammatory events, few, if any, general correlations of chemical structures and physical characteristics with biologic activities would be expected. Nevertheless, some general features seem to be commonly associated with a large number of active drugs. It should be emphasized that these generalizations are neither necessary nor sufficient, but they may reflect on certain physicochemical requirements for *in vivo* efficacy.

As described below, a large proportion of nonsteroidal anti-inflammatory–analgesic drugs are aryl acidic molecules or their metabolic precursors. Most of them have two to three aromatic or heteroaromatic rings, either fused or linear and preferably nonplanar. To this hydrophobic structure is attached an acidic function, in the form of a carboxylic or enolic group, with a pK_a ranging from 3 to 6. The presence of chlorine, fluorine, or other pseudohalogen equivalents are often activity-enhancing. Their molecular weights are in the range of 250–350 and they are slightly soluble in an aqueous medium. These drugs are generally well absorbed and are often extensively ($>95\%$) serum protein bound. There are two or more high affinity hydrophobic binding sites for these drugs per molecule of serum albumin; the ε-amino residues of lysine in albumin are likely involved in the binding of the acidic anti-inflammatory compounds. These hydrophobic and electrostatic interactions can be studied by the extrinsic Cotton effect produced in circular dichroism spectra.

For aryl propionic acids, a high degree of stereospecificity is shown by the chiral center at the α-carbon atom. Biologic activity is generally associated with the $(S)(+)$ isomer. The $(R)(-)$ isomer is either inactive or weakly active *in vivo* (60) and *in vitro* (61).

The preferred nonplanar conformation of the aryl groups was originally proposed on the basis of well-defined structure–activity relationships in the indomethacin (62) (62.**5**) and fenamate series (63) (see Section 7.2). After prostaglandin cyclooxygenase was identified as an important site of action of anti-inflammatory aryl acids, a refined "receptor contour," which readily accommodates both arachidonic acid (the substrate of cyclooxygenase) and various potent anti-inflammatory drugs, was de-

rived from X-ray projection and computer modeling (64) (Fig. 62.9). These hypothetical "receptor contours" have served as useful working models in designing new analogs.

The acidic function is not essential for either anti-inflammatory activity *in vivo* or for cyclooxygenase inhibition *in vitro*. Several nonacidic or nonfunctionalized heteroaryl structures have displayed potent activities (see Section 8 below). Conceivably the hydrophobic binding site for nonacidic inhibitors on cyclooxygenase may overlap but not necessarily be identical with that for aryl acids.

The combination of an ionic head group with a hydrophobic aryl moiety in many anti-inflammatory drugs suggests that they may interact with the bi-layer cell membranes. Physical measurements, e.g., NMR., electron spin resonance, fluorescence probes, and differential scanning calorimetry, have been used to investigate the mode of interaction of anti-inflammatory drugs with phospholipid components in liposome vesicles (65).

5 PHARMACODYNAMICS

Because most anti-inflammatory drugs are administered orally on a chronic basis and often in conjunction with other medications, the importance of pharmacodynamics to both efficacy and tolerance is well appreciated. The application of a "prodrug" concept to gain pharmacodynamic advantages has also received increasing attention recently. A brief discussion of absorption, distribution, metabolism, drug interactions, and possible manipulation of these parameters follows.

5.1 Absorption

All anti-inflammatory agents are well absorbed in the gastrointestinal tract. Peak

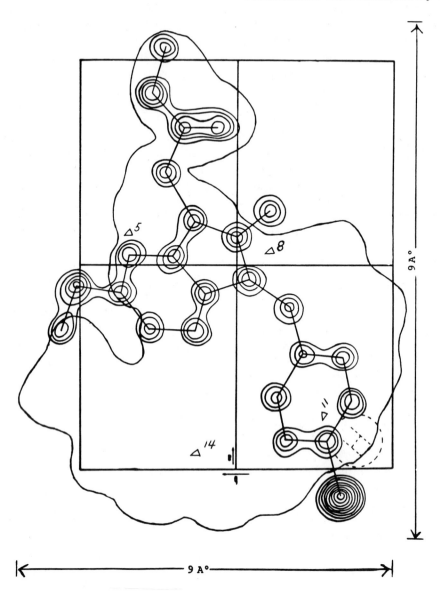

Fig. 62.9 The superposition of the X-ray projection of a noncoplanar anti-inflammatory molecule over a computer-modeled hypothetical binding site of arachidonic acid in cyclooxygenase (64). The relative positions of four double bonds △ 5, 8, 11, and 14 in arachidonic acid are indicated.

plasma levels of 1–70 μg/ml are usually reached in less than 2 hr. Slight retardation in the presence of antacids or food has been noted. Suppository formulations are also widely used in Europe and some countries abroad. On the other hand, many anti-inflammatory drugs are less effective when given topically for dermatologic or ocular inflammation. Better pharmaceutical vehicles for aryl acidic compounds in these applications are therefore needed.

To improve patient convenience and compliance, there is an increasing interest in developing drugs with a long serum half-life to support a twice or once daily schedule. Special pharmaceutical preparations such as liquid formulations and sustained-release capsules or devices are also used.

5.2 Distribution

Most anti-inflammatory drugs are extensively bound to plasma proteins and well distributed in various tissues. A two-compartment open model is generally used to describe their *in vivo* dispositions (65). The concentration in synovial fluid increases slowly after a single dose, then decreases at a rate with similar half-life to the terminal half-life in plasma. There are two interesting aspects particularly related to aryl acids.

5.2.1 SELECTIVE CONCENTRATION IN GASTRIC MUCOSA AND INFLAMED TISSUE (67–69). Aryl acids are absorbed and distributed in their un-ionized form. The degree of ionization, which contributes to local accumulation, is determined by the pK_a of the compound and the pH of the extracellular fluid. In more acidic media, such as gastric juice (pH ~ 2) and inflamed tissue (pH ≤ 6.8), the weakly acidic aryl acids predominantly assume the undissociated form and are readily absorbed. Once taken into the nearly neutral tissue compartments, aryl acids dissociate to corresponding anions and accumulate. Thus there is a tendency for anti-inflammatory aryl acids to accumulate in the parietal cells of stomach and in the

inflamed tissue. This pattern of preferential tissue distribution may contribute to the gastrointestinal irritation, as well as the efficacy, of these drugs (Fig. 62.10). Obviously a nonacidic agent will not accumulate in the gastric mucosa in the same manner. A nonacidic derivative, such as a metabolically labile ester or amide, of aryl acids presumably will also circumvent the initial localization in the gastric mucosa. However, the active acidic molecule liberated after absorption still may redistribute by systemic routes to the gastrointestinal tract. Thus only the local irritation, not the systemic ulcerogenic effect, of active aryl acids can be avoided with its derivatives.

5.2.2 ENTEROHEPATIC RECIRCULATION. Many hydrophobic aryl acids, particularly those with higher molecular weight (> 300), and their acyl glucuronide conjugates are secreted via the bile duct to the lower intestine (Fig. 62.11). The glucuronides are readily cleaved to regenerate the free acid, which is then reabsorbed. This enterohepatic recirculation increases the bioavailability of the free drug to the systemic circulation but also exposes the intestinal endothelium repeatedly to the irritation of the active drug. Indeed, at least in the case of indomethacin, a fortyfold variation of ulcerogenicity of the drug is directly proportional to the extent of enterohepatic recirculation in each of the five species, mouse, rat, guinea pig, dog, and monkey (70). The enterohepatic recirculation of indomethacin in man is not very extensive.

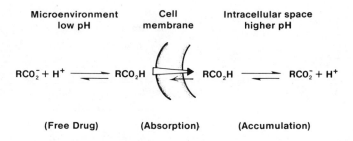

Fig. 62.10 Tissue accumulation of acidic drugs.

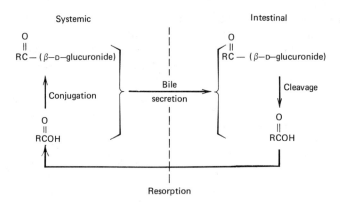

Fig. 62.11 Enterohepatic recirculation of acidic drugs.

5.3 Metabolism

With the usual daily dosage of 100 mg–3 g, most anti-inflammatory drugs are readily metabolized in the liver, kidney, intestine, or other tissues, and excreted by both the urinary and biliary routes (71). Common metabolic conversions are hydroxylation of aryl and alkyl groups, followed by glucuronide formation of carboxyl and hydroxyl groups. Oxidative O-demethylation and deacylation may also occur. Other individual reactions specific to certain chemical structures are mentioned below.

In vivo hydrolysis of ester and amide derivatives and oxidative degradation of alcohol and homologs to generate the active carboxylic acid group have been used in several cases of prodrugs.

5.4 Drug Interactions

Since anti-inflammatory drugs are often given concomitantly with other therapeutic agents, possible drug interactions are routinely investigated (72, 73).

5.4.1 DISPLACEMENT FROM PROTEIN BINDING SITES. Competitive displacement of anti-coagulants from their binding sites in serum albumin has been observed (74) with salicylates and phenylbutazone, for example, but not with indomethacin and some anti-

inflammatory drugs in spite of their high affinity for serum albumin. Obviously some structure specificity in competitive binding is involved.

5.4.2 ANTAGONISTIC PHARMACOLOGICAL ACTIONS. Varying degrees of competitive antagonism between aspirin, sodium salicylate, diflunisal, and indomethacin, for example, have been noted in cyclooxygenase inhibition *in vitro* but not in the carrageenin paw edema assay. On the other hand, a reduction of the gastrointestinal irritation of potent anti-inflammatory aryl acids *in vivo* by sodium salicylate, diflunisal, and other agents (see below), without any loss of anti-inflammatory potency, has been demonstrated in several laboratories. The nature of this apparent protection of gastrointestinal tract remains to be elucidated.

The activity of loop diuretics, furosemide and ethacrynic acid, is mediated by an increase in the level of PGE_2 in the kidney through inhibition of PGE_2 degradative enzymes, 15-hydroxy prostaglandin dehydrogenase, and 9-keto reductase. Their diuretic effect is counteracted by prostaglandin cyclooxygenase inhibitors which reduce the formation of all prostaglandins (75, 76).

A competition of two drugs at the common receptor site is another possible mechanism of drug interactions.

5.4.3 ALTERATION OF DRUG METABOLISM. Induction of the synthesis of hepatic microsomal enzymes (e.g., by salicylates) and competitive inhibition at the site of metabolizing enzymes by two similar drugs may also affect the duration and potency of antirheumatic agents.

5.4.4 COMPETITION FOR CLEARANCE MECHANISMS. A competition of organic acids for the renal anion secretory transport mechanism may also lead to a pharmacokinetic interaction of two different drugs, e.g., furosemide and indomethacin. Probenecid generally inhibits renal clearance of acidic β-lactam antibiotics and some anti-inflammatory drugs. It may also decrease biliary excretion of indomethacin. The net result is an elevation of the plasma drug level (77).

6 COMMON SIDE EFFECTS

The incidence of side effects of antiarthritic drugs often reaches 40% or higher of the patient population. Most of these are minor or transient discomforts, such as dyspepsia, headache, or dizziness. Since similar complaints are frequently made by arthritic patients on placebo treatment during double-blind controlled trials, the occurrence of these side effects may be partly related to the general indisposition of chronically ill patients. Nevertheless, several potential side effects have been commonly associated with antiarthritic therapy. In some cases of gastrointestinal and renal toxicities, the underlying mechanism may be related to the same suppression of prostaglandin synthesis involved in anti-inflammatory actions.

6.1 Gastrointestinal Irritation

Rheumatic diseases are sometimes accompanied by gastrointestinal problems, such as motility disorder, vascular lesions, and malabsorption. These conditions may be further complicated by drug therapy. In varying degrees nonsteroidal anti-inflammatory–analgesic drugs can produce gastric ulceration and hemorrhage. Aspirin in particular disrupts the gastric "mucosal barrier" against the back-diffusion of hydrogen ions into the tissues (78, 79) (Fig. 62.12). This action may be attributed to several factors, such as weakening of the mucus protective layer, damage to mucus-

FOCAL DAMAGE OF GASTRIC MUCOSAL BARRIER

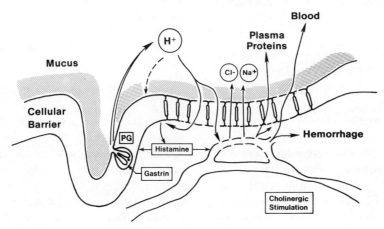

Fig. 62.12 Drug-induced back-diffusion of hydrogen ions and gastric ulceration.

secreting cells, release of histamine, and increase of capillary permeability. Recognized biochemical actions of aspirin contributing to ulceration are inhibitions of the biosynthesis of mucus glycoprotein (80) and prostaglandins. Both PGE_2 and PGI_2 regulate gastric acid secretion and maintain mucosal blood flow (81, 82). Indeed, stable analogs of PGE_2 and PGI_2 reduce the gastric irritation by NSAIDS (83). The possible correlation of physicochemical properties, e.g., lipophilicity or electronic factors, of several families of NSAIDS with their ulcerogenic activities is being analyzed (84).

Improvements in gastrointestinal tolerance have been made by several experimental approaches:

1. Synthesizing novel chemical structures with a more favorable therapeutic index of intrinsic activity/ulcerogenicity, e.g., ibuprofen and diflunisal.

2. Using metabolically labile derivatives or "prodrugs" to circumvent initial local irritation by an active drug, e.g., benorylate or sulindac.

3. Reducing enterohepatic recirculation of the active drug, e.g., the sulfide metabolite of sulindac.

4. Using a combination with other pharmacological agents, such as stable PGE analogs, acetaminophen, sodium salicylate, cimetadine (H_2-receptor inhibition), and anticholinergics, to counteract the perturbation of prostaglandin metabolism or gastric acid secretion (83).

5. Restoration of impaired mucus production is another possibility.

6.2   Renal Toxicity

As prostaglandin synthesis inhibitors, aspirin, phenylbutazone, indomethacin, and other cyclooxygenase inhibitors decrease renal blood flow and the excretion of sodium and water. This effect is more pro-

nounced in patients with impairment of renal function and is not significant in normal subjects (85).

Renal papillary edema and necrosis are commonly seen in the chronic safety assessment of anti-inflammatory–analgesic agents at higher dose levels. A narrow safety margin would restrict the chronic usage of the drug. Nephropathy in man has been observed with high dose or chronic administration of analgesics like acetaminophen (86).

6.3   Hepatic Toxicity

Since the liver is a major site of oxidative metabolism and conjugation of most anti-inflammatory agents, disorders of hepatic functions, such as a transient elevation of serum transaminase activities, are seen in some cases, especially at higher doses or with longer-acting drugs (87).

6.4   Hematologic Disorders (87)

Low incidence of agranulocytosis has long been associated with pyrazolones. Antirheumatic drugs, D-penicillamine, gold, and especially levamisole have a propensity to cause leukopenia and agranulocytosis. Indeed, bone marrow suppression is a common potential side effect of immunoregulants. Renal dysfunction, proteinuria, and skin rash are other potential side effects associated with these drugs, especially sulfhydryl or thiourea derivatives.

6.5   Cartilage Degeneration

At relatively high concentrations *in vitro*, many anti-inflammatory drugs uncouple oxidative phosphorylation and inhibit the incorporation of ^{35}S into glycosaminoglycan. The significance of these properties to their anti-inflammatory actions is uncertain, but any retardation of cartilage metabolism may have a detrimental effect in chronic joint diseases like osteoarthritis. Depression of sulfated glycosaminoglycan metabolism on human osteoarthritis cartilage by sodium salicylate and several other drugs has been observed (88). Because of the experimental difficulty of precise sampling of human cartilage and establishing basal levels of biosynthetic activities, a reliable and quantitative comparison of various drugs is still lacking.

7 ARYL ACIDIC DRUGS

In the field of therapeutics, certain chemical structural types are sometimes associated with specific pharmacological actions. Analogous to tricyclic amines in mental health and aralkylamines as antihistamines, a large group of aryl and aralkyl acids have been found in the past two decades to be nonsteroidal anti-inflammatory–analgesic drugs. Together, they are conveniently called NSAIDS. The extensive effort devoted to NSAIDS by laboratories worldwide has produced numerous clinical candidates, mostly with similar pharmacological characteristics. Since the chemical and biologic properties of these have been comprehensively reviewed in Ref. 3 in 1974, only more recent information is highlighted in this general survey. At present, more than 20 of these are already available commercially, and many others are steadily being developed in the clinic. The medical acceptance for each new NSAID as they emerge clearly indicates the need for better therapy.

The anti-inflammatory–analgesic actions of NSAIDS, however, provide only symptomatic relief of the disease. The current research interest is gradually shifting toward new approaches in the hope of achieving a more fundamental therapy. Thus the gradual phasing out of an era of NSAID research in the near future is anticipated.

7.1 Salicylic Acid Derivatives

7.1.1 ASPIRIN AND SALICYLATES. The use of salicylates for inflammatory conditions dates back to antiquity. The active ingredient in willow bark was eventually identified as salicylic acid and later synthesized in 1860. The acetylation of salicylic acid to give a less irritating O-acetyl derivative, aspirin, by Felix Hoffman in 1899, marked an early example of structure modifications in medicinal chemistry and the beginning of a long reign of aspirin as the treatment of first choice in arthritis until very recently (89).

Aspirin is readily absorbed and deacetylated *in vivo* to salicylic acid. Both aspirin and salicylic acid are active anti-inflammatory agents but only aspirin is considered to produce significant analgesia. There are also differences in their mechanisms of action (90–92). The irreversible inactivation of cyclooxygenase by aspirin through transacetylation (Fig. 62.13) of the lysyl amino group in the enzyme is important to its activity (93, 94). On the other hand, salicylic acid is chemically incapable of acylating enzymes. Since it is a virtually inactive inhibitor of prostaglandin biosynthesis, the anti-inflammatory action of salicylic acid may depend more on other mechanisms such as the inhibition of leukocyte emigration (91).

Aspirin and salicylic acid have been found to be inhibitors of a variety of metabolic pathways such as fibrinolysis, oxidative phosphorylation, transaminases, and dehydrogenases (89). In view of the high concentrations, $0.1 \, \text{m}M$ or higher, needed to achieve a significant degree of inhibition, these relatively nonspecific actions may have a secondary effect on efficacy and toxicity only.

Numerous attempts have been made to seek a superior aspirin. The objectives are threefold: higher potency, better tolerance, and longer duration of action. The simplicity of the aspirin molecule has defied exten-

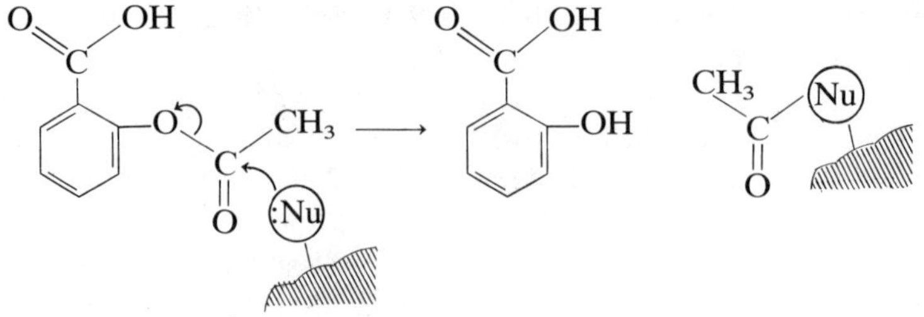

(Nu) : Serum albumin   (Lys-NH$_2$)
       Cyclooxygenase   (irreversible inactivation)
       Platelet membrane

Fig. 62.13   Transacetylation of biopolymers by aspirin.

sive synthetic efforts to discern any quantitative structure–activity relationship toward the design of a superior analog. As a consequence, considerable development in pharmaceutical formulation has been carried out to improve the pharmacokinetics of aspirin and derivatives. The outcome of these multiple approaches are exemplified by a complex salt, trilisate, an ester, benorylate (62.**10**), and a new chemical analog, diflunisal (62.**11**).

Trilisate is a complex salt of salicylic acid with choline and magnesium (95). The insoluble nature of the complex is reported to give less gastrointestinal irritation, higher plasma level of salicylate, and a longer duration of action than aspirin.

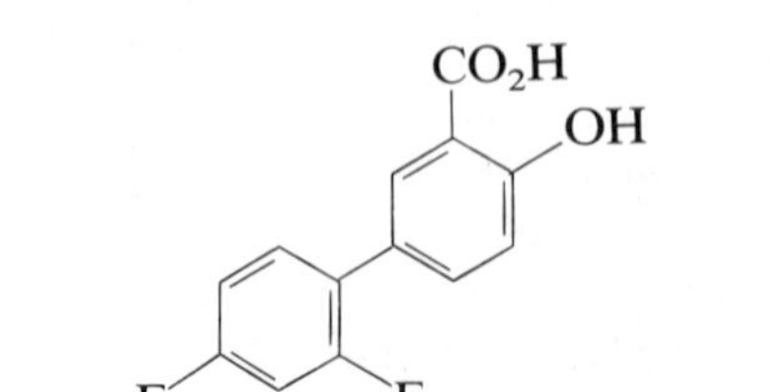

62.**10**   Benorylate

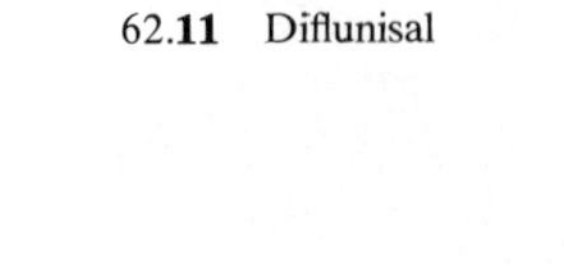

62.**11**   Diflunisal

7.1.2 BENORYLATE.   Benorylate is the N-acetyl-p-aminophenol ester of aspirin (62.**10**). Benorylate is largely absorbed intact and reported to cause less gastrointestinal bleeding than aspirin (96). It is hydrolyzed *in vivo* to give N-acetyl-p-aminophenol and salicylic acid and to provide a complement of anti-inflammatory, analgesic, and antipyretic activities. The plasma level of 8 g of benorylate is comparable to that of 4.8 g of aspirin. A slight delay in the onset of antipyretic activity was noted.

Not surprisingly, the pharmacodynamics of benorylate is highly species dependent. The multiple metabolic pathways of benorylate, some of which yield inactive metabolites only, also complicate the optimal delivery of the two active ingredients *in vivo*. Nevertheless, similar "chemical" formulation of two active compounds by covalent bond coupling, either directly or through a metabolically labile linkage, may be used in other cases to gain possible advantages in:

1. Chemical novelty and patentability.
2. Additive or synergistic effect of two drugs.
3. Reduced exposure of gastrointestinal mucosa to active drugs during absorption.
4. Patient compliance and convenience in multiple drug therapy.

5. A modified absorption and early disposition characteristics, such as delayed onset or sustained release, as compared with a physical mixture of active drugs.

7.1.3 DIFLUNISAL. Diflunisal, 5-(2,4-difluorophenyl)salicyclic acid (62.**11**), is a rare and novel salicylate which fulfills the three objectives for a superior salicylate mentioned above. The discovery of diflunisal culminated an extensive synthetic effort, including the biologic evaluation of 500 salicylates (98). An early recognition of the activity-enhancing tendency of a 5-phenyl group on salicylic acid and the fruitful application of fluoro substituents in anti-inflammatory agents led to the investigation of diflunisal and its congeners. The purposeful deletion of the *O*-acetyl group circumvents the transacetylation of aspirin and associated potential side effects. Interestingly, with 5-aryl salicylates the *O*-acetyl group is no longer needed for better absorption or analgesia (99). Diflunisal is four times more potent and much less irritating than aspirin, and has a duration of action of 8 hr in man (100). Diflunisal is a moderately active reversible cyclooxygenase inhibitor with minimal platelet inhibitory effect at therapeutic doses (101) (Table 62.5).

The *O*-carbonate ester of diflunisal (62.**12**) is also nonacylating and nearly as active as diflunisal. Among 5-heteroaryl salicylates, only the 5-(1-pyrryl) analog (62.**13**) has moderate anti-inflammatory activity (102). In a separate study, fendosal (62.**14**), which has a bulky aryl-substituted

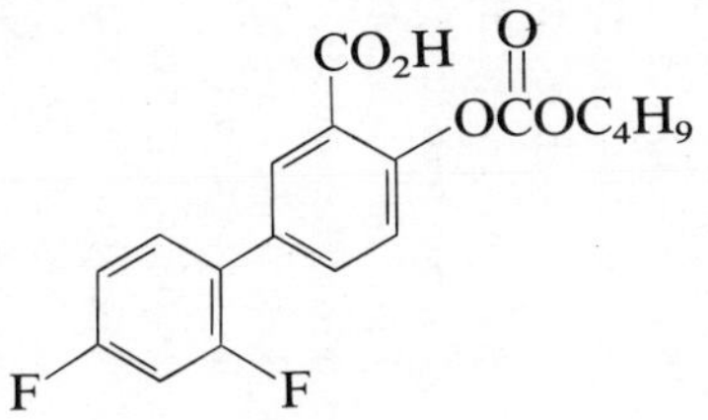

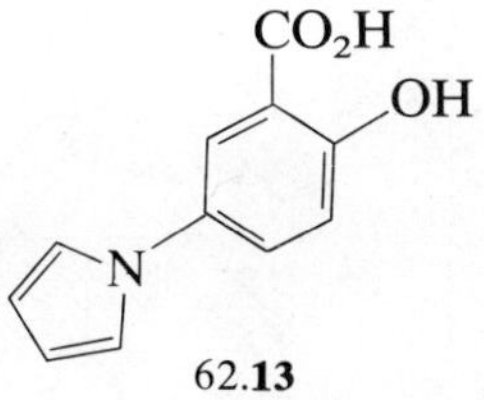

62.**13**

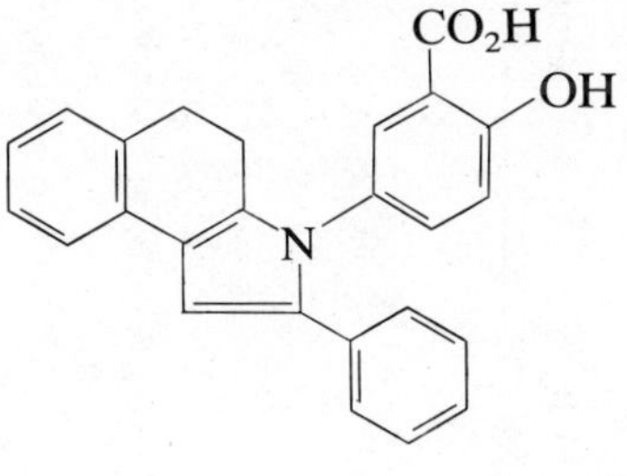

62.**14** Fendosal

pyrryl at C_5, possesses an analgesic activity comparable to that of diflunisal (103).

The binding site of diflunisal on cyclooxygenase is probably similar to that of indomethacin, overlapping but not identical to the binding site of aspirin. The marked increase in molecular dimension and hydrophobicity of diflunisal and fendosal may well bring their pharmacodynamics and modes of action closer to those of fenamates or other aryl acids.

7.2 Fenamates

Fenamates (104) are a family of *N*-arylanthranilic acids first discovered by their pronounced activity in the UV erythema assay in guinea pigs. The pharmacological profile of three clinically useful fenamates, mefenamic acid (62.**15**), flufenamic acid (62.**16**), and meclofenamic acid (62.**17**) are compared in Table 62.6. Mefenamic acid has a modest anti-inflammatory activity and is mainly used as a short-term analgesic. Notable side effects of mefenamic acid and flufenamic acid are diarrhea (15% of patients) and occasional hematologic complications (87).

62.**12**

Table 62.6 Pharmacological Profile of Some NSAIDS[a]

Drug	Carrageenin-Edema[b] Inhibition Indomethacin = 1	Adjuvant Arthritis[c] Inhibition Indomethacin = 1	Relative Ulcerogenicity[d]	Other Properties[e]
Section 7.1				
Aspirin	$\frac{1}{30}$	$\frac{1}{150}$	I	
Diflunisal (62.**11**)	$\frac{1}{4}$	$\frac{1}{30}$	III	Alg > Asp, modest Apyr
Fendosal (62.**14**)	$\frac{1}{15}$	$\frac{1}{20}$	III	Alg > Asp, modest Apyr
Section 7.2				
Mefenamic acid (62.**15**)	$\frac{1}{30}$	$\frac{1}{100}$	II	Moderate Alg
Flufenamic acid (62.**16**)	$\frac{1}{10}$	$\frac{1}{20}$	I	UV $\frac{1}{2}$ × Ind
Meclofenamic acid (62.**17**)	$\frac{1}{6}$	$\frac{1}{6}$	I	UV 4 × Ind
Clonixin (62.**19**)	$\frac{1}{20}$			Alg with some central action
Section 7.3				
Indomethacin (62.**5**)	1	1	I	Inactive *in vitro* or topically.
Sulindac (62.**31**)	$\frac{1}{2}$	$\frac{1}{2}$	II	Activity *in vivo* by sulfide metabolite
Section 7.4				
Ibuprofen (62.**37**)	$\frac{1}{10}$	$\frac{1}{100}$	I	Plet-aggr 10^{-7} M or 0.06 mg/kg
Flurbiprofen (62.**44**)	5	1	I	
Naproxen (62.**52**)	1	$\frac{1}{7}$	II	UV ED$_{50}$ 1 mg/kg, Apyr 25 mg/kg
Fenoprofen (62.**38**)	~$\frac{1}{10}$		II	
Ketoprofen (62.**55**)	$1\frac{1}{2}$	1	I	
Suprofen (62.**56**)	$\frac{1}{2}$	<1	III	UV 10 × Ind, Apyr $\frac{1}{2}$ × Ind
Carprofen (62.**54**)	~1	~1	III	Alg ~ $\frac{1}{3}$ Ind, Apyr ~ Ind
Pirprofen (62.**46**)	1	~1	II	
Benoxaprofen (62.**48**)	$\frac{1}{3}$		III	Moderate PGSI
R-803 (62.**50**)	$\frac{1}{4}$		II	
Y-9213 (62.**51**)	$\frac{1}{3}$			Alg
Tolmetin (62.**28**)	$\frac{1}{3}$		II	Alg in severe pains
Zomepirac (62.**29**)	2			Alg > asp, low Apyr
Indoprofen (62.**47**)	2	~1		Alg > Ind, some effects on nervous function
Pranoprofen (62.**49**)	3	2	II	

Compound	b	c	Ulcerogenicity[d]	Comments
Alclofenac (62.45)	$\frac{1}{20}$		I	
Diclofenac (62.61)	$\frac{2}{3}$		I	
Fenclofenac (62.62)	$\frac{1}{40}$	$\frac{1}{15}$	II	
Fenbufen (62.43)	$\frac{1}{30}$	$\frac{1}{20}$	II	Moderate Alg, Apyr. Inactive PGSI. Acetic acid metabolite $\frac{1}{5}\times$Ind in PGSI
Fenclorac (62.40)	$\frac{1}{3}$	<1	I	
Etodolic acid (62.64)	$\frac{1}{8}$	$\frac{1}{3}$	II	α-OH metabolite $\frac{1}{3}$ as active
Isoxepac (62.59)	$\frac{1}{2}$	$\frac{1}{4}$	III	12×prodolic acid in potency
Oxepinac (62.58)	2	>1	III	
Tiopinac (62.60)	2	2	III	Alg 1–3×Ind
Y-9213 (62.51)	$\frac{1}{3}$			Weak PGSI
Section 7.5				
Phenylbutazone (62.6)	$\frac{1}{15}$	$\frac{1}{50}$	I	Uricosuric, lysosome membrane stabilization
Oxyphenbutazone (62.67)	$\frac{1}{15}$		I	
Azapropazone (62.68)	$\frac{1}{20}$	$\sim\frac{1}{100}$	II	
Isoxicam (62.72)	$\frac{1}{20}$	$\frac{1}{4}$		
Piroxicam (62.71)	$\frac{1}{2}$	$\frac{1}{3}$	III	Long duration action
R-805 (62.74)	>1	>1		Inactive Gran
Section 7.6				
Flumizole (62.77)	~ 3			PGSI 2×Ind, poorly absorbed p.o.
Proquazone (62.81)	~ 1	$\frac{1}{4}$	II	Alg, Apyr~Ind
Ciproquazone (62.82)	$\frac{1}{8}$	$\frac{1}{50}$	III	PGSI $\frac{1}{4}\times$Ind, blocking Ind. Induced GI lesions in rats

[a] The relative potency of these compounds are estimated from published data. Considerable variations are sometimes noted. Actual dose levels for several compounds in mg/kg p.o. are in tables. With a few exceptions, their peripheral analgesic and antipyretic activities are generally of the same order as their anti-inflammatory activity in the carrageenin edema assay.

[b] Indomethacin ED_{50} = 2.3 mg/kg p.o., protocol. See Section 3.2.1.

[c] Indomethacin ED_{50} = 0.25 mg/kg p.o., regular protocol. See Section 3.2.4.

[d] The "relative ulcerogenicity" is estimated by the ratio of (minimal ulcerogenic dose)/(ED_{50} in the carrageenin edema assay) to indicate the therapeutic safety margin in animal models. Since several versions of acute and subacute, gastric hemorrhage, and intestinal perforation assays are used in different laboratories, and since the precision and predicative value of these GI irritation models are also uncertain, only a rough scale is used here: the therapeutic ratio for score I, II, and III is <3, <10 and <30, respectively. Higher score indicates possible greater safety margin in man. The correlation of these scores with clinical observations remains to be established.

[e] Abbreviations: Alg, analgesia; Apyr, antipyretic activity; Gran, cotton pellet granuloma inhibition; PGSI, prostaglandin synthesis inhibition in vitro; Plet-Aggr, platelet aggregation inhibition; UV, UV erythema inhibition; Asp, aspirin; Ind, indomethacin.

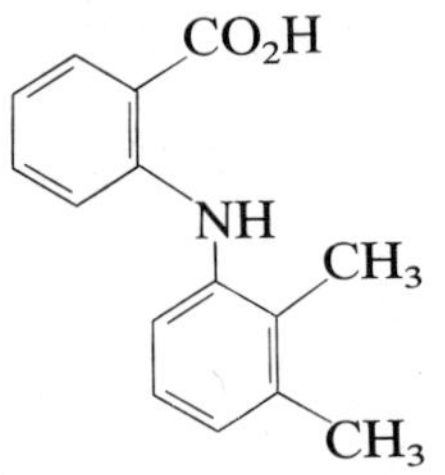

62.**15** Mefenamic acid

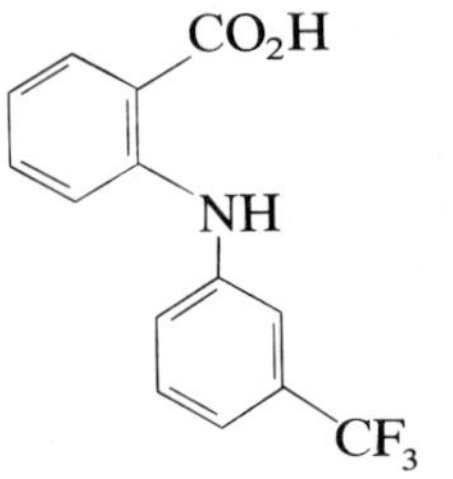

62.**16** Flufenamiz acid

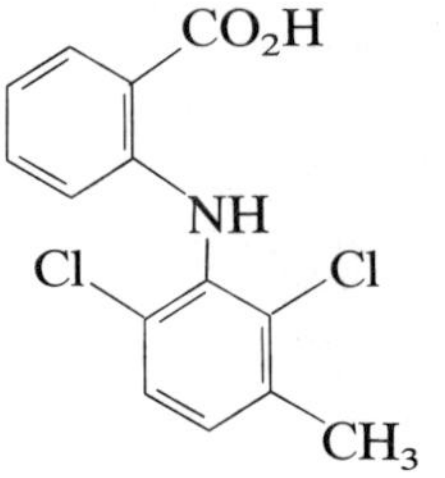

62.**17** Meclofenamic acid

Heterocyclic isosters of fenamates are exemplified by niflumic acid (105) (62.**18**), which is limited by its gastrointestinal intolerance, and clonixin (62.**19**) which is more active as an analgesic in animal models, possibly acting both peripherally and centrally in the nervous system (106, 107). A newer congener, flunixin (62.**20**), three to five times more potent than clonixin, is under development.

Another substituted aza analog developed independently is the analgesic glaphenine (62.**21**) used widely in Europe (109). Glaphenine is a combination of 8-chloroquinoline and anthranilic acid. The trifluoromethyl analog (floctafenine) and other hydroxy alkyl esters have also been investigated (110). Floctafenine (62.**22**) 200 mg is slightly more potent than

propoxyphene 65 mg in postsurgery patients (111). These compounds have only weak anti-inflammatory activities.

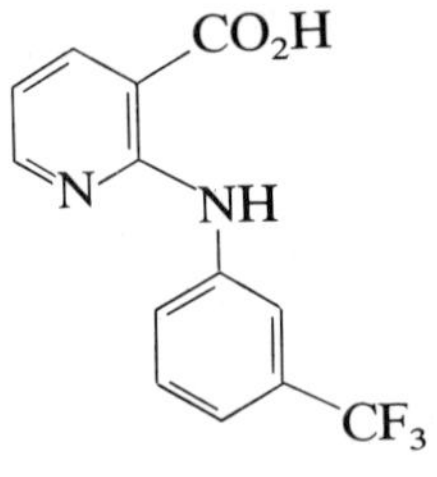

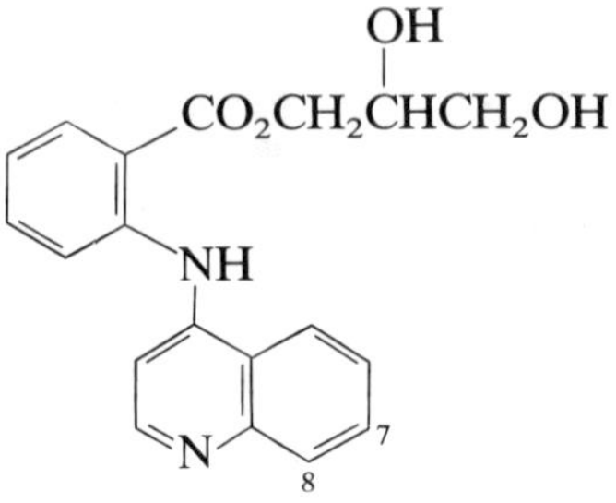

62.**21** 7-Cl: glaphenine
62.**22** 8-CF$_3$: floctafenine

It is of interest to note that the m-CF$_3$ substituent, originally found to be optimal for activity in flufenamic acid, has been retained in the two aza analogs, niflumic acid (62.**18**) and flunixin (62.**20**), as well. A m-CF$_3$ group in the anilino moiety is chemically and metabolically stable. For example, the principal metabolic conversions of flufenamic acid involves ring hydroxylation at the 4 and 4′ positions, followed by glucuronide conjugation. No significant extent of defluorination has been observed.

One may also compare the differences in chemical features in salicylates, fenamates, and aryl acetic acids and their biochemical properties. The stereochemistry of active fenamates has the noncoplanar arrangement of two hydrophobic aromatic moieties similar to that found in many NSAIDS. The weakly basic hydrogen bonding anilino group is analogous to the phenolic group in

62.**18** Niflumiz acid

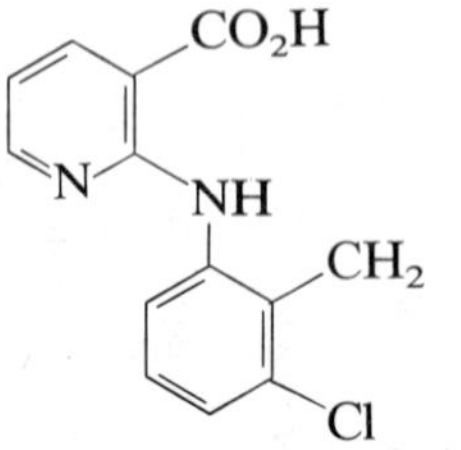

62.**19** Clonixin

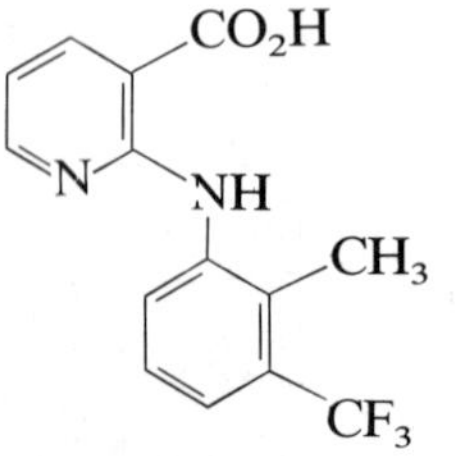

62.**20** Flunixin

salicylate, but the orientation of the *N*-phenyl group differs from the stereochemistry of diflunisal. Fenamates bind strongly to albumin, and other protein sites, in a manner different from that of indomethacin analogs (112). Fenamates are potent cyclooxygenase inhibitors and, unlike other NSAIDS, modest prostaglandin antagonists *in vitro* (113).

7.3 Indomethacin, Sulindac, and Congeners

7.3.1 DISCOVERY OF INDOMETHACIN (62.**5**).

The chemical and biologic studies of indomethacin, sulindac, and related compounds have been summarized in a recent review (114).

The original 1-benzylindole-3-acetic acid lead was discovered in an attempt to use structures related to serotonin metabolites for anti-inflammatory activity. After laboratory evaluation of 350 indole derivatives and clinical trials of two prototypes, indomethacin was finally discovered as a potent antiarthritic agent. Its pharmacological profile is shown in Table 62.5. In the clinic, indomethacin is used at 75–150 mg. t.i.d. or 100 mg in suppository for various rheumatic disorders. Two common side effects are gastrointestinal irritation and headache.

Since 1964 indomethacin has been used widely and has remained a clinical standard in the evaluation of newer NSAIDS. It has also served as a valuable research tool in numerous biochemical–pharmacological experiments, especially in prostaglandin research. As a potent inhibitor of the biosynthesis of prostaglandins, indomethacin was used frequently to decide the possible involvement of prostaglandins in various biologic processes *in vitro* and *in vivo*.

7.3.2 STRUCTURE–ACTIVITY RELATIONSHIP OF INDOMETHACIN ANALOGS. The structure–activity relationship of indomethacin

analogs was progressively developed from several medicinal chemical concepts. A systematic chemical modification effort was facilitated by the use of model compounds, which showed parallel structure–activity relationships, and by the additivity of activity-enhancing effects of substituents at different parts of the molecule.

Parallel changes of anti-inflammatory activity were observed in derivatives of methyl *N*-benzylindole acetate, *N*-benzoylindole acetic acid, and the indene isostere, 1-benzylidenylindene acetic acid (62.**23**). The additive effect of ring or side chain substituents indicates that the configurational and physicochemical properties of the parent molecule predominate; each substituent contributes almost independently to optimal drug action. This is reminiscent of the stepwise increment of potency of hydrocortisone by Δ^1, 9αF, and 16α-CH$_3$ substitutions. Thus combinations of preferred (1) indole (or indene) substituents, e.g., 5-MeO, F, Me$_2$N, 5-MeO-6-F, or 2-methyl, with (2) benzoyl (benzyl or benzylidenyl) substituents, e.g., *p*-Cl, F, or CH$_3$S, and (3) acetic acid modifications, e.g., H vs. α-CH$_3$ or CO$_2$H vs. CO$_2$CH$_3$, generally give expected activities. Many carboxyl equivalents (e.g., tetrazole), precursors (e.g., aldehyde or alcohol), and metabolically labile derivatives (e.g., esters or amides), investigated are generally less active than the carboxylic acid itself.

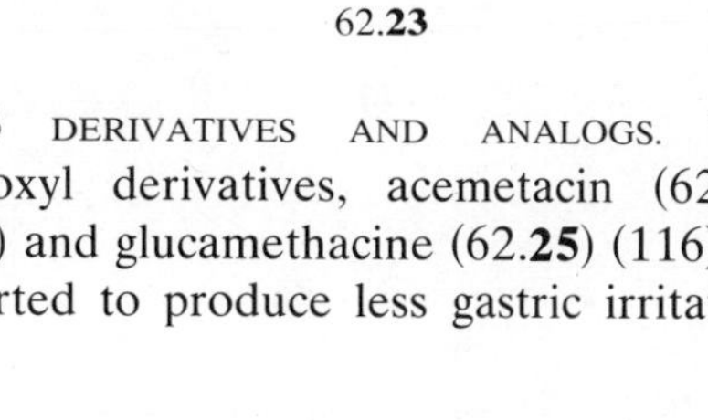

62.**23**

7.3.3 DERIVATIVES AND ANALOGS. Two carboxyl derivatives, acemetacin (62.**24**) (115) and glucamethacine (62.**25**) (116) are reported to produce less gastric irritation.

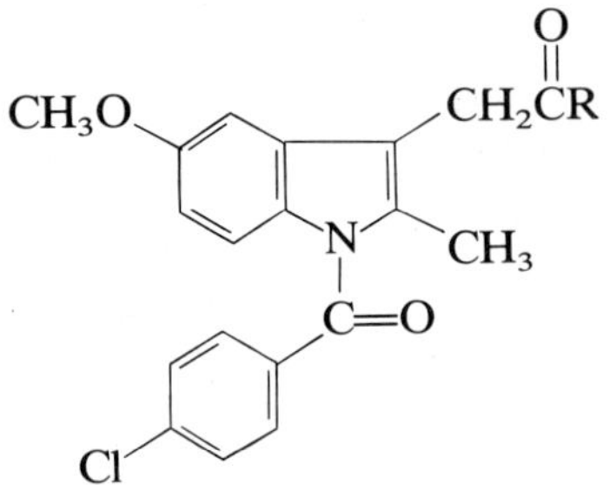

62.24 R = OCH$_2$CO$_2$H: acemetacin
62.25 R = D-glucosamine (amide): glucamethacine

Both drugs are not active as cyclo-oxygenase inhibitors *per se* and are converted to indomethacin and other inactive metabolites *in vivo*. As new chemical derivatives, they are used at three to four times the dosage of indomethacin.

Many analogs of indomethacin have been synthesized and are generally disappointing. Compounds showing clinical activities are MK-825 (62.**26**) (114), cinmetacin (62.**27**) (117, 118), and analogs (119), all of which are less potent ($\frac{1}{10}$–$\frac{1}{2}$ × indomethacin) but possibly less irritating. Investigation of

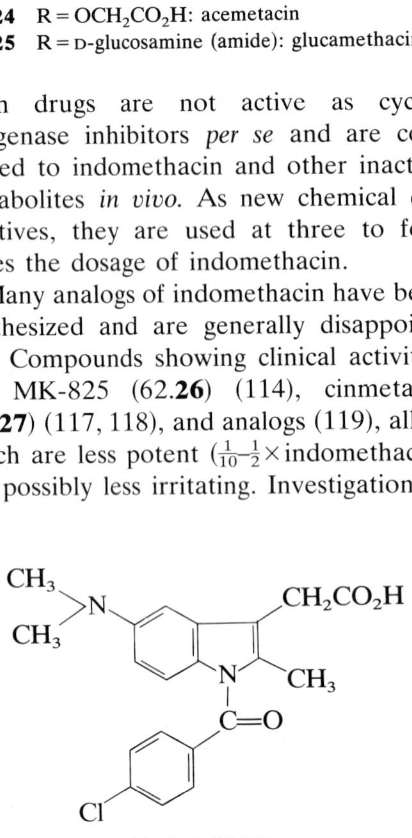

62.**26** MK-825

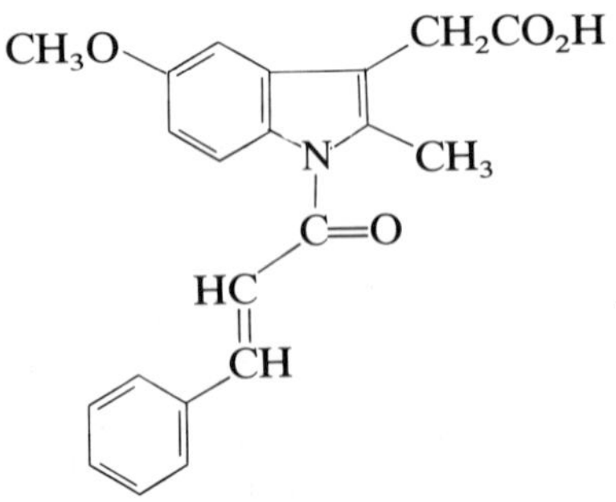

62.**27** Cinmetacin

a group of pyrrole acids modeled after indomethacin has led to the discovery of tolmetin (62.**28**) (120) and zomepirac (62.**29**) (121, 122). (See Section 7.4.)

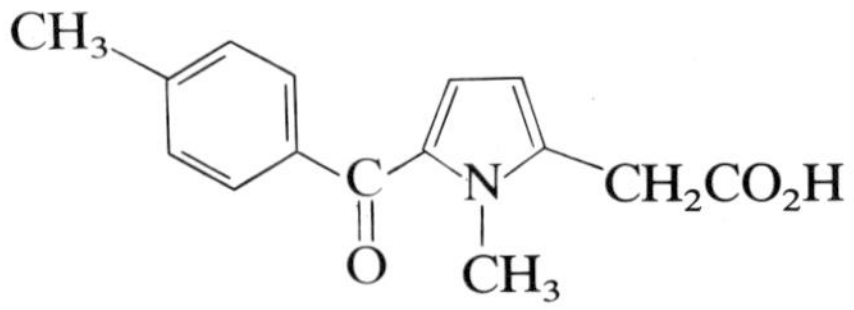

62.**28** Tolmetin

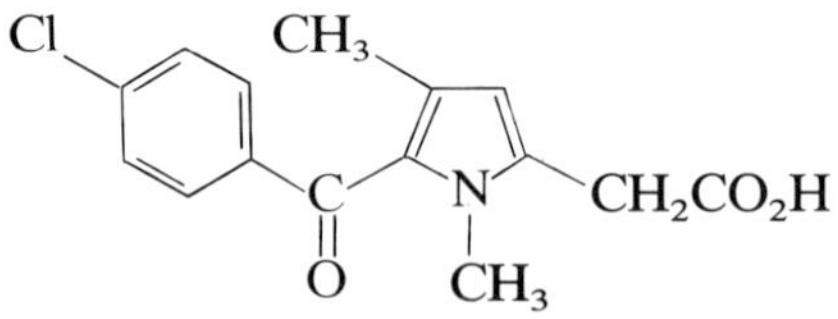

62.**29** Zomepirac

7.3.4 STEREOCHEMISTRY AND MECHANISM OF ACTION. A consistent correlation of two stereochemical aspects with optimal biological activity was noted with indomethacin analogs. First, when a chiral center is created by changing the side chain acetic acid to α-propionic acid, bioactivity is generally associated with the (S)(+) enantiomer (112). This stereospecificity has since been shown to be generally valid for many aryl-α-propionic acids. Second, as shown by X-ray crystallography of indomethacin and the rigid indene isosteres, the two phenyl moieties in indomethacin analogs are noncoplanar and in the *cis* form. This preferred configuration has been refined with CNDO calculation and computer modeling to give a hypothetical receptor contour for indomethacin, which also accommodates arachidonic acid (62.**30**), the substrate of cyclooxygenase (Fig. 62.9).

Indomethacin, like other NSAIDS, probably does not exert its anti-

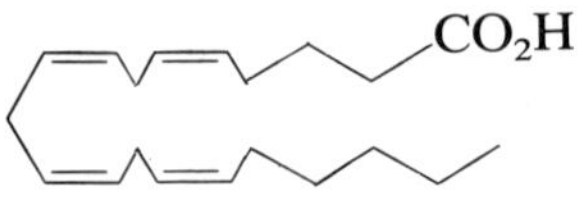

62.**30** Arachidonic acid

inflammatory–analgesic action by a single biochemical mechanism (124). Among more than a score of *in vitro* biochemical activities shown by indomethacin so far, only the inhibition of cyclooxygenase in the arachidonic acid cascade fulfills the following criteria considered significant in the mechanism of action:

1. Independent biochemical evidence to associate cyclooxygenase metabolites with the inflammatory process.

2. Inhibition of the enzyme *in vitro* at concentrations comparable to or below the plasma/tissue levels of indomethacin ($5 \times 10^{-7} M$) at normal therapeutic doses.

3. Parallelism between the ranking order of enzyme inhibition *in vitro* and anti-inflammatory potency *in vivo* for a group of NSAIDS with similar biologic properties.

Of special interest is the observation that the *in vivo* stereospecificity for (S)-(+) enantiomers of aryl-α-propionic acids is also true in the inhibition of cyclo-oxygenase *in vitro*. No discrimination of optical isomers has been observed with other proposed biochemical mechanisms, e.g., the uncoupling of oxidative phosphorylation.

Indomethacin has also been shown to inhibit several pathways associated with the arachidonic acid cascade such as phospholipase A_2 of polymorphonuclear leukocytes (125), the release of arachidonic acid (126), and 15-hydroxy prostaglandin dehydrogenase (127) at low concentrations under certain experimental conditions.

7.3.5 SULINDAC. In the search for an indomethacin analog with a better patient tolerance, the indene isostere (MK-715) (62.**23**) was found to be less irritating to the GI tract and apparently free of CNS in man. Further improvement of MK-715 led to the discovery of sulindac (Fig. 62.14, 62.**31**) (128). Sulindac has a stereochemistry similar to that of indomethacin. Compared with other substituents, the 5-fluoro group enhances analgesia in this series of compounds. The *p*-methylsulfinyl group was introduced to increase the solubility of indene derivatives manyfold, and to provide a center of metabolism to minimize the accumulation of any single metabolite in the urine. The overall pharmacological profile of sulindac is shown in Table 62.6. It is approximately half as potent as indomethacin in anti-inflammatory and antipyretic assays but is slightly more active as an analgesic agent (129). At 300–400 mg b.i.d. it is much better tolerated in man in all five indications, rheumatoid arthritis, osteoarthritis, gout, ankylosing spondylitis, and acute shoulder pain (130).

Extensive laboratory data indicate that sulindac is a reversible prodrug; its biologic activities are mediated via an active sulfide metabolite (62.**32**) which is reversibly produced in different tissue compartments and has a long serum half-life of 16.4 hr.

Evidence supporting the reversible prodrug concept follows (131):

1. Potency is a function of metabolism. Sulindac has no intrinsic activity *in vitro*. It is weakly active when applied locally, e.g., in topical and ocular inflammation, where metabolic conversions are minimal. The sulfide metabolite is fully active in all cases. The *in vivo* potency of sulindac given orally gradually approaches that of its sulfide metabolite as the duration of the *in vivo* assay is increased to allow the buildup of the sulfide metabolite.

2. After oral administration of either sulindac or the sulfide, the efficacy is correlated with the concentration of the sulfide, but not sulindac, in the plasma and synovial fluid in the rat paw edema and canine synovitis models, respectively.

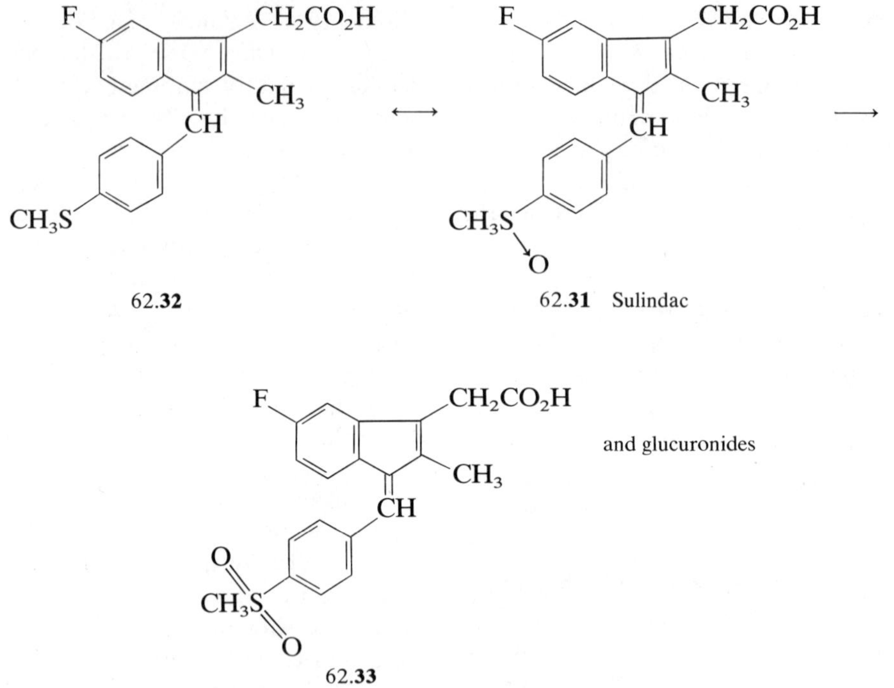

62.**32**   62.**31** Sulindac

and glucuronides

62.**33**

Fig. 62.14 Principal metabolites of sulindac.

The possible therapeutic advantages of using sulindac as a reversible prodrug are as follows:

1. Circumventing the initial exposure of gastric mucosa to the active drug.
2. Reducing the amount of the active metabolite in bile secretion during enterohepatic recirculation.
3. Optimizing tissue distribution of sulindac and the sulfide to increase efficacy and, possibly, to reduce side effects (e.g. less disturbance of renal functions).

7.3.6 METABOLISM OF INDOMETHACIN AND SULINDAC. Indomethacin undergoes metabolic O-demethylation and/or deacylation. The acyl glucuronide of these metabolites and unchanged indomethacin are mainly excreted in the urine. Indomethacin, like many NSAIDS, also undergoes an enterohepatic recirculation, i.e., bile duct secretion followed by intestinal reabsorption

(132). The extent of enterohepatic recirculation varies in different species (70).

With sulindac metabolic conversions involve mainly valency changes of the sulfur atom. The methylsulfinyl group is irreversibly oxidized to the sulfone (62.**33**) and reversibly reduced to the sulfide (62.**32**). All three compounds are more than 93% protein bound (Fig. 62.14). The glucuronide of sulindac and sulfone are major metabolites in urinary and biliary excretions.

The long action of the sulfide is sustained by (1) its accumulation in the tissue, (2) its lack of urinary excretion, and (3) the enterohepatic recirculation of sulindac which is reduced again to the sulfide.

The relative concentration of sulindac and the sulfide in different tissue compartments is a function of the local enzymatic redox capacity and distribution characteristics of the more hydrophilic sulindac vs. the more lipophilic sulfide. The pharmacodynamics of such a reversible prodrug is very different from that of most prodrugs, e.g. benorylate and acemetacin, which are irreversibly activated.

7.3.7 SYNTHESIS OF ACYL GLUCURONIDES. The glucuronide of indomethacin (62.**34**) is both acid- and alkali-labile. A synthetic procedure using a protected intermediate of glucuronic acid which can be deblocked under neutral conditions has been developed (133).

The glucuronide of sulindac and its sulfide metabolite are slightly more stable. They can be synthesized in moderate yields by partial acid hydrolysis of a readily prepared glucuronide derivative (134).

These two procedures may be used for the synthesis of other acyl glucuronides.

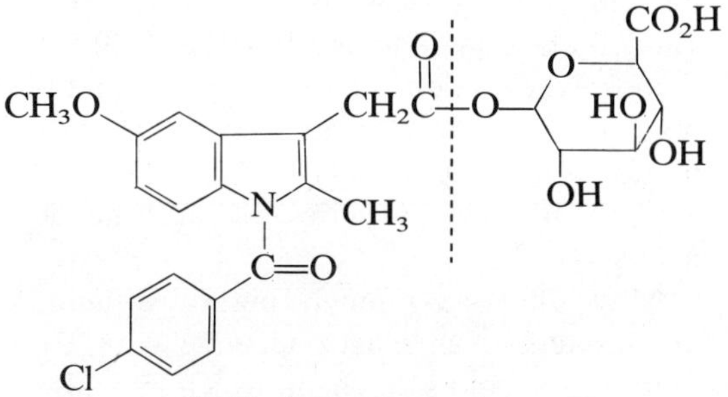

62.**34** Indomethacin glucuronide

7.4 Phenylpropionic Acids

Substituted phenyl-α-propionic acids constitute the largest family of aryl acidic antiinflammatory agents. More than 20 generic names have been registered. The endings "profen" and "fenac" are generally used to denote phenylpropionic and phenylacetic acids, respectively.

The synthetic chemistry and structure–activity relationship of many phenyl propionic acids reported before 1973 have been reviewed in detail (135). The development of this large family of congeners is a tribute to the ingenuity of numerous chemists in pursuing a broad and rewarding lead. The

effectiveness of several medicinal chemical concepts, such as the application of a metabolic precursor or a cyclic analog of the chiral propionic side chain, halogen and electronegative substituents of an aromatic ring, heteroaryl isosteres, an angular linkage, or less rigid seven-membered ring to achieve a noncoplanar configuration, is also well demonstrated.

In recent years, clinicians have been inundated with many "phenylpropionics." However, in spite of their general similarity in biologic activities, several have shown some distinct advantages and are considered to be valuable contributions to therapy.

7.4.1 GENERAL CHEMICAL CHARACTERISTICS. The basic chemical features and structure–activity relationship of "phenylpropionics" may be discussed in terms of three structure moieties: the propionic acid side chain, phenyl substitutents (X), and a second hydrophobic group (Ar).

The preference for (S)-(+) configuration of the propionic side chain has been discussed above (60). Similar stereospecificity for more potent compounds is shown in a cyclized analog, the indancarboxylic acid clidenac (62.**35**) (TAI-284,35) (136). Clidenac is comparable to indomethacin in activity. It is ca. 10 times less potent than the uncyclized model, MK-830 (62.**36**) (60), but is better tolerated in safety assessment.

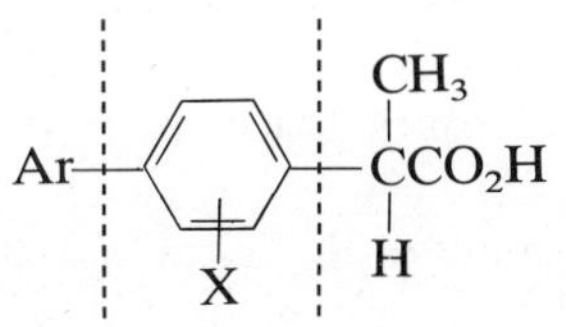

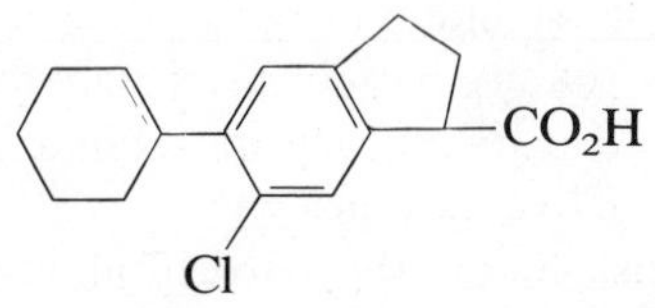

62.**35** Clidenac

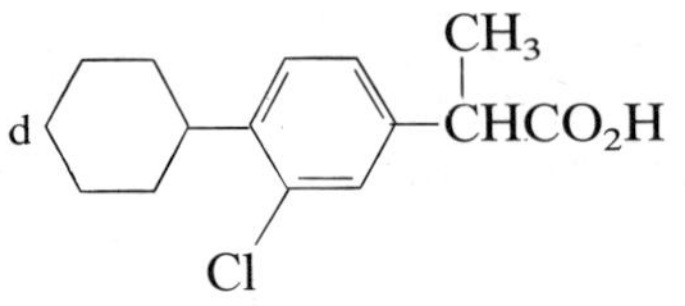

62.**36**   MK-830

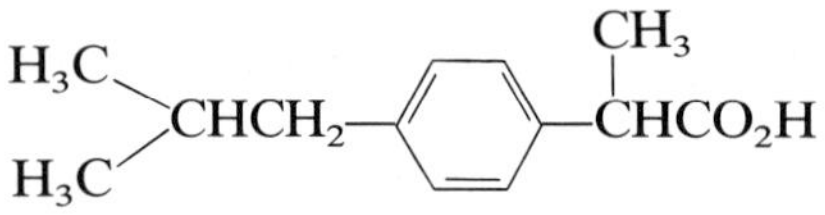

62.**37**   Ibuprofen

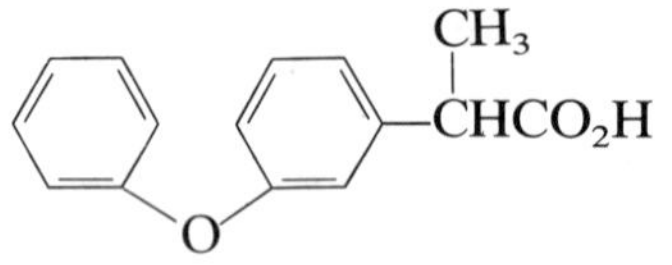

62.**38**   Fenoprofen

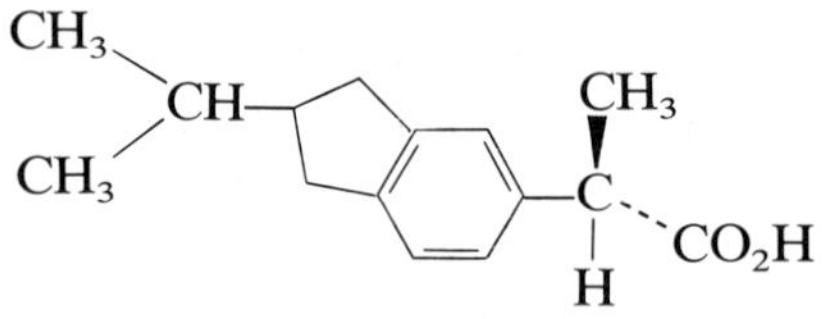

62.**39**

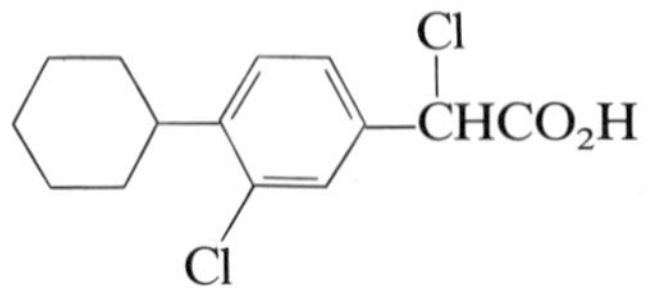

62.**40**   Fenclorac

The stereospecificity of the α-propionic acid side chain is apparently less important in moderately potent agents like ibuprofen (62.**37**), fenoprofen (62.**38**), and a series of diastereoisomeric indan-5-acetic acids (e.g., 62.**39**), which are twice as potent as ibuprofen (137).

Replacement of the α-methyl in MK-830 by a chloro group gives a less irritating fenclorac (62.**40**) (138), which is one-third as potent as indomethacin. The α-chloro group is readily metabolized to α-hydroxy *in vivo*. The α-hydroxy metabolite is one-third as active as fenclorac.

In most series, the corresponding acetic acid analog is less potent. Some carboxyl

derivatives, e.g., esters and amides, and carboxyl precursors, e.g., hydroxy ethyl and butyric acid, which are metabolically convertible to the active carboxylic acid side chain, have also been used. A carbonyl propionic acid side chain, readily introduced by succinylation of the aromatic ring, has been independently studied by several laboratories. Bucloxic acid (62.**41**) (139), fenbufen (62.**42**) (140, 141), and furobufen (62.**43**) (142) are three examples. These aryl ketobutyric acids are generally comparable to phenylbutazone in animal models, being less potent than the corresponding aryl α-propionic acids. The activity of fenufen and furobufen have been attributed to their major metabolite *in vivo*, the corresponding acetic acid. Being an inactive prodrug, fenbufen appears to be less irritating to the gastrointestinal tract than phenylbutazone in clinical trials (140). A carboxyl equivalent, 5-tetrazolyl, is metabolically more stable (no glucuronide formation) but is generally less active when applied to several series of aryl acetic acids.

Most effective phenyl ring substituents are limited to an electronegative F or Cl, meta to the acid side chain, which may also

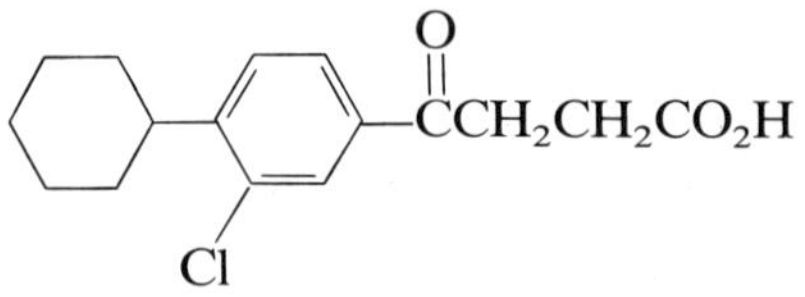

62.**41**   Bucloxic acid

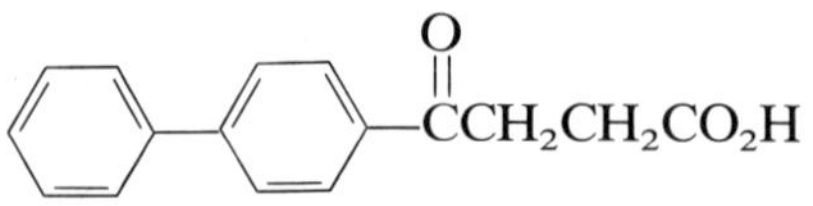

62.**42**   Fenbufen

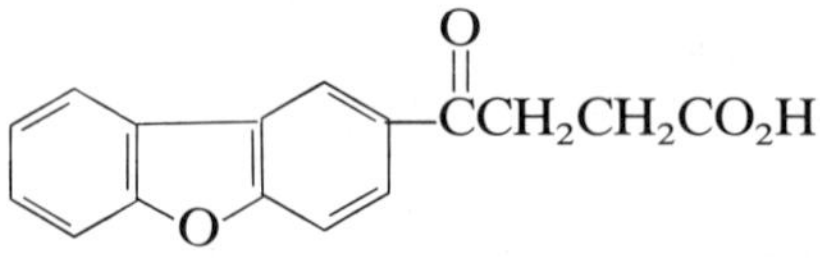

62.**43**   Furobufen

exert a steric effect to favor a nonplanar arrangement of the second hydrophobic group.

A variety of second hydrophobic substituents at C_4 have been found effective. A group of clinically active structures and their pharmacological profiles are listed in Table 62.6. Linear aliphatic or aromatic substituents studied initially are isobutyl (ibuprofen, 62.**37**) (143), phenyl (flurbiprofen, 62.**44**) (144), and allyloxy (alclofenac, 62.**45**) (145). Cyclohexyl derivative MK-830 (62.**36**) (60) set an early mark of being 10–20 times as potent as indomethacin in the carrageenin edema assay but was too irritating for clinical application. Various heteroaryl groups introduced more recently are illustrated by pirprofen (62.**46**) (146), indoprofen (62.**47**) (147), benoxaprofen (62.**48**) (148), pranoprofen (62.**49**) (149), R-803 (62.**50**) (150), and a potent analgesic agent, Y-9213 (62.**51**)

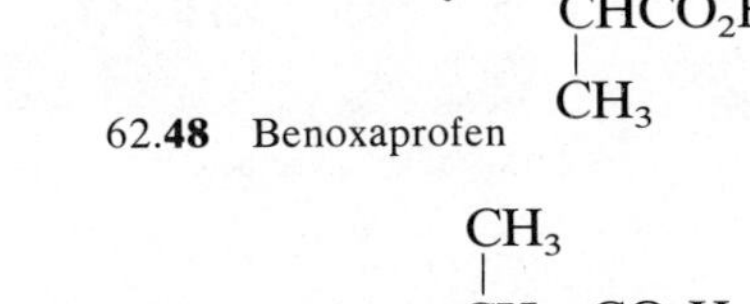

62.**48** Benoxaprofen

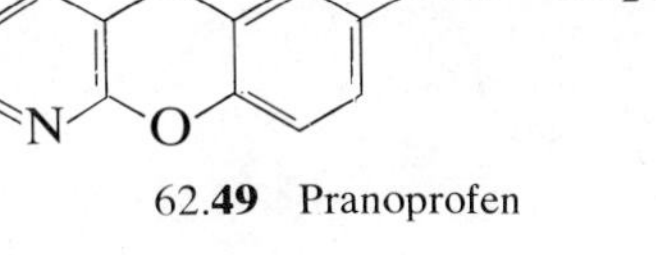

62.**49** Pranoprofen

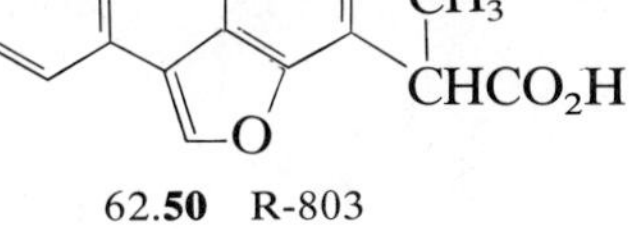

62.**50** R-803

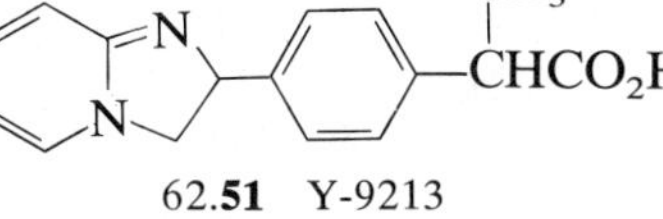

62.**51** Y-9213

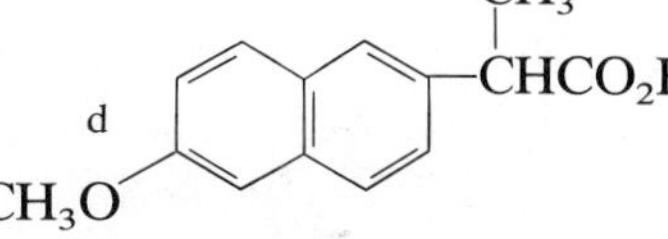

62.**52** Naproxen

(151). A benzo substituent was studied earlier to give the naphthalene derivative, naproxen (62.**52**) (152). Clinically effective tricyclic analogs are the phenothiazine derivative, metiazinic acid (62.**53**) (153), and the carbazole derivative, carprofen (62.**54**) (154). A notable variation of the linear biaryl arrangement is to attach the second hydrophobic group through an angular carbonyl or ether linkage at C_3. Active drugs derived from this approach are the 3-benzoyl (ketoprofen, 62.**55**) (155), 3-thenoyl (suprofen, 62.**56**) (156), and 3-phenoxy (fenoprofen, 62.**38**) (157) analogs. Tolmetin (62.**23**) (120, 123), zomepirac (62.**29**) (122), and triaprofenic acid (62.**57**) (158) are heteroaryl analogs of this type. Cyclization of ketoprofen with a seven-membered ring to maintain a nonplanar

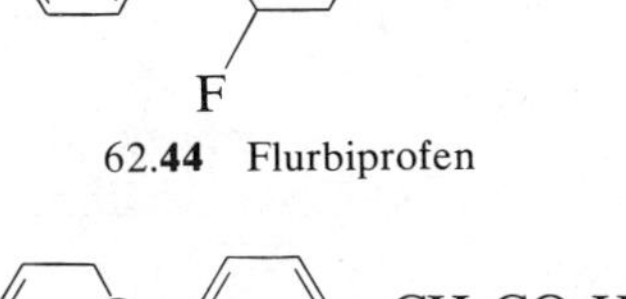

62.**44** Flurbiprofen

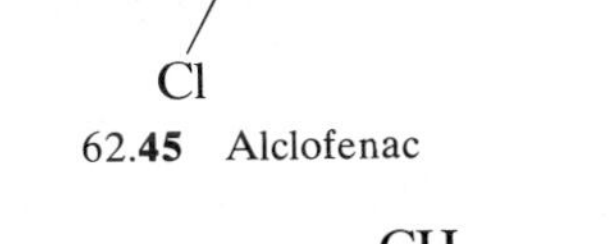

62.**45** Alclofenac

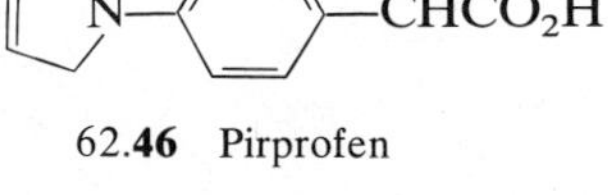

62.**46** Pirprofen

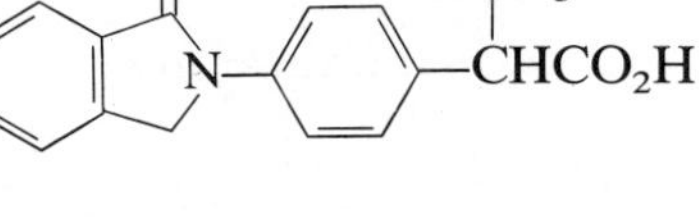

62.**47** Indoprofen

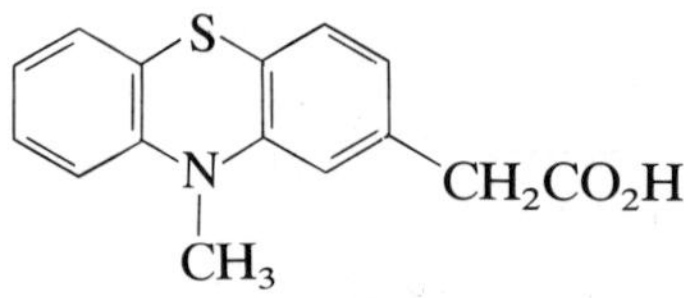

62.**53**   Metiazinic acid

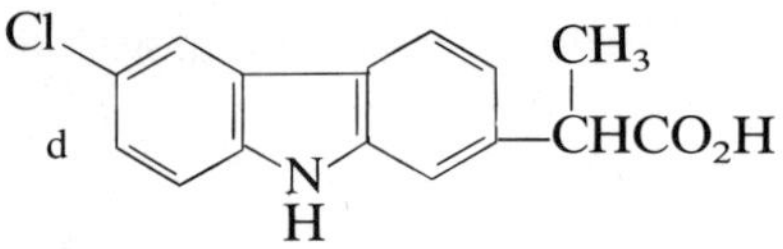

62.**54**   Carprofen

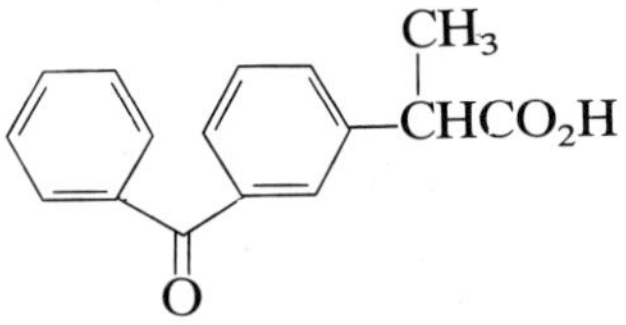

62.**55**   Ketoprofen

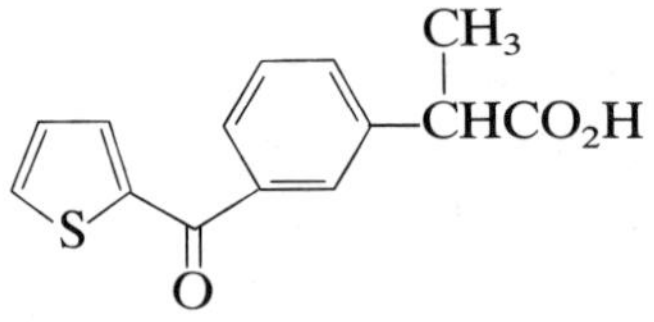

62.**56**   Suprofen

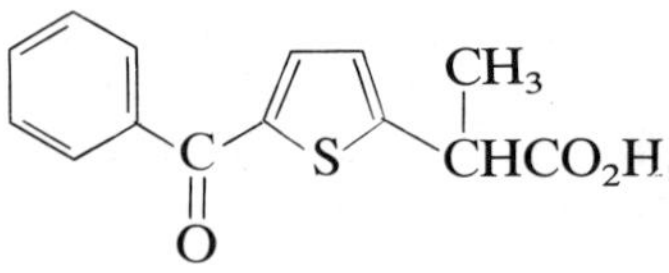

62.**57**   Tiaprofenic acid

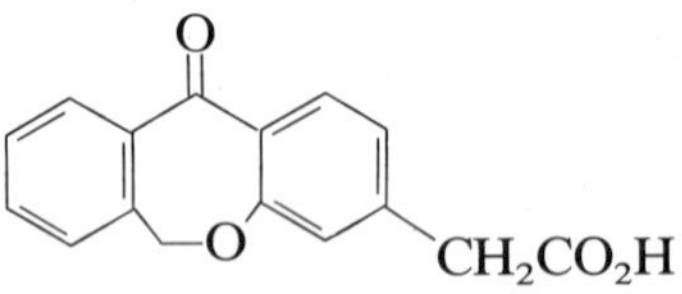

62.**58**   Oxepinac

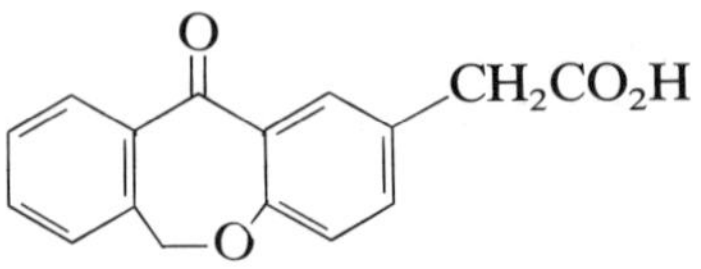

62.**59**   Isoxepac

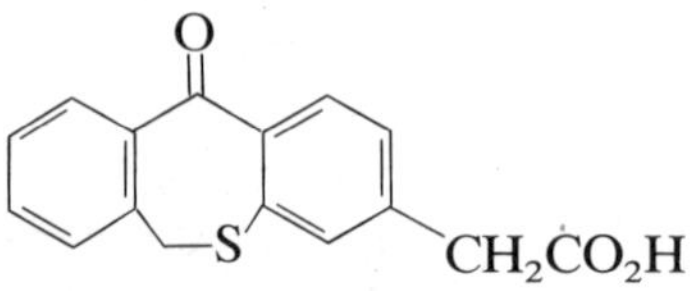

62.**60**   Tiopinac

configuration gives oxepinac (62.**58**) (159, 160), isoxepac (62.**59**) (161), and tiopinac (62.**60**) (162). These compounds are one to two times as active as indomethacin in antiinflammatory and analgesic assays, and are much less ulcerogenic in animal models. Tiopinac (62.**60**) is also less efficient than indomethacin in the inhibition of prostaglandin synthetase, a factor that may contribute to its improved GI tolerance (163). The overall clinical safety of tiopinac remains to be ascertained. An interesting structure–activity relationship has emerged from three independent studies of these tricyclic compounds. Among 2–300 analogs investigated, the dibenzoxepins appear to be slightly more potent than the dibenzothiepins. 3-Substituted dibenzooxepins and dibenzothiepins, with the acid side chain para to the carbonyl bridge, are twice as active as 2-substituted analogs. The dextrorotatory enantiomer of the α-propionic acid analog of tiopinac is almost five times more potent but is appreciably more irritating. Other position isomers, thiophene isosteres (164),

propanol, and ester side chains are less potent. Translocation of the oxygen or sulfur atom and the methylene group of the central ring caused a dramatic ten to fortyfold decrease in potency in oxepinac and tiopinac, respectively. The changing conformation of the central seven-membered ring associated with structural modifications has been followed to some extent by NMR analysis.

The broad scope of active biaryl arrangements is indicated by the potent C_2-substituted phenyl acetic acid, diclofenac (62.**61**) (165), which may also be considered as a hybrid of fenamate and phenyl-

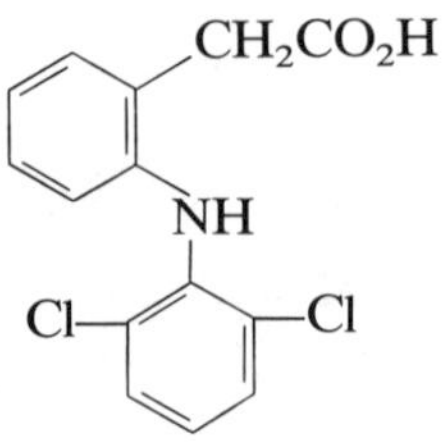

62.**61**   Diclofenac

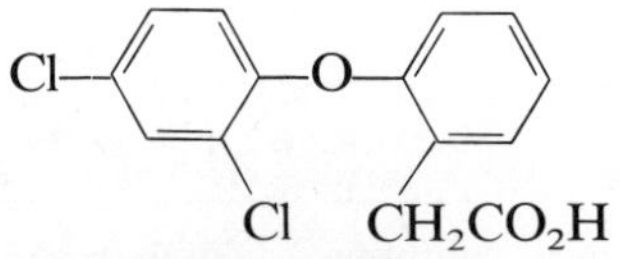

62.**62** Fenclofenac

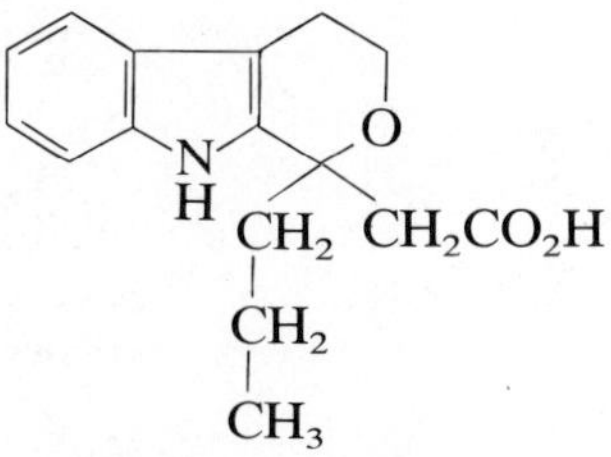

62.**63** Prodolic acid

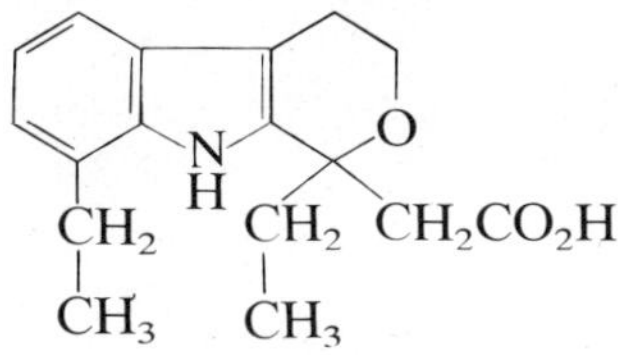

62.**64** Etodolic acid

acetic acid. A moderately active C_2-dichlorophenoxy analog is fenclofenac (62.**62**) (166). Other complex structures are prodolic acid (62.**63**) (167) and etodolic acid (62.**64**) (168). The increased serum level and potency (12X) of etodolic acid has been attributed to the 8-ethyl group, which may block the catabolism of the nucleus. Obviously there are many potentially active variations of the general theme, and more novel structures are still being developed. The relative merit of these second-generation active compounds will largely depend on their novel mechanism of action or improvements in both efficacy and tolerance in long-term animal and clinical studies.

7.4.2 BIOLOGIC PROPERTIES. With few exceptions, the pharmacological profiles of numerous aryl acetic or propionic acids are very similar (see Table 62.6). Most of them are also fatty acid cyclooxygenase inhibitors. A few have been shown to be reversible inhibitors competitive with the substrate arachidonic acid. They are generally active in the carrageenin paw edema, UV erythema, and adjuvant arthritis assays. Many are more potent than phenylbutazone, and some are comparable to or several times more active than indomethacin in these animal models. It seems that higher doses of phenylpropionic acids are sometimes required in the clinic. Their analgesic activities are mostly peripheral in nature. However, a greater degree of analgesia for severe pain is claimed for zomepirac (62.**29**) and Y-9213 (62.**51**), suggesting possibly altered biochemical properties. Their ulcerogenic potentials in animals also vary; many have more favorable therapeutic indexes than indomethacin and phenylbutazone in acute anti-inflammatory and ulcerogenic assays. Since the predictive value of acute gastric hemorrhage and intestinal perforation assays is semiquantitative at best, more definitive clinical comparisons at equieffective dosages of newer agents are not yet complete. Potency differences among many drugs are mainly in dosage size, rather than overall clinical efficacy. Varying degrees of patient tolerance and duration of action (mostly t.i.d.) have been noted.

The metabolism of substituted phenylpropionic acids involves mainly aromatic or aliphatic hydroxylation followed by glucuronide conjugation of the hydroxy and/or carboxyl group. When a racemic mixture, e.g., ibuprofen, is used, asymmetric metabolism *in vivo* yields a mixture of chiral metabolites. The glucuronides are excreted in the urine and, especially in the case of higher molecular weight aryl acids, undergo an enterohepatic recirculation.

7.4.3 CLINICAL EXPERIENCES (Table 62.7). Ibuprofen is widely used as an aspirin-like antiarthritic drug in the U.S. At 1.2–2.4 g t.i.d. it is a well-tolerated analgesic agent with moderate anti-inflammatory efficacy. It is used as a racemic mixture, since both optical isomers

Table 62.7 Clinical Usage of Some NSAIDS

NSAID	Plasma Level		Average Daily Doses	
	Concn., μg/ml	Half-life, hr	Number	Total Amount
Section 7.1				
Aspirin	150–300	0.25	4	4–8 g
Benorylate (62.**10**)			2	8 g
Diflunisal (62.**11**)			2	0.7–1 g
Section 7.2				
Mefenamic acid (62.**15**)	10–15	4	3	1.5 g
Flufenamic acid (62.**16**)	3–6	4	3	600 mg
Section 7.3				
Indomethacin (62.**5**)	1–3	2	3	75–100 mg
Sulindac (62.**24**)			2	300–400 mg
Active metabolite (62.**25**)	2–6	16		
Section 7.4				
Ibuprofen (62.**37**)	25–50	1–2	3–4	1.6–2.4 g
Fenoprofen (62.**38**)	20–50	2–3	3–4	1.2–2.4 g
Tolmetin (62.**30**)	20–80	0.5–1	3	0.8–1.6 g
Pirprofen (62.**46**)		5	3	3–4 g
Naproxen (62.**52**)	25–75	13	2	500–750 mg
Ketoprofen (62.**55**)	0.5–6	1	3	150 mg
Flurbiprofen (62.**44**)	2–12	6	3–4	150–300 mg
Diclofenac (62.**61**)	0.5–4	4	3–4	75–150 mg
Alclofenac (62.**45**)	50–150	1.25	3–4	3–4 g
Carprofen (62.**54**)	<10	15	3–4	150–300 mg
Section 7.5				
Phenylbutazone (62.**6**)		72	3	300–400 mg
Oxyphenbutazone (62.**67**)		72	3	300–400 mg
Azapropazone (62.**68**)		12	4	1.2 g
Piroxicam (62.**71**)		45	1	20–40 mg

are equipotent in the UV erythema assay. The recently introduced flurbiprofen is its more potent congener with a (*S*)-(+) stereochemical configuration. Flurbiprofen has a pharmacological profile similar to that of indomethacin, but with fewer CNS side effects.

Naproxen has a long serum half-life of 12–15 hr and is given 250 mg twice daily. The b.i.d. dosing schedule is more convenient to patients and leads to better compliance with therapy. It is comparable to full doses of aspirin in rheumatoid arthritis, and more effective than ibuprofen. It causes moderate GI disturbances.

Tolmetin is about 0.4 times the potency of indomethacin in the carrageenin edema assay. In the clinic it is used at 0.8–1.6 g day and is relatively well tolerated by rheumatoid arthritis patients (123). Zomepirac is a more potent congener still under clinical investigation as an analgesic–anti-inflammatory agent. It is active orally at 100–200 mg as a potent analgesic for severe pains in cancer patients. Compared with indomethacin, these pyrrole analogs have somewhat fewer CNS side effects. Headaches or dizziness occurred in 15% of tolmetin-treated patients. Gastrointestinal discomfort is a major complaint (123).

Fenoprofen is the calcium salt of the *dl* acid. At 2.4 g q.i.d. it is as effective as naproxen. The incidence of its GI disturbances is between those of aspirin and ibuprofen.

Ketoprofen is given 150 mg t.i.d. with a clinical efficacy comparable to that of ibuprofen but with more side effects.

In addition to aspirin-like anti-inflammatory–analgesic activities, alclofenac has been reported to reduce the abnormal parameters in rheumatoid arthritis patients, e.g., acute-phase proteins, erythrocyte sedimentation rate, and rheumatoid factor (145). These changes are usually seen only with corticosteroids and "antirheumatic" agents (see below) and not with NSAIDS. Alclofenac is dealkylated and dihydroxylated *in vivo*. An epoxide was postulated as a possible intermediate. The mechanism of action of alclofenac (and its metabolites) is not clear. At 3 g/day alcofenac is comparable to 150 mg indomethacin in long-term trials with similar gastrointestinal side effects. The most important adverse reaction of alclofenac is an allergic type skin rash.

Another unusual aryl alknoic acid is clozic (62.**65**), originally developed as a congener of the antilipidemic drug clofibrate (62.**66**). Like indomethacin, clozic inhibits the synthesis of acute phase proteins and connective tissue turnover in adjuvant arthritic rats (169). However, clozic has neither analgesic effect nor anti-inflammatory activity in animal models. It is re-

ported to improve the clinical state of rheumatoid arthritis patients, accompanied by a fall in erythrocyte sedimentation rate, serum C-reactive protein and fibrinogen, after 2 months of treatment in preliminary clinical trials (170).

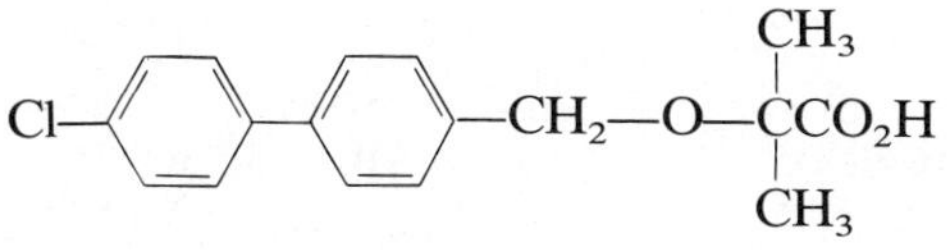

7.5 Enolic and Other Acidic Agents (171, 172)

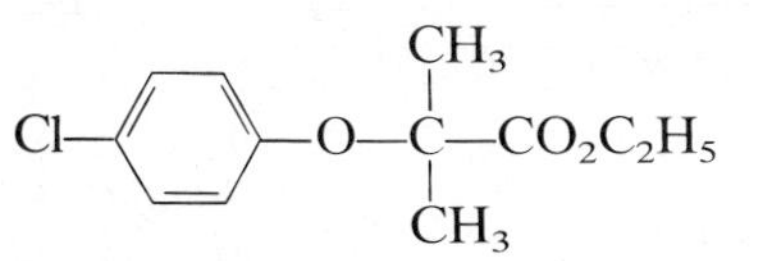

Another group of aromatic anti-inflammatory agents possesses ionizable protons from an enolic or potentially enolic β-diketones. The acidity of these compounds, pK_a 4–7, is comparable to various carboxylic groups. The slower rate of glucuronide conjugation of the enolic group prolongs the half-life of these compounds *in vivo*. The presence of two aryl moieties provides the lipophilic characteristics for protein binding and tissue distribution. Two prominent groups are pyrazolidinediones, e.g., phenylbutazone (62.**6**) (173) and azapropazone (62.**68**) (174, 175), and hydroxybenzothiazines (176), e.g., piroxicam (62.**71**) (177). The pharmacological profiles of these compounds are generally similar to those NSAIDS possessing a carboxylic acid function. They are also prostaglandin synthesis inhibitors. However, some biochemical differences in their modes of action have been noted.

7.5.1 PYRAZOLIDINEDIONES (172, 173). The serendipitous discovery of phenylbutazone in the clinic as a potent anti-inflammatory agent in the 1940s was perhaps the second milestone, since aspirin, in the progress of NSAIDS. It also served as a valuable reference standard in the development of pharmacological assays for newer NSAIDS. The acidity of phenylbutazone, pK_a 4.5, the long half-life, 72 hr in man, and the non-planar arrangement of the two phenyl rings, in retrospect, all signify important clues in the search for newer agents. In spite of their apparent chemical differences, the similarity in stereochemical configurations

62.**65** Clozic

62.**66** Clofibrate

between phenylbutazone, indomethacin, and fenamates was noted.

The pharmacological profiles of phenylbutazone and other enolic compounds are summarized in Table 62.6 Gastrointestinal irritation and low incidence of hematologic disorders like agranulocytosis are major side effects.

Two principal metabolites of phenylbutazone are formed in the liver; one by hydroxylation of the butyl side chain and the other by hydroxylation of the para position of one of the phenyl rings. The latter compound is oxyphenbutazone (62.**67**), which has a potency comparable to that of phenylbutazone but is slightly better tolerated.

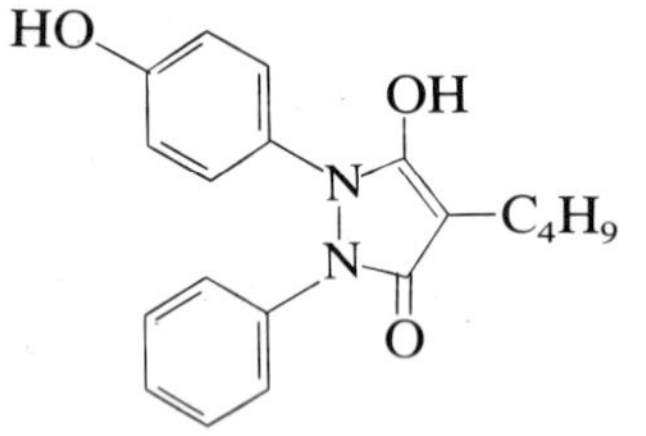

62.**67**   Oxyphenbutazone

Increasing the acidity of phenylbutazone analogs decreases their serum half-life but increases their uricosuric activity. Sulfinpyrazone (62.**3**), with a pK_a of 2.8 is used as a uricosuric agent. It also inhibits platelet aggregation *in vivo*. The corresponding sulfide metabolite is more active *in vitro* as an inhibitor of prostaglandin synthetase and platelet aggregation.

Phenylbutazone is only moderately active in various animal models (see Table 62.6). Possibly because of its long half-life and tissue accumulation the clinical efficacy of 400–600 mg phenylbutazone per day is generally considered to be equivalent to that of 100–150 mg indomethacin and more effective than many phenylpropionic acids. Studies related to phenylbutazone and various analogs have been extensively reviewed.

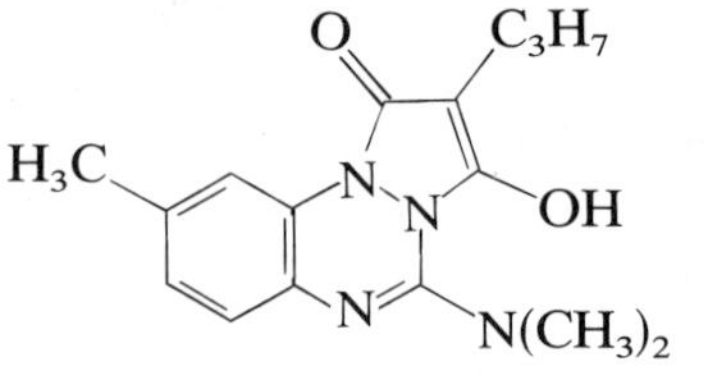

62.**68**   Azapropazone

A pyrazolo benzotriazinedione derivative, azapropazone (62.**68**), may be considered as a complex ring-fused pyrazolidinedione. It is similar to phenylbutazone in potency in animal assays (174). It has a short half-life in man, $8\frac{1}{2}$–12 hr, and is used at 600–1200 mg/day to achieve an anti-inflammatory effect comparable to that of phenylbutazone. Side effects in man include modest incidence of gastric symptoms and exanthema with pruritis. The chemical reactivity of azapropazone toward various nucleophiles *in vitro* has been noted. Azapropazone has been reported to stabilize lysosome membrane *in vitro* (175).

7.5.2   4 - HYDROXY - 1,2 - BENZOTHIAZINES. Following earlier studies of 2-aryl-1,3-indandiones and 1,3-dioxoisoquinoline-4-carboxanilides as anti-inflammatory agents, the 1,2-benzothiazine analogs were found to be highly potent compounds (176, 177). The acidic enolate anion is stabilized by internal hydrogen bonding with the amide proton. Their pK_a values, as measured in 2:1 dioxane–water, are in the range of 5–6. These studies led to investigation of the 4-hydroxy analog W 7477 (62.**69**), which is comparable to phenylbutazone in potency (178, 179). More important, continuation of the effort culminated with the development of sudoxicam (62.**70**), and piroxicam (62.**71**), which are *N*-heterocyclic (2-thiazolyl) and (2-pyridyl) carboxamides of 4-hydroxy-2*H*-1,2-benzothiazine 1,1-dioxide, respectively (180). The enolate of piroxicam may be stabilized in two tautomeric forms.

In the carrageenin edema and adjuvant arthritis models, piroxicam is approximately 0.4 times as potent as indomethacin

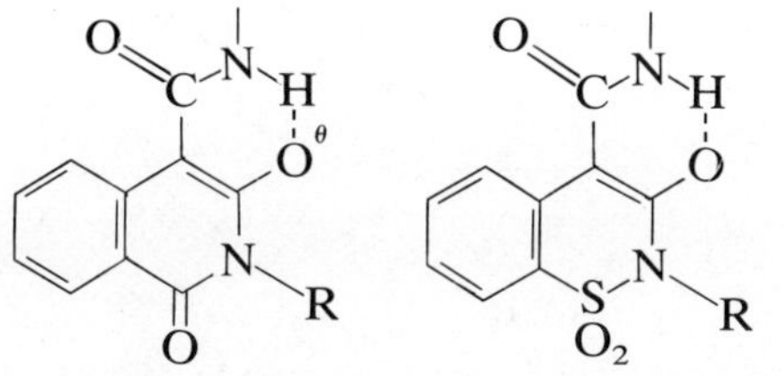

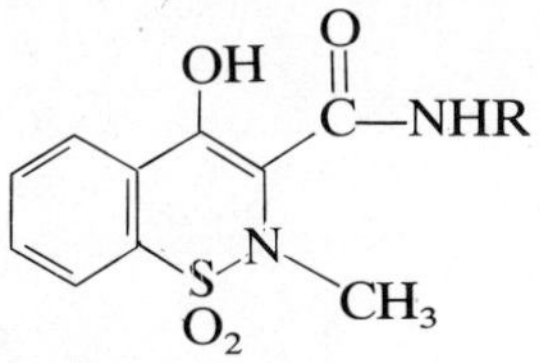

62.**69** R =

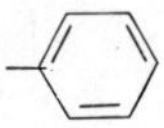

62.**70** R =

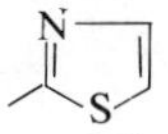

62.**71** R =

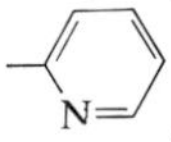

62.**72** R =

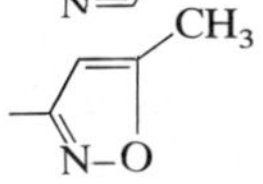

and 14 times as phenylbutazone. It is also a prostaglandin synthetase inhibitor. The metabolism of piroxicam involves mainly hydroxylations in the phenyl and pyridyl rings, hydrolysis of the N-pyridyl amide linkage, and conjugation of these metabolites. The plasma half-life of piroxicam varies extensively in different species. It is shorter in the rat and monkey (6–8 hr) than in the dog and man (35–50 hr). Thus a single 20–40 mg daily dose of piroxicam in man leads to stable plasma concentrations which are maintained throughout the day (181). In man and monkey, plasma concentrations of sudoxicam are not affected by concurrent administration of aspirin, presumably without significant interactions. An initial clinical study of sudoxicam was terminated by some hepatotoxicity observed in patients. The clinical efficacy of piroxicam in rheumatoid arthritis, osteoarthritis, and ankylosing spondylitis is comparable to other NSAIDS. No serious side effects have been reported.

The overall drug efficacy is related to its (intrinsic potency) × (area under the curve of plasma level) over a period of time. The successful application of piroxicam as a 20–40 mg once a day therapy clearly exemplifies the importance of pharmacokinetic considerations in drug development.

The 5-methyl-3-isoxolyl analog, isoxicam (62.**72**), was independently developed as a moderately active (3 × phenylbutazone) and long-acting anti-inflammatory agent with a low degree of ulcerogenicity in animals (182).

7.5.3 SULFONAMIDES (183). The bioequivalence of sulfonamide, RSO_2NH_2, with carboxylic acid, RCO_2H, is well demonstrated by the classical example of using sulfonilamide as an antagonist of p-aminobenzoic acid. However, in the study of aryl acidic NSAIDS replacement of the carboxyl (pK_a 3–5) by sulfonamide (pK_a 8–10) invariably loses activity. Stimulated by the highly electronegative (Hammet $\sigma = 1.3$) and lipophilic ($\pi = 0.95$) characters of the CF_3SO_2 group, a series of fluoroalkane sulfonyl anilides $RC_6H_4NHSO_2R_f$ were investigated. Both the acidity and lipophilicity of these compounds can be progressively increased from $R_f = CH_2F$, to CHF_2, to CF_3, although no correlation was discernible with their biologic activities. Diflumidone sodium (62.**73**), was comparable to phenylbutazone in anti-inflammatory potency but showed hepatotoxicity in preliminary clinical trials. A successor, R-805 (62.**74**), was found to possess greater potency in animal models (184).

In conjunction with their potential application as plant growth regulants, approxi-

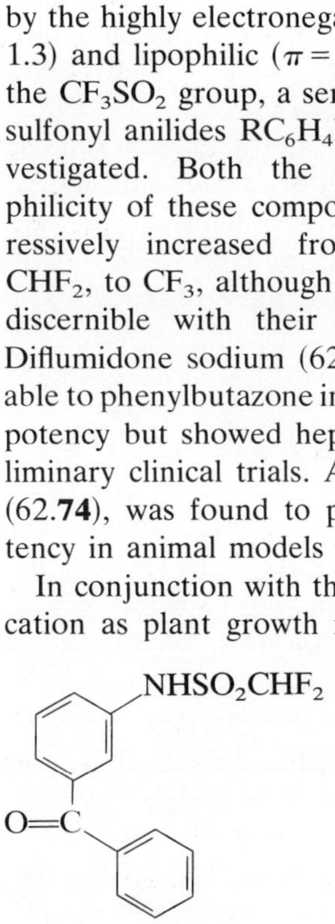

62.**73** Diflumidone

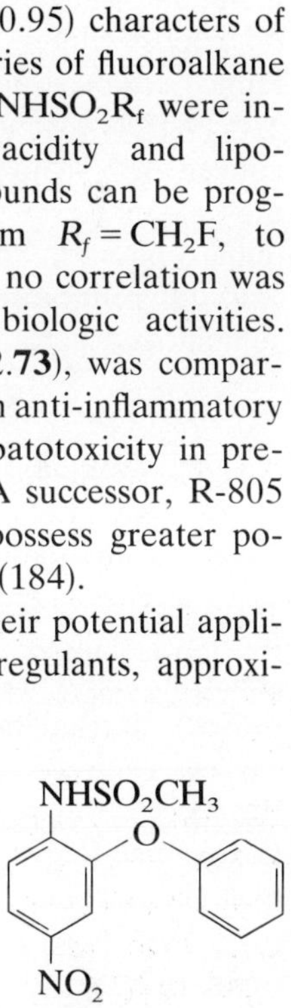

62.**74** R-805

mately 2500 compounds, including a diverse series of heterocyclic isosteres, have been synthesized and screened for anti-inflammatory activity (185, 186).

8   NONACIDIC ANTI-INFLAMMATORY AGENTS (187, 188)

Following an extensive study of anti-inflammatory aryl acids, a number of nonacidic compounds have also been found to have promising activities. Compared with aryl acids, their pharmacological profiles are more structure-dependent and they generally produce less gastrointestinal irritation. Even without a carboxyl group, some are potent prostaglandin synthetase inhibitors. The pharmacokinetics, e.g., oral absorption, serum protein binding, and tissue distribution, of nonacidic agents are much less pH dependent. Some nonacidic structures may also circumvent the usual metabolic patterns of aryl acids and thus offer possibilities for more selective systemic or topical applications.

A variety of nonacidic agents may be conveniently categorized as anti-inflammatory–analgesic substituted triaryls and quinazolinones. A miscellaneous group with different biochemical properties is also summarized here.

8.1   Substituted Triaryls

Several combinations of three aryl groups, such as two phenyl and a five-membered heterocycle, in a fused or angular stereochemical configuration have been found to possess anti-inflammatory activities. The earliest example in this group is indoxole (62.**75**), 2,3-di-*p*-anisyl indole (189). Indoxole was found to have phenylbutazone-like activities but caused photosensitivity in man. Two more potent analogs are bimetopyrol (62.**76**) (190) and flumizole (62.**77**) (191). Flumizole is poorly soluble in water.

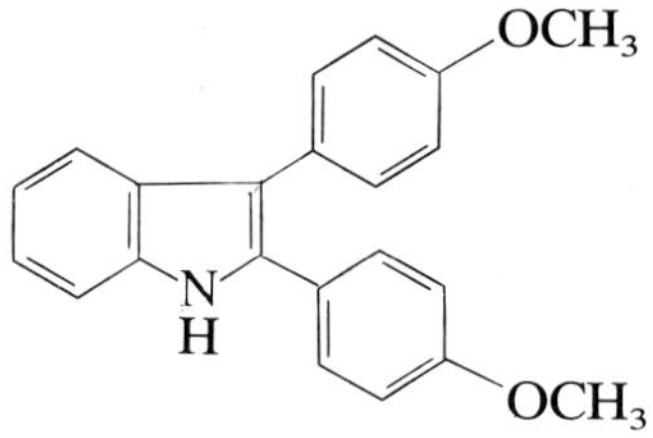

62.**75**   Indoxole

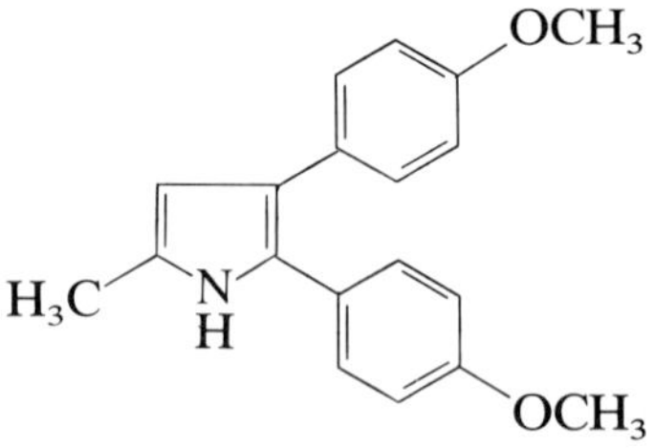

62.**76**   Bimetopyrol

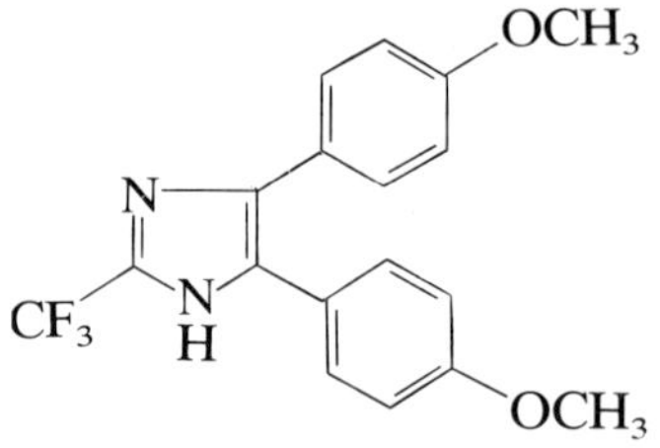

62.**77**   Flumizole

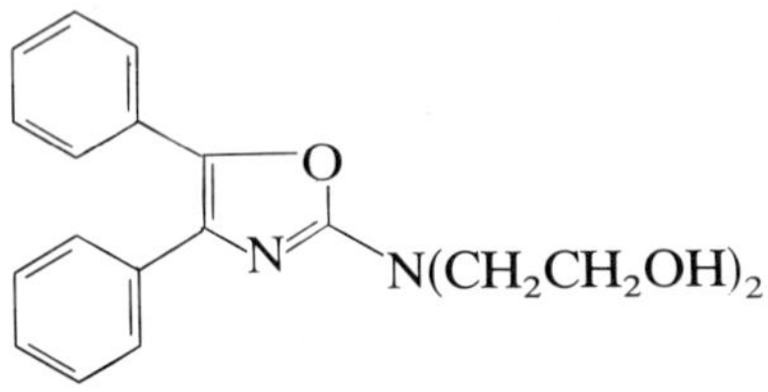

62.**78**   Ditazole

Its potency in the rat paw edema assay is variable but estimated to be higher than indomethacin.

Ditazole (62.**78**) is a less active anti-inflammatory–analgesic agent which also inhibits platelet aggregation (192). Ditazole has the interesting property of entering preferentially into the brain after i.v. injection in rats (193).

Thiabendazole (62.**79**), an anthelmintic and antifungal agent, also has moderate anti-inflammatory and analgesic activities.

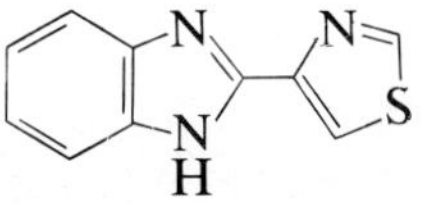

62.**79** Thiabendazole

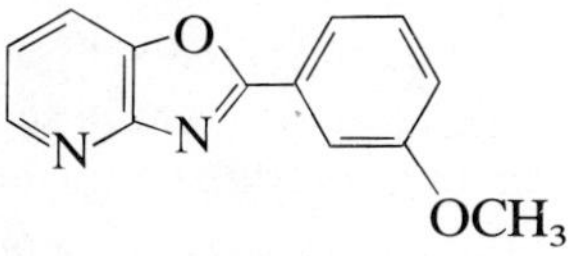

62.**80**

Further examination of this type of phenyl heteroaryls led to the synthesis of 2-substituted phenyl oxazolopyridines (62.**80**) (194). Several members in this series are comparable to indomethacin as cyclo-oxygenase inhibitors *in vitro*, and as topical anti-inflammatory agents in the guinea pig UV erythema assay. Among these, several are rapidly inactivated *in vivo* and are devoid of systemic activity as well as side effects (188).

8.2 Quinazolinones

The activity of quinazolinones was observed early. Among various analogs studied proquazone (62.**81**) is active in animal models at 5 mg/kg (195, 196) and effective against rheumatoid arthritis in man at 300 mg t.i.d. (197). Some gastrointestinal disturbances are also noted. It is four times more potent than aspirin as an analgesic agent with a comparable duration of action. A similar analog is ciproquazone (SL 573,

62.**81** Proquazone

62.**82**), which is comparable to phenylbutazone in potency at 50–100 mg/kg (198). SL-573 is a reversible inhibitor of prostaglandin synthetase *in vitro* at 1 μg/ml. It protects the enzyme against irreversible inactivation by aspirin (199).

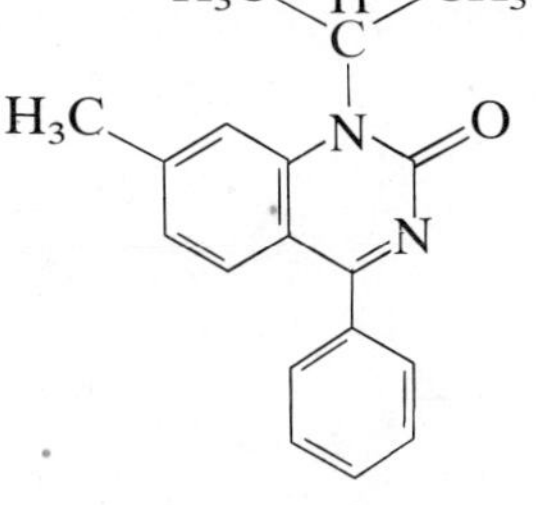

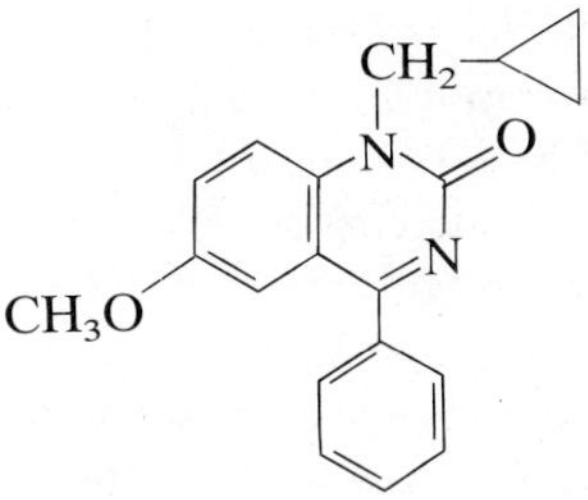

62.**82** Ciproquazone

8.3 Others

Diftalone (62.**83**) is a nonacidic moderately active anti-inflammatory compound (200). It is used at 0.5–1 g doses in the clinic with little gastrointestinal blood loss. Plasma concentrations of diftalone, and possibly its therapeutic activity, in some patients are decreased by induction of hepatic microsomal enzymes after repeated administration (201).

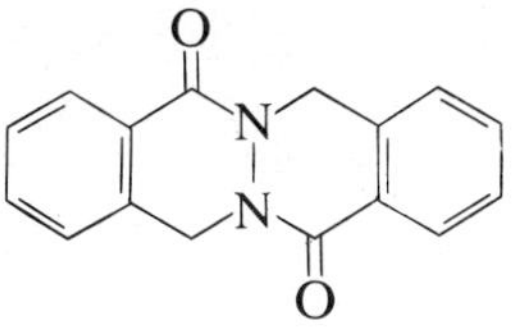

62.**83** Diftalone

Tribenoside (62.**84**) is an unique saccharide derivative possessing a wide spectrum of pharmacological activities (202). It is considered as a vasoprotective agent with modest anti-inflammatory and analgesic properties. It also enhances microcirculation, wound healing, and membrane stability. Its antirheumatic potential remains to be established (203).

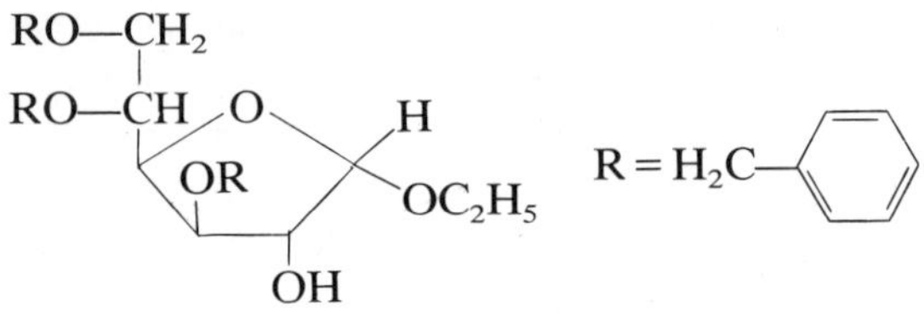

62.**84** Tribenoside

$R = H_2C$—⟨benzene ring⟩

The nicotinoyl indole, nictindole (L-8027, 62.**85**), became of interest as a research tool by virtue of its inhibition of thromboxane synthetase at 10^{-4} M in $vitro$ (204). At slightly higher levels it also inhibits cyclooxygenase. The in $vivo$ anti-inflammatory activity of nictindole is comparable to that of phenylbutazone. No special advantage seems to be attributable to its inhibition of thromboxane synthetase. 1-(Carboxyheptyl)imidazole (62.**86**) is a more selective thromboxane synthetase inhibitor in $vitro$ at 1 μM (204).

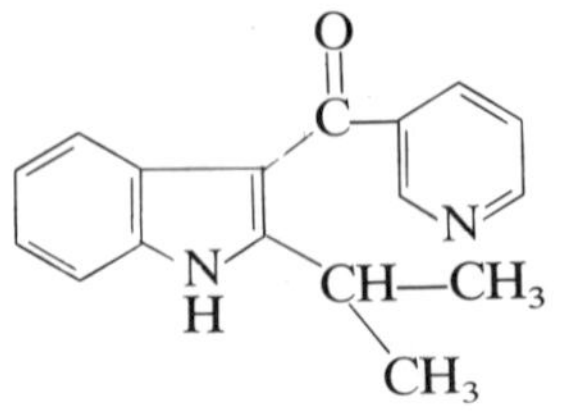

62.**85** Nictindole

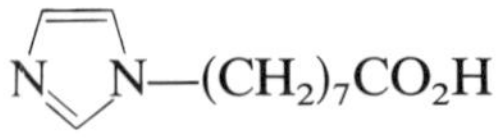

62.**86**

9 ANTIRHEUMATICS

The anti-inflammatory–analgesic NSAIDS discussed above provide symptomatic relief of the pain and swelling associated with arthritic diseases. They may slow down but do not stop or reverse the progression of the underlying pathogenic process. The laboratory search for therapeutic agents with more fundamental actions has long been stymied by the lack of understanding

of the complex pathogenic mechanisms of arthritis and by the lack of really useful animal models. In recent years extensive investigations of rheumatoid arthritis have generated hypotheses of the pathogenesis cycle (Fig. 62.5) (205).

A vicious circle is propelled by a persistent immunologic response, generating immune complex (rheumatoid factor) of an autoimmune nature. The ensuing complement fixation and cellular responses involving lymphocytes, PMN, and macrophages lead to the release of inflammatory mediators and the degradative lysosomal hydrolases. Thus an immune-based inflammatory and degenerative cycle is perpetrated. This type of working hypothesis has helped to relate various abnormal cellular and humoral parameters observed in rheumatic patients and to rationalize the possible mode of action of several classes of drugs whose antirheumatic effects were discovered in the clinic. Because of the slow onset of their beneficial effects, they have been collectively termed slow-acting antirheumatic drugs or SAARDS. The discovery of these clinical leads, in spite of their side effects, has provided an optimism and encouragement to antirheumatic research (206, 207).

9.1 Gold Preparations (206, 207)

The rationale for chrysotherapy in the treatment of rheumatoid arthritis was based on the similarity of some manifestations between tuberculosis and rheumatoid arthritis in early clinical observations. Gold thioglucose (62.**87**) was first used in 1927 to relieve joint pain but the efficacy of gold

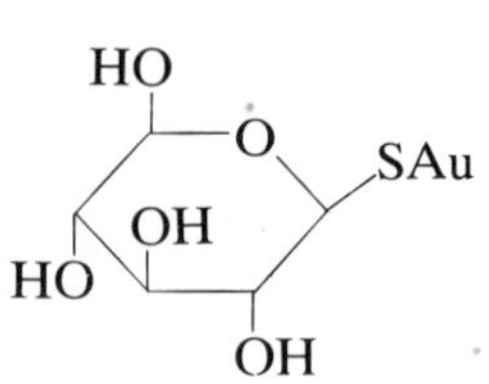

62.**87** Gold thioglucose

$$CO_2HCH(SAu)CH_2CO_2H$$

62.**88**   Sodium aurothiomalate

preparations in treating rheumatoid arthritis was not firmly established until a large-scale double-blind study with sodium aurothiomalate (62.**88**) by the British Empire Rheumatism Council in 1961. Positive radiological evidence showed that chrysotherapy significantly slowed the progression of the disease in joints.

The mechanism of action of gold derivatives is not clear. Because gold compounds interact with various proteins, the following actions related to inflammation have been observed:

1. Stabilization of collagen vs. collagenases.
2. Inhibition of lysosomal enzymes.
3. Prevention of denaturation of macroglobulins and formation of antigen–antibody complexes.
4. Uncoupling of oxidative phosphorylation.
5. Inhibition of leukocyte chemotaxis.

In the adjuvant arthritis assay, gold sodium thiomalate inhibits the development of both primary and secondary lesions at 5–10 mg/kg.

The systemic toxicity in man of gold compounds involve skin, mucous membranes, liver, kidney, and other organs. Various forms of dermatitis often appear after a cumulative dose of 300–400 mg. More serious but less frequent side effects are blood dyscrasias, hepatitis, and nephrotic syndromes such as proteinuria and hematuria. Ocular toxicities have also been observed.

An orally absorbed gold preparation auranofin (SK & F D-39162) (62.**89**) has been developed recently (208). Low oral doses of a gold preparation given daily are more convenient and may produce more steady blood levels and less renal gold accumulation than weekly injection of higher doses. In laboratory systems auranofin inhibits the production of antibodies and the release of lysosomal enzymes from phagocytizing PMN leukocytes, and inhibits PMN-mediated antibody-dependent cellular cytotoxicity of target cells. It also inhibits adjuvant arthritis in rats on oral administration. At doses of 3 mg b.i.d. auranofin was found to be clinically effective with gastrointestinal disturbances as main adverse effects (209).

In man auranofin increases serum albumin/globulin ratios and decreases α-2 globulin, rheumatoid factor titers, sedimentation rate, and the level of IgG. These chemical and immunologic parameters, as

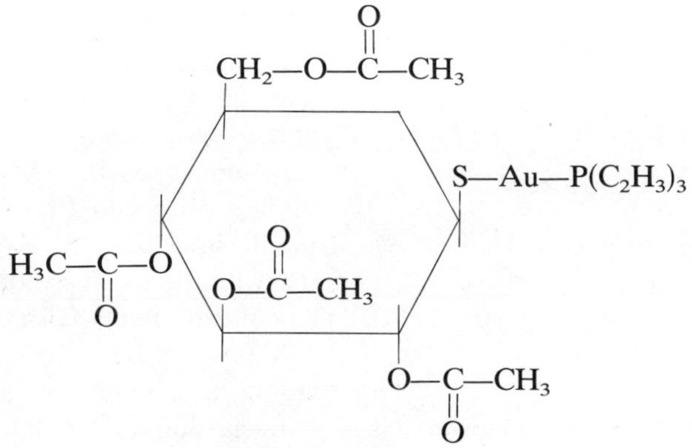

62.**89**   Auranofin

well as clinical improvements in joint swelling and functions, persisted 2–3 months after the treatment was stopped (210).

9.2 Antimalarials

9.2.1 CHLOROQUINE. Chronic adminstration of the antimalarial chloroquine diphosphate (62.**90**) (211) at 250 mg daily produces a useful suppression of disease activities in two out of three rheumatoid arthritis patients, though not in other types of arthritis. Significant reductions of the erythrocyte sedimentation rate (ESR) and rheumatoid factor (RF) titer are achieved but no changes in radiological manifestations are observed. Unfortunately, the usefulness of chloroquine is limited by its dose-related ocular toxicities; both corneal and retinal changes have been reported. It also causes occasional gastrointestinal disturbances and skin rashes. Chloroquine is also useful in mild cases of systemic lupus erythematosus (SLE). It exacerbates psoriasis.

The mode of action of chloroquine is unknown. It is lysosomotropic and accumulates in lysosomes to inhibit hydrolytic enzymes. It stabilizes lysosomal membrane *in vitro* and affects various membrane-related cellular responses. *In vivo*, chloroquine may protect cartilage and collagen against degradation. It is neither analgesic nor anti-inflammatory in animal models at nontoxic levels.

Hydroxychloroquine has similar properties.

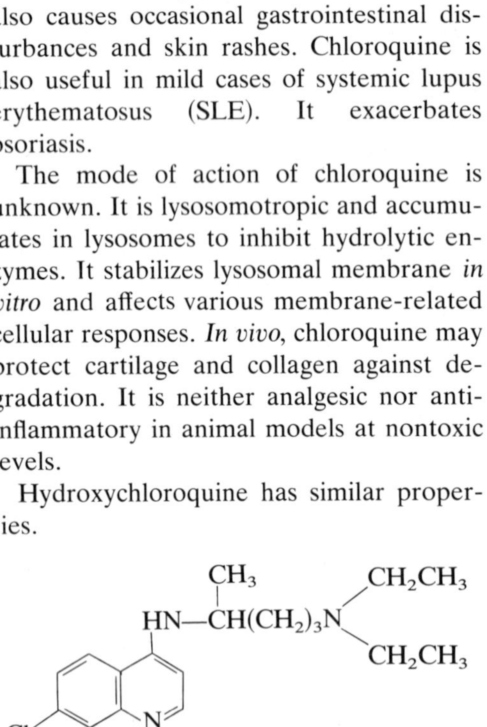

62.**90** Chloroquine

9.2.2 DAPSONE (212, 213). Dapsone is an established antimalarial and antileprotic agent. It suppresses inflamma-tion in the carrageenin edema, cotton pellet granuloma, and adjuvant arthritis models at 100–200 mg/kg, and inhibits zymosan-induced release of lysosomal hydrolases from rat peritoneal macrophages at $>10^{-5}\,M$. The antipyretic and peripheral analgesic activities of dapsone are similar to those produced by phenylbutazone. Dapsone does not appear to be ulcerogenic in rats. It has been reported to be an effective antirheumatic agent in man; however, further development of dapsone derivatives is shadowed by the potential carcinogenic effect of dapsone in animals.

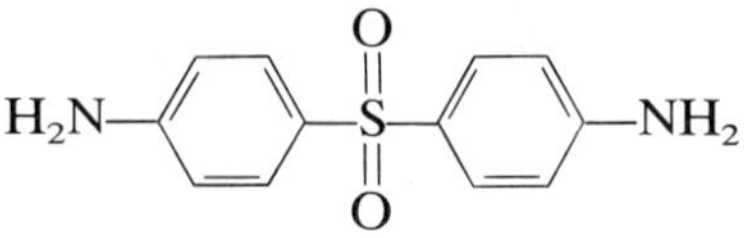

62.**91** Dapsone

9.3 D-Penicillamine and Other Sulfhydryl Compunds

9.3.1 D-PENICILLAMINE. D-Penicillamine (62.**92**) (214) is a degradation product of penicillin originally developed to promote urinary copper excretion for the treatment of Wilson's disease in man. It dissociates macroglobulins, e.g., rheumatoid factor (RF) *in vitro*. However, *in vivo* the reduction of circulating RF is achieved only after 6 months of therapy and is not correlated with the clinical response (215). The effectiveness of D-penicillamine has been demonstrated in multiple well-controlled studies. At 0.5–1 g daily it reduces the pain and duration of morning stiffness, and increases grip strength, articular index, and functional capacity. The maximum improvement is produced after 4–6 months of treatment in 75% of rheumatoid arthritic (R.A.) patients. It is comparable to gold in its clinical effects (216, 217).

Many serious toxicities of D-penicillamine are immunologic in nature. Proteinuria due to immune-complex nephritis occurs in 15% of patients. Skin rashes and thrombocytopenia are other common side

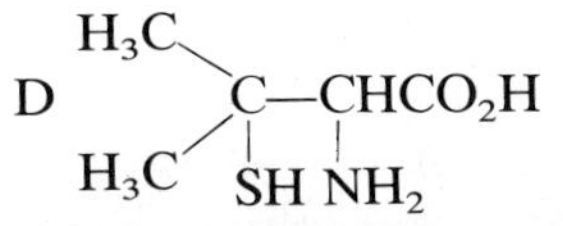

62.**92**   D-Penicillamine

effects. D-Penicillamine also induces a low incidence of SLE, myasthenia gravis, and other autoimmune syndromes (218).

Attempts to find a less toxic D-penicill-amine have long been hampered by the lack of suitable laboratory models and a poor understanding of the mechanism of its antirheumatic action. D-Penicillamine has shown a variety of *in vitro* actions. A synergistic inhibition of mitogen-induced lymphocyte proliferation by D-penicillamine and copper salts was noted recently (219). However, their significance to the *in vivo* beneficial effects remains unclear. In animal studies, D-penicillamine is inactive in the acute anti-inflammatory–analgesic assays. It has no effect on the primary lesions of adjuvant arthritis but exacerbates the disease when given just prior to the development of the secondary lesions (from tenth day postinjection of the adjuvant). It appears that D-penicillamine may enhance the cell-mediated immunity in the protocol (220). Similar enhancement of delayed hypersensitivity is seen in the pertussis pleurisy assay in sensitized animals (221). Cell-mediated immune responses are depressed in R.A. patients. An increase of their skin reaction to tuberculin after treatment with D-penicillamine has also been noted. Whether this type of immune stimulation would facilitate the removal of persistent antigenic substance and suppress the chronic inflammation in R.A. remains to be determined.

9.3.2 MERCAPTOPYRIDOXINE   DERIVATIVES. Some of the *in vitro* properties of D-penicillamine may be attributable to its sulfhydryl group. Among a few sulfhydryl compounds explored in early clinical experiments, the 5-mercaptomethyl analog of pyridoxine (62.**93**) and its disulfide,

pyrithioxin (62.**94**), have been found to possess D-penicillamine-like efficacy as well as side effects (222, 223).

A new analog, the 4-mercaptomethyl-5-vinyl analog of pyridoxine (MK-159, 62.**95**), is comparable to phenylbutazone in the adjuvant arthritis assay and is more potent than 5-mercaptopyridoxine (62.**93**) in suppressing inflammation induced by a dermal lymphokine in guinea pig assays (224).

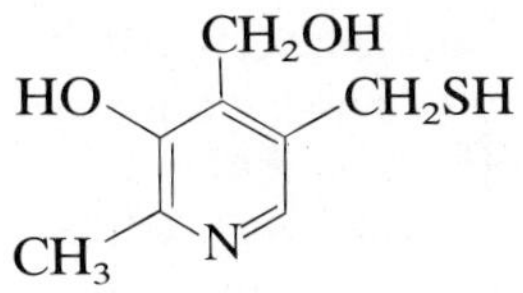

62.**93**   5-MP

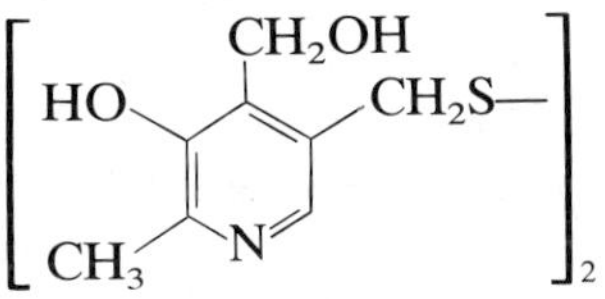

62.**94**   Pyrithioxin

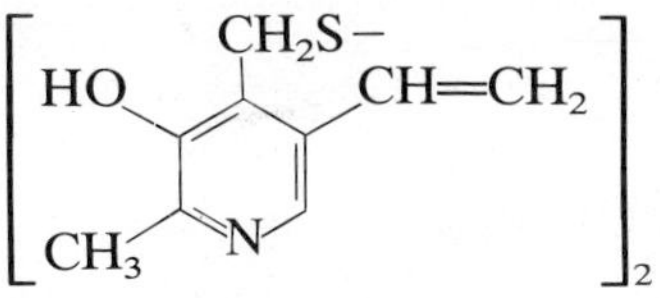

62.**95**   MK-159

9.4   Immunostimulants

9.4.1 LEVAMISOLE (62.**96**).   Levamisole is a broad-spectrum anthelmintic agent with immunostimulatory properties (225). Its delayed antirheumatic action in man is similar to that of D-penicillamine, both in efficacy and in time course. Levamisole responders have significant relief of pain and reduction in the duration of morning stiffness, number of tender joints, and joint swelling, accompanied by reduction in ESR and RF titer. Peak effects are reached after 4 months of treatment. There are also significant depression of total white cell count

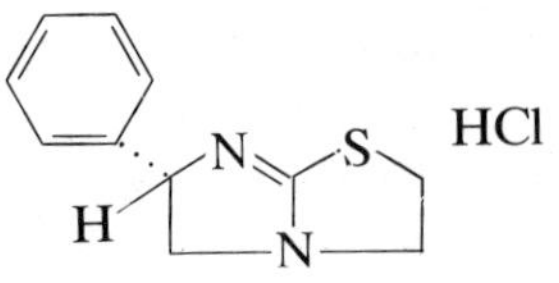

62.**96** Levamisole

and IgG level and a rise in hemoglobin
(226, 227).

Levamisole also produces serious adverse
reactions. An upredictable and dangerous
leukopenia limits its use. Other side effects
such as rashes, mouth ulcers, nausea, and
disturbance of taste are similar to those
produced by D-penicillamine.

As an immune stimulant, levamisole enhances the secondary lesions of adjuvant
arthritis and the inflammatory response in
pertussis vaccine pleurisy. It restores the
depressed delayed hypersensitivity skin
reactions to tuberculin in old age and in
cancer patients and enhances macrophage
phagocytosis. Some reported effects of
levamisole on lymphocyte function and
other immunologic systems are highly sensitive to variations of dosage and experimental conditions. Some of the *in vivo*

effects may also be attributable to its
metabolite(s).

Levamisole is well absorbed orally and
extensively metabolized. Four initial
metabolic transformations have been identified (228). These are hydroxylation at the
para position of the phenyl ring and at C_2,
dehydrogenation of the dihydroimidazole
ring (Δ^5), and hydrolysis of the pseudo-
thiourea linkage. Combinations of these
conversions and subsequent oxidation,
methylation, and conjugation of the intermediates lead to a multitude of metabolites
(Fig. 62.15). Their biologic properties remain to be clarified.

The curious structural overlap of anthel-
mintics with potential antiarthritics is
further demonstrated by the anthelmintic–
antifungal thiabendazole (62.**79,** see Section 8.1 above) (229), R-17934 (62.**97**)
(230), and frenazole (62.**98**) (231). Some
immunostimulatory activity of thiabendazole and frenazole in laboratory systems
has been reported. R-17934 was reported
to inhibit microtubule assembly and tumor
metastasis.

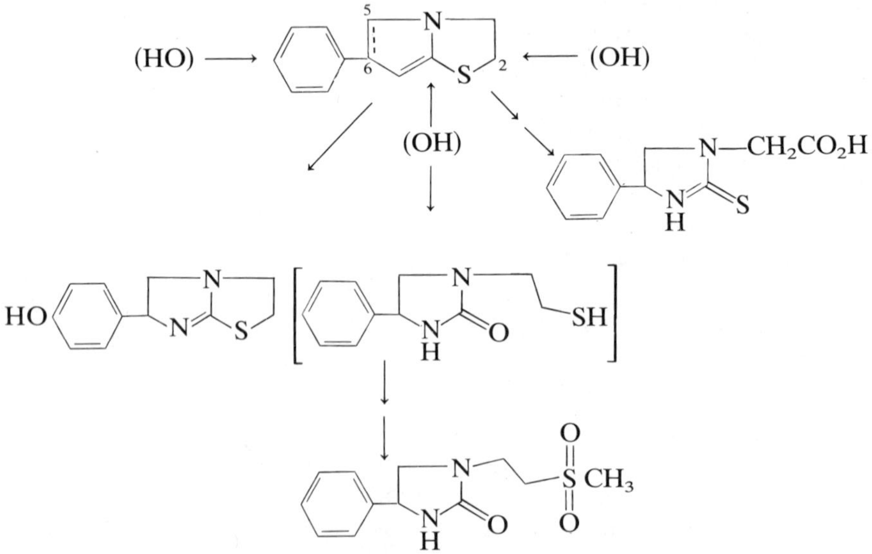

Levamisole metabolites

Fig. 62.15 Metabolism of levamisole.

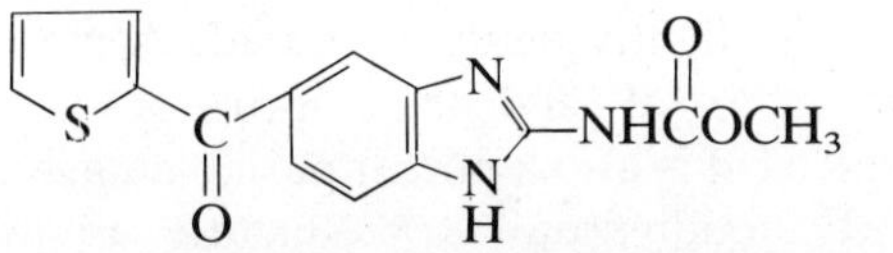

62.**97** R-17934

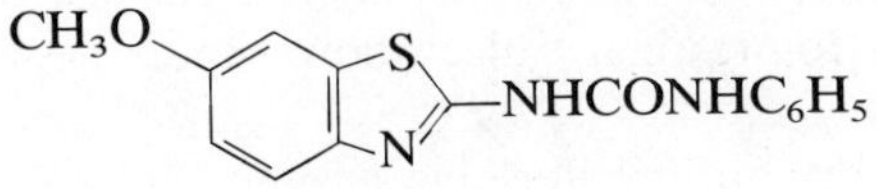

62.**98** Frenazole

9.5 Immunosuppressants

Considering the immunologic nature of chronic inflammation, the therapeutic potential of immunosuppressants including corticosteroids, alkylating agents, and antimetabolites has been well investigated (232, 233). Since many immunologic processes are cell surface phenomena, agents affecting the function of membrane components, such as inhibitors of microtubules, colchicine, and vinblastin, may also be considered as immunosuppressants in a broad sense.

As in cancer therapy, the clinical application of these potent cytotoxic drugs is limited by their low therapeutic indexes and potential side effects. Depression of host resistance to bacterial and viral infections and increasing tumorogenesis are the most serious concerns. With the progressive development in immunology, more selective and safer immunoregulants, e.g., the natural product cyclosporin A, will undoubtedly be discovered in the coming years.

9.5.1 ALKYLATING AGENTS. Among numerous alkylating agents (234), chlorambucil (62.**99**) and cyclophosphamide (62.**100**) are

62.**99** Chlorambucil

most commonly used in rheumatoid arthritis (235). In addition to potential toxicities mentioned above, alopecia and cystitis are the main side effects of cyclophosphamide. Several cytotoxic metabolites from the oxidative cleavage of the ring in cyclophosphamide have been identified, e.g., 62.**101** and 62.**102** (236).

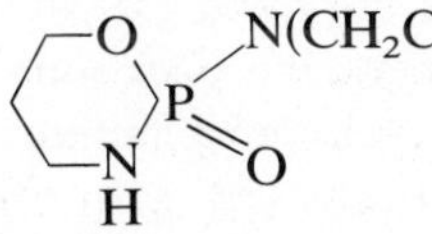

62.**100** Cyclophosphamide

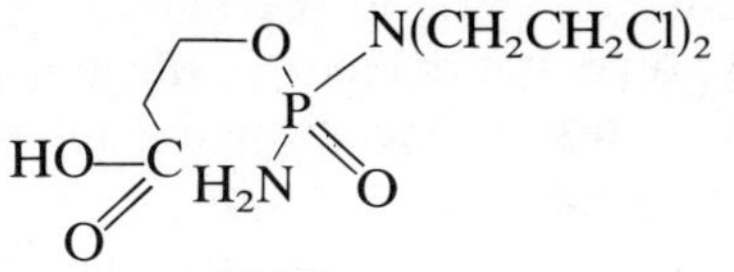

62.**101**

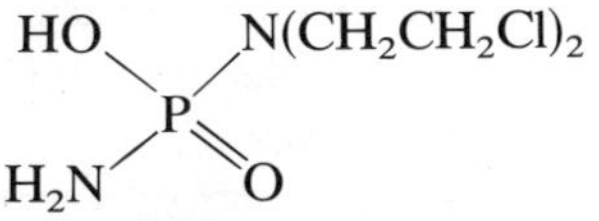

62.**102**

Cytoxan metabolites

Alkylating agents are "cycle nonspecific," being effective against both dividing and intermitotic cells. Their antiproliferative effect on leukocytes and connective tissue cells may also contribute to their overall beneficial and toxic effects. Two sites of action of alkylating agents can be distinguished, within the cell nucleus and at the cell membrane. Factors influencing the relative specificity of alkylating agents are the following:

1. Chemical reactivity of the alkylating group (e.g., ethylenimine, epoxide, activated olefin, sulfhydryl reagents).
2. Physicochemical characteristics of the backbone, which influences the pharmacokinetics and membrane permeability of the drug.

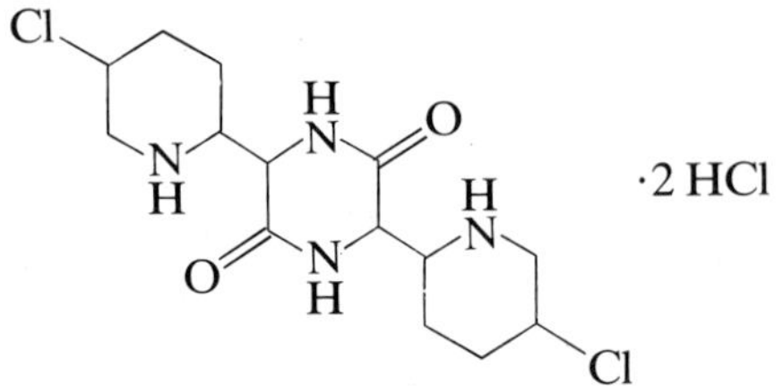

62.**103**   593A

For example, antibiotic 593A (62.**103**) with a diketopiperazine backbone is effective against cyclophosphamide-resistant leukemia L1210 cells (237). In principle, a nonpermeable alkylating agent may inactivate enzymes or receptors on the cell surface but not DNA in the nucleus. It may achieve a greater degree of cellular specificity by virtue of the changing membrane characteristics of different cell types. Chemical ligands, e.g., peptides, carbohydrates, and lipids with specificity for cell surface receptors may also be used as backbone structures for selective alkylating, or irreversible, inactivators.

9.5.2 ANTIMETABOLITES. The purine antimetabolite, 6-mercaptopurine (6-MP, 62.**104**) is useful in the treatment of chronic inflammation (238). Azathioprine

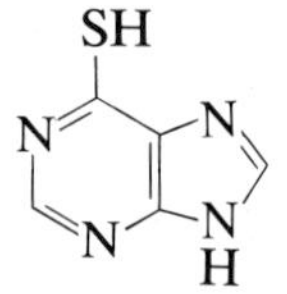

62.**104**   6-MP 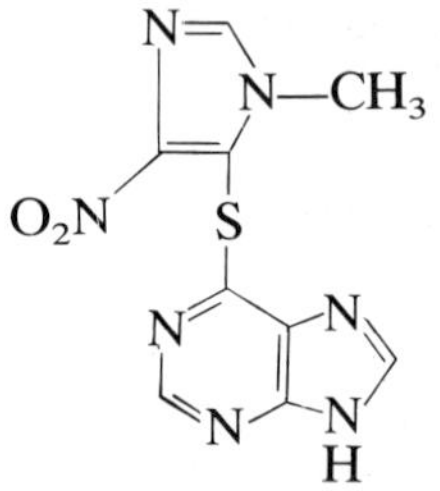   62.**105**   Azathioprine

(62.**105**), which liberates 6-MP *in vivo* by the action of plasma or cellular sulfhydryl groups, is equally effective at 3 mg/kg daily

and is slightly better tolerated. A metabolite of 6-MP and azathioprine, 6-thioinosinic acid is also a potent purine antagonist.

The dihydrofolate reductase inhibitor methotrexate (62.**106**) has been used in severe arthritis. A wider application is discouraged by its serious side effects, oral and gastrointestinal ulceration and hepatic damage.

The antiproliferative antimetabolites are "cycle-specific"; i.e., they are primarily active against cells in the S (DNA synthetic) or M (mitotic) phase of their cell cycle. A generalized leukopenia is produced by clinically effective doses, but they appear to be more toxic to stimulated lymphocytes and suppress the elaboration of lymphokines. In addition, 6-MP and azathioprine also suppress nonimmunologic inflammations in the animal models.

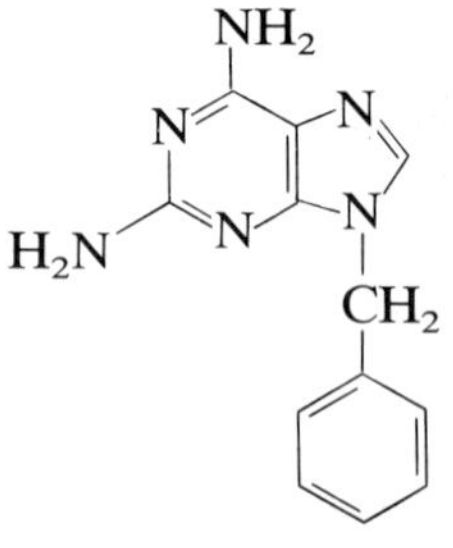

62.**107** 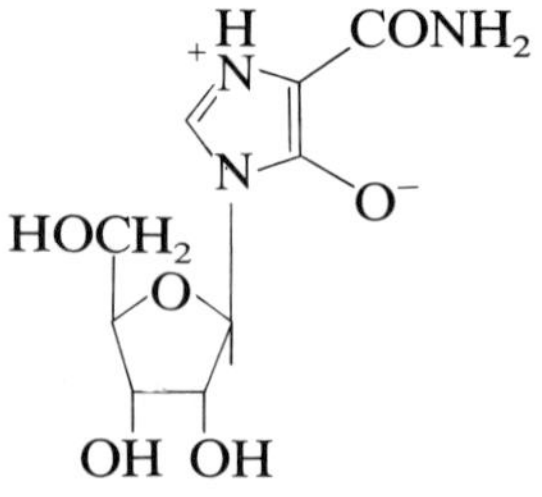   62.**108**   Bredinin

Other purine and pyrimidine antimetabolites, such as 2-amino-9-benzyl adenosine (62.**107**) analogs (239) and antibiotic bredinin (62.**108**) (240), have been reported to possess immunosuppressive activity in various laboratory models.

9.5.3 MICROTUBULAR INHIBITORS (241, 242). Colchicine (62.**4**), an alkaloid from *Colchicum autumnale*, is an established

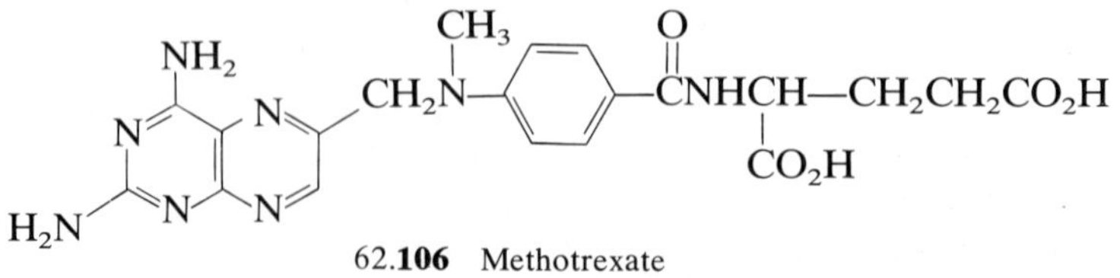

62.**106**   Methotrexate

treatment for acute gout. Various derivatives have also been found to inhibit rat paw edema or canine synovitis induced by injection of a suspension of microcrystalline sodium urate. The methoxytropane moiety and the nitrogen function of colchicine are deemed essential. In the carrageenin edema assay colchicine and its *N*-desacetyl-*N*-methyl derivative are active orally at 33 mg/kg. Both compounds also suppress the reverse passive Arthus reaction in the rat at 2 mg/kg i.p. (243).

As one of the oldest agents in arthritis therapy, colchicine (62.**4**), given in multiple small doses of 0.5–1 mg p.o. or i.v., provides dramatic relief to acute attacks of gouty arthritis and pseudogout (244). Its primary mode of action is inhibition of microtubule assembly, which is important to the organization and function of cell membranes. As a consequence, colchicine causes impaired locomotion of inflammatory cells and interferes with their membrane functions, such as phagocytosis, release of mediators, prostaglandins, and collagenase, and the transport mechanism. It also blocks the capping of membrane-bound immunoglobulins on the lymphocyte surface. It inhibits the generation of the spindle apparatus required for mitosis and thus has a direct antiproliferative effect.

Major side effects of colchicine are gastrointestinal disturbances, bone marrow depression, and alopecia.

Other microtubule inhibitors, such as vinblastin (62.**109**) and podophyllotoxin (62.**110**) (246), have similar activities and are slightly more toxic. A benzimidazole microtubule inhibitor R-17934 (62.**97**) is mentioned in Section 9.4 above (230).

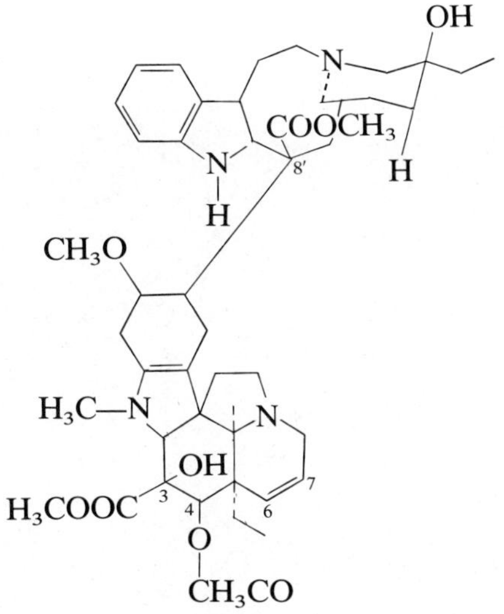

9.5.4   CYCLOSPORIN A.   Cyclosporin A is a fungal metabolite discovered from the random screening of fermentation broths. It is a cyclic undecapeptide containing unnatural amino acids (62.**111**) (247). Cyclosporin A inhibits reversibly an early stage of T-lymphocyte transformation without concomit-

62.**109**   Vinblastin

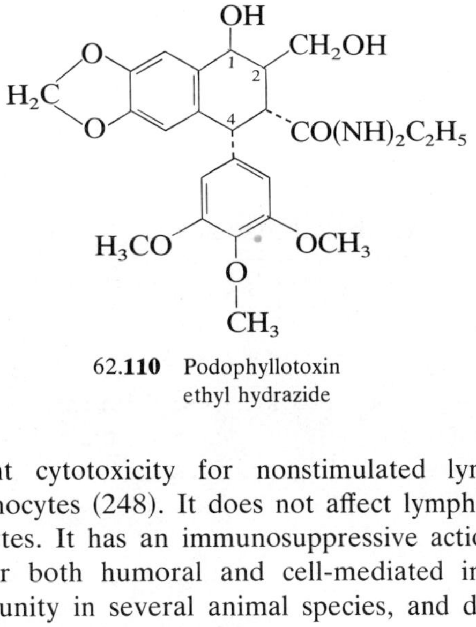

62.**110**   Podophyllotoxin
ethyl hydrazide

ant cytotoxicity for nonstimulated lymphocytes (248). It does not affect lymphocytes. It has an immunosuppressive action for both humoral and cell-mediated immunity in several animal species, and depresses chronic inflammation without producing severe bone marrow toxicity (249). Cyclosporin A is orally absorbed in an olive oil preparation and prolongs the survival of skin and heart grafts in animals at 15–25 mg/kg doses. However, serious hepatotoxicity was observed in transplantation patients (250). The potential antiarthritic application of this possibly more selective immunosuppressant remains to be ascertained.

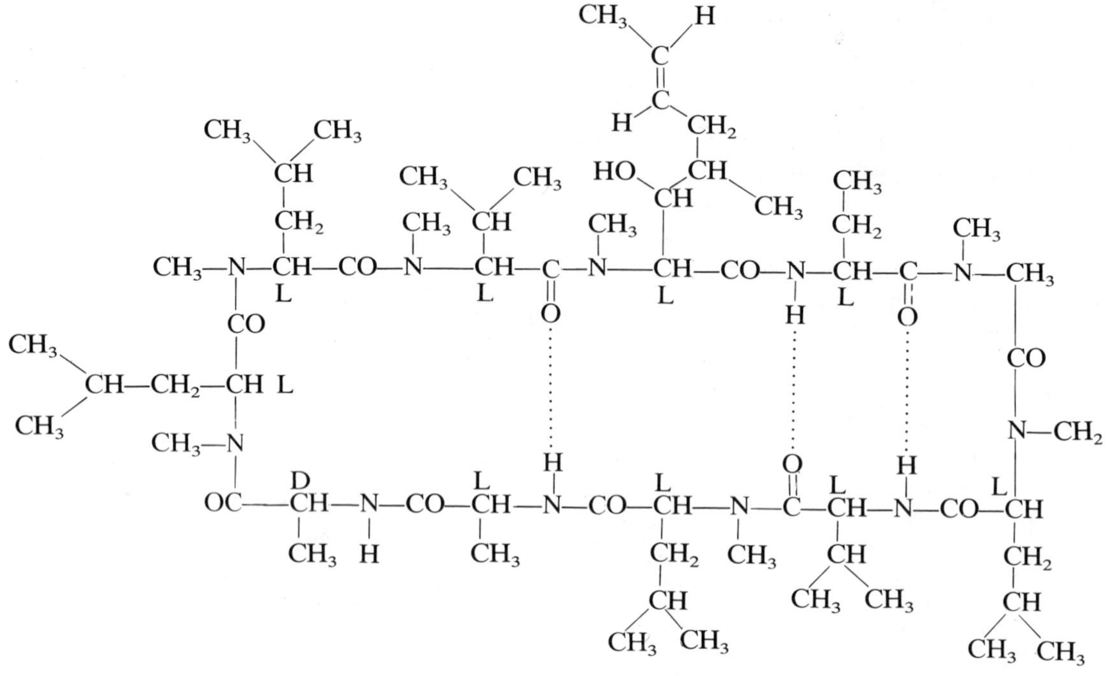

62.**111**   Cyclosporin A

10   NATURAL PRODUCTS

Natural products (251), either of animal or plant origin, have been used since ancient civilizations as anti-inflammatory agents. They also provide some insight into biologic as well as chemical studies. Salicylates, colchicine, and corticosteroids are classical examples. Although the discovery and development of various synthetic chemicals such as NSAIDS have dominated the field in recent decades, an increasing number of natural products have been identified as anti-inflammatory substances in laboratory models. As techniques in the production, evaluation, isolation, and structural elucidation of complex natural products are steadily improved, more progress in this field is anticipated. The failure by random screening of synthetic chemicals to find selectively active inhibitors of several important inflammatory pathways, such as the complement cascade, proteases, mem-

brane receptors, and cellular interactions, also suggests that it may require a complex molecule, e.g., peptides, saccharides, lipids, and their variants, to compete effectively with the macromolecular substrate at binding site and to achieve the desired specificity. The discovery of pepstatin (62.**112**) (252), muramyl dipeptide (62.**113**) (253), and cyclosporin A (62.**111**) (247) are a few examples.

10.1   Animal Origin

Aside from polypeptide ACTHs, adrenocortical hormones, and catecholamines, few chemically defined structures have shown significant anti-inflammatory effects.

10.1.1   VITAMINS, AMINO ACIDS, AND LIPIDS. Various activities in laboratory models have been observed with vitamins. Ascorbic acid inhibits β-glucuronidase *in vitro* and adjuvant arthritis but is inactive in the

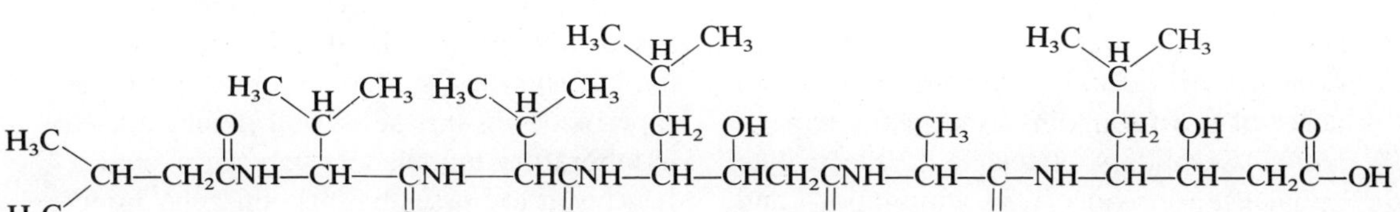

62.**112**   Pepstatin

carrageenin edema and UV erythema assays (254). Tocopherol (62.**114**) stabilizes the membranes of rat liver lysosomes, erythrocytes, and leukocytes. It also scavenges free radicals in biochemical systems. However, its *in vivo* activity has not been very impressive in several conventional anti-inflammatory models (255). Vitamins K_1 and K_3 have also shown activity in the granuloma and edema assays in the rat (256). Clinical studies of vitamin B_{12} and calciferol were inconclusive.

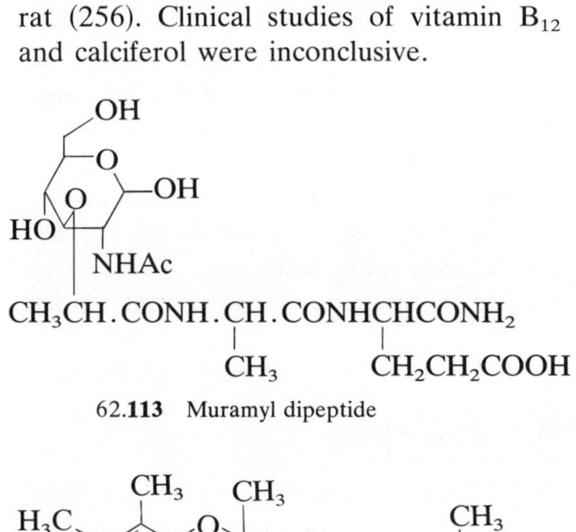

62.**113**   Muramyl dipeptide

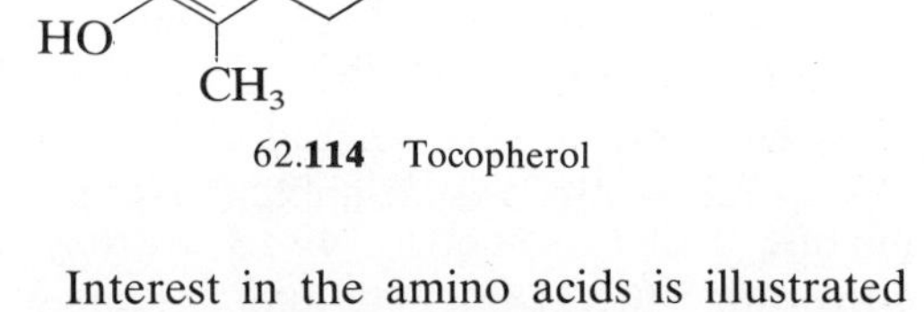

62.**114**   Tocopherol

Interest in the amino acids is illustrated by studies with histidine, tryptophan, and cysteine. The concentration of histidine in the serum of rheumatoid arthritis patients is abnormally low. However, the initial observation of the possible antirheumatic effect of histidine was not confirmed in a subsequent controlled clinical trial (257).

Many NSAIDS displace tryptophan from its binding site to circulating proteins. Tryptophan itself has shown weak anti-inflammatory effects in animal models (258). The possible involvement of sulfhydryl groups in cell membrane and immunoglobulins in inflammation stimulated the investigation of cysteine, a lower homolog of the antirheumatic D-penicillamine. Sporadic activities were obtained with cysteine and N-acetylcysteine at ≥ 200 mg/kg in several animal models.

A group of alkoxyglycerols found in fish liver oils and egg yolk, batyl (62.**115**) and selachyl (62.**116**) alcohols, are modestly active orally in the granuloma pouch assay (259). N-(2-Hydroxyethyl)palmitamide was identified as the anti-inflammatory substance in the phospholipid fraction of egg yolk (250). A controlled clinical trial at an oral does of 1.8 g per day in rheumatoid arthritis patients showed that it is less active than a daily doses of 3 g of aspirin (261).

Contrary to their pro-inflammatory effects, prostaglandins, e.g., PGE_2, have been reported to possess anti-inflammatory

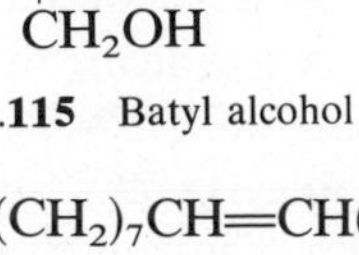

$$CH_2OC_{18}H_{37}$$
$$|$$
$$CH_2OH$$
$$|$$
$$CH_2OH$$

62.**115**   Batyl alcohol

$$CH_2OCH_2(CH_2)_7CH=CH(CH_2)_7CH_3$$
$$|$$
$$CHOH$$
$$|$$
$$CH_2OH$$

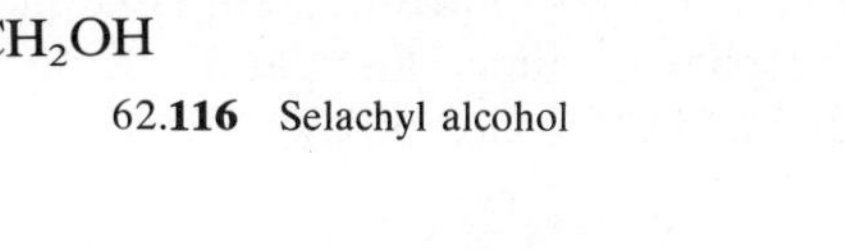

62.**116**   Selachyl alcohol

activities in laboratory models. The confusion may arise from very high (0.5–10 mg) doses of prostaglandins used in the experiments. Secondary effects, e.g., electrolyte imbalance, adrenocortical stimulation, and vascular disturbances, may produce nonspecific or toxic manifestations. On the other hand, judicial alterations of the prostaglandin feedback mechanism, the tissue levels of different prostaglandins, and the ratio of cyclic nucleotides may also result in some net anti-inflammatory responses. The potential beneficial effect of PGI_2 (prostacyclin), which inhibits platelet aggregation and adhesion, remains to be clarified.

10.1.2 PEPTIDES AND ENZYMES. Aprotinin (Trasylol) is a basic polypeptide consisting of 58 amino acids and three disulfide bridges. It inhibits a variety of proteases including trypsin, chymotrypsin, plasmin, and leukocytic proteases. It also inhibits the release of bradykinin *in vivo*. Aprotinin is clinically useful in treating acute pancreatitis but only modestly effective in arthritic patients by multiple injections (262).

Several proteolytic enzyme preparations are used to reduce acute inflammatory responses following surgery or athletic injuries. Trypsin and chymotrypsin are absorbed from the gastrointestinal tract and orally effective.

Superoxide dismutases (SOD, orgotein) are a group of metalloproteins capable of destroying the harmful superoxide free radicals produced by enzymes such as xanthine oxidase (263).

$$2O_2^- + 2H^+ \xrightarrow{\text{SOD}} H_2O_2 + O_2$$

The pathological effects of superoxide radical anion and free radicals derived from it have been investigated extensively in recent years. Free radicals play an active and nonspecific role in inflammatory processes such as the destruction of enzymes and membrane components, stimulation of macrophage functions and leukocyte chemotaxis, and degradation of connective tissue and hyaluronic acid in the synovial fluid. The anti-inflammatory effect of superoxide dismutase is well demonstrated in laboratory models and veterinary clinics. It is given to horses by intramuscular injection of 5 mg doses for several days. In human patients it produces good responses in chronic interstitial cystitis. Clinical trials in arthritis patients are still in progress. As a metalloprotein it has very weak immunogenic activity and appears to be well tolerated.

10.1.3 CARTILAGE AND BONE MARROW EXTRACTS. Several poorly defined extracts of cartilage and bone marrow have been reported to stimulate cartilage metabolism in cartilage tissue culture and in rats. Rumalon ®, commercially available abroad, is an aqueous extract containing 6.5 mg of peptides, nucleotides, oligosaccharides, and minerals and 3 mg *m*-cresol per milliliter. Weekly intramuscular injections of 2–3 ml of the preparation in patients with degenerative hip disease for a year or longer have been claimed to provide clinical and radiological improvements (264). The mechanism of action of these extracts is not clear.

10.2 Plant Origin

10.2.1 FLAVONOIDS. The flavonoids (265), 2- or 3-phenyl-γ-pyrone derivatives, are widespread pigments in the plant kingdom. Many of them have been examined in biologic systems. Rutin (62.**117**) inhibits paw edema induced by egg white at 100 mg/kg s.c. Its hydroxylation products, a mixture of isomeric *O*-(β-hydroxyethyl)rutin (62.**118**), and other related flavonoids have been found to inhibit edema and granuloma formation induced by a variety of irritants, e.g., serotonin and bradykinin, at similar doses i.p. or s.c. Certain flavonoids have been reported to stabilize lysosome membranes *in vitro* and *in vivo*. They reduce the damage of ery-

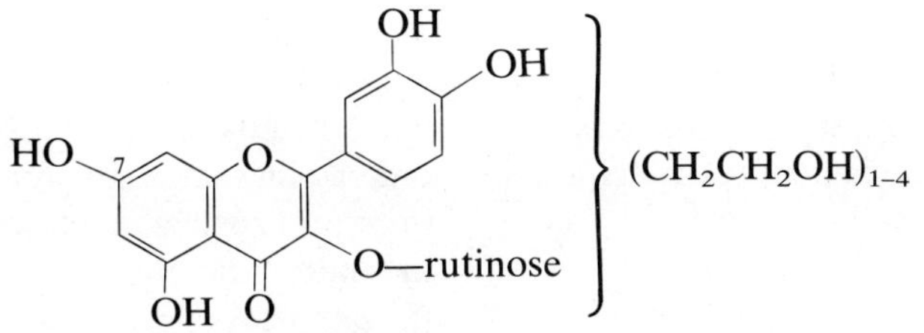

62.**117**   Rutin

62.**118**

throcyte membrane and the leakage of endothelial wall produced in phospholipase edema in rats. β-(O-hydroxyethyl)rutin also increases the plasma steroid level by stimulation of the adrenal cortex. The mechanisms of action of flavonoids apparently are very complex.

Several structures related to phenyl- or benzochromone and coumarin are potent nonacidic inhibitors of prostaglandin synthetase *in vitro* (113, 188).

A phosphorylated derivative, polyphloretin phosphate (PPP), is a prostaglandin antagonist (266). Phloretin is an acyclic analog of flavonoids and the aglycone of phlorizin. PPP antagonizes the actions of PGE_2 and $PGF_{2\alpha}$ in various *in vitro* and *in vivo* systems, including the contraction of smooth muscle, hypotensive effect, and increase of intraocular pressure. It inhibits rat paw edema and guinea pig lung inflammation, and it reduces capillary permeability. At low doses ($\sim 1 \mu g/ml$) PPP and diphloretin phosphate also prevent the inactivation of PGE_2 and $PGF_{2\alpha}$ by PG 15-OH dehydrogenase and thus potentiate the effect of prostaglandins (267).

A group of coumarin derivatives have been reported to increase vascular permeability and stimulate phagocytosis and proteolysis, partly through a membrane effect. They inhibit carrageenin edema at *ca.* 40 mg/kg i.p. but are less effective orally.

10.2.2 TRITERPENOIDS. An active substance in horse chestnut, escin (62.**119**), restores abnormal permeability and inhibits the early exudative phase of edema induced by a variety of irritants and in local Arthus reactions (268).

A constitutent of licorice, glyzrrehetinic acid (62.**120**), and its 3-hemisuccinate are active anti-inflammatory agents in several edema and granuloma assays. The antirheumatic effect of glyzyrrehetinic acid in man was found unsatisfactory, but the 3-hemisuccinate was reported to promote the healing of gastric ulcers (269).

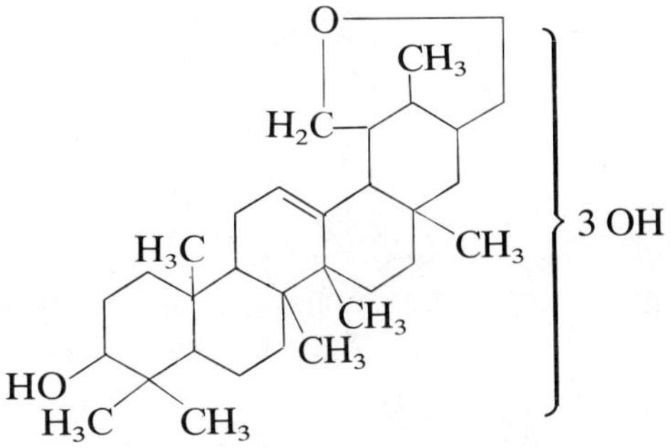

62.**119**   Escin

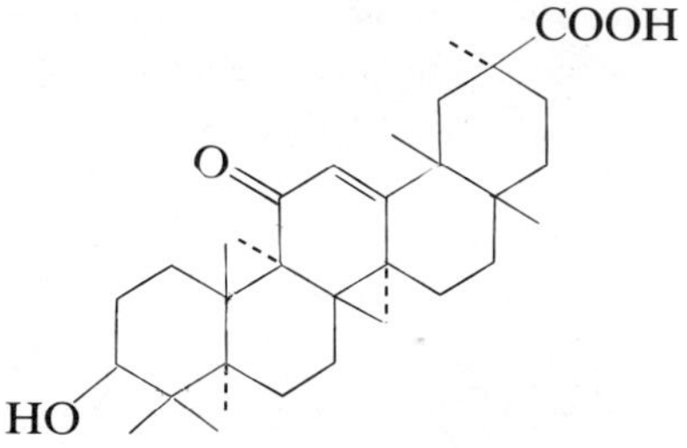

62.**120**   Glyzyrrehetinic acid

11   OTHER APPLICATIONS OF ANTI-INFLAMMATORY AGENTS

In addition to the treatment of various arthritic conditions, anti-inflammatory agents are useful, or potentially useful, in a number of chronic or acute inflammatory disorders. Furthermore, some pathological consequences of excessive prostaglandin production are remedied by prostaglandin synthetase inhibitors.

11.1   Dermatologic Lesions

Most inflammatory skin disorders, dermatitis and erythema, are treated with topical steroids. To promote the penetration of drugs through the outer layer of epidermis (stratum corneum) special pharmaceutical formulations and a nonporous occlusive dressing are often used. Although the amount of steroids applied locally is limited, the residual systemic side effects and local tissue atrophy are still of some concern. Some NSAIDS have been formulated in 1–5% concentrations in creamy or aqueous vehicles, but are generally effective in sunburn and nonimmunologic inflammation only (270, 271).

Thus three basic requirements for an improved topical anti-inflammatory agent are efficacy vs. both immune and nonimmune mediated inflammation, ability to penetrate the outer skin layer, and a low degree of systemic toxicity.

One approach to minimize the systemic side effect of topical anti-inflammatory agents is to use chemical structures that are rapidly metabolized and detoxified systemically. It is a strategy equivalent to the reverse of the "prodrug" concept. An example toward this goal is a group of 2-aryloxazolopyridines (e.g., 62.**80**). These compounds are active *in vitro* as potent cyclooxygenase inhibitors and active in the UV erythema and croton oil induced mouse ear edema assays when applied topically, but are devoid of efficacy and toxicity in various inflammatory models when given orally or parentally. Their facile metabolic inactivation can readily be demonstrated by incubation with liver homogenate *in vitro* (195).

11.2   Ocular Inflammation

Ocular inflammatory disorders may have either immunologic or nonimmunologic origins. Prostaglandins of the E series are mediators mainly for nonimmune uveitis (272). They potentiate histamine-induced increase in vascular permeability of the conjunctiva. Topical administration of several NSAIDS, e.g., ketoprofen and indomethacin, suppresses external ocular inflammation induced by arachidonic acid and internal inflammation induced by paracentesis in the rabbit eye. They are generally much less effective against allergic uveitis (273).

The eye, as a therapeutic target organ, is almost like an *in vitro* system largely isolated from the influence of systemic circulation. The relative sensitivity of the PG synthetase system from different ocular tissues, conjunctiva, anteria uvea, and retina, to inhibition by indomethacin and other drugs varies over a wide range (274). The efficacy of a topical agent also depends on some unique distribution, tissue penetration, and metabolic factors in the ocular system.

More effective nonsteroidal ocular anti-inflammatory agents remain to be developed.

11.3   Periodontal Disease (275)

The most prevalent form of periodontal disease is chronic periodontitis, a slowly progressing inflammatory lesion. The deposit of bacterial plaque on the teeth stimulates an inflammatory reaction, involving both immunologic and nonimmunologic pathways, which causes the damage of gingival and periodontal tissue. The humoral and cellular events taking place are remarkably similar to those well known in degenerative arthritis (276). For example, clinical treatment with levamisole, which potentiates cell-mediated immunity (see Section 9.4.1 above), was reported to

promote the development of and exacerbate existing gingivitis in man (277). The
potential applications of anti-inflammatory
agents in the prevention and treatment of
chronic periodontitis are obvious.

11.4   Other Prostaglandin-mediated Disorders

11.4.1   PRIMARY DYSMENORRHEA. Prostaglandins play an essential role in the pain
and discomforts in primary dysmenorrhea.
The efficacy of indomethacin naproxen, and
other NSAIDS in relieving the symptoms
were reported in a number of clinical
studies (278, 279). Both mefenamic acid
and ibuprofen have already been approved
for this application.

11.4.2   DUCTUS ARTERIOSUS. The ductus
arteriosus is maintained in the open or relaxed state in fetal life by the action of
prostaglandins, primarily PGE_2, and is normally closed by constriction soon after birth
(280). Failure of closure of the ductus occurs in up to 50% of underweight premature infants, and may lead to fatal heart
failure. Potent prostaglandin synthesis inhibitors like indomethacin (at 0.1 mg/kg)
have been successfully used to correct this
defect (281). Renal and platelet dys-
functions may be potential side effects
(282).

11.4.3   MISCELLANEOUS. Prostaglandin synthetase inhibitors have also been used with
success in the treatment of Bartter's syndrome in early childhood, which is associated with abnormal renal prostaglandin
metabolism and growth failure (283). Indomethacin appears to be effective in the
treatment of the pericarditis associated with
hemodialysis (284). Its protective action in
traumatic shock (285) and prostaglandin-
induced diarrhea, and possible benefit in
Hodgkin's disease and hypercalcemia in
cancer have also been investigated (286,
287). The potential application of small

doses of aspirin and other prostaglandin
synthesis inhibitors in preventing thrombo-
sis due to platelet aggregation has also received some attention.

12   FUTURE TRENDS

As mentioned in Section 3, the most significant advances in arthritic therapy, salicylates, cortisone, gold preparations, and D-
penicillamine, for example, were direct
clinical observations. Each of these clinical
discoveries became a valuable guide for
laboratory researchers to gain some insight
of the disease and to develop better animal
models. Time and again, this process has
led to the development of superior agents.
In recent years, advances in biochemistry
and immunology have further facilitated
our understanding of drug actions. A trend
toward more rational therapy in arthritis
has become increasingly evident.

Although most NSAIDS inhibit cyclooxygenase, newer aspects in the arachidonic acid cascade (Fig. 62.16), e.g.,
thromboxane, prostacyclin (PGI_2), oxygen
radicals, and metabolites in the lipoxygenase pathway, may offer biochemical
approaches toward more selective and
more effective anti-inflammatory analgesic
agents (113, 288).

The influence of arachidonic acid
metabolites is not limited to acute pain and
inflammation only. They are also intimately
involved in various aspects of immunologic
responses contributing to the pathogenesis
cycle in rheumatoid arthritis, such as vascular permeability, production of antibodies
and complement, cellular infiltration and
proliferation, phagocytosis by PMN and
macrophage, release of mediators and
lysosomal enzymes, and tissue damage.
Prostaglandins are also secreted by macrophages along with other inflammatory and
immunologic mediators. A pivotal role of
macrophage in antigen processing and in
the control of lymphocyte proliferation and

The Arachidonic Acid Cascade

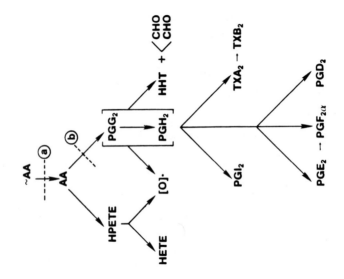

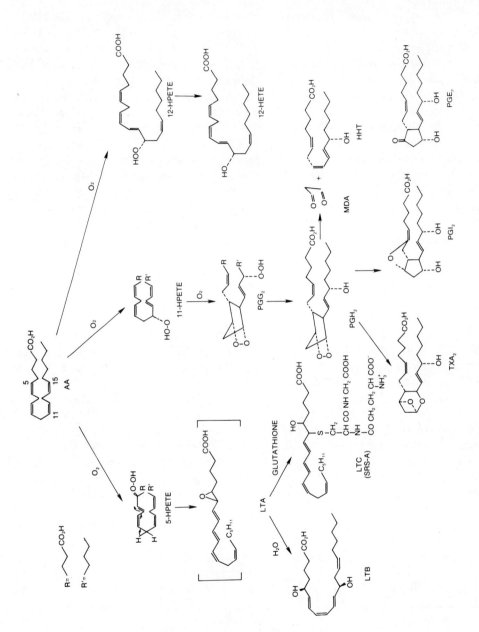

Fig. 62.16 Potential biochemical targets for drug intervention in the arachidonic acid cascade; sites of inhibition by corticosteroids (a) and many NSAIDS (b) are indicated. Abbreviations: AA, arachidonic acid; HPETE, 12*l*-hydroperoxy-5,8,10,14-eicosatetraenoic acid; HETE, 12*l*-hydroxy-5,8,10,14-eicosatetraenoic acid; HHT, 12*l*-hydroxyhepta-5,8,10-trienoic acid. The stereochemistry of LTB and LTC are being defined.

responses was recognized recently. Thus we see a close relationship between these pharmacological mediators and immunologic responses. These findings may facilitate the discovery of new immunoregulatory agents.

Antirheumatic therapy through immunosuppression by corticosteroids, antimetabolites, and cytotoxic agents was extensively studied in the past decade. To circumvent severe toxicities of most immunosuppressants, the alternative approach of achieving antirheumatic effects through immunostimulation has captured much attention and imagination recently. Experience gained in the use of immune adjuvants, such as muramyl dipeptide (113), glycolipids, and interferon inducers in immunotherapy of cancer and infectious diseases may be extended to other immunodeficiency disorders. In the laboratory, a group of SAARDS (see Section 9 above) have become valuable prototypes to guide the chemical search for new immunoregulatory agents with similar antirheumatic action, but with fewer side effects. Many *in vitro* and *in vivo* immunologic models, each reflecting some specific participation by subsets of T and B lymphocytes and macrophages, are now available. The possible correlation of these assays with rheumatoid arthritis is not clear, but a popular pharmacological approach is to use their responses to SAARDS as criteria. In other words, SAARDS are being used to determine the relevance of specific immunologic models, which in turn will be used in search for selective immunoregulants or immunostimulants for antirheumatic therapy (289).

At a more fundamental level, the search for novel biomembrane regulators offers another potentially fruitful area of antiarthritic research. Many important events in the pathogenesis cycle of rheumatoid arthritis take place at the cell membrane. Antigen recognition, the complement cascade, chemotaxis, cell-mediated cyto-

toxicity, release of hydrolases, and the actions of prostaglandins, plasmin, and kinin systems are all surface-mediated reactions. Just to indicate a few examples, specific chemical structures, such as the PMN chemotactic factor f-Met-Leu-Phe (290) and the macrophage stimulator Tuftsin (Ala-Lys-Pro-Arg) (291), and the biochemical nature of their interaction with specific cell receptors are being unraveled. The potential application of their analogs have already been demonstrated (292, 293). Further elucidation of the binding site in immunoglobulins for membrane Fc receptors may also provide the necessary structural information for medicinal chemists to design immune regulators.

The membrane-stabilizing effect of corticosteroids has been related to their inhibition of the release of lysosomal enzymes, the initiation of arachidonic cascade, and lymphocyte functions. These biochemical effects can be evaluated in PMN, macrophage, and lymphocyte cultures. In addition, the biophysical interaction of drugs with membrane components can be investigated with liposomes in terms of bilayer fluidity, membrane potential, and conformational changes by NMR, ESR, or other physical techniques. Thus a renewed effort to search for novel membrane stabilizers or regulators would seem timely.

In the clinic, the incidence of arthritic disorders has been correlated with the genetic makeup of patients. The association of ankylosing spondylitis and rheumatoid arthritis with histocompatibility antigens, B-27 and D-4, respectively, may be related to genetic differences of cell membrane characteristics (294, 295). Interestingly, some determinants involved in T cell–B cell recognition and antigen processing by macrophages have also been shown in the laboratory to be controlled by major histocompatibility genes (296). The emerging new concepts of cell surface phenomena and new knowledge on the structure–function relationship of membrane constituents may well provide the basis for a rational approach to new immunopharmacological agents.

Finally, taking a broader view, rheumatoid arthritis and osteoarthritis are the two major arthritic disorders treated by NSAIDS. The more fundamental action of SAARDS, e.g., gold and D-penicillamine, in severe rheumatoids has already stimulated an intensive search for safer immunoregulants. In view of the recent progress in the biochemistry and animal models related to osteoarthritis, the emergence of a new generation of selective antidegenerative agents to complement the anti-rheumatic immunoregulants in the future may well be expected. For example, in an experimental canine osteoarthritis model (297) there are three distinct phases in the slow development of joint lesions. A possible correlation of some early and focal biochemical changes of cartilage with later lesions was recognized. Thus one might use early biochemical parameters to project the long-term benefit of antidegenerative drugs.

In conclusion, significant development in antiarthritis therapy will surely be made in the next two decades, not only to relieve the symptomatic discomfort and slow down the degenerative processes, but to alter the basic pathogenic course of these chronic, debilitating disorders as well.

REFERENCES

1. M. Rocha e Silva, in *Inflammation*, J. R. Vane and S. H. Ferreira, Eds., *Handbook of Experimental Pharmacology*, Vol. 50/I, Springer-Verlag, New York, 1978, p. 6.

2. G. P. Rodnan, C. McEwen, and S. L. Wallace, *Primer on the Rheumatic Diseases* 7th ed., The Arthritis Foundation, Atlanta, Ga., 1973.

3. R. A. Scherrer and M. W. Whitehouse, Eds., *Antiinflammatory Agents*, Vols. 1, 2, Academic, New York, 1974.

4. J. R. Vane and S. H. Ferreira, Eds., *Inflammation, Handbook of Experimental Pharmacology*, Vol. 50/I, Springer-Verlag, New York, 1978.

5. J. R. Vane and S. H. Ferreira, Eds., *Antiinflammatory Drugs*, Springer-Verlag, New York, 1978.

6. J. L. Hollander, Eds., *Arthritis and Allied Conditions*, 8th ed., Lea and Febiger, Philadelphia, 1972.

7. W. Muller, H. G. Hanwerth, and K. Fehr, Eds., *Rheumatoid Arthritis, Pathogenetic Mechanisms and Consequences in Therapeutics*, Academic, New York, 1971.

8. J. L. Gordon and B. L. Hazelman, Eds., *Rheumatoid Arthritis, Cellular Pathology and Pharmacology*, North-Holland, New York, 1977.

9. I. H. Lepow and P. A. Ward, Eds., *Inflammation, Mechanisms and Control*, Academic, New York, 1972.

10. B. W. Zweifach, L. Grant, and R. T. McCluskey, Eds., *The Inflammatory Process*, 2nd ed., Academic, New York, 1973.

11. Gabor Katona and Jose R. Blengio, Eds., *Inflammation and Antiinflammatory Therapy*, Spectrum, New York, 1975.

12. M. E. Rosenthal and H. C. Mansmann, Eds., *Immunopharmacology*, Spectrum, New York, 1975.

13. A. Bertelli, Ed., *New Antiinflammatory and Antirheumatic Drugs*, Vol. II, No. 1, J. R. Prous, Barcelona, Spain, 1977.

14. P. Bresloff, "Miscellaneous Antirheumatic Drugs and Their Possible Modes of Actions," in *Advances in Drug Research*, Vol. II, N. J. Harper and Alma B. Simmonds, Eds., Academic, New York, 1977.

15. Harry J. Robinson and John R. Vane, Eds., *Prostaglandin Synthetase Inhibitors*, Raven Press, New York, 1974.

16. B. Samuelsson and R. Paoletti, Eds., *Advances in Prostaglandin and Thromboxane Research*, Vols. 1, 2, Raven Press, New York, 1976.

17. F. Benti, B. Samuelsson, and G. P. Velo, Eds., *Prostaglandins and Thromboxanes*, Plenum, New York, 1977.

18. B. Samuelsson, M. Goldyne, E. Granstrom, M. Hamberg, S. Hammarstrom, and C. Malmsten, "Prostaglandins and Thromboxanes," in Annual Review of Biochemistry, Vol. 47, E. Snell, P. Boyer, A. Meister, and C. Richardson, Eds., Annual Reviews, Palo Alto, Calif., 1978, pp. 997.

19. D. A. Brewerton, *J. R. Soc. Med.* **71**, 331 (1978).

20. J. R. Klinenberg, *Med. Clin. North Am.*, **61**, 299 (1977).

21. J. A. Markensan and P. E. Phillips, *Arthritis Rheum.*, **21**, 266 (1978).

22. J. R. Ward and S. G. Atchesan, *Med. Clin. North Am.*, **61,** 313 (1977).

23. H. Hart and B. P. Manmion, *Ann. Rheum. Dis.*, **36,** 3 (1977).

24. J. A. Sachs and D. A. Brewerton, *Brit. Med. Bull.*, **34,** 275 (1978).

25. J. W. Hollingsworth and R. S. Saykaly, *Med. Clin. North Am.*, **61,** 217 (1977).

26. P. A. Dieppe, P. Crocker, E. C. Huskisson, and D. A. Willoughby, *Lancet,* **1976-I,** 266.

27. H. R. Schumacher, A. P. Smolyo, R. L. Tse, and K. Maurer, *J. Intern. Med.*, **87,** 411 (1977).

28. H. Muir, *Ann. Rheum. Dis.*, **36,** 199 (1977).

29. R. W. Moskowitz, D. S. Howell, V. M. Goldberg, O. Muniz, and J. C. Pita, *Arth. Rheum.*, **22,** 155 (1979).

30. G. Wilhelmi, *Pharmacology*, **16,** 268 (1978).

31. K. F. Swingle, "Evaluation for Antiflammatory Activity" in *Antiinflammatory Agents*, Vol. 2, R. A. Scherrer and M. W. Whitehouse, Eds., Academic, New York, 1974, p. 33.

32. J. R. Vane, *Nature*, **231,** 232 (1971).

33. K. Komoriya, H. Ohmori, A. Azuma, S. Kurozumi, and Y. Hashimoto, *Prostaglandins*, **16,** 557 (1978).

34. I. M. Goldstein, C. L. Malmsten, H. Kindahl, H. B. Kaplan, O. Radmark, B. Samuelsson, and G. Weissmann, *J. Exp. Med.*, 787 (1978).

35. I. L. Bonta and M. J. Pannham, *Biochem. Pharmacol.*, **27,** 1611 (1978).

36. P. Needleman, *Biochem. Pharmacol.*, **27,** 1515 (1978).

37. S. H. Ferreira, S. Moncada, and J. R. Vane, *Brit. J. Pharmacol.*, **49,** 86 (1973).

38. G. P. Lewis, *J. Reticuloendothelial Soc.*, **22,** 389 (1977).

39. S. R. Turner, J. A. Tainen, and W. S. Lynn, *Nature*, **257,** 680 (1975).

40. R. J. Flower and G. J. Blackwell, *Nature*, **278,** 456 (1979).

41. P. A. Ward, E. R. Unanue, S. J. Goralnick, and G. F. Schreiner, *J. Immunol.*, **119,** 416 (1977).

42. V. J. Stecher and G. L. Chinea, *Agents Actions*, **8,** 258 (1978).

43. P. Davies and A. C. Allison, in *Immunobiology and the Macrophage*, D. S. Nelson, Ed., Academic, New York, 1976, p. 427.

44. H. U. Schorlemmer, P. Davies, W. Hylton, M. Gugig, and A. C. Allison, *Brit. J. Exp. Pathology*, **58,** 315 (1977).

45. R. J. Bonney, P. Davies, F. Kuehl, Jr., and J. L. Humes, *Eur. J. Rheum. Inflam.*, **1,** 308 (1978).

46. E. Reich, D. B. Rifkin, and E. Shaw, Eds., *Proteases and Biological Control,* Cold Spring Harbor Laboratory, 1975.

47. R. B. Zurier and K. Krakauer, in Ref. 4, p. 293.

48. R. J. Gryglewski, *Agents Action*, **S3,** 17 (1977).

49. C. A. Winter, E. A. Risley, and G. W. Nuss, *Proc. Soc. Exp. Biol. Med.*, **111,** 544 (1962).

50. R. Vinegar, J. F. Truax, and S. L. Selph, *Fed. Proc.*, **35,** 2447 (1976).

51. D. V. Doyle, C. J. Dunn, and D. A. Willoughby, *Europ. J. Rheum. Inflam.*, **1,** 212 (1978).

52. S. Tsurufugi, K. Sugio, and Y. Endo, *Biochem. Pharm.*, **26,** 1131 (1977).

53. C. A. Winter, in *Non-Steroidal Anti-inflammatory Drugs*, S. Garattini and M. N. G. Dukes, Eds., Excerpta Medica, Amsterdam, 1965, p. 190.

54. T. Koga, S. Kotani, T. Narita, and C. M. Pearson, *Int. Archs. Allergy Appl. Immun.*, **51,** 206 (1976).

55. C. Steffen, W. Kovac, T. A. Endler, J. Menzel, and J. Smolen, *Immunology*, **32,** 161 (1977).

56. D. Brackertz, G. F. Mitchell, and I. R. MacKay, *Arthritis Rheum.*, **20,** 841 (1977).

57. A. R. Poole and R. R. A. Coombs, *Int. Archs. Allergy Appl. Immun*, **54,** 97 (1977).

58. H. R. Schumacher, P. Phelps, and C. Agudelo, *J. Rheum.*, **1,** 102 (1974).

59. G. L. Floersheim, K. Brune, and K. Seiler, *Agents Actions*, **3,** 24 (1973).

60. T. Y. Shen, *Angew. Chem. Int. Ed.*, **11,** 460 (1972).

61. T. Y. Shen in *Prostaglandin Synthetase Inhibitors*, H. J. Robinson and J. R. Vane, Eds., Raven Press, New York, 1974, p. 379.

62. T. Y. Shen, in *Topics in Medicinal Chemistry*, J. L. Rabinowitz and R. M. Meyerson, Eds., Vol. 1, Wiley-Interscience, New York, 1967, p. 29.

63. R. A. Scherrer, in *Antiinflammatory Agents*, R. A. Scherrer and M. W. Whitehouse, Eds., Academic, New York, 1974, p. 35.

64. P. Gund and T. Y. Shen, *J. Med. Chem.*, **20,** 1146 (1977).

65. T. Y. Shen, in *Advances in Inflammation Research*, G. Weissmann, Ed., Vol. 1, Raven Press, New York, 1979, p. 535.

66. G. D. Champion and G. G. Graham, *Aust. N. Z. J. Med.*, **8:** Suppl. 1, 94 (1978).

67. K. Brune and P. Graf, *Biochem. Pharmacol.*, **27,** 525 (1978).

68. K. Brune, A. Schweitzer, and H. Eckert, *Biochem. Pharmacol.*, **26,** 1735 (1977).

69. K. Brune, P. Graf, and K. D. Rainsford, *Drugs Exp. Clin. Res.*, **2,** 155 (1977).

70. D. E. Duggan, K. F. Hooke, R. M. Noll, and K. C. Kwan, *Biochem. Pharmacol.*, **25**, 1749 (1975).

71. R. E. Ober, "Metabolism of Selected Anti-inflammatory Compounds," in Ref. 3, Vol. 2, p. 327.

72. I. H. Raisfeld, *Ann. Rev. Med.*, **24**, 385 (1973).

73. A. S. Nies, *Med. Clin. N. Amer.*, **58**, 965 (1974).

74. J. Koch-Weser and E. M. Sellers, *New Engl. J. Med.*, **294**, 526 (1976).

75. H. E. Williamson, G. R. Gaffney, W. A. Bourland, D. B. Farley, and D. E. Van Orden, *J. Pharmacol. Exp. Ther.*, **204**, 130 (1978).

76. B. Noordewier, V. G. Stygles, J. B. Hook, and R. Z. Gussin, *J. Pharmacol. Exp. Ther.*, **204**, 461 (1978).

77. N. Baber, L. Halliday, R. Sibeon, T. Littler, and M. L'E. Orme, *Clin. Pharmacol. Ther.*, **24**, 298 (1978).

78. T. E. Chvasta and A. R. Cooke, *J. Lab. Clin. Med.*, **79**, 302 (1972).

79. K. D. Rainsford, *Agents Actions*, **5**, 326 (1975).

80. K. D. Rainsford, *Biochem. Pharmacol.*, **27**, 877 (1978).

81. A. Bennett and B. P. Curwain, *Brit. J. Pharm.*, **60**, 499 (1977).

82. B. J. R. Whittle, N. K. Boughton-Smith, S. Moncada, and J. R. Vane, *Prostaglandins*, **15**, 953 (1978).

83. P. H. Guth, D. Aures, and G. Paulsen, *Gastroenterology*, **76**, 88 (1979).

84. K. D. Rainsford, *Agents Actions*, **8**, 587 (1978).

85. J. C. McGiff and P. Y-K. Wong, *Fed. Proc.*, **38**, 89 (1979).

86. M. W. Whitehouse and K. D. Rainsford, *Agents Actions*, **S3**, 171 (1977).

87. E. C. Huskisson, *Semin. Arthritis Rheum.* **7**, 1 (1977).

88. L. S. McKenzie, B. A. Horsburgh, P. Ghosh, and T. K. R. Taylor, *Ann. Rheum. Dis.*, **36**, 369 (1977).

89. M. J. H. Smith and P. K. Smith, Eds., *The Salicylates*, Wiley-Interscience, New York, 1966.

90. B. B. Vargaftig, *J. Pharm. Pharmacol.*, **30**, 101 (1978).

91. M. J. H. Smith, *Agents Actions*, **8**, 427 (1978).

92. J. R. Vane, *Agents Actions*, **8**, 430 (1978).

93. G. J. Roth, N. Stanford, and P. W. Majerus, *Proc. Natl. Acad. Sci. U.S.*, **72**, 3073 (1975).

94. J. W. Burch, N. Stanford, and P. W. Majerus, *J. Clin. Invest.*, **61**, 314 (1978).

95. S. Cassell, D. Furst, S. Dromgoole, and H. Paulus, *Arthritis Rheum.*, **22**, 384 (1979).

96. D. N. Croft, J. H. P. Cuddigan, and C. Sweetland, *Brit. Med. J.*, **2**, 546 (1972).

97. D. L. Beales, H. C. Burry, and R. Grahame, *Brit. Med. J.*, **2**, 483 (1972).

98. J. Hannah, W. V. Ruyle, H. Jones, A. R. Matzuk, K. W. Kelly, B. E. Witzel, W. J. Holtz, R. A. Houser, T. Y. Shen, and L. H. Sarett, *Brit. J. Clin. Pharm.*, **4** (Suppl. 1), 7 (1977).

99. J. Hannah, W. V. Ruyle, H. Jones, A. R. Matzuk, K. W. Kelly, B. E. Witzel, W. J. Holtz, R. A. Houser, T. Y. Shen, L. H. Sarett, V. J. Lotti, E. A. Risley, C. G. Van Arman, and C. A. Winter, *J. Med. Chem.*, **21**, 1093 (1978).

100. P. J. DeSchepper, T. B. Tjandramaga, M. DeRoo, L. Verhaest, C. Daurio, S. L. Steelman, and K. F. Tempero, *Clin. Pharmacol. Ther.*, **23**, 669 (1978).

101. P. W. Majerus and N. Stanford, *Brit. J. Clin. Pharmacol.*, **4**: Suppl. 1, 15 (1977).

102. H. Jones, M. W. Fordice, R. B. Greenwald, J. Hannah, A. Jacobs, W. V. Ruyle, G. L. Walford, and T. Y. Shen, *J. Med. Chem.*, **21**, 1100 (1978).

103. S. S. Bloomfield, T. P. Barden, and J. Mitchell, *Clin. Pharmacol. Ther.*, **23**, 390 (1978).

104. R. A. Scherrer, in Ref. 3, Vol. 1, p. 45.

105. J. R. Boisser, J. M. Lwolf, and F. Hertz, *Therapie*, **25**, 43 (1970).

106. A. S. Watnick, R. I. Taber, and I. Tobachnick, *Arch. Int. Pharmacodyn. Ther.*, **190**, 78 (1971).

107. B. Katchen, S. Buxbaum, J. Meyer, and J. Ning, *J. Pharmacol. Exp. Ther.*, **184**, 453 (1973).

108. J. S. Finch and S. J. Repasky, *Pharmacologist*, **18**, 174 (1976).

109. A. Allais, G. Rousseau, P. Girault, J. Mathieu, M. Peterfalvi, D. Brancerni, G. Azadian-Boulanger, L. Chifflot, and R. Jequier, *Chem. Ther.*, **65** (1966).

110. J. K. Stenport, *Curr. Ther. Res.*, **18**, 303 (1975).

111. M. E. Morris and I. W. D. Henderson, *Clin. Pharmacol. Ther.*, **23**, 383 (1978).

112. T. Y. Shen, *Angew Chem. Int. Ed.*, **11**, 460 (1972).

113. T. Y. Shen in Ref. 5, p. 323 and references cited therein.

114. T. Y. Shen and C. A. Winter, in *Advances in Drug Research*, Vol. 12, N. J. Harper and A. B. Simmonds, Eds., Academic, New York, 1978, p. 90.

115. L. Fisnerova, J. Grimova, V. Rabek, and Z. Roubal, *Cesk. Farm.*, **26**, 227 (1977); through *Chem. Abstr.*, **88**, 62247 (1978).

116. E. Paroli, P. Nencini, and M. C. Anania, *Arzneim.-Forsch.*, **28**, 819 (1978).

117. H. Yamamoto, C. Saito, T. Okamoto, H. Awata, T. Inukai, A. Hirohashi, and Y. Yukawa, *Arzneim.-Forsch.*, **19,** 981 (1969).

118. H. Yamamoto and M. Nakao, *J. Med. Chem.*, **12,** 176 (1969).

119. T. Komatsu, C. Saito, H. Awata, Y. Sakai, T. Inukai, H. Kurokawa, and H. Yamamoto, *Arnzeim.-Forsch.*, **23,** 1690 (1973).

120. J. R. Carson, D. N. McKinstry, and S. Wong, *J. Med. Chem.*, **14,** 646 (1971).

121. J. R. Carson and S. Wong, *J. Med. Chem.*, **16,** 172 (1973).

122. S. Wong, J. F. Gardocki, and T. P. Pruss, *J. Pharmacol. Exp. Ther.*, **185,** 127 (1973).

123. R. N. Brogden, R. C. Heel, T. M. Speight, and G. S. Avery, *Drugs*, **15,** 429 (1978).

124. R. J. Flower, *Pharmacol. Rev.*, **26,** 33 (1974).

125. L. Kaplan, J. Weiss, and P. Elsbach, *Proc. Natl. Acad. Sci. U.S.*, **75,** 2955 (1978).

126. K. Ohuchi and L. Levine, *Prostaglandins Med.*, **1,** 421 (1978).

127. H. S. Hansen, *Prostaglandins*, **8,** 95 (1974).

128. T. Y. Shen, in *Clinoril in the Treatment of Rheumatic Disorders*, E. C. Huskisson and P. Franchimont, Eds., Raven Press, New York, 1976, p. 1.

129. C. G. Van Arman, E. A. Risley, G. W. Nuss, H. B. Hucker, and D. E. Duggan, in *Clinoril in the Treatment of Rheumatic Disorders*, E. C. Huskisson and P. Franchimont, Eds., Raven Press, New York, 1976, p. 9.

130. R. J. Bower, E. R. Umbenhauer, and V. Hecus, in *Advan. Inflam. Res.*, Vol. 1, G. Weissmann, B. Samuelsson, and R. Paoletti, eds., Raven Press, New York, 1979, p. 559.

131. D. E. Duggan, K. F. Hooke, E. A. Risley, T. Y. Shen, and C. G. Van Arman, *J. Pharmacol. Exp. Ther.*, **201,** 8 (1977).

132. K. C. Kwan, G. O. Breault, E. R. Umberhauer, F. G. McMahon, and D. E. Duggan, *J. Pharmacokinet. Biopharm.*, **4,** 255 (1976).

133. R. L. Bugianesi and T. Y. Shen, *Carbohydr. Res.*, **19,** 179 (1971).

134. H. Jones, R. L. Bugianesi, and T. Y. Shen, *J. Carbohydr. Nucleosides Nucleotides*, **3,** 369 (1976).

135. P. F. Juby in Ref. 3, Vol. 1, p. 92.

136. S. Noguchi, S. Kishimoto, I. Minamida, and M. Obayashi, *Chem. Pharm. Bull.*, **22,** 529 (1974).

137. J. M. Teulon, J. C. Cognacq, F. Hertz., J. M. Lwoff, F. Foulow, F. Baert, M. J. Brienne, L. Lacombe, and J. Jacques, *J. Med. Chem.*, **21,** 901 (1978).

138. G. W. Nuss, R. D. Smyth, C. H. Breder, M. J. Hitchings, G. N. Mir, and N. H. Reavey-Cantwell, *Agents Actions*, **6,** 735 (1976).

139. J. Navarro, M. Stoliaroff, J. M. Savy, C. Berny, and M. Brunaud, *Arzneim.-Forsch.*, **24,** 1368 (1974).

140. I. De Salcedo, L. F. Arias, and B. P. Greenberg, *Curr. Ther. Res.*, **18,** 295 (1975).

141. R. L. Tolman, J. E. Birnbaum, F. S. Chiccarelli, J. Panagides, and A. E. Sloboda, in *Advances in Prostaglandin and Thromboxane Research*, B. Samuelsson and R. Paoletti, Eds., Raven Press, New York, 1976, p. 133.

142. R. Martel, J. Rochefort, J. Klicius, and T. Dobson, *Can. J. Physiol. Pharmacol.*, **52,** 669 (1974).

143. S. S. Adams, K. F. McCullough, and J. S. Nicholson, *Arch. Int. Pharmacodyn.*, **178,** 115 (1969).

144. S. S. Adams, K. F. McCullough, and J. S. Nicholson, *Arzneim.-Forsch.*, **25,** 1786 (1975).

145. R. N. Brogden, R. C. Heal, T. M. Speight, and G. S. Avery, *Drugs*, **14,** 241 (1977).

146. R. W. J. Carney, J. J. Chart, R. Goldstein, N. Howie, and J. Wojtkunski, *Experientia*, **29,** 938 (1973).

147. A. Buttinoni, A. Cuttica, J. Franceschini, V. Mandelli, G. Orsini, N. Passerini, C. Turba, and R. Tommasini, *Arzneim.-Forsch.*, **23,** 1100 (1973).

148. C. H. Cashin, W. Dawson, and E. A. Kitchen, *J. Pharm. Pharmacol.*, **29,** 330 (1977).

149. M. Nakanishi, *Japan J. Pharmacol.*, **24:** Suppl. 140 (1974).

150. K. F. Swingle, R. A. Scherrer, and T. J. Grant, *Arch. Int. Pharm. Ther.*, **214,** 240 (1975).

151. Y. Maruyama, K. Anami, and Y. Katow, *Arzneim.-Forsch.*, **28,** 2102 (1978).

152. I. T. Harrison, B. Lewis, P. Nelson, W. Rooks, A. Roszkowiski, A. Tomolonis, and J. H. Fried, *J. Med. Chem.*, **13,** 203 (1970).

153. M. Messer, D. Farge, J. C. Guyonnet, C. Jeanmart, and L. Julou, *Arzneim.-Forsch.*, **19,** 1193 (1969).

154. L. O. Randall and H. Baruth, *Arch. Int. Pharmacodyn.*, **220,** 94 (1976).

155. L. Julou, J.-C. Guyonnet, R. Ducrot, C. Garret, M.-C. Bardon, G. Maignan, and J. Pasquet, *J. Pharmacol.*, **2,** 259 (1971).

156. C. J. E. Niemegeers, J. A. A. Van Bruggen, and P. A. J. Janssen, *Arzneim.-Forsch.*, **25,** 1505 (1975).

157. R. C. Nickander, R. J. Kraay, and W. S. Marshall, *Fed. Prod.*, **30,** 563 (1971).

158. A. V. Camp, *Scand. J. Rheumatol.*, **4**: Suppl. 8, 96 (1975).

159. D. E. Aultz, G. C. Helsley, D. Hoffman, A. R. McFadden, H. B. Lassman, and J. C. Wilker, *J. Med. Chem.*, **20**, 66 (1977).

160. T. Yoshioka, M. Kitagawa, M. Oki, S. Kubo, H. Tagawa, K. Ueno, W. Tsukada, M. Tsubokawa, and A. Kasahara, *J. Med. Chem.*, **21**, 633 (1978).

161. H. B. Lassman, *Pharmacologist*, **17**, 226 (1975).

162. J. Ackrell, Y. Antonio, F. Franco, R. Landerso, A. Leon, J. M. Muchowski, M. L. Maddox, P. H. Nelson, W. H. Rooks, A. P. Roszkowski, and M. B. Wallach, *J. Med. Chem.*, **21**, 1035 (1978).

163. D. V. K. Murtly and M. Kruseman-Aretz, *Fed. Proc. Fed. Am. Soc. Exp. Biol.*, **37**, 622 (1978).

164. D. E. Aultz, A. R. McFadden, and H. B. Lassman, *J. Med. Chem.*, **20**, 456 (1977).

165. R. Ziel and P. Krupp, *Int. J. Clin. Pharmacol.*, **12**, 186 (1975).

166. D. C. Atkinson and E. Leach, *Agents Actions*, **6**, 657 (1976).

167. R. Martel, J. Klicius, and F. Herr, *Pharmacologist*, **16**, 291 (1974).

168. C. A. Demerson, L. G. Humber, and A. H. Phillipp, *J. Med. Chem.*, **19**, 391 (1976).

169. M. E. J. Billingham, J. S. Lowe, M. A. Perry, E. H. Turner, and T. M. Twose, in *Proc. Int. Congr. Inflamm., Bologna, October* 1978, *Abstr.*, p. 205.

170. B. McConkey, T. J. Constable, R. S. Amos, P. J. G. Forster, and M. E. J. Billingham, in *Proc. Int. Congr. Inflamm., Bologna, October* 1978, *Abstr.*, p. 133.

171. J. G. Lombardino, in Ref. 3, Vol. 1, p. 129.

172. M. W. Whitehouse, *Prog. Drug Res.*, **8**, 321 (1965).

173. H. K. von Rechenberg, *Phenylbutazone*, 2nd ed., Arnold, London, 1962.

174. U. Jahn and R. W. Adrian, *Arzneim.-Forsch.*, **19**, 36 (1969).

175. R. B. Capstick and D. A. Lewis, *Drugs Exp. Clin. Res.*, **2**, 79 (1977).

176. J. G. Lombardino, E. H. Wiseman, and W. M. McLamore, *J. Med. Chem.*, **14**, 1171 (1971).

177. J. G. Lombardino, E. H. Wiseman, and J. Chiaini, *J. Med. Chem.*, **16**, 493 (1973).

178. G. DiPasquale, C. L. Rassaert, R. S. Richter, and L. V. Tripp, *Arch. Int. Pharmacodyn.*, **203**, 92 (1973).

179. H. Zinnes, N. A. Lindo, J. C. Sircar, M. L. Schwartz, J. Shavel, Jr., and G. DiPasquale, *J. Med. Pharm. Chem.*, **16**, 44 (1973).

180. E. H. Wiseman, Y. H. Chang, and J. G. Lombardino, *Arzneim.-Forsch.*, **26**, 1300 (1976).

181. E. H. Wiseman, Y. H. Chang, and D. C. Hobbs, *Clin. Pharmacol. Ther.*, **18**, 441 (1975).

182. C. L. Rassaert, G. DiPasquale, and S. O'Donoghue, *Agents Actions*, **5**, 128 (1975).

183. G. G. I. Moore, in Ref. 3, Vol. 1, p. 159.

184. R. L. Vigdahl and R. H. Tukey, *Biochem. Pharmacol.*, **26**, 307 (1977).

185. K. F. Swingle, R. R. Hamilton, J. K. Harrington, and D. C. Kvam, *Arch. Int. Pharmacodyn. Ther.*, **189**, 129 (1971).

186. K. F. Swingle, J. K. Harrington, R. R. Hamilton, and D. C. Kvam, *Arch. Int. Pharmacodyn. Ther.*, **192**, 16 (1971).

187. T. Y. Shen in Ref. 3, Vol. 1, p. 179.

188. T. Y. Shen, *Drugs Exp. Clin. Res.*, **2**, 1 (1977).

189. J. Szmuszkovicz, E. M. Glenn, R. V. Heinzelman, J. B. Hester, Jr., and G. A. Youngdale, *J. Med. Chem.*, **9**, 527 (1966).

190. K. Tamaka, Y. Iizuka, N. Yashida, K. Tomita, and H. Masuda, *Experientia*, **28**, 937 (1972).

191. J. G. Lombardino and E. H. Wiseman, *J. Med. Chem.*, **17**, 1182 (1974).

192. L. Caprino, F. Borrelli, and R. Falchetti, *Arzneim.-Forsch.*, **23**, 1972 (1973).

193. F. Marcussi, R. Riva, R. Gomeni, G. Zavattini, P. Salva Lacombe, and E. Mussini, *J. Pharm. Sci.*, **67**, 705 (1978).

194. R. L. Clark, A. A. Pessolano, B. Witzel, T. Lanza, T. Y. Shen, C. G. VanArman, and E. A. Risley, *J. Med. Chem.*, **21**, 1158 (1978).

195. R. V. Coombs, R. P. Danna, M. Denzer, G. E. Hardtmann, B. Huegi, G. Koletar, J. Koletar, H. Ott, E. Jukniewicz, J. W. Perrine, E. I. Takesue and J. H. Trapold, *J. Med. Chem.*, **16**, 1237 (1973).

196. E. J. Takesue, J. W. Perrine, and J. H. Trapold, *Arch. Int. Pharmacodyn.*, **221**, 122 (1976).

197. M. Schattenkirchner and Z. Fryda-Kaurimski, *Curr. Ther. Res.*, **24**, 905 (1978).

198. T. Komatsu, H. Awata, Y. Sakai, T. Inukai, M. Yamamoto, S. Inaba, and H. Yamamoto, *Arzneim.-Forsch.*, **22**, 1958 (1972).

199. Y. Yanagi and T. Komatsu, *Biochem. Pharmacol.*, **25**, 937 (1976).

200. P. Schiatti, D. Selva, E. Arrigoni-Martelli, L. J. Lerner, A. Diena, A. Sardi, and G. Maffii, *Arzneim.-Forsch.*, **24**, 2003 (1974).

201. J. C. Garnham, L. Saunders, D. M. Stainton-Ellis, C. Franklin, G. Volans, R. Turner, and T. Natunen, *J. Pharm. Pharm.*, **30**, 407 (1978).

202. R. Jaques, *Pharmacology*, **15**, 445 (1977).

203. G. Wilhelmi, *Arzneim.-Forsch.*, **28**, 1724 (1978).

204. R. J. Gryglewski, A. Zmuda, A. Dembinska-

Kiec, and E. Krecioch, *Pharmacol. Res. Commun.*, **9,** 106 (1977).

204. (a) T. Yoshimoto, S. Yamamoto, and O. Hayaishi, *Prostaglandins,* **16,** 529 (1978).

205. N. J. Zvaifleu, in Ref. 6, p. 302.

206. P. Bresloff, in *Advances in Drug Research*, Vol. 11, N. J. Harper and A. B. Simmonds, Eds., Academic, New York, 1977, p. 1.

207. D. T. Walz, M. S. DiMartino, and B. M. Sutton, in Ref. 3, Vol. 1, p. 209.

208. B. M. Sutton, E. McGusty, D. T. Walz, and M. S. DiMartino, *J. Med. Chem.,* **15,** 1095 (1972).

209. D. T. Walz, M. S. DiMartino, and L. W. Chakrin, *J. Pharmacol. Exp. Ther.,* **197,** 142 (1976).

210. F. Berglöf, K. Berglöf, and D. T. Walz, *J. Rheumatol.,* **5,** 68 (1878).

211. E. C. Huskisson in Ref. 5, p. 399.

212. R. B. Capstick and D. A. Lewis, *Drugs Exp. Clin. Res.,* **2,** 79 (1977)

213. A. L. Lewis, D. K. Gemmell, and W. S Stimson, *Agents Actions,* **8,** 578 (1978).

214. E. Munthe, *Penicillamine Research in Rheumatic Disease*, Fabritius and Sonner, Oslo, 1976.

215. I. A. Jaffe, *Arthritic Rheum.,* **8,** 1064 (1965).

216. I. A. Jaffe, *Arthritis Rheum.,* **13,** 435 (1970).

217. E. C. Huskisson and E. D. Hart, *Ann. Rheum. Dis.,* **31,** 402 (1972).

218. P. A. Kendall, *Lancet,* **1976-II,** 862.

219. P. E. Lipsky and M. Ziff, *J. Immunol.,* **120,** 1006 (1978).

220. P. A. Kendall and D. Hutchins, *Immunol.,* **35,** 189 (1978).

221. E. Arrigoni-Martelli, E. Bramm, E. C. Huskisson, D. A. Willoughby, and P. A. Dieppe, *Agents Actions,* **6,** 613 (1976).

222. I. A. Jaffe, E. C. Huskisson, and D. P. Jacobus, private communications.

223. I. A. Jaffe, U.S. Pat. 3,852,454 (1974).

224. T. Y. Shen, H. Jones, C. P. Dorn, Jr., P. Bailey, and D. P. Jacobus, unpublished.

225. G. Renoux, *Pharm. Ther. A,* **2,** 397 (1978).

226. L. A. Runge, R. S. Pinals, S. H. Lourie, and R. H. Tomar, *Arthritis Rheum.,* **20,** 1445 (1977).

227. J. Scott, P. A. Dieppe, and E. C. Huskisson, *Ann. Rheum. Dis.,* **37,** 259 (1978).

228. G. Graziani and G. L. DeMartin, *Drugs Exp. Clin. Res.,* **2,** 221 (1977).

229. E. J. Lovett, III and J. Lundy, *Transplantation,* **24,** 93 (1977).

230. M. J. DeBrabander, R. M. L. Van de Veire, F. E. M. Aerts, M. Borgers, and P. A. J. Jenssen, *Can. Res.,* **36,** 905 (1976).

231. R. L. Stone, R. N. Wolfe, C. G. Culbertson, and C. J. Poget, *Fed. Proc.,* **35,** 333 (1976).

232. K. Brune and M. W. Whitehouse, in Ref. 5, p. 531.

233. T. Y. Shen, in M. E. Rosenthale and H. C. Mansmann, Jr., Eds., *Immunopharmacology*, Spectrum Publications, New York, 1975, p. 85.

234. K. Brune, *Agents Actions,* **7**: Suppl. 3, 149 (1977).

235. A. C. Allison, *Proc. Roy. Soc. Med.,* **63,** 1077 (1970).

236. M. W. Whitehouse, F. W. J. Beck, M. M. Dröge, and R. F. Struck, *Agents Actions,* **4,** 34 (1974).

237. C. O. Gitterman, E. L. Rickes, D. E. Wolf, J. Medas, Jr., S. B. Zimmerman, T. M. Stoudt, and T. C. Demney, *J. Antibiot.,* **23,** 305 (1970).

238. Y. H. Chang, *Arthritis Rheum.,* **20,** 1135 (1977).

239. R. J. Wojnar and R. J. Brittain, *Agents Actions,* **5,** 152 (1975).

240. H. Iwata, H. Iwaki, T. Masukawa, S. Kasamatsu, and H. Okamoto, *Experientia,* **33,** 502 (1977).

241. Soifer, Ed., "The Biology of Cytoplasmic Microtubules," *Ann. N.Y. Acad. Sci.,* **253** (1975).

242. T. J. Fitzgerald, in Ref. 3, Vol. 1, p. 295.

243. Y. H. Chang, *J. Pharmacol. Exp. Ther.,* **194,** 154 (1975).

244. I. Spilberg, *Arthritis Rheum.,* **18,** 129 (1975).

245. S. L. Wallace, *Arthritis Rheum.,* **18,** 847 (1975).

246. C. F. Brewer, J. D. Loike, S. B. Horwitz, H. Steinlich, and W. J. Gensler, *J. Med. Chem.,* **22,** 215 (1979).

247. A. Ruegger, M. Kuhn, H. Lichti, H.-R. Loosli, R. Huguenin, C. Quiquerez and A. Wartburg, *Helv. Chim. Acta.,* **59,** 1075 (1976).

248. J. F. Borel, C. Feurer, C. Magnee, and H. Stahelin, *Immunology,* **32,** 1017 (1977).

249. R. Y. Calne, D. J. G. White, K. Rolles, D. P. Smith, and B. M. Herbertson, *Lancet,* **1978-I,** 1183.

250. R. L. Powles, A. J. Barrett, H. Clink, H. E. M. Kay, J. Sloane, and T. J. McElwain, *Lancet,* **1978-II,** 1327.

251. M. J. H. Smith and A. W. Ford-Hutchinson, in Ref. 5, p. 661.

252. H. Umezawa in *Method Enzymology*, Vol. 45, L. Lorand, Ed., Academic, New York, 1976, p. 678.

253. A. Adam, M. Devys, V. Souvannavong, P. Lefrancier, J. Chody, and E. Lederer, *Biochem. Biophys. Res. Commun.,* **72,** 339 (1976).

254. F. A. Dolbeare and K. A. Martlage, *Proc. Soc. Exp. Biol. Med.,* **139,** 540 (1972).

255. J. L. Taylor and J. H. Brown, *Proc. Soc. Exp. Biol. Med.*, **145,** 32 (1974).

256. P. Görog, I. B. Kovács, L. Szporny, and G. Fekete, *Arzneim.-Forsch.*, **18,** 227 (1968).

257. R. S. Pinals and D. A. Gerber, *Arthritis Rheum.*, **16,** 126 (1973).

258. R. Hirschelmann and H. Bekemeier, *Acta Biol. Med. Germ.*, **31,** 899 (1973).

259. R. G. Burford and C. W. Gowdey, *Arch. Int. Pharmacodyn.*, **173,** 56 (1968).

260. F. A. Kuehl, T. A. Jacob, O. H. Ganley, R. E. Ormond, and M. A. P. Meisinger, *J. Am. Chem. Soc.*, **79,** 5577 (1957).

261. F. Perlik and K. Masek, in *Future Trends in Inflammation*, G. P. Velo, D. A. Willoughby, and J. P. Giroud, Eds., Piccin Medical Books, Padua, 1974, p. 301.

262. J. Trapnell, C. C. Rigby, C. H. Talbot, and E. H. L. Duncan, *Brit. J. Surg.*, **61,** 177 (1974).

263. I. Fridovich, *Ann. Rev. Biochem.*, **43,** 147 (1975).

264. C. W. Denko, *Agents Actions*, **8,** 268 (1978).

265. M. Gabor, in Ref. 5, p. 698.

266. K. E. Eakins, J. D. Miller, and M. M. Karim, *J. Pharmacol. Exp. Ther.*, **176,** 441 (1971).

267. P. A. Ganesan and S. M. M. Karim, *J. Pharmacol.* **25,** 229 (1973).

268. G. Vogel, M. K. Marek and R. Oertner, *Arzneim.-Forsch.*, **20,** 699 (1970).

269. M. W. Whitehouse, in *Progress in Drug Research*, Vol. 8, E. Jucker, Ed., Birkhauser, Basel-Stuttgart, 1965, p. 321.

270. D. S. Snyder and W. H. Eaglstein, *Brit. J. Dermatol.*, **90,** 91 (1974).

271. W. L. Morrison, B. S. Paul, and J. A. Parrish, *J. Invest. Dermacol.*, **68,** 120 (1977).

272. K. E. Eakins and P. Bhattacherjee, *Exp. Eye Res.*, **24,** 299 (1977).

273. P. Conquet, B. Plazonnet, and J. C. LeDouarec, *Invest. Ophthalmol.*, **14,** 772 (1975).

273. (a) P. D. Gautheron, V. J. Lotti and J. C. LeDouarec, *Agents Actions*, **8,** 629 (1978).

274. P. Bhattacherjee and B. R. Hammond, *Exp. Eye Res.*, **21,** 499 (1975).

275. N. S. Taichman and W. P. McArthur, in *Annual Reports in Medicinal Chemistry*, Vol. 10, R. V. Heinzelman, Ed., Academic, New York, 1975, p. 228.

276. J. M. A. Wilton, H. H. Renggi, and T. Lehner, *Clin. Exp. Immunol.*, **27,** 152 (1977).

277. L. Ivanyi and T. Lehner, *Scand. J. Immunol.*, **6,** 219 (1977).

278. A. Schwartz, U. Zor, H. R. Lindner, and S. Naor, *Obstet. Gynecol.*, **44,** 709 (1974).

279. M. O. Pulkkinen, M. R. Henzel, and A. I. Csapo, *Prostaglandins*, **15,** 543 (1978).

280. W. F. Friedman, M. J. Kirschklau, M. P. Printz, P. T. Pitlick, and S. E. Kirkpatrick, *New Engl. J. Med.*, **295,** 526 (1976).

281. M. A. Keymann, A. M. Rudolph, and N. H. Silverman, *New Engl. J. Med.*, **295,** 530 (1976).

282. R. E. Bowden, J. R. Gill, N. Radfar, A. A. Taylor, and H. R. Keiser, *J. Am. Med. Assoc.*, **239,** 117 (1978).

283. J. M. Littlewood, M. R. Lee, and S. R. Meadow, *Arch. Dis. Childhood*, **53,** 43 (1978).

284. A. N. W. Minuth, G. A. Nottebohm, G. Eknoyan, and W. N. Suki, *Arch. Int. Med.*, **135** (1975).

285. S. Halevy and B. M. Altura, *Circ. Shock*, **3,** 299 (1976).

286. J. A. Dodge, I. Hamdi, and S. Walker, *Arch. Dis. Child.*, **52,** 800 (1977).

287. G. K. Morris and J. R. A. Mitchett, *Brit. Med. J.*, **i,** 535 (1977).

288. T. Y. Shen, *Eur. J. Rheumatol. Inflam.*, **1,** 167 (1978).

289. T. Y. Shen, *Extrait Actual. Chim. Ther.*, 213 (1978).

290. E. Schiffmann, B. A. Corcoran, and S. M. Wahl, *Proc. Natl. Acad. Sci. U.S.*, **72,** 1059 (1975).

291. V. A. Jajjar and K. Kishioka, *Nature*, **228,** 672 (1970).

292. S. H. Zigmond, *J. Cell. Biol.*, **77,** 269 (1978).

293. Y. Stabinsky, P. Gottlieb, V. Zakuth, Z. Spirer, and M. Fridkin, *Biochem. Biophys. Res. Commun.*, **83,** 599 (1978).

294. D. A. Brewerton, *Arthritis Rheum.*, **19,** 656 (1976).

295. A. J. McMichael, T. Sasazuki, H. O. McDevitt, and R. O. Payne, *Arth. Rheum.*, **20,** 1037, (1977).

296. S. Z. Ben-Sasson, M. F. Lipscomb, T. F. Tucker, and J. W. Uhr, *J. Immunol*, **119,** 1493 (1977).

297. C. McDevitt, E. Gilbertson, and H. Muir, *J. Bone Joint Surg.*, **59,** 24 (1977).

CHAPTER SIXTY THREE

Anti-inflammatory Steroids

MANFRED E. WOLFF

Department of Pharmaceutical Chemistry
School of Pharmacy
University of California
San Francisco, California 94143, USA

CONTENTS

1273

1 INTRODUCTION

The subject of steroid structure–activity relationships is as old as the history of steroids themselves, for the early isolations of testosterone, progesterone, and estradiol were monitored by bioassay. Development of this field was spurred by the hope of obtaining valuable new drugs in the 1950s and 1960s. This was particularly true for the anti-inflammatory steroids, following the discovery of the antiarthritic properties of cortisone (63.**1**) by Hench and co-workers (1).

Remarkably, no synthetic corticoid more active than cortisone itself was found in the first few years of the search. This led to the pessimistic view in some quarters that the naturally occurring adrenal steroids, cortisone and cortisol (63.**2**), were unique, analogous to the vitamins that had been studied in the preceding decade, and that man could not improve upon nature in

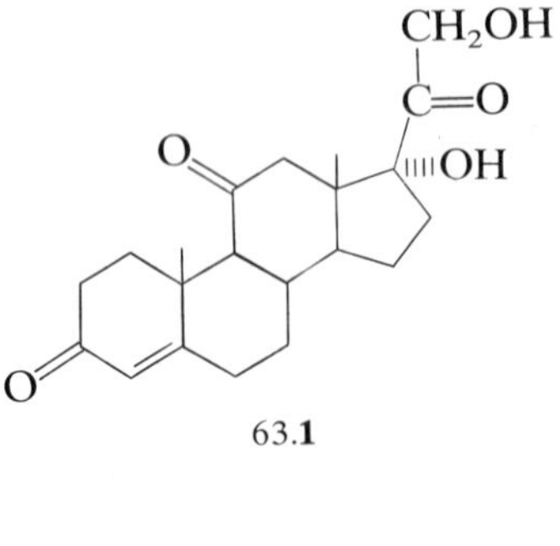

63.**2**

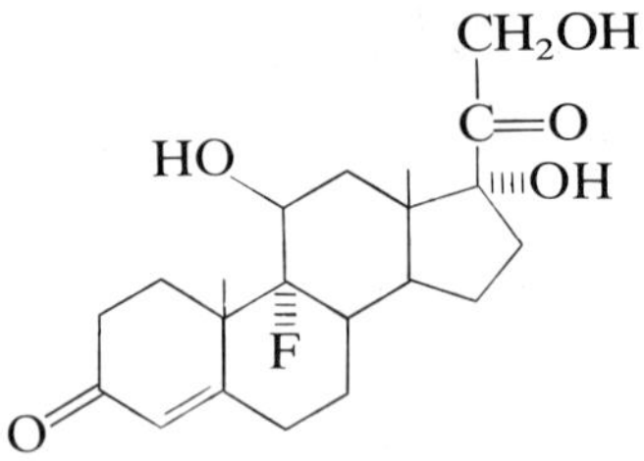

63.**3**

63.**1**

designing anti-inflammatory steroids. This attitude was swept away by Fried and Sabo (2) in 1953 when they described the synthesis of 9α-fluorocortisol (63.**3**) and reported that it had a potency 10 times greater than that of cortisol itself. Hundreds of other highly active compounds were prepared in the ensuing years and steroid chemists invested much time and thought in trying to answer the fascinating question of how structural changes in steroids bring about corresponding changes in biological activity.

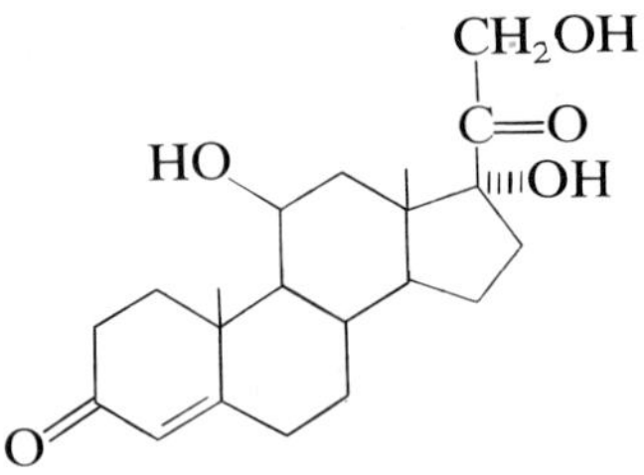

We know today that structural changes in steroids can bring about potency alterations in animal pharmacology through a number of mechanisms. The processes that are affected include pharmacokinetic parameters such as drug absorption and drug distribution (Part I, Chapter 2), as well as drug metabolism to more or less active metabolites (Part I, Chapters 3 and 4). There is now a large body of literature dealing with these phenomena that makes predictive thinking possible in these areas. Less well understood are other mechanisms that are involved in the effect of structural changes on pharmacological activity in steroids. These include the effect of steroid structure on receptor affinity and the manner in which changes in the steroid agonist affect intrinsic activity through alterations in gene expression.

Comprehensive reviews dealing with the pharmacological structure–activity relationships of anti-inflammatory steroids have been published (3–6). Almost all anti-inflammatory steroids are based on the pregnane ring system (63.**4**).

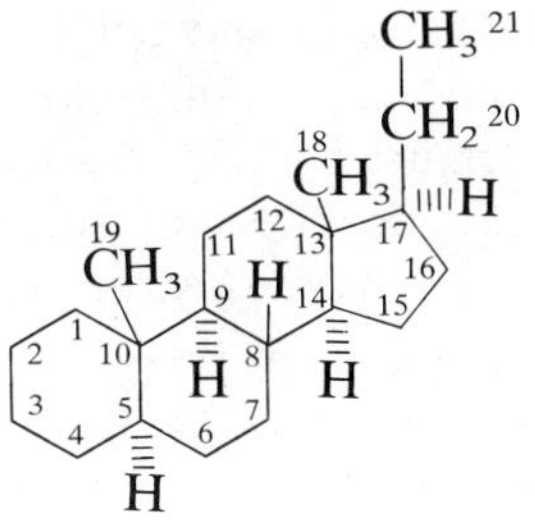

63.4

Abbreviated names for compounds employed in this chapter are as follows:

6α-Methylprednisolone (63.**7**) 6α-Methyl-11β, 17, 21-trihydroxypregna-1, 4-diene-3, 20-dione.

Dexamethasone (63.**9**) 9-Fluoro-11α, 17, 21-trihydroxy-16α-methylpregna-1, 4-diene-3, 20-dione

Betamethasone (63.**14a**) 9-Fluoro-11β, 17, 21-trihydroxy-16β-methylpregna-1, 4-diene-3, 20-dione

9α-Fluorocortisol (63.**3**) 9-Fluoro-11β, 17, 21-trihydroxypregn-4-ene-3, 20-dione

Dichlorisone 9, 11β-Dichloro-17, 21-dihydroxypregn-4-ene-3, 20-dione

Corticosterone (63.**21**) 11β, 21-Dihydroxypregn-4-ene-3, 20-dione

6α-Fluorocortisol (63.**55**) 6α-Fluoro-11β, 17, 21-trihydroxypregn-4-ene-3, 20-dione

Prednisolone (63.**6**) 11β, 17, 21-Trihydroxypregna-1, 4-diene-3, 20-dione

Cortisol (63.**2**) 11β, 17, 21-Trihydroxypregn-4-ene-3, 20-dione

Deoxycorticosterone (63.**11**) 21-Hydroxypregn-4-ene-3, 20-dione

Cortexolone 17, 21-Dihydroxypregn-4-ene-3, 20-dione

Progesterone (63.**10**) Pregn-4-ene-3, 20-dione

Prednisone (63.**5**) 17, 21-Dihydroxypregna-1, 4-diene-3, 11, 20-trione

Cortisone (63.**1**) 17, 21-Dihydroxypregn-4-ene-3, 11, 20-trione

21-Deoxydexamethasone (63.**34**) 9-Fluoro-11β, 17-dihydroxy 16α-methylpregna-1, 4-diene-3, 20-dione

Paramethasone (63.**37**) 6α-Fluoro-11β, 17, 21-trihydroxy-16α-methylpregna-1, 4-diene-3, 20-dione

Fluocinolone (63.**23**) $6\alpha,9$-Difluoro-11β, 16α, 17, 21-tetrahydroxypregna-1, 4-diene-3, 20-dione

Fluocinolone acetonide (63.**13a**) 6α, 9-Fluoro-11β, 21-dihydroxy-16α, 17-[(1-methylethylidene)bis(oxy)]pregna-1, 4-diene-3, 20-dione

6α-Fluoro-16α-hydroxycortisol 6α-Fluoro-11β, 16α, 17, 21-tetrahydroxypregn-4-ene-3, 20-dione

Flurandrenolide 6α-Fluoro-11β, 21-dihydroxy-16α, 17-[(1-methylethylidene)-bis(oxy)]pregn-4-ene-3, 20-dione

Triamcinolone acetonide (63.**12**) 9-Fluoro-11β, 21-dihydroxy-16α, 17-[(1-methylethylidene)bis(oxy)]pregna-1, 4-diene-3, 20-dione

9α-Fluoroprednisolone (63.**31**) 9-Fluoro-11β, 17, 21-trihydroxypregna-1, 4-diene-3, 20-dione

Flumethasone (63.**58**) 6α, 9α-Difluoro-16α-methyl-11β, 17, 21-trihydroxy-1, 4-pregnadiene-3, 20-dione

2 CLINICAL USE OF ANTI-INFLAMMATORY STEROIDS

Anti-inflammatory steroids are used in six major classes of disease:

1. Collagen diseases, e.g., rheumatoid arthritis, lupus erythematosus.

2. Allergic diseases, e.g., asthma, hay fever, drug sensitivity.

3. Dermatologic diseases, e.g., atopic dermatitis, poison ivy, neurodermatitis, urticaria.

4. Hematologic diseases, e.g., acquired hemolytic anemia, idiopathic thrombocytopenic leukemia.

5. Miscellaneous diseases, e.g., gout, congenital adrenal hyperplasia, bursitis, sarcoidosis, pulmonary emphysema.

6. Neoplastic disease, discussed in Part II, Chapter 24, page 642.

The background underlying the use of anti-inflammatory steroids has been fully considered in the preceding chapter (Chapter 62), dealing with the nonsteroidal anti-inflammatory agents. Section 2 of Chapter 62 considers anti-inflammatory diseases and their pathogenesis. Section 3 deals with laboratory models and biochemical assays for inflammation. The *in vivo* models described in Section 3.2, especially the carrageenian-induced paw edema in rats and the granuloma formation models, are extensively used in the assay of anti-inflammatory steroids. Section 11 of Chapter 62 discusses the application of anti-inflammatory agents to dermatologic lesions and to ocular inflammation. The concepts discussed in these sections apply also to the use of anti-inflammatory steroids for these conditions.

3 SIDE EFFECTS OF ANTI-INFLAMMATORY STEROIDS

With few exceptions, the side effects of synthetic derivatives of cortisol are those seen in Cushing's syndrome, caused by excess biosynthesis of adrenal corticoids. They include the following undesirable actions:

1. In high doses anti-inflammatory agents produce protein catabolism and a negative nitrogen balance.

2. High doses of anti-inflammatory agents cause gluconeogenesis and are antagonistic to the action of insulin.

3. High doses of anti-inflammatory steroids cause increases in fat synthesis and redeposition of fat in certain areas. The facial redeposition of fat results in the characteristic "moon face" seen in Cushing's syndrome.

4. Some anti-inflammatory steroids cause sodium retention and enhanced loss of urinary potassium. In addition, loss of bone calcium resulting in osteoporosis is a serious side effect of some of these compounds, especially in patients undergoing long-term therapy.

5. Enhanced secretion of HCl due to anti-inflammatory steroids can lead to gastric ulceration in long-term patients.

6. Many anti-inflammatory steroids produce CNS effects which are manifested as enhanced mental alertness and euphoria, leading to the symptoms of mania in extreme cases.

7. The pituitary and hypothalamus are suppressed by high levels of anti-inflammatory steroids.

8. The production of purple patches on the skin and in the mucous membranes (purpura) is caused by high doses of anti-inflammatory steroids.

Most of the hundreds of anti-inflammatory steroids that have been synthesized in the quarter century that has elapsed since the work of Fried and Sabo have been prepared in the hope of increasing potency and of decreasing side effects. As can be seen in Table 63.1, excellent progress has been made in reducing sodium retention, potassium loss, and the resulting effects on hypertension. CNS stimulation and appetite stimulation vary greatly with the particular analog under consideration. In some cases the two effects have been eliminated entirely, whereas they are actually enhanced in others. For many of the side effects, including the production of peptic ulcer,

Table 63.1 Comparative Clinical Effects of Anti-inflammatory Steroids[a]

Effect	Cortisone (63.1)	Cortisol (63.2)	Prednisone (63.5)	Prednisolone (63.6)	6α-Methyl-prednisolone (63.7)	Tri-amcinolone (63.8)	Dexa-methasone (63.9)
Edema	+ + + +	+ + +	+	+ +	+	0	+
Weakness, K$^+$ depletion	+ + +	+ +	+	+	+	+ +	+
Hypertension	+ +	+	+	+ +	+	+	+
Mental stimulation	+ + +	+	+ +	+ +	+	0 to −	+ + + +
Increased appetite and weight gain	+ +	+ +	+ +	+ +	+	−	+ + + +
Peptic ulcer production	+ +	+	+ + +	+ + +	+ +	+ + +	+ +
Purpura	+	+	+ + +	+ + +	+ +	+ + +	+ +
Moon face	+ + +	+ +	+ +	+ +	+ +	+ + +	+ +
Hirsutism	+ +	+ +	+ +	+ +	+ +	+ + + +	+
Skin effects	+	+	+	+	+	+ + + +	+
Osteoporosis	+ + +	+ +	+ + +	+ + +	+ + +	+ + +	+ +
Diabetes	+ +	+ +	+ + +	+ + + +	+ + +	+ +	+
Infection increase	+ +	+ +	+ +	+ +	+ +	+ +	+ +
Topical effect	+	+ + +	+	+ + +	+ +	+ + +	+ +
Adrenal atrophy	+ + +	+ + +	+ + +	+ + +	+ + +	+ + +	+ + +

[a] Data from Ref. 3.

purpura, "moon face," hirsutism, osteoporosis, diabetes, adrenal atrophy, and enhanced susceptibility to infection, little or no reduction has been achieved in many newer analogs. Therefore, although some of the novel corticoids to be discussed in this chapter have extremely high anti-inflammatory potencies (in some cases, more than 1000 times that of cortisol), the incidence of side effects has been so high that only a few of such compounds have been successfully introduced into the clinic.

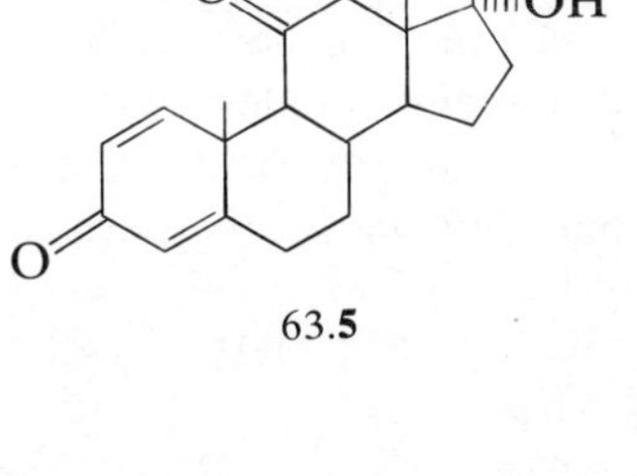

63.5

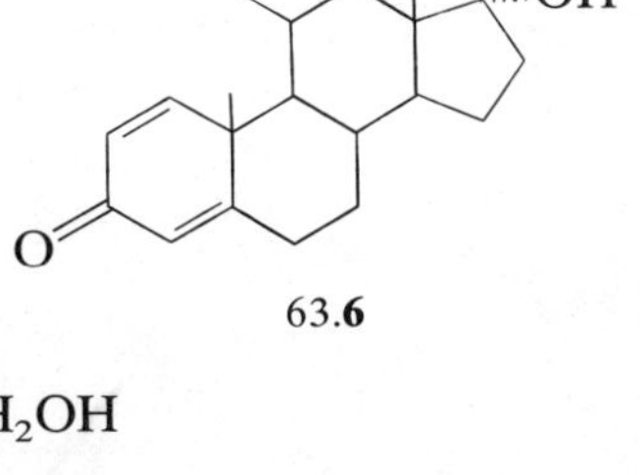

63.6

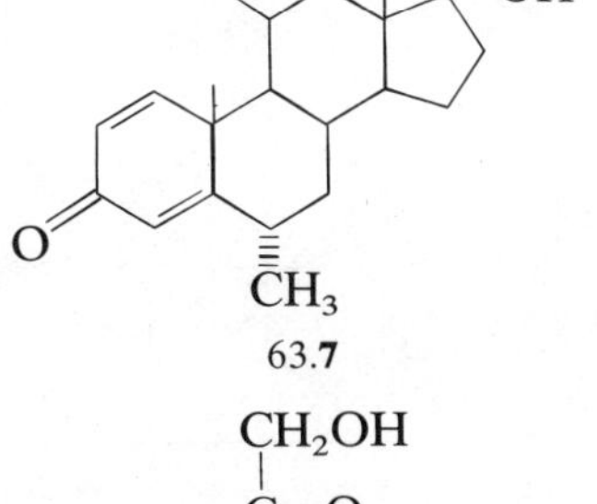

63.7

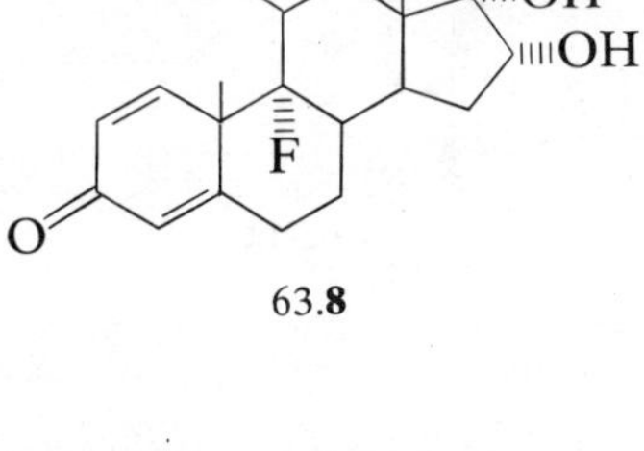

63.8

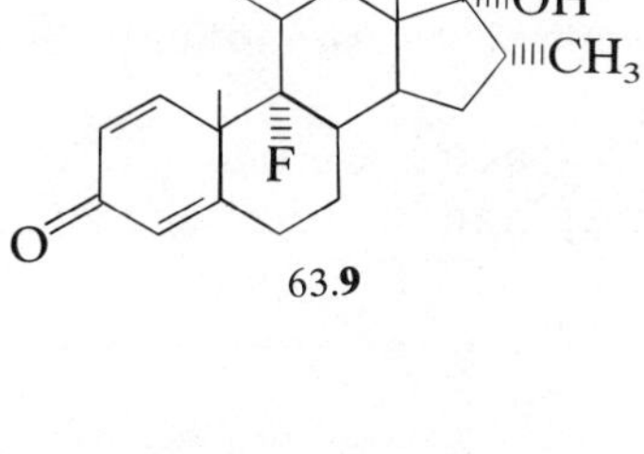

63.9

4 EFFECTS ON ABSORPTION

4.1 Intestinal Absorption

Schedl and Clifton (8) showed that the absorption of steroids by the perfused rat small intestine is strongly correlated with the polarity of the compound. The least polar compound in the study, progesterone (63.**10**), was absorbed almost completely under the condition of the study, whereas the introduction of polar atoms, and particularly hydroxyl groups, reduced the extent of absorption (Table 63.2). Acetylation of the hydroxyl groups invariably increased the extent of absorption. Although absorption is thus readily correlated with the physical properties of the steroid and therefore appears to be a diffusion-controlled process rather than active transport, these figures had no relationship to relative oral clinical potencies. Thus it seems likely that the rate of intestinal absorption is not a controlling factor in the activity of the steroids.

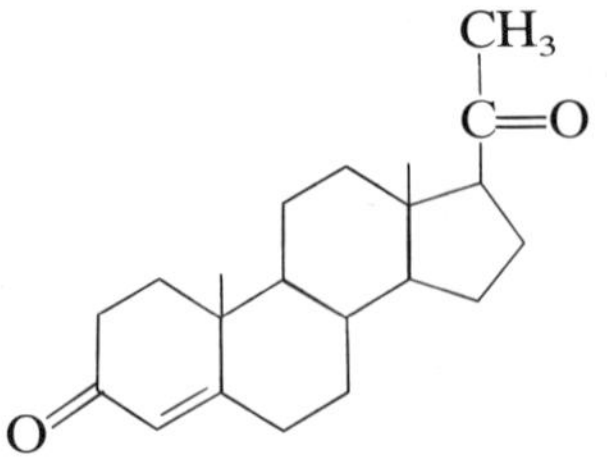

Table 63.2 Steroid Absorption by Perfused Rat Small Intestine[a]

Steroid	% Absorbed	Acetate Derivative
Progesterone (63.**10**)	93.9	—
Deoxycorticosterone (63.**11**)	83.7	—
Corticosterone (63.**21**)	46.5	—
Cortisol (63.**2**)	21.0	29.9
Triamcinolone (63.**8**)	11.5	—

[a] Data from Ref. 8.

lone (63.**8**) are absorbed from a topical site of application and that the radioactivity appears in the urine (9). The more potent analogs of cortisol are all effective when applied topically, although large quantities can produce systemic effects (10).

In the early 1960s it was found that triamcinolone acetonide (63.**12**) was 10 times as active topically as triamcinolone (63.**8**) itself, but only equiactive systemically (11). As pointed out by Popper and Watnick (4), to be topically effective the steroid must penetrate the keratin layer of the stratum corneum of the skin before it can exert its effect on the squamous cell layer of the epidermis. But to reach the general circulation and produce systemic side effects, the steroid must later penetrate the barrier between the epidermis and the dermis. Thus for a useful topical agent it is desirable for the compound to *remain in the epidermis* and to migrate only slowly into the dermis.

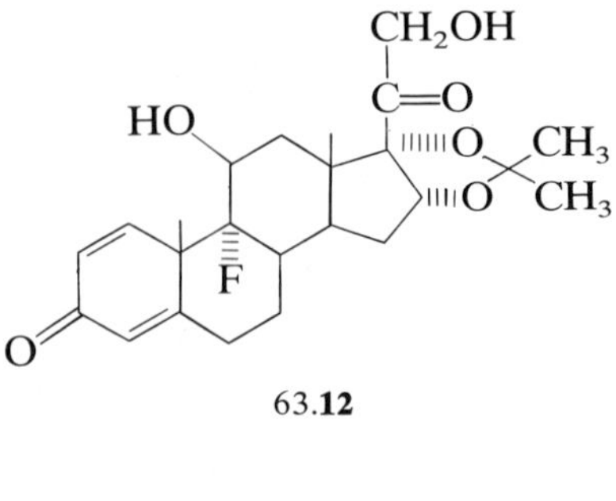

63.**10**

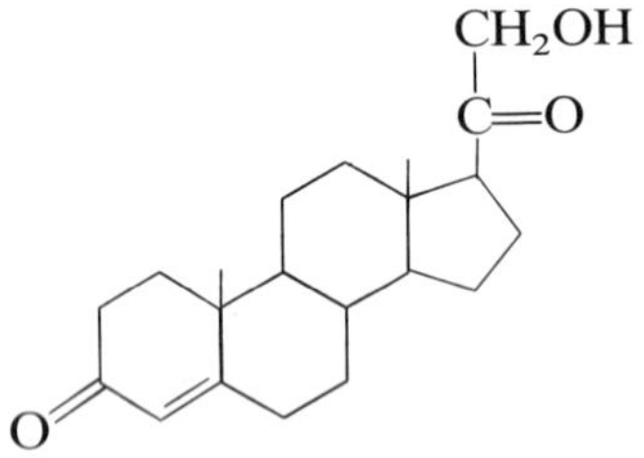

63.**11**

4.2 Percutaneous Absorption

Using ^{14}C-labeled steroids, it has been shown that cortisol (63.**2**) and triamcino-

63.**12**

This property is fostered by the presence of lipophilic groups and by the absence of hydroxy groups in the steroid (4a). The conversion of one or two hydroxyl groups in anti-inflammatory steroids to more lipophilic derivatives, such as esters or ketals, is an effective way to produce locally active anti-inflammatory agents, as in the case of triamcinolone already cited.

4.2.1 16α,17α-KETALS. 16α, 17α-ketals are fomed by the reaction of 16α,17α-dihydroxy steroids and the appropriate ketones or aldehydes in the presence of an acid catalyst, to give a new pentacyclic ring. Unlike other dioxolanes which are readily hydrolyzed by dilute acid to afford the parent constituents, these steroidal dioxolanes are unusually stable. This led Fried et al. (12) to conclude that the compounds are active *per se*, and not as a result of hydrolysis *in vivo* to the parent compound. As has been mentioned, triamcinolone acetonide displays a dissociation between topical and systemic activity. The 6α-fluoro derivative, fluocinolone acetonide (63.**13a**), is also used extensively as a topical agent.

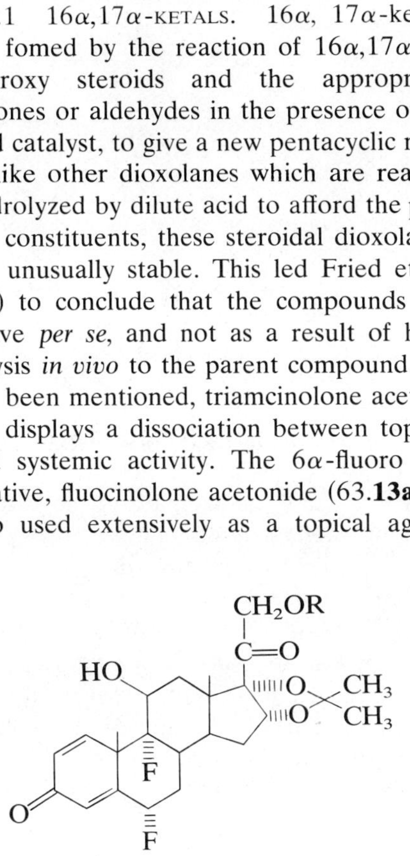

63.**13a** R = H
63.**13b** R = Ac

These compounds can be made even more lipophilic by the preparation of 21-esters. Thus fluocinonide (63.**13b**), the 21-acetate of fluocinolone acetonide, is about five times as active as the latter compound (13). Other ketals that have anti-inflammatory activity are the 17,21-acetonides, but these have not found clinical application.

4.2.2 ESTERS. The evaluation of a number of 17-esters, 21-esters, and 17,21-diesters of betamethasone (63.**14a**) was carried out by McKenzie and Atkinson (14) (Table 63.3). The least active compounds are the unesterified parent and the highly polar monophosphate ester (63.**14b**). In all three series shown, activity seems to have a parabolic dependence on the π value of the esterifying acid, as would be expected on the basis of the absorption process already discussed. Betamethasone 17-valerate

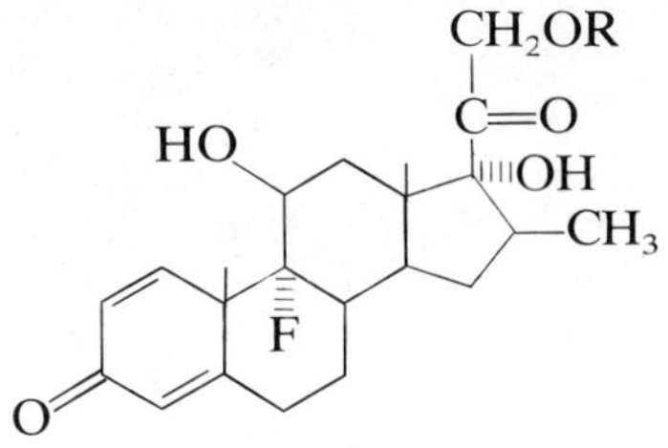

63.**14**

a   R = H
b   R = P(O)(ONa)$_2$
c   R = Ac
d   R = C(O)C$_3$H$_7$
e   R = C(O)C$_4$H$_9$
f   R = C(O)C$_5$H$_{11}$
g   R = C(O)C$_{15}$H$_{31}$

(63.**15c**) is a widely used topical anti-inflammatory agent and the related 17-benzoate (63.**15d**) is also in clinical use. Betamethasone 17,21-dipropionate is also in clinical use as a topical anti-inflammatory steroid. Even the weakly active 21-deoxyprednisolone (63.**17**), which has

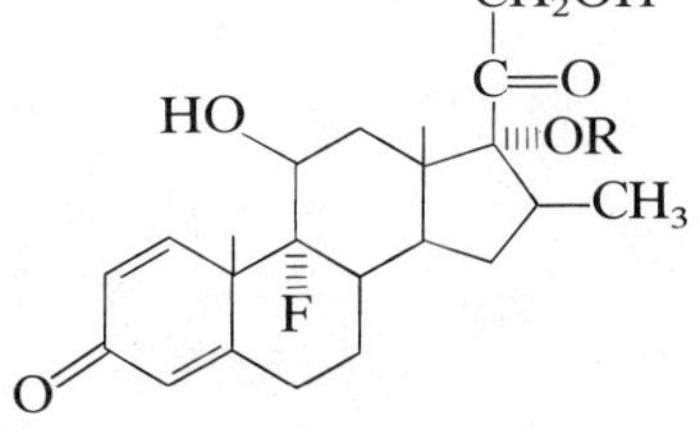

63.**15**

a   R = Ac
b   R = C(O)C$_3$H$_7$
c   R = C(O)C$_4$H$_9$
d   R = C(O)C$_6$H$_5$

Table 63.3 Relative Potencies of Betamethasone and Some of Its Esters in Vasocon-striction Assays against Fluocinolone Acetonide[a]

Compound No.	Compound	Relative Potency[b]
63.**14a**	Betamethasone alcohol	0.8
63.**14b**	Betamethasone 21-disodium phosphate	0.9
63.**14c**	Betamethasone 21-acetate	18
63.**14d**	Betamethasone 21-butyrate	85
63.**14e**	Betamethasone 21-valerate	26
63.**14f**	Betamethasone 21-hexanoate	123
63.**14g**	Betamethasone 21-palmitate	0.1
63.**15a**	Betamethasone 17-acetate	114
63.**15b**	Betamethasone 17-butyrate	168
63.**15c**	Betamethasone 17-valerate	360
63.**16a**	Betamethasone 17,21-ethylorthoformate	1
63.**16b**	Betamethasone 17,21-ethylorthopropionate	402
63.**16c**	Betamethasone 17,21-ethylorthovalerate	150

[a] Data from Ref. 14.
[b] Fluocinolone acetonide 63.**13a** = 100.

25% of the systemic activity of cortisol (15), gives a clinically useful compound upon conversion to the 17-propionate (4).

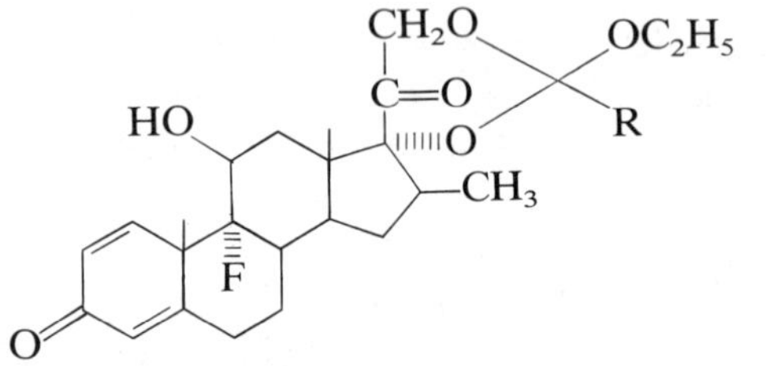

63.**16a**   R = H
63.**16b**   R = C$_2$H$_5$
63.**16c**   R = C$_4$H$_9$

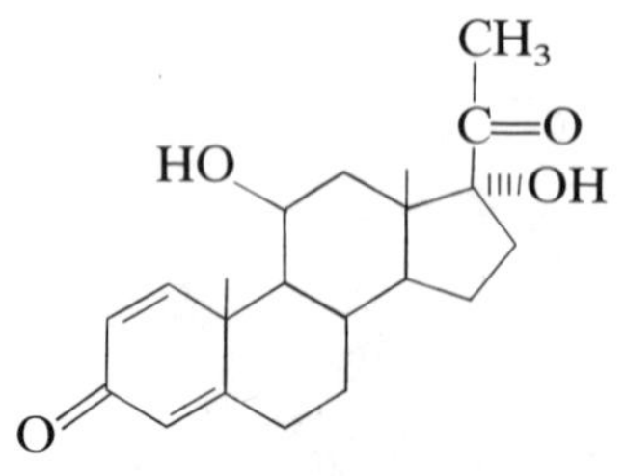

63.**17**

4.3 Intra-articular Administration

Arthritic and inflammatory conditions afflicting skeletal joints may be treated by intra-articular injections in which a hypodermic needle is passed through the synovial membrane and a dose of cortico-steroid is injected into the joint cavity. The specific local anti-inflammatory effect lasts from 5 to 21 days or longer. Water-soluble esters of anti-inflammatory steroids are rapidly cleared from the joint and have a very short duration of action under these circumstances. Conversely, aqueous micro-crystalline suspensions of ketals and esters of anti-inflammatory steroids dissolve suffi-cient quantities to permit local action in the joint but do not enter the systemic circula-tion in amounts needed to exert substantial systemic effect. In addition to tri-amcinolone acetonide, branched esters that hydrolyze slowly, such as triamcinolone hexacetonide (16) (63.**18**) and dexa-methasone 21-trimethylacetate (17) (63.**19**), are useful for this purpose. 6α-Methyl-

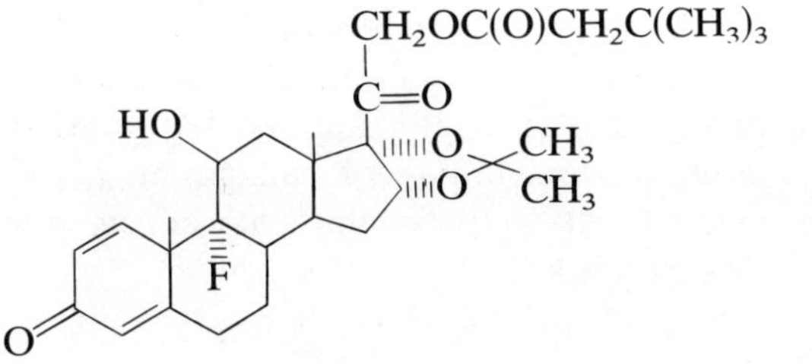

63.**18**

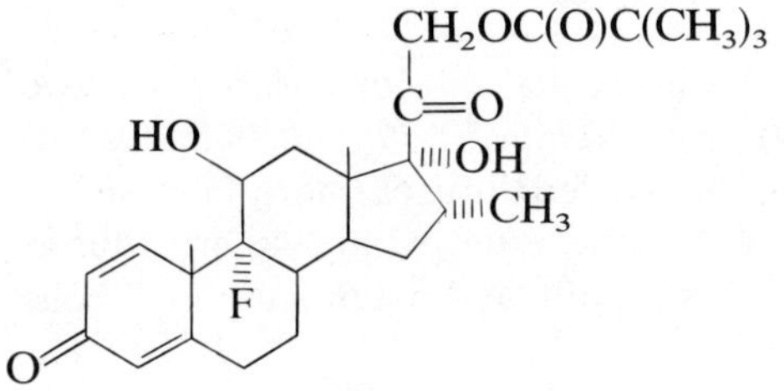

63.**19**

prednisolone acetate (18) and betametha-sone 17,21-dipropionate (19) also are active long enough to be useful.

4.4 Water-soluble Esters

The incorporation of ionic groups into anti-inflammatory steroids at the 21 position results in water-soluble steroids that have rapid onset of action but are of fleeting duration. The esters employed include the 21-phosphate disodium salts and the 21-hemisuccinate sodium salts. There is extensive evidence indicating that such esters rapidly hydrolyze to the active 21 alcohols (19a) and therefore only represent solubilizing groups. Such compounds can be used for ophthalmic purposes as well as for intravenous administration. Moreover, they may be incorporated in long-acting depot preparations in order to add a rapid-acting component.

4.5 Corneal Penetration

Schoenwald and Ward (19b) determined the permeability rates across excised rabbit cornea for 11 steroids. They derived a parabolic relationship between log permeability and octanol–water partition coefficient with an optimum at log P_0 of 2.9 (close to dexamethasone acetate).

5 EFFECTS ON DRUG DISTRIBUTION

Only about 5% of cortisol in plasma is circulated in the unbound state. The remainder is bound to two major moieties in serum: serum albumin and corticosteroid binding globulin (CBG). This subject has been reviewed by Westphal (20). Serum albumin is present in higher concentration ($5500 \times 10^{-7} M$ in human serum) whereas the concentration of CBG in human serum is $8 \times 10^{-7} M$. However, the equilibrium association constant (K_{aff}) for cortisol–CBG is $3 \times 10^{-7} M^{-1}$, about 10^3 greater than that for cortisol–serum albumin.

There is good evidence to support the notion that the steroids are complexed to these proteins primarily by hydrophobic bonds (21, 22). This implies that the steroid interacts primarily with nonpolar portions of the protein. The affinity of steroids to serum albumin decreases with an increasing number of hydrophilic or polar groups in the molecule (23). The hydrophobic effect depends on the displacement of ordered water from two surfaces, and it is clear that the presence of a hydrophilic group on one of the surfaces will interfere with this process. The type of substituent group is obviously important, since on this basis, a hydroxyl group should interfere more with binding than would a more lipophilic fluorine congener. The stereochemistry of the derivative is also significant; 11β-hydroxyprogesterone (63.**20**) has higher affinity for serum albumin than does the 11α epimer. This has led to the suggestion (24) that the steroids are bound to albumin on their α face.

Binding of steroids to human and rat CBG is also diminished by the presence of

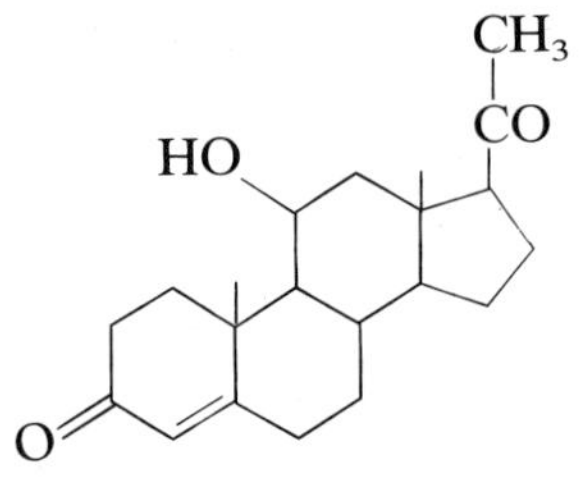

63.**20**

polar groups (25). Interestingly, the order of binding for rabbit CBG is cortisol (63.**2**) > corticosterone (63.**21**) > progesterone (63.**10**) and thus opposite to the order one would predict from the polarity of substituents (25). This is evidence for structural specificity in steroid–CBG binding, and it suggests the presence of a "binding site" on the protein with specific structural requirements for optimum binding.

This concept of a specific binding site is also in harmony with the reduction of binding to CBG on introduction of numerous substituents into the cortisol structure, irrespective of the polarity of the group (26). A study (27) that illustrates this difference compared the binding to CBG of cortisol, dexamethasone (63.**9**), and its 16β-methyl epimer (betamethasone, 63.**14a**). It was found that all the steroids are bound extensively to serum albumin, whereas only cortisol is bound to CBG.

The effect of protein binding on biologic activity is not simple to assess. On the one hand, CBG-bound cortisol is biologically inactive (28), and decreased protein binding would lead to enhanced activity on this basis. On the other hand, it has been shown (29) that CBG protects cortisol against

63.**21**

metabolic degradation by rat liver homogenate. Since the two phenomena tend to cancel each other, it is impossible to state *a priori* the magnitude of changes in pharmacological activity due to effects on plasma binding.

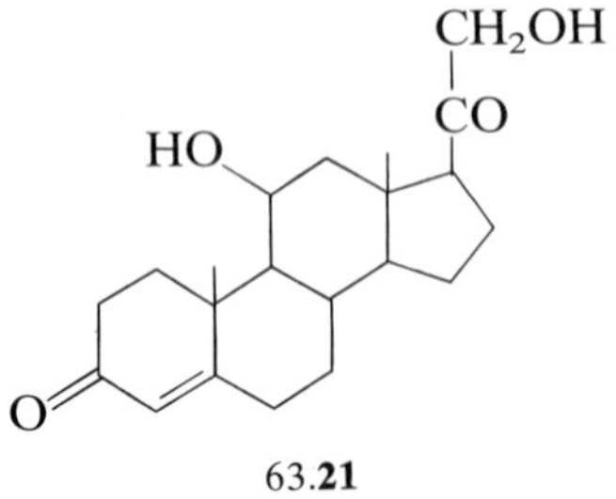

6   EFFECTS ON DRUG METABOLISM

The plasma half-life of cortisol is between 80 and 100 mins. After the administration of ^{14}C-labeled cortisol, more than 90% appears in the urine within 48 hr. Thus cortisol is rapidly and extensively metabolized (30).

Five major routes exist for the metabolism of corticoids to neutral products in the human (30) (Fig. 63.1). Each involves an initial attack at a different location in the molecule: oxidation of the 11β-hydroxy group, reduction of the 4,5 double bond, reduction of the C-20 ketone, hydroxylation at C-6, and degradation of the two-carbon side chain to the 17-ketone. About three-quarters of the metabolites of cortisol are the foregoing neutral species; oxidation at C-21 to C-21 carboxylic acids (30a) accounts for the remainder of the products (31) (Fig. 63.2). All these metabolic changes result in inactive or nearly inactive compounds, and only the oxidation of the 11β-alcohol to the 11-ketone is a reversible process (Fig. 63.1). Therefore, any group that stabilizes a corticoid to metabolic transformation will necessarily enhance the potency of the resulting compound, even if it has no effect, or a negative effect, on some other process such as receptor affinity.

In general, synthetic corticosteroids are metabolized by the same routes as cortisol (Figs. 63.1 and 63.2), but the rate of metabolism is usually slower (Table 63.4) and the proportion of each metabolite is different. Steroids with the greatest number of substituents generally have the slowest rate of metabolism. Groups that appear to

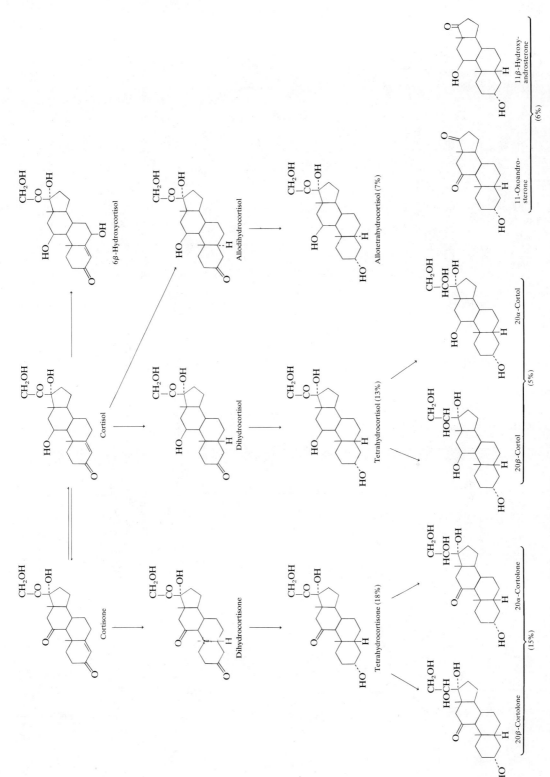

Fig. 63.1 Metabolism of corticosteroids (figures in parentheses denote percentage of administered dose of cortisol recovered as urinary metabolites).

1283

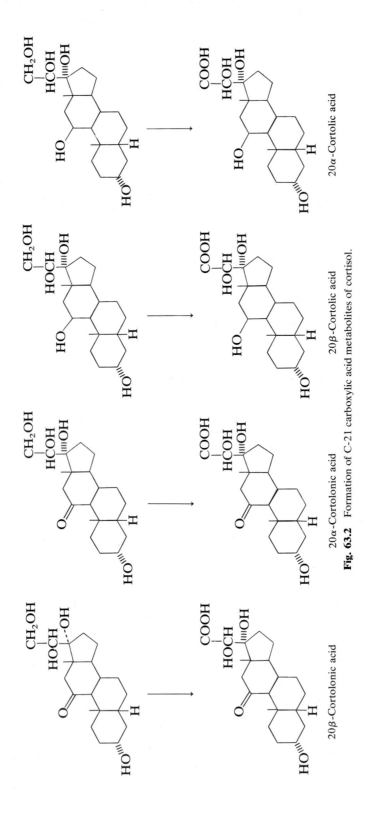

20α-Cortolic acid 20β-Cortolic acid 20α-Cortolonic acid 20β-Cortolonic acid

Fig. 63.2 Formation of C-21 carboxylic acid metabolites of cortisol.

Table 63.4 Half-lives of Corticosteroids in Dog Plasma

Steroid	Half-life, min	Ref.
Cortisol (63.**2**)	44–52	35–39
Prednisone (63.**5**)	38	38
9α-Fluorocortisol (63.**3**)	58	38
Dexamethasone (63.**9**)	60	39
Prednisolone (63.**6**)	60–71	35–39
6α-Methyl-prednisolone (63.**7**)	81	36
6α-Methyl-9α-fluoro-prednisolone (63.**22**)	110	36
Triamcinolone (63.**8**)	116	26, 40

activate by effects on metabolism include 2β-methyl, which stabilizes the resulting molecule to the action of the 4,5-reductase (32) and to the action of 20-keto reductases (33). Similarly, 6α-methyl protects the A ring against metabolic destruction (33). Again, the introduction of 16α-hydroxyl, as in triamcinolone (63.**8**), prolongs the half-life (34). The 16α-methyl and 16β-methyl groups have similar action. Triamcinolone is unusual in that it is metabolized principally to the 6β-hydroxy derivative (34).

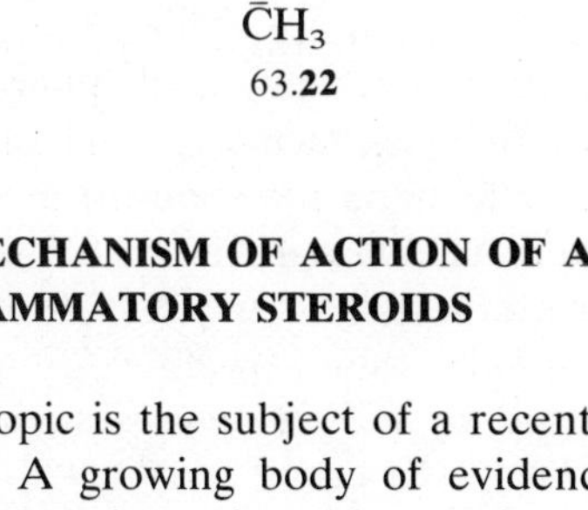

63.**22**

7 MECHANISM OF ACTION OF ANTI-INFLAMMATORY STEROIDS

This topic is the subject of a recent review (34a). A growing body of evidence indicates that induction of protein synthesis mediates the action of steroid hormones on growth, differentiation, and metabolism in target tissues (41). The initial events involve binding to a steroid-specific protein and attachment of the resulting complex to the genome.

Cytoplasmic receptors characterized by specificity in binding steroid hormones with high affinity have been demonstrated for all the physiological steroids (42). The situation regarding such receptors for anti-inflammatory steroids is complex. Cortisol and its congeners exert pronounced effects on a diversity of tissues. In the liver they stimulate the synthesis of enzymes such as tryptophan pyrrolase (42a) and tyrosine aminotransferase (TAT) (42b). Both these enzymes are probably involved in gluconeogenesis, one of the primary effects of cortisol.

The anti-inflammatory effect, by contrast, is apparently due to the induction of totally different proteins. Like nonsteroidal anti-inflammatory drugs (Chapter 62), the anti-inflammatory steroids can prevent prostaglandin biosynthesis. Unlike nonsteroidal anti-inflammatory drugs, anti-inflammatory steroids have no inhibitory effect on cyclooxygenase. Instead, they exert their action by inhibiting the release of phospholipids required for the biosynthesis of prostaglandins (43–50) (Fig. 63.3).

Vane and co-workers (51, 52) have shown that stimulation of release of thromboxane A$_2$ (TXA$_2$) (Part II, Chapter 33) by agents such as histamine, 5-hydroxytryptamine, and rabbit aorta contracting substance-releasing factor (RCS-RF), but not by arachidonic acid, is inhibited by anti-inflammatory steroids. Their potency in this action closely parallels their anti-inflammatory activity. Moreover, Vane's work has demonstrated that the mechanism of action of anti-inflammatory steroids involves the inhibition of phospholipase A$_2$ activity and thus of arachidonate release within the lung.

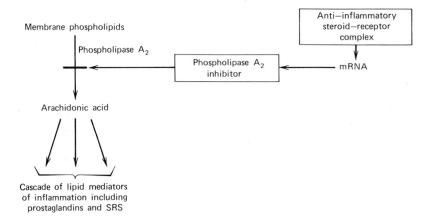

Fig. 63.3 Mechanism of action of anti-inflammatory steroids.

Recently, Flower and Blackwell (53) concluded that the antiphospholipase action of steroids is induced by a mechanism essentially similar to that mediating their other metabolic actions. The steroid first combines with a cytoplasmic receptor in the lung. The amounts of steroid required to saturate the lung receptors (10–20 pmol/mg protein) are higher than those reported for other tissues whereas the actual binding (fmol/mg protein) is lower. Hence either the lung has an exceptionally high concentration of receptors or the affinity of the steroid for the lung receptors is lower than is the case with other receptors. Inhibitors of RNA biosynthesis as well as of protein biosynthesis block the anti-inflammatory effects of the steroids in these preparations. Thus steroids appear to induce the synthesis of a factor that blocks phospholipase A_2. This factor is presumably a peptide or protein, for its biosynthesis is prevented by cycloheximide. Hence anti-inflammatory steroids can prevent biosynthesis of a whole cascade of lipid mediators of inflammation, including the prostaglandins and slow-reacting substance A (SRS-A) or leukotriene C (54, 55), which are derived from arachidonic acid (Fig. 63.3) (see Chapter 62).

8 EFFECTS ON DRUG RECEPTOR AFFINITY

The effect of structural alteration in steroids on receptor affinity, which could only be guessed at prior to 1960, has received increasing study as the fascinating story of steroid receptors has unfolded (42). However, the receptor affinity of a given steroid is not the sole or even the major determinant of its pharmacological potency. This can be appreciated readily from the data of Wolff et al. (56) (Table 63.5) relating to the glucocorticoid receptor of rat hepatoma cells. Whereas 9α-F (63.**3**) and 9α-Cl cortisol (63.**23b**) have essentially the same receptor affinity, their pharmacological activity differs by a factor of 2. The enhanced pharmacological potency of the 9α-F derivative is thus only partially accounted for at the receptor affinity level, and one or a combination of other major processes (intrinsic activity, drug distribution, and effects on metabolism) must also be affected. The data in Table 63.5 indicate that intrinsic activity is in fact also affected by the 9α substituent, since TAT induction is enhanced by the 9α-F substituent relative to the 9α-Cl group.

A similar situation is seen in the data of

Table 63.5   Comparison of Receptor Affinity and Intrinsic Activity of 9α-Substituted Cortisol Derivatives in Hepatoma Tissue Culture Cells[a]

Compound	Log K_{aff}	$-$Log $M_{1/2}$ TAT[b] Induction	Relative Potency (Glycogen Deposition, Rats)
9α-H (63.**2**)	7.69	6.68	1
9α-F (63.**23a**)	8.35	7.57	10
9α-Cl (63.**23b**)	8.24	5.77	4.7
9α-Br (63.**23c**)	6.16	3	0.3
9α-OMe (63.**23g**)	5.92	2	0

[a] Data from Ref. 56.

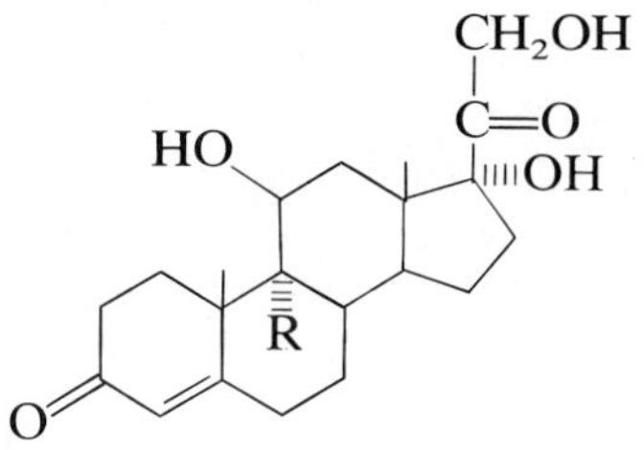

63.**23**

a   R = F
b   R = Cl
c   R = Br
d   R = I
e   R = OH
f   R = CH$_3$
g   R = OCH$_3$
h   R = OC$_2$H$_5$
i   R = SCN

Table 63.6   Receptor Binding and Biologic (Clauberg) Activity in Progestational Steroids[a]

Compound	Receptor Binding, %	Clauberg Activity, %
6α-Methylprogesterone (63.**24**)	26	150
Chlormadinone (63.**25**)	50	6000
6α-Methyl-17α-acetoxy-progesterone (63.**26**)	90	5500
6α-Fluoroprogesterone (63.**27**)	130	200
19-Norprogesterone (63.**28**)	168	600
Progesterone (63.**10**)	100	100

[a] Data from Ref. 57.

Smith et al. (57) (Table 63.6) regarding the progesterone receptor. Whereas 6-substituents and the 17α-acetoxy group actually decrease the receptor binding of progesterone, Clauberg activity is markedly enhanced. Decreased metabolic inactivation may be responsible for this, although more data are needed. Even the 19-nor modification, which substantially increases receptor binding, increases biologic activity only by a factor of 6, whereas the most powerful enhancing groups (Table 63.6) raise activity by a factor of 60.

Nevertheless, the relationship between chemical constitution and receptor binding is of great interest, since receptor binding is a *sine qua non* for biological activity. In a systematic study of the thermodynamics of binding of 29 different corticoids to the glucocorticoid receptor of rat hepatoma cells, Wolff et al. (56) formulated a concept of the nature of the steroid receptor interaction that rationalizes the thermodynamic properties of the steroid receptor binding process and affords a basis for predicting the binding affinity of any glucocorticoid derivative.

The temperature dependence of binding of these glucocorticoids to the rat HTC receptor was determined and a second-degree polynomial equation was fitted to the data points obtained (Fig. 63.4). The enthalpic and entropic terms of binding were calculated. As was the case for other steroid-protein interactions (58), both enthalpy and entropy decreased as the temp-

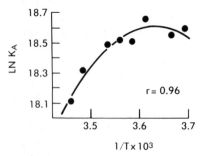

63.24   63.25   63.26

63.27   63.28

erature was increased (Table 63.7). It was concluded that the steroid receptor binding forces are mainly hydrophobic in character. Both the steroid and receptor are extensively hydrated and the displacement of water molecules upon binding is a principal driving force. This is reflected by the positive entropy (ΔS), negative enthalpy (ΔH), and negative heat capacity (ΔC_p) of association, since these phenomena are characteristic of the hydrophobic effect. From the temperature dependence of the rate constant (Fig. 63.5), the enthalpy of activation was found to be 12.8 kcal/mol and the en-

tropy of activation to be 17.2 eu, indicating that the driving force for the formation of the transition state is also the hydrophobic effect. It is noteworthy that if the formation of ligand–protein hydrogen bonds and other oriented structures were of paramount importance in the transition state, the entropy of activation would be negative, rather than positive. Hydrogen bonding presumably contributes very little to the overall driving force for ligand–protein interactions since the net differences in free energy between hydrogen bonding for ligand–protein in the bound state and hydrogen bonding between ligand, protein, and water in the unbound state are probably small.

From a consideration of the relationship between surface area of proteins and its contribution to hydrophobic bonding (59, 60), it could be shown (56) that the energy of binding could best be accounted for if the *entire steroid were enveloped on both sides by the receptor*. The steroid appears as a "hamburger patty" enveloped on both sides by the "hamburger bun" of the receptor.

Fig. 63.4 Plot of ln K_A versus $1/T$ for corticosterone binding to the rat HTC cell glucocorticoid receptor (T in °K). Adapted from Ref. 56.

Table 63.7 Calculated Values of the Enthalpic and Entropic Terms for Corticosterone Binding to the Rat HTC Glucocorticoid Receptor[a]

Term	Temperature,°C				
	0	5	10	15	20
ΔH, cal/mol	1200	0	−1000	−2200	−3200
ΔS, eu	29	24	20	15	12

[a] Data from Ref. 56. The polynomial function employed was $1.62 \times 10^7(1/T^2) + 118{,}000(1/T) - 195 = \ln K_a$.

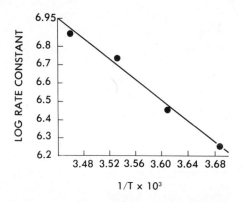

Fig. 63.5 Plot of the log of the association rate constant versus $1/T$ (°K) for dexamethasone binding to glucocorticoid receptors. Adapted from Ref. 56.

Interestingly, Anderson et al. (61) have recently proposed a similar picture of the binding of another nonprotein ligand to a protein. This is the case of the complex between glucose and hexokinase, an enzyme possessing a deep cleft between two lobes. They concluded that a dramatic conformational change occurs in hexokinase as glucose binds to the bottom of the cleft: the two lobes of hexokinase come together, engulfing the sugar (Fig. 63.6). These workers propose that glucose is sufficiently surrounded by the enzyme in this closed conformation that it cannot leave its binding site, which provides an explanation for the

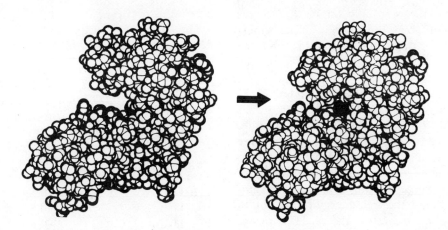

Fig. 63.6 Computer graphics display of the binding of glucose by hexokinase. Left, free hexokinase. Right, the enzyme substrate complex: the two lobes of hexokinase come together engulfing the sugar. Adapted from Anderson et al. (61).

Table 63.8   Free Energy Contribution to Binding to the Rat HTC Glucocorticoid Receptor per Substituent of Progesterone[a]

Substituent	Free Energy kcal/mol	Fried Glycogen Deposition Enhancement Factor (Rat)
Δ^1	−0.29	3–4
6α-F	−0.36	—
6α-CH$_3$	−1.09	2–3
9α-F	−0.57	10
9α-Cl	−0.71	3–5
9α-Br	+1.89	0.4
9α-OCH$_3$	+2.21	—
11β-OH	−0.89	—
11β-OH → 11-keto	+2.23	—
11-keto	+1.67	—
16α-CH$_3$	−0.11	—
16β-CH$_3$	−0.21	—
16α-OH + acetonide	−0.35	—
17α-OH	+0.49	1–2
21-OH	−0.56	4–7

[a] Data from Ref. 56.

observation (62) that the off-rate of glucose from its hexokinase complex is slow (58 sec^{-1}). It is noteworthy that far slower off-rates are characteristic of steroid–receptor complexes.

Another interesting point relates to the question of whether the steroid interacts with the receptor only on its β face, as suggested by Bush (63). The thermodynamic data indicate that this is not the case and that all of the steroid is in contact with receptor.

From a comparison of the binding of 22 corticoids, the approximate free energy increments of each substituent group were calculated (Table 63.8) (56). These free energy group increments can be added to approximate the binding constants of steroids whose binding constants are unknown. Thus the free energy of binding of fluocinolone (63.**29**) to the rat HTC receptor relative to progesterone is calculated as follows for substituents in fluocinolone in excess of the progesterone skeleton.

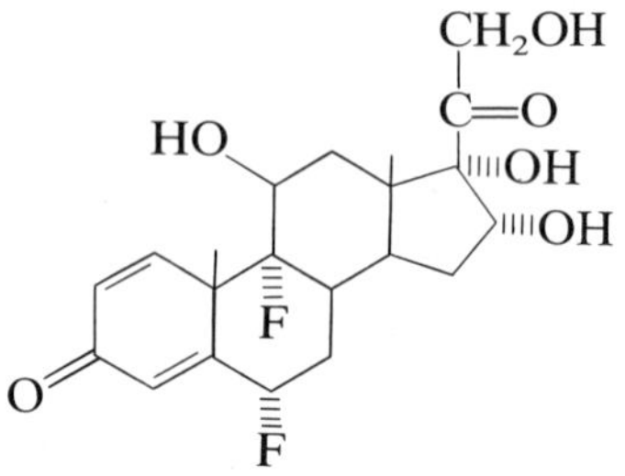

63.**29**

Substituent	ΔG Binding Contribution, kcal/mol
Δ^1	−0.29
6α-Fluoro	−0.36
9α-Fluoro	−0.57
11β-Hydroxy	−0.89
16α-Hydroxy	+0.86
17α-Hydroxy	+0.49
21-Hydroxy	−0.56
Total	−1.32

This calculation predicts that fluocinolone would bind to the receptor with a free energy of −1.32 kcal/mol more negative than progesterone, in fair agreement with the experimental value of −1.65 kcal/mol. These free energy increments may be compared with the pharmacological enhancement factors of Fried (64) (Table 63.8) (also see Section 9). It is seen that there is little correlation between the two parameters, indicating again that other variables, such as the inhibition of metabolic destruction, are of major importance.

The conformation of the A ring (65) has a pronounced effect on the binding of the steroid to the receptor. The difference in the C-3 to C-17 distance from progesterone in the steroids was employed as a measure of the A ring conformation, since this distance is strongly influenced by such conformational changes. It appeared that binding was greater as the distance decreased. The inclusion of a fluoro group at C-9 or a double bond at C-2 had the greatest effects on the A ring conformation. Other substituents had varying effects on the direction and magnitude of changes in the A ring conformation.

The effect of 9α-methoxy and 9α-bromo substituents stand apart in these binding studies. They result in derivatives with low binding affinities (Table 63.5), yet the surface area increases, owing to the respective 9α substituent. Evidently, the size of these substituents prevents the proper engagement of the steroid within the receptor site or induces a conformational change in the receptor such that binding is significantly altered.

A multiple regression analysis relating the above four parameters with the logarithm of the dissocation constant was made. The surface area (SA) employed for each derivative was the summation of the Bondi surface of each substituent present over that of a progesterone skeleton. The second parameter (P) is a de novo variable representing the interaction of polar groups

with the receptor. For each hydroxyl group present in the C-11 and/or C-21 position a value of +1 is assigned to account for the specific favorable interaction with the hydrogen bond acceptor in the receptor. If no group resides in these positions a value of 0 is assigned. A value of −1 is assigned for the presence of each C-17 or C-16 polar group to account for the consequences of placing a polar group in a nonpolar region and a value of −2 is given for the presence of an 11-keto functionality to express the conformational change associated with a sp^3 to sp^2 transformation and the undesirable dipole–dipole interaction of the 11-keto group with the hydrogen bond acceptor of the receptor apparently in that position. A total of these values is used for the second parameter, denoted as the polar interaction term. The third parameter (tilt) expresses the conformation of the A ring through the C-3 to C-17 distance in angstroms. The fourth parameter (X) expresses the size limitation at the 9α position. The value employed is the maximum of the function $(0, R_X − R_{Cl})$ where R_X is the distance in angstroms that a substituent radially extends from the pregnane ring system. An excellent correlation was found relating these four parameters to the logarithm of the equilibrium dissociation constant:

$$\log K_D = -0.022(\pm 0.002)SA$$
$$-0.59(\pm 0.05)P$$
$$+1.50(\pm 0.35)\text{tilt}$$
$$+6.10(\pm 0.49)X$$
$$-6.52$$

For this equation, n, the number of data points, is 29; r, the multiple correlation coefficient, is 0.97; s, the standard deviation of the regression, is 0.26; and F, a measure of the significance of the regression, is 106. Each parameter is significant at better than the 0.999 level. Shown in Fig. 63.7 is a plot of the calculated versus the observed logarithm of the equilibrium dissociation constant.

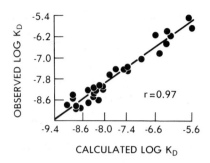

Fig. 63.7 Plot of observed logarithms of the equilibrium dissociation constant versus the values calculated from the QSAR equation. Adapted from Ref. 56.

An examination of the physical significance of this equation is of interest, since it should reflect the thermodynamic contributions of the substituents. The equation represents the effects of substituents on the K_D of progesterone, given by the intercept (−6.52). By multiplying by $2.303RT$, the equation is transormed to

$$\Delta G_{assoc}\ (\text{cal}) = -27(\pm 2)SA\ (\text{cal/Å})$$
$$-734(\pm 62)P\ (\text{cal/P})$$
$$+1865(\pm 435)\text{tilt}\ (\text{cal/Å})$$
$$+7585(\pm 609)X\ (\text{cal/Å})$$
$$-8143\ (\text{cal})$$

giving the thermodynamic equivalent of each parameter. The surface area term shows a contribution of 27 cal/Å², in good agreement with the temperature-corrected value of 22.5 cal/Å², based on the work of Chothia (59). The absolute value of 0.76 kcal per P unit agrees well with the values ranging from −0.89 kcal (attractive) + 0.86 kcal (repulsive) for hydroxyl groups (Table 63.8) and with the figure of −600 cal per hydrogen bond in the binding of trisaccharides to lysosome (66). The high value of the X term indicates the disruptive effect on binding owing to the introduction of a group larger than the corresponding "pocket" in the receptor.

A study by Ahmad and Mellors (81) indicated that the binding of steroid analogs to specific cytosol receptor proteins is correlated with the steroidal parachors although a quantitative relationship was not derived. Parachor is a molar parameter defined as the product of the molar volume and the fourth root of surface tension (66a). Hence parachor and surface area are strongly cross-correlated.

9 EFFECT OF STRUCTURAL CHANGE ON PHARMACOLOGICAL ACTION

9.1 Pharmacological Tests

In Table 63.9 are listed various pharmacological tests for anti-inflammatory steroids. Granuloma tests measure the ability of the rat to encapsulate a cotton pellet and are a measure of the anti-inflammatory effect. The liver glycogen deposition test is an index of glucocorticoid action that usually is well correlated with the anti-inflammatory effect. The other tests in Table 63.9 reflect the diverse action of these steroids. Nonsteroidal anti-inflammatory agents are poorly active in the granuloma tests, indicating the difference in their mode of action.

Table 63.9 Biologic Evaluation of Anti-inflammatory Steroids

Method	Species	Ref.
Granuloma (pellet)	Rat	66b, 67
Granuloma (pouch)	Rat	68, 69
Thymus involution	Rat	66b, 67, 70
Adrenal suppression	Rat	67
Adrenal steroid concentration	Rat	71
Body weight depression	Rat	66b, 67
Eosinopenia	Mouse	72
	Dog	69
Liver glycogen deposition	Rat	73
	Mouse	66b
Ulcerogenesis	Rat	66b, 74
Sodium retention	Rat	75

Table 63.10 Some Anti-inflammatory Steroids With Atypically Poor Correlation Between Human and Animal Data[a]

Compound	Anti-inflammatory Potency	
	Animals	Human
Cortisol (63.**2**)	1.0	1.0
Corticosterone (63.**21**)	0.3	Inactive
Δ^6-Cortisone (63.**30**)	0.5	Inactive
16α-Methylcortisol (63.**31**)	1.2	3
2α-Methylcortisol (63.**32**)	4.5	~1
Triamcinolone 16,17-acetonide (63.**12**)	75–80	4
21-Deoxy-16α-methyl-9α-fluoroprednisolone (63.**33**)	21	4–5
Betamethasone (63.**14a**)	58	30–35
Dexamethasone (63.**9**)	154	30

[a] Data from Ref. 3.

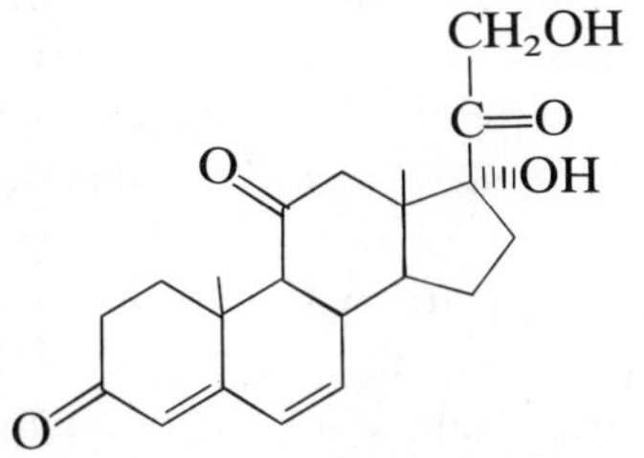

63.**30**

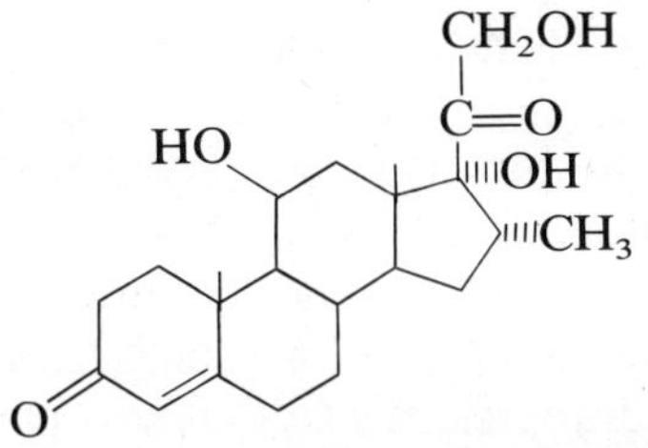

63.**31**

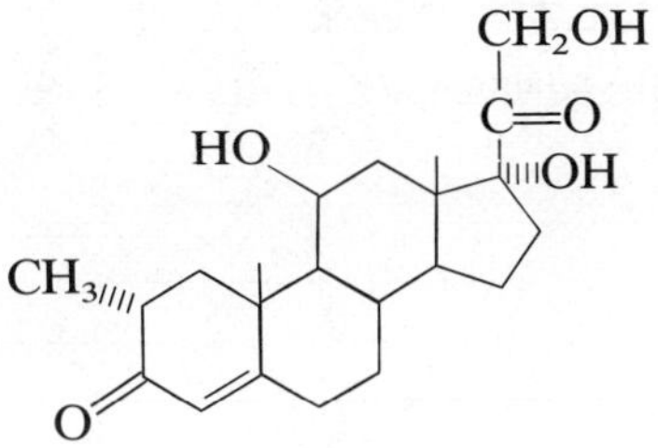

63.**32**

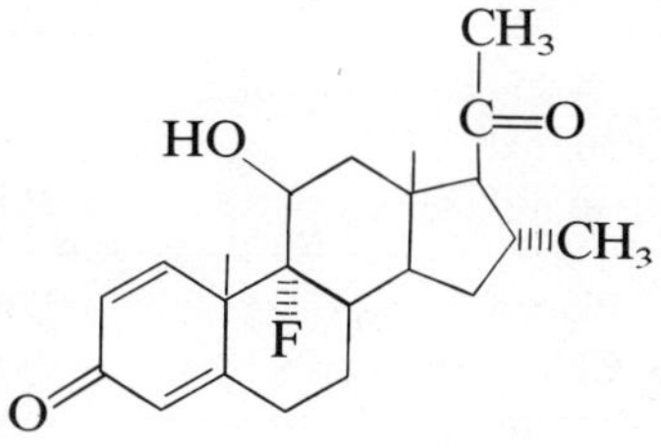

63.**33**

Animal data do not always predict potency in humans with accuracy. A number of examples are shown in Table 63.10 (3). At least a part of the problem lies in the fact that the rat secretes corticosterone (63.**21**), which is inactive as an anti-inflammatory in humans, rather than cortisol. The important drugs triamcinolone acetonide (63.**12**) and dexamethasone (63.**9**) are much more potent in rats than in humans.

9.2 QSAR Analyses of Pharmacological Action

In Section 8 we considered the application of QSAR techniques to a single process underlying steroid action, namely, drug receptor binding. In this section we examine the attempts that have been made to express the gross pharmacological activity of anti-inflammatory steroids through QSAR techniques.

As already noted, pharmacological activity represents the summation of a number of processes including absorption, metabolism, drug receptor affinity, intrinsic activity, and drug distribution. The effect of a given substituent, such as a 9α substituent, on these combined processes is difficult to parameterize; a single parameter for a substituent can represent only its *average* effect. Therefore, QSAR analyses of gross pharmacological activity are necessarily less accurate than those relating to a single process such as drug receptor binding. On the other hand, since pharmacological activity is the goal of drug design, the attempts described in this section have considerable interest. Such studies represent only approaches to the correlation of activity with structure and have not given final answers. Yet because they are relatively rigid molecules in which the effects of structural change are easily understood in steric and electronic terms, and because we know something of their mechanism of action, steroids represent a fruitful area in QSAR.

9.2.1 USE OF *de novo* CONSTANTS. The earliest QSAR analysis of anti-inflammatory steroids, and indeed one of the first QSAR analyses of any kind, was carried out by Fried and Borman (64) in an examination of compounds obtained by introducing halogen, hydroxyl or alkyl groups, or unsaturation into certain positions of the steroid molecule. These workers discovered the remarkable fact that each substituent affects the activity of the molecule almost independently of the presence of other activity modifying groups. The effect of each substituent was assigned a numerical value, a *de novo* constant termed an *enhancement factor* (Table 63.11). Multiplication of the biologic activity of a parent compound by the enhancement factors for the substituent groups gives the activity of the final analog. For example, Table 63.12 (76) illustrates the calculation of the potencies of a sequence of steroids starting with 11β-hydroxyprogesterone and culminating in triamcinolone. The ranges obtained are in good agreement

Table 63.11   Fried–Borman Enhancement Factors for Various Functional Groups[a]

Functional Group	Glycogen Deposition, Rat	Anti-inflammatory, Rat (Granuloma)	Effect on Urinary Sodium[b]
9α-Fluoro	10	7–10	+ + +
9α-Chloro	3–5	3	+ +
9α-Bromo	0.4[c]		+
12α-Fluoro	6–8[d]		+ +
12α-Chloro	4[c]		
1-Dehydro	3–4	3–4	−
6-Dehydro	0.5–0.7		+
2α-Methyl	3–6	1–4	+ +
6α-Methyl	2–3	1–2	− − −
16α-Hydroxyl	0.4–0.5	0.1–0.2	− − − − −
17α-Hydroxyl	1–2	4	−
21-Hydroxyl	4–7	25	+ +
21-Fluoro	2	2	− −

[a] Data from Ref. 64.
[b] + = Retention, − = Excretion.
[c] In 1-dehydrosteroids this value is 4.
[d] In the presence of a 17α-hydroxyl group this value is <0.01.

Table 63.12   Fried–Borman Calculation of Activities of Triamcinolone (63.8) Using Enhancement Factors[a]

Functional Group	Resulting Compound	Glycogen Deposition		Anti-inflammatory (Granuloma)		Effect on Urinary Sodium[b]	
		Calculated	Found	Calculated	Found	Calculated	Found
	11β-Hydroxypro-gesterone (63.**20**)		0.1		<0.01		
9α-Fluoro	9α-Fluoro-11β-hydroxy-progesterone (63.**34**)	1	0.85	<0.1	<0.1	+ + +	+ + +
21-Hydroxy	9α-Fluorocorti-costerone	4–7	4.6	<2.5	2.7	+ + + + +	+ + + + +
17α-Hydroxy	9α-Fluorocortisol (63.**3**)	4–14	11	11	13	+ + + +	+ + +
1-Dehydro	9α-Fluoroprednisolone (63.**34a**)	12–56	28	33–44	20	+ + +	+ + + +
16α-Hydroxy	Triamcinolone (63.**8**)	4.8–28	13	3.3–8.8	4	– –	– –

[a] Data from Ref. 76.
[b] +, Retention; –, excretion.

with the bioassay figures and their 95% confidence limits. Fried and Borman were unable to derive similar quantitative expressions for salt retaining activity, although the action of the various substituents on salt retention could be expressed in semiquantitative terms (Table 63.11). The effect in this case is additive rather than multiplicative.

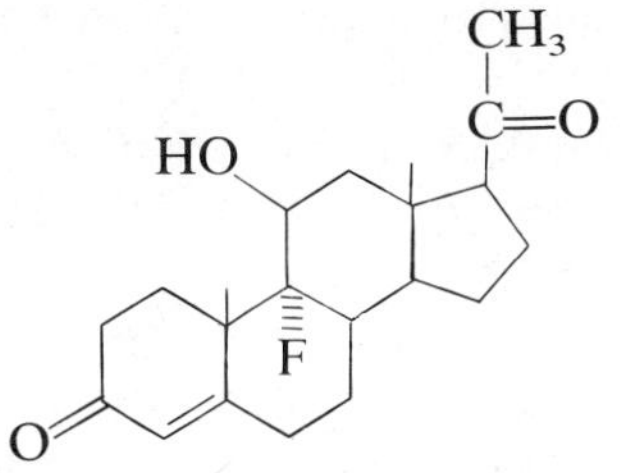

63.**34**

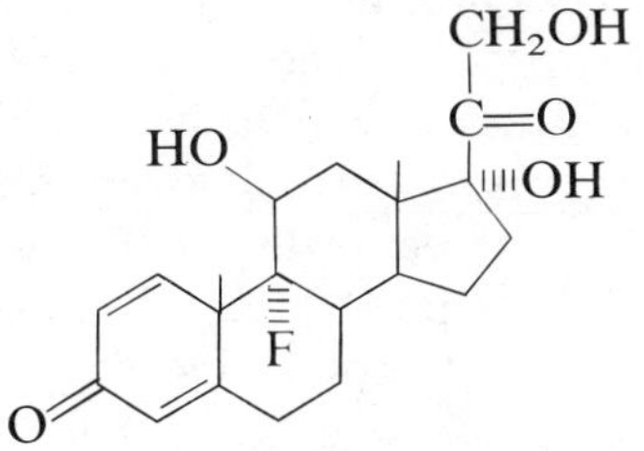

63.**34a**

Other workers have added additional enhancement factors to those listed in Table 63.11. In Table 63.13 additional values are given including those for activity in man. Although activities in man and the rat are

Table 63.13   Enhancement Factors for Important Corticoid Substituents[a]

Group	Anti-inflammatory (Rat)	Anti-inflammatory (Man)
1-Dehydro	3	4
2α-CH$_3$	4.5	0.7
6-Dehydro	0.5	Variable[b]
6α-CH$_3$	2	1.3
6α-F	8	2.5
9α-F	8	10
16α-CH$_3$	1.5	2
16β-CH$_3$	1.8	2.5
16-Methylene	1.5	—
16α-OH	0.2	0.5
16,17-Acetonide	8	1, (oral)[c]
21-F	2	—
21-Deoxy	0.1	<0.1

[a] Taken from Ref. 3, p. 73.
[b] Usually <1.
[c] Topical effect is high.

Table 63.14   Adrenocorticoid Activity Enhancement Factors[a]

Group	Glycogen Deposition	Thymolytic
9α-F	3.3	3.9
1-Dehydro	2.3	2.8
6α-Methyl	2.4	2.9
16α-Hydroxy	0.4	0.3
16,17-Acetonide	~2	~2.5

[a] From Ref. 77.

similar for many substituents, a major species difference is seen for the 2α-methyl group and the 6α-fluoro group. In Table 63.14 are listed enhancement factors from another laboratory (77), in which the 9α-fluoro substituent has a value of 3–4 rather than 7–10. A Fujita–Ban analysis on 44 corticoids was carried out by Justice (77a).

9.2.2   HANSCH TYPE ANALYSES.   Wolff and Hansch (78) carried out the first multiparameter regression analysis for steroids in an analysis of the anti-inflammatory activity of 9α-substituted cortisol derivatives. A series of seven active compounds, the 9α-F (63.**23a**), 9α-Cl (63.**23b**), 9α-Br (63.**23c**), 9α-I (63.**23d**), 9α-OH (63.**23e**), and 9α-CH$_3$ (63.**23f**) cortisol derivatives as well as cortisol itself, were analyzed. The results were applied to the inactive 9α-methoxy (63.**23g**), 9α-ethoxy (63.**23h**), and 9α-SCN (63.**23i**) compounds. It was found that activity was correlated with the inductive effect (σ_I), the size of substituents (molar reactivity, P_E), and π, giving the equation

$$\log A = 0.07 + 0.76\pi - 0.22 \log P_E + 2.78\sigma_I$$

For this equation n, the number of data points, is 7; s, the standard deviation, is 0.33; and r, the coefficient of correlation, is 0.96. The equation suggests that the activity of the compound rises with increasing electron withdrawal, decreasing size, and increasing hydrophobic bonding of the 9α

substituent. Moreover, it correctly predicts that the methoxy, ethoxy, and thiocyano compounds have little or no activity. The inverse relationship between the radius of the 9α-halogen atom and the magnitude of adrenocorticoid activity had already been noted by Fried (79), but Fried and Borman argued that the low activity of the 9α-hydroxy and 9α-methoxy compounds, which also have relatively small substituents, indicates "that it is the electronegativity of the substituent rather than its size that determines its enhancement properties." It is noteworthy that the quantitative multiparameter regression technique shows it is perfectly possible for the inverse relationship with increasing size to exist, even though a qualitative examination of the data led the earlier workers to conclude otherwise. Fried and Borman (76) suggested that the function of the electron-withdrawing group at C-9 was to increase the acidity of the neighboring 11β-hydroxy group and that "the corticoid activity of an 11β-hydroxysteroid increases with increasing acidity of the 11β-hydroxy group." They further speculated that "protein steroid binding at the site of action could be a function of the acidity of the 11β-hydroxy group." Newer developments concerning this possibility are described in Section 9.3.2.

The significance of the π parameter is more difficult to delineate. The increase in activity with increasing hydrophobicity could be due to better transport to the site of action for the more lipophilic compounds and/or to hydrophobic interactions at the active site. In a reexamination of this problem Coburn and Solo (80) found that the activity of 9α-substituted cortisols is well correlated with σ_I and a simple steric factor such as molar refractivity (MR), provided that the 9α-hydroxylated compound is excluded from the series. They suggested that compounds containing strongly hydrated 9α-substituents would have a larger effective bulk than is found in the unhydrated species and hence a lower predicted activity. In another reexamination, Ahmad and Mellors (81) found that molar parachor gives a better fit than π in single parameter equations but not in a three parameter equation.

9.3   Some Steric and Electronic Factors Affecting Anti-inflammatory Activity

In the following we discuss a number of studies using the techniques of extended Hückel theory (EHT) and geometry optimization through energy minimization to determine the preferred conformation of steroid molecules. In some cases it is possible to compare these theoretical results with the findings of X-ray crystallography. Also discussed are electronic structure examinations using CNDO/2 molecular orbital calculations. Although none of these examinations has provided a comprehensive understanding of the effect of structural change on biologic activity, a few underlying principles are beginning to emerge.

9.3.1   EFFECT OF STRUCTURAL CHANGE ON STEROID CONFORMATION. Some steroids have greater flexibility than others. The introduction of unsaturation into the steroid molecule tends to increase its flexibility. In the case of many anti-inflammatory steroids the presence of unsaturation at C-4 and C-1 produces compounds that may exist as a range of conformers oscillating over a broad energy minimum, or as several conformers of nearly equal energy separated by a significant barrier. This flexibility complicates the question of interatomic distances between such key atoms as O-3 and O-20 and the effect of structural change on these distances.

An obvious point of interest in this connection is the conformation of the side chain of glucocorticoids, since this portion of the molecule includes the key O-20 and O-21 oxygen functions. In principle, a 360° rotation of the side chain is possible, but it is obvious that steric factors will tend to favor only selected conformations. Numerous investigators have studied this matter by chemical (82), physicochemical (83, 84), quantum chemical (85), crystallographic (86, 87), and energy minimization (88) methods. Most of these analyses have indicated that O-20 approximately eclipses C-16. In the energy minimization work of Schmit and Rousseau (88) significant differences were found relative to the crystallographic studies cited. They suggested that one reason for the discrepancy between energy optimized and X-ray diffraction data could be the influence of intermolecular hydrogen bonds and packing forces in the crystal. Moreover, as they pointed out, in certain cases two independent crystallographic structures are observed, indicating that the crystallographic data do not necessarily give an unambiguous picture of side chain conformation. The most important factor influencing the position of the C-20 carbonyl is the presence or absence of a 17α-hydroxyl group, according to the study of Schmit and Rousseau (88).

Weeks et al. (89) examined the structures of six corticosteroids and noted a correlation between the degree of bowing of the fused ring system toward the α face and the anti-inflammatory activity. The presence of a C-1 double bond and a 9α-fluoro group brought about these changes. (Fig. 63.8). It is clear that bowing could only be one of several factors affecting biologic activity since 9α-chlorocortisol (90) is about four times as active as cortisol, but is not bowed more than cortisol, whereas 9α-methoxy-cortisol (91) is inactive but is bowed more than cortisol. Schmit and Rousseau (92) undertook a Free–Wilson (93) analysis of the effect of various substituents on the conformation of the steroid based on predicted energy minimization structure (not the X-ray structure). In accord with

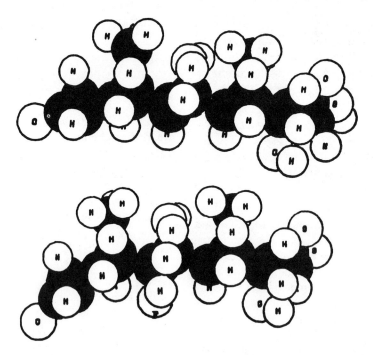

Fig. 63.8 PROPHET computer graphics representation of cortisol (63.**1**) and 9α-fluorocortisol (63.**3**) based on X-ray coordinates. Carbon atoms are black; all other elements are open circles. The greater "tilt" of the A ring in 9α-fluorocortisol relative to the BCD ring plane is readily seen. Adapted from Ref. 94.

the X-ray results, they found that the curvature of the entire steroid molecule (A/D angle) is increased 30% by a C-1 double bond and 14% by an 11β-hydroxy substituent. It is decreased 14% by a 17α-hydroxy substitution. These results parallel the biologic data in rats.

A geometry minimization study by Marsh et al. (94) indicated that the conformational effect of the 9α-fluoro group is due to its effect on B, C, and D rings which then induces a conformational change in the A ring.

Dideberg et al. (95) analyzed the crystal structure data of 20 corticoids. On the basis of their results they suggested that the distance between the atoms on the receptor capable of binding the steroid at O-3 and O-20 is 16.5 Å.

9.3.2 EFFECTS OF STRUCTURAL CHANGE ON ELECTRONIC CHARACTERISTICS OF THE STEROID. As noted, the electronic effect

of the 9α substituent was already invoked by Fried in attempting to explain how substitution at C-9 could modify biologic activity. More recently the electron densities in portions of cortisol, 6α-fluorocortisol, and 9α-fluorocortisol were calculated using X-ray structures and the CNDO/2 method by Kollman et al. (96).

They concluded that hydrogen bonding differences due to electron density changes engendered by the 9α-substituent could not fully account for the observed activity differences. Moreover, Divine and Lack (97) showed that the hydrogen bonding ability of the hydroxyl proton of 9α-substituted 11β-hydroxyprogesterone derivatives decreases in the order F≅Cl> Br>H. If the cortisols behave similarly, there must be additional factors explaining the greater glucocorticoid activity of 9α-fluoro cortisol relative to 9α-chlorocortisol, which has only four times the activity of cortisol itself.

9.4 Summary of the Results of Theoretical Studies

Theoretical studies have shown that a given structural change in an anti-inflammatory steroid affects not one but a multitude of factors. The introduction of a 9α-fluoro substituent, for example, alters the conformation of the entire steroid molecule and increases the acidity and hydrogen bonding capacity of the 11β-hydroxyl group. These changes influence receptor binding, protein binding, and metabolic stability. The sum of these effects is manifested as the observed increase in biologic activity. The action of structural changes on only one individual processes, receptor binding, can be predicted with accuracy (19). Gross pharmacological activity has been predictable for two decades using the technique of

Table 63.15   Relative Potencies of Glucocorticoids (I)[a]

Compound	Relative Activity in Adrenalectomized Rat		
	Granuloma	Thymolytic	Glycogen Deposition
Cortisol 21-acetate	1.0	1.0	1.9
Cortisone 21-acetate	0.5	0.5	1.0
Prednisione 21-acetate	1.0	0.9	5.2
Prednisolone 21-acetate	2.7	4.0	9.9
6α-Methylprednisolone (63.**7**)	6.0	3.0	26.0
9α-Fluoroprednisolone (63.**34a**)	17.7	4.4	53.9
Triamcinolone (63.**8**)	2.6	3.6	34.0
Triamcinolone acetonide (63.**12**)	48.5	37.7	216.
$6\alpha,9\alpha$-Difluoro-16α-hydroxy-cortisol $16\alpha,17\alpha$-acetonide (63.**35**)	103.	22.0	143.
Fluocinolone (63.**29**)	19.7	8.5	88.3
Fluocinolone acetonide (63.**13a**)	446.	263.	276.
6α-Chloro-9α-fluoro-16α-hydroxyprednisolone $16\alpha,17\alpha$-acetonide 21-acetate (63.**36**)	123.	188.	114.
Paramethasone (63.**37**)	63.6	45.1	46.2
Dexamethasone (63.**9**)	104.	47.0	181.
Betamethasone (63.**14a**)	35.8	11.7	118.

[a] Data from Ref. 98.

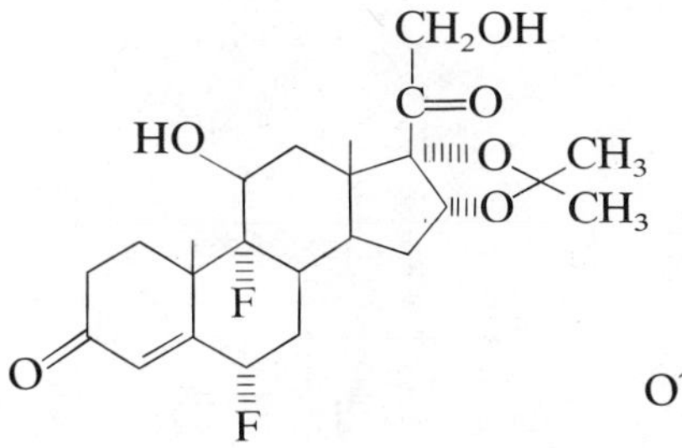

63.35

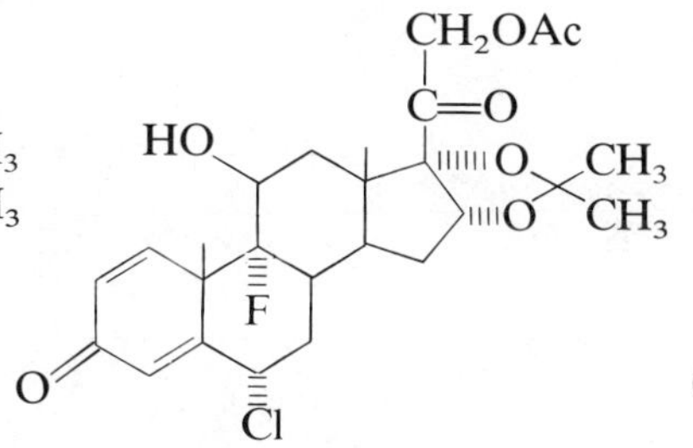

63.36

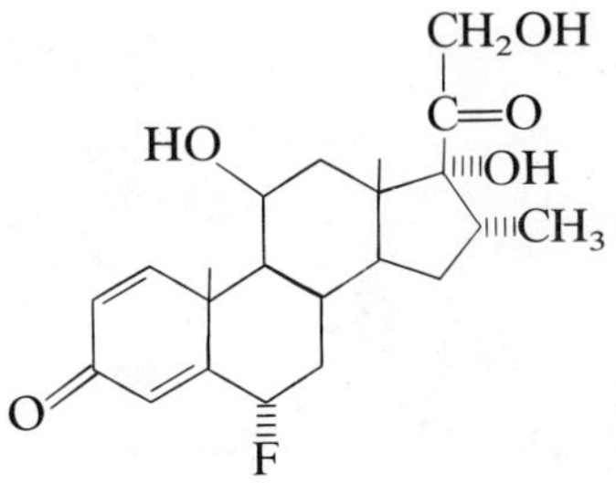

63.37

Table 63.16 Relative Potencies of Glucocorticoids (II)[a]

Steroid	Glycogen Deposition	Thymolytic
Cortisol (63.**2**)	1.0	1.0
16α-Hydroxycortisol (63.**38**)	0.4	0.3
16α-Hydroxycortisol 16,17-acetonide (63.**39**)	2.0	2.2
Prednisolone (63.**6**)	4.1	2.3
16α-Hydroxyprednisolone (63.**40**)	0.9	1.3
16α-Hydroxyprednisolone 16,17-acetonide (63.**41**)	13.0	17.0
6α-Methylcortisol (63.**42**)	9.5	5.8
16α-Hydroxy-6α-methylcortisol (63.**43**)	1.1	1.2
16α-Hydroxy-6α-methyl-cortisol 16,17-acetonide (63.**44**)	10.0	14.0
9α-Fluorocortisol (63.**3**)	6.1	5.6
16α-Hydroxy-9α-fluorocortisol (63.**45**)	7.9	2.4
16α-Hydroxy-9α-fluorocortisol 16,17-acetonide (63.**46**)	14.0	14.0
6α-Methyl-9α-fluorocortisol (63.**47**)	9.0	9.8
16α-Hydroxy-6α-methyl-9α-fluorocortisol (63.**48**)	2.8	4.2
16α-Hydroxy-6α-methyl-9α-fluorocortisol 16,17-acetonide (63.**49**)	15.0	29.0
6α-Methylprednisolone (63.**7**)	8.4	10.0
16α-Hydroxy-6α-methylprednisolone (63.**50**)	2.0	2.2
16α-Hydroxy-6α-methylprednisolone 16,17-acetonide (63.**51**)	24.0	28.0
9α-Fluoroprednisolone (63.**34a**)	13.0	16.0
Triamcinolone (63.**8**)	6.1	3.9
Triamcinolone acetonide (63.**12**)	32.0	33.0
6α-Methyl-9α-fluoroprednisolone (63.**22**)	16.0	25.0
16α-Hydroxy-6α-methyl-9α-fluoroprednisolone (63.**52**)	4.9	5.5
16α-Hydroxy-6α-methyl-9α-fluoroprednisolone 16,17-acetonide (63.**53**)	21.0	70.0

[a] Data from Ref. 77.

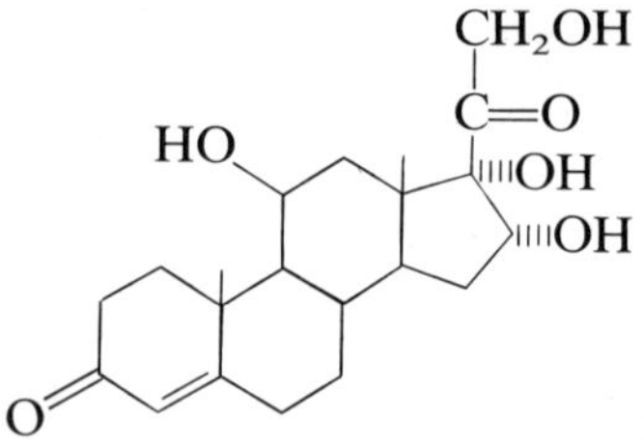

63.**38**

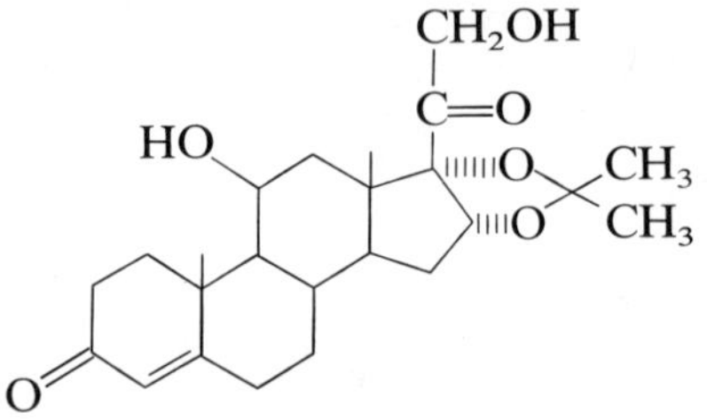

63.**39**

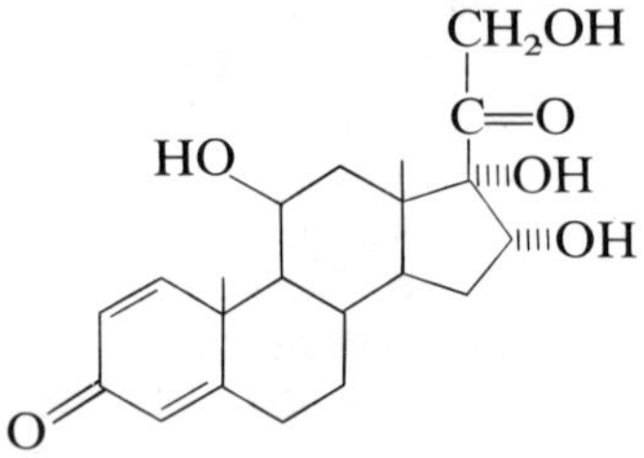

63.**40**

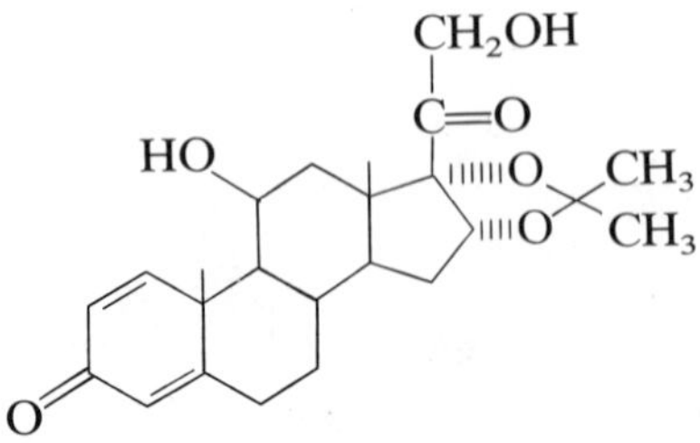

63.**41**

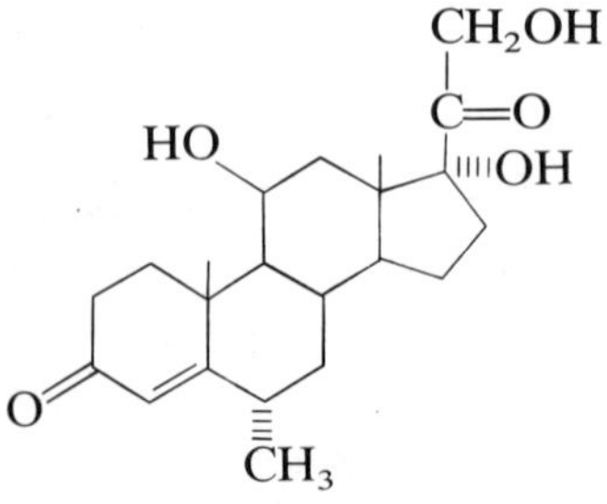

63.**42**

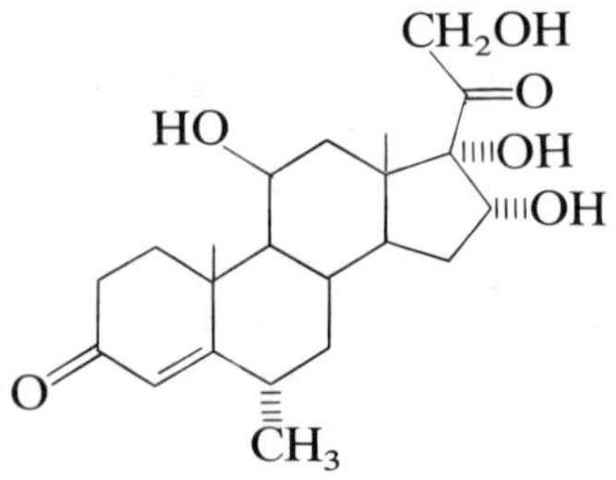

63.**43**

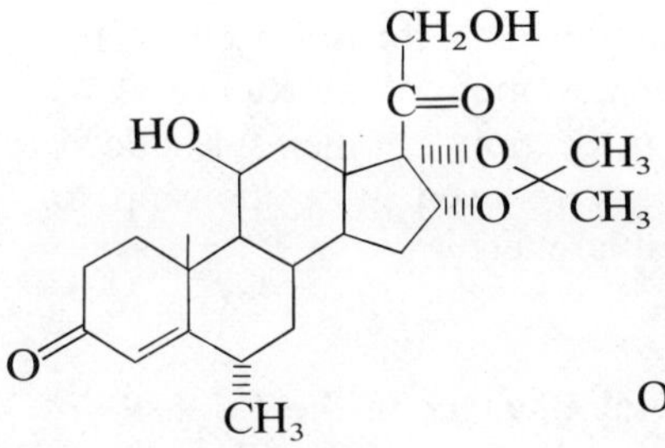

63.**44**

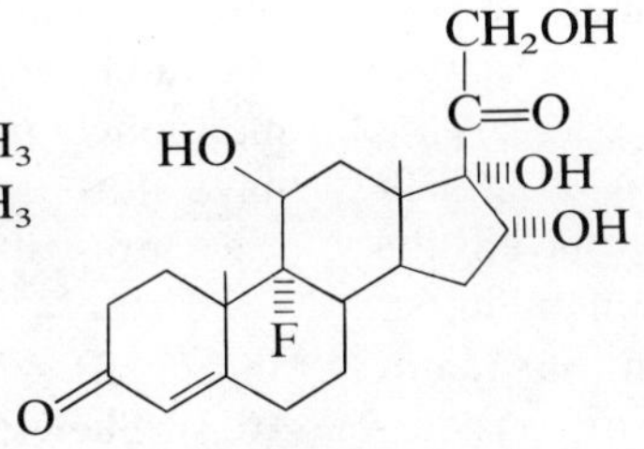

63.**45**

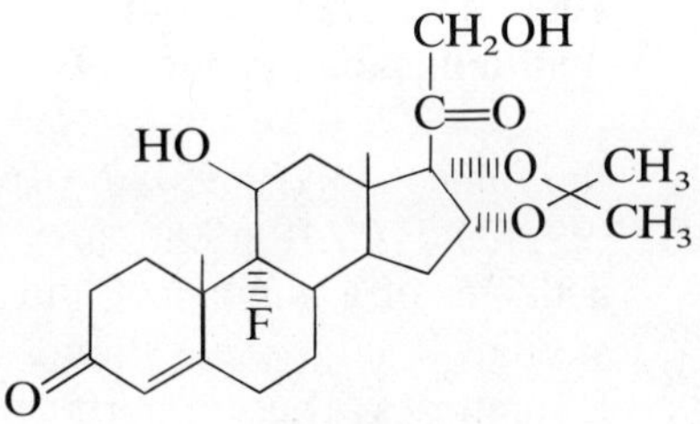

63.**46**

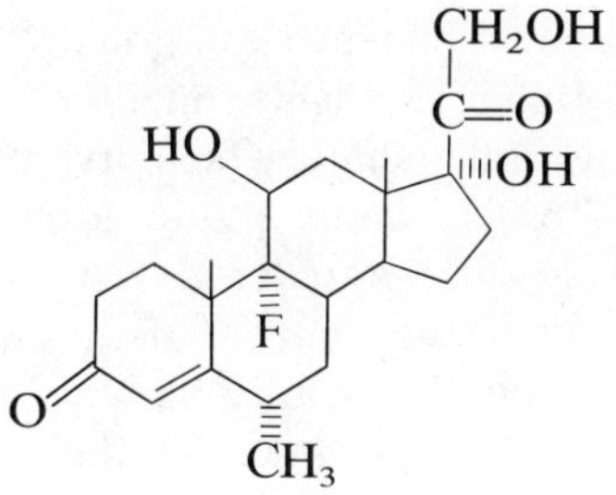

63.**47**

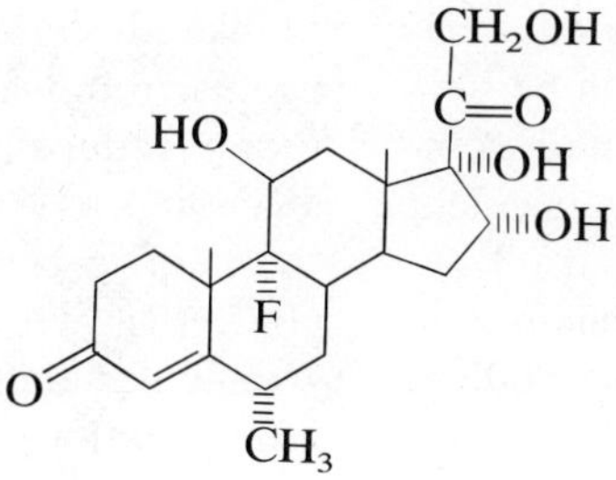

63.**48**

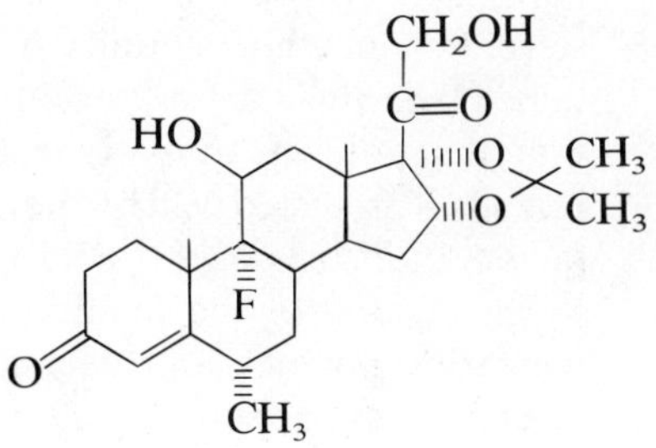

63.**49**

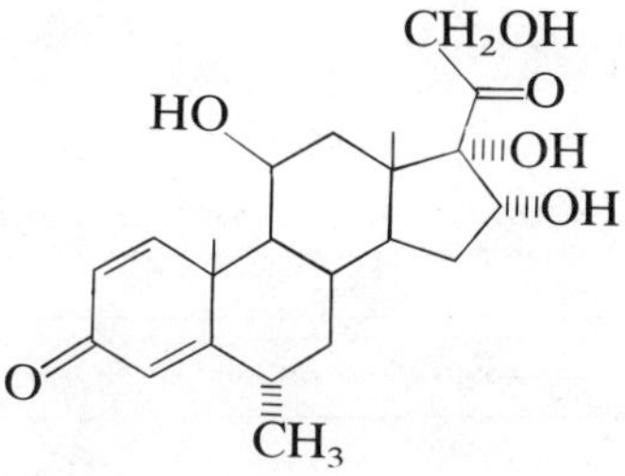

63.**50**

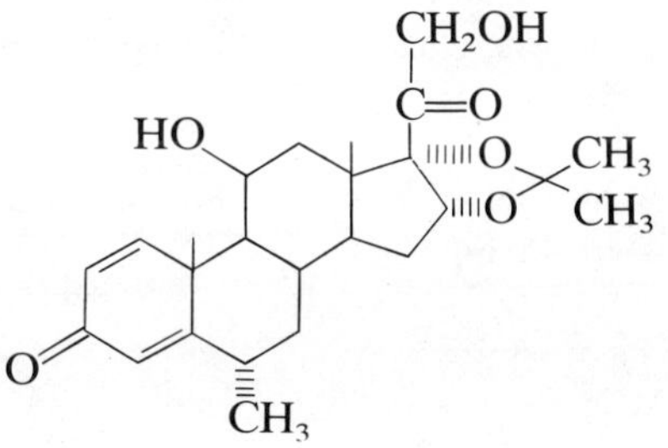

63.**51**

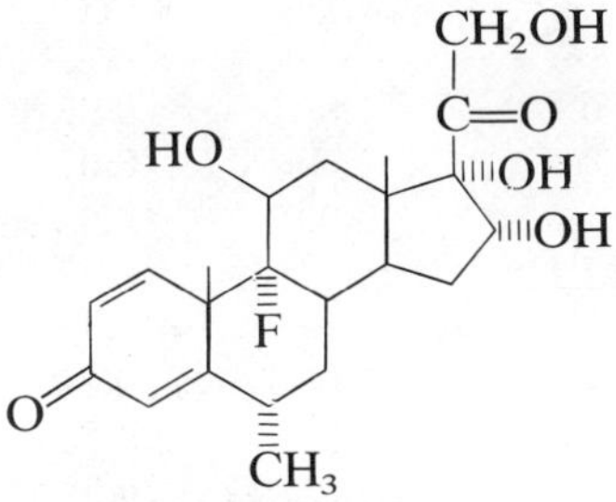

63.**52**

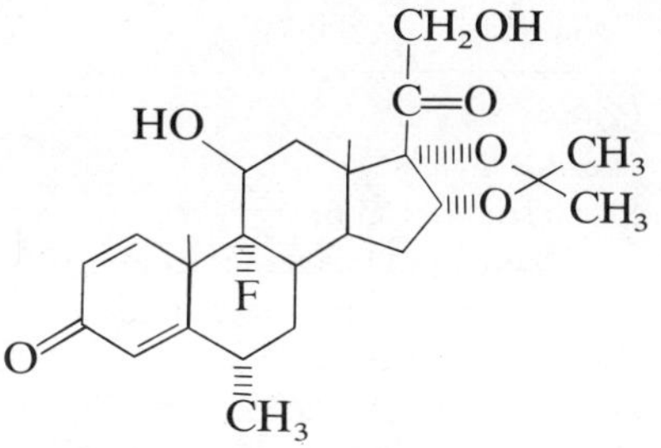

63.**53**

Fried and Borman (76). QSAR studies on metabolic stability, drug distribution, and intrinsic activity remain for the future. Combining all these relationships using mathematical modeling techniques may lead to a complete quantitative theory of anti-inflammatory steroid design in the next two decades.

10 EFFECT OF INDIVIDUAL STRUCTURAL CHANGES ON ANTI-INFLAMMATORY ACTIVITY

In this section we examine the SAR at each position in the steroid nucleus. First, however, it is useful to make an overview of the more important changes.

10.1 Overview of Major Changes in Anti-inflammatory Steroids

In Tables 63.15 (98), 63.16 (77), 63.17 (99), and 63.18 (99a) are displayed the activities of a number of anti-inflammatory steroids in large-scale studies in four major laboratories. These reports are of considerable interest. They make it possible to compare the activities of clinically important steroids and other steroids from data obtained by a single laboratory. It can be seen that the potency of polysubstituted compounds is predicted well by the enhancement factors of Tables 63.11, 63.13, and 63.14.

The success of the medicinal chemist in increasing potency and decreasing sodium retention is apparent in Table 63.17. Flumethasone acetate, the 21-acetate of 63.59, is 424 times as active as cortisol in the granuloma assay and has no more

sodium retention than cortisol itself—a remarkable achievement. Unfortunately, as mentioned in Section 3, other side effects have not been reduced in relationship to the therapeutic effect.

10.2 Skeletal Changes in the Cortisol Molecule

Unlike the situation in the progestational agents, removal of the 19-angular methyl group reduces anti-inflammatory activity. 19-Norcortisol (63.**62**) has only $\frac{3}{10}$ the activity of cortisol in the granuloma test. (100, 101). However, if the removal of the 19-angular methyl group is accompanied by aromatization of the A ring as in 63.**63**, the compound retains activity equal to cortisol in the granuloma test (102).

D-Homocortisone acetate (63.**64**) is less

Table 63.17 Effect of 6α-Fluoro and 9α-Fluoro Substitution on Activity of Cortisol Derivatives[a]

	Relative Activity		
Compound	Granuloma	Glycogen Deposition	Sodium Retention (DOCA = 1.0)
Cortisol (63.**2**)	1.0	1.0	<0.02
16α-Methylcortisol (63.**31**)	0.8	1.4	<0.02
Prednisolone (63.**6**)	3.1	3.0	<0.02
16α-Methylprednisolone acetate (63.**54**)[b]	8.7	24.0	<0.02
9α-Fluorocortisol acetate (63.**3**)[b]	8.0	12.6	5.0
Dexamethasone (63.**9**)	164.0	251.0	<0.02
2α-Methylcortisol acetate (63.**32**)[b]	2.8	5.8	2.7
9α-Fluoroprednisolone acetate (63.**31**)[b]	16.5	50.0	20.0
6α-Fluorocortisol acetate (63.**55**)[b]	8.7	10.9	Slight
6α-Fluoro-16α-methylcortisol (63.**37**)	6.1	36.0	<0.02
6α-Fluoroprednisolone acetate (63.**56**)[b]	25.0	100.0	Slight
Paramethasone acetate (63.**57**)[b]	50.0	150.0	<0.02
6α,9α-Difluorocortisol acetate (63.**58**)[b]	8.0	63.0	4.0
Flumethasone acetate (63.**59**)[b]	424.0	677.0	<0.02
6α-Fluoro-2α-methylcortisol acetate (63.**60**)[b]	23.0	60.0	3.0
6α,9α-Difluoroprednisolone acetate (63.**61**)[b]	66.0	443.0	2.5

[a] Data from Ref. 99.
[b] 21-acetate.

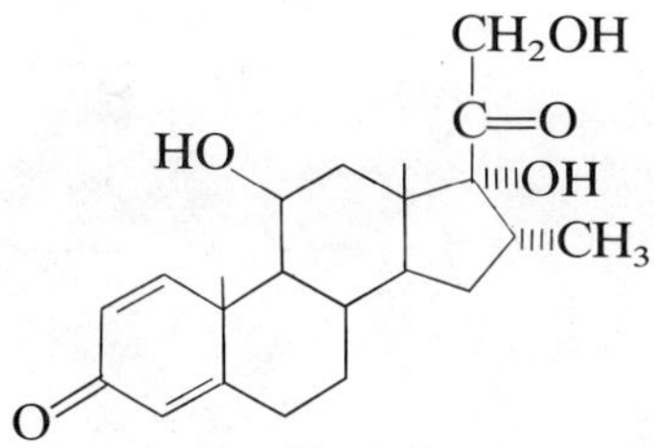

63.**54**

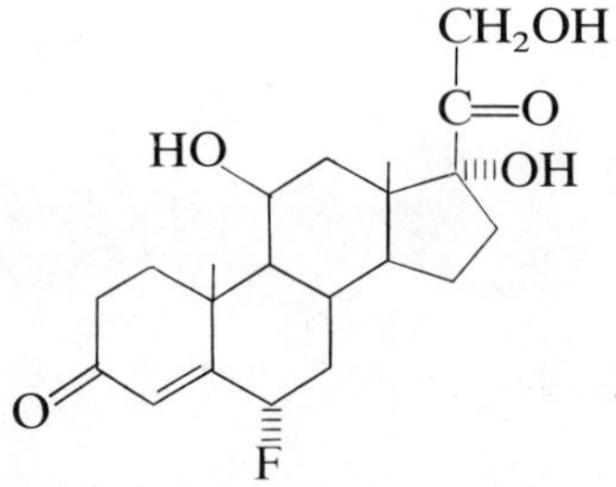

63.**55**

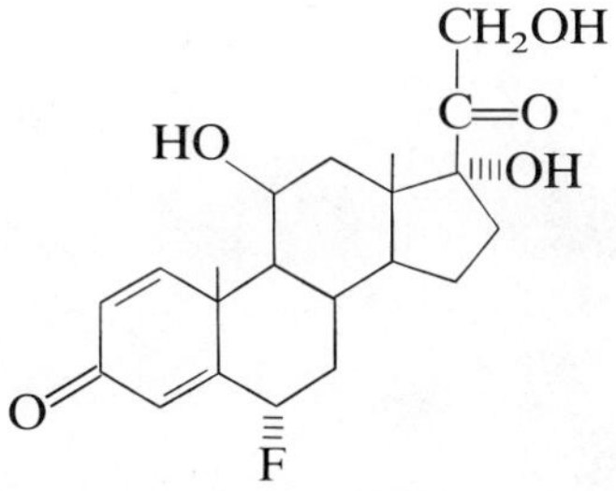

63.**56**

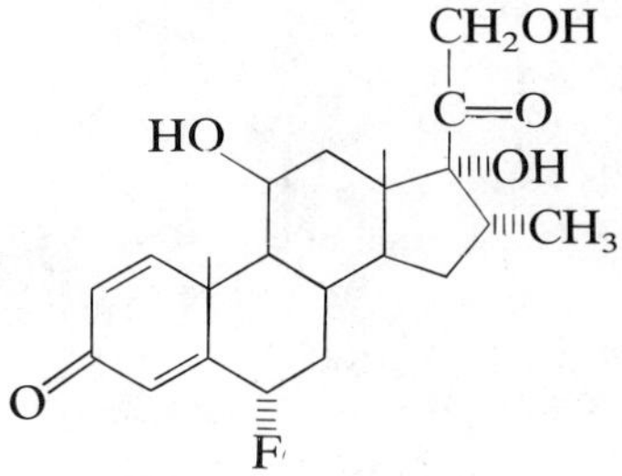

63.**57**

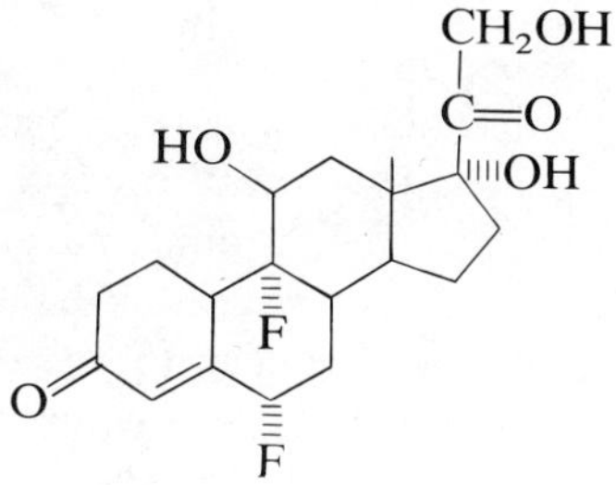

63.**58**

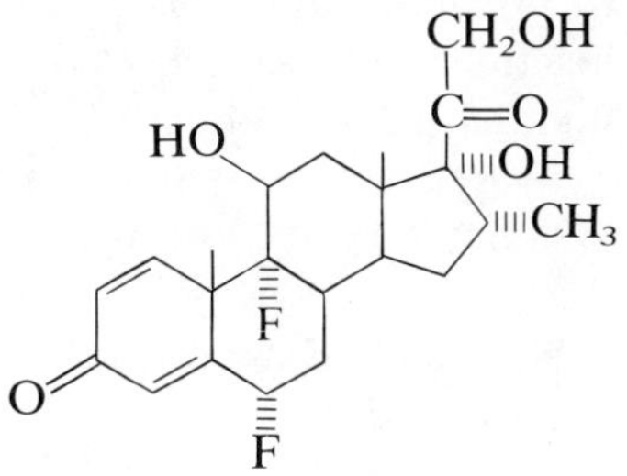

63.**59**

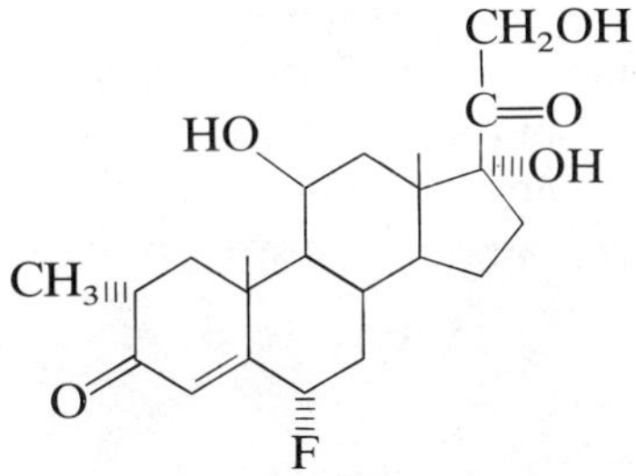

63.**60**

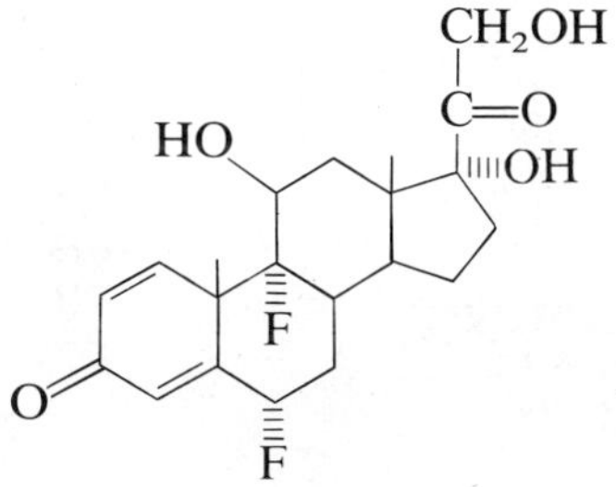

63.**61**

active than cortisol but retains some corti-cal hormone activity (103). Contraction of the A ring to A-norcortisol (63.**65**) gives an inactive compound (104).

The A ring can be modified by isosteric replacement to afford a heterocycle like 2-oxacortisol acetate (63.**66**), which has one-quarter of the activity of cortisol. The in-troduction of a 9α-chloro group and a

16α-methyl group gives 63.**67**, which is equal to cortisol in activity (105).

10.3 Alterations at C-1

The introduction of a double bond at C-1 leads to enhanced anti-inflammatory activi-ty, as has already been discussed, but a

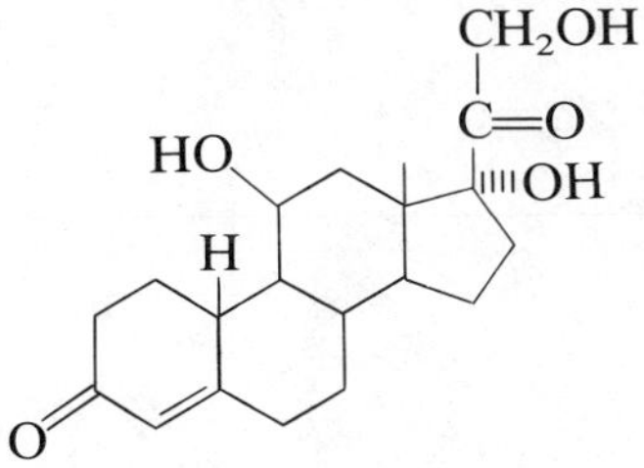

63.**62**

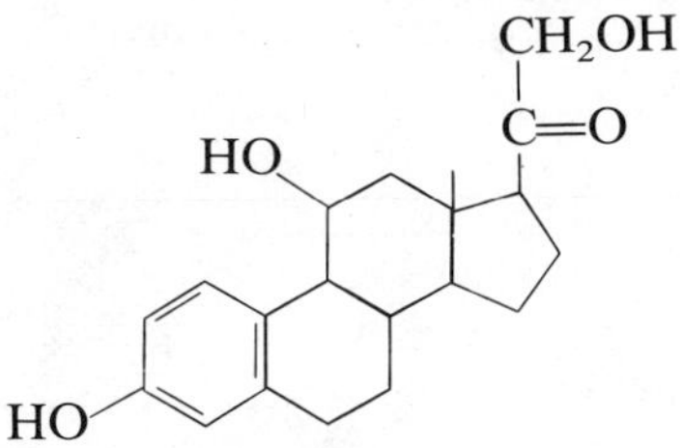

63.**63**

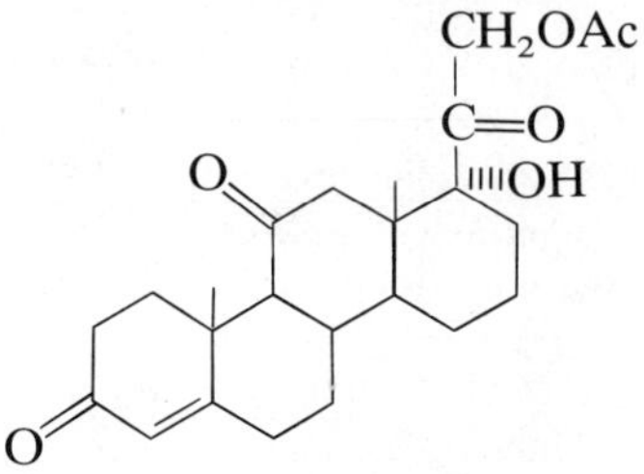

63.**64**

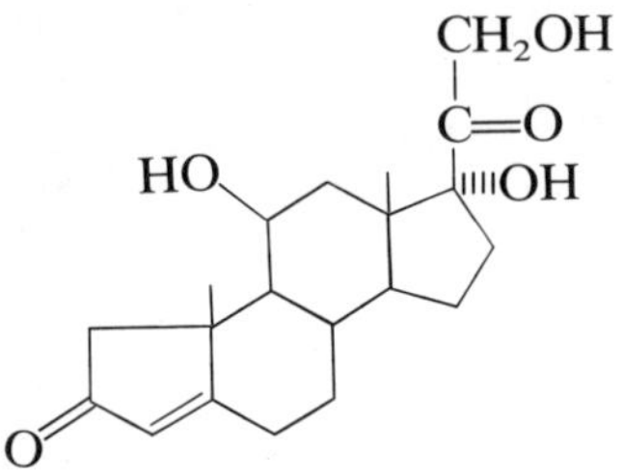

63.**65** 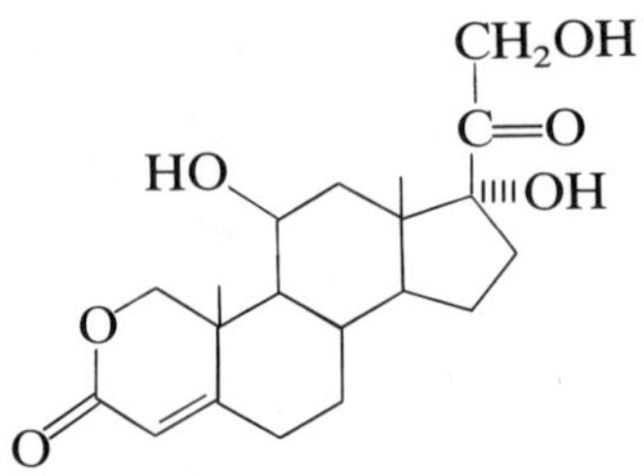   63.**66** 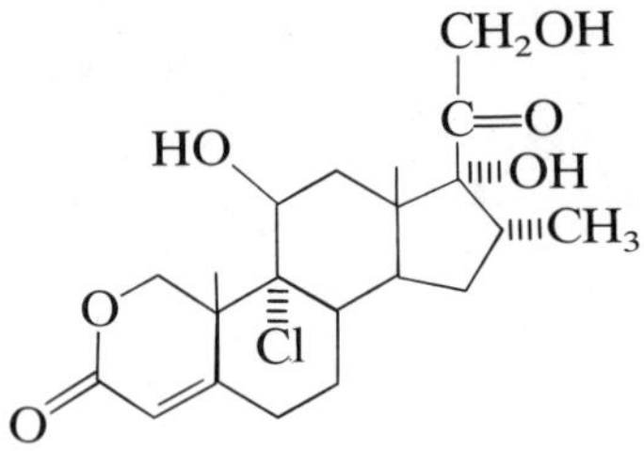   63.**67**

hydroxyl group in this position leads to an inactive product. Thus 1ξ-hydroxy-9α-fluorocortisol, obtained by microbial hydroxylation, is virtually inactive in anti-inflammatory assays (106).

Table 63.18 Human Topical Anti-inflammatory Potency[a]

Compound	Activity
Cortisol (63.**2**)	1
Cortisol 17-butyrate	280
Cortisol 17-valerate	100–200
Dexamethasone (63.**9**)	10–20
Dexamethasone 21-acetate	10–20
Dexamethasone 21-phosphate	10
Prednisolone (63.**6**)	1–2
Prednisolone 21-acetate	3
Prednisolone 17-valerate	2
Flurandrenolone	12
Flurandrenolone acetate	100–300
Flurandrenolide	1–2
Triamcinolone (63.**8**)	2
Triamcinolone acetonide (63.**12**)	40–400
Betamethasone (63.**14a**)	3–5
Betamethasone 21-acetate (63.**14c**)	18–33
Betamethasone 17-valerate (63.**15c**)	500
Fluorometholone (63.**83**)	30–40
Fluoroprednisolone (63.**56**)	4–6
Fluocinolone (63.**29**)	100–300
Fluocinolone acetonide (63.**13a**)	600–800
Fluocinonide (63.**13b**)	1600
Flumethasone pivalate (63.**59**)[b]	800
Halcinonide (63.**86**)	790
Desonide (63.**41**)	380

[a] Data in the human vasoconstrictor assay from Ref. 99a.
[b] Pivalate ester.

10.4 Alterations at C-2

The introduction of a 2α-methyl group into cortisol and its analogs (107) increases granuloma activity in rats about fourfold, but this enhancement is not observed in man (108). The 2α-methyl group also produces a marked increase in sodium retention. The 2α-methyl group exerts its effect through a reduced rate of reduction of the Δ^4,3-ketone system (109). It is likely that metabolism in other positions, such as at C-11 and C-20, is also retarded. By contrast, introduction of a 2α-fluoro group reduces the biologic activity in several tests (110, 111).

10.5 Alterations at C-3

Almost all active anti-inflammatory steroids have a carbonyl group at C-3, but some exceptions exist. One is the ring A phenol (63.**63**) discussed in Section 10.2.

2'-Phenylpregn-4-ene[3,2-c]pyrazoles of corticoids are more potent anti-inflam-

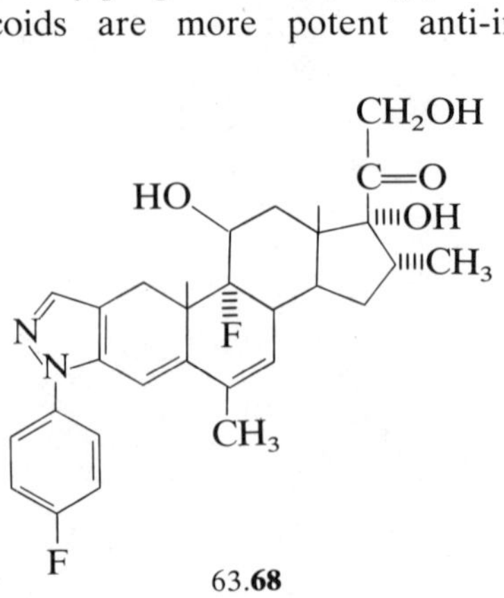

63.**68**

matory agents than their parent Δ^4,3-keto steroids. Activity can be enhanced still further by *p*-fluorophenyl substitution of the pyrazole ring, as in 63.**68**, which has 2000 times the potency of cortisol (112–114). The pyrazole derivatives do not exhibit mineralocorticoid activity. They have high affinity for cytoplasmic glucocorticoid receptors (114a).

10.6 Alterations at C-4

The Δ^4 double bond is important but not essential for anti-inflammatory activity. Thus the 5α-pregnan-3-one (63.**68a**) derived from triamcinolone 16α,17α-acetonide is more active than cortisol in glycogen deposition (115). Since 5α-steroids have approximately the same shape as the corresponding Δ^4 compounds it appears that reduction of the Δ^4 double bond in this manner still allows receptor binding but results in a hundred fold decrease in the activity of the compound.

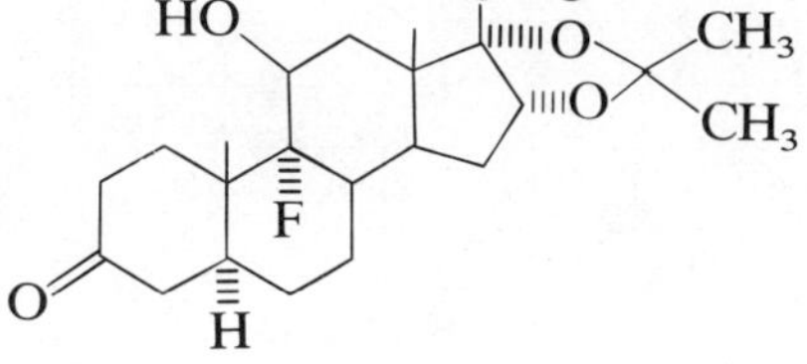

63.**68a**

4-Methylcortisol acetate is inactive in the granuloma and glycogen deposition tests (116). The reported anti-inflammatory activity of 4-fluorocortisol is very low (117). Allen et al. prepared 4-methyl and 4-ethyl derivatives of 9α-fluorocortisol and the 4-methyl derivative of 9α-fluoroprednisolone (118). In all cases the 4-methyl analog was less potent than the parent compound and the 4-ethyl derivative was even weaker.

10.7 Alterations at C-6

In general polar substituents such as hydroxy or oxo in the 6α-position decrease biologic activity, whereas 6α-substituted hydrophobic substituents, such as alkyl groups or halogens, tend to increase activity. 6β-Substituents of any type impair biologic activity, except as noted in Section 10.9. Thus 6β-hydroxycortisol 6,21-diacetate has less than one-third the thymolytic potency of its parent compound (119) and 6α-hydroxycortisone is less active than cortisone in the granuloma test (120). 6-Oxocortisone 21-acetate is only weakly active (121).

The enhancing activity of the 6α-methyl group has been mentioned in a number of preceding sections of this chapter. The closely related 6-methylene group, as in 6-methylene 16α-methylprednisolone, impairs activity (122). 6α-Chloro groups (123) enhance activity markedly in 6α-chlorocortisol acetate, but have no effect on cortisone or prednisone (124), perhaps because the group interferes with reduction of the 11-keto moiety. The 6α-fluoro group is very similar to the 9α-fluoro group in enhancing the activity of corticoids (125). 6β-Chloro and 6β-fluoro (126) groups give weakly active or inactive products when substituted in cortisone. Introduction of 6α-fluoromethyl groups into prednisolone and 9α-fluoroprednisolone affords compounds that are still active as anti-inflammatory steroids (127). The more polar 6α-methoxy group drastically reduces thymolytic activity when introduced into 9α-fluoroprednisolone (128).

Although the introduction of a 6,7-double bond has little effect on the activity of cortisol (129), Δ^6-6-chloroprednisolone is about twice as active as prednisolone in arthritis (130). When the 6-azido group was introduced into 9α-unsubstituted Δ^6-corticosteroids to give Δ^6-6-azidocortisol, systemic anti-inflammatory activity was increased five to eight times, whereas the

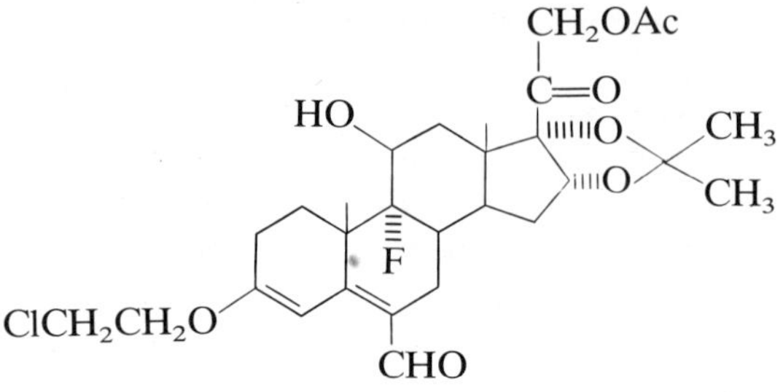

63.**69**

corresponding change in 9α-fluorocorti-
coids left potency unaffected (131). A 6-
formylpregnadiene derivative (63.**69**), upon
oral administration, had a relative potency
of 680 compared with cortisol acetate in
the granuloma pouch assay (131a).

10.8 Alterations at C-7

Both 7α and 7β substituents reduce anti-
inflammatory activity. 7α-Methyl and 7β-
methyl cortisol derivatives are less active
than the parent compound (132). Introduction of a methylthio, ethylthio, acetylthio,
or thiocyano group into the 7α position
of cortisol or cortisone reduces the activity
of the resulting compound (133).

10.9 6,7-Disubstituted Compounds

6α,7α-Dihydroxycortisone 21-acetate is
much less active than cortisone acetate in
the granuloma and thymolytic tests (134).
The epoxide 6α,7α-epoxycortisone is about
$\frac{1}{10}$ as active as cortisol in the glycogen deposition test (122). However, the introduction of a 6,7-difluoromethylene substituent
can give rise to highly active compounds
(135). Both the 6α,7α-difluoromethylene
derivatives and the 6β,7β-derivatives are
active. Compound 63.**70** has 1400 times
the systemic anti-inflammatory activity of
cortisol on subcutaneous administration.
The high potency of both α and β isomers
was taken as evidence that the 6,7 region of

the steroid is not in contact with the receptor, although the opposite case could be
argued equally well.

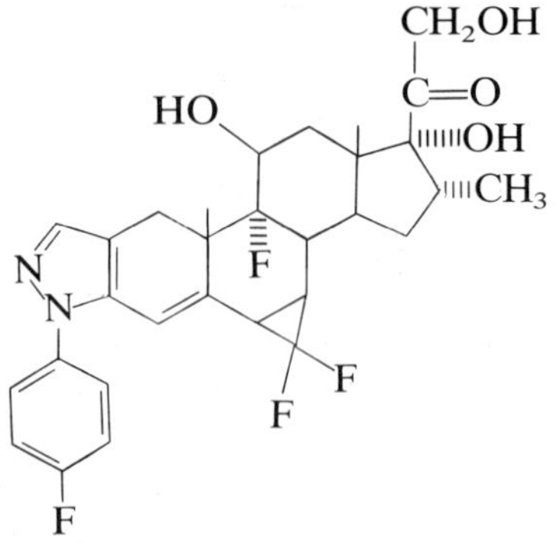

63.**70**

10.10 Alterations at C-8

The introduction of an 8(9) double bond
into prednisolone derivatives gives products
of somewhat lower anti-inflammatory potency than the parent compound (136).
Thus 6α-fluoro-8(9)-dehydroprednisolone
acetate (63.**71**) has 2.3 times the thymolytic
activity of cortisol.

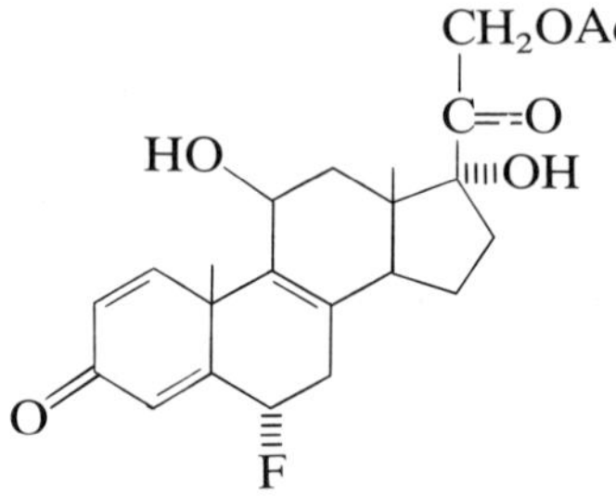

63.**71**

10.11 Alterations at C-9

Modifications at C-9 are discussed in Sections 9.2 and 9.3.

10.12 Alterations at C-10

Modifications at C-10 are discussed in Section 10.2.

10.13   Alterations at C-11

The C-11 oxygen group is not essential for anti-inflammatory activity if enough other enhancing groups are present in the molecule. Thus the 16,17-acetonide (63.**71a**) is an active anti-inflammatory steroid in spite of the absence of a C-11 oxygen group (137). However, changes at C-11 profoundly affect biologic activity. The 11α-hydroxy epimer of cortisol is inactive in the glycogen deposition test (138). 12β-Hydroxyprednisolone 11β,12β-acetonide is much less active than cortisol in the granuloma and thymolytic assays (139). Converting the 11β-hydroxy group to a tertiary alcohol through the formation of 11α-methylcortisol 21-acetate gives an inactive compound (140).

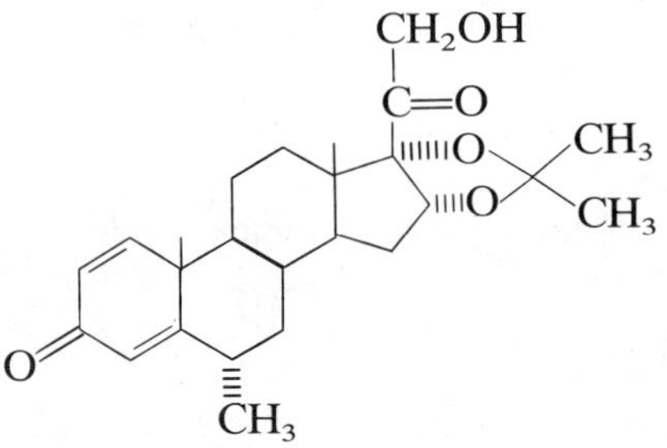

63.**71a**

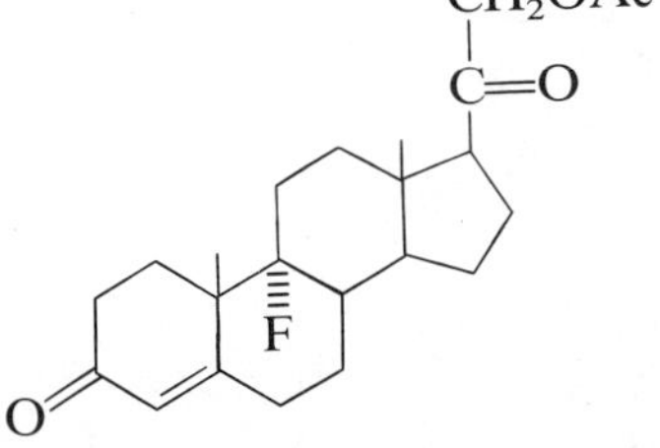

63.**71b**

The introduction of a 9α-fluoro atom into deoxycorticosterone acetate (DOCA) gives a 9α-fluorinated steroid lacking an 11β-hydroxy group (63.**71b**) that has 12 times the mineralocorticoid action of

DOCA. However, 63.**71b** has only 5–10% the anti-inflammatory action of cortisol (141). This is an indication that some of the enhancing effect of the 9α-fluoro group is due to its action on the 11β-OH group.

An especially interesting series of compounds is the 9α,11β-dihalocorticoids. These derivatives lack the 11-oxygen atom and yet have useful anti-inflammatory activity. The 11β-fluoro-9α-bromo derivative (63.**72**) has less than one-quarter the activity of cortisol in the granuloma assay (142) but dichlorisone acetate (21-acetate of 63.**73**) is a useful topical anti-inflammatory steroid (143). However, 9,11-dichloro-steroids undergo solvolysis as shown in the formation of 63.**74** from 63.**73** (144). Thus the activity of 11β-chlorosteroids may be due to their conversion to the 11β-hydroxy compounds *in vivo*. In support of this is the poor activity of 63.**72**, which would not be expected to undergo such a solvolysis since fluoroine is a poor leaving group. 16α-Methylation causes a major increase in potency of dichlorosone, which is unexpected on the basis of the enhancement factor of this group. However, the 16α-methyl compound undergoes the solvolysis to the corresponding 11β-hydroxy derivative much more readily than the parent 63.**73**. This also provides evidence that some of the activity of the 9,11-dichlorosteroids is due to the solvolysis reaction shown (145). Thus these compounds do not unequivocally represent highly active 11-deoxy anti-inflammatory steroids, as has sometimes been claimed.

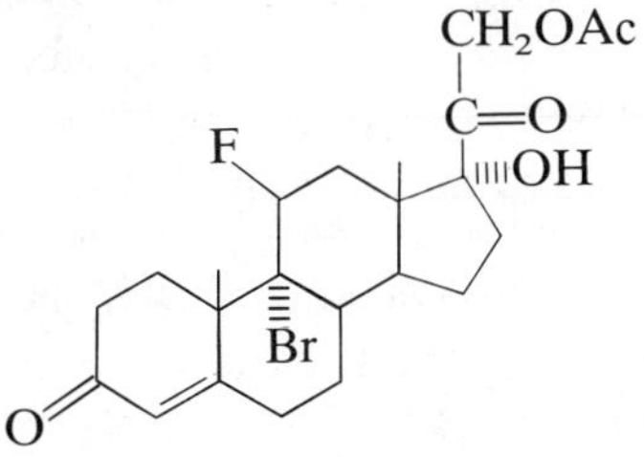

63.**72**

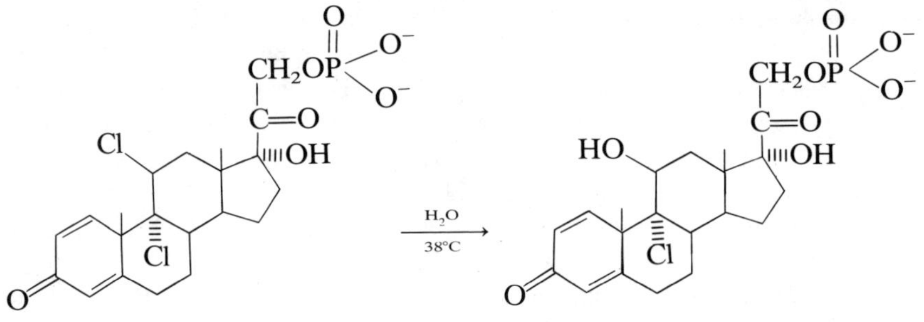

63.**73**

63.**74**

10.14 Alterations at C-12

12α-Hydroxycorticosterone has $\frac{1}{10}$ the activity of cortisol in the glycogen deposition test (146). 12α-Methyl-11-oxodeoxycorticosterone is less active in the glycogen deposition test than the corresponding compound lacking the 12α-methyl group (147). The effect of the 12α-halo substituent in corticoids was used by Fried (79) in an effort to understand the action of 9α halogens. He reasoned that if the enhancement produced by a 9α-halogen is due to an inductive effect, similar enhancement would be expected from a 12α-halogen, since the 9α and 12α positions are equivalent with respect to their electronic effect on C-11. It was shown that the liver glycogen and sodium retention activities of 12α-halo-11β-hydroxyprogesterones paralleled those of the corresponding 9α-halo-11β-hydroxyprogesterones (148, 149). Again, Taub et al. (146) showed that 9α- and 12α-fluoro groups produced equivalent activity enhancement in the glycogen deposition test when substituted in corticosterone and 1-dehydrocorticosterone, and that 9α- and 12α-hydroxy groups cause similar reduction in activity in corticosterone.

Surprisingly, 12α-chlorocortisone is inactive in the liver glycogen and sodium retention assays (150), whereas the 9α-chloro analog has a glycogen deposition activity of 3.5 times cortisone acetate (2). Fried and Borman hypothesized that hydrogen bonding from the 17α-hydroxyl group to the

12α-halogen is responsible for the loss of activity (64). To test this hypothesis they synthesized the 9α- and 12α-fluoro-16α-hydroxycortisol derivatives 63.**75a** and 63.**75b** and their respective acetonides 63.**76a** and 63.**76b**. It was found that the acetonides 63.**76a** and 63.**76b** have equivalent biologic activity (10 times hydrocortisone) in the glycogen deposition test. On the other hand, the parent steroid 73.**75b** has only $\frac{1}{10}$ the activity of 63.**75a**. Thus masking the 17α-hydroxyl group restores the 12α-halogen to parity with the 9α-halogen as an enhancing group.

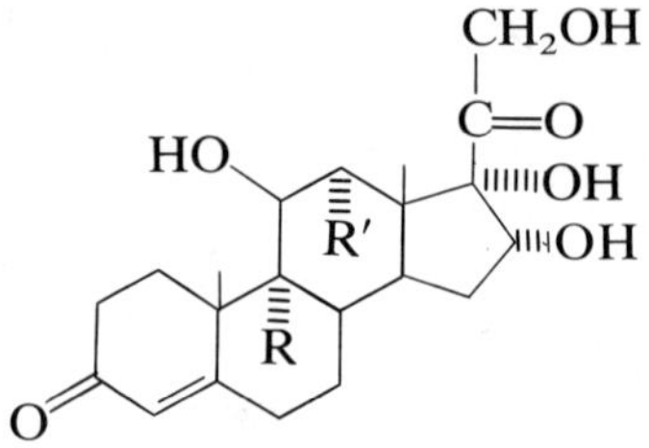

63.**75a**   R = F, R′ = H
63.**75b**   R = H, R′ = F

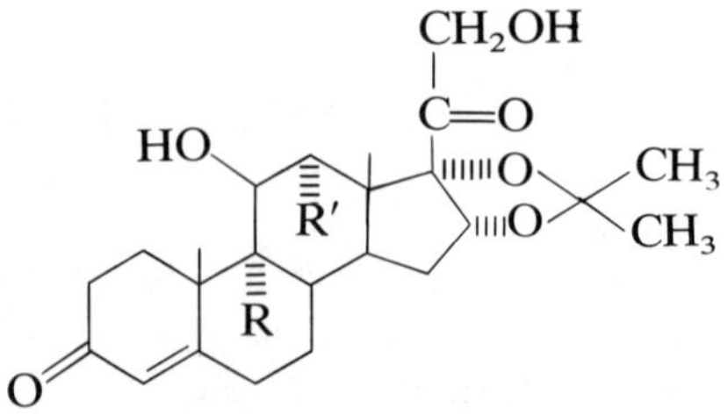

63.**76a**   R = F, R′ = H
63.**76b**   R = H, R′ = F

One matter that has not been discussed adequately in this theory is why the hydrogen bond formation between a 17α-hydroxy group, which is not even needed for activity in the rat, and the 12α-halogen should impair activity. One possible explanation would be through a conformational effect on the steroid molecule. This would be an interesting area to explore through X-ray crystallography.

10.15   Alterations at C-15

Methyl groups can be substituted in the 15α position of anti-inflammatory steroids with enhancement factors of approximately 0.5 on both anti-inflammatory action and sodium retention. A 15β-methyl group has little effect on glycogen deposition. Parent steroids substituted with the 15β-fluoro group include cortisol, prednisolone, 9α-fluorocortisol, and 9α-fluoroprednisolone (152). Bioassays suggest a small increase in anti-inflammatory activity owing to the 15β-fluoro group and a 97–99% reduction in sodium retention.

10.16   Alterations at C-16

The effect of introducing 16α-methyl, 16α-hydroxy, and 16α,17α-acetonides has already been discussed. 16α-Fluoro derivatives of prednisolone and 9α-fluoroprednisolone having 16 times and 75 times the anti-inflammatory·activity of cortisol were reported by Magerlein et al (153). This group also enhances the activity of 6α-fluoroprednisolone derivatives (154). By contrast, the 16β-fluoro group in cortisol, 9α-fluorocortisol, or 9α-fluoroprednisolone produces compounds with decreased anti-inflammatory activity (155). Likewise, loss of activity is seen upon introduction of a 16β-methoxy group (155). The 16β-acetoxy group abolishes the glucocorticoid action of 9α-fluorocortisol or 9α-fluoro-

63.**77**

prednisolone (156). Introduction of the 16α-chloro group into 9α-fluorocorticoids greatly increases anti-inflammatory and glycogenic activity (157). 16α-Chloro-6α,9α-difluoroprednisolone 21-acetate has 1100 times the activity of cortisol (63.**77**) (157). 16α-Ethyl substitution is similar to 16α-methyl and 16α-hydroxyl substitution in eliminating effects on electrolytes (158).

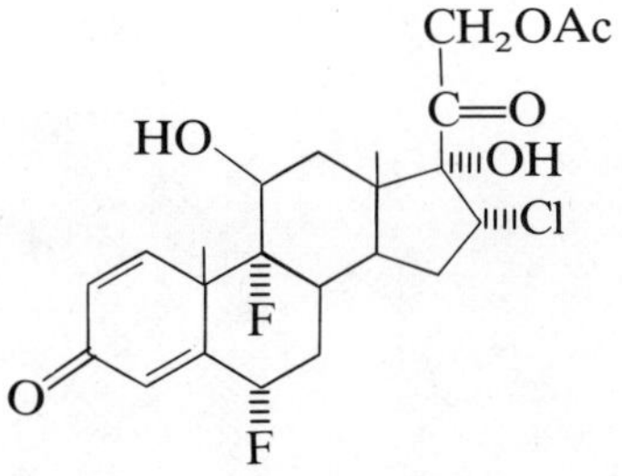

Beal and Pike (159) synthesized the 16α-fluoromethyl derivative of 9α-fluoroprednisolone 21-acetate. It is highly active as an anti-inflammatory agent and produces mild electrolyte excretion similar to 16α-methyl steroids. The 16α-methoxy derivative of cortisol exhibits twice the thymolytic activity of the parent compound (160).

Isomeric 16-methylene and Δ^{15},16-methyl steroids (161) show interesting differences in activity. The Δ^{15},16-methyl compound (63.**78**) has 156 times the oral activity of cortisol in the granuloma test and produces sodium retention. By contrast, the isomeric 16-methylene compound (63.**79**) has only one-third the anti-inflammatory action of 63.**78** and produces sodium excretion. The 16β-methoxy group reduces the anti-inflammatory potency of

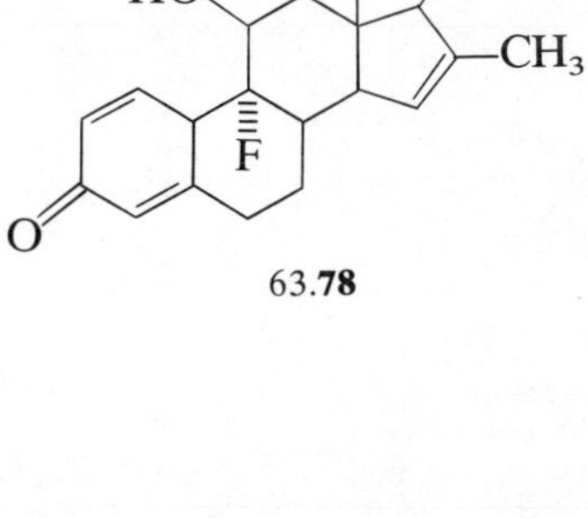

63.**78**

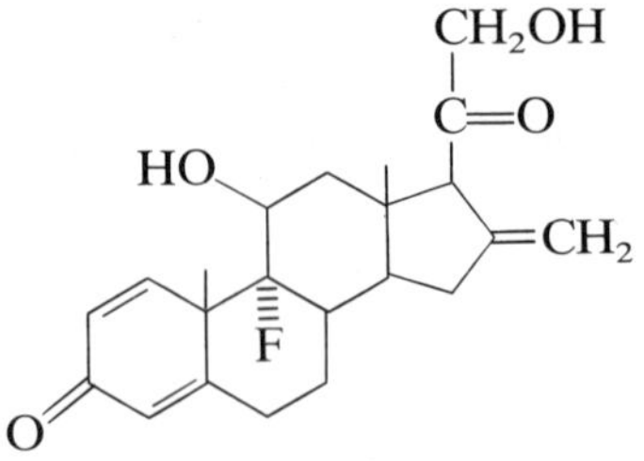

63.**79**

9α-fluorocortisone 21-acetate (155). 16,16-Dimethylprednisone 21-acetate is inactive in the systemic granuloma test (162).

10.17 Alterations at C-17

The 17α-hydroxy group is not essential for activity. 17α-Methylcorticosterone 21-acetate has nearly half the activity of cortisol in the glycogen deposition assay (163). The introduction of fluorine, chlorine, or bromine into the 17α-position of 11-dehydrocorticosterone gives compounds of inferior activity (164–166). The activity of 16,17-ketals has already been discussed.

10.18 Alterations at C-20

Ketalization of the C-20 carbonyl group of corticoids with ethylene glycol gives ketals that retain biologic activity although it is lower than in the parent compound (167). The most active compound is the 9α-fluoro-6α-methylprednisone derivative 63.**80**, which is four times as potent as tri-

63.**80**

amcinolone. Whether the compound must first be hydrolyzed to the 20-ketone is not known, although it is stable in weak acid and enzymatic hydrolysis in liver brei did not occur. The related bismethylenedioxy compound (63.**81**) is more active than cortisol itself but the activity is lower than that of the parent steroid (168).

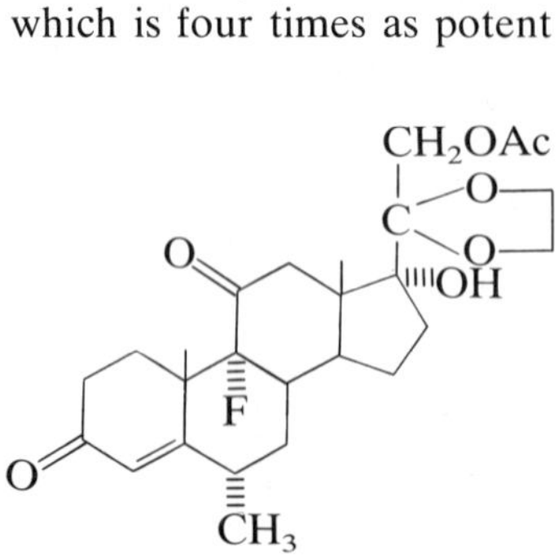

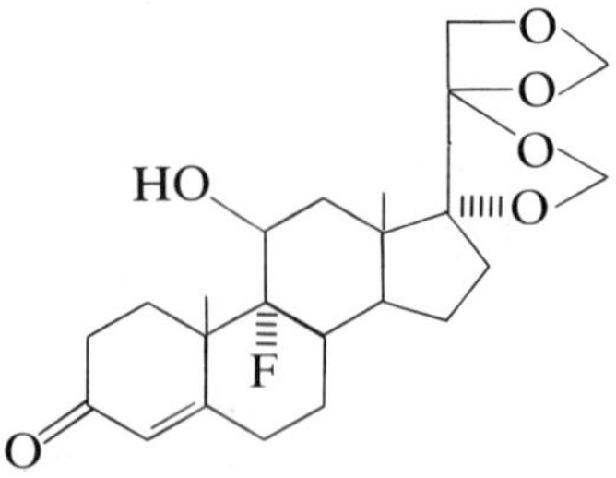

63.**81**

10.19 Alterations at C-21

Reduction of cortisol to 21-deoxycortisol gives a compound having about one-third the thymolytic activity of its parent (169). If activating groups are introduced into the molecule clinically useful opthalmic anti-inflammatory steroids such as medrysone (63.**82**) result. Medrysone has good anti-inflammatory activity with relatively little effect on intraocular pressure (170).

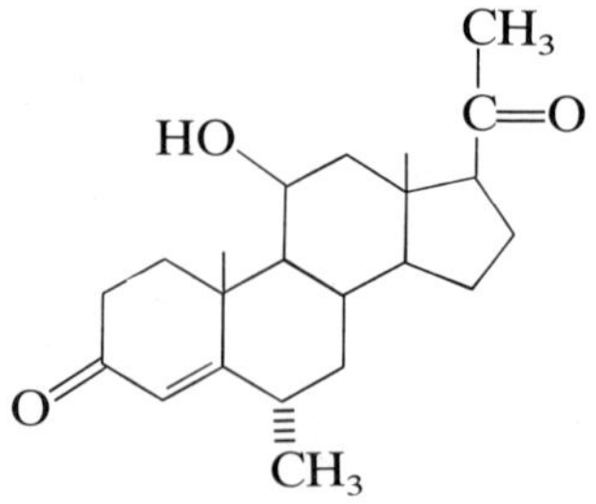

63.**82**

Fluorometholone (63.**83**) is an efficacious topical agent (171) and also has little tendency to increase intraocular pressure when used as an anti-inflammatory agent in ocular diseases (172). The propionate and butyrate 17-monoesters of 6α,9α-difluoro-21-deoxyprednisolone have high topical

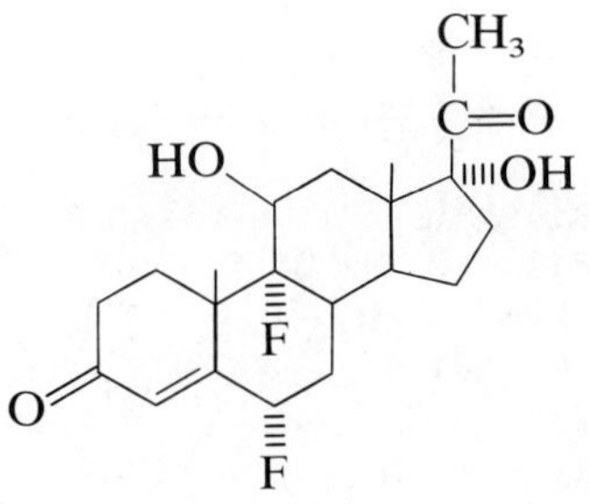

63.**83**

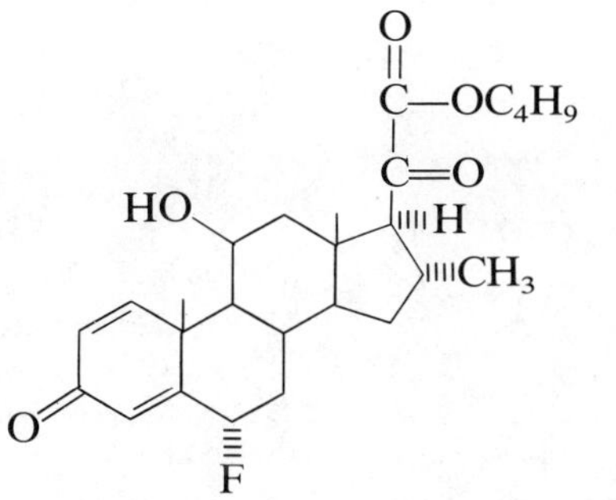

63.**84**

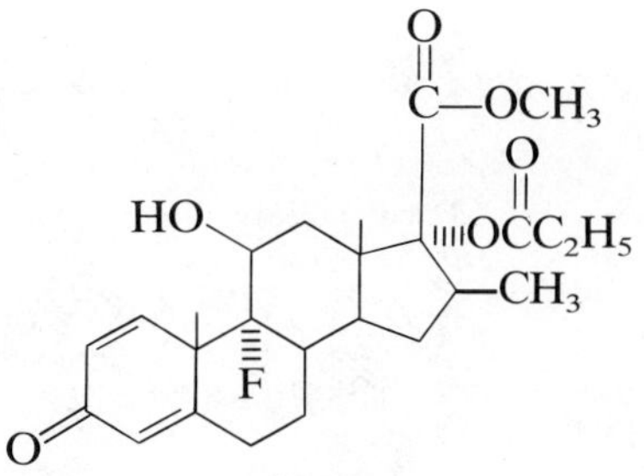

63.**85**

anti-inflammatory activity (172a) (refer also to Section 4.2.2 and Ref. 4).

Oxidation of cortisol to the 21-aldehyde gives a product that retains its anti-inflammatory activity (173), but it is not known whether this is due to reduction back to the primary alcohol.

A steroid containing a 21-carboxylic acid ester, fluocortin butyl (63.**84**), shows significant activity on human skin, but little or no systemic action in rats (173a). Related diesters of 17α-hydroxyandrostane-17β-carboxylic acids, such as 63.**85**, are active topically (174).

The introduction of an additional methyl group at C-21 to produce a secondary alcohol gives compounds with about ½ the activity of the parent structure (175, 176). The related 20,21-diketone 63.**86** is also active (176a). Replacement of the hydroxyl group at C-21 by a fluorine atom (177) doubles anti-inflammatory activity. The effect of substitution of the 21-hydroxyl function by chlorine in steroids with a 16α,17α-acetonide group depends greatly

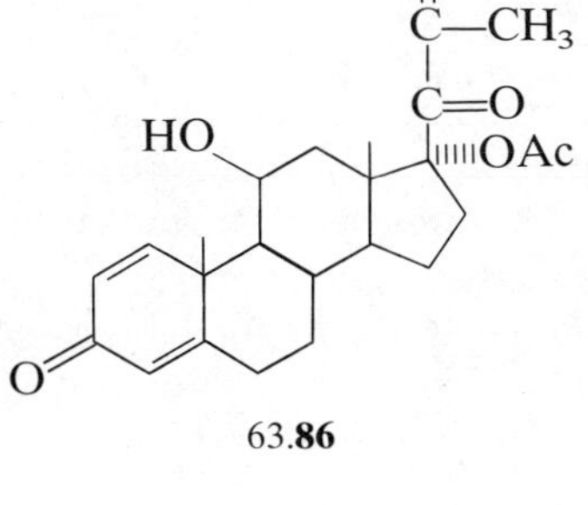

on other molecular substituents (178). When the 9α-fluoro substituents is present in the parent compound a useful compound, halcinonide (63.**87**), results. The introduction of diazo and azido groups into prednisolone gives compounds that retain moderate amounts of activity (179, 180).

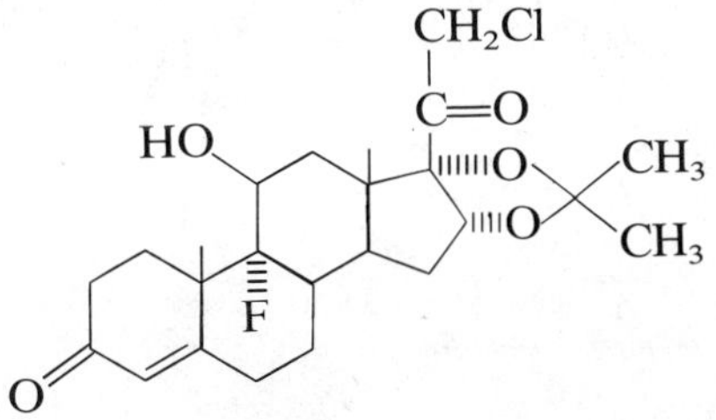

63.**87**

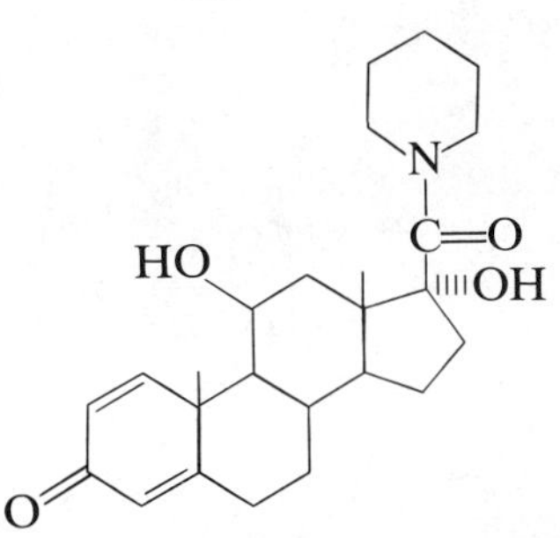

63.**88**

An amide at C-20 as in (63.**88**) gives steroids that retain more than half the activity of the parent compound in the liver glycogen test (181). However, sulfur-containing substituents at C-21, such as 21-mercapto, 21-methylthio, 21-thiocyano, and 21-acetylthio, give corticoids that are not of biologic interest (182).

63.**86**

REFERENCES

1. P. S. Hench, E. C. Kendall, C. H. Slocumb, and H. F. Polley, *Proc. Staff Meet., Mayo Clinic*, **24,** 181 (1949).

2. J. Fried and E. F. Sabo, *J. Am. Chem. Soc.*, **75,** 2273 (1953).

3. L. H. Sarrett, A. A. Patchett, and S. Steelman, in *Progress in Drug Research*, Vol. 5, E. Jucker, Ed., Birkhauser Verlag, Basel, 1963, pp. 13–153.

4. T. L. Popper and A. S. Watnick, in *Antiinflammatory Agents*, Vol. 1, R. A. Scherer and M. W. Whitehouse, Eds., Academic, New York, 1974, pp. 245–294.

4a. J. Wepierre and J.-P. Marty, *Trends Pharmacol. Sci.*, 23 (1979).

5. P. S. Chen, Jr. and P. Borrevang, in *Handbook of Experimental Pharmacology*, Vol. 20, Part II, Frank A. Smith, Ed., Springer Verlag, Berlin, 1970, pp. 193–252.

6. M. E. Wolff, in *Monographs on Endocrinology*, Vol. 12, J. Baxter and G. Rousseau, Eds., Springer Verlag, Berlin, 1979, pp. 97–107.

7. J. L. Hollander, *J. Am. Med. Assoc.*, **92,** 306 (1960).

8. H. T. Schedl and J. A. Clifton, *Gastroenterology*, **41,** 491 (1961).

9. S. B. Malkinson and M. B. Kirschenbaum, *Arch. Dermatol.*, **88,** 427 (1963).

10. J. R. Scholtz and D. H. Nelson, *Clin. Pharmacol. Ther.*, **6,** 498 (1965).

11. C. H. Demos, V. A. Place, and J. M. Ruegsegger, *Abstr. 1st Int. Congr. Endocrinol., Copenhagen, 1960*, p. 759.

12. J. Fried, W. B. Kessler, P. Grabowich, and E. F. Sabo, *J. Am. Chem. Soc.*, **80,** 23–38 (1958).

13. V. A. Place, J. Giner-Velazquez, and K. H. Burdick, *Arch. Dermatol.*, **101,** 531 (1970).

14. A. W. McKenzie and R. M. Atkinson, *Arch. Dermatol.*, **89,** 741 (1964).

15. I. Ringler, *Methods Hormone Res.*, **3,** 261 (1964).

16. P. H. Kendall, *Ann. Phys. Med.*, **9,** 55 (1967).

17. A. Verhaeghe, R. Lebeurre, M. Hennion, and T. Cheval, *Lille Med.*, **10,** 211 (1965).

18. M. Pearlgood, *J. R. Coll. Gen. Pract.*, **21,** 410 (1971).

19. E. J. Collins, J. Aschenbrenner, and M. Nakahama, *Steroids*, **20,** 543 (1972).

19a. Cf. L. E. Hare, K. C. Yeh, C. A. Ditzler, F. G. McMahon, and D. E. Duggan, *Clin. Pharmacol, Therp.*, **18,** 330 (1975) and references cited therein.

19b. R. D. Schoenwald and R. C. Ward, *J. Pharm. Sci.*, **67,** 786 (1978).

20. U. Westphal, *Steroid Protein Interactions*, Springer Verlag, New York, 1971.

21. U. Westphal, *J. Am. Oil Chem. Soc.* **41,** 481 (1964).

22. H. E. Smith, R. G. Smith, D. O. Toft, J. R. Neergaard, E. P. Burrows, and B. W. O'Malley, *J. Biol. Chem.*, **249,** 5924 (1974).

23. K. B. Eik-Nes, J. A. Schellman, C. Lumry, and L. T. Samuels, *J. Biol. Chem.*, **206,** 411 (1954).

24. U. Westphal and B. D. Ashley, *J. Biol. Chem.*, **234,** 2847 (1959).

25. U. Westphal, *Arch. Biochem. Biophys.*, **118,** 556 (1967).

26. J. R. Florini and D. A. Buyske, *J. Biol. Chem.* **236,** 247 (1961).

27. E. A. Peets, M. Staub, and S. Symchowicz, *Biochem. Pharmacol.*, **28,** 1655 (1969).

28. W. R. Slaunwhite, Jr., G. N. Lockie, N. Back, and A. A. Sandberg, *Science*, **135,** 1062 (1962).

29. A. A. Sandberg and W. R. Slaunwhite Jr., *J. Clin. Invest.*, **42,** 51 (1963).

30. K. Fotherby and F. James, in, *Advances in Steroid Biochemistry and Pharmacology*, M. H. Briggs and G. A. Christie, Eds., Academic New York, 1972.

30a. E. Gerhards, B. Nieuweboer, G. Schulz, and H. Gibian, *Acta Endocrinol.* **68,** 98 (1971).

31. H. L. Bradlow, B. Zumoff, C. Monder, H. J. Lee, and L. Hellman, *J. Clin. Endocrinol. Metab.*, **37,** 811 (1973).

32. G. M. Tomkins and P. J. Michael, *J. Biol. Chem.*, **225,** 13 (1957).

33. E. M. Glenn, R. O. Stafford, S. C. Lyscer, and B. J. Bowman, *Endocrinol.*, **61,** 128 (1957).

34. J. R. Florini, L. L. Smith, and D. A. Buyske, *J. Biol. Chem.*, **236,** 1038 (1961).

34a. M. K. Jasani, in *Handbook of Experimental Pharmacology*, Vol. 50, Part 2, *Antiinflammatory Drugs*, Springer Verlag, Berlin, 1979, pp. 598–660.

35. E. J. Collins, A. A. Forist, and E. B. Nodolski, *Proc. Soc. Exp. Biol. Med.*, **93,** 369 (1956).

36. W. E. Dulin, L. E. Barnes, E. M. Glenn, S. C. Lyster, and E. J. Collins, *Metabolism*, **7,** 398 (1958).

37. F. Kuipers, R. S. Ely, E. R. Hughes, and V. C. Kelley, *Proc. Soc. Exp. Biol. Med.*, **95,** 187 (1957).

38. R. H. Silber and E. R. Morgan, *Clin. Chem.*, **2,** 170 (1956).

39. R. H. Silber, *Ann. N.Y. Acad. Sci.*, **82,** 821 (1956).

40. R. S. Ely, A. K. Done, and V. C. Kelley, *Proc. Soc. Exp. Biol. Med.*, **91,** 503 (1956).

41. D. Feldman, J. W. Funder, and I. S. Edelman, *Am. J. Med.* **53**, 545 (1972).

42. R. J. B. King and W. I. P. Mainwaring, *Steroid-Cell Interactions*, University Park Press, Baltimore, 1974.

42a. W. E. Knox and V. H. Auerbach, *J. Biol. Chem.*, **214**, 307 (1955).

42b. E. C. C. Lynn and W. E. Knox, *Biochem. Biophys. Acta*, **26**, 85 (1957).

43. R. J. Gryglewski, B. Panczenko, R. Korbut, A. Grodzinska, and A. Oczekiewicz, *Prostaglandins*, **10**, 343 (1975).

44. A. H. Tashjian, E. F. Voekel, J. McDonough, and L. Levine, *Nature*, **258**, 739 (1976).

45. F. Kantrowitz, D. W. Robinson, M. B. McGuire, and L. Levine, *Nature*, **258**, 737 (1976).

46. N. Floman and U. Zor, *Invest. Ophthal. Visual Sci.*, **16**, 69 (1977).

47. S. C. Hong and L. Levine, *Proc. Natl. Acad. Sci. U.S.*, **73**, 1730 (1976).

48. S. T. Tam, S. C. Hong, and L. Levine, *J. Pharm. Exp. Ther.*, **203**, 162 (1977).

49. G. P. Lewis and P. J. Piper, *Nature*, **254**, 308 (1975).

50. S. Hammarstrom et al., *Science*, **197**, 994 (1977).

51. F. P. Nijkamp, R. J. Flower, S. Moncada, and J. R. Vane, *Nature*, **263**, 479 (1976).

52. G. J. Blackwell, R. J. Flower, F. P. Nijkamp, and J. R. Vane, *Brit. J. Pharmacol.* **62**, 79 (1978).

53. R. J. Flower and G. J. Blackwell, *Nature*, **278**, 456 (1979).

54. K. M. Bach, J. F. Brashler, and R. R. Gorman, *Prostaglandins*, **14**, 21 (1977).

55. B. A. Jakschick, S. Falkenhein, and C. W. Parker, *Proc. Natl. Acad. Sci. U.S.*, **74**, 4577 (1977).

56. M. E. Wolff, J. Baxter, P. A. Kollman, D. L. Lee, I. D. Kuntz, E. Bloom, D. Matulich, and J. Morris, *Biochemistry*, **7**, 3201 (1978).

57. H. E. Smith, R. G. Smith, D. O. Toft, J. R. Neergaard, E. P. Burrows, and B. W. O'Malley, *J. Biol. Chem.*, **249**, 5924 (1974).

58. U. Westphal, *Arch. Biochem. Biophys.*, **118**, 556 (1967).

59. C. Chothia, C., *Nature* **248**, 338 (1974); **254**, 304 (1975).

60. J. Janin and C. Chothia, *J. Mol. Biol.* **100**, 197 (1976).

61. C. M. Anderson, F. H. Zucker, and T. A. Steitz, *Science*, **204**, 375 (1979).

62. P. R. Ehrlich and R. W. Holm, *Science*, **138**, 652 (1962).

63. I. E. Bush, *Pharmacol. Rev.*, **14**, 317 (1962).

64. J. Fried and A. Borman, *Vitamins and Hormones*, **16**, 303 (1958).

65. C. M. Weeks, W. L. Duax, and M. E. Wolff, *J. Am. Chem. Soc.*, **95**, 2865 (1973).

66. J. A. Rupley, L. Butler, M. Gerring, F. J. Hartdegen, and R. Pecoraro, *Proc. Natl. Acad. Sci. U.S.*, **57**, 1083 (1967).

66a. S. Sudgen, *J. Chem. Soc.*, **125**, 1177 (1924).

66b. S. L. Steelman and E. R. Morgan, *Inflammation and Diseases of Connective Tissue*, Saunders, Philadelphia and London, 1961, p. 350.

67. R. H. Silber, *Ann. N.Y. Acad. Sci.*, **82**, 821 (1959).

68. A. Robert and J. E. Nezamis, *Acta Endocrinol.*, **25**, 105 (1957).

69. S. Tolksdorf, *Ann. N.Y. Acad. Sci.*, **82**, 829 (1959).

70. N. R. Stephenson, *J. Pharm. Pharmacol.* **12**, 411 (1960).

71. F. G. Peron and R. I. Dorfman, *Endocrinology*, **64**, 431 (1959).

72. S. Tolksdorf, M. L. Battin, J. W. Cassidy, R. M. MacLeod, F. H. Warren, and P. L. Perlman, *Proc. Soc. Exp. Med.*, **92**, 207 (1957).

73. R. O. Stafford, L. E. Barnes, B. J. Bowman, and M. M. Meinzinger, *Proc. Soc. Exp. Biol. Med.*, **91**, 67 (1956).

74. A. Robert and J. E. Nezamis, *Proc. Soc. Exp. Biol. Med.*, **99**, 443 (1950).

75. F. Marcus, L. P. Romanoff, and G. Pincus, *Endocrinology*, **50**, 286 (1952).

76. Ref. 64, p. 368.

77. I. Ringler, S. Mauer, and E. Heyder, *Proc. Soc. Exp. Biol. Med.*, **107**, 451 (1961).

77a. J. B. Justice, Jr., *J. Med. Chem.*, **21**, 465 (1978).

78. M. E. Wolff and C. Hansch, *Experientia*, **29**, 1111 (1973).

79. J. Fried, *Cancer*, **10**, 752 (1957).

80. R. A. Coburn and A. J. Solo, *J. Med. Chem.*, **19**, 748 (1976).

81. P. Ahmad and A. Mellors, *J. Steroid Biochem.*, **7**, 19 (1976).

82. S. Rakhit and C. R. Engel, *Can. J. Chem.* **40**, 2163 (1962).

83. N. L. Allinger and M. A. DaRooge, *J. Am. Chem. Soc.*, **83**, 4256 (1961).

84. K. M. Wellman and C. Djerassi, *J. Am. Chem. Soc.*, **87**, 60 (1965).

85. L. B. Kier, *J. Med. Chem.*, **11**, 915 (1968).

86. A. Cooper and W. L. Duax, *J. Pharm. Sci*, **58,** 1159 (1969).

87. W. L. Duax, C. M. Weeks, D. C. Rohrer, Y. Osawa and M. E. Wolff, *J. Steroid Biochem.*, **6,** 195 (1975).

88. J. P. Schmit and G. G. Rousseau, *J. Steroid Biochem.*, **9,** 909 (1978).

89. C. M. Weeks, W. L. Duax, and M. E. Wolff, *J. Am. Chem. Soc.*, **95,** 2865 (1973).

90. C. M. Weeks, W. L. Duax, and M. E. Wolff, *Acta Crystallogr.*, **B30,** 2516 (1974).

91. C. M. Weeks, W. L. Duax, and M. E. Wolff, *Acta Crystallogr.*, **B32,** 261 (1976).

92. J. P. Schmit and G. G. Rousseau, *J. Steroid Biochem.*, **9,** 921 (1978).

93. S. M. Free and J. W. Wilson, *J. Med. Chem.*, **7,** 395 (1964).

94. F. J. Marsh, D. L. Lee, P. K. Weiner, P. Kollman, and M. E. Wolff, Unpublished studies.

95. O. Dideberg, L. Dupont, and H. Campsteyn, *J. Steroid Biochem.*, **7,** 757 (1976).

96. P. A. Kollman, D. D. Gianinni, W. L. Duax S. Rothenberg, and M. E. Wolff, *J. Am. Chem. Soc.*, **95,** 2869 (1973).

97. A. B. Divine and R. E. Lack, *J. Chem. Soc., C*, **1966,** 1902.

98. L. J. Lerner, A. R. Turkheimer, A. Bianchi, A. Singer, and A. Borman, *Proc. Soc. Exp. Biol. Med.*, **116,** 385 (1964).

99. W. E. Dulin, F. L. Schmidt, and S. C. Lyster, *Proc. Soc. Exp. Biol. Med.*, **104,** 345 (1960).

99a. O. J. Lorenzetti, *Curr. Ther. Res.*, **25,** 92 (1979).

100. B. J. Magerlein and J. A. Hogg, *J. Am. Chem. Soc.*, **82,** 2226 (1958).

101. A. Zaffaroni, H. J. Ringold, G. Rosenkranz, F. Sondheimer, G. H. Thomas, and C. Djerassi, *J. Am. Chem. Soc.*, **80,** 6110 (1958).

102. B. J. Magerlein and J. A. Hogg, *J. Am. Chem. Soc.*, **79,** 1508 (1957).

103. R. O. Clinton, H. C. Newmann, A. J. Mason, S. C. Laskowski, and R. G. Christiansen, *J. Am. Chem. Soc.*, **80,** 3395 (1958).

104. R. Hirschmann, G. A. Bailey, R. Walker, and J. M. Chemerda, *J. Am. Chem. Soc.*, **81,** 2822 (1959).

105. R. Hirschmann, N. G. Steinberg, and R. Walker, *J. Am. Chem. Soc.*, **84,** 1270 (1962).

106. W. J. McAleer, M. A. Kozlowski, T. H. Stoudt, and J. M. Chemerda, *J. Org. Chem.*, **23,** 508 (1958).

107. J. A. Hogg, F. H. Lincoln, R. W. Jackson, and W. P. Schneider, *J. Am. Chem. Soc.*, **77,** 6401 (1955).

108. G. W. Liddle, J. E. Richard, and G. M. Tomkins, *Metabolism*, **5,** 384 (1956).

109. E. M. Glenn, R. O. Stafford, S. C. Lyster, and B. J. Bowman, *Endocrinology*, **61,** 28 (1957).

110. A. H. Nathan, B. J. Magerlein, and J. Λ. Hogg, *J. Org. Chem.*, **24,** 1517 (1959).

111. H. M. Kissman, A. S. Hoffman, J. F. Poletto, and M. J. Weiss, *J. Med. Pharm. Chem.*, **5,** 950 (1962).

112. R. Hirschmann, N. G. Steinberg, T. Buchschacher, J. H. Fried, G. J. Kent, M. Tishler, and S. L. Steelman, *J. Am. Chem. Soc.*, **85,** 120 (1963).

113. R. Hirschmann, N. G. Steinberg, E. F. Schoenwaldt, W. J. Paleveda, and M. Tishler, *J. Med. Chem.*, **7,** 352 (1964).

114. J. H. Fried, H. Mrozik, G. E. Arth, T. S. Bry, N. G. Steinberg, M. Tishler, R. Hirschmann, and S. L. Steelman, *J. Am. Chem. Soc.*, **85,** 236 (1963).

114a. S. S. Simons, Jr. E. B. Thompson, and D. F. Johnson, *Biochem. Biophys. Res. Commun.*, **86,** 793 (1979).

115. A. E. Hydorn, L. J. Lerner, and J. Schwartz, *Steroids*, **6,** 247 (1965).

116. N. G. Steinberg, R. Hirschmann, and J. M. Chemerda, *Chem. Ind.* (London), **1958,** 975.

117. B. J. Magerlein, J. E. Pike, R. W. Jackson, G. E. Vandenberg, and F. Kagan, *J. Org. Chem.*, **20,** 2982 (1964).

118. W. S. Allen, C. C. Pidacks, R. E. Schaub, and M. J. Weiss, *J. Org. Chem.*, **26,** 5046 (1961).

119. M. Hayano and R. I. Dorfman, *Arch. Biochem. Biophys.*, **50,** 218 (1954).

120. S. Bernstein and R. Littel, *J. Org. Chem.*, **25,** 313 (1960).

121. F. Sondheimer, O. Mancera, and G. Rosenkranz, *J. Am. Chem. Soc.*, **76,** 5020 (1954).

122. G. E. Arth, personal communication.

123. H. J. Ringold, O. Mancera, C. Djerassi, A. Bowers, E. Batras, H. Martinez, E. Necoechea, J. Edwards, M. Velasco, C. C. Campillow, and R. I. Dorfman, *J. Am. Chem. Soc.*, **80,** 6464 (1958).

124. R. I. Dorfman, H. J. Ringold, and F. A. Kincl, *Chemotherapia*, **5,** 294 (1962).

125. W. E. Dulin, F. L. Schmidt, and S. C. Lyster, *Proc. Soc. Exp. Biol. Med.*, **104,** 345 (1960).

126. E. M. Glenn, R. O. Stafford, S. C. Lyster, and D. J. Bowman, *Endocrinology*, **61,** 128 (1957).

127. P. F. Beal, R. W. Jackson, and J. E. Pike, *J. Org. Chem.*, **27,** 1752 (1962).

128. M. Heller and S. Bernstein, *J. Org. Chem.*, **26**, 3876 (1961).

129. G. W. Liddle, J. E. Richard, and G. M. Tomkins, *Metabolism*, **5**, 384 (1956).

130. E. Ortega, C. Rodriguez, L. J. Strand, and E. Segre, *The Endocrine Soc., 57th Ann. Meet. Program Abstr.*, 302 (1975).

131. M. J. Green, S. C. Bisara, H. L. Herzog, R. Rausser, E. L. Shapiro, H. J. Shue, B. Sutton, R. L. Tiberi, M. Monahan, and E. J. Collins, *J. Steroid Biochem.*, **5**, 599 (1975).

132. R. E. Beyler, A. E. Oberster, F. Hoffman, and L. H. Sarett, *J. Am. Chem. Soc.*, **82**, 170 (1960).

133. R. E. Schaub and M. J. Weiss, *J. Org. Chem.*, **26**, 3915 (1961).

134. J. A. Zderic, H. Carpio, and C. Djerassi, *J. Org. Chem.*, **24**, 909 (1959).

135. I. T. Harrison, C. Beard, L. Kirkham, B. Lewis, I. M. Jamieson, W. Rooks, and J. H. Fried, *J. Med. Chem.*, **11**, 868 (1968).

136. S. Mauer, E. Heyder, and I. Ringler, *Proc. Soc. Exp. Biol. Med.*, **107**, 345 (1962).

137. C. Bianchi, A. David, B. Ellis, V. Petrow, S. Waddington-Feather, and E. J. Woodward, *J. Pharm. Pharmacol.* **13**, 355 (1961).

138. A. Segaloff and B. M. Horwitt, *Science*, **118**, 220 (1953).

139. J. A. Zderic, H. Carpio, and C. Djerassi, *J. Am. Chem. Soc.*, **82**, 466 (1960).

140. R. E. Beyler, F. Hoffman, and L. H. Sarett, *J. Am. Chem. Soc.*, **82**, 178 (1960).

141. A. Wettstein, *Carbon-Fluorine Compounds; Chemistry, Biochemistry, and Biological Activities*, Ciba Symposium, Elsevier, Amsterdam, 1971, p. 291.

142. R. I. Dorfman, F. A. Kincl, and H. J. Ringold, *Endocrinology*, **68**, 616 (1961).

143. C. H. Robinson, L. Finckenor, E. P. Oliveto, and D. Gould, *J. Am. Chem. Soc.*, **81**, 2191 (1959).

144. N. Murrill, R. Grocela, W. Gabert, O. Gnoj, and H. L. Herzog, *Steroids*, **8**, 233 (1966).

145. H. L. Herzog, R. Neri, S. Symchowicz, I. I. A. Tabachnick, and J. Black, *Proceedings of the Second International Congress on Hormonal Steroids, Milan, May 23–28, 1966*, Excerpta Medica Foundation, Amsterdam, pp. 525–529.

146. D. Taub, R. D. Hoffsommer, and N. L. Wendler, *J. Am. Chem. Soc.*, **79**, 452 (1957).

147. B. G. Christensen, R. G. Strachan, M. R. Trenner, D. H. Arison, R. Hirschmann, and J. M. Chemerda, *J. Am. Chem. Soc.*, **82**, 3995 (1960).

148. J. E. Herz, J. Fried, and E. F. Sabo, *J. Am. Chem. Soc.*, **78**, 2017 (1956).

149. J. Fried, W. B. Kessler, and A. Borman, *Ann. N.Y. Acad. Sci.*, **71**, 494 (1958).

150. J. Fried, J. E. Herz, E. F. Sabo, and M. H. Morrison, *Chem. Ind.*, (London), **1956,** 1232.

151. J. Fried, *Inflammation and Diseases of Connective Tissue*, Saunders, Philadelphia, 1961, p. 353.

152. D. E. Ayer, *J. Med. Pharm. Chem.*, **6**, 608 (1963).

153. B. J. Magerlein, R. D. Birkenmeyer, and F. Kagan, *J. Am. Chem. Soc.*, **82**, 1252 (1960).

154. B. J. Magerlein, F. H. Lincoln, R. D. Birkenmeyer, and F. Kagan, *J. Med. Chem.*, **7**, 748 (1964).

155. W. T. Moreland, R. G. Berg, D. P. Cameron, C. E. Maxwell, J. S. Buckley, and B. G. Laubauch, *Chem. Ind.*, (London), 1084 (1960).

156. S. Bernstein, M. Heller, and S. M. Stolar, *J. Am. Chem. Soc.*, **81**, 1256 (1959).

157. F. Kagan, R. B. Birkenmeyer, and B. J. Magerlein, *J. Med. Chem.*, **7**, 751 (1964).

158. E. P. Oliveto and L. Weber, *Chem. Ind.* (London), **1961,** 514.

159. P. F. Beal and J. E. Pike, *J. Org. Chem.*, **26**, 3887 (1961).

160. M. Heller, S. M. Stollar, and S. Bernstein, *J. Org. Chem.*, **27**, 328 (1962).

161. D. Taub, R. D. Hoffsommer, H. L. Slates, C. H. Kuo, and N. L. Wendler, *J. Org. Chem.*, **29**, 3486 (1964).

162. R. D. Hoffsommer, H. L. Slates, D. Taub, and N. L. Wendler, *J. Org. Chem.*, **24**, 1617 (1959).

163. C. R. Engel, *Can. J. Chem.*, **35**, 131 (1957).

164. R. Deghenghi and C. R. Engel, *J. Am. Chem. Soc.*, **82**, 3201 (1960).

165. H. L. Herzog, M. J. Gentles, H. H. Marshall, and E. B. Hernshberg, *J. Am. Chem. Soc.*, **82,** 3691 (1960).

166. C. R. Engel, R. M. Heogerle, and R. Deghenghi, *Can. J. Chem.*, **38**, 1199 (1960).

167. W. S. Allen, H. M. Kissman, S. Mauer, I. Ringler, and M. J. White, *J. Med. Pharm. Chem.*, **5**, 133 (1962).

168. R. E. Beyler, F. Hoffman, R. M. Moriarty, and L. H. Sarett, *J. Org. Chem.*, **26**, 2421 (1961).

169. R. I. Dorfman and A. S. Dorfman, *Endocrinology*, **69**, 283 (1961).

170. G. L. Spaeth, *Arch. Opthamol.*, **75**, 784 (1966).

171. C. A. Schlagel, *J. Pharm. Sci.*, **54**, 335, (1965).

172. W. D. Fairbarn and J. C. Thorson, *Arch. Ophthamol.*, **86**, 138 (1971).

172a. R. Vitali, S. Gladiali, G. Falconi, G. Celasco, and R. Gardi, *J. Med. Chem.*, **20,** 853 (1977).

173. W. J. Leanza, J. P. Conbere, E. F. Rogers, and K. Pfister, *J. Am. Chem. Soc.*, **76,** 1691 (1954).

173a. H. Laurent, E. Gerhards, and R. Wiechert, *J. Steroid Biochem.*, **6,** 185 (1975).

174. B. W. Bain, P. J. May, G. H. Phillips, and E. A. Woolett, *J. Steroid Biochem.*, **5,** 299, (1974).

175. M. Tanabe and B. Bigley, *J. Am. Chem. Soc.*, **83,** 756 (1961).

176. J. G. Llaurado, *Acta Endocrinologica*, **38,** 137 (1961).

176a. S. Kuzuna, M. Obayashi, S. Morimoto and K. Kiyohisa, *Yakugaku Zasshi*, **99,** 871 (1979).

177. J. E. Herz, J. Fried, T. Grabowich, and E. F. Sabo, *J. Am. Chem. Soc.*, **78,** 4812 (1956).

178. M. Heller, R. H. Lenhard, and S. Bernstein, *Steroids*, **5,** 615 (1965).

179. B. G. Christensen, N. G. Steinberg, and R. Hirschmann, *Chem. Ind.* (London), **1961,** 1259.

180. E. W. Boland, *Am. J. Med.*, **31,** 581 (1961).

181. R. I. Dorfman, A. S. Dorfman, E. J. Agnello, S. K. Figdor, and G. D. Laubach, *Acta Endocrinol.*, **37,** 577 (1961).

182. R. E. Schaub and M. E. Weiss, *J. Org. Chem.*, **26,** 1223 (1961).

Index